Ellenberg & Rifkin's

DIABETES MELLITUS

Ellenberg & Rifkin's

DIABETES MELLITUS

sixth edition

Daniel Porte, Jr., MD
Professor of Medicine
University of California, San Diego
VA San Diego Health Care System
San Diego, California
Emeritus Professor of Medicine
University of Washington
Seattle, Washington

Robert S. Sherwin, MD
C.N.H. Long Professor of Medicine
Director, Diabetes Endocrinology Research Center
Associate Director, General Clinical Research Center
Yale University School of Medicine
New Haven, Connecticut

Alain Baron, MD
Senior Vice President, Clinical Research
Amylin Pharmaceuticals, Inc.
San Diego, California

Professor of Medicine
Indiana University School of Medicine
Indianapolis, Indiana

McGraw-Hill
Medical Publishing Division

New York   Chicago   San Francisco   Lisbon   London   Madrid
Mexico City   Milan   New Delhi   San Juan   Seoul   Singapore
Sydney   Toronto

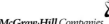

McGraw-Hill

A Division of The McGraw·Hill Companies

Ellenberg & Rifkin's Diabetes Mellitus, Sixth Edition

1 2 3 4 5 6 7 8 9 0   KGP/KGP   0 9 8 7 6 5 4 3 2

ISBN: 0-8385-2178-9

This book was set in Times Roman by The Clarinda Company.
The editors were James Shanahan, Susan Noujaim, and Barbara Holton.
The production supervisor was Richard Ruzycka.
The index was prepared by Katherine Pitcoff.
Quebecor World Kingsport was the printer and binder.

This book is printed on acid-free paper.

Cataloging-in-Publication Data is on file for this book at the Library of Congress.

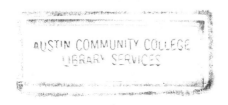

CONTENTS

CONTRIBUTORS

Bo Ahren, MD, PhD
Professor of Medicine
Department of Medicine
Lund University
Lund, Sweden

Lloyd P. Aiello, MD, PhD
Assistant Professor of Ophthalmology
Joslin Diabetes Center
Boston, Massachusetts

Cameron M. Akbari, MD
Attending Vascular Surgeon and Co-director
Noninvasive Vascular Lab
Beth Israel Deaconess Medical Center
Assistant Professor of Surgery
Harvard Medical School
Boston, Massachusetts

K George MM Alberti, DPhil, BM, Bch, FRCP, FRCPath
Professor and Dean of Medicine
St. Mary's Hospital Campus
Imperial College
London, England

John M. Amatruda, MD
Vice President, Metabolic Disorders Research
Bayer Corporation,
West Haven, Connecticut
Professor of Medicine, Adjunct
Yale University School of Medicine
New Haven, Connecticut

Stephanie A. Amiel, FRCP
Professor of Diabetic Medicine
Kings College School of Medicine
London, England

Shereen Arent, JD
National Director of Legal Advocacy
American Diabetes Association
Alexandria, Virginia

Eric S. Bachman, PhD., MD
Instructor in Medicine
Beth Israel Deaconess Medical Center
Harvard Medical School
Boston, Massachusetts

Francisco J. Baigorri, MD
Private Practice
Miami, Florida

Jamie S. Barkin MD, FACG, FACP
Professor of Medicine
Division of Gastroenterology
Mt. Sinai Medical Center
Miami Beach, Florida

Joyce P. Barnett, MS, RD, LD
Assistant Professor, Department of Clinical Nutrition
The University of Texas Southwestern Medical Center at
  Dallas
Dallas, Texas

Eugene J. Barrett, MD, PhD
Madge Jones Professor of Medicine and Pediatrics
Director, University of Virginia Diabetes Center
University of Virginia, Health Science Center
Charlottesville, Virginia

Denis G. Baskin, PhD
Research Professor of Medicine and Biological Structure
University of Washington
Senior Research Career Scientist
Division of Metabolism, Endocrinology and Nutrition
VA Puget Sound Health Care System
Seattle, Washington

Peter H. Bennett, MB, FRCP
Senior Investigator
National Institute of Diabetes & Digestive and Kidney
  Diseases
Phoenix, Arizona

Clifton Bogardus, MD
Chief, Clinical Diabetes & Nutrition Section
Chief, Phoenix Epidemiology & Clinical Research
   Branch
National Institute of Diabetes, Digestive and Kidney
   Diseases, National Institutes of Health
Phoenix, Arizona

Michael Brownlee, MD
Anita and Jack Saltz Professor of Diabetes Research
Professor of Medicine and Pathology
Diabetes Research Center
Albert Einstein College of Medicine
Bronx, New York

Maria Luiza Avancini Caramori, MD, PhD
Post-Doctoral Associate, Department of Pediatrics
University of Minnesota,
Minneapolis, Minnesota

Joan I. Casey, MD, FRCPC
Professor/Assistant Dean of Students,
Department of Internal Medicine
Albert Einstein College of Medicine
Program Director Emeritus/Vice Chairman
Montefiore Medical Center
Bronx, New York

Ronald E. Chance, PhD
Lilly Research Lab (Retired)
Lilly Corporation Center
Indianapolis, Indiana

Andrew D. Cherniak, PhD
Research Assistant Professor
Program in Molecular Medicine
Department of Biochemistry and Molecular Pharmacology
University of Massachusetts Medical Center
Worcester, Massachusetts

Alan D. Cherrington, PhD
Charles H. Best Professor and Chair
Department of Molecular Physiology & Biophysics
Vanderbilt University School of Medicine
Nashville, Tennessee

Deborah A. Chyun, PhD, RN
Assistant Professor
Yale University School of Nursing
New Haven, Connecticut

William C. Coleman, DPM
Section Head, Podiatry
Department of Orthopedics
Ochsner Clinic Foundation
New Orleans, Louisiana

Bruce R. Conway, PhD
Program in Molecular Medicine
Department of Biochemistry and Molecular Biology
University of Massachusetts Medical Center
Worcester, Massachusetts

Philip E. Cryer, MD
Irene E. and Michael M. Karl Professor of Endocrinology
   and Metabolism
Washington University School of Medicine
Chief of Endocrinology, Diabetes and Metabolism
Barnes-Jewish Hospital
St. Louis, Missouri

Brian P. Currie, MD, MPH
Assistant Professor, Department of Medicine
Albert Einstein College of Medicine
Medical Director
Montefiore Medical Center
Bronx, New York

Michael P. Czech, PhD
Professor and Chair, Program in Molecular Medicine
Department of Biochemistry
University of Massachusetts Medical School
Worcester, Massachusetts

David A. D'Alessio, MD
Associate Professor, Department of Medicine
University of Cincinnati
Cincinnati VA Medical Center
Cincinnati, Ohio

Michael R. DeFelippis, PhD
Lilly Research Lab
Lilly Corporation Center
Indianapolis, Indiana

Ralph A. DeFronzo, MD
Professor of Medicine and Chief, Diabetes Division
Deputy Director, University of Texas Health Science Center
South Texas Veterans Health Care System, Audie L.
   Murphy Division
San Antonio, Texas

Kevin Docherty, BSc, PhD
MacLeod Smith Professor of Biochemistry
Department of Molecular and Cell Biology
University of Aberdeen
Institute of Medical Sciences
Aberdeen, Scotland

Sharon L. Dooley, MD, MPH
Professor, Maternal-Fetal Medicine
Northwestern University
Chicago, Illinois

Elia J. Duh, MD
Assistant Professor
Wilmer Eye Institute
Johns Hopkins University School of Medicine
Baltimore, Maryland

Elizabeth Delionback Ennis, MD
Clinical Assistant Professor
Endocrinology and Metabolism
University of Alabama at Birmingham
Birmingham, Alabama

Tomris Erbas, MD
Fellow, The Strelitz Diabetes Research Institutes
East Virginia Medical School
Norfolk, Virginia

Mark L. Evans, MD
Diabetes Endocrine Research Center
Yale University School of Medicine
New Haven, Connecticut

Eva L. Feldman, MD, PhD
Professor, Department of Neurology
University of Michigan
Director, JDRF Center for the Study of Complications in
  Diabetes
Attending Physician
University of Michigan Health System
Ann Arbor, Michigan

Daniel W. Foster, MD
Donald W. Seldin Distinguished Chair in Internal Medicine
Chairman, Department of Internal Medicine
The University of Texas Southwestern Medical Center at
  Dallas
Dallas, Texas

Bruce H. Frank, PhD
Lilly Research Lab (Retired)
Lilly Corporation Center
Indianapolis, Indiana

Om P. Ganda, MD
Associate Professor of Medicine
Harvard Medical School
Senior Physician
Joslin Diabetes Center and Beth-Israel Deaconess Medical
  Center
Boston, Massachusetts

Abhimanyu Garg, MD
Chief, Division of Nutrition and Metabolic Diseases
The University of Texas Southwestern Medical Center at
  Dallas
Dallas, Texas

John E. Gerich, MD
Professor, Department of Medicine, Physiology and
  Pharmacology
University of Rochester School of Medicine
Rochester, New York

Douglas A. Greene, MD
Executive Vice President, Clinical Sciences & Product
  Development
Merck Pharmaceuticals
Rahway, New Jersey

Margaret Grey, DrPH, FAAN, CDE
Associate Dean for Research Affairs
Independence Foundation Professor of Nursing
Yale University School of Nursing
New Haven, Connecticut

Angelika C. Gruessner, PhD
Associate Professor of Surgery
Department of Surgery
University of Minnesota
Minneapolis, Minnesota

Rainer WG Gruessner, MD, PhD
Professor of Surgery
Department of Surgery
University of Minnesota
Minneapolis, Minnesota

Jeffrey B. Halter, MD
Professor of Medicine
University of Michigan Geriatric Center
Ann Arbor, Michigan

Peter J. Havel, DVM, PhD
Associate Professor, Department of Nutrition
University of California, Davis
Davis, California

Robert R. Henry, MD
Professor of Medicine
University of California, San Diego
Chief, Diabetes/Metabolism Section
VA San Diego Healthcare System
San Diego, California

Robert V. Hogikyan, MD
Clinical Assistant Professor of Internal Medicine
University of Michigan Medical School
Director, Extended Care Program,
VA Ann Arbor Healthcare System
Ann Arbor, Michigan

Silvio E. Inzucchi, MD
Associate Professor of Medicine
Clinical Director, Section of Endocrinology
Yale University School of Medicine
Director, Yale Diabetes Center
Attending Staff, Yale-New Haven Hospital
New Haven, Connecticut

Charles A. Janeway, Jr., MD
Howard Hughes Medical Institute
Chevy Chase, Maryland
Professor of Medicine
Yale University School of Medicine
New Haven, Connecticut

Steven E. Kahn, MB, ChB
Professor of Medicine
Division of Metabolism, Endocrinology and Nutrition
University of Washington
Associate Chief of Staff for Research and Development
Veterans Affairs Puget Sound Health Care System
Seattle, Washington

Norman M. Kaplan, MD
Clinical Professor of Internal Medicine
The University of Texas Southwestern Medical Center at
    Dallas
Dallas, Texas

Jes K. Klarlund, PhD
Assistant Professor,
Program in Molecular Medicine
Department of Biochemistry and Molecular Biology
University of Massachusetts Medical Center
Worcester, Massachusetts

Ronald Klein, MD, MPH
Professor, Department of Ophthalmology and Visual
    Sciences
The University of Wisconsin-Madison Medical School
Madison, Wisconsin

William C. Knowler, MD, DrPH
Chief, Diabetes and Arthritis Epidemiology Section
National Institute of Diabetes, Digestive and Kidney
    Diseases
Phoenix, Arizona

Gregory S. Korbutt, PhD
Associate Professor of Surgery
Surgical-Medical Research Institute
Department of Surgery
University of Alberta
Edmonton, Alberta, Canada

Robert A. Kreisberg, MD
Associate Vice-President for Clinical Affairs
University of South Alabama
Mobile, Alabama

Yolanta T. Kruszynska, MRCP(UK), PhD
Associate Professor of Medicine, Department of Medicine
University of California, San Diego
San Diego, California

Pierre J. Lefèvre, MD, PhD, FRCP, MAE
Emeritus Professor of Medicine, Department of Medicine
Division of Diabetes, Nutrition & Metabolic Disorders
University of Liege, Medical School
Liege, Belgium

Åke Lernmark, PhD
Robert H. Williams Professor of Medicine
Department of Medicine
Adjunct Professor
Department of Immunology
University of Washington
Seattle, Washington

William C. Little, MD
Professor of Internal Medicine
Chief of Cardiology
Wake Forest University School of Medicine
Winston-Salem, North Carolina

James N. Livingston, DVM, PhD
Director, Diabetes Research
Bayer Corporation
West Haven, Connecticut

Frank W. LoGerfo, MD
William V. McDermott Professor of Surgery
Harvard Medical School
Chief, Division of Vascular Surgery
Beth Israel Deaconess Medical Center
Boston, Massachusetts

Robert Matz, MD
Professor of Medicine
Medical Director of Quality Assurance and Improvement
Attending Physician
Mt. Sinai Hospital and Medical Center
New York, New York

Michael Mauer, MD
Professor, Department of Pediatrics
Co-Director, Pediatric Nephrology
University of Minnesota
Minneapolis, Minnesota

J. Denis McGarry, PhD†
Professor, Internal Medicine and Biochemistry
The University of Texas Southwestern Medical Center at
    Dallas
Dallas, Texas

Boyd E. Metzger, MD
Professor of Medicine
Northwestern University, Feinberg School of Medicine
Attending Physician
Northwestern Memorial Hospital
Chicago, Illinois

Mary Courtney Moore, PhD
Department of Molecular Physiology & Biophysics
Vanderbilt University Medical Center
Nashville, Tennessee

Sunder Mudaliar, MD
Assistant Clinical Professor of Medicine
University of California, San Diego
Staff Physician, Diabetes/Metabolism Section
VA San Diego Healthcare System
San Diego, California

Hindrik Mulder, PhD
Section for Molecular Signaling,
Department of Cell and Molecular Biology
Biomedical Research Center
Lund University
Lund, Sweden

Ramachandra G. Naik, MD
Consultant Endocrinologist
Department of Endocrinology and Metabolism
Bombay Hospital and Medical Research Center
Mumbai, India

David M. Nathan, MD
Professor, Department of Medicine
Harvard Medical School
Director, Diabetes Center and General Clinical Research
    Center
Massachusetts General Hospital
Boston, Massachusetts

Christopher B. Newgard, PhD
Randolf and Gifford Touchstone Chair in Diabetes
    Research
Center for Diabetes Research
Professor of Biochemistry and Internal Medicine
The University of Texas Southwestern Medical Center at
    Dallas
Dallas, TX

†Deceased

Irina Obrosova, PhD
Assistant Research Scientist
University of Michigan Medical Center
Ann Arbor, Michigan

Edward S. Ogata, MD
Professor, Department of Obstetrics and Gynecology
Feinberg School of Medicine
Northwestern University
Chicago, Illinois

Jerrold M. Olefsky, MD
Professor of Medicine
University of California, San Diego
VA San Diego Health Care System
San Diego, California

John E. Olerud, MD
Professor, Department of Medicine
Head, Division of Dermatology
University of Washington
Seattle, Washington

Jerry P. Palmer, MD
Director, Endocrinology, Metabolism, and Nutrition
    Section
Primary and Specialty Medical Care
DVA Puget Sound Health Care System
Director
Diabetes Endocrinology Research Center and Diabetes
    Care Center
Professor of Medicine, University of Washington
Seattle, Washington

Michael A. Pfeifer, MD, MS, CDE, FACE
Medical Product Leader
Metabolism/Medical Affairs
Aventis Pharmaceuticals
Bridgewater, New Jersey

Richard L. Phelps, MD
Assistant Professor of Clinical Medicine
Department of Medicine
Division of Endocrinology and Metabolism
Northwestern University Medical School
Chicago, Illinois

Rodica Pop-Busci, MD, PhD
Assistant Professor of Medicine
Department of Endocrinology and Metabolism
Medical College of Ohio
Toledo, Ohio

Daniel Porte, Jr., MD
Professor of Medicine
University of California, San Diego
VA San Diego Health Care System
San Diego, California
Emeritus Professor of Medicine
University of Washington
Seattle, Washington

Ray V. Rajotte, PhD
Professor, Departments of Surgery and Medicine
Director, Surgical-Medical Research Institute
Director, Islet Transplantation Group
Univerity of Alberta
Edmonton, Alberta
Canada

Philip Raskin, MD
Professor, Department of Internal Medicine
The University of Texas Southwestern Medical Center at
    Dallas
Medical Director, University Diabetes Treatment Center
Parkland Health and Hospital System
Dallas, Texas

Gina R. Rayat, PhD
Surgical-Medical Research Institute,
Department of Surgery, University of Alberta,
Alberta, Edmonton,
Canada

Marian J. Rewers, MD, PhD, MPH
Professor, Pediatrics and Preventive Medicine
Clinical Director
The Barbara Davis Center for Childhood Diabetes
University of Colorado Health Sciences Center
Denver, Colorado

James W. Russell, MD, MS
Assistant Professor, Department of Neurology
University of Michigan
GRECC Scientist
Ann Arbor Veterans Administration
Attending Physician
University of Michigan Health System
Ann Arbor, Michigan

Lester B. Salans, MD
Clinical Professor of Medicine,
Department of Medicine, Section of Endocrinology
Mt. Sinai School of Medicine
New York, New York

Christopher D. Saudek, MD
Professor of Medicine
Johns Hopkins University School of Medicine
Baltimore, Maryland

Andre J. Scheen, MD, PhD
Professor of Internal Medicine, Department of Medicine
University of Liege, Medical School
Head, Division of Diabetes, Nutrition and Metabolic
    Disorders
Head
Division of Clinical Pharmacology
University Hospital
Liege, Belgium

Michael W. Schwartz, MD
Professor and Head
Section of Clinical Nutrition
Division of Metabolism, Endocrinology and Nutrition
University of Washington and Harborview Medical Center
Seattle, Washington

Randy Seeley, MD
Associate Professor
Department of Psychiatry
University of Cincinnati, Ohio

Clay F. Semenkovich, MD
Professor, Department of Medicine
Professor, Department of Cell Biology & Physiology
Washington University School of Medicine
St. Louis, Missouri

Eleazar Shafrir, PhD
Professor of Biochemistry
Hebrew University-Hadassah Medical School
Jerusalem, Israel

Harry Shamoon, MD
Professor of Medicine
Associate Dean for Clinical Research
Albert Einstein College of Medicine
Bronx, New York

Robert S. Sherwin, MD
C.N.H. Long Professor of Internal Medicine
Director, Diabetes Endocrinology Research Center
Associate Director, General Clinical Research Center
Yale University School of Medicine
New Haven, Connecticut

Zhi-Qing Shi, MD, PhD
Research Scientist, Department of Metabolic Disorders
Amgen, Inc.
Thousand Oaks, California
Adjunct Professor, Department of Physiology
University of Toronto
Toronto, Canada

Gerald I. Shulman, MD, PhD
Investigator, Howard Hughes Medical Institute
Professor of Internal Medicine and Cellular & Molecular
    Physiology
Director, General Clinical Research Center
Yale University School of Medicine
New Haven, Connecticut

Bernard L. Silverman, MD
Department of Pediatrics
Northwestern University Medical School
Chicago, Illinois

Jay S. Skyler, MD
Professor of Medicine, Pediatrics and Psychology
University of Miami School of Medicine
Miami, Florida

Daniel Steinberg, MD, PhD
Research Professor, Department of Medicine
University of California, San Diego
La Jolla, California

Donald F. Steiner, MD
Professor, Department of Biochemistry and Molecular
    Biology
Senior Investigator, Howard Hughes Medical Institute
The University of Chicago
Chicago, Illinois

Martin J. Stevens, MD, MBBCh
Associate Professor, Division of Endocrinology &
    Metabolism,
Department of Internal Medicine
Attending Physician
The University of Michigan Health System
Ann Arbor, Michigan

Suzanne M. Strowig, MSN, RN
Faculty Associate, Department of Internal Medicine
The University of Texas Southwestern Medical Center at
    Dallas
Dallas, Texas

David E.R. Sutherland, MD, PhD
Professor, Department of Surgery
Head, Division of Transplantation
University of Minnesota
Minneapolis, Minnesota

Gerald J. Taborsky, Jr., PhD
Research Professor of Medicine
Division of Metabolism, Endocrinology and Nutrition
University of Washington
Senior Research Career Scientist
VA Puget Sound Health Care System
Seattle, Washington

William V. Tamborlane, MD
Professor and Chief of Pediatric Endocrinology
Department of Pediatric Endocrinology
Yale University School of Medicine
New Haven, Connecticut

P. Antonio Tataranni, MD
Head, Obesity, Diabetes & Energy Metabolism Unit
Director, Clinical Research Unit, Clinical Diabetes &
    Nutrition Section
National Institutes of Health
Phoenix, Arizona

Douglas E. Vaughan, MD
Professor of Medicine and Pharmacology
Chief, Division of Cardiovascular Medicine
Vanderbilt University
Nashville, Tennessee

Barbara VanRenterghem, PhD
Department of Biochemistry and Molecular Biology
University of Massachusetts Medical Center
Worcester, Massachusetts

Aaron I. Vinik, MD, PhD, FCP, FACP
Director, Diabetes Research Institute
Scientific Director, Department of Medicine
Professor of Medicine, Eastern Virginia Medical School
Norfolk, Virginia

Mladen Vranic, MD, DSc, FRCP(C), FRSC
Professor, Department of Physiology and Medicine
University of Toronto
Toronto, Ontario, Canada

Elizabeth A. Walker, DNSc, RN
Associate Professor of Medicine
Director, Prevention & Control Component, The Diabetes
    Research & Training Center
Albert Einstein College of Medicine
Bronx, New York

David H. Wasserman, PhD
Professor, Department of Molecular Physiology &
    Biophysics
Vanderbilt University
Nashville, Tennessee

Gretchen Wells, MD, PhD
Assistant Professor of Internal Medicine
Wake Forest University School of Medicine
Winston-Salem, North Carolina

Per Westermark, MD, PhD
Professor and Chairman, Department of Genetics and
    Pathology
Uppsala University
Sweden

F. Susan Wong, MB, PhD, MRCP
Wellcome Trust Senior Fellow in Clinical Science,
    Department of Pathology & Microbiology
University of Bristol
Honorary Medical Staff
Bristol Royal Infirmary
Bristol, England

Stephen C. Woods, PhD
Professor, Department of Psychiatry
Director, Obesity Research Center
University of Cincinnati
Cincinnati, Ohio

Judith Wylie Rosett, EdD, RD
Professor of Epidemiology and Social Medicine
Albert Einstein College of Medicine
Bronx, New York

Lawrence H. Young, MD
Professor, Department of Internal Medicine
Yale University School of Medicine
Attending Staff
Yale-New Haven Hospital
New Haven, Connecticut

PREFACE

This new edition reflects the many changes and rapid developments in the field of diabetes mellitus. The sixth edition adds a new editor as well as new authors and topics, but maintains our focus by asking the authors to present those areas of the greatest significance and general use to the field. We believe that we have produced a book which covers the complete spectrum of what has become an increasingly important medical epidemic affecting more than 135 million patients around the world. The scientific basis for the disease remains the focus of the first half of the book and reflects the rapid increase in scientific developments in our understanding of carbohydrate and lipid metabolism. Here the impact of these exciting and novel biological insights, which are so important to clinical pathophysiology and treatment, is heavily emphasized. This is most readily seen in the completely revised chapters on the molecular and cellular biology of the β-cell, the mechanisms of insulin action, and the biochemical mechanisms of microvascular disease. The impact of the revolution in the molecular understanding of disease is also evident in many other contributions such as the new chapter on vascular thrombosis and endothelial dysfunction, the molecular mechanisms and genetic engineering of insulin secreting cells, and the chapters on the pathophysiology and genetics of type 2 diabetes, the immunology relevant to diabetes, and the pathophysiology and genetics of type 1 diabetes. Change is also reflected by our adding six entirely new chapters and 22 new authors. Thus the book continues to evolve at the same rapid rate as the field.

In the pathophysiology area there has been extensive revision of our view of integrated metabolism and major updates on the mechanism involved in the complications of the disease plus several new chapters on the specific mechanisms for the eye, kidney, and nerve complications of the disease. The impact of the explosion of understanding of how body weight and adiposity are regulated is presented from both a basic perspective of the process to the clinical significance of the interaction between obesity and type-2 diabetes. Reflecting the final agreement between European and American organizations including the American Diabetes Association, National Institute of Health, and World Health Organization, the terminology type 1 and 2 diabetes is used throughout the text and the updated standards for the diagnosis and classification of these forms of diabetes are presented in the new chapter on this topic.

Clinical aspects of diagnosis, treatment and management are the focus of the other half of the book which also contains a number of new chapters and authors. The major recognition of the importance of good plasma glucose control to diabetes complications is strongly represented for both type 1 and 2 diabetes and new treatment modalities and pharmaceutical agents for both forms of the disease are presented and their use discussed. Chapters on patients with complications also focus on specific diagnostic tools and their use for the prevention and management of each complication including discussion of the newer methods and treatments which most critically address these associated disorders. Reflecting the increasing recognition of cardiovascular disease to the shortened life expectancy of this patient population there are several new chapters on the mechanisms of macrovascular disease and the impact of all of the major risk factors on its clinical manifestations including hypertension, dyslipidemia and endothelial and hematological dysfunction. In each of these areas potential treatments are reviewed and compared, and where possible, related to mechanisms and outcomes. Finally, there are chapters on the behavioral, economic and educational factors that are so important to patient well being and comfort. In addition we look to the future with a chapter on new treatments on the horizon that are playing such an important role in the rate of change of everyday clinical practice and that reflect the enormous interest of the biotechnical and pharmaceutical industry in the field. Thus clinicians will find the biochemical and physiological basis of disease available to them as new treatments are developed that are based on this fundamental understanding of disease. At the same time scientists who wish to develop these new treatments will have the missing elements of present day treatment approaches clearly enunciated in the clinical sections of the book to assist them in understanding how the biochemical and physiological mechanisms express themselves clinically at the present time. We hope this book will prove useful to all those interested in any and all aspects of this protean medical problem.

As is always true, we are indebted to our authors for their untiring effort to provide the most complete, most efficient information in their chapters and their forbearance with the comments of their editors during this process. We also wish to recognize the loss of our dear friend and founding editor, Harold Rifkin, whose philosophy to do what we can to help patients remains our guiding light. We also wish to acknowledge and thank the staff of our new publisher, McGraw-Hill, for their help and support in bringing this book to you and express our immense appreciation to the loyal and dedicated assistants at our institutions, Tessa Trowbridge, Bethany Heintz and Kathleen Catalano who were critical to all of the administrative details that are so necessary, allowing the editors to focus on the intellectual challenge of this project.

The editors dedicate this book to Eunice Porte, Leslie Sherwin, Marilyn Baron, and Bibi Rifkin for their loving patience, understanding, and support.

Ellenberg & Rifkin's

DIABETES
MELLITUS

Integrated Fuel Metabolism

Gerald I. Shulman

Eugene J. Barrett

Robert S. Sherwin

INTRODUCTION

Regulation of fuel metabolism in humans involves a complex interplay between hormones, exogenous nutrients, and interorgan exchanges of substrates designed to maintain a constant and adequate supply of fuel for all organs of the body. The key regulatory hormone orchestrating the exchange and distribution of substrate between tissues under fed and fasting conditions is insulin (see Chaps. 3 through 5). Glucagon, catecholamines, cortisol, and growth hormone play major roles in energy regulation during times of acute glucose requirements, such as during exercise, under stress, or in response to hypoglycemia (see Chaps. 9, 27, and 31). The major organs involved in maintaining fuel homeostasis are the liver and kidney, by virtue of their unique ability to produce glucose; the brain, due to its almost total dependence on glucose as an energy source; and the muscle and adipose tissue, due to their ability to respond to insulin and store energy in the form of glycogen and fat, respectively.

The purpose of this introductory chapter is to review how humans utilize energy and the means by which the body manages its energy stores during times of feeding, fasting, and exercise. In addition, a brief overview of the impact of diabetes on these processes is presented.

FORMS OF ENERGY

Ultimately, all animals sustain life from the energy released by the breaking of carbon-carbon bonds formed in plants during photosynthesis. Cellulose is the principal form of this stored energy in the biosphere. It consists of polymers of glucose joined by $\beta 1,4$ linkages. In contrast to the $\alpha 1,4$ linkages that occur between glucose molecules in glycogen and other edible starches, cellulose is not digestible by humans. However, most ruminants harbor cellulase-producing bacteria in their digestive tracts which can degrade cellulose to glucose and therefore take advantage of this abundant energy supply. Energy in foodstuffs exists in three forms: (1) carbohydrate, (2) protein, and (3) fat, which in turn consist of three basic units: sugars, amino acids, and free fatty acids. It is self-evident, glycogen is the main storage form for carbohydrate in humans. It is a macromolecule (10^6–10^8 kd) consisting of branching chains of glucose bonded by $\alpha 1,4$ or $\alpha 1,6$ linkages. It is stored by most cells, with the highest concentrations occurring in liver and muscle. Glycogen is highly hydrophilic, with 1–2 grams of water stored with each gram of glycogen. Storage of energy in the form of glycogen is therefore relatively inefficient on a weight basis, yielding not the theoretical 4 cal/g of dry carbohydrate but rather only 1–2 calories for each gram of hydrated glycogen. Unlike carbohydrate, protein is not accumulated in humans as a primary energy reserve. Instead, each molecule of protein serves other important biological functions. In the healthy adult human eating a weight-maintaining diet, amino acids derived from ingested protein replenish those proteins that have been oxidized in normal daily protein turnover. Once these protein requirements have been met, any excess protein is either oxidized to carbon dioxide or, if there is energy excess, this excess protein is ultimately converted to glycogen or triglyceride. Like glycogen, most proteins are significantly hydrated and therefore the energy stored per gram of protein is less than the 4 cal/g of dry protein. In contrast to glycogen and protein, fat is stored in a nonaqueous environment and therefore yields an energy level very close to its theoretical 9.4 cal/g of triglyceride. This greater efficiency of energy storage provided by fat is crucial for all animals in that it allows for greater mobility and prolongs survival during famine.

FUEL STORAGE

A healthy adult human uses approximately 1 cal/min or 1500–1800 cal/d to meet basal energy requirements.[1] Energy expenditure may increase as much as two- to threefold with exposure to a cold environment or during the performance of heavy exercise.[2] Table 1-1 provides an estimate of the amount of energy stored in glycogen, protein, and fat in a normally proportioned 70-kg human. As can be seen, if glycogen were the sole source of calories, liver and muscle stores would be rapidly depleted, furnishing calories for less than 1 day's resting energy expenditure. Body protein mass is much larger with nearly half contained within skeletal muscle ($\sim$6 kg). This potentially could provide $\sim$10–15 days' worth of energy. However, energy stored as protein serves important enzymatic, structural, regulatory, and locomotive functions, which if compromised would be very detrimental to survival. On the other hand, whole-body triglyceride stores (mostly in adipose tissue) are normally sufficiently large to provide fuel for several months of

TABLE 1-1. Approximate Distribution of Body Fuels and Their Potential Energy In a 70-kg Adult Human

	Kilograms	Kilocalories
Adipose tissue triglyceride	12	108,000
Muscle protein (dry weight)	6	24,000
Carbohydrate (dry weight)		
Muscle glycogen	0.3	1200
Liver glycogen	0.1	400

survival depending on the level of physical activity. Therefore, while humans have two large storage depots of potential energy (protein and fat), fat serves as the major expendable fuel source. Thus, when less energy is taken in than is required to meet metabolic demands, the body initially draws on its limited quantities of hepatic glycogen, but soon adapts so it can draw on its fat reserves to meet energy demands, thereby minimizing its loss of body protein stores. Similarly, when more energy is ingested than is being oxidized, excess calories are stored as glycogen and/or fat. There also exists a hierarchy for energy interconversion that is unidirectional in that amino acids can be converted to glucose and fat, and glucose can be converted to fat; however fat, once formed, can only be stored or oxidized.

FUEL UTILIZATION

There are three main priorities that humans have for fuel utilization. The first priority is accorded to maintaining a stable supply of substrate for central nervous system function. The brain has little stored energy in glycogen or triglyceride and therefore depends on the liver (and under some circumstances the kidney) for a constant supply of energy. In the fed state and early in fasting the brain derives essentially all of its energy for function from glucose oxidation. Most other major organs of the body (muscle, liver, and heart) fill their energy needs at this time by oxidizing fatty acids. However, the blood–brain barrier is impermeable to fatty acids, restricting their use by the brain.[3] As a continuous supply of glucose is required to meet the energy demands of the nervous system, humans have evolved elaborate, redundant mechanisms to maintain plasma glucose concentrations within a narrow range between 55 and 140 mg/dL under both fed and fasted conditions. Lower glucose concentrations impair brain function, whereas high glucose concentrations exceed the renal glucose reabsorption threshold, resulting in wasting of this valuable energy source. In contrast, fatty acids and the water-soluble by-products of incomplete fatty acid oxidation, β-hydroxybutyrate and acetoacetate, can vary in concentration by 10- and 100-fold, respectively, depending on the fed/fasted conditions.[4] During prolonged fasting (>2 days) plasma β-hydroxybutyrate and acetoacetate concentrations rise sufficiently to supply much of the brain's oxidative fuel needs.[5] Thus the brain indirectly uses fatty acids as an energy source.

The second priority for the body is to maintain its protein reserves (i.e., contractile proteins, enzymes, nervous tissue, etc.) in times of fasting and replenish them during feeding. This has obvious survival benefits.[6]

The final priority is to replenish its limited liver and muscle glycogen reserves following a meal. Once these stores are full, any excess energy in the form of carbohydrate and protein is converted

to fat. Muscle glycogen is the most readily available form of energy for muscle contraction, especially when intense bursts of physical activity are required, and therefore maintaining an adequate supply of muscle glycogen at all times also has obvious survival benefits in times of fight or flight.[7]

METABOLISM DURING FEEDING

Three mechanisms exist to maintain normoglycemia following carbohydrate ingestion.[8] They are: (1) suppression of hepatic glucose production, (2) stimulation of hepatic glucose uptake, and (3) stimulation of glucose uptake by peripheral tissues, predominantly muscle (Fig. 1-1). Insulin is the primary signal that orchestrates the storage and metabolism of glucose.[9] While glucose is the dominant mediator of insulin secretion, stimulation of insulin secretion with meals involves coordination of multiple effectors (see Chap. 4). This becomes apparent when comparing the insulin response between identical amounts of glucose given intravenously versus orally.[10] Oral glucose raises insulin severalfold higher than comparable glycemia achieved by giving intravenous glucose. This differential insulin response is due to the secretion of multiple incretins from the pancreas and gastrointestinal tract [of which gastrointestinal peptide (GIP) and glucagon-like peptide (GLP-1) appear to be most important], as well as to signals from the central nervous system (parasympathetic innervation of the β cells of the pancreas) in response to local GI stimulation.[11] The incretins and neural signals prime the β cells so as to increase the release of insulin following meal-induced increases in blood glucose. This "priming" of insulin release is absent when blood glucose increases as a result of increased hepatic glycogenolysis in response to stress, thereby avoiding potentially detrimental hyperinsulinemia under these conditions.

The rise in portal vein insulin and glucose concentrations in conjunction with a reduction in portal vein glucagon concentration following a carbohydrate-containing meal suppresses hepatic glucose production and net hepatic glucose uptake ensues.[12] In this manner the liver buffers the entry of glucose from the portal vein into the systemic circulation and minimizes plasma glucose excursions, while at the same time promoting glucose storage. Once the meal is absorbed and blood glucose returns to baseline, the liver resumes net glucose production to maintain normoglycemia. Depending on the size of the carbohydrate load, anything from a quarter to a third of the ingested exogenous glucose load is taken up by the liver.[12–14] It should be emphasized that since the liver is not only decreasing its production of glucose, but also taking up a significant amount of glucose, the contribution of the liver to postprandial glucose homeostasis is substantial and approaches that of muscle. Glucose taken up by the liver during the meal is predominantly stored as glycogen.[15] Using ^{13}C NMR spectroscopy to noninvasively monitor hepatic glycogen content in humans, recent studies have demonstrated that hepatic glycogen stores peak 4–6 hours following a meal.[16] As a result, when meals are ingested at 4- to 6-hour intervals (e.g., breakfast, lunch, and dinner), hepatic glycogen increases throughout the day in a stepwise fashion while most of the glucose required for metabolism is derived from exogenous glucose absorption[17] (Fig. 1-2). Having reached its peak at around midnight, hepatic glycogenolysis supplies glucose for the brain and other glucose-requiring tissues during sleep.

Recent studies have demonstrated that liver glycogen is synthesized by both a direct (glucose → glucose-6-phosphate → glucose-

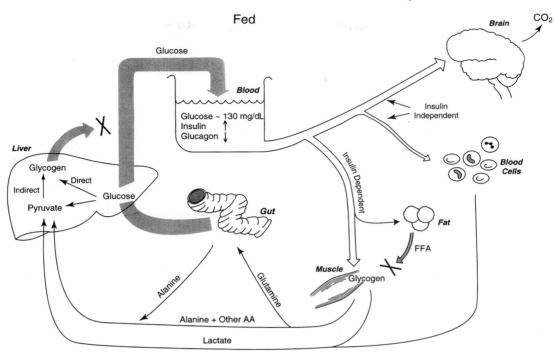

FIGURE 1-1. Whole body fuel metabolism in the fed state following a carbohydrate meal.

1-phosphate → UDP-glucose → glycogen) and an indirect [three-carbon units (lactate, alanine, glycerol, pyruvate) → glucose-6-phosphate → glucose-1-phosphate → UDP-glucose → glycogen] gluconeogenic pathway.[18–20] When a meal is ingested following an overnight fast, these pathways contribute roughly equally to hepatic glycogen synthesis. However, the relative contribution of these pathways appears to depend on many factors, including the composition of diet, the level of glycemia achieved during the meal, and the relative concentrations of insulin and glucagon. Specifically, a high-carbohydrate diet, hyperglycemia, and insulin promote the direct pathway,[21] whereas reduced carbohydrate intake, lower glucose levels, and elevations in circulating glucagon stimulate the indirect pathway.[22,23] One of the recent controversies regarding hepatic glycogen synthesis has been the source of the three carbon units that are used for the indirect pathway of hepatic glycogen synthesis. While muscle, skin, and erythrocytes are all potentially important sources of lactate and alanine for the indirect pathway of hepatic glycogen synthesis, recent studies in dogs and humans have demonstrated that following a glucose meal the liver takes up enough glucose to account for all of the glycogen synthesized by both the direct and indirect pathways.[15] These observations might be explained by either hepatocyte heterogeneity in that periportal cells may be predominantly gluconeogenic and perivenous hepatocytes may be predominately glycolytic, or by substrate cycling between glycolysis and gluconeogenesis within all hepatocytes. Recent studies in rats, in which the relative fluxes for glycogen synthesis in periportal and perivenous hepatocytes have been examined, are consistent with the latter mechanism.[24,25]

Glucose escaping the splanchnic (liver and gut) circulation is cleared predominantly by muscle where most is stored as glycogen.[12,26] The remaining glucose is metabolized via the glycolytic pathway and then is either oxidized or recycled back to the liver as three-carbon intermediates. The uptake of glucose into muscle as well as adipose tissue is predominantly mediated by a rise in in-

sulin concentration and to a lesser extent by the mass effect of hyperglycemia *per se*. Insulin promotes translocation of the GLUT-4 transporter to the plasma membrane and thereby stimulates glucose uptake by muscle and fat.[27,28] In addition, insulin modulates the subsequent metabolism of glucose by increasing the activity of glycogen synthase,[29] thereby promoting glucose storage, and by increasing the activity of pyruvate dehydrogenase,[30] thereby increasing glucose oxidation as well.

While adipose tissue typically represents a large component of the peripheral mass (~12 kg), glucose utilization by adipocytes in humans represents a relatively small sink for ingested glucose. There is relatively little *de novo* free fatty acid synthesis from glucose in human adipocytes, likely due to the relative lack of citrate lyase.[31] The glucose that is metabolized by adipocytes does, however, serve an important role for triglyceride synthesis in that it is used to generate α-glycerol phosphate, which is required for triglyceride synthesis. In times of caloric and carbohydrate excess the liver (which has abundant amounts of citrate lyase) synthesizes fatty acids *de novo* from glucose, esterifies the fatty acids to triglyceride, and exports them to the periphery in the form of very low density lipoprotein (VLDL) particles (Fig. 1-3). The triglyceride in VLDL is hydrolyzed by endothelial lipoprotein lipase to fatty acids. Subsequently, the fatty acids are reesterified and stored as triglyceride in the myocyte and adipocyte.

The larger the meal, the greater is the rate of glucose uptake by liver, muscle, and adipose tissue, a phenomenon explained by the higher levels of circulating insulin and glucose that are generated. In contrast, the brain continues to use glucose, its major oxidative fuel, at a constant rate. GLUT-1 and GLUT-3 transporters facilitate brain glucose uptake (i.e., transport across the blood–brain barrier and into neurons, respectively) independent of insulin (see Chap. 8).[32,33]

While the metabolic changes that follow glucose ingestion have been studied extensively, the humoral and substrate response to protein, fat, and mixed meals have not been as well defined. In-

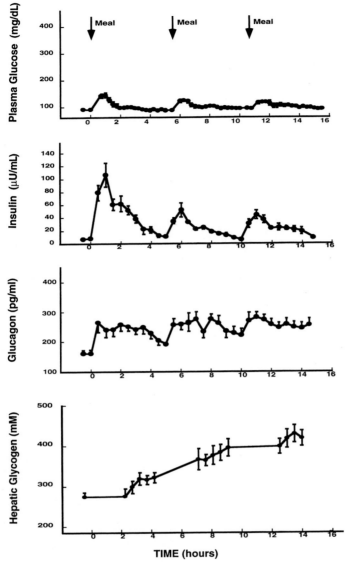

FIGURE 1-2. Hepatic glycogen concentration time course throughout a day in which three identical mixed meals are ingested at: 8:00 AM, 1:00 PM, and 6:00 PM.

marked for the branched-chain amino acids. As a result, these amino acids constitute the main substrate for the immediate repletion of muscle nitrogen after protein ingestion. In muscle, branched-chain amino acids have a unique capacity to directly promote net protein accumulation, predominantly by inhibiting protein breakdown and to some extent through stimulation of protein synthesis.[35,36] Again, the increased secretion of insulin plays a major role in promoting net protein anabolism postprandially when the concentrations of amino acids are elevated following protein feeding. Recent studies have demonstrated that low-dose insulin infusions, recreating the relatively small rise in plasma insulin seen with protein ingestion, lower plasma amino acid concentrations in fasted humans and decrease the rate of net amino acid release from muscle.[37] This is accompanied by suppression of the rate of whole-body and muscle protein degradation.[38–40] Whole-body protein synthesis, measured as the nonoxidative disposal of leucine, does not increase,[38,40] nor does muscle protein synthesis.[39,41] As a result, the improved body and muscle nitrogen balance that accompany even modest increases in plasma insulin *per se* can be attributed to a specific action of insulin to retard proteolysis. Though no increase in overall protein synthesis has been seen either in the whole body, muscle, or splanchnic tissue in response to physiologic increases in plasma insulin, almost certainly the synthesis of some proteins will have been induced while that of others is repressed. It is noteworthy, however, that the combined presence of hyperinsulinemia and hyperaminoacidemia as is seen during protein feeding not only blocks proteolysis but also stimulates protein synthesis.[42,43] Carbohydrate in a mixed meal, along with protein, further augments insulin secretion beyond the effect of protein alone. This can further facilitate uptake of amino acids by muscle and enhance protein anabolism. It is noteworthy that some amino acids (e.g., arginine and leucine) are strong insulin secretagogues and after protein meals are ingested, insulin release is stimulated, even when the meal is lacking carbohydrate. Under these conditions glucagon plays a critical biological role in preventing potential hypoglycemia by maintaining hepatic glucose production in the face of hyperinsulinemia.[34]

Finally, with regard to fat metabolism, insulin has three major anabolic actions that combine to promote net triglyceride accumulation in adipose tissue (Fig. 1-3). Following a fat-containing meal, the triglyceride is hydrolyzed to free fatty acids by lipases in the duodenum, absorbed in the small intestine, and reesterified into chylomicron triglyceride, which then enters the systemic circulation via the lymphatics. Insulin, secreted in response to the carbohydrate and/or protein components of the meal, stimulates lipoprotein lipase (LPL) activity and promotes fat and muscle storage of both exogenously derived triglyceride as well as that produced endogenously.[44] LPL in the capillary endothelium hydrolyzes triglycerides in chylomicrons and VLDL to free fatty acids, which are then transferred to the adipocyte for reesterification into triglyceride. This effect is complemented by insulin's potent inhibitory effect on hormone-sensitive lipase within the fat cell. This lipase normally catalyzes the hydrolysis of stored triglyceride. By this dual mechanism insulin markedly decreases plasma free fatty acid concentrations and stores fat. Finally, insulin stimulates glucose uptake into the adipocyte by stimulating GLUT-4 translocation from the cytoplasm to the plasma membrane, in a fashion similar to that which occurs in the myocyte. Alpha-glycerophosphate formed from glucose is required for the reesterification of fatty acids into triglyceride. Adipocytes lack glycerol kinase and therefore, unlike liver and kidney, are unable to phosphorylate glycerol directly.[45]

gested protein in the meal is hydrolyzed by proteolytic enzymes and peptidases in the gastrointestinal tract to amino acids, which are then actively transported across the gastrointestinal epithelium into the portal vein. The absorbed amino acids serve two main functions: they can either be oxidized to yield energy or incorporated into protein. As protein, amino acids are readily accessible to meet later fuel needs, but only at the sacrifice of functioning proteins. Therefore, it is necessary to eat a sufficient amount of protein-containing foods daily in order to maintain whole-body protein mass. The liver removes a large fraction of amino acids that enter portal blood following a meal, particularly the gluconeogenic amino acids. The branched-chain amino acids (leucine, isoleucine, and valine) are more likely to escape hepatic extraction and are removed mainly by muscle.[34] This is shown by a switch in the net balance of amino acids across the muscle bed from a net output postabsorptively to a net uptake after feeding. The uptake is most

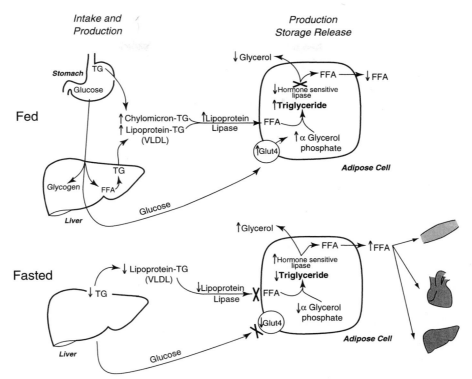

FIGURE 1-3. Fat metabolism in the fed state following a fat-containing mixed meal (top panel) and in the fasted state (bottom panel).

Thus, following a meal, insulin is the primary hormonal factor that controls the storage and metabolism of ingested metabolic fuels. Under conditions of mixed meal ingestion when substrate is available in the form of glucose, amino acids, and free fatty acids, an increase in plasma insulin concentration will augment their net storage as glycogen, protein, and fat, respectively. This is accomplished by the inhibition of glycogenolysis, proteolysis, and lipolysis as well as by facilitating the incorporation of substrates into storage depots. It is noteworthy that the dose-response relationships are such that the processes involving breakdown of energy stores are much more sensitive to insulin than those involved with energy accumulation. Thus, small meals (associated with smaller insulin responses) serve mainly to conserve depots by affecting breakdown, whereas larger meals (and concomitant greater insulin responses) are generally required for the direct stimulation of storage mechanisms.

METABOLISM AFTER AN OVERNIGHT FAST

The period after an overnight fast and preceding the ingestion of the morning meal serves as a useful reference point because it represents the period of transition from the fed to the fasted state. At this time the concentrations of insulin, glucagon, and metabolic substrates that were altered by meal ingestion during the preceding day have returned to baseline, and a relative steady state ensues in which the rate of fuel consumption is closely matched by the release of endogenous fuels from storage depots (Fig. 1-4).

After an overnight fast, the decline in circulating insulin leads to a marked decrease in glucose uptake by peripheral insulin-sensitive tissues (e.g., muscle) and a shift toward the use of free fatty acids by these tissues that are mobilized from fat stores. Nevertheless, the average adult continues to consume glucose at a rate of 7–10 g/h. Total body stores of free glucose, which exist mostly in the extracellular space, amount to only 15–20 grams or about 2 hours' worth of glucose fuel. However, it is even less than that if one takes into consideration a more physiologic excursion going from a fasting plasma glucose concentration of ~90 mg/dL to ~55 mg/dL, the lowest level of plasma glucose that allows normal brain function. Thus the maintenance of circulating glucose concentration in the face of this ongoing glucose use, particularly by the brain, requires that glucose be produced at rates sufficient to match its ongoing consumption. Here again, insulin is the key regulator of the transition from the fed to fasted state, and as in the fed state the liver is at the center of this adaptive mechanism. Four to five hours after a meal (perhaps longer for a very large meal), the liver begins to break down its stores of glycogen and release it as free glucose. This is accomplished by virtue of a reduction in circulating insulin and is supported by the presence of glucagon in the portal circulation. Both the liver and kidney contain significant amounts of glucose-6-phosphatase, and therefore they are the only organs capable of releasing significant amounts of glucose derived from glycogenolysis or gluconeogenesis into the bloodstream. Muscle tissue, which comprises ~25–30% of body mass and contains most of the body's reserves of glycogen (~300 grams versus ~100 grams in liver under fed conditions), lacks glucose-6-phosphatase and therefore is incapable of directly contributing to the maintenance of plasma glucose concentration.

The hepatic processes that provide most of the glucose needed to meet whole-body glucose requirements consist of glycogenolysis and gluconeogenesis. Recent human ^{13}C NMR studies have demonstrated that net hepatic glycogenolysis and gluconeogenesis

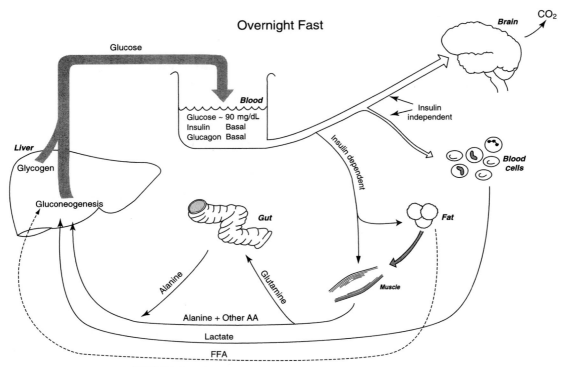

FIGURE 1-4. Whole-body fuel metabolism in the postabsorptive state.

contribute about 50% each to rates of whole-body glucose production during the first several hours of a fast.[46,47] This relatively high level of gluconeogenic activity early in a fast is consistent with other recent studies demonstrating the importance of the gluconeogenic (indirect) pathway for repletion of hepatic glycogen. This suggests that gluconeogenesis is a life-sustaining process that is never completely suppressed, and that when an individual ingests a meal, gluconeogenic flux is directed into hepatic glycogen stores (indirect pathway) along with contributions from the direct pathway. Once the meal is absorbed, the gluconeogenic flux is redirected toward hepatic glucose delivery.

In the first several hours of a fast the brain consumes more than half ($\sim$4–5 g/h) of the glucose produced by the liver, which amounts to about 180 g/d. Other obligate anaerobic tissues consisting of the formed elements of blood (erythrocytes, leukocytes, and bone marrow) and the renal medulla metabolize glucose but convert it primarily to lactate and pyruvate, which recycle back to the liver to form glucose (Cori cycle). About 20% of the glucose utilized daily in this cycle is remade into glucose. It is noteworthy that neither the Cori cycle nor the glucose-alanine cycle in muscle (see below) yields new carbon skeletons for *de novo* glucose synthesis. Rather, they serve an important role for energy and nitrogen (glucose-alanine cycle) transfer between muscle and liver. Operation of these cycles allows the transfer of energy from the liver to the peripheral tissues. The energy for glucose synthesis derived from oxidation of fat in the liver is delivered to the peripheral tissues, where the energy is gained from the metabolism of glucose to lactate.

After an overnight fast the body is in negative nitrogen balance; i.e., the rate of whole-body protein degradation exceeds the rate of whole-body protein synthesis. The amino acids that furnish the nitrogen, measured as urinary nitrogen loss, arise principally from muscle and splanchnic tissues. Organ balance studies[9] in

overnight-fasted humans have shown that muscle, which represents the major reservoir of body protein, like the whole body, is in negative nitrogen balance as reflected by a net loss of both essential and total amino acids. The splanchnic bed removes many of these amino acids, especially alanine and other gluconeogenic amino acids. Yet despite removing nitrogen from the circulating plasma, splanchnic tissues themselves are in negative protein balance. Indeed, the observed net loss of tissue protein mass is more dramatic from the liver in animals undergoing fasts of short duration.[48]

As a result of the uptake of gluconeogenic amino acids by the splanchnic bed, there is a net transfer of amino acid carbon and nitrogen to liver. This provides carbon for gluconeogenesis and net glucose production by the liver, and nitrogen for ureagenesis. Alanine and glutamine are particularly important in this process. They are released from muscle in amounts ($\sim$50% of total amino acid release) that significantly exceed their representation in muscle tissue proteins ($\sim$10–13% of total amino acid residues in muscle protein). Alanine is produced in muscle by transamination of pyruvate derived from glucose and the catabolism of other muscle-derived amino acids (e.g., branched-chain amino acids). Glutamate is produced by transamination of α ketoglutarate supplied by the TCA cycle, and glutamine is produced by the action of glutamine synthase adding a second amino group to glutamate.[49] The intestine uses some of the glutamine taken up by the splanchnic bed as an oxidative fuel.[50] The amino groups are released into portal blood either as alanine or ammonia. On a molar basis, alanine is the principal amino acid taken up by the liver. Within the postabsorptive liver, alanine carbon is principally converted to glucose. As the alanine carbon backbone is essentially derived from glucose in peripheral tissues, a metabolic "glucose-alanine cycle" operates between the liver and periphery, analogous to the Cori cycle. The glucose-alanine cycle provides a nontoxic alternative to ammonia for transfer of amino acid groups derived from muscle amino acid catabolism to the liver for conversion to urea. Glutamine is removed by the kidney, as well as by the liver and gut. In the kidney it serves a dual purpose of supplying carbon for renal gluconeogenesis and amino groups for ammoniagenesis. The latter process is of particular importance in maintaining body acid-base balance during fasting.[51,52] Combined, alanine and glutamine account for more than 40% of the amino acid carbon provided to the splanchnic organs and kidneys for use in glucose production.

Finally, the fall in insulin levels after an overnight fast permits the release of free fatty acids and glycerol from fat stores (Fig. 1-3). This response appears to be more pronounced in visceral than peripheral fat depots (see Chap. 26). While the rate of lipolysis and magnitude of the decline in insulin is of sufficient magnitude to supply extracerebral tissues such as muscle, heart, and liver with free fatty acids and hepatic tissues with glycerol for gluconeogenesis, these changes are not of sufficient magnitude to stimulate appreciably the rate of hepatic conversion of free fatty acid to ketones.

EARLY ADAPTATION TO STARVATION

Since the glycogen stores in the liver are typically limited to approximately 70 grams after an overnight fast, while glucose utilization occurs at a rate of approximately 7–10 g/h, hepatic glycogen stores are largely dissipated early in the course of fasting.[47,53] Thus the initial phase of starvation is characterized by a relative increase in the rate of gluconeogenesis in order to meet the ongoing tissue demands for glucose (mainly from the central nervous system). The dependence of glucose production on protein stores is reflected by an increase in urinary nitrogen excretion in the early phase of starvation. During the first 24 hours of a fast, urinary nitrogen excretion averages 4–7 g/m² in the absence of nitrogen intake.[53] This amounts to approximately 50–75 grams of protein ($\sim$1 g N/6.25 g protein) for the average 70-kg person. Similar results are obtained using isotopic tracer methods to estimate total body rates of protein oxidation.[54] Therefore, regardless of whether simple urinary nitrogen balance is measured or a tracer method is used, the results suggest that about 50 grams of protein are oxidized in the 24 hours following a meal. Since the tissue protein content does not exceed 20% by weight for any tissue, 50–75 grams of protein translates into 250–375 grams of tissue or the equivalent of $\frac{1}{2}$–$\frac{3}{4}$ pound of lean body mass lost on the first day of a fast.

The increase in gluconeogenesis is mediated by adaptations in both hepatic and peripheral insulin-responsive tissues. In muscle, the release of alanine and other glycogenic amino acids increases in conjunction with an acceleration of proteolysis.[54] At the same time the rate of hepatic conversion of gluconeogenic amino acids into glucose is augmented.[55] The increase in glucose synthesis from amino acids is not, however, solely due to increased precursor availability, since plasma levels of alanine and other glycogenic amino acids decline.[56] Taken together, these observations suggest that intrahepatic gluconeogenic mechanisms are stimulated as well, which enhances the efficiency of this process. Recent data suggest that peroxisome proliferator activated receptor α (PPARα) and the transcriptional coactivator PGC-1 are likely important factors mediating the adaptive response of liver during fasting.[57,58] An additional factor contributing to glucose homeostasis is the increased release of fatty acids and glycerol from triglyceride stores in adipose tissue and muscle due to activation of hormone-sensitive li-

pase. The increased availability of glycerol provides the liver with an additional substrate for gluconeogenesis. The increased availability of fatty acids to peripheral tissues limits glucose transport into skeletal muscle, thus preserving glucose for the central nervous system and other obligate glucose-utilizing tissues and diminishing the demands for gluconeogenesis and proteolysis. Early *in vitro* studies found that fatty acids reduced insulin-stimulated glucose uptake in isolated cardiac myocytes through a reduction in pyruvate dehydrogenase activity, resulting in an increase in intracellular citrate concentrations and inhibition of hexokinase activity.[59,60] More recent studies in humans have found that fatty acids cause insulin resistance in skeletal muscle by directly interfering with insulin activation of glucose transport activity.[61,62] Recent data suggest that this is likely occurring through fatty acid activation of a serine/threonine kinase cascade, leading to increased serine phosphorylation of IRS-1/IRS-2, which in turn leads to decreased IRS-1/IRS-2 tyrosine phosphorylation and decreased activation of phosphatidylinositol 3-kinase, a necessary step for insulin-stimulated glucose transport in skeletal muscle.[63] This fatty acid–induced decrease in insulin-stimulated glucose metabolism, while protective under fasting conditions, plays an important pathologic role in mediating the insulin resistance associated with obesity and type 2 diabetes.

At the same time, the fatty acids in the circulation are also delivered to the liver where they generate energy by undergoing β oxidation. This is accomplished by a fall in the insulin/glucagon ratio in the portal circulation, which inhibits acetyl CoA carboxylase, thereby decreasing intracellular malonyl CoA concentrations, which in turn activates carnitine palmityl transferase, thereby promoting mitochondrial fatty acid oxidation[64] (see Chap. 2). In this way both the increase in supply of fatty acids and the activation of enzymes of the fat oxidation pathway are synchronized. Thus oxidation of fatty acids by muscle spares glucose for use by the central nervous system, whereas their oxidation by the liver serves to activate gluconeogenesis by furnishing the energy and reducing power required for glucose synthesis.

The metabolic adaptations in the early stages of starvation (namely increased gluconeogenesis, proteolysis, and lipolysis) coincide with and are mainly orchestrated by a decline in insulin secretion below levels seen in the overnight fasted condition, as well as by a modest increase in portal vein glucagon concentrations.[65] Insulin deficiency promotes all aspects of the metabolic response, whereas the effect of glucagon is confined to the liver. Specifically, the decline in insulin promotes protein and fat breakdown and thus the delivery of gluconeogenic amino acids from muscle and glycerol from fat stores to the liver, while the activation of intrahepatic gluconeogenic processes is promoted by both the rise in glucagon and fall in insulin in the portal circulation. Hypoinsulinemia further contributes to glucose homeostasis by reducing glucose metabolism by extracerebral tissues (e.g., muscle) and by increasing the availability of fatty acids for oxidative metabolism by muscle and liver and ketones for muscle and the central nervous system (Fig. 1-5).

TRANSITION FROM BRIEF TO PROLONGED FASTING

As the duration of fasting progresses, the body shifts from utilization of protein for gluconeogenesis to utilization of fat for ketogenesis and the brain shifts from oxidation of glucose to oxidation of β-hydroxybutyrate and acetoacetate to meet most of its energy requirements[4,66] (Fig. 1-5). From examination of the potential energy

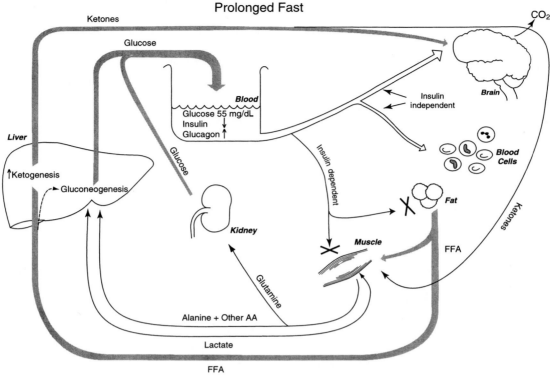

FIGURE 1-5. Whole-body fuel metabolism in the fasted state.

stores (Table 1-1) it is clear that a fasting human could survive for only a few weeks if he/she was totally dependent on protein utilization to meet whole-body energy as well as glucose requirements, and therefore a major reduction in nitrogen metabolism must take place in order to allow for prolonged survival.[4,66] This alteration in substrate utilization is reflected in urea and ammonia excretion data in humans undergoing a prolonged fast; in these subjects urea excretion decreases from 10–15 g/d during the initial days of a fast to less than 1 g/d after 6 weeks of fasting.[66,67] Since urea is the major osmolyte in the urine that requires excretion, this reduction in urea production lessens the amount of obligatory water excretion and therefore decreases the daily water requirement during a prolonged fast. The increase in ketone production by the liver, together with the capacity of the brain to utilize the increased levels of ketones in the circulation, permits humans to extend their survival time during a prolonged fast from weeks to months as long as an adequate water supply and fat stores are available.[68,69] During this transition the liver decreases its rate of gluconeogenesis, mostly due to diminished substrate delivery,[67] while the kidney increases its contribution, which may reach as much as 40% of whole-body glucose production.[66] The latter most likely represents an adaptive process that allows the body to handle the excess protons generated from fat oxidation. Under these conditions the excess protons are converted to ammonia in the kidney and excreted in the urine. In fact, previous studies have shown increased renal gluconeogenesis during acidosis and a strong correlation between ammoniagenesis and gluconeogenesis.[52] During the first few weeks of a fast, plasma alanine levels fall markedly to less than one-third of postabsorptive concentrations due to a marked fall in muscle alanine release[70] (Fig. 1-6). This amino acid as well as lactate are the principal substrates for hepatic gluconeogenesis. The fact that substrate availability is limiting for gluconeogenesis during a prolonged fast has been demonstrated by a rise in plasma glucose concentration following an infusion of small amounts of alanine under these conditions.[70]

In contrast to alanine, the plasma levels of fatty acids double in the first 3–7 days of fasting, after which they remain stable[65,66] (Fig. 1-6). The increased delivery of fatty acids to the liver facilitates a marked acceleration of hepatic ketogenesis that occurs in the first few days of fasting (see Chap. 2). Peak rates of ketone production (approximately 100 g/d) are achieved by the third day, and are

FIGURE 1-6. Time course for substrates (glucose, alanine, free fatty acids, β-hydroxybutyrate, acetoacetate) and urea nitrogen excretion during a prolonged fast.

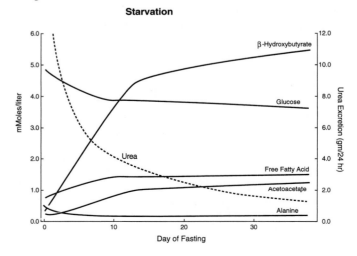

maintained thereafter.[66,69] Despite relatively stable rates of ketone production by the liver, the circulating levels of ketoacids continue to rise throughout the next few weeks as their extraction by peripheral tissues progressively declines.[71] As a result, the central nervous system is supplied with an increasing supply of these water-soluble fat-derived substrates, which eventually account for over one-half of the brain's energy requirements.[5] The following sequence of events is orchestrated by the accompanying changes in insulin and glucagon concentrations produced during fasting: (1) accelerated delivery of fatty acids from adipose tissue; (2) increased hepatic oxidation of the fatty acids delivered from the circulation, which leads to the formation of keto acids ("ketogenic capacity"); and (3) a reduction in the removal of ketones by peripheral tissues.[72,73] Hypoinsulinemia activates each of these steps, whereas glucagon plays a key role by enhancing the ketogenic capacity of the liver. In this way ketones ultimately supplant the brain's dependency on glucose and thus provide a means of limiting the brain's gluconeogenic demands, thereby preserving protein stores, a factor critical for survival. In addition, the metabolism of ketones can provide a significant proportion of the energy demands of other body tissues, especially the heart and skeletal muscle.[4] It has been suggested that the use of such lipid-derived fuels during prolonged starvation may be directly linked to the conservation of body protein stores;[74] however, the precise mechanisms underlying protein sparing in the face of hypoinsulinemia remain to be elucidated. As the fast progresses and fat stores are depleted, leptin levels also decrease, which serves as another protective signal to the body.[75] This decrease in leptin concentration has a profound effect on neuroendocrine function and the gonadal axes, which results in a decrease in LH/FSH oscillations and anovulation. In this way nature protects the starving mother from the additional nutritional demands associated with pregnancy in times of famine.

In summary, the body has evolved powerful adaptive mechanisms that ensure an adequate substrate supply in the form of glucose and ketones to the brain at all times, including times of prolonged fasting, to ensure adequate CNS function. Even under the most strenuous conditions of a prolonged fast, humans do not experience loss of consciousness from decreased substrate supply to brain. Instead, death under these conditions typically occurs when fat stores are depleted and protein breakdown is of sufficient magnitude to cause severe respiratory muscle protein wasting, which in turn leads to atelectasis and terminal pneumonia.[76]

ENERGY METABOLISM DURING AND FOLLOWING RECOVERY FROM EXERCISE

Muscle energy requirements during intense exercise can increase by over 10-fold. This increased energy demand is met by mobilizing energy stores locally from muscle glycogen and triglyceride, as well as systemically from liver glycogen and adipose tissue triglyceride (see Chap. 31). Depending on the intensity of the activity, these substrate supplies are used in differing amounts. If the power demands are great (e.g., running a sprint), anaerobic metabolism of muscle glycogen meets the need for rapid supply of energy, whereas if the power requirements are low, such as when jogging, most of the energy requirements are met by oxidation of fat and glucose derived from the circulation. Overall, muscle derives two molecules of ATP for every molecule of glucose from muscle glycogen or glucose that is glycolyzed to lactate, and ~8 molecules of ATP when glucose is metabolized to pyruvate and con-

verted to alanine. While anaerobic metabolism of glucose by muscle produces only a fraction of the 38 molecules of ATP generated when glucose is completely oxidized, it has the major advantage of being able to provide energy more quickly to meet the increased metabolic demands of an intense workload even before oxygen, glucose, or fatty acid delivery from blood increases. However, due its inherent inefficiency muscle glycogen stores are rapidly depleted by even brief periods of anaerobic metabolism, limiting this type of activity to providing short bursts of energy.

During aerobic exercise of longer duration, glycogenolysis and gluconeogenesis in the liver supply sufficient glucose to the muscle to account for approximately 40% of the increase in fuel consumption with free fatty acids providing the remainder.[77,78] As the duration of exercise lengthens, glucose utilization by the muscle declines and fatty acid oxidation progressively increases, becoming the dominant oxidative fuel. Glucose uptake by exercising muscle can increase 7- to 40-fold; however, circulating glucose remains relatively stable with hepatic glucose production rising to match the increased need. An increase in portal vein glucagon concentration in conjunction with a decline in portal vein insulin concentration is the main signal for this increased hepatic glucose production.[79] Studies performed in exercising, hepatically denervated dogs suggest that activation of the sympathetic nervous system is not essential for the maintenance of accelerated rates of glucose production during exercise.[80] The increase in muscle glucose uptake is accompanied by an exercise-induced translocation in GLUT-4 transporter from the cytoplasm to the plasma membrane that is insulin independent[81,82] and likely mediated by activation of AMP kinase.[83–85] As liver and muscle glycogen stores are typically depleted after a few hours of exercise, with time hepatic gluconeogenesis becomes more important for maintaining these high rates of hepatic glucose production. Alanine and lactate derived from the glucose-alanine cycle and the glucose-lactate cycle provide substrate for this increased hepatic gluconeogenesis.[78] In addition, these cycles play an important role in redistributing glycogen from resting muscle to exercising muscle during and after prolonged exercise. After prolonged arm exercise, release of lactate by leg muscle is six- to sevenfold greater than in the preexercise basal state.[86] Similarly, after leg exercise, output of lactate by forearm muscle increases.[78] These studies suggest that the glucose-lactate cycle redistributes glycogen from resting muscle to fuel those muscles in use during prolonged exercise.[87] During recovery, muscle glycogenolysis and lactate release from previously resting muscle continue and lactate is cycled to the liver where it is converted to glucose so it can be subsequently taken up by recovering muscle, thereby replenishing glycogen stores in previously exercised muscle.[87,88] In this way the body ensures an adequate supply of emergency fuel for the next fight-or-flight response.

IMPACT OF DIABETES ON FUEL HOMEOSTASIS

The metabolic derangements associated with diabetes largely reflect the magnitude of the deficiency in insulin concentration and/or insulin action present. Mild deficiency leads to an impairment in the capacity to effectively increase the storage of ingested fuels (e.g., postprandial hyperglycemia), whereas in its most severe form the deficiency causes a marked acceleration of catabolic processes, including gluconeogenesis, lipolysis, ketogenesis, and proteolysis. In the latter circumstance, the catabolic state in the hyperglycemic patient with insulin-dependent diabetes actually resembles that seen in starving nondiabetic subjects with reduced glucose levels and thus may be viewed as a state of accelerated starvation. This should not be surprising considering that the hormonal milieu of diabetes and starvation share common features, namely, insulin deficiency in conjunction with relative or absolute glucagon excess.

Fed State

As reviewed earlier, the ingestion of glucose triggers a variety of homeostatic responses in nondiabetic subjects (suppression of hepatic glucose production, stimulation of glucose uptake by hepatic and peripheral tissues), all of which serve to minimize the rise in circulating glucose concentrations. Because these responses are to a large extent dependent on insulin action, diabetes, even in its mildest forms, is invariably accompanied by postprandial hyperglycemia.

In diabetic patients who retain some capacity for endogenous insulin secretion [e.g., type 2 diabetes mellitus (T2DM)], postprandial hyperglycemia is closely related to the fasting glucose level and is accounted for both by a delay in the suppression of endogenous[89,90] and by an impaired ability of peripheral tissues to remove the glucose released from the splanchnic bed, reflecting defects in insulin action in both hepatic and peripheral tissues[91,92] (see Chaps. 24 and 25). However, the magnitude of the postprandial glucose excursion is generally less pronounced in T2DM compared to that seen in untreated type 1 diabetes mellitus (T1DM) patients who lack functioning β cells. The absence of an insulin portal-peripheral gradient in T1DM leads to a more severe derangement, particularly at the level of the liver, which is manifest by a gross defect in suppression of hepatic glucose production following glucose ingestion.[93] Moreover, the liver of the patient with T1DM fails to appropriately take up glucose in response to a rising circulating glucose level. This is manifest by a severe defect in the capacity of the liver to store glucose as glycogen following meal ingestion as has recently been demonstrated by NMR spectroscopy in T1DM patients.[17] This increases delivery of glucose to peripheral tissues, where the capacity of muscle (and adipose) tissue to remove glucose is also severely compromised by the lack of an insulin secretory response, as well as by the development of impaired insulin action resulting from chronic insulin deprivation and hyperglycemia (glucose toxicity).[94,95] The multifaceted nature of the disturbance (i.e., liver plus periphery) in the T1DM patient leads to a gross defect in the efficiency of metabolic glucose disposal. The resulting hyperglycemia is partially "compensated" for by increased renal glycosuria.

The diabetic state also leads to impaired metabolic handling of ingested protein and fat. After protein ingestion, postprandial elevations of circulating amino acids are exaggerated in T1DM patients, mainly due to increased levels of branched-chain amino acids.[34] This is largely due to a reduction in the net uptake of branched-chain amino acids by muscle tissue, a finding consistent with the known capacity of insulin to inhibit the release of branched-chain amino acids from muscle.[37,39] Protein feeding also alters glucose homeostasis in insulin-deficient T1DM subjects due to amino acid stimulation of glucagon release that is not matched by an increase in portal vein insulin. As a result hepatic glucose production, and in turn plasma glucose, increases. Finally, the ingestion of fat-containing foods may lead to increased or prolonged

FIGURE 1-7. Whole-body fuel metabolism in diabetic ketoacidosis.

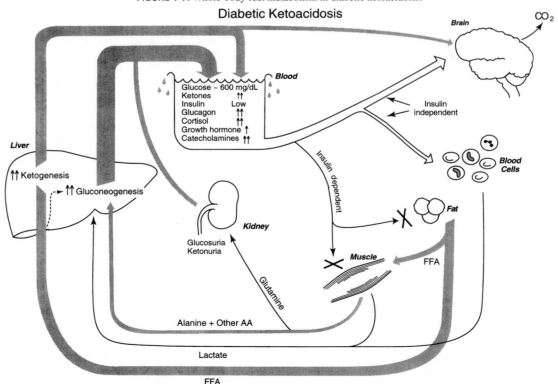

elevations of plasma triglycerides in both T2DM and T1DM patients because of defective triglyceride removal (see Chap. 47). This is because the disposal of exogenous triglycerides (packaged in chylomicrons) is mediated by the activity of the insulin-sensitive enzyme lipoprotein lipase.[44] The alteration in triglyceride removal is most evident during ingestion of mixed meals, when the discrepancies between insulin levels in nondiabetic and diabetic individuals are most pronounced. Taken together, these observations suggest that the scope of the metabolic disorder associated with insulin deficiency or deficient insulin action during feeding may not be restricted to glucose intolerance, but may involve protein and fat intolerance as well.

Fasted State

The presence of relative or absolute insulin deficiency after an overnight fast leads to an elevation of circulating glucose levels in the basal state. In patients with T2DM, fasting insulin concentrations may be normal or even elevated, but only because of insulin resistance and at the expense of fasting hyperglycemia. In such patients, hepatic glucose production is generally elevated in proportion to the magnitude of the hyperglycemia.[95] In patients with T1DM, portal insulin deficiency is more pronounced and this, in conjunction with ongoing glucagon secretion, consistently increases hepatic glucose production (see Chap. 7). Because glucose uptake in the fasting state mainly takes place in non-insulin-sensitive tissues (e.g., the brain), total body glucose uptake actually tends to be increased (due to the mass action effect of hyperglycemia), underscoring the key role of the liver in determining the fasting glucose level in diabetes.

Increased rates of hepatic glucose production in both T2DM and T1DM can be attributed to increased rates of gluconeogenesis,[96] which may be due to both intrahepatic mechanisms and increased substrate delivery through recycling of gluconeogenic precursors (e.g., lactate, alanine, and glycerol).[91,94–97] The former changes can be mostly attributed to decreased portal vein insulin:glucagon ratios, whereas the latter changes are to a large extent attributable to accelerated fat mobilization. Insulin deficiency leads to the generation of glycerol from activation of lipolysis that is used by the liver for gluconeogenesis and to the generation of free fatty acids, which impair glucose oxidation in muscle, thereby promoting the recycling of lactate and pyruvate to the liver.[61]

In the extreme situation of complete β-cell failure, an ever-increasing fasting plasma glucose concentration fails to elicit a secretory response (Fig. 1-7). This hyperglycemia, glycosuria, and volume depletion stimulate the secretion of a variety of counterregulatory hormones (glucagon, catecholamines, growth hormone, and cortisol), which greatly augment hepatic gluconeogenesis and ketogenesis, which in turn result in glucose and ketone overproduction.[98,99](see Chap. 9). Under these conditions, the breakdown of protein and triglyceride stores is dramatically increased, leading to the accelerated delivery of amino acids, lactate, glycerol, and free fatty acids to the liver, where under the influence of hyperglucagonemia and increased free fatty acid oxidation they are rapidly converted to glucose and ketones. Because of the combined effects of hypoinsulinemia and insulin resistance produced by the elevated levels of counterregulatory hormones, compensatory increases in glucose removal (other than renal) virtually cease.[100,101] The clinical correlate of this sequence of events is profound hyperglycemia and hyperketonemia, as is observed in diabetic ketoacidosis (see Chap. 34).

REFERENCES

1. Ravussin E, Lillioja S, Anderson TE, *et al*: Determinants of 24-hour energy expenditure in man. Methods and results using a respiratory chamber. *J Clin Invest* 1986;78:1568.
2. Sims EA, Danforth E Jr.: Expenditure and storage of energy in man. *J Clin Invest* 1987;79:1019.
3. Pardridge WM, Oldendorf WH: Transport of metabolic substrates through the blood–brain barrier. *J Neurochem* 1977;28:5.
4. Cahill GF Jr.: Starvation in man. *N Engl J Med* 1970;282:668.
5. Owen OE, Morgan AP, Kemp HG, *et al*: Brain metabolism during fasting. *J Clin Invest* 1967;46:1589.
6. Benedict FG: *A Study of Prolonged Fasting*. Carnegie Institute, 1915:Publication No. 203.
7. Bergstrom J, Hultman E: Muscle glycogen synthesis after exercise: an enhancing factor localized to the muscle cells in man. *Nature* 1966;210:309.
8. DeFronzo RA: Lilly lecture 1987. The triumvirate: Beta-cell, muscle, liver. A collusion responsible for NIDDM. *Diabetes* 1988;37:667.
9. Cahill GF Jr.: The Banting Memorial Lecture 1971. Physiology of insulin in man. *Diabetes* 1971;20:785.
10. Tillil H, Shapiro ET, Miller MA, *et al*: Dose-dependent effects of oral and intravenous glucose on insulin secretion and clearance in normal humans. *Am J Physiol* 1988;254:E349.
11. Rasmussen H, Zawalich KC, Ganesan S, *et al*: Physiology and pathophysiology of insulin secretion. *Diabetes Care* 1990;13:655.
12. Katz LD, Glickman MG, Rapoport S, *et al*: Splanchnic and peripheral disposal of oral glucose in man. *Diabetes* 1983;32:675.
13. Felig P, Wahren J, Hendler R: Influence of oral glucose ingestion on splanchnic glucose and gluconeogenic substrate metabolism in man. *Diabetes* 1975;24:468.
14. Ferrannini E, Bjorkman O, Reichard GA Jr., *et al*: The disposal of an oral glucose load in healthy subjects. A quantitative study. *Diabetes* 1985;34:580.
15. Moore MC, Cherrington AD, Cline G, *et al*: Sources of carbon for hepatic glycogen synthesis in the conscious dog. *J Clin Invest* 1991;88:578.
16. Taylor R, Magnusson I, Rothman DL, *et al*: Direct assessment of liver glycogen storage by ^{13}C nuclear magnetic resonance spectroscopy and regulation of glucose homeostasis after a mixed meal in normal subjects. *J Clin Invest* 1996;97:126.
17. Hwang JH, Perseghin G, Rothman DL, *et al*: Impaired net hepatic glycogen synthesis in insulin-dependent diabetic subjects during mixed meal ingestion. A ^{13}C nuclear magnetic resonance spectroscopy study. *J Clin Invest* 1995;95:783.
18. Katz J, McGarry JD: The glucose paradox. Is glucose a substrate for liver metabolism? *J Clin Invest* 1984;74:1901.
19. McGarry JD, Kuwajima M, Newgard CB, *et al*: From dietary glucose to liver glycogen: The full circle round. *Annu Rev Nutr* 1987;7:51.
20. Shulman GI, Landau BR: Pathways of glycogen repletion. *Physiol Rev* 1992;72:1019.
21. Shulman GI, DeFronzo RA, Rossetti L: Differential effect of hyperglycemia and hyperinsulinemia on pathways of hepatic glycogen repletion. *Am J Physiol* 1991;260:E731.
22. Rossetti L, Rothman DL, DeFronzo RA, *et al*: Effect of dietary protein on in vivo insulin action and liver glycogen repletion. *Am J Physiol* 1989;257:E212.
23. Roden M, Perseghin G, Petersen K, *et al*: The roles of insulin and glucagon in the regulation of hepatic glycogen synthesis and turnover in humans. *J Clin Invest* 1996;97:1.
24. Cline GW, Shulman GI: Quantitative analysis of the pathways of glycogen repletion in periportal and perivenous hepatocytes in vivo. *J Biol Chem* 1991;266:4094.
25. Cline GW, Shulman GI: Mass and positional isotopomer analysis of glucose metabolism in periportal and pericentral hepatocytes. *J Biol Chem* 1995;270:28062.
26. Shulman GI, Rothman DL, Jue T, *et al*: Quantitation of muscle glycogen synthesis in normal subjects and subjects with non-insulin-dependent diabetes by ^{13}C nuclear magnetic resonance spectroscopy. *N Engl J Med* 1990;322:223.
27. Kahn BB, Horton ES, Cushman SW: Mechanism for enhanced glucose transport response to insulin in adipose cells from chronically hyperinsulinemic rats. Increased translocation of glucose transporters from an enlarged intracellular pool. *J Clin Invest* 1987;79:853.

28. Klip A, Ramlal T, Young DA, *et al*: Insulin-induced translocation of glucose transporters in rat hindlimb muscles. *FEBS Lett* 1987; 224:224.

29. Bogardus C, Lillioja S, Stone K, *et al*: Correlation between muscle glycogen synthase activity and in vivo insulin action in man. *J Clin Invest* 1984;73:1185.

30. Mandarino LJ, Wright KS, Verity LS, *et al*: Effects of insulin infusion on human skeletal muscle pyruvate dehydrogenase, phosphofructokinase, and glycogen synthase. Evidence for their role in oxidative and nonoxidative glucose metabolism. *J Clin Invest* 1987;80:655.

31. Bjorntorp P, Sjostrom L: Carbohydrate storage in man: Speculations and some quantitative considerations. *Metabolism* 1978;27:1853.

32. Flier JS, Mueckler M, McCall AL, *et al*: Distribution of glucose transporter messenger RNA transcripts in tissues of rat and man. *J Clin Invest* 1987;79:657.

33. Maher F, Vannucci S, Takeda J, *et al*: Expression of mouse-glut3 and human-glut3 glucose transporter proteins in brain. *Biochem Biophys Res Comm* 1992;182:703.

34. Wahren J, Felig P, Hagenfeldt L: Effect of protein ingestion on splanchnic and leg metabolism in normal man and in patients with diabetes mellitus. *J Clin Invest* 1976;57:987.

35. Sherwin RS: Effect of starvation on the turnover and metabolic response to leucine. *J Clin Invest* 1978;61:1471.

36. Buse MG, Reid SS: Leucine: a possible regulator of protein turnover in muscle. *J Clin Invest* 1975;56:1250.

37. Pozefsky T, Felig P, Tobin LD, *et al*: Amino acid balance across tissues of the forearm in postabsorptive man. Effects of insulin at two dose levels. *J Clin Invest* 1969;48:2273.

38. Tessari P, Trevisan R, Inchiostro S, *et al*: Dose-response curves of effects of insulin on leucine kinetics in humans. *Am J Physiol* 1986;251:E334.

39. Louard RJ, Fryburg DA, Gelfand RA, *et al*: Insulin sensitivity of protein and glucose metabolism in human forearm skeletal muscle. *J Clin Invest* 1992;90:2348.

40. Fukagawa NK, Minaker KL, Rowe JW, *et al*: Insulin-mediated reduction of whole body protein breakdown. Dose response effects on leucine metabolism in postabsorptive man. *J Clin Invest* 1985;76:2306.

41. McNurlan MA, Essen P, Thorell A, *et al*: Response of protein synthesis in human skeletal muscle to insulin: An investigation with L-[2H5]phenylalanine. *Am J Physiol* 1994;267:E102.

42. Castellino P, Luzi L, Simonson DC, *et al*: Effect of insulin and plasma amino acid concentrations on leucine metabolism in man. Role of substrate availability on estimates of whole body protein synthesis. *J Clin Invest* 1987;80:1784.

43. Kettlehut IC, Wing SS, Goldberg AL: Endocrine regulation of protein breakdown in skeletal muscle. *Diabetes Metab Rev* 1988;4:751.

44. Eckel RH, Yost TJ: Weight reduction increases adipose tissue lipoprotein lipase responsiveness in obese women. *J Clin Invest* 1987;80:992.

45. Robinson J, Newsholme EA: Glycerol kinase activities in rat heart and adipose tissue. *Biochem J* 1967;104:2C.

46. Petersen KF, Cline GW, Gerard DP, *et al*: Contribution of net hepatic glycogen synthesis to disposal of an oral glucose load in humans. *Metabolism* 2001;50:598.

47. Rothman DL, Magnusson I, Katz LD, *et al*: Quantitation of hepatic glycogenolysis and gluconeogenesis in fasting humans with ^{13}C NMR. *Science* 1991;254:573.

48. Addis T, Poo LJ, Lew W: The quantities of protein lost by the various organs and tissues of the body during a fast. *J Biol Chem* 1936; 115:111.

49. Goodman MN, Lowell B, Belur E, *et al*: Sites of protein conservation and loss during starvation, influence of adiposity. *Am J Physiol* 1984;246:E383.

50. Garber AJ, Karl IE, Kipnis D: Alanine and glutamine synthesis and release from skeletal muscle. *J Biol Chem* 1976;251:836.

51. Cahill GF Jr., Aoki TT, Smith RJ: Amino acid cycles in man. *Curr Top Cell Regul* 1981;18:389.

52. Goodman AD, Fuisz RE, Cahill GF: Renal gluconeogenesis in acidosis, alkalosis, and potassium deficiency: Its possible role in regulation of renal ammonia production. *J Clin Invest* 1966;45:612.

53. O'Connell RC, Morgan AP, Aoki TT, *et al*: Nitrogen conservation in starvation: Graded responses to intravenous glucose. *J Clin Endocrinol Metab* 1974;39:555.

54. Fryburg DA, Barrett EJ, Louard RJ, *et al*: Effect of starvation on human muscle protein metabolism and its response to insulin. *Am J Physiol* 1990;259:E477.

55. Chiasson JL, Liljenquist JE, Lacy WW, *et al*: Gluconeogenesis: methodological approaches in vivo. *Fed Proc* 1977;36:229.

56. Felig P, Marliss E, Owen OE, *et al*: Role of substrate in the regulation of hepatic gluconeogenesis in fasting man. *Adv Enzyme Regul* 1969; 7:41.

57. Kersten S, Seydoux J, Peters JM, *et al*: Peroxisome proliferator-activated receptor alpha mediates the adaptive response to fasting. *J Clin Invest* 1999;103:1489.

58. Yoon JC, Puigserver P, Chen G, *et al*: Control of hepatic gluconeogenesis through the transcriptional coactivator PGC-1. *Nature* 2001; 413:131.

59. Randle PJ, Garland PB, Hales C, *et al*: The glucose fatty-acid cycle: its role in insulin sensitivity and the metabolic disturbances of diabetes mellitus. *Lancet* 1963;i:785.

60. Randle PJ, Garland PB, Newsholme EA, *et al*: The glucose fatty acid cycle in obesity and maturity onset diabetes mellitus. *Ann NY Acad Sci* 1965;131:324.

61. Roden M, Price TB, Perseghin G, *et al*: Mechanism of free fatty acid-induced insulin resistance in humans. *J Clin Invest* 1996;97:2859.

62. Dresner A, Laurent D, Marcucci M, *et al*: Effect of free fatty acids on glucose transport and IRS-1-associated phosphatidylinositol 3-kinase activity. *J Clin Invest* 1999;103:253.

63. Griffin ME, Marcucci MJ, Cline GW, *et al*: Free fatty acid-induced insulin resistance is associated with activation of protein kinase C theta and alterations in the insulin signaling cascade. *Diabetes* 1999; 48:1270.

64. McGarry JD, Mannaerts GP, Foster DW, *et al*: A possible role for malonyl-CoA in the regulation of hepatic fatty acid oxidation and ketogenesis. *J Clin Invest* 1977;60:265.

65. Marliss EB, Aoki TT, Unger RH, *et al*: Glucagon levels and metabolic effects in fasting man. *J Clin Invest* 1970;49:2256.

66. Owen OE, Felig P, Morgan AP, *et al*: Liver and kidney metabolism during prolonged starvation. *J Clin Invest* 1969;48:574.

67. Felig P, Owen OE, Wahren J, *et al*: Amino acid metabolism during prolonged starvation. *J Clin Invest* 1969;48:584.

68. Cahill GF Jr.: Starvation in man. *Clin Endocrinol Metab* 1976;5:397.

69. Garber AJ, Menzel PH, Boden G, *et al*: Hepatic ketogenesis and gluconeogenesis in humans. *J Clin Invest* 1974;54:981.

70. Felig P: The glucose-alanine cycle. *Metabolism* 1973;22:179.

71. Owen OE, Reichard GA Jr.: Human forearm metabolism during progressive starvation. *J Clin Invest* 1971;50:1536.

72. McGarry JD, Foster DW: Hormonal control of ketogenesis. *Adv Exp Med Biol* 1979;111:79.

73. Sherwin RS, Hendler RG, Felig P: Effect of diabetes mellitus and insulin on the turnover and metabolic response to ketones in man. *Diabetes* 1976;25:776.

74. Sherwin RS, Hendler RG, Felig P: Effect of ketone infusions on amino acid and nitrogen metabolism in man. *J Clin Invest* 1975; 55:1382.

75. Ahima RS, Prabakaran D, Mantzoros C, *et al*: Role of leptin in the neuroendocrine response to fasting. *Nature* 1996;382:250.

76. Garrow JS, Fletcher K, Halliday D: Body composition in severe infantile malnutrition. *J Clin Invest* 1965;44:417.

77. Ahlborg G, Felig P, Hagenfeldt L, *et al*: Substrate turnover during prolonged exercise in man. Splanchnic and leg metabolism of glucose, free fatty acids, and amino acids. *J Clin Invest* 1974;53:1080.

78. Ahlborg G, Felig P: Lactate and glucose exchange across the forearm, legs, and splanchnic bed during and after prolonged leg exercise. *J Clin Invest* 1982;69:45.

79. Wasserman DH, Spalding JA, Lacy DB, *et al*: Glucagon is a primary controller of hepatic glycogenolysis and gluconeogenesis during muscular work. *Am J Physiol* 1989;257:E108.

80. Wasserman DH, Williams PE, Lacy DB, *et al*: Hepatic nerves are not essential to the increase in hepatic glucose production during muscular work. *Am J Physiol* 1990;259:E195.

81. Sternlicht E, Barnard RJ, Grimditch GK: Exercise and insulin stimulate skeletal muscle glucose transport through different mechanisms. *Am J Physiol* 1989;256:E227.

82. Wallberg HH, Constable SH, Young DA, *et al*: Glucose transport into rat skeletal muscle: Interaction between exercise and insulin. *J Appl Physiol* 1988;65:909.

83. Merrill GF, Kurth EJ, Hardie DG, *et al*: AICA riboside increases AMP-activated protein kinase, fatty acid oxidation, and glucose uptake in rat muscle. *Am J Physiol* 1997;273(6 Pt 1):E1107.

84. Bergeron R, Russell RR 3rd, Young LH, *et al*: Effect of AMPK activation on muscle glucose metabolism in conscious rats. *Am J Physiol* 1999;276(5 Pt 1):E938.

85. Goodyear LJ: AMP-activated protein kinase: a critical signaling intermediary for exercise-stimulated glucose transport? *Exerc Sport Sci Rev* 2000;28:113.

86. Ahlborg G, Wahren J, Felig P: Splanchnic and peripheral glucose and lactate metabolism during and after prolonged arm exercise. *J Clin Invest* 1986;77:690.

87. Krssak M, Petersen KF, Bergeron R, *et al*: Intramuscular glycogen and intramyocellular lipid utilization during prolonged exercise and recovery in man: a ^{13}C and ^{1}H nuclear magnetic resonance spectroscopy study. *J Clin Endocrinol Metab* 2000;85:748.

88. Maehlum S, Hastmark AT, Hermansen L: Synthesis of muscle glycogen during recovery after prolonged severe exercise in diabetic subjects. Effect of insulin deprivation. *Scand J Clin Lab Invest* 1978; 38:35.

89. Firth RG, Bell PM, Marsh HM, *et al*: Postprandial hyperglycemia in patients with noninsulin-dependent diabetes mellitus. Role of hepatic and extrahepatic tissues. *J Clin Invest* 1986;77:1525.

90. Mitrakou A, Kelley D, Mokan M, *et al*: Role of reduced suppression of glucose production and diminished early insulin release in impaired glucose tolerance. *N Engl J Med* 1992;326:22.

91. DeFronzo RA, Ferrannini E, Koivisto V: New concepts in the pathogenesis and treatment of noninsulin-dependent diabetes mellitus. *Am J Med* 1983;74:52.

92. Olefsky JM, Ciaraldi TP, Kolterman OG: Mechanisms of insulin resistance in non-insulin-dependent (type II) diabetes. *Am J Med* 1985; 79:12.

93. Wahren J, Felig P, Cerasi E, *et al*: Splanchnic and peripheral glucose and amino acid metabolism in diabetes mellitus. *J Clin Invest* 1972; 51:1870.

94. DeFronzo RA, Hendler R, Simonson D: Insulin resistance is a prominent feature of insulin-dependent diabetes. *Diabetes* 1982;31:795.

95. DeFronzo RA, Simonson D, Ferrannini E: Hepatic and peripheral insulin resistance: a common feature of type 2 (non-insulin-dependent) and type 1 (insulin-dependent) diabetes mellitus. *Diabetologia* 1982; 23:313.

96. Magnusson I, Rothman DL, Katz LD, *et al*: Increased rate of gluconeogenesis in type II diabetes mellitus. A ^{13}C nuclear magnetic resonance study. *J Clin Invest* 1992;90:1323.

97. Gerich JE, Nurjhan N: Gluconeogenesis in type 2 diabetes. *Adv Exp Med Biol* 1993;334:253.

98. Press M, Tamborlane WV, Sherwin RS: Importance of raised growth hormone levels in mediating the metabolic derangements of diabetes. *N Engl J Med* 1984;310:810.

99. Shamoon H, Hendler R, Sherwin RS: Altered responsiveness to cortisol, epinephrine, and glucagon in insulin-infused juvenile-onset diabetics. A mechanism for diabetic instability. *Diabetes* 1980;29:284.

100. Barrett EJ, DeFronzo RA, Bevilacqua S, *et al*: Insulin resistance in diabetic ketoacidosis. *Diabetes* 1982;31:923.

101. DeFronzo RA, Matsuda M, Barrett EJ: Diabetic ketoacidosis. *Diabetes Reviews* 1994;2:209.

CHAPTER 2

Ketogenesis

J. Denis McGarry
Daniel W. Foster

PHYSIOLOGICAL AND CLINICAL OVERVIEW

In the normal, fed state the ketone bodies, acetoacetic acid and 3-hydroxybutyric acid, play little role in body metabolism. Production rates by the liver and plasma concentrations are low. The primary circulating substrates are diet-derived glucose and mobilized free fatty acids (FFA). On the other hand, if food is unavailable, the ketones rapidly take on major importance as an alternative energy source, particularly for the brain.[1] It is a peculiarity of the central nervous system that it cannot use plasma FFA as a metabolic fuel, in contrast to most other tissues in the body. Because the great bulk of stored energy is in the form of triglyceride contained in the adipose tissue mass (and because reserve stores of carbohydrate in the form of glycogen are extremely limited, sufficient to sustain energy needs for less than 24 hours), it follows that a mechanism to convert fat into a form of substrate the brain can use for energy is critical. The process involved is *ketogenesis,* the conversion of long-chain fatty acids into acetoacetate and 3-hydroxybutyrate by the liver. These four-carbon substrates protect the central nervous system in two ways, one directly and the other indirectly. Directly, the brain oxidizes the ketoacids so efficiently that normal function is unimpaired even in the face of plasma glucose levels sufficient to cause sweating, nervousness, chest pain, and mental confusion, provided plasma ketone concentrations are in the low millimolar range. Indirectly, acetoacetate and 3-hydroxybutyrate are used effectively in a variety of other tissues (together with FFA), preempting their need for glucose and thereby conserving the hexose for use by the brain.[2] It is clear, therefore, that the primary utility of ketogenesis is to provide universally oxidizable substrate for energy purposes.

Two other functions of the ketoacids have also received attention. On the basis of the observation that infusion of 3-hydroxybutyrate results in diminished urinary nitrogen loss in starved humans, it has been widely assumed that the ketones somehow limit muscle breakdown, thereby providing protection against the deleterious effect of a prolonged negative nitrogen balance. Two mechanisms have been assumed. First, by limiting demands for glucose as described previously, the drive for gluconeogenesis (which of necessity is fueled by muscle amino acids) is diminished. Second, ketone bodies have been thought to have a direct inhibitory effect on proteolysis in muscle. However, it has been shown that although sodium acetoacetate diminishes amino acid release from muscle, free acetoacetic acid does not. Because

sodium bicarbonate sufficient to produce the same alkalinizing effect as sodium acetoacetate also diminishes amino acid release, it may turn out that the anions derived from the ketoacids have no regulatory effect on muscle breakdown. The only other known function of acetoacetate and 3-hydroxybutyrate is as precursors for lipid synthesis in the cerebral tissue of neonates.[3]

Although the increased production of acetoacetate and 3-hydroxybutyrate that characterizes starvation is a beneficial adaptive response, larger accumulations of ketones are dangerous. This is because they are powerful organic acids capable of producing a profound metabolic acidosis. This point is illustrated by the fact that untreated diabetic and alcoholic ketoacidoses, the major pathologic ketotic states, are potentially fatal illnesses. The physiological ketosis of fasting or prolonged starvation, on the other hand, never progresses to a life-threatening acidosis. The pathologic transition is prevented by the presence of an intact pancreatic β cell (Fig. 2-1). When plasma FFA and ketone concentrations rise, there is a modulation of free fatty acid mobilization from adipose tissue. The major mechanism is probably a fatty acid and ketone-induced stimulation of insulin release from the pancreas, which serves to attenuate lipolysis,[4,5] although a direct antilipolytic effect of ketone bodies on the adipocyte has also been postulated. In any event, ketogenesis is limited because of insufficient fatty acids to allow maximal rates of ketone production in the liver; thus a metabolic acidosis does not occur.

In the sections that follow, current understanding of the mechanisms by which ketogenesis is controlled will be discussed in some depth. Because the system is complicated, it may be helpful to give a brief anticipatory summary at this point. Details will subsequently be added.

It has already been pointed out that the substrate for ketone body formation is long-chain fatty acids. These fatty acids are ordinarily derived from adipose tissue but can also arise from hepatic triglycerides. For practical purposes (in the absence of certain inborn errors of amino acid metabolism such as maple syrup urine disease), accelerated ketone body production does not occur unless the rate of FFA delivery to the liver is increased. On the other hand, increased fatty acid delivery alone is not sufficient to induce rapid ketogenesis; the second necessary component is an activation of hepatic fatty acid oxidative capacity. The required changes in adipose and hepatic tissues are initiated by alterations in plasma concentrations of glucagon and insulin: a low glucagon:insulin ratio, characteristic of the fed state, inhibits free fatty acid release from

SIMPLE STARVATION

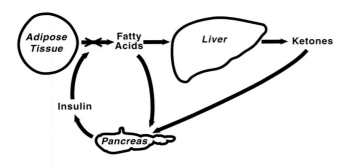

TYPE I DIABETES

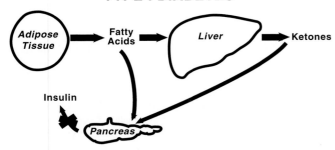

FIGURE 2-1. Feedback control of ketogenesis during fasting by insulin. As described in the text, the ketogenic sequence is initiated by a fall in plasma insulin and a rise in plasma glucagon. Free fatty acids are mobilized from adipose tissue stores and transported to the liver, which has been activated for ketone body production. In simple starvation, as plasma fatty acid and ketone concentrations rise, insulin release from the pancreas is stimulated. This blunts (but does not normalize) lipolytic activity in the fat cell such that plasma free fatty acid levels are fixed at about 0.7–1.0 mmol—sufficient to allow moderate production of acetoacetate and 3-hydroxybutyrate by the liver, but insufficient to allow the maximum rates of production required to develop ketoacidosis. In type 1 diabetic subjects, the protective insulin feedback loop cannot operate because of β-cell destruction in the islets of Langerhans. As a consequence, plasma FFA reach much higher concentrations, driving ketone production to maximal rates, thereby leading to the ketoacidotic state. Experimentally, ketone bodies can directly suppress lipolysis, but this is likely of lesser importance because FFA levels are very high in diabetic ketoacidosis despite markedly elevated ketone concentrations.

adipose tissue stores and deactivates the β-oxidative sequence for free fatty acids, which controls the ketogenic rate in the liver. Change to a high glucagon: insulin ratio, as occurs in fasting or diabetes, is characterized by enhanced lipolysis and activation of hepatic fatty acid oxidation. In the liver, a critical factor is the level of malonyl CoA, the first committed intermediate in long-chain fatty acid synthesis. When malonyl CoA concentrations are high, rates of fatty acid oxidation are repressed through inhibition of the carnitine palmitoyl transferase I (CPT I) reaction. This enzyme regulates entry of FFA into the mitochondrion and thus controls ketogenesis. Conversely, when malonyl CoA levels are low, derepression of the transferase allows ketogenesis to proceed at rates directly proportional to delivery of the fatty acyl substrate. Put in other terms, activation of the ketogenic machinery by a fall in malonyl CoA concentration shifts the control of ketogenesis from

the hepatic enzymic machinery to the rate of delivery of free fatty acids.

It is critical to understand that the liver is fully operational for acetoacetate and 3-hydroxybutyrate formation after a short period of fasting (i.e., there is little difference in the potential for ketone body synthesis between a short fast and completely uncontrolled diabetes). The severe ketoacidosis seen in the latter state (and in alcoholic ketoacidosis) is due solely to plasma fatty acid concentrations much higher than those seen during a fast. In the diabetic state limitation of lipolysis is precluded by the inability of the pancreas to respond to rising FFA and ketone levels with appropriate release of insulin; in alcoholic ketoacidosis, alteration of FFA release from fat depots in response to hormones appears to be abnormal. Interactions between fat metabolism in adipose and hepatic tissues should become clearer from the discussion that follows.

RELATIONSHIP BETWEEN ADIPOSE TISSUE AND LIVER IN KETOGENESIS

As noted previously, the primary substrate for ketone body formation is free fatty acids. Although under certain circumstances these may be derived from hepatic triglycerides, their major source is adipose tissue. Because it can be easily shown that a precursor-product relationship exists between plasma free fatty acids and circulating ketone bodies, it was initially felt that rates of hepatic ketogenesis were simply the passive consequence of the rate of delivery of free fatty acids to the liver. According to this formulation no regulatory control was exerted in the hepatocyte, which remained poised to make ketones once substrate became available. Supporting evidence for this view came from the experimental observation that if the triglyceride stores of adipose tissue were depleted by systematic semistarvation, acute ketosis disappeared in rats made diabetic by pancreatectomy.[6] It was also noted that in the mild ketosis (2–5 mmol) of starvation, plasma free fatty acid concentrations were generally around 1 mmol,[7] although in full-blown ketoacidosis ketone concentrations in the range of 17–20 mmol were accompanied by fatty acid levels of 2–4 mmol.[8] On the basis of these observations, the simple lipolytic theory for the control of ketogenesis became broadly accepted.

It subsequently became apparent that such a theory was inadequate. Three major observations indicated that a substantial change in the pattern of liver metabolism was also required for ketogenesis to attain maximal rates. First, FFA levels in plasma could be elevated *in vivo* to levels equivalent to those seen in diabetic ketoacidosis without inducing ketosis in normal animals.[9,10] Second, developed ketosis could be reversed under circumstances in which plasma FFA concentrations were kept high and unchanged.[11,12] Third, and most important, if livers were removed from normal, fed rats and perfused with high concentrations of oleic acid, production of acetoacetic and 3-hydroxybutyric acids was only minimally stimulated. On the other hand, livers taken from fasted or diabetic animals, given the same concentration of oleic acid, produced ketone bodies at rates five- to tenfold higher than those seen in nonketotic rats.[13] It thus became clear that biochemical changes were required in both adipose tissue and liver for major ketogenesis to supervene. Conceptually, adipose tissue would be considered the substrate storage site, and liver would represent the conversion machinery. As will become apparent in the subsequent discussion, regulation of the two sites can occur in coupled or independent fashion. Activation of each is necessary, but not sufficient, to induce maximal ketogenic rates.

HORMONAL CONTROL OF KETOGENESIS

For many years it was thought that a relative or absolute deficiency of insulin was in itself sufficient for full activation of the ketogenic process. After all, insulin deficiency was known to be a characteristic of diabetes mellitus, and it had long been recognized that plasma insulin concentrations fell with the progression of a fast in inverse proportion to the rise of plasma ketones.[7] That this formulation might be oversimplified was suggested by two sets of observations. First, Unger[14] showed that diabetes was characterized not only by insulin deficiency, but by a relative or absolute excess of glucagon; therefore it was a bihormonal metabolic disorder. Second, a series of experiments carried out *in vitro* indicated that the α cell hormone had ketogenic activity in isolated liver preparations.[15,16] The roles of the two hormones in the ketogenic process were then examined using intact rats as the experimental model.[17] Fed, nonketotic animals were infused with either anti-insulin serum (AIS) or glucagon for short periods of time (1–3 hours). AIS infusion rapidly produced severe hyperglycemia, elevated plasma levels of FFA, and a prompt rise in plasma ketones. Thus by binding to insulin and preventing its biologic activity, AIS induced a state of early diabetic ketoacidosis. Glucagon, by contrast, caused only a minimal elevation of plasma glucose concentrations and no change in FFA or ketone body levels. Although glucagon is known to be a potent initiator of glycogenolysis in the liver (glycogen stores in these rats were dissipated), it did not cause hyperglycemia. The reason is quite straightforward. As glycogenolysis supervened, a transient rise in plasma glucose occurred, which in turn stimulated insulin release from the pancreas. This insulin accelerated the efficient disposition of glucose in muscle and adipose tissue; in effect, glucagon caused transfer of stored carbohydrates from liver to peripheral tissues in the absence of hyperglycemia.

Up to this point the findings were not unexpected, and were fully in accord with predictions. The second part of the experiment, however, produced results that elucidated the independent roles of insulin and glucagon in the regulation of ketogenesis. At the end of the infusion periods, livers were removed from the experimental animals and placed in an *in vitro* perfusion system. Oleic acid was added to bring the FFA concentration to 0.7 mmol in the perfusion media, approximately the level seen with fasting. Under these circumstances, livers taken from animals treated with AIS produced ketone bodies at an accelerated rate when compared with control livers from nontreated animals. This was fully expected, because the livers were taken from animals that were ketotic *in vivo*. Surprisingly, however, perfusion of livers from glucagon-treated animals (which were not ketotic) produced acetoacetate and 3-hydroxybutyrate at rates comparable to those in animals made experimentally diabetic. Thus, a ketogenic liver had been produced in a nonketotic animal. Measurements of hormones in plasma showed that in AIS-treated rats, insulin concentrations were low and glucagon concentrations were high. In the glucagon-treated animals, levels of the α-cell hormone were elevated into the patho-

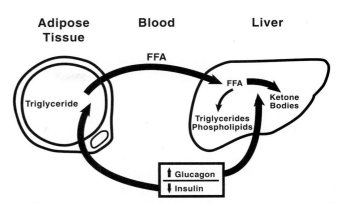

FIGURE 2-2. Bihormonal model for the control of ketogenesis. *(Reprinted with permission from the American Diabetes Association, Inc., from McGarry JD: Lilly lecture. New perspectives in the regulation of ketogenesis.* Diabetes *1979;28:517.)*

physiologic range, but in contrast to the AIS experiment, plasma insulin levels were also high. The latter observation meant, contrary to the generally held view, that the switch in the metabolic profile of the liver to fatty acid oxidation and ketone formation did not require an insulin-deficient state *in vivo* for its induction.

Why was the glucagon-treated animal not ketotic? The answer turned out to be quite simple: It was deficient in substrate. Recall that measured FFA concentrations after glucagon were low; this was because glucagon-induced hyperglycemia had produced an insulin response and insulin has a powerful antilipolytic effect. Correctness of this interpretation was proved by showing that experimental elevation of plasma FFA concentrations caused the glucagon-treated animals to develop a brisk ketosis. It was thus proposed[17] that the hepatic ketogenic machinery was under the same bihormonal control as had been postulated for glucose homeostasis by Unger.[14]

Current understanding of the system, based on the previously mentioned experiments, is shown in Fig. 2-2. According to this model, insulin deficiency acts primarily at the level of the adipocyte to provide long-chain fatty acid substrate for ketone body formation in the liver; in the presence of insulin, lipolysis is blocked and ketosis does not occur because of substrate deficiency. Glucagon, on the other hand, is thought to act primarily on the liver to activate fatty acid oxidation and ketone formation at the expense of triglyceride synthesis. Although emphasis has been placed on the independent roles of insulin and glucagon, it should not be concluded that insulin deficiency has no effect on the liver. Considerable evidence has accrued to indicate that the glucagon:insulin ratio is more important than absolute concentrations of either hormone in determining metabolic events within the hepatocyte. It should also not be inferred that insulin and glucagon are the only hormones involved in the regulation of ketogenesis. Although they doubtless represent the primary signals, a variety of other hormones, particularly catecholamines, have been shown to exert effects similar to those of glucagon.

Does the model developed in the rat apply to humans? The evidence is quite strong that it does. For example, Gerich and associates[18] showed that hyperglycemia and ketonemia in type 1 diabetic patients withdrawn from insulin were almost completely inhibited when glucagon secretion was blocked by infusion of somatostatin.

Further, it was shown that diabetic subjects pretreated with glucagon had enhanced ketogenic responses compared with control subjects given the same level of infused fatty acids.[19] Finally, patients with glucagon-producing tumors have small but definitely increased ketone concentrations as a consequence of their disease.[20] It thus seems safe to conclude that the overall thrust of the model is correct.

BIOCHEMICAL ASPECTS

The enzymatic pathway for the production of acetoacetate and 3-hydroxybutyrate can conveniently be divided into two sections. The first, collectively called the β-oxidative sequence for fatty acid oxidation, involves the generation of acetyl CoA from long-chain fatty acids. The second concerns the synthesis of the two ketones from acetyl CoA. Four enzymes are involved in the latter portion of the pathway, as indicated by the following reactions (called the HMG-CoA cycle):

$$2 \text{ Acetyl CoA} \leftrightharpoons \text{acetoacetyl CoA} + \text{CoA} \tag{2-1}$$

$$\text{Acetoacetyl CoA} + \text{acetyl CoA} \rightarrow$$
$$\text{Hydroxymethylglutaryl CoA} + \text{CoA} \tag{2-2}$$

$$\text{Hydroxymethylglutaryl-CoA} \rightarrow$$
$$\text{Acetoacetate} + \text{Acetyl CoA} \tag{2-3}$$

$$\text{Acetoacetate} + \text{NADH} + \text{H}^+ \leftrightharpoons$$
$$\text{3-Hydroxybutyrate} + \text{NAD}^+ \tag{2-4}$$

Reactions 1 through 4 are catalyzed by the enzymes acetoacetyl CoA thiolase (E.C.2.3.1.9), HMG-CoA synthase (E.C.4.1.3.5), HMG-CoA lyase (E.C.4.1.3.4), and D-3-hydroxybutyrate dehydrogenase (E.C.1.1.1.30), respectively. All are located in the mitochondria. The rate-limiting enzyme is considered to be HMG-CoA synthase, which is present in high concentrations only in liver mitochondria. The other three enzymes are found in significant quantities in a variety of extrahepatic tissues. (Note that most tissues contain another isoform of HMG-CoA synthase in the extramitochondrial compartment, but this is involved in the process of cholesterol biosynthesis.) It had become clear by the late 1960s that neither the amount nor the activity of these enzymes changed sufficiently to account for the increased ketogenic capacity of the liver in ketotic states. Other studies focused on alternative routes of acetyl CoA disposal as playing a key role. Thus, it was considered that a deficiency of oxaloacetate (thought to be characteristic of all ketotic states) diverted acetyl CoA from citrate formation to the ketogenic sequence. Although disposal of acetyl CoA can, under certain circumstances, modulate absolute rates of ketone formation, it was possible to show that high rates of ketone synthesis can be produced in situations where tricarboxylic acid cycle activity is not suppressed, but stimulated. These experiments indicated that the primary regulatory role was not exerted through alterations in acetyl CoA disposal, but rather by changes in the series of reactions leading to the generation of acetyl CoA from long-chain fatty acids.

As shown in Fig. 2-3, when a long-chain fatty acid is taken up by the hepatocyte it has two major routes of metabolism. Either it

FIGURE 2-3. Fatty acid metabolism in the liver. Fatty acids are taken up by the liver in concentration-dependent fashion. Following esterification to coenzyme A, the fatty acid may be utilized for triglyceride (and phospholipid) formation and leave the liver as very low density lipoproteins. Alternatively, fatty acyl CoA can be transported inside the mitochondrion for oxidation to ketone bodies and CO_2. Transport across the inner mitochondrial membrane requires esterification to carnitine under the influence of the enzyme carnitine palmitoyl transferase I (CPT I) present on the outer membrane. This reaction appears to be the rate-limiting step for fatty acid oxidation and ketogenesis. Inside the mitochondrion, the acyl CoA derivative is reformed under the influence of carnitine palmitoyl transferase II (CPT II). The capacity for fatty acid oxidation is fixed and large relative to activity of the Krebs tricarboxylic acid cycle. Therefore, the bulk of fatty acids entering the matrix will be converted into ketone bodies.

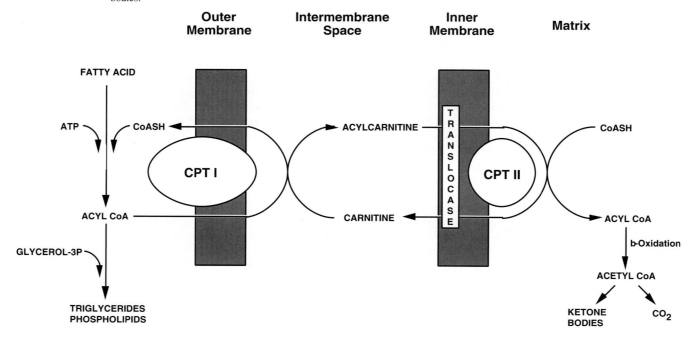

can be esterified with glycerol-3-phosphate to form triglycerides (and phospholipids) or it enters the mitochondrion for oxidation to acetyl CoA and ketone bodies. In the fed, nonketotic state, the bulk of fatty acids traverse the esterification pathway. With fasting or diabetes, the distribution changes as ketone body production is accelerated; a much larger fraction of the fatty acids taken up enter the oxidative pathway at the expense of esterification.[13] It was initially believed that regulation was exerted on the esterification wing of the pathway, but this was disproved in an experiment wherein fatty acid oxidation was blocked acutely in the perfused liver by the inhibitor (+)-decanoylcarnitine, with the result that flux of fatty acids into esterification was immediately restored to normal.[21] This experiment indicated that there was nothing intrinsically wrong with the esterification sequence and strongly suggested that primary control of ketogenesis was exerted on the oxidative pathway. The site of such control was initially deduced from studies comparing the metabolism of oleic acid (representative of long-chain fatty acids) and the medium-chain fatty acid, octanoate.[13,22] Coenzyme A derivatives of long-chain fatty acids are unable to penetrate the inner mitochondrial membrane. For transfer to occur there must be an esterification with carnitine, a reaction catalyzed by the enzyme carnitine palmitoyl transferase I (CPT I). Long-chain fatty acyl CoA is resynthesized by a reversal of the carnitine esterification reaction inside the mitochondrion under the influence of the enzyme carnitine palmitoyl transferase II (CPT II). In contrast to their long-chain analogues, medium-chain fatty acids are freely permeable across the inner mitochondrial membrane and have no need for esterification to carnitine. When livers from fed and fasted animals were perfused with oleic acid, rates of ketone formation in fasted livers were five- to sevenfold greater than in the control organs. When octanoic acid was used as substrate, ketogenic rates in the two types of liver were equivalent. Moreover, infusion of octanoate into normal fed rats promptly induced ketosis, but long-chain fatty acids had no such effect.[22] It thus became clear that the regulatory site was the carnitine palmitoyl transferase system of enzymes, the first specific step in the fatty acid oxidative sequence.

The mechanism whereby this enzyme system is regulated emerged in 1977. Solution of the problem provided understanding not only of the control of ketogenesis, but of two other longstanding observations: the fact that when rates of fatty acid oxidation are high (fasting, uncontrolled diabetes), fatty acid synthesis is low, and the demonstration that ketotic states are always associated with hepatic glycogen depletion. A relationship between glucose and lipid metabolism in the liver was implicit in the observation that starvation ketosis is immediately reversed by the ingestion of small amounts of carbohydrate. The initial hypothesis was that when glucose was available to the liver, a glycolytic metabolite would act to suppress the carnitine palmitoyl transferase step. It was presumed that the concentration of this metabolite would fall in parallel with glycogen stores when the liver was exposed to a high glucagon:insulin ratio. The hypothesis turned out to be correct in principle, but the controlling intermediate was not a participant in the glycogenolytic-gluconeogenic pathway. Rather, it was malonyl CoA, the primary substrate for long-chain fatty acid synthesis, which is derived via citrate from ingested or stored carbohydrate.[23] It was already known that malonyl CoA levels in liver fluctuated in direct proportion to the rate of fatty acid synthesis.[24] Its position as the first committed intermediate in long-chain fatty acid synthesis made it an attractive candidate as a regulator of fatty acid oxidation. Thus, when malonyl CoA levels were high, assuring vigorous

fatty acid synthesis, it would be logical to expect that rates of fatty acid oxidation should be low (to avoid a futile cycle of long-chain fatty acid synthesis and breakdown). When added to liver homogenates, malonyl CoA powerfully inhibited the oxidation of oleic acid and did so at physiologically relevant concentrations. The block in fatty acid oxidation was immediately reversed upon removal of malonyl CoA and was not reproduced with other CoA esters such as acetyl CoA, propionyl CoA, or methylmalonyl CoA.[23] When tested with mitochondrial fractions, malonyl CoA was shown to block the oxidation of oleate, palmitate, and palmitoyl CoA (which requires the action of both transferases), but did not inhibit the oxidation of palmitoyl carnitine (which requires only the action of CPT II), or of octanoate (which is carnitine-independent).[25] In studies with mitochondrial membranes, it was shown directly that only CPT I was inhibited by malonyl CoA and that the inhibitor acts in pseudocompetitive fashion against the long-chain acyl CoA substrate in the reaction.[26] The Ki is 1–2 μmol both in rat and human (fetal) liver.

Support for the key role of malonyl CoA came from experiments in which rates of fatty acid oxidation were manipulated over wide ranges. Under these circumstances it could be shown that malonyl CoA concentrations followed the predicted course; i.e., when malonyl CoA levels were high, rates of fatty acid synthesis were brisk and fatty acid oxidation was inhibited.[27] When malonyl CoA levels were at their nadir, fatty acid oxidation was maximal and fatty acid synthesis ceased. These interrelationships persisted in a smoothly-related fashion as the system was manipulated from one extreme to the other. Such observations meshed nicely with the previously mentioned role of glucagon in inducing ketogenesis and the demonstration that glucagon treatment of intact animals or its addition to isolated hepatocytes precipitously dropped malonyl CoA concentrations.[28,29] It is now known that glucagon acts by causing cyclic AMP–mediated phosphorylation of key enzymes in the glycolytic sequence such that citrate concentrations fall, imposing a limitation on substrate available for malonyl CoA formation. In addition, glucagon is thought to inhibit acetyl CoA carboxylase, the enzyme catalyzing the formation of malonyl CoA from acetyl CoA.

As in most metabolic pathways, the primary control mechanism for fatty acid oxidation and ketogenesis (in this case fluctuation in hepatic malonyl CoA levels) is modulated by other regulatory components. Three such factors are now recognized. First, in all ketotic states, hepatic concentrations of carnitine (the transfer molecule for long-chain fatty acids across the membrane restriction barrier) rise to high levels.[30] This further accelerates CPT I activity by a mass-action effect. Second, long-chain fatty acyl CoAs, like glucagon, inhibit acetyl CoA carboxylase, assuring a maximal fall in malonyl CoA generation and an increase in fatty acid oxidation as the liver is flooded with fatty acids secondary to uncontrolled diabetes.[31] Although glucagon is considered to be the primary regulator of the process, long-chain fatty acyl CoAs function synergistically in a backup role. Third, ketotic states are characterized not only by cessation of hepatic malonyl CoA synthesis, but also by reduced sensitivity of liver CPT I to this inhibitory molecule.[32–35] Teleologically, the latter phenomenon might be viewed as an amplification mechanism for control of CPT I activity over and above that imparted simply by changes in tissue malonyl CoA content. Also noteworthy is that upon reversal of the ketotic state (refeeding after a fast or treatment of diabetic animals with insulin) it takes several hours for normal malonyl CoA sensitivity of liver

CPT I to be restored.[34,35] This might be nature's way of ensuring that hepatic fatty acid oxidation is not immediately shut down under such conditions, but continues at a rate sufficient to support gluconeogenic carbon flow and thus repletion of hepatic glycogen stores via the so-called indirect pathway.[35,36] Presumably, under these conditions the fatty acid substrate derives not so much from plasma (as adipose tissue lipolysis is rapidly suppressed by the rising insulin concentration), but from triglyceride stores accumulated in the liver during the prior period of insulin deficiency.

OVERVIEW

Against this background, the overall features of the model, schematically depicted in Fig. 2-4, can now be reviewed.[37] With the ingestion of carbohydrate (or an ordinary mixed meal of carbohydrate, fat, and protein), glucagon concentrations are low and insulin concentrations are high, with the result that hepatic malonyl CoA concentrations are elevated, fatty acid synthesis is brisk, and the opposing pathway of fatty acid oxidation is blocked. Under these circumstances the physiologic role of malonyl CoA can be viewed as a mechanism to ensure unidirectional flow of carbon from glucose (or other precursors of pyruvate), into the sequence long-chain fatty acid → triglyceride → very low density lipoprotein through suppression of the activity of CPT I, thereby preventing the futile reoxidization of newly synthesized fatty acids. In the absence of food or in uncontrolled diabetes, insulin is deficient and glucagon concentrations are high. This results in a fall in malonyl CoA synthesis, with the consequence that lipogenesis slows and CPT I becomes activated. Fatty acid oxidation is further enhanced by the rise in tissue carnitine (mechanism not yet determined). Simultaneously, low plasma insulin levels allow activation of lipolysis such that ample free fatty acid substrate is now available to the derepressed hepatic ketogenic machinery. As fatty acyl CoA levels in the liver rise, backup inhibition of acetyl CoA carboxylase is assured. With carbohydrate feeding or the administration of insulin, the glucagon:insulin ratio falls and the entire sequence is ultimately reversed.

Increased oxidation of fatty acids in the liver, initiated by the fall in malonyl CoA concentrations, is the primary cause of all ketotic states. However, it should be emphasized that rates of ketone use in peripheral tissues are not unlimited. Once these processes are saturated, plasma ketone levels rise disproportionately to synthetic rates. Such saturation never occurs in the ketosis of fasting, but is characteristic of alcoholic and diabetic ketoacidoses.

Solution of the control of ketogenesis took several decades and the work of many investigators. It is quite remarkable that at the heart of the mystery was a simple molecule, malonyl CoA. It functions not only to regulate the opposing pathways of fatty acid synthesis and oxidation, but also represents a key link between carbohydrate and lipid metabolism in the liver. Evidence is accumulating that the malonyl CoA–CPT I interaction also plays a regulatory role in "fuel crosstalk" in a variety of nonhepatic tissues, in particular heart and skeletal muscle.[38,39] The dominant form of CPT I expressed in myocytes is the so-called M (for muscle) variant, which is a separate gene product from the L (for liver) type enzyme.[40] Curiously, compared with L-CPT I, M-CPT I is about 100 times more sensitive to inhibition by malonyl CoA. It is of interest that both heart and skeletal muscle contain acetyl CoA carboxylase activity, and that in both sites the concentration of malonyl CoA changes reciprocally with the rate of fatty acid oxidation under different nu-

tritional and experimental conditions.[38–40] Since neither tissue expresses significant levels of fatty acid synthase, it seems likely that the function of malonyl CoA in heart and skeletal muscle cells is solely for the regulation of fatty acid oxidation.[38,39] Finally, the possibility has been raised that malonyl CoA inhibition of CPT I activity represents an important component of glucose-stimulated insulin secretion by the pancreatic β cell.[41,42]

EPILOGUE

It is noteworthy that interest in the mitochondrial carnitine palmitoyl transferase enzyme system has suddenly begun to grow at an exponential rate. Several reasons for this renaissance can be discerned. First, as discussed previously, it is now clear that CPT I represents a pivotal site in the overall regulation of mammalian fatty acid metabolism. Second, there is growing momentum in the pharmaceutical industry to design drugs that will selectively suppress the activity of CPT I in liver and thus act as hypoglycemic agents.[43] Third, inherited defects in mitochondrial fatty acid transport, some with pathologic consequences, are now being documented more and more frequently.[44] Finally, and quite remarkably, this complex, membrane-bound dual enzyme system, known to be present in essentially all tissues of the body but discussed solely in operational terms for most of the past 30 years, has only recently proved amenable to analysis at the molecular level.[40] Although further discussion on this point is beyond the scope of the present review, exciting new insight into structure–function–regulatory relationships surrounding the CPT enzymes and the control of their respective genes can be expected in the near future.

REFERENCES

1. Owen OE, Morgan AP, Kemp HG, *et al*: Brain metabolism during fasting. *J Clin Invest* 1967;46:1589.
2. Cahill GF Jr.: Starvation in man. *N Engl J Med* 1970;282:668.
3. Webber RJ, Edmond J: The *in vivo* utilization of acetoacetate, D-(–)-3-hydroxybutyrate, and glucose for lipid synthesis in brain in the 18-day-old rat. Evidence for an acetyl-CoA bypass for sterol synthesis. *J Biol Chem* 1979;254:3912.
4. Madison LL, Mebane D, Unger RH: The hypoglycemic action of ketones, 2. Evidence for a stimulatory feedback of ketones on the pancreatic β-cell. *J Clin Invest* 1964;43:408.
5. Dobbins RL, Chester MW, Daniels MB, *et al*: Circulating fatty acids are essential for efficient glucose-stimulated insulin secretion after prolonged fasting in humans. *Diabetes* 1998;47:1613.
6. Scow RO, Chernick SS: Hormonal control of protein and fat metabolism in the pancreatectomized rat. *Recent Prog Horm Res* 1960; 16:497.
7. Owen OE, Felig P, Morgan AP, *et al*: Liver and kidney metabolism during prolonged starvation. *J Clin Invest* 1969;48:574.
8. Alberti KGMM, Hockaday TDD, Turner RC: Small doses of intramuscular insulin in the treatment of diabetic "coma." *Lancet* 1973;2:515.
9. Seyffert WA Jr., Madison LL: Physiologic effects of metabolic fuels on carbohydrate metabolism. Acute effect of elevation of plasma free fatty acids on hepatic glucose output, peripheral glucose utilization, serum insulin, and plasma glucagon levels. *Diabetes* 1967;16:765.
10. Crespin SR, Greenough WB, Steinberg D: Stimulation of insulin secretion by infusion of free fatty acids. *J Clin Invest* 1969;48:1934.
11. Williamson DH, Veloso D, Ellington EV, *et al*: Changes in the concentrations of hepatic metabolites on administration of dihydroxyacetone or glycerol to starved rats and their relationship to the control of ketogenesis. *Biochem J* 1969;114:575.
12. Bieberdorf FA, Chernick SS, Scow RO: Effect of insulin and acute diabetes on plasma FFA and ketone bodies in the fasting rat. *J Clin Invest* 1970;49:1685.

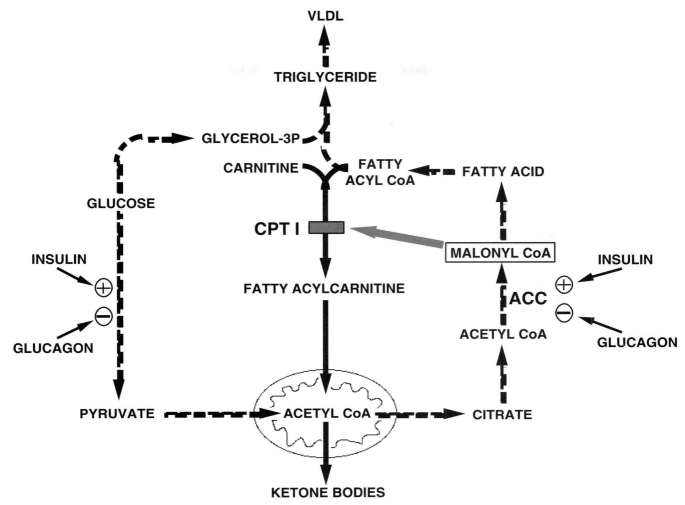

FIGURE 2-4. Relationship between fatty acid synthesis and oxidation in liver. In the normal, fed state (high insulin:glucagon ratio) fatty acid synthesis from glucose is active, resulting in an elevated level of malonyl CoA. This causes suppression of CPT I activity such that newly formed fatty acyl CoA molecules are directed away from oxidation and into the esterification pathway leading to very low density lipoprotein (VLDL) production. Conversely, in starvation or uncontrolled diabetes (low insulin:glucagon ratio) fatty acid synthesis ceases because of inhibition of glycolysis and the acetyl CoA carboxylase (ACC) reaction. The concomitant fall in malonyl CoA concentration allows derepression of CPT I such that fatty acids mobilized from fat depots and entering the liver can readily react with carnitine and enter the β-oxidation pathway, allowing efficient production of ketone bodies. Note that pyruvate is a poor ketogenic substrate because its ability to generate acetyl CoA is low compared with that of fatty acids. For simplicity, CPT I has been placed outside the mitochondrion though it actually resides on the outer mitochondrial membrane.

13. McGarry JD, Foster DW: The regulation of ketogenesis from oleic acid and the influence of antiketogenic agents. *J Biol Chem* 1971;246:6247.

14. Unger RH: Role of glucagon in the pathogenesis of diabetes: The status of the controversy. *Metabolism* 1978;27:1691.

15. Bewsher PD, Ahsmore J: Ketogenic and lipolytic effects of glucagon on liver. *Biochem Biophys Res Comm* 1966;24:431.

16. Williamson JR, Browning ET, Thurman RG, *et al*: Inhibition of glucagon effects in perfused rat liver by (1)decanoylcarnitine. *J Biol Chem* 1969;244:5055.

17. McGarry JD, Wright PH, Foster DW: Hormonal control of ketogenesis. Rapid activation of hepatic ketogenic capacity in fed rats by antiinsulin serum and glucagon. *J Clin Invest* 1975;55:1202.

18. Gerich JE, Lorenzi M, Bier DM, *et al*: Prevention of human diabetic ketoacidosis by somatostatin. Evidence for an essential role of glucagon. *N Engl J Med* 1975;292:985.

19. Schade DS, Eaton RP: Glucagon regulation of plasma ketone body concentration in human diabetes. *J Clin Invest* 1975;56:1340.

20. Boden G, Owen OE, Rezvani I, *et al*: An islet cell carcinoma containing glucagon and insulin. Chronic glucagon excess and glucose homeostasis. *Diabetes* 1977;26:128.

21. McGarry JD, Meier JM, Foster DW: The effects of starvation and refeeding on carbohydrate and lipid metabolism *in vivo* and in the perfused rat liver. The relationship between fatty acid oxidation and esterification in the regulation of ketogenesis. *J Biol Chem* 1973;248:270.

22. McGarry JD, Foster DW: The regulation of ketogenesis from octanoic acid. The role of the tricarboxylic acid cycle and fatty acid synthesis. *J Biol Chem* 1971;246:1149.

23. McGarry JD, Mannaerts GP, Foster DW: A possible role for malonyl-CoA in the regulation of hepatic fatty acid oxidation and ketogenesis. *J Clin Invest* 1977;60:265.

24. Guynn RW, Veloso D, Veech RL: The concentration of malonyl-coenzyme A and the control of fatty acid synthesis *in vivo*. *J Biol Chem* 1972;247:7325.

25. McGarry JD, Mannaerts GP, Foster DW: Characteristics of fatty acid oxidation in rat liver homogenates and the inhibitory effect of malonyl-CoA. *Biochim Biophys Acta* 1978;530:305.

26. McGarry JD, Leatherman GF, Foster DW: Carnitine palmitoyltransferase I: The site of inhibition of hepatic fatty acid oxidation by malonyl-CoA. *J Biol Chem.* 1978;253:4128.

27. McGarry JD, Takabayashi Y, Foster DW. The role of malonyl-CoA in the coordination of fatty acid synthesis and oxidation in isolated rat hepatocytes. *J Biol Chem* 1978;253:8294.

28. Cook GA, Nielsen RC, Hawkins RA, *et al*: Effect of glucagon on hepatic malonyl coenzyme A concentration and on lipid synthesis. *J Biol Chem* 1977;252:4421.

29. Cook GA, King MT, Veech RL: Ketogenesis and malonyl coenzyme A content of isolated rat hepatocytes. *J Biol Chem* 1978;253:2529.

30. McGarry JD, Robles-Valdes C, Foster DW: The role of carnitine in hepatic ketogenesis. *Proc Natl Acad Sci USA* 1975;72:4385.

31. McGarry JD, Foster DW: Effects of exogenous fatty acid concentration on glucagon-induced changes in hepatic fatty acid metabolism. *Diabetes* 1980;29:236.

32. Cook GA, Otto DA, Cornell NW: Differential inhibition of ketogenesis by malonyl-CoA in mitochondria from fed and starved rats. *Biochem J* 1980;192:955.

33. Saggerson ED, Carpenter CA: Effects of fasting, adrenalectomy and streptozotocin-diabetes on sensitivity of hepatic carnitine acyltransferase to malonyl CoA. *FEBS Lett* 1981;129:225.

34. Grantham BD, Zammit VA: Restoration of the properties of carnitine palmitoyltransferase I in liver mitochondria during refeeding of starved rats. *Biochem J* 1986;239:485.

35. Grantham BD, Zammit VA: Role of carnitine palmitoyltransferase I in the regulation of hepatic ketogenesis during the onset and reversal of chronic diabetes. *Biochem J* 1988;249:409.

36. McGarry JD, Kuwajima M, Newgard CB, *et al*: From dietary glucose to liver glycogen—the full circle round. *Annu Rev Nutr* 1987;7:51.

37. McGarry JD, Foster DW: Regulation of hepatic fatty acid oxidation and ketone body production. *Annu Rev Biochem* 1980;49:395.

38. Kantor PF, Dyck JRB, Lopaschuk GD: Fatty acid oxidation in the reperfused ischemic heart. *Am J Med Sci* 1999;318:3.

39. Ruderman NB, Saha AK, Vavvas D, *et al*: Malonyl-CoA, fuel sensing, and insulin resistance. *Am J Physiol.* 1999;276:E1.

40. McGarry JD, Brown NF: The mitochondrial carnitine palmitoyltransferase system—from concept to molecular analysis. *Eur J Biochem* 1997;244:001.

41. Prentki M, Vischer S, Glennon MC, *et al*: Malonyl-CoA and long-chain acyl-CoA esters as metabolic coupling factors in nutrient-induced insulin secretion. *J Biol Chem* 1992;267:5802.

42. Chen S, Ogawa A, Ohneda M, *et al*: More direct evidence for a malonyl-CoA-carnitine palmitoyltransferase I interaction as a key event in pancreatic β-cell signalling. *Diabetes* 1994;43:878.

43. Wolf HPO: Aryl-substituted 2-oxirane carboxylic acids: A new group of antidiabetic drugs. In: Bailey CJ, Flatt PR, eds. *New Antidiabetic Drugs*. Smith-Gordon:1990;217.

44. Bonnefont J-P, Demaugre F, Prip-Buus C, *et al*: Carnitine palmitoyltransferase deficiencies. *Mol Genet Metab* 1999;68:424.

CHAPTER 3

The Molecular and Cell Biology of the Beta Cell

Kevin Docherty

Donald F. Steiner

INTRODUCTION

The discovery of insulin in 1921[1] ushered in the modern era of diabetes therapy and at the same time opened many new areas for biochemical and physiological investigation—activities that continue to flourish. Insulin is a small globular protein (MW ~5800 kd) consisting of two peptide chains, designated A and B, linked together by two disulfide bonds (Fig. 3-1).[2] It is produced and secreted by the β (beta) cells of the islets of Langerhans and acts by binding to a receptor molecule located on the plasma membrane of its target tissues. The receptor is a large integral membrane protein consisting of two polypeptide chains, the alpha and beta subunits, each present in two copies forming a heterotetramer ($\alpha_2\beta_2$). Although the molecular mechanism of signal transduction by the insulin receptor continues to be intensively investigated (see Chapt. 5), it is now clear that the receptor initiates a series of intracellular chemical events, including tyrosine phosphorylations on various targets, that lead to increased use and storage of glucose, as well as enhanced nitrogen retention and somatic growth (in immature organisms).

Both insulin and its receptor are derived from single-chain precursor molecules that are each encoded in a single autosomal gene. Biosynthesis results in the production of proinsulin, or proreceptor. These molecules are then processed posttranslationally to yield the mature proteins which are either stored for secretion, as in the case of insulin, or in the case of the receptor, transferred to the plasma membrane via small constitutive or unregulated vesicles. A great deal of information has accumulated in recent years on the structure and expression of the insulin gene. This chapter will describe the insulin gene, the molecular mechanisms underlying the biosynthesis and conversion of proinsulin, and the regulation of these processes by glucose and other factors. The clinical relevance of proinsulin and C peptide will be reviewed, and islet amyloid peptide (IAPP) or amylin, a newly identified neuropeptide product of the β cell that is cosecreted with insulin and is a major constituent of islet amyloid deposits in type 2 diabetes mellitus (T2DM), will be discussed.

INSULIN STRUCTURE

Insulin occurs in all vertebrates (Fig. 3-1), and two-chain insulin-like substances have been found in the nervous or digestive systems of several invertebrates.[3] These include a growth-promoting hormone of the light green cells in the snail *Lymnaea*,[4] an insulin-like brain peptide from the silkworm *Bombyx mori*,[5] an insulin-like peptide from the locust,[6] and the recently discovered multiple insulin-related genes in *Caenorhabditis elegans*.[7] Vertebrates also have insulin-like growth factors (IGF-I and -II), single-chain peptides related to proinsulin, which interact with growth hormone, insulin, and other hormones to regulate both somatic and tissue growth. These forms are found only in vertebrates and are believed to have arisen via gene duplication from the insulin gene early in vertebrate evolution.[8] Many tissues express a receptor—the IGF-I receptor—that is closely similar in structure to the classic insulin receptors, but which preferentially binds IGF-I and also IGF-II. A separate IGF-II binding receptor that also binds mannose-6-P lacks tyrosine kinase activity and appears to serve as an IGF scavenger.[9] Other less closely related members of the insulin superfamily include ovarian relaxin[10] and several recently discovered relaxin-like hormones.[11,12]

Certain structural features of insulin have been highly conserved throughout vertebrate evolution, including the positions of the three disulfide bonds, the N-terminal and C-terminal regions of the A chain, and the hydrophobic residues in the C-terminal region of the B chain (see Fig. 3-1). These residues influence receptor binding and are also intimately associated with maintaining the native three-dimensional structure of the hormone, as revealed by the x-ray crystallographic studies of Baker and coworkers.[13] The structure of a porcine insulin monomer is shown in Fig. 3-2. In this high-resolution (0.15-nm) representation, all the amino acid side chains are shown in their normal orientations and the putative receptor binding region is outlined. Nuclear magnetic resonance (NMR) studies[14] provide support for the conclusion that the structure of the insulin monomer in solution is closely similar to that in the crystals. Human and most other mammalian insulins form hexamers in the presence of zinc, and it is this form that exists in the rhombohedral Zn-insulin crystals.

Other recent studies have led to new insights regarding the location of the receptor binding region(s) in the insulin molecule, especially studies with several naturally occurring human insulin mutants involving residues A3, B24, and B25[15] and with despentapeptide insulin, in which the last five residues of the B chain have been deleted,[16] as well as with certain insulins with crosslinks between B29 and A1.[17] These data suggest that during receptor binding, the flexible C-terminal region of the B chain is reoriented, exposing underlying residues, such as A3 valine. Recent NMR data on various insulin derivatives in solution[14,18,19] also confirm the importance of significant conformational changes in the C terminus

Human Insulin

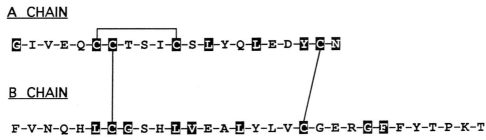

A CHAIN

G-I-V-E-Q-C-C-T-S-I-C-S-L-Y-Q-L-E-D-Y-C-N

B CHAIN

F-V-N-Q-H-L-C-G-S-H-L-V-E-A-L-Y-L-V-C-G-E-R-G-F-F-Y-T-P-K-T

FIGURE 3-1. Amino acid sequence of human insulin. Invariant residues in over 70 other vertebrate insulins are enclosed in boxes.

of the B chain in receptor binding. A question that remains unanswered is whether the insulin molecule interacts with more than one site on the receptor molecule in order to achieve the typical high affinity binding isotherm and curvilinear Scatchard.[20]

BIOSYNTHESIS OF INSULIN

The precursor of insulin is preproinsulin (Fig. 3-3), which consists of a single chain of 110 amino acids having a hydrophobic

FIGURE 3-2. View of a monomer of porcine insulin. The side chains of all the amino acids are shown: the A chain is dark gray and the B chain is light gray. The dashed outline delineates the approximate region on the surface of the insulin monomer which is believed to contact the receptor upon binding. (*Computer graphic representation kindly provided by Dr. Bing Xiao, University of York.*)

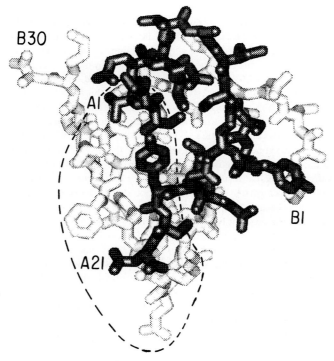

24-amino-acid N-terminal prepeptide or signal peptide in most mammalian species.[21,22] The signal peptide facilitates the transfer of proinsulin from the cytosolic compartment, where protein chain elongation occurs, into the secretory pathway. Interactions involving signal recognition particle (SRP) and the SRP receptor in the membrane of the rough endoplasmic reticulum (RER) lead to the translocation of the nascent peptide into its internal compartments, or cisternae.[23,24] During translocation the signal sequence is rapidly removed by the signal peptidase, a protease located on the inner surface of the RER membrane,[24] to give rise to proinsulin, which then folds and undergoes rapid formation of disulfide bonds, catalyzed by the enzyme protein-thiol reductase, to gain its native structure. Proinsulin is a stable precursor that includes the insulin B and A chains within a single 9000-kd polypeptide chain.[25–27] Newly formed proinsulin is then transported to the *cis* region of the Golgi apparatus for further processing and packaging (Fig. 3-4), while the signal peptide is rapidly degraded in the RER and is not a secretory product.

During the intracellular maturation of secretory granules, proinsulin is cleaved to yield insulin and a 31-residue (in humans and several other mammals) connecting peptide fragment designated the C peptide. Both insulin and C peptide are stored in mature secretion granules along with small amounts of residual proinsulin and its intermediate cleavage forms[28] as well as various other minor secretory products.[29] Due to the time required for transit from the RER to the immature granules, conversion of proinsulin to insulin begins only about 20 minutes after peptide chain synthesis is completed, and it then proceeds as a pseudo first-order process with a half time of 30–60 minutes. It requires neither energy nor continued protein synthesis once initiated in the granules. Mature β-cell secretory granules contain only low percentages (1–2%) of proinsulin and intermediate materials, and as a consequence, secreted insulin normally contains only small amounts of these precursor-related peptides.[30] Newly synthesized insulin and proinsulin are selectively released to a slight extent, but the bulk of the secreted material normally consists of stored preformed hormone and C peptide.[30–32]

Numerous studies have confirmed that like other cells that elaborate secretory proteins, newly synthesized proinsulin passes via the Golgi apparatus into the β-cell secretory granules (Fig. 3-4). Immunocytochemical studies using monoclonal antibodies specific for uncleaved proinsulin have demonstrated that newly formed clathrin-clad granules in the *trans* Golgi cisternae

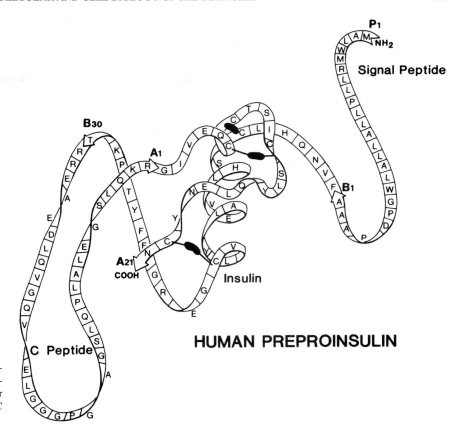

HUMAN PREPROINSULIN

FIGURE 3-3. Schematic structure of human preproinsulin. Removal of the first 24 amino acids (signal peptide) gives rise to proinsulin. Cleavage after B30 (**T**) and before A1 (**G**) gives rise to insulin and C peptide.

are rich in proinsulin, confirming that conversion to insulin occurs principally during the maturation of these secretory "progranules."[33,34] Energy is required for the intracellular translocation of secretory proteins from RER through the Golgi apparatus, and is associated with the budding and/or fusion of small non-clathrin clad vesicles that transport secretory proteins from the *cis* through the *trans* Golgi cisternae.[35,36] Because proteolytic conversion itself does not require energy, it is likely that proinsulin processing is initiated in the *trans* compartment of the Golgi apparatus or in newly formed secretory granules, or progranules, as these leave the Golgi region, and that it continues for several hours within these granules as they collect and mature biochemically in the cytosol (Fig. 3-4).

The major proteolytic cleavages required for converting proinsulin to insulin are summarized in Fig. 3-5. In early studies it was shown that the conjoint action of trypsin and carboxypeptidase B can give rise to the naturally occurring pancreatic products C peptide and native insulin, essentially quantitatively converting proinsulin to insulin *in vitro*,[37] a process used in some commercial processes for making recombinant human insulin via proinsulin.[38]

The Prohormone Convertases and Proinsulin Processing

The identification of the proinsulin convertases has lead to the solution of the longstanding puzzle as to the nature of the endoproteases responsible for the cleavage of prohormones characteristi-

cally at paired basic residues. Two novel calcium-dependent endoproteases (PC2 and PC3/PC1) related to subtilisin, a bacterial serine protease, and to kexin, a yeast-mating pheromone convertase, were found by polymerase chain reaction strategies applied to human insulinoma cDNA and to AtT20 cells.[39,40] PC3/PC1 was present at lower levels in the human insulinoma but at higher levels in ACTH-secreting AtT20 cells. PC2 consists of 638 residues, and PC3/PC1 contains 753 residues. Their structures are shown diagrammatically in Fig. 3-6.

A related human protease, furin, that was identified serendipitously, was initially believed to be a growth factor receptor due to the presence of a cysteine-rich domain and a putative transmembrane segment.[41,42] However, this protease also contains a catalytic domain similar to that of PC3/PC1, PC2, and kexin, having the characteristic catalytic Ser-Asp-His triad of active site residues (Fig. 3-5). Subsequent studies have shown that furin, like yeast kexin, is localized to the *trans* Golgi region, and that it is expressed ubiquitously in tissues, where it serves to process a variety of precursors secreted via constitutive pathways, such as insulin receptor precursors and other growth factors, clotting factor precursors, and viral envelope glycoproteins.[43]

PC2 and PC3 lack transmembrane localization domains and are optimally active at pH 5.5.[44] They are expressed (in varying amounts) only in neuroendocrine tissues such as the islets of Langerhans, pituitary, adrenal medulla, and many regions of the brain, but not at appreciable levels in other nonendocrine tissues such as liver, spleen, intestine, kidney, or muscle.[40,45] Moreover, antisera to PC2 and PC3 indicate that the β cells, as well as the other cell types of the islets of Langerhans, express one or both of

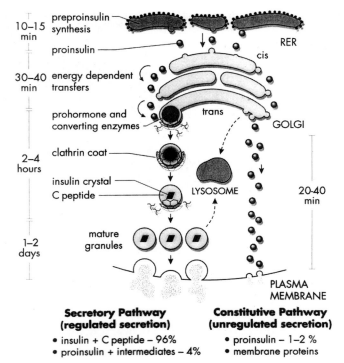

10–15 min — preproinsulin synthesis

proinsulin

RER

cis

30–40 min — energy dependent transfers

prohormone and converting enzymes

trans

GOLGI

2–4 hours — clathrin coat

insulin crystal

C peptide

LYSOSOME

20–40 min

1–2 days — mature granules

PLASMA MEMBRANE

Secretory Pathway (regulated secretion)
- insulin + C peptide – 96%
- proinsulin + intermediates – 4%

Constitutive Pathway (unregulated secretion)
- proinsulin – 1–2 %
- membrane proteins

FIGURE 3-4. Schematic model of the insulin biosynthetic machinery of the β cell. Preproinsulin is synthesized in the rough endoplasmic reticulum (**RER**) and is then rapidly cleaved to proinsulin (within 1–2 minutes). In the intracisternal spaces of the RER, proinsulin folds and forms the native disulfide bonds of insulin. After being transported to the Golgi apparatus by an energy-requiring vesicular mechanism, proinsulin is efficiently sorted (>99%) into clathrin-coated early granules arising in the *trans* Golgi network. These granules are rich in proinsulin and contain the converting proteases, PC2 and PC3, and carboxypeptidase E. Processing to proinsulin occurs mainly, if not exclusively, in these early secretory granules, giving rise to the more condensed mature granules, which lack the clathrin coat. The mature granule-dense cores consist almost entirely of insulin, often in crystalline arrays, while the granule-soluble phase that surrounds the inclusion consists mainly of C peptide and small amounts of proinsulin. The release of newly synthesized proinsulin and insulin begins about 1 hour after synthesis in the RER, and hence granules must undergo a maturation process that renders them competent for secretion. Nongranular routes of secretion of proinsulin or insulin comprise only a few percent of total secretion in normal islets. Exocytosis of granules is regulated by glucose and many other factors, and in both humans and dogs results in the release of insulin and C peptide in equimolar proportions under both basal and stimulated conditions.

these proteases. Immunogold labeling of both proinsulin and PC2 in newly formed β-cell secretory vesicles has confirmed the colocalization of the enzyme and its putative substrate.[46]

Various studies indicate that PC2 cleaves proinsulin preferentially at the Lys Arg ↓ Gly sequence at the junction of the C peptide and the A chain, and PC3 cleaves mainly at the Arg Arg ↓ Glu sequence in the B chain-C peptide junction.[46] These and other findings support the proposed identity of PC3 and PC2 with the calcium-dependent type 1 and type 2 insulinoma granule proinsulin processing activities, respectively, described by Davidson, Bailyes, and Bennett and all their coworkers.[47–49] Sizonenko and Halban[50] have reported that rat/mouse proinsulin II, which has Met

rather than Lys at B29, four residues upstream (P4 position) of the B chain-C peptide cleavage site, is processed more slowly at this site in normal islets. These results and others suggest that both PC3 and PC2 cleavage, like that of furin, is augmented by basic residues at the fourth position upstream from the cleavage site (designated P4) in some of its substrates, and this could account for observed cleavage of rat/mouse proinsulins at the A-chain junction (Arg Gln Lys Arg ↓ Gly) by PC3 in early studies.[46]

More recent studies confirm that both PC2 and PC3 participate in the processing of proinsulin and indicate that their action is most likely sequential, with PC3 acting initially to produce 32,33 split proinsulin, which is a preferred substrate for PC2 cleavage at the remaining C peptide-A chain junction. This is illustrated schematically in Fig. 3-5. Recent studies of insulin biosynthesis in islets from a PC2 null mouse strain[51] have confirmed the importance of PC2 for proinsulin processing.[52] The pancreatic proinsulin content in these mice is significantly elevated (~35% vs. ~5% in wild-type or heterozygotes) and circulating levels of proinsulin approach 60%. Pulse-chase labeling studies show that the rates of proinsulin processing are reduced by about threefold and significant accumulations of des 31,32 proinsulin intermediate, resulting from PC3 action, are evident.[52] In normal human islets of Langerhans, significant levels of des 31,32 proinsulin accumulate during pulse-chase studies.[53] This occurs because human proinsulin lacks a P4 basic amino acid at the C peptide-A chain junction, which slows PC2 cleavage at this site, while the B chain-C peptide site has a lysine as the P4 residue. As a consequence of this simple structural difference, in humans the des 31,32 intermediate form makes up a considerable proportion of normal circulating insulin-like components, in addition to intact proinsulin.[52–54]

PC2 has also been shown to be expressed at high levels in the α cells, where it appears to act alone in the processing of proglucagon to release only glucagon as the major hormonal product.[55,56] Glucagon-like peptide 1 (GLP-1$_{[7–37]}$), another endocrine product derived from proglucagon by selective proteolysis in the intestinal L cells, has been shown to be an important incretin, augmenting insulin secretion in response to ingested fuels, and opposite to glucagon, which is an insulin counterregulatory hormone. (see chapt. 6 and 7) The L-cell processing enzyme has been tentatively identified as PC3, since PC3 has been shown to carry out the cleavages leading to the release of GLP-1 and GLP-2, but not of glucagon from proglucagon.[57,58] In the PC2 null mice proglucagon processing is markedly impaired, leading to a lack of circulating mature glucagon and resulting in chronic hypoglycemia and α cell hyperplasia.[51] PC2 is also the major convertase expressed in the islet somatostatin-producing delta cells, and consequently processing of prosomatostatin to somatostatin 14 is blocked. Instead, somatostatin 28 accumulates in the PC2 nulls. The pancreatic polypeptide (PP)–-producing gamma cells also are rich in PC2, and so the processing of proPP may also be impaired. All of these results and others indicate that PC2 and PC3 are major secretory granule-processing enzymes and are responsible for processing many neuroendocrine precursors.[46,59] For further information on the prohormone convertase family of processing enzymes, see references 60–63.

Another important component of the processing machinery, carboxypeptidase E (CPE), a carboxypeptidase B-like enzyme, was first identified in islets but is expressed in many other neuroendocrine tissues, including brain (Fig. 3-5). This enzyme has been

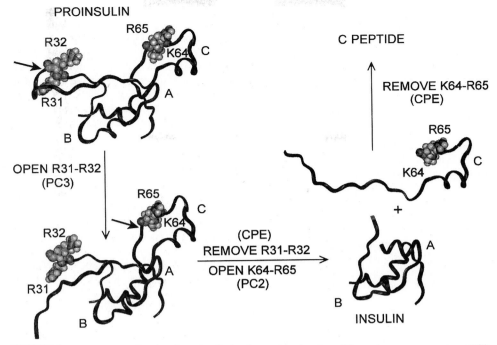

FIGURE 3-5. The cleavage of proinsulin to insulin by the combined action of the prohormone convertases PC2, PC3/PC1, and carboxypeptidase H. This scheme is based on evidence, cited in the text, that PC3 cleavage at the B chain-C peptide junction precedes cleavage by PC2 at the C peptide-A chain junction. The conformation shown for proinsulin is based on modeling studies to optimize binding to the convertases during cleavage.[284] Note that the interaction with PC2 requires unwinding of the N-terminal alpha helix of the A chain to allow the A2 Ile residue to move out from the hydrophobic core of the insulin moiety, where it normally resides with the A19 Tyr, to enter the active site of PC2 (subside S2').

extensively studied both in terms of its enzymatic properties as well as its biosynthesis.[64] These studies have shown that it is clearly distinct from the classical pancreatic carboxypeptidases A and B, but is structurally homologous to these enzymes, suggesting that it arose from a common ancestral exopeptidase.[64] The CPE^fat mutation is a spontaneously occurring loss of function mutation in

CPE that causes a metabolic syndrome characterized by obesity, mild diabetes, and hyperproinsulinemia.[65] CPE activity is absent in the islets and reduced[66] in brains of these mice. Interestingly, absence of CPE leads to impaired convertase action, perhaps due in part to the accumulation of cleaved intermediates extended C-terminally with basic residues.[67]

FIGURE 3-6. Schematic structures of the proinsulin processing prohormone convertases PC2 and PC3/PC1. The various subregions are designated as follows: signal peptides (**SP**), proregion (**PRO**), catalytic domain (**CAT**), P or homeo B domain (**P**), and amphipathic helix (**AH**). The catalytic Asp, His, Asn (Asp), and Ser residues, cleavage sites (**?**) and a potential integrin-binding sequence (**RGD**) are shown. C-terminal shortening of PC2 occurs in the secretory granules.

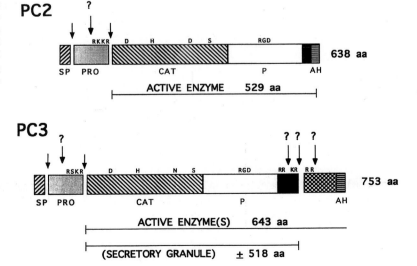

Secretory Granule Formation

In β cells the "progranules" characteristically are less dense than the mature granules and have a uniform density throughout.[33,68] Evidence suggests that newly synthesized proinsulin enters these granules as a sol rather than an aggregate. Various changes take place as these progranules mature in the cytoplasm of the cell, including the proteolytic conversion of proinsulin to insulin and the condensation of the insulin with Ca and Zn ions.[69,70] The dense central core of mature insulin-secretory granules is crystalline with repeat-unit spacings closely similar to those of ordinary zinc insulin crystals.[71,72] Thus as insulin is liberated from proinsulin, it tends to crystallize with zinc that is concentrated by the β cells. The role of zinc in secretory granule formation is not well understood.[73] Most of the zinc in islets is present in the β granules and is liberated proportionately with insulin during secretion.[74] Mature islet secretory granule cores seem to contain only insulin, while the C-peptide liberated in the conversion process remains in solution in the clear fluid space surrounding the dense crystalline core.[72] The C peptide does not cocrystallize with insulin, but low levels of proinsulin do cocrystallize with insulin such that granule cores normally contain 1–2% of intact or partially processed precursor,[72] mainly des 31,32 intermediate in man.[54]

The pH of the interior of the mature secretory granule is approximately 5.0,[33,34] an optimal pH for both proinsulin conversion and insulin crystallization. In contrast, the *trans* Golgi and newly formed secretory granules are more nearly neutral, which may favor receptor-mediated sorting mechanisms, such as those involved in the sorting of lysosomal enzymes into endosomes via mannose-6-P receptors. Thus the biosynthesis of insulin via preproinsulin and proinsulin and their intracellular handling, proteolysis, and ultimate storage as insulin in secretory granules, is a remarkably well-integrated process, at both the molecular and cell biological levels, within the β cells.[74,75] This well-poised mechanism is disturbed in islet cell tumors, which often show unregulated release of insulin and other hormones together with excessive amounts of proinsulin. Measurements of proinsulin levels are thus useful adjuncts in the diagnosis of islet cell tumors (see Chap. 58).[76,77]

C Peptide as a Product of Proinsulin Transformation

C peptide accumulates along with insulin in essentially equimolar amounts[28,78] and is secreted along with the hormone by exocytosis of the granule contents.[75,78] Recent studies suggest that a small proportion (2–3%) of newly synthesized C peptide may be released constitutively,[79] presumably due to budding of small clathrin-coated vesicles from newly formed secretory granules. Because mammalian C peptides exhibit a 15-fold higher rate of mutation acceptance than the corresponding insulins, it seems likely that this region in the proinsulin molecule does not have any specific hormonal function. Nonetheless, it has been suggested that low-dose (biosynthetic) C peptide infusion may influence human muscle microcirculation as well as renal function by unknown mechanisms.[80]

The renewal and regulation of the granular stores of insulin and C peptide in the β cells is an important aspect of normal homeostasis. Calcium-dependent exocytosis of preformed storage granules[81] appears to be the major source of both basal and glucose-stimulated insulin and C peptide release *in vivo*.[75] The chief positive effector in maintaining this storage compartment is glucose, augmented by cyclic AMP, which appears to be generated by a mechanism closely coupled to glucose metabolism in the β cell.[82–84] Secretion is not a direct stimulus to insulin biosynthesis, as can be proven by blocking secretion by lowering external calcium levels or using inhibitors such as diazoxide. These agents do not impair the biosynthetic response to glucose.[28] However, when inhibition of secretion is prolonged, intracellular degradation (autophagy) of granules occurs.[34,75]

Clinical Relevance of Proinsulin and C Peptide

The measurement of the secretion rate of insulin *in vivo* is complicated by its rapid plasma half-life, which is in turn determined in part by the pool of available insulin receptors in the liver and peripheral tissues. A large proportion of normal insulin metabolism, beyond renal disposal, appears to result from receptor-mediated endocytosis, followed by intracellular degradation of the hormone in liver and other target tissues, perhaps as modulated by still other factors such as hepatic glucose metabolism.[85] As a consequence the relationship between circulating insulin levels and the rates of secretion of the hormone from the pancreas is complex and difficult to assess. It is further complicated in the insulin-treated diabetic by the presence of insulin antibodies and pools of residual bound and free hormone, even after withdrawal of insulin therapy.

The C peptide, on the other hand, represents a cosecreted product that is directly related stoichiometrically to insulin on a one-to-one basis and is far less complicated to measure. It is not extracted significantly by the liver, and its metabolic clearance rate is independent of its plasma concentration over a wide concentration range. Whether a receptor exists for C peptide is an unsettled topic, but its prolonged half-life and kinetically accessible distribution characteristics suggest that it is probably biologically inert and is mainly excreted by the kidney. No effects of metabolic state have been observed on C-peptide distribution or turnover. By a deconvolutional analysis that corrects for distribution beyond plasma compartments, Polonsky and coworkers have shown that peripheral C-peptide levels can be used to derive true secretion rates for insulin *in vivo* under a variety of conditions, including the presence of insulin antibodies.[85]

C-peptide measurement has proven helpful in the diagnosis of hypoglycemia due to insulinoma and/or surreptitious administration of insulin. In the former case, failure to suppress C-peptide levels during insulin-induced hypoglycemia (levels below 50% of baseline when blood glucose falls below 40 mg/dL) strongly suggests insulinoma. In contrast, factitious insulin administration should be suspected when very high insulin concentrations are accompanied by normal or suppressed C-peptide levels.

Proinsulin is normally secreted in much smaller amounts than insulin or C peptide (usually 3–5%). However, its rate of metabolism is much slower than that of insulin because of its reduced insulin receptor affinity (approximately 3% that of insulin). But some proinsulin intermediates, particularly des 64,65 proinsulin (cleaved at the C peptide-A chain junction), exhibit potencies approaching that of insulin and hence are more rapidly metabolized. Whether for this reason or others, several recent studies have determined that circulating proinsulin-like material (PLM) is mainly composed of intact proinsulin and des 31,32 proinsulin (cleaved at the B chain-C peptide junction), both being low-potency, slow-turnover forms. These forms make up a small proportion (10–20%) of normal fasting plasma but may account for as much as 50% of circulating insulin components in type 2 diabetes.[86] This finding has lead to suggestions that conversion of proinsulin to insulin may be impaired in the diabetic β cell and high proinsulin levels may tend to obscure the extent of bioactive insulin deficiency, based on simple plasma insulin radioimmunoassays (which fail to distinguish between active insulin and these less active biosynthetic intermediates). Whether this circulating imbalance may also be due in part to more rapid insulin disposal in the diabetic (due to receptor upregulation) remains an issue that requires further clarification. Nonetheless, there appears to be some basis for believing that elevated secretion of proinsulin-related materials may be a concomitant of β-cell decompensation, although the mechanistic basis for this phenomenon is not well understood (see Chap. 21). Recent studies of the effects of prolonged exposure of β cells to elevated fatty acids on insulin biosynthesis indicate inhibition of maturation of not only proinsulin, but also of the convertases, resulting in secretion of increased proportions of proinsulin.[87]

Proinsulin is stable in the circulation and is cleared mainly by the kidney. Hence renal failure is usually accompanied by markedly elevated proinsulin levels. Elevated proinsulin is frequently found in patients with insulinomas. More than 80% of benign adenomas and almost all islet cell carcinomas manifest elevated proinsulin levels that are not suppressed by hypoglycemia.[76] Biosynthetic human proinsulin has been tested in clinical trials as a potential long-acting form of insulin. These studies unfortunately revealed a slight excess of cardiac mortality in the proinsulin group and were discontinued.[38] Whether lower, more physiologic proportions of proinsulin in combination with insulin (and C peptide) might have superior therapeutic characteristics than insulin alone remains a possibility deserving further exploration. Recent studies suggest the existence of high-affinity proinsulin-specific receptors on vascular endothelial[88] and intestinal crypt[89] cells.

STRUCTURE AND EVOLUTION OF THE INSULIN GENE

The gene for insulin was among the first to be isolated. Its structure in man[90] is summarized in Fig. 3-7. The insulin gene has been cloned from a wide range of species including primates, rodents, birds, fish, and amphibians.[91,92] Its structure is highly conserved among species and consists of three exons and two introns. Exon 1 is located in the 5′ untranslated region of the gene. Exon 2 contains sequences encoding the signal peptide, the insulin B chain and part of the C peptide, while exon 3 encodes the remainder of the C peptide, the insulin A chain and the 3′ untranslated sequences.[90] The length and sequence of the introns are highly variable among species. However, the relative length of intron 1 is always less than that of intron 2, and it is located in the 5′ untranslated region while intron 2 interrupts the gene between the first and second nucleotides of the codon for amino acid 7 of the C peptide.

Only one insulin gene is present in most species studied, with the exception of rat, mouse, and *Xenopus*, which have two nonallelic insulin genes. Intron 2 is absent from the rat and mouse insulin I genes. The second gene of rodents (i.e., rat and mouse insulin I) arose from a process of reverse transcription of a partially spliced germ line transcript.[93] The RNA transcript involved was

initiated from a site upstream of the normal physiological promoter of the insulin II gene; thus the insulin I gene is homologous to the insulin II gene within about 500 bp upstream of the transcription start site. The rat and mouse insulin I and II genes are expressed equally in normal islets,[94] though not in fetal yolk sac[95] or in some rat insulinoma-derived cells.[96] Both alleles of the mouse insulin I and II genes are active in embryonic tissue but only the paternal alleles for both genes are active in the yolk sac.[97] This suggests that the maternal alleles undergo selective imprinting in extrapancreatic tissue during embryonic development, raising questions about the role of such extrapancreatic expression.

The single-copy human gene is located on the short arm of chromosome 11 in band p15.[98,99] It is flanked on the 5′ side by a unique polymorphic region composed of tandem repeats that lie beyond the upstream regulatory region and does not seem to influence its expression but provides a useful marker for genetic linkage analysis.[100] Earlier reported correlations of the presence of larger (Class 3) versus smaller (Class 1 or Class 2) repeats in this region with the incidence of type 2 diabetes were confounded by ethnic differences in the distribution of tandem repeats. Further analyses of larger populations failed to support this conclusion, but have revealed that Class 1 alleles and genotypes are significantly more frequent in Caucasians with type 1 diabetes than type 2 diabetics or controls.[101] This allele may thus be a marker for a nearby susceptibility gene for type 1 diabetes mellitus (T1DM).

REGULATION OF INSULIN GENE TRANSCRIPTION

DNA Sequences and Transcription Factors Controlling Transcription of the Insulin Gene

β-cell-specific expression of the insulin gene is dependent on DNA sequences located within a region of approximately 400 base pairs immediately upstream of the transcription start site.[102–106] This region is highly conserved among species and contains a number of regulatory elements as depicted in Fig. 3-8.[107] The transcription factors that bind to these promoter elements play an important role in (1) restricting expression of the insulin gene to β cells, (2) silencing the insulin gene in non β cells, (3) determining when and where the insulin gene is expressed during islet cell ontogeny, and (4) regulating expression of the insulin gene in response to changes in nutrient status. Transcription factors, some of which bind to the insulin promoter, also play an important role in lineage determination in the developing pancreas while defects in these transcription factors may be related to the development of diabetes mellitus.

Of the regulatory sequences depicted in Fig. 3-8, the two E-box elements GCCATCTGC (E1 and E2) are particularly important. Transcription factors that bind E boxes consist of heterodimers between a ubiquitous class A and a tissue-specific class B member of the basic helix loop helix (bHLH) family. These proteins contain a conserved basic DNA-binding domain and two amphipathic helices separated by a loop structure that are required for dimerization. Class A bHLH members include the E2A gene products E12 and E47, while class B family members include BETA2/NeuroD, MyoD, and myogenin. Other class B proteins, such as Id, emc, and hairy, which lack a basic DNA-binding domain, can form inactive heterodimers with class A proteins.[107]

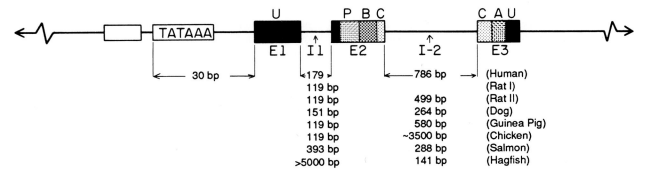

FIGURE 3-7. Diagrammatic representation of the structure of the insulin gene in vertebrates. Exons (**E**) appearing in mature preproinsulin mRNA are shown as bars and the sizes of the two introns or intervening sequences (**I**) in various species are tabulated below. **U**, Untranslated region; **P**, prepeptide coding region; **B**, B-chain coding region; **C**, C-peptide coding region; and **A**, A-chain coding region. A typical TATA box signaling transcription initiation is shown approximately 30 base pairs upstream from the messenger start site, preceded by a promoter region (unfilled box). The human insulin gene, abbreviated INS, is located on the short arm of chromosome 11 in the region p15.[98,99]

The E1 element located at approximately −100 is highly conserved among insulin genes. It is critical for insulin gene expression, since mutagenesis has a drastic effect on insulin promoter activity.[108] The E1 element binds a heterodimer of the ubiquitously expressed E2A gene product E47 and BETA2, which is also known as NeuroD.[109,110] BETA2/NeuroD is expressed in islets of Langerhans, brain, and intestine (where it is thought to regulate the secretin gene).[109] The importance of BETA2/NeuroD is emphasized by inactivation of the gene in mice: mice homozygous for the *BETA2/NeuroD* gene deletion develop severe diabetes and die 3–5 days after birth.[111] On the other hand, mice lacking the *E2A* gene exhibit normal levels of insulin, suggesting functional redundancy among members of the class A bHLH family.[112]

The E2 region, located at around −230, is not as well conserved as the E1 region. In the rat insulin I gene the sequence of the E2 box is identical to that of the E1 box, and it binds a similar factor, i.e., E47/BETA2. The E2 box of the human insulin gene differs from the E1 box. It has an imperfect E box, CACCGG, which binds E47/BETA2 but only weakly. However, it binds the ubiquitously expressed bHLH factor USF (upstream stimulating factor) with high affinity.[113] On the 5′ side of the E2 box is an element (C2) containing a number of CAGG sequences. This C2 element binds

an islet cell–specific factor RIPE3b1,[114] which was originally shown to bind to the C1 element located between the A1 and E1 boxes of the rat insulin II gene.[115] RIPE3b1 has yet to be cloned and characterized.

The A box elements have the consensus sequence C(C/T)TAATG. There are four in the human insulin gene at positions −82 (A1), −140 (A2), −215 (A3) and −319 (A5). The A box binds a transcription factor PDX1, which was previously known as IPF1,[116] IDX1,[117] STF1,[118] and IUF1.[119] Expression of PDX1 in the adult is restricted to β cells of the pancreas and to somatostatin-expressing cells of the pancreas and small intestine. PDX1 belongs to the *Antennapedia* class of homeodomain proteins and is highly homologous to the *XlHbox* 8 from *Xenopus laevis*.[120] Mice homozygous for a targeted mutation in the *pdx1* gene selectively lack a pancreas.[121] These and other findings suggest that PDX1 functions both in the early specification of the primitive gut to a pancreatic fate and in the maturation of the pancreatic β cell.[122,123] The human *pdx1* gene, located on chromosome 13q/12, encodes a 283-amino-acid protein with a central homeodomain flanked by two proline-rich domains.[124] The transactivation domain is located at the NH2-terminus of the protein.[125,126] The mechanisms whereby PDX1 binding to the A box activates the

FIGURE 3-8. Schematic depicting the arrangement of regulatory sequences in the human insulin gene promoter. The scale at the bottom represents base pairs upstream of the transcription start site. The boxes on the dark line denote sequence elements, and when the name of the element and sequence are known, they are given. Above the boxes the transcription factors are schematically represented. The factor IEF1 is a heterodimer of BETA2/E47.

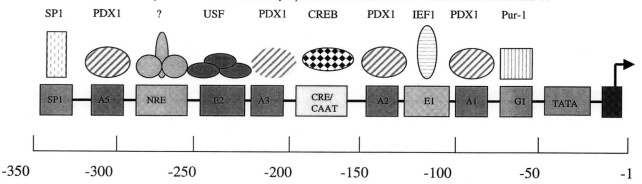

insulin gene is not well understood. It synergizes with bHLH proteins bound to the E1 element and with the homeodomain factor Pbx.[127,128] The interaction with Pbx involves a conserved pentapeptide sequence, FPWMK, located amino terminal to the homeodomain. Some preliminary data on the sequences regulating the PDX1 gene have been published. A regulatory sequence that binds HNF3β has been mapped to a DNase hypersensitive regions at about −2 kb,[129] while the bHLH protein USF binds to a regulatory site close to the promoter, at −104.[130]

Other putative regulatory elements that are conserved among species include a cyclic AMP–responsive element (CRE) and an enhancer core sequence that could bind C/EBP. In the rat insulin I gene a G-rich sequence binds a factor, Pur-1, that is ubiquitously expressed.[131] A STAT5 binding site that may mediate the effects of growth hormone has been mapped to the sequence between −330 and −322 in the rat insulin I gene.[132] And a complex negative regulatory element has been identified between −258 and −279 of the human insulin gene.[133] This element binds a number of proteins[134] and contains a palindromic repeat sequence that may function as a negative glucocorticoid response element.[135]

The human insulin gene contains variable numbers of tandem repeats (VNTRs) of the sequence 5′ TCTGGGGAGAGGGG 3′ located upstream of −365.[100] Termed the insulin-linked polymorphic region (ILPR), this region has been shown to exhibit transcriptional activity,[136] possibly through the binding of the transcription factor Pur-1 to G-rich sequences.[137] Interestingly, the ILPR has the ability to adopt an altered DNA structure. This has been characterized as a quadriplex involving interactions between the G residues on the top strand,[138–140] while the C-rich strand forms hairpin structures.[141] The quadriplex structure is present *in vivo*[142] and in DNA assembled in chromosomes *in vitro*.[143] The structure is present when the insulin gene is actively transcribed, while mutations that destabilize the structure lower the transcriptional activity of the gene. Further regulatory sequences, including a steroid-responsive element[144] and a RIPE3b1 binding site,[145] may reside upstream of the ILPR.

Nutrient and Hormonal Control of Insulin Gene Expression

The biosynthesis and secretion of insulin by pancreatic β cells is controlled primarily by the circulating glucose levels. Metabolism of glucose is essential for its stimulatory effect as only metabolizable analogues are effective. Hexose phosphorylation in β cells by a high-K_m glucokinase is the rate-limiting step for sugar metabolism. Glucokinase is thus regarded as the β cell glucose sensor conferring concentration dependence and specificity to the insulin secretory response to sugars.[146] Metabolism of glucose results in an increase in the intracellular ATP/ADP ratio, which causes closure of the ATP-sensitive K^+ channel in the plasma membrane. The consequent depolarization causes opening of the voltage-dependent Ca^{2+} channel, and the increase in intracellular Ca^{2+} initiates the events that lead to exocytosis of the insulin granule contents (see Chap. 4). Hormones such as glucagon-like peptide I (7-37) (GLP-I) that activate adenylate cyclase stimulate insulin secretion by amplifying the response to glucose, primarily by increasing the sensitivity of the secretory apparatus to Ca^{2+}.[147] Insulin has also been shown to activate insulin secretion by an autocrine mechanism involving an increase in $[Ca^{2+}]_i$ and activation of protein kinase C.[148]

Glucose can also stimulate insulin secretion in a K_{ATP}–channel independent manner. Thus, in the presence of diazoxide that inhibits the closure of K_{ATP} channels by glucose, the plasma membrane potential (Äυ) is depolarized by K^+, causing an increase in cytosolic Ca^{2+} to permissive levels.[149] It is thought that at this permissive level of Ca^{2+}, glucose can stimulate the activity of Ca^{2+}-sensitive dehydrogenases in the mitochondrial matrix. The resultant increased flow through the TCA cycle generates a mitochondrial factor distinct from ATP. This factor has been identified as glutamate, which leaves the mitochondria and interacts directly with insulin secretory granules to promote exocytosis.[150,151]

Following the release of insulin it is important that the β cell replenishes its stores. There are several stages at which this can occur: transcription of the insulin gene, preRNA processing, transport into the cytoplasm and turnover of mRNA, and translation of preproinsulin mRNA.[152] The major acute (<2 hours) control of insulin production is exerted at the level of translation. This is in keeping with the requirement to replenish insulin stores rapidly following insulin secretion in response to elevated circulating glucose levels. Over longer periods (>6 hours) glucose stimulates transcription of the insulin gene, and, at least in the mouse, it also regulates the level of preRNA splicing.[153]

In recent years it has become clear that the cells within islets communicate with each other through connexin-like molecules, such that the overall response to nutrient stimulation reflects the integrated action of β cells with individually differing behaviours.[154] Thus an increase in glucose concentrations not only stimulates gene expression and proinsulin biosynthesis within individual β cells, but also increases the number of cells that respond to glucose.[155] The following account of events should therefore be viewed in the context of this synergistic response.

Evidence that glucose affects insulin mRNA levels initially came from *in vivo* experiments in which rats fasted for 4 days exhibited decreased insulin mRNA levels which could be restored to normal on refeeding or injection of glucose.[156] *In vitro* studies[157] confirmed that this occurred through stabilization of insulin mRNA and through effects on the rate of transcription of the insulin gene.[158] Insulin mRNA is relatively stable, with a half-life of about 30 hours; however, its half-life was almost threefold longer in islets incubated in 17 mmol glucose compared with 3 mmol glucose.[159] Direct effects of glucose on gene transcription were demonstrated by using transcription run-on assays or transfection of plasmid constructs containing insulin promoter fragments joined to a reporter gene encoding chloramphenicol acetyl transferase (CAT) or firefly luciferase.[160–162]

A glucose-responsive element was originally mapped to the E2/A4/A3 (−196 to −247) region of the rat insulin I gene promoter in transfected neonatal rat islets.[161] Part of this response results from the binding at the E2 site of a protein complex that includes the bHLH protein E47 (probably BETA2/E47). Subsequent studies suggested that multiple regulatory elements interact with each other to elicit a full transcriptional response to glucose.[163] It has also been shown that the binding of the yet-to-be-characterized factor RIPE3b1 to its recognition sequence (the C1 box) in the rat insulin II promoter may be regulated by glucose.[164] The fact that RIPE3b1 DNA-binding activity is inhibited by the oxidizing agent diamide and the alkylating agent N-ethylmaleimide suggests that changes in the redox state of the cell may contribute to the regulation of the insulin promoter by nutrients.[165]

There is also very strong evidence that the homeodomain transcription factor PDX1 plays a major role in linking nutrient metabolism in the β cell to the regulation of the insulin gene.[166–168]

Melloul and colleagues[166] demonstrated that glucose stimulated the DNA binding activity of a factor (GSF) which was subsequently identified as PDX1.[169] Glucose activation of PDX1 occurred rapidly (within 10–15 minutes) and involved phosphorylation of the transcription factor.[167] The effects of glucose could not be mimicked by cyclic AMP–elevating agents or tumor-promoting phorbol esters, suggesting that neither cyclic AMP–dependent protein kinase nor protein kinase C was involved. The mechanism by which glucose stimulates PDX1 DNA binding activity and insulin promoter activity has recently been elucidated. It involves a stress-activated protein kinase pathway in which SAPK2 (also known as RK/p38) plays a critical role,[170] although this has been disputed.[171] SAPK2 is a member of an expanding family of MAP kinase-related kinases that are activated in response to adverse stimuli such as heat, osmotic shock, ultraviolet light, and DNA-damaging reagents, and by proinflammatory cytokines that are produced under conditions of stress.[172] In β cells, activation of the SAPK2 pathway by glucose involves phosphatidylinositol-3-kinase (PI-3-kinase), while activation by stress (e.g., treatment with sodium arsenite) is independent of PI-3-kinase. Interestingly, activation of recombinant PDX1 by SAPK2 in vitro is associated with an increase in molecular mass from 31 kd to 46 kd. This increase in mass is also seen in vivo, where the 31-kd form of PDX1 is present in the cytoplasm of low glucose treated islets. Upon transfer to high glucose, PDX1 is rapidly (within 10–15 minutes) converted to an active phosphorylated 46-kd form that is present predominantly in the nucleus.[173,174] Other metabolizable nutrients that induce insulin secretion (including xylitol, fructose, and pyruvate), as well as insulin itself, activated PDX1 DNA-binding activity and insulin promoter through PI-3-kinase.[175] It is unclear whether the effects of glucose and insulin are additive or whether glucose activates PI-3-kinase and insulin gene transcription by stimulating insulin secretion that then acts via an autoregulatory loop.[176]

Glucose and other nutrients stimulate the biosynthesis of proinsulin[177,178] and a number of other proteins, including the secretory granule membrane protein SGM110[179] and chromogranin A.[180] There may be a general, but relatively weak, stimulatory effect on the synthesis of a large number of islet proteins, along with a rapid and strong stimulation of proinsulin biosynthesis.[181] The biosynthesis of proinsulin is coupled to secretion insofar as many insulin secretagogues also stimulate proinsulin biosynthesis. However, the transducing systems differ in a number of respects. First, glucose-stimulated insulin release is inhibited in a Ca^{2+}-free medium, whereas biosynthesis is still activated. Second, tolbutamide and phosphodiesterase inhibitors, such as isobutylmethylxanthine (IBMX), potentiate glucose-stimulated insulin release by increasing islet cyclic AMP levels, but do not affect proinsulin biosynthesis. Third, the threshold for glucose-stimulated insulin secretion (4.2–5.6 mmol) is higher than that for proinsulin synthesis (2.5–3.9 mmol). The point of divergence appears to occur early in the β-cell metabolic signaling pathway.[182]

The molecular mechanisms whereby glucose stimulates translation of preproinsulin mRNA are not well understood. Translation initiation factors may be involved. The activity of the guanine exchange factor eIF2B is stimulated rapidly (within 15 minutes) and over the same range of glucose concentrations that stimulate proinsulin synthesis.[183] EIF2B facilitates the exchange of GTP between inactive and active forms of eIF-2, the factor involved in mediating the binding of the initiator Met-tRNA to the 40S ribosomal subunit. In other systems the activity of eIF2B is modulated by phosphorylation of its subunit eIF2α; however, in islets, glucose stimulates eIF2B by an alternative mechanism that does not involve phosphorylation of eIF2α. Another factor, eIF4E-BP1, which is also known as PHAS-1, is phosphorylated in response to glucose in β cells.[184] EIF4E-BP1 is a protein that binds and inhibits the activity of eIF4E, a component of the mRNA cap site recognition complex. Phosphorylation of eIF4E-BP1 causes it to dissociate from eIF4E. Glucose-stimulated phosphorylation of eIF4E-BP1 is dependent on the presence of amino acids, and may be mediated via insulin acting on the β cell. Thus, as for effects on insulin secretion and gene transcription, insulin release from the β cells may activate an insulin-receptor signaling pathway to autoregulate its own biosynthesis. The activated eIF4E forms part of a complex that in addition to recognizing the mRNA cap site, also unwinds secondary structure within the 5′ untranslated region of the mRNA. The selective effects of glucose on proinsulin may therefore be based on the presence of stem loop structures within the 5′UTR of preproinsulin mRNA.[185]

The Insulin Gene and Diabetes Mellitus

There are several aspects of the regulation of insulin gene expression and β-cell transcription factors that may relate to a better understanding of the development of type 1 (T1DM) and type 2 diabetes mellitus (T2DM). As a result of a genome-wide search, a number of loci (around 18) that confer susceptibility to T1DM have been described.[186] Of these, the T1DM 1 locus within the major histocompatibility complex on chromosome 6p21, and the T2DM 2 locus within the insulin gene region on chromosome 11p15 have the most powerful effects. The T2DM 2 locus has been further mapped and identified as allelic variations in the insulin VNTR. There are two main classes of VNTR allele: class I (26–36 repeats) and class III (140–200 repeats). The class I VNTRs confer an increased risk of T1DM, while class III VNTRs are dominantly protective.[187] As described above, the VNTR (or ILPR) is transcriptionally active in β cells,[188,189] with the shorter class I allele appearing to exhibit stronger transcriptional activity than the class III allele,[190] although not in all studies.[188] The reason why the class III allele should provide protection against T1DM has proved puzzling until it was recently discovered that insulin mRNA (along with that of other β cell autoantigens such as GAD, ICA69 and IA2) was expressed at low levels in human fetal thymus.[191,192] In the thymus, as opposed to the β cell, the class III allele was associated with higher insulin mRNA levels. Expression of the insulin gene in the thymus may serve to enhance immune tolerance to proinsulin, which is a major autoantigen in T1DM, by deletion of autoreactive thymocytes or the generation of regulatory T lymphocytes. This would provide a plausible explanation for the protective influence of the class III VNTR allele in T1DM.

A number of lines of evidence suggest that the homeodomain protein PDX1 is a potential factor contributing to the pathogenesis of diabetes mellitus.[193] The key role of this transcription factor in islet cell ontogeny is emphasized by the demonstration that in mouse gene inactivation models[121] and in a human subject with a homozygous mutation in the pdx1 gene the pancreas fails to develop.[194] In the adult, PDX1 is expressed primarily in the β cell, where it regulates expression of a number of genes that are preferentially expressed in the β cell, including insulin, GLUT-2, glucokinase, and islet amyloid polypeptide. It also mediates the activation of the insulin gene by glucose (see above). In β cells cultured for prolonged periods in high glucose, expression of the insulin gene is repressed,[195] as is expression of PDX1,[196] and another insulin gene regulatory protein, RIPE3b1.[197] This suggests that the glucotoxic effects of prolonged hyperglycemia on the β cell, as seen in T2DM, may be mediated in part by repression of PDX1.[198]

Mutations in PDX1 have been found in patients with maturity onset diabetes of the young (MODY4),[199] a monogenic early onset form of T2DM. Three other forms of MODY have been described with mutations in the genes encoding glucokinase (MODY2),[200] and the transcription factors HNF1α (MODY3) and HNF4α (MODY1).[201] The discovery of mutations in PDX1,[202,203] HNF1α, and HNF4α in MODY families stresses the importance of transcription factors in the pathogenesis of certain forms of T2DM. This is further emphasized by the finding that heterozygous (+/−) pdx1 mice injected intraperitoneally with 20 mmol glucose remained hyperglycemic for up to 2 hours, while normal control mice returned to euglycemia within this time period.[204] As well as regulating development of the endocrine pancreas, PDX1 also appears to play a key role in glucose homeostasis in the adult.(See Chapt. 21).

MUTATIONS IN THE INSULIN GENE

H.S. Tager and his associates were the first to identify a structurally abnormal insulin in the circulation and pancreas of a patient with mild diabetes associated with elevated insulin levels.[205] These and similar studies have led to the definition of a new clinical syndrome of familial mild hyperinsulinemic diabetes that is now considered to be a form of MODY, but often resembles T2DM.[206,207] Affected individuals have high circulating immunoreactive insulin levels and decreased C peptide:insulin ratios, resulting most likely from the delayed turnover, in vivo, of circulating insulin variants due to their impaired receptor binding properties.[208] The disorder is inherited in an autosomal dominant fashion within families, consistent with the Mendelian distribution of a defective allele.

In all cases studied a single nucleotide substitution occurs in only one of the two insulin gene alleles, leading to a single amino acid replacement within the insulin molecule.[207,209,210] The abnormal insulins generated by these missense mutations are all characterized by a very low binding potency, below 5% of normal, as demonstrated by direct assays.[211,212] However, the replacements occur at different sites within the insulin molecule [at residues B24 (Phe → Ser), B25 (Phe → Leu), and A3 (Val → Leu)], and the affected individuals thus far have all been heterozygous for the defective gene. It is evident from the high incidence of mild diabetes or glucose intolerance among the affected individuals in these families that the presence of a defective insulin allele can be a significant predisposing factor to the development of diabetes.

Other insulin variants have been identified that give rise to elevated circulating proinsulin, with or without clinically significant carbohydrate intolerance.[213,214] These families also exhibit an autosomal dominant pattern of inheritance, and in several cases the defect has been localized to the C peptide-A chain conversion site in the proinsulin molecule, where the arginine of the Lys-Arg pair recognized by the converting enzyme has been replaced by another amino acid (histidine or leucine), rendering this site uncleavable.[215,216] A very rare form of hyperproinsulinemia in which a point mutation changes the histidine at position 10 of the B chain to aspartic acid has also been identified in one family.[217,218] This is a

particularly interesting mutation since the resultant proinsulin molecule retains the normal paired basic residues, but is not processed efficiently due to a defect in its sorting into secretory granules, which leads to its increased secretion as intact proinsulin via constitutive pathways.[219,220] In this case the insulin (or proinsulin) has approximately fourfold elevated relative receptor binding potency and there is no evidence of its association with diabetes.

The study of insulin variants has led to significant revisions in previous theories regarding the location of the receptor binding region in the insulin molecule, as discussed earlier, and has also provided direct evidence that receptor-mediated uptake and degradation of insulin[221–223] is a major pathway of insulin metabolism in vivo. The frequency of insulin gene mutations in diabetic populations appears to be quite low, probably less than 0.1% of patients.

Recent studies using the new technique of SSCP (single strand conformational polymorphism) analysis to characterize variability in the insulin gene in 100 African-Americans with T2DM have revealed the existence of significant variations in the promoter region and exons 1, 2, and 3.[224,225] No significant variants were found in any of the coding sequences, although a silent G to A substitution (allele frequency, 6%) was detected in the codon for Ala10 of the signal peptide. Several promoter variants were also found, some of which exhibited significantly reduced insulin promoter activity (38–44% of normal). Thus naturally occurring promoter variants that reduce insulin gene expression may contribute to a small proportion of diabetics in some ethnic groups. (See reference 15 for more information on insulin gene mutations.)

IAPP/AMYLIN: A NEW SECRETORY PRODUCT OF THE β CELL

Evidence has accumulated indicating that β cells secrete small amounts of a number of other peptides and proteins in addition to insulin. Some of these are unique to the islet β cells, while others, such as chromogranin A, are expressed in other neuroendocrine cells and neoplasms.[29,226] The role of these accessory secretory proteins is not understood, but they may have roles in normal physiology or in the formation and organization of the secretory granule and/or the processing of prohormones.

Considerable recent attention has been focused on one of these in particular, a novel neuropeptide-like molecule known as islet amyloid polypeptide (IAPP), or amylin (Fig. 3-9). This peptide was first identified as a major protein constituent of the amyloid

FIGURE 3-9. Primary structure of human islet amyloid polypeptide (IAPP or amylin).

Human IAPP

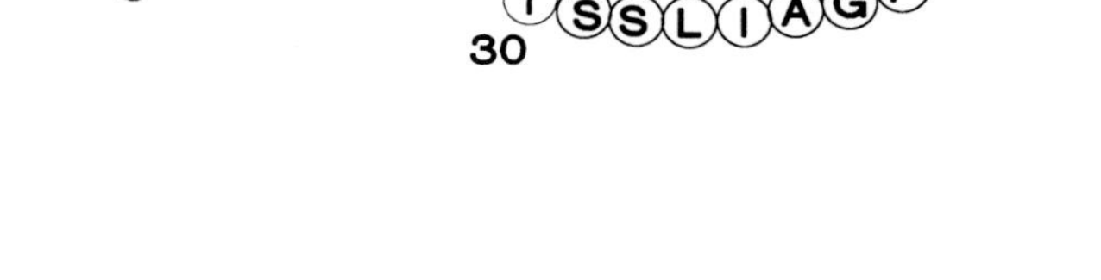

A.

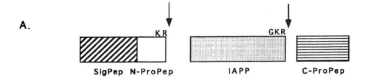

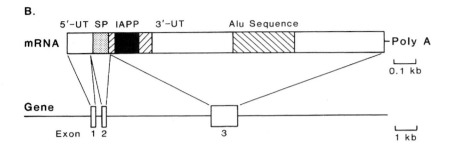

B.

C.

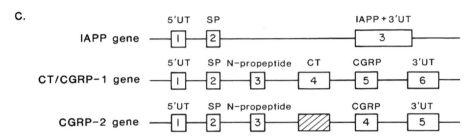

FIGURE 3-10. A. Schematic structure of the precursor of human islet amyloid polypeptide (IAPP). The arrows indicate the cleavage sites for generating the mature IAPP sequence. **B.** Schematic representation of the mRNA encoding preproIAPP, indicating its relation to the exons of the IAPP gene. **C.** Comparison of IAPP and CGRP gene structures. The ancestral gene of this superfamily may have been organized similarly to that of the CGRP-2 gene. **5′UT,** 5 untranslated region; **SP,** signal peptide; **CT,** calcitonin.

deposits that occur in the islets of elderly diabetics (those having type 2 diabetes, previously called non-insulin-dependent diabetes mellitus) and in many benign insulinomas of the pancreas, as well as in the normal pancreata of elderly individuals (see Chap. 17).[227–230] The presence of amyloid-like material was first observed in diabetic human pancreata as early as 1901 by the pathologist Opie,[231] but it was not until 1986 that this material was successfully extracted for analysis.[227] When soluble extracts were analyzed, they were found to consist of a single peptide, IAPP, which when sequenced turned out to be related to the 37-amino-acid neuroendocrine peptides calcitonin gene-related peptide (CGRP) 1 and 2 (Fig. 3-10).[227–230] The CGRP-1 is a second product of the calcitonin type I gene, derived through an alternative splicing event that occurs mainly in neural tissues.[232–234] As a result of this process, a calcitonin-encoding exon (exon 4) is replaced by another encoding CGRP (exon 5) to produce an mRNA encoding a preproprotein that gives rise to CGRP via proteolytic processing at paired basic residues.[233]

The decoding of the amino acid sequence of IAPP led to the identification of both the cDNA and the chromosomal gene encoding this hormone-like polypeptide in man.[234–238] In addition, cDNAs encoding IAPP precursors from a number of mammalian species have been described.[235,236,239] PreproIAPP is a typical neuroendocrine precursor having a signal peptide followed by a short propeptide ending in Lys.Arg before the IAPP sequence, which is then followed by Gly.Lys.Arg and another short propeptide region (Fig. 3-10A). The glycine residue at the C terminus of the IAPP

domain in the precursor is the hallmark signal for carboxyamidation, a feature also seen in the CGRPs.[235,239] Comparison of the sequences of several mammalian IAPPs and CGRPs revealed extensive sequence similarities, but also canonical sequence differences. This pattern suggests that separate, but related, tissue receptors may exist for these peptides. The single gene encoding IAPP in man (Fig. 3-10C) is located on the short arm of chromosome 12,[237,238] which is believed to be an evolutionary homologue of chromosome 11, where the CGRP-1 and -2 genes are located.[232] Thus the available evidence strongly supports the divergence of IAPP, CGRP, and calcitonin from a common ancestral gene.

Biosynthesis and Levels of IAAP in Islets

The IAPP precursor is transferred along with proinsulin into newly forming secretory vesicles in the *trans* Golgi of the β cells, where it is then processed by the same enzymatic machinery as proinsulin to release the mature 37-residue carboxyamidated peptide. It is then stored in the insulin granules and subsequently secreted together with insulin.[240] Very low levels of IAPP mRNA have also been detected in the stomach and other regions of the gastrointestinal tract, in the lung, and also in the dorsal root ganglia of the spinal cord.[241]

The relative levels of IAPP in the β cell appears to be only a few percent of the level of insulin. High-performance liquid chromatography (HPLC) analysis of freshly isolated rat islets shows amounts of IAPP that are in the range of 1–2% those of insulin.[29]

Biosynthetic labeling experiments in islets have also corroborated these low levels of IAPP expression relative to insulin [R. Carroll and D.F. Steiner, unpublished results]. Most studies[242–244] agree that the levels of IAPP are in the range of 0.2–3% of the level of insulin in normal adult rat islets or normal human pancreas. Studies with isolated rat islets have shown that IAPP secretion is stimulated by glucose and that IAPP amounts to about 5% of the amount of insulin released in 1 hour at 16.7 mmol glucose (see Chap. 21).[244]

The question of whether IAPP inhibits insulin secretion from the islets of Langerhans has been controversial because the doses required for this effect in most studies are relatively high. However, recent studies on IAPP knockout mice lend support to this idea.[245] Both male and female IAPP $^{-/-}$ mice have normal basal levels of circulating insulin and glucose, but males exhibit an increased insulin response to glucose administration and more rapid glucose disappearance in oral and IV glucose tolerance tests. These findings indicate an autocrine or paracrine suppression of insulin secretion by IAPP under normal physiological conditions. Interestingly, male IAPP-deficient mice showed a 20% increase in body mass, possibly as a consequence of increased insulin secretion or an effect of IAPP on food intake[246,247] (see Chap. 10).

IAPP inhibits insulin-stimulated glucose uptake and glycogen synthesis in rat muscle *in vitro*, an effect it shares with CGRP.[248,249] In whole animals, efforts to modify glucose tolerance with IAPP infusion have met with mixed success but usually require supraphysiologic doses of IAPP. In IAPP knockout mice, insulin sensitivity was not altered in insulin tolerance tests.[245] Other observed effects of IAPP are vasodilation, an effect it shares with CGRP, and lowering of serum ionized calcium, an effect it shares with calcitonin. IAPP can produce hyperglycemia in rats, evidently through mobilization of muscle glycogen to lactate, and thus might synergize with glucagon to enhance its hyperglycemic effects. This hyperglycemic effect has not been observed in humans treated with IAPP. Its major *in vivo* effect is a strong inhibition of gastric emptying and inhibition of glucagon secretion[250,251] at physiologic levels, which is under consideration as a potential treatment for diabetes.

In summary, studies thus far suggest that IAPP may exert a mild insulinostatic effect in the islets. It also has a glucagonostatic effect which may be mediated via the CNS through efferent vagal activity.[251] Because of its structural relatedness to CGRP, IAPP at pharmacological levels may interact with CGRP receptors to produce some of the peripheral effects that have been attributed to it. Recent efforts to identify amylin receptors indicate the existence of a novel mechanism for regulating its actions via receptor activity–modifying proteins, or RAMPs, which interact with certain calcitonin receptor isoforms to generate high-affinity IAPP receptors.[252–254] Seven helix receptors with high intrinsic IAPP binding affinity have not yet been unambiguously identified, but binding is high in the nucleus accumbens and several other brain areas[255,256] that are accessible via the systemic circulation. However, much further study will be required to clarify the mechanism and physiological significance of these observations.

Mechanisms of Amyloid Formation

Several studies[257–259] have indicated that islet amyloid formation occurs more prominently in spontaneously diabetic animals and preferentially in certain species, including man and several species of nonhuman primates, as well as cats and raccoons. Interestingly, the IAPP sequences in these species differ most significantly in the region that has been defined as amyloidogenic (residues 20–29) in studies of Glenner and associates[260] and of Westermark and coworkers[261] (see Chap. 17).[239] Synthetic peptides from this region had the greatest tendency to form fibrillar stacked β pleated sheet structures similar to those occurring in amyloid. Although in normal β cells, IAPP is localized within the insulin secretory granules,[262,263] fibrillar immunoreactive amyloid deposits have been noted primarily extracellularly, although some have been reported within the cytoplasm of β cells of some patients with T2DM by Clark and colleagues.[264] Others have noted the proximity of amyloid deposits to the β cells, suggesting that it has arisen from these cells either by secretion or some other means of deposition.[261,265] Clark and associates[266] have found IAPP immunoreactivity in lysosomes and lipofuscin bodies within the β cells of the islets of both normal and diabetic individuals and have suggested that amyloid may begin to form during the intracellular degradation of secretory granules, as occurs in the normal turnover of unused secretory products, a process known as crinophagy.

Transgenic mice overexpressing the human isoform of IAPP in their β cells *in vivo* by driving expression with the rat insulin I gene promoter have been reported to form amyloid deposits in some strains, but not in others.[267–270] However, when cultured *in vitro* at elevated glucose concentrations or implanted under the renal capsule in nude mice, islets from transgenic mice expressing human IAPP produce extracellular deposits typical of amyloid fibrils.[270–272] Human islets implanted in nude mice also rapidly develop islet amyloid deposits, especially with hyperglycemia,[273] raising a possible caveat to some human islet transplantation strategies in diabetes. One possible factor in *in vivo* fibril formation is the degree of elevation of the level of expression of hIAPP in the mouse β cells. More recent studies have shown that high-fat diets and hyperglycemia favor the formation of islet amyloid deposits in hIAPP transgenic mice.[274] The intragranular environment also influences the formation of hIAPP fibrils;[275] hence alterations associated with hyperglycemia and/or diabetes may favor the nucleation of deposits.

Just why diabetes leads to amyloid deposition remains unclear,[276] but the reason may be related to hypersecretion of IAPP associated with hyperglycemia in conjunction with other as yet unknown factors that may enhance β fibril accumulation, such as disturbed islet microcirculation. Although earlier studies failed to reveal any abnormalities in the predicted sequence of IAPP precursors in 25 type 2 diabetic patients,[277] a more recent study has reported a Ser → Gly mutation at position 20 of IAPP in 4.1% of Japanese patients with type 2 diabetes.[278] Thus abnormalities in the structure of IAPP or its precursor forms may occur, but are likely to be a minor contributing factor to diabetes. A more interesting possibility is that altered proteolytic processing of proIAPP by PC2 and PC3 may occur under certain conditions,[279–281] giving rise to incompletely processed intermediate products with altered aggregation properties and/or bioactivity. Amyloid deposits occur in the islets during normal aging and appear to be similar to those in diabetic subjects, but are usually much less abundant.[282, 283]

REFERENCES

1. Bliss M: *The Discovery of Insulin.* University of Chicago Press:1982.
2. Sanger F: Chemistry of insulin. *Science* 1959;129:1340.

3. Falkmer S, El-Salhy M, Titlbach M: Evolution of the neuroendocrine system in vertebrates: A review with particular reference to the phylogeny and postnatal maturation of the islet parenchyma. In: Falkmer S, Håakanson R, Sundler F, eds. *Evolution and Tumour Pathology of the Neuroendocrine System*. Elsevier:1984;59.

4. Smit A, Geraerts W, Meester I, *et al*: Characterization of a cDNA clone encoding molluscan insulin-related peptide II of *Lymnaea stagnalis*. *Eur J Biochem* 1991;199:699.

5. Kawakami A, Iwami M, Nagasawa H, *et al*: Structure and organization of four clustered genes that encode bombyxin, as insulin-related brain secretory peptide of the silkmoth *Bombyx mori*. *Proc Natl Acad Sci USA* 1989;86:6843.

6. Lagueux M, Lwoff L, Meister M, *et al*: cDNAs form neurosecretory cells of brains of *Locusta migratoria* (Insecta, Orthoptera) encoding a novel member of the superfamily of insulins. *Eur J Biochem* 1990; 187:249.

7. Duret L, Guex N, Peitsch MC, *et al*: New insulin-like proteins with atypical disulfide bond pattern characterized in *Caenorhabditis elegans* by comparative sequence analysis and homology modeling. *Genome Res* 1998;8:348.

8. Chan S, Cao Q-P, Steiner D: Evolution of the insulin superfamily: Cloning of a hybrid insulin/insulin-like growth factor cDNA from amphioxus. *Proc Natl Acad Sci USA* 1990;87:9319.

9. Ludwig T, Eggenschwiler J, Fisher P, *et al*: Mouse mutants lacking the type 2 IGF receptor (IGF2R) are rescued from perinatal lethality in *Igf2* and *Igf1r* null backgrounds. *Dev Biol* 1996;177:517.

10. Bryant-Greenwood G, Schwabe C: Human relaxins: Chemistry and biology. *Endocrinol Rev* 1994;15:5.

11. Adham I, Burkhardt E, Benahamed M, *et al*: Cloning of a cDNA for a novel insulin-like peptide of the testicular Leydig cells. *J Biol Chem* 1993;268:26668.

12. Conklin D, Lofton-Day CE, Haldeman BA, *et al*: Identification of INSL5, a new member of the insulin superfamily. *Genomics* 1999; 60:50.

13. Baker E, Blundell T, Cutfield J, *et al*: The structure of 2Zn pig insulin crystals at 1.5 Å resolution. *Philos Trans Roy Soc Lond* 1988; 319:369.

14. Weiss MA, Frank B, Khait I, *et al*: NMR and photo-CIDNP studies of human proinsulin and prohormone processing intermediates with application to endopeptidase recognition. *Biochemistry* 1990;29:8389.

15. Steiner D, Tager H, Nanjo K, *et al*: Familial syndromes of hyperproinsulinemia and hyperinsulinemia with mild diabetes. In: Scriver CR, Beaudet AL, Sly WS, *et al* (eds). *The Metabolic and Molecular Bases of Inherited Disease*, 7th ed. McGraw-Hill:1995;897.

16. Hua Q-X, Kochoyan M, Weiss M: Structure and dynamics of des-pentapeptide-insulin in solution: the molten-globule hypothesis. *Proc Natl Acad Sci USA* 1992;89:2379.

17. Brandenburg D, Wollmer A: The effect of a non-peptide interchain cross-link on the reoxidation of reduced insulin. *Hoppe-Seylers Z Physiol Chem* 1993;354:613.

18. Hua Q-X, Shoelson S, Kochoyan N, *et al*: Receptor binding redefined by a structural switch in a mutant human insulin. *Nature* 1991;354:238.

19. Kline A, Justice R: Complete sequence-specific ^{1}H NMR assignments for human insulin. *Biochemistry* 1990;29:2906.

20. Schaffer L: A model for insulin binding to the insulin receptor. *Eur J Biochem* 1994;221:1121.

21. Chan S, Keim P, Steiner D: Cell-free synthesis of rat preproinsulins: characterization and partial amino acid sequence determination. *Proc Natl Acad Sci USA* 1976;73:1964.

22. Lomedico P, Chan S, Steiner D, *et al*: Immunological and chemical characterization of bovine preproinsulin. *J Biol Chem* 1977;252:7971.

23. Steiner D, Quinn P, Chan S, *et al*: Processing mechanisms in the biosynthesis of proteins. *Proc Natl Acad Sci USA* 1980;343:1.

24. Sanders S, Schekman R: Polypeptide translocation across the endoplasmic reticulum membrane. *J Biol Chem* 1992;267:13791.

25. Steiner DF, Oyer PE: The biosynthesis of insulin and a probable precursor of insulin by a human islet cell adenoma. *Proc Natl Acad Sci USA* 1967;57:473.

26. Chance R, Ellis R, Bromer W: Porcine proinsulin: characterization and amino acid sequence. *Science* 1968;161:165.

27. Steiner DF, Clark JL, Nolan C, *et al*: Proinsulin and the biosynthesis of insulin. *Rec Prog Horm Res* 1969;25:207.

28. Steiner DF, Kemmler W, Clark JL, *et al*: The biosynthesis of insulin. In: Steiner DF, Freinkel N, eds. *Handbook of Physiology-Endocrinology I*. Williams & Wilkins:1972;175.

29. Nishi M, Sanke T, Nagamatsu S, *et al*: Islet amyloid polypeptide. A new beta cell secretory product related to islet amyloid deposits. *J Biol Chem* 1990;265:4173.

30. Sando H, Borg J, Steiner D: Studies on the secretion of newly synthesized proinsulin and insulin from isolated rat islets of Langerhans. *J Clin Invest* 1972;51:1476.

31. Sando H, Grodsky G: Dynamic synthesis and release of insulin and proinsulin from perifused islets. *Diabetes* 1973;22:354.

32. Gold G, Gishizky M, Grodsky G: Evidence that glucose "marks" β cells resulting in preferential release of newly synthesized insulin. *Science* 1982;218:56.

33. Orci L, Ravazzola M, Amherdt M, *et al*: Direct identification of prohormone conversion site in insulin-secreting cells. *Cell* 1985;42:671.

34. Orci L: The insulin cell: its cellular environment and how it processes (pro)insulin. *Diabetes Metab Rev* 1986;2:71.

35. Wattenberg B, Rothman J: Multiple cytosolic components promote intra-Golgi protein transport: resolution of a protein acting at a late state, prior to membrane fusion. *J Biol Chem* 1986;61:2208.

36. Chappell T, Welch W, Schlossman D, *et al*: Uncoating ATPase is a member of the 70-kilodalton family of stress proteins. *Cell* 1986;45:3.

37. Kemmler W, Peterson JD, Steiner DF: Studies on the conversion of proinsulin to insulin. I. Conversion *in vitro* with trypsin and carboxypeptidase B. *J Biol Chem* 1971;246:6786.

38. Galloway JA, Hooper SA, Spradlin CT, *et al*: Biosynthetic human proinsulin—review of chemistry, *in vitro* and *in vivo* receptor binding, animal and human pharmacology studies, and clinical experience. *Diabetes Care* 1992;15:666.

39. Smeekens SP, Steiner DF: Identification of a human insulinoma cDNA encoding a novel mammalian protein structurally related to the yeast dibasic processing protease kex2. *J Biol Chem* 1990;265:2997.

40. Smeekens SP, Avruch AS, LaMendola J, *et al*: Identification of a cDNA encoding a second putative prohormone convertase related to PC2 in AtT20 cells and islets of Langerhans. *Proc Natl Acad Sci USA* 1991;88:340.

41. van de Ven W, Voorberg J, Fontijn R, *et al*: Furin is a subtilisin-like proprotein processing enzyme in higher eukaryotes. *Mol Biol Rep* 1990;14:265.

42. Barr P, Mason O, Landsberg K, *et al*: cDNA and gene structure for a human subtilisin-like protease with cleavage specificity for paired basic amino acid residues. *DNA Cell Biol* 1991;10:319.

43. Hosaka M, Nagahama M, Kim W-S, *et al*: Arg-x-lys/arg-arg motif as a signal for precursor cleavage catalyzed by furin within the constitutive secretory pathway. *J Biol Chem* 1991;266:12127.

44. Halban P, Irminger J: Sorting and processing of secretory proteins. *Biochem J* 1994;299:1.

45. Seidah N, Marcinkiewicz M, Benjannet S, *et al*: Cloning and primary sequence of a mouse candidate prohormone convertase PC1 homologous to PC2, furin, and kex2: distinct chromosomal localization and messenger RNA distribution in brain and pituitary compared to PC2. *Mol Endocrinol* 1991;5:111.

46. Smeekens SP, Montag AG, Thomas G, *et al*: Proinsulin processing by the subtilisin-related proprotein convertases furin, PC2, and PC3. *Proc Natl Acad Sci USA* 1992;89:8822.

47. Davidson H, Rhodes C, Hutton J: Intraorganellar calcium and pH control proinsulin cleavage in the pancreatic β cell via two distinct site-specific endopeptidases. *Nature* 1988;333:93.

48. Bailyes E, Shennan K, Seal A, *et al*: A member of the eukaryotic subtilisin family (PC3) has the enzymatic properties of the type I proinsulin-converting endopeptidase. *Biochem J* 1992;285:391.

49. Bennett DL, Bailyes EM, Nielsen E, *et al*: Identification of the type 2 proinsulin processing endopeptidase as PC2, a member of the eukaryote subtilisin family. *J Biol Chem* 1992;267:15229.

50. Sizonenko SV, Halban PA: Differential rates of conversion of rat proinsulins I and II. Evidence for slow cleavage at the B-chain/C-peptide junction of proinsulin II. *Biochem J* 1991;278:621.

51. Furuta M, Yano H, Zhou A, *et al*: Defective prohormone processing and altered pancreatic islet morphology in mice lacking active SPC2. *Proc Natl Acad Sci USA* 1997;94:6646.

52. Furuta M, Carroll R, Martin S, *et al*: Incomplete processing of proinsulin to insulin accompanied by elevation of des-31,32 proinsulin intermediate in islets of mice lacking active PC2. *J Biol Chem* 1998;273:3431.

53. Sizonenko S, Irminger J-C, Buhler L, *et al*: Kinetics of proinsulin conversion in human islets. *Diabetes* 1993;42:933.

54. Hartling SG: Proinsulin in subjects with hyperglycaemia and in first degree relatives of patients with IDDM. *Danish Med Bull* 1999;46:291.

55. Rouillé Y, Westermark G, Martin SK, *et al*: Proglucagon is processed to glucagon by prohormone convertase PC2 in α-TC1-6 cells. *Proc Natl Acad Sci USA* 1994;91:3242.

56. Rouillé Y, Bianchi M, Irminger J-C, *et al*: Role of the prohormone convertase PC2 in the processing of proglucagon to glucagon. *FEBS Lett* 1997;413:119.

57. Rouillé Y, Martin S, Steiner D: Differential processing of proglucagon by the subtilisin-like prohormone convertases PC2 and PC3 to generate either glucagon or glucagon-like peptide. *J Biol Chem* 1995;270:26488.

58. Rouillé Y, Kantengwa S, Irminger J-C, *et al*: Role of the prohormone convertase PC3 in the processing of proglucagon to glucagon-like peptide 1. *J Biol Chem* 1997;272:32810.

59. Thomas L, Leduc R, Thorne B, *et al*: Kex2-like endoproteases PC2 and PC3 accurately cleave a model prohormone in mammalian cells: evidence for a common core of neuroendocrine processing enzymes. *Proc Natl Acad Sci USA* 1991;88:5297.

60. Zhou A, Webb G, Zhu X, *et al*: Proteolytic processing in the secretory pathway. *J Biol Chem* 1999;274:20745.

61. Rouillé Y, Duguay S, Lund K, *et al*: Proteolytic processing mechanisms in the biosynthesis of neuroendocrine peptides: the subtilisin-like proprotein convertases. *Front Neuroendocrinol* 1995;16:322.

62. Seidah N, Mbikay M, Marcinkiewicz M, *et al*: The mammalian precursor convertases: paralogs of the subtilisin/kexin family of calcium-dependent serine proteinases. In: Hook V, ed. *Proteolytic and Cellular Mechanisms in Prohormone Processing*. RG Landes:1998;49.

63. Muller L, Lindberg I: The cell biology of the prohormone convertases PC1 and PC2. *Prog Nucl Acid Res Mol Biol*. Academic Press:2000;69.

64. Fricker L: Peptide-processing exopeptides: amino- and carboxypeptidases involved with peptide biosynthesis. *Peptide Biosynthesis and Processing*. CRC Press:1992; p.199-230.

65. Naggert J, Fricker L, Varlamov O, *et al*: Hyperproinsulinemia in obese *fat/fat* mice is associated with a point mutation in the carboxypeptidase E gene and reduced carboxypeptidase activity in the pancreatic islets. *Nat Genet* 1995;10:135.

66. Dong W, Fricker LD, Day R: Carboxypeptidase D is a potential candidate to carry out redundant processing functions of carboxypeptidase E based on comparative distribution studies in the rat central nervous system. *Neuroscience* 1999;89:1301.

67. Day R, Lazure C, Basak A, *et al*: Prodynorphin processing by proprotein convertase 2. Cleavage at single basic residues and enhanced processing in the presence of carboxypeptidase activity. *J Biol Chem* 1998;273:829.

68. Munger B: A light and electron microscopic study of cellular differentiation in the pancreatic islets of the mouse. *Am J Anat* 1958;103:275.

69. Arvan P, Castle D: Sorting and storage during secretory granule biogenesis: looking backward and looking forward. *Biochem J* 1998;332:593.

70. Kuliawat R, Prabakaran D, Arvan P: Proinsulin endoproteolysis confers enhanced targeting of processed insulin to the regulated secretory pathway. *Mol Biol Cell* 2000;11:1959.

71. Greider M, Howell S, Lacy P: Isolation and properties of secretory granules from rat islets of Langerhans. II. Ultrastructure of the beta granule. *J Cell Biol* 1969;41:162.

72. Michael J, Carroll R, Swift H, *et al*: Studies on the molecular organization of rat insulin secretory granules. *J Biol Chem* 1987;262:16531.

73. Emdin S, Dodson G, Cutfield J, *et al*: Role of zinc in insulin biosynthesis. Some possible zinc-insulin interactions in the pancreatic B-cell. *Diabetologia* 1980;19:174.

74. Steiner DF, Bell GI, Tager HS: Chemistry and biosynthesis of pancreatic protein hormones. In: DeGroot L, ed. *Endocrinology*. WB Saunders:1995;1296.

75. Halban PA: Structural domains and molecular lifestyles of insulin and its precursors in the pancreatic beta cell. *Diabetologia* 1991;34:767.

76. Rubenstein A, Steiner D, Horwitz D, *et al*: Clinical significance of circulating proinsulin and C-peptide. *Recent Prog Horm Res* 1977;33:435.

77. Cohen R, Given B, Licinio-Paixao J, *et al*: Proinsulin radioimmunoassay in the evaluation of insulinomas and familial hyperproinsulinemia. *Metabolism* 1986;35:1137.

78. Rubenstein A, Clark J, Melani F, *et al*: Secretion of proinsulin C-peptide by pancreatic β cells and its circulation in blood. *Nature* 1969;224:697.

79. Kuliawat R, Arvan P: Protein targeting via the "constitutive-like" secretory pathway in isolated pancreatic islets: passive sorting in the immature granule compartment. *J Cell Biol* 1992;118:521.

80. Johansson B-L, Linde B, Wahren J: Effects of C-peptide on blood flow, capillary diffusion capacity and glucose utilization in the exercising forearm of type 1 (insulin-dependent) diabetic patients. *Diabetologia* 1992;35:1151.

81. Grodsky G: Insulin and the pancreas. In: Harris RS, Munson PL, Diczfalvsy E, eds. *Vitamins and Hormones*. Academic Press:1970;37.

82. Valverde I, Garcia-Morales P, Ghiglione M, *et al*: The stimulus-secretion coupling of glucose-induced insulin release. LIII. Calcium-dependency of the cyclic AMP response to nutrient secretagogues. *Horm Metab Res* 1983;15:62.

83. Theler J-M, Mollard P, Guerineau N, *et al*: Video imaging of cytosolic Ca^{2+} in pancreatic β-cells stimulated by glucose, carbachol, and ATP. *J Biol Chem* 1992;267:18110.

84. Meglasson M, Matschinsky F: Pancreatic islet glucose metabolism and regulation of insulin secretion. *Diabetes Metab Rev* 1986;2:163.

85. Polonsky KS, O'Meara NM: Secretion and metabolism of insulin, proinsulin, and C-peptide. In: DeGroot L, ed. *Endocrinology*. WB Saunders:1995;1354.

86. Ward W, LaCava E, Paquette T, *et al*: Disproportionate elevation of immunoreactive proinsulin in type 2 (non-insulin-dependent) diabetes mellitus and in experimental insulin resistance. *Diabetologia* 1987;30:698.

87. Furukawa H, Carroll RJ, Swift HH, *et al*: Long-term elevation of free fatty acids leads to delayed processing of proinsulin and prohormone convertases 2 and 3 in the pancreatic β-cell line MIN6. *Diabetes* 1999;48:1395.

88. Faehling M, Fussgaenger R, Jehle P: High affinity binding sites for proinsulin on human umbilical vein endothelial cells (HUVEC). *Diabetologia* 1999;42:259.

89. Jehle P, Lutz M, Fussgaenger R: High affinity binding sites for proinsulin in human IM-9 lymphoblasts. *Diabetologia* 1996;39:421.

90. Bell G, Pictet R, Rutter W, *et al*: Sequence of the human insulin gene. *Nature* 1980;284:26.

91. Steiner DF, Chan SJ, Welsh JM, *et al*: Structure and evolution of the insulin gene. *Ann Rev Genet* 1985;19:463.

92. Bell G, Seino S: The organization and structure of the insulin gene. In: Okamoto H, ed. *Molecular Biology of the Islets of Langerhans*. Cambridge University Press:1990;9.

93. Soares M, Schon E, Henderson A, *et al*: RNA-mediated gene duplication: the rat preproinsulin I gene is a functional retroposon. *Mol Cell Biol* 1985;5:2090.

94. Giddings S, Carnaghi L: The two nonallelic rat insulin mRNAs and pre-mRNAs are regulated coordinately *in vivo*. *J Biol Chem* 1988;263:3845.

95. Giddings S, Carnaghi L: Rat insulin II gene expression by extraplacental membranes. A non-pancreatic source for fetal insulin. *J Biol Chem* 1989;264:9462.

96. Fiedorek FT Jr., Carnaghi LR, Giddings SJ: Selective expression of the insulin I gene in rat insulinoma-derived cell lines. *Molec Endocrinol* 1990;4:990.

97. Giddings SJ, King CD, Harman KW, *et al*: Allele specific inactivation of insulin 1 and 2, in the mouse yolk sac, indicates imprinting. *Nat Genet* 1994;6:310.

98. Owerbach D, Bell G, Rutter W, *et al*: The insulin gene is located on the short arm of chromosome 11 in humans. *Diabetes* 1981;30:267.

99. Harper M, Ullrich A, Saunders G: Localization of the human insulin gene to the distal end of the short arm of chromosome 11. *Proc Natl Acad Sci USA* 1981;78:4458.

100. Bell G, Selby M, Rutter W: The highly polymorphic region near the human insulin gene is composed of simple tandemly repeating sequences. *Nature* 1982;295:31.

101. Julier C, Hyer R, Davies J, *et al*: Insulin-IGF2 region on chromosome 11p encodes a gene implicated in HLA-DR4-dependent diabetes susceptibility. *Nature* 1991;354:155.

102. Philippe J: Structure and pancreatic expression of the insulin and glucagon genes. *Endocr Rev* 1991;12:252.

103. Walker MD: Insulin gene regulation. In: *Handbook of Experimental Pharmacology, Vol. 92: Insulin*. Cautrecasas P, Jacobs S, eds. Springer Verlag:1990;93.

104. Clark AR, Docherty K: The insulin gene. In: Ashcroft FM, Ashcroft SJ, eds. *Insulin, Molecular Biology to Pathology*. Oxford University Press:1992;37.

105. Stein R: Factors regulating insulin gene transcription. *Trends Endocrinol Metab* 1993;4:96.

106. German M, Ashcroft S, Docherty K, *et al*: The insulin gene promoter: a simplified nomenclature. *Diabetes* 1995;44:1002.

107. Kingston RE: Transcription control and differentiation: the HLH family, c-myc and C/EBP. *Curr Opin Cell Biol* 1989;1:1081.

108. Karlsson O, Edlund T, Moss LB, *et al*: A mutational analysis of the insulin gene transcription control region: expression in beta cells is dependent on two related sequences within the enhancer. *Proc Natl Acad Sci USA* 1987;84:8819.

109. Naya FJ, Stellrecht CM, Tsai MJ: Tissue-specific regulation of the insulin gene by a novel basic helix-loop-helix transcription factor. *Genes Dev* 1995;9:1009.

110. Lee JE, Hollenberg SM, Snider L, *et al*: Conversion of *Xenopus* ectoderm into neurons by NeuroD, a basic helix loop helix protein. *Science* 1995;268:836.

111. Naya FJ, Huang H-P, Qiu Y, *et al*: Diabetes, defective pancreatic morphogenesis, and abnormal enteroendocrine differentiation in BETA2/NeuroD-deficient mice. *Genes Dev*. 1997;11:2323.

112. Itkin-Ansari P, Bain G, Beattie GM, *et al*: E2A gene products are not required for insulin gene expression. *Endocrinology* 1996;37:3540.

113. Read ML, Smith SB, Docherty K: The insulin enhancer binding site 2 (IEB2; FAR) box of the insulin gene regulatory region binds at least three factors that can be distinguished by their DNA binding characteristics. *Biochem J* 1995;309:231.

114. Read ML, Masson MR, Docherty K: A RIPE3b1-like factor binds to a novel site in the human insulin promoter in a redox-dependent manner. *FEBS Letts* 1997;418:68.

115. Shieh S-Y, Tsai M-J: Cell-specific and ubiquitous factors are responsible for the enhancer activity of the rat insulin II gene. *J Biol Chem* 1991;266:16708.

116. Ohlsson H, Karlsson K, Edlund T: IPF1, a homeodomain-containing transactivator of the insulin gene. *EMBO J* 1993;12:4251.

117. Miller CP, McGehee Jr RE, Habener JF: IDX-1: a new homeodomain transcription factor expressed in rat pancreatic islets and duodenum that transactivates the somatostatin gene. *EMBO J* 1994;13:1145.

118. Leonard J, Peers B, Johnson T, *et al*: Characterisation of somatostatin transactivating factor-1, a novel homeobox factor that stimulates somatostatin expression in pancreatic islet cells. *Mol Endocrinol* 1993;7:275.

119. Boam DSW, Docherty K: A tissue specific nuclear factor binds to multiple sites in the human insulin gene enhancer. *Biochem J* 1989;264:233.

120. Peshavaria M, Gamer L, Henderson E, *et al*: XlHbox 8, an endoderm-specific *Xenopus* homeodomain protein, is closely related to a mammalian insulin gene transcription factor. *Mol Endocrinol* 1994;8:806.

121. Jonsson J, Carlsson L, Edlund T, *et al*: Insulin promoter factor 1 is required for pancreas development in mice. *Nature* 1994;371:606.

122. Jonsson J, Ahlgren U, Edlund T, *et al*: IPF1, a homeodomain protein with a dual function in pancreas development. *Int J Dev Biol* 1995;39:789.

123. Guz Y, Montminy MR, Leonard J, *et al*: Expression of murine STF-1, a putative insulin gene transcription factor, in β cells of pancreas, duodenum epithelium and pancreatic exocrine and endocrine progenitors during ontogeny. *Development* 1995;121:11.

124. Inoue H, Riggs AC, Tanizawa Y, *et al*: Isolation, characterisation and chromosomal mapping of the human insulin promoter factor-1 (IPF-1) gene. *Diabetes* 1996;45:789.

125. Peshavaria M, Henderson E, Sharma A, *et al*: Functional characterisation of the transactivation properties of the PDX-1 homeodomain protein. *Mol Cell Biol* 1997;17:3987.

126. Lu M, Miller CP, Habener JF: Functional regions of the homeodomain protein IDX-1 required for transactivation of the rat somatostatin gene. *Endocrinology* 1996;137:2959.

127. Peers B, Leonard J, Sharma S, *et al*: Insulin expression in pancreatic islet cells relies on cooperative interactions between the helix loop helix factor E47 and the homeobox factor STF-1. *Mol Endocrinol* 1994;8:1798.

128. Peers B, Sharma S, Johnson T, *et al*: The pancreatic islet factor STF-1 binds cooperatively with Pbx to a regulatory element in the somatostatin promoter: importance of the FPWMK motif and of the homeodomain. *Mol Cell Biol* 1995;5:7091.

129. Wu KL, Gannon M, Peshavaria M, *et al*: Hepatocyte nuclear factor 3β is involved in pancreatic β-cell specific expression of the *pdx1* gene. *Mol Cell Biol* 1997;17:6002.

130. Sharma S, Leonard J, Lee S, *et al*: Pancreatic islet expression of the homeobox factor STF-1 relies on an E-box motif that binds USF. *J Biol Chem* 1996;271:2294.

131. Kennedy GC, Rutter WJ: Pur-1, a zinc-finger protein that binds to purine-rich sequences, transactivates an insulin promoter in heterologous cells. *Proc Natl Acad Sci USA* 1992;89:11498.

132. Galsgaard ED, Gouilleux F, Groner B, *et al*: Identification of a growth hormone responsive STAT-5 binding element in the rat insulin I gene. *Mol Endocrinol* 1996;10:652.

133. Boam DSW, Clark AR, Docherty K: Positive and negative regulation of the human insulin gene by multiple trans-acting factors. *J Biol Chem* 1990;265:8285.

134. Clark AR, Wilson ME, Leibiger I, *et al*: A silencer and an adjacent positive element interact to modulate the activity of the human insulin promoter. *Eur J Biochem* 1995;232:627.

135. Goodman PA, Medina-Martinez O, Fernandez-Mejia C: Identification of the human insulin negative regulatory element as a negative glucocorticoid response element. *Mol Cell Endocrinol* 1996;120:139.

136. Kennedy GC, German MS, Rutter WJ: The minisatellite in the diabetes susceptibility locus IDDM2 regulates insulin transcription. *Nat Genet* 1995;9:293.

137. Bennett ST, Lucassen AM, Gough SCL, *et al*: Susceptibility to human type 1 diabetes at IDDM2 is determined by tandem repeat variations at the insulin gene minisatellite locus. *Nat Genet* 1995;9:28.

138. Hammond-Kosack MCU, Dobrinski B, Lurz R, *et al*: The human insulin linked polymorphic region exhibits an altered DNA structure. *Nucl Acids Res* 1992;20:231.

139. Hammond-Kosack MCU, Docherty K: A consensus repeat sequence from the human insulin gene linked polymorphic region adopts multiple quadriplex structures *in vitro*. *FEBS Lett* 1992;301:79.

140. Catasti P, Chen X, Moyzis RK, *et al*: Structure-function correlations of the insulin-linked polymorphic region. *J Mol Biol* 1996;264:534.

141. Catasti P, Chen X, Deaven LL, *et al*: Cytosine-rich strands of the insulin minisatellite adopt hairpins with intercalated cytosine(+) centre dot cytosine pairs. *J Mol Biol* 1997;272:369.

142. Hammond-Kosack MCU, Kilpatrick MW, Docherty K: Analysis of the human insulin gene linked polymorphic region *in vivo*. *J Mol Endocrinol* 1992;9:221.

143. Hammond-Kosack MCU, Kilpatrick MW, Docherty K: The human insulin gene linked polymorphic region adopts a quadriplex structure in chromatin assembled *in vitro*. *J Mol Endocrinol* 1993;10:121.

144. Clark AR, Wilson NE, London NJM, *et al*: Identification and characterisation of a thyroid hormone/retinoic acid response element upstream of the human insulin gene. *Biochem J* 1995;309:863.

145. Ohtani K, Shimizu H, Kato Y: Identification and characterisation of a glucose-responsiveness region upstream of the human insulin gene in transfected HIT-T15 cells. *Biochem Biophys Res Commun* 1998;242:446.

146. Ashcroft SJH: Glucoreceptor maechanisms and the control of insulin release and biosynthesis. *Diabetologia* 1980;18:5.

147. Ashcroft FM, Ashcroft SJH: Mechanisms of insulin secretion. In: Ashcroft FM, Ashcroft SJH, eds. *Insulin, Molecular Biology to Pathology*. Oxford University Press:1992;97.

148. Aspinwall CA, Qian W-J, Roper MG, *et al*: Roles of insulin receptor substrate-1, phosphatidylinositol 3-kinase, and release of intracellular Ca^{2+} stores in insulin-stimulated insulin secretion in β cells. *J Biol Chem* 2000;275:22331.

149. Gembal M, Gilon P, Henquin JC: Evidence that glucose can control insulin release independently from its action on ATP-sensitive K^+ channels in mouse β cells. *J Clin Invest* 1992;89:1288.

150. Maechler P, Wollheim CB: Mitochondrial glutamate acts as a messenger in glucose-induced insulin exocytosis. *Nature* 1999;402:685.

151. Wollheim CB: Beta-cell mitochondria in the regulation of insulin secretion: a new culprit in type II diabetes. *Diabetologia* 2000;43:265.

152. Docherty K, Clark AR: Nutrient regulation of insulin gene expression. *FASEB J* 1994;8:20.

153. Wang JH, Shen LP, Najafi H, *et al*: Regulation of insulin preRNA splicing by glucose. *Proc Natl Acad Sci USA* 1997;94:4360.

154. Charollais A, Gjinovci A, Huarte J, *et al*: Junctional communication of pancreatic β cells contributes to the control of insulin secretion and glucose tolerance. *J Clin Invest* 2000;106:235.

155. Schuit RC, In'tVeld PA, Pipeleers DG: Glucose stimulates proinsulin biosynthesis by a dose-dependent recruitment of pancreatic beta cells. *Proc Natl Acad Sci USA* 1988;85:3865.

156. Giddings SJ, Chirgwin J, Permutt MA: The effect of fasting and feeding on preproinsulin messenger RNA in rats. *J Clin Invest* 1981;67:952.

157. Brundstedt J, Chan SJ: Direct effect of glucose on the preproinsulin mRNA level in isolated pancreatic islets. *Biochem Biophys Res Commun* 1982;106:1383.

158. Nielsen DA, Welsh M, Casadaban MJ, *et al*: Control of insulin gene expression in pancreatic β cells and in an insulin-secreting cell line,

RIN-5F cells. I. Effects of glucose and cyclic AMP on the transcription of insulin mRNA. *J Biol Chem* 1985;260:13585.

159. Welsh M, Nielsen DA, MacKrell AJ, et al: Control of insulin gene expression in pancreatic b cells and in an insulin-secreting cell line, RIN-5F cells. II. Regulation of insulin mRNA stability. *J Biol Chem* 1985;260:13590.

160. Efrat S, Surana M, Fleischer N: Glucose induces insulin gene transcription in a murine pancreatic β-cell line. *J Biol Chem* 1991;266: 11141.

161. German MS, Moss LG, Rutter WJ: Regulation of insulin gene expression by glucose and calcium in transfected primary islet cultures. *J Biol Chem* 1990;265:22063.

162. Goodison S, Kenna S, Ashcroft SJH: Control of insulin gene expression by glucose. *Biochem J* 1992;285:563.

163. German M, Wang J: The insulin gene contains multiple transcriptional elements that respond to glucose. *Mol Cell Biol* 1994;14: 4067.

164. Sharma A, Stein R: Glucose-induced transcription of the insulin gene is mediated by factors required for b cell type specific expression. *Mol Cell Biol* 1994;14:871.

165. Read ML, Masson MR, Docherty K: A RIPE3b1-like factor binds to a novel site in the human insulin promoter in a redox-dependent manner. *FEBS Lett* 1997;418:68.

166. Melloul D, Ben-Neriah Y, Cerasi E: Glucose modulates the binding of an islet-specific factor to a conserved sequence within the rat I and human insulin promoters. *Proc Natl Acad Sci USA* 1993;90:3865.

167. Macfarlane WM, Read ML, Gilligan M, et al: Glucose modulates the binding activity of the β cell transcription factor, IUF1, in a phosphorylation-dependent manner. *Biochem J* 1994;303:625.

168. Petersen HV, Serup P, Leonard J, et al: Transcriptional regulation of the human insulin gene is dependent on the homeodomain protein STF1/IPF1 acting through the CT boxes. *Proc Natl Acad Sci USA* 1994;91:10465.

169. Marshak S, Totary H, Cerasi E, et al: Purification of the β-cell glucose-sensitive factor that transactivates the insulin gene differentially in normal and transformed islet cells. *Proc Natl Acad Sci USA* 1996;93:15057.

170. Macfarlane WM, Smith SB, James RFL, et al: The p38/reactivating kinase mitogen-activated protein kinase cascade mediates the activation of the transcription factor insulin upstream factor 1 and insulin gene transcription by glucose in pancreatic β cells. *J Biol Chem* 1997; 272:20936.

171. Rafiq I, da Sila Xavier G, Hooper S, et al: Glucose-stimulated preproinsulin gene expression and nuclear translocation of pancreatic duodenum homeobox-1 require activation of phosphatidylinositol 3-kinase but not p38 MAPK/SAPK2. *J Biol Chem* 2000;275:15977.

172. Cohen P: The search for physiological substrates of MAP and SAP kinases in mammalian cells. *Trends Cell Biol* 1997;7:353.

173. Macfarlane WM, McKinnon CM, Felton-Edkins ZM, et al: Glucose stimulates translocation of the homeodomain transcription factor PDX1 from the cytoplasm to the nucleus in pancreatic β cells. *J Biol Chem* 1999;274:1011.

174. Rafiq I, Kennedy HJ, Rutter GA: Glucose-dependent translocation of insulin promoter factor-1 (IPF-1) between the nuclear periphery and the nucleoplasm of single MIN6 β-cells. *J Biol Chem* 1998;273:23241.

175. Wu H, MacFarlane WM, Tadayyon M, et al: Insulin stimulates PDX1 DNA-binding and insulin promoter activity in pancreatic β cells. *Biochem J* 1999;344:813.

176. Leibiger IB, Leibiger B, Moede T, et al: Exocytosis of insulin promotes insulin gene transcription via the insulin receptor/PI 3-kinase/p70S⁶ kinase and CAMKinase pathways. *Mol Cell* 1998;1:933.

177. Permutt MA, Kipnis DM: Insulin biosynthesis. 1. On the mechanism of glucose stimulation. *J Biol Chem* 1972;247:1194.

178. Itoh N, Okamoto H: Translational control of proinsulin synthesis by glucose. *Nature* 1980;283:100.

179. Grimaldi KA, Siddle K, Hutton JC: Biosynthesis of insulin secretory granule membrane proteins. *Biochem J* 1987;245:567.

180. Guest PC, Rhodes CJ, Hutton JC: Regulation of the biosynthesis of insulin-secretory-granule proteins. *Biochem J* 1989;257:431.

181. Guest PC, Bailyes EM, Rutherford NG, et al: Insulin secretory granule biogenesis. Co-ordinate regulation of the biosynthesis of the majority of constituent proteins. *Biochem J* 1991;274:73.

182. Skelly RH, Bollheimer LC, Wicksteed BL, et al: A distinct difference in the metabolic stimulus-response coupling pathways for regulating proinsulin biosynthesis and insulin secretion that lies at the level of a requirement for fatty acyl moieties. *Biochem J* 1998;331:553.

183. Gilligan M, Welsh G, Flynn A, et al: Glucose stimulates the activity of the guanine exchange factor eIF-2B in isolated rat islets of Langerhans. *J Biol Chem* 1996;271:2121.

184. Xu G, Marshall CA, Lin T-A, et al: Insulin mediates glucose-stimulated phosphorylation of PHAS-1 by pancreatic beta cells. *J Biol Chem* 1998;273:4485.

185. Knight SW, Docherty K: RNA-protein interactions in the 5′ untranslated region of preproinsulin mRNA. *J Mol Endocrinol* 1992;8:225.

186. Davies JL, Kawaguchi Y, Bennett ST, et al: A genome-wide search for human type 1 diabetes susceptibility genes. *Nature* 1994;371:130.

187. Bennet ST, Todd JA: Human type I diabetes and the insulin gene: principles of mapping polygenes. *Ann Rev Genet* 1996;30:343.

188. Kennedy GC, German MS, Rutter WJ: The minsatellite in the diabetes susceptibility locus IDDM2 regulates insulin transcription. *Nat Genet* 1995;9:293.

189. Bennett ST, Lucassen AM, Gough SCL, et al: Susceptibility to human type 1 diabetes at IDDM2 is determined by tandem repeat variations at the insulin gene minisatellite locus. *Nat Genet* 1995;9:284.

190. Owerbach D, Gabbay KH: The search for IDDM susceptibility genes. The next generation. *Diabetes* 1996;45:544.

191. Pugliese A, Zeller M, Fernandez A Jr., et al: The insulin gene is transcribed in the human thymus and transcription levels correlate with allelic variation at the INS VNTR susceptibility locus for type 1 diabetes. *Nat Genet* 1997;15:293.

192. Vafiadis P, Bennet ST, Todd JA, et al: Insulin expression in human thymus is modulated by INS VNTR alleles at the IDDM2 locus. *Nat Genet* 1997;15:289.

193. Stoffers DA, Thomas MK, Habener JF: Homeodomain protein IDX-1. A master regulator of pancreas development and insulin gene expression. *Trends Endocrinol Metab* 1997;8:145.

194. Stoffers DA, Zinkin NT, Stanojevic V, et al: Pancreatic agenesis attributable to a single nucleotide deletion in the human *IPF1* gene coding sequence. *Nat Genet* 1997;15:106.

195. Olson KL, Redmon JB, Towle HC, et al: Chronic exposure of HIT cells to high glucose concentrations paradoxically decreases insulin gene transcription and alters binding of insulin gene regulatory protein. *J Clin Invest* 1993;92:514.

196. Olson KL, Sharma A, Peshavaria M, et al: Reduction of insulin gene transcription in HIT-T15 β cells chronically exposed to a supraphysiological glucose concentration is associated with a loss of STF-1 transcription factor expression. *Proc Natl Acad Sci USA* 1995;92:9127.

197. Sharma A, Olson LK, Robertson RP, et al: The reduction of insulin gene transcription in HIT-T15 β cells chronically exposed to high glucose concentration is associated with the loss of RIP3b1 and STF-1 transcription factor expression. *Mol Endocrinol* 1995;9:1127.

198. Robertson RP, Olson LK, Zhang H-J: Differentiating glucose toxicity from glucose densensitisation: a new message from the insulin gene. *Diabetes* 1994;4:1085.

199. Stoffers DA, Ferrer J, Clarke WL, et al: Early-onset type-II diabetes mellitus (MODY4) linked to *IPF1*. *Nat Genet* 1997;17:138.

200. Froguel P, Zouali H, Vionnet N, et al: Familial hyperglycaemia due to mutations in glucokinase: definition of a subtype of diabetes mellitus. *N Engl J Med* 1993;328:697.

201. Hattersley AT: Maturity-onset diabetes of the young; clinical heterogeneity explained by genetic heterogeneity. *Diabetes Med* 1998; 15:15.

202. Macfarlane WM, Frayling TM, Ellard S, et al: Missense mutations in insulin promoter factor-1 gene predispose to type 2 diabetes. *J Clin Invest* 1999;104:R33.

203. El Habib H, Stoffers DA, Chèvre J-C, et al: Defective mutations in the insulin promoter factor-1 (IPF-1) gene in late-onset type 2 diabetes mellitus. *J Clin Invest* 1999;104:R41.

204. Dutta S, Bonner-Weir S, Montminy M, et al: Regulatory factor linked to late-onset diabetes? *Nature* 1998;392:560.

205. Tager H, Given B, Baldwin D, et al: A structurally abnormal insulin causing human diabetes. *Nature* 1979;281:122.

206. Haneda M, Polonsky KS, Bergenstal RM, et al: Familial hyperinsulinemia due to a structurally abnormal insulin. Definition of an emerging new clinical syndrome. *N Engl J Med* 1984;310:1288.

207. Nanjo K, Sanke T, Miyano M, et al: Diabetes due to secretion of a structurally abnormal insulin (insulin Wakayama). Clinical and functional characteristics of [LeuA3] insulin. *J Clin Invest* 1986;77:514.

208. Shoelson S, Polonsky K, Zeidler A, et al: Human insulin B24 (Phe → Ser). Secretion and metabolic clearance of the abnormal insulin in man and in a dog model. *J Clin Invest* 1984;73:1351.

209. Kwok SC, Steiner DF, Rubenstein AH, *et al*: Identification of a point mutation in the human insulin gene giving rise to a structurally abnormal insulin (insulin Chicago). *Diabetes* 1983;32:872.

210. Haneda M, Chan SJ, Kwok SC, *et al*: Studies on mutant human insulin genes: identification and sequence analysis of a gene encoding [SerB24]insulin. *Proc Natl Acad Sci USA* 1983;80:6366.

211. Assoian R, Thomas N, Kaiser E, *et al*: [Leu^{B24}] insulin and [Ala^{B24}] insulin: altered structures and cellular processing of B24-substituted insulin analogs. *Proc Natl Acad Sci USA* 1982;79:5147.

212. Shoelson S, Fickova M, Haneda M, *et al*: Identification of a mutant human insulin predicted to contain a serine-for-phenylalanine substitution. *Proc Natl Acad Sci USA* 1983;80:7390.

213. Gabbay KH, Bergenstal RM, Wolff J, *et al*: Familial hyperproinsulinemia: partial characterization of circulating proinsulin-like material. *Proc Natl Acad Sci USA* 1979;76:2881.

214. Kanazawa Y, Hayashi M, Ikeuchi M, *et al*: Familial proinsulinemia: A rare disorder of insulin biosynthesis. In: Baba S, Kaneko T, Yanaihara N, eds. *Proinsulin, Insulin, C-Peptide*. Excerpta Medica:1979;262.

215. Robbins DC, Blix PM, Rubenstein AH, *et al*: A human proinsulin variant at arginine 65. *Nature* 1981;291:679.

216. Robbins DC, Shoelson SE, Rubenstein AH, *et al*: Familial hyperproinsulinemia. Two cohorts secreting indistinguishable type II intermediates of proinsulin conversion. *J Clin Invest* 1984;73:714.

217. Gruppuso PA, Gorden P, Kahn CR, *et al*: Familial hyperproinsulinemia due to a proposed defect in conversion of proinsulin to insulin. *N Engl J Med* 1984;311:629.

218. Chan SJ, Seino S, Gruppuso PA, *et al*: A mutation in the B chain coding region is associated with impaired proinsulin conversion in a family with hyperproinsulinemia. *Proc Natl Acad Sci USA* 1987;84:2194.

219. Gross DJ, Halban PA, Kahn CR, *et al*: Partial diversion of a mutant proinsulin (B10 aspartic acid) from the regulated to the constitutive secretory pathway in transfected AtT-20 cells. *Proc Natl Acad Sci USA* 1989;86:4107.

220. Carroll RJ, Hammer RE, Chan SJ, *et al*: A mutant human proinsulin is secreted from islets of Langerhans in increased amounts via an unregulated pathway. *Proc Natl Acad Sci USA* 1988;85:8943.

221. Terris S, Hofmann C, Steiner DF: Mode of uptake and degradation of 125I-labelled insulin by isolated hepatocytes and H4 hepatoma cells. *Can J Biochem* 1979;57:459.

222. Terris S, Steiner DF: Binding and degradation of 125I-insulin by rat hepatocytes. *J Biol Chem* 1975;250:8389.

223. Terris S, Steiner DF: Retention and degradation of 125I-insulin by perfused livers from diabetic rats. *J Clin Invest* 1976;57:885.

224. Olansky L, Janssen R, Welling C, *et al*: Variability of the insulin gene in American blacks with NIDDM. Analysis by single-strand conformational polymorphisms. *Diabetes* 1992;41:742.

225. Olansky L, Welling C, Giddings S, *et al*: A variant insulin promoter in non-insulin-dependent diabetes mellitus. *J Clin Invest* 1992;89:1596.

226. Hutton JC: The insulin secretory granule. *Diabetologia* 1989;32:271.

227. Westermark P, Wernstedt C, Wilander E, *et al*: A novel peptide in the calcitonin gene related peptide family as an amyloid fibril protein in the endocrine pancreas. *Biochem Biophys Res Commun* 1986;140:827.

228. Clark A, Cooper GJ, Lewis CE, *et al*: Islet amyloid formed from diabetes-associated peptide may be pathogenic in type-2 diabetes. *Lancet* 1987;2:231.

229. Westermark P, Wernstedt C, Wilander E, *et al*: Amyloid fibrils in human insulinoma and islets of Langerhans of the diabetic cat are derived from a neuropeptide-like protein also present in normal islet cells. *Proc Natl Acad Sci USA* 1987;84:3881.

230. Cooper GJ, Willis AC, Clark A, *et al*: Purification and characterization of a peptide from amyloid-rich pancreases of type 2 diabetic patients. *Proc Natl Acad Sci USA* 1987;84:8628.

231. Opie E: The relation of diabetes mellitus to lesions of the pancreas: Hyaline degeneration of the islands of Langerhans. *J Exp Med* 1901;5:527.

232. Breimer LH, MacIntyre I, Zaidi M: Peptides from the calcitonin genes: molecular genetics, structure and function. *Biochem J* 1988;255:377.

233. Amara SG, Jonas V, Rosenfeld MG, *et al*: Alternative RNA processing in calcitonin gene expression generates mRNAs encoding different polypeptide products. *Nature* 1982;298:240.

234. Crenshaw EB III, Russo AF, Swanson LW, *et al*: Neuron-specific alternative RNA processing in transgenic mice expressing a metallothionein-calcitonin fusion gene. *Cell* 1987;49:389.

235. Sanke T, Bell GI, Sample C, *et al*: An islet amyloid peptide is derived from an 89-amino acid precursor by proteolytic processing. *J Biol Chem* 1988;263:17243.

236. Leffert JD, Newgard CB, Okamoto H, *et al*: Rat amylin: cloning and tissue-specific expression in pancreatic islets. *Proc Natl Acad Sci USA* 1989;86:3127.

237. Mosselman S, Hoppener JW, Zandberg J, *et al*: Islet amyloid polypeptide: identification and chromosomal localization of the human gene. *FEBS Lett* 1988;239:227.

238. Nishi M, Sanke T, Seino S, *et al*: Human islet amyloid polypeptide gene: complete nucleotide sequence, chromosomal localization, and evolutionary history. *Molec Endocrinol* 1989;3:1775.

239. Betsholtz C, Svensson V, Rorsman F, *et al*: Islet amyloid polypeptide (IAPP): cDNA cloning and identification of an amyloidogenic region associated with the species-specific occurrence of age-related diabetes mellitus. *Exp Cell Res* 1989;183:484.

240. Nagamatsu S, Nishi M, Steiner DF: Biosynthesis of islet amyloid polypeptide. Elevated expression in mouse beta TC3 cells. *J Biol Chem* 1991;266:13737.

241. Ferrier GJ, Pierson AM, Jones PM, *et al*: Expression of the rat amylin (IAPP/DAP) gene. *J Molec Endocrinol* 1989;3:R1.

242. Nakazato M, Asai J, Kangawa K, *et al*: Establishment of radioimmunoassay for human islet amyloid polypeptide and its tissue content and plasma concentration. *Biochem Biophys Res Commun* 1989; 164:394.

243. Asai J, Nakazato M, Miyazato M, *et al*: Regional distribution and molecular forms of rat islet amyloid polypeptide. *Biochem Biophys Res Commun* 1990;169:788.

244. Kanatsuka A, Makino H, Ohsawa H, *et al*: Secretion of islet amyloid polypeptide in response to glucose. *FEBS Lett* 1989;259:199.

245. Gebre-Medhin S, Mulder H, Pekny M, *et al*: Increased insulin secretion and glucose tolerance in mice lacking islet amyloid polypeptide (amylin). *Biochem Biophys Res Commun* 1998;250:271.

246. Lutz TA, Del Prete E, Scharrer E: Reduction of food intake in rats by intraperitoneal injection of low doses of amylin. *Phys Behav* 1994; 55:891.

247. Morley JE, Flood JF: Amylin decreases food intake in mice. *Peptides* 1991;12:865.

248. Leighton B, Cooper GJ: Pancreatic amylin and calcitonin gene-related peptide cause resistance to insulin in skeletal muscle *in vitro*. *Nature* 1988;335:632.

249. Cooper GJ, Leighton B, Dimitriadis GD, *et al*: Amylin found in amyloid deposits in human type 2 diabetes mellitus may be a hormone that regulates glycogen metabolism in skeletal muscle. *Proc Natl Acad Sci USA* 1988;85:7763.

250. Gedulin BR, Rink TJ, Young AA: Dose-response for glucagonostatic effect of amylin in rats. *Metabolism* 1997;46:67.

251. Silvestre RA, Rodriguez-Gallardo J, Jodka C, *et al*: Selective amylin inhibition of the glucagon response to arginine is extrinsic to the pancreas. *Am J Physiol* 2001;280:E443.

252. Christopoulos G, Perry K, Morfis M, *et al*: Multiple amylin receptors arise from receptor activity-modifying protein interaction with the calcitonin receptor gene product. *Mol Pharmacol* 1999;56:235.

253. Muff R, Bühlmann N, Fischer JA, *et al*: An amylin receptor is revealed following co-transfection of a calcitonin receptor with receptor activity modifying proteins-1 or -3. *Endocrinology* 1999;140: 2924.

254. Tilakaratne N, Christopoulos G, Zumpe ET, *et al*: Amylin receptor phenotypes derived from human calcitonin receptor/RAMP coexpression exhibit pharmacological differences dependent on receptor isoform and host cell environment. *J Pharmacol Exp Ther* 2000;294:61.

255. Christopoulos G, Paxinos G, Huang XF, *et al*: Comparative distribution of receptors for amylin and the related peptides calcitonin gene related peptide and calcitonin in rat and monkey brain. *Canadian J Physiol Pharmacol* 1995;73:1037.

256. van Rossum D, Menard DP, Fournier A, *et al*: Autoradiographic distribution and receptor binding profile of [125I]Bolton Hunter-rat amylin binding sites in the rat brain. *J Pharm Exp Ther* 1994;270:779.

257. Howard CF Jr.: Diabetes in *Macaca nigra*: metabolic and histologic changes. *Diabetologia* 1974;10(Suppl):671.

258. Westermark P: On the nature of the amyloid in human islets of Langerhans. *Histochemistry* 1974;38:27.

259. Yano BL, Johnson KH, Hayden DW: Feline insular amyloid: histochemical distinction from secondary systemic amyloid. *Vet Pathol* 1981;18:181.

260. Glenner GG, Eanes ED, Wiley CA: Amyloid fibrils formed from a segment of the pancreatic islet amyloid protein. *Biochem Biophys Res Commun* 1988;155:608.

261. Westermark P, Johnson KH, O'Brien TD, *et al*: Islet amyloid poly-peptide—a novel controversy in diabetes research. *Diabetologia* 1992;35:297.

262. Johnson KH, O'Brien TD, Hayden DW, *et al*: Immunolocalization of islet amyloid polypeptide (IAPP) in pancreatic beta cells by means of peroxidase-antiperoxidase (PAP) and protein A-gold techniques. *Am J Pathol* 1988;130:1.

263. Lukinius A, Wilander E, Westermark GT, *et al*: Co-localization of islet amyloid polypeptide and insulin in the B cell secretory granules of the human pancreatic islets. *Diabetologia* 1989;32:240.

264. Clark A, Wells CA, Buley ID, *et al*: Islet amyloid, increased A-cells, reduced B-cells and exocrine fibrosis: quantitative changes in the pancreas in type 2 diabetes. *Diabetes Res* 1988;9:151.

265. Westermark P: Fine structure of islets of Langerhans in insular amyloidosis. *Virchows Archiv - A: Pathology - Pathologische Anatomie* 1973;359:1.

266. Clark A, Edwards CA, Ostle LR, *et al*: Localisation of islet amyloid peptide in lipofuscin bodies and secretory granules of human B-cells and in islets of type-2 diabetic subjects. *Cell Tiss Res* 1989;257:179.

267. Fox N, Schrementi J, Nishi M, *et al*: Human islet amyloid polypeptide transgenic mice as a model of non-insulin-dependent diabetes mellitus (NIDDM). *FEBS Lett* 1993;323:40.

268. Yagui K, Yamaguchi T, Kanatsuka A, *et al*: Formation of islet amyloid fibrils in beta-secretory granules of transgenic mice expressing human islet amyloid polypeptide/amylin. *Eur J Endocrinol* 1995;132:487.

269. Janson J, Soeller WC, Roche PC, *et al*: Spontaneous diabetes mellitus in transgenic mice expressing human islet amyloid polypeptide. *Proc Natl Acad Sci USA* 1996;93:7283.

270. de Koning EJ, Morris ER, Hofhuis FM, *et al*: Intra- and extracellular amyloid fibrils are formed in cultured pancreatic islets of transgenic mice expressing human islet amyloid polypeptide. *Proc Natl Acad Sci USA* 1994;91:8467.

271. Westermark G, Arora MB, Fox N, *et al*: Amyloid formation in response to beta cell stress occurs *in vitro*, but not *in vivo*, in islets of transgenic mice expressing human islet amyloid polypeptide. *Mol Med* 1995;1:542.

272. Westermark G, Westermark P, Eizirik DL, *et al*: Differences in amyloid deposition in islets of transgenic mice expressing human islet amyloid polypeptide versus human islets implanted into nude mice. *Metabolism* 1999;48:448.

273. Westermark P, Eizirik DL, Pipeleers DG, *et al*: Rapid deposition of amyloid in human islets transplanted into nude mice. *Diabetologia* 1995;38:543.

274. Verchere CB, D'Alessio DA, Palmiter RD, *et al*: Islet amyloid formation associated with hyperglycemia in transgenic mice with pancreatic beta cell expression of human islet amyloid polypeptide. *Proc Natl Acad Sci USA* 1996;93:3492.

275. Westermark P, Li ZC, Westermark GT, *et al*: Effects of beta cell granule components on human islet amyloid polypeptide fibril formation. *FEBS Lett* 1996;379:203.

276. Porte Jr D, Kahn SE: Hyperproinsulinemia and amyloid in NIDDM. Clues to etiology of islet β-cell dysfunction? *Diabetes* 1989;38:1333.

277. Nishi M, Bell GI, Steiner DF: Islet amyloid polypeptide (amylin): no evidence of an abnormal precursor sequence in 25 type 2 (non-insulin-dependent) diabetic patients. *Diabetologia* 1990;33:628.

278. Sakagashira S, Sanke T, Hanabusa T, *et al*: Missense mutation of amylin gene (S20G) in Japanese NIDDM patients. *Diabetes* 1996;45:1279.

279. Hou X, Ling Z, Quartier E, *et al*: Prolonged exposure of pancreatic beta cells to raised glucose concentrations results in increased cellular content of islet amyloid polypeptide precursors. *Diabetologia* 1999;42:188.

280. Wang J, Xu J, Finnerty J, *et al*: The prohormone convertase enzyme 2 (PC2) is essential for processing of pro-islet amyloid polypeptide at the N-terminal cleavage site. *Diabetes* 2001;50:534.

281. Melato M, Antonutto G, Ferronato E: Amyloidosis of the islets of Langerhans in relation to diabetes mellitus and aging. *Beitrage zur Pathologie* 1977;160:73.

282. Westermark P, Wilander E: The influence of amyloid deposits on the islet volume in maturity onset diabetes mellitus. *Diabetologia* 1978;15:417.

283. Maloy AL, Longnecker DS, Greenberg ER: The relation of islet amyloid to the clinical type of diabetes. *Hum Pathol* 1981;12:917.

284. Lipkind G, Steiner D: Predicted structural alterations in proinsulin during its interactions with prohormone convertases. *Biochemistry* 1999;38:890.

Beta-Cell Function and Insulin Secretion

Bo Ahren

Gerald J. Taborsky, Jr.

In this chapter we shall describe the mechanisms by which the beta cells (B cells, β cells) of the islets of Langerhans of the pancreas synthesize and secrete insulin in response to changes in the metabolic state of the organism. Although insulin is made by the same peptide synthetic mechanisms as in other cells, β cells are unique in that insulin synthesis is stimulated by increases in the blood glucose level. Furthermore, β cells possess a complex set of mechanisms (Fig. 4-1) by which glucose metabolism controls membrane electrical activity, calcium uptake, and insulin release. The β cell is also remarkable in its sensitivity to a host of other plasma metabolites, hormones, and neurotransmitters that participate in the control of peripheral metabolism. The β cell integrates input from these stimuli to synthesize and secrete the amount of insulin needed to regulate plasma nutrient levels and systemic metabolic processes under a full range of physiologic conditions.

ANATOMY OF THE ISLETS OF LANGERHANS

β Cells and Other Endocrine Cells

In all mammalian species, pancreatic β cells are found in the islets of Langerhans,[1] which are discrete clusters of endocrine cells scattered throughout the pancreas but found most abundantly in the tail of the pancreas. Although both pancreatic endocrine and exocrine cells are important for fuel absorption and metabolism, their nearly universal anatomical association remains largely unexplained. The islets number from 100,000–2,500,000 per pancreas, vary in size from about 50–300 μm in diameter, and contain from hundreds to a few thousand hormone-secreting endocrine cells. A delicate connective tissue sheath separates the islet cells from the acinar cells of the surrounding exocrine pancreas. Islets receive sympathetic and parasympathetic nerves and are maintained by an arterial blood supply that branches into a rich, intraislet capillary bed. Venous efferents from smaller islets pass through neighboring pancreatic exocrine acini before emptying into the portal venous system; efferents from larger islets pass directly to the portal system. Islet hormones therefore arrive in high concentrations in the liver and parts of the exocrine pancreas before reaching peripheral tissues. Because the liver degrades and clears a large fraction of the insulin that it receives, peripheral insulin levels are considerably lower than found in the portal vein.

The islets are a densely packed collection of peptide-secreting endocrine cells, all of which are involved in metabolic regulation.

The insulin-secreting β cells are the most abundant and constitute from 70–90% of islet endocrine cells. The less numerous α cells (or A cells) secrete glucagon and make up the bulk of the remaining cells. The remaining islet cells include δ cells (or D cells), which secrete somatostatin, and F cells, which secrete pancreatic polypeptide (PP). In rodent islets, but less obviously in human islets, β cells tend to be located in a central core with α cells nearer the islet's surface along with δ and F cells. The various islet secretory cells are packed very closely together with a common, but very narrow, extracellular space that may allow hormones secreted by one cell to diffuse directly to other cells and affect their behavior in a "paracrine" manner. Further intraislet communication and coordination between islet cell types is also possible via cell-cell gap junctions, which can conduct small molecules and bioelectrical signals.

All islet cell types share the classic features of other peptide-secreting cells. The β cells are from 10–15 μm in diameter and have a prominent nucleus, rough endoplasmic reticulum (RER), and Golgi apparatus. As described in Chap. 5, these structures synthesize, package, and store the peptide hormones in numerous membrane-bound secretory granules (known as secretory vesicles), which share the cytoplasmic space with a large complement of mitochondria. Although the various islet cell types are remarkably similar in most details, the appearance of the quarter-micron-diameter (250 nm) secretory granules differs. The insulin in β-cell granules appears as electron-dense crystals surrounded by an electron-lucent halo. Glucagon in α-cell granules more nearly fills the granular space with an electron-dense spherical core. The cores of δ- and F-cell granules are spherical but much less dense in appearance.

Circulatory, Neural, and Intraislet Inputs

The islet arterial blood supply is carried through a neurovascular stalk before breaking into arterioles. The arterioles pass through the non-β-cell rim before bifurcating into fenestrated capillaries, which pass into the β-cell–rich islet interior. Morphological work[2] suggests that β cells are polarized such that afferent capillaries first pass the cell side, which is presumably enriched with various membrane receptors. After passing several β cells in this manner, the capillaries turn back toward the islet surface and pass the secretory poles of the β cells, where insulin is secreted and diffuses into the capillary. Plasma containing freshly secreted insulin is then carried to the receptor poles of α cells, and then δ cells (and F cells) as the capillaries approach the islet's surface. Glucagon

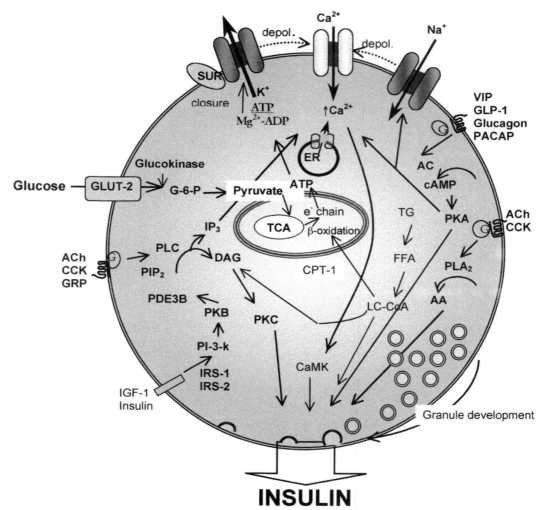

FIGURE 4-1. A simplified schematic view of signaling pathways in the β cell activated by external stimuli. All illustrated receptors are not always expressed in the same β cells. Abbreviations: AA = arachidonic acid, AC = adenylate cyclase, ACh = acetylcholine, ADP = adenosine diphosphate, ATP = adenosine trisphosphate, CaMK = calmodulin kinase, cAMP = cyclic adenosine monophosphate, CCK = cholecystokinin, CPT-1 = carnitine palmitoyl transferase-1, DAG = diacylglycerol, ER = endoplasmic reticulum, FFA = free fatty acid, G-6-P = glucose-6-phosphate, GLP-1 = glucagon-like peptide-1, GLUT-2 = glucose transporter 2, GRP = gastrin-releasing polypeptide, IGF-1 = insulin-like growth factor-1, IP$_3$ = inositol-1,4,5-trisphosphate, IRS-1 = insulin receptor substrate-1, IRS-2 = insulin receptor substrate-2, LC-CoA = long-chain coenzyme A, PACAP = pituitary adenylate cyclase–activating polypeptide, PDE3B = phosphodiesterase 3B, PI-3-K = phosphatidylinositol-3-kinase, PIP$_2$ = phosphatidyl inositol-4,5-biphosphate, PKA = protein kinase A, PKB = protein kinase B, PKC = protein kinase C, PLA$_2$ = phospholipase A$_2$, PLC = phospholipase C, SUR = sulfonylurea receptor, TCA = tricarboxylic acid cycle, TG = triglyceride pool, VIP = vasoactive intestinal polypeptide. For further details, see text.

and somatostatin (and pancreatic polypeptide) are secreted and enter the plasma stream by diffusing into superficial venules lying underneath the islet's capsule. The implication of this vascular arrangement is that β cells, which are stimulated by glucagon and inhibited by somatostatin, may respond to circulating, but not locally secreted, glucagon and somatostatin. Superficial α and δ cells, on the other hand, may respond to locally secreted insulin, which reaches them either by the intraislet capillary circulation or by diffusion (a paracrine effect).

Parasympathetic and sympathetic nerves of the autonomic nervous system also pass through the islet's neurovascular stalk. These nerves do not form classical synapses with islet cells, but do have specialized release sites as they pass near islet cells. Via these nerves, the central nervous system modulates islet hormone release using a variety of neurotransmitter receptor mechanisms; muscarinic receptors for acetylcholine (ACh) released from parasympathetic nerves can potentiate glucose-induced insulin release. Activation of α-adrenergic receptors by norepinephrine (from sympathetic nerves) and epinephrine (from the adrenal medulla) inhibits insulin secretion, while activation of β-adrenergic receptors (by the same neurohormone) stimulates insulin secretion. β cells also possess a variety of receptors for neuropeptides that may be coreleased with the classical autonomic neurotransmitters. For example, in some species galanin inhibits, and vasoactive intestinal polypeptide (VIP), pituitary adenylate cyclase–activating polypeptide (PACAP) and gastrin-releasing polypeptide (GRP) stimulate, insulin secretion (see Chap. 8). Islets are also innervated by sensory nerves, which contain the neuropeptides, substance P, and calcitonin gene-related peptide (CGRP). These sensory nerves reach the spinal cord via the splanchnic nerves.[3] Studies with the neurotoxin capsaicin, which destroys small unmyelinated sensory nerve fibers, result in a potentiation of glucose-stimulated insulin secretion in mice, suggesting that they tonically restrain insulin secretion.[4]

INTRACELLULAR CONTROL OF INSULIN SYNTHESIS AND SECRETION

Synthesis and Packaging in Secretory Granules

As in other peptide-secreting cells, β cells synthesize insulin via a complex process (see Chap. 3) that begins with transcription of the DNA insulin gene to messenger RNA (mRNA) in the cell nucleus. Glucose stimulates the transcription of both human and rodent insulin genes, as does glucagon-like peptide 1(GLP-1).[5] Some of this stimulation occurs through a cyclic AMP response element in the insulin gene promoter,[6] and some stimulation occurs through trans-activation factors,[7] such as islet duodenum homeobox-1 (IDX-1), pancreas duodenum homeobox–containing transcription factor-1 (PDX-1), and fibroblast growth factor (FGF), and signals from developmental morphogenic proteins known as hedgehogs (Hh).[7–9]

In the ribosomes of the RER, the mRNA is translated to the large peptide preproinsulin. This process is stimulated by glucose through phosphorylation of two translation factors, called eIF-2B and PHAS-1/eIF-4E-BP.[10,11] Glucose's stimulation of translation makes a significant contribution to preproinsulin synthesis.[10,12] After preproinsulin is formed, the signal sequence (necessary for inserting the peptide into the RER) is cleaved, and the resulting proinsulin is transported to the Golgi apparatus by small membrane-bound vesicles. As the Golgi apparatus concentrates and packages the proinsulin into secretory granules, converting enzymes begin to cleave proinsulin to yield insulin and C peptide. Mature secretory granules contain equimolar amounts of mature insulin and C peptide, with residual amounts of unconverted proinsulin and proinsulin intermediates. The membrane-bound granules also concentrate zinc ions, which are essential for crystallizing the insulin, as well as protons that control the activity of the converting enzymes. Secretory granules have specific membrane proteins important for their docking to the plasma membrane. In addition they contain high levels of calcium, the monoamines, dopamine, and serotonin, as well as the 36-amino-acid peptide islet amyloid polypeptide (IAPP). IAPP is a fibrillogenic peptide which is the main constituent of the amyloid seen in islets of subjects with type 2 diabetes mellitus (T2DM).[13] However, fibrils are not normally found in the secretory granules, because intragranular factors prevent fibril formation.[14]

Once formed, granules enter a large cytoplasmic granule storage pool. Only 1% of this pool is available for immediate release upon stimulation of the cell, probably because it is located immediately adjacent to the plasma membrane.[15] The release of these granules is thought to constitute the first phase of insulin secretion seen within a few minutes after stimulation with glucose. This readily releasable pool of granules is refilled from the large reserve pool, which is thought to account for the second phase of insulin secretion.[16] Granules undergo translocation from the reserve pool by

microtubules and microfilaments.[17] The fusion of the granules with the plasma membranes requires ATP, is triggered by Ca^{2+}, and shows similarities to granule-membrane fusion in neurons.[18] In the β cells, the secretory granular membrane protein synaptobrevin, and the plasma membrane proteins, syntaxin and N-ethylmaleimide–sensitive factor attachment protein-25 (SNAP-25), play major roles in this fusion. Furthermore, the granule protein, synaptotagmin, seems to be responsible for the Ca^{2+} sensitivity of exocytosis in β cells.[15,19] Older granules that are not secreted are degraded by fusion with lysosomes.

Intracellular Signals That Control Insulin Release

Once insulin is synthesized and packaged in granules, its exocytotic release is controlled by complex interactions of several signaling pathways within the β cell. This complexity allows integration of complex metabolic and physiologic information, resulting in an insulin secretory rate appropriate for regulating metabolism. Figure 4-1 classifies the major players in this regulation. Although these players will be familiar to students of other neural and secretory cells, it is safe to say that the pancreatic islet β cell is unique in the specialized way it uses these systems and in the degree to which these systems interact with each other. To a remarkable degree, this single cell is responsive to all types of neurohumoral and metabolic inputs, whereas other neurosecretory cells are generally specialized to respond to only a few inputs.

The most important function of the β cell is to respond to elevations of extracellular glucose by secreting enough insulin to restore a normal plasma glucose level. This basic pathway begins with mechanisms for glucose uptake and metabolism, which controls membrane ion fluxes and electrical activity. In turn these raise the cytoplasmic free Ca^{2+}, which controls the rate of the exocytosis of insulin. This basic glucose-controlled secretory pathway for the β cell is modulated by other regulatory factors, including nutrients, hormones, or neurotransmitters.

Once stimulated by glucose, β-cell insulin secretion can be augmented or inhibited by various neurohumoral inputs. Glucagon and other peptide hormones, as well as β-adrenergic agonists, augment insulin secretion via the cyclic AMP messenger system. Parasympathetic activation of muscarinic receptors augments secretion via the phosphoinositide messenger system. Inhibitory receptors for several neurohumoral agents such as galanin, somatostatin (Ss), and α-adrenergic agonists interact at several points in these processes. Insulin secretion is also controlled by pathways activated by insulin and IGF-1, and finally, intracellular lipolysis is of importance through the formation of lipid signals affecting exocytosis.

The following paragraphs describe these subsystems and how they respond to each other and to exogenous stimuli. After over 50 years of intense scrutiny, the β cell has only recently revealed some of these major findings. The full story will certainly be more complex and may remain confused by significant differences between the "β cells" from different species and from different transformed model β-cell lines used in the laboratory. The coverage here will of necessity be broad and pass over many secondary, albeit important, interactions and effects.

Glucose Uptake and Metabolism

The β cell's specialization for regulating blood glucose levels in the normal range (roughly 90 mg/dL or 5 mmol) begins at the first two steps. Glucose is transported into the β cell by the same insulin-insensitive facilitated transporter, GLUT-2, which is also found in the liver.[20] Although there are other glucose transporters in β cells, GLUT-2 carriers provide the high-capacity, low-affinity transport needed to nearly equilibrate glucose concentrations across the cell membrane to support the β cell's very high metabolic rate. The initial phosphorylation of glucose is by an islet-specific, low-affinity glucokinase with high capacity,[21] mutations of which are diabetogenic in certain populations of patients with maturity-onset diabetes of the young (MODY).[22] Although also present, hexokinase, which has a higher affinity for glucose, is largely inhibited. Thus, low-affinity glucokinase becomes the predominant path and effectively desensitizes β-cell glycolysis to glucose stimulation such that half-maximal and maximal levels of glycolytic metabolism, although higher than in most other cells, require much higher levels of glucose. This in effect raises the threshold for subsequent metabolic signaling to other cellular subsystems.[21] Following phosphorylation of glucose and further metabolism, pyruvate is formed that is taken up by the mitochondria for oxidation. In fact, more than 90% of glucose-derived carbons are oxidized in the mitochondria.[23] Through metabolism in the tricarboxylic acid cycle and transfer of reducing equivalents to the electron transport chain, ATP is generated. This will raise the cellular ATP:ADP ratio, which is a key mechanism for the closure of the specific K_{ATP} channels.

Membrane Ion Fluxes and Electrical Activity: K_{ATP} Channels and Ca Channels

Since it was first discovered in 1968,[24] the triggering of β-cell membrane electrical activity by glucose metabolism is now understood to be an obligate step in the stimulus-secretion coupling of glucose-induced insulin secretion. The key metabolic-ionic link is the ATP-sensitive potassium channel (K_{ATP}),[25–27] which also renders hypothalamic neurons, vascular smooth muscle, and myocardial cells sensitive to their metabolic states. The β-cell K_{ATP} channels are octamer complexes composed of four pore-forming Kir6.2 subunits, which form an inward rectifier K^+ channel comprised of 390 amino acids and four sulfonylurea receptor (SUR1) subunits.[28–30]

β-Cell K_{ATP} channels are tonically open and maintain the β-cell resting membrane potential near the potassium equilibrium potential (near −60 mV). The channels, however, have two important receptors regulated by β-cell metabolism. One receptor is the Kir6.2 subunit, which binds free ATP (or free ADP, but at tenfold lower affinity) and closes the channel, thus allowing the cell to depolarize. SUR1, the second receptor subunit, binds nucleotide diphosphates in the presence of Mg^{2+} (such as Mg-ADP) and increases channel opening, competing with the closing effect of free ATP. Thus, increasing glucose levels will convert more ADP to ATP through glycolytic and oxidative metabolism so that the opening effect of Mg-ADP is reduced to reveal the closing effect of free ATP.[31,32] The net closure of K_{ATP} channels depolarizes the β-cell membrane.

Studies in genetically engineered mice either expressing a dominant negative form of Kir6.2 in the β cells or lacking Kir6.2 have demonstrated that the K_{ATP} channels are the major determinant of the resting membrane potential in the β cells and that normal insulin secretion after glucose requires these channels. Furthermore, even though Kir6.2 knockout mice develop only mild glucose intolerance, fasting hyperglycemia is seen in aged and obese mice lacking Kir6.2.[30] Interestingly, a mutation of either the SUR1 gene or, less commonly, the Kir6.2 gene, both of which are located on chromosome 11, causes defective function of K_{ATP} channels, which is associated with the persistent hyperinsulinemic hypoglycemia of infancy.[30,33]

K_{ATP} Channels are also targets for clinically important antidiabetic compounds, sulfonylureas, because they close K_{ATP} channels by binding to the SUR1,[23,34] as do the newly developed antidiabetic agents repaglinide and nateglinide.[35,36]

The depolarization due to closing of K_{ATP} channels opens voltage-dependent calcium (Ca) channels. At a threshold level of glucose near 5 mmol, the glucose-induced membrane depolarization (to about −60mV) is sufficient to trigger the opening of voltage-dependent L-type calcium channels in the β-cell membrane. This admits extracellular Ca^{2+} into the intracellular pool of free Ca^{2+}, where it interacts directly with the insulin exocytotic machinery to fuse the insulin secretory granules to the plasma membrane and release insulin.

The opening of Ca^{2+} channels is, however, coordinated to produce rhythmic oscillations[37] of membrane potential consisting of trains of Ca^{2+} action potentials (at frequencies between 4 and 12 spikes per second) superimposed on depolarized "plateau" potentials. At low, suprathreshold levels of glucose (~6 mmol) the plateaus are brief (about 1–2 seconds long) and separated by "silent phases" lasting about 10 seconds. At levels of glucose that are half-maximal for insulin secretion, the plateaus last longer (5–10 seconds) and the silent phases are brief (about 5 seconds). At maximal levels of glucose (>15 to 20 mmol), the silent phases are abolished altogether and the cell remains depolarized and spikes persistently. The rhythmic pacing of Ca^{2+} uptake during the bursts of Ca^{2+} spikes is paralleled by oscillations of the free Ca^{2+} level with the cells that are synchronized throughout the islet by electrical coupling.[38,39] The progressive increase in the Ca spiking activity as glucose increases underlies the increase of Ca^{2+} uptake seen in Ca^{2+} flux studies. The cause of the modulation is the progressive closure of K_{ATP} channels as the glucose metabolic rate increases with the increased glucose stimulation.

One hypothesis[40] is that the spike-and-burst pattern results from two functionally distinct L-type Ca^{2+} channels (drawn as a single channel for simplicity in Fig. 4-1). The spike channel activates rapidly and is closed almost as rapidly (within tens of milliseconds) by the rapid accumulation of intracellular calcium. The plateau Ca^{2+} channel also activates rapidly to produce the persistent plateau depolarization, but closes much more slowly (in seconds) in a depolarization-dependent manner to finally terminate the plateau. Both Ca^{2+} channels appear to contribute to the Ca^{2+} uptake required for insulin secretion. Another class of β-cell K^+ channel (not shown in Fig. 4-1) is the delayed rectifier K channel, which, as for nerve action potentials, assists in repolarizing the Ca^{2+} spike.[41]

Calcium Metabolism

The calcium accumulated during the spiking plateau phase is pumped out of the cell by membrane Ca-ATPase pumps. In addition, free Ca^{2+} is taken up and stored by the cell's endoplasmic reticulum (ER), where it can be released when inositol-1,4,5-trisphosphate (IP₃) and its related compounds activate specialized Ca^{2+} channels in the membrane of the ER. By providing additional substrate for the generation of IP₃, glucose metabolism may further increase free Ca^{2+} levels. The parallel pathway increasing the formation of cyclic AMP may also be of importance for the increase in cytoplasmic Ca^{2+} after glucose activation because it has been demonstrated that cyclic AMP, through activation of protein kinase A (PKA), increases cytoplasmic Ca^{2+} by opening the voltage-dependent L-type Ca^{2+} channels.[42]

An important consequence of the complexity of the calcium metabolic machinery is slow oscillations of free Ca^{2+} level, which occur with a period of 5–10 minutes, roughly 10–20 times slower than the frequency of the bursts of electrical activity described above. The oscillations may be of glycolytic origin, but membrane ionic channels and the phosphoinositide system are likely participants as well. The oscillations are observed as slow fluctuations of the intensity of membrane electrical activity,[43] intermediary metabolism, cytoplasmic free Ca^{2+} level, and insulin secretory activity.[44] These *in vitro* observations may explain the oscillations of islet secretory activity observed *in vivo*.[45,46]

Insulin Secretion

The actual release of insulin occurs by exocytosis, a process in which the granule membrane fuses with the cell membrane. The membranes are disrupted at the point of fusion and the insulin crystal is discharged to the extracellular space, leaving the granule membrane and its proteins inserted into the cell's plasma membrane. The process of exocytosis is the rate-limiting step for physiologic insulin secretion, but its regulation is just now becoming understood. As in other secretory cells, cytoplasmic free Ca^{2+} concentration appears to be of paramount importance, yet the precise site of action and cofactors required for secretion are now only becoming known for a few model secretory systems. It is clear, however, for β cells, that several "second messenger" systems are critically important for controlling the secretory steps and for setting the sensitivity of the release sites to the prevailing free Ca^{2+} level. Furthermore, studies[47] indicate a yet to be identified signal(s) that depends on glucose metabolism that bypasses the Ca^{2+} metabolism step and allows glucose to potentiate the effects of Ca^{2+} on secretory rate.

To summarize the basic pathway for glucose-induced insulin secretion: First, glucose depolarizes β cells and triggers membrane electrical activity, which brings extracellular Ca^{2+} into the cell through voltage-gated Ca^{2+} channels. Second, glucose may generate IP_3, which mobilizes Ca^{2+} from intracellular stores in the ER. Third, glucose inhibits the pumping of Ca^{2+} from the cytoplasm back to the extracellular space. Fourth, by an unknown pathway, glucose metabolism sensitizes the secretory machinery to the prevailing cytoplasmic Ca^{2+} level, allowing insulin secretion independent of changes in the K_{ATP}-channel activity or cytoplasmic Ca^{2+} level.[48]

Calcium Messenger System

Raising cytoplasmic Ca^{2+} augments exocytosis through the activation of serine/threonine protein kinases. The mediators of this activation appear to be a family of proteins called calmodulins (CaMs). Of these, the Ca^{2+}/CaM-dependent protein kinase II (CaMK II) has been explored in most detail[49] with four isoforms found in islets.[50] Inhibition of CaMK II impairs nutrient-induced insulin secretion.[51] Ca^{2+} also activates the myosin light-chain kinase (MLCK) and inhibition of MLCK may help to impair glucose-stimulated insulin secretion.[52]

Phosphoinositide Messenger System

Glucose increases production of diacylglycerol (DAG) and inositol-1,4,5-trisphosphate (IP_3) perhaps by providing additional phospholipid substrate or by activating membrane phospholipases. DAG and IP_3 are also formed by hydrolysis of phosphatidylinositol-biphosphate (PIP_2) through the action of phospholipase C (PLC), which is of particular importance for eliciting insulin secre-

tion after activation of muscarinic or cholecystokinin (CCK) receptors.[53] Several PLC isoforms have been identified in β cells (PLC-β_1, PLC-β, PLC-γ, and PLC-δ) and PLC activation is triggered by guanosine triphosphate-binding proteins. As in other cell types, DAG remains membrane-bound and activates protein kinase C (PKC). This family of enzymes acts as serine/threonine kinases to phosphorylate various β-cell proteins. Several different PKC isoenzymes may exist in the β cells, including the conventional forms that are Ca^{2+}-responsive (PKC-α, PKC-β, and PKC-γ), forms that are Ca^{2+}-unresponsive but DAG-dependent (PKC-δ, PKC-ε, PKC-η, and PKC-θ), and forms that are both Ca^{2+}-unresponsive and DAG-independent (PKC-ξ, PKC-λ, and PKC-μ).[49,54] When PKC isoenzymes are activated, they translocate to the plasma membrane and phosphorylate β-cell proteins, which in turn modulate ion channels and augment cell metabolism, which affects insulin secretion. PKC is involved in the responses to activation of muscarinic receptors.[55]

IP_3, which is also formed through PKC activation, on the other hand, is soluble and is released into the cytoplasm, unlike DAG, where it interacts with the endoplasmic reticulum to release stored calcium. Various isomers and breakdown products of IP_3, as well as other polyphosphoinositides such as inositol hexakisphosphate (IP_6),[56] have been described in a growing list of phospholipid metabolites that may modulate insulin secretion.

The main role of IP_3 is in transducing input to the β cells of secretagogues that activate PLC, like acetycholine[57] or CCK.[58] This enhances glucose-induced insulin secretion, but does not stimulate release in the absence of glucose. In addition to mobilizing ER Ca^{2+}, muscarinic activation activates a membrane Na^+ channel,[59] which may explain its depolarizing effects on β cells.[42] Also, the peptide secretagogues GLP-1 and PACAP have been shown to increase the β-cell uptake of Na^+.[60–62] The increased cytosolic Na^+ may increase the uptake of Ca^{2+}, thereby increasing cytosolic Ca^{2+}. The importance of Na^+-induced insulin secretion for these secretagogues is illustrated by findings that removal of extracellular Na^+ reduces their insulin secretory ability.[60,62]

Cyclic AMP Messenger System

Activation of adenylate cyclase by various peptidergic (glucagon, GLP-1, PACAP, VIP) and β-adrenergic stimuli converts ATP to cyclic AMP. Each of these stimuli has a receptor linked to adenylate cyclase by guanine-binding proteins (G proteins). cAMP in turn binds to the regulatory subunit of PKA, activating its catalytic subunit, which phosphorylates proteins. There are two different forms of PKA. One form has a regulatory subunit that is cytosolic, whereas the other type interacts with proteins in the plasma membrane and in the secretory granule. PKA phosphorylates GLUT-2, K_{ATP} channels, and L-type Ca^{2+} channels, all of which are involved in insulin secretion.[63–65] However, activation of PKA is not sufficient to elicit insulin secretion after stimulation with glucose, but rather appears to potentiate the effect of other pathways. cAMP also can directly activate the exocytosis process since it augments insulin secretion in the absence of raised cytoplasmic Ca^{2+}.[42]

Intracellular cAMP is also regulated by its phosphodiesterases (PDEs), which degrade the cyclic nucleotide. Three different isoforms of PDE (PDE1, PDE2, and PDE3) are expressed in islets. The most important of these is PDE3, which in turn exists in two different subtypes, PDE3A and PDE3B.[66] PDE3 is activated by protein kinase B (PKB), which in turn is activated by phosphoinositide-3-kinase (PI-3-K). Both these enzymes are expressed in the β cells.[67,68] The inhibitory actions of IGF-1 on insulin secretion may be mediated by activation of PDE through PI-3-K and PKB and the subsequent reduction of intracellular levels of cAMP.

Arachidonic Acid Messenger System

Glucose, muscarinic activation, and CCK have been shown to activate phospholipase A_2 (PLA$_2$), which hydrolyzes plasma membrane phospholipids, resulting in formation of arachidonic acid (AA).[69–71] At least two different isozymes of PLA$_2$ are expressed in the β cells: a Ca^{2+}-dependent and a Ca^{2+}-independent form, which seem to be of importance for insulin secretion under different conditions. Thus, activation by the muscarinic agonist stimulates the Ca^{2+}-dependent PLA$_2$, whereas activation by CCK stimulates both the Ca^{2+}-dependent and Ca^{2+}-independent forms.[71] The formed AA directly increases cytoplasmic calcium and results in the formation of prostaglandins and eicosanoids, which in turn can affect insulin secretion. Therefore, the AA messenger system may also be of importance for insulin secretion, although its relative contribution to the insulin responses to muscarinic activation and CCK is probably less than the PLC pathway.

Lipid Messenger System

Lipid-derived signals are also important for insulin secretion. These signals are long-chain acyl CoA (LC-CoA) derived from triglycerides stored in the β cells,[72,73] and they augment the fusion of granules with the plasma membrane during exocytosis through activation of PKC.[73] Neurohormonal agents may therefore regulate the exocytosis of insulin through activating or inhibiting LC-CoA formation. One target for these agents is the hormone-sensitive lipase (HSL) which is expressed in the β cells.[74] HSL is activated by PKA; therefore, agents increasing cAMP might augment insulin secretion through HSL-mediated formation of LC-CoA, as has been proposed for GLP-1.[75]

Insulin Messenger System

The insulin receptor is also expressed in the β cells.[76] Since previous data showed that exogenous insulin inhibits insulin secretion, it was thought that the β cells exhibit autocrine inhibition like some other secreting cells. However, the generation of β-cell–specific insulin-receptor–deleted mice have challenged this view. These mice develop a defective insulin response to glucose and progressive impairment of glucose tolerance.[77] Although the relevance of these findings for the physiological regulation of insulin secretion remains to be established, these mouse studies indicate that insulin's action on its β-cell receptors is important for maintaining normal β-cell function.[78]

Inhibitory Receptors

The β cell bears receptors for a number of physiologically important inhibitory neurohumoral signals that are superimposed on the stimulatory pathways described. α-Adrenergic stimulation does not appear to act via adenylate cyclase[79] as in many other systems but has clear effects that hyperpolarize β cells and inhibit insulin secretion, apparently at the release site.[80] The hyperpolarization may be due to the activation of low-conductance G protein–linked potassium channels[81] that may also be activated by galanin.[82] Although both galanin[83] and somatostatin[84] activate K$_{ATP}$ channels, it is not clear that these effects are critical since galanin[85] and somatostatin[86] also act directly on the secretory machinery to block insulin release. The adipocyte hormone leptin has also been shown to directly restrain insulin secretion.[87] This effect is induced by opening K$_{ATP}$ channels, activation of PDE to breakdown cAMP, or activation of transcription factors.[87–89]

EXTRACELLULAR CONTROL OF INSULIN SECRETION

Basal Insulin Secretion

Basal insulin secretion is defined *in vivo* as that which occurs in the absence of any exogenous stimulation of insulin release. The basal insulin level is usually measured in the morning after an overnight fast because by then the postabsorptive stimulation of insulin release is clearly over and the circulating levels of metabolic and gut hormone secretagogues are related to endogenous, rather than exogenous, signals. Even though the plasma glucose levels after an overnight fast are low (80–100 mg/dL), they maintain the basal insulin secretion *in vivo*,[90] perhaps by potentiating the insulin response to the low levels of other secretagogues. Recent data suggest that the elevated levels of plasma free fatty acids seen during fasting also help maintain basal insulin secretion.[91,92] The definition of basal insulin secretion *in vitro* is somewhat arbitrary because it is dependent on the insulin secretagogues present in the buffer. These secretagogues are mandatory; *in vitro* insulin secretion stops in their absence.

Although many investigators assume that basal insulin secretion is constant, others have provided evidence for periodic oscillations in the basal insulin level with periods of 9–14 minutes.[45,93] The first report of large oscillations in peripheral plasma insulin was from studies in rhesus monkeys;[94] smaller oscillations were later found in humans.[95] Oscillations in plasma levels of secretagogues are not the stimulus for the periodicity of basal insulin secretion; the same phenomenon can be demonstrated *in vitro* when secretagogue levels are held constant.[96] The synchronization of the pancreatic β cell apparently involves intrapancreatic ganglia and nerves, because the oscillations can be reduced by either nicotinic antagonists or neurotoxins.[97,98] These oscillations in plasma insulin are perturbed in T2DM,[99,100] and can be partially restored by inhibiting the β cell for a period.[101]

Secretagogues and Inhibitors of Insulin Secretion

Metabolites

Glucose

Although many agents stimulate insulin release, glucose is the most critical for three reasons (Table 4-1). First, insulin is the major controller of carbohydrate metabolism. For example, during fasting the low levels of glucose (80–100 mg/dL) reduce the plasma insulin level to between 5 and 10 μU/mL, allowing glycogenolysis, proteolysis, and lipolysis to release stored fuels into the circulation. Conversely, during feeding, the high level of glucose (100–200 mg/dL) increases the plasma insulin level to 30–150 μU/mL, which not only inhibits the release of stored fuels but also increases the tissue uptake and storage of incoming nutrients. Second, physiologic levels of glucose stimulate insulin release through most of its physiologic range. Thus, changes of plasma glucose level must be taken into account when interpreting insulin secretion. Even the low levels of glucose present during fasting maintain insulin secretion. Third, because glucose plays a central role in β-cell metabolism, glucose can influence the insulin

TABLE 4-1. Major Secretagogues and Inhibitors of Insulin Release

Secretagogue/Inhibitor	Type	Circulating Concentrations	Effect	Physiologic State
Glucose	Metabolite	5–20 mmol	↑↑↑	Carbohydrate feeding
Amino acids	Metabolite	0.1–10 mmol	↑↑	Protein feeding
Free fatty acids	Metabolite	100–1000 μmol	0	Fasting
GIP	GI hormone	10^1–10^2 pmol	↑↑	Carbohydrate or fat meal
CCK	GI hormone	1–10^1 pmol	↑	Protein meal (?)
GLP-1(7–36)-NH$_2$	GI hormone	10^1–10^2 pmol	↑↑	Carbohydrate meal
Epinephrine	Stress hormone	0.2–20 nmol	↓↓	Stress
Neurotransmitters		Synaptic concentrations*		
Acetylcholine	Parasympathetic neurotransmitter	Unknown	↑↑	Feeding
VIP	Parasympathetic neurotransmitter	Unknown	↑	Feeding (?)
Norepinephrine	Sympathetic neurotransmitter	Unknown	↓	Stress
Galanin	Sympathetic neurotransmitter	Unknown	↓↓	Stress (?)

*Neurotransmitters are released locally, achieving concentrations at the β cell that are not currently measurable.

responses to other secretagogues and to subsequent stimulation. Part of the potentiating effects of glucose may be mediated by its effect of increasing insulin synthesis. Thus glucose has a permissive as well as a regulatory role for insulin secretion.

Amino Acids

Most amino acids can stimulate insulin release, but their potencies vary with species, ambient glucose level, and amino acid type. The mixed amino acids in a pure protein meal stimulate insulin release, but less potently than a pure carbohydrate meal. The insulin released during protein meals promotes the uptake and storage of amino acids as muscle protein and slows muscle proteolysis, which supplies gluconeogenic amino acids during fasting. Amino acids stimulate glucagon release, which counteracts the hypoglycemic action of the secreted insulin.[102]

Fats

Early studies suggested that acute increases of triglycerides, free fatty acids (FFAs), and ketones had negligible effects on insulin release in humans. The carbohydrate and protein components of the mixed meal help to stimulate insulin release, which suppresses both lipolysis and FFA mobilization, favoring net storage of ingested triglycerides for the next period of fasting. However, ingested fats slow the absorption of other nutrients that directly stimulate the β cell, such as protein and carbohydrate. Thus mixed meals of varying fat content are not ideal for assessing β-cell function.

More recent studies have revealed both stimulatory and inhibitory effects of FFAs and islet triglycerides on insulin secretion.[73] One stimulatory effect of FFAs is to maintain basal insulin secretion during starvation, when plasma glucose levels are very low.[92] Another stimulatory effect of plasma FFAs is the partial mediation of the increased basal insulin secretion seen in obesity and other insulin-resistant states.[91,103] In contrast, several in vitro[104–106] and in vivo studies[107] suggest that chronic, pathologic elevations of plasma FFAs may contribute to impaired insulin secretion, a phenomenon called lipotoxicity.[108] Certain studies have focused on the accumulation of islet triglycerides as critical for lipotoxicity.[108] This lipotoxicity can extend beyond the inhibition of insulin secretion to include inhibition of insulin biosynthesis[104,109] and the death of susceptible β cells,[106,108] perhaps mediated by islet triglyceride–dependent generation of nitric oxide (NO),[110] a mechanism thought to be involved in the death of islet β cells in type 1 diabetes mellitus (T1DM).

Hormones

Gastrointestinal Hormones

A variety of gastrointestinal hormones are released during meals to coordinate gastric emptying, gastrointestinal motility, exocrine pancreatic secretion, and gallbladder contraction. These gastrointestinal hormones also potentiate substrate-induced insulin release. The hormones responsible for the extra insulin released by the oral versus intravenous administration of glucose have been termed incretins. Of the many gut hormones evaluated as candidate incretins, the three detailed below have received the strongest support (see Chap. 6).

Gastric Inhibitory Polypeptide

Gastric inhibitory polypeptide (GIP) is a 43-amino-acid polypeptide isolated from endocrine cells of the duodenum and jejunum with the ability to inhibit gastric acid secretion. GIP is one of the few gut hormones released by carbohydrate ingestion. This release (1) is triggered by intraluminal carbohydrate, not circulating glucose, (2) proportional to the oral glucose load,[111] and (3) dependent on the absorption of glucose across the intestinal mucosa.[111] These findings suggest that the release of GIP is triggered by the activation of a glucose sensor within the intestine. Many gut hormones, including GIP, are released by fat and protein ingestion. The effectiveness of GIP to stimulate insulin release is dependent on the plasma glucose level (it has thus been renamed glucose-dependent insulinotropic polypeptide [GIP]). Therefore, fat-stimulated GIP release causes little rise of plasma insulin, whereas carbohydrate-stimulated GIP release causes significant insulin release, more than that produced by equivalent levels of glucose alone. Infusions of the human form of GIP that reproduce GIP levels during a mixed meal clearly stimulate insulin release.[112] Antibodies that bind and neutralize GIP attenuate, but do not abolish, the insulin response to oral glucose, both supporting a physiologic role for GIP as an incretin and indicating that other factors also participate in the incretin effect. A physiologic incretin effect of GIP is also suggested by studies showing that GIP antagonists attenuate meal-induced insulin release in rats[113] and that mice with gene deletion of the GIP receptor have impaired insulin responses to oral glucose.[114]

Cholecystokinin

Cholecystokinin (CCK) is a 33-amino-acid peptide isolated from the duodenum and proximal jejunum with the ability to contract the gallbladder. A much shorter but equally potent form, CCK-8, is found in the nerves of both gut and brain. Both CCKs can stimulate the secretion of digestive enzymes and metabolic hormones such as insulin, as well as inhibit food intake and delay gastric emptying.[115] These actions coordinate the flow and processing of nutrients. CCK is released in response to the ingestion of fat and protein, but not carbohydrates.[116] Evidence in favor of an incretin action of CCK includes the presence of CCK$_A$ receptors on islet β cells and the finding that the levels of CCK achieved during mixed meals appear sufficient to potentiate amino acid–stimulated insulin release. However, potent antagonists of the CCK$_A$ receptor have little effect upon meal-stimulated insulin release in humans, calling into question a major role for CCK as an incretin.

GLP-1[7-36 Amide]

L cells of the distal small intestine release a peptide encoded by the preproglucagon gene. This peptide is a truncated, amidated form of glucagon-like peptide 1, GLP-1[7-36 amide].[117] The plasma concentration of this peptide increases during mixed and carbohydrate[118] meals in humans. Although the quantities released are less than those of GIP, GLP-1[7-36 amide] is such a potent glucose-sensitive potentiator of insulin secretion[119] that it is currently thought to be a major incretin. Direct experimental support for this concept comes from studies showing that GLP-1 antagonists or immunoneutralization of GLP-1 impairs oral glucose tolerance in primates.[120] Likewise, transgenic male mice with a knockout of the GLP-1 receptor have both impaired insulin secretion to oral glucose and impaired glucose tolerance.[121] In addition to the incretin effect, evidence is accumulating that GLP-1 helps maintain the normal levels of insulin content[122] and β-cell mass,[123] which are important for insulin responses to other nonincretin stimuli. These latter observations have prompted studies of GLP-1 or analogs for treatment of T2DM.[124,125]

Gut Neuropeptides

Although the polypeptides discussed above are gastrointestinal hormones, there are many others in the gastrointestinal tract that are localized to nerves, not endocrine cells. Examples are vasoactive intestinal polypeptide (VIP) and the related peptide, pituitary adenylate cyclase–activating peptide (PACAP). Because part of the incretin effect may be mediated by the complex neural activation of the gastrointestinal tract that accompanies meals, it is possible that some of these gut neuropeptides may also serve an incretin function. Indeed, transgenic mice with a knockout of the PACAP 1 receptor have impaired insulin responses to gastric glucose.[126] Further, recent work suggests that nerves in the myenteric plexus of the adjacent duodenum innervate intrapancreatic ganglia,[127,128] raising the possibility that the intrapancreatic ganglia may be part of the enteric nervous system of the gut, and as such may be activated during feeding.

Stress Hormones

Epinephrine

The sympathetic neurohormone epinephrine is secreted from the adrenal medulla in response to stress. Such stresses include physical disturbances of homeostasis such as hypoglycemia, hypotension, and hypoxia, as well as the accompanying or preceding emotional responses of fear and/or anxiety. The epinephrine released during stress activates an α$_2$-adrenergic inhibitory receptor as well as a β-adrenergic stimulatory receptor on the β cell. This

simultaneous activation results in little net change of basal insulin release, yet substantial inhibition of the acute insulin response to glucose (see Chap. 8).

Others

The pituitary hormones ACTH, growth hormone, TSH, prolactin, and vasopressin and the adrenal and thyroid hormones cortisol and thyroxin, are also released under stress. These hormones are not major, acute modulators of insulin release, although growth hormone and cortisol have long-term direct or indirect effects on insulin secretion in the hours or days following a major stressful event.[129]

Neurotransmitters

Parasympathetic

Acetylcholine (ACh) is the classic postganglionic neurotransmitter of parasympathetic nerves, including those that innervate the pancreas. ACh stimulates insulin release via the M3 subtype of the muscarinic receptor[130–132] that can be blocked by atropine. Activation of the parasympathetic nerves of the pancreas can be produced (1) experimentally by electrical activation of the vagus nerve, (2) physiologically by both the cephalic and intestinal phases of feeding, and (3) pathophysiologically by hypoglycemia. The action of ACh to stimulate insulin release is glucose dependent,[133] so that during hypoglycemic stress the vagal activation produces little stimulation of insulin release. In contrast, during carbohydrate feeding, equivalent vagal activation would be expected to produce significant neurally induced stimulation of insulin secretion. Old evidence, primarily in rats,[134] and newer evidence in humans[135] suggest that pancreatic parasympathetic nerves mediate the cephalic phase of insulin release. This phase occurs before the absorption of ingested glucose. More recent data suggest that pancreatic parasympathetic nerves may also be important for the insulin response during absorption,[136,137] contrary to the traditional view that ingested metabolites are the primary stimuli for absorptive insulin secretion.

Parasympathetic nerves in the pancreas may also release neuropeptides such as VIP and PACAP. Both have been found in postganglionic parasympathetic-like fibers innervating pancreatic islets, and VIP has been measured in the pancreatic venous effluent during electrical activation of the vagus.[138] Infusion of exogenous VIP[138] stimulates glucagon and insulin secretion as well as increasing pancreatic blood flow and the flow of pancreatic exocrine juice.

Sympathetic

Norepinephrine is the classic postganglionic neurotransmitter for the sympathetic neurons that innervate the pancreas. Norepinephrine, like epinephrine, is a dual agonist activating both α$_2$-adrenergic inhibitory receptors and β-adrenergic stimulatory receptors on the β cell. The net effect of norepinephrine on insulin secretion *in vivo* is usually inhibition of glucose-stimulated insulin release with little change of basal insulin release. Intrapancreatic norepinephrine can be released experimentally by electrical activation of sympathetic nerves and pathophysiologically by hypoglycemic stress.[139]

Sympathetic nerves in the pancreas may also release other neurotransmitters such as neuropeptide Y (NPY) and galanin. NPY fibers innervate the islets of many species, whereas the sympathetic galaninergic innervation of the islet[140] seems restricted to the dog.[141] In the dog, but not the primate, galanin is released into the pancreatic venous blood during electrical activation of sympathetic nerves,[142,143] and infusion of exogenous galanin impairs both basal and stimulated insulin release.[140,144] NPY has minor effects on insulin secretion but may stimulate glucagon secretion.[145]

Intraislet Peptides

Older evidence suggests an interaction between the different islet cell types. For example, the δ-cell peptide somatostatin may be a paracrine controller of glucagon release.[146] However, evidence of its role as a paracrine controller of insulin release is less well established. Likewise, insulin appears to be a local endocrine controller of glucagon release[147] via the portal circulation from the β-cell core to the α-cell mantle of the normal islet.[148] However, glucagon does not appear to be a physiologic modulator of insulin release within the islet. β cells make and release islet amyloid polypeptide (IAPP) in addition to insulin. Although the physiologic role of IAPP remains unclear, a pathophysiologic role for this peptide has been suggested in type 2 diabetes,[13,149] since amyloid fibrils are cytotoxic to β cells[150] (see Chap. 21).

Effects of Glucose on Insulin Secretion

Although glucose clearly stimulates insulin release, the simplicity of that statement belies the complexity of glucose's direct effects on insulin secretion and the dominant role that glucose plays in controlling the β-cell response to other secretagogues, both of which are detailed below.

First- and Second-Phase Insulin Release

The magnitude of the insulin response to glucose is related not only to the absolute level of glucose, but also to the rate of change of glucose level. Thus an abrupt increase of glucose level elicits a rapid and transient burst of insulin secretion, called the first or acute phase of insulin response, that subsides within 10 minutes (Fig. 4-2). The second-phase response begins when glucose levels increase slowly and progressively for up to 4 hours of glucose exposure. The separation of these two phases of insulin release has been demonstrated most clearly by exposing the isolated rat pancreas to a large stepwise increase of glucose, but it can also be demonstrated in humans during hyperglycemic glucose clamp studies.

The first-phase insulin response to glucose is not prevented by blockade of insulin synthesis *in vitro*, nor is its magnitude dependent on the prestimulus glucose level *in vivo*. This acute release of insulin may be due to release of insulin granules that are directly adjacent or "marginated" to the β-cell membrane. In contrast, the magnitude and timing of the second-phase insulin response are dependent upon the prestimulus glucose level *in vivo*. The second-phase response is probably due to the release of more internal insulin granules as well as some that are not preformed, because at least part of this second-phase response is dependent on the synthesis of new insulin. This newly synthesized insulin is preferentially released during the period of continuous glucose stimulation, a phenomenon observed during stimulation of many other granular secretory processes.

Although these two distinct phases of insulin release do occur in humans following intravenous glucose administration, they are not readily apparent during a carbohydrate meal. During a carbohydrate meal, absorption of glucose into the circulation is not fast enough to produce a rapid increase in the plasma glucose level. However, the rate sensitivity that characterizes the first-phase insulin response to glucose is probably physiologically important even during less abrupt changes of plasma glucose. For example, feedback-controlled insulin infusion studies suggest that a rapid response of the β cell to an increasing plasma glucose level is necessary to prevent excessive hyperglycemia during a carbohydrate meal, as well as to prevent the development of hypoglycemia following the meal[151] due to the late and excessive release of insulin and its relatively long duration of action. Recent studies have reemphasized the importance of the early insulin response to meals for the preservation of normal glucose tolerance. Thus prevention of this early insulin response in healthy humans results in glucose intolerance,[152] and impairment of this insulin response is associated with glucose intolerance both in individuals at high risk[153] and in those individuals who already have[154] T2DM. The addition of a cephalic phase of insulin response improves the glucose intolerance seen during intragastric installation of glucose in healthy subjects,[155] and infusion of rapid-acting insulin early during the meal corrects the glucose intolerance seen in type 2 diabetes.[156]

Potentiation

Glucose not only stimulates insulin secretion directly, but also influences the magnitude of the insulin response to other, nonglucose, secretagogues. Thus the acute insulin response to gut hormones, amino acids, and other secretagogues is larger when the ambient glucose level is higher (Fig. 4-3). Although the intracellular signals that subserve potentiation are not clear, it is likely that constant stimulation by glucose increases not only the synthesis of new insulin, but also the transport of insulin granules toward the cell membrane, making them available for acute release by

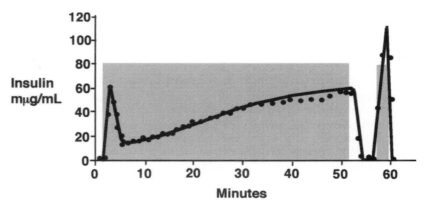

FIGURE 4-2. First- and second-phase response to glucose. Immediately after the stepwise increase of perfusate glucose concentration (300 mg/dL; **first shaded area**), there is a transient burst of insulin release (first phase), which can persist for 2–5 minutes in vitro. Thereafter, there is a slow but progressive increase of insulin secretion (second phase), which continues for the duration of the original exposure to the high glucose level (5–52 minutes). *Priming*: Prior exposure (2–52 minutes) of the pancreas to glucose (300 mg/dL, **first shaded area**) produces a first-phase insulin response (57–59 minutes) to an equivalent stepwise increase of glucose (300 mg/dL, **second shaded area**) that is significantly enhanced. *(Reprinted with permission from Grodsky GM, Landahl H, Curry D: The Structure and Metabolism of the Pancreatic Islets. Pergamon:1970.)*

Insulin mμg/mL

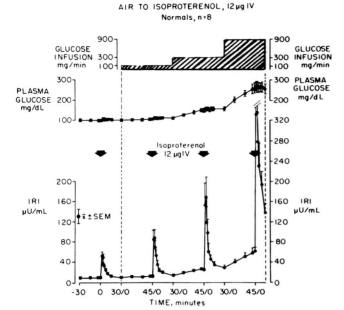

FIGURE 4-3. *Potentiation*: The effect of increasing the ambient glucose level on the magnitude of acute insulin response (AIR) to isoproterenol. *(Reprinted with permission from Halter, et al.[157])*

secretagogues other than glucose. This potentiating effect has not only been demonstrated *in vitro* using pharmacologic amounts of nonglucose secretagogues, but it is also an important physiologic mechanism for the control of insulin release *in vivo*. For example, the amino acids absorbed during a mixed protein/carbohydrate meal stimulate more insulin secretion because the glucose level is elevated by the digestion and absorption of the carbohydrate. Further, in research settings, the measurement of glucose's ability to potentiate non-glucose-induced secretion has provided clear evidence of defects in β-cell function in T2DM[157] (see Chap. 21).

Priming

In addition to directly stimulating and potentiating insulin secretion, glucose also has a priming effect on the β cell. That is, previous exposure to high levels of glucose can enhance the insulin response to subsequent stimulation even though the glucose levels have returned to normal (Fig. 4-2). Thus the β cell's acute response to glucose or other secretagogues is conditioned by its "memory" of prior glucose stimulation. The amount of subsequent priming is increased with the magnitude and duration of the original glucose exposure; it is decreased by lengthening the time between the end of that exposure and subsequent stimulation.[158] The priming effect is not dependent upon the original insulin secretion itself, because blockade of that insulin release still permits priming of subsequent insulin responses.[158] The priming effect is apparently dependent on intracellular glucose metabolism, because some glycolytic intermediates can also produce priming. Because prior exposure to glucose also increases the subsequent acute insulin response to arginine in humans, the priming effect probably increases the slope of glycemic potentiation. Priming may also account for the dramatic differences in the insulin responsiveness between fasted and recently fed individuals, and probably contributes to the effects of antecedent diet on the insulin response to an oral glucose tolerance test (see below).

Desensitization

Chronic exposure of the β cells to high glucose levels ultimately leads to a decrease in the sensitivity of the β cells to stimulation by glucose. *In vitro* this desensitization appears after 4–8 hours of exposure, when insulin secretion is decreased to 25% of maximal.[159] Desensitization may be due to a downregulation of the glycolytic enzymes within the β cell, but this is not the only mechanism, because chronic exposure of β cells to nonglucose stimuli also produces desensitization. Likewise, the reduced insulin secretion is not due to a significant reduction of total insulin content or to a decrease in the rate of insulin synthesis.[159] Desensitization may, however, be related to depletion of insulin from a very responsive subset of β cells, leaving insulin to be secreted from progressively fewer responsive β cells. Indeed studies suggest the presence of sets of β cells within the islet that have different thresholds and sensitivities for stimulation by glucose.[160] There is also evidence of early hypersensitivity of the β cell to glucose stimulation, perhaps mediated by increases of glucokinase activity. Such increased glucokinase activity may produce overstimulation of β cells despite modest hyperglycemia, and therefore result in a later loss of glucose responsiveness.

Desensitization can also occur *in vivo* after exposure to either 2 days of marked hyperglycemia in normal rats or 6 weeks of minimal hyperglycemia in partially pancreatectomized rats.[161] After such exposure, the first-phase insulin response to glucose in the subsequently isolated and perfused pancreas is nearly abolished. Restoration of euglycemia in partially pancreatectomized rats lessens the impairment of the first-phase insulin response.[162] Even short periods of extremely low glucose *in vitro* can reverse the suppressive effects of long periods of hyperglycemia *in vivo* on the acute insulin response to glucose. Interestingly, such *in vitro* exposure does not reverse the suppressive effect of hyperglycemia on the second phase of the insulin response. Those data suggest that the chronic hyperglycemia present in T2DM may exacerbate the defect in glucose-stimulated insulin secretion.[163] It is interesting that many type 2 diabetic patients retain some of their second-phase insulin response to glucose; in contrast, this response is almost completely lost in most animal models with chronic hyperglycemia (see Chap. 21).

In Vivo Measures of Insulin Secretion and β-Cell Function

When determining the function of the pancreatic β cell, it is critical to relate the amount of insulin secretion to the amount of glucose stimulation that the β cell receives. For example, if the plasma insulin level has increased appropriately in response to an increase in plasma glucose, then the efficiency or function of the β cell has not really changed. Alternatively, if insulin secretion has increased more than expected for the increase of ambient glucose level, then β-cell function has increased. Several *in vivo* measurements, such as fasting plasma glucose level, oral and intravenous glucose tolerance tests, and fasting insulin level, have been used to suggest changes of β-cell function. However, these measures either do not adequately take into account the insulin level at which the glucose level is measured or, conversely, the ambient glucose level at which the insulin level is measured. Although they may reveal some information either about the amount of insulin released or its effect on plasma glucose, they may not provide reliable information about how efficiently the pancreatic β cell reacts to glucose as a stimulus—that is, β-cell function. Other measures or calculated parameters, such as the acute insulin response (AIR) to glucose, the slope of glycemic potentiation, AIR_{max}, and PG_{50} (discussed later), do relate the insulin responses to the ambient glucose level and therefore provide better insight into the function or efficiency of the pancreatic β cell. The use and limitation of each index is discussed below.

Fasting Glucose Levels

The concentration of glucose in the plasma of fasting individuals is a very insensitive indicator of β-cell function. For example, loss of two-thirds of the β cells induced by partial pancreatectomy produces no significant change of the fasting glucose level[164,165] (Table 4-2). Conversely, the increase of β-cell function that occurs in obesity does *not* lower fasting glucose levels. However, if the β-cell dysfunction is severe (total pancreatectomy or autoimmune

or chemical destruction of most β cells), then fasting hyperglycemia will result. Thus the fasting glucose level reflects only impairments of β-cell function that are severe enough to prevent the increase of insulin secretion that usually compensates for losses of β-cell mass or defects in insulin action.

Oral Glucose Tolerance Test

The insulin released by the ingestion of carbohydrate aids in the clearance of the absorbed glucose from plasma. Thus in the oral glucose tolerance test (OGTT), plasma glucose levels at specified times after a standard oral glucose load (usually 75 g) are used to assess the adequacy of insulin secretion. However, the relationship between the insulin and glucose levels is time-dependent, because the insulin released early in the test influences the glucose values later in the test. Thus only the early part of the OGTT can be used

TABLE 4-2. Indices of Insulin Secretion and β-Cell Function in Normal and Pathophysiologic States

	Fasting Plasma Glucose (mg/dL)	K_G (%/min)	Insulin Sensitivity $\left(\dfrac{\times 10^{-4}\mathrm{min}^{-1}}{\mu U/mL}\right)$	Fasting Plasma Insulin (μU/mL)	AIR_G (μU/mL)	AIR_{NG}[†] (μU/mL)	Slope of Glycemic Potentiation (μU/mg)	AIR_{max} (μU/mL)	PG_{50} (mg/dL)	Ref.
■ INSULIN RESISTANCE										
Experimental										
Control (human)	98 ± 2	2.0 ± 0.2	4.6 ± 0.5	11 ± 1	80 ± 23	63 ± 8	1.24 ± 0.22	301 ± 39	178 ± 9	175
Nicotinic acid	101 ± 2	1.5 ± 0.1*	1.7 ± 0.3*	23 ± 3*	121 ± 23*	115 ± 24*	1.45 ± 0.29	384 ± 53*	172 ± 6	
Naturally occurring										
Control (human)	98 ± 2	1.8 ± 0.2	5.0 ± 0.8	10 ± 1	2.1 ± 0.8‡	32 ± 5	0.77 ± 0.15	—	—	208
Obesity	96 ± 2	1.4 ± 0.2	2.8 ± 0.7*	27 ± 3*	8.8 ± 1.9*‡	52 ± 9	1.59 ± 0.13*	—	—	
■ INSULIN SENSITIVITY										
Naturally occurring										
Control (elderly man)	95 ± 4	1.4 ± 0.1	2.4 ± 0.3	9 ± 1	56 ± 11	63 ± 12	0.91 ± 0.17	254 ± 41	174 ± 11	214
Exercise-trained (elderly)	97 ± 3	1.4 ± 0.2	3.3 ± 0.3*	7 ± 1*	38 ± 8*	50 ± 8	0.73 ± 0.15*	186 ± 30*	158 ± 9	
■ β-CELL LOSS										
Experimental										
Control (dog)	112 ± 4	—	0.34 ± 0.10§	11 ± 2	42 ± 9	23 ± 3	0.34 ± 0.05	113 ± 13	249 ± 30	164
65% Pancreatectomy	115 ± 5	—	0.21 ± 0.02§	11 ± 1	32 ± 5	13 ± 2*	0.04 ± 0.01*	28 ± 7*	170 ± 20*	
Control (rat)	103 ± 2	—	—	61 ± 4	121 ± 13	95 ± 10	3.9 ± 0.8	—	—	162
90% Pancreatectomy	119 ± 3*	—	—	59 ± 5	12 ± 2*	43 ± 9*	0.2 ± 0.2*	—	—	
■ β-CELL DAMAGE										
Experimental										
Control (baboon)	84 ± 4	2.0 ± 0.2	4.1 ± 1.5	27 ± 3	88 ± 24	68 ± 19	1.8 ± 0.5	—	—	
Streptozocin	85 ± 4	1.8 ± 0.3	2.7 ± 0.4*	36 ± 8	61 ± 26	67 ± 15	0.1 ± 0.1*	—	—	190
■ β-CELL DYSFUNCTION										
Experimental										
Control (human)	89 ± 2	1.9 ± 0.2	7.8 ± 1.1	7 ± 1	38 ± 7	34 ± 4	65 ± 13	146 ± 26	157 ± 11	239
Somatostatin analog	102 ± 5*	1.0 ± 0.1*	6.6 ± 1.2	2 ± 1*	9 ± 4*	41 ± 8	32 ± 7*	>152 ± 32	>200 ± 14*	
■ β-CELL LOSS, DAMAGE, DYSFUNCTION										
Naturally occurring										
Control (human)	92 ± 2	1.7 ± 0.6	5.3 ± 0.6	11 ± 1	53 ± 16	46 ± 4	0.98 ± 0.21	256 ± 35	—	219
HLA-siblings of type I diabetics	91 ± 2	1.6 ± 0.1	3.0 ± 0.2*	11 ± 1	45 ± 7	42 ± 4	0.91 ± 0.08	210 ± 20*	—	
Control (human)	93 ± 1	—	—	14 ± 3	—	57 ± 13	1.1 ± 0.2	450 ± 93	192 ± 20	176
Type II diabetes	232 ± 25*	—	—	15 ± 2	—	35 ± 8	0.2 ± 0.05*	83 ± 4*		234
± 8										

* Significantly different from control.

—, Measurement not performed in cited study.

[†] NG, nonglucose stimuli.

[‡] Units $= \dfrac{\mu U \cdot min \cdot dL}{mL \cdot mg}$

[§] Units of insulin sensitivity $= \dfrac{mL \cdot Kg^{-1} \cdot min^{-1}}{\mu U/mL}$

to estimate β-cell function. One such estimate is the insulinogenic index, which is the early increment of plasma insulin divided by the early increment of plasma glucose. This index provides a crude measure of β-cell function useful in epidemiologic studies.[166] However, low insulinogenic values do not necessarily reflect just β-cell defects, since part of the early insulin release is in turn stimulated by activation of the parasympathetic nervous system and the release of gastrointestinal hormones that occurs during digestion. Impairment of gastrointestinal function can therefore influence both the insulinogenic index and the OGTT by reducing gastrointestinal hormone release and by reducing the rate of glucose absorption. Further, the rate of clearance of glucose from plasma is dependent not only on the amount of insulin secreted, but also on the sensitivity of liver and muscle to insulin. Both stress and obesity can produce insulin resistance, resulting in impaired glucose tolerance in the face of a normal or even an enhanced insulin response. Thus the ability of other factors besides insulin secretion to influence the plasma glucose levels during the oral glucose tolerance test makes it difficult, if not impossible, to assess the adequacy of β-cell function. Only when the impairment of glucose tolerance is severe, as in diabetes, can the OGTT be used to infer an impairment of the pancreatic β cell's ability to recognize glucose.[167]

Intravenous Glucose Tolerance Test

The rapid intravenous injection of a bolus of glucose (usually 5–25 g) results in a rapid peak of the plasma glucose level (between 2 and 4 minutes) followed by a slower, nearly exponential fall in the plasma glucose level. The rate of the fall during the first 10 minutes of the test is largely influenced by the mixing and distribution of glucose, but the natural logarithm of the rate of the fall between 10 and 30 minutes can be used to define the glucose disappearance constant, K_G, which is related to glucose uptake and is therefore an index of glucose tolerance.

The intravenous glucose tolerance test (IVGTT) avoids some of the previously mentioned problems with the OGTT. Because the glucose is administered intravenously, abnormalities in glucose absorption and gastrointestinal function do not affect plasma glucose levels. Further, activation of the parasympathetic nervous system and release of gastrointestinal hormones do not occur during IV injection of glucose, but only during its oral ingestion. One serious problem remains, however. Changes in the sensitivity of peripheral tissues to the action of secreted insulin do influence the plasma glucose profile during the IVGTT. In fact, an estimate of insulin sensitivity can be obtained from the plasma glucose profile, providing that one adequately accounts for the timing and magnitude of the insulin response.[168] In addition, the rate of glucose fall is dependent on the mass-action effect of glucose to accelerate its own disposal, a factor that may change in pathophysiologic states. Thus, K_G is a combined measure influenced not only by the timing and magnitude of the insulin response to the bolus injection of glucose, but also the sensitivity of tissues to the effects of both glucose and insulin to accelerate glucose uptake. When K_G is 1.7 or greater, neither insulin secretion nor insulin action is likely to be markedly impaired. If K_G is between 1.0 and 1.7, then insulin secretion, insulin action, or both are impaired. Only when K_G is less than 1.0 is a reduction of β-cell function always indicated; however, it is usually already evidenced by fasting hyperglycemia (Table 4-2).

Fasting Insulin Levels

The plasma insulin level in a normal weight, overnight-fasted individual is approximately 5–15 μU/mL. Insulin action has a clear effect on this measure of insulin release. The fasting insulin level can be low (for example, 3–5 μU/mL) in well-trained, lean athletes[169] who are very sensitive to insulin; it can be high (15–40 μU/mL) in obese subjects who are insulin-resistant (Table 4-2). The fasting plasma glucose level is also a major determinant of fasting insulin levels. For example, fasting insulin levels decrease progressively during 8 days of starvation, despite the insulin resistance associated with starvation, because the plasma glucose levels decrease progressively. In contrast, β-cell mass is usually not a determinant of the fasting insulin level. For example, partial pancreatectomy does not lead to a significant decrease in the fasting insulin level.[164,165] Likewise, streptozocin can produce significant β-cell damage without lowering the fasting insulin level.[170] Apparently the remaining β cells increase their basal secretory rate to compensate. Moreover, in type 2 diabetes and even in some type 1 diabetic patients, fasting insulin levels can be within the normal range, reflecting adequate basal insulin secretion. However, these "normal" fasting insulin levels present in the diabetic state do not take into account the marked differences in the fasting glucose level between diabetic and normal individuals.[157,171] When the fasting insulin levels are compared at the matched hyperglycemic levels of diabetes, it becomes apparent that diabetic patients have a major impairment of β-cell function.[157,171] Thus fasting insulin levels reflect changes in insulin sensitivity and in the fasting plasma glucose level, but do not usually reflect reductions in β-cell mass or β-cell function. Some insight into β-cell function can be derived from the combination of fasting insulin and glucose values when interpreted in the context of insulin sensitivity.[172]

First-Phase Insulin Response to Glucose

The acute or first-phase insulin response to glucose is a large and transient increase of the plasma insulin level. The acute response can be elicited by either an intravenous bolus of glucose like that used for the IVGTT or the rapid rise of glucose that occurs at the start of a hyperglycemic clamp.[173] Even though glucose levels remain elevated during the hyperglycemic clamp, insulin levels fall, reaching a nadir at 10 minutes, which defines the end of the first phase.[174] The magnitude of this acute insulin response (AIR) to glucose, unlike most other insulin responses, is *independent* of the prestimulus glucose level *in vivo*. This feature allows comparison of insulin responses without the need to experimentally match the basal glucose levels between groups. For example, the β-cell dysfunction present in type 2 diabetes is reflected by the absence of the AIR to glucose (see Chap. 21) despite the presence of fasting hyperglycemia. Less severe β-cell loss or dysfunction that does not produce fasting hyperglycemia, such as two-thirds pancreatectomy or low-dose streptozocin, results in a transient reduction of the AIR to glucose that usually resolves despite continuing β-cell dysfunction.[164,170] Conversely, changes in insulin sensitivity are usually reflected by changes in the AIR to glucose. Obesity[168] and the accompanying insulin resistance[175] are associated with an enhanced AIR to glucose. In summary, the magnitude of the AIR to glucose is not determined by the prestimulus plasma glucose levels. The changes of the AIR to glucose usually reflect changes in insulin sensitivity and can reflect early reductions in β-cell mass and β-cell function.

Second-Phase Insulin Response to Glucose

Sustained hyperglycemia elicits a second phase of insulin secretion that is dependent on both the glucose level and the duration of the hyperglycemia. Thus quantitation of this second-phase insulin response requires a fixed glucose level like that achieved during the hyperglycemic clamp technique. The second-phase insulin response is usually measured from the nadir following termination of the first phase of the insulin response. During the second-phase response, plasma insulin levels increase linearly with time for at least 2 hours.[174] The magnitude of the second-phase insulin response is also influenced by the prestimulus glucose level, like many other insulin responses, and therefore is less useful than the first-phase response in comparing β-cell function between groups with differing fasting glucose levels.

Acute Insulin Response to Nonglucose Stimuli

The magnitude of AIR to nonglucose stimuli such as amino acids, neurotransmitters, and gut hormones is dependent on the prestimulus glucose level. As the glucose level is raised from 100 to 250 mg/dL, the AIR increases in an almost linear fashion (Figs. 4-3 and 4-4). The slope of the straight line relating the magnitude of AIR to the ambient plasma glucose level at which it was measured is defined as the *slope of glycemic potentiation*. As the plasma glucose level is increased above 250 mg/dL, the relationship between AIR and the plasma glucose level is no longer linear, exhibiting a progressively decreasing slope as the glucose levels approach 450 mg/dL. Above 450 mg/dL, there is usually no further increase in AIR. This maximal acute insulin response (AIR_{max}) is a critical parameter for characterizing this curve and thus β-cell function (see below). Because a standard Michaelis-Menten equation does not fit this curve, one cannot calculate the analogous

value of K_m. However, an alternative parameter, the glucose level giving a half-maximal response (PG_{50}), provides an estimate of the β-cell sensitivity to glucose (see below).

Slope of Glycemic Potentiation

The slope of glycemic potentiation has been used as an index of β-cell function. However, a decrease in slope could be due to either of two causes: a decrease in the overall capacity of the pancreas to secrete insulin, or a decrease in the sensitivity of the individual β cells to respond to the potentiating effects of glucose. For example, partial pancreatectomy, which by definition decreases overall β cell mass and thus the maximal capacity of the pancreas to secrete insulin, also decreases the slope of glycemic potentiation, despite evidence that the glucose sensitivity of the remaining β cells is increased, not decreased.[164] Conversely, treatment with an insulin inhibitory analog of somatostatin, octreotide (SMS-201,995), which decreases the sensitivity of the β cell to glucose, markedly reduces the slope of potentiation despite evidence that the maximal capacity of the β cell to secrete insulin is not decreased. The important point is that although the slope of glycemic potentiation can be a useful measure of β-cell function, it is a combined measure that is influenced by both changes in insulin secretory capacity and by changes in sensitivity of the β cell to the potentiating effects of glucose. To determine which of these two factors is responsible for the changes in slope, one must complete the dose–response curve and from it calculate the parameters AIR_{max} and PG_{50}.

AIR_{max}

The ability of glucose to potentiate the acute insulin response to nonglucose stimuli is limited. In normal humans it is maximal at a glucose level of approximately 450 mg/dL (Fig. 4-4). This maximal acute insulin response (AIR_{max}) is a measure of the insulin secretory capacity of the pancreas. AIR_{max} is a very sensitive indicator of β-cell loss, damage, or dysfunction. Thus, AIR_{max} is markedly reduced in type 2 diabetic patients[176] and even in nonhyperglycemic animals with two-thirds pancreatectomy (Table 4-2).[164] Conversely, AIR_{max} is increased, but to a smaller extent, in states of increased β-cell function such as experimentally induced insulin resistance.[175]

PG_{50}

β-Cell sensitivity to the potentiating effects of glucose can be estimated by the parameter PG_{50}, which is calculated from the dose–response curve relating AIR to nonglucose stimuli to the plasma glucose level. This dose–response curve must include the maximal acute insulin response to a nonglucose stimulus, because PG_{50} is defined as the ambient glucose level at which the half-maximal AIR response occurs (Fig. 4-4). Although PG_{50}, as opposed to the slope of glycemic potentiation, is an index of the sensitivity of the individual β cells to the potentiating effects of glucose, PG_{50} and glucose sensitivity are inversely related. Thus, if the calculated PG_{50} increases, then the sensitivity of the β cells to the potentiating effects of glucose has decreased. Further, because the calculation of this parameter, as opposed to slope of glycemic potentiation, involves normalization to the AIR_{max}, PG_{50} provides an index of sensitivity that is independent of changes in the overall capacity of the pancreas to secrete insulin. For example, partial pancreatectomy, which markedly reduces β-cell mass and thus AIR_{max}, decreases PG_{50},[164] reflecting an actual increase in the sensitivity of the remaining β cells to the potentiating effects of glucose. Conversely, treatment with a somatostatin analog that does not decrease AIR_{max} produces a significant increase of PG_{50}, indicating

FIGURE 4-4. Relationship between magnitude of acute insulin response (AIR) to arginine and the prestimulus glucose level in normal human subjects, illustrating calculation of the slope of glycemic potentiation, AIR_{max}, and PG_{50}. *(Reprinted with permission from Ward, et al.[176])*

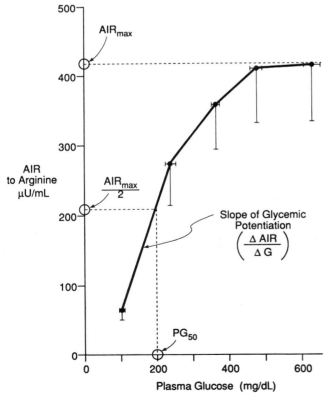

a marked decrease in the sensitivity of the β cell to the potentiating defects of glucose. Finally, type 2 diabetic patients who have a marked reduction in AIR_{max}, due presumably to a combination of β-cell loss and β-cell dysfunction, have a normal PG_{50}, suggesting that the residual functioning β cells are normally sensitive to the potentiating effects of glucose.[176]

Proinsulin : Insulin Ratio

In the normally functioning β cell, the vast majority (>95%) of proinsulin is converted to insulin and C peptide before release. However, in certain states this conversion is less complete, resulting in both greater pancreatic content and increased circulating levels of proinsulin relative to insulin. In practice, insulin is usually measured with radioimmunoassays using antibodies that cross-react with proinsulin and its degradation intermediates. Thus, immunoreactive insulin (IRI) can be a measure of the combination of insulin and proinsulin-like molecules; selective antibodies or special separation techniques are required to measure proinsulin by itself in order to calculate a PI : IRI ratio. This PI : IRI ratio is the percentage of all molecules containing insulin that are comprised of true proinsulin. The PI : IRI in extracts of the pancreas is less than 5%. Presumably, most of the proinsulin and insulin are already in releasable β-cell granules, because the PI:IRI ratio in plasma after acute stimulation of the β cell is similar.[177] In theory, agents that produce other types of acute stimulation or inhibition of the β cell should not change the ratio significantly, because they would be expected to influence the secretion of proinsulin and insulin equally. This concept ignores, however, the plasma clearance of proinsulin, which is markedly slower than that of insulin. This differential clearance accounts for a higher PI : IRI (15%) obtained from the plasma of fasting human subjects.[177] Thus, one should not compare fasting to stimulated PI : IRI ratios to infer a change of the β-cell function.

The effect of drugs and physiologic or pathophysiologic states on the fasting PI : IRI in plasma has been used to infer changes of the intracellular processing of insulin and, therefore, of β-cell function; decreased PI : IRI is interpreted as more efficient β-cell

function, whereas increased PI : IRI is interpreted as impaired β-cell function. This interpretation is supported by several pieces of experimental evidence. First, drugs that impair β-cell function, such as glucocorticoids[171,177] and streptozocin,[178] increase the plasma PI : IRI. Second, type 2 diabetic patients who have other evidence of β-cell impairment have increased PI : IRI.[177] Increases of PI : IRI do not appear to be secondary to the increased secretory demand on a normal β cell because partial pancreatectomy, obesity, and drug-induced insulin resistance, all of which increase secretory demand, do not increase the PI : IRI ratio. However, increased demand on an already impaired β cell may increase the PI : IRI ratio simply by accelerating proinsulin release before full processing can occur.[179] Thus an increased PI : IRI has been used to suggest impaired β-cell function in individuals at high risk for development of type 2 diabetes.[180]

Adaptive Changes of Insulin Secretion

β-Cell Adaptation to Insulin Resistance

Introduction

Resistance to the action of secreted insulin leads to a compensatory increase of insulin release. When β cells are functioning normally, the extra insulin released is usually sufficient to overcome the resistance to insulin's action and to prevent marked fasting hyperglycemia and glucose intolerance. The normal relationship between insulin secretion and insulin action is hyperbolic[181,182] (Fig. 4-5), implying that their product is a constant called the disposition index.[181] Changes in insulin secretion that fully compensate for changes in insulin resistance result in movement along this hyperbolic line and maintenance of glucose tolerance. Therefore, this hyperbolic function has been called an isotolerance line.[182] Only when the insulin resistance is extreme (as in congenital receptor loss with acanthosis nigricans) or when the capacity of the β cell to secrete insulin is severely impaired (as in type 2 diabetes) does insulin resistance result in fasting hyperglycemia. More modest reductions in insulin secretory capacity

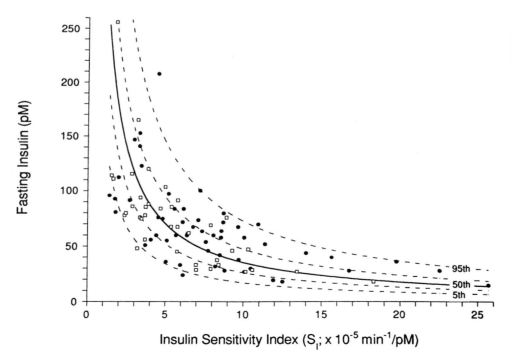

FIGURE 4-5. Hyperbolic relationship between the fasting plasma insulin level and the insulin sensitivity index in normal human subjects. *(Reprinted with permission from Kahn, et al.[182])*

result in glucose intolerance without fasting hyperglycemia, a characteristic of groups at high risk for progression to type 2 diabetes. However, in most individuals insulin resistance is accompanied by an increase in several indices of insulin secretion, particularly the fasting plasma insulin level, and is therefore rarely accompanied by fasting hyperglycemia.

Drug-Induced Insulin Resistance

Certain drugs and hormones such as growth hormone, glucocorticoids, and nicotinic acid[183] can produce a rapid and reversible insulin resistance which is accompanied by a compensatory increase of insulin secretion. However, growth hormone and corticosteroids have direct inhibitory effects on the β cell that prevent complete compensation and thus produce mild hyperglycemia. In contrast, nicotinic acid has minimal direct effects on the β cell and markedly reduces insulin action (Table 4-2).[175] In humans, 2 weeks of treatment with nicotinic acid doubles the fasting insulin level with no change of the fasting plasma glucose level, and nearly doubles the acute insulin response to glucose and nonglucose secretagogues. The slope of glucose potentiation increases slightly as does AIR_{max}, with no change of PG_{50} or PI:IRI. Thus, the β cells appear to increase their secretion of insulin by increasing their overall secretory capacity. Perhaps the higher and more prolonged glucose levels during meals, suggested by glucose intolerance, may mediate this increase of AIR_{max}.

Gene-Induced Insulin Resistance

Certain genetic knockouts of the insulin receptor, its signaling molecules, or the insulin-sensitive glucose transporter (GLUT-4) cause insulin resistance and hyperinsulinemia. For example, knocking out the insulin receptor in the liver produces hepatic insulin resistance and hyperinsulinemia, the latter due to both decreased hepatic insulin clearance and increased insulin secretion.[184] Knocking out insulin receptor substrate-1 (IRS-1) produces muscle insulin resistance,[185,186] hyperinsulinemia,[187] and a β-cell hyperplasia[188,186] that is also seen in obesity. Knocking out insulin receptor substrate-2 (IRS-2) produces liver insulin resistance[188] and a transient hyperinsulinemia. A heterozygous, global knockout of GLUT-4 causes insulin resistance and hyperinsulinemia.[189] Thus the genetic disruption of certain insulin signaling pathways causes insulin resistance resulting in a compensatory hyperinsulinemia. Indeed, earlier studies of drug-induced insulin resistance had demonstrated this compensatory hyperinsulinemia.[175]

Surprisingly, genetic disruption of the insulin signaling pathway selectively in muscle[190–192] does not cause hyperinsulinemia despite the current view that muscle is quantitatively the most important tissue for insulin-mediated glucose disposal.

Finally, in some knockout mice with insulin resistance, the hyperinsulinemia is transient or does not occur at all because of defects in β-cell function. Thus the transient hyperinsulinemia of IRS-2 knockout mice is followed by diabetes[188] because β-cell hyperplasia, normally seen in response to sustained insulin resistance, is mediated through IRS-2.[193] Thus knockout mice with defects in both insulin action and β-cell function develop diabetes,[187,188] whereas those with defects in insulin action alone develop compensatory β-cell hyperplasia and hyperinsulinemia.

Obesity-Related Insulin Resistance

Experimental Obesity Lesions of the ventromedial hypothalamus (VMH) produce obesity and insulin resistance in rats. Their fasting glucose levels are normal, and their fasting insulin levels and AIR are elevated. Although the more sophisticated tests of islet function have not been performed in VMH-lesioned animals, the AIR to nonglucose secretagogues is also elevated, suggesting that the slope of glycemic potentiation might be increased.

Although the origin of this hyperinsulinemia in VMH-lesioned animals has not been definitively established, three observations suggest that increased parasympathetic tone to the pancreas contributes to this hyperinsulinemia. First, the rise of plasma insulin level immediately following the actual lesioning is rapid enough to be neurally mediated. Second, this acute increase of insulin can be reversed by vagotomy. Third, autotransplantation of the pancreas, which severs extrinsic pancreatic nerves, also lowers the plasma insulin level. It is interesting, however, that part of the hypersecretion persists even when the pancreas is isolated and perfused in vitro.[194] This residual hypersecretion can be reversed by atropine, suggesting that intrinsic cholinergic stimulation of insulin secretion is also increased.[195] There is also evidence for decreased sympathetic tone to the pancreas in VMH-lesioned animals,[196] which should enhance insulin secretion. Recent studies suggest that increased parasympathetic activity can decrease pancreatic sympathetic tone.[197]

Certain strains of mice and rats develop obesity by inheritance of a recessive gene. In *ob/ob* mice there is a defect in the coding for an adipocyte protein,[198] leptin, that has satiety effects in *ob/ob* and wild-type but not *db/db* mice.[199] Zucker (*fa/fa*) rats and other obese rats overexpress the *ob* protein leptin,[200] but like *db/db* mice, are resistant to its action because of a defect in the leptin receptor. These mice and rats are also insulin resistant. In the *fa/fa* rats, fasting glucose levels are near normal, but fasting insulin levels and AIR to secretagogues are markedly exaggerated. Although the mechanism for the hyperinsulinemia has not been established, increased vagal tone has been suggested: The animals are hyperresponsive to vagal stimulation and vagotomy partially decreases their hyperinsulinemia.[201] Zucker fatty (*fa/fa*) rats have decreased pancreatic sympathetic tone,[202] as do the VMH-lesioned rats. This decreased pancreatic sympathetic tone may contribute to their hyperinsulinemia.

Obesity can also be induced by high-energy diets in approximately one-half of outbred Sprague Dawley rats; the other half are resistant to this diet-induced obesity (DIO). These DIO rats have increased carcass fat,[203] presumed insulin resistance, and hyperinsulinemia.[203] Rats with DIO have decreased pancreatic sympathetic tone,[203,204] as do the VMH-lesioned and Zucker fatty rats. This decreased sympathetic tone may contribute to their hyperinsulinemia. The role of pancreatic parasympathetic tone in the hyperinsulinemia of DIO has not been examined.

Both *fa/fa* and VMH-lesioned rats eventually develop enlarged islets, either as a response to chronic parasympathetic stimulation or as a response to the chronic need for increased insulin secretion secondary to their chronic insulin resistance. This hypertrophy may result in increased insulin secretory capacity and thus increased AIR_{max}.

Naturally Occurring Obesity Human obesity is also characterized by insulin resistance.[205] The fasting glucose level is normal in the vast majority of obese subjects, but the fasting insulin levels are usually elevated in proportion to the amount of excess body fat and the degree of insulin resistance[206] (see Chaps. 21 and 22 and Table 4-2). Drugs such as thiazolidinediones, which reduce insulin resistance, reduce this basal hyperinsulinemia.[207] The insulin responses to acute secretagogues and the slope of glycemic potentiation are increased in obese subjects,[208] but the PI:IRI is unchanged (see Fig. 4-6 and Table 4-2).[209] Cross-sectional data obtained from human subjects of varying degrees of obesity[182] suggest that AIR_{max} is also increased, consistent with the enlarged islets found during autopsy of obese humans.

Although the mechanism of hyperinsulinemia in human obesity is still being debated, most believe it to be secondary to increased insulin secretion. Such increased secretion may be due to the increased ratio of pancreatic parasympathetic to sympathetic tone discussed above for the rodent models of obesity. Other potential causes include glucose intolerance that can accompany insulin resistance. These prolonged elevations of plasma glucose after meals may prime the β cells, producing an increase in their sensitivity to the potentiating effects of glucose. There is also evidence that plasma FFAs are elevated in the obese subjects and they contribute to the hyperinsulinemia observed in this state.[91,103] Finally, another potential cause of hyperinsulinemia is related not to insulin secretion, but to the clearance of insulin: In obese humans, the insulin resistance is associated with reduced removal of insulin from plasma.[206,210,211]

Just as weight gain produces insulin resistance, both long-term weight loss and exercise increase insulin sensitivity. Exercise increases the amount of glucose uptake at a given insulin level, resulting in an increase of whole-body measures of insulin sensitivity. This increased insulin sensitivity persists for a few days after the exercise, but is lost after 2 weeks of relative inactivity.[212] As a result of this increased sensitivity to insulin's action on glucose disposal and a decrease of the fasting glucose level, insulin secretion decreases.[169,212] In animals, the decrease of insulin secretion is accompanied by a decrease of proinsulin and glucokinase mRNA, suggesting a decrease in islet glucose metabolism and insulin synthesis.[213] In well-trained humans, fasting plasma insulin levels can be very low (3–5 μU/mL), as is the AIR to glucose[169] or nonglucose secretagogues. As little as a week of exercise training can decrease insulin secretion in the elderly, without any change of weight or body composition. Long-term exercise training in the elderly produces a decrease of AIR_{max} with no change in PG_{50},[214] suggesting that the reduction of insulin secretion in response to exercise may be due to a reduction of insulin secretory capacity.

Adaptation to Partial β-Cell Loss or Dysfunction

Experimental β-Cell Loss or Dysfunction

Partial Pancreatectomy One can remove up to 80% of the pancreas and yet not produce the fasting hyperglycemia characteristic of diabetes. However, 80% suppression of insulin with an insulin-selective analogue of somatostatin does produce marked hyperglycemia.[215] The combined data imply that after pancreatectomy, the remaining β cells increase their secretion of insulin to compensate for the β-cell loss, whereas during somatostatin analogue infusion, all β cells are inhibited. Indeed, studies demonstrate that two-thirds pancreatectomy in dogs produced no reduction of the fasting insulin level or PI:IRI and only a small reduction of AIR_G.[164] The AIR_{max} was, however, markedly reduced in proportion to the β-cell loss (Fig. 4-7).[164] Interestingly, PG_{50} appeared to be decreased,[164] suggesting that sensitivity of the remaining β cells to the potentiating effects of glucose was enhanced, perhaps accounting for the maintenance of near-normal basal insulin and glucose level. Studies of islets isolated from rats several weeks after 60% pancreatectomy demonstrate the suspected increase in the sensitivity of the remaining β cells to glucose. Although fasting hyperglycemia is

FIGURE 4-7. **A**. Effect of two-thirds pancreatectomy (**px**) on the slope of glycemic potentiation and AIR_{max} in dogs. **B**. Effect of two-thirds pancreatectomy on PG_{50}, an index of β-cell sensitivity to the potentiating effect of glucose. Note that the data in A have been normalized to their respective maximal responses and replotted in B to illustrate the leftward shift in the dose–response curves. (**Solid line**, animals before px; **dashed line**, animals 1 and 6 weeks after px.) *(Reprinted with permission from Ward, et al.[164])*

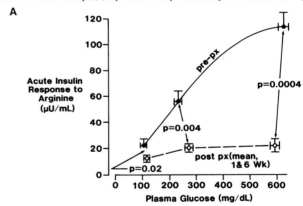

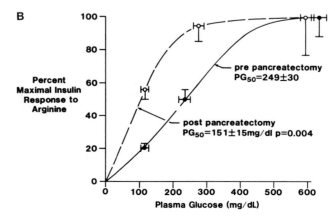

FIGURE 4-6. Effect of obesity on the slope of glycemic potentiation. *(Reprinted with permission from Beard, et al.[208])*

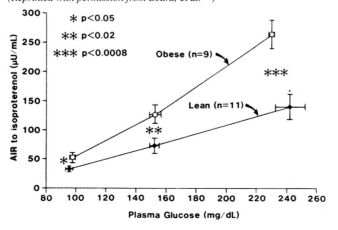

not required for this increased sensitivity to occur, the mechanism still may involve stimulation of the residual β cells by abnormally elevated glucose levels following meals.

A series of partial pancreatectomy studies in young rats suggests another mechanism for compensatory insulin secretion: regrowth of islets. A 90% pancreatectomy resulted in a tripling of the pancreatic remnant weight and insulin content over the next 2 months.[165] However, the importance of this mechanism of compensation in adult animals remains to be established.

β-Cell Toxins   β-Cell toxins such as alloxan and streptozocin have been used extensively to produce animal models of diabetes. The amount of β-cell damage is dose and age dependent. When streptozocin is given to neonatal rats, it produces severe transient hyperglycemia that evolves into a mild persistent hyperglycemia. The pancreata of these animals seem insensitive to the acute stimulatory effects of glucose *in vitro*.[216] The β cells can mount a small insulin response to arginine, but it is maximal at low levels of glucose.[216] Thus the dose–response curve is attenuated and shifted to the left, demonstrating a decrease of insulin secretory capacity and suggesting an increase in the sensitivity of the remaining β cells to the potentiating effects of glucose, similar to that seen in partially pancreatectomized animals.

Low doses of streptozocin given to baboons do not increase fasting plasma glucose, decrease fasting plasma insulin,[170] or increase PI : IRI.[178] However, K_G, AIR to glucose and arginine, and the slope of glycemic potentiation all decrease initially (Table 4-2).[170] Two months later, however, most indices return toward normal with the exception of the slope of glycemic potentiation, which remains markedly impaired (Fig. 4-8).[170] Thus the reduced

FIGURE 4-8. Effect of subdiabetogenic doses of streptozocin (STZ) on the slope of glycemic potentiation in baboons. Stage 1 (—), normal animals before STZ; stage 2 (– –), animals 1 week after STZ; stage 3 (- - - -), animals 8 weeks after STZ. *(Reprinted with permission from McCulloch, et al.[170])*

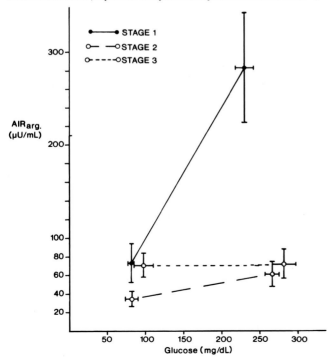

slope of glycemic potentiation may be an indicator of persistent β-cell damage.[170]

Naturally Occurring β-Cell Loss or Dysfunction

Subclinical Type 1 Diabetes   The risk of developing type 1 diabetes is 0.1–0.3% in the general population but 10–15% among first-degree relatives of type 1 diabetic individuals. The risk is 20–30% in HLA-identical siblings of type 1 diabetic patients and 30–40% in monozygotic twins of a person with type 1 diabetes.[217] In addition to the genetic factors that increase the risk of developing type 1 diabetes, there are other factors, such as environmental ones, that increase the risk.

Many of those predisposed to type 1 diabetes have islet dysfunction years before presentation of clinical diabetes, suggesting that the autoimmune process has either reversibly impaired or even destroyed a significant percentage of β cells (see Chap. 20). This islet dysfunction is manifested by a reduced AIR to glucose,[218] and a relative reduction in the slope of glycemic potentiation and AIR_{max}.[219] Certain studies suggest that the β-cell destruction can be progressive not only because of continued autoimmune attack on the remaining β cells, but also because of the increasing demand placed on the dwindling number of β cells. This concept has led to attempts to arrest or delay the development of type 1 diabetes by treatment of high-risk subjects either with immune suppressants or with agents that rest the β cell.[220] There are major therapeutic trials in progress to prevent or delay development of type 1 diabetes in high-risk individuals.[221] To identify those at high risk for development of this disease, most workers have focused on the detection of autoantibodies generated by antigens released from destroyed β cells. The combination of the standard islet cell antibody[222] with autoantibodies against glutamic acid decarboxylase (GAD-65)[223] and a newer islet cell antibody (ICA 512) improves the prediction of risk[224] since it increases the association with a markedly decreased AIR_G.[224] (see Chap. 20).

Type 1 Diabetes   In type 1 diabetes, the β-cell damage is so extensive that there are few β cells left to compensate. The compensation, if present, shows up in some type 1 diabetic patients as fasting plasma insulin or C-peptide levels that are within the normal range; in others, these values are low despite the marked stimulation by fasting hyperglycemia. In most patients, the endogenous insulin and C-peptide responses to secretagogues are low.

Some type 1 diabetic patients go into remission, a so-called "honeymoon" period, usually within a few months of the institution of insulin treatment and the resultant improvement in glycemic control. During this honeymoon phase, the requirement for exogenous insulin decreases and C-peptide levels usually rise, indicating a resurgence of endogenous insulin secretion from the residual β cells. The mechanism responsible for this improvement in insulin secretion is unknown. One theory is that chronic severe hyperglycemia overdrives the residual β cells and desensitizes or exhausts them. Then, treatment with exogenous insulin lowers the plasma glucose level, reducing the drive and allowing the residual β cells to recover and to regain partial function. Unfortunately, the honeymoon period is usually transient, perhaps because of continuing autoimmune damage of the residual β-cell population.

Type 2 Diabetes   The pathophysiology of the hyperglycemia and the compensated insulin secretion of T2DM is described in detail in Chap. 21. Therefore, only a brief outline will be given here. Near-total β-cell loss, a prominent feature of type 1 diabetes, is not a major feature of type 2 diabetes. Morphometric studies suggest that type 2 diabetic patients have lost at most 50% of their β cells. Because a 50% β-cell loss in experimental animals does not produce the fasting hyperglycemia seen in type 2 diabetes, additional factors, such as a dysfunction of the remaining β cells or concomitant insulin resistance, must contribute. Part of the β-cell dysfunction, particularly in the late stages of type 2 diabetes, may be due to the formation of the islet amyloid[13,149] via its inhibitory and eventually cytotoxic effect on β cells.[150]

In animals with selective impairment of insulin secretion, the resulting hyperglycemia is the dominant factor that maintains the fasting insulin and acute insulin responses to nonglucose secretagogues in the normal range.[215] The same is true in patients with T2DM. For example, when the glucose levels of type 2 diabetics is lowered to those of normal individuals, the basal insulin level and the acute insulin responses to nonglucose stimuli become clearly abnormal.[158] Indices of β-cell function that are independent of plasma glucose level or that account for the effect of hyperglycemia also reveal a marked impairment of insulin secretion: PI : IRI is increased, AIR to glucose is absent, and the slope of glycemic potentiation and AIR_{max} are both markedly reduced; PG_{50} is normal.[176,177] Thus there is a major reduction in the capacity of type 2 diabetic patients to secrete insulin despite normal sensitivity of the β cells to the potentiating effects of glucose.

Controversy exists regarding the primacy of the contribution of defects in insulin sensitivity versus insulin secretion to the development of T2DM. Although both defects are present, type 2 diabetes rarely occurs without impaired insulin secretion, and studies of first-degree relatives of type 2 diabetic patients report β-cell dysfunction as an early lesion in this disease.[225] Further, careful studies in groups at high risk for the development of T2DM reveal that they have an impairment of insulin secretion relative to the amount of their insulin resistance.[153,226–231] Many investigators believe that subjects with mild defects in insulin secretion do not present with clinical type 2 diabetes until they become sufficiently insulin resistant. In Western societies a common form of insulin resistance occurs in late middle age associated with increased abdominal obesity. This insulin resistance is thought to increase the demand for insulin secretion to the point where the defective β cell is unable to compensate.[182,232–235] This attractive model of type 2 diabetes pathogenesis was confirmed earlier in primates with combinations of β-cell toxins and agents causing insulin resistance,[170] and more recently in mice with a gene knockout which impairs both insulin secretion and action.[187,188,193]

CONCLUSIONS

In vivo, pancreatic β cells adjust their output of insulin to compensate for changes in the sensitivity of tissues to insulin or for changes in β-cell number or function. Both the defect that elicits the compensatory response, and the compensatory response of the β cells themselves, can be reflected in indices of insulin secretion and β-cell function (Table 4-2). However, two generalizations are worthy of emphasis. First, the compensatory insulin response to insulin resistance is best reflected in the increase of the fasting insulin level. The usual accompanying glucose intolerance suggests that the compensation is not complete, but rather just sufficient to prevent fasting hyperglycemia. Second, the compensatory insulin response to partial β-cell loss or dysfunction usually normalizes

the fasting insulin level, excluding its use as an index of β-cell loss or dysfunction. The slope of glycemic potentiation and AIR_{max} are, however, decreased in approximate proportion to the degree of β-cell loss or dysfunction, thus providing clear evidence of a defect.

The important implication of this last conclusion relates to the detection of latent diabetes in susceptible individuals. It seems likely that those measures of islet dysfunction that either take into account the ambient glucose level (slope of glycemic potentiation, PG_{50}, and AIR_{max}) or are independent of it (AIR to glucose) could detect β-cell dysfunction in individuals before it is severe enough to result in the fasting hyperglycemia characteristic of diabetes. In addition, relating these measures to the degree of insulin resistance has allowed the identification of individuals with subtler β-cell defects.[236] Currently, major effort is being expended to identify individuals at high risk for development of both type 1 and type 2[237,238] diabetes, because they are candidates for the therapeutic trials that might delay or prevent the onset of clinical diabetes.

REFERENCES

1. Howell SL: The mechanism of insulin secretion. *Diabetologia* 1984; 26:319.
2. Bonner-Weir S: Morphological evidence for pancreatic polarity of beta-cell within islets of Langerhans. *Diabetes* 1988;37:616.
3. Brunicardi FC, Shavelle DM, Andersen DK: Neural regulation of the endocrine pancreas. *Int J Pancreatol* 1995;18:177.
4. Karlsson S, Scheurink AJ, Steffens AB, et al: Involvement of capsaicin-sensitive nerves in regulation of insulin secretion and glucose tolerance in conscious mice. *Am J Physiol* 1994;267:R1071.
5. Skoglund G, Hussain MA, Holz GG: Glucagon-like peptide 1 stimulates insulin gene promoter activity by protein kinase A-independent activation of the rat insulin I gene cAMP response element. *Diabetes* 2000;49:1156.
6. Philippe J, Missotten M: Functional characterization of a cAMP-responsive element of the rat insulin I gene. *J Biol Chem* 1990;265: 1465.
7. Macfarlane WM, Shepherd RM, Cosgrove KE, et al: Glucose modulation of insulin mRNA levels is dependent on transcription factor PDX-1 and occurs independently of changes in intracellular Ca^{2+}. *Diabetes* 2000;49:418.
8. Thomas MK, Lee JH, Rastalsky N, et al: Hedgehog signaling regulation of homeodomain protein islet duodenum homeobox-1 expression in pancreatic beta-cells. *Endocrinology* 2001;142:1033.
9. Hart AW, Baeza N, Apelqvist A, et al: Attenuation of FGF signalling in mouse beta-cells leads to diabetes. *Nature* 2000;408:864.
10. Gilligan M, Welsh GI, Flynn A, et al: Glucose stimulates the activity of the guanine nucleotide-exchange factor eIF-2B in isolated rat islets of Langerhans. *J Biol Chem* 1996;271:2121.
11. Xu G, Marshall CA, Lin TA, et al: Insulin mediates glucose-stimulated phosphorylation of PHAS-I by pancreatic beta cells. An insulin-receptor mechanism for autoregulation of protein synthesis by translation. *J Biol Chem* 1998;273:4485.
12. Wicksteed B, Herbert TP, Alarcon C, et al: Cooperativity between the preproinsulin mRNA untranslated regions is necessary for glucose-stimulated translation. *J Biol Chem* 2001;276:22553.
13. Hoppener JWM, Ahren B, Lips CJM: Mechanisms of disease: Islet amyloid and type 2 diabetes mellitus. *N Engl J Med* 2000;343:411.
14. Janciauskiene S, Eriksson S, Carlemalm E, et al: B cell granule peptides affect human islet amyloid polypeptide (IAPP) fibril formation in vitro. *Biochem Biophys Res Commun* 1997;236:580.
15. Daniel S, Noda M, Straub SG, et al: Identification of the docked granule pool responsible for the first phase of glucose-stimulated insulin secretion. *Diabetes* 1999;48:1686.
16. Rorsman P, Eliasson L, Renstrom E, et al: The cell physiology of biphasic insulin secretion. *News Physiol Sci* 2000;15:72.
17. Klenchin VA, Martin TF: Priming in exocytosis: Attaining fusion-competence after vesicle docking. *Biochimie* 2000;82:399.
18. Calakos N, Scheller RH: Synaptic vesicle biogenesis, docking, and fusion: A molecular description. *Physiol Rev* 1996;76:1.

19. Lang J, Fukuda M, Zhang H, *et al*: The first C2 domain of synaptotagmin is required for exocytosis of insulin from pancreatic beta-cells: Action of synaptotagmin at low micromolar calcium. *EMBO J* 1997; 16:5837.

20. Takeda J, Kayano T, Fukomoto H, *et al*: Organization of the human GLUT2 (pancreatic beta-cell and hepatocyte) glucose transporter gene. *Diabetes* 1993;42:773.

21. Matschinsky F: Glucokinase as glucose sensor and metabolic signal generator in pancreatic β-cells and hepatocytes. *Diabetes* 2000;39: 647.

22. Permutt MA, Chiu KC, Tanizawa Y: Gluckokinase and NIDDM. *Diabetes* 1992;41:1367.

23. Schuit F, De Vos A, Farfari S, *et al*: Metabolic fate of glucose in purified islet cells. Glucose-regulated anaplerosis in beta cells. *J Biol Chem* 1997;272:18572.

24. Dean PM, Matthews EK: Electrical activity in pancreatic islet cells. *Nature* 1968;219:389.

25. Cook DL, Hales CN: Intracellular ATP directly blocks K^+ channels in pancreatic B-cells. *Nature* 1984;311:271.

26. Cook DL, Satin LS, Ashford ML, *et al*: ATP-sensitive K^+ channels in pancreatic b-cells: Spare channel hypothesis. *Diabetes* 1988;37:495.

27. Ashcroft SJ, Ashcroft FM: Properties and functions of ATP-sensitive K-channels. *Cell Signal* 1990;2:197.

28. Babenko AP, Aguilar-Bryan L, Bryan J: A view of sur/KIR6.X, K_{ATP} channels. *Annu Rev Physiol* 1998;60:667.

29. Ashcroft FM, Gribble FM: Correlating structure and function in ATP-sensitive K^+ channels. *Trends Neurosci* 1998;21:288.

30. Seino S, Iwanaga T, Nagashima K, *et al*: Diverse roles of K(ATP) channels learned from Kir6.2 genetically engineered mice. *Diabetes* 2000;49:311.

31. Ghosh A, Ronner P, Cheong E, *et al*: The role of ATP and free ADP in metabolic coupling during fuel-stimulated insulin release from islet β-cells in the isolated perfused rat pancreas. *J Biol Chem* 1991;266: 22887.

32. Hopkins WF, Fatherazi S, Peter-Riesch B, *et al*: Two sites for adenine-nucleotide regulation of ATP-sensitive potassium channels in mouse pancreatic β-cells and HIT cells. *J Membr Biol* 1992;129:287.

33. Cartier EA, Conti LR, Vandenberg CA, *et al*: Defective trafficking and function of K_{ATP} channels caused by a sulfonylurea receptor 1 mutation associated with persistent hyperinsulinemic hypoglycemia of infancy. *Proc Natl Acad Sci USA* 2000;98:2882.

34. Gribble FM, Ashcroft FM: Sulfonylurea sensitivity of adenosine triphosphate-sensitive potassium channels from beta cells and extrapancreatic tissues. *Metabolism* 2000;49:3.

35. Wolffenbuttel BH: Repaglinide—a new compound for the treatment of patients with type 2 diabetes. *Neth J Med* 1999;55:229.

36. Dunn CJ, Faulds D: Nateglinide. *Drugs* 2000;60:607, discussion 616.

37. Cook DL, Satin LS, Hopkins WF: Pancreatic B-cells are bursting, but how? *Trends Neurosci* 1991;14:411.

38. Santos RM, Rosario LM, Nadal A, *et al*: Widespread synchronous $[Ca^{2+}]i$ oscillations due to bursting electrical activity in single pancreatic islets. *Pflugers Arch* 1991;418:417.

39. Valdeolmillos M, Nadal A, Soria B, *et al*: Fluorescence digital image analysis of glucose-induced $[Ca^{2+}]i$ oscillations in mouse pancreatic islets of Langerhans. *Diabetes* 1993;42:1210.

40. Cook DL: Electrical bursting in islet β cells. *Nature* 1992;357:28.

41. Rorsman P, Trube G: Calcium and delayed potassium currents in mouse pancreatic beta-cells under voltage-clamp conditions. *J Physiol (Lond)* 1986;374:531.

42. Ammala C, Ashcroft FM, Rorsman P: Calcium-independent potentiation of insulin release by cyclic AMP in single beta-cells. *Nature* 1993;363:356.

43. Cook DL: Isolated islets of Langerhans have slow oscillations of electrical activity. *Metabolism* 1983;32:681.

44. Longo EA, Tornheim K, Deeney JT, *et al*: Oscillations in cytosolic free Ca^{2+}, oxygen consumption and insulin secretion in glucose stimulated rat pancreatic islets. *J Biol Chem* 1991;266:9314.

45. Weigle DS: Pulsatile secretion of fuel-regulatory hormones. *Diabetes* 1987;36:764.

46. Tornheim K: Are metabolic oscillations responsible for normal oscillatory insulin secretion? *Diabetes* 1997;46:1375.

47. Gembal M, Gilon P, Henquin JC: Evidence that glucose can control insulin release independently from its action on ATP-sensitive K^+ channels in mouse β-cells. *J Clin Invest* 1992;89:1288.

48. Henquin JC: Triggering and amplifying pathways of regulation of insulin secretion by glucose. *Diabetes* 2000;49:1751.

49. Jones PM, Persaud SJ: Protein kinases, protein phosphorylation and the regulation of insulin secretion from pancreatic β-cells. *Endocr Rev* 1999;19:429.

50. Breen MA, Ashcroft SJ: Human islets of Langerhans express multiple isoforms of calcium/calmodulin-dependent protein kinase II. *Biochem Biophys Res Commun* 1997;236:473.

51. Wenham RM, Landt M, Walters SM, *et al*: Inhibition of insulin secretion by KN-62, a specific inhibitor of the multifunctional Ca^{2+}/calmodulin-dependent protein kinase II. *Biochem Biophys Res Commun* 1992;189:128.

52. Hagiwara S, Sakurai T, Tashiro F, *et al*: An inhibitory role for phosphatidylinositol 3-kinase in insulin secretion from pancreatic β cell line MIN6. *Biochem Biophys Res Commun* 1995;214:51.

53. Zawalich WS, Zawalich KC: Regulation of insulin secretion by phospholipase C. *Am J Physiol* 1996;271:E409.

54. Rasmusaln H, Jeales M, Calle R, et al: Diacylglycerol production, Ca^{2+} influx, and protein kinase C activation in sustained cellular responses. *Endocr Rev* 1995;16:649.

55. Karlsson S, Ahren B: Cholecystokinin-stimulated insulin secretion and protein kinase C in rat pancreatic islets. *Acta Physiol Scand* 1991; 142:397.

56. Efanov AM, Zaitsev SV, Berggren PO: Inositol hexakisphosphate stimulates non-Ca^{2+}-mediated and primes Ca^{2+}-mediated exocytosis of insulin by activation of protein kinase C. *Proc Natl Acad Sci USA* 1997;94:4435.

57. Peter-Riesch B, Fathi M, Schlegel W, *et al*: Glucose and carbachol generate 1,2-diacylglycerols by different mechanisms in pancreatic islets. *J Clin Invest* 1988;81:1154.

58. Karlsson S, Ahren B: Cholecystokinin and the regulation of insulin secretion. *Scand J Gastroenterol* 1992;27:161.

59. Henquin JC, Garcia MC, Bozem M, *et al*: Muscarinic control of pancreatic B cell function involves sodium-dependent depolarization and calcium influx. *Endocrinology* 1988;122:2134.

60. Fridolf T, Ahren B: GLP-1(7-36)amide-stimulated insulin secretion in rat islets is sodium- dependent. *Biochem Biophys Res Commun* 1991; 179:701.

61. Kato M, Ma HT, Tatemoto K: GLP-1 depolarizes the rat pancreatic beta cell in a Na(+)-dependent manner. *Regul Pept* 1996;62:23.

62. Filipsson K, Karlsson S, Ahren B: Evidence for contribution by increased cytoplasmic Na^+ to the insulinotropic action of PACAP38 in HIT-T15 cells. *J Biol Chem* 1998;273:32602.

63. Thorens B, Deriaz N, Bosco D, *et al*: Protein kinase A-dependent phosphorylation of GLUT2 in pancreatic beta cells. *J Biol Chem* 1996;271:8075.

64. Inagaki N, Tsuura Y, Namba N, *et al*: Cloning and functional characterization of a novel ATP-sensitive potassium channel ubiquitously expressed in rat tissues, including pancreatic islets, pituitary, skeletal muscle, and heart. *J Biol Chem* 1995;270:5691.

65. Leiser M, Fleischer N: cAMP-dependent phosphorylation of the cardiac-type alpha 1 subunit of the voltage-dependent Ca^{2+} channel in a murine pancreatic beta-cell line. *Diabetes* 1996;45:1412.

66. Zhao AZ, Zhao H, Teague J, *et al*: Attenuation of insulin secretion by insulin-like growth factor 1 is mediated through activation of phosphodiesterase 3B. *Proc Natl Acad Sci USA* 1997;94:3223.

67. Gao Z, Konrad RJ, Collins H, *et al*: Wortmannin inhibits insulin secretion in pancreatic islets and beta-TC3 cells independent of its inhibition of phosphatidylinositol 3-kinase. *Diabetes* 1996;45:854.

68. Stenson Holst L, Mulder H, Manganiello V, *et al*: Protein kinase B is expressed in pancreatic B cells and activated upon stimulation with insulin-like growth factor 1. *Biochem Biophys Res Commun* 1998;250:181.

69. Konrad RJ, Jolly YC, Major C, *et al*: Carbachol stimulation of phospholipase A2 and insulin secretion in pancreatic islets. *Biochem J* 1992;287:283.

70. Simonsson E, Karlsson S, Ahren B: Ca^{2+}-independent phospholipase A2 contributes to the insulinotropic action of cholecystokinin-8 in rat islets: Dissociation from the mechanism of carbachol. *Diabetes* 1998; 47:1436.

71. Simonsson E, Ahren B: Phospholipase A2 and its potential regulation of islet function. *Int J Pancreatol* 2000;27:1

72. Prentki M, Corkey BE: Are the B-cell signaling molecules malonyl-CoA and cytosolic long-chain Acyl-CoA implicated in multiple tissue defects of obesity and NIDDM? *Diabetes* 1996;45:273.

73. McGarry JD, Dobbins RL: Fatty acids, lipotoxicity and insulin secretion. *Diabetologia* 1999;42:128.

74. Mulder H, Holst LS, Svensson H, *et al*: Hormone-sensitive lipase, the rate-limiting enzyme in triglyceride hydrolysis, is expressed and active in beta-cells. *Diabetes* 1999;48:228.

75. Yaney GC, Civelek VN, Richard AM, *et al*: Glucagon-like peptide 1 stimulates lipolysis in clonal pancreatic beta-cells (HIT). *Diabetes* 2001;50:56.

76. Harbeck MC, Louie DC, Howland J, *et al*: Expression of insulin receptor mRNA and insulin receptor substrate 1 in pancreatic islet beta-cells. *Diabetes* 1996;45:711.

77. Kulkarni RN, Bruning JC, Winnay JN, *et al*: Tissue-specific knockout of the insulin receptor in pancreatic beta cells creates an insulin secretory defect similar to that in type 2 diabetes. *Cell* 1999;96:329.

78. Mauvais-Jarvis F, Kahn CR: Understanding the pathogenesis and treatment of insulin resistance and type 2 diabetes mellitus: What can we learn from transgenic and knockout mice? *Diabetes Metab* 2000; 26:433.

79. Ullrich S, Wollheim CB: Islet cyclic AMP levels are not lowered during alpha 2-adrenergic inhibition of insulin release. *J Biol Chem* 1984; 259:4111.

80. Cook DL, Perara E: Islet electrical pacemaker response to alpha-adrenergic stimulation. *Diabetes* 1982;31:985.

81. Rorsman P, Bokvist K, Ammala C, *et al*: Activation by adrenaline of a low-conductance G protein dependent K^+ channel in mouse pancreatic B cells. *Nature* 1991;349:77.

82. Drews G, Debuyser A, Nenquin M, *et al*: Galanin and epinephrine act on distinct receptors to inhibit insulin release by the same mechanisms including an increase in K^+ permeability of the B-cell membrane. *Endocrinology* 1990;126:1646.

83. Dunne MJ, Bullett MJ, Li GD, *et al*: Galanin activates nucleotide-dependent K^+ channels in insulin-secreting cells via a pertussis toxin-sensitive G-protein. *EMBO J* 1989;8:413.

84. de Weille JR, Schmid-Antomarchi H, Fosset M, *et al*: Regulation of ATP-sensitive K^+ channels in insulinoma cells: activation by somatostatin and protein kinase C and the role of cAMP. *Proc Natl Acad Sci USA* 1989;86:2971.

85. Ullrich S, Wollheim CB: Galanin inhibits insulin secretion by direct interference with exocytosis. *FEBS Lett* 1989;247:401.

86. Draznin B, Leitner JW, Sussman KE: A unique control mechanism in the regulation of insulin secretion. Secretagogue-induced somatostatin receptor recruitment. *J Clin Invest* 1985;75:1510.

87. Kieffer TJ, Habener JF: The adipoinsular axis: effects of leptin on pancreatic beta-cells. *Am J Physiol Endocrinol Metab* 2000;278:E1.

88. Zhao AZ, Bornfeldt KE, Beavo JA: Leptin inhibits insulin secretion by activation of phosphodiesterase 3B. *J Clin Invest* 1998;102:869.

89. Ahren B, Havel PJ: Leptin inhibits insulin secretion induced by cellular cAMP in a pancreatic B cell line (INS-1 cells). *Am J Physiol* 1999; 277:R959.

90. Flattem N, Igawa K, Shiota M, *et al*: Alpha and beta cell responses to small changes in plasma glucose in the conscious dog. *Diabetes* 2001; 50:367.

91. Boden G, Chen X, Iqbal N: Acute lowering of plasma fatty acids lowers basal insulin secretion in diabetic and nondiabetic subjects. *Diabetes* 1998;47:1609.

92. Stein DT, Esser V, Stevenson BE, *et al*: Essentiality of circulating fatty acids for glucose-stimulated insulin secretion in the fasted rat. *J Clin Invest* 1996;97:2728.

93. Lefebvre PJ, Paolisso G, Scheen AJ, *et al*: Pulsatility of insulin and glucagon release: physiological significance and pharmacological implications. *Diabetologia* 1987;30:443.

94. Goodner CJ, Walike BC, Koerker DJ, *et al*: Insulin, glucagon, and glucose exhibit synchronous, sustained oscillations in fasting monkeys. *Science* 1977;195:177.

95. Lang DA, Matthews DR, Peto J, *et al*: Cyclic oscillations of basal plasma glucose and insulin concentrations in human beings. *N Engl J Med* 1979;301:1023.

96. Stagner JI, Samols E, Weir GC: Sustained oscillations of insulin, glucagon, and somatostatin from the isolated canine pancreas during exposure to a constant glucose concentration. *J Clin Invest* 1980;65: 939.

97. Stagner JI, Samols E: Perturbation of insulin oscillations by nerve blockade in the *in vitro* canine pancreas. *Am J Physiol* 1985;248: E516.

98. Stagner JI, Samols E: Modulation of insulin secretion by pancreatic ganglionic nicotinic receptors. *Diabetes* 1986;35:849.

99. Polonsky KS, Given BD, Hirsch LJ, *et al*: Abnormal patterns of insulin secretion in non-insulin-dependent diabetes mellitus. *N Engl J Med* 1988;318:1231.

100. Lang DA, Matthews DR, Burnett M, *et al*: Brief, irregular oscillations of basal plasma insulin and glucose concentrations in diabetic man. *Diabetes* 1981;30:435.

101. Laedtke T, Kjems L, Porksen N, *et al*: Overnight inhibition of insulin secretion restores pulsatility and proinsulin/insulin ratio in type 2 diabetes. *Am J Physiol* 2000;279:E520.

102. Unger RH, Orci L: Physiology and pathophysiology of glucagon. *Physiol Rev* 1976;56:778.

103. Boden G, Chen X, Rosner J, *et al*: Effects of a 48-h fat infusion on insulin secretion and glucose utilization. *Diabetes* 1995;44:1239.

104. Zhou YP, Grill VE: Long-term exposure of rat pancreatic islets to fatty acids inhibits glucose-induced insulin secretion and biosynthesis through a glucose fatty acid cycle. *J Clin Invest* 1994;93:870.

105. Zhou YP, Ling ZC, Grill VE: Inhibitory effects of fatty acids on glucose-regulated B-cell function: association with increased islet triglyceride stores and altered effect of fatty acid oxidation on glucose metabolism. *Metabolism* 1996;45:981.

106. Shimabukuro M, Zhou YT, Levi M, *et al*: Fatty acid-induced beta cell apoptosis: A link between obesity and diabetes. *Proc Natl Acad Sci USA* 1998;95:2498.

107. Lee Y, Hirose H, Ohneda M, *et al*: Beta cell lipotoxicity in the pathogenesis of non-insulin-dependent diabetes mellitus of obese rats: Impairment in adipocyte-beta-cell relationships. *Proc Natl Acad Sci USA* 1994;91:10878.

108. Unger RH: Lipotoxicity in the pathogenesis of obesity-dependent NIDDM. *Diabetes* 1995;44:863.

109. Bollheimer LC, Skelly RH, Chester MW, *et al*: Chronic exposure to free fatty acid reduces pancreatic beta cell insulin content by increasing basal insulin secretion that is not compensated for by a corresponding increase in proinsulin biosynthesis translation. *J Clin Invest* 1998;101:1094.

110. Shimabukuro M, Ohneda M, Lee Y, *et al*: Role of nitric oxide in obesity-induced beta cell disease. *J Clin Invest* 1997;100:290.

111. Schirra J, Katschinski M, Weidmann C, *et al*: Gastric emptying and release of incretin hormones after glucose ingestion in humans. *J Clin Invest* 1996;97:92.

112. Jia X, Brown JC, Ma P, *et al*: Effects of glucose-dependent insulinotropic polypeptide and glucagon-like peptide-I-(7-36) on insulin secretion. *Am J Physiol* 1995;268:E645.

113. Tseng CC, Kieffer TJ, Jarboe LA, *et al*: Postprandial stimulation of insulin release by glucose-dependent insulinotropic polypeptide (GIP). *J Clin Invest* 1996;98:2440.

114. Miyawaki K, Yamada Y, Yano Y, *et al*: Glucose intolerance caused by a defect in the entero-insular axis: A study in gastric inhibitory polypeptide receptor knockout mice. *Proc Natl Acad Sci USA* 1999; 96:14843.

115. Liddle RA, Morita ET, Conrad CK, *et al*: Regulation of gastric emptying in humans by cholecystokinin. *J Clin Invest* 1986;77:992.

116. Hopman WP, Jansen JB, Lamers CB: Comparative study of the effects of equal amounts of fat, protein, and starch on plasma cholecystokinin in man. *Scand J Gastroenterol* 1985;20:843.

117. Holst JJ, Orskov C, Nielsen OV, *et al*: Truncated glucagon-like peptide I, an insulin-releasing hormone from the distal gut. *FEBS Lett* 1987;211:169.

118. Kreymann B, Ghatei MA, Williams G, *et al*: Glucagon-like peptide-1 7-36: A physiological incretin in man. *Lancet* 1987;2:1300.

119. Mojsov S, Weir GC, Habener JF: Insulinotropin: Glucagon-like peptide I (7-37) co-encoded in the glucagon gene is a potent stimulator of insulin release in the perfused rat pancreas. *J Clin Invest* 1987;79:616.

120. D'Alessio DA, Vogel R, Prigeon R, *et al*: Elimination of the action of glucagon-like peptide 1 causes an impairment of glucose tolerance after nutrient ingestion by healthy baboons. *J Clin Invest* 1996;97:133.

121. Scrocchi LA, Brown TJ, MaClusky N, *et al*: Glucose intolerance but normal satiety in mice with null mutation in the glucagon-like peptide 1 receptor gene. *Nat Med* 1996;2:1254.

122. Pederson RA, Satkunarajah M, McIntosh CH, *et al*: Enhanced glucose-dependent insulinotropic polypeptide secretion and insulinotropic action in glucagon-like peptide 1 receptor −/− mice. *Diabetes* 1998;47:1046.

123. Xu G, Stoffers DA, Habener JF, *et al*: Exendin-4 stimulates both beta-cell replication and neogenesis, resulting in increased beta-cell mass and improved glucose tolerance in diabetic rats. *Diabetes* 1999;48: 2270.

124. Ahren B, Larsson H, Holst JJ: Effects of glucagon like peptide-1 on islet function and insulin sensitivity in noninsulin-dependent diabetes mellitus. *J Clin Endocrinol Metab* 1997;82:473.

125. Nauck MA, Bartels E, Orskov C, *et al*: Additive insulinotropic effects of exogenous synthetic human gastric inhibitory polypeptide and glucagon-like peptide-1 (7-36) amide infused at near-physiological insulinotropic hormone and glucose concentrations. *J Clin Endocrinol Metab* 1993;76:912.

126. Jamen F, Persson K, Bertrand G, *et al*: PAC1 receptor-deficient mice display impaired insulinotropic response to glucose and reduced glucose tolerance. *J Clin Invest* 2000;105:1307.

127. Kirchgessner AL, Gershon MD: Innervation of the pancreas by neurons in the gut. *J Neurosci* 1990;10:1626.

128. Kirchgessner AL, Liu MT: Pituitary adenylate cyclase activating peptide (PACAP) in the enteropancreatic innervation. *Anat Rec* 2001; 262:91.

129. Gerich JE: Lilly lecture 1988. Glucose counterregulation and its impact on diabetes mellitus. *Diabetes* 1988;37:1608.

130. Verspohl EJ, Tacke R, Mutschler E, *et al*: Muscarinic receptor subtypes in rat pancreatic islets: Binding and functional studies. *Eur J Pharmacol* 1990;178:303.

131. Boschero AC, Szpak-Glasman M, Carneiro EM, *et al*: Oxotremorine-m potentiation of glucose-induced insulin release from rat islets involves M3 muscarinic receptors. *Am J Physiol* 1995;268:E336.

132. Iismaa TP, Kerr EA, Wilson JR, *et al*: Quantitative and functional characterization of muscarinic receptor subtypes in insulin-secreting cell lines and rat pancreatic islets. *Diabetes* 2000;49:392.

133. Bergman RN, Miller RE: Direct enhancement of insulin secretion by vagal stimulation of the isolated pancreas. *Am J Physiol* 1973;225:481.

134. Strubbe JH, Steffens AB: Rapid insulin release after ingestion of a meal in the unanesthetized rat. *Am J Physiol* 1975;229:1019.

135. Teff K: Oral sensory stimulation improves glucose tolerance in humans: Effects on insulin, C-peptide, and glucagon. *Am J Physiol* 1996; 270:R1371.

136. Benthem L, Mundinger T, Taborsky G: Meal-induced insulin secretion in dogs is mediated by both branches of the autonomic nervous system. *Am J Physiol* 2000;278:E603.

137. D'Alessio DA, Kieffer TJ, Taborsky GJ, *et al*: Activation of the parasympathetic nervous system is necessary for normal meal-induced insulin secretion in Rhesus macaques. *J Clin Endocrinol Metab* 2001;86:1253.

138. Holst JJ, Fahrenkrug J, Knuhtsen S, *et al*: Vasoactive intestinal polypeptide in the pig pancreas: Role of VIPergic nerves in control of fluid and bicarbonate secretion. *Regul Pept* 1984;8:245.

139. Havel PJ, Veith RC, Dunning BE, *et al*: Pancreatic noradrenergic nerves are activated by neuroglucopenia but not hypotension or hypoxia in the dog: Evidence for stress-specific and regionally-selective activation of the sympathetic nervous system. *J Clin Invest* 1988;82: 1538.

140. Dunning BE, Ahren B, Veith RC, *et al*: Galanin: A novel pancreatic neuropeptide. *Am J Physiol* 1986;251:E127.

141. Verchere CB, Kowalyk S, Shen GH, *et al*: Major species variation in the expression of galanin messenger ribonucleic acid in mammalian celiac ganglion. *Endocrinology* 1994;135:1052.

142. Dunning BE, Taborsky GJ Jr: Galanin release during pancreatic nerve stimulation is sufficient to influence islet function. *Am J Physiol* 1989; 256:E191.

143. Dunning BE, Havel PJ, Veith RC, *et al*: Pancreatic and extrapancreatic galanin release during sympathetic neural activation. *Am J Physiol* 1990;258:E436.

144. McDonald TJ, Dupre J, Tatemoto K, *et al*: Galanin inhibits insulin secretion and induces hyperglycemia in dogs. *Diabetes* 1985;34:192.

145. Dunning BE, Ahren B, Bottcher G, *et al*: The presence and actions of NPY in the canine endocrine pancreas. *Regul Pept* 1987;18:253.

146. Taborsky GJ Jr: Evidence of a paracrine role for pancreatic somatostatin in vivo. *Am J Physiol* 1983;245:E598.

147. Maruyama H, Hisatomi A, Orci L, *et al*: Insulin within islets is a physiologic glucagon release inhibitor. *J Clin Invest* 1984;74:2296.

148. Samols E, Bonner-Weir S, Weir GC: Intra-islet insulin-glucagon-somatostatin relationships. *J Clin Endocrinol Metab* 1986;15:33.

149. Kahn SE, Andrikopoulos S, Verchere CB: Islet amyloid: A long-recognized but underappreciated pathological feature of type 2 diabetes. *Diabetes* 1999;48:241.

150. Lorenzo A, Rabbaboni B, Weir GC, *et al*: Pancreatic islet cell toxicity of amylin associated with type 2 diabetes mellitus. *Nature* 1994;368: 756.

151. Albisser AM, Leibel BS, Ewart TG, *et al*: An artificial endocrine pancreas. *Diabetes* 1974;23:389.

152. Calle-Escandon J, Robbins DC: Loss of early phase release in humans impairs glucose tolerance and blunts thermic effect of glucose. *Diabetes* 1987;36:1167.

153. Ahren B, Pacini G: Impaired adaptation of first phase insulin secretion in postmenopausal women with glucose intolerance. *Am J Physiol* 1997;273:E701.

154. Mitrakou A, Kelley D, Mokam M, *et al*: Role of reduced suppression of glucose production and diminished early insulin release in impaired glucose tolerance. *N Engl J Med* 1992;326:22.

155. Teff KL, Engleman K: Oral sensory stimulation improves glucose tolerance in humans: Effects on insulin, C-peptide, and glucagon. *Am J Physiol* 1996;270:R1371.

156. Bruttomesso D, Pianta A, Mari A, *et al*: Restoration of early rise in plasma insulin levels improves the glucose tolerance of type 2 diabetic patients. *Diabetes* 1999;48:99.

157. Halter JB, Graf RJ, Porte D Jr: Potentiation of insulin secretory responses by plasma glucose levels in man: Evidence that hyperglycemia in diabetes compensates for impaired glucose potentiation. *J Clin Endocrinol Metab* 1979;48:946.

158. Grill V: Time and dose dependencies for priming effect of glucose on insulin secretion. *Am J Physiol* 1981;240:E24.

159. Bolaffi JL, Bruno L, Heldt A, *et al*: Characteristics of desensitization of insulin secretion in fully in vitro systems. *Endocrinology* 1988; 122:1801.

160. Stefan Y, Meda P, Neufeld M, *et al*: Stimulation of insulin secretion reveals heterogeneity of pancreatic B cells in vivo. *J Clin Invest* 1987; 80:175.

161. Leahy JL, Bonner-Weir S, Weir GC: Minimal chronic hyperglycemia is a critical determinant of impaired insulin secretion after an incomplete pancreatectomy. *J Clin Invest* 1988;81:1407.

162. Rossetti L, Shulman GI, Zawalich W, *et al*: Effect of chronic hyperglycemia on in vivo insulin secretion in partially pancreatectomized rats. *J Clin Invest* 1987;80:1037.

163. Unger RH, Grundy S: Hyperglycaemia as an inducer as well as a consequence of impaired islet cell function and insulin resistance: Implications for the management of diabetes. *Diabetologia* 1985;28:119.

164. Ward WK, Wallum BJ, Beard JC, *et al*: Reduction of glycemic potentiation. Sensitive indicator of beta-cell loss in partially pancreatectomized dogs. *Diabetes* 1988;37:723.

165. Bonner-Weir S, Trent DF, Weir GC: Partial pancreatectomy in the rat and subsequent defect in glucose-induced insulin release. *J Clin Invest* 1983;71:1544.

166. Hanson RL, Pratley RE, Bogardus C, *et al*: Evaluation of simple indices of insulin sensitivity and insulin secretion for use in epidemiologic studies. *Am J Epidemiol* 2000;151:190.

167. National Diabetes Data Group: Classification and diagnosis of diabetes mellitus and other categories of glucose intolerance. *Diabetes* 1979;28:1039.

168. Bergman RN: Toward physiological understanding of glucose tolerance. Minimal-model approach. *Diabetes* 1989;38:1512.

169. LeBlanc J, Nadeau A, Richard D, *et al*: Studies on the sparing effect of exercise on insulin requirements in human subjects. *Metabolism* 1981;30:1119.

170. McCulloch DK, Raghu PK, Johnston C, *et al*: Defects in beta-cell function and insulin sensitivity in normoglycemic streptozocin-treated baboons: A model of preclinical insulin-dependent diabetes. *J Clin Endocrinol Metab* 1988;67:785.

171. Kahn SE, Horber FF, Prigeon RL, *et al*: Effect of glucocorticoid and growth hormone treatment on proinsulin levels in humans. *Diabetes* 1993;42:1082.

172. Matthews DR, Hosker JP, Rudenski AS, *et al*: Homeostasis model assessment: Insulin resistance and beta cell function from fasting plasma glucose and insulin concentrations in man. *Diabetologia* 1985;84:412.

173. DeFronzo RA, Tobin JD, Andres R: Glucose clamp technique: A method for quantifying insulin secretion and resistance. *Am J Physiol* 1979;237:E214.

174. Elahi D: In praise of the hyperglycemic clamp. A method for assessment of beta-cell sensitivity and insulin resistance. *Diabetes Care* 1996;19:278.

175. Kahn SE, Beard JC, Schwartz MW, et al: Increased beta-cell secretory capacity as mechanism for islet adaptation to nicotinic acid-induced insulin resistance. *Diabetes* 1989;38:562.

176. Ward WK, Bolgiano DC, McKnight B, et al: Diminished B cell secretory capacity in patients with noninsulin-dependent diabetes mellitus. *J Clin Invest* 1984;74:1318.

177. Ward WK, LaCava EC, Paquette TL, et al: Disproportionate elevation of immunoreactive proinsulin in type 2 (non-insulin-dependent) diabetes mellitus and experimental insulin resistance. *Diabetologia* 1987;30:698.

178. Kahn SE, McCulloch DK, Schwartz MW, et al: Effect of insulin resistance and hyperglycemia on proinsulin release in a primate model of diabetes mellitus. *J Clin Endocrinol Metab* 1992;74:192.

179. Alarcon C, Leahy JL, Schuppin GT, et al: Increased secretory demand rather than a defect in the proinsulin conversion mechanism causes hyperproinsulinemia in a glucose-infusion rat model of non-insulin-dependent diabetes mellitus. *J Clin Invest* 1995;95:1032.

180. Larsson H, Ahern B: Relative hyperproinsulinemia as a sign of islet dysfunction in women with impaired glucose tolerance. *J Clin Endocrinol Metab* 1999;84:2068.

181. Bergman RN, Phillips LS, Cobelli C: Physiologic evaluation of factors controlling glucose tolerance in man. Measurement of insulin sensitivity and B-cell glucose sensitivity from the response to intravenous glucose. *J Clin Invest* 1981;68:1456.

182. Kahn SE, Prigeon RL, McCulloch DK, et al: Quantification of the relationship between insulin sensitivity and beta-cell function in human subjects. Evidence for a hyperbolic function. *Diabetes* 1993;42:1663.

183. Larsson H, Ahren B: Insulin resistant subjects lack islet adaptation to acute dexamethasone-induced reduction in insulin sensitivity. *Diabetologia* 1999;42:936.

184. Michael MD, Kulkarni RN, Postic C, et al: Loss of insulin signaling in hepatocytes leads to severe insulin resistance and progressive hepatic dysfunction. *Mol Cell* 2000;6:87.

185. Yamauchi T, Tobe K, Tamemoto J, et al: Insulin signalling and insulin actions in the muscles and livers of insulin-resistant, insulin receptor substrate 1-deficient mice. *Mol Cell* 1996;16:3074.

186. Kido Y, Burks DJ, Withers D, et al: Tissue-specific insulin resistance in mice with mutations in the insulin receptor, IRS-1, and IRS-2. *J Clin Invest* 2000;23:32.

187. Terauchi Y, Iwamoto K, Tamemoto H, et al: Development of non-insulin-dependent diabetes mellitus in the double knockout mice with disruption of insulin receptor substrate-1 and β cell glucokinase genes. Genetic reconstitution of diabetes as a polygenic disease. *J Clin Invest* 1997;99:861.

188. Kubota N, Tobe K, Terauchi Y, et al: Disruption of insulin receptor substrate 2 causes type 2 diabetes because of liver insulin resistance and lack of compensatory beta-cell hyperplasia. *Diabetes* 2000;49:1880.

189. Stenbit AE, Tsao TS, Li J, et al: GLUT4 heterozygous knockout mice develop muscle insulin resistance and diabetes. *Nat Med* 1997;3:1096.

190. Bruning JC, Michael MD, Winnay JN, et al: A muscle-specific insulin receptor knockout exhibits features of the metabolic syndrome of NIDDM without altering glucose tolerance. *Mol Cell* 1998;2:559.

191. Kim JK, Michael MD, Previs SF, et al: Redistribution of substrates to adipose tissue promotes obesity in mice with selective insulin resistance in muscle. *J Clin Invest* 2000;105:1791.

192. Zisman A, Perone OD, Abel ED, et al: Targeted disruption of the glucose transporter 4 selectively in muscle causes insulin resistance and glucose intolerance. *Nat Med* 2000;6:924.

193. Withers DJ, Burks DJ, Towery HH, et al: IRS-2 coordinates IGF-1 receptor-mediated beta-cell development and peripheral insulin signalling. *Nat Genet* 1999;23:32.

194. Rohner-Jeanrenaud F, Jeanrenaud B: Consequences of ventromedial hypothalamic lesions upon insulin and glucagon secretion by subsequently isolated perfused pancreases in the rat. *J Clin Invest* 1980;65:902.

195. Rohner-Jeanrenaud F, Jeanrenaud B: Possible involvement of the cholinergic system in hormonal secretion by the perfused pancreas from ventromedial-hypothalamic lesioned rats. *Diabetologia* 1981;20:217.

196. Vander Tuig JG, Knehans AW, Romsos DR: Reduced sympathetic nervous system activity in rats with ventromedial hypothalamic lesions. *Life Sci* 1982;30:913.

197. Benthem L, Mundinger TO, Taborsky JGJ: Parasympathetic inhibition of sympathetic neural activity to the pancreas. *Am J Physiol* 2001;280:E378.

198. Zhang Y, Proenca R, Maffel M, et al: Positional cloning of the mouse obese gene and its human homologue. *Nature* 1994;372:425.

199. Campfield LA, Smith FJ, Guisez Y, et al: Recombinant mouse OB protein: Evidence for a peripheral signal linking adiposity and central neural networks. *Science* 1995;269:546.

200. Murakami T, Shima K: Cloning of rat obese cDNA and its expression in obese rats. *Biochem Biophys Res Commun* 1995;209:944.

201. Rohner-Jeanrenaud F, Hochstrasser AC, Jeanrenaud B: Hyperinsulinemia of preobese and obese fa/fa rats is partly vagus nerve mediated. *Am J Physiol* 1983;244:E317.

202. Levin BE, Triscari J, Sullivan AC: Studies of origins of abnormal sympathetic function in obese Zucker rats. *Am J Physiol* 1983;245:E87.

203. Levin BE, Triscari J, Hogan S, et al: Resistance to diet-induced obesity: Food intake, pancreatic sympathetic tone, and insulin. *Am J Physiol* 1987;252:R471.

204. Levin BE: Reduced norepinephrine turnover in organs and brains of obesity-prone rats. *Am J Physiol* 1995;268:R389.

205. Olefsky JM, Kolterman OG: Mechanisms of insulin resistance in obesity and noninsulin-dependent (type II) diabetes. *Am J Med* 1981;70:151.

206. Jones CN, Abbasi F, Carantoni M, et al: Roles of insulin resistance and obesity in regulation of plasma insulin concentrations. *Am J Physiol* 2000;278:E501.

207. Nolan JJ, Ludvik B, Beerdsen P, et al: Improvement of glucose tolerance and insulin resistance in obese subjects treated with troglitazone. *N Engl J Med* 1994;3:1188.

208. Beard JC, Ward WK, Halter JB, et al: Relationship of islet function to insulin action in human obesity. *J Clin Endocrinol Metab* 1987;65:59.

209. Shiraishi I, Iwamoto Y, Kuzuya T, et al: Hyperinsulinaemia in obesity is not accompanied by an increase in serum proinsulin/insulin ratio in groups of human subjects with and without glucose intolerance. *Diabetologia* 1991;34:737.

210. Faber OK, Christensen K, Kehlet H, et al: Decreased insulin removal contributes to hyperinsulinemia in obesity. *J Clin Endocrinol Metab* 1981;53:618.

211. Jones CN, Pei D, Staris P, et al: Alterations in the glucose-stimulated insulin secretory dose-response curve and in insulin clearance in nondiabetic insulin-resistant individuals. *J Clin Endocrinol Metab* 1997;82:1834.

212. King DS, Dalsky GP, Clutter WE, et al: Effects of lack of exercise on insulin secretion and action in trained subjects. *Am J Physiol* 1988;254:E537.

213. Koranyi LI, Bourey RE, Slentz CA, et al: Coordinate reduction of rat pancreatic islet glucokinase and proinsulin mRNA by exercise training. *Diabetes* 1991;40:401.

214. Kahn SE, Larson VG, Beard JC, et al: Effect of exercise on insulin action, glucose tolerance, and insulin secretion in aging. *Am J Physiol* 1990;258:E937.

215. Taborsky GJ Jr, Porte D Jr: Endogenous hyperglycemia restores the insulin release impaired by somatostatin analog. *Am J Physiol* 1981;240:E407.

216. Leahy JL, Bonner-Weir S, Weir GC: Abnormal insulin secretion in a streptozocin model of diabetes. Effects of insulin treatment. *Diabetes* 1985;34:660.

217. McCulloch DK, Palmer JP, Benson EA: Beta cell function in the preclinical period of insulin-dependent diabetes. *Diabetes Metab Rev* 1987;3:27.

218. Ganda OP, Srikanta S, Brink SJ, et al: Differential sensitivity to beta-cell secretagogues in "early," type I diabetes mellitus. *Diabetes* 1984;33:516.

219. Johnston C, Raghu P, McCulloch DK, et al: Beta-cell function and insulin sensitivity in nondiabetic HLA-identical siblings of insulin-dependent diabetics. *Diabetes* 1987;36:829.

220. Keller RJ, Eisenbarth GS, Jackson RA: Insulin prophylaxis in individuals at high risk of type I diabetes. *Lancet* 1993;34:927.

221. Wilson DM, Buckingham B: Prevention of type 1a diabetes mellitus. *Pediatr Diabetes* 2001;2:17.

222. Schatz D, Krischer J, Horne G, *et al*: Islet cell antibodies predict insulin-dependent diabetes in United States school age children as powerfully as in unaffected relatives. *J Clin Invest* 1994;93:2403.

223. Vold B, Maclaren N: GAD65 autoantibodies increase the predictability but not the sensitivity of islet cell and insulin autoantibodies for developing insulin dependent diabetes mellitus. *J Autoimmun* 1994;7:865.

224. Yu L, Cuthbertson DD, Maclaren N, *et al*: Expression of GAD65 and islet cell antibody (ICA512) autoantibodies among cytoplasmic ICA+ relatives is associated with eligibility for the Diabetes Prevention Trial-Type 1. *Diabetes* 2001;50:1735.

225. Pimenta W, Korytkowski M, Mitrakou A, *et al*: Pancreatic beta-cell dysfunction as the primary genetic lesion in NIDDM. Evidence from studies in normal glucose-tolerant individuals with a first-degree NIDDM relative. *JAMA* 1995;273:1855.

226. Ward WK, Johnston CL, Beard JC, *et al*: Abnormalities of islet B-cell function, insulin action, and fat distribution in women with histories of gestational diabetes: Relationship to obesity. *J Clin Endocrinol Metab* 1985;61:1039.

227. Kahn SE: The importance of β-cell failure in the development and progression of type 2 Diabetes. *J Clin Endocrinol Metab* 2001;86:4047.

228. Cavaghan MK, Ehrmann DA, Byrne MM, *et al*: Treatment with oral antidiabetic agent troglitazone improves B cell responses to glucose in subjects with impaired glucose tolerance. *J Clin Invest* 1997;100:530.

229. Ehrmann DA, Sturis J, Byrne MM, *et al*: Insulin secretory defects in polycystic ovary syndrome. Relationship to insulin sensitivity and family history of non-insulin-dependent diabetes mellitus. *J Clin Invest* 1995;96:520.

230. Buchanan TA, Xiang AH, Kjos SL, *et al*: Antepartum predictors of the development of type 2 diabetes in Latino women 11–26 months after pregnancies complicated by gestational diabetes. *Diabetes* 1999;48:2430.

231. Elbein SC, Wegner K, Kahn SE: Reduced beta-cell compensation to the insulin resistance associated with obesity in members of caucasian familial type 2 diabetic kindreds. *Diabetes Care* 2000;23:221.

232. Weir GC: Non-insulin-dependent diabetes mellitus: interplay between β-cell inadequacy and insulin resistance. *Am J Med* 1982;73:461.

233. Porte DJ: Banting lecture 1990. Beta cells in type 2 diabetes mellitus. *Diabetes* 1990;40:166.

234. Kahn SE: Regulation of B-cell function in vivo: from health to disease. *Diabetes Rev* 1996;4:372.

235. Polonsky KS, Sturis J, Bell GL: Seminars in Medicine of the Beth Israel Hospital. Non-insulin dependent diabetes is a genetically programmed failure of the beta cell to compensate for insulin resistance. *N Engl J Med* 1996;334:777.

236. Kahn SE: The importance of β-cell failure in the development and progression of type 2 Diabetes. *J Clin Endocrinol Metab* 2001;86:4047.

237. The Diabetes Prevention Program Research Group: The Diabetes Prevention Program. Design and methods for a clinical trial in the prevention of type 2 diabetes. *Diabetes Care* 1999;22:623.

238. Chiasson JL, Gomis R, Hanefeld M, *et al*: The Study to Prevent Non-Insulin-Dependent Diabetes Mellitus Trial: an international study on the efficacy of an alpha-glucosidase inhibitor to prevent type 2 diabetes in a population with impaired glucose tolerance: Rationale, design, and preliminary screening data. *Diabetes Care* 1998;21:1720.

239. Kahn SE, Klaff LJ, Schwartz MW, *et al*: Treatment with a somatostatin analogue decreases pancreatic B-cell and whole body sensitivity to glucose. *J Clin Endocrinol Metab* 1990;71;994.

Mechanisms of Insulin Action

Jes K. Klarlund

Andrew D. Cherniack

Bruce R. Conway

Barbara VanRenterghem

Michael P. Czech

Although the hormone insulin and its specific cell membrane receptor share characteristics with many peptide growth factors and their receptors, insulin plays a unique role in human biology. Its absence uniquely causes major abnormalities in multiple metabolic pathways and is lethal. In adults, the major actions of insulin lead to increased synthesis of protein, glycogen, and fat, thereby promoting muscle strength and energy reserves when food is available. The signaling systems that mediate these anabolic responses to insulin regulate key controlling enzymes in these respective metabolic pathways. In general, these regulated enzymes are stimulated or inhibited by insulin through phosphorylation of protein serine/threonine residues or by dephosphorylation of such sites. Because the insulin receptor is a tyrosine kinase, the general underlying feature of insulin signaling is switching the initial receptor-mediated tyrosine phosphorylation to modulation of protein serine/threonine protein kinases and protein serine/threonine phosphate phosphatases. Over the past several years it has been recognized that one switch is the proto-oncogene product p21 ras, which binds guanosine triphosphate (GTP) in response to insulin and initiates activation of Raf protein kinases and in turn a cascade of other serine/threonine protein kinases (for reviews, see references 1 and 2). This pathway appears to play a major role in mediating effects of insulin on cell proliferation. Another switching mechanism involves the activation of a lipid kinase, phosphatidylinositol-3-kinase (PI-3-kinase), which catalyzes the formation of 3′ polyphosphoinositides that in turn initiate recruitment and activation of the serine/threonine protein kinases Akt (also denoted protein kinase B) and certain protein kinase C isoforms (for reviews, see references 237–240). Many of the metabolic effects of insulin appear to be regulated by this pathway. This new information allows us for the first time to trace the molecular circuitry of insulin signaling pathways from the receptor tyrosine kinase through downstream events that regulate metabolic pathways.

Activation of the Raf protein kinase cascade and Akt by insulin leads to extensive protein phosphorylations on serine/threonine residues in target cells within minutes of exposure to the hormone. This stimulation of protein phosphorylation by insulin in ^{32}P-labeled cells is quantitatively greater than the enzyme dephosphorylations that also occur, and can be easily visualized by electrophoretic analysis of whole-cell extracts. Several major proteins are targets of such phosphorylation in addition to the above protein serine/threonine kinases themselves, including the forkhead transcription factor (X5 and X6), S6 ribosomal protein,[3] ATP citrate lyase,[4,5] acetyl CoA carboxylase,[6,7] PHAS,[8–10] and several unidentified species. The insulin receptor is also serine/threonine phosphorylated in response to insulin binding in intact cells.[11] Although increased serine/threonine phosphorylation of cellular proteins is a major effect of insulin, in many instances the physiologic effect on these proteins has not been determined. However, recent exciting data indicate that insulin-mediated phosphorylation of PHAS dramatically modulates its activity and plays a major role in increasing protein synthesis. Also, phosphorylation of forkhead in response to insulin appears to play a major role in regulating transcription of hepatic enzymes involved in gluconeogenesis.[242]

New information has also yielded insights into how enzyme dephosphorylations may occur in response to cell signaling by insulin. Such dephosphorylations include that of glycogen synthase, which increases the activity of the enzyme, leading to increased glycogen deposition,[12] and hormone-sensitive lipase, which inhibits its activity and the hydrolysis of triglyceride stores.[13] Similarly, pyruvate dehydrogenase is dephosphorylated and activated in response to insulin,[14] leading to increased synthesis of acetyl CoA and fatty acids. Regulation of protein serine/threonine phosphate phosphatases appears to involve their recruitment to target enzymes. This recruitment may result from the action of one or more protein serine kinases on regulatory subunits of the protein phosphatase 1.[15] However, recent results show rather normal insulin responsiveness of glycogen synthase activity in mice where such a major regulatory subunit is ablated through gene knockout techniques.[244] Thus there may be other phosphatases involved in these insulin actions. The identity of such hypothetical insulin-sensitive phosphatases is an important area of future investigation. In addition, decreased protein kinase activity in response to insulin has been established as a possible mechanism of protein dephosphorylation, as discussed below in reference to glycogen synthase regulation.

Taken together, the above considerations indicate that understanding the molecular basis of insulin's actions will depend on defining the many molecular elements involved in linking the insulin receptor tyrosine kinase to target protein serine/threonine phosphorylations and dephosphorylations. This review summarizes our current understanding of such signaling elements, using insulin's actions on glucose transport, protein synthesis, and glycogen synthesis to exemplify their mechanisms of action.

THE INSULIN RECEPTOR

The insulin receptor is a large heterotetrameric transmembrane glycoprotein that is expressed in nearly all vertebrate tissues at levels ranging from as few as 40 receptors per cell in circulating erythrocytes to over 200,000 receptors per cell in adipocytes.[18,19] The receptor is composed of two 723-amino-acid polypeptide α subunits that are each linked to a β subunit (620 amino acids) and to each other by disulfide bonds, forming a functional dimeric protein complex (Fig. 5-1).[18–21] The extracellular α subunits contain the insulin binding domain,[22–24] and the transmembrane β subunits contain the insulin-regulated tyrosine kinase domain.[25,26] Both subunits are derived from a single prophor by proteolytic processing at a site consisting of four basic amino acids.[27–29] Noncovalent dimerization of ligand-bound receptor tyrosine kinases is generally observed,[30,31] but the insulin receptor (along with the closely related IGF-1 receptor and insulin-related receptor[32,33]) is unique in that the unbound receptor is maintained in the basal state as a covalent dimer.[34]

The insulin receptor gene is located on the short arm of human chromosome 19, near the low-density lipoprotein (LDL) receptor gene, and encodes a 4.2-kb mRNA, despite its 150-kb length.[35] The large size of the insulin receptor gene may lead to an increased susceptibility to random mutation, and hence to receptors with altered

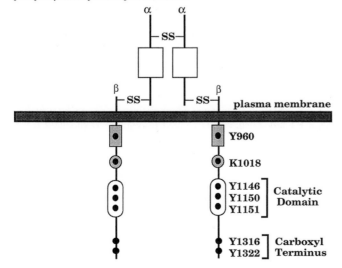

FIGURE 5-1. Structural features of the insulin receptor. The insulin receptor is a heterotetramer with two α and two β subunits linked by interchain disulfide bonds (—SS—). The α and β subunits are synthesized as a single polypeptide prior to proteolytic cleavage. The α subunits reside entirely on the extracellular surface. Numbering of individual amino acid residues are as in HIR-A, Ex11–.[10] **Open rectangles**, ligand-binding domains. **Filled rectangles**, juxtamembrane region. **Filled circles**, ATP-binding region. **Open oval**, regulatory region (Y xx YY). All tyrosines (**Y**) shown can be phosphorylated upon receptor activation.

biochemical activity. Alternative splicing of the receptor mRNA at exon 11 produces two nearly identical isoforms differing by 12 amino acids at the carboxyl-terminus of the α subunit.[36,37] These receptor variants are termed HIR-A (human insulin receptor, variant A, Ex11₂, lacking the 12 amino acids of exon 11) and HIR-B (Ex11₁). Although these isoforms are reported to exhibit subtle biochemical and physiologic differences,[38,39] changes in receptor protein isoform expression levels have not been consistently found in patients with diabetes mellitus.[29,40]

The binding of insulin to its receptor occurs with a stoichiometry of between 1 and 2 insulin molecules per receptor, and displays negative cooperativity as determined by Scatchard analysis.[41] Identification of the insulin-binding site or sites has been an important goal due to the implications such a finding has on the design of insulin analogs for therapeutic use. Although the exact sequences of the insulin receptor that directly associate with hormone are still being defined, the ligand-binding domain has been broadly mapped to the first 500 amino acids of the α subunit.[42–44] Use of various techniques such as affinity labeling, epitope mapping, *in vitro* mutagenesis, and construction of IGF-1/insulin receptor chimeras has allowed the identification of hormone-binding determinants within distinct regions of the α-subunit amino terminus.[19] Mutations in other regions of the α subunit can also adversely affect insulin binding, indicating that the hormone-binding site is created by the three-dimensional structure of the α subunit and does not rely solely on a linear segment of primary amino acid sequence.[18]

Once insulin is bound to the receptor, the β subunits undergo rapid autophosphorylation on tyrosine residues in the intracellular juxtamembrane domain (Y960, numbering of HIR-A, Ex11₂),[27] the regulatory region within the kinase domain (Y1146, Y1150, Y1151), and the carboxyl terminus (Y1316, Y1322).[18,19,29] Tyrosine autophosphorylation appears to occur through a transmechanism in which insulin binding to the α subunit of one αβ dimer stimulates the phosphorylation of the adjacent covalently bound β subunit.[45] Hormone binding appears to relieve an inhibitory constraint imposed by the extracellular domain of the receptor on its tyrosine kinase activity. This observation is based on several studies showing that proteolytic cleavage or mutagenesis of the extracellular domain results in constitutive receptor tyrosine kinase activity.[46–49] Consistent with these findings, crystallographic studies have shown that in the absence of insulin, the receptor's cytoplasmic domains bind and block its own active sites via a cis-inhibitory mechanism. This inhibition is relieved by insulin binding, which induces a conformational change in the receptor such that trans-tyrosine autophosphorylation and activation can occur.[50] Thus the insulin receptor behaves as a classic allosteric enzyme with both regulatory (α) and catalytic (β) subunits. Further analysis of the insulin receptor tyrosine kinase domain in the tyrosine phosphorylated state by x-ray crystallography has revealed a major change in the conformation of an inhibitory loop that blocks catalytic activity of the kinase (325). Thus the action of autophosphorylation of the receptor kinase to increase tyrosine kinase activity of the receptor can be explained at high resolution.

The autophosphorylation of the regulatory region increases the activity of the receptor tyrosine kinase 10- to 20-fold, leading to greatly increased tyrosine phosphorylation of cellular proteins, such as IRS-1 and Shc.[51,52] The activation of the receptor tyrosine kinase also permits transmission of the insulin signal to metabolic pathways, such as glucose transport, glycogen synthesis, protein synthesis, and lipid metabolism, within the cell.[19] The receptor is also phosphorylated on both serine and threonine residues by cellular kinases both in the basal state and after stimulation by phorbol esters, cyclic AMP analogs, and prolonged insulin treatment.[53,54] These phosphorylation events are often inhibitory to the receptor tyrosine kinase,[54,55] and provide an additional level of control that may play an important role in altering receptor activity in both physiologic and pathologic states. The combination of hormone binding, tyrosine autophosphorylation, and serine/threonine phosphorylation appear to comprise a complex network of regulatory mechanisms for maintaining appropriate insulin receptor function.

Numerous mutational studies have been performed to address the contribution of various domains and individual amino acid residues on ligand–receptor binding, receptor activation mechanisms, and intracellular signaling pathways, as well as receptor regulation and internalization. Although much of this information remains controversial, there have been some notable findings. Among these discoveries is that the tyrosine kinase activity of the receptor is essential for the metabolic and growth-promoting actions of insulin and for receptor internalization. Introduced mutations at the conserved lysine residue (K1018) in the kinase ATP-binding pocket abolish receptor tyrosine kinase activity and signaling,[26] and naturally occurring receptor mutations in this region have been found in cells of insulin-resistant individuals.[56–58] Numerous studies have also found that autophosphorylation of the regulatory region within the kinase domain is essential for regulating the kinase activity of the receptor towards endogenous substrates, such as IRS-1, and for the generation of metabolic signals, particularly glucose transport and glycogen synthesis, from the receptor (reviewed in reference 59).

In addition to signal transduction, the insulin receptor mediates internalization of itself bound to hormone. Endocytosis of this complex leads to insulin degradation and recycling of receptors back to the plasma membrane.[19] It appears that signaling by the insulin receptor in endosomes may be limited,[246] and is not required for its action on glucose utilization.[247] Interestingly, both the PI-3-kinase and MAP kinase pathways may be involved in regulating insulin receptor endocytosis and downstream trafficking.[248] Other proteins implicated are the GTPase Ral[249] and sorting nexins.[250] Although the mechanism by which the hormone–receptor complex is internalized is still under investigation, available evidence indicates the existence of more than one pathway for this process.[60,61] Aggregation of receptors into coated pits is a common initial endocytic step for many receptors, and is likely also a major pathway used by the insulin receptor.[61–63] In cases of prolonged insulin

stimulation, as is seen in patients with type 2 diabetes mellitus (T2DM),[64] receptors are degraded along with hormone, resulting in receptor downregulation and attenuation of the insulin signal.[65,66] These cases of hyperinsulinemic downregulation have been reported to cause selective loss of the HIR-A variant, as these receptors are preferentially occupied, internalized, and degraded.[37,39,67] Although insulin receptor internalization may not be required for full insulin action,[18] the internalized receptor is still catalytically active.[68] Impaired receptor internalization has been observed in cells of patients with T2DM,[64] suggesting that some element of the insulin signaling pathway is defective and may contribute to the disease state.

INSULIN RECEPTOR SUBSTRATES

In addition to the multisite tyrosine phosphorylation of the β subunit of the receptor, several endogenous candidate substrates for the insulin receptor tyrosine kinase have been identified in insulin-responsive tissues such as muscle, adipose tissue, and liver. These putative substrates appear to initiate events that lead to protein serine/threonine kinase and protein serine/threonine phosphate phosphatase regulation. The proteins in intact cells that are tyrosine phosphorylated (Table 5-1) in response to insulin include the first identified insulin receptor substrate, referred to as IRS-1,[73,76] and the Src homology collagen (Shc) protein, which has several forms.[69] Several isoforms of IRS-1 have now been identified, including IRS-2,[251] IRS-3,[252] and IRS-4.[253] The insulin-dependent tyrosine phosphorylation of several other substrates has also been reported, including Gab-1,[254] APS,[255,256] CAP,[257] Grb10,[258,259] and pp62Dok.[260] The full functional significance of these latter substrates is in the process of being determined. Therefore, we shall emphasize the best characterized tyrosine phosphorylated substrates (IRS-1 and related isoforms, and Shc) in this section and the next.

IRS-1 was initially identified as a 185-kd phosphoprotein present in antiphosphotyrosine immunoprecipitates from insulin-stimulated Fao hepatoma cells.[73] It is rapidly tyrosine phosphorylated in response to insulin in a dose-dependent manner. IRS-1 has been identified in virtually all insulin-sensitive cell types examined including rat myoblasts, Chinese hamster ovary cells, and adipocytes from rat, mouse, and humans (reviewed in reference 74). IRS-1 was successfully purified from liver extracts,[75] and

Table 5-1. Cellular Targets of Tyrosine Phosphorylation in Response to Insulin

Phosphoprotein	Role of Tyrosine Phosphorylation	Possible Physiologic Role of Phosphoprotein
Insulin receptor	Receptor kinase activation	Tyrosine phosphorylate substrates and initiate insulin actions
Insulin receptor substrate (IRS) proteins 1–4	Binding of SH2-containing proteins	
	Binding and activation of PI-3-K	Activation of Akt
	Binding and activation of SHP2	Activation of p21ras
	Binding and activation of Grb-2	Activation of p21ras
	Binding and activation of Nck	Actin polymerization
Gab-1	Binding of Grb2	Activation of p21ras
	Binding of PI-3-kinase	Activation of Akt
	Binding of PLC	Activation of PKC
c-Cbl	Binding of C3G	Activation of TC10 and Actin polymerization
APS	Binding of c-Cbl	Insulin receptor degradation
pp62Dok		Negative regulator of P21ras/MAP kinase
Grb10		Negative regulator of insulin receptor kinase

sufficient amino acid sequences of peptides were obtained to allow cloning of the full-length cDNA from a rat liver library.[76] Comparison of IRS-1 cDNA clones from the rat liver, mouse 3T3-L1 adipocytes,[77] and human skeletal muscle[78] reveals striking similarity at the nucleotide and amino acid level. Analysis of the IRS-1 amino acid sequence reveals a number of potential functionally important motifs, including a possible nucleotide-binding site near the amino-terminus and a pleckstrin homology (PH) domain between amino acid residues 7 and 120. PH domains are found in a variety of signaling molecules[79] and have been postulated to mediate protein–protein or protein–lipid interactions. In the case of IRS-1, the PH domain has been shown to be crucial for its proper engagement with the insulin receptor.[261,262] The PH domain appears to act in tandem with an adjacent domain, the PTB domain, in specifically orienting its association with the insulin receptor for optimal tyrosine phosphorylation.[263] PTB domains are known to bind directly to phosphotyrosine-containing peptides,[264,265] and in the case of the insulin receptor, tyrosine 960 in its juxtamembrane domain has been identified as the binding site for the IRS-1 PTB module.[266] Amino acid residues N-terminal to this tyrosine phosphate participate in defining the specificity of PTB domain binding. The PTB domains of the IRS isoforms are highly similar in amino acid sequence. Thus the combined actions of the PH and PTB domains of all the IRS proteins are thought to direct the physical association of these substrates to the insulin receptor. In addition, interactions of these domains with the insulin receptor are likely highly regulated by signaling mechanisms designed to control the strength of the signals emanating from the receptor.[267]

The most prominent feature of the IRS-1 molecule is the presence of at least 20 potential tyrosine phosphorylation sites, including 6 that occur in a repetitive motif YMXM, and 3 that present within a YXXM motif. Multiple potential tyrosine phosphorylation sites are also a prominent feature of the structures of the other IRS proteins.[268] Recent studies have unveiled a specialized functional role for tyrosine phosphorylated YXXM/YMXM motifs in the recognition of a specific protein domain homologous to a region of the Src tyrosine kinase referred to as the Src homology (SH)2 domain. SH2 domains are present in many intracellular signaling molecules, and bind with high affinity to specific phosphotyrosine motifs, thus creating the basis for specific protein–protein interactions within the cell. Moreover, several SH2-containing proteins possess intrinsic catalytic activities that appear to be regulated upon binding to specific phosphotyrosine motifs. IRS-1 also contains at least 35 potential serine or threonine phosphorylation sites, including recognition motifs for cyclic AMP–dependent protein kinase, protein kinase C, casein kinase II, and cdc2 kinase. IRS-1 is highly phosphorylated on serine and threonine residues; however, the exact residues and the functional significance of these phosphorylations in the intact cell are currently being defined.[269] Insulin action reportedly enhances phosphorylation of IRS-1 at a casein kinase II site.[80] Insulin also appears to initiate a feedback inhibition loop whereby the downstream protein serine/threonine kinase Akt phosphorylates IRS to cause inhibition of its function.[270]

The presence of multiple phosphorylated tyrosyl residues on IRS proteins, each with a selective binding specificity for PTB- or SH2-containing proteins, provides a mechanism for divergence of the insulin signal. According to this paradigm, tyrosine phosphorylation of IRS-1 and its isoforms provides a stage for the assembly of multimolecular signaling complexes and represents a potential pivotal point at which insulin-mediated metabolic and mitogenic

responses might diverge.[70-72] Because EGF and PDGF receptors fail to phosphorylate IRS-1,[73] such a mechanism also provides a level of specificity regarding the molecular events unique to insulin action. Several signaling molecules have been demonstrated to bind, in an insulin-dependent manner, to specific phosphotyrosine motifs on IRS-1 and its isoforms. These proteins include the p85/p110 type PtdIns 3′ kinase, which is required for the activation of one major switch mechanism to activate protein serine/threonine kinases. A second set of interacting proteins include the growth factor receptor–bound protein-2 (Grb2), the protein tyrosine phosphatase Syp/SHP2, and the adaptor Shc, all of which are involved in activating a second major pathway through the proto-oncogene GTPase p21Ras. How these proteins may contribute to the downstream actions of insulin will be briefly described.

The p85/p110-type PtdIns 3′ kinase is one of several lipid kinases responsible for the phosphorylation of phosphoinositides on the 3-position of the D-myo-inositol ring. This enzyme produces PtdIns(3)P, but also the multiphosphorylated PtdIns(3,4)P2 and PtdIns(3,4,5)P3 products. The physiologic role of these novel phospholipids has been studied extensively, and several downstream effector domains characterized, including FYVE and PX domains [PtdIns(3)P][271] and certain PH domains [PtdIns(3,4)P2 and PtdIns(3,4,5)P3].[272] The p85/p110-type PtdIns 3′ kinase activation has been linked to several biologic actions, including glucose transport regulation, glycogen synthesis, growth factor–stimulated mitogenesis, and cellular growth. The enzyme is comprised of a 110-kd catalytic subunit (p110) and an 85-kd regulatory subunit (p85), which contains two SH2 domains and a single SH3 domain. PtdIns 3′ kinase was the first enzymatic activity shown to associate with tyrosine phosphorylated IRS-1.[76] More recently, *in vitro* studies indicate that phosphotyrosines at positions 608 and 939 of IRS-1[81] preferentially bind to the SH2 domains of p85, thus enhancing PtdIns 3′ kinase activity. This IRS-mediated pathway is illustrated in Fig. 5-2A. It is clear that binding of this lipid kinase is a major

FIGURE 5-2. Elements of the PI-3-kinase pathway. **A.** The insulin receptor catalyzes tyrosine phosphorylation of IRS proteins which recruit the p85 regulatory subunit of PI-3-kinase to the membrane, where the catalytic p110 subunit phosphorylates PtdIns(4,5)P2 to produce PtdIns(3,4,5)P3. **B.** Membrane-bound PtdIns(3,4,5)P3 attracts the protein serine/threonine kinases PDK1 and Akt to the membrane through binding their PH domains, where PDK1 phosphorylates and activates Akt. Other protein kinases are also phosphorylated and activated by PDK1, while substrates of Akt include the protein kinase GSK3, transcription factors forkhead and CREB, and the apoptosis-related protein BAD.

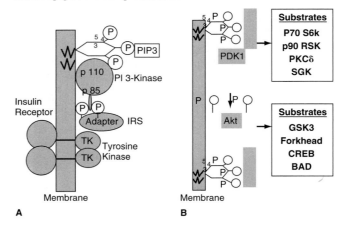

function of all the IRS proteins, and that activation of its downstream protein serine/threonine kinases represents a major pathway for the regulation of metabolic processes by insulin in its target tissues.[268]

Another cellular component capable of binding specifically to IRS-1 is Grb2,[81] a protein first characterized by its ability to bind directly to tyrosine-phosphorylated EGF receptors.[82] Grb2 is devoid of catalytic activity and is comprised of a single SH2 domain flanked by two distinct protein–binding domains that share significant homology to a region of the Src tyrosine kinase referred to as the SH3 domain. SH3 domains recognize proline-rich sequences, thus mediating specific protein–protein interactions.[83,84] The SH2/SH3-containing Grb2 molecule is particularly interesting, because it binds the ras activating protein, Son-of-sevenless (Sos).[85,86] Therefore, one possible consequence of insulin-dependent formation of IRS-1:Grb2:Sos complexes is the activation of ras.[69] It has been suggested that IRS-1 is indispensable for insulin-stimulated mitogenesis and cell-cycle progression[87]; however, gene knockout experiments demonstrate that IRS-1 is not required for insulin-mediated responses to be observed in intact animals.[88,89] The ability of insulin to stimulate mitogen-activated protein kinase in livers of normal mice and those homozygous for the IRS-1 knockout was indistinguishable. Moreover, replacement of the specific Grb2 recognition site on IRS-1 (tyrosine 895) with phenylalanine fails to abrogate insulin-induced mitogenesis.[90] These results provide evidence for an IRS-1–independent pathway that contributes to the mitogenic response that may involve Grb2 association with other putative insulin receptor substrates such as other IRS protein isoforms or Shc.

The microtubule-activated GTPase dynamin also binds to the SH3 domain(s) of Grb2 through a proline-rich region present in its COOH-terminal domain.[91–93] Evidence suggests that the dynamin GTPase activity is increased upon binding to the Grb2 SH3 domain.[91] Insulin stimulation results in the formation of a heterotrimeric complex between IRS-1 and Grb2:dynamin. GTPase activity is stimulated when a phosphotyrosine peptide containing the Grb2 binding site of IRS-1 is added to the dynamin:Grb2 complex in a cell-free system.[94] The precise role that the dynamin plays in receptor-mediated signaling events remains unclear; however, several recent reports suggest a functional role in receptor-mediated endocytosis[95] and clathrin-coated vesicle function.[96] Mutations within the GTP binding site of dynamin block receptor-mediated endocytosis at a stage following coat assembly and preceding the sequestration of ligand into deeply invaginated coated pits.[95] The next critical step is to precisely define the functional role, if any, of IRS-1:Grb2:dynamin complex formation in the insulin-induced endocytic event.

A third SH2-containing molecule capable of binding to phosphorylated IRS-1 in response to insulin is the protein tyrosine phosphatase, Syp/SHPTP2/SHP2.[81,97] SHP2 contains two SH2 domains, both of which are believed to mediate binding to tyrosine-phosphorylated IRS-1.[98] A systematic analysis of the relative binding affinities of various IRS-1 phosphopeptides for the amino- and carboxy-terminal SH2 domains of SHP2 revealed preferential binding of phosphotyrosine residues 1172 and 1222, respectively.[98,99] These IRS-1 phosphopeptides specifically stimulate SHP2 phosphatase activity up to 50-fold *in vitro*, suggesting that SHP2 represents a second enzymatic activity regulated upon association with IRS-1. Recent investigations using a catalytically inactive SHP2 mutant, which still binds IRS-1, demonstrate that insulin-dependent formation of the IRS-1:SHP2 complex may con-

tribute to insulin-induced ras activation;[100,101] however, the molecular mechanism for this role of SHP2 has yet to be elucidated.[273]

SHP2 also binds directly to the SH2 domain of Grb2 in response to PDGF.[102] This interaction is presumably a reflection of PDGF-induced tyrosine phosphorylation of SHP2.[102,103] Insulin receptor activation does not result in the tyrosine phosphorylation of SHP2,[97] a finding consistent with the inability to detect a complex of SHP2 and Grb2 after insulin treatment.[101] In any event, the ability of SHP2 to associate with IRS-1 in an insulin-dependent manner suggests this protein may be one of many participants in the cascade of events mediating the biologic actions of insulin.

Several variant sequences in the IRS genes have been reported to be increased in prevalence among patients with T2DM, for example the Gly to Arg72 substitution in IRS-1 that seems to have a pathogenic role.[104,274–278] The regulation of insulin signaling through IRS-1 has been studied in several models of diabetes, including the insulin-deficient streptozocin (STZ)-treated rat and the insulin-resistant ob/ob mouse.[74,105] These studies demonstrate that IRS-1 phosphorylation parallels that of insulin receptor phosphorylation, suggesting that the tyrosine kinase activity of the receptor is rate-limiting in the cascade of events following insulin administration to diabetic animals. Furthermore, in diabetic animals the level of IRS-1 protein is differentially regulated in liver and muscle. In the liver, IRS-1 protein is increased in hypoinsulinemic states and decreased in hyperinsulinemic states, whereas the converse is observed in muscle. Collectively, these data suggest that IRS-1 is centrally located within the insulin-signaling pathway and, by virtue of its ability to assemble multimeric protein complexes, is uniquely positioned to orchestrate biologic responses to insulin. Recent studies using cells with low endogenous levels of IRS-1, such as oocytes[106] and 32-D myeloid progenitor cells,[107] provide evidence that IRS-1 is critical for the restoration of insulin-dependent cell-cycle progression. Furthermore, IRS-1–deficient mice exhibit impaired growth and development as well as some resistance to the glucose-lowering effect of insulin.[279–282] Insulin signaling is also dramatically impaired in mice with only one allele each of the insulin receptor and IRS-1 genes.[283] Therefore, IRS-1 appears to be necessary for normal growth and metabolism. Similarly, it is likely that IRS-2 also contributes significantly to glucose homeostasis, based on studies with IRS-2–deficient mice, and this includes significant effects both in the peripheral tissues,[284–286] and in the β cells[287] of the pancreas which produce and secrete insulin. Taken together, these studies of mice with ablated IRS genes fully support a central role of IRS-1 and IRS-2 in the mechanisms by which insulin signals to its target cells.

INSULIN ACTION THROUGH THE PI-3-KINASE SIGNALING PATHWAY

The generation of cellular 3′ phophoinositides by activation of the p85/p110 type PI-3-kinase through its recruitment to insulin receptor substrate proteins represents a major triggering event for a multitude of insulin's actions. These include many physiologically important metabolic effects, such as its regulation of glucose transport in muscle and fat, as well as its enhancement of glycogen synthesis and protein synthesis. The insulin-activated PI-3-kinase acts preferentially on PtdIns(4,5)P2 to yield the signaling lipid PtdIns(3,4,5)P3, as depicted in Fig. 5-2A. This mediator, as well as PtdIns(3,4)P2 that is generated either by phophosphorylation of PtdIns(4)P or dephosphorylation of PtdIns(3,4,5)P3, appears in the inner leaflet of the plasma membrane very rapidly upon insulin stimulation. This cell surface localization has been established through the use of PH domains that have high affinity and selectivity for binding PtdIns(3,4,5)P3 or PtdIns(3,4,5)P3 and PtdIns(3,4)P2.[288–290] Phosphorylation of PtdIns to generate PtdIns(3)P also probably occurs in response to insulin, but this adds little to the total pool of PtdIns(3)P present in unstimulated cells. Thus the PI-3-kinase pathway of insulin signaling is thought to reflect downstream events initiated by the two 3′ polyphosphoinositides described above.

The major downstream effector proteins of PtdIns(3,4,5)P3 and PtdIns(3,4)P2 in response to insulin are thought to be the protein kinases PDK1 and Akt.[291] As shown in Fig. 5-2B, both protein kinases are thought to localize to the plasma membrane through binding of their PH domains to these phosphoinositides. There is evidence that the higher affinity of the PDK1 PH domain for phosphoinositide compared to that of Akt renders the former protein kinase membrane-bound even in the absence of insulin.[292] According to this scheme, Akt is recruited to PtdIns(3,4,5)P3 at the plasma membrane, thus allowing it to become a substrate for PDK1. Phosphorylation of Akt at threonine 308 by PDK1 and serine 473 by an unknown protein kinase causes activation of its protein kinase activity. The active form of Akt can presumably move to the cytoplasm as well as migrate to the nucleus, where it can phosphorylate substrates.

The PI-3-kinase cascade leads to the activation of multiple protein serine/threonine kinases based on the fact that both PDK1 and Akt can phosphorylate and activate several such enzymes (Fig. 5-2B). PDK1, for example, acts on the serum- and glucocorticoid-induced kinases,[293] p70 S6K protein kinase,[294] p21-activated protein kinase,[295] and p90 RSK protein kinase,[296] and two protein kinase C isoforms.[297] Akt, on the other hand, phosphorylates and inactivates the protein kinase GSK3,[298,299] which modulates glycogen synthase as discussed in detail in a later section. These protein kinases downstream of PDK1 and Akt each potentially have multiple substrates which can potentially regulate multiple cellular processes. Thus a tremendous diversity of cell functions can be regulated by the production of 3′ polyphosphoinositides in response to insulin. These include nuclear functions. For example, the phosphorylation of the transcription factor forkhead by Akt occurs acutely in response to the hormone,[300,301] but other kinases may also be critical to regulation of forkhead.[302] Recent evidence suggests that hepatic gluconeogenesis may in part be inhibited by insulin through this forkhead-mediated mechanism which regulates gene expression.[303] Three other examples of signaling downstream of PDK1 are the regulation of glucose transport, glycogen synthesis, and protein synthesis, as discussed in detail below.

REGULATION OF GLUCOSE TRANSPORT

One of the most dramatic and important biologic functions of insulin *in vivo* is the rapid stimulation of glucose transport across muscle and fat cell membranes. This effect has been extensively studied both *in vivo* and in isolated cell systems, where effects of insulin in the 10- to 30-fold range are readily observed. Only fat and muscle cells exhibit this extraordinary responsiveness to insulin with respect to glucose uptake, and only these cell types express a particular glucose transporter protein isoform, GLUT-4[108] (also known as the insulin-regulated glucose transporter). In the absence of insulin, almost all of the GLUT-4 transporter is se-

questered in intracellular, tubulovesicular endosomal membrane structures, as visualized by immunoelectron microscopy.[109,110] Fractionation of fat or muscle cells in the basal state leads to a low-density microsome preparation that is rich in GLUT-4 transporter protein. Addition of insulin to intact muscle or fat cells rapidly redistributes the GLUT-4 from the low-density microsomes to the plasma membrane fraction.[111–113] Cell surface localization of GLUT-4 in response to insulin is confirmed by immunoelectron microscopy.[109,110] A variety of independent techniques have further documented this major effect of insulin to cause GLUT-4 transporters to localize at the cell surface membrane, where they can catalyze glucose transport.[113–116] It is not known whether additional effects of insulin are involved in regulating glucose uptake, such as an increase in the intrinsic catalytic activity of glucose transporter proteins.[117]

Data now available related to insulin action on glucose transport suggest two possible mechanisms whereby intracellular GLUT-4 in endosomal membranes may redistribute to the plasma membrane. The first possibility is that sequences within the GLUT-4 molecule cause intracellular retention of the protein by binding to putative intracellular membrane receptor species. According to this concept, such GLUT-4 receptors might prevent GLUT-4 from traveling back to the plasma membrane via endosomal recycling pathways. Consistent with this hypothesis, several laboratories have recently identified domains within the GLUT-4 transporter that appear to be necessary for intracellular sequestration. Three groups have identified the 30-amino-acid COOH-terminus of GLUT-4 as the major sequestration signal.[118–120] Sequences within the middle region of GLUT-4 have also been suggested as influencing intracellular localization by two laboratory groups.[118,121] It is not clear why earlier indications of a role for N-terminal sequences of GLUT-4 in maintaining its unique cellular localization[122] have not been observed by other laboratories.[118–120] However, experiments with chimera glucose transporters expressed in cultured adipocytes do appear to suggest some influence of the N-terminal region of GLUT-4 on its trafficking.[304]

Recently, a dileucine motif has been identified as the element within the COOH-terminal 30 amino acids of GLUT-4 that may be responsible for its sequestration signal.[123,124] Other nearby acidic sequences may also be involved.[305] Mutation of these leucines (residues 489 and 490) to alanines abolishes the ability of the GLUT-4 COOH-terminus to direct intracellular localization, although this may not be the case in cultured adipocytes.[304] These experiments were conducted by utilizing chimera transporter constructs, linking regions of GLUT-4 to domains of the ubiquitously expressed GLUT-1 transporter isoform. GLUT-1 is predominantly a cell surface protein even in the basal state. Thus, substituting the 30-amino-acid COOH-terminus of GLUT-4, but not the dialanine mutant construct, confers an intracellular localization to this transporter chimera. It remains to be determined whether other domains of GLUT-4 act in concert with the dileucine motif, but the latter is clearly an important functional element. Importantly, these data lead to the hypothesis that an as-yet-unidentified receptor for this dileucine motif plays a role in GLUT-4 sequestration within the endosomal compartment. Furthermore, insulin action may cause disruption of this interaction between GLUT-4 and its dileucine receptor to cause release of GLUT-4 into the membrane recycling pathway. This hypothesis requires rigorous evaluation and testing in future studies.

A second mode by which insulin may regulate GLUT-4 redistribution to the plasma membrane is the stimulation of bulk intracellular membrane flow to the cell surface. According to this hypothesis, GLUT-4 present in intracellular membrane compartments would be moved with these membranes as they translocate to the plasma membrane. This concept is consistent with several studies that indicate the major effect of insulin is to stimulate exocytosis of GLUT-4 from intracellular vesicles, although an insulin effect to inhibit endocytosis of GLUT-4 has also been observed.[8,125,126] Estimations of the kinetics of endocytosis versus exocytosis of GLUT-4 in basal and insulin-stimulated cells indicate that GLUT-4 continuously recycles between plasma membrane and intracellular membranes in both conditions.

Further support for the concept that insulin causes bulk membrane movement to the cell surface has been recently reported. First, many other receptors and transporter proteins, such as GLUT-1, are also depleted in intracellular membranes upon insulin action, suggesting an effect even on proteins that lack the dileucine motif.[127,128] Second, components that are involved in membrane docking and fusion events, such as Rab and guanine nucleotide dissociation inhibitor (GDI) proteins, are markedly modulated by insulin.[129,130] Both Rab4 and the GDI2 isoform are released from endosomal membranes to the cytoplasm upon insulin action. This is consistent with the notion that insulin causes membrane movements and fusions, resulting in the rapid cycling of these proteins. Similar data have been presented for the synaptobrevin protein.[131] The membrane proteins thought to be involved in the trafficking and fusion of GLUT-4–containing vesicles have recently been discussed in a review format.[306] Finally, insulin causes a decreased amount of GLUT-4 vesicle mass when these membranes are purified from control versus stimulated adipocytes.[307] Taken together, these results are consistent with the notion that insulin receptor signaling causes major changes in the dynamics of membrane recycling pathways and exocytosis of GLUT-4, causing increased concentrations of GLUT-4 and other proteins in these compartments at the cell surface.

The mechanisms by which insulin might cause intracellular membrane movements are not understood. However, recent data suggest the possibility that regulation of PI-3-kinase activity by insulin plays a key role in regulating glucose transporter redistribution to the plasma membrane. Important studies in yeast suggest that the product of the VPS34 gene, which displays PI-3-kinase activity, is an important element in membrane trafficking to the vacuole.[132] Moreover, in mammalian cells it has been demonstrated that PDGF receptor trafficking to the lysosome depends upon its ability to bind PI-3-kinase.[133] Taken together, these data indicate that PI-3-kinase activity, presumably through 3' phosphoinositide reaction products, plays a major role in membrane trafficking phenomena in mammalian systems. Furthermore, several laboratories have demonstrated that insulin action on glucose transporter translocation is inhibited by highly specific PI-3-kinase inhibitors.[134–136] Dominant negative regulators of PI-3-kinase also block insulin action on glucose transport.[308] These data directly implicate, although do not prove, that the increased PI-3-kinase activity observed in the presence of insulin is necessary for GLUT-4 translocation.

Recent data have converged to strongly implicate Akt as a necessary signaling element downstream of PI-3-kinase in GLUT-4 regulation by insulin. First, expression of membrane-directed Akt in cultured adipocytes leads to sustained GLUT-4 translocation, mimicking the action of insulin.[309] Secondly, a triple mutant dominant negative construct of Akt is inhibitory to insulin action on GLUT-4 when expressed in such adipocytes.[310] Finally, mice with ablated genes for each of two isoforms of this protein kinase have been prepared. The double knockout is lethal, and the Akt1 knockout mouse shows no sign of deficient insulin action on glucose uptake in fat.[311] However, mice lacking the gene encoding Akt2, the predominant isoform in fat, show insulin resistance and a defective responsiveness of glucose transport to insulin in both muscle and fat cells.[312] Taken together, these results indicate that Akt likely plays a major role in mediating the action of insulin on GLUT-4 translocation. However, it should also be noted that very recent reports indicate there may be a PI-3-kinase–independent signaling pathway that operates in conjunction with Akt to cause GLUT-4 translocation. This pathway may involve binding of CAP to the insulin receptor, thereby attracting c-Cbl to the complex.[313] This in turn recruits the exchange factor C3G, which can activate the GTP-binding protein TC10.[314] This PI-3-kinase pathway may be required to mobilize F-actin filaments thought to be necessary for some step in the movement of GLUT-4–containing vesicles to the plasma membrane.[315–319] Further studies will be required to clarify the role of this pathway in regulating GLUT-4.

REGULATION OF PROTEIN SYNTHESIS

It has long been recognized that insulin and other growth factors increase the rate of protein synthesis.[195,196] Insulin stimulation appears to act primarily on the process of initiation of translation, in that insulin increases the number of initiated ribosomes.[197–199] The binding of ribosomes to mRNA is facilitated by complexes of eukaryotic initiation factors (eIF).[200] There are two steps in the initiation of translation where insulin might exert its effect. These are the attachment of the initiator methionyl-tRNA (met-tRNA$_i$) to the ribosome and the binding of mRNA.

The delivery of the initiator met-tRNA$_i$ to ribosomes is mediated by the initiation factors eIF-2 and eIF-2B. The heterotrimeric G protein eIF-2 binds to met-tRNA$_i$ in a GTP-dependent manner.[196] Following the formation of the ribosomal 80S initiation complex, eIF-2–bound GTP is hydrolyzed to GDP and the GDP·eIF-2 is released from the ribosome. Until its bound GDP is exchanged for GTP, eIF-2 cannot bind another met-tRNA$_i$. This GDP to GTP exchange is catalyzed by the guanine nucleotide exchange factor eIF-2B (formally called GEF).[196] Phosphorylation on serine 51 of the eIF-2 subunit has been shown to inhibit its ability to bind eIF-2B, which subsequently impedes translation.[201] It has been reported that insulin decreases eIF-2α phosphorylation in calf chondrocytes.[202] Yet in Swiss 3T3 fibroblast, insulin or other growth factors have no effect on eIF-2 phosphorylation.[203] However, insulin apparently does increase the activity of eIF-2B in Swiss 3T3 fibroblasts.[203] In vitro eIF-2B is a substrate for casein kinase 1 and 2 and GSK-3, but it is disputed whether these phosphorylations have an effect on exchange activity.[204–206] Likewise, it is not yet known if insulin changes the phosphorylation state of eIF-2B in vivo.

The initiation complex involved in binding mRNA is eIF-4F, which is composed of three polypeptides, eIF-4E, eIF-4A, and p220. Initiation factor eIF-4E recognizes the 5' 7-methylguanosine cap structure; eIF-4A is an RNA helicase, and p220 (also known as eIF-4γ) is believed to be an RNA-binding protein. The binding of eIF-4F to RNA is followed by the binding of eIF-4B, which appears to stimulate the helicase activity of eIF-4A.[200,207] Three of these initiation factors, eIF-4E, p220, and eIF-4B, have been shown to be phosphorylated in response to insulin.[208,209] Although the functions of p220 and eIF-4B phosphorylations are not known, mutating the major phosphorylation site of eIF-4E, serine 53, to an alanine results in the protein failing to bind to initiation complexes.[210] Thus a mechanism may exist where insulin exerts control over translation through the phosphorylation olf these initiation factors.

A major breakthrough in determining how insulin controls the initiation of protein synthesis came with the discovery that the eIF-4E binding protein, 4E-BP1, is identical to the MAPK substrate PHAS.[8] PHAS is a 12.4-kd heat- and acid-soluble protein that is phosphorylated in response to insulin. Moreover, serine 64, the major site in PHAS that is phosphorylated by insulin *in vivo*, is also phosphorylated by MAPK *in vitro*, indicating that MAPK phosphorylates PHAS directly upon insulin stimulation.[10,211] In its unphosphorylated state, PHAS/4E-BP1 can bind to eIF-4E, but eIF-4E does not bind PHAS/4E-BP1 phosphorylated by MAPK *in vitro* or PHAS/4E-BP1 from insulin-treated adipose tissue. Furthermore, when eIF-4E is complexed to PHAS/4E-BP1, it no longer can bind to a 7 methyl GDP resin. Finally, PHAS/4E-BP1 can inhibit cap-dependent, but not cap-independent, translation *in vitro*.[8,9] Taken together, these data suggest that in unstimulated cells, eIF-4E is bound to PHAS/4E-BP1, which inhibits translation initiation. Insulin stimulation results in the phosphorylation of PHAS/4E-BP1, which dissociates eIF-4E from PHAS/4E-BP1. This allows eIF-4E to bind to 5′ caps and initiate translation.[8]

A major breakthrough in understanding how this pathway is regulated in intact cells resulted from experiments showing that the protein kinase mTOR, the target of rapamycin inhibition, accounts for phosphorylation of PHAS in intact cells.[320] This mTOR protein kinase is downstream of PI-3-kinase, evidenced by its inhibition by wortmannin.[321] Furthermore, it was demonstrated that activation of Akt in intact cells leads to enhanced mTOR activity related to PHAS phosphorylation.[321] What is as yet unresolved is which protein kinases downstream of Akt directly phosphorylate mTOR in intact cells, and how they are apparently activated by Akt. Nonetheless, these new results clearly place control of protein synthesis by insulin within the PI-3-kinase/PDK1/Akt pathway.

REGULATION OF GLYCOGEN SYNTHESIS

A major consequence of insulin stimulation of muscle, fat, and liver is the rapid synthesis of glycogen.[212–214] The rate-limiting step of glycogen metabolism is catalyzed by the enzyme glycogen synthase. Skeletal muscle glycogen synthase is an 80- to 84-kd protein that contains at least nine different serines that have been shown to be phosphorylated *in vivo*.[213,215] Seven of these sites are clustered at the C-terminus of the protein, and the other two are located in the N-terminal region. Over 30 years ago, it was shown that the activity of glycogen synthase is inhibited by phosphorylation, and that insulin stimulates glycogen synthase through dephosphorylation.[216,217] Insulin is believed to activate glycogen synthase by decreasing the phosphorylation of a C-terminal region that contains three serine residues, C30, C34, and C38.[218] A 24-hour insulin stimulation of rabbits has also been reported to dephosphorylate the N-terminal phosphorylation site serine N7.[214,219] Thus it is apparent that in order for insulin to activate glycogen synthase, it must either activate phosphatases, inhibit kinases, or both.

The major phosphatase responsible for the dephosphorylation of glycogen synthase is protein phosphatase-1 (PP1).[220] In skeletal muscle, a glycogen-bound isoform of PP1, PP1G, is involved in regulating glycogen synthase in response to insulin. PP1G consists of two subunits, a 37-kd catalytic (C) subunit and a 160-kd G

subunit required for the enzyme to interact with glycogen particles.[221–223] Phosphorylation of the G subunit occurs at two separate sites, designated as site 1 and site 2. Site 2 is not phosphorylated in response to insulin, and its phosphorylation results in the dissociation of PP1G from glycogen particles, which subsequently decreases PP1G activity towards glycogen synthase.[222] Phosphorylation at site 1 is stimulated by insulin and results in an increase in the rate at which PP1G dephosphorylates glycogen synthase.[15] In rat skeletal muscle, the kinase that phosphorylates the G subunit site 1 in response to insulin may be the p90 isoform of ribosomal protein S6 kinase,[224] which is sometimes called MAP kinase-activated protein kinase-1 (MAPKAPK-1). This kinase itself is activated by phosphorylation catalyzed by MAPK, which thus was postulated to link the dephosphorylation of glycogen synthase in skeletal muscle to the activation of p21ras by the insulin receptor.[193] Remarkably, however, mice that have had the gene for the G targeting subunit ablated have recently been found to exhibit no apparent phenotype.[322] Moreover, their muscle glycogen synthase is readily activated by insulin. These new results confound the above postulates, and suggest there is another phosphatase involved in insulin action on glycogen synthase.

Another way in which glycogen synthase may be activated is through the inhibition of kinases that phosphorylate it. Although at least six different kinases can phosphorylate glycogen synthase, the three primary C-terminal serines believed to be dephosphorylated in response to insulin are all substrates for glycogen-synthase kinase-3 (GSK3).[214,225] There are two isoforms of GSK3, α and β, which are 90% identical in their kinase domains.[226] Besides glycogen synthase, GSK3 can phosphorylate a wide variety of other substrates, such as inhibitor 2 of PP1,[227] type II regulatory subunit of cyclic AMP–dependent protein kinase,[228] eukaryotic protein synthesis initiation factor (eIF-2B),[206] and the transcription factors c-jun and c-myc.[229,230]

Originally, GSK3 was thought to be constitutively activated. However, the α isoform of GSK3 was recently found to be identical to ATP citrate lyase kinase, which has been shown in rat fat cells to be deactivated by insulin.[231] Further studies have shown that the GSK3α from skeletal muscle is phosphorylated by both p70 and p90 S6 kinases *in vitro*, and that this phosphorylation inhibits 80% of the GSK3 activity.[232] It has also been reported that in both CHO cells overexpressing the insulin receptor (CHOT) and in rat skeletal muscle L6 cells, wortmannin, which can inhibit p70 and p90 S6 kinase in some cells, blocks insulin's ability to deactivate GSK3. Moreover, insulin-stimulated GSK3 deactivation is not blocked by rapamycin, which inhibits p70 but not p90 S6 kinase.[233,234] Thus the activity of GSK3, like PP1, is influenced by p90 S6 kinase and the ras-MAPK pathway. However, EGF also activates MAPK and p90 S6 kinase, yet it fails to activate glycogen synthase.[214,235] Thus another pathway is required to fulfill this role.[17] Again, the PI-3-kinase pathway appears to be the key to glycogen synthase regulation because wortmannin is found to inhibit insulin signaling to this enzyme. Furthermore, Akt has been shown to phosphorylate and inactivate GSK3,[289,299] leading to the hypothesis that this inhibition contributes to glycogen synthase activation by insulin.

THE RAS–PROTEIN KINASE SIGNALING PATHWAY

The GTP-binding protein p21ras is the normal product of the first oncogene found in human neoplastic tissue. It exists in activated forms in approximately one-third of human tumors, and it is therefore not surprising that p21ras is now one of the most extensively studied proteins.[143–149] Four similar ras proteins have been identified, H-p21ras, K-p21rasA, K-p21rasB, and N-p21ras, each of which can function as an oncogene when carrying certain mutations, and a somewhat more distantly related nontransforming R-p21ras has also been identified. The protein p21ras is located at the plasma membrane, and this localization is essential for its biologic function.[150] Although inactive when bound to GDP, when bound to GTP, p21ras triggers a large number of cellular responses. The structural basis for the difference in activities of p21ras bound to the two nucleotides has been studied in great detail. Mutational analysis has shown that amino acids in the region 32–40 are of particular importance for interaction of p21ras with downstream effectors, and this has therefore been termed the effector region. Crystallographic analysis of p21ras bound to GDP or GTP has revealed that the effector region and another small region differ significantly in conformation in the two forms. Thus it is thought that interaction of the effector domain with critical cellular targets is crucial to transmission of downstream signals. Interestingly, p21ras has now been demonstrated to be involved in at least some of the intracellular signaling pathways of insulin.[140–142,151–154]

In the continuous presence of insulin, maximal GTP loading of p21ras is achieved after 2–5 minutes at 37°C.[155] This is followed by a deactivation phase, and the GTP content of p21ras returns to basal levels after 20–30 minutes. The nucleotide content of p21ras is determined by two reactions. It has an intrinsic weak GTPase activity, which converts bound GTP to GDP. This reaction can be enhanced up to 50-fold by the presence of certain proteins such as GAP and neurofibromin.[156] These proteins can therefore be seen as deactivators of p21ras, and inhibition of their activities may result in activation of p21ras. Such a mechanism appears to exist in T lymphocytes,[157] but may not be of significance in the p21ras response in insulin-sensitive tissues. The activities of GDP/GTP exchange factors offer a different route of p21ras activation. These factors cause the release of bound GDP from p21ras, followed by the spontaneous binding of GTP. Pulse-chase experiments using permeabilized cells have demonstrated that p21ras activation by insulin is brought about by increased exchange activities, rather than by decreases of GTPase activities.[158] Two closely related exchange factors, Son-of-sevenless (Sos) 1 and 2, are present in insulin-sensitive tissues,[159] as is a newly discovered exchange factor, C3G.[160] Sos is rapidly phosphorylated on serine and threonine after stimulation with insulin, but the role of this phosphorylation is at present unclear.

Insulin may cause p21ras activation primarily through tyrosine phosphorylation of the Shc family of proteins.[161,162] These proteins are ubiquitously expressed as three forms in cells. They all contain a carboxy-terminal SH2 domain, and have a glycine- and proline-rich region of homology to collagen in their amino terminal regions. As yet, no catalytic activity has been ascribed to Shc. Shc tyrosine phosphorylation results in the formation of complexes with Grb2 and Sos,[155,163] and such complexes could result in p21ras activation simply by recruiting Sos to its substrate, p21ras, at the cell membrane. Current results implicate a complex array of components involved in positioning Sos to interact with p21ras at the membrane,[164,165] as shown in Fig. 5-3. It is also possible that the intrinsic exchange activity of Sos is modulated in response to insulin, perhaps as a consequence of complex formation or as a result of phosphorylation.

The search for downstream targets for p21ras has been extensive, and recent progress has greatly enhanced our understanding

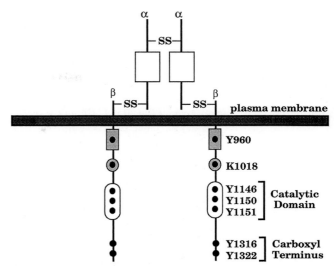

FIGURE 5-3. Hypothetical model of components involved in causing GTP loading of p21ras and activation of downstream targets by insulin. **A.** According to this model, insulin-receptor activation causes tyrosine phosphorylation of itself, recruiting Shc through its SH2 domain. The bound Shc is tyrosine phosphorylated by the receptor or by another tyrosine kinase, recruiting Grb2/Sos complexes through the SH2 domain of Grb2. The presence of a necessary component (**B**) that binds the N-terminal domain of Sos is suggested by recent results using truncation mutants of Sos.[164,16] **B.** Activation of p21ras leads to activation of the protein serine/threonine kinase Raf-1, which initiates a cascade that activates MAP kinase. MAP kinase regulates the protein kinase p90[RSK], and together they phosphorylate and regulate a transcription factor involved in controlling gene expression.

of the processes controlled by p21ras. Raf-1 is a 74-kd serine/threonine kinase that in mutated form acts as an oncogene.[166] The kinase domain resides in the carboxy-terminal part of the molecule, whereas the amino-terminal part is considered important in regulating the kinase activity, because mutations in this region activate the oncogenic potential of Raf-1. A prolonged search for a ligand that might bind to the regulatory domain of Raf-1 resulted in the discovery that it binds to p21ras specifically in the GTP-bound, biologically active form.[1] Mutations in the effector domain of p21ras that render it biologically inactive in cells also abolish Raf-1 binding. Binding of Raf-1 directly to p21ras explains the translocation from the cytosol to the cell membrane that Raf-1 undergoes in response to growth factors. Once bound to p21ras at the cell membrane, Raf-1 is activated. This appears not to be simply the result of binding to p21ras, because Raf-1 is not activated when bound to p21ras *in vitro*. When a membrane targeting signal is added to the carboxy-terminal part of Raf-1, the kinase was found to be constitutively active after transfection into COS-1 cells.[167,168] This was the case even when dominant negative mutants of p21ras were cotransfected, indicating that activation of Raf-1 is independent of p21ras function once the Raf kinase has been recruited to the plasma membrane. Thus the role of activated p21ras may simply be to cause Raf-1 to translocate to the membrane, after which other processes occur to activate the kinase. Also, under certain conditions Raf-1 dissociates from p21ras in detergent extracts of hormone-stimulated cells, while remaining activated.[167] Recent results indicate that Raf-1 phosphorylation and dephosphorylation correlate with active and less active forms of the enzyme, suggesting that the role of p21ras-mediated recruitment of Raf-1 to the membrane is to promote its phosphorylation and activation.[323]

Also, chaperone proteins such as 14-3-3 appear to be involved in the regulation of Raf-1 activity. The exact molecular events that lead to Raf-1 activation are still unclear, however.[324]

The substrate specificity of Raf-1 is quite limited and the only known cellular target is a protein kinase, MAP kinase (MEK). This kinase was first isolated as an activator of yet another protein kinase, the mitogen-activated protein kinase (MAPK). MEK is activated by phosphorylation on serines by Raf-1. Curiously, MEK phosphorylates MAPK at both a threonine and a tyrosine located in a Thr-Glu-Tyr motif. Thus MEK has the rather unusual property of being able to phosphorylate both an aliphatic and an aromatic amino acid. By mutational analysis and by selective dephosphorylation with protein phosphatases, phosphorylation of both the tyrosine and threonine has been demonstrated to be required for activation of MAPK.[2,169–177] In the cell, activation of MAPK is transient even in the continued presence of insulin, and the time course is similar to that of p21ras activation.[178] Thus a cascade of phosphorylation and activation events occur with these kinases.[2,169–177] Using dominant negative mutants of p21ras, the activation of this cascade by insulin has been shown to be dependent on p21ras function.

Although both Raf-1 and MEK have restricted substrate specificities, MAPK appears to phosphorylate numerous cellular targets. There are several isoforms of MAPK,[2,169–177] but appreciable differences in substrate specificity have not been demonstrated. Interestingly, upstream signaling elements such as Sos, Raf-1, and MEK are phosphorylated by MAPK.[179,180] This may constitute negative feedback mechanisms, but this idea awaits experimental confirmation. Many targets for MAPK are in the nucleus. In several systems, MAPK is targeted to the nucleus from the cytoplasm in response to external signaling factors, and this presumably constitutes an important mechanism by which extracellular signals regulate nuclear events.[181–184] The c-jun, c-myc, elk-1, and NF-IL6 transcription factors are phosphorylated and activated by MAPK.[185–190] The activities of several enzymes are modulated by MAPK phosphorylation. Phospholipase A$_2$, which catalyzes the rate-limiting step in the synthesis of prostaglandins and leukotrienes, has been shown to be activated by MAPK phosphorylation.[191] A tyrosine phosphatase, tyrosine phosphatase 2C, is deactivated by MAPK.[192] MAPK also can activate two serine kinases, p90[rsk] and MAPKAP-2.[193,194] At our current state of understanding, it seems likely that insulin action on the ras/MAP kinase pathway is related to regulation of transcription factors and nuclear events that mediate its effects on cell proliferation and perhaps other important processes through the regulation of protein expression levels.

CONCLUSIONS

Our overall understanding of the mechanisms of insulin action has been significantly extended over the past several years, leading to the identification and characterization of two important signaling pathways, p21ras/MAP kinase and PI-3-kinase/PDK1/Akt. Each of these pathways is initiated by the insulin receptor tyrosine kinase and downstream tyrosine-phosphorylated substrate proteins, which act as scaffolds for downstream signaling proteins. Each of these pathways also leads to switching of the signaling mode from tyrosine kinase (receptor) to protein serine/threonine kinases that act on target proteins to modulate cellular processes. In the case of the

p21ras pathway, it appears that the protein serine/threonine kinases may act primarily to modulate gene expression and cell proliferation, while the protein kinases downstream of the PI-3-kinase pathway acutely regulate a large number of metabolic processes as well as gene transcription. Classic insulin-sensitive pathways regulated by these latter protein kinases include glucose transport, glycogen synthesis, gluconeogenesis, and protein synthesis. A third insulin-signaling pathway involving CAP/c-Cb1/TC10 may also play a significant role in the regulation of glucose transport in fat and muscle, and will be an important topic for future investigation. Much work is required to clarify a number of details in connecting the protein kinases known to mediate insulin action to the proteins and processes they regulate. Furthermore, it is also recognized that protein serine/threonine phosphatase activity is involved in key insulin responses such as the activation of glycogen synthase. The underlying mechanisms of this regulation will also require substantial additional research to bring us to a full understanding of insulin action.

REFERENCES

1. Avruch J, Zhang XF, Kyricakis JM: Raf meets Ras: Completing the framework of a signal transduction pathway. *Trends Biochem Sci* 1994;19:279.
2. Marshall CJ: MAP kinase kinase, MAP kinase kinase and MAP kinase. *Curr Opin Genet Dev* 1994;4:82.
3. Smith CJ, Rubin CS, Rosen OM: Insulin treated 3T3-L1 adipocytes and cell-free extracts derived from them incorporate 32P into ribosomal protein S6. *Proc Natl Acad Sci USA* 1980;77:2641.
4. Alexander MC, Palmer JC, Pointer RH, *et al*: Insulin-stimulated phosphorylation of ATP-citrate lyase in isolated hepatocytes. Stoichiometry and relation to the phosphoenzyme intermediate. *J Biol Chem* 1982;257:2049.
5. Pucci DS, Ramakrishna S, Benjamin WB: ATP-citrate lyase phosphorylation of acetyl coenzyme A carboxylase within intact rat epididymal fat-cells. *J Biol Chem* 1983;258:12907.
6. Writers LA, Tipper JP, Bacon GW: Stimulation of site-specific phosphorylation of acetyl coenzyme A carboxylase by insulin and epinephrine. *J Biol Chem* 1983;258:5643.
7. Brownsey RW, Hughes WA, Denton RM: Demonstration of the phosphorylation of acetylcoenzyme A carboxylase within intact rat epididymal fat-cells. *Biochem J* 1977;168:441.
8. Pause A, Belsham GJ, Gingras AC, *et al*: Insulin-dependent stimulation of protein synthesis by phosphorylation of a regulator of 5′-cap function. *Nature* 1994;371:762.
9. Lin T-A, Kong X, Haystead TAJ, *et al*: PHAS-1 as a link between mitogen-activated protein kinase and translation initiation. *Science* 1994;266:653.
10. Haystead TA, Haystead CM, Hu C, *et al*: Phosphorylation of PHAS-I by mitogen-activated protein (MAP) kinase. Identification of a site phosphorylated by map kinase in vitro and in response to insulin in rat adipocytes. *J Biol Chem* 1994;269:23185.
11. Kasuga M, Zick Y, Blith DL, *et al*: Insulin stimulation of phosphorylation of the beta subunit of the insulin receptor. Formation of both phosphoserine and phosphotyrosine. *J Biol Chem* 1982;257:9891.
12. Roach PJ, Rosell-Perez M, Larner J: Muscle glycogen synthase in vivo state: Effects of insulin administration on the chemical and kinetic properties of the purified enzyme. *FEBS Lett* 1977;80:95.
13. Stralfors P, Bjorgell P, Belfrage P: Hormonal regulation of hormone-sensitive lipase in intact adipocytes: Identification of phosphorylated sites and effects on the phosphorylation by lipolytic hormones and insulin. *Proc Natl Acad Sci USA* 1984;81:3317.
14. Denton RM, Randle PJ, Bridges BJ, *et al*: Regulation of mammalian pyruvate dehydrogenase. *Mol Cell Biochem* 1975;9:27.
15. Dent P, Lavoinne A, Narkielny S, *et al*: The molecular mechanism by which insulin stimulates glycogen synthesis in mammalian skeletal muscle. *Nature* 1990;348:302.

16. Fingar DC, Birnbaum MJ: Characterization of the mitogen-activated protein kinase/90-kilodalton ribosomal protein S6 kinase signaling pathway in 3T3-L1 adipocytes and its role in insulin-stimulated glucose transport. *Endocrinology* 1994;134:728.

17. Robinson LJ, Razzack ZF, Lawrence JC Jr, *et al*: Mitogen-activated protein kinase activation is not sufficient for stimulation of glucose transport or glycogen synthase in 3T3-L1 adipocytes. *J Biol Chem* 1993;268:26422.

18. Kahn CR, Folli F: Molecular determinants of insulin action. *Horm Res* 1993;39:93.

19. White MF, Kahn CR: The insulin signaling system. *J Biol Chem* 1994;269:1.

20. Czech MP: The nature and regulation of the insulin receptor: Structure and function. *Annu Rev Physiol* 1985;47:357.

21. Kahn CR, White MF: The insulin receptor and the molecular mechanism of insulin action. *J Clin Invest* 1988;82:1151.

22. Yip CC, Yeung CWT, Moule ML: Photoaffinity labelling of insulin receptor of rat adipocyte plasma membrane. *J Biol Chem* 1978;253:1743.

23. Massague J, Pilch PF, Czech MP: Electrophoretic resolution of three major insulin receptor structures with unique subunit stoichiometries. *Proc Natl Acad Sci USA* 1978;77:7137.

24. Jacobs S, Hazum E, Shechter Y, *et al*: Insulin receptor: Covalent labelling and identification of subunits. *Proc Natl Acad Sci USA* 1979; 76:4918.

25. Kasuga M, Karlsson FA, Kahn CR: Insulin stimulates the phosphorylation of the 95,000 dalton subunit of its own receptor. *Science* 1982; 215:185.

26. Rosen OM: After insulin binds. *Science* 1987;237:1452.

27. Ullrich A, Bell JR, Chen EY, *et al*: Human insulin receptor and its relationship to the tyrosine kinase family of oncogenes. *Nature* 1985; 313:756.

28. Ebina Y, Ellis L, Jarnagin K, *et al*: The human insulin receptor cDNA: The structural basis for hormone-activated transmembrane signalling. *Cell* 1985;40:747.

29. Lee J, Pilch PF: The insulin receptor: Structure, function and signalling. *Am J Physiol* 1994;266:C319.

30. Ullrich A, Schlessinger J: Signal transduction by receptors with tyrosine kinase activity. *Cell* 1990;61:203.

31. Schlessinger J, Ullrich A: Growth factor signalling by receptor tyrosine kinases. *Neuron* 1992;9:383.

32. Ullrich A, Gray A, Tam AW, *et al*: Insulin-like growth factor-1 receptor primary structure: Comparison with insulin receptor suggests structural determinants that define functional specificity. *EMBO J* 1986;5:2503.

33. Shier P, Watt VM: Primary structure of a putative receptor for a ligand of the insulin family. *J Biol Chem* 1989;264:14605.

34. Massague J, Czech MP: Role of disulfides in the subunit structure of the insulin receptor. Reduction of class 1 disulfides does not impair transmembrane signalling. *J Biol Chem* 1982;257:6729.

35. Yang-Feng TL, Francke U, Ullrich A: Gene for human insulin receptor: Localization to site on chromosome 19 involved in pre-B-cell leukemia. *Science* 1985;228:728.

36. Seino S, Bell GI: Alternative splicing of human insulin receptor messenger RNA. *Biochem Biophys Res Comm* 1989;159:312.

37. Yamaguchi Y, Flier JS, Yokota A, *et al*: Functional properties of 2 naturally occurring isoforms of the human insulin receptor in Chinese hamster ovary cells. *Endocrinology* 1991;129:2058.

38. McClain DA: Different ligand affinities of the two human insulin receptor splice variants are reflected in parallel changes in sensitivity for insulin action. *Mol Endocrinol* 1991;5:734.

39. Vogt B, Carrascosa JM, Ermel B, *et al*: The two isotypes of the human insulin receptor (HIR-A and HIR-B) follow different internalization kinetics. *Biochem Biophys Res Comm* 1991;177:1013.

40. Benecke H, Flier JS, Moller DE: Alternatively spliced variants of the insulin receptor protein. Expression in normal and diabetic human tissues. *J Clin Invest* 1992;89:2066.

41. DeMeyts P, Roth J, Neville DM Jr, *et al*: Insulin interactions with its receptors: Experimental evidence for negative cooperativity. *Biochem Biophys Res Comm* 1973;55:154.

42. DeMeyts P, Gu JL, Shymko RM, *et al*: Identification of a ligand binding region of the human insulin receptor encoded by the second exon of the gene. *Mol Endocrinol* 1990;4:409.

43. Yip C: The insulin-binding domain of insulin receptor is encoded by exon 2 and exon 3. *J Cell Biochem* 1992;48:19.

44. Schumaker R, Soos MA, Schlessinger J, *et al*: Signaling competent receptor chimeras allow mapping of major insulin receptor binding domain determinants. *J Biol Chem* 1991;268:1087.

45. Lee J, O'Hare T, Pilch PF, *et al*: Insulin receptor autophosphorylation occurs asymmetrically. *J Biol Chem* 1993;268:4092.

46. Ellis L, Morgan DO, Clauser E, *et al*: A membrane-anchored cytoplasmic domain of the human insulin receptor mediates a constitutively elevated insulin-independent uptake of 2-deoxyglucose. *Mol Endocrinol* 1987;1:15.

47. Shoelson SE, White MF, Kahn CR: Tryptic activation of the insulin receptor. Proteolytic truncation of the α-subunit releases the β-subunit from inhibitory control. *J Biol Chem* 1988;263:4852.

48. Clark S, Eckardt G, Siddle K, *et al*: Changes in insulin-receptor structure associated with trypsin-induced activation of the receptor tyrosine kinase. *Biochem J* 1991;276:27.

49. Lebwohl DE, Nunez I, Chan M, *et al*: Expression of inducible membrane-anchored insulin receptor kinase enhances deoxyglucose uptake. *J Biol Chem* 1991;266:386.

50. Hubbard SR, Wei L, Ellis L, *et al*: Crystal structure of the tyrosine kinase domain of the human insulin receptor. *Nature* 1994;372:746.

51. White MF, Shoelson SE, Keutmann H, *et al*: A cascade of tyrosine autophosphorylation in the β-subunit activates the phosphotransferase of the insulin receptor. *J Biol Chem* 1988;263:2969.

52. Flores-Riveros JR, Sibley E, Kastelic T, *et al*: Substrate phosphorylation catalyzed by the insulin receptor tyrosine kinase. Kinetic correlation to autophosphorylation of specific sites in the beta subunit. *J Biol Chem* 1989;264:21557.

53. Stadtmauer L, Rosen OM: Increasing the cAMP content of IM-9 cells alters the phosphorylation state and protein kinase activity of the insulin receptor. *J Biol Chem* 1986;261:3402.

54. Takayama S, White MF, Kahn CR: Phorbol ester-induced serine phosphorylation of the insulin receptor decreases its tyrosine kinase activity. *J Biol Chem* 1988;263:3440.

55. Roth RA, Beaudoin J: Phosphorylation of purified insulin receptors by cAMP kinase. *Diabetes* 1987;36:123.

56. Yamamoto-Honda R, Koshio O, Tobe K, *et al*: Phosphorylation state and biological function of a mutant human insulin receptor Val1996. *J Biol Chem* 1990;265:14777.

57. Moller DE, Benecke H, Flier JS: Biologic activities of naturally occurring human insulin receptor mutations. Evidence that metabolic effects of insulin can be mediated by a kinase-deficient insulin receptor mutant. *J Biol Chem* 1991;266:10995.

58. Cama A, Quon MJ, de la Luz Sierra M: Substitution of isoleucine for methionine at position 1153 in the beta-subunit of the human insulin receptor. A mutation that impairs receptor tyrosine kinase activity, receptor endocytosis, and insulin action. *J Biol Chem* 1992;267:8383.

59. Tavare JM, Siddle K: Mutational analysis of insulin receptor function: Consensus and controversy. *Biochim Biophys Acta* 1993;1178:21.

60. Wiley HS: Anomalous binding of EGF to A431 cells is due to the effect of high receptor densities and a saturable endocytotic system. *J Cell Biol* 1988;107:801.

61. McClain DA, Olefsky JM: Evidence for two independent pathways of insulin receptor internalization in hepatocytes and hepatoma cells. *Diabetes* 1988;37:806.

62. Pilch PF, Shia MA, Benson RJJ, *et al*: Coated vesicles participate in the receptor-mediated endocytosis of insulin. *J Cell Biol* 1983;96:133.

63. Carpentier JL: The cell biology of the insulin receptor. *Diabetologia* 1989;32:627.

64. McClain DA: Mechanism and role of insulin receptor endocytosis. *Am J Med Sci* 1992;304:192.

65. Backer JM, Kahn CR, White MF: The dissociation and degradation of internalized insulin occur in the endosomes of rat hepatoma cells. *J Biol Chem* 1990;265:14828.

66. Doherty JJ, Kay DG, Lai WH, *et al*: Selective degradation of insulin within rat liver endosomes. *J Cell Biol* 1990;110:35.

67. Mosthaf L, Grako K, Dull TJ, *et al*: Functionally distinct insulin receptors generated by tissue-specific alternative splicing. *EMBO J* 1990; 9:2409.

68. Khan MN, Baquiran G, Brule C, *et al*: Internalization and activation of the rat liver insulin receptor kinase in vivo. *J Biol Chem* 1989; 264:12931.

69. Skolnik EY, Lee C-H, Batzer A, *et al*: The SH2/SH3 domain-containing protein Grb2 interacts with tyrosine-phosphorylated IRS-1 and Shc: Implications for insulin control of ras signalling. *EMBO J* 1993;12:1929.

70. Wang LM, Keegan AD, Li W, *et al*: Common elements in interleukin 4 and insulin signaling pathways in factor-dependent hematopoietic cells. *Proc Natl Acad Sci USA* 1993;90:4032.

71. Lavan BE, Lienhard GE: The insulin-elicited 60-kDa phosphotyrosine protein in rat adipocytes is associated with phosphatidylinositol 3-kinase. *J Biol Chem* 1993;268:5921.

72. Sung CK, Sanchez-Margalet V, Goldfine ID: Role of p85 subunit of phosphatidylinositol 3-kinase as an adaptor molecule linking the insulin receptor, p62, and GTPase-activating protein. *J Biol Chem* 1994; 269:503.

73. White MF, Maron R, Kahn CR: Insulin rapidly stimulates tyrosine phosphorylation of a Mr-185,000 protein in intact cells. *Nature* 1985; 318:183.

74. Kahn CR, White MF, Shoelson SE, *et al*: The insulin receptor and its substrate: Molecular determinants of early events in insulin action. *Recent Prog Horm Res* 1993;48:291.

75. Rothenberg PL, Lane WS, Karasik A, *et al*: Purification and partial sequence analysis of pp185, the major cellular substrate of the insulin receptor tyrosine kinase. *J Biol Chem* 1991;266:8302.

76. Sun XJ, Rothenberg P, Kahn CR, *et al*: Structure of the insulin receptor substrate IRS-1 defines a unique signal transduction protein. *Nature* 1991;352:73.

77. Keller SR, Aebersold R, Garner CW, *et al*: The insulin-elicited 160 kDa phosphotyrosine protein in mouse adipocytes is an insulin receptor substrate 1: Identification by cloning. *Biochim Biophys Acta* 1993; 1172:323.

78. Araki E, Sun X-J, Haag BJ 3d, *et al*: Human skeletal muscle insulin receptor substrate-1. Characterization of the cDNA, gene, and chromosomal localization. *Diabetes* 1994;42:1041.

79. Mayer BJ, Ren R, Clark KL, *et al*: A putative modular domain present in diverse signaling proteins. *Cell* 1993;73:629.

80. Tanasijevic MJ, Myers MG Jr, Thoma RS, *et al*: Phosphorylation of the insulin receptor substrate IRS-1 by casein kinase II. *J Biol Chem* 1993;268:18157.

81. Sun XJ, Crimmins DL, Myers MG Jr, *et al*: Pleiotropic insulin signals are engaged by multisite phosphorylation of IRS-1. *Mol Cell Biol* 1993;13:7418.

82. Lowenstein EJ, Daly RJ, Batzer AG, *et al*: The SH2 and SH3 domain-containing protein Grb2 links receptor tyrosine kinases to ras signaling. *Cell* 1992;70:431.

83. Cicchetti P, Mayer BJ, Thiel G, *et al*: Identification of a protein that binds to the SH3 region of abl and is similar to Bcr and GAP-rho. *Science* 1992;257:803.

84. Ren R, Mayer BJ, Cicchetti P, *et al*: Identification of a ten-amino acid proline-rich SH3 binding site. *Science* 1993;259:1157.

85. Egan SE, Giddings BW, Brooks MW, *et al*: Association of Sos ras exchange protein with Grb2 is implicated in tyrosine kinase signal transduction and transformation. *Nature* 1993;363:45.

86. Buday L, Downward J: Epidermal growth factor regulates p21ras through the formation of a complex of receptor, Grb2 adapter protein, and Sos nucleotide exchange factor. *Cell* 1993;73:611.

87. Myers MG Jr, Sun XJ, White MF: The IRS-1 signaling system. *Trends Biochem Sci* 1994;19:289.

88. Tamemoto H, Kadowaki T, Tobe K, *et al*: Insulin resistance and growth retardation in mice lacking insulin receptor substrate-1. *Nature* 1994;372:182.

89. Araki E, Lipes MA, Patti ME, *et al*: Alternative pathway of insulin signalling in mice with targeted disruption of the IRS-1 gene. *Nature* 1994;372:186.

90. Myers MG Jr, Wang LM, Sun XJ, *et al*: Role of IRS-1-Grb2 complexes in insulin signaling. *Mol Cell Biol* 1994;14:3577.

91. Gout I, Dhand R, Hiles ID, *et al*: The GTPase dynamin binds to and is activated by a subset of SH3 domains. *Cell* 1993;75:25.

92. Miki H, Miura K, Matuoka K, *et al*: Association of Ash/Grb2 with dynamin through the Src homology 3 domain. *J Biol Chem* 1994; 269:5489.

93. Seedorf K, Kostka G, Lammers R, *et al*: Dynamin binds to SH3 domains of phospholipase Cg and Grb2. *J Biol Chem* 1994;269:16009.

94. Ando A, Yonezawa K, Gout I, *et al*: A complex of Grb2-dynamin binds to tyrosine phosphorylated insulin receptor substrate-1 after insulin treatment. *EMBO J* 1994;13:3033.

95. Van der Bliek AM, Redelmeier TE, Damke H, *et al*: Mutations in human dynamin block an intermediate stage in coated vesicle formation. *J Cell Biol* 1993;122:553.

96. Schmid SL: Coated-vesicle formation in vitro: Conflicting results using different assays. *Trends Cell Biol* 1993;3:145.

97. Kuhne MR, Pawson T, Lienhard GE, *et al*: The insulin receptor substrate-1 associates with the SH2-containing phosphotyrosine phosphatase Syp. *J Biol Chem* 1993;268:11479.

98. Sugimoto S, Wandless TJ, Shoelson SE, *et al*: Activation of the SH2-containing protein tyrosine phosphatase, SH-PTP2, by phosphotyrosine-containing peptides derived from insulin receptor substrate-1. *J Biol Chem* 1994;269:13614.

99. Case RD, Piccione E, Wolf G, *et al*: SH-PTP2/Syp SH2 domain binding specificity is defined by direct interactions with platelet-derived growth factor beta-receptor, epidermal growth factor receptor, and insulin receptor substrate-1-derived phosphopeptides. *J Biol Chem* 1994;269:10467.

100. Milarski KL, Saltiel AR: Expression of catalytically inactive Syp phosphatase in 3T3 cells blocks stimulation of mitogen-activated protein kinase by insulin. *J Biol Chem* 1994;269:21239.

101. Noguchi T, Matozaki T, Horita K, *et al*: Role of SH-PTP2, a protein-tyrosine phosphatase with Src homology 2 domains, in insulin-stimulated ras activation. *Mol Cell Biol* 1994;14:6674.

102. Li W, Nishimura R, Kashishian A, *et al*: A new function for a phosphotyrosine phosphatase: Linking Grb2-Sos to a receptor tyrosine kinase. *Mol Cell Biol* 1994;14:509.

103. Feng GS, Hui CC, Pawson T: SH2-containing phosphotyrosine phosphatase as a target of protein-tyrosine kinases. *Science* 1993; 259:1607.

104. Almind K, Bjorbaek C, Vestergaard H, *et al*: Amino acid polymorphisms of insulin receptor substrate-1 in non-insulin-dependent diabetes mellitus. *Lancet* 1993;342:828.

105. Saad MJA, Araki E, Miralpeix M, *et al*: Regulation of insulin receptor substrate 1 in liver and muscle of animal models of insulin resistance. *J Clin Invest* 1992;90:1839.

106. Chuang LM, Myers MG Jr, Seidner GA, *et al*: Insulin receptor substrate-1 mediates insulin- and insulin-like growth factor 1-stimulated maturation of Xenopus oocytes. *Proc Natl Acad Sci USA* 1993;90:5172.

107. Wang LM, Myers MG Jr, Sun XJ, *et al*: IRS-1: Essential for insulin- and IL-4-stimulated mitogenesis in hematopoietic cells. *Science* 1993;261:1591.

108. Mueckler M: Facilitative glucose transporters. *Eur J Biochem* 1994; 219:713.

109. Slot JW, Geuze HJ, Gigengack S, *et al*: Immuno-localization of the insulin regulatable glucose transporter in brown adipose tissue of the rat. *J Cell Biol* 1991;113:123.

110. Bornemann A, Ploug T, Schmalbruch H: Subcellular localization of GLUT4 in nonstimulated and insulin-stimulated soleus muscle of rat. *Diabetes* 1992;41:215.

111. Cushman SW, Wardzala LJ: Potential mechanism of insulin action on glucose transport in the isolated rat adipose cell. *J Biol Chem* 1980; 255:4758.

112. Suzuki K, Kono T: Evidence that insulin causes translocation of glucose transport activity to the plasma membrane from an intracellular storage site. *Proc Natl Acad Sci USA* 1980;77:2542.

113. Marette A, Burdett E, Douen A, *et al*: Insulin induces the translocation of GLUT4 from a unique intracellular organelle to transverse tubules in rat skeletal muscle. *Diabetes* 1992;41:1562.

114. Czech MP, Buxton JM: Insulin action on the internalization of the GLUT4 glucose transporter in insolated rat adipocytes. *J Biol Chem* 1993;268:9187.

115. Kanai F, Nishioka Y, Hayashi H, *et al*: Direct demonstration of insulin-induced GLUT4 translocation to the surface of intact cells by insertion of a c-myc epitope into an exofacial GLUT4 domain. *J Biol Chem* 1993;268:14523.

116. Holman GD, Kozka IJ, Clark AE, *et al*: Cell surface labeling of glucose transporter isoform GLUT4 by bis-mannose photolabel. *J Biol Chem* 1990;265:18172.

117. Czech MP, Clancy BM, Pessino A, *et al*: Complex regulation of simple sugar transport in insulin-responsive cells. *Trends Biochem Sci* 1992;17:197.

118. Czech MP, Chawla A, Woon CW, *et al*: Exofacial epitope-tagged glucose transporter chimeras reveal COOH-terminal sequences governing cellular localization. *J Cell Biol* 1993;123:127.

119. Marshall BA, Murata H, Hresko RC, *et al*: Domains that confer intracellular sequestration of the GLUT4 glucose transporter in Xenopus oocytes. *J Biol Chem* 1993;268:26193.

120. Verhey KJ, Hausdorff SF, Birnbaum MJ: Identification of the carboxy terminus as important for the isoform-specific subcellular targeting of glucose transporter proteins. *J Cell Biol* 1993;123:137.

121. Asano T, Takata K, Katagiri H, *et al*: Domains responsible for the differential targeting of glucose transporter isoforms. *J Biol Chem* 1992; 267:19636.

122. Piper RC, Tai C, Kulesza P, *et al*: GLUT-4 NH$_2$ terminus contains a phenylalanine-based targeting motif that regulates intracellular sequestration. *J Cell Biol* 1993;121:1221.

123. Corvera S, Chawla A, Chakrabarti R, *et al*: A double leucine within the GLUT4 glucose transporter COOH-terminal domain functions as an endocytosis signal. *J Cell Biol* 1994;126:979.

124. Verhey KJ, Birnbaum MJ: A Leu-Leu sequence is essential for COOH-terminal targeting signal of GLUT4 glucose transporter in fibroblasts. *J Biol Chem* 1994;269:2353.

125. Yang J, Holman GD: Comparison of GLUT4 and GLUT1 subcellular trafficking in basal and insulin-stimulated 3T3-L1 cells. *J Biol Chem* 1993;268:4600.

126. Jhun BH, Rampal AL, Liu H, *et al*: Effects of insulin on steady state kinetics of GLUT4 subcellular distribution in rat adipocytes. *J Biol Chem* 1992;267:17710.

127. Clancy B, Czech MP: Hexose transport and membrane redistribution of glucose transporter isoforms in response to cholera toxin, dibutyryl cyclic AMP and insulin in 3T3-L1 adipocytes. *J Biol Chem* 1990; 265:12434.

128. Zorzano A, Wilkinson W, Kotliar N, *et al*: Insulin-regulated glucose uptake in rat adipocytes is mediated by two transporter isoforms present in at least two vesicle populations. *J Biol Chem* 1989;264:12358.

129. Cormont M, Tanti JF, Zahraoui A, *et al*: Insulin and okadaic acid induce Rab4 redistribution in adipocytes. *J Biol Chem* 1993;268:19491.

130. Shisheva A, Buxton J, Czech MP: Differential intracellular localizations of GDP dissociation inhibitor isoforms. *J Biol Chem* 1994; 269:23865.

131. Corley CC, Trimble WS, Leinhard GE: Members of the VAMP family of synaptic vesicle proteins are components of glucose transporter-containing vesicles from rat adipocytes. *J Biol Chem* 1992;267:11681.

132. Schu PV, Takegawa K, Fry MJ, *et al*: Phosphatidylinositol 3-kinase encoded by yeast VPS34 gene essential for protein sorting. *Science* 1993;260:88.

133. Joly M, Kazlauskas A, Fay FS, *et al*: Disruption of PDGF receptor trafficking by mutation of its PI-3 kinase binding sites. *Science* 1994; 263:684.

134. Kanai F, Ito K, Todaka M, *et al*: Insulin-stimulated GLUT4 translocation is relevant to the phosphorylation of IRS-1 and the activity of PI3-kinase. *Biochem Biophys Res Comm* 1993;195:762.

135. Okada T, Kawano Y, Sakakibara T, *et al*: Essential role of phosphatidylinositol 3-kinase in insulin-induced glucose transport and antilipolysis in rat adipocytes. *J Biol Chem* 1994;269:3568.

136. Cheatham B, Vlahos CJ, Cheatham L, *et al*: Phosphatidylinositol 3-kinase activation is required for insulin stimulation of pp70 S6 kinase, DNA synthesis, and glucose transporter translocation. *Mol Cell Biol* 1994;14:4902.

137. Kelly KL, Ruderman NB, Chen KS: Phosphatidylinositol-3-kinase in isolated rat adipocytes. Activation by insulin and subcellular distribution. *J Biol Chem* 1992;267:3423.

138. Kublaoui B, Jongsoon L, Pilch PF: Dynamics of signaling during insulin-stimulated endocytosis of its receptor in adipocytes. *J Biol Chem* 1995;270:59.

140. Kozma L, Baltensperger K, Klarlund J, *et al*: The Ras signaling pathway mimics insulin action on glucose transporter translocation. *Proc Natl Acad Sci USA* 1993;90:4460.

141. Manchester J, Kong X, Lowry OH, *et al*: Ras signaling in the activation of glucose transport by insulin. *Proc Natl Acad Sci USA* 1994; 91:4644.

142. Hausdorff SF, Frangioni JV, Birnbaum MJ: Role of p21^{ras} in insulin-stimulated glucose transport in 3T3-L1 adipocytes. *J Biol Chem* 1994; 269:21391.

143. Burgering BM, Pronk GJ, Medema JP, *et al*: Role of p21ras in growth factor signal transduction. *Biochem Soc Trans* 1993;21:888.

144. Feig LA: Guanine-nucleotide exchange factors: A family of positive regulators of Ras and related GTPases. *Curr Opin Cell Biol* 1994; 6:204.

145. Khosravi-Far R, Der CJ: The Ras signal transduction pathway. *Cancer Metastasis Rev* 1994;13:67.

146. Lowry DR, Willumsen BM: Function and regulation of Ras. *Annu Rev Biochem* 1993;62:851.

147. McCormick F: Activators and effectors of ras p21 proteins. *Curr Opin Genet Dev* 1994;4:71.

148. Medema RH, Bos JL: The role of p21ras in receptor tyrosine kinase signaling. *Crit Rev Oncog* 1993;4:615.

149. Moodie SA, Wolfman A: The 3Rs of life: Ras, Raf and growth regulation. *Trends Genet* 1994;10:44.

150. Willumsen BM, Christensen A, Hubbert NL, *et al*: The p21 ras C-terminus is required for transformation and membrane association. *Nature* 1984;310:583.

151. Benito M, Porras A, Nebreda AR, *et al*: Differentiation of 3T3-L1 fibroblasts to adipocytes induced by transfection of ras oncogenes. *Science* 1991;253:565.

152. Medema RH, Wubbolts R, Bos JL: Two dominant inhibitory mutants of p21Ras interfere with insulin-induced gene expression. *Mol Cell Biol* 1991;11:5963.

153. De Vries-Smits AM, Burgering BM, Leevers SJ, *et al*: Involvement of p21ras in activation of extracellular signal-regulated kinase 2. *Nature* 1992;357:602.

154. Jhun BH, Meinkoth JL, Leitner JW, *et al*: Insulin and insulin-like growth factor-I signal transduction requires p21ras. *J Biol Chem* 1994;269:5699.

155. Sasaoka T, Draznin B, Leitner JW, *et al*: Evidence for a functional role of Shc proteins in mitogenic signaling induced by insulin, insulin-like growth factor-1, and epidermal growth factor. *J Biol Chem* 1994;269:10734.

156. Boguski MS, McCormick F: Proteins regulating Ras and its relatives. *Nature* 1993;366:643.

157. Downward J, Graves JD, Warne PH, *et al*: Stimulation of p21^{ras} upon T-cell activation. *Nature* 1990;346:719.

158. Medema RH, deVries-Smits AM, van der Zon GCM, *et al*: Ras activation by insulin and epidermal growth factor through enhanced exchange of guanine nucleotides on p21^{ras}. *Mol Cell Biol* 1993;13:155.

159. Bowtell D, Fu P, Simon M, *et al*: Identification of murine homologues of the Drosophila son of sevenless gene: Potential activators of ras. *Proc Natl Acad Sci USA* 1992;89:6511.

160. Tanaka T, Morishita T, Hashimoto Y, *et al*: C3G, a guanotide-releasing protein expressed ubiquitously, binds to the Src homology 3 domains of Crk and GRB2/ASH proteins. *Proc Natl Acad Sci USA* 1994; 91:3443.

161. Pellichi G, Lafrancone L, Grignani F, *et al*: A novel transforming protein (SHC) with an SH2 domain is implicated in mitogenic signal transduction. *Cell* 1992;70:93.

162. Pronk GJ, McGlade J, Pelicci G, *et al*: Insulin-induced phosphorylation of the 46 and 52 kDa Shc proteins. *J Biol Chem* 1993;268:5748.

163. Pronk GJ, de Vries-Smits AMM, Buday L, *et al*: Involvement of Shc in insulin- and epidermal growth factor-induced activation of p21^{ras}. *Mol Cell Biol* 1994;14:1575.

164. Karlovich CA, Bonfini L, McCollam, *et al*: In vivo functional analysis of the Ras exchange factor son of sevenless. *Science* 1995;268:576.

165. McCollam L, Bonfini L, Karlovich CA, *et al*: Functional roles for the pleckstrin and Dbl homology regions in the Ras exchange factor son-of-sevenless. *J Biol Chem* 1995;270:15954.

166. Li P, Wood K, Mamon H, *et al*: Raf-1: A kinase currently without a cause, but not lacking in effects. *Cell* 1991;64:479.

167. Leevers SJ, Paterson HF, Marshall CM: Requirement for Ras in Raf activation is overcome by targeting Raf to the plasma membrane. *Nature* 1994;369:411.

168. Stokoe D, MacDonald SG, Cadwallader K, *et al:* Activation of Raf as a result of recruitment to the plasma membrane. *Science* 1994;264:1463.

169. Blenis J: Signal transduction via the MAP kinases: Proceed at your own RSK. *Proc Natl Acad Sci USA* 1993;90:5889.

170. Cohen P: Dissection of the protein phosphorylation cascades involved in insulin and growth factor action. *Biochem Soc Trans* 1993;21:555.

171. Crews CM, Erikson RL: Extracellular signals and reversible protein phosphorylation: What is Mek of it all. *Cell* 1993;74:215.

172. Davis RJ: The mitogen-activated protein kinase signal transduction pathway. *J Biol Chem* 1993;268:14553.

173. Blumer KJ, Johnson GL: Diversity in function and regulation of MAP kinase pathways. *Trends Biochem Sci* 1994;19:236.

174. Johnson GL, Vaillancourt RR: Sequential protein kinase reactions controlling cell growth and differentiation. *Curr Opin Cell Biol* 1994; 6:230.

175. Kazlauskas A: Receptor tyrosine kinases and their targets. *Curr Opin Genet Dev* 1994;4:5.

176. Marshall CJ: MAP kinase kinase kinase, MAP kinase kinase and MAP kinase. *Curr Opin Genet Dev* 1994;4:82.

177. Williams NG, Roberts TM: Signal transduction pathways involving the Raf protooncogene. *Cancer Metastasis Rev* 1994;13:105.

178. Ray LB, Sturgill TW: Rapid stimulation by insulin of a serine/threonine kinase in 3T3-L1 adipocytes that phosphorylates microtubule-associated protein 2 in vitro. *Proc Natl Acad Sci USA* 1987;84:1502.

179. Cherniack A, Klarlund JK, Czech MP: Phosphorylation of the Ras nucleotide exchange factor son-of-sevenless by mitogen-activated protein kinase. *J Biol Chem* 1994;269:4717.

180. Anderson NG, Li P, Marsden LA, et al: Raf-1 is a potential substrate for the mitogen-activated protein kinase in vivo. *Biochem J* 1991; 277:573.

181. Chen RH, Sarnecki C, Blenis J: Nuclear localization and regulation of erk and rsk-encoded protein kinases. *J Mol Cell Biol* 1992;12:915.

182. Gonzalez FA, Seth A, Raden DL, et al: Serum-induced translocation of mitogen-activated protein kinase to the cell surface ruffling membrane and to the nucleus. *J Cell Biol* 1993;122:1089.

183. Lenormand P, Sardet C, Pages G, et al: Growth factors induce nuclear translocation of MAP kinases (p42mapk and p44mapk) but not of their activator MAP kinase kinase (p45mapkk) in fibroblasts. *J Cell Biol* 1993;122:1079.

184. Traverse S, Gomez N, Paterson H, et al: Sustained activation of the mitogen-activated protein (MAP) kinase cascade may be required for differentiation of PC12 cells. Comparison of the effects of nerve growth factor and epidermal growth factor. *Biochem J* 1992;288:351.

185. Pulverer BJ, Kyriakis JM, Avruch J, et al: Phosphorylation of c-jun mediated by MAP kinases. *Nature* 1991;353:670.

186. Derijard B, Hibi M, Wu IH, et al: JNK1: A protein kinase stimulated by UV light and HaRas that binds and phosphorylates the c-jun activation domain. *Cell* 1994;76:1025.

187. Seth A, Alvarez E, Gupta S, et al: A phosphorylation site located in the NH_2 terminal domain of c-Myc increases transactivation of gene expression. *J Biol Chem* 1991;266:23521.

188. Gille H, Sharrocks AD, Shaw PE: Phosphorylation of transcription factor p62TCF by MAP kinase stimulates ternary complex formation at fos-promotor. *Nature* 1992;358:414.

189. Janknecht R, Ernst WH, Pingoud V, et al: Activation of ternary complex factor Elk-1 by MAP kinases. *EMBO J* 1993;12:5097.

190. Nakajima T, Kinoshita S, Sasagawa T, et al: Phosphorylation at threonine-235 by a ras-dependent mitogen-activated protein kinase cascade is essential for transcription factor NF-IL6. *Proc Natl Acad Sci USA* 1993;90:2207.

191. Lin LL, Wartman M, Lin AY, et al: $cPLA_2$ is phosphorylated and activated by MAP kinase. *Cell* 1993;72:269.

192. Peraldi P, Zhao Z, Filloux C, et al: Protein-tyrosine-phosphatase 2C is phosphorylated and inhibited by 44-kDa mitogen-activated protein kinase. *Proc Natl Acad Sci USA* 1994;91:5002.

193. Sturgill TW, Ray LB, Erikson E, et al: Insulin-stimulated MAP-2 kinase phosphorylates and activates ribosomal protein S6 kinase II. *Nature* 1988;334:715.

194. Stokoe D, Campbell DG, Nakielny S, et al: MAPKAP kinase-2, a novel protein kinase activated by mitogen-activated protein kinase. *EMBO J* 1992;11:3985.

195. Kimball SR, Vary TC, Jefferson LJ: Regulation of protein synthesis by insulin. *Annu Rev Physiol* 1994;56:321.

196. Redpath NT, Proud CG: Molecular mechanisms in the control of translation by hormones and growth factors. *Biochim Biophys Acta* 1994;1220:147.

197. Lyons RT, Nordeen SK, Young DA: Effects of fasting and insulin administration on polyribosome formation in rat epididymal fat cells. *J Biol Chem* 1980;255:6330.

198. Morgan HE, Jefferson LS, Wolpert EB, et al: Regulation of protein synthesis in heart muscle, 2. Effect of amino acid levels and insulin on ribosomal aggregation. *J Biol Chem* 1971;246:2163.

199. Stirewalt WS, Wool IG, Cavicchi P: The relation of RNA and protein synthesis to the sedimentation of muscle ribosomes: Effect of diabetes and insulin. *Proc Natl Acad Sci USA* 1967;57:1885.

200. Sonnenberg N: mRNA translation: Influence of 5′ and 3′ untranslated regions. *Curr Opin Genet Dev* 1994;4:310.

201. Rowlands AG, Panniers R, Henshaw EC: The catalytic mechanism of guanine nucleotide exchange factor action and competitive inhibition by phosphorylated eukaryotic initiation factor 2. *J Biol Chem* 1988; 263:5526.

202. Towle CA, Mankin HJ, Avruch J, et al: Insulin promoted decrease in the phosphorylation of protein synthesis initiation factor eIF-2. *Biochem Biophys Res Comm* 1984;121:134.

203. Welsh GI, Proud CG: Regulation of protein synthesis in Swiss 3T3 fibroblasts. Rapid activation of the guanine-nucleotide-exchange factor by insulin and growth factors. *Biochem J* 1992;284:19.

204. Dholakia JN, Wahba AJ: Phosphorylation of the guanine nucleotide exchange factor from rabbit reticulocytes regulates its activity in polypeptide chain initiation. *Proc Natl Acad Sci USA* 1988;85:51.

205. Oldfield S, Proud CG: Purification, phosphorylation and control of the guanine-nucleotide-exchange factor from rabbit reticulocyte lysates. *Eur J Biochem* 1992;208:73.

206. Welsh GI, Proud CG: Glycogen synthase kinase-3 is rapidly inactivated in response to insulin and phosphorylates eukaryotics initiation factor eIF-2B. *Biochem J* 1993;294:625.

207. Sonnenberg N: Remarks on the mechanism of ribosome binding to eukaryotic mRNAs. *Gene Expr* 1993;3:317.

208. Morley SJ, Traugh JA: Stimulation of translation in 3T3-L1 cells in response to insulin and phorbol ester is directly correlated with increased phosphate labelling of initiation factor (eIF-) 4F and ribosomal protein S6. *Biochimie* 1993;75:985.

209. Manzella JM, Rychlik W, Rhoads RE, et al: Insulin induction of ornithine decarboxylase. Importance of mRNA secondary structure and phosphorylation of eukaryotic initiation factors eIF-4B and eIF-4E. *J Biol Chem* 1991;266:2383.

210. Joshi-Barve S, Rychlik W, Rhoads RE: Alteration of the major phosphorylation site of eukaryotic protein synthesis initiation factor 4E prevents its association with the 48 S initiation complex. *J Biol Chem* 1990;265:2979.

211. Hu C, Pang S, Kong X, et al: Molecular cloning and tissue distribution of PHAS-I, an intracellular target for insulin and growth factors. *Proc Natl Acad Sci USA* 1994;91:3730.

212. Bak JF: Insulin receptor function and glycogen synthase activity in human skeletal muscle. *Dan Med Bull* 1994;41:179.

213. Cohen P: Dissection of protein phosphorylation cascades involved in insulin and growth factor action. *Biochem Soc Trans* 1993;21:555.

214. Lawrence JC Jr: Signal transduction and protein phosphorylation in the regulation of cellular metabolism by insulin. *Annu Rev Physiol* 1992;54:177.

215. Browner MF, Nakano K, Bang AG, et al: Human muscle glycogen synthase cDNA: A negatively charged protein with an asymmetric charge distribution. *Proc Natl Acad Sci USA* 1989;86:1443.

216. Friedman DL, Larner J: Studies on UDPG-α-glucan transglucosylase by a phosphorylation-dephosphorylation reaction sequence. *Biochemistry* 1963;2:669.

217. Craig JW, Larner J: Influence of epinephrine and insulin on uridine diphosphate glucose-α-glucan transferase and phosphorylase in muscle. *Nature* 1964;202:971.

218. Parker PJ, Caudwell FB, Cohen P: Glycogen synthase from rabbit skeletal muscle. Effect of insulin on the state of phosphorylation of the seven phosphoserine residues in vivo. *Eur J Biochem* 1983; 130:227.

219. Sheorain VS, Juhl H, Bass M, et al: Effects of epinephrine, diabetes, and insulin on rabbit skeletal muscle glycogen synthase. Phosphorylation site occupancies. *J Biol Chem* 1984;259:7024.

220. Ingebritsen TS, Stewart AA, Cohen P: The protein phosphatases involved in cellular regulation. 6. Measurement of type-1 and type-2 protein phosphatases in extracts of mammalian tissues: An assessment of their physiological roles. *Eur J Biochem* 1983;132:297.

221. Hubbard MJ, Cohen P: On target with a new mechanism for the regulation of protein phosphorylation. *Trends Biochem Sci* 1993;18:172.

222. Hubbard MJ, Cohen P: Regulation of protein phosphatase-1G from rabbit skeletal muscle. 1. Phosphorylation by cAMP-dependent protein kinase at site 2 releases catalytic subunit from the glycogen-bound holoeonzyme. *Eur J Biochem* 1989;186:701.

223. Stralfors P, Hiraga A, Cohen P: The protein phosphatases involved in cellular regulation. Purification and characterization of the glycogen-bound form of protein phosphatase-1 from rabbit skeletal muscle. *Eur J Biochem* 1985;149:295.

224. Lavoinne A, Erikson E, Maller JL, et al: Purification and characterization of the insulin-stimulated protein kinase from rabbit skeletal muscle: Close similarity to S6 kinase II. *Eur J Biochem* 1991;199:723.

225. Rylatt DB, Aitkin A, Bilham J, *et al*: Glycogen synthase from rabbit skeletal muscle. Amino acid sequence at the sites phosphorylated by glycogen synthase kinase-3, and extension of the N-terminal sequence containing the site phosphorylated by phosphorylase kinase. *Eur J Biochem* 1980;107:529.

226. Woodget JR: Molecular cloning and expression of glycogen synthase kinase-3/factor A. *EMBO J* 1990;9:2431.

227. Hemmings BA, Resink TJ, Cohen P: Reconstitution of a Mg-ATP-dependent protein phosphatase and its activation through a phosphorylation mechanism. *FEBS Lett* 1982;150:319.

228. Hemmings BA, Aitken A, Cohen P, *et al*: Phosphorylation of the type-II regulatory subunit of cyclic-AMP-dependent protein kinase by glycogen synthase kinase 3 and glycogen synthase kinase 5. *Eur J Biochem* 1982;127:473.

229. Boyle WJ, Smeal T, Defize LH, *et al*: Activation of protein kinase C decreases phosphorylation of c-jun at sites that negatively regulate its DNA-binding activity. *Cell* 1991;64:573.

230. Saksela K, Makela TP, Hughes K, *et al*: Activation of protein kinase C increases phosphorylation of the L-myc trans-activator domain at a GSK-3 target site. *Oncogene* 1992;7:347.

231. Woodgett JR, Plyte SE, Pulverer BJ, *et al*: Roles of glycogen synthase kinase-3 in signal transduction. *Biochem Soc Trans* 1993;21:905.

232. Sutherland C, Cohen P: The α-isoform of glycogen synthase kinase from rabbit skeletal muscle is inactivated by p70 S6 kinase or MAP kinase-activated protein kinase-1 in vitro. *FEBS Lett* 1994;338:37.

233. Welsh GI, Foulstone EJ, Young SW, *et al*: Wortmannin inhibits the effects of insulin and serum on the activities of glycogen synthase kinase-3 and mitogen-activated protein kinase. *Biochem J* 1994;303:15.

234. Cross DS, Alessi DR, Vandenheede JR, *et al*: The inhibition of glycogen synthase kinase-3 by insulin or insulin-like growth factor 1 in the rat skeletal muscle cell line L6 is blocked by wortmannin, but not by rapamycin: Evidence that wortmannin blocks activation of the mitogen-activated protein kinase pathway in L6 cells between Ras and Raf. *Biochem J* 1994;303:21.

235. Lin TA, Lawrence JC Jr: Activation of ribosomal protein S6 kinase does not increase glycogen synthesis or glucose transport in rat adipocytes. *J Biol Chem* 1994;269:21255.

236. Heller-Harrison RA, Morin M, Guilherme A, *et al*: Insulin-mediated targeting of phosphatidylinositol 3-kinase to glut-4 containing vesicles. *J Biol Chem* 1996;271:10200.

237. Fruman DA, Meyers RE, Cantley LC: Phosphoinositide kinases. *Annu Rev Biochem* 1998;67:481.

238. Rameh LE, Cantley LC: The role of phosphoinositide 3-kinase lipid products in cell function. *J Biol Chem* 1999;274:8347.

239. Leevers SJ, Vanhaesebroeck B, Waterfield MD: Signalling through phosphoinositide 3-kinases: The lipids take centre stage. *Curr Opin Cell Biol* 199;11:219.

240. Meier R, Hemmings BA: Regulation of protein kinase B. *J Recept Signal Transduct Res* 1999;19:121.

241. Unterman TG: Insulin/IGF signaling and HNF-3/forkhead proteins. *Science* 1998;279:787.

242. Kops GJ, de Ruiter ND, De Vries-Smits AM, *et al*: Direct control of the Forkhead transcription factor AFX by protein kinase B. JOURNAL? YEAR? VOL. NO. OPENING PAGE.

243. Hall RK, Yamasaki T, Kucera T, *et al*: Regulation of phosphoenolpyruvate carboxykinase and insulin-like growth factor-binding protein-1 gene expression by insulin. The role of winged helix/forkhead proteins. *J Biol Chem* 2000;275:30169.

244. Suzuki Y, Lanner C, Kim JH, *et al*: Insulin control of glycogen metabolism in knockout mice lacking the muscle-specific protein phosphatase PP1G/RGL. *Mol Cell Biol* 2001;21:2683.

245. Till JH, Ablooglu AJ, Frankel M, *et al*: Crystallographic and solution studies of an activation loop mutant of the insulin receptor tyrosine kinase: Insights into kinase mechanism. *J Biol Chem* 2001;276:10049.

246. Wiley HS, Burke PM: Regulation of receptor tyrosine kinase signaling by endocytic trafficking. *Traffic* 2001;2:12.

247. Kao AW, Ceresa BP, Santeler SR, *et al*: Expression of a dominant interfering dynamin mutant in 3T3L1 adipocytes inhibits GLUT4 endocytosis without affecting insulin signaling. *J Biol Chem* 1998;273:25450.

248. Sasaoka T, Wada T, Ishihara H, *et al*: Synergistic role of the phosphatidylinositol 3-kinase and mitogen-activated protein kinase cascade in the regulation of insulin receptor trafficking. *Endocrinology* 1999;140:3826.

249. Nakashima S, Morinaka K, Koyama S, *et al*: Small G protein Ral and its downstream molecules regulate endocytosis of EGF and insulin receptors. *EMBO J* 1999;18:3629.

250. Phillips SA, Barr VA, Haft DH, *et al*: Identification and characterization of SNX15, a novel sorting nexin involved in protein trafficking. *J Biol Chem* 2001;276:5074.

251. Sun XJ, Wang LM, Zhang Y, *et al*: Role of IRS-2 in insulin and cytokine signalling. *Nature* 1995;377:173.

252. Lavan BE, Lane WS, Lienhard GE: The 60-kDa phosphotyrosine protein in insulin-treated adipocytes is a new member of the insulin receptor substrate family. *J Biol Chem* 1997;272:11439.

253. Lavan BE, Fantin VR, Chang ET, *et al*: A novel 160-kDa phosphotyrosine protein in insulin-treated embryonic kidney cells is a new member of the insulin receptor substrate family. *J Biol Chem* 1997;272:21403.

254. Holgado-Madruga M, Emlet DR, Moscatello DK, *et al*: A Grb2-associated docking protein in EGF-and insulin-receptor signalling. *Nature* 1996;379:560.

255. Moodie SA, Alleman-Sposeto J, Gustafson TA: Identification of the APS protein as a novel insulin receptor substrate. *J Biol Chem* 1999;274:11186.

256. Ahmed Z, Pillay TS: Functional effects of APS and SH2-B on insulin receptor signalling. *Biochem Soc Trans* 2001;29:529.

257. Baumann CA, Brady MJ, Saltiel AR: Activation of glycogen synthase by insulin in 3T3-L1 adipocytes involves c-Cbl-associating protein (CAP)-dependent and CAP-independent signaling pathways. *J Biol Chem* 2001;276:6065.

258. Hansen H, Svensson U, Zhu J, *et al*: Interaction between the Grb10 SH2 domain and the insulin receptor carboxyl terminus. *J Biol Chem* 1996;271:8882.

259. He W, Rose DW, Olefsky JM, *et al*: Grb10 interacts differentially with the insulin receptor, insulin-like growth factor I receptor, and epidermal growth factor receptor via the Grb10 Src homology 2 (SH2) domain and a second novel domain located between the pleckstrin homology and SH2 domains. *J Biol Chem* 1998;273:6860.

260. Wick MJ, Dong LQ, Hu D, *et al*: Insulin receptor-mediated p62{superdok} tyrosine phosphorylation at residues 362 and 398 plays distinct roles for binding GAP and Nck and is essential for inhibiting insulin-stimulated activation of Ras and Akt. *J Biol Chem* 2001;267:42843.

261. Yenush L, Makati KJ, Smith-Hall J, *et al*: The pleckstrin homology domain is the principal link between the insulin receptor and IRS-1. *J Biol Chem* 1996;271:24300.

262. Burks DJ, Pons S, Towery H, *et al*: Heterologous pleckstrin homology domains do not couple IRS-1 to the insulin receptor. *J Biol Chem* 1997;272:27716.

263. Jacobs AR, LeRoith D, Taylor SI: Insulin receptor substrate-1 PH and PTB domains are both involved in plasma membrane targeting. *J Biol Chem* 2001;276:40795.

264. Margolis B: The PI/PTB domain: a new protein interaction domain involved in growth factor receptor signaling. *J Lab Clin Med* 1996;128:235.

265. Shoelson SE: SH2 and PTB domain interactions in tyrosine kinase signal transduction. *Curr Opin Chem Biol* 1997;1:227.

266. Eck MJ, Dhe-Paganon S, Trub T, *et al*: Structure of the IRS-1 PTB domain bound to the juxtamembrane region of the insulin receptor. *Cell* 1996;85:695.

267. Aguirre V, Werner ED, Giraud J, *et al*: Phosphorylation of SER307 in IRS-1 blocks interactions with the insulin receptor and inhibits insulin action. *J Biol Chem* 2002;277:1531.

268. White MF: The IRS-signaling system: a network of docking proteins that mediate insulin and cytokine action. *Recent Prog Horm Res* 1998;53:119.

269. Aguirre V, Uchida T, Yenush L, *et al*: The c-Jun NH(2)-terminal kinase promotes insulin resistance during association with insulin receptor substrate-1 and phosphorylation of Ser(307). *J Biol Chem* 2000;24;275:9047.

270. Li J, DeFea K, Roth RA: Modulation of insulin receptor substrate-1 tyrosine phosphorylation by an Akt/phosphatidylinositol 3-kinase pathway. *J Biol Chem* 1999;274:9351.

271. Corvera S: Phosphatidylinositol 3-kinase and the control of endosome dynamics: New players defined by structural motifs. *Traffic* 2001;2:859.

272. Czech MP: PIP2 and PIP3: complex roles at the cell surface. *Cell* 2000;100:603.

273. Xu H, Goldfarb M: Multiple effector domains within SNT1 coordinate ERK activation and neuronal differentiation of PC12 cells. *J Biol Chem* 2001;276:13049.

274. El Mkadem SA, Lautier C, Macari F, *et al*: Role of allelic variants Gly972Arg of IRS-1 and Gly1057Asp of IRS-2 in moderate-to-severe insulin resistance of women with polycystic ovary syndrome. *Diabetes* 2001;50:2164.

275. Wang H, Rissanen J, Miettinen R, *et al*: New amino acid substitutions in the IRS-2 gene in Finnish and Chinese subjects with late-onset type 2 diabetes. *Diabetes* 2001;50:1949.

276. Baroni MG, Arca M, Sentinelli F, *et al*: The G972R variant of the insulin receptor substrate-1 (IRS-1) gene, body fat distribution and insulin-resistance. *Diabetologia* 2001;44:367.

277. Stumvoll M, Fritsche A, Volk A, *et al*: The Gly972Arg polymorphism in the insulin receptor substrate-1 gene contributes to the variation in insulin secretion in normal glucose-tolerant humans. *Diabetes* 2001;50:882.

278. Sesti G: Insulin receptor substrate polymorphisms and type 2 diabetes mellitus. *Pharmacogenomics* 2000;1:343.

279. Araki E, Lipes MA, Patti ME, *et al*: Alternative pathway of insulin signalling in mice with targeted disruption of the IRS-1 gene. *Nature* 1994;372:186.

280. Tamemoto H, Kadowaki T, Tobe K, *et al*: Insulin resistance and growth retardation in mice lacking insulin receptor substrate-1. *Nature* 1994;372:182.

281. Yamauchi T, Tobe K, Tamemoto H, *et al*: Insulin signalling and insulin actions in the muscles and livers of insulin-resistant, insulin receptor substrate 1-deficient mice. *Mol Cell Biol* 1996;16:3074.

282. Sesti, G, Frederici, M, Hribal, ML, Lauro, R. Defects of the insulin receptor substrate (IRS) system in human metabolic disorders. FASEB 2001;15:2099.

283. Bruning JC, Winnay J, Bonner-Weir S, *et al*: Development of a novel polygenic model of NIDDM in mice heterozygous for IR and IRS-1 null alleles. *Cell* 1997;88:561.

284. Withers DJ, Gutierrez JS, Towery H, *et al*: Disruption of IRS-2 causes type 2 diabetes in mice. *Nature* 1998;391:900.

285. Withers DJ, Burks DJ, Towery HH, *et al*: Irs-2 coordinates Igf-1 receptor-mediated beta-cell development and peripheral insulin signalling. *Nat Genet* 1999;23:32.

286. Fasshauer M, Klein J, Ueki K, *et al*: Essential role of insulin receptor substrate-2 in insulin stimulation of Glut4 translocation and glucose uptake in brown adipocytes. *J Biol Chem* 2000;275:25494.

287. Burks DJ, White MF: IRS proteins and beta-cell function. *Diabetes* 2001;50(Suppl 1):S140.

288. Oatey PB, Venkateswarlu K, Williams AG, *et al*: Confocal imaging of the subcellular distribution of phosphatidylinositol 3,4,5-trisphosphate in insulin- and PDGF-stimulated 3T3-L1 adipocytes. *Biochem J* 1999;344(Pt 2):511.

289. Klarlund JK, Guilherme A, Holik JJ, *et al*: Signaling by phosphoinositide-3,4,5-trisphosphate through proteins containing pleckstrin and Sec7 homology domains. *Science* 1997;275:1927.

290. Langille SE, Patki V, Klarlund JK, *et al*: ADP-ribosylation factor 6 as a target of guanine nucleotide exchange factor GRP1. *J Biol Chem* 1999;274:27099.

291. Blume-Jenson, P, Hunter T: Oncogenic kinase signaling. *Nature* 2001;411:355.

292. Currie RA, Walker KS, Gray A, *et al*: Role of phosphatidylinositol 3,4,5-trisphosphate in regulating the activity and localization of 3-phosphoinositide-dependent protein kinase-1. *Biochem J* 1999;337(Pt 3):575.

293. Biondi RM, Kieloch A, Currie RA, *et al*: The PIF-binding pocket in PDK1 is essential for activation of S6K and SGK, but not PKB. *EMBO J* 2001;20:4380.

294. Balendran A, Currie R, Armstrong CG, *et al*: Evidence that 3-phosphoinositide-dependent protein kinase-1 mediates phosphorylation of p70 S6 kinase *in vivo* at Thr-412 as well as Thr-252. *J Biol Chem* 1999;274:37400.

295. King CC, Gardiner EM, Zenke FT, *et al*: p21-Activated kinase (PAK1) is phosphorylated and activated by 3-phosphoinositide-dependent kinase-1 (PDK1). *J Biol Chem* 2000;275:41201.

296. Jensen CJ, Buch MB, Krag TO, *et al*: 90-kDa ribosomal S6 kinase is phosphorylated and activated by 3-phosphoinositide-dependent protein kinase-1. *J Biol Chem* 1999;274:27168.

297. Balendran A, Hare GR, Kieloch A, *et al*: Further evidence that 3-phosphoinositide-dependent protein kinase-1 (PDK1) is required for the stability and phosphorylation of protein kinase C (PKC) isoforms. *FEBS Lett* 2000;484:217.

298. Cohen P, Alessi DR, Cross DA: PDK1, one of the missing links in insulin signal transduction? *FEBS Lett* 1997;410:3.

299. Cohen P: The Croonian Lecture 1998. Identification of a protein kinase cascade of major importance in insulin signal transduction. *Philos Trans R Soc Lond B Biol Sci* 1999;354:485.

300. Nakae J, Park BC, Accili D: Insulin stimulates phosphorylation of the forkhead transcription factor FKHR on serine 253 through a Wortmannin-sensitive pathway. *J Biol Chem* 1999;274:15982.

301. Kops GJ, Burgering BM: Forkhead transcription factors are targets of signalling by the proto-oncogene PKB (C-AKT). *J Anat* 2000;197(Pt 4):571.

302. Nakae J, Kitamura T, Ogawa W, *et al*: Insulin regulation of gene expression through the forkhead transcription factor Foxo1 (Fkhr) requires kinases distinct from Akt. *Biochemistry* 2001;40:11768.

303. Yeagley D, Guo S, Unterman T, *et al*: Gene- and activation-specific mechanisms for insulin inhibition of basal and glucocorticoid-induced insulin-like growth factor binding protein-1 and phosphoenolpyruvate carboxykinase transcription. Roles of forkhead and insulin response sequences. *J Biol Chem* 2001;276:33705.

304. Verhey KJ, Yeh JI, Birnbaum MJ: Distinct signals in the GLUT4 glucose transporter for internalization and for targeting to an insulin-responsive compartment. *J Cell Biol* 1995;130:1071.

305. Shewan AM, Marsh BJ, Melvin DR, *et al*: The cytosolic C-terminus of the glucose transporter GLUT4 contains an acidic cluster endosomal targeting motif distal to the dileucine signal. *Biochem J* 2000;350(Pt 1):99.

306. Pessin JE, Thurmond DC, Elmendorf JS, *et al*: Molecular basis of insulin-stimulated GLUT4 vesicle trafficking. Location! Location! Location! *J Biol Chem* 1999;274:2593.

307. Guilherme A, Emoto M, Buxton JM, *et al*: Perinuclear localization and insulin responsiveness of GLUT4 requires cytoskeletal integrity in 3T3-L1 adipocytes. *J Biol Chem* 2000;275:38151.

308. Guilherme A, Emoto M, Buxton JM, *et al*: Perinuclear localization and insulin responsiveness of GLUT4 requires cytoskeletal integrity in 3T3-L1 adipocytes. *J Biol Chem* 2000;275:38151.

309. Kohn AD, Summers SA, Birnbaum MJ, *et al*: Expression of a constitutively active Akt Ser/Thr kinase in 3T3-L1 adipocytes stimulates glucose uptake and glucose transporter 4 translocation. *J Biol Chem* 1996;271:31372.

310. Wang Q, Somwar R, Bilan PJ, *et al*: Protein kinase B/Akt participates in GLUT4 translocation by insulin in L6 myoblasts. *Mol Cell Biol* 1999;19:4008.

311. Cho H, Thorvaldsen JL, Chu Q, *et al*: Akt1/pkb alpha is required for normal growth but dispensable for maintenance of glucose homeostasis in mice. *J Biol Chem* 2001;276:38349.

312. Cho H, Mu J, Kim JK, *et al*: Insulin resistance and a diabetes mellitus-like syndrome in mice lacking the protein kinase Akt2 (PKB beta). *Science* 2001;292:1728.

313. Baumann CA, Ribon V, Kanzaki M, *et al*: CAP defines a second signalling pathway required for insulin-stimulated glucose transport. *Nature* 2000;407:147.

314. Chiang SH, Baumann CA, Kanzaki M, *et al*: Insulin-stimulated GLUT4 translocation requires the CAP-dependent activation of TC10. *Nature* 2001;410:944.

315. Omata W, Shibata H, Li L, *et al*: Actin filaments play a critical role in insulin-induced exocytotic recruitment but not in endocytosis of GLUT4 in isolated rat adipocytes. *Biochem J* 2000;346(Pt 2):321.

316. Wang Q, Bilan PJ, Tsakiridis T, *et al*: Actin filaments participate in the relocalization of phosphatidylinositol 3-kinase to glucose transporter-containing compartments and in the stimulation of glucose uptake in 3T3-L1 adipocytes. *Biochem J* 1998;331(Pt 3):917.

317. Kanzaki M, Pessin JE: Insulin-stimulated GLUT4 translocation in adipocytes is dependent upon cortical actin remodeling. *J Biol Chem* 2001;276:42436.

318. Jiang ZY, Chawla A, Bose, A, *et al*: A PI 3-kinase-independent insulin signaling pathway to N-WASP/Arp2-3/F-actin required for GLUT4 glucose transporter recycling. *J Biol Chem* 2002;277:509.

319. Patki V, Buxton J, Chawla A, *et al*: Insulin action on GLUT4 traffic visualized in single 3T3-11 adipocytes by using ultra-fast microscopy. *Mol Biol Cell* 2001;12:129.

320. Brunn GJ, Hudson CC, Sekulic A, *et al*: Phosphorylation of the translational repressor PHAS-I by the mammalian target of rapamycin. *Science* 1997;277:99.

321. Scott PH, Brunn GJ, Kohn AD, *et al*: Evidence of insulin-stimulated phosphorylation and activation of the mammalian target of rapamycin mediated by a protein kinase B signaling pathway. *Proc Natl Acad Sci USA* 1998;95:7772.

322. Suzuki Y, Lanner C, Kim JH, *et al*: Insulin control of glycogen metabolism in knockout mice lacking the muscle-specific protein phosphatase PP1G/RGL. *Mol Cell Biol* 2001;21:2683.

323. Tzivion G, Luo Z, Avruch J: A dimeric 14-3-3 protein is an essential cofactor for Raf kinase activity. *Nature* 1998;394:88.

324. Kerkhoff E, Rapp UR: The Ras-Raf relationship: an unfinished puzzle. *Adv Enzyme Regul* 2001;41:261.

325. Hubbard SR, Till JH. Protein tyrosine kinase structure and function. *Annu Rev Biochm* 2000;69:373.

Incretins: Glucose-Dependent Insulinotropic Polypeptide and Glucagon-Like Peptide 1

David D'Alessio

THE INCRETIN EFFECT

Healthy humans have the capacity to ingest and efficiently assimilate large amounts of carbohydrate with relatively minor changes in circulating glucose concentrations. This precise control of glycemia despite widely varying intake is due in large measure to the rapid secretion of appropriate amounts of insulin after meals. Insulin secretion in response to eating is a complex process that is regulated by the interaction of substrate and neural and hormonal stimuli. The gastrointestinal (GI) tract plays an important role in the disposition of carbohydrate meals by secreting insulinotropic peptides that effectively connect substrate absorption to insulin secretion, a process that is critical for adjusting pancreatic β cell output to a given load of nutrients. These GI peptides were termed **incretins** by investigators in the early part of the last century to signify that they stimulated internal or endocrine secretions of the pancreas, in contrast to **excretins**, hormones that stimulated pancreatic exocrine secretion. Thus incretins represent one of the earliest classes of hormones to be described and their study, especially as they relate to normal and abnormal glucose tolerance, has a long history.[1]

Although the presence of insulinotropic substances in the mucosa of the intestine had been known for many years, it was not until the advent of radioimmunoassay (RIA) and the ability to measure circulating insulin levels that the importance of incretins was clearly demonstrated. The observation that circulating insulin levels are significantly higher after glucose is ingested, compared to when it is administered intravenously (IV), was made by several groups and termed the **incretin effect**.[2,3] Insulin secretion during progressively increasing oral glucose loads increases linearly, despite peak plasma glucose levels that vary only slightly. This indicates that plasma glucose levels *per se* constitute a relatively fixed proportion of the stimulus to the β cell, and this fraction becomes smaller as the load of ingested glucose increases (Fig. 6-1). Thus stimuli other than glucose effect the increase in meal-induced insulin release and influence the overall β-cell output. Incretin hormones, released in proportion to meal size, augment glucose-stimulated insulin secretion, a synergy that links insulin secretion to the quantity of ingested nutrients. When calculated as the difference between plasma insulin and/or C-peptide levels after oral glucose and isoglycemic IV glucose infusions, the incretin effect accounts for 30–60% of the β-cell output following glucose ingestion in healthy humans.[2,4]

Beyond regulating the amount of insulin secreted during meal absorption, incretins prime the β-cell response to glucose, inducing the rapid release of insulin characteristic of the normal postprandial response. The combination of stimuli activated by food ingestion triggers a brisk islet cell response that does not require, and in fact preempts, large increases in plasma glucose. The importance of a primed, rapid pattern of insulin release after eating is exemplified by studies of persons with impaired glucose tolerance (IGT) in whom a sluggish early insulin response to carbohydrate meals is associated with exaggerated glycemic excursions and late prandial hyperinsulinemia. The integrity of the incretin effect in IGT is not well characterized, but persons with type 2 diabetes mellitus (T2DM), have only a minimal augmentation of insulin release with oral versus IV glucose, constituting a marked impairment in the incretin effect[5] (Fig. 6-2). Whether the abnormal incretin effect in persons with diabetes is due to specific abnormalities in the release or action of incretin hormones, or is simply another consequence of generalized β-cell dysfunction is a question presently under investigation. However, given the major contribution of the incretin effect to normal glucose tolerance, its loss undoubtedly contributes to the delayed and attenuated insulin secretion that is a hallmark of diabetes.

The two major characteristics used to define an incretin are: (1) that it is released following nutrient, particularly carbohydrate, ingestion and (2) that concentrations reached after meals stimulate insulin secretion.[2] There are currently two known hormones that meet these criteria: *glucose-dependent insulinotropic polypeptide (GIP)* and *glucagon-like peptide 1 (GLP-1)*. Recent studies suggest that both of these peptides are necessary for normal glucose tolerance. Consideration of incretins in relation to diabetes is timely because recent evidence raises the possibility that abnormalities of incretin function may contribute to the pathogenesis of diabetes. In addition, there are ongoing efforts to exploit the incretin pathways to treat diabetic patients. This chapter will review the physiology of the two major incretins, their integration into the insulin response to meals, and the relation of these peptides to the pathophysiology of diabetes.

GLUCOSE-DEPENDENT INSULINOTROPIC POLYPEPTIDE (GIP)

Brown and Pederson discovered and isolated GIP based on the ability of extracts of the porcine upper intestine to suppress gastric acid secretion in dogs.[6,7] Originally called gastric inhibitory polypeptide, this 42-amino-acid peptide has significant homology

FIGURE 6-1. The incretin effect. Plasma concentrations of glucose (**top**) and C peptide (**bottom**) during 25-g (left), 50-g (middle), and 100-g (right) oral glucose loads (**filled circles**) and isoglycemic intravenous glucose infusions (**open circles**). Plasma glucose concentrations are similar for the three doses of oral glucose, demonstrating the precision of normal glucose homeostasis, and matched in each case by IV glucose, providing equivalent levels of glycemic stimulus during both sets of studies. Insulin secretion, as reflected by plasma C-peptide levels, is greater for oral glucose in comparison with intravenous glucose, and the magnitude of this difference increases with the dose of oral glucose. *(Reprinted with permission from Nauck* et al.[4]*)*

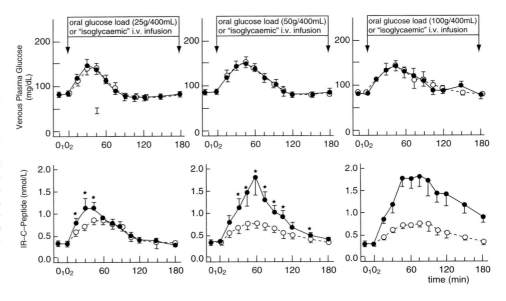

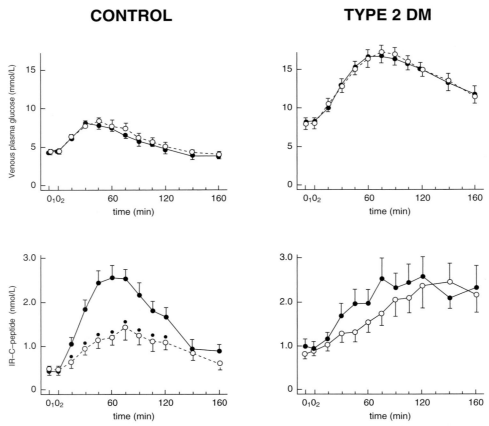

FIGURE 6-2. Reduced incretin effect in subjects with type 2 diabetes. Plasma glucose (**top**) and C peptide (**bottom**) concentrations in persons with type 2 diabetes, and nondiabetic controls, during 50-g glucose ingestion (**filled circles**) and glucose infusions to glycemic levels matching those following oral glucose (**open circles**). In the control subjects insulin secretion, as reflected in plasma insulin and C peptide levels, is substantially greater following oral compared to IV glucose. However, in the diabetic subjects there is no difference overall in the integrated insulin and C peptide responses during oral and IV glucose loading. *(Reprinted with permission from Nauck* et al.[5]*)*

with peptides in the secretin family of regulatory peptides and the sequence is highly conserved across mammalian species, suggesting an important physiologic role.[7] Soon after the structure of GIP was elucidated, the peptide was demonstrated to augment glucose-stimulated insulin secretion, and once specific RIAs became available to measure GIP in plasma, it became apparent that GIP is secreted into the circulation after meal consumption.[1,6] Based on these findings, GIP was classified as an incretin and subsequent work indicates that this is the primary function of this hormone, while a physiologic role in the regulation of gastric function has not been clearly demonstrated. For these reasons the peptide was renamed glucose-dependent insulinotropic polypeptide.

Distribution, Synthesis, and Secretion of GIP

GIP is synthesized by endocrine K cells that are most prevalent in the mucosa of the duodenum and upper jejunum, and these cells are the only known source of GIP in humans.[6–8] The GIP gene encodes preproGIP, a prohormone that is processed into the bioactive molecule.[7] The nucleic acid and protein sequences of GIP are highly conserved across mammalian species, with homology of 40 of the 42 amino-acid residues between the human and porcine peptides, and a similar degree of homology between rats and humans.[6,7] Expression

of the GIP gene is stimulated by oral glucose or enteral infusion of lipid in rats,[7] and the effect of glucose to increase proGIP mRNA is also seen in an intestinal cell line,[9] suggesting that direct contact of nutrients with the K cells stimulates GIP synthesis. Rats made diabetic by injection of streptozocin have increased intestinal GIP mRNA and peptide levels relative to control animals, indicating that GIP synthesis may be increased in diabetes.[10]

Ultrastructural examination of K cells reveals the characteristic intracellular secretory granules that typify endocrine cells. Indeed, GIP secretion occurs in a regulated manner and enteral nutrients are the primary stimulus. Both carbohydrate and lipids are potent activators of K-cell secretion, while the observed response to protein ingestion or amino acids in the gut has been more variable. Importantly, intravenous delivery of glucose, amino acids, or lipids does not stimulate GIP release, indicating that luminal interaction of substrates with the gut mucosa is critical for this process.[6,7] GIP secretion in response to enteral glucose is proportional to the amount of glucose administered[11] and is dependent on the absorption of glucose by the intestinal mucosa.[6,7] Schirra and colleagues demonstrated that following ingestion of a glucose-containing drink, GIP was released throughout the entire period of gastric emptying and ceased only after delivery of glucose to the duodenum was complete (left panels of Fig. 6-3).[11] Carbo-

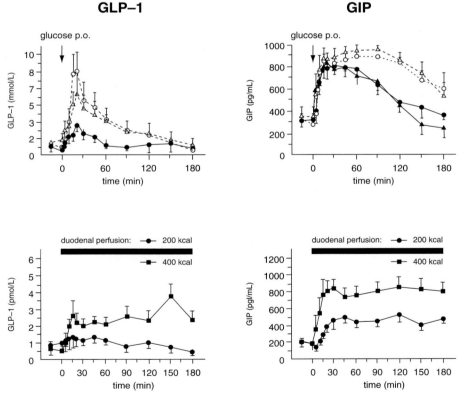

FIGURE 6-3. Secretion of incretin hormones in response to oral and intraduodenal glucose. GLP-1 and GIP secretion in response to 50 g (**solid symbols**) and 100 g (**open symbols**) of oral glucose are shown in the top two panels. Plasma levels of the incretins increase rapidly following glucose ingestion and the concentrations of GIP and GLP-1 are more elevated in response to the larger dose of glucose. The lower panel shows plasma levels of GLP-1 and GIP in response to different rates of intraduodenal glucose. The release of GIP shows a dose-response relationship with the amount of glucose infused, while the pattern of GLP-1 release suggests a threshold of glucose delivery required to initiate secretion. *(Reprinted with permission from Schirra et al.[11])*

hydrate-stimulated GIP release is inhibited by pharmacologic inhibition of α-glucosidases, which limits glucose absorption in the upper gut, and phlorhizin, an inhibitor of mucosal glucose transport.[2] Sucrose and galactose also stimulate GIP release, while fructose does not.[12]

Stimulation of GIP release by triglycerides is dependent on intraluminal hydrolysis, absorption of fatty acids, and the packaging of reesterified triglycerides into chylomicrons.[2,6] GIP release in response to fat increases with the quantity of lipid ingested, and fat is a more potent stimulus of GIP than glucose on a per-gram basis.[13] It is likely that the mechanisms of glucose- and lipid-induced GIP secretion are distinct, and possibly derived from separate populations of cells.[2,7] Consistent with this observation, the addition of fat to a glucose meal greatly accentuates the GIP response. Taken as a whole, the available data indicate that GIP secretion is regulated directly by the products of meal digestion in a dose-dependent manner. This supports the concept advanced by Ebert and Creutzfeldt that GIP acts as a quantitative signal of nutrient absorption to the endocrine pancreas.[12]

Following release into the circulation, GIP is metabolized by the enzyme dipeptidyl peptidase IV, a ubiquitous protease that cleaves specifically between residues 2 and 3, leaving GIP-[3–42].[7,14] This conversion occurs rapidly, so that the circulating half-life of full-length GIP is only several minutes, and is inactivating because GIP[3–42] does not stimulate insulin secretion.

Signaling Through the GIP Receptor

A single GIP receptor has been identified and is currently believed to mediate all of the physiologic effects of the peptide. The GIP receptor has seven-transmembrane domains and substantial homology with receptors in the secretin-VIP receptor family, particularly the glucagon and GLP-1 receptors.[8,15,16] The GIP receptor is expressed in both α and β cells of the pancreatic islet,[17] the upper GI tract, adipocytes, adrenal cortex, pituitary, and a variety of brain regions.[8] Both full-length GIP[1–42] and several GIP congeners, truncated at the N- and C-terminus bind to the GIP receptor with high affinity, but none of the related peptides from the glucagon family interact with this receptor.[7,15]

Ligand binding to the GIP receptor activates adenylyl cyclase through stimulatory GTP-binding proteins and GIP induces dose-dependent increases in intracellular cyclic AMP.[15,16] The potentiation of glucose-, and depolarization-stimulated exocytosis from β cells by GIP is mediated primarily via the protein kinase A signaling pathway.[18] There remains some question as to whether or not GIP also acts through other signaling pathways in the β cell, and the details of the intracellular effects of incretins is an active area of ongoing research.

Recent work demonstrates that the GIP receptor is susceptible to homologous desensitization.[10,19,20] Both in vitro, as well as in intact animals, extended exposure to GIP attenuates the insulinotropic effect of the peptide. The mechanism for agonist-mediated desensitization of the GIP receptor is multifactorial and involves both uncoupling of the receptor from G proteins and an increased turnover of activated G proteins. Ligand-induced desensitization of the GIP receptor, in the context of the increased circulating GIP levels reported by many groups to occur in type 2 diabetic subjects (see below), has been advanced as an explanation for the diminished incretin effect seen in diabetes.

The Incretin Function of GIP

GIP is insulinotropic in the presence of glucose concentrations greater than 5–6 mmol.[2,6] This action has been demonstrated in a broad range of experimental models including cell lines, cultured pancreatic islets, isolated perfused pancreas, and a variety of animals. In humans both porcine and synthetic human GIP stimulate insulin secretion when infused to concentrations mimicking those occurring after meals. A key point is that GIP-stimulated insulin secretion occurs only when glucose levels are elevated above fasting. This glucose dependence is common to most endogenous insulinotropic peptides and neurotransmitters, and functionally serves as protection against hypoglycemia. The tight coupling of GIP secretion to glucose absorption by the gut, the potency of postprandial concentrations of peptide, and the dependence of GIP action on the ensuing hyperglycemia have become the hallmarks of incretin physiology.

Beyond the fact that infusions of GIP to humans in amounts estimated to be physiologic augment glucose-stimulated insulin release, the role of GIP as an incretin has been demonstrated by several classic experimental methods in rodents. Removal of circulating GIP with a specific antiserum abolished the insulinotropic effect of exogenous GIP and caused glucose intolerance with diminished insulin secretion during enteral glucose loading.[2,6] Similarly, administration of GIP[7–30 amide], a competitive antagonist of the GIP receptor, significantly attenuated the insulin response to a typical meal.[21] Most recently, a line of mice was created with a targeted gene deletion of the GIP receptor.[22] These animals had normal fasting glucose and insulin levels and responses to intraperitoneal glucose loads that were comparable to wild-type control mice. However, in response to oral glucose loading the GIP-receptor-knockout mice had significant glucose intolerance and impaired insulin secretory responses (Fig. 6-4). Interestingly, when these animals were made insulin-resistant by chronic feeding of a high-fat diet, their glucose intolerance worsened, in contrast to high-fat-fed control mice that maintained normal glycemic excursions following oral glucose. This experiment demonstrated that absence of the GIP receptor impairs the normal augmentation of insulin secretion induced by insulin resistance. Taken together, these studies in rodents indicate that the incretin action of GIP is necessary for normal glucose tolerance and suggest that GIP may play a role in adapting insulin secretion to changes in insulin sensitivity.

Other Effects of GIP

The GIP receptor is expressed on pancreatic α as well as β cells, but the role of GIP in the control of glucagon secretion is not clear. GIP stimulates exocytosis in isolated rat α cells[23] and increases glucagon release from the isolated perfused pancreas.[6] However, in humans infusion of GIP does not change plasma glucagon concentrations significantly.[24] It is possible that other effects of GIP, such as stimulation of insulin release, counteract direct effects to stimulate the α cell. Regardless, current information indicates that there is little overall effect of GIP on glucagon levels in vivo.

The GIP receptor is expressed in adipose tissue and evidence exists to suggest that GIP has regulatory effects on lipid metabolism.[7,25] In isolated adipocytes or adipocyte cell lines, GIP potentiates the effects of insulin to promote glucose uptake and augment lipogenesis, inhibits glucagon-stimulated lipolysis, and increases lipoprotein lipase activity.[25] In animals, GIP administration promotes the clearance of postprandial triglyceride-rich lipoproteins.

Thus the hypothesis that GIP, synthesized and secreted in response to ingested fat, plays an important role in lipid anabolism has some support in animal studies.[25] However, a physiologic role for GIP to regulate lipid metabolism in humans has yet to be convincingly demonstrated.

Since GIP was initially isolated based on its activity to inhibit acid secretion in denervated gastric pouches, it is ironic that an important physiologic role for GIP in gastric function has yet to be demonstrated.[6,7] It is possible that GIP contributes to the suppression of gastric acid secretion that occurs after consumption of a fat meal. The most likely mechanism for decreased acid production is via stimulation of gastric somatostatin release.[6,7] Recently GIP has been shown to increase intestinal glucose transport during enteral glucose infusion in isolated rat intestine,[26] a finding that was confirmed in intact rats by administration of a GIP antagonist that inhibited glucose transport relative to controls.[27] These results suggest a broad role for GIP to increase glucose metabolism by increasing both substrate absorption and disposition through its actions on the gut and pancreatic islet.

GIP in Diabetes

Because GIP plays an important role in the normal physiology of insulin secretion after nutrients are ingested, a number of investigators have considered whether or not abnormalities in GIP secretion or action contribute to glucose intolerance or diabetes. There have been important incongruities among some of these studies and it is not likely that GIP has a prominent role in the pathogenesis of glucose intolerance and diabetes in humans. However, when all the evidence is considered, a plausible case can be made that abnormalities in the GIP axis contribute to the impaired incretin effect in at least some diabetic subjects.

It is unlikely that GIP is involved in the metabolic abnormalities seen in type 1 diabetes. In newly diagnosed patients with T1DM, GIP secretion after meals is lower than in nondiabetic controls but returns to normal over several months.[13] However, in neither newly diagnosed patients nor individuals with longstanding type 1 diabetes is there a correlation between GIP concentrations in the plasma and β cell function. Type 1 diabetic subjects retaining some insulin secretory capacity respond to exogenous GIP, but have subnormal responses relative to controls, in all likelihood due to decreased islet mass and abnormal β-cell function. The molecular species of GIP found in diabetic patients are qualitatively comparable to controls, and there seems to be no effect of glycemic control or intensity of insulin treatment on the GIP response to ingested nutrients in persons with T1DM. Based on these data, the notion that K-cell secretion of GIP is regulated in a feedback manner by insulin, as had been suggested previously, seems doubtful.

Many studies have found that persons with type 2 diabetes have increased plasma concentrations of GIP following glucose or meal ingestion, compared with nondiabetic individuals.[12,13] However, GIP hypersecretion has not been a uniform finding in diabetic subjects,[13,24] and there is no obvious explanation for this discrepancy among studies. It is plausible that increased meal-induced GIP secretion occurs only in subgroups of diabetic individuals, a possibility suggested by several studies including large numbers of subjects.[12,13] Studies of nondiabetic obese subjects indicate that obesity *per se* does not alter postprandial GIP levels or clearance of GIP, and GIP does not seem to contribute to the hyperinsulinemia seen in obese persons.[28,29] Similarly to subjects with type 1 diabetes, neither glycemic control nor treatment with insulin or oral agents affects nutrient-stimulated GIP in type 2 diabetic patients.[29,30] Thus there is no clear explanation for the common finding of augmented secretion of GIP after meals in at least a substantial proportion of diabetic individuals. A recent examination of healthy first-degree relatives of type 2 diabetic patients demonstrated that integrated GIP release over 24 hours, including three meals, was increased by 20–25% relative to persons with no family history of diabetes.[31] These findings suggest that changes in GIP secretion may precede the onset of impaired glucose tolerance, and raise the possibility that increased incretin secretion could develop to compensate for early β-cell dysfunction.

Several studies have assessed the insulinotropic effect of GIP in type 2 diabetes using infusions of synthetic human GIP. Overall these studies demonstrate that GIP increases glucose-stimulated insulin secretion in diabetic subjects but the relative magnitude of this response is significantly less than that of control subjects.[13,24] For example, Nauck and colleagues found that in a group of well compensated type 2 diabetic subjects the incremental C-peptide response to GIP during a hyperglycemic clamp was only 46% of the response seen in nondiabetic individuals.[24] However, in a small study of diabetic subjects with more severe β-cell defects, the insulinotropic effect of GIP was completely absent.[32] Interestingly, several point mutations of the GIP receptor have been discovered, some of which diminish GIP-stimulated cyclic AMP generation,[33,34] and it has been suggested that this might account for a decreased GIP effect in diabetic subjects. However, the frequency of these mutant forms is not different among type 2 diabetic and nondiabetic subjects, and so is unlikely to explain any general impairment of the incretin function of GIP among subjects with diabetes. The important issue is whether an impaired response to GIP is a specific defect of the diabetic β cell, or simply another manifestation of the overall insulin secretory defects seen in diabetic patients. While one group of investigators has calculated "normal" sensitivity to GIP of diabetic subjects when considered in the context of generalized β-cell dysfunction, this remains an undecided question.[35] Interestingly, it appears that islet sensitivity to GIP is decreased in older humans, and it has been suggested that this may contribute to glucose intolerance seen with aging.[36]

GLUCAGON-LIKE PEPTIDE 1 (GLP-1)

When the structure of proglucagon (ProG) was determined in the early 1980s, it became apparent that peptides other than glucagon were produced from this prohormone. Based on the nucleotide and amino acid sequence of ProG, the glucagon-like peptides GLP-1 and GLP-2 were deduced. GLP-1 has significant sequence homology to glucagon but a very different physiologic role. Like GIP, GLP-1 is secreted after meals and is a potent stimulus to glucose-stimulated insulin secretion. Recent studies have proven that GLP-1 has a physiologic role as an incretin. Moreover, administration of this peptide to persons with type 2 diabetes causes marked improvements in insulin secretion and glucose disposition, raising the possibility that GLP-1 or analogues could be useful in the treatment of these patients.

Distribution, Synthesis, and Secretion of GLP-1

In humans, proglucagon is synthesized by pancreatic α cells, L cells located in the intestinal mucosa, and a population of neurons located in the hindbrain.[1,37,38] These cells all transcribe identical

ProG mRNA that is translated to a common prohormone (see Chap. 7). Processing of ProG in the pancreatic islet yields glucagon with little production of GLP-1, while L cells make GLP-1, GLP-2, and virtually no glucagon.[1,38] This tissue-specific processing of ProG is due at least in part to the presence of prohormone convertase 1 (PC1/3) in L cells, but not α cells, since PC1/3 cleaves GLP-1 from ProG.[37] Within the ProG molecule, putative dibasic cleavage sites occur on either end of the 37-amino-acid moiety GLP-1[1–37]. However, L cells process ProG almost entirely into the truncated peptides, GLP-1[7–36 amide] and GLP-1[7–37], and these are the species for which biologic activity has been demonstrated. In humans and other mammals, approximately 80% of intestinally derived GLP-1 is the amidated form, GLP-1[7–36 amide].

In contrast to the GIP-producing K-cells located most prominently in the duodenum and upper jejunum, L cells are most prevalent in the lower gut. On average, 70–90% of the intestinal GLP-1 is synthesized in the lower jejunum, ileum, and colon.[1] GLP-1 levels in the circulation increase after ingestion, but not IV infusion, of nutrients.[11,39,40] Like GIP, glucose and lipids are the most potent stimuli to GLP-1 release, with some question as to whether or not protein or amino acids are stimulatory. Unlike GIP, the release of GLP-1 does not seem to be dependent on nutrient absorption in the intestine, but appears to be linked to the rate at which nutrients are delivered to the gut (left panels of Fig. 6-3).[11]

Despite the marked difference in the distribution of the two peptides along the gut, secretion of GLP-1 and GIP after mixed or glucose meals occurs in parallel (Fig. 6-3).[11,40] The rapid release of GLP-1 in response to food intake is somewhat paradoxical in light of the distal location of the majority of L cells and raises questions as to the mechanism of nutrient-stimulated GLP-1 secretion. One possibility is suggested by the observation that in rats, increased ProG synthesis in response to refeeding after a fast seems to be localized to upper but not lower intestinal L cells.[41] From these data it could be inferred that in fact nutrient-stimulated GLP-1 secretion may be accounted for by the minority of L cells in the upper gut. Alternatively, there is evidence that a neural pathway from the upper to lower gut mediates GLP-1 release,[37] and it appears that vagal cholinergic and peptidergic signaling contributes to the coupling of intestinal nutrients with GLP-1 secretion in rats. This finding is supported by one study in healthy humans given cholinergic blocking agents,[42] and another showing a normal GLP-1 response of subjects with proximal ileostomies, in whom the majority of L cells do not come in contact with luminal nutrients.[43] However, GLP-1 secretion is normal, or even accentuated, in subjects with total gastrectomy and surgical disruption of the abdominal vagi.[44] So, while there are several aspects of nutrient-stimulated GLP-1 secretion to suggest neural coupling, the specific pathways involved are not clear. Interestingly GIP has been shown to evoke GLP-1 secretion in several *in vitro* models,[37] suggesting that GIP could act as a humoral stimulus of GLP-1 release. However, in humans IV infusions of even supraphysiologic amounts of GIP do not increase plasma GLP-1 concentrations.[45] A recent examination of the canine gut indicates that there is substantial overlap among GIP-secreting K cells and L cells, with a high frequency of jejunal L cells immediately adjacent to K cells.[46] This finding presents the possibility of paracrine stimulation of GLP-1 secretion by GIP as an alternative to nutrient-, endocrine-, or neurally-mediated mechanisms. Despite the interesting possibilities suggested by studies addressing the mechanism(s) of nutrient-stimulated GLP-1 secretion, this issue remains an open and important question. Efforts to understand the process of GLP-1 release are driven by the possibility that factors enhancing endogenous release of the peptide could be useful in stimulating insulin secretion and promoting glucose tolerance in diabetes.

Similarly to GIP, GLP-1 is rapidly metabolized in the circulation by dipeptidylpeptidase (DPP) IV.[14] This enzyme is present on capillary endothelial cells located diffusely throughout mammalian tissues and in plasma. DPP IV cleaves the N-terminal His-Ala from GLP-1[7–36 amide] leaving GLP-1[9–36 amide], and this process occurs with a half-life of approximately 1–2 minutes for intact GLP-1 in mammalian plasma.[1,37] Because the N-terminus of GLP-1 is essential for its insulinotropic effect, metabolism by DPP IV likely inactivates this action. In fact GLP-1[9–36 amide] may be a competitive antagonist of the GLP-1 receptor, an effect that has been reported both *in vitro* and *in vivo*.[1] GLP-1[9–36 amide] is renally cleared with a half-life of approximately 5–10 minutes, so it is the primary circulating GLP-1 species in the postprandial circulation.[47]

Signaling Through the GLP-1 Receptor

A specific GLP-1 receptor was cloned from pancreatic islet cells[1,37] and is the only known mediator of GLP-1 signaling in mammals. The mRNA for this receptor has been unequivocally demonstrated in specific regions of the brain, stomach, and lung, as well as pancreatic β cells. Additionally, some investigators have reported that the GLP-1 receptor is synthesized by islet α cells, hepatocytes, skeletal muscle cells and renal parenchymal cells, but these findings have not been uniform. Binding of radiolabeled GLP-1 to adipocytes, and the expression of the GLP-1 receptor in a preadipocyte cell line suggests that fat tissue also contains specific GLP-1 binding sites.

Like the GIP receptor, the GLP-1 receptor is a member of the secretin-VIP family of seven-membrane-spanning, G-protein coupled receptors. Ligand binding by this receptor is highly specific and there is little affinity for glucagon or GIP. However, exendin-4 and exendin[9–39], peptides homologous to GLP-1 found in the venom of the Gila monster (*Heloderma suspectum*), are a naturally-occurring GLP-1 receptor agonist and antagonist, respectively.[48] Similarly to GIP, GLP-1 mediates its effects on the β cell through activation of adenylyl cyclase and formation of intracellular cyclic AMP. Foremost among these effects are: synergism with glucose to close K_{ATP} channels, augmentation of glucose-induced increases in intracellular calcium, and promotion of secretory granule exocytosis at a site distal to the elevation of intracellular calcium.[49] While protein phosphorylation by protein kinase A (PKA) is central to the intracellular transmission of the GLP-1 signal, recent work indicates that PKA-independent processes are also important.[50]

Ligand binding leads to internalization and degradation of the GLP-1 receptor. There is evidence from studies of β-cell lines and normal islets in culture that the GLP-1 receptor also undergoes homologous and heterologous desensitization since protracted incubation with GLP-1, or activation of the protein kinase C pathway, decreases generation of cyclic AMP and downstream effects of the peptide. It has been suggested that overlapping desensitization through signaling pathways that promote β-cell secretion acts as a means of preventing excessive insulin release.[51] However, it is unclear what role ligand-induced desensitization has *in vivo*, or whether this effect would lead to tachyphylaxis in the presence of prolonged elevations of circulating GLP-1.

Incretin Actions of GLP-1

Administration of GLP-1 to animals and humans increases insulin secretion during hyperglycemia (right panels of **Fig. 6-4**),[1,39] and this effect occurs at concentrations of GLP-1 that are similar to those observed in the circulation after meals. Similarly to GIP, the insulin stimulatory effect of GLP-1 is glucose-dependent and is substantially diminished at glucose levels less than 5.5 mmol. The effect of GLP-1 to promote insulin release is additive to that of GIP, suggesting that the two incretin hormones act together in regulating postprandial insulin secretion.[45]

In addition to acting as an acute insulin secretagogue, GLP-1 has several other actions that enhance the release of insulin. GLP-1 increases insulin biosynthesis, and stimulates the transcription of other β-cell genes including glucokinase and the GLUT-2 glucose transporter.[37,52] Exendin-4, a GLP-1 receptor agonist, induces β-cell neogenesis and expansion in rats.[53] Finally, GLP-1 increases the capacity of individual β cells to respond to stimulation by glucose, and this effect to activate glucose-insensitive cells has been termed induction of glucose competence.[1] Taken together, these findings suggest a broad role for GLP-1 to promote β-cell function.

Several recent reports have conclusively established a role for GLP-1 as a physiologic incretin. Rats given exendin[9–39], a specific GLP-1 receptor antagonist, during enteral glucose feeding had increased postmeal glycemia coincident with attenuated insulin release, compared to control animals.[1] Similar results were reported in nonhuman primates given either exendin[9–39] or an anti-GLP-1 monoclonal antibody, and in these studies interference with the action of GLP-1 caused a rightward shift in the insulin response curve such that insulin secretion was decreased during the early phases of nutrient absorption, but rose later in the study, possibly in response to the higher levels of glucose.[54] Consistent with these findings, male mice with a targeted gene deletion of the GLP-1 receptor have abnormal glucose tolerance and attenuated insulin release after glucose ingestion[55] (**Fig. 6-4**). Interestingly, these animals have increased circulating levels of GIP and an accentuated insulin secretory response to GIP,[56] raising the possibility that the incretin effect is part of a closed-loop regulatory system. Thus substantial experimental evidence demonstrates an important role for GLP-1 in mediating the insulin response to meals, and indicates that this gut peptide is necessary for normal glucose tolerance.

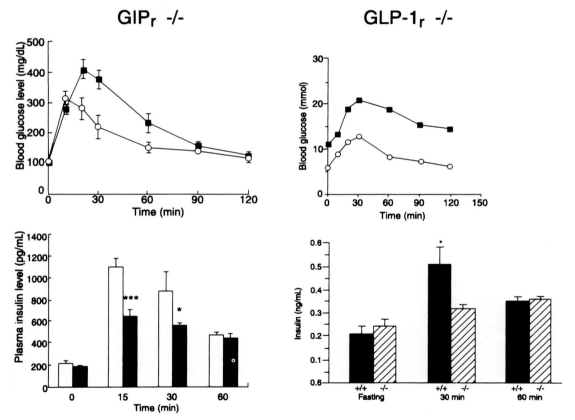

FIGURE 6-4. Glucose tolerance (**top**) and insulin secretion (**bottom**) in mice with targeted gene deletions of the GIP (**left panel**) and GLP-1 (**right panel**) receptors. GIP-receptor-knockout mice (**solid squares**) have an increased glucose excursion during oral glucose loading compared to control mice (**open circles**). Despite the increased plasma glucose levels, insulin secretion in the mice lacking the GIP receptors (**black bars**) is lower than controls (**white bars**). The GLP-1-receptor-knockout mice (**solid squares**) also have impaired glucose tolerance following oral glucose administration compared to control animals (**open circles**). Similarly to the GIP knockouts there is a decrement in insulin secretion during the oral glucose tolerance test (GLP-1r -/- **hatched bars**) (controls **black bars**). These data demonstrate that signaling through both the GIP and GLP-1 receptors is necessary for a normal incretin effect, with appropriate insulin secretion and glucose tolerance in response to enteral glucose. (*Reprinted with permission from Miyawaki et al[22] and Scrocchi et al.[55]*)

In addition to abnormalities in the insulin and glucose responses to ingested glucose, GLP-1-receptor-deficient mice have fasting hyperglycemia and impaired insulin secretion in response to parenteral glucose.[55] While this latter finding is puzzling at first glance since an incretin factor should be secreted and act during nutrient absorption, recent studies in vitro,[57] and in humans,[58] suggest that basal levels of GLP-1 may play a role in β-cell function. The observation that GLP-1 receptor knockout mice have decreased pancreatic insulin and insulin mRNA content[56] is also consistent with the notion that basal, or unstimulated levels of GLP-1 have important effects on β-cell function. These cumulative data suggest that GLP-1 may have important effects on insulin biogenesis and release beyond its action as an acute secretagogue.

Other Actions of GLP-1

Similarly to GIP, GLP-1 has been shown to have effects on tissues other than the pancreatic β cell. In general, these possible alternative functions of GLP-1 have not been as conclusively established as are the effects of the peptide as an insulin secretagogue. Nonetheless, these extrainsular effects of GLP-1 involve other processes in the regulation of nutrient, particularly carbohydrate, metabolism, and so are consistent with the known incretin function of the hormone. Therefore a reasonable case can be made that GLP-1 has a broad physiologic role in minimizing fluctuations in blood glucose levels.

In contrast to GIP, GLP-1 lowers fasting and postprandial glucagon concentrations in humans and animals.[1,39] Of note, only a minority of α cells expresses the GLP-1 receptor,[59] and among these cells relative expression is lower than that of the GIP receptor.[17] Similar to findings in vivo, GLP-1 stimulates insulin secretion and inhibits glucagon release from isolated human islets.[60] However, GLP-1 has little effect on glucagon secretion from cultured α cells from disrupted islet cell preparations, and actually stimulates glucagon release from isolated, purified α cells.[23] The different responses to GLP-1 in animals and intact islets compared to isolated α cells imply that paracrine actions of insulin and/or somatostatin are the primary mechanisms by which GLP-1 regulates glucagon secretion. Similarly to the β cell, the α cell seems to be tonically regulated by GLP-1 since glucagon levels increase when the GLP-1 receptor antagonist exendin[9–39] is administered in the fasting state when GLP-1 is at basal levels.[54,58] With the addition of a glucagonostatic effect to its incretin action, GLP-1 can be seen as coordinating the secretion of islet hormones in the postprandial state to restrain elevations in blood glucose.

Doses of GLP-1 estimated to mimic postprandial plasma concentrations inhibit antral contractions, increase pyloric tone, and substantially lower the rate of gastric emptying of both liquid and solid meals.[61] This effect is sufficient to minimize the rise in meal-induced glucose and insulin levels. Supraphysiologic doses of GLP-1 virtually abolish gastric emptying. The effects of GLP-1 on gastric motility, as well as its inhibition of gastric acid secretion, are likely mediated through vagal afferent signals emanating from nerve terminals in the gastrointestinal lining.[62,63] While it is likely that regulation of gastric function is a normal part of the physiologic action of GLP-1, this has not been proven. In nonhuman primates given the GLP-1 receptor antagonist exendin[9–39] during oral glucose tolerance tests, no difference in delivery of carbohydrate to the intestine was noted,[54] suggesting that with small liquid meals the effect of GLP-1 to slow gastric emptying may be small.

Administration of GLP-1 into the cerebroventricular system of rats decreases food intake[64] raising the possibility that this incretin may also play a regulatory role in satiety or body weight regulation. Short-term infusion of GLP-1 to humans suppresses consumption of a subsequent lunch[65,66] suggesting that the satiety effects of GLP-1 are mediated by peripherally, rather than centrally, derived peptide. It is possible that effects of GLP-1 on food intake are mediated through the same neural circuits that regulate gastric emptying. Currently there is some debate as to whether or not long-term administration of GLP-1 causes weight loss, and this remains an important question for future investigation.

Several reports suggest that GLP-1 increases glucose disposal independent of its effects on islet hormones. In type 1 diabetic subjects infused with constant rates of IV insulin, the amount of glucose required to maintain euglycemia was 15–20% higher when GLP-1 was also given, suggesting that GLP-1 increased glucose disposal independent of changes in insulin concentration.[67] Subsequently, it was shown that infusions of GLP-1 increased the rate of glucose disappearance in healthy subjects given IV glucose, and that this effect was due to increases in both insulin secretion and glucose effectiveness, an index of insulin-independent glucose disposition.[68] No specific process has yet been discovered to explain these findings, although it appears that GLP-1 does not affect insulin sensitivity in humans.[68,69] In vitro studies indicate that GLP-1 can increase glucose transport in adipocytes and preadipocytes,[70,71] and promote glycogen synthesis in both muscle and hepatocyte preparations.[1] However, to date none of the in vitro and in vivo results have been corroborated in a manner that provides a mechanism for these actions of GLP-1. Therefore, the physiologic importance of extra-islet effects of GLP-1 on glucose metabolism remains controversial.

GLP-1 in Diabetes

Because of its importance for glucose tolerance, and because diabetic persons appear to have a defective incretin augmentation of insulin secretion, the adequacy of GLP-1 secretion in type 2 diabetes has been examined in several studies. While some groups have suggested that GLP-1 secretion is increased in type 2 diabetes,[72,73] others have come to the opposite conclusion, that GLP-1 secretion is impaired in diabetic individuals.[74] These studies have used different assays of plasma GLP-1, so the lack of consensus may be due to technical discrepancies. However, it seems more likely that these differences are the result of the relatively small sample sizes studied with distinct characteristics that could independently affect the results. For example, it is not clear whether obesity, antidiabetic treatment, or duration of diabetes alters GLP-1 secretion; but any of these (or other parameters) could confound the results of a small study. Given that GLP-1 secretion has not been consistently observed to be impaired in diabetic subjects, it is probably safe to conclude that decreased release of this incretin does not play an etiologic role in the vast majority of cases of T2DM. This conclusion is supported by the fact that nondiabetic, but high-risk, members of families with diabetes have normal GLP-1 secretion.[31]

GLP-1 improves hyperglycemia, sometimes dramatically, in diabetic subjects, and this is due in great part to its effects on the release of the islet hormones. Continuous IV administration of GLP-1 to poorly controlled type 2 diabetic patients decreased blood glucose concentrations to near normal levels within 3–4 hours,

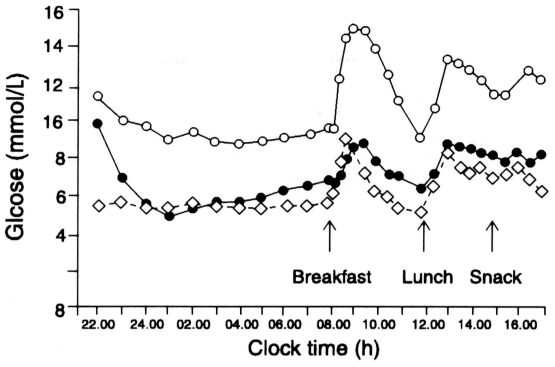

FIGURE 6-5. Plasma glucose concentrations in type 2 diabetic subjects infused with saline (**open circles**), or GLP-1 (**filled circles**). Values from untreated control subjects are also shown (**open diamonds**). Administration of GLP-1 rapidly lowered fasting glucose to normal levels in the diabetic subjects, and greatly improved glucose tolerance with meal ingestion. *(Reprinted with permission from Rachman et al.[79])*

coincident with increased insulin and decreased glucagon levels.[75] In addition, fasting hyperglycemia was significantly improved in a group of type 1 diabetic subjects with minimal insulin secretory reserve given IV GLP-1, most likely due to suppressed glucagon secretion.[76] However, the most prominent effect of GLP-1 in diabetic individuals is stimulation of the β cell. Even in low doses GLP-1 improves the responsiveness of the β cell to glucose in persons with impaired glucose tolerance,[77] an effect that may pertain to persons with mild diabetes as well.[78] Pharmacologic doses of GLP-1 are almost uniformly insulinotropic in subjects with type 2 diabetes,[24,79] in marked contrast to the relative ineffectiveness of GIP to stimulate insulin release in this population. Continuous IV administration of GLP-1 to persons with T2DM normalized fasting and postprandial glucose levels for nearly a full day (Fig. 6-5).[79] That this effect was due primarily to improvements in insulin secretion is supported by a recent study demonstrating that GLP-1 did not change insulin-independent glucose disposal in diabetic persons.[80]

The principal mechanism(s) by which GLP-1 exerts insulinotropic effects in diabetic subjects is not clear. Furthermore, it is not known why GLP-1, but not GIP, retains these properties in people with T2DM given the similarities in intracellular cell signaling between the two incretins. In aged rats with glucose intolerance, 48 hours of GLP-1 administration increased the expression of several genes—proinsulin, glucokinase, and the GLUT-2 glucose transporter—that are important in β-cell function.[52] In this study there was an associated increase in the rapidity and magnitude of the insulin response that corrected the glucose intolerance of these aged animals. This suggests that some of the effects of GLP-1 to improve dysfunctional insulin secretion may result from stimula-

tion of the synthesis of key proteins. Understanding the processes through which GLP-1 renews insulin secretion in persons with diabetes is likely to provide important insights into the pathology of the β cell in this condition and as well as generating targets for novel therapeutics.

Because of the potent effects of IV GLP-1 in improving blood glucose levels in persons with diabetes, there has been much interest in using this peptide or an analogue in treating these patients. One major advantage of GLP-1 over many of the currently available agents used in treating diabetes is that its insulinotropic effect is glucose-dependent and so hypoglycemia is not likely to be a major side effect. GLP-1 has been administered to diabetic patients by subcutaneous injection before meals to decrease postprandial blood glucose excursions,[81,82] but the doses used in these studies were pharmacologic and most likely caused significant inhibition of gastric emptying, sometimes associated with symptoms of nausea. Buccal preparations containing GLP-1 have also been shown to deliver peptide to the circulation and represent another potential mode of administration.[83] However, the problem with both subcutaneous and buccal delivery of GLP-1 is that because of the rapid metabolism of the peptide by DPP IV, the effects are short-lived. Continuous subcutaneous infusion of GLP-1 via a portable pump to subjects with type 2 diabetes caused significant improvements in their glycemic levels for up to 1 week and was well tolerated.[84] Several approaches to minimize the metabolism of GLP-1 to GLP-1[9–36 amide] and extend its time of action are currently being pursued.[85] DPP IV-resistant analogues of GLP-1 have been given to animals and shown to have increased potency compared to the native peptide. Additionally, DPP IV inhibitors are available and have been used to augment the effectiveness of endogenous GLP-1. Other means of harnessing GLP-1 receptor signaling to improve glucose homeostasis include the use of longer acting or more potent parenteral analogues of GLP-1,[86] and genetically-engineered cells that can continuously secrete GLP-1.[87] These strategies, and the possibility of developing orally active GLP-1 receptor activators, are under current investigation.

OTHER INSULINOTROPIC PEPTIDES

Several other peptides synthesized in the GI tract affect β-cell function and have been examined for physiologic roles in meal-induced insulin secretion.[2,88] Among these, cholecystokinin (CCK), gastrin, and secretin are secreted after food ingestion, are insulinotropic, and have clear endocrine functions, and so received significant attention as potential incretins. The CCK_A receptor is present on pancreatic islets and CCK increases insulin secretion *in vitro*. However, in humans, nutrient protein and fat, and not glucose, are the primary stimulus to CCK release, making it an unlikely candidate to mediate glucose-stimulated insulin secretion. Furthermore, CCK is not insulinotropic in humans when given in physiologic amounts and administration of CCK receptor antagonists does not alter postprandial insulin levels in healthy humans. Interestingly, pharmacologic doses of CCK potentiate insulin secretion and decrease postprandial glycemia in type 2 diabetic subjects.[89] Similarly to CCK, secretin stimulates insulin secretion only at plasma levels that are clearly pharmacologic and so is not likely to play a physiologic role as an incretin. Gastrin also stimulates insulin secretion at levels significantly above what are normally measured following meals. However, in several disease states hypergastrinemia is common, so it is possible that this peptide may affect insulin secretion in specific patients.[2] Somatostatin-28 (S-28) is released from the upper GI tract in response to protein- and fat-containing meals. Plasma levels peak in the later phases of nutrient absorption, and in physiologic amounts S-28 inhibits insulin release. This peptide has therefore been proposed as a decretin that slows β-cell secretion as carbohydrate delivered from the gut wanes.[88]

There are a number of neural peptides produced in the GI tract that are also contained in neurons innervating the pancreatic islets.[90] While not true incretins, it is likely that signaling via these autonomic transmitters plays a role in insulin secretion in response to meals. Pituitary adenylate cyclase activating polypeptide (PACAP), vasoactive intestinal polypeptide (VIP), and gastrin-releasing peptide (GRP) are contained in parasympathetic neurons and likely play a role in neurally mediated insulin secretion. As an example, mice with targeted gene deletion of the PAC1 receptor, an important target for PACAP, have impaired insulin secretion and increased plasma glycemia in response to gastric glucose loads.[91] This finding suggests that signaling through neural pathways that release PACAP is activated by glucose in the GI tract and promotes insulin release, and is consistent with a large body of literature implicating the autonomic nervous system in physiologic insulin secretion. It is clear that in humans and other mammals neurally mediated insulin secretion occurs soon after food consumption, before sufficient nutrients have been absorbed to change circulating levels of glucose and other substrates. Although it comprises a relatively small amount of the total postprandial insulin released, this early, or cephalic-phase, insulin secretion has been shown to be important for normal glucose tolerance.[90] The contribution of neural signals to insulin secretion during the absorptive phase of meals is not as clearly established, but it is plausible that parasympathetic cholinergic or peptidergic inputs synergize with substrates and incretins to regulate the β cell.

SUMMARY

Insulin secretion during nutrient ingestion and absorption is finely controlled by the interactions of hyperglycemia, neural signals, and incretins. The incretin effect is essential for normal glucose tolerance, and it appears that the contributions of both GIP and GLP-1 are important in this regard. It is not surprising that GIP and GLP-1 have additional activity beyond the stimulation of insulin release, and it appears that these extra-incretin actions tend to complement the incretin effect by promoting nutrient assimilation and/or glucose homeostasis. Major questions remain as to the role of the incretins in normal physiology. Central among these are the specific roles, as well as the interactions, of GIP and GLP-1, the nature of nutrient-K/L-cell coupling leading to incretin release, and the mechanisms and physiologic significance of the extra-islet effects of incretins. In addition, there are important areas for future research relating the incretins and diabetes. For example, the cause of the impaired incretin effect in type 2 diabetes and the ultimate contribution of this defect on postprandial glycemia has not yet been determined, but is likely to provide both pathogenetic and therapeutic insights. Understanding the apparent loss of β-cell responsiveness to GIP, but not GLP-1, in type 2 diabetes may explain the decreased incretin effect in these patients. In addition, this line of inquiry has the potential to uncover important intra-β-cell signaling pathways and sites of dysfunction. Finally, there are numerous exciting possibilities currently under investigation for harnessing the incretin pathways to improve insulin secretion and glucose tolerance. Thus the long history of research devoted to enteric hormones and their regulation of insulin secretion may soon result in tangible benefits for patients with diabetes.

REFERENCES

1. Kieffer TJ, Habener JF: The glucagon-like peptides. *Endocr Rev* 1999;20:876.
2. Creutzfeldt W, Nauck M: Gut hormones and diabetes mellitus. *Diabetes Metab Rev* 1992;8:149.
3. Dupre J: Influences of the gut on the endocrine pancreas. In: Samols E, ed. *The Endocrine Pancreas.* Raven Press:1991;253.
4. Nauck MA, Homberger E, Siegel EG, *et al*: Incretin effects of increasing glucose loads in man calculated from venous insulin and C-peptide responses. *J Clin Endocrinol Metab* 1986;63:492.
5. Nauck M, Stockmann F, Ebert R, *et al*: Reduced incretin effect in type 2 (non-insulin-dependent) diabetes. *Diabetologia* 1986;29:46
6. Pederson R: Gastric inhibitory polypeptide. In: Walsh JH, Dockray GJ, eds. *Gut Peptides.* Raven Press:1995;217.
7. Wolfe MM BM, Kieffer TJ, Tseng C-C: Glucose-dependent insulinotropic polypeptide (GIP): Incretin vs. enterogastrone. In: Greeley GH, ed. *Gastrointestinal Endocrinology.* Humana Press:1999;439.
8. Usdin TB, Mezey E, Button DC, *et al*: Gastric inhibitory polypeptide receptor, a member of the secretin-vasoactive intestinal peptide receptor family, is widely distributed in peripheral organs and the brain. *Endocrinology* 1993;133:2861.
9. Kieffer TJ, Huang Z, McIntosh CH, *et al*: Gastric inhibitory polypeptide release from a tumor-derived cell line. *Am J Physiol* 1995;269: E316.
10. Tseng CC, Boylan MO, Jarboe LA, *et al*: Chronic desensitization of the glucose-dependent insulinotropic polypeptide receptor in diabetic rats. *Am J Physiol* 1996;270:E661.

11. Schirra J, Katschinski M, Weidmann C, *et al*: Gastric emptying and release of incretin hormones after glucose ingestion in humans. *J Clin Invest* 1996;97:92.

12. Ebert R, Creutzfeldt W: Gastrointestinal peptides and insulin secretion. *Diabetes Metab Rev* 1987;3:1.

13. Krarup T: Immunoreactive gastric inhibitory polypeptide. *Endocrinol Rev* 1988;9:122.

14. Mentlein R: Dipeptidyl-peptidase IV (CD26)—role in the inactivation of regulatory peptides. *Regul Pept* 1999;85:9.

15. Wheeler MB, Gelling RW, McIntosh CH, *et al*: Functional expression of the rat pancreatic islet glucose-dependent insulinotropic polypeptide receptor: ligand binding and intracellular signaling properties. *Endocrinology* 1995;136:4629.

16. Gremlich S, Porret A, Hani EH, *et al*: Cloning, functional expression, and chromosomal localization of the human pancreatic islet glucose-dependent insulinotropic polypeptide receptor. *Diabetes* 1995;44:1202.

17. Moens K, Heimberg H, Flamez D, *et al*: Expression and functional activity of glucagon, glucagon-like peptide 1, and glucose-dependent insulinotropic peptide receptors in rat pancreatic islet cells. *Diabetes* 1996;45:257.

18. Ding WG, Gromada J: Protein kinase A-dependent stimulation of exocytosis in mouse pancreatic beta-cells by glucose-dependent insulinotropic polypeptide. *Diabetes* 1997;46:615.

19. Tseng CC, Zhang XY: Role of regulator of G protein signaling in desensitization of the glucose-dependent insulinotropic peptide receptor. *Endocrinology* 1998;139:4470.

20. Tseng CC, Zhang XY: Role of G protein-coupled receptor kinases in glucose-dependent insulinotropic polypeptide receptor signaling. *Endocrinology* 2000;141:947.

21. Tseng CC, Kieffer TJ, Jarboe LA, *et al*: Postprandial stimulation of insulin release by glucose-dependent insulinotropic polypeptide (GIP). Effect of a specific glucose-dependent insulinotropic polypeptide receptor antagonist in the rat. *J Clin Invest* 1996;98:2440.

22. Miyawaki K, Yamada Y, Yano H, *et al*: Glucose intolerance caused by a defect in the entero-insular axis: a study in gastric inhibitory polypeptide receptor knockout mice. *Proc Natl Acad Sci USA* 1999;96:14843.

23. Ding WG, Renstrom E, Rorsman P, *et al*: Glucagon-like peptide I and glucose-dependent insulinotropic polypeptide stimulate Ca^{2+}-induced secretion in rat alpha-cells by a protein kinase A-mediated mechanism. *Diabetes* 1997;46:792.

24. Nauck MA, Heimesaat MM, Orskov C, *et al*: Preserved incretin activity of glucagon-like peptide 1 (7–36 amide) but not of synthetic human gastric inhibitory polypeptide in patients with type 2 diabetes mellitus. *J Clin Invest* 1993;91:301.

25. Morgan LM: The metabolic role of GIP: physiology and pathology. *Biochem Soc Trans* 1996;24:585.

26. Cheeseman CI, Tsang R: The effect of GIP and glucagon-like peptides on intestinal basolateral membrane hexose transport. *Am J Physiol* 1996;271:G477.

27. Tseng CC, Zhang XY, Wolfe MM: Effect of GIP and GLP-1 antagonists on insulin release in the rat. *Am J Physiol* 1999;276:E1049.

28. Roust LR, Stesin M, Go VL, *et al*: Role of gastric inhibitory polypeptide in postprandial hyperinsulinemia of obesity. *Am J Physiol* 1988;254:E767.

29. Jones IR, Owens DR, Moody AJ, *et al*: The effects of glucose-dependent insulinotropic polypeptide infused at physiological concentrations in normal subjects and type 2 (non-insulin-dependent) diabetic patients on glucose tolerance and B-cell secretion. *Diabetologia* 1987;30:707.

30. Jones IR, Owens DR, Luzio S, *et al*: The glucose dependent insulinotropic polypeptide response to oral glucose and mixed meals is increased in patients with type 2 (non-insulin-dependent) diabetes mellitus. *Diabetologia* 1989;32:668.

31. Nyholm B, Walker M, Gravholt CH, *et al*: Twenty-four-hour insulin secretion rates, circulating concentrations of fuel substrates and gut incretin hormones in healthy offspring of type II (non-insulin-dependent) diabetic parents: evidence of several aberrations. *Diabetologia* 1999;42:1314.

32. Elahi D, McAloon-Dyke M, Fukagawa NK, *et al*: The insulinotropic actions of glucose-dependent insulinotropic polypeptide (GIP) and glucagon-like peptide-1 (7–37) in normal and diabetic subjects. *Regul Pept* 1994;51:63.

33. Kubota A, Yamada Y, Hayami T, *et al*: Identification of two missense mutations in the GIP receptor gene: a functional study and association analysis with NIDDM: no evidence of association with Japanese NIDDM subjects. *Diabetes* 1996;45:1701.

34. Almind K, Ambye L, Urhammer SA, *et al*: Discovery of amino acid variants in the human glucose-dependent insulinotropic polypeptide (GIP) receptor: the impact on the pancreatic beta cell responses and functional expression studies in Chinese hamster fibroblast cells. *Diabetologia* 1998;41:1194.

35. Holst JJ, Gromada J, Nauck MA: The pathogenesis of NIDDM involves a defective expression of the GIP receptor. *Diabetologia* 1997;40:984.

36. Meneilly GS, Ryan AS, Minaker KL, *et al*: The effect of age and glycemic level on the response of the beta-cell to glucose-dependent insulinotropic polypeptide and peripheral tissue sensitivity to endogenously released insulin. *J Clin Endocrinol Metab* 1998;83:2925.

37. Brubaker PL DD: Intestinal proglucagon-derived peptides. In: Greeley GH, ed. *Gastrointestinal Endocrinology*. Humana Press:1999;493.

38. Fehmann H-C, Goke R, Goke B: Cell and molecular biology of the incretin hormones glucagon-like peptide-1 and glucose-dependent insulin releasing polypeptide. *Endocrinol Rev* 1995;16:390.

39. Kreymann B, Ghatei MA, Williams G, *et al*: Glucagon-like peptide-1 7–36: A physiological incretin in man. *Lancet* 1987;2:1300.

40. Herrmann C, Goke R, Richter G, *et al*: Glucagon-like peptide-1 and glucose-dependent insulin-releasing polypeptide plasma levels in response to nutrients. *Digestion* 1995;56:117

41. Hoyt EC, Lund PK, Winesett DE, *et al*: Effects of fasting, refeeding, and intraluminal triglyceride on proglucagon expression in jejunum and ileum. *Diabetes* 1996;45:434.

42. Balks HJ, Holst JJ, von zur Muhlen A, *et al*: Rapid oscillations in plasma glucagon-like peptide-1 (GLP-1) in humans: cholinergic control of GLP-1 secretion via muscarinic receptors. *J Clin Endocrinol Metab* 1997;82:786.

43. D'Alessio DA, Thirlby R, Laschansky EC, *et al*: Response of GLP-1 to nutrients in humans. *Digestion* 1993;54:377.

44. Miholic J, Orskov C, Holst JJ, *et al*: Emptying of the gastric substitute, glucagon-like peptide-1 (GLP-1), and reactive hypoglycemia after total gastrectomy. *Dig Dis Sci* 1991;36:1361.

45. Nauck MA, Bartels E, Orskov C, *et al*: Additive insulinotropic effects of exogenous synthetic human gastric inhibitory polypeptide and glucagon-like peptide-1-(7–36) amide infused at near-physiological insulinotropic hormone and glucose concentrations. *J Clin Endocrinol Metab* 1993;76:912.

46. Damholt AB, Kofod H, Buchan AM: Immunocytochemical evidence for a paracrine interaction between GIP and GLP-1-producing cells in canine small intestine. *Cell Tissue Res* 1999;298:287.

47. Deacon CF, Nauck MA, Toft-Nielsen M, *et al*: Both subcutaneously and intravenously administered glucagon-like peptide 1 are rapidly degraded from the NH$_2$-terminus in type II diabetic patients and in healthy subjects. *Diabetes* 1995;44:1126.

48. Montrose-Rafizadeh C, Yang H, Rodgers BD, *et al*: High potency antagonists of the pancreatic glucagon-like peptide-1 receptor. *J Biol Chem* 1997;272:21201.

49. Gromada J, Holst JJ, Rorsman P: Cellular regulation of islet hormone secretion by the incretin hormone glucagon-like peptide 1. *Pflugers Arch* 1998;435:583.

50. Bode HP, Moormann B, Dabew R, *et al*: Glucagon-like peptide 1 elevates cytosolic calcium in pancreatic beta-cells independently of protein kinase A. *Endocrinology* 1999;140:3919.

51. Thorens B, Widmann C: Signal transduction and desensitization of the glucagon-like peptide-1 receptor. *Acta Physiol Scand* 1996;157:317.

52. Wang Y, Perfetti R, Greig NH, *et al*: Glucagon-like peptide-1 can reverse the age-related decline in glucose tolerance in rats. *J Clin Invest* 1997;99:2883.

53. Xu G, Stoffers DA, Habener JF, *et al*: Exendin-4 stimulates both beta-cell replication and neogenesis, resulting in increased beta-cell mass and improved glucose tolerance in diabetic rats. *Diabetes* 1999;48:2270.

54. D'Alessio DA, Vogel RE, Prigeon RL, *et al*: Elimination of the action of glucagon-like peptide 1 causes an impairment of glucose tolerance after nutrient ingestion by healthy baboons. *J Clin Invest* 1996;97:133.

55. Scrocchi LA, Brown TJ, MacLusky N, *et al*: Glucose intolerance but normal satiety in mice with a null mutation in the glucagon-like peptide 1 receptor gene. *Nat Med* 1996;2:1254.

56. Pederson RA, Satkunarajah M, McIntosh CH, *et al*: Enhanced glucose-dependent insulinotropic polypeptide secretion and insulinotropic action in glucagon-like peptide 1 receptor −/− mice. *Diabetes* 1998;47:1046.

57. Serre V, Dolci W, Schaerer E, *et al*: Exendin-(9–39) is an inverse agonist of the murine glucagon-like peptide-1 receptor: implications for

basal intracellular cyclic adenosine 3',-monophosphate levels and beta-cell glucose competence. *Endocrinology* 1998;139:4448.

58. Schirra J, Sturm K, Leicht P, *et al*: Exendin(9–39)amide is an antagonist of glucagon-like peptide-1(7–36)amide in humans. *J Clin Invest* 1998;101:1421.

59. Heller RS, Kieffer TJ, Habener JF: Insulinotropic glucagon-like peptide I receptor expression in glucagon-producing alpha-cells of the rat endocrine pancreas. *Diabetes* 1997;46:785.

60. Fehmann HC, Hering BJ, Wolf MJ, *et al*: The effects of glucagon-like peptide-I (GLP-I) on hormone secretion from isolated human pancreatic islets. *Pancreas* 1995;11:196.

61. Schirra J, Houck P, Wank U, *et al*: Effects of glucagon-like peptide-1(7–36)amide on antro-pyloro-duodenal motility in the interdigestive state and with duodenal lipid perfusion in humans. *Gut* 2000;46:622.

62. Imeryuz N, Yegen BC, Bozkurt A, *et al*: Glucagon-like peptide-1 inhibits gastric emptying via vagal afferent-mediated central mechanisms. *Am J Physiol* 1997;273:G920.

63. Wettergren A, Wojdemann M, Holst JJ: Glucagon-like peptide-1 inhibits gastropancreatic function by inhibiting central parasympathetic outflow. *Am J Physiol* 1998;275:G984.

64. Turton MD, O'Shea D, Gunn I, *et al*: A role for glucagon-like peptide-1 in the central regulation of feeding. *Nature* 1996;379:69.

65. Flint A, Raben A, Astrup A, *et al*: Glucagon-like peptide 1 promotes satiety and suppresses energy intake in humans. *J Clin Invest* 1998;101:515.

66. Gutzwiller JP, Goke B, Drewe J, *et al*: Glucagon-like peptide-1: a potent regulator of food intake in humans. *Gut* 1999;44:81.

67. Gutniak M, Orskov C, Holst J, *et al*: Antidiabetogenic effect of glucagon-like peptide-1(7–36) in normal subjects and patients with diabetes mellitus. *N Engl J Med* 1992;326:1316.

68. D'Alessio DA, Kahn SE, Leusner CR, *et al*: Glucagon-like peptide 1 enhances glucose tolerance both by stimulation of insulin release and by increasing insulin-independent glucose disposal. *J Clin Invest* 1994;93:2263.

69. Orskov L, Holst JJ, Moller N, *et al*: GLP-1 does not acutely affect insulin sensitivity in healthy man. *Diabetologia* 1996;39:1227.

70. Oben J, Morgan L, Fletcher J, *et al*: Effect of the entero-pancreatic hormones, gastric inhibitory polypeptide and glucagon-like polypeptide-1 (7–36) amide, on fatty acid synthesis in explants of rat adipose tissue. *J Endocrinol* 1991;130:267.

71. Egan JM, Montrose-Rafizadeh C, Wang Y, *et al*: Glucagon-like peptide 1 (7–36)amide enhances insulin-stimulated glucose metabolism in 3T3-LI adipocytes: One of several potential extrapancreatic sites of GLP-1 action. *Endocrinology* 1994;135:2070.

72. Orskov C, Jeppesen J, Madsbad S, *et al*: Proglucagon products in plasma of noninsulin-dependent diabetics and nondiabetic controls in the fasting state and after oral glucose and intravenous arginine. *J Clin Invest* 1991;87:415.

73. Fukase N, Manaka H, Sugiyama H, *et al*: Response of truncated glucagon-like peptide-1 and gastric inhibitory polypeptide to glucose ingestion in non-insulin dependent diabetes mellitus. *Acta Diabetol* 1995;32:165.

74. Vaag AA, Holst JJ, Volund A, *et al*: Gut incretin hormones in identical twins discordant for non-insulin-dependent diabetes mellitus (NIDDM)—evidence for decreased glucagon-like peptide 1 secretion

75. Nauck MA, Kleine N, Orskov C, *et al*: Normalization of fasting hyperglycemia by endogenous glucagon-like peptide 1 (7–36 amide) in type 2 (non-insulin-dependent) diabetic patients. *Diabetologia* 1993;36:741.

76. Creutzfeldt W, Orskov C, Kleine N, *et al*: Glucagonostatic actions and reduction of fasting hyperglycemia by exogenous glucagon-like peptide I (7–36) amide in type I diabetic patients. *Diabetes Care* 1996;19:580.

77. Byrne MM, Gliem K, Wank U, *et al*: Glucagon-like peptide 1 improves the ability of the beta-cell to sense and respond to glucose in subjects with impaired glucose tolerance. *Diabetes* 1998;47:1259.

78. Ahren BO, Larsson H, Holst JJ: Effects of glucagon-like peptide-1 on islet function and insulin sensitivity in noninsulin-dependent diabetes mellitus. *J Clin Endocrinol Metab* 1997;82:473.

79. Rachman J, Barrow BA, Levy JC, *et al*: Near-normalisation of diurnal glucose concentrations by continuous administration of glucagon-like peptide-1 (GLP-1) in subjects with NIDDM. *Diabetologia* 1997;40:205.

80. Vella A, Shah P, Basu R, *et al*: Effect of glucagon-like peptide 1(7–36) amide on glucose effectiveness and insulin action in people with type 2 diabetes. *Diabetes* 2000;49:611.

81. Dupre J, Behme MT, Hramiak IM, *et al*: Glucagon-like peptide I reduces postprandial glycemic excursions in IDDM. *Diabetes* 1995;44:626.

82. Gutniak MK, Linde B, Holst JJ, *et al*: Subcutaneous injection of the incretin hormone glucagon-like peptide 1 abolishes postprandial glycemia in NIDDM. *Diabetes Care* 1994;17:1039.

83. Gutniak MK, Larsson H, Sanders SW, *et al*: GLP-1 tablet in type 2 diabetes in fasting and postprandial conditions. *Diabetes Care* 1997;20:1874.

84. Toft-Nielsen MB, Madsbad S, Holst JJ: Continuous subcutaneous infusion of glucagon-like peptide 1 lowers plasma glucose and reduces appetite in type 2 diabetic patients. *Diabetes Care* 1999;22:1137.

85. Holst JJ, Deacon CF: Inhibition of the activity of dipeptidyl-peptidase IV as a treatment for type 2 diabetes. *Diabetes* 1998;47:1663.

86. Greig NH, Holloway HW, De Ore KA, *et al*: Once daily injection of exendin-4 to diabetic mice achieves long-term beneficial effects on blood glucose concentrations. *Diabetologia* 1999;42:45.

87. Burcelin R, Rolland E, Dolci W, *et al*: Encapsulated, genetically engineered cells, secreting glucagon-like peptide-1 for the treatment of non-insulin-dependent diabetes mellitus. *Ann NY Acad Sci* 1999;875:277.

88. Ebert R: Gut signals for islet hormone release. *Eur J Clin Invest* 1990;20(Suppl 1):20.

89. Ahren B, Holst JJ, Efendic S: Antidiabetogenic action of cholecystokinin-8 in type 2 diabetes. *J Clin Endocrinol Metab* 2000;85:1043.

90. Ahren B: Autonomic regulation of islet hormone secretion—implications for health and disease. *Diabetologia* 2000;43:393.

91. Jamen F, Persson K, Bertrand G, *et al*: PAC1 receptor-deficient mice display impaired insulinotropic response to glucose and reduced glucose tolerance. *J Clin Invest* 2000;105:1307

during oral glucose ingestion in NIDDM twins. *Eur J Endocrinol* 1996;135:425.

CHAPTER 7

Glucagon

John M. Amatruda

James N. Livingston

INTRODUCTION

Glucagon, through its effects on the liver, is an important regulator of glucose and lipid metabolism in health and disease. Murlin and Kimball discovered glucagon in 1923, and the peptide was first purified and its biological actions studied in the 1940s and 1950s. Proof of its hormonal status was not available until the development of a radioimmunoassay for glucagon in 1959. In the 1960s and 1970s, the α (alpha) cell was shown to be a vital component of the islets of Langerhans and glucagon was found to play an essential role in the overproduction of glucose and ketones in diabetes. By 1985, the role of glucagon in health and disease was largely understood.

In the 1980s and '90s, most research focused on the molecular and cell biology of glucagon including the preproglucagon gene, its distribution and regulation, the processing of the prohormone, and the cloning and characterization of the glucagon receptor. In addition, newer *in vivo* techniques and animal models have refined our knowledge of the importance of glucagon in glucose homeostasis. This chapter will review the regulation and function of glucagon at the molecular, cellular, and physiological levels.

THE GLUCAGON GENE AND ITS PRODUCTS

Preproglucagon Gene

The preproglucagon gene apparently arose from the duplication of an ancestral gene over 800 million years ago.[1] The gene for preproglucagon is located on the long arm of chromosome 2[2,3] and has six exons of which four encode the 5'-untranslated region, the signal peptide, the preprohormone, and the 3' untranslated region.[4] Control of the preproglucagon gene is through six identified promoters, which include G1 through G4, CRE (cyclic AMP response element), and ISE (intestine-specific enhancer) (Fig. 7-1).[5] The promoter activity depends on the tissue in which the gene is being expressed. For example, the G1 promoter, a ~40 nucleotide element located near the TATA box, is acted on by homeoproteins to direct α-cell expression,[6–11] whereas G2 and G3 promoters are enhancers that are active in islets as well as in other cells.[12,13] The G3 element may mediate the suppressive insulin response found in studies of glucagon gene expression in islets.[14] The CRE is located near the G3 element and responds to cyclic AMP–mediated events. The presence of this promoter is consistent with the finding in α cells that elevation of cyclic AMP increases preproglucagon gene expression.[15–17]

Less is understood about the control of preproglucagon gene expression in sites other than the α cell. For example, intestinal L cells appear to use the ISE promoter element, although other upstream elements are also required.[5,18]

TISSUE EXPRESSION OF PREPROGLUCAGON

Preproglucagon can be demonstrated in a variety of cells. The most important sites of production are the α cells in pancreatic islets and L cells in the jejunum, ileum, and to a lesser extent in the duodenum and large bowel. Other locations of preproglucagon expression are specific neurons in the brain (hypothalamus, cerebral cortex, amygdaloid nuclei, and medulla oblongata)[19] and "a cells" in the gastric fundus of the dog.[20]

There are a number of peptides that can be produced from preproglucagon. The peptides generated depend on posttranslational processing of the preprohormone at dibasic amino acid sites.[21–25] Enzymes called prehormone convertases, which process prohormones, are involved in the cleavage of preproglucagon to glucagon. Two of the convertases, PC2 and PC1/3, are found in high concentrations in islet cells. PC2 is thought to convert preproglucagon to glucagon in α cells,[26] whereas PC1/3 generates glucagon-like peptides (GLPs) in the intestine.[27] Mice with a deficiency of PC2 generated by knockout experiments have fasting hypoglycemia consistent with a deficiency in circulating glucagon.[28]

Figure 7-2 shows the different peptides generated from preproglucagon by α cells in pancreatic islets or by L cells in the intestine. Depending on the tissue, a number of peptides have been identified from preproglucagon processing.[29] These peptides include GRPP (glicentin-related pancreatic peptide), glucagon, IP-1 (intervening peptide-1), GLP-1, IP-2 (intervening peptide-2), and GLP-2. In the α cell, the glicentin fragment, which contains sequences for GRPP, glucagon, and IP-1, is first processed to oxyntomodulin, a fragment that contains glucagon and IP-1. This latter peptide is further processed to form glucagon. Small amounts of oxyntomodulin representing about 10–15% of the glucagon content can be found in α cells. A large C-terminal fragment of preproglucagon is also present and has the sequences of GLP-1 and GLP-2. However, the α cell cannot efficiently generate GLP-1 or GLP-2 from this fragment.

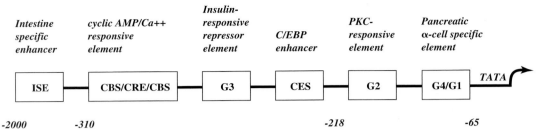

FIGURE 7-1. DNA control elements for the rat glucagon gene. **ISE**, intestine-specific enhancer; **CBS**, CAP-binding site; **CRE**, cyclic AMP response element; **CES**, C/EBP enhancer site; **G1–G4**, major α cell/islet enhancers; **TATA**, TATA box. *(Modified from Kieffer et al.[29])*

In L cells, the processing of preproglucagon generates GLP-1, GLP-2, and glicentin, which in this cell type is further processed into oxyntomodulin and GRPP.[29] Unlike the α cell, the L cell cannot generate glucagon from oxyntomodulin. Overall, these findings with α cells and L cells point to a remarkably cell-specific processing of preproglucagon to generate an array of gene products fashioned for the needs of a particular tissue.

The processing of preproglucagon in the brain generally corresponds to the processing in the intestine.[30–35] Interestingly, however, glucagon can be found in fetal brain, but this processing ability disappears as the brain matures.

A miniglucagon has been reported in plasma that represents the 19–29 amino acid fragment of glucagon.[36] The short half-life of the fragment and the failure to find significant amounts in the circulation suggests that miniglucagon is produced from glucagon at the surface of the hepatocyte, where the fragment is purported to act.[37] Studies of the effects of miniglucagon on liver indicate that the fragment has different actions than glucagon, although the importance of these effects is not clear, nor has a possible physiological role for this fragment been established.[37]

GLUCAGON SYNTHESIS AND SECRETION

The rate-limiting step in the synthesis of glucagon by α cells is the production of preproglucagon. The elevation of cyclic AMP increases preproglucagon gene expression with the consequent increase in preprohormone production. This effect of cyclic AMP

FIGURE 7-2. Processing of the proglucagon to peptides in intestinal L cells and pancreatic α cells. **GLP**, glucagon-like peptide; **GRPP**, glicentin-related pancreatic peptide; **IP**, intervening peptide. *(Modified from Kieffer et al.[29])*

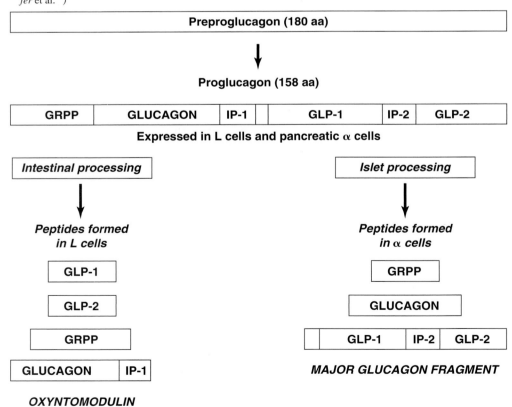

may demonstrate synergy with elevations in Ca^{++} to increase the production rate to levels greater than either alone.[38,39] Membrane depolarization in which calcium/calmodulin-dependent kinase II participates is also part of this process.

In contrast to agents that increase glucagon synthesis, insulin is reported to inhibit preproglucagon gene expression in α cells.[40] This inhibitory effect is thought to be mediated by an insulin response element in the preproglucagon gene that corresponds to the previously identified enhancer-like element, G3.[41]

Expression of preproglucagon in L cells has been monitored by the synthesis and secretion of GLP-1.[29] Intestinal cell cultures have shown that cyclic AMP–mediated responses stimulate GLP-1 synthesis and release.[18,42–44] The release of GLP-1 from L cells involves a rapid response to hormonal and neural signals and a slower response to direct contact with nutrients.[29]

The secretion of glucagon from α cells is under a complex control system that responds acutely to nutritional and hormonal signals. This acute response is geared to immediate changes in fuel homeostasis.[45] Because of the complexities in this control system and the likelihood that multiple, parallel changes will occur in a number of regulatory systems in response to metabolic alterations, it is difficult to distinguish direct effects on glucagon secretion from indirect effects. For example, a stimulus that causes insulin release may also be associated with a drop in plasma glucagon. In this case, it is difficult to know if the effect is from a direct action on the α cell or an indirect effect from β-cell stimulation and a consequent increase in insulin secretion, which in itself will reduce glucagon secretion.

The signals to the α cell that regulate glucagon secretion can be divided into neural signals from the nerve endings that surround the pancreatic islet; signals from circulating hormones, especially those from the gut or from other cells in the islets; or signals from fuels, particularly glucose and amino acids. Figure 7-3 illustrates the role of the central nervous system in the regulation of glucagon

secretion in response to hypoglycemia. The neural signals are delivered by adrenergic, cholinergic, peptidergic, and purinergic nerves, and link areas in the hypothalamus to the islets through the autonomic nervous system. Thus stimulation of the ventromedial nucleus in the hypothalamus produces glucagon release while inhibiting insulin release, the latter of which further enhances glucagon secretion.[46] Likewise, stimulation of the lateral hypothalamus also increases glucagon release.[47]

The release of norepinephrine from sympathetic nerve endings in pancreatic islets activates α_2- and β_2-adenoreceptors on α cells and increases glucagon secretion.[48,49] Parasympathetic innervation of the islet increases glucagon secretion by the release of acetylcholine and the consequent activation of M_1 and M_3 muscarinic receptors on α cells.[48,50]

Peptidergic stimulation of α cells involves a growing list of neuropeptides. Glucagon secretion is stimulated by a pancreatic sympathetic neuropeptide like galanin[51] or a parasympathetic neuropeptide like vasoactive intestinal peptide (VIP).[52] More recently, PACAP-27 and PACAP-38 (pituitary adenylate cyclase activating polypeptide), two forms of a neuropeptide related to VIP, were found in human pancreas and shown to cause glucagon secretion.[53]

Gastrointestinal neuropeptides that have activity on α cells include gastrin and cholecystokinin (CCK).[54] Both peptides apparently act on the CCK-B/G receptor in α cells to stimulate glucagon release. α-Cell function may be altered by serotonin and prostaglandins[55] as well as GLP-1, which inhibits glucagon secretion *in vivo*.[56,57] However this effect may be secondary to the potent stimulatory effects GLP-1 has on insulin secretion,[58–60] since *in vitro* experiments on isolated islets show a stimulation of glucagon secretion.[16,17]

Besides neuropeptides from the gut, somatostatin, a peptide produced in the brain, in the GI tract, and in pancreatic islets, is a potent inhibitor of glucagon secretion.[61] The binding of somato-

FIGURE 7-3. Control of glucagon secretion by hypoglycemia. Low plasma glucose has direct and indirect effects on glucagon secretion by the α cell. The indirect effects are through the autonomic system that acts both on the α cell and β cell. A direct effect of low plasma glucose on the α cell is illustrated. The importance of a reduction in insulin secretion for enhanced glucagon secretion is shown.

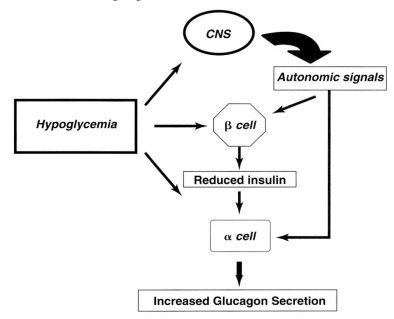

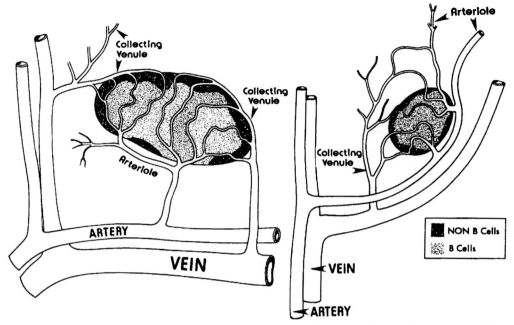

FIGURE 7-4. Diagram of islet microcirculation in large (left) and small (right) islets. β Cells are shown in the core of the islets and the α cells and other non-β cells are in the periphery. *(Modified from Unger et al.[68])*

statin to the somatostatin receptor SSTR2 is responsible for this effect.[62] Since δ (delta) cells in the islets secrete somatostatin, the somatostatin effect on glucagon secretion has generally been considered part of the islet's paracrine system.

Argument against a paracrine effect is that the amount of somatostatin in the venous effluent is much greater than the amount needed to maximally inhibit glucagon release.[63] Thus, in order for the α cell to function properly, it must be shielded from the majority of somatostatin produced by the islet δ cells.

Insulin is a major regulator of glucagon secretion. Evidence for this regulation has been gathered from perfusion of rat islets with an insulin antibody to neutralize the insulin effects. Antibody perfusion results in a rapid increase in glucagon secretion.[64] The islet arrangement of the α and β cells and islet microcirculation play a role in this regulation (Fig. 7-4).[64,65] The β cells are located within the interior of the islet, whereas α cells and other non-β cells are located on the periphery. In the rat the afferent blood vessels enter the islet and pass through to the cortex where they branch to perfuse β cells. The effect of this arrangement is that α cells are exposed to potentially high local concentrations of insulin released by β cells. The effect of insulin on glucagon secretion is possibly one of the most important controls imposed on the α cell. Abnormalities in this control may contribute to the pathophysiology of diabetes by, for example, the increase in glucagon secretion that has been reported in cases where insulin secretion is impaired.[66,67]

Secretin and IGF-1 (insulin-like growth factor-1) are other hormones associated with a negative effect on glucagon secretion,[68,69] whereas hormones associated with an increase in glucagon secretion include cortisol, oxytocin, vasopressin, growth hormone, and β-endorphin.[70,71] The effects of various agents on glucagon secretion are summarized in Table 7-1.

One of the most powerful regulators of glucagon secretion is the plasma level of glucose. A fall in plasma glucose below euglycemia results in a rise in glucagon to protect against hypo-

glycemia.[72,73] Much of this effect is believed to be secondary to the decrease in insulin that accompanies the fall in glucose and to autonomic changes associated with hypoglycemia.[48]

Amino acids also influence the secretion of glucagon, an effect that is observed in human subjects and in studies of perfused pancreas.[74] Except for branched-chain amino acids, glucagon secretion is stimulated by essentially all amino acids to varying degrees.[75] Arginine is a potent stimulator that has been used to test α-cell function. However, less is known about the role of amino acids in glucagon release than the effects of other secretagogues. Because relatively high amino acid concentrations are needed to produce an effect on glucagon secretion, amino acids may not be important physiologic regulators of α-cell secretion.[68] There is some evidence, however, that preventing the decrease in plasma

TABLE 7-1. Nonnutrient Agents That Regulate Glucagon Secretion

Glucagon Secretion	
Increase	*Decrease*
Epinephrine	Insulin
Norepinephrine	Somatostatin
Acetylcholine	GLP-1 (*in vivo*)
Galanin	Secretin
VIP	IGF-1
PACAP-27	
PACAP-38	
Gastrin	
CCK	
Cortisol	
Oxytocin	
Growth hormone	
β-Endorphin	

amino acids during insulin-induced hypoglycemia enhances the glucagon response.[76]

Free fatty acids (FFA) are another fuel that can influence glucagon secretion. At high concentrations, FFA inhibits glucagon release while stimulating insulin secretion.[77] Further studies have shown that relatively small changes in FFA in the physiological range can influence the plasma level of glucagon.[78] However, it is generally believed that the role of glucose predominates over the role of FFA in the regulation of glucagon secretion.[79]

THE GLUCAGON RECEPTOR AND GLUCAGON SIGNALING

The action of glucagon begins with the binding of the hormone to a cell surface receptor. Following its cloning and sequencing, the receptor was shown to be a G-protein-coupled receptor in the family of receptors that includes GLP-1, gastrointestinal peptide (GIP), secretin, PACAP, growth hormone releasing factor (GHF), calcitonin, parathyroid hormone (PTH), and VIP.[29] The amino acid sequence identity of the glucagon receptor to the other receptor members varies between 27% and 49%.

The gene for the receptor is located on chromosome 17.[80] There is apparently only one gene that encodes the receptor and differentially spliced variants have not been identified.[81] Based on mRNA profiling of rat tissues, the glucagon receptor gene is expressed in liver, kidney, heart, adipose tissue, duodenum, stomach, and brain.[82] Of these, the liver is recognized as the major site of expression. Functional glucagon receptors have been identified in adipose tissue, kidney, pancreatic islets, brain, heart, and intestinal tract.[83]

The cloned human glucagon receptor contains 477 amino acids. The third intracellular loop of the receptor that associates with G proteins is relatively short. The extracellular portion of the receptor that binds glucagon has been studied by making chimeric receptors between sequences of glucagon and GLP-1 receptors.[84] These studies show that a portion of the amino terminal extracellular domain and the first and third extracellular loops are required for glucagon binding, whereas the third, fourth, and sixth transmembrane segments contribute to the specificity of the binding reaction for glucagon. From these findings it appears that most of the extracellular portion of the glucagon receptor participates in binding glucagon. Although the cell surface portions of the receptor are the main binding determinants, glucagon binding can be inhibited by small molecules that act at nonsurface sites on the receptor to perturb its structure.[85] For example, small compounds that insert at the transmembrane site, Leu 388, block glucagon binding and inhibit glucagon action. These compounds have potential to treat type 2 diabetic subjects by reducing the relative overstimulation of glucagon that is a factor in the excessive production of glucose found in this disease.

The molecular events involved in glucagon action are shown in Fig. 7-5. Following binding of glucagon, the glucagon receptor interacts with a G-coupled protein to generate an increase in cyclic AMP through the adenylate cyclase system.[86,87] The finding that GTP was required during glucagon stimulation of the cyclase system led to the important discovery that GTP-coupled proteins are needed to mediate the actions of seven transmembrane receptors.[88] The GTP-coupled protein that functionally links the glucagon receptor to adenylate cyclase is Gs, a trimeric protein in its unstimulated state. The interaction of the glucagon receptor complex with Gs provokes the exchange of GDP in the nucleotide-binding site for GTP. The α-subunit of the Gs trimer is then liberated to interact with and activate adenylate cyclase to produce cyclic AMP from ATP.[89] Termination of this activation occurs with the slow hydrolysis of GTP to GDP by the GTPase activity inherent in the α-subunit.[90]

A less studied signaling pathway for glucagon action is through an increase in Ca^{++}.[91] It is not clear if the increase in

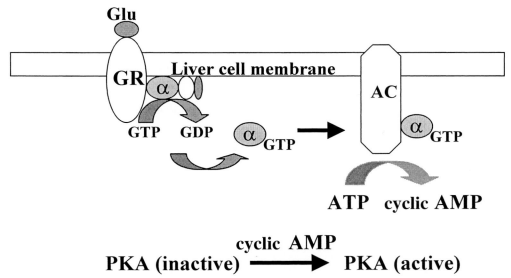

FIGURE 7-5. Activation of the liver adenylate cyclase system by glucagon (**Glu**). Binding of glucagon to the glucagon receptor (**GR**) causes the exchange of guanosine diphosphate (**GDP**) for guanosine triphosphate (**GTP**) in the α-subunit of the GTP-binding protein. This freed subunit activates adenylate cyclase (**AC**) to produce cyclic AMP from adenosine triphosphate (**ATP**). Cyclic AMP in turn activates protein kinase A (**PKA**) which phosphorylates enzymes that control glucose metabolism in the glycogenolytic, glycolysis, and gluconeogenesis pathways.

Ca^{++} is secondary to the effects of glucagon on cyclic AMP levels or if it involves another signaling system. This second pathway may be the IP-3 system, which is coupled to G∝q or G11.[92] Regardless, the best-documented system for glucagon action is the activation of the adenylate cyclase system and an increase in cyclic AMP levels.

METABOLIC EFFECTS OF GLUCAGON

The action of cyclic AMP starts with its binding to regulatory subunits of inactive protein kinase A (PKA). The binding activates the catalytic subunits by allowing them to dissociate from the regulatory subunits that restrain catalytic activity.[93] The freed catalytic subunits migrate to target proteins and phosphorylate serine and threonine residues in specific amino acid motifs. The changes in the phosphorylation state of proteins is a well recognized regulatory process for acutely modifying the activity and function of a large number of different proteins.

Reversal of these effects includes the action of phosphodiesterases that reduce the level of cyclic AMP through hydrolysis to AMP. This is reputedly the mechanism by which insulin inhibits the actions of glucagon in the liver cell (i.e., by activating a phosphodiesterase to lower cyclic AMP levels).[94] A second level of reversal is the conversion of the phosphorylated protein to its nonphosphorylated form by the actions of protein phosphatases.

GLUCAGON ACTION ON LIVER ENZYMES

Glucagon is a major contributor to the regulation of liver enzymes involved in glucose metabolism. This regulation is through elevations in cyclic AMP levels, although some effects of the hormone may be mediated through the Ca^{++}, IP-3 system. Both systems provide similar overall effects on liver glucose metabolism.[95]

Among the metabolic systems controlled by cyclic AMP are glycogenolysis, glycolysis, and gluconeogenesis (Fig. 7-6). As illustrated, the overall consequence of unimpeded glucagon stimulation is an increase in hepatic glucose production, resulting from elevated glycogen breakdown (glycogenolysis), an increase in the synthesis

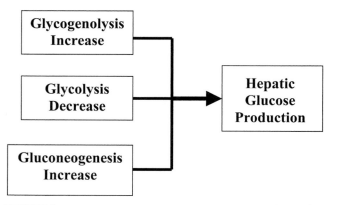

FIGURE 7-6. Effects of glucagon on the metabolic pathways that produce an increase in hepatic glucose production.

of glucose from gluconeogenic precursors (gluconeogenesis), and a decrease in the rate of glucose catabolism (glycolysis). Because three different pathways are involved, the changes induced by glucagon in each must be exquisitely coordinated. These changes can be divided into short-term and long-term. The short-term changes, which acutely alter the catalytic activities of key enzymes, are mediated by protein phosphorylation or by allosteric regulation. The long-term changes result from the regulation of gene expression for particular enzymes in the glycolytic and gluconeogeneic pathways. Both types of regulation are carried out by the cyclic AMP system and both play important roles in glucagon regulation of glucose metabolism.

Glycogenolysis

Glucagon's effect on glycogenolysis is geared to provide a rapid increase in hepatic glucose production that counteracts dropping plasma glucose levels. The action of glucagon begins with an elevation in cyclic AMP, which activates protein kinase A, to set in motion the cascade shown in Fig. 7-7. The first step in glycogenolysis is the phosphorylation and consequent activation of phosphorylase b kinase. Active phosphorylase b kinase then catalyzes the phosphorylation of inactive phosphorylase b to generate its active form, phosphorylase a. This phosphorylation is on serine-14, which provides enough conformational change to activate the enzyme.[96] Phosphorylase a cleaves glycogen at its nonreducing end to generate glucose-1-phosphate, which is available for energy production or for glucose formation. Since the activity of phosphorylase a is the rate-limiting step in liver glycogenolysis, activation of phosphorylase regulates the amount of glucose generated from glycogen. A specific phosphatase converts the active a form back to the inactive phosphorylase b form. Insulin provides an important inhibitory action on this system by reducing the level of cyclic AMP through an increase in phosphodiesterase activity.[94]

Glycolysis and Gluconeogensis

These two pathways are mirror images of each other, but with important distinctions. Since both pathways have interlocking control systems, they will be discussed together.

In order to increase hepatic glucose production, glucagon must inhibit glycolysis and increase gluconeogenesis. A key regulatory step acted on by glucagon that impacts both pathways is the modulation of the two separate catalytic activities mediated by the bifunctional enzyme 6-phosphofructose-2-kinase/fructose-2,6 bisphosphatase (Fig. 7-8). The overall consequence of bifunctional enzyme activity is to regulate the level of fructose-2,6 bisphosphate. This phosphorylated sugar has major effects on both glycolysis and gluconeogenesis through its acute allosteric regulation of two enzymes, 6-phosphofructose-1 kinase (glycolysis) and fructose-1,6 bisphosphatase (gluconeogenesis). The overall effect is that a high level of fructose-2,6 bisphosphate stimulates glycolysis and a low level allows gluconeogenesis to proceed.

As Fig. 7-8 shows, the bifunctional enzyme catalyzes two opposing reactions, one of which (the kinase activity) forms fructose-2,6 bisphosphate from fructose-6 phosphate, and the second (the phosphatase activity) hydrolyzes the bisphosphate sugar back to fructose-6 phosphate. The net effect is determined by cyclic AMP–dependent phosphorylation of the enzyme.[97,98] When the bifunctional enzyme is phosphorylated, its phosphatase activity predominates, which reduces the level of fructose-2,6 bisphosphate through its hydrolysis to fructose-6 phosphate. In contrast, in the

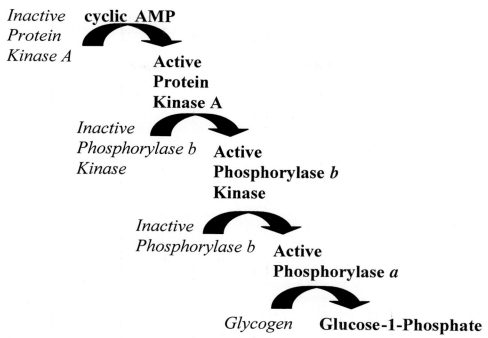

FIGURE 7-7. Steps in the cyclic AMP–mediated increase in glycogenolysis.

FIGURE 7-8. Changes in glycolysis and gluconeogenesis induced by cyclic AMP. Cyclic AMP acting on the bi-functional enzyme 6-phosphofructose-2-kinase (**F-6 kinase**)/fructose-2,6 bisphosphatase (**F-2,6 Pase**) regulates the level of fructose-2,6 bisphosphate. The level of this phosphorylated sugar regulates the rates of glycolysis and gluconeogenesis as shown. Glucagon produces an increase in cyclic AMP and insulin produces a decrease in cyclic AMP.

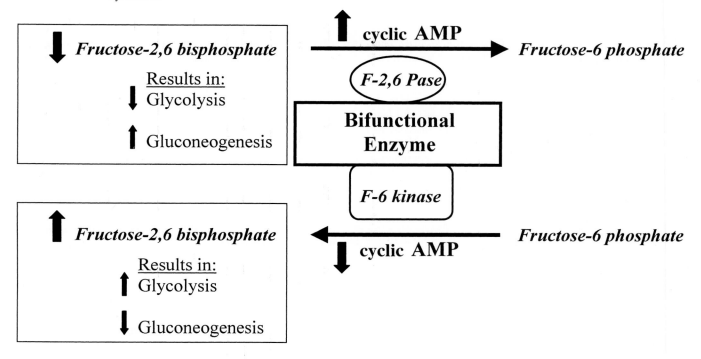

presence of low cyclic AMP, the nonphosphorylated form of the enzyme dominates, and thus generates fructose-2,6 bisphosphate from fructose-6 phosphate.

The key rate-controlling enzyme in glycolysis that is regulated by fructose-2,6 bisphosphate is 6-phosphofructose-1 kinase. Thus a decrease in fructose-2,6 bisphosphate from high cyclic AMP levels results in a decrease in 6-phosphofructose-1 kinase activity and a corresponding decrease in glycolysis. When cyclic AMP levels are low, an increase in fructose-2,6 bisphosphate occurs with a consequent allosteric-mediated increase in 6-phosphofructose-1 kinase activity that promotes glycolysis.

Gluconeogenesis is controlled by the enzymatic activity of fructose-1,6 bisphosphatase. In turn its activity is controlled by the level of fructose-2,6 bisphosphate, but in an opposite manner to glycolysis. Thus high levels of fructose-2,6 bisphosphate inhibit this enzyme and reduce the rate of gluconeogensis, whereas low levels allow the enzyme to act and thereby increase glucose production. Various physiologic states regulate glucose metabolism in liver through changes in fructose-2,6 bisphosphate. For example, in the fed state (low glucagon and high insulin), the levels of fructose-2,6 bisphosphate are increased, which increases glycolysis and inhibits gluconeogensis. In contrast, a decrease in fructose-2,6 bisphosphate occurs in the starved state (high glucagon and low insulin) or in poorly controlled diabetes, both of which result in an increase in gluconeogenesis and a decrease in glycolysis.

Other processes also impact on the activities of these pathways. For example, gluconeogenesis is increased by an elevation in the activity of pyruvate carboxylase that occurs during glucagon stimulation. This increase in activity is not mediated through changes in cyclic AMP or by other phosphorylation mechanisms. Glucagon may increase the activity at this step by accelerating pyruvate entry into mitochondria or through mechanisms that involve Ca^{++} or other changes in mitochondrial systems.[99]

Another regulatory point is pyruvate dehydrogenase (PDH), an enzyme complex that generates acetyl CoA in the mitochondria from pyruvate. The importance of this enzyme lies in its competition for pyruvate with pyruvate carboxylase. When PDH activity predominates in this competition, gluconeogenesis is reduced. How glucagon regulates this system is unclear, but the hormone may decrease the activity of the Ca^{++}-sensitive PDH phosphatase,[100] which in turn will reduce PDH activity by trapping the enzyme in its phosphorylated form.

A cytosolic enzyme, pyruvate kinase (L form), also influences the flow of carbon from glucose-6-phosphate to pyruvate. By contributing to the availability of pyruvate, this enzyme helps determine whether glucose is produced, or simply used as fuel during glycolysis. It is clear that the increase in cyclic AMP generated by glucagon stimulation causes an inhibitory phosphorylation of pyruvate kinase and reduces glycolysis.[99] This reduction allows phosphoenolpyruvate to be diverted to the gluconeogenic pathway.

Long-Term Regulation

The acute changes in enzyme activities are supplemented by longer-term changes in the levels of five important enzymes. However, like the acute changes, the long-term changes from glucagon stimulation are mediated by changes in cyclic AMP levels.[95] Depending on the pathway involved, the expression of the genes is either increased or decreased by elevated cyclic AMP. Three of the enzymes are in the glycolytic pathway and include glucokinase, 6-

phosphofructose-1 kinase and pyruvate kinase. With glucagon elevation, the levels of all three enzymes are reduced, which provides an important means of sustaining the reduction in the glycolytic response.

Two enzymes in the gluconeogenic pathway, phosphoenolpyruvate carboxykinase and fructose-1,6 bisphosphatase, are elevated through a cyclic AMP–mediated increase in the expression of their respective genes. This is an especially important mechanism to increase the activity of phosphoenolpyruvate carboxykinase, since the activity of this key enzyme is not regulated acutely by phosphorylation or allosteric mechanisms.

In summary, the regulation of hepatic glucose metabolism by glucagon is complex because of the need to orchestrate the activities of three different metabolic pathways. This orchestration results in the production of glucose rather than its use to expand the glycogen depot or in the support of fatty acid synthesis. Acutely, hepatic glucose production is derived from the breakdown of glycogen, which begins to wane after 1–2 hours.[101] With more chronic stimulation, hepatic glucose production is sustained by gluconeogenesis, which becomes the major source of glucose after an overnight fast. Acute and chronic regulatory mechanisms are used to provide these changes in glycolysis and gluconeogensis. Phosphorylation of key enzymes and allosteric controls are imposed to achieve acute regulation while chronic regulation is achieved by changes in the expression of genes that code for key enzymes.

GLUCAGON IN GLUCOREGULATION AND KETOGENESIS

To further understand glucagon's role in glucose regulation, it is necessary to understand its relationship with insulin. Specifically, insulin antagonizes the effects of glucagon on the liver by inhibiting the cyclic AMP system. An unopposed action of insulin on the liver results in a decrease in glycogenolysis, an increase in glycolysis with increases in glycogen and glucose-supported fatty acid synthesis, and a decrease in gluconeogenesis. Because of this antagonism, the ratio of glucagon to insulin is important since it establishes the overall net effect. Thus when insulin is high and glucagon low (e.g., after a high carbohydrate meal), hepatic glucose production is low and glycogen and triglyceride production is high.[95] In contrast, in the postabsorptive state, glucagon predominates over insulin to provide glucose and maintain euglycemia. For example, in the basal (fasting) state, 75% of the hepatic glucose production is dependent on glucagon action.[102,103]

Abnormalities in this ratio are especially important in diabetes. In type 1 diabetic subjects, low or absent insulin fails to balance the effects of glucagon, which when left unrestrained overstimulates the liver to produce excessive glucose and ketones. In contrast, type 2 diabetic subjects may have significant amounts of insulin, but the presence of insulin resistance contributes to a functional imbalance between the two hormones that supports inappropriate hepatic glucose production.

Lipids

Ketones are an energy source that does not depend on carbohydrate or protein metabolism to supply energy for the central nervous system during starvation.[104] Glucagon acting on the liver promotes ketogenesis by the fall in fructose-2,6 bisphosphate, which in turn reduces the rate of lipogenesis. This reduction is followed by a reduction in malonyl CoA that inhibits carnitine palmitoyl transferase-1, the enzyme that esterifies fatty acyl CoA to fatty acylcarnitine.[105] This form of the fatty acid enters mitochondria and undergoes oxidation to ketones. These events occur in situations like diabetes or starvation in which insulin levels are very low and glucagon levels are high. An elevation in plasma free fatty acid levels occurs in such states, which provide enough substrate to generate large amounts of ketone bodies that can supply over half of the energy requirements of the brain.

IN VIVO EFFECTS OF GLUCAGON IN ANIMALS AND MAN

Glucose Production

In the postabsorptive state (i.e., 5–14 hours after a meal) plasma glucose levels are stable and a normal human uses approximately 1.8–2.6 mg glucose/kg/min. Approximately 60% of this is used by the brain and the rest by other tissues, including the formed elements of the blood.[106] The liver is the major source of glucose in the postabsorptive state, with the kidneys contributing a minor component.[107,108]

Because the liver is the major source of glucose in the fasting state, fasting plasma glucose and hepatic glucose output are closely related. As discussed in detail above, glucagon regulates these processes through its regulation of gluconeogenesis and glycogenolysis (Fig. 7-9).[109–115] Approximately 66% of the basal glucose output of the canine liver is dependent on glucagon.[114] In

dogs, increasing plasma glucagon fourfold increases hepatic glucose output approximately fourfold. This effect is primarily due to an increase in glycogenolysis with no effect on gluconeogenesis (Fig. 7-10).[115]

The converse (i.e., the effect of selective glucagon deficiency with insulin held constant) is to decrease hepatic glucose output by 70%, requiring glucose infusion to prevent hypoglycemia. This acute effect is due to a decrease in glycogenolysis with no effect of gluconeogenesis. The lack of effect on gluconeogenesis in both cases is at least partly due to the constant insulin infusion that limited substrate supply to the liver (Fig. 7-11).[115]

The dose–response relationship between hepatic glucose output and hepatic sinusoidal glucagon is illustrated in Fig. 7-12.[115] This curve shows the sensitivity of hepatic glucose output to small, physiologic changes in glucagon.

Studies in man largely confirm those in dogs. In overnight fasted humans, isolated glucagon suppression with serum glucose maintained at basal levels leads to suppression of hepatic glucose output of 71% in normal control subjects and 58% in patients with type 2 diabetes (Fig. 7-13).[116] Under these conditions, even though gluconeogenesis accounts for 70% of hepatic glucose output,[117] glycogenolysis accounts for almost all of the increase in hepatic glucose output after an acute, physiologic increase in glucagon.[118] The onset of glucagon action is rapid, with the one-half maximum activation and deactivation occurring in approximately 4.0 minutes.[119]

In the postabsorptive period in man, suppression of glucagon secretion with somatostatin and replacement of insulin leads to a reduction of plasma glucose by ~33% and a reduction in hepatic glucose output of about 50%.[120] Hypoglycemia is prevented be-

FIGURE 7-9. The relationship between hepatic glucose production and fasting plasma glucose in normal weight diabetic subjects (**open circles**) and in age- and weight-matched control subjects (**closed circles**). *(Reproduced with permission from DeFronzo.[109])*

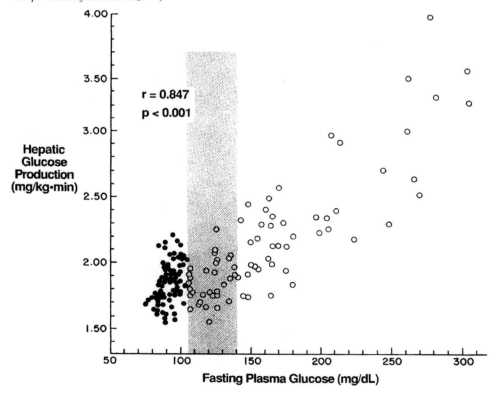

FIGURE 7-10. The effect of a selective increase in glucagon on hepatic glucose output, glycogenolysis (**GLY**), and gluconeogenesis (**GNG**) in conscious dogs. All dogs received somatostatin and a portal vein infusion of insulin and glucagon. The closed symbols represent the experiments in which portal vein glucagon was increased and insulin held constant. The open symbols represent control experiments in which glucagon and insulin were held constant and glucose was infused to match the increase in plasma glucose seen in the experimental group. *(Reproduced with permission from Cherrington.[115])*

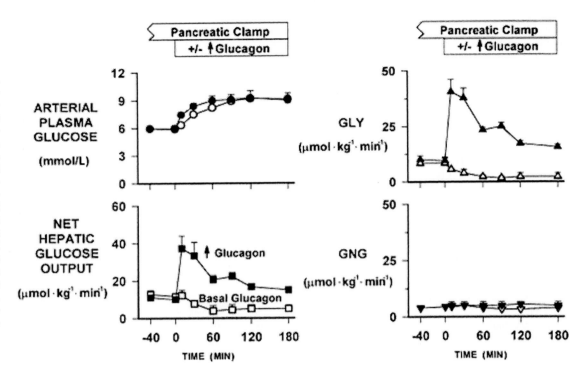

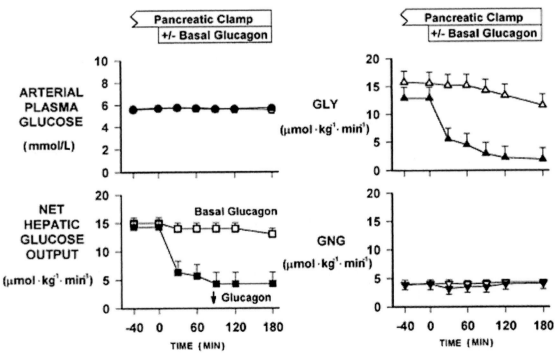

FIGURE 7-11. The effect of a selective decrease in glucagon on plasma glucose, hepatic glucose output, glycogenolysis (**GLY**), and gluconeogenesis (**GNG**). Conscious dogs were infused with somatostatin and portal vein insulin and glucagon at basal concentrations. In the control experiments (**open symbols**), insulin and glucagon were held constant. In the experimental group (**closed symbols**), no glucagon was infused and complete glucagon deficiency resulted. *(Reproduced with permission from Cherrington.[115])*

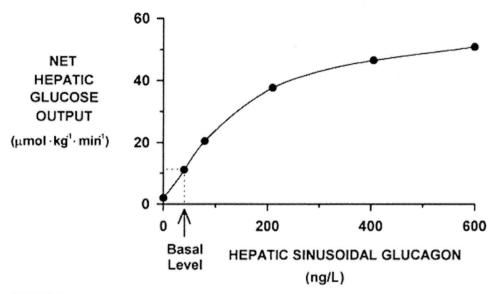

FIGURE 7-12. The dose–response relationship between the liver sinusoidal glucagon level and net hepatic glucose output in overnight fasted dogs. *(Reproduced with permission from Cherrington.[115])*

cause of an approximately eightfold increase in plasma epinephrine. Similar results are observed with fasting plus somatostatin with insulin replacement.[121]

The ability of glucagon to maintain increased glucose production through its glycogenic action only lasts for approximately 2 hours in normal dogs[122] and humans.[123] In man, as in dogs, the large majority of glucose production in this time period is from glycogenolysis. Higher glucagon levels over a longer period increase gluconeogenesis.[124] Several mechanisms have been postulated for the waning effect of glucagon after 2 hours, including the suppressive effect of the increase in plasma glucose, an increase in plasma insulin levels induced by the hyperglycemia, a depletion of liver glycogen, and intrahepatic regulation. While all may be important, the waning of glucose output is seen in studies in which glucose and insulin are fixed.[125] In addition, while glycogen is clearly not depleted, the role of a 25–36% decrease in glycogen stores on glycogenolysis is unknown.[115,118]

In contrast to the waning effect on glycogenolysis, the effect of glucagon on gluconeogenesis persists and increases in importance with time (Fig. 7-14).[126,127] This may explain the proposed role for hyperglucagonemia in the sustained hyperglycemia of diabetes.[116] Another factor may be the pulsatile release of glucagon and insulin. Under conditions of episodic release, the effects of glucagon on hepatic glucose production are sustained[128–131] and the ketogenic effects of glucagon also persist.[112,132]

Following a meal when glucose is being absorbed from the intestine, there is little need for the liver to release glucose. It is therefore not surprising that in normal humans glucagon is suppressed in the postprandial state.[133–135] This is likely due to the effect of hyperglycemia and hyperinsulinemia, both of which are known to suppress glucagon secretion.[116] The complete suppression of he-

patic glucose output occurs within 30 minutes of a meal, with a steady increase from 1–4 hours after the meal that mirrors the plasma glucagon:insulin ratio.[136]

Importantly, glucagon is not suppressed by carbohydrate ingestion in patients with diabetes.[137–139] This lack of suppression of glucagon results in higher postprandial glucose due to higher rates of hepatic glucose release.[140] The hyperglucagonemia of diabetes thus contributes to hyperglycemia in both the fasting and postprandial states.

COORDINATE CONTROL OF GLUCOSE AND LIPID METABOLISM BY GLUCAGON, INSULIN, AND GLUCOSE

Glucose Production

The ratio of insulin to glucagon and the glucose level in the portal circulation all contribute to the control of hepatic glucose output.[115,137,141] While the effects of insulin on the liver are due to both direct effects on glycogenolysis and gluconeogenesis and indirect effects on glycolysis and gluconeogenesis from the inhibition of peripheral lipolysis,[115] the effects of glucagon on the liver are almost exclusively direct. Recently an effect of glucagon on lipolysis in human adipocytes was demonstrated,[142] but the importance of this effect of glucagon *in vivo* is controversial.[143] In humans, hyperglycemia itself inhibits hepatic glucose output primarily by inhibiting glycogen phosphorylase, while insulin primarily stimulates glycogen synthase and enhances glycogen cycling.[144] With insulin held constant at basal levels and glucose elevated, suppression of glucagon leads to a marked decrease in glycogen turnover,

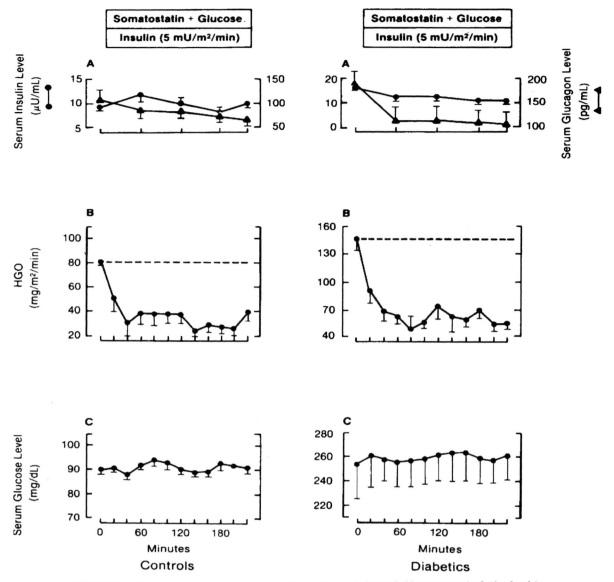

FIGURE 7-13. The effects of somatostatin with insulin replaced and glucose held constant at the fasting level (selective glucagon deficiency) on hepatic glucose output (**HGO**) in control subjects (**left panels**) and patients with type 2 diabetes (**right panels**). *(Reproduced with permission from Baron et al.[116])*

a fivefold increase in glycogen synthesis, and a decrease in the contribution of gluconeogenesis to glycogen synthesis.[145] This supports the important antagonist roles of glucagon and insulin.

Ketogenesis

Ketogenesis is also stimulated by glucagon. Ketogenesis depends on the free fatty acids delivered to the liver and the "ketogenic set" of the liver as determined by the glucagon:insulin ratio.[105] A high glucagon:insulin ratio reduces acetyl CoA carboxylase activity and the intracellular concentration of malonyl CoA. This reduces fatty acid synthesis and stimulates ketogenesis by increasing the activity of carnitine acyltransferase. (Fig. 7-15). The enhanced carnitine acyltransferase activity seen in ketotic animals was shown to be from an increase in carnitine acyltransferase I activ-

ity.[146] In patients with type 1 diabetes, somatostatin infusion during insulin withdrawal markedly attenuated the appearance of hyperglycemia and ketoacidosis (Fig. 7-16).[147] Alanine levels rose dramatically in the presence of somatostatin, most likely because gluconeogenesis is inhibited. These data suggest that over the time period of the study, glucagon is necessary for the appearance of severe hyperglycemia and ketoacidosis. Similar studies have been performed following the withdrawal of continuous subcutaneous insulin infusions with and without somatostatin.[148,149] In dogs, in the absence of glucagon, somatostatin-induced hypoinsulinemia fails to cause hyperglycemia. Dogs given somatostatin plus glucagon to restore glucagon levels to normal become hyperglycemic.[111] In alloxan diabetic dogs, somatostatin reduces glucose levels by ~200 mg/100 mL in the absence of exogenous insulin.[111]

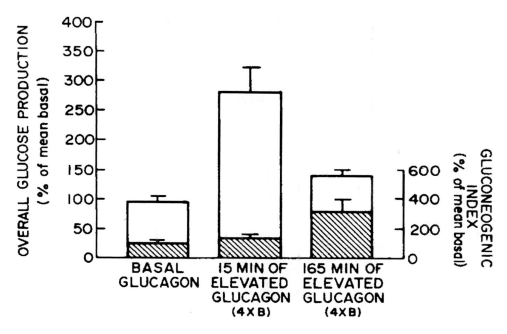

FIGURE 7-14. The early and late effects of hyperglucagonemia with insulin held constant on overall glucose production and the conversion of lactate and alanine into glucose (gluconeogenic index) in conscious overnight fasted dogs. *(Reproduced with permission from Cherrington et al.[126])*

FIGURE 7-15. The biochemical basis for insulin-glucagon interactions on fuel metabolism in the liver. Glucagon increases and insulin decreases cyclic AMP in the liver. This leads to both direct and indirect effects on enzymes that control glycogenolysis and glycogenesis, gluconeogenesis, lipid synthesis, and ketogenesis. Glycogen synthesis and glycogenolysis are controlled directly by cyclic AMP–mediated phosphorylation and dephosphorylation of glycogen synthase and glycogen phosphorylase. In addition, approximately 50% of the carbon incorporated into glycogen comes from new glucose synthesis via gluconeogenesis.[174] The relative flux of carbon into oxidative pathways (i.e., glycolysis vs. glucose production), is determined by the intracellular concentration of fructose-2,6 bisphosphate.[99] Glucagon decreases and insulin increases fructose-2,6 bisphosphate. Gluconeogenesis is also regulated by transcriptional regulation of rate-limiting enzymes in gluconeogenesis. Glucagon increases the transcription of phosphoenolpyruvate carboxykinase (PEPCK) and insulin decreases it. Glucagon and insulin also regulate lipolysis and lipid synthesis through cyclic AMP. The level of malonyl CoA formed during lipogenesis in turn inhibits carnitine palmitoyl transferase 1 (CPT-1), which is the rate-limiting enzyme for the transport of fatty acids into mitochondria for oxidation.[146] Thus in the presence of insulin, lipid synthesis is enhanced and lipid oxidation is inhibited. *(with permission from Unger RH, Foster DW: DIABETES MELLITUS In: Wilson JD, Foster DW, Kronenberg HM, Larsen PR. Williams Textbook of Endocrinology, 6th ed. Saunders:1998;1004.)*

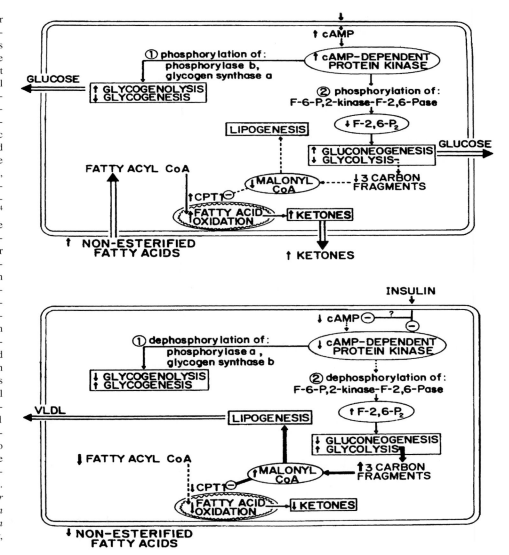

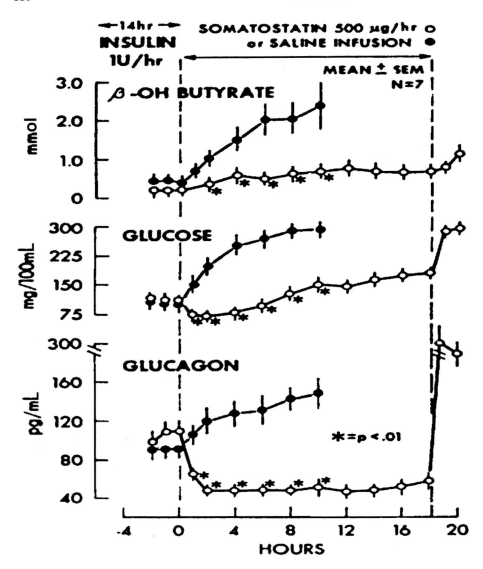

FIGURE 7-16. The effect of somatostatin on plasma β-hydroxybutyrate (**β-OH Butyrate**), glucose, and glucagon levels after acute withdrawal of insulin in 7 patients with type 1 diabetes. *(Reproduced with permission from Gerich et al.[147])*

GLUCAGON AND DIABETES

Glucagon levels are increased throughout the day in poorly controlled patients with type 1 and type 2 diabetes.[150–152] The magnitude of increase is the same in obese and nonobese type 2 diabetics (Fig. 7-17).[151] Glucagon levels are grossly elevated in patients with ketoacidosis,[152] hyperosmolar coma,[153] and poorly controlled diabetes.[154] Good control of diabetes with insulin restores plasma glucagon levels to normal.[155,156] In animals, restoration of euglycemia with phlorhizin normalized the suppression of glucagon by glucose.[157] The hyperglucagonemia of diabetes likely results from both the lack of insulin suppression of glucagon secretion in the islet and the effect of chronic hyperglycemia which, through unknown mechanisms, leads to desensitization of the α cells to glucose suppression of glucagon secretion.[154] Patients with total pancreatectomy have decreased levels of gluconeogenesis and increased plasma gluconeogenic amino acids.[158]

Patients with glucagon-producing islet cell tumors or glucagonomas have diabetes (67%) or impaired glucose tolerance (23%), necrolytic migratory erythema and stomatitis (64%), weight loss (56%), and anemia (44%).[159–161] Patients often have low levels of gluconeogenic amino acids (26%), which is most likely responsible for the rash.[162] The severity of the diabetes is variable, which may be at least partly due to the differential ability to mount an insulin response to the glucagon-induced increase in hepatic glucose output.[163]

As mentioned above, the importance of glucagon in the hyperglycemia of patients with diabetes is at least partially shown by the suppression of glucagon. This leads to a 58% decrease in hepatic glucose output[116] in patients with type 2 diabetes, and normalizes glucose in patients with type 1 diabetes.[164] Failure of glucagon suppression also contributes to postprandial hyperglycemia in patients with type 2 diabetes.[140]

Glucagon Deficiency

Mice with the glucagon receptor gene removed by homologous recombination have glucose levels in the fed and fasted state that are reduced by approximately 20 mg/dL below control animals [unpublished observations]. These knockout animals also have normal liver glycogen levels, elevated levels of gluconeogenic amino acids

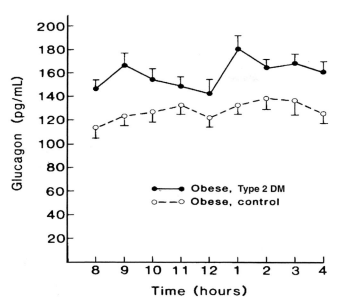

FIGURE 7-17. Mean plasma glucagon concentrations in obese individuals with normal glucose tolerance (**open circles**) and obese individuals with type 2 diabetes (**closed circles**). Meals were consumed at 0800 hours and at noon. (*Reproduced with permission from Reaven et al.[151]*)

and cholesterol, very high plasma glucagon levels, and normal insulin levels, body weight, fertility, life span and gross pathology. These findings argue that glucagon action is not necessary for survival and reproduction. While not specifically measured, it is likely that severe hypoglycemia is prevented by other counterregulatory hormones. Previous reports of severe hypoglycemia due to glucagon deficiency are likely due to other confounding factors.

A glucagon receptor antagonist given to humans has been shown to decrease the glucose response to a glucagon infusion. Six-teen normal volunteers were infused with somatostatin and replacement insulin in the absence or presence of hyperglucagonemia. Glucose production increased twofold in the presence of glucagon and this effect was completely blocked by the glucagon antagonist.[165] While it is possible that glucagon receptor antagonists may prove useful in the treatment of type 2 diabetes, additional studies in humans will be necessary to substantiate this utility.

Hypoglycemia

Glucagon plays a primary role in the prevention and correction of hypoglycemia along with epinephrine, growth hormone, cortisol, and in normal individuals, the suppression of insulin (Fig. 7-18). The primacy of glucagon in the prevention of hypoglycemia has been shown during a fast and during exercise in humans.[166–169] In addition, glucagon deficiency leads to a 30% reduction in the nadir plasma glucose concentration following a 75-gram oral glucose tolerance test.[170] Adrenergic blockade and epinephrine deficiency had no effect. Combined glucagon and epinephrine deficiency led to hypoglycemia, with nadir glucose values ~30% lower than glucagon deficiency alone.

Studies of glucose counterregulation from insulin-induced hypoglycemia indicate that glucagon deficiency alone reduces the recovery from hypoglycemia by approximately 40%, while isolated growth hormone or epinephrine deficiency or α- and β-adrenergic blockade have little effect. In the absence of glucagon, however, epinephrine deficiency leads to profound impairment of recovery from hypoglycemia.[171] In normal volunteers[172] and in type 1 diabetic patients, the glucagon response to hypoglycemia is suppressed by high concentrations of insulin within the physiologic range.[173] Thus, at the site of the liver, increases in plasma glucagon along with decreases in plasma insulin are the primary mechanisms for maintenance of normal plasma glucose. In the absence of glucagon or in the presence of nonsuppressed insulin (i.e., insulin-induced hypoglycemia), catecholamines become primary.

FIGURE 7-18. Idealized plasma glucose curves during insulin-induced hypoglycemia in normal subjects during control studies (**solid lines**) and as modified (**dashed lines**) by: (**A**) somatostatin infusion; (**B**) somatostatin plus growth hormone infusion; (**C**) somatostatin plus glucagon infusion; (**D**) phentolamine plus propranolol infusion or studies in patients with bilateral adrenalectomy; (**E**) somatostatin plus phentolamine and propranolol infusion; and (**F**) somatostatin infusion in bilaterally adrenalectomized patients.

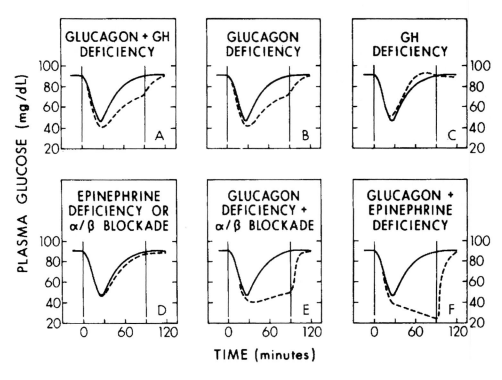

In summary, the secretion of glucagon and insulin are coordinately regulated and their metabolic effects provide a coordinate regulation of hepatic glucose, amino acid, and lipid metabolism. While insulin's effects are on both the liver and the periphery, glucagon's metabolic effects are exclusively on the liver. These effects occur through cyclic AMP–mediated events to enhance glycogenolysis, gluconeogenesis, and ketogenesis. The importance of glucagon in the regulation of fasting and postprandial glucose as well as ketogenesis in normal and diabetic humans is well documented. Future efforts will focus on the role of inhibiting glucagon secretion or glucagon action in the treatment of patients with both type 2 and type 1 diabetes.

REFERENCES

1. Campbell RM, Scanes CG: Evolution of the growth hormone-releasing factor (GRF) family of peptides. *Growth Regul* 1992;2:175.
2. Tricolli HAV, Bell GI, Shows TB: The human glucagon gene is located on chromosome 2. *Diabetes* 1984;33:200.
3. Schroeder WT, Lopez SC, Harper ME, et al: Localization of the human glucagon gene (GCG) to chromosome segment 2136-37. *Cytogenet Cell Genet* 1984;38:76.
4. Bell GI: The glucagon superfamily: precursor structure and gene organization. *Peptides* 1986;7(Suppl 1):27.
5. Jin T, Drucker DJ: The proglucagon gene upstream enhancer contains positive and negative domains important for tissue-specific proglucagon gene transcription. *Mol Endocrinol* 1995;9:1306.
6. Philippe J, Drucker DJ, Knepel W, et al: Alpha cell-specific expression of the glucagon gene is conferred to the glucagon promoter element by the interactions of DNA-binding proteins. *Mol Cell Biol* 1988;8:4877.
7. Morel C, Cordier-Bussat M, Philippe J: The upstream promoter element of the glucagon gene G1 confers pancreatic a cell-specific expression. *J Biol Chem* 1995;270:3046.
8. Hussain MA, Lee J, Miller CP, et al: POU domain transcription factor brain 4 confers pancreatic a-cell-specific expression of the proglucagon gene through interaction with a novel proximal promoter G1 element. *Mol Cell Biol* 1997;7:7186.
9. Laser B, Meda P, Constant I, et al: The caudal-related homeodomain protein Cdx-2/3 regulates glucagon gene expression in islet cells. *J Biol Chem* 1996;271:28984.
10. Jin T, Drucker DJ: Activation of proglucagon gene transcription through a novel promoter element by the caudal-related homeodomain protein cdx-2/3. *Mol Cell Biol* 1996;16:19.
11. Jin T, Trinh DKY, Wang F, et al: The caudal homeobox protein cdx-2/3 activates endogenous proglucagon gene expression in InRl—G9 islet cells. *Mol Endocrinol* 1997;11:203.
12. Philippe J: Hepatocyte-nuclear factor 3b gene transcripts generate protein isoforms with different transactivation properties on the glucagon gene. *Mol Endocrinol* 1995;9:368.
13. Diedrich T, Furstenau U, Knepel W: Glucagon gene G3 enhancer: evidence that activity depends on combination of an islet specific factor and a winged helix protein. *Biol Chem* 1997;378:89.
14. Philippe J, Morel C, Cordier-Bussat M: Islet-specific proteins interact with the insulin-response element of the glucagon gene. *J Biol Chem* 1995;270:3039.
15. Moens K, Heimberg H, Flamez D, et al: Expression and functional activity of glucagon, glucagon-like peptide 1, and glucose-dependent insulinotropic peptide receptors in rat pancreatic islet cells. *Diabetes* 1996;45:257.
16. Heller RS, Kieffer TJ, Habener JF: Insulinotropic glucagon-like peptide 1 receptor expression in glucagon-producing a-cells of the rat endocrine pancreas. *Diabetes* 1997;46:785.
17. Ding W-G, Renstrom E, Rorsman P, et al: Glucagon-like peptide 1 and glucose dependent insulinotropic polypeptide stimulate Ca^{2+}-induced secretion in rat a-cells by a protein kinase A-mediated mechanism. *Diabetes* 1997;46:792.
18. Drucker DJ, Jin T, Asa SL, et al: Activation of proglucagon gene transcription by protein kinase-A in a novel mouse enteroendocrine cell line. *Mol Endocrinol* 1994;8:1646.
19. Bernstein HG: Glucagon-like peptides in the CNS of man: localization and possible functional importance. *Folia Histochem Cytobiol* 1984;22:191.
20. Baetens D, Rufener C, Srikant CB, et al: Identification of glucagon-producing (A-Cells) in dog gastric mucosa. *J Cell Biol* 1976;69:455.
21. Novak U, Wilks A, Buell C, et al: Identical mRNA for preproglucagon in pancreas and gut. *Eur J Biochem* 1987;164:553.
22. Drucker DJ, Mojsov S, Habener JF: Cell-specific post-translational processing of preproglucagon expressed from a metallothionine-glucagon fusion gene. *J Biol Chem* 1986;261:9637.
23. Mojsov S, Heinrich G, Wilson IB, et al: Preproglucagon gene expression in pancreas and intestine diversifies at the level of post-translational processing. *J Biol Chem* 1986;261:11880.
24. Lee YC, Brubaker PL, Drucker DJ: Developmental and tissue-specific regulation of proglucagon gene expression. *Endocrinology* 1990;127:2217.
25. Steiner DF: The proprotein convertases. *Curr Opin Chem Biol* 1998;2:31.
26. Rothenberg ME, Eilertson CD, Klein K, et al: Processing of mouse proglucagon by recombinant prohormone convertase 1 and immunopurified prohormone convertase 2 in vitro. *J Biol Chem* 1995;270:10136.
27. Ørskov C, Holst JJ, Knuhtsen S, et al: Glucagon-like peptides GLP-1 and GLP-2, predicted products of the glucagon gene, are secreted separately from pig small intestine but not pancreas. *Endocrinology* 1986;119:1467.
28. Furuta M, Yano H, Zhou A, et al: Defective prohormone processing and altered pancreatic islet morphology in mice lacking active SPC2. *Proc Natl Acad Sci USA* 1997;94:6646.
29. Kieffer TJ, Habener JF: The glucagon-like peptides. *Endocrine Reviews* 1999;20:876.
30. Lui EY, Asa SL, Drucker DJ, et al: Glucagon and related peptides in fetal rat hypothalamus in vivo and in vitro. *Endocrinology* 1990;126:110.
31. Van Delft J, Uttenthal LO, Hermida OG, et al: Identification of amidated forms of GLP-1 in rat tissues using a highly sensitive radioimmunoassay. *Regul Pept* 1997;70:191.
32. Kreymann B, Ghatei MA, Burnet P, et al: Characterization of glucagon-like peptide-1-(7–36)amide in the hypothalamus. *Brain Res* 1989;502:325.
33. Larsen PJ, Tang-Christensen M, Holst JJ: Distribution of glucagon-like peptide-1 and other preproglucagon-derived peptides in the rat hypothalamus and brainstem. *Neuroscience* 1997;77:257.
34. Blache P, Kervran A, Bataille D: Oxyntomodulin and glicentin: brain-gut peptides in the rat. *Endocrinology* 1988;123:2782.
35. Yoshimoto S, Hirota M, Ohboshi C: Identification of glucagon-like peptide-1(7–36) amide in rat brain. *Ann Clin Biochem* 1989;26:169.
36. Mallat A, Pavoine C, Dufour M, et al: A glucagon fragment is responsible for the inhibition of the liver Ca^{2+} pump by glucagon. *Nature* 1987;325:620.
37. Bataille D: Preproglucagon and its processing. In: Lefebvre PJ, ed. *Handbook of Experimental Pharmacology*. Glucagon III Springer-Verlag::1996;123:31.
38. Gajic D, Drucker DJ: Multiple cis-acting domains mediate basal and adenosine 3′, 5′-monophosphate-dependent glucagon gene transcription in a mouse neuroendocrine cell line. *Endocrinology* 1993;132:1055.
39. Schwaninger M, Lux G, Blume R, et al: Membrane depolarization and calcium influx induce glucagon gene transcription in pancreatic islet cells through the cyclic AMP-responsive element. *J Biol Chem* 1993;268:5168.
40. Philippe J, Morel C, Cordier-Bussat M: Islet specific proteins interaction with the insulin-response element of the glucagon gene. *J Biol Chem* 1995;270:3039.
41. Philippe J: Insulin regulation of the glucagon gene is mediated by an insulin-responsive DNA element. *Proc Natl Acad Sci USA* 1991;88:7224.
42. Drucker DJ, Brubaker PL: Proglucagon gene expression is regulated by a cyclic AMP-dependent pathway in rat intestine. *Proc Natl Acad Sci USA* 1989;86:3953.
43. Saifia S, Chevrier AM, Bosshard A, et al: Galanin inhibits glucagon-like peptide-1 secretion through pertussis toxin-sensitive G protein and ATP-dependent potassium channels in rat ileal L-cells. *J Endocrinol* 1998;157:33.
44. Damholt AB, Buchan AMJ, Kofod H. Glucagon-like-peptide-1 secretion from canine L-cells is increased by glucose-dependent-insulinotropic peptide but unaffected by glucose. *Endocrinology* 1998;139:2085.
45. Unger RH, Eisentraut AM: Entero-insular axis. *Arch Int Med* 1969;123:261.

46. Frohman LR, Bermardis LL: Effect of hypothalamic stimulation on plasma glucose, insulin, and glucagon levels. *Am J Physiol* 1971;221:1596.

47. Helman AM, Giraud P, Nicolaidis S, *et al*: Glucagon release after stimulation of the lateral hypothalamic area in rats: Predominant B-adrenergic transmission and involvement of endorphin pathways. *Endocrinology* 1983;113:1.

48. Taborsky GJ Jr, Ahren B, Havel PJ: Autonomic mediation of glucagon secretion during hypoglycemia: implications for impaired a-cell responses in type 1 diabetes. *Diabetes* 1998;47:995.

49. Lacey RJ, Berrow NS, Scarpello JH, *et al*: Selective stimulation of glucagon secretion by beta 2-adrenoceptors in isolated islets of Langerhans of the rat. *Br J Pharmacol* 1991;103:1824.

50. Iismaa TP, Kerr EA, Wilson JR, *et al*: Quantitative and functional characterization of muscarinic receptor subtypes in insulin-secreting cell lines and rat pancreatic islets. *Diabetes* 2000;49:392.

51. Dunning B, Ahren B, Veith R, *et al*: Galanin: a novel pancreatic neuropeptide. *Am J Physiol* 1986;251:E127.

52. Lindkaer S, Jensen J, Fahrenkrug J, *et al*: Secretory effects of VIP on isolated perfused porcine pancreas. *Am J Physiol* 1978;235:E387.

53. Filipsson K, Tornoe K, Holst J, *et al*: Pituitary adenylate cyclase-activating polypeptide stimulates insulin and glucagon secretion in humans. *J Clin Endocrinol Metab* 1997;82:3093.

54. Saillan-Barreau C, Dufresne M, Clere P, *et al*: Evidence for a functional role of the cholecystokinin-B/gastrin receptor in the fetal and adult pancreas. *Diabetes* 1999;48:2015.

55. Dobbs RE: Control of glucagon secretion: Nutrients, gastroenteropancreatic hormones, calcium and prostaglandins. In: Unger RH, Orci L, eds. *Glucagon: Physiology, Pathophysiology and Morphology of the Pancreatic A-Cells.* Elsevier:1981;115.

56. Fridolf T, Bottcher G, Sundler F, *et al*: GLP-1 and GLP-1(7–36) amide: influences on basal and stimulated insulin and glucagon secretion in the mouse. *Pancreas* 1991;6:208.

57. Komatsu R, Matsuyama T, Namba M, *et al*: Glucagonostatic and insulinotropic action of glucagon-like peptide 1 (7-36) amide. *Diabetes* 1989;38:902.

58. Mojsov S, Weir GC, Habener JF: Insulinotropin: glucagon-like peptide-1(7-37) co-encoded in the glucagon gene is a potent stimulator of insulin release in the perfused rat pancreas. *J Clin Invest* 1987;79:616.

59. Holst JJ, Ørskov C, Van Nielsen O, *et al*: Truncated glucagon-like peptide I, an insulin-releasing hormone from the distal gut. *FEBS Lett* 1987;211:169.

60. Kreymann B, Ghatei MA, Williams G, *et al*: Glucagon-like peptide-1 (7–36); a physiological incretin in man. *Lancet* 1987;2:1300.

61. Mandarino L, Stenner D, Blanchard W, *et al*: Selective effects of somatostatin-14, -25 and -28 on *in vitro* insulin and glucagon secretion. *Nature* 1981;291:76.

62. Kumar U, Sasi R, Suresh S, *et al*: Subtype-selective expression of the five somatostatin receptors (hSSTR1-5) in human pancreatic cells: a quantitative double-label immunohistochemical analysis. *Diabetes* 1999;48:77.

63. Kawai K, Ipp I, Orci L, *et al*: Circulating somatostatin acts on the islets of Langerhans by way of a somatostatin-poor compartment. *Science* 1982;218:477.

64. Maruyama H, Hisatomi A, Orci L, *et al*: Insulin within islets is a physiologic glucagon release inhibitor. *J Clin Invest* 1984;74:2296.

65. Samols E, Stagner JI, Ewart RBL, *et al*: The order of islet microvascular cellular perfusion is B→A→D in the perfused rat pancreas. *J Clin Invest* 1988;82:350.

66. Unger RH, Aguilar-Parada E, Muller WA, *et al*: Studies of pancreatic alpha cell function in normal and diabetic subjects. *J Clin Invest* 1970;49:837.

67. Muller WA, Faloona CR, Unger RH: The effect of experimental insulin deficiency on glucagon secretion. *J Clin Invest* 1971;50:1992.

68. Unger RH, Orci L: Glucagon. In: Porte D Jr, Sherwin RS, eds. *Diabetes Mellitus,* 5th ed. Appleton & Lange:1997;115.

69. Mauras N, Horber FF, Haymond MW: Low dose recombinant human insulin-like growth factor-I fails to affect protein anabolism but inhibits islet cell secretion in humans. *J Clin Endocrinol Metab* 1992;75:1192.

70. Dunning BE, Moltz JH, Fawcett CP: Effects of oxytocin and vasopressin on release of insulin and glucagon from pancreatic islets *in vitro. Neuroendocrinol Lett* 1982;4:89.

71. Wallin LA, Fawcett CP, Rosenfeld CR: Oxytocin stimulates glucagon and insulin secretion in fetal and neonatal sheep. *Endocrinology* 1989;125:2289.

72. Cryer P, Gerich J: Relevance of glucose counterregulatory systems to patients with diabetes: critical roles of glucagon and epinephrine. *Diabetes Care* 1983;6:95.

73. DeFeo P, Perriello G, Torlone E, *et al*: Evidence against important catecholamine compensation for absent glucagon counterregulation. *Am J Physiol* 1991;260:E203.

74. Assan R, Attali J, Ballerio G, *et al*: Glucagon secretion induced by natural and artificial amino acids in the perfused rat pancreas. *Diabetes* 1977;26:300.

75. Rocha D, Faloona G, Unger R: Glucagon-stimulating activity of twenty amino acids in dogs. *J Clin Invest* 1972;51:2346.

76. Nair KS, Welle SL, Tito J: Effect of plasma amino acid replacement on glucagon and substrate responses to insulin-induced hypoglycemia in humans. *Diabetes* 1990;39:376.

77. Madison L, Seyffert W, Unger R, *et al*: Effects of plasma free fatty acids on plasma glucagon and serum insulin concentrations. *Metabolism* 1968;17:301.

78. Gerich J, Langlois M, Schneider V, *et al*: Effects of alterations of plasma free fatty acid levels on pancreatic glucagon secretion in man. *J Clin Invest* 1974;53:1284.

79. Luyckx A, Lefebvre P: Free fatty acids and glucagon secretion. In: Lefebvre PJ, ed. *Glucagon II.* Springer-Verlag:1983;43.

80. Lok S, Kuijper J, Jelinek L, *et al*: The human glucagon receptor encoding gene: structure, cDNA sequence and chromosomal location. *Gene* 1994;140:203.

81. Christophe J: Glucagon receptors: from genetic structure and expression to effector coupling and biological responses. *Biochim Biophys Acta* 1995;1241:45.

82. Svoboda M, Tastenoy M, Vertongen P, *et al*: Relative quantitative analysis of glucagon receptor mRNA in rat tissue. *Mol Cell Endocrin* 1994;105:131.

83. Iwanij V: The glucagon receptor gene: organization and tissue distribution. In: Lefebvre PJ, ed. *Glucagon III.* Springer-Verlag:1996;53.

84. Buggy J, Livingston J, Rabin D, *et al*: Glucagon/glucagon-like peptide-1 receptor chimeras reveal domains that determine specificity of glucagon binding. *J Biol Chem* 1995;270:7474.

85. Livingston J, Macdougall M, Ladouceur G, *et al*: BAY 27-9955, a novel, non-peptide antagonist of glucagon binding to the glucagon receptor. *Diabetes* 1999;(Suppl 1)48:A199.

86. Pohl S, Birnbaumer L, Robell M: The glucagon sensitive adenylyl cyclase system in plasma membranes of rat liver: I. Properties. *J Biol Chem* 1971;246:1849.

87. Gilman AG: Guanine nucleotide-binding regulatory proteins and dual control of adenylate cyclase. *J Clin Invest* 1984;73:1.

88. Rodbell M, Birnbaumer L, Pohl S, *et al*: The glucagon-sensitive adenyl cyclase system in plasma membranes of rat liver. V. An obligatory role of guanyl nucleotides in glucagon action. *J Biol Chem* 1971;246:1877.

89. Iyengar R, Rich K, Herberg J, *et al*: Glucagon receptor-mediated activation of Gs is accompanied by subunit dissociation. *J Biol Chem* 1988;263:15348.

90. Freissmuth M, Casey P, Gilman A: G proteins control diverse pathways of transmembrane signaling. *FASEB J* 1989;3:2125.

91. Mine T, Kojima I, Ogata E: Evidence of cyclic AMP-independent action of glucagon on calcium mobilization in rat hepatocytes. *Biochim Biophys Acta* 1988;970:166.

92. Wakelam M, Murphy G, Hruby V, *et al*: Activation of two signal-transduction systems in hepatocytes by glucagon. *Nature* 1986;323:68.

93. Ciudad CJ, Villa J, Moor MA, *et al*: Effects of glucagon and insulin on the cyclic AMP binding capacity of hepatocyte cyclic AMP-dependent protein kinase. *Mol Cell Biochem* 1987;73:37.

94. Conti M: Phosphodiesterases and cyclic nucleotide signaling in endocrine cells. *Mol Endocrinol* 2000;14:1317.

95. Pilkis SJ, Claus TH: Hepatic gluconeogenesis/glycolysis: regulation and structure/function relationships of substrate cycle enzymes. *Ann Rev Nutr* 1991;11:465.

96. Sprang SR, Acharya KR, Goldsmith EJ, *et al*: Structural changes in glycogen phosphorylase induced by phosphorylation. *Nature* 1988;336:215.

97. Hers HG, Van Schaftingen E: Fructose-2,6 bisphosphate 2 years after its discovery. *Biochem J* 1982;206:1.

98. Claus TH, Park CR, Pilkis SJ: Glucagon and gluconeogenesis. In: Lefebvre PJ, ed. *Handbook of Experimental Pharmacology.* Springer-Verlag:1983;315.

99. Chen J-LJ, Babcock DF, Lardy HA: Norepinephrine, vasopressin, glucagon, and A23187 induced efflux of calcium from an exchangeable pool in isolated rat hepatocytes. *Proc Natl Acad Sci USA* 1978;75:2234.

100. Tóth B, Bollen M, Stalmans W: Acute regulation of hepatic protein phosphatases by glucagon, insulin and glucose. *J Biol Chem* 1988; 263:14061.

101. Felig P, Wahren J, Hendler R: Influence of physiologic hyperglucagonemia on basal and insulin inhibited splanchnic glucose output in normal man. *J Clin Invest* 1976;58:761.

102. Cherrington AD, Lacy WW, Chiasson JL: Effect of glucagon on glucose production during insulin deficiency in the dog. *J Clin Invest* 1978;62:664.

103. Liljenquist JE, Mueller CL, Cherrington AD, *et al*: Hyperglycemia per se (insulin and glucagon withdrawn) can inhibit hepatic glucose production in man. *J Clin Endocrinol Metab* 1979;48:171.

104. Cahill CF Jr.: Starvation in man. *N Engl J Med* 1970;282:668.

105. McGarry JD, Foster DW: Regulation of hepatic fatty acid oxidation and ketone body production. *Ann Rev Biochem* 1980;49:395.

106. Cryer PE, Polonsky KS: Glucose homeostasis and hypoglycemia. In: Wilson JD, Foster DW, Kronenberg HM *et al*, eds. *Williams Textbook of Endocrinology*. WB Saunders:1998;941.

107. Rothman DL, Magnusson I, Katz LD, *et al*: Quantitation of hepatic glycogenolysis and gluconeogenesis in fasting humans with 13C NMR. *Science* 1991;254:573.

108. Stumvoll M, Chintalapudi U, Perriello G, *et al*: Uptake and release of glucose by the human kidney. Postabsorptive rates and responses to epinephrine. *J Clin Invest* 1995;96:2528.

109. DeFronzo RA: The triumvirate: beta cell, muscle, liver. A collusion responsible for NIDDM. *Diabetes* 1988;37:667.

110. Sakurai H, Dobbs R, Unger RH: Somatostatin-induced changes in insulin and glucagon secretion in normal and diabetic dogs. *J Clin Invest* 1974;54:1395.

111. Dobbs RE, Sakuri H, Faloona GR: Glucagon: Role in the hyperglycemia of diabetes mellitus. *Science* 1975;187:544.

112. Gerich JE, Lorenzi M, Bier DM, *et al*: Prevention of human diabetic ketoacidosis by somatostatin. Evidence for an essential role of glucagon. *N Engl J Med* 1975;292:985.

113. Sakurai H, Dobbs RE, Unger RH: The role of glucagon in the pathogenesis of the endogenous hyperglycemia of diabetes mellitus. *Metabolism* 1975;24:1287.

114. Cherrington AD, Lacy WW, Chiasson JL: Effect of glucagon on glucose production during insulin deficiency in the dog. *J Clin Invest* 1978;62:664.

115. Cherrington AD: Control of glucose uptake and release by the liver *in vivo*. *Diabetes* 1999;48:1198.

116. Baron AD, Schaeffer L, Shragg P, *et al*: Role of hyperglucagonemia in maintenance of increased rates of hepatic glucose output in type II diabetes. *Diabetes* 1987;36:274.

117. Magnusson I, Rothman DL, Katz LD, *et al*: Increased rate of gluconeogenesis in type II diabetes mellitus. A 13C nuclear magnetic resonance study. *J Clin Invest* 1992;90:1323.

118. Magnusson I, Rothman DL, Gerard DP, *et al*: Contribution of hepatic glycogenolysis to glucose production in humans in response to a physiological increase in plasma glucagon concentration. *Diabetes* 1995;44:185.

119. Dobbins RL, Davis SN, Neal D, *et al*: Rates of glucagon activation and deactivation of hepatic glucose production in conscious dogs. *Metabolism* 1998;47:135.

120. Rosen SG, Clutter WE, Berk MA, *et al*: Epinephrine supports the postabsorptive plasma glucose concentration and prevents hypoglycemia when glucagon secretion is deficient in man. *J Clin Invest* 1984;73:405.

121. Boyle PJ, Shah SD, Cryer PE: Insulin, glucagon, and catecholamines in prevention of hypoglycemia during fasting. *Am J Physiol* 1989; 256:E651.

122. Cherrington AD, Diamond MP, Green DR, *et al*: Evidence for an intrahepatic contribution to the waning effect of glucagon on glucose production in the conscious dog. *Diabetes* 1982;31:917.

123. Magnusson I, Rothman DL, Gerard DP, *et al*: Contribution of hepatic glycogenolysis to glucose production in humans in response to a physiological increase in plasma glucagon concentration. *Diabetes* 1995;44:185.

124. Chhibber VL, Soriano C, Tayek JA: Effects of low-dose and high-dose glucagon on glucose production and gluconeogenesis in humans. *Metabolism* 2000;49:39.

125. El-Refai M, Bergman RN: Glucagon-stimulated glycogenolysis: time-dependent sensitivity to insulin. *Am J Physiol* 1979;236:E246.

126. Cherrington AD, Williams PE, Shulman GI, *et al*: Differential time course of glucagon's effect on glycogenolysis and gluconeogenesis in the conscious dog. *Diabetes* 1983;30:180.

127. Lecavalier L, Bolli G, Cryer P, *et al*: Contributions of gluconeogenesis and glycogenolysis during glucose counterregulation in normal humans. *Am J Physiol* 1989;256:E844.

128. Rizza R, Verdonk C, Miles J, *et al*: Effect of intermittent endogenous hyperglucagonemia on glucose homeostasis in normal and diabetic man. *J Clin Invest* 1979;63:1119.

129. Rizza RA, Gerich JE: Persistent effect of sustained hyperglucagonemia on glucose production in man. *J Clin Endocrinol Metab* 1979;48:352.

130. Fradkin J, Shamoon H, Felig P, *et al*: Evidence for an important role of changes in rather than absolute concentrations of glucagon in the regulation of glucose production in humans. *J Clin Endocrinol Metab* 1980;50:698.

131. Paolisso G, Scheen AJ, Albert A, *et al*: Effects of pulsatile delivery of insulin and glucagon in humans. *Am J Physiol* 1989;257:E686.

132. Keller U, Chiasson JL, Liljenquist JE, *et al*: The roles of insulin, glucagon, and free fatty acids in the regulation of ketogenesis in dogs. *Diabetes* 1977;26:1040.

133. Tse TF, Clutter WE, Shah SD, *et al*: Neuroendocrine responses to glucose ingestion in man. Specificity, temporal relationships, and quantitative aspects. *J Clin Invest* 1983;72:270.

134. Butler RC, Rizza RA: Contribution to postprandial hyperglycemia and effect on initial splanchnic glucose clearance of hepatic glucose cycling in glucose-intolerant or NIDDM patients. *Diabetes* 1991; 40:73.

135. Dineen S, Alzaid A, Miles J, *et al*: Metabolic effects of the nocturnal rise in cortisol on carbohydrate metabolism in normal humans. *J Clin Invest* 1993;92:2283.

136. Taylor R, Magnusson I, Rothman DL, *et al*: Direct assessment of liver glycogen storage by 13C nuclear magnetic resonance spectroscopy and regulation of glucose homeostasis after a mixed meal in normal subjects. *J Clin Invest* 1996;97:126.

137. Unger RH: Role of glucagon in the pathogenesis of diabetes: the status of the controversy. *Metabolism* 1978;27:1691.

138. Lefebvre PJ, Liyckx AS: Glucagon and diabetes: a reappraisal. *Diabetologia* 1979;16:347.

139. Gerich JE, Tsalikian E, Lorenzi M, *et al*: Normalization of fasting hyperglucagonemia and excessive glucagon responses to intravenous arginine in human diabetes mellitus by prolonged infusion of insulin. *J Clin Endocrinol Metab* 1975;41:1178.

140. Dineen S, Alzaid A, Turk D, *et al*: Failure of glucagon suppression contributes to postprandial hyperglycaemia in IDDM. *Diabetologia* 1995;38:337.

141. Lefèbvre, PJ. Glucagon and Diabetes. In: Glucagon III, Lefèbvre, PJ. ed. Handbook of Experimental Pharmacology, Springer-Verlag: 1996;123:115.

142. Perea A, Clemente F, Martinell J, *et al*: Physiological effect of glucagon in human isolated adipocytes. *Horm Metab Res* 1995; 27:372.

143. Jeng CY, Sheu WH, Jaspan JB, *et al*: Glucagon does not increase plasma free fatty acid and glycerol concentrations in patients with noninsulin-dependent diabetes mellitus. *J Clin Endocrinol Metab* 1993;77:6.

144. Petersen KF, Laurent D, Rothman DL, *et al*: Mechanism by which glucose and insulin inhibit net hepatic glycogenolysis in humans. *J Clin Invest* 1998;101:1203.

145. Roden M, Price TB, Perseghin G, *et al*: The roles of insulin and glucagon in the regulation of hepatic glycogen synthesis and turnover in humans. *J Clin Invest* 1996;97:2859.

146. Amatruda, JM, Lockwood DH, Margolis S, *et al*: (14C)Palmitate uptake in isolated rat liver mitochondria: Effects of fasting, diabetes mellitus, and inhibitors of carnitine acyltransferase. *J Lipid Res* 1978;19:688.

147. Gerich JE, Lorenzi M, Bier DM, *et al*: Prevention of human diabetic ketoacidosis by somatostatin. Evidence for an essential role of glucagon. *N Engl J Med* 1975;292:985.

148. Scheen AJ, Krzentowski G, Castillo M, *et al*: A 6-hour nocturnal interruption of a continuous subcutaneous insulin infusion: 2. Marked attenuation of the metabolic deterioration by somatostatin. *Diabetologia* 1983;24:319.

149. Scheen AJ, Gillet J, Rosenthaler J, *et al*: Sandostatin, a new analogue of somatostatin, reduces the metabolic changes induced by the nocturnal interruption of continuous subcutaneous insulin infusion in

type 1 (insulin-dependent) diabetic patients. *Diabetologia* 1989;32: 801.

150. Unger RH, Orci L: Glucagon and the A cell. Physiology and pathophysiology. *N Engl J Med* 1981;304:1518.

151. Reaven GM, Chen YD, Golay A, *et al*: Documentation of hyperglucagonemia throughout the day in nonobese and obese patients with noninsulin-dependent diabetes mellitus. *J Clin Endocrinol Metab* 1987;64:106.

152. Muller WA, Faloona GR, Unger RH: Hyperglucagonemia in diabetic ketoacidosis. Its prevalence and significance. *Am J Med* 1973;54:52.

153. Lindsey CA, Faloona GR, Unger RH: Plasma glucagon in nonketotic hyperosmolar coma. *JAMA* 1974;229:1771.

154. Lefebvre PJ: Glucagon and its family revisited. *Diabetes Care* 1995; 18:715.

155. Raskin P, Pietri A, Unger R: Changes in glucagon levels after four to five weeks of glucoregulation by portable insulin infusion pumps. *Diabetes* 1979;28:1033.

156. Kawamori R, Shichiri M, Kikuchi M, *et al*: Perfect normalization of excessive glucagon responses to intravenous arginine in human diabetes mellitus with the artificial beta cell. *Diabetes* 1980;29:762.

157. Starke A, Grundy S, McGarry JD, *et al*: Correction of hyperglycemia with phloridzin restores the glucagon response to glucose in insulin-deficient dogs: implications for human diabetes. *Proc Natl Acad Sci USA* 1985;82:1544.

158. Vigili de Kreutzenberg S, Maifreni L, Lisato G, *et al*: Glucose turnover and recycling in diabetes secondary to total pancreatectomy: effect of glucagon infusion. *J Clin Endocrinol Metab* 1990;70:1023.

159. Stacpoole PW: The glucagonoma syndrome: clinical features, diagnosis, and treatment. *Endocr Rev* 1981;2:347.

160. Wermers RA, Fatourechi V, Wynne AG, *et al*: The glucagonoma syndrome. Clinical and pathologic features in 21 patients. *Medicine* 1996;75:53.

161. Soga J, Yakuwa Y: Glucagonomas/diabetico-dermatogenic syndrome (DDS): a statistical evaluation of 407 reported cases. *J Hepatobiliary Pancreat Surg* 1998;5:312.

162. Norton JA, Kahn CR, Schiebinger R, *et al*: Amino acid deficiency and the skin rash associated with glucagonoma. *Ann Intern Med* 1979;91:213.

163. Henry JG, Xue N, Kinder BK, *et al*: A 73-year-old man with hyperglycemia, skin rashes, anemia and weight loss. *J Clin Endocrinol Metab* 1996;81:2428.

164. Raskin P, Unger RH: Hyperglucagonemia and its suppression. Importance in the metabolic control of diabetes. *N Engl J Med* 1978; 299:433.

165. Petersen KF, Sullivan JT, Amatruda JM, *et al*: The effects of a specific glucagon antagonist on glucagon stimulated glucose production. (Abstract) European Association for the Study of Diabetes, Brussels: 1999.

166. Rosen SG, Clutter WE, Berk MA, *et al*: Epinephrine supports the postabsorptive plasma glucose concentration and prevents hypoglycemia when glucagon secretion is deficient in man. *J Clin Invest* 1984;73:405.

167. Boyle PJ, Shah SD, Cryer PE: Insulin, glucagon, and catecholamines in prevention of hypoglycemia during fasting. *Am J Physiol* 1989; 256:E651.

168. Hirsch IB, Marker JC, Smith LJ, *et al*: Insulin and glucagon in prevention of hypoglycemia during exercise in humans. *Am J Physiol* 1991;260:E695.

169. Marker JC, Hirsch IB, Smith LJ, *et al*: Catecholamines in prevention of hypoglycemia during exercise in humans. *Am J Physiol* 1991;260: E705.

170. Tse TF, Clutter WE, Shah SD, *et al*: Mechanisms of postprandial glucose counterregulation in man. Physiologic roles of glucagon and epinephrine vis-a-vis insulin in the prevention of hypoglycemia late after glucose ingestion. *J Clin Invest* 1983;72:278.

171. Cryer PE: Glucose counterregulation in man. *Diabetes* 1981;30:261.

172. Liu D, Moberg E, Kollind M, *et al*: A high concentration of circulating insulin suppresses the glucagon response to hypoglycemia in normal man. *J Clin Endocrinol Metab* 1991;73:1123.

173. Liu DT, Adamson UC, Lins PE, *et al*: Inhibitory effect of circulating insulin on glucagon secretion during hypoglycemia in type I diabetic patients. *Diabetes Care* 1992;15:59.

174. Salhanick AI, Chang CL, Amatruda JM: Hormone and substrate regulation of glycogen accumulation in primary cultures of rat hepatocytes. *Biochem J* 1989;261:985.

Role of the CNS in Glucose Regulation

Mark L. Evans

Alan D. Cherrington

Mary Courtney Moore

Robert S. Sherwin

INTRODUCTION

The human brain is an extremely active metabolic organ. Despite making up only 2% of adult body weight, it receives about 800 mL/min (15%) of the cardiac output and consumes approximately 50 mL/min of oxygen, representing 20% of the body's resting glucose consumption. Although early measurements may have underestimated the glycogen content of brain tissue, the energy stored as glycogen is only sufficient to fuel the brain for a few minutes if it were the sole energy supply.[1] The central nervous system (CNS) is thus largely dependent on circulating glucose as its predominant source of energy, with cognitive performance becoming impaired during moderate hypoglycemia. If the blood glucose falls low enough, coma or even permanent brain injury or death may eventually occur.[2]

In contrast to most tissues of the body, brain parenchyma is separated from the bloodstream by the endothelial blood–brain barrier. In order to reach and fuel neurons, glucose from the bloodstream must traverse luminal and abluminal membranes of endothelial cells and possibly also through astrocyte foot processes to enter the extracellular fluid (ECF) of the brain. Although there is some simple nonsaturable diffusion of glucose across the blood–brain barrier, most transport across these membranes is effected by the facilitative glucose transporter GLUT-1 (Fig. 8-1). GLUT-1 is also referred to as the red blood cell transporter, and in contrast to GLUT-4 is insensitive to the actions of insulin. GLUT-1 exists in both glycosylated (55 kd) and nonglycosylated (45 kd) forms in the CNS in the endothelium and astrocytic compartments, respectively, although the functional significance of these differences is uncertain. Glucose in the brain ECF may then enter into neurons by the facilitative transporter GLUT-3.

Glucose levels in brain are lower than in plasma, suggesting that the blood–brain barrier limits the supply of glucose for the central nervous system, with most estimates of ECF glucose being between 20% and 30% of plasma values. CSF glucose values are higher than in ECF, with typical values being 50–70% of plasma glucose.

Although the main fuel supply for brain tissue is undoubtedly glucose originating from the bloodstream, there is increasing evidence that neurons may be able to metabolize nonglucose fuels. A number of alternate substrates may support neuronal metabolism in brain slice studies in which the blood–brain barrier is absent. During *in vivo* human studies, lactate and the ketone β-hydroxybutyrate have been demonstrated to support, at least in part, brain metabolism and cognitive functioning during hypoglycemia.[3–5] For some of these substrates, the physiological relevance of their metabolism by brain tissue is questionable. However, lactate appears to be a genuine brain fuel, with some *in vitro* studies even suggesting that lactate may be preferred over glucose by neurons.[6] In contrast to glucose, lactate levels in the brain ECF are higher than plasma lactate values (suggesting that lactate is synthesized locally) and brain ECF glucose values.[7] The significance of glycogen stores in astrocytes is uncertain. One possibility is that astrocytic glycogen stores act as a buffer against a sudden rise in neuronal energy requirements during local brain activation, but with lactate rather than glucose being released. Whatever the exact metabolic pathways involved in fueling neurons, it seems likely that astrocytic and neuronal metabolism are coupled. It is important to emphasize, however, that regardless of the exact pathway(s) involved within the CNS, glucose from the bloodstream is the predominant source of energy to support neuronal metabolism and function.

The main energy-consuming activities of the CNS are biosynthesis and transport—mostly of ions and neurotransmitters. In particular, an important energy-requiring activity is the clearance of neurotransmitters such as glutamate from the ECF. Glutamate is the main excitatory neurotransmitter in the CNS but may produce brain toxicity if extracellular levels are high and/or sustained. A glutamate-glutamine cycle exists so that glutamate released from neurons is rapidly taken up by astrocytes and subsequently converted to glutamine. The uptake of glutamate is driven by the cell membrane sodium-potassium pump (Na^+,K^+-ATPase), a process dependent on ATP derived from glucose. The glutamine produced in astrocytes is then transported back into neurons for conversion into glutamate and storage in secretory vesicles for subsequent release.[8] Thus the glutamate-glutamine cycle requires a sufficient supply of glucose to maintain astrocytic functioning and this appears to be associated with anaerobic glycolysis and release of lactate from glia. During profound hypoglycemia, the lack of energy for these homeostatic mechanisms may result in rises in glutamate and aspartate in brain interstitial fluid. These excitotoxins act on

Blood-Brain Glucose Transport

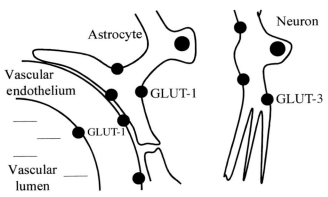

FIGURE 8-1. Glucose transport from vascular lumen to neurons involves the facilitative glucose transporters GLUT-1 and GLUT-3 in endothelium/glial cells and neurons, respectively. *(Reproduced from Borg et al.[26])*

specific receptors such as the NMDA glutamate receptor to trigger further downstream effects that may eventually result in brain damage by cell apoptosis or necrosis. It is unclear whether the more moderate hypoglycemia seen during the day-to-day management of diabetes causes a similar perturbation of excitatory neurotransmitters. Indeed, it is possible that milder degrees of hypoglycemia are accompanied by an adaptive reduction in neurotransmission that would protect the brain against excessive accumulation of excitotoxins at the expense of impaired function.

The central nervous system has a key regulatory role in glucose homeostasis. In particular, the brain is important in initiating and coordinating protective counterregulatory responses in the face of a falling blood glucose. This role is probably a consequence of the central nervous system's metabolic dependence on glucose so the brain will tend to protect its own fuel supply. In health, blood glucose is normally maintained within a relatively narrow range. A number of rare medical conditions such as insulin-secreting tumors of the pancreas may overcome or suppress these defenses and cause hypoglycemia, but by far the most significant cause of hypoglycemia in clinical practice is the treatment of diabetes with insulin or insulin secretagogues. As described later in this chapter, the risk of hypoglycemia in diabetes may be further increased by defects in the defensive counterregulatory responses triggered by the central nervous system in response to a low glucose concentration (See Chapter 31).

ROLE OF THE CNS IN THE RESPONSE TO HYPOGLYCEMIA

Counterregulatory Defenses Against Hypoglycemia

A hierarchy of defensive counterregulatory neurohumoral responses is triggered by a fall in blood glucose. The cessation of insulin secretion from the healthy pancreas is an important early step in nondiabetic subjects,[9] and the subsequent release of the hormone glucagon acts in concert with the fall in insulin to increase glucose production by the liver.[10] The precise mechanisms responsible for the activation of glucagon release from pancreatic α cells is

not clear, but they may be dependent on both local pancreatic detection of hypoglycemia and on central brain-dependent control via pancreatic innervation, as well as stimulation of circulating catecholamines.

Increased glucagon and decreased insulin release in response to a falling blood glucose are a potent combination that will tend to rapidly restore normal blood glucose levels in healthy subjects. Other counterregulatory neurohumoral changes also occur during hypoglycemia. In particular, the catecholamines epinephrine and (to a lesser extent) norepinephrine are released from the adrenal medulla under the control of preganglionic sympathetic neurons. In addition to this direct release of norepinephrine from the adrenal medulla, norepinephrine also appears in the bloodstream as a consequence of the increase in autonomic sympathetic outflow to other target tissues, resulting in some spillover from synapses into the circulation. In general, catecholamines, both in the circulation and by direct neural innervation, will act quickly to decrease glucose uptake into peripheral tissues and increase endogenous glucose output (from liver and perhaps also kidney) both directly and indirectly by increasing the supply of gluconeogenic precursors and free fatty acids from muscle and adipose tissue.[11]

Cortisol also rises during hypoglycemia, probably via a sequence of events involving activation of parvocellular neurons in the hypothalamic paraventricular nucleus, subsequent release of CRH from projections of these neurons in the median eminence, and subsequent ACTH release from corticotroph cells in the anterior pituitary. Growth hormone is released from the anterior pituitary during hypoglycemia, mainly as a result of changes in releasing factors from hypothalamic areas (i.e., GHRH) and/or a fall in inhibitory factors such as somatostatin. Cortisol and growth hormone exert a number of both direct and indirect effects to decrease glucose uptake into peripheral tissues and to promote endogenous glucose production.[12,13] However, these changes take time to occur, and therefore their actions are important when hypoglycemia is sustained. A number of other neuroendocrine changes also occur during hypoglycemia, such as increased endorphin and vasopressin release, although the significance of these is unclear.

These neurohumoral responses will tend to diminish, prevent, or correct a falling blood glucose by direct metabolic effects to antagonize the effects of insulin. These metabolic defense systems are complemented by the generation of symptoms—both those believed to be associated directly with the neurohumoral responses (such as heart palpitations from increased adrenergic drive and sweating linked to activation of cholinergic sympathetic fibers) and those resulting from brain neuroglycopenia such as behavioral changes. In patients with diabetes who have been suitably educated, these symptoms may warn of impending hypoglycemia and allow appropriate actions to correct blood glucose that depend on cognitive areas of the brain being able to function sufficiently to do what is necessary. Clearly, if blood glucose has fallen too low, these cognitive areas may not function sufficiently to effect rescue of blood glucose and severe hypoglycemia requiring third-party rescue may occur.

One symptom worthy of special mention is hunger, which not only warns of low glucose, but will also provoke eating to aid correction of blood glucose. The exact mechanisms by which hunger is generated during hypoglycemia are unknown, but it is worthy of note that many of the areas of the brain thought to be involved in glucose homeostasis, such as the ventromedial and lateral hypothalamic areas, are also thought to be important in control of appetite and satiety.

Sensing of Hypoglycemia

In order for the above protective responses to occur, the body must first detect hypoglycemia. The exact site or sites at which a low glucose level is detected and which of these sites, if any, is dominant remains controversial. However, considerable evidence suggests that brain areas play a critical role in sensing low blood glucose.

Outside the brain, pancreatic glucose sensing is important in nondiabetic subjects for triggering the cessation of insulin release, and this in turn is probably the dominant influence resulting in increased glucagon release during hypoglycemia. It is noteworthy in this regard that intraislet blood flow occurs to a large extent from the β-cell–rich core out into the periphery, the predominant location of α cells. Glucose-sensing mechanisms are undoubtedly present in the liver and/or portal vein, although the exact role that these areas may play in the generation of counterregulatory defenses against hypoglycemia is unclear. In support of a role for sensors in the hepatic area, adrenomedullary responses to (but not glucose recovery from) hypoglycemia were blunted by hepatic denervation in dogs.[14] Similarly, adrenomedullary responses to a systemic hypoglycemic challenge were blunted when portal vein (and liver) glucose levels were maintained by selective portal glucose infusion,[15] although it is possible that the arterioportal glucose gradient created might have acted as a feeding signal[16] to suppress counterregulatory responses to hypoglycemia,[17] as we will describe more fully later in this chapter.

In contrast, other work has suggested that hepatic/portal glucose sensors play a minimal role in sensing hypoglycemia. Studies in dogs in which the vagal nerve was cooled to reduce hepatic afferent neural transmission, or in human recipients of liver transplants with resulting hepatic denervation, showed no impairment of counterregulatory hormonal responses to hypoglycemia.[18–21] Furthermore, oral ingestion of glucose augmented rather than suppressed counterregulatory responses to a controlled hypoglycemic challenge in healthy male subjects, suggesting that portal glucose sensors had little role in sensing hypoglycemia.[22] In summary, the contribution of hepatic sensors to counterregulatory responses to hypoglycemia remains unclear. Even if liver or portal vein areas have a significant role in detecting hypoglycemia, it seems likely that these sensors act via coordinating CNS areas to trigger distal counterregulatory responses.

Much of the investigation of brain hypoglycemia sensing has employed either local delivery of nonmetabolizable glucose analogues to create local glucopenia (or the converse strategy of maintaining glucose levels within candidate sensing areas) or lesioning studies. Biggers and associates[23] used arterial catheterization of canine carotid and vertebral arteries to create a model in which brain glucose levels could be selectively maintained at euglycemia in the presence of systemic hypoglycemia. When brain glucose levels were maintained euglycemic, counterregulatory responses (catecholamines, cortisol, pancreatic polypeptide, and glucagon) were attenuated, suggesting that the predominant hypoglycemia sensor lay within the cerebral circulation. Subsequent selective infusion of either vertebral or carotid arteries suggested that both circulations contributed to the sensing area(s).[23]

The exact areas involved in CNS hypoglycemia sensing remain a source of debate. Studies by Borg and colleagues[24–26] suggest that the ventromedial hypothalamus (VMH) is an important area. Lesioning of rat VMH reduced counterregulatory responses to a systemic hypoglycemic challenge.[24] Subsequent studies used mi-

crodialysis techniques to deliver substrates directly into the hypothalamus, with counterregulatory responses being triggered by local VMH perfusion of the nonmetabolizable glucose analogue 2-deoxyglucose, or attenuated by VMH delivery of glucose during systemic hypoglycemia (Fig. 8-2).[25,26] As described below, a number of groups have identified and characterized neurons that respond to changes in blood glucose in the ventromedial (and lateral) hypothalamus.

In contrast, a number of studies have suggested that sensing areas around the brain stem may be predominant. Delivery of the antimetabolic glucose analogue 5-thioglucose (5TG) into the fourth ventricle was more effective in eliciting feeding and hyperglycemic responses than lateral ventricle injection. Acute blockade of the cerebral aqueduct abolished responses to injection of 5TG into the lateral ventricles, but injection into the fourth ventricle did not.[27] Using direct microinjection of 5TG into the brain parenchyma, a number of brain sites around the fourth ventricle were identified that triggered feeding and/or hyperglycemic responses. In contrast, a number of candidate hypothalamic areas showed no response to local delivery of 5TG.[28] Analogous to the hypothalamus, neurons with the ability to increase or decrease activity in response to changes in ambient glucose have also been identified in brain stem areas such as the nucleus tractus solitarius and area postrema.[29]

Despite the controversy about the relative importance of the different hypoglycemia sensing sites, it seems most likely that a redundancy of hypoglycemia sensors exists. A number of different sensing areas, both within the brain and possibly outside the CNS, are capable of detecting a low glucose and contributing to counterregulatory responses. Counterregulatory responses to systemic hypoglycemia may represent a coordinated response to complementary information from a number of different sensors.

Mechanisms of Brain Hypoglycemia Sensing

Although the exact mechanisms utilized by the CNS to detect low glucose remain to be defined, it seems to be a fall in cerebral metabolism that triggers counterregulatory responses. Studies

FIGURE 8-2. Delivery by microdialysis of D-glucose (but not nonmetabolizable L-glucose) into the ventromedial hypothalamus in rats,[2] obtunded counterregulatory responses to a systemic hypoglycemic challenge, suggesting that it is a fall in glucose levels in this area of the brain that initiates counterregulatory responses.

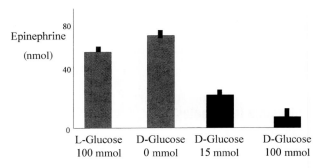

Hypoglycemia Sensing in the VMH

Borg et al JCI 1997

described earlier in the chapter examined the effects of infusion of the nonglucose substrates lactate or β-hydroxybutyrate during hypoglycemia. Counterregulatory responses were attenuated when blood glucose was lowered in the presence of elevated levels of either of these substrates, both capable of fueling brain areas. These studies suggest that it is a fall in cerebral metabolism in specialized brain areas that is the signal initiating counterregulatory responses, rather than a fall in glucose *per se*. In keeping with this view, local delivery of lactate into the VMH region was also sufficient to blunt counterregulatory hormone release during hypoglycemia.

Changes in CNS metabolism are probably detected by specialized neurons that have the ability to alter activity as ambient glucose levels change. The activity of most neurons is unaffected by changes in glucose, unless levels fall too low or so high as to cause a generalized metabolic decompensation. However, it has long been recognized that a subset of neurons from certain brain areas is capable of altering activity in response to changes in ambient glucose levels. Oomura and associates[30] first described glucose-responsive neurons in the VMH that increased activity in response to a rise in glucose, and another subset of neurons in the lateral hypothalamus that were inhibited by a rise in glucose. Although these neurons were initially referred to as GR (for glucose responsive) and GS (for glucose sensitive), respectively, the acronyms are not consistently used, with GS being used to describe generic glucose-sensing neurons, for example. More recently GR and GS neurons have been described in both hypothalamic and brain stem areas such as the area postrema and the nearby nucleus tractus solitarius.[31] Silver and Erecinska[32] reported that 30% of lateral hypothalamic neurons responded to changes in glucose. A rise in glucose inhibited activity in neurons termed types 1, 2, and 3, depending on the sensitivity to glucose, or increased activity in neurons labeled as type 4. Similarly, 40% of VMH neurons behaved like type 4 neurons, with an increase in activity with a rise in glucose levels.[32]

Further work is needed to determine how the metabolic signal of low glucose is transformed into neuronal electrical activity. One intriguing possibility is that some of the mechanisms utilized by glucose-sensing β cells of the pancreas may be used in brain hypoglycemia-sensing areas. For example, in the classic pathway of β-cell glucose sensing, specialized cell surface potassium channels (potassium ATP channels) allow the changes in energy supply as ATP to be converted into alterations in cell membrane polarization. Similar potassium ATP channels as well as glucokinase have been detected in glucose-sensing neurons from both the ventromedial hypothalamus[33] and brain stem glucose-sensing areas.[34]

Information about changes in blood and brain glucose levels may allow the central nervous system to contribute to a number of different homeostatic functions such as central control of endogenous glucose production, insulin secretion, and appetite/feeding pathways. Sensing of hypoglycemia may thus represent one end of a continuum of nutritional signaling, with sensory information from both GR and GS neurons and perhaps also peripheral glucose sensors being processed to allow a coordinated response to a threatened fuel supply.

Defective CNS Defenses Against Hypoglycemia in Diabetes

As described above, the CNS has a critical role to play in defending against hypoglycemia and thus protecting its own fuel supply. In diabetes, a number of defenses may be altered, both within and outside the CNS, leading to an increased risk of severe hypoglycemia.

Diabetic patients treated with insulin or insulin secretagogues are unable to reduce insulin release into blood in response to a falling blood glucose, resulting in an absolute or relative excess of insulin compared with nondiabetic subjects. In addition, most type 1 diabetic patients develop deficient glucagon responses to hypoglycemia within the first 5 years after diagnosis. Deficient glucagon (and insulin) responses to a falling blood glucose mean that patients are dependent on centrally driven catecholamine responses as the most important neurohumoral response to prevent hypoglycemia.[35] Unfortunately, a number of diabetic subjects develop additional defects in catecholamine responses to hypoglycemia. The combination of deficient glucagon and adrenomedullary/catecholaminergic responses and the associated loss of symptomatic awareness of hypoglycemia significantly increases the risk of severe hypoglycemia.[36,37] (See Chapter 31).

The exact mechanisms involved in abnormal counterregulation in diabetes are unknown. Abnormal glucagon responses that develop in most insulin-deficient patients most likely result from local pancreatic changes, although a central brain adaptation may contribute. The former may be, at least in part, a consequence of the loss of local islet insulin secretion, and its inhibitory effect on α-cell secretion. Normally, insulin secretion and intraislet insulin levels paradoxically fall in response to insulin-induced hypoglycemia, but in the insulin-deficient diabetic pancreas, exogenous insulin results in a rise in islet insulin levels that would be expected to suppress glucagon release. Deficient catecholamine defenses against hypoglycemia are believed to be a consequence of an adaptation occurring in those brain areas that sense low glucose and/or initiate counterregulatory defenses. Thus the mechanisms for these two abnormalities may, at least in part, be different. Important risk factors for abnormal counterregulation are intensified glycemic control, longer duration of diabetes, and a history of hypoglycemia *per se*.

There is considerable evidence that the hypoglycemia that occurs as a consequence of treatment of diabetes may itself result in a downregulation of counterregulatory responses to a subsequent hypoglycemic episode. Healthy volunteers exposed to two episodes of relatively mild hypoglycemia display temporary deficits in counterregulatory responses to hypoglycemia on the following day (Fig. 8-3).[38] Subsequent work from a number of groups has confirmed that antecedent hypoglycemia can result in a downregulation of subsequent responses to low blood glucose in both healthy and diabetic subjects. In keeping with this hypothesis, defective counterregulation in type 1 diabetes may be improved, at least in part, by scrupulous avoidance of hypoglycemia.[39]

The mechanisms by which antecedent hypoglycemia can downregulate counterregulatory responses to a subsequent hypoglycemic episode are uncertain. One possibility is that an adaptation in blood–brain glucose transport occurs in response to antecedent hypoglycemia, allowing the brain to maintain better local glucose levels during hypoglycemia. In keeping with this, a number of animal studies have reported increases in endothelial GLUT-1[40–42] and/or the neuronal glucose transporter GLUT-3[43] following periods of prolonged hypoglycemia.

In human studies, brain glucose uptake has been assessed either by measuring arteriovenous differences in glucose across the brain or noninvasively by using brain imaging techniques. In keeping with the animal data described above, net global brain glucose uptake measured by the difference between arterial and jugular bulb glucose levels was preserved during hypoglycemia in healthy human volunteers previously subjected to 56 hours of interprandial

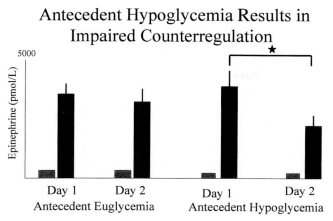

Antecedent Hypoglycemia Results in Impaired Counterregulation

Heller + Cryer Diabetes 1991

FIGURE 8-3. Hypoglycemia itself downregulates responses to subsequent hypoglycemia. The figure shows baseline and peak epinephrine responses to a brief hypoglycemic challenge in healthy subjects on two successive days. A period of 2 hours of moderate (3 mmol/L) hypoglycemia (but not euglycemia) on the afternoon of day 1 was sufficient to downregulate epinephrine responses to a subsequent hypoglycemic challenge on day 2. *(Reproduced from Heller et al.[38])*

hypoglycemia.[44] Similarly, a study of type 1 diabetic subjects showed that those with good glycemic control and frequent hypoglycemia were able to preserve brain glucose uptake during hypoglycemia.[45] In contrast, positron emission tomography (PET) scanning using a 1-^{11}C-glucose tracer technique demonstrated no global increase in glucose uptake after 24 hours of interprandial hypoglycemia in healthy volunteers.[46]

One possibility is that regional changes in glucose metabolism in glucose-sensing areas may not be apparent with these measures of global brain glucose metabolism. Using ^{18}F-fluorodeoxyglucose (FDG) as a tracer during PET scanning, Cranston and associates[47] reported that regional FDG brain uptake in an area including the ventromedial hypothalamus behaved differently during hypoglycemia in type 1 diabetic subjects with or without impaired counterregulatory defects. In animal studies regional brain metabolism can be examined by using microdialysis or microinjection techniques. Direct delivery by microdialysis of the glucose analogue 2-deoxyglucose (2DG) into the ventromedial hypothalamus in rats simulates local glucopenia and results in a counterregulatory-type response. In this model, the blood–brain barrier is effectively bypassed and substrate is delivered directly into the brain ECF. In animals previously exposed to chronic hypoglycemia, counterregulatory hormonal responses to 2DG delivery were obtunded, suggesting that at least part of the adaptation occurs downstream of blood–brain barrier glucose transport.[48]

An alternate, although not necessarily competing, hypothesis is that the rise in glucocorticoids that occurs as part of the counterregulatory response may activate a negative feedback loop that downregulates counterregulatory responses to a subsequent hypoglycemic challenge. Davis and colleagues[49] infused insulin and dextrose for two episodes of 120 minutes during the morning and afternoon in healthy subjects on day 1 and examined responses to a controlled hypoglycemic challenge on the next day (Fig. 8-4). When blood glucose was allowed to fall to 50 mg/dL (2.8 mmol/L) during the day 1 episodes, counterregulatory responses on day 2 were suppressed compared to when blood glucose was maintained

at 90 mg/dL (5 mmol/L) on day 1. When cortisol was infused on day 1 at a dose that mimicked the response seen with day 1 hypoglycemia (together with insulin and dextrose to maintain constant glucose levels), counterregulatory responses on day 2 were partially suppressed. These results suggest the downregulation of counterregulation by antecedent hypoglycemia may be in part mediated by cortisol.[49] A subsequent study by the same group of researchers examined patients with primary adrenocortical failure who underwent a similar 2-day experiment with two periods of controlled hypoglycemia on day 1 with an infusion of cortisol to mimic basal levels only. Responses to hypoglycemia were similar on both day 1 and day 2, suggesting that the absence of a glucocorticoid response to the low blood glucose on day 1 had prevented downregulation of counterregulation with hypoglycemia, although it should be noted that responses in general were less robust than those of a healthy control group.[50] However, the finding of downregulation with glucocorticoids is not universal. Shum and associates[51] demonstrated no effects of 4 days of corticosterone treatment on neuroendocrine responses to a subsequent hypoglycemic challenge in healthy rats. In contrast, antecedent hypoglycemia or even just exposure to high insulin levels with blood glucose maintained over the previous 4 days resulted in attenuated neurohumoral responses to hypoglycemia.[51]

If glucocorticoids are part of the mechanism by which hypoglycemia impairs counterregulatory responses to subsequent hypoglycemia, what might the teleological explanation be? In general, glucocorticoids display a complex series of interactions with stress responses (for review, see reference 52). Glucocorticoids have a permissive or stimulatory role on some aspects of the stress response. For example, deficient glucocorticoid secretion in Addison's syndrome results in impaired responses to a variety of insults as diverse as cardiovascular disruption, sepsis, and infection. On the other hand, glucocorticoids have also been demonstrated to have a role in limiting stress responses that prevent overstimulation, and in preparing the stress axis for future insults, possibly acting via brain steroid receptors. In clinical hypoglycemia, this may

FIGURE 8-4. Glucocorticoids released during hypoglycemia may modulate the downregulation of counterregulatory responses to a subsequent hypoglycemic challenge. Figure shows epinephrine responses to hypoglycemia on day 2 after one of three antecedent treatments given on day 1 (described in text). *(Reproduced from Davis et al.[49])*

Glucocorticoids May Mediate Hypoglycemia-Induced Impairment of Counterregulation

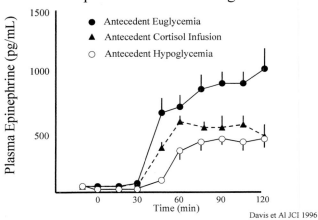

Davis et Al JCI 1996

be further complicated by the contribution of other components of the hypophysio-adrenal axis such as brain release of CRH that may also modulate stress responses.

It is possible that a number of different adaptations in the diabetic brain including, but not restricted to, alterations in brain glucose transport and feedback from the hypothalamic-pituitary-adrenal axis contribute to impaired CNS defenses against hypoglycemia. Other putative adaptive mechanisms that have been suggested include alterations in brain metabolic pathways in sensing areas, local blood flow, local substrate fluxes (and in particular changes in brain lactate and/or glycogen metabolism), and changes in neurotransmitter pathways.

ROLE OF THE CNS IN THE RESPONSE TO HYPERGLYCEMIA

DeFronzo and colleagues[53] showed decades ago that when glucose was delivered through a peripheral vein in the human, the plasma glucose (221 mg/dL) and insulin levels (101 μU/mL) rose, but splanchnic glucose uptake was minimal. When in the same subjects glucose was given orally and the glucose infusion rate was reduced to maintain the same arterial glucose level, net splanchnic glucose uptake increased more than fourfold (Fig. 8-5). Although the plasma insulin level was increased modestly in the oral group relative to the IV-only group, it is now known that the insulin increment could not explain the larger increase in net splanchnic glucose uptake. Based on their findings, the investigators suggested that a gut factor may play an important role in signaling the liver to take up and store glucose following feeding. Subsequent work in animal models in other laboratories determined that enhancement of net hepatic glucose uptake (NHGU) was evident with portal glucose infusion, and not just with enteral glucose delivery, dispelling the notion that gut factors could be responsible for the findings.[54–56]

Studies were therefore carried out to try and understand whether the CNS could play a role in the response to oral/portal glucose delivery. It would now appear that glucose uptake and storage by the liver are regulated by three factors: the plasma insulin/glucagon levels, the plasma glucose level, and a signal generated by entry of glucose into the body via the portal vein. In a series of studies employing the conscious dog, it was shown that with insulin increased to fourfold basal, the rate at which the liver took up glucose correlated linearly with the hepatic glucose load (i.e., the rate at which glucose was delivered to the liver).[57] Administering a small portion of the glucose infusion into the hepatic portal vein shifted the dose–response curve to the left. Thus when the arterial plasma glucose level ranged between 100 and 200 mg/dL, the "portal" signal was responsible for most of the NHGU.

Significance of the Portal Signal in Disposition of a Glucose Load

When the glucose load to the liver was doubled and the insulin level was varied, there was a curvilinear relationship between the insulin level and NHGU[58] (Fig. 8-6). Once again, infusion of a small amount of glucose into the hepatic portal vein to activate the portal signal shifted the dose–response curve to the left. In fact, the ability of this signal to augment NHGU was equivalent to the effect of a fourfold rise in plasma insulin. Experiments were then carried out in which the insulin level was increased fourfold and the glucose load to the liver was doubled, but the magnitude of the por-

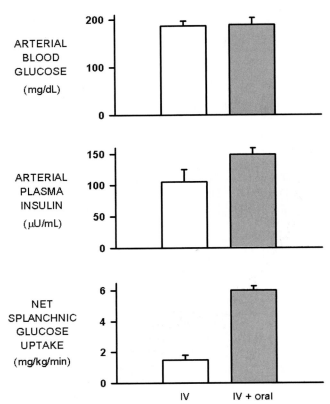

FIGURE 8-5. Normal human volunteers received an intravenous glucose infusion continuously for 4 hours so that they achieved steady-state glucose (221 mg/dL) and insulin (101 μU/mL) concentrations (IV group). An additional group (IV + oral) received an intravenous glucose infusion to achieve similar hyperglycemia and hyperinsulinemia to the IV group. After steady-state glucose concentrations were reached, they ingested glucose 1.2 g/kg, and the peripheral glucose infusion rate was adjusted to maintain their plasma glucose at ~220 mg/dL. Net splanchnic glucose uptake was significantly enhanced by oral glucose ingestion, an effect not solely attributable to the relatively small differential in insulin concentrations between groups. *(Redrawn from DeFronzo et al.[53])*

tal vein and peripheral vein glucose infusion rates was varied so as to create a range of arterial-portal (A-P) glucose gradients. There was a curvilinear dose–response relationship between the A-P glucose gradient and the fractional uptake of glucose by the liver (Fig. 8-6),[59] such that the signal was most effective with a low glucose load and, in fact, saturated at an A-P gradient of about 20 mg/dL, a physiologic gradient observed in the postprandial state.

It was further demonstrated that the portal signal, while augmenting glucose uptake by the liver, decreased muscle glucose uptake.[60] Thus, instead of regulating whole-body glucose clearance, in this way it tended to control the distribution of glucose between the liver and muscle (Fig. 8-7). The suggestion was also made that the portal signal had a mild incretin effect, thereby raising the plasma insulin level and thus also promoting whole-body glucose clearance.[61–63] This is consistent with data demonstrating a relationship between hepatoportal glucose sensors and insulin secretion. Hepatic vagotomy attenuated insulin secretion following intraportal or intraperitoneal glucose administration in the rat, but it did not decrease insulin release following peripheral intravenous glucose injection.[64,65] Moreover, injection of glucose into the portal vein decreased the afferent firing rate in the hepatic branch of

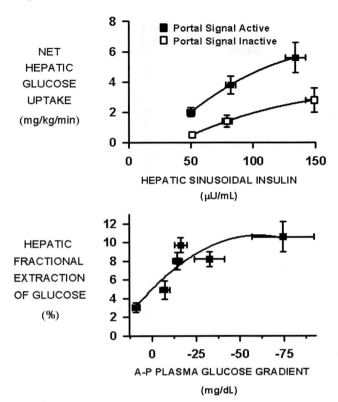

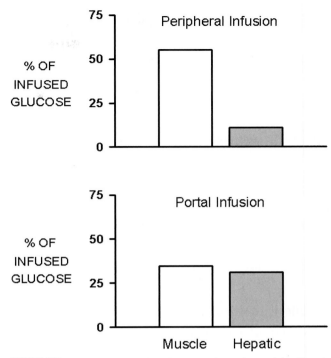

FIGURE 8-6. Net hepatic glucose uptake is enhanced by portal vein versus peripheral glucose infusion over a wide range of insulin concentrations (**top panel**). With the hepatic glucose load at twofold basal and plasma insulin at fourfold basal, net hepatic fractional extraction of glucose is directly related to the magnitude of the negative arterial-portal vein glucose gradient, an effect that saturates above a gradient of approximately −20 mg/dL (**bottom panel**). (*Top panel: redrawn from Myers* et al.[58] *Bottom panel: redrawn from Pagliassotti* et al.[59])

FIGURE 8-7. The portal signal is an important determinant of the disposition of a glucose load. During peripheral glucose delivery, the net hepatic glucose uptake accounts for only approximately 10% of the infused glucose, and muscle accounts for more than 50%. In the presence of the portal signal, the percentage of the glucose load taken up by skeletal muscle and liver is almost equal. (*Derived from data in Adkins-Marshall BA* et al: *Interaction between insulin and glucose-delivery route in regulation of net hepatic glucose uptake in conscious dogs*. Diabetes *1990;39:87*.)

the vagus nerve, but at the same time it increased the firing rate of the vagal pancreatic efferents, an effect ablated by sectioning the hepatic branch of the vagus.[66]

This synchronized pattern of response led to the hypothesis that the portal signal involves the CNS. Certain evidence has now accumulated to support this hypothesis. The speeds of onset and offset of the response of the liver to an alteration in the portal signal are rapid. A maximal response to the portal signal was seen within 15 minutes[67] (Fig. 8-8) and the response was lost equally rapidly.[68,69] Thus the speed of the response is consistent with neural signaling. In addition, in the presence of a fourfold increase in plasma insulin and a doubling of the hepatic glucose load, the ability of portal glucose infusion to modify hepatic and muscle glucose uptake was eliminated by hepatic denervation.[70] These data provide strong support for neural involvement in the effect of the portal signal on hepatic and muscle glucose uptake.

The Afferent Limb of the Portal Signal

It is worth considering how the body monitors the difference in the arterial and portal vein glucose levels. It must first be noted that increasing the portal glucose level by infusing glucose through a peripheral vein does not trigger the portal signal. The signal is only manifest when the portal glucose level exceeds the arterial glucose

level, as it does during glucose feeding. It would appear that the arterial glucose level provides a reference point against which the portal glucose level can be viewed. It seems clear that the latter is perceived by the portal glucose sensors described by Niijima and his colleagues.[71–73] It is less clear, however, where the arterial glucose level is sensed. It could be monitored in the liver, the brain, or the carotid bodies.[17,74–76]

FIGURE 8-8. The effect of the glucose portal signal is rapid, with maximal enhancement of NHGU by 15 minutes. In contrast, the effect of insulin on NHGU is slow. When hyperinsulinemia is combined with the portal signal, the response is more rapid than the response to insulin in the absence of the portal signal. (*Redrawn from Pagliassotti* et al.[67])

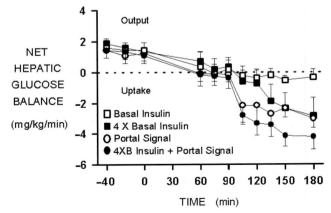

The role of CNS glucose sensors in providing the reference information was assessed by Hsieh and associates.[76] The insulin level in conscious dogs was increased fourfold, along with a doubling of the hepatic glucose load in the presence of the portal signal to fully activate NHGU. The glucose level in the head was then increased by glucose infusion through catheters in the carotid and vertebral arteries, to a point where it was slightly above the portal glucose level. There was no impact on NHGU, suggesting that arterial glucose sensing in this context was taking place outside the CNS. Matsuhisa and colleagues[17] tried a similar approach, but only used unilateral glucose infusion. They observed a small reduction in NHGU, suggesting brain sensors may be involved, but their study has some limitations[76] that prevent a definitive conclusion from being drawn. On the other hand, using similar conditions to those in their first study, Hsieh and coworkers[75] infused glucose into the hepatic artery so as to eliminate the intrahepatic arterial-portal glucose gradient. This resulted in a complete abolition of the effect of the portal signal on NHGU, strongly suggesting that the arterial-portal glucose comparison is made within the liver.

The Efferent Limb of the Portal Signal

The portal signal increased the activation of glycogen synthase in the dog and enhanced hepatic glycogen deposition in the dog and rat.[67,77] Based on work by Shimazu and associates[78] and Jungermann and colleagues[79,80] it appears likely that activation of the liver in response to the portal signal would involve an augmentation of parasympathetic input and/or a diminution of sympathetic signaling. Shimazu and associates[78] noted that electrical stimulation of the lateral hypothalamus (LH, primarily parasympathetic in nature) resulted in an increase in glycogen synthase activity and hepatic glycogen concentrations. Vagal, but not splanchnic, nerve stimulation produced similar effects.[81] Shiota and coworkers[82] therefore carried out a study in which they gave alpha- and beta-blockers portally, along with acetylcholine (ACh), in an attempt to examine the impact of these regulators on NHGU in conscious dogs. Insulin was increased to fourfold basal in the presence of a twofold rise in the hepatic glucose load (but without any portal glucose infusion). NHGU increased twice as much in the dogs receiving ACh and adrenergic blockers as it did in the control dogs. On the other hand, there was a marked rise in hepatic arterial flow in the experimental group that complicated data interpretation. Since no such change in hepatic artery flow occurs in response to portal glucose infusion, it raises the possibility that this effect of ACh on NHGU was associated with a nonspecific vascular event. Concomitantly, however, Stumpel and Jungermann,[79] using the perfused rat liver, also came to the conclusion that the efferent limb of the portal signal involved the parasympathetic nervous system.

Cardin and colleagues[83] next employed a vagus nerve cooling technique to determine whether removal of vagal efferent input would reduce or eliminate the effect of the portal signal on NHGU. Vagal cooling would reduce firing in the vagal afferents, thereby intensifying portal signaling. Thus any effect of vagal cooling to reduce NHGU would be attributable to a diminution in efferent activity and presumably ACh release. Somewhat surprisingly, vagal cooling was without effect on NHGU despite the fact that it caused a maximal increase in heart rate,[83] thereby validating its effectiveness. These data thus suggest that the efferent limb of the response involves a change in the level of a neural mediator other than acetylcholine. Among the possibilities are norepinephrine, neu-ropeptide Y, and other mediators associated with the sympathetic nervous system. It thus appears at this time as if the efferent signal reaches the liver through nonparasympathetic efferent fibers.

SUMMARY

In summary, the brain has a critical role to play in maintaining blood glucose levels within narrow limits in order to promote efficient fuel metabolism and to support optimal brain function. A number of defensive counterregulatory responses that protect against falling blood glucose are initiated and/or controlled by the CNS. The exact brain areas and pathways involved in these responses have not been fully identified, but specialized hypothalamic and/or brain stem areas containing nutrient-sensitive neurons probably play an important role. In diabetes, treatment regimens with insulin or insulin secretagogues may overcome or interfere with these defenses and result in hypoglycemia. The mechanisms for these deficits in counterregulation are unknown, but it is assumed that at least part of these adaptations ultimately act to alter the function of specialized brain hypoglycemia-sensing areas.

During carbohydrate feeding it would appear that afferent nerve signaling regarding both the level of hepatic arterial glucose and the level of hepatic portal vein glucose is communicated to the CNS, where it results in a modification of sympathetic or some other input to the liver, which then activates NHGU. Many questions remain about the role of the CNS in coordinating the response of the body to nutrient intake. The significance of the portal signal in humans needs to be verified, and the nature of the afferent sensing and efferent signaling needs to be clarified. Likewise, the significance of the signal in the context of fat and protein ingestion needs to be examined. It seems clear, however, that the CNS plays an important role in coordinating the distribution of incoming nutrients to the various tissues of the body.

REFERENCES

1. Clarke DD, Sokoloff L: Circulation and energy metabolism of the brain. In: Siegel GJ, Agranoff BW, Albers RW *et al*, eds. *Basic Neurochemistry: Molecular, Cellular and Medical Aspects.* Lippincott-Raven:1998;637.
2. Auer RN, Hugh J, Cosgrove E, *et al*: Neuropathologic findings in three cases of profound hypoglycemia. *Clin Neuropathol* 1989;8:63.
3. Amiel SA, Archibald HR, Chusney G, *et al*: Ketone infusion lowers hormonal responses to hypoglycaemia: Evidence for acute cerebral utilization of a non-glucose fuel. *Clin Sci (Colch)* 1991;81:189.
4. Maran A, Cranston I, Lomas J, *et al*: Protection by lactate of cerebral function during hypoglycaemia. *Lancet* 1994;343:16.
5. Veneman T, Mitrakou A, Mokan M, *et al*: Effect of hyperketonemia and hyperlacticacidemia on symptoms, cognitive dysfunction, and counterregulatory hormone responses during hypoglycemia in normal humans. *Diabetes* 1994;43:1311.
6. Tabernero A, Vicario C, Medina JM: Lactate spares glucose as a metabolic fuel in neurons and astrocytes from primary culture. *Neurosci Res* 1996;26:369.
7. Wallace E, Maggs D, Spencer D, *et al*: High lactate concentration in human brain ECF: An alternative fuel during hypoglycemia? *Diabetes* 1995;44:154A.
8. Martin DL: The role of glia in the inactivation of neurotransmitters. In: Kettenmann H, Ransom BR, eds. *Neuroglia.* Oxford University Press:1995;732.
9. Yalow R, Berson S: Dynamics of insulin secretion in hypoglycemia. *Diabetes* 1965;14:341.

10. Stevenson RW, Steiner KE, Davis MA, *et al*: Similar dose responsiveness of hepatic glycogenolysis and gluconeogenesis to glucagon in vivo. *Diabetes* 1987;36:382.

11. Chu CA, Sindelar DK, Neal DW, *et al*: Comparison of the direct and indirect effects of epinephrine on hepatic glucose production. *J Clin Invest* 1997;99:1044.

12. De Feo P, Perriello G, Torlone E, *et al*: Demonstration of a role for growth hormone in glucose counterregulation. *Am J Physiol* 1989; 256:E835.

13. De Feo P, Perriello G, Torlone E, *et al*: Contribution of cortisol to glucose counterregulation in humans. *Am J Physiol* 1989;257:E35.

14. Lamarche L, Yamaguchi N, Peronnet F: Hepatic denervation reduces adrenal catecholamine secretion during insulin-induced hypoglycemia. *Am J Physiol* 1995;268:R50.

15. Hevener AL, Bergman RN, Donovan CM: Novel glucosensor for hypoglycemic detection localized to the portal vein. *Diabetes* 1997; 46:1521.

16. Tordoff MG, Friedman MI: Hepatic portal glucose infusions decrease food intake and increase food preference. *Am J Physiol* 1986;251: R192.

17. Matsuhisa M, Morishima T, Nakahara I, *et al*: Augmentation of hepatic glucose uptake by a positive glucose gradient between hepatoportal and central nervous systems. *Diabetes* 1997;46:1101.

18. Perseghin G, Regalia E, Battezzati A, *et al*: Regulation of glucose homeostasis in humans with denervated livers. *J Clin Invest* 1997; 100:931.

19. Jackson PA, Pagliassotti MJ, Shiota M, *et al*: Effects of vagal blockade on the counterregulatory response to insulin-induced hypoglycemia in the dog. *Am J Physiol* 1997;273:E1178.

20. Joseph SE, Lomas J, Pernet A, *et al*: Denervated liver and kidney show defective glucose counterregulation to hypoglycaemia in man. *Diabet Med* 1998;15:S11.

21. Joseph SE, Pernet A, Hopkins E, *et al*: Hepatic innervation is not required for catecholamine responses to hypoglycaemia in man. *Diabet Med* 1998;15:S12.

22. Heptulla RA, Tamborlane WV, Ma TY, *et al*: Oral glucose augments the counterregulatory hormone response during insulin-induced hypoglycemia in humans. *J Clin Endocrinol Metab* 2001;86:645.

23. Biggers DW, Myers SR, Neal D, *et al*: Role of brain in counterregulation of insulin-induced hypoglycemia in dogs. *Diabetes* 1989;38:7.

24. Borg WP, During MJ, Sherwin RS, *et al*: Ventromedial hypothalamic lesions in rats suppress counterregulatory responses to hypoglycemia. *J Clin Invest* 1994;93:1677.

25. Borg WP, Sherwin RS, During MJ, *et al*: Local ventromedial hypothalamus glucopenia triggers counterregulatory hormone release. *Diabetes* 1995;44:180.

26. Borg MA, Sherwin RS, Borg WP, *et al*: Local ventromedial hypothalamus glucose perfusion blocks counterregulation during systemic hypoglycemia in awake rats. *J Clin Invest* 1997;99:361.

27. Ritter RC, Slusser PG, Stone S: Glucoreceptors controlling feeding and blood glucose: Location in the hindbrain. *Science* 1981;213: 451.

28. Ritter S, Dinh TT, Zhang Y: Localization of hindbrain glucoreceptive sites controlling food intake and blood glucose. *Brain Res* 2000;856: 37.

29. Yettefti K, Orsini JC, Perrin J: Characteristics of glycemia-sensitive neurons in the nucleus tractus solitarii: Possible involvement in nutritional regulation. *Physiol Behav* 1997;61:93.

30. Oomura Y, Ono T, Ooyama H, *et al*: Glucose and osmosensitive neurones of the rat hypothalamus. *Nature* 1969;222:282.

31. Funahashi M, Adachi A: Glucose-responsive neurons exist within the area postrema of the rat: In vitro study on the isolated slice preparation. *Brain Res Bull* 1993;32:531.

32. Silver IA, Erecinska M: Glucose-induced intracellular ion changes in sugar-sensitive hypothalamic neurons. *J Neurophysiol* 1998;79:1733.

33. Lee K, Dixon AK, Richardson PJ, *et al*: Glucose-receptive neurones in the rat ventromedial hypothalamus express KATP channels composed of Kir6.1 and SUR1 subunits. *J Physiol* 1999;515:439.

34. Dallaporta M, Perrin J, Orsini JC: Involvement of adenosine triphosphate-sensitive K$^+$ channels in glucose-sensing in the rat solitary tract nucleus. *Neurosci Lett* 2000;278:77.

35. Gerich J, Davis J, Lorenzi M, *et al*: Hormonal mechanisms of recovery from insulin-induced hypoglycemia in man. *Am J Physiol* 1979; 236:E380.

36. Clarke WL, Cox DJ, Gonder-Frederick LA, *et al*: Reduced awareness of hypoglycemia in adults with IDDM. A prospective study of hypoglycemic frequency and associated symptoms. *Diabetes Care* 1995; 18:517.

37. Gold AE, MacLeod KM, Frier BM: Frequency of severe hypoglycemia in patients with type I diabetes with impaired awareness of hypoglycemia. *Diabetes Care* 1994;17:697.

38. Heller SR, Cryer PE: Reduced neuroendocrine and symptomatic responses to subsequent hypoglycemia after one episode of hypoglycemia in nondiabetic humans. *Diabetes* 1991;40:223.

39. Cranston I, Lomas J, Maran A, *et al*: Restoration of hypoglycaemia awareness in patients with long-duration insulin-dependent diabetes. *Lancet* 1994;344:283.

40. Kumagai AK, Kang YS, Boado RJ, *et al*: Upregulation of blood-brain barrier GLUT1 glucose transporter protein and mRNA in experimental chronic hypoglycemia. *Diabetes* 1995;44:1399.

41. McCall AL, Fixman LB, Fleming N, *et al*: Chronic hypoglycemia increases brain glucose transport. *Am J Physiol* 1986;251:E442.

42. Simpson IA, Appel NM, Hokari M, *et al*: Blood-brain barrier glucose transporter: Effects of hypo- and hyperglycemia revisited. *J Neurochem* 1999;72:238.

43. Uehara Y, Nipper V, McCall AL: Chronic insulin hypoglycemia induces GLUT-3 protein in rat brain neurons. *Am J Physiol* 1997;272: E716.

44. Boyle PJ, Nagy RJ, O'Connor AM, *et al*: Adaptation in brain glucose uptake following recurrent hypoglycemia. *Proc Natl Acad Sci USA* 1994;91:9352.

45. Boyle PJ, Kempers SF, O'Connor AM, *et al*: Brain glucose uptake and unawareness of hypoglycemia in patients with insulin-dependent diabetes mellitus. *N Engl J Med* 1995;333:1726.

46. Segel SA, Fanelli CG, Dence CS, *et al*: Blood-to-brain glucose transport, cerebral glucose metabolism, and cerebral blood flow are not increased after hypoglycemia. *Diabetes* 2001;50:1911.

47. Cranston I, Reed LJ, Marsden PK, *et al*: Changes in regional brain (18)F-fluorodeoxyglucose uptake at hypoglycemia in type 1 diabetic men associated with hypoglycemia unawareness and counterregulatory failure. *Diabetes* 2001;50:2329.

48. Borg MA, Borg WP, Tamborlane WV, *et al*: Chronic hypoglycemia and diabetes impair counterregulation induced by localized 2-deoxyglucose perfusion of the ventromedial hypothalamus in rats. *Diabetes* 1999;48:584.

49. Davis SN, Shavers C, Costa F, *et al*: Role of cortisol in the pathogenesis of deficient counterregulation after antecedent hypoglycemia in normal humans. *J Clin Invest* 1996;98:680.

50. Davis SN, Shavers C, Davis B, *et al*: Prevention of an increase in plasma cortisol during hypoglycemia preserves subsequent counterregulatory responses. *J Clin Invest* 1997;100:429.

51. Shum K, Inouye K, Chan O, *et al*: Effects of antecedent hypoglycemia, hyperinsulinemia, and excess corticosterone on hypoglycemic counterregulation. *Am J Physiol Endocrinol Metab* 2001; 281:E455.

52. Sapolsky RM, Romero LM, Munck AU: How do glucocorticoids influence stress responses? Integrating permissive, suppressive, stimulatory, and preparative actions. *Endocr Rev* 2000;21:55.

53. DeFronzo RA, Ferrannini E, Hendler R, *et al*: Influence of hyperinsulinemia, hyperglycemia, and the route of glucose administration on splanchnic glucose exchange. *Proc Natl Acad Sci USA* 1978;75: 5173.

54. Ishida T, Chap Z, Chou J, *et al*: Differential effects of oral, peripheral intravenous, and intraportal glucose on hepatic glucose uptake and insulin and glucagon extraction in conscious dogs. *J Clin Invest* 1983; 72:590.

55. Adkins BA, Myers SR, Hendrick GK, *et al*: Importance of the route of intravenous glucose delivery to hepatic glucose balance in the conscious dog. *J Clin Invest* 1987;79:557.

56. Bergman RN, Beir JR, Hourigan PM: Intraportal glucose infusion matched to oral glucose absorption. Lack of evidence for "gut factor" involvement in hepatic glucose storage. *Diabetes* 1982;31:27.

57. Myers SR, Biggers DW, Neal DW, *et al*: Intraportal glucose delivery enhances the effects of hepatic glucose load on net hepatic glucose uptake in vivo. *J Clin Invest* 1991;88:158.

58. Myers SR, McGuinness OP, Neal DW, *et al*: Intraportal glucose delivery alters the relationship between net hepatic glucose uptake and the insulin concentration. *J Clin Invest* 1991;87:930.

59. Pagliassotti MJ, Myers SR, Moore MC, *et al*: Magnitude of negative arterial-portal glucose gradient alters net hepatic glucose balance in conscious dogs. *Diabetes* 1991;40:1659.

60. Galassetti P, Shiota M, Zinker BA, *et al*: A negative arterial-portal venous glucose gradient decreases skeletal muscle glucose uptake. *Am J Physiol* 1998;275:E101.

61. Fery F, Deviere J, Balasse EO: Metabolic handling of intraduodenal vs. intravenous glucose in humans. *Am J Physiol Endocrinol Metab* 2001;281:E261.

62. Dunning BE, Moore MC, Ikeda T, *et al*: Evidence for a neurally mediated incretin effect of portal vs. peripheral glucose infusion in conscious dogs. (Submitted).

63. Moore MC, Hsieh PS, Neal DW, *et al*: Nonhepatic response to portal glucose delivery in conscious dogs. *Am J Physiol Endocrinol Metab* 2000;279:E1271.

64. Sakaguchi T, Hayashi Y: Reflex secretion of insulin evoked by hepatic portal injection of D-glucose anomers in the rat. *Biomed Res* 1981; 2:222.

65. Lee KC, Miller RE: The hepatic vagus nerve and the neural regulation of insulin secretion. *Endocrinology* 1985;117:307.

66. Nagase H, Inoue S, Tanaka K, *et al*: Hepatic glucose-sensitive unit regulation of glucose-induced insulin secretion in rats. *Physiol Behav* 1993;53:139.

67. Pagliassotti MJ, Holste LC, Moore MC, *et al*: Comparison of the time courses of insulin and the portal signal on hepatic glucose and glycogen metabolism in the conscious dog. *J Clin Invest* 1996;97:81.

68. Hsieh PS, Moore MC, Neal DW, *et al*: Rapid reversal of the effects of the portal signal under hyperinsulinemic conditions in the conscious dog. *Am J Physiol* 1999;276:E930.

69. Hsieh PS, Moore MC, Neal DW, *et al*: Hepatic glucose uptake rapidly decreases after removal of the portal signal in conscious dogs. *Am J Physiol* 1998;275:E987.

70. Adkins-Marshall B, Pagliassotti MJ, Asher JR, *et al*: Role of hepatic nerves in response of liver to intraportal glucose delivery in dogs. *Am J Physiol* 1992;262:E679.

71. Niijima A: Glucose-sensitive afferent nerve fibres in the hepatic branch of the vagus nerve in the guinea-pig. *J Physiol* 1982;332:315.

72. Niijima A, Fukuda A, Taguchi T, *et al*: Suppression of afferent activity of the hepatic vagus nerve by anomers of D-glucose. *Am J Physiol* 1983;244:R611.

73. Niijima A: Glucose-sensitive afferent nerve fibers in the liver and their role in food intake and blood glucose regulation. *J Auton Nerv Syst* 1983;9:207.

74. Koyama Y, Coker RH, Denny JC, *et al*: Role of carotid bodies in control of the neuroendocrine response to exercise. *Am J Physiol Endocrinol Metab* 2001;281:E742.

75. Hsieh PS, Moore MC, Neal DW, *et al*: Importance of the hepatic arterial glucose level in generation of the portal signal in conscious dogs. *Am J Physiol Endocrinol Metab* 2000;279:E284.

76. Hsieh PS, Moore MC, Marshall B, *et al*: The head arterial glucose level is not the reference site for generation of the portal signal in conscious dogs. *Am J Physiol* 1999;277:E678.

77. Cardin S, Emshwiller M, Jackson PA, *et al*: Portal glucose infusion increases hepatic glycogen deposition in conscious unrestrained rats. *J Appl Physiol* 1999;87:1470.

78. Shimazu T, Matsushita H, Ishikawa K: Cholinergic stimulation of the rat hypothalamus: Effects of liver glycogen synthesis. *Science* 1976; 194:535.

79. Stumpel F, Jungermann K: Sensing by intrahepatic muscarinic nerves of a portal-arterial glucose concentration gradient as a signal for insulin-dependent glucose uptake in the perfused rat liver. *FEBS Lett* 1997;406:119.

80. Jungermann K, Gardemann A, Beuers U, *et al*: Regulation of liver metabolism by the hepatic nerves. *Adv Enzyme Regul* 1987;26:63.

81. Shimazu T: Regulation of glycogen metabolism in liver by the autonomic nervous system. V. Activation of glycogen synthetase by vagal stimulation. *Biochim Biophys Acta* 1971;252:28.

82. Shiota M, Jackson P, Galassetti P, *et al*: Combined intraportal infusion of acetylcholine and adrenergic blockers augments net hepatic glucose uptake. *Am J Physiol Endocrinol Metab* 2000;278:E544.

83. Cardin S, Edgerton DS, Farmer B, *et al*: Lack of involvement of the parasympathetic nervous system in the hepatic response to portal glucose delivery. *Diabetes* 2001;50:A326.

Stress-Induced Activation of the Neuroendocrine System and Its Effects On Carbohydrate Metabolism

Peter J. Havel

Gerald J. Taborsky, Jr.

BASIC NEUROENDOCRINE CONTROL OF PLASMA GLUCOSE

Maintenance of plasma glucose levels within a narrow range, both in the basal state and during and after meals, is the responsibility of a neuroendocrine control system. In the basal state, the basic feedback loop (Fig. 9-1) depends on the liver as a source of glucose and peripheral tissues as the site of glucose utilization. In the basal state, the brain is the most important site of utilization since it metabolizes 80% of the glucose produced after an overnight fast. Insulin and glucagon secretion from the pancreatic islet by the plasma glucose level is the major feedback regulator for maintaining glucose at steady-state levels (Fig. 9-1). Most individuals have adequate islet mass and α and β cells that have sufficient glucose sensitivity to secrete the amount of insulin and glucagon needed. Furthermore, the hepatic sensitivity to insulin and glucagon and the peripheral sensitivity to insulin are such that this amount of insulin and glucagon achieves fasting plasma glucose levels between 60 and 100 mg/dL. However, the islet, liver, and peripheral tissues are sensitive to circulating and locally released neuroendocrine controllers. Therefore, the basic islet-glucose feedback loop can be modulated by these neuroendocrine factors, which usually results, during stress, in regulation at a higher steady-state plasma glucose concentration.

MECHANISMS FOR HYPERGLYCEMIA

Due to the brain's absolute requirement for glucose, there are redundant neuroendocrine mechanisms to maintain adequate delivery of glucose to the brain between meals. Recognition that the neuroendocrine control system functions to ensure adequate glucose to maintain brain function helps one understand the mechanisms for stress hyperglycemia and their redundancy. In the simplest view there are only two ways to achieve hyperglycemia: increase the rate of glucose production by the liver or decrease the rate of glucose utilization by peripheral tissues (Fig. 9-2). Since the rate of glucose utilization by the brain is not dependent on insulin (Fig. 9-2), it is relatively constant. Thus only approximately 20% of total glucose utilization in the basal state can be modulated, and in practical terms, reduction of *basal* glucose utilization makes at most a small contribution to the *initiation* of hyperglycemia during

stress. Therefore, it is the increased hepatic production of glucose, primarily by glycogenolysis, that is responsible for the initiation of hyperglycemia during stress. Increased hepatic glucose production is characteristic of stress; for example, of the nine individual stresses discussed later in the chapter, all have increased hepatic glucose production at some point during the stress. Whether they also are characterized by fasting hyperglycemia depends on the individual stress and its effects on glucose utilization. Some stresses are characterized by impaired glucose utilization, which as the glucose level rises during stress, makes an increasing contribution to the maintenance of the hyperglycemia (Fig. 9-2). Other stresses are characterized by increased glucose utilization that nearly parallels the increase of hepatic glucose production. If glucose production and glucose utilization are increased simultaneously, then glucose turnover will increase with only minor changes of the plasma glucose level. Therefore, it is not the absolute rates of glucose production or utilization that are responsible for hyperglycemia during stress, but rather it is the imbalance between glucose production and its utilization. For this reason, it is possible for absolute glucose turnover to be increased, normal, or even decreased during stress hyperglycemia. However, total glucose turnover is usually increased during stress whether or not hyperglycemia is present. This concept is important since it is often assumed that the hyperglycemia itself is an index of carbohydrate utilization during stress. This is not the case, and recognition of this potential problem will be important to the consideration of the mechanisms for stress hyperglycemia in nondiabetic subjects and treatment of stress hyperglycemia in diabetic patients.

REGULATION OF GLUCOSE PRODUCTION AND UTILIZATION BY NEUROENDOCRINE FACTORS

Two types of neuroendocrine control factors achieve the regulation of hepatic glucose production. One type produces quick, minute-to-minute changes in hepatic glucose output. This type includes the endocrine pancreatic hormones, insulin and glucagon, and the neuroendocrine amines, epinephrine and norepinephrine (Fig. 9-3). These are short-term regulators of glycogenolysis and gluconeogenesis. Insulin inhibits hepatic glucose output from the liver, whereas glucagon, epinephrine, and norepinephrine stimulate hepatic glucose mobilization. It is the balance between these

BASAL GLUCOSE FEEDBACK LOOP

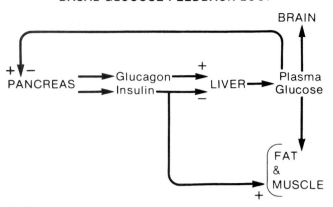

FIGURE 9-1. This basal glucose feedback loop is the underlying regulator of plasma glucose to maintain an adequate supply of glucose to the brain. Note the key role of the endocrine pancreas in this loop. *(Reprinted with permission from Pfeifer, et al.[163])*

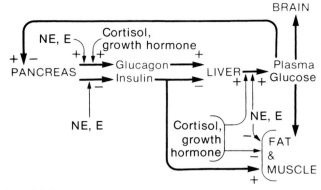

FIGURE 9-3. Neuroendocrine changes in stress hyperglycemia. Note that the basal feedback loop is modulated in the pancreas, liver, and insulin-sensitive tissues. Brain remains sensitive only to plasma glucose level and cerebral blood flow. Also note the key role of epinephrine (**E**) and norepinephrine (**NE**) in restraining the insulin response to hyperglycemia.

opposing factors which determines the amount of glucose that the liver produces. The second type of neuroendocrine factors determines the sensitivity of the liver to these short-term regulators of glycogenolysis and gluconeogenesis. These are the hormones cortisol, thyroxine, growth hormone (GH), and estrogens (Fig. 9-3). They alter the sensitivity of the liver to regulation by the short-term regulatory factors. Many of these long-term regulators appear to be more permissive than regulatory; that is, the pathologic excess or lack of such factors alters hepatic glucose production, but fluctuations of their plasma concentration within the usual physiologic range has no major effect.

Many of these same neuroendocrine factors are also important to the regulation of glucose utilization in peripheral tissues and thus to regulation of glucose turnover (Fig. 9-2). Insulin, epinephrine, and norepinephrine can have rapid actions on glucose utilization by affecting the ongoing processes of glucose transport without requiring changes in the rate of new protein synthesis. Cortisol, thyroxine, GH, and estrogens are slower regulators of insulin-sensitive glucose uptake, perhaps because many of their actions are mediated through gene regulation and protein synthesis. Finally, release of cytokines during certain types of stress can have direct actions on muscle to increase glucose uptake. The glu-

cose uptake of tissues such as brain, red blood cells, gut, endothelial connective tissue, and bone cells appears to be relatively insensitive to hormonal, neural, or cytokine factors. It is the glucose utilization of adipose tissue and muscle that is primarily regulated by the neuroendocrine system. Due to its mass, changes of muscle glucose utilization tend to be responsible for measured changes in whole-body glucose utilization. The glucose utilization rate of brain and the other insulin-insensitive tissues is nearly constant because this uptake process is nearly saturated at glucose levels greater than 100 mg/dL.

One important difference among these various neuroendocrine factors is the control of their secretion. Only the secretion of insulin and glucagon is sensitive to changes of plasma glucose concentration in the physiologic range. Thus hyperglycemia increases the secretion of insulin and decreases the secretion of glucagon (Fig. 9-1). Those hormonal changes will decrease glucose production by the liver and increase glucose utilization by peripheral tissues, restoring euglycemia (Fig. 9-1). Thus this feedback control system makes it difficult to achieve lasting hyperglycemia unless the sensitivity of the islet β cell to stimulation by glucose is impaired. The action of several neuroendocrine factors to decrease the β cell's sensitivity to stimulation by glucose and to decrease the α cell's sensitivity to suppression by glucose is what allows them to produce sustained hyperglycemia (Fig. 9-3).

Neuroendocrine factors can also change the sensitivity of the liver and peripheral tissues to insulin and glucagon (Fig. 9-2), but this effect by itself is not sufficient to produce lasting hyperglycemia. Again, an impairment of α- and β-cell sensitivity to glucose is required. For example, in obesity many tissues are resistant to the actions of insulin, including its ability to suppress hepatic glucose output and to increase glucose uptake in adipose tissue and muscle. Despite this impairment of insulin action, fasting hyperglycemia is not usually found in obese subjects because the islet increases its secretion of insulin. Thus the obese individual is characterized by an insulin resistance both at the liver and at the peripheral tissues that is compensated by elevated basal and stimulated insulin secretion, leading to normal basal glucose levels and normal glucose responses to ingested nutrients. This example illustrates that alterations in peripheral or hepatic insulin sensitivity, by themselves, will not necessarily lead to significant hyperglycemia unless the islet sensitivity to glucose is reduced.

FIGURE 9-2. A simplified view of stress hyperglycemia. Hyperglycemia can be due to either increased glucose output from the liver or decreased use by insulin-sensitive tissues. Note that both mechanisms are usually used.

STRESS HYPERGLYCEMIA

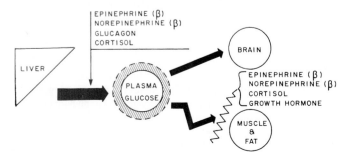

GENERAL CONSIDERATIONS IN STRESS HYPERGLYCEMIA

The primary role of the metabolic response to stress is to increase substrate flux to tissues that need it. The brain is the major glucose user in the fasting state and its rate of utilization is not dependent on insulin. Therefore, maintenance of adequate central glucose delivery is solely dependent on the plasma glucose concentration and adequate cerebral blood flow. Accordingly, stress hyperglycemia can be viewed as a means of ensuring adequate delivery of glucose to the brain during stress. During conditions of normal cerebral blood flow, glucose uptake into the central nervous system (CNS) is sufficient if plasma glucose levels are above 70 mg/dL. Increased hepatic production of ketone bodies during a prolonged fast and use of ketones by the brain can reduce its obligatory need for carbohydrate by approximately 50% without interfering with neuronal function. However, any further reduction of brain glucose uptake compromises brain function and eventually leads to neuronal death. Thus, even during a prolonged fast, any compromise of cerebral blood flow will produce the need for stress hyperglycemia to compensate for a reduced rate of glucose delivery to the brain. Again, the neuroendocrine system is the key to producing this hyperglycemia. Since the brain is dependent on a continuous supply of glucose, it is not surprising that stress hyperglycemia is regulated centrally. In addition, since the CNS need for glucose is so critical, it is not surprising that redundant neuroendocrine mechanisms exist to produce hyperglycemia during stress.

Thus, there are different afferent inputs to the central nervous system that can signal the need for increased carbohydrate flux to the brain. Some of these are psychological factors involved in the perception of imminent stress. A number of others are related to physiologic factors that reflect the adequacy of substrate and oxygen delivery to the brain. These latter systems include oxygen and pH chemoreceptors in the carotid bodies, pressure sensors in the carotid sinus and the aortic arch, temperature receptors and pain receptors in the skin, and glucose receptors in the liver and brain. The signals from these peripheral receptors are carried by afferent neurons to the brain stem and relayed to higher centers where they are integrated. One of these centers, the hypothalamus, is critical for the integration and coordination of those autonomic efferent responses that influence carbohydrate metabolism and cause stress hyperglycemia. These autonomic responses stimulate hepatic glucose production, impair peripheral glucose utilization, and impair the islet responsiveness to glucose. All three changes are usually present during most types of stress, but it is the third change that is critical in allowing sustained hyperglycemia to occur. The adipose tissue hormone leptin is a humoral signal to the CNS that provides information regarding nutritional status. It also appears to regulate basal autonomic outflow and may influence the neuroendocrine response to certain stresses. Circulating leptin concentrations are proportional to body fat content, but acutely decrease and increase in response to reductions of energy intake, or overfeeding.[1,2] Leptin receptors in the CNS are localized primarily in the hypothalamus, and leptin acts there to regulate long-term energy homeostasis via its actions to decrease food intake and increase energy expenditure.[3,4] The effects of exogenous leptin on appetite,[5] food intake,[6] food-seeking behavior,[7] and energy expenditure[8] are more pronounced when endogenous leptin levels are low (e.g., during fasting or energy restriction) than when they are elevated (e.g., during overfeeding or obesity). Thus leptin appears to play its major physiologic role in increasing appetite and decreasing energy expenditure during the adaptation to fasting or energy restriction.[2,4]

There is also evidence that leptin has an important role in regulating the hypothalamic-pituitary-endocrine axis (hypothalamic-pituitary axis [HPA] and thyroid and reproductive axes) during its adaptation to periods of negative energy balance.[9] For example, the activation of the HPA (via increased adrenocorticotropic hormone [ACTH] and glucocorticoid secretion) and downregulation of the thyroid and reproductive axes (decreased thyroid-stimulating hormone [TSH], gonadotropins, and reproductive and thyroid hormones) that occur during fasting in mice are attenuated when exogenous leptin is administered to prevent the normal fasting-induced fall of circulating leptin.[10] In addition, sympathoadrenal activity decreases during fasting or energy restriction in rodents[11] and humans,[12] and the decrease of leptin production during fasting contributes to the reduction of energy expenditure by decreasing sympathetic nervous system (SNS) outflow to brown adipose tissue in rodents.[8,13,14] Consistent with this observation, administration of exogenous leptin activates the SNS in fasting rodents[15-17] and non-human primates.[18] Furthermore, leptin-induced SNS activation can influence glucose homeostasis at least in part through its effects on insulin and glucagon secretion.[19,20] Although the role of leptin in mediating fasting-induced changes in neuroendocrine function is relatively straightforward, its role in mediating the effects of fasting on the neuroendocrine activation induced by stress is complex. Leptin may mediate the effect of fasting on the neuroendocrine responses to certain stresses, but during other types of stress, leptin is unlikely to have a role.

For example, cardiac surgery in humans decreases circulating leptin levels, which may in turn potentiate the HPA response to the surgical stress. In addition, patients with sepsis[21] or burn injury[22] lose their diurnal rhythm of cortisol, perhaps because of the loss of their diurnal pattern of circulating leptin. These patients receive continuous parenteral or enteral feeding, disrupting the diurnal leptin pattern that is dependent on the timing[23] and magnitude[24] of insulin responses to meals.

Several studies examining the role of leptin in the neuroendocrine response to stress have reported that leptin inhibits the HPA response to stress in rodents that is induced by physical restraint[25] or exposure to ether, but not stress induced by cold exposure.[26] The problem with extrapolating these results to deduce a physiological role for the fasting-induced decrease of leptin to augment HPA activation during stress is that HPA responses to many stresses are reduced, not increased, in fasted animals.[27]

One exception appears to be the stress of neuroglucopenia. Fasting augments the cortisol and ACTH responses to the neuroglucopenia produced by insulin-induced hypoglycemia in mice.[28] Exogenous leptin administration inhibits those responses as well as the cortisol response to the neuroglucopenia induced by 2-deoxy-D-glucose in the rat.[29] In contrast, even though the sympathoadrenal (epinephrine) response to insulin-induced hypoglycemia is augmented in the fasted compared to the fed state,[30] leptin is unlikely to be the mediator, because during fasting endogenous leptin inhibits and exogenous leptin stimulates sympathetic outflow.

In summary, the fall of endogenous leptin may help mediate the increase of basal corticosterone and the decrease of sympathetic tone seen during fasting or energy restriction. It may also have a similar action on the HPA response to certain stresses (e.g., neuroglucopenia), but not to other types of stress. This complex interaction between the leptin system and neuroendocrine activation during stress warrants further study.

NEUROENDOCRINE SIGNALS INVOLVED IN STRESS-INDUCED HYPERGLYCEMIA

The classic description of neuroendocrine activation during stress includes increased secretion of epinephrine, norepinephrine, cortisol, GH, and glucagon, and decreased secretion of insulin. These neuroendocrine changes produce hyperglycemia by interfering with all of the important mechanisms responsible for the regulation of plasma glucose (Fig. 9-3). This neuroendocrine pattern can be reproduced by stimulation of the ventromedial hypothalamus. In nonstressed individuals, normal activities such as standing, walking, or running can also activate the sympathetic nervous system and the glucose-mobilizing hormones. As a result, there is a stimulation of hepatic glucose production. However, during these normal activities, there is not the impairment of glucose utilization in the peripheral tissues, and therefore no hyperglycemia is seen as during stress (Fig. 9-2). In fact, there is a simultaneous increase of glucose utilization secondary to increased muscular activity during exercise (Fig. 9-4). Thus hyperglycemia in such circumstances is unusual.

This form of sympathetic arousal is coordinated with muscular activity to keep the plasma glucose concentration within relatively narrow limits despite a marked increase of turnover rate (Fig. 9-4). If carbohydrate is ingested during exercise, one might expect that the exercise-induced sympathetic activation would inhibit the insulin response to the ingested glucose and thereby impair insulin-mediated glucose uptake. Thus the rate of glucose utilization might not increase enough to counterbalance the rate of glucose absorption, resulting in hyperglycemia. However, the ability of glucose to suppress the activation of the sympathetic nervous system appears to be enhanced during exercise, and prevention of the small decline in plasma glucose that occurs during strenuous exercise reduces the degree of sympathetic activation.[1] The sensitivity of the central glucose sensors is dependent on the physiologic state. Because of this increased sensitivity, carbohydrate ingestion during exercise may reduce sympathetic activation and allow sufficient insulin secretion and action to prevent hyperglycemia.

Exercise is an example of a situation in which activation of the somatic motor system leads to an increase in glucose removal that is independent of insulin secretion. This increase in glucose use is counterbalanced by a neuroendocrine-mediated increase in hepatic glucose production, so that plasma glucose levels remain constant despite a marked increase of glucose turnover (Fig. 9-4). In many types of stress, the same neuroendocrine activation increases hepatic glucose production (Fig. 9-5). However, without the exercise-induced increase in peripheral glucose utilization, hyperglycemia occurs (Fig. 9-5). Indeed, stress-induced neuroendocrine activation, by itself, impairs insulin secretion and impairs insulin-mediated glucose uptake (Fig. 9-3). Many stresses including hypoxia, hypotension, myocardial infarction, trauma, surgery, and the early stages of burn trauma, cold exposure, and sepsis cause impaired glucose utilization. Although different stresses can activate different afferent signals to the brain, the efferent responses usually involve sympathetic activation and increased secretion of glucose-mobilizing hormones. Thus there is a close similarity between the mechanisms for the metabolic responses to different stresses. However, as discussed below, there are real and important differences in metabolism that depend upon the particular type of stress and its etiology. Therefore, each form of stress hyperglycemia must be evaluated independently in regard to the mechanisms of its production and the rationale for treatment.

CLINICAL FORMS OF STRESS-INDUCED HYPERGLYCEMIA

Hypoxia

Acute hypoxia can produce the classic activation of the sympathetic nervous system seen during other types of stress. Both plasma norepinephrine and epinephrine are increased during acute, severe hypoxia (6–7% inspired O_2) but not during moderate hypoxia (10–12% inspired O_2).[31,32] Thus there is a clear threshold for activation of the sympathetic nervous system by hypoxia, and

FIGURE 9-4. Basal and exercise-induced glucose turnover. A schematic of glucose production by the liver (**left arrow**), glucose use by the brain, muscle, and fat (**right arrows**), and the effect on plasma glucose concentration (**circle**) after an overnight fast (**solid lines**) and during moderate exercise (**dashed lines**). Note that during exercise there is a simultaneous increase in hepatic glucose production and muscle glucose use, so that plasma glucose level remains constant despite a marked increase in glucose turnover. The stresses of acute cold exposure and cold acclimation show a similar stimulation of both hepatic glucose production and glucose use with little change of plasma glucose level.

FIGURE 9-5. Hyperglycemia during hypoxia. The activation of the neuroendocrine system during hypoxia increases hepatic glucose production (**left, dashed arrow**) and increases the plasma glucose level (**dashed circle**). Hyperglycemia does not cause the expected increase of glucose use by muscle and adipose tissue (**right arrow**) because the neuroendocrine activation impairs insulin-stimulated glucose uptake. The stresses of hypotension, myocardial infarction, mild sepsis, and early burn and other types of trauma show a similar stimulation of hepatic glucose production, restraint of glucose use, and hyperglycemia.

Exercise

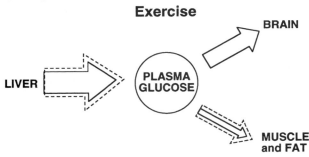

Hypoxia

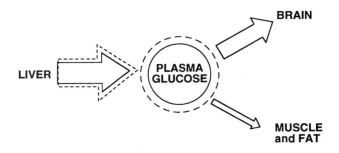

severe hypoxia is required to produce this activation. When the hypoxia is severe, the sympathetic response to acute hypoxia is pronounced, with total catecholamine levels exceeding 1000 pg/mL. Although cytokines may be involved in mediating the sympathetic responses to certain other stresses, there is little evidence that they contribute during hypoxia. It is more likely that they are released from tissue damaged by anoxia after an episode of ischemia and reperfusion.[33] Despite the magnitude of the general sympathetic activation, the noradrenergic nerves to the pancreas are not usually activated by hypoxic stress.[34] In addition, the effect of sympathoadrenal activation on pancreatic hormone secretion and metabolism can be different than expected because there is evidence for β-adrenergic receptor dysfunction during hypoxia.[31] Thus the α-adrenergic actions of circulating epinephrine and locally released norepinephrine predominate.

In addition to sympathetic activation, acute severe hypoxia can elicit the secretion of other counterregulatory hormones. Thus ACTH, glucocorticoid, and glucagon secretion are also increased. The stimulation of glucagon secretion produced by hypoxia is not mediated by the β-adrenergic action of catecholamines as it seems to be in other stresses, but rather by α-adrenergic mechanisms.[35] These findings are consistent with the β-adrenergic receptor dysfunction seen in hypoxia.

The inhibition of glucose-induced insulin released during hypoxia is consistent with marked sympathetic activation (Fig. 9-3). However, the inhibition is more than would be expected for the circulating levels of epinephrine. For example, epinephrine infusion in normal subjects can abolish the acute insulin response to glucose, but usually produces only a mild impairment of the acute insulin response to arginine. The marked inhibition of both glucose and arginine-induced insulin secretion during hypoxia is reminiscent of selective activation of inhibitory α-adrenergic receptors. The lack of an opposing stimulatory action of β-adrenergic receptor activation would explain the marked inhibition of insulin release seen during hypoxia. Direct evidence for such dysfunction includes abolition of the acute insulin response to isoproterenol, a selective β-adrenergic agonist, during hypoxia.[36] β-Adrenergic effects on other organs (e.g., lipolysis in adipose tissue and chronotropism in the heart) are also impaired.[31]

These sympathetic and hormonal changes seen during hypoxia result in insulin resistance (Fig. 9-2), carbohydrate intolerance, and hyperglycemia (Fig. 9-5). The magnitude of the hyperglycemia depends, however, on the severity of the hypoxia and the age of the subject.[31] In animals, the threshold for the hyperglycemic effects of hypoxia are similar to those for activation of the sympathetic nervous system (i.e., a P_{O_2} of between 30 and 40 mm Hg). These hyperglycemic effects are more pronounced in the young and may help protect the developing brain from hypoxic damage.[37]

Hypotension

During hypotension the central problem is that the blood flow decreases to the point where delivery of oxygen and substrate is inadequate to support tissue metabolic demands. Under these conditions, glucose has an advantage over other substrates since it can be partially metabolized even when tissue oxygen levels are low. However, during anaerobic metabolism of glucose, lactic acid accumulates, and this build-up is exacerbated by its reduced removal secondary to hypoperfusion. Since tissue glucose uptake is increased simply by increasing its plasma level, the hyperglycemia in-

duced by hypotension may represent a compensatory mechanism to maintain adequate fuel delivery during hypoperfusion. The pattern of increased hepatic glucose production and hyperglycemia during hypotension is similar to that seen during hypoxia (Fig. 9-5). Adequate glucose delivery is critical for both brain and cardiac function since the brain is dependent on glucose as its primary metabolic fuel and the heart becomes dependent on glucose during hypoperfusion. Despite such compensatory mechanisms, fuel delivery may still be inadequate if the hypotension is both severe and prolonged. This decompensated phase of hypotension, known as shock, is characterized by persistent vasodilation, acute respiratory distress, loss of consciousness, and multiple organ failure and death.

Hyperglycemia has been found in a number of clinical situations in which hypotension is present. For example, hyperglycemia is present in injured combat soldiers in shock, as well as in patients with heart failure and associated hypotension or shock. Although the interpretation of these clinical studies is complicated by the presence of stresses in addition to hypotension, several of these complications can be ruled out as causes of hyperglycemia. First, the moderate hypoperfusion secondary to moderate hypotension (arterial blood pressure of 50 mm Hg) is usually not severe enough to impair glucose utilization by the brain, or to impair insulin secretion from the pancreas. Second, the local and systemic acidosis seen in hemorrhagic hypotension is not responsible for the hyperglycemic response, because hypotension simulated by unloading the carotid baroreceptors, in the absence of acidosis, can also elicit substantial hyperglycemia.[38] Finally, it is unlikely that cytokines have a role in the hyperglycemic response to moderate hypotension, since they are only released in large quantities during shock.

Cytokines do have a role in shock, but it is related more to vasodilation. During severe shock, tumor necrosis factor alpha (TNF-α) is released from macrophages,[39] stimulating nitric oxide production from the vasculature.[40] This nitric oxide produces a hypocontractility of vascular smooth muscle resulting in hypotension during shock that persists despite marked sympathetic activation. Clinical studies have suggested an association between TNF-α and IL-1 levels and the multiple organ failure and mortality of hemorrhagic shock.[41]

The general mechanisms by which hypotension leads to hyperglycemia can be deduced by reading the available literature. Both central neural pathways and peripheral sympathetic pathways are involved. Elegant neuroanatomic studies have shown that only certain brain areas are activated during hemorrhagic hypotension, most of these in proportion to the degree of hypotension.[42] These discrete brain areas presumably control the peripheral autonomic response to hypotension that includes activation of the sympathetic nervous system. Catecholamines have a well-recognized role in defending blood pressure. Catecholamines also contribute to the hyperglycemia of hypotension since combined adrenalectomy and splanchnic sympathectomy abolished this hyperglycemic response.[43]

The endocrine pancreas also has a substantial role in hyperglycemia, since pancreatic hormone secretion changes in a direction that would produce glycogenolysis (Fig. 9-5) and hyperglycemia in normal animals[44] (Fig. 9-3). Insulin release is usually inhibited by hypotension, especially the insulin response to secretagogues. Since glucose is a major insulin secretagogue, such inhibition allows hyperglycemia to persist. The α2-adrenergic effects of catecholamines are presumed to mediate this inhibition of insulin release. If so, circulating epinephrine is the likely mediator since the local noradrenergic nerves to the pancreas are not activated by moderate hypotension.[34] Indeed, elimination of the epinephrine response to hypotension by adrenalectomy reverses the inhibition of insulin release.[45] During marked hypotension, it is also possible that severe hypoperfusion of the pancreas could impair insulin secretion.

Glucagon secretion is also increased during marked hemorrhagic hypotension and undoubtedly contributes to the hyperglycemic response. This stimulation of glucagon secretion is mediated by sympathoadrenal mechanisms since combined adrenalectomy and splanchnic sympathectomy abolished this glucagon response.[43] Increased vasopressin secretion during hypotension may also stimulate glucagon secretion; experiments with vasopressin antagonists, which have implicated vasopressin in the defense of blood pressure during hypotension, also suggest a role for vasopressin in stimulating glucagon secretion during hypotension. Finally, both ACTH and cortisol secretion increase in response to hypotension,[46] but their role in the hyperglycemic response is unknown.

It is also important to recognize that the high levels of circulating catecholamines present during hypotension can directly stimulate liver glycogenolysis and thereby increase the plasma glucose level. There are also suggestions that vasopressin has a similar direct action on the liver. Glucocorticoids may also play an important role in allowing the liver to respond since adrenalectomy increases the morbidity associated with hemorrhage and this effect is prevented by glucocorticoid replacement.[47] Finally, hepatic sympathetic nerves may directly contribute since hepatic denervation reduces the hyperglycemic response to hypotension.[48,49] Thus there are many mechanisms, both direct and indirect, whereby the sympathetic activation produced in response to hypotension can defend brain metabolism by causing hyperglycemia, just as it defends blood pressure by causing vasoconstriction.

Hypoglycemia

The administration of excess insulin or overproduction of endogenous insulin (e.g., insulinoma) induces hypoglycemia by increasing peripheral glucose use and by suppressing hepatic glucose production (Fig. 9-6). Because lowering the plasma glucose level reduces brain glucose uptake and because the central nervous system is dependent on glucose as its primary metabolic fuel, systemic hypoglycemia induces a state of central glucose deficiency known as neuroglucopenia. Traditionally, central glucose receptors were thought to be the sole stimulus for activation of the neuroendocrine system. Recent evidence suggests the participation of hepatic portal vein glucose sensors.[50,51] This activation does not produce the hyperglycemia seen in other types of stress, but rather it prevents the development of more severe hypoglycemia and eventually restores euglycemia (Fig. 9-7), by stimulating hepatic glucose production and by impairing insulin's stimulation of peripheral glucose uptake.

The neuroendocrine activation includes increased activity of the hypothalamic-pituitary-adrenal axis as reflected by increases of circulating ACTH and glucocorticoids. Hypoglycemia also stimulates the secretion of growth hormone from the anterior pituitary gland. Both glucocorticoids and growth hormone impair insulin's action to stimulate peripheral glucose uptake. In addition, glucocorticoids help sustain increased hepatic glucose production by inducing gluconeogenic enzymes. Both hormones have a relatively slow onset of action and thus do not contribute significantly to the rapid reversal of hypoglycemia[52] (see Chap. 31). In contrast, glucagon and epinephrine have rapid actions to stimulate hepatic glucose production, and thus mediate the acute restoration of euglycemia. In addition, epinephrine, like glucocorticoids and GH, impairs insulin-stimulated glucose uptake. Available evidence suggests that glucagon is the primary factor mediating rapid glucose recovery, and that epinephrine becomes critical only when the glucagon response is impaired (see Chap. 31). Other mechanisms including the sympathetic nerves to the liver might also contribute to glucose recovery, because they are activated during central neuroglucopenia;[53] however, their contribution is currently unknown. The sympathetic nerves innervating the kidney are also activated during hypoglycemia[54] and may contribute to glucose counterregulation by stimulating gluconeogenesis in the kidney.

There is evidence that both the sympathetic and parasympathetic nerves that innervate the pancreas are activated during hypoglycemia, and that this autonomic neural activation, together with the sympathetic neurohormone epinephrine, mediates the glucagon response.[55–57] Although it has been known for 70 years that hypoglycemia activates the adrenal medulla,[58] it has only recently been

FIGURE 9-6. Induction of hypoglycemia. The injection of large amounts of insulin suppresses hepatic glucose production (**left, dashed arrow**) and markedly increases glucose use by muscle and fat (**lower right, dashed arrow**), which combine to markedly lower plasma glucose (**dashed circle**). The fall in the plasma glucose level reduces glucose uptake by the brain (**upper right, dashed arrow**). The stress of severe sepsis produces a similar suppression of hepatic glucose production, stimulation of glucose use, and fall of plasma glucose level.

FIGURE 9-7. Recovery from hypoglycemia. The low plasma glucose level following insulin injection activates the neuroendocrine system and thereby stimulates hepatic glucose production (**left, dashed arrow**). These neuroendocrine factors also impair insulin-stimulated muscle glucose use, which helps, with the falling insulin level, to restore glucose use toward normal (**lower right arrow**). Both these effects help return plasma glucose toward basal levels (**dashed circle**).

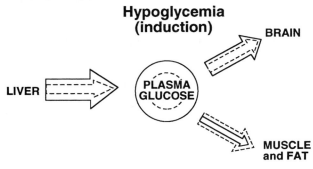

Hypoglycemia (induction)

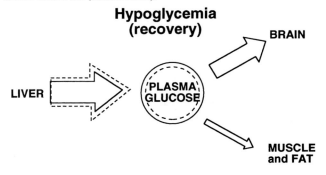

Hypoglycemia (recovery)

demonstrated that hypoglycemia also activates the sympathetic nerves of the pancreas. For example, neuroglucopenia induced by administration of the nonmetabolizable glucose analog 2-deoxy-D-glucose increases the spillover of norepinephrine from the sympathetic nerves of the pancreas, demonstrating their activation during neuroglucopenia.[34] This activation is due to a central reflex and is specific for neuroglucopenia. Two other stresses, hypotension and hypoxia, do not increase pancreatic norepinephrine spillover.[34] Activation of pancreatic sympathetic nerves has also been demonstrated during insulin-induced hypoglycemia. In dogs, this activation releases the peptidergic neurotransmitter galanin[59] as well as norepinephrine from the pancreas.[60]

Pancreatic parasympathetic nerves are known to be activated during the ingestion of food and this activation contributes to meal-induced insulin secretion.[61–63] However, neuroglucopenia is the only stress known to activate the pancreatic parasympathetic nerves.[55] Current indices of the activity of pancreatic parasympathetic nerves are less direct than the use of pancreatic norepinephrine release to assess sympathetic activation. The problem is that the parasympathetic neurotransmitter acetylcholine is rapidly degraded in plasma, and therefore, its release from the pancreas is extremely difficult to measure. However, pancreatic polypeptide (PP), a peptide hormone produced by the F cells of the endocrine pancreas, is known to be under strong parasympathetic control and is therefore a useful index of the activity of pancreatic parasympathetic nerves.[64] The secretion of PP increases dramatically during hypoglycemia in rodents,[65,66] monkeys,[67] and humans.[68] This increased PP secretion is blocked by either surgical vagotomy or cholinergic antagonists, demonstrating that the PP response to hypoglycemia is mediated by parasympathetic cholinergic activation. Thus, there is evidence that all three autonomic inputs, sympathetic neurohormone (adrenal catecholamine) secretion, sympathetic nerves, and parasympathetic nerves (Fig. 9-8), are activated during hypoglycemia.[55,69] Furthermore, since all three autonomic inputs are known to stimulate glucagon secretion,[55] activation of these neural inputs would contribute to the glucagon response to hypoglycemia. Therefore, autonomic activation is likely to contribute to glucose recovery through the stimulation of glucagon secretion.

Despite this evidence for autonomic mediation of the glucagon response, it is known that exposure of the islet to low glucose concentrations can directly stimulate glucagon secretion,[70] even in the absence of neural activation, suggesting that autonomic neural activation may not be required to increase glucagon secretion during systemic hypoglycemia. In accord with this observation, a number of early studies, primarily in humans, did not find a significant autonomic contribution to the glucagon response to hypoglycemia.[69] In many of these experiments one or two, but usually not all three, of the autonomic inputs to the pancreas were pharmacologically blocked or surgically ablated.[55,69] However, if there is redundancy in the autonomic stimulation of glucagon secretion, then this partial blockade would be insufficient to prevent autonomic mediation of the glucagon response.

In more recent experiments, the activation of all three autonomic inputs to the pancreas has been interrupted in order to assess the autonomic contribution to the glucagon response to insulin-induced hypoglycemia. In several of these studies ganglionic antagonists, such as hexamethonium or trimethaphan, were used to pharmacologically impair the activation of the autonomic inputs to the pancreas, because activation of all three inputs involves neurotransmission across nicotinic ganglia (Fig. 9-8). Ganglionic

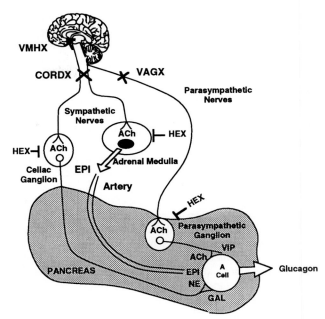

FIGURE 9-8. Three autonomic inputs to the islet. (1) Preganglionic sympathetic nerves travel in the spinal cord and innervate the celiac ganglia, which supply the postganglionic sympathetic fibers that innervate the pancreas. These nerves release norepinephrine (**NE**), and in some species, galanin (**GAL**). (2) Preganglionic parasympathetic nerves travel in the vagus and innervate intrapancreatic, parasympathetic ganglia, which send postganglionic parasympathetic fibers to the islet and exocrine tissue. These nerves release acetylcholine (**ACh**) and vasoactive intestinal peptide (**VIP**). (3) Preganglionic sympathetic nerves from the spinal cord innervate the adrenal medulla and stimulate the release of the sympathetic neurohormone epinephrine (**EPI**), which reaches the islet via the arterial circulation. Each of these three autonomic inputs to the pancreas is activated by hypoglycemic stress; other stresses rarely activate autonomic inputs besides the sympathetic neurohormone epinephrine. These redundant autonomic pathways can be blocked (⊣) either at the ganglionic level by a nicotinic antagonist like hexamethonium (**HEX**), or by surgical disruption (X) of the preganglionic parasympathetic nerves traveling in the vagus (**VAGX**) and preganglionic sympathetic nerves traveling in the spinal cord (**CORDX**), or by lesioning the autonomic control centers in the ventromedial hypothalamus (**VMHX**). The islet effects of NE and ACh, but not the neuropeptides GAL or VIP, can be blocked by adrenergic and muscarinic antagonists.

blockers were found to significantly impair the glucagon response to insulin-induced hypoglycemia in dogs,[71] mice,[66] and rhesus monkeys.[67] In other studies, the combined surgical interventions of vagotomy and sympathectomy in anesthetized dogs[71] or electrolytic lesions of the ventromedial hypothalamus in rats[72] markedly reduced glucagon responses to hypoglycemia. Using a different approach, it was shown that preventing central, but not peripheral, hypoglycemia impaired both parasympathetic (PP) and sympathoadrenal (epinephrine) responses and abolished the glucagon responses to hypoglycemia.[73] Thus, evidence from a variety of animal studies suggested that autonomic neural activation mediates a significant portion of the glucagon response to hypoglycemia.

The hypothesis of redundant autonomic stimulation of glucagon secretion during hypoglycemia has gained recent support. For example, neither methylatropine nor α- and β-adrenergic blockade alone significantly reduced the glucagon response to hypoglycemia in conscious rats, whereas together they inhibited the response by 75%.[74] In mice, there is partial redundancy, because either atropine or combined adrenergic blockade alone significantly reduced the increase of plasma glucagon during insulin-induced hypoglycemia, whereas together they completely prevented the response.[66] Furthermore, there is also redundancy within the sympathoadrenal system itself in dogs since neither adrenalectomy nor surgical denervation of the pancreas alone inhibited the increase of glucagon secretion during hypoglycemia in vagotomized animals, but the two interventions together eliminated the glucagon response.[75] Although the older evidence for autonomic mediation of the glucagon response to hypoglycemia in humans was less compelling, studies with ganglionic blockade[76] and two studies of patients with chronic autonomic disease[77,78] suggested autonomic mediation. Furthermore, hypoglycemia-associated autonomic failure in human subjects (see Chap. 31), which reduces both parasympathetic and sympathoadrenal (epinephrine) responses, was also shown to reduce the glucagon response to a subsequent episode of hypoglycemia.[79] In contrast, combined adrenergic and muscarinic blockade did not affect the glucagon response to insulin-induced hypoglycemia in humans,[80,81] suggesting either that the response is not autonomically mediated or alternatively that neuropeptides, such as vasoactive intestinal peptide (VIP), participate in the neural mediation of the glucagon response to hypoglycemia. Indeed, VIP is localized in pancreatic nerves, is released from the pancreas during vagal nerve stimulation, and stimulates glucagon secretion.[82] Classical muscarinic or adrenergic antagonists would not block the effects of neuropeptides on glucagon secretion.

More recently, a definitive study was conducted to investigate the autonomic neural contribution to the glucagon response to hypoglycemia in humans.[68] In this study the ganglionic blocker trimethaphan was infused to impair the activation of all three autonomic inputs to the pancreas in nondiabetic human subjects. Ganglionic blockade was verified by marked reductions in the plasma epinephrine, norepinephrine, and PP responses to hypoglycemia. During ganglionic blockade, the glucagon response to matched levels of hypoglycemia was reduced by 80% (Fig. 9-9). Thus this study demonstrated in humans, as previously documented in animals, that activation of the autonomic nervous system mediates the majority of the glucagon response to hypoglycemia.

Since the glucagon response to insulin-induced hypoglycemia is impaired in type 1 diabetes mellitus, the possibility that autonomic defects may cause part of this impairment has recently been suggested.[57] Alternative explanations for the impairment of the glucagon response in diabetes include impaired α-cell recognition of hypoglycemia[83] or defects related to β-cell loss in type 1 diabetes.[84–87] The problem with the autonomic explanation is that classic diabetic autonomic neuropathy (DAN) is thought to occur primarily in diabetes of long duration (>15 years), whereas loss of the glucagon response to insulin-induced hypoglycemia can occur relatively early in the course of the disease (within the first 5 years). However, more sensitive tests of autonomic function have demonstrated autonomic impairments that occur well before the classical criteria for DAN.[57] Thus, it remains possible that the progressive loss of the glucagon response to insulin-induced hypoglycemia seen in conventionally treated patients with type 1 diabetes is related to a concomitant impairment of the autonomic inputs to the islet.

Further, with the advent of intensive insulin treatment, there appears to be a more rapid loss of the glucagon response to insulin-induced hypoglycemia. Since intensive insulin treatment is associated with increased episodes of hypoglycemia[88] and since prior

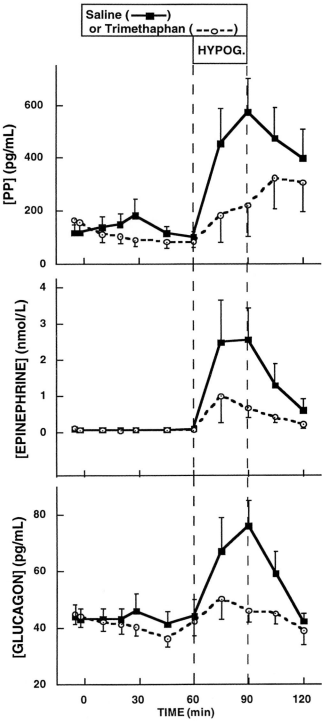

FIGURE 9-9. Pancreatic polypeptide, epinephrine, and glucagon concentrations in the peripheral plasma of seven women before, during, and after a period of 2.5 mmol/L hypoglycemia (**HYPOG; vertical dashed lines**) during either a saline infusion (**solid squares**) or ganglionic blockade with trimethaphan (**open circles**). *(Adapted from Taborsky, et al.[57])*

hypoglycemia can diminish the autonomic response to insulin-induced hypoglycemia,[79,89,90] it appears that the rapid loss of the glucagon response to insulin-induced hypoglycemia in intensively treated patients may be secondary to a hypoglycemia-associated autonomic failure.

Finally, while marked β-cell loss is associated with rapid loss of the glucagon response to insulin-induced hypoglycemia in an animal model of type 1 diabetes,[91] β-cell destruction may also be associated with loss of islet nerves. Thus, older data[92] and very recent data[93] suggest rapid loss of islet sympathetic nerves in BB diabetic rats. Whether this early sympathetic islet neuropathy contributes to the loss of the glucagon response to insulin-induced hypoglycemia is currently untested, but it clearly demonstrates that not all forms of diabetic autonomic neuropathy are slow in onset.

In conclusion, hypoglycemia activates some of the same neuroendocrine mechanisms activated by other stresses. In addition, it activates both the sympathetic and the parasympathetic nerves innervating the pancreas. Evidence from experiments in non-diabetic animals demonstrates that combined autonomic activation redundantly mediates the majority of the glucagon response to hypoglycemia in a number of species. More recent evidence from human studies supports a similar mechanism.[68] The glucagon response in turn is critical for the rapid stimulation of hepatic glucose production during hypoglycemia, which helps restore euglycemia. Because the glucagon response to hypoglycemia is impaired in type 1 diabetes, autonomic defects, in addition to β-cell and α-cell defects, may contribute to this impairment.

Cold Stress

The exposure of many warm-blooded animals, including humans, to a cold environment for a period of hours (acute cold exposure) produces a neural, hormonal, and metabolic stress response that helps meet the new demands for increased thermogenesis and conservation of body heat. If the environmental challenge is not too severe and the animal's compensatory systems are intact, then a sustained fall in body core temperature will be avoided despite a lowering of skin temperature. In these animals, continued exposure to a cold environment for weeks will produce acclimation to the cold environment characterized by replacement of shivering thermogenesis with nonshivering thermogenesis. In contrast, if the cold environment is too severe or if the animal's thermoregulatory system has been impaired, body temperature will drop, resulting in hypothermia. Each of these states, acute cold exposure, cold acclimation, and hypothermia, is characterized by specific neural, hormonal, and metabolic responses. Acute cold exposure is most similar to the other acute stress states previously discussed.

Acute cold exposure activates the sympathetic nervous system as reflected by an increase of plasma norepinephrine. The activation of the adrenal medulla, however, is not a central feature of the response, being elevated primarily during more severe forms of cold exposure. Pituitary stress hormones including GH, ACTH, and TSH can be elevated if the cold exposure is severe. Surprisingly, thyroid hormones are usually not elevated despite their acknowledged role in energy production (for explanation, see below). Glucocorticoids are elevated. Acute cold exposure consistently stimulates glucagon secretion either without a significant change of basal insulin or with a significant decrease of the plasma insulin level. Acute, moderate cold exposure produces little change of plasma glucose or plasma free fatty acids despite clear increases in oxygen consumption and despite increases of both free fatty acid and glucose turnover like those seen during exercise (Fig. 9-4). More severe cold exposure can sometimes produce increases of both the plasma glucose and free fatty acid levels.

Hepatic glucose production is usually increased during acute cold exposure (Fig. 9-4). Presumably, the increase of glucagon coupled with the restraint of insulin secretion contributes to the stimulation of hepatic glucose production. Catecholamines may also contribute, but epinephrine, the most glycogenolytic of the two major endogenous catecholamines, is usually not elevated. The sympathetic nerves of the liver may be activated,[94] as are nerves innervating adipose tissue and muscle. The increase of hepatic glucose production is usually matched by an increase of glucose utilization during cold stress (Fig. 9-4). It is likely that the shivering seen during acute cold exposure increases glucose uptake since muscle contraction, as it does during exercise, can increase glucose uptake in the absence of an increase of plasma insulin.

The increase of sympathetic nervous activity during acute cold exposure may be more related to thermoregulation than to increased hepatic glucose production. In animals that have brown fat, locally released norepinephrine can dramatically increase heat production from this tissue. In animals and adult humans who do not have brown fat, norepinephrine can still increase heat production via β-adrenergic mechanisms. Activation of the sympathetic nerves innervating skin and the extremities during cold exposure causes the peripheral vasoconstriction that is essential for heat conservation.

Chronic exposure to cold for a period of 4–6 weeks results in a sustained increase of oxygen consumption and heat production, which characterizes acclimation to the cold. However, plasma norepinephrine, plasma glucagon levels, and several other stress hormones tend to return to control levels after 4–6 weeks of cold exposure. Further, insulin secretion, which can be inhibited during acute exposure, tends to normalize during chronic cold exposure. Likewise, shivering, which characterizes the physical response to acute cold exposure, is diminished or absent during chronic cold exposure and is replaced by nonshivering thermogenesis. Although the levels of stress hormones decline during chronic cold exposure, their actions on metabolism and thermogenesis are enhanced. For example, the thermogenic response to exogenous catecholamine infusion is markedly increased in cold-acclimated animals. The role of thyroid hormones in mediating this increased sensitivity is unclear because T_3 levels are decreased in cold-acclimated humans, yet T_3 production, secretion, clearance, and turnover rate are all increased.

The increase in stress hormone secretion seen during acute cold exposure and in stress hormone action seen during cold acclimation are both impaired by hypothermia, in proportion to the decrease in core temperature. During severe hypothermia the decrease in organ temperature appears to directly suppress transmitter release from neurons, hormone secretion from endocrine glands, and substrate release from the adipose tissue, muscle, and liver. For example, hypothermia is used clinically to suppress metabolism in children during open heart surgery. A variety of measurements made in this clinical situation suggest that an impairment of insulin secretion, insulin action, and glucose metabolism leads to glucose intolerance and hyperglycemia (Fig. 9-10). However, it is not clear from these studies whether these changes of carbohydrate metabolism are due to anesthesia or hypothermia *per se*. Studies in animals have clarified the mechanisms for these effects. In general, hypothermia impairs insulin secretion. Whether or not this is a direct effect of hypothermia to induce hypofunction of pancreatic β cells or an effect mediated by circulating catecholamines may depend on the level of hypothermia achieved. For example, severe hypothermia can directly impair insulin secretion from isolated perfused pancreas, whereas the acute cold stress accompanying more moderate hypothermia increases plasma catecholamine levels that mediate a part of the impairment of insulin secretion.

Hypothermia

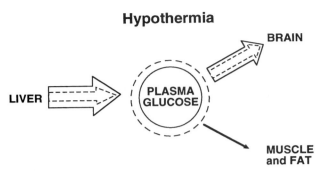

FIGURE 9-10. Hypothermia and glucose turnover. The decrease of body and organ temperature during hypothermia slows all metabolic processes including hepatic glucose production (**left, dashed arrow**) and glucose use by both brain (**upper right, dashed arrow**) and peripheral tissues (**lower right arrow**). The plasma glucose level can be unchanged or sometimes increased (**dashed circle**). However, carbohydrate tolerance is always severely impaired because of the marked reduction of glucose use (**right arrows**).

The resistance to insulin action in hypothermic animals and humans probably has two causes: a direct suppressive effect of hypothermia on insulin-sensitive tissues dominant during severe hypothermia, and a β-adrenergically mediated inhibition of insulin-stimulated glucose uptake dominant during moderate hypothermia. This impaired insulin action, combined with impaired insulin secretion, produces severe glucose intolerance in hypothermic subjects (Fig. 9-10). Indeed, patients undergoing hypothermia for surgery become markedly hyperglycemic when given relatively modest glucose infusions. Even without exogenous glucose, most hypothermic animals and patients are at least mildly hyperglycemic despite a direct suppressive effect of hypothermia on hepatic glucose production.

During more severe hypothermia, these neural and hormonal factors may be directly suppressed by the effects of low organ temperature on secretory mechanisms. It should also be noted that anesthesia usually impairs the sympathetic activation that protects against hypothermia. This concept has two important implications. First, a level of cold exposure which would induce a stress response sufficient to maintain the core temperature in a conscious animal may result in moderate hypothermia in anesthetized animals. Second, studies of cold exposure in anesthetized animals tend to find less activation of the sympathetic nervous system, less stimulation of stress hormones and metabolism, and more direct suppressive effects of hypothermia.

Myocardial Infarction

Acute myocardial infarction (MI) has been associated with stress hormone responses and stress hyperglycemia, as in hypoxia (Fig. 9-5). Thus there is evidence that plasma catecholamines are elevated in patients admitted for MI. Although plasma norepinephrine levels can be significantly higher than controls, the epinephrine levels are more consistently elevated.[95] The elevation of plasma catecholamines is short-lived; it may normalize in 1–2 days after hospital admission. The adrenal cortical hormone cortisol is also increased within 6 hours of MI. The magnitude of the cortisol response is related to the size of the infarct and predicts mortality.[96] The mechanism for the increasing cortisol is unclear because ACTH seems to be suppressed after MI despite elevations of both arginine vasopressin (AVP) and corticotropin-releasing hormone

(CRH). Cortisol, AVP, and CRH fall toward normal between 1 and 3 days after MI.[97] GH levels are elevated for the first week after uncomplicated MI. Plasma glucagon levels are also increased after MI and insulin secretion is impaired. As expected, these changes in stress hormone levels are accompanied by either mild hyperglycemia or glucose intolerance.

The mechanism of the increase of stress hormones during myocardial infarction is multifactorial. Although it is likely that the chest pain and general anxiety experienced by a patient undergoing an acute MI contributes significantly to the sympathetic activation detected immediately after the episode, direct experimental tests of this hypothesis in humans have suggested that cardiac ischemia rather than angina increases plasma norepinephrine.[98] Nonetheless, the anxiety associated with a spontaneous MI can also contribute to the catecholamine response to MI. However, this contribution is relatively selective. Anxiety and fear usually result in increases of plasma epinephrine rather than norepinephrine. Because epinephrine is the more potent of the two endogenous catecholamines in producing hyperglycemia, the addition of significant anxiety and fear to the other factors during MI has a disproportionate influence on the amount of stress hyperglycemia produced.

In myocardial infarction patients with concomitant heart failure, the plasma catecholamines on the day of admission and the few days thereafter are markedly higher than in patients who do not experience heart failure with the MI,[95] and heart failure without MI can increase plasma catecholamines and AVP.[99] It is likely that both the increased myocardial damage associated with heart failure as well as the hypotension present in patients with heart failure contribute to the higher elevations of plasma catecholamines and AVP seen in these patients.[95,100] In addition, the stress of hypoxia may also contribute in some severe cases of heart failure since this stress can independently activate the sympathetic nervous system and produce hyperglycemia. However, the threshold for the hypoxia-induced activation is high (see above), suggesting that severe heart failure would probably be necessary to impair oxygen delivery to the point where hypoxia *per se* would contribute significantly to the other factors that activate the sympathetic nervous system during myocardial infarction.

Recent studies suggest that cytokines are released in response to myocardial infarction, but their potential role in mediating the stress hormone response to MI has not been investigated. Certain cytokines may, however, mediate the tissue damage that is usually produced by MI. Interleukin-8 shows a transient rise during the very early phase of MI and has been suggested to attract and stimulate neutrophils, which may cause myocardial damage.[101] IL-6 levels are also elevated in MI patients upon hospital admission, but unlike IL-8, IL-6 levels remain elevated for weeks after an MI.[102] Although the role of IL-6 in MI is unclear, it does stimulate the production of certain acute-phase proteins which may predispose to coronary thrombosis. Finally, there is evidence that circulating levels of tumor necrosis factor are elevated after MI. TNF levels peak within the first 24 hours after admission, and the magnitude of the TNF response is related to the creatine kinase response,[103] an index of infarct size. The elevations of TNF may contribute to cardiac tissue damage by activating leukocytes. Other studies find elevations of TNF only in severe MI accompanied by heart failure but not during uncomplicated MI.[104] Thus, certain cytokines are elevated after MI. Since elevations of cytokines have been associated with the hormonal responses to other stresses, their potential role in contributing to the neuroendocrine and metabolic response to MI deserves investigation.

Although there is little debate that the release of cytokines during myocardial infarction is detrimental, the effect of neuroendocrine activation during MI can be viewed in two different ways. The potential benefit of such activation may come from the hyperglycemia subsequently produced, since the heart itself becomes dependent on glucose as fuel during periods of hypoperfusion. Additionally, MI accompanied by heart failure may produce a significant hypotension, during which increased levels of circulating glucose may compensate for the decreased cerebral perfusion rate. In contrast, others have viewed the neuroendocrine activation that accompanies MI as maladaptive. The increased circulating, and perhaps local, levels of catecholamines might increase heart rate and thus cardiac work when the delivery of the necessary metabolic fuel is already compromised. Further, elevated catecholamines increase the risk of fibrillation.

Surgery

Major surgery produces a response characterized by activation of the sympathetic nervous system and hyperglycemia (Fig. 9-5). A variety of old and new studies demonstrate that both clinical and experimental surgery increase the release of the neurotransmitter norepinephrine from sympathetic nerves and the sympathetic neurohormone epinephrine from the adrenal medulla in proportion to the severity of the surgical stress.[105] Surgical stress also increases the release of cortisol from the adrenal cortex. The pancreatic hormone glucagon is increased, while insulin secretion shows relative inhibition. These neural and hormonal changes are the major contributors to the elevation of plasma glucose and lactate levels seen during surgical stress.

Although it is often thought that the general anesthetics used during major surgery prevent the recognition of pain, it is clear that nociceptive stimulation is a major factor in the sympathetic activation that occurs during surgical stress. For example, early experiments in animals have shown laparotomy produces an increase of plasma catecholamines that is reversed by the analgesic morphine.[106] This action of morphine is blocked by the opioid antagonist naloxone. In addition, morphine does not reverse the rise of plasma catecholamines induced by central glucopenia,[107] demonstrating that its action is specific for nociceptive stress. Other early studies in humans suggest that activation of pain afferents during surgery causes activation of the sympathetic nervous system. For example, the catecholamine response to surgery on the lower half of the body is reduced by low spinal anesthesia,[108] which would be expected to block the afferent signals coming from the site of surgery but not the higher efferent sympathetic outflow. Recent studies on the effects of either high-dose opioid anesthesia or epidural anesthesia confirm and extend these findings. In brief, high-dose opioid anesthesia significantly reduces the sympathetic activation, the increase of stress hormones, and the metabolic responses accompanying cardiac bypass surgery on infants.[109] Likewise, the plasma catecholamine response to vascular surgery on the lower extremities is markedly reduced by epidural anesthesia.[110] Taken together, these studies emphasize that despite the unconsciousness induced by general anesthesia, nociceptive receptors are activated during surgery and send afferent signals to the brain, resulting in a classic stress response. Opiates can block the neurotransmission of these signals either at the spinal cord or brain.

The clinical implications of these findings have only recently been recognized and documented. The evidence suggests that neuroendocrine responses to surgery are maladaptive and result in significant morbidity and mortality. In adults, suppression of the neuroendocrine response to surgery is associated with a decreased incidence of hypertension, arterial thrombosis, postoperative cardiovascular failure, and death.[111] In newborns, suppression of the stress response decreases the incidence of sepsis, disseminated cardiovascular coagulation, and postoperative death.[109]

Although carefully designed animal and clinical studies suggest that nociceptive activation causes a stress response during surgery, common surgical procedures are frequently much more complex, being complicated by the effects of various anesthetics as well as other stresses that are associated with particular diseases. For example, different types of anesthetics vary in their suppressive effects on the sympathetic activation and hyperglycemia produced by stress. Pentobarbital anesthesia in dogs abolishes both the moderate plasma catecholamine response and moderate hyperglycemia produced by central glucopenia in conscious animals.[112] In contrast, low-dose halothane, which produces full surgical anesthesia, allows both a plasma catecholamine and plasma glucose response to moderate glucopenia similar to that of the conscious animal.[113] Equally important is the dose of anesthetic. Studies with halothane and other inhalation anesthetics suggest that higher doses, not surprisingly, produce a progressive suppression of certain neural reflexes, probably including the sympathetic response to surgical stress. Finally, nociception is not the only stimulus present; many surgeries are often complicated by the presence of other stresses. For example, surgical procedures that produce substantial blood loss are complicated by the stress of hemorrhagic hypotension (see above). In addition, major thoracic or abdominal surgery can produce heat loss, and since many anesthetics impair autonomic thermoregulation, mild hypothermia can result.[114] Indeed, in pediatric cardiac surgery, hypothermia is intentional and beneficial. Nonetheless, hypothermia can be a stress in itself (see above). Also, vascular bypass operations, most notably cardiopulmonary bypass, can occasionally result in release of inflammatory cytokines associated with use of bypass pumps[115] or the reperfusion of ischemic tissue. Finally, surgery in the gastrointestinal tract has the potential for infection secondary to the release of endogenous bacteria and endotoxins from the gut, and postsurgical infections from exogenous organisms can significantly complicate the stress response following surgery (see below).

After the surgery is over and the anesthetic has been discontinued, the stress response can in fact increase, because much of the nociceptive stimulation is still present but the suppressive effects of the anesthesia are not. Therefore, there can be a large increase in plasma catecholamines, cortisol, and other stress hormones during the immediate postsurgery period. The rapid action of catecholamines and the delayed effects of cortisol and growth hormone can sometimes lead to hyperglycemia but more often to glucose intolerance (Fig. 9-2), either of which may resolve when the nociceptive stimulation of the counterregulatory hormones wanes. Therefore, analgesics in the postoperative period would be expected to reduce plasma catecholamines,[116] GH, and cortisol levels and accelerate the restoration of normal glucose tolerance, in addition to reducing the morbidity and mortality. Indeed, recent studies have emphasized the need and potential strategies to reduce postsurgical stress during early recovery. Several of the studies, cited above, that demonstrated low postoperative complication rates included the administration of postoperative analgesics, some under patient control. Thus, the understanding of the mechanism of the stress response to surgery is beginning to have significant clinical impact.

Sepsis

The glucose response to sepsis can be qualitatively different depending on the time elapsed since the initial septic insult and its magnitude. Sepsis quickly produces a transient hyperglycemia[117,118] similar to that of hypoxia (Fig. 9-5), which eventually resolves. Thereafter, plasma glucose can be normal if the sepsis is mild. Despite this euglycemia, glucose utilization is usually increased[119,117] without a significant increase of insulin. Hepatic glucose production is also increased, but the counterregulatory hormones glucagon, epinephrine, or cortisol are not. It appears that both the increase of glucose production and utilization (Fig. 9-4) may be mediated by cytokines secreted from macrophages in response to infection.[120] One such cytokine, TNF, is released in response to bacterial endotoxins and can increase the metabolic clearance rate of glucose.[121,122] Although it may not be the exclusive mediator of the increased glucose turnover observed during sepsis,[123] TNF in turn stimulates the release of certain interleukins (IL-1 and IL-6) which may help mediate its hypotensive effects and perhaps some of its effect on glucose uptake.

During more chronic moderate infection, glucose production can be depressed.[124] Such depression occurs despite a doubling or tripling of glucagon, cortisol, and plasma catecholamine levels. However, the elevated level of plasma catecholamines supports even this low level of glucose production. Infusions of medium doses of TNF can reproduce these effects on glucose metabolism and counterregulatory hormone secretion.

When the infection is severe, hypoglycemia can ensue, probably due to a further direct suppressive effect of endotoxin or cytokines on hepatic glucose production coupled with a further, stimulatory effect of TNF[121] and/or high plasma insulin[125] on peripheral glucose uptake. Glucose production is suppressed in this state in a manner similar to that which occurs during induction of hypoglycemia by insulin injection (Fig. 9-6). During chronic moderate sepsis, these effects occur despite increased circulating levels of glucagon and plasma catecholamines.

Although shock is widely thought to cause the mortality seen in severe sepsis, it is not well recognized that hypoglycemia can also contribute. Thus prevention of hypoglycemia by exogenous glucose infusion decreases the incidence of mortality in anesthetized animals with extreme sepsis. Animals that are able to mount a sufficient counterregulatory response to offset the suppressive effects of endotoxins and cytokines on hepatic glucose production and prevent hypoglycemia usually survive severe sepsis. Those that are not able to mount such a response die. High doses of either endotoxin or TNF,[121,122] in addition to reproducing the hypotension characteristic of severe sepsis, can also reproduce the hypoglycemia. Furthermore, immunoneutralization of TNF reduces the lethal effect of endotoxin,[126] suggesting a pathogenic role for TNF in the fatal combination of hypotension and hypoglycemia of severe sepsis. Such studies dramatically illustrate the importance of glucose counterregulatory mechanisms in severe sepsis.

In summary, sepsis initially produces a transient hyperglycemia (Fig. 9-5) mediated by the low levels of macrophage factors released in response to the infection. If the sepsis is not quickly resolved, the secretion of the classic stress hormones is stimulated in an attempt to counterregulate the suppressive effects of accumulating levels of endotoxins and cytokines on hepatic glucose production so a precarious balance of euglycemia is struck (Fig. 9-4). As sepsis worsens and marked endotoxemia occurs, the activity of the sympathetic nervous system and the release of glucagon and cortisol are increased further, but may be overwhelmed, producing hypotension, hypoglycemia (Fig. 9-6), and eventually death.

Burns

Major burns produce a catabolic state reflected by a prolonged increase of the resting metabolic rate proportional to the area of the burn.[127] The metabolic rate normalizes over 1–2 months following serious burns.[127] The increase in oxygen consumption is not due to increased thyroid hormone levels, which are in fact suppressed in burn patients.[127] Hepatic glucose production is also usually increased in burn victims and accounts for the 1–2 weeks of mild hyperglycemia seen after severe burns (50% or more of the body surface area)[127] (Fig. 9-11). The rate of glucose utilization is also usually elevated after burns[128]; this sometimes accounts for the euglycemia seen in the face of increased glucose production following less severe burns. The turnover of gluconeogenic amino acids (e.g., alanine) is increased after burns[128] and reflects accelerated net protein catabolism in peripheral tissues. This negative nitrogen balance and the potential loss of muscle are significant clinical problems in burn patients.

Levels of stress hormones are usually elevated after severe burns. Thus plasma catecholamine levels are increased,[128] reflecting activation of the sympathetic nerves and the adrenal medulla. Both ACTH and glucocorticoids are increased markedly in burn stress[128] as is vasopressin. Baseline glucagon levels are also consistently elevated[127,128] as are glucagon responses to the amino acid arginine. In contrast, GH and its mediator, insulin-like growth factor 1 (IGF-1), are low in burn patients[129] for unknown reasons.

It is likely that most of the stress hormones contribute in different ways to the hypermetabolism and increased glucose production characteristic of burn stress. For example, combined adrenergic blockade tends to normalize resting metabolic rate, suggesting a significant contribution of increased sympathetic tone to the elevated metabolic rate of burn patients.[124] Platelet-activating factor

FIGURE 9-11. Burn (late) and glucose turnover. After the acute stress response to burn subsides, a later hypermetabolic phase ensues. It is characterized by increased glucose production by the liver (**left, dashed arrow**) and increased glucose utilization both by muscle and injured tissues (**lower right, dashed arrow**). Increased glucose turnover is therefore present late in burn stress, usually accompanied by a mild hyperglycemia (**dashed circle**). Protein turnover is also increased, which supplies the amino acids for gluconeogenesis and tissue repair, but which also can eventually lead to muscle wasting. The stress of severe trauma can show a similar hypermetabolic phase late, after the acute stress response subsides.

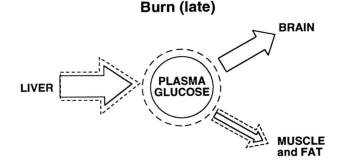

Burn (late)

(PAF) may mediate the activation of the sympathetic nervous system since a PAF antagonist reduces the plasma catecholamine response to burn stress.[130] Cytokines released from activated macrophages may contribute to the activation of the sympathetic nervous system, the increased secretion of counterregulatory hormones, and the hypermetabolism of burn stress. Indeed, plasma levels of IL-6 and IL-2 are elevated in proportion to the area of the burn,[131] while elevations of TNF-α may be more related to the common complication of sepsis.[132]

The stimulation of hepatic glucose production by elevated glucagon levels clearly makes a substantial contribution to the hyperglycemia of burn stress since suppression of glucagon secretion not only reverses the elevated rate of glucose production, but also necessitates the infusion of glucose to prevent hypoglycemia.[128] The sympathetic nervous system also contributes since PAF antagonists, which reduce the plasma catecholamine but not the glucagon response to burn stress, prevent part of the hyperglycemic response as well. Finally, the high plasma levels of glucocorticoids probably contribute to the increased glucose production, both indirectly by increasing proteolysis and thereby the plasma levels of gluconeogenic amino acids, and directly by inducing gluconeogenic enzymes. Suppressed GH secretion may allow increased proteolysis and plasma amino acid levels. Indeed, recently GH treatment has been used to limit protein catabolism[133] and accelerate donor skin healing.[134] Both of these beneficial effects may be due to stimulation of protein synthesis via IGF-1.[135]

Despite the elevated levels of catecholamines, plasma insulin levels are normal or even elevated in burn stress. These elevated levels of plasma insulin contribute significantly to the increased glucose uptake observed in burn stress, since suppression of insulin secretion with somatostatin leads to a significant fall in the metabolic clearance rate for glucose.[128] Despite the clear effect of elevated insulin on glucose uptake, the other major anabolic effects of insulin (i.e., inhibition of lipolysis and proteolysis) do not appear to be fully expressed, as indicated by increased plasma levels of free fatty acids and increased turnover of plasma alanine. Perhaps sympathetic stimulation of adipose tissue and glucocorticoid stimulation of muscle proteolysis partially overcomes these expected inhibitory effects of insulin.

Although burn stress can be characterized by the features listed above, it is important to recognize that these responses can also be due to the presence of other stress. For example, severe burns can produce an acute shock-like hypotension, which by itself (see above) can activate the sympathetic nervous system. Indeed, volume and electrolyte replacement, which help reverse hypotension, are recognized as essential for the management of burns. In addition, the loss of large amounts of burned skin removes an important barrier to infection and frequently leads to sepsis. Recently, it has been recognized that the inflammatory response to burns itself can result in sepsis without external infection, due to translocation of gut bacteria. As reviewed above, sepsis evokes a set of stress responses that include some of those described for burn stress. Thus, the potential presence and contribution of sepsis complicates the interpretation of clinical studies of burn stress.

Trauma

Major trauma such as multiple large-bone fractures, multiple organ injuries, or head injury can quickly cause a stress response similar to those produced by many other stresses (Fig. 9-5). Later, it produces a catabolic state like that of burn stress (Fig. 9-11).

Trauma usually activates the sympathetic nervous system. In head injury patients, the degree of elevation of plasma norepinephrine and epinephrine is correlated with the size of brain injury as assessed by CT scan.[136] In multiple-system trauma, the degree of elevation of norepinephrine and sometimes epinephrine is associated with the severity of the injury.[137] Trauma acutely elevates plasma ACTH and cortisol levels, but these can normalize within a week of the injury. In contrast, GH is suppressed during major trauma,[138] as it appears to be in burn stress. The pancreatic hormone glucagon is elevated by trauma, and plasma insulin levels are depressed.[139]

Trauma produces mild to marked fasting hyperglycemia, depending on the severity of the injury.[139,140] The degree of hyperglycemia increases with the age of the subject, probably secondary to the insulin resistance found in the elderly. When mild hyperglycemia is present, there is still a large increase in glucose turnover due to elevation of hepatic glucose production that is partially offset by an increase of non-insulin-mediated uptake (Fig. 9-11). The turnover of amino acids is also increased in major trauma as it is in burn stress. This results in significant negative nitrogen balance in these patients. Studies simulating the hormonal pattern observed during major trauma suggest that the early suppression of insulin secretion significantly augments the ability of cortisol and glucagon to produce whole-body nitrogen loss.[141] Although the role of GH in the negative nitrogen balance of major trauma has not been extensively studied, the inhibition of GH secretion during major trauma may make a significant contribution. Other stresses associated with negative nitrogen balance also have low GH levels, and GH treatment significantly ameliorates the negative nitrogen balance.[133] Indeed, the suggestion has been made that GH improves nitrogen balance, but probably at the expense of hyperglycemia in major trauma patients.[138]

One mechanism for the stimulation of the autonomic nervous system and activation of the stress response appears to be the pain associated with major trauma. As in surgical stress, such nociceptive stimulation can lead to neural, hormonal, and metabolic responses even during impaired cerebral cortical function and loss of consciousness. In addition, if the patient were conscious, the anxiety associated with major trauma would be expected to activate the sympathetic nervous system, primarily the adrenal medulla.

Depending on the type of trauma there can be stimuli, in addition to the pain associated with the trauma, that contribute to the activation of the neuroendocrine system. These include the surgery sometimes necessary to repair organ or limb injury. Also, severe head and neck injuries can sometimes result in impaired autonomic regulation of blood pressure and body temperature, resulting in the additional stress of hypotension or hypothermia.

The stress response to major trauma can be prevented by reversing or blocking the set of stimuli specific for that trauma and its associated complications. For example, analgesics can be expected to reduce the nociceptive stimulation caused by both the original trauma and the subsequent surgery, and therefore may reduce the neuroendocrine response. Furthermore, maintenance of body temperature and blood pressure would prevent the effects of hypothermia or hypotension. However, blocking or reversing the stimuli for neuroendocrine activation is not the only way to correct the negative nitrogen balance found in trauma patients. Administering exogenous insulin would help decrease net amino acid mobilization from muscle and reduce hyperglycemia. Growth hormone administration may also decrease protein turnover and muscle wasting via IGF-1. However, the positive effect of GH on nitrogen balance may be at the expense of further hyperglycemia, since GH directly antagonizes the action of insulin on glucose uptake.

STRESS-INDUCED HYPERGLYCEMIA IN DIABETES MELLITUS

Type 1 Diabetes Mellitus (T1DM)

Type 1 diabetes mellitus is characterized by an islet lesion leading to markedly impaired insulin secretion with eventual death and loss of almost all of the islet β cells. It often presents as diabetic coma with ketoacidosis, which was thought to indicate almost total permanent destruction of the islet β cells at the time of diagnosis. However, it is now apparent that restoration of some islet cell function is quite common. It is the restoration of this function that is responsible for the "honeymoon" phase. This restoration could be due to recovery from a virally induced or autoimmune type of injury. However, neuroendocrine findings during acute ketoacidosis suggest that a type of stress response is responsible for part of the abnormalities found in the acute ketoacidosis syndrome, and reduced neuroendocrine stress hormones may also be important to this improvement.

Elevated levels of catecholamines, cortisol, GH, and glucagon are characteristic of diabetic ketoacidosis.[142] Treatment with intravenous fluids alone without insulin will reduce the hyperglycemia, fatty acid mobilization, and ketogenesis (Fig. 9-12).[143] These findings suggest that elevation of these counterregulatory hormones is responsible for converting rather severe insulin deficiency without ketoacidosis to decompensated hyperglycemia with ketoacidosis. Confirming this concept, it has been shown that β-adrenergic blocking agents are effective in reducing elevated fatty acid mobilization in ketoacidosis.[142] Because many type 1 diabetic patients present to the physician without ketoacidosis, we have suggested that insulin deficiency of the magnitude usually observed is a necessary but not a sufficient explanation for the ketoacidosis syndrome. We believe that volume depletion and ac-

FIGURE 9-12. The effect of intravenous fluid therapy without insulin in severe diabetic hyperglycemia. Note the marked suppression of norepinephrine (**NE**), epinephrine (**E**), and glucose (**BG**), indicating volume depletion as an important cause of the marked elevation of these and other counterregulatory hormones in decompensated diabetes. The levels eventually achieved by fluid therapy alone are shown as the equilibrium value. *(Modified with permission from Waldhause W, Kleinberger G, Korn A, et al: Severe hyperglycemia: Effects of rehydration on endocrine derangements and blood glucose concentration.* Diabetes *1979;28:577.)*

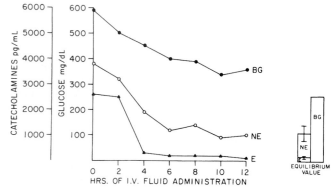

tivation of baroreceptor-mediated stimulation of the autonomic nervous system and the hypothalamopituitary axis are necessary additional factors in initiating ketoacidosis.

We have suggested that β-cell injury leads to impaired insulin secretion that is partially compensated by the hyperglycemia that follows. When the hyperglycemia becomes of sufficient magnitude to lead to glycosuria and electrolyte loss, it is the subsequent volume depletion associated with this excretion of glucose that activates the counterregulatory hormones epinephrine, glucagon, GH, and cortisol to produce the full-blown diabetic ketoacidosis syndrome. Of course, any other stimulus to the sympathetic system, such as trauma or burn, would lead to the same problems in underinsulinized patients. This concept may explain why low-dose insulin has become so effective in the treatment of ketoacidosis. It may be partly because such therapy is usually associated with vigorous replacement of fluid and electrolyte losses. This treatment minimizes volume depletion and restores elevated counterregulatory hormones toward normal.[143] Such fluid replacement reduces the insulin resistance induced by these hormones and possibly allows for improved insulin secretion from residual β cells. Thus, ketoacidosis in type 1 diabetes would be characterized as a sequence of events in which insulin deficiency leads to hyperglycemia, which leads to glycosuria, volume depletion, activation of the autonomic and pituitary hypothalamic axes, mobilization of fatty acids, increased hepatic glucose and ketone production, and ketoacidosis. In this context, diabetes mellitus is a form of stress, and there is a vicious cycle in which the underlying pancreatic abnormality leads to hyperglycemia, which leads to a neuroendocrine stress response, which leads to more hyperglycemia and eventual ketoacidosis. This phenomenon is more likely to occur in type 1 diabetes because of the efficient excretion of glucose in the younger age group coupled with the greater severity of insulin deficiency. In some circumstances, it would appear that ketoacidosis could occur even in the presence of "normal" levels of basal insulin being overwhelmed by increased levels of catecholamines, GH, cortisol, and glucagon. We have documented such an instance in which a patient who had basal insulin levels that were apparently normal, but in fact were low given the associated hyperglycemia (Fig. 9-13). This patient went from hyperglycemia and glycosuria without ketosis to full-blown ketoacidosis without any further change in plasma insulin.[144] This would seem to indicate that ketoacidosis can develop because of increased stimulation of lipolysis rather than further insulin deficiency.

Some experimental efforts have been directed to the study of whether psychologic stress can influence ketoacidosis in susceptible patients. Based upon the observation that poorly controlled type I diabetic patients develop elevated ketone body levels during stress interviews, two difficult-to-manage patients with recurrent acidosis thought to be related to psychological factors in their environment were treated with oral propranolol therapy.[145] The rationalization was that catecholamine-induced lipolysis would be prevented, so that episodes of poor diabetes control would not be associated with ketoacidosis. In these two patients, this treatment was associated with marked reduction of the frequency of hospitalization for ketoacidosis, in contrast to other forms of therapy directed at reducing the environmental stress factors in these patients' lives. This form of therapy has obvious problems because of its potential to enhance hypoglycemia unawareness in insulin-treated patients and is not recommended as therapy for such individuals. However, it does indicate, as do the findings during stress interviews, that type 1 diabetic patients are particularly sensitive to

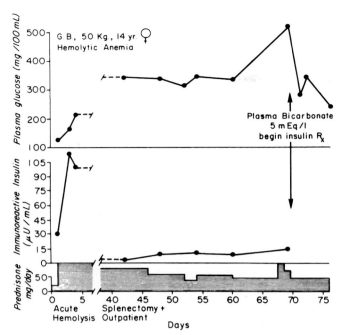

FIGURE 9-13. Ketoacidosis in a patient with sustained insulin secretion. Note the effect of high-dose prednisone to exaggerate hyperglycemia minimally, until insulin secretion fails to keep up between days 5 and 40. Acidosis does not develop until day 69 without any further decline in basal insulin. After splenectomy and discontinuance of prednisone, hyperglycemia completely disappeared. *(Reprinted with permission from Porte, et al.[142])*

activation of the autonomic and hypothalamopituitary systems. Attempts to quantitate this phenomenon in insulin-treated, type 1 diabetic patients have been made and are consistent with such a hypothesis. It has been shown, for example, that hyperglycemia induced by cortisol, epinephrine, or glucagon is exaggerated in type 1 diabetic patients, and this is particularly true during periods of relatively poor diabetes control.[146] For this reason, a variety of stress states are associated with increased need for insulin in such patients. It is also commonly observed that deterioration of diabetes control is likely during episodes of sepsis, burn, hypoxia, hypotension, or vascular accidents in insulin-treated diabetic patients. The presumption is that although normal subjects will have impaired insulin secretion during these stress states, the islet will tend to adapt to some degree due to the ability of β-adrenergic stimulation and glucose to modulate the α-adrenergic effects of catecholamines on the islet. Although the same adrenergic effects to increase hepatic glucose mobilization and impair peripheral insulin-mediated glucose uptake will be observed in type 1 diabetic patients, the simultaneous modulation of this phenomenon by β-adrenergic and glucose stimulation of insulin secretion does not occur, and more severe glycemia would be predicted. Treatment of these distorted relationships in type 1 diabetes mellitus will be discussed later.

Potential Role in the Etiology of Type 1 Diabetes*

Islet injury and destruction are now known to precede the onset of clinical hyperglycemia and take place over a much longer period

---

*Reprinted from ref. 151, pp. 533–534, courtesy of Marcel Decker, Inc.

of time than is clinically apparent. This immune injury is indicated by the presence of islet cell antibodies and insulin autoantibodies, which appear several years before the diagnosis of type I diabetes mellitus[147,148] (see Chap. 20). In addition, reduced insulin responses to intravenous glucose also appear months to years prior to severe hyperglycemia.[149]

The reasons for the activation of this destructive process are unknown but are believed to represent the activation of an autoimmune state followed by an imbalance between T-helper and T-suppressor cells and the susceptibility or resistance of islet β cells to injury.[150] Because some stress hormones (particularly cortisol) are known to modulate the immune system and others to alter islet β-cell activity (epinephrine, glucagon, cortisol), there has been speculation regarding the potential role of such modulation on the development and progress of islet injury.[151] Thus, neurohormonal changes associated with stress have been proposed as one of the environmental factors that interact with hereditary factors known to be associated with risk of the development of type I diabetes. It has been suggested that lymphokines produced by activated macrophages and helper T cells are toxic to insulin-secreting islet β cells and therefore the regulation of antigen-presenting cells and/or regulation of helper T-cell production of interleukin (IL-1), interferon-gamma (IFN-γ), or tumor necrosis factor (TNF) could increase destruction of β cells.[150] Hormonal regulation of suppressor cells that normally minimize or prevent immune injury is another potential mechanism by which stress hormones (particularly cortisol) and the sympathetic nerves may contribute to the likelihood of autoimmune β-cell destruction of type 1 diabetes. For example, it has been shown that suppressor T cells are more sensitive to glucocorticoids than T-helper cells.[152] Thus at moderate cortisol dosages, immune injury could be increased by steroids. An example of this phenomenon may be the increased rate of development of an autoimmune form of diabetes induced in mice by low-dosage streptozocin when they are housed 10 to a cage compared with mice housed 1 to a cage, because crowded housing is associated with higher circulating adrenal steroid levels.[153] A similar phenomenon may explain why cyclophosphamide-treated NOD mice (a model of type 1 diabetes) have an increased prevalence of diabetes.[154] Cyclophosphamide, which is known to be an immune suppressant, markedly increases the eventual development of diabetes in this mouse model of autoimmunity and diabetes. Evidence presented so far suggests that this is best explained by postulating a toxic effect of the drug on suppressor T-cell function.[155,156]

As an alternative, immune-related damage of islet β cells has been shown to be related to the insulin-secretory activity of these cells at the time of exposure to IL-1.[150] Thus, increased secretion of insulin seems to be followed by an enhanced ability of IL-1 to impair β-cell function. Because increased β-cell secretion of insulin has been found during physical stress and infection, it has been postulated that the β cells would be more sensitive to injury at these times. This increase in insulin level is usually associated with insulin resistance. Glucocorticoids, GH, and the catecholamines all cause insulin resistance, and it has been hypothesized that they are the cause of insulin resistance during stress. Because catecholamines also impair insulin secretion, the activity level of the β cell of a stressed individual can be highly varied. However, the temporal pattern of the stress response can often be characterized by an early excess of catecholamines and a late excess of glucocorticoids and GH.[157] Therefore, the early response to stress may be characterized by reduced insulin secretion, while the later recovery phase is often characterized by insulin resistance, and a compensatory increase in β-cell activity with increased insulin secretion. In fact, studies *in vitro* and *in vivo* have suggested that the sensitivity to both immune[158] and nonimmune[159] injury may be increased when insulin secretion is increased. Thus, an alternative explanation for the increased sensitivity of crowded mice to low-dosage streptozocin discussed above could be related to an increased sensitivity of activated islet β cells to injury rather than a decrease in suppressor T-cell function. Such changes in islet β-cell secretory activity could explain why type 1 diabetes occurs with greater frequency in the fall and winter than during spring and summer. This was originally thought to be due to the increased likelihood of a specific infection that causes islet destruction, but the association is without relation to any specific infection. Thus it may be that the neurohumoral stress response to infection causes insulin resistance and increased islet β-cell insulin activity, which in turn sensitizes the β cell to autoimmune injury. The increased activity of the β cell during puberty[160] may provide a similar explanation for the increased incidence of type 1 diabetes in susceptible subjects at that time of life. Reducing islet number by pancreatectomy (another way of activating residual β cells) has been found to increase the likelihood of permanent diabetes in stressed rats.[161] Thus there are a variety of mechanisms by which stress could contribute to the onset of type 1 diabetes.

A role for psychological stress in the causes and/or onset of human type 1 diabetes has also been postulated. Major life events have been found to be more frequent in diabetic children prior to diagnosis than in controls,[162] but no prospective study has been carried out.

Type 2 Diabetes Mellitus (T2DM)

During this discussion of stress hyperglycemia, we have emphasized the key role that the islet β cells must play in any hyperglycemic state. Due simply to the feedback nature of islet regulation, it appears that increased hepatic glucose production and/or decreased peripheral glucose use alone or together cannot lead to sustained hyperglycemia unless the islet fails to adapt. Therefore, on theoretical grounds one would expect that hyperglycemia in type 2 diabetes mellitus must be associated with an abnormality of islet function. Nevertheless, the presence of such an islet abnormality has been somewhat controversial (see Chap. 21). This is because during standard oral glucose tolerance testing, insulin levels appear to be normal or even hypernormal in many type 2 diabetic patients. The apparent presence of normal amounts of insulin is partly related to the fact that control groups of equivalent body weight have not always been used to evaluate the appropriateness of the insulin response. In addition, insulin secretory responses to a variety of nonglucose stimulants are normal in many type 2 diabetic patients. Thus if the fasting plasma glucose level is less than 200 mg/dL, most of these patients have normal basal insulin levels for body weight, and there are apparently normal insulin responses to intravenous arginine, secretin, isoproterenol, and tolbutamide.[163] Only an abnormal response to intravenous glucose can be consistently demonstrated. However, it is now recognized that the responses to nonglucose stimulants are only normal because of the associated hyperglycemia. Thus there is a persistent and important impairment of islet sensitivity to glucose in type 2 diabetes that reduces the insulin response to all stimuli, but the hyperglycemia compensates for a reduced response to the nonglucose inputs (see Chap. 21).[164] Thus any stimulus that tends to impair insulin action or accelerate hepatic glucose production will be more effective in elevating glucose in type 2 patients because it would require a greater degree of hyperglycemia for the islet-cell adaptation to occur. In addition, it has now become apparent that islet β cells are probably more sensitive to the inhibitory actions of epinephrine in type 2 diabetes because the ability of epinephrine to impair islet function is also glucose-sensitive.[165] An increase in sensitivity to norepinephrine in type 2 diabetes has been demonstrated.[166] In normal individuals, the initial suppression of basal insulin by epinephrine can be reversed by a relatively modest hyperglycemia. This restores basal insulin secretory rates to pretreatment levels and modulates the hyperglycemia induced by epinephrine. In type 2 diabetes, much greater degrees of hyperglycemia are required to modulate the effects of epinephrine. Thus the same amount of stress hormone during baroreceptor, chemoreceptor, pain receptor, or psychological stimulation would be expected to produce greater increments of glycemia in such patients.[167] These impairments of the islet responses to glucose with their attendant effects on the sensitivity of islet β cells to nonglucose stimulants probably explains why some type 2 diabetic patients develop ketoacidosis during stress due to burn, trauma, surgery, or vascular occlusive events and transiently require insulin treatment. Not only is there increased mobilization of fatty acids from stress hormones, but there is simultaneously an exaggerated impairment of insulin secretion. After the stress activation of the neuroendocrine system is over and catecholamine and other counterregulatory hormone levels decline, these same patients may be able to maintain reasonable blood sugar levels with their usual diet or oral drug therapy.

Potential Role in the Etiology of T2DM

Studies have suggested that glucose recognition by a number of neuroendocrine cells may be abnormal and have raised the possibility that a glucose-sensing defect may be the explanation for some of the abnormal neuroendocrine findings in this syndrome.[168] The poor suppression of glucagon by glucose, the elevation of catecholamines unrelated to any ketoacidosis, and the supersensitivity to exercise-induced increases in GH or its paradoxical increase by oral glucose in some individuals with mild hyperglycemia may be part of the underlying disease. Although this abnormality may be due to other intrinsic structural or metabolic defects, there is also the possibility that neuroendocrine factors known to influence the islet response to glucose are also involved. Thus, increased insulin release may be observed in type 2 diabetes during the infusion of the α-adrenergic receptor blocking agent phentolamine, implying increased α-adrenergic receptor activity or sensitivity in such subjects.[169]

We have shown that infusion of a synthetic somatostatin analogue in dogs produces hyperglycemia and selective impairment of glucose-induced insulin release quite analogous to that found in type 2 diabetes.[106] A similar phenomenon has been observed with infusion of the neuropeptide galanin, which is present in pancreatic nerves of some species.[170] Thus a variety of inhibitory β-cell neuroendocrine factors can produce a syndrome that resembles type 2 diabetes. A mouse model of diabetes and obesity (ob ob) has been found to be supersensitive to catecholamines and stress. It has been suggested that this change is a key factor in the development of diabetes in this animal model.[171]

Although none of these findings are conclusive, it is apparent that activation of neuroendocrine systems that impair glucose sensitivity of the islet β cell can produce a syndrome quite similar to type 2 diabetes. There is accumulating evidence that such activation may be an important part of the hyperglycemia observed in type 2 diabetes. Regardless of etiologic considerations, it is clear that stress hyperglycemia in such patients is almost certain to be more severe and to be less well counteracted than in normal subjects. This will have important treatment and therapeutic implications, which will be discussed later.

CLINICAL MANAGEMENT OF STRESS-INDUCED HYPERGLYCEMIA

Normal Subjects

Metabolic adaptation to an environmental stress may be beneficial or harmful. The stress responses that occur in normal animals or humans are not necessarily beneficial for long-term survival. In fact, maladaptive responses may be a significant cause of long-term morbidity and mortality in humans. Recommendations for the treatment of stress hyperglycemia must be based on the concept that the hyperglycemic response is more harmful than helpful. This determination will vary with the clinical state and with the degree of hyperglycemia observed. Because the central nervous system is dependent upon maintenance of at least 50% of its usual basal glucose flux, assessment of CNS needs for glucose and its adequate provision is a key determinant of treatment. Thus, glucose concentration, cerebral blood flow, and cerebral oxygenation are all critical parameters to be evaluated. One of the most efficient ways of increasing glucose flux to the central nervous system is to increase its concentration in the circulation, and this presumably underlies the biologic response of stress hyperglycemia. It is not possible to increase this flux by increasing insulin because the uptake of glucose by the CNS is insulin-independent. Therefore, if insulin is administered and plasma glucose levels fall, CNS use of glucose will remain stable or decline. In hypovolemic and hypotensive states, in patients with cerebrovascular occlusive disease or with myocardial infarction and low cardiac output, or in hypoxic states, reversal of the hyperglycemia is contraindicated unless the plasma glucose levels rise to what are considered to be toxic levels. What must be kept in mind is that the delivery rate or flux of glucose provided to the central nervous system and not the glucose level is the key parameter that will determine the adequacy of fuel delivery. In the absence of significant glycosuria and/or electrolyte imbalance, detrimental effects of hyperglycemia are minimal, and short of these complications, hyperglycemia in such states should not be treated because it is enhancing glucose delivery to the central nervous system.

In conditions in which nutrient need in peripheral tissues is increased—such as burn, trauma, or cold stress—and when there is no reduction of flow or glucose delivery to the central nervous system, hyperglycemia is not necessary for high rates of glucose uptake. In these instances, the need for carbohydrate is related to a general need for substrate by injured body tissues, most of which are insulin-sensitive. Thus, the delivery of glucose can be accelerated by the use of insulin alone or with glucose without depriving the CNS of adequate fuel. In this case, the potentially harmful side effects of glycosuria, electrolyte loss, hyperosmolarity, and increased gluconeogenesis can be avoided. In patients with myocardial infarction, it has been suggested that the ischemic myocardial tissue may benefit from increased glucose uptake and decreased fatty acid mobilization.[172,173] When one administers insulin, it must be remembered that as the blood glucose falls, those tissues that are insulin-insensitive will receive less glucose. Therefore, cerebral blood flow needs to be assessed to be sure that it is adequate before giving insulin to patients with MI. It is likely that the injured heart tissue remains insulin-sensitive, and therefore glucose uptake by

cardiovascular muscle is likely to increase despite a decrease of plasma glucose. However, this is not known for certain, and it may be advisable to give glucose along with the insulin to maintain significant amounts of hyperglycemia while accelerating glucose uptake in insulin-sensitive tissues.

One must remember that under these circumstances potassium uptake will also be accelerated. Any change of serum potassium may influence cardiac contractility or cardiac rhythmicity. Thus the use of glucose, insulin, and potassium solutions has been recommended, but there are potential risks as well as benefits. Because simple elevation of plasma glucose levels may not be effective in increasing glucose uptake in an insulin-sensitive tissue in the absence of additional insulin, provision of insulin may be critical. Thus the elevation of catecholamines during infarction may be playing a critical role in limiting the uptake of glucose by the heart. Insulin treatment may be simply reversing an insulin deficiency state. This issue is still at present unresolved, and therefore the level of glucose and or the level of insulin may both be important. This may even vary from patient to patient and could explain some of the controversy regarding the benefits of such therapy.

Some forms of stress hyperglycemia are characterized by hyperglycemia that appears to be of no useful purpose. That is, the hyperglycemia appears to be an unnecessary response to a perceived threat, which in primitive humans might have been associated with increased muscular activity and nutrient demand but is not so in present circumstances. This leads to an imbalance between an increased glucose production and unaltered use, leading to hyperglycemia. This would also be true of most pain-related syndromes, particularly those in which significant amounts of trauma have not occurred and there is no need for increased glucose use or nutrient support for injured tissues. This can be the case in the postoperative period after surgical procedures in which tissue damage or injury has been relatively minor. Treatment under such circumstances is indicated whenever hyperglycemia is severe, and there appears to be no real contraindication. A similar situation occurs in hypothermia in which total body metabolism is reduced. In the absence of extra glucose administration, hyperglycemia is unusual. However, if glucose is given to hypothermic humans, rather severe hyperglycemia can occur. In this case, treatment to reduce this glucose level is unlikely to have any harmful side effects. Usually all that is necessary is to stop the administration of exogenous glucose. More important is the prevention of this hyperglycemic syndrome by not giving glucose to hypothermic patients.

In summary, treatment of stress hyperglycemia resolves itself into three separate approaches: (1) maintenance of the hyperglycemia for those conditions in which there is a real or potential deficiency of central nervous system uptake that can be reversed by maintaining or even increasing the hyperglycemia; (2) increasing glucose turnover by administering glucose and insulin or insulin alone, for those conditions in which an increase of glucose use by insulin-sensitive tissues is desired; or (3) no treatment in those conditions in which there is no change of nutrient need. If hyperglycemia becomes severe, it can be treated with insulin alone, because the extra glucose being produced is not providing any needed function.

T1DM Patients

General treatment concepts in type 1 diabetic patients are no different than those in normal subjects. Stress hyperglycemia in the diabetic patient has the same implications as it does in the normal population, but there are circumstances during which euglycemia is not desirable and hyperglycemia should be promoted. Again, these are conditions in which central nervous system glucose uptake is impaired. This includes hypoxia, hypotension, cerebrovascular occlusive disease, and cardiovascular states in which reduced cerebral blood flow is present. Under most conditions, hepatic glucose production will increase and hyperglycemia will be present despite the administration of the usual amounts of insulin. However, this may not always be the case, because there may be simultaneous reduction in nutrient intake, and a considerable amount of insulin administration is related to nutrient ingestion. Therefore, it may be necessary to reduce insulin dose in type 1 diabetic subjects during this form of stress.

In burns, trauma, MI, or surgery related to trauma or in which traumatic injury is likely to be extensive, the need for increased nutrient delivery to peripheral tissues in a type 1 diabetic patient is similar to that in normal subjects. Again, the need for increased substrate use may be severe, and although euglycemia may be achieved by reducing caloric intake, this is not the desirable treatment. As in the normal individual, carbohydrate, fat, and protein either orally or intravenously should be given along with sufficient additional insulin to maintain euglycemic levels. Thus, in conditions in which catabolic protein loss is undesirable and gluconeogenesis is to be suppressed, sufficient exogenous calories should be given to meet metabolic needs even if these are increased over basal levels. In order to suppress hepatic glucose production, it may be necessary to administer large amounts of intravenous carbohydrate. If hyperglycemia occurs, then additional insulin should be given along with the additional carbohydrate rather than restricting carbohydrate calories, because the goal is to promote nitrogen uptake in injured tissues while sparing protein resources from gluconeogenesis.

In trying to anticipate insulin need during surgical procedures, a number of approaches have been taken. In general terms, insulin should be administered as a basal amount plus an amount in proportion to expected caloric intake. Basal insulin needs are real, and therefore insulin should always be administered every day. In uncomplicated surgical procedures, we have tended to reduce long-acting insulin to approximately 50% of the usual dose and to cover additional caloric need by monitoring plasma glucose before and after the surgery. Plasma glucose levels are to be maintained between 150 and 200 mg/dL. Under complex surgical conditions, long-acting insulins have not been used, and the patients have been switched to six hourly injections of subcutaneous regular insulin or to continuous intravenous insulin infusion along with sufficient carbohydrate to provide at least 600 cal/24 h, preferably 1000 calories or more per 24 hours (see Chap. 37). Insulin dosage must be individualized because insulin sensitivity varies considerably from patient to patient. Because counterregulatory hormones are suppressed by many anesthetics, it may be the postoperative phase in which insulin resistance will be most severe. Normal prehepatic basal insulin secretory rates for a lean individual are approximately 15–25 U/d in the basal state. One can estimate insulin need on the basis of this requirement. Approximately an equal amount of insulin appears to be required to maintain normal glucose homeostasis during the provision of a 2000- to 2500-calorie diet. These considerations can lead to rough estimates of insulin need in lean type 1 diabetic patients to be 40–50 U/d.

The major problem in type 1 diabetes is the inability to anticipate the impact of neuroendocrine control mechanisms upon plasma glucose. It is clear that stress produces increased glucose

levels and a tendency towards ketosis in poorly controlled type 1 diabetic patients. In some patients, the impact of the environment seems to be particularly important in the regulation of plasma glucose. Whether some individuals are particularly sensitive to environmental influences, whether individuals vary widely in their autonomic and hypothalamic responses to perceived injury, or whether there is wide variability in the sensitivity of various individuals to catecholamines, cortisol, or GH is unknown. However, it is clear that it is difficult to predict in any patient what emotional trauma or surgical stress will produce in the way of altered glucose homeostasis. As mentioned earlier, in a few instances it has been possible to ameliorate severe psychological stress by treating patients prophylactically with propranolol to prevent recurrent episodes of ketoacidosis. Treatment with other types of more selective blocking agents in an attempt to improve diabetes control has not been attempted as yet. However, the emphasis on improved diabetes control by the use of open-loop insulin infusion devices would seem to require not only careful control of nutrient intake but attempts to modify autonomic influences on carbohydrate metabolism as the other major area of therapeutic intervention that will need to be addressed. The recent recognition of hypoglycemia-associated autonomic failure (see Chap. 31) has revealed that autonomic counterregulation may be expected to vary from day to day in some patients. Thus autonomic excess and/or deficiency may be quite common and contribute significantly to hypo- and hyperglycemia.

T2DM Patients

In type 2 diabetes, plasma glucose is reregulated to a stable level which is greater than in the normal population. However, the usual regulatory mechanisms for maintaining a constant plasma glucose level remain intact although impaired. That is, insulin secretion is still present, and it responds to glucose. The sensitivity of this response is reduced, and therefore any nutrient challenge or challenge from an increased output of counterregulatory hormones will result in greater degrees of hyperglycemia for longer periods of time. However, as in the normal individual, these mechanisms will tend to stabilize plasma glucose levels even during stress. Thus with mild forms of stress, the reregulated plasma glucose level will tend to remain constant. The degree to which hyperglycemia will be increased by a particular stress in a type 2 diabetic patient is difficult to anticipate. This is because it will depend upon the sensitivity of that individual to all of the stress-related hormones, the basic nature of his or her islet impairment, and the responsiveness of the counterregulatory hormones to the stressful event. Very little is known regarding changes in sensitivity or responsiveness of this system in type 2 diabetes; however, there are studies suggesting that psychological stress may increase plasma glucose.[174] Nevertheless, because glucose sensitivity of the islets is clearly impaired and many of these subjects are insulin-resistant to begin with, it seems clear that greater degrees of glycemic increments are going to occur if the stress produces similar elevations of stress hormones. Presumably, this sensitivity will depend upon the degree of hyperglycemia prior to the stressful event. Individuals under relatively poor control will therefore be expected to become much worse and perhaps be unable to reregulate due to the increased glycosuria. If so, volume depletion and increased stress hormone responses will occur. This is presumably the explanation for the development of ketoacidosis during sepsis, trauma, and surgical interventions in relatively poorly controlled type 2 diabetic patients (see Chap. 34). On the other hand, the use of oral hypoglycemic agents to lower plasma glucose and to improve islet function and peripheral sensitivity to insulin results in a patient who has reregulated plasma glucose to a more normal value. In this case, it has been the general experience that maintaining the individual on oral agents allows reasonable responses to the modest stress associated with elective surgical procedures, without the need to switch to insulin (see Chap. 37).

Thus, the major treatment decision that must be made in the type 2 diabetic patient is whether or not to stop an oral agent and to institute insulin treatment. Well-controlled patients will manage quite well during elective surgery and other minor stressful situations. However, in any poorly controlled patient during episodes of bacterial sepsis, MI, burn, major trauma, and so on, the stress response may overwhelm the islet or produce a stimulus that is beyond the ability of the impaired islet to counterregulate. Thus, severe degrees of hyperglycemia and ketoacidosis are not uncommon in type 2 diabetes during stress and may even occur in normal individuals with very severe stress. In this case, insulin treatment must be instituted. Insulin treatment should be given to any poorly controlled patient who is about to go to surgery or to any patient if a major traumatic event can be anticipated, such as a major surgical procedure. The treatment of such patients with insulin does not predict that they will require insulin after the stressful period. Thus, the discovery of severe hyperglycemia and even ketoacidosis during stress in an individual who on clinical grounds would be suspected of type 2 diabetes (onset over age 50 or a major degree of obesity) does not indicate the permanent need for insulin. Such patients may respond quite well to the usual therapeutic approaches to type 2 diabetes when the stressful event is over. Once the decision has been made to treat a type 2 diabetic patient with insulin, then the evaluation and treatment of stress hyperglycemia is similar to that for the type 1 diabetic patient discussed earlier.

SUMMARY AND CONCLUSIONS

Neural regulation of the pancreatic islet in conjunction with other hormonal glucoregulatory systems is an important component of plasma glucose regulation, which contributes significantly to the normal disposition of exogenous nutrients and to defining the glycemic response to environmental stress. The neuroendocrine system tends to modulate the intrinsic regulatory control system for plasma glucose, which involves the liver, peripheral tissues, and the islet as the primary nutrient and substrate sensors. The sensitivity and function of all three elements of this system are responsive to neuroendocrine control. Neural and endocrine influences are important to hepatic glucose production and to the use and disposition of fuels in adipose tissue and muscle, as well as to islet function. Stress responses that occur in normal animals or humans may or may not be beneficial for long-term survival. Thus evaluation of the impact of the hyperglycemia found under such circumstances must be made prior to a treatment decision. Although maladaptive responses may be a significant cause of long-term morbidity and mortality in humans, there are many circumstances under which hyperglycemia may be beneficial or even essential for survival. Treatment will depend on which category of hyperglycemic response one can place the particular patient into. Is this hyperglycemia related to the need for the central nervous system to increase glucose uptake and substrate utilization? Is this hyperglycemia related to a need for peripheral tissues to increase glucose uptake for repair or anabolic processes? Or is this hyperglycemia an inappropriate or excessive response to some perceived or actual threat from the environment in which the hyperglycemia is useless or perhaps even detrimental to health? This will be a critical decision affecting treatment.

A number of physiologic and psychological types of stress have been discussed, and it is clear that although there is a general pattern to the neuroendocrine changes found, each stress state represents a unique set of circumstances with specific metabolic disturbances. At times it is difficult to distinguish the stress response of a normal individual from idiopathic diabetes mellitus, particularly type 2 diabetes mellitus. In the short term, the therapeutic decision is not related to the etiology of the hyperglycemia, but in the long term this may be a critical issue in the development of a suitable treatment protocol. Thus treatment considerations vary from patient to patient and depend upon the nature of the stress and the specific response to that stress in the individual case. Associated conditions play an important role in this evaluation. In the final analysis, the question that must be asked is, "Is the hyperglycemic state more harmful than helpful and will the contemplated treatment be beneficial and decrease risk?" An understanding of the neuroendocrine response system for stress and its actions upon substrate-using systems is an essential prerequisite for this decision. In diabetes mellitus, neuroendocrine abnormalities are common. Even in the apparently unstressed individual, increased sensitivity or increased levels of stress-related hormones and neural inputs may contribute either etiologically or pathophysiologically to the hyperglycemia observed. At times, a pathophysiologic separation of stress hyperglycemia and type 2 diabetes is not possible. Both involve alterations of the regulation of hepatic glucose output and peripheral sensitivity of tissues to insulin, as well as alterations of islet function. Therefore, regardless of etiologic significance, neuroendocrine control systems must be taken into account in the diagnosis, evaluation, and treatment of any hyperglycemic state in humans.

REFERENCES

1. Havel PJ: Role of adipose tissue in body-weight regulation: Mechanisms regulating leptin production and energy balance. *Proc Nutr Soc* 2000;59:359.
2. Harris RB: Leptin—much more than a satiety signal. *Annu Rev Nutr* 2000;20:45.
3. Schwartz MW, Woods SC, Porte D Jr., et al: Central nervous system control of food intake. *Nature* 2000;404:661.
4. Havel PJ: Peripheral signals conveying metabolic information to the brain: Short-term and long-term regulation of food intake and energy homeostasis. *Exp Biol Med.* 2001;226:963.
5. Keim NL, Stern JS, Havel PJ: Relation between circulating leptin concentrations and appetite during a prolonged, moderate energy deficit in women. *Am J Clin Nutr* 1998;68:794.
6. Sindelar DK, Havel PJ, Seeley RJ, et al: Low plasma leptin levels contribute to diabetic hyperphagia in rats. *Diabetes* 1999;48:1275.
7. Figlewicz DP, Higgins MS, Ng-Evans SB, et al: Leptin reverses sucrose-conditioned place preference in food-restricted rats. *Physiol Behav* 2001;73:229.
8. Doring H, Schwarzer K, Nuesslein-Hildesheim B, et al: Leptin selectively increases energy expenditure of food-restricted lean mice. *Int J Obes Relat Metab Disord* 1998;22:83.
9. Ahima RS, Saper CB, Flier JS, et al: Leptin regulation of neuroendocrine systems. *Front Neuroendocrinol* 2000;21:263.
10. Ahima RS, Prabakaran D, Mantzoros C, et al: Role of leptin in the neuroendocrine response to fasting. *Nature* 1996;382:250.
11. De Boer S, Koopmas S, Slangen J, et al: Effects of fasting on plasma catecholamine, corticosterone and glucose concentrations

under basal and stress conditions in individual rats. *Physiol Behav* 1989;45:989.

12. O'Dea K, Esler M, Leonard P, *et al*: Noradrenaline turnover during under and over-eating in normal weight subjects. *Metabolism* 1982; 31:896.

13. Scarpace PJ, Matheny M, Pollock BH, *et al*: Leptin increases uncoupling protein expression and energy expenditure. *Am J Physiol* 1997; 273:E226.

14. Scarpace PJ, Matheny M: Leptin induction of UCP1 gene expression is dependent on sympathetic innervation. *Am J Physiol* 1998;275: E259.

15. Collins S, Kuhn CM, Petro AE, *et al*: Role of leptin in fat regulation. *Nature* 1996;380:677.

16. Haynes WG, Morgan DA, Walsh SA, *et al*: Receptor-mediated regional sympathetic nerve activation by leptin. *J Clin Invest* 1997; 100:270.

17. Haynes WG, Sivitz WI, Morgan DA, *et al*: Sympathetic and cardiorenal actions of leptin. *Hypertension* 1997;30:619.

18. Tang-Christensen M, Havel PJ, Jacobs RR, *et al*: Central administration of leptin inhibits food intake and activates the sympathetic nervous system in rhesus macaques. *J Clin Endocrinol Metab* 1999;84: 711.

19. Ahren B, Havel PJ: Leptin increases circulating glucose, insulin and glucagon via sympathetic neural activation in fasted mice. *Int J Obes Relat Metab Disord* 1999;23:660.

20. Havel PJ, Pelleymounter MA: Acute adrenergically mediated increases of circulating glucose and lactate after leptin administration in rhesus monkeys. *Obesity Res.* 1997;5(suppl 1):17S.

21. Bornstein SR, Licinio J, Tauchnitz R, *et al*: Plasma leptin levels are increased in survivors of acute sepsis: associated loss of diurnal rhythm, in cortisol and leptin secretion. *J Clin Endocrinol Metab* 1998;83:280.

22. Hobson K, Havel P, McMurtry A, *et al*: Circulating leptin and cortisol after burn injury: loss of diurnal pattern. *J Clin Endocrinol Metab* Paper is in press to Annals of Surgery (submitted), 2001.

23. Schoeller DA, Cella LK, Sinha MK, *et al*: Entrainment of the diurnal rhythm of plasma leptin to meal timing. *J Clin Invest* 1997;100:1882.

24. Havel PJ, Townsend R, Chaump L, *et al*: High-fat meals reduce 24-h circulating leptin concentrations in women. *Diabetes* 1999;48:334.

25. Heiman ML, Ahima RS, Craft LS, *et al*: Leptin inhibition of the hypothalamic-pituitary-adrenal axis in response to stress. *Endocrinology* 1997;138:3859.

26. Hochol A, Nowak KW, Belloni AS, *et al*: Effects of leptin on the response of rat pituitary-adrenocortical axis to ether and cold stresses. *Endocr Res* 2000;26:129.

27. Akana SF, Strack AM, Hanson ES, *et al*: Regulation of activity in the hypothalamo-pituitary-adrenal axis is integral to a larger hypothalamic system that determines caloric flow. *Endocrinology* 1994;135: 1125.

28. Giovambattista A, Chisari AN, Gaillard RC, *et al*: Food intake-induced leptin secretion modulates hypothalamo-pituitary-adrenal axis response and hypothalamic Ob-Rb expression to insulin administration. *Neuroendocrinology* 2000;72:341.

29. Nagatani S, Thompson RC, Foster DL: Prevention of *glucoprivic* stimulation of corticosterone secretion by leptin does not restore high frequency luteinizing hormone pulses in rats. *J Neuroendocrinol* 2001;13:371.

30. Vollmer RR, Balcita JJ, Sved AF, *et al*: Adrenal epinephrine and norepinephrine release to hypoglycemia measured by microdialysis in conscious rats. *Am J Physiol* 1997;273:R1758.

31. Baum D, Porte DJ: Stress hyperglycemia and the adrenergic regulation of pancreatic hormones in hypoxia. *Metabolism* 1980;29:1176.

32. Thoresen M, Dahlin I, Lundberg JM, *et al*: Neuropeptide Y and catecholamine release in the piglet during hypoxia: enhancement by theophylline. *J Dev Physiol* 1992;18:187.

33. Metinko AP, Kunkel SL, Standiford TJ, Strieter RM: Anoxia-hyperoxia induces monocyte-derived interleukin-8. *J Clin Invest* 1992;90:791.

34. Havel PJ, Veith RC, Dunning BE, *et al*: Pancreatic noradrenergic nerves are activated by neuroglucopenia but not hypotension or hypoxia in the dog: Evidence for stress-specific and regionally-selective activation of the sympathetic nervous system. *J Clin Invest* 1988;82: 1538.

35. Baum D, Porte D, Ensinck J: Hyperglucagonemia and α-adrenergic receptor in acute hypoxia. *Am J Physiol* 1979;237:E404.

36. Baum D, Porte DJ: Beta adrenergic receptor dysfunction in hypoxic inhibition of insulin release. *Endocrinology* 1976;98:359.

37. Tuor UI, Simone CS, Arellano R, *et al*: Glucocorticoid prevention of neonatal hypoxic-ischemic damage: Role of hyperglycemia and antioxidant enzymes. *Brain Res* 1993;604:165.

38. Jarhult J, Holst JJ: Reflex adrenergic control of endocrine pancreas evoked by unloading of carotid baroreceptors in cats. *Acta Physiol Scand* 1978;104:188.

39. Zingarelli B, Squadrito F, Altavilla D, *et al*: Role of tumor necrosis factor-α in acute hypovolemic hemorrhagic shock in rats. *Am J Physiol* 1994;266:H1512.

40. Thiemermann C, Szabo C, Mitchell JA, *et al*: Vascular hyporeactivity to vasoconstrictor agents and hemodynamic decompensation in hemorrhagic shock is mediated by nitric oxide. *Proc Natl Acad Sci USA* 1993;90:267.

41. Roumen RMH, Hendriks T, van der Ven-Jongekrijg J, *et al*: Cytokine patterns in patients after major vascular surgery, hemorrhagic shock, and severe blunt trauma. *Ann Surg* 1993;218:769.

42. Savaki HE, Macpherson H, McCulloch J: Alterations in local cerebral glucose utilization during hemorrhagic hypotension in the rat. *Circ Res* 1982;50:633.

43. Jarhult J: Role of the sympatho-adrenal system in hemorrhagic hyperglycemia. *Acta Physiol Scand* 1975;93:25.

44. Cherrington AD, Stevenson RW, Steiner KE, *et al*: Insulin, glucagon, and glucose as regulators of hepatic glucose uptake and production in vivo. *Diabetes Metab Rev* 1987;3:307.

45. Andersson PO, Farnebo LO, Fredholm BB, *et al*: Metabolic and hormonal adjustments during hemorrhage in cats after interference with the sympatho-adrenal system. *Acta Physiol Scand* 1982;114:111.

46. Lilly MP, Engeland WC, Gann DS: Pituitary-adrenal responses to repeated small hemorrhage in conscious dogs. *Am J Physiol* 1986; 251:R1200.

47. Darlington DN, Chew G, Ha T, *et al*: Corticosterone, but not glucose, treatment enables fasted adrenalectomized rats to survive moderate hemorrhage. *Endocrinology* 1990;127:766.

48. Lautt WW: Afferent and efferent neural roles in liver function. *Prog Neurobiol* 1983;21:323.

49. Briand R, Yamaguchi N, Gagne J: Plasma catecholamine and glucose concentrations during hemorrhagic hypotension in anesthetized dogs. *Am J Physiol* 1989;257:R317.

50. Donovan CM, Hamilton-Wessler M, Halter JB, *et al*: Primacy of liver glucosensors in the sympathetic response to progressive hypoglycemia. *Proc Natl Acad Sci USA* 1994;91:2863.

51. Hevener AL, Bergman RN, Donovan CM: Portal vein afferents are critical for the sympathoadrenal response to hypoglycemia. *Diabetes* 2000;49:8.

52. Gerich JE: Lilly lecture 1988. Glucose counterregulation and its impact on diabetes mellitus. *Diabetes* 1988;37:1608.

53. Mundinger TO, Boyle MR, Taborsky GJ Jr: Activation of hepatic sympathetic nerves during hypoxic, hypotensive and glucopenic stress. *J Auton Nerv Syst* 1997;63:153.

54. Cersosimo E, Garlick P, Ferretti J: Renal glucose production during insulin-induced hypoglycemia in humans. *Diabetes* 1999;48:261.

55. Havel PJ, Taborsky GJ Jr.: The contribution of the autonomic nervous system to changes of glucagon and insulin secretion during hypoglycemic stress. *Endocr Rev* 1989;10:332.

56. Havel PJ, Taborsky GJ Jr.: The contribution of the autonomic nervous system to increased glucagon secretion during hypoglycemic stress: Update, 1994. *Endocr Rev Monographs* 1994;2:201.

57. Taborsky GJ Jr., Ahren B, Havel PJ: Autonomic mediation of glucagon secretion during hypoglycemia: Implications for impaired alpha-cell responses in type 1 diabetes. *Diabetes* 1998;47:995.

58. Cannon WB, McLuer MA, Bliss SW: Studies on the condition of activity in endocrine glands. XIII. A sympathetic and adrenal mechanism for mobilizing sugar in hypoglycemia. *Am J Physiol* 1924; 69:46.

59. Dunning BE, Taborsky GJ Jr: Galanin—sympathetic neurotransmitter in endocrine pancreas? *Diabetes* 1988;37:1157.

60. Havel PJ, Mundinger TO, Veith RC, *et al*: Corelease of galanin and NE from pancreatic sympathetic nerves during severe hypoglycemia in dogs. *Am J Physiol* 1992;263:E8.

61. Ahren B, Holst JJ: The cephalic insulin response to meal ingestion in humans is dependent on both cholinergic and noncholinergic mechanisms and is important for postprandial glycemia. *Diabetes* 2001;50: 1030.

62. D'Alessio DA, Kieffer TJ, Taborsky GJ, *et al*: Activation of the para-sympathetic nervous system is necessary for normal meal-induced insulin secretion in Rhesus macaques. *J Clin Endocrinol Metab* 2001; 86:1253.

63. Benthem L, Mundinger T, Taborsky G: Meal-induced insulin secretion in dogs is mediated by both branches of the autonomic nervous system. *Am J Physiol* 2000;278:E603.

64. Schwartz TW: Pancreatic polypeptide: A hormone under vagal control. *Gastroenterology* 1983;85:1411.

65. Havel PJ, Parry SJ, Curry DL, *et al*: Autonomic nervous system mediation of the pancreatic polypeptide response to insulin-induced hypoglycemia in conscious rats. *Endocrinology* 1992;130:2225.

66. Havel PJ, Akpan JO, Curry DL, *et al*: Autonomic control of pancreatic polypeptide and glucagon secretion during neuroglucopenia and hypoglycemia in mice. *Am J Physiol* 1993;265:R246.

67. Havel PJ, Valverde C: Autonomic mediation of glucagon secretion during insulin-induced hypoglycemia in rhesus monkeys. *Diabetes* 1996;45:960.

68. Havel PJ, Ahren B: Activation of autonomic nerves and the adrenal medulla contributes to increased glucagon secretion during moderate insulin-induced hypoglycemia in women. *Diabetes* 1997;46:801.

69. Palmer JP, Porte D Jr.: Neural control of glucagon secretion. In: Lefebvre PJ, ed. *Glucagon II*. Springer-Verlag:1983;115.

70. Gerich JE: Glucose in the control of glucagon secretion. In: Lefebvre PJ, ed. *Handbook of Experimental Pharmacology*. Springer-Verlag: 1983; 3.

71. Havel PJ, Veith RC, Dunning BE, *et al*: Role for autonomic nervous system to increase pancreatic glucagon secretion during marked insulin-induced hypoglycemia in dogs. *Diabetes* 1991;40:1107.

72. Borg WP, During MJ, Sherwin RS, *et al*: Ventromedial hypothalamic lesions in rats suppress counterregulatory responses to hypoglycemia. *J Clin Invest* 1994;93:1677.

73. Biggers DW, Myers SR, Neal D, *et al*: Role of brain in counterregulation of insulin-induced hypoglycemia in dogs. *Diabetes* 1989;37:7.

74. Havel PJ, Parry SJ, Stern JS, *et al*: Redundant parasympathetic and sympathoadrenal mediation of increased glucagon secretion during insulin-induced hypoglycemia in conscious rats. *Metabolism* 1994; 43:860.

75. Havel PJ, Mundinger TO, Taborsky GJ Jr: Pancreatic sympathetic nerves increase glucagon secretion during severe hypoglycemia in dogs. *Am J Physiol* 1996;270:E20.

76. Coiro V, Passeri M, Rossi G, *et al*: Effect of muscarinic and nicotinic-cholinergic blockade on the glucagon response to insulin-induced hypoglycemia in normal men. *Horm Metab Res* 1989;21:102.

77. Long RG, Albuquerque RH, Prata A, *et al*: Responses of pancreatic and gastrointestinal hormones and growth hormone to oral and intravenous glucose and insulin hypoglycemia in Chagas' disease. *Gut* 1980;21:772.

78. Sasaki K, Matsuhashi A, Murabayashi S, *et al*: Hormonal response to insulin-induced hypoglycemia in patients with Shy-Drager syndrome. *Metabolism* 1983;32:977.

79. Heller SR, Cryer PE: Reduced neuroendocrine and symptomatic responses to subsequent hypoglycemia after 1 episode of hypoglycemia in nondiabetic humans. *Diabetes* 1991;40:223.

80. Towler DA, Havlin CE, Craft S, *et al*: Mechanism of awareness of hypoglycemia: Perception of neurogenic (predominantly cholinergic) rather than neuroglycopenic symptoms. *Diabetes* 1993;42:1791.

81. Hilsted J, Frandsen H, Holst JJ, *et al*: Plasma glucagon and glucose recovery after hypoglycemia: The effect of total autonomic blockade. *Acta Endocrinol* 1991;125:466.

82. Havel PJ, Dunning BE, Verchere CB, *et al*: Evidence that vasoactive intestinal polypeptide is a parasympathetic neurotransmitter in the endocrine pancreas in dogs. *Regul Pept* 1997;71:163.

83. Gerich J, Langlois M, Noacco C, *et al*: Lack of glucagon response to hypoglycemia in diabetes: Evidence for an intrinsic pancreatic alpha cell defect. *Science* 1973;182:171.

84. Unger RH: Insulin-glucagon relationships in the defense against hypoglycemia. *Diabetes* 1983;32:575.

85. Samols E: Glucagon and insulin secretion. In: Lefebvre PJ, ed. *Handbook of Experimental Pharmacology*. Springer-Verlag:1983; 485.

86. Liu DT, Adamson UC, Lins P-ES, *et al*: Inhibitory effect of circulating insulin on glucagon secretion during hypoglycemia in type 1 diabetic patients. *Diabetes Care* 1992;15:59.

87. Fukuda M, Tanaka A, Tahara Y, *et al*: Correlation between minimal secretory capacity of pancreatic B-cells and stability of diabetic control. *Diabetes* 1988;37:81.

88. The Diabetes Control and Complications Trial Research Group: Hypoglycemia in the diabetes control and complications trial. *Diabetes* 1997;46:271.

89. Davis SN, Shavers C, Davis B, *et al*: Prevention of an increase in plasma cortisol during hypoglycemia preserves subsequent counter-regulatory responses. *J Clin Invest* 1997;100:429.

90. Powell AM, Sherwin RS, Shulman GI: Impaired hormonal responses to hypoglycemia in spontaneously diabetic and recurrently hypoglycemic rats. *J Clin Invest* 1993;92:2667.

91. Jacobs RJ, Dziura J, Morgen JP, *et al*: Time course of the defective alpha-cell response to hypoglycemia in diabetic BB rats. *Metabolism* 1996;45:1422.

92. Tominaga M, Maruyama H, Vasko MR, *et al*: Morphologic and functional changes in sympathetic nerve relationships with pancreatic alpha-cells after destruction of beta-cells in rats. *Diabetes* 1987;36:365.

93. Mei Q, Mundinger TO, Kung, D, Baskin DG, *et al*: Fos expression in rat celiac ganglia: An index of the activation of post-ganglionic sympathetic nerves: *Am J Physiol* 2001;281:E655.

94. Young JB, Landsberg L: Effect of diet and cold exposure on norepinephrine turnover in pancreas and liver. *Am J Physiol* 1979;236:E524.

95. McAlpine HM, Morton JJ, Leckie B, *et al*: Neuroendocrine activation after acute myocardial infarction. *Br Heart J* 1988;60:117.

96. Bain RJ, Fox JP, Jagger J, *et al*: Serum cortisol levels predict infarct size and patient mortality. *Int J Cardiol* 1992;37:145.

97. Donald RA, Crozier IG, Foy SG, *et al*: Plasma corticotrophin releasing hormone, vasopressin, ACTH and cortisol responses to acute myocardial infarction. *Clin Endocrinol (Oxf)* 1994;40:499.

98. Remme WJ, de Leeuw PW, Bootsma M, *et al*: Systemic neurohumoral activation and vasoconstriction during pacing-induced acute myocardial ischemia in patients with stable angina pectoris. *Am J Cardiol* 1991;68:181.

99. Spes CH, Angermann CE, Gerzer R, *et al*: Plasma hormones in patients with chronic heart failure before and early after orthotopic heart transplantation. *Z Kardiol* 1991;80:580.

100. Sigurdsson A, Held P, Swedberg K: Short- and long-term neurohormonal activation following acute myocardial infarction. *Am Heart J* 1993;126:1068.

101. Abe Y, Kawakami M, Kuroki M, *et al*: Transient rise in serum interleukin-8 concentration during acute myocardial infarction. *Br Heart J* 1993;70:132.

102. Miyao Y, Yasue H, Ogawa H, *et al*: Elevated plasma interleukin-6 levels in patients with acute myocardial infarction. *Am Heart J* 1993;126: 1299.

103. Lissoni P, Pelizzoni F, Mauri O, *et al*: Enhanced secretion of tumour necrosis factor in patients with myocardial infarction. *Eur J Med* 1992;1:277.

104. Latini R, Bianchi M, Correale E, *et al*: Cytokines in acute myocardial infarction: selective increase in circulating tumor necrosis factor, its soluble receptor, and interleukin-1 receptor antagonist. *J Cardiovasc Pharmacol* 1994;23:1.

105. Chernow B, Alexander HR, Smallridge RC, *et al*: Hormonal responses to graded surgical stress. *Arch Intern Med* 1987;147:1273.

106. Taborsky GJ Jr., Porte D Jr.: Endogenous hyperglycemia restores the insulin release impaired by somatostatin analog. *Am J Physiol* 1981; 240:E407.

107. Taborsky GJ Jr., Halter JB, Porte D Jr.: Morphine suppresses plasma catecholamine responses to laparotomy but not to 2-deoxyglucose. *Am J Physiol* 1982;252:E317.

108. Pflug AE, Halter JB: Effect of spinal anesthesia on adrenergic tone and the neuroendocrine responses to surgical stress in humans. *Anesthesiology* 1981;55:120.

109. Anand KJS, Hickey PR: Halothane-morphine compared with high-dose sufentanil for anesthesia and postoperative analgesia in neonatal cardiac surgery. *N Engl J Med* 1992;326:1.

110. Breslow MJ, Parker SD, Frank SM, *et al*: The PIRAT Study Group: Determinants of catecholamine and cortisol responses to lower extremity revascularization. *Anesthesiology* 1993;79:1202.

111. Yeager MP, Glass DD, Neff RK, *et al*: Epidural anesthesia and analgesia in high-risk surgical patients. *Anesthesiology* 1987;66:729.

112. Taborsky GJ Jr., Halter JB, Baum D, *et al*: Pentobarbital anesthesia suppresses basal and 2-deoxy-glucose stimulated plasma catecholamines. *Am J Physiol* 1984;247:R905.

113. Havel PJ, Flatness DE, Halter JB, *et al*: Halothane anesthesia does not suppress sympathetic activation produced by neuroglucopenia. *Am J Physiol* 1987;252:E667.

114. Carli F, Webster J, Nandi P, et al: Thermogenesis after surgery: Effect of perioperative heat conservation and epidural anesthesia. *Am J Physiol* 1992;263:E441.

115. Dauber IM, Parsons PE, Welsh CH, et al: Peripheral bypass-induced pulmonary and coronary vascular injury. Association with increased levels of tumor necrosis factor. *Circulation* 1993;88:726.

116. Bachmann-Mennenga B, Biscoping J, Kuhn DF, et al: Intercostal nerve block, interpleural analgesia, thoracic epidural block or systemic opioid application for pain relief after thoracotomy? *Eur J Cardiothorac Surg* 1933;7:12.

117. Spitzer JJ, Bagby GJ, Meszaros K, et al: Altered control of carbohydrate metabolism in endotoxemia. *Prog Clin Biol Res* 1989;286:145.

118. Van der Poll T, Romijn JA, Endbert E, et al: Tumor necrosis factor mimics the metabolic response to acute infection in healthy humans. *Am J Physiol* 1991;261:E457.

119. Hargrove DM, Bagby GJ, Lang CH, et al: Adrenergic blockade does not abolish elevated glucose turnover during bacterial infection. *Am J Physiol* 1988;254:E16.

120. Old LJ: Tumor necrosis factor. *Science* 1985;230:630.

121. Evans DA, Jacobs DO, Wilmore DW: Tumor necrosis factor enhances glucose uptake by peripheral tissues. *Am J Physiol* 1989;257:R1182.

122. Sakurai Y, Zhang X-J, Wolfe RR: Short-term effects of tumor necrosis factor on energy and substrate metabolism in dogs. *J Clin Invest* 1993; 91:2437.

123. Bagby GJ, Lang CH, Skrepnik N, et al: Regulation of glucose metabolism after endotoxin and during infection is largely independent of endogenous tumor necrosis factor. *Circ Shock* 1993;39:211.

124. Durkot MJ, Wolfe RR: Effects of adrenergic blockade on glucose kinetics in septic and burned guinea pigs. *Am J Physiol* 1981;241: R222.

125. Wolfe RR, Shaw JHF: Glucose and FFA kinetics in sepsis: Role of glucagon and sympathetic nervous system activity. *Am J Physiol* 1985;248:E236.

126. Beutler B, Milsark IW, Cerami AC: Passive immunization against cachectin/tumor necrosis factor protects mice from lethal effect of endotoxin. *Science* 1985;229:869.

127. Vaughan GM, Becker RA, Unger RH: Nonthyroidal control of metabolism after burn injury: Possible role of glucagon. *Metabolism* 1985; 34:637.

128. Jahoor F, Herndon DN, Wolfe RR: Role of insulin and glucagon in the response of glucose and alanine kinetics in burn-injured patients. *J Clin Invest* 1986;78:807.

129. Jeffries MK, Vance ML: Growth hormone and cortisol secretion in patients with burn injury. *J Burn Care Rehabil* 1992;13:391.

130. Lang C, Dobrescu C: Attenuation of burn-induced changes in hemodynamics and glucose metabolism by the PAF antagonist SRI 63-675. *Eur J Pharmacol* 1988;156:207.

131. Kowal VA, Walenga JM, Hoppensteadt D, et al: Interleukin-2 and interleukin-6 in relation to burn wound size in the acute phase of thermal injury. *J Am Coll Surg* 1994;178:357.

132. de Brandt JP, Chollet-Martin S, Hernvann A, et al: Cytokine response to burn injury: Relationship with protein metabolism. *World J Surg* 1994;16:30.

133. Ziegler TR, Young LS, Ferrari-Baliveriera E, et al: Use of human growth hormone combined with nutritional support in a critical care unit. *J Parenter Enteral Nutr* 1990;14:574.

134. Herndon DN, Barrow RE, Kunkel KR, et al: Effects of recombinant human growth hormone on donor-site healing in severely burned children. *Ann Surg* 1990;212:424.

135. Gore DC, Honeycutt D, Jahoor F, et al: Effects of exogenous growth hormone on whole-body and isolated-limb protein kinetics in burned patients. *Arch Surg* 1991;126:38.

136. Kido DK, Cox C, Hamill RW, et al: Traumatic brain injuries: Predictive usefulness of CT. *Radiology* 1992;182:777.

137. Woolf PD, McDonald JV, Feliciano DV, et al: The catecholamine response to multisystem trauma. *Arch Surg* 1992;127:899.

138. Jeevanandam M, Ramias L, Shamos RF, et al: Decreased growth hormone levels in the catabolic phase of severe injury. *Surgery* 1992; 111:495.

139. Meguid MM, Brennan MF, Aoki TT, et al: Hormone-substrate interrelationships following trauma. *Arch Surg* 1974;109:776.

140. Margulies DR, Hiatt JR, Vinson D Jr, et al: Relationship of hyperglycemia and severity of illness to neurologic outcome in head injury patients. *Am Surg* 1994;60:387.

141. Bessey PQ, Lowe KA: Early hormonal changes affect the catabolic response to trauma. *Ann Surg* 1993;218:476, discussion 489.

142. Porte D Jr, Robertson RP: Control of insulin secretion by catecholamines, stress, and the sympathetic nervous system. *Fed Proc* 1973;32:1792.

143. Waldhausl W, Kleinberger G, Korn A, et al: Severe hyperglycemia: Effects of rehydration on endocrine derangements and blood glucose concentration. *Diabetes* 1979;28:577.

144. Porte D Jr: Sympathetic regulation of insulin secretion and its relation to diabetes mellitus. *Arch Int Med* 1969;123:252.

145. Baker L, Barcai A, Kaye R, et al: Beta adrenergic blockade and juvenile diabetes: Acute studies and long-term therapeutic trial. Evidence for the role of catecholamines in mediating diabetic decompensation following emotional arousal. *J Pediatrics* 1969;75:19.

146. Shamoon H, Hendler R, Sherwin RS: Altered responsiveness to cortisol, epinephrine, and glucagon in insulin-infused juvenile-onset diabetics. A mechanism for diabetic instability. *Diabetes* 1980;29: 284.

147. Palmer J, Lernmark A: Pathophysiology of type I (insulin-dependent) diabetes. In: Rifkin JH, Porte D, eds. *Diabetes Mellitus, Theory and Practice.* Elsevier:1990;414.

148. Tarn AC, Smith CP, Spenser KM, et al: Type I (insulin-dependent) diabetes: A disease of slow clinical onset? *Br Med J* 1987;294:342.

149. Srikanta S, Ganda OP, Gleason RE, et al: Pre-type I diabetes: Linear loss of beta cell response to intravenous glucose. *Diabetes* 1984;33: 717.

150. Nerup J, Mandrup-Poulson T, Molvig J, et al: Mechanisms of pancreatic β-cell destruction in type I diabetes. *Diabetes Care* 1988;11:16.

151. Taborsky GJJ, Porte DJ: Stress-induced hyperglicemia and its relation to diabetes mellitus. In: Brown MR, Koob GF, Rivier C, eds. *Stress: Neurobiology and Neuroendocrinology.* Marcel Dekker:1991;519.

152. Bradley LM, Mishell RI: Differential effects of glucocorticosteroids on the functions of helper and suppressor T lymphocytes. *Proc Natl Acad Sci USA* 1981;78:3155.

153. Mazelis AG, Albert D, Crisa C, et al: Relationship of stressful housing conditions to the onset of diabetes mellitus induced by multiple, subdiabetogenic doses of streptozotocin in mice. *Diabetes Res* 1987;6: 195.

154. Harada M, Makino S: Promotion of spontaneous diabetes in nonobese diabetes-prone mice by cyclophosphamide. *Diabetologia* 1982;27: 604.

155. Juenaga K, Yoon JW: Association of β-cell specific expression of endogenous retrovirus with development of insulitis and diabetes in NOD mouse. *Diabetes* 1988;37:1722.

156. Charlton B, Bacelj A, Slattery RM, et al: Evidence for suppression in spontaneous autoimmune diabetes mellitus. *Diabetes* 1989;38:441.

157. Wolfe RR: Acute versus chronic response to burn injury. *Circ Shock* 1981;8:105.

158. Spinas GA, Palmer JP, Mandrup-Poulsen T, et al: The bimodal effect of interleukin-1 on rat pancreatic beta-cells—stimulation followed by inhibition—depends upon dose, duration of exposure and ambient glucose concentration. *Diabetologia* 1988;31:168.

159. West DB, Seino Y, Woods SC, et al: Ventromedial hypothalamic lesions increase pancreatic sensitivity to streptozotocin in rats. *Diabetes* 1980;29:948.

160. Block CA, Paed FC, Clemons SAP, et al: Puberty decreases insulin sensitivity. *J Pediatr* 1987;110:481.

161. Capponi R, Kawanda ME, Varela C, et al: Diabetes mellitus by repeated stress in rats bearing chemical diabetes. *Horm Metab Res* 1980;12:411.

162. Robinson N, Fuller JH: Role of life events and difficulties in the onset of diabetes mellitus. *J Psychol Res* 1985;29:583.

163. Pfeifer MA, Halter JB, Porte DJ: Insulin secretion in diabetes mellitus. *Am J Med* 1981;70:579.

164. Halter JB, Porte DJ: Current concepts of insulin secretion. In: Rifkin HAR, Bowie P, eds. *Diabetes Mellitus: Diagnosis and Treatment.* Robert J. Brady Co.:1981;33.

165. Halter JB, Beard JC, Porte DJ: Islet function and stress hyperglycemia: Plasma glucose and epinephrine interaction. *Am J Physiol* 1984;247: E47.

166. Bruce DG, Chisholm DJ, Storlien LH, et al: The effects of sympathetic nervous system activation and psychological stress on glucose metabolism and blood pressure in subjects with type 2 (non-insulin-dependent) diabetes mellitus. *Diabetologia* 1992;35:835.

167. Goetsch VL, Van Dorsten B, Pbert LA, *et al*: Acute effects of laboratory stress on blood glucose in noninsulin-dependent diabetes. *Psychosom Med* 1993;55:492.

168. Porte DJ, Robertson RP, Halter JB, *et al*: Neuroendocrine recognition of glucose: The glucoreceptor hypothesis and the diabetic syndrome. In: Katsuki Y, Sato M, Takagi SF, eds. *International Symposium on Food Intake and Chemical Senses*. University of Tokyo Press:1977; 331.

169. Robertson RP, Halter JB, Porte D Jr: A role for alpha adrenergic receptors in abnormal insulin secretion in diabetes mellitus. *J Clin Invest* 1976;57:791.

170. Dunning BE, Ahren B, Veith RC, *et al*: Galanin: A novel pancreatic neuropeptide. *Am J Physiol* 1986;251:E127.

171. Surwit RS, Feinglos MN: Stress and autonomic nervous system in type II diabetes: A hypothesis. *Diabetes Care* 1988;11:83.

172. Opie LH, Stubbs WA: Carbohydrate metabolism in cardiovascular disease. *Clin Endocrinol Metab* 1976;5:703.

173. Rogers WJ, Stanley AW Jr, Breinig JB, *et al*: Reduction of hospital mortality rate of acute myocardial infarction with glucose-insulin-potassium infusion. *Am Heart J* 1976;92:441.

174. Goetsch VL, Wiebe DJ, Veltum LG, *et al*: Stress and blood glucose in type II diabetes mellitus. *Behav Res Ther* 1990;28:531.

Food Intake and Energy Balance

Stephen C. Woods

Randy J. Seeley

Denis G. Baskin

Michael W. Schwartz

INTRODUCTION

Over the past two decades, knowledge of the biological controls of eating and the regulation of body adiposity has advanced at an unprecedented pace. This denouement of sorts is due in part to technological innovations that enable us to probe the workings of individual cells and molecules, as well as to an enormous investment of funds for basic research by government and industry. While this explosion of new information may one day lead to novel therapeutic approaches that limit energy intake[1-7] and thereby lower body weight, the prevalence of obesity continues to increase in spite of this wealth of new information, as does the incidence of obesity-related health consequences including non-insulin-dependent diabetes mellitus or type 2 diabetes mellitus (T2DM).[4] Our intent in this chapter is to summarize and discuss what is new and exciting in the realm of the neuroendocrine control of energy homeostasis, focusing on food intake, and to suggest avenues for novel therapeutic strategies.

FOOD INTAKE

Food intake is a complex behavior with multiple levels and kinds of regulatory control.[8] In addition to providing the calories necessary to enable the body to grow and function, food also provides appropriate micronutrients (vitamins and minerals), macronutrients (carbohydrates, fats, and proteins), and a certain amount of water. Food intake occurs in distinct bouts or meals, and different controllers influence the onset and the offset of meals. Food intake addresses acute energy needs as well as long-term energy storage as fat depots. Finally, whereas regulation of food intake is related directly to energy or caloric homeostasis, food intake is also influenced by other kinds of needs. For example, when individuals are ill or incapacitated, or preoccupied with other behaviors, they often eat less food despite the stimulus of reduced fat or reduced fat stores. The integration of all of these needs relies upon neural and hormonal signals arising in many sites within the body and impinging upon regulatory control areas of the brain. As discussed below, many signals important in the regulation of blood glucose are also critical to the regulation of energy intake. In this chapter, we focus first on the control of individual meal initiation and cessation, and later on the complex array of neuropeptides (as well as other neurotransmitters) thought to be important in the overall regulation of energy stores.

MEALS

Most animals, including humans, adopt an eating schedule that accommodates their idiosyncratic environmental conditions. In most individuals, distinct patterns can be discerned (e.g., consuming three meals a day, at the same time each day). However, because obligatory activities (such as working or going to school) and constraints (the probable presence of predators at certain times of day for some species) vary widely among individuals, most adapt by developing unique eating patterns (the size and timing of meals) that provide necessary nutrients and otherwise optimize fitness.[9] In spite of this variation among individuals, most members of a species develop and maintain a rather consistent body weight as adults,[10-12] and this is also true of humans. The control system that allows meal patterns to vary while adjusting daily caloric intake to meet energy needs and maintain body weight is elegant. A key feature is that whereas meal size has been found to be controlled by physiologic signals important in energy homeostasis, meal onset has not (see below). Hence, meals can be initiated at times that are convenient, or that have proven successful in the past, or that are imposed by the environment, and the individual is still able to obtain and eat adequate calories each day to maintain his or her weight. The explanation, as documented below, is that if an individual's weight begins to decrease slightly, he or she will eat larger meals when the opportunity arises and thereby regain lost weight by increasing meal size. Conversely, an individual whose weight begins to increase due to overconsumption of food will tend to eat smaller meals until the increment is lost.

Meal Initiation

Historically, the prevailing belief was that meal initiation (and perhaps its subjective analogue, hunger) is regulated by important changes in key metabolic parameters. Early in the 20th century, Cannon and his colleagues postulated that contractions of the stomach signaled dwindling energy supplies and compelled an individual to seek and eat food.[13] The concept of "hunger pangs" emanating from the stomach has considerable face validity and has persisted in common parlance in spite of a wealth of evidence indicating that, if anything, signals related to gastric contractions are more numerous and robust after rather than before meals. Further, individuals who are incapable of sensing stomach contractions experience normal hunger and meal initiation. Perhaps the most popular belief concerning the cause of meal initiation was based on Jean Mayer's glucostatic hypothesis. Early in this century blood glucose was thought to be a critical determinant of meals,[14] and this concept was formalized and popularized by Mayer.[15,16] In its original version, the glucostatic hypothesis stated that hunger and eating are initiated when blood glucose decreases to a threshold level, and meals are terminated when blood glucose returns to a higher and hence safer level. Later versions of the hypothesis recognized the fact that individuals with type 1 diabetes mellitus (T1DM) have both elevated blood glucose and hunger and food intake. Hence the predominant incarnation of the hypothesis is that meal onset and offset are determined by the level of metabolic utilization of glucose by sensory cells located in the hypothalamus. These glucose-sensing cells were postulated by Mayer to be insulin sensitive. It is now recognized that there are glucose-sensitive neurons in many places in the brain, including the hypothalamus, and that some of these in turn are in fact also sensitive to insulin.[17] Recent evidence also indicates that the level of circulating glucose is detected by sensory nerves located in the hepatic portal vein and that the signal is relayed to the brain via the vagus nerves.[18]

It is reasonable to speculate that the tendency to take food would be linked causally to the ebb and flow of metabolic fuels in the blood. That is, when readily available energy becomes relatively depleted from the blood, potentially threatening the ongoing nourishment of critical tissues, eating is initiated and the circulating energy supply becomes repleted. "Depletion-repletion" logic has been applied successfully to the understanding of water and salt ingestion as they apply to the maintenance of blood volume.[19,20] A key point, however, is that under usual circumstances, the supply of energy in the blood does not decrease to anywhere near the threshold necessary to trigger eating. Rather, individuals initiate meals even though ample energy is readily available. It is true that if the amount of energy derived from glucose is greatly decreased, either by drugs that deplete it from the blood (exogenous insulin[21–23]) or drugs that prevent its cellular oxidation (e.g., 2-deoxy-D-glucose, or 2-DG[21,24]), an emergency situation occurs as the brain detects its requisite fuel supply dwindling. One result is that animals seek and ingest food.[25] Likewise, if fat utilization is experimentally compromised,[26,27] the source of usable fuel by the liver is challenged, the liver sends critical neural messages to the brain, and animals also seek and ingest food.[25,28]

Several observations argue against the notion that meals are triggered in response to depletion of metabolic substrates. Eating is in fact a relatively inefficient way to get calories into the blood rapidly. Unless pure glucose is available (rare in natural settings), foods must be processed and digested in the stomach, passed to the intestine where they are further processed, and then absorbed into the blood. When the glucose supply to the brain is compromised by administering insulin or 2-DG systemically, the initial response is increased glucagon and epinephrine secretion.[29] Hence the first line of defense is to mobilize stored carbohydrate. Eating also occurs, but after a considerable lag.[21] In this light, the induced eating can be considered more as a hedge against future excursions of

hypoglycemia than as a means of reversing the present one. It also seems maladaptive to require an individual to attain dangerously low levels of glucose prior to the initiation of every meal, nor is it clear what the consequences would be if glucose availability dipped to the threshold for initiating meals at a time when it was inconvenient or impossible to eat. It is now generally recognized that this protective system is probably activated to the point of initiating a meal only in extreme metabolic emergencies rather than as part of normal food intake regulation.[21,25,30]

In spite of the contrary evidence, the glucostatic hypothesis has enjoyed tremendous popularity over the years. Renewed interest in the hypothesis arose when it became possible to monitor blood glucose continuously by means of an indwelling intravenous catheter. Using this technique, Campfield and Smith[31,32] observed that blood glucose starts decreasing beginning a few minutes prior to the initiation of "spontaneous" meals in freely feeding rats. More recently the same researchers reported a similar phenomenon in humans.[33] This is an important observation because, at least in rats, every observed spontaneous meal was preceded by the small (approximately 12%) but reliable decline of plasma glucose.[34] The premeal decline of blood glucose reverses just prior to the actual initiation of eating, and if food is removed at that point (and no eating occurs), glucose returns to the baseline that was present before the decline began. Campfield and Smith have interpreted the premeal glucose decline as providing a signal that is monitored by the brain.[32,35,36] When the parameters of the decline are "correct," a meal is initiated. If metabolic conditions preclude the decline meeting the "correct" parametric criteria, no meal is initiated. In their schema, Campfield and Smith believe that the brain is the initiator of the decline of plasma glucose. Consistent with this, there is a small increase of plasma insulin at the start of the premeal decline of glucose which is dependent on an intact vagus nerve,[31,32] and cutting the vagus disrupts the relationship between changes of glucose and the start of meals.[35] This body of research suggests that small, physiological fluctuations of glucose can provide important signals that the brain uses to help determine ingestive responses.

Analogous to decreases of blood glucose, other metabolic events occur prior to, and hence are predictive of, the onset of meals. Implanted thermistors allow body temperature to be monitored continuously in freely moving and feeding animals. Just prior to spontaneous meals, the body temperature of rats begins to increase.[37] When the meal begins, temperature continues to increase and then declines as the meal is terminated. Likewise, metabolic rate as assessed by indirect calorimetry reportedly decreases prior to the start of spontaneous meals, and increases as eating begins.[38,39] All of these parameters (blood glucose, temperature, metabolic rate, and no doubt others as well) begin a gradual change 10–15 minutes before meals begin, and all are therefore highly correlated with meal onset. With a slightly different time course, laboratory rats increase their activity (e.g., running in a wheel) prior to spontaneous meals.[40–43] These phenomena have generally been viewed as supporting the hypothesis that animals eat because these changes are occurring; i.e., that the decrease of blood glucose or of metabolic rate, or the exercise-induced use of fuels, is causally related to meal onset. However, a compelling case can also be made that, based on factors such as habit or opportunity, other factors determine when a meal is going to start, and that as part of the overall meal initiation process the brain elicits metabolic changes to prepare the body to receive the food.[44,45] As an example, a premeal decline of blood glucose can limit the magnitude of the otherwise much larger postprandial increase of blood glucose.

In this schema, individuals do not initiate meals because one or another tissue's supply of available energy is about to be compromised, but rather one eats in response to learned cues and various environmental or sensory stimuli. The timing of meals can therefore be quite idiosyncratic and dictated by an individual's lifestyle, convenience, and opportunity. This schema can account for the extreme variability of meal patterns among individuals in a society, but it cannot in itself account for the remarkable ability of individuals to maintain neutral energy balance and a constant level of adiposity.

To summarize, although it is possible that meal-related fluctuations in blood glucose and other parameters are the initiators and terminators of meals, the bulk of evidence is to the contrary. The brain and liver are quite efficient at controlling the provision of what is needed by various tissues, and as a result adequate amounts of utilizable fuels (glucose and fats) are generally always available to tissues via the blood. Major fluctuations in the circulating levels of these fuels generally occur only during and after meals, as ingested energy passes from the gut into the circulation, and from the circulation into tissues and energy storage organs. Decreases of plasma fuels below levels adequate to meet tissue requirements are rare in normal, free-feeding individuals, although they can be experimentally induced. Under usual circumstances, therefore, neither meal initiation nor meal termination is likely to occur as a response to fluctuations of metabolic fuels. Rather, meal initiation is based on idiosyncratic factors (such as habit and convenience) and meal termination is based, at least in part, on gastrointestinal peptides secreted during the ingestion of food, as discussed below.

Meal Termination

As ingested food interacts with receptors in the gastrointestinal tract, it elicits the secretion of enzymes and generates neural and hormonal signals that help orchestrate the digestive process and customize it to the contents of the meal that is being consumed. In the early 1970s, Gibbs and colleagues provided the first solid evidence that some of these same signals originating in the gut additionally provide information to the brain that helps determine when the meal will end.[46] Specifically, they found that when the gut peptide cholecystokinin (CCK) is administered to animals prior to a meal, the animals eat less food, with larger doses of CCK causing greater suppression of meal size. This basic phenomenon has been replicated in dozens of labs using many species (including humans),[47,48] and it can be elicited by doses of CCK that do not cause signs of illness or malaise in animals or humans.[47,48] After receiving CCK, humans report that they stop eating sooner because they feel full.

As potent and selective agonists and antagonists to CCK receptors became available, two important new findings emerged. The first is that CCK acts uniquely at the CCK-A receptor to reduce meal size.[49–51] Consistent with this, when antagonists to the CCK-A receptor are administered prior to a meal, individuals eat larger meals.[49,50] This key observation implies that endogenous CCK normally contributes to the termination of meals, and it further suggests that when exogenous CCK is administered, it combines with endogenously secreted CCK to terminate the meal prematurely. The second finding is that CCK combines with other factors that limit meal size, such as gastric distension, in a synergistic manner. Hence the ability of a small dose of exogenous CCK to reduce meal size is greatly enhanced when the stomach is slightly distended.[52,53] This observation is presumably related to the fact that

many individual sensory nerve fibers passing from the stomach and intestine to the central nervous system express more than one kind of sensory ending.[54] The possibility that one branch of a sensory neuron is sensitive to molecules such as CCK, whereas another branch of the same neuron is sensitive to stomach distension, can thus be considered. There is in fact evidence that isolated sensory axons integrate information from both CCK and gastric distension,[52,53] and that the integrity of these axons (that travel in the vagus nerve) is essential for the ability of exogenous CCK to reduce meal size.[55,56]

CCK is but one of several peptides secreted from the gut during a meal that reduces meal size. Others include members of the bombesin family of peptides (bombesin, gastrin-related peptide [GRP], and neuromedin-B),[48,57] glucagon,[58] somatostatin,[59] enterostatin,[60,61] and apolipoprotein A-IV.[62,63] For many of these, administration of the appropriate antagonists or antibodies causes increased meal size, implying that these peptides contribute to the termination of normal meals (see reference 64). This is important because humans (as well as rats, the species in which meal size has been most extensively investigated) are general omnivores and will eat a broad spectrum of foods. The specific cocktail of peptides secreted from the gut that helps mediate the digestion and absorption of each meal can vary considerably since the various peptides are differentially responsive to different mixes or amounts of specific macro- and micronutrients. Signals comprised of combinations of peptides that gradually accumulate and stop the meal would be especially functional for omnivores. Accordingly, combinations of CCK and bombesin,[65] and of CCK and glucagon,[66] have been reported to interact to reduce meal size in rats.

In addition to those peptides secreted by the gut during meals that help to determine when meals end, the pancreatic hormone amylin (also known as islet amyloid polypeptide [IAPP]) also serves this function. Amylin is cosecreted with insulin in response to glucose and other nutrients, and, like insulin, its levels in the blood are directly proportional to body fat content.[67–69] Also like insulin, amylin is rapidly and efficiently transported through the blood-brain barrier into the brain,[70,71] where it interacts with receptors in the hypothalamus and area postrema of the brain stem.[72–74] In the periphery, amylin is a potent inhibitor of gastric emptying.[75] The systemic administration of exogenous amylin causes a dose-dependent decrease of food intake and body weight,[76–79] and amylin-deficient knockout mice weigh more than wild-type controls.[80] When administered directly into the brain, amylin decreases food intake and body weight at doses far lower than are required when it is given systemically. These data are consistent with the hypothesis that amylin has a central site of action.[81] Like both insulin and leptin, amylin reduces food intake without making animals ill,[82,83] and the central administration of insulin plus amylin causes a synergistic reduction of food intake.[84] Therefore, both intestinal (e.g., CCK and others) and pancreatic (e.g., amylin) are secreted during meals and contribute to satiety. Presumably all of these signals relay information to the brain that is related to the caloric content and make-up of food presented to the intestines during a meal. Importantly, low levels of amylin and CCK combine synergistically to reduce meal size,[85] suggesting that all of these meal-related signals interact in controlling food intake and the subjective sensation of feeling full after a meal.

In summary, evidence suggests that under normal circumstances, the physiological controls over meals are directed mainly at meal offset rather than onset. Individuals are therefore able to adapt to a wide range of environments and consequently to accommodate imposed constraints as to when meals will occur. Ingestion of sufficient nutrients, and maintenance of appropriate levels of stored fat, is assured via regulation of how much is consumed once a meal begins. Several gut peptides secreted during the digestion and absorption of meals function as signals to the brain and act to limit meal size.

EATING AND THE REGULATION OF BODY WEIGHT

A strong interrelationship exists between body fat stores (adiposity) and food intake. All things being equal, consuming more than sufficient calories to maintain weight each day leads to increased stored energy and vice versa. Forced or voluntary overeating for several days elicits weight gain as inevitably as dieting or food restriction elicits weight loss (Fig. 10-1). In this light, body weight (mainly body adiposity) can be considered to be at the mercy of food intake. The other side of the same coin, however, is equally relevant to understanding the relationship between food intake and body fuel stores. For example, when an otherwise weight-stable adult eats insufficient food for a period of time and consequently loses weight, he or she will likely overeat when ample food once again becomes available (or when the enthusiasm for dieting wanes). Likewise, if an individual consumes excess calories to the point of weight gain for a prolonged interval, there will be an increasing tendency to eat less food and thus help return body weight and body fat stores to their preintervention levels. Viewed in this light, food intake would seem to be controlled by the amount of stored body fat. There are many reviews of these phenomena.[10,86–90] Understanding the causal factors that interrelate food intake and body adiposity is an important goal and the subject of considerable ongoing research.

The link between body fat and food intake was formalized a half century ago when Kennedy postulated that signals propor-

FIGURE 10-1. Weight-matched rats were divided into three groups. Overfed and restricted rats received three meals per day by gavage to achieve body weights that were significantly above or below, respectively, those of ad lib-fed controls. After 140 days, the gavage feeding was discontinued and all three groups had ad lib food. The formerly overfed rats stopped eating for several days, whereas the formerly restricted rats became hyperphagic. Within 2 weeks, the weights of all 3 groups had converged and were not statistically different from one another. This is an example of long-term regulation of body weight. (*Redrawn from Bernstein* et al.[204])

tional to body fat influence the control of appetite and feeding by the brain.[91] Thus Kennedy's lipostatic hypothesis stated that adiposity is regulated by a negative feedback system in which food intake is controlled in part by the amount of total stored body fat. While the existence of a link between energy intake and body energy stores has never been questioned, an important issue over the intervening years has been the nature of the signal or signals that indicate how much fat is present in the body. Because body fat is located in multiple storage depots dispersed widely throughout the body, several possibilities exist by which body fat might be monitored by the brain. For example, sensory nerves could innervate and hence provide information from each fat depot, with the accumulated information from multiple sites integrated within the brain into a reliable "total adiposity" signal. Although this is plausible in principle, adipose tissue is only sparsely innervated, and the majority of the fibers innervating fat depots are motor, controlling the release of stored energy when it is acutely needed. A second possibility is that a single fat depot is sufficiently representative of all of the others that it serves as a bellwether of sorts. In this schema, the brain need only receive a signal from this sentinel depot. Such a depot could theoretically be located anywhere, including within the brain itself. Pursuing this possibility, Nicolaidis and his colleagues have hypothesized that specialized cells within the hypothalamus serve this function and are ideally situated to influence all aspects of energy homeostasis.[38,39] Unlike other brain cells, this "adipose-tissue homunculus" is postulated to function analogously to peripheral adipocytes and therefore to be sensitive to insulin. In point of fact, cells in the ventral hypothalamus have been found to be insulin-sensitive in that their electrical activity varies with the local application of insulin and other metabolic signals.[17,92] More recently, neurons specifically sensitive to intracellular levels of malonyl CoA as a metabolic signal have been proposed. Malonyl CoA is a precursor for fatty-acid synthesis and its levels increase following inhibition of the enzyme fatty-acid synthase. Consistent with this hypothesis, fatty-acid synthase inhibitors potently reduce food intake, apparently via a mechanism whereby brain levels of malonyl CoA are increased.[93] There is also evidence for an energy homunculus being located in the liver (or at least within the influence of the hepatic branches of the vagus nerves).[28,94] While there seems little doubt that signals related both to stored energy and to ongoing energy utilization can arise in both the brain and the liver (and presumably other tissues as well), it is not clear how much they contribute to the control of meals. Further, there is compelling evidence for a third signaling pathway, one with a strong influence on overall energy homeostasis, that utilizes hormones secreted in the periphery in proportion to the total amount of fat in the body.

Circulating Adiposity Signals

When two experimental animals are joined surgically at the flank such that a small proportion of the circulation exchanges between them (termed parabiotic animals), the existence of circulating adiposity signals is revealed. In a typical such experiment, two otherwise normal animals with similar body weight (either two lean or two obese rats or mice) are parabiotically joined. In this situation, each animal eats normally and maintains its customary (presurgical) body weight. These control experiments indicate that the parabiotic procedure itself is tolerated and that both normal-weight and obese animals can still maintain their body weight. Contrary to this, when an obese animal is parabiotically joined with a lean part-

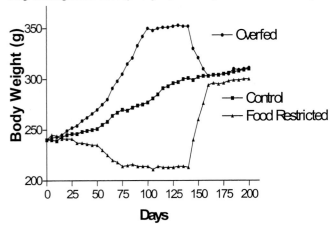

ner, their respective body weights diverge rather than converging. The obese partner often gains a little weight, but the dramatic effect occurs with the lean partner, which may stop eating all together and which loses body weight precipitously.[95] Unless the two partners are separated, the lean animal might starve itself to death. Such experiments have been interpreted to indicate that a circulating signal proportional to body fat passes between the two parabiotic partners. The relatively high titer of the signal entering the lean animal from its obese partner is hypothesized to provide a false message that too much fat exists in the lean animal's body. The lean animal consequently responds to this increased signal by reducing its food intake and losing weight. Hence a circulating signal can have a powerful influence over eating behavior, and an important implication of this is that the administration of the exogenous signal can effectively elicit weight loss.

The best candidates for circulating indicators of body fat are several peptide hormones that are secreted from peripheral organs in proportion to body adiposity and that are transported into the brain from the circulation. The two most investigated are leptin, which is secreted from adipose tissue, and insulin, which is secreted from the β cells of the pancreas. Both are synthesized and secreted in direct proportion to the amount of fat in the body. In the section below, we review the evidence that each of these peptides satisfies criteria for being an adiposity signal to the brain.

Insulin as an Adiposity Signal

To be considered an adiposity signal, a compound should be secreted in proportion to body fat, should have access to appropriate areas of the nervous system, and should influence food intake and body weight in predictable ways.[11,90,96,97] Insulin was the first hormone proven to have these properties (see reviews in references 98 and 99). Insulin is, of course, the body's predominant controller of blood glucose, and its secretion from the pancreas is controlled in large part by ambient glucose. Nonetheless, the responsiveness of the β cells to glucose (and to most other secretagogues as well) is proportional to body fat.[100–102] A fatter individual has higher basal insulin and secretes proportionally more insulin to a given increase of blood glucose than does a lean individual. Hence, plasma insulin reflects both acute metabolic needs as well as body fat content. Circulating insulin gains direct access to areas of the brain with a reduced blood-brain barrier (such as the circumventricular organs). Perhaps more importantly, brain capillary endothelial cells contain insulin receptors, and insulin penetrates into the brain from the blood via a receptor-mediated, intracellular transport process (see reviews in references 99, 103, and 104). Hence, circulating insulin has access to neurons and glial cells throughout the brain.

Insulin receptors are expressed in brain regions important in the control of energy homeostasis such as the ventral hypothalamus.[105–108] Insulin receptors are also expressed in other brain regions (e.g., the olfactory bulbs and the hippocampus) where their function is less well understood. Within the hypothalamus, the arcuate nuclei (ARC) have particularly high densities of insulin receptors, and the ARC is the location of at least two major types of neurons that potently influence food intake (see below). Hence these cells have the capacity to detect and respond to insulin and are therefore also indirectly sensitive to body adiposity.

When exogenous insulin is administered directly into the brain (into the ARC itself, into nearby ventral hypothalamus, or into the cerebrospinal fluid in the adjacent third ventricle), animals behave as if they are overweight (i.e., they eat less food and lose weight)

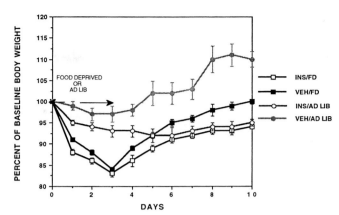

FIGURE 10-2. Weight-matched rats were divided into four groups, two being food restricted for days 1 through 3 and the other two having ad lib food. All four groups had ad lib food after day 3. One of the restricted groups and one of the ad lib-fed groups received insulin (10 mU/d) infusion into the third cerebral ventricle throughout via osmotic minipumps (**INS/FD; INS/AD LIB**); the other restricted and ad lib-fed groups received a third ventricular infusion of physiological saline (**VEH/FD; VEH/AD LIB**). The ad lib-fed rats receiving saline gained weight over the 10 days of the experiment, whereas the ad lib-fed rats receiving insulin ate less food and lost weight. Both restricted groups lost weight over the 3 days without food, and those getting insulin lost significantly more weight after 1 and 2 days. When food was returned at the end of the third day, both groups were significantly hyperphagic. However, the formerly restricted rats getting insulin ate only enough to reach the same body weight plateau as the other insulin group, whereas the formerly restricted rats receiving saline gained more weight and were approaching the weight of the other saline group by the end of the experiment. Hence rats receiving insulin into the brain ended up at a lower body weight than saline-infused controls, and they achieved the same absolute weights whether they had to eat less (nonrestricted group) or more (restricted group) to achieve it. *(Reproduced from Chavez et al.[123])*

(Fig. 10-2).[109–114] This response develops over several hours and is proportional to the amount of insulin administered. Conversely, when local concentrations of insulin are reduced (by administering antibodies to insulin into the brain), animals eat more food[115] and gain weight.[116] Consistent with these observations, mice with targeted deletion of the insulin receptor in neuronal tissue have enhanced food intake and body weight gain, particularly on a high-fat diet.[117] Recent data suggest that insulin's neuronal effects involve downstream molecules such as the product of the *tubby* gene (Tub) and IRS-2 since activation of insulin receptors phosphorylates these proteins, and since mice with genetic alterations of these proteins have obese phenotypes.[118,119]

These findings support the hypothesis that insulin is an adiposity signal to the brain. A key prediction of this hypothesis is that an experimentally-induced elevation of plasma insulin should result in a decrease of food intake since brain insulin would be anticipated to increase secondarily and proportionally to the increment in the blood. This has been difficult to investigate in a simple way, because when plasma insulin is experimentally increased, it causes a rapid decrease in blood glucose (and frank hypoglycemia), which itself causes animals to eat more food.[22,23,30] This scenario of an increase of plasma insulin in the absence of an *a priori* increase of plasma glucose would not normally occur. Rather, elevations of endogenous insulin typically occur in response to already elevated blood glucose, and function to reduce glucose to normal levels as opposed to eliciting hypoglycemia. When circulating insulin is experimentally elevated and hypoglycemia is circumvented, animals eat less food.[120-122] Conversely, conditions associated with low circulating insulin (e.g., fasting and uncontrolled T1DM) are associated with hyperphagia. These observations support the hypothesis that insulin's effects in the brain and in peripheral tissues oppose one another where energy homeostasis is concerned. Thus, whereas systemically-acting insulin promotes fat deposition, centrally-acting insulin functions as an adiposity signal that limits weight gain. Moreover, insulin-induced weight loss is not due to toxic or aversive effects, since when it is administered into the brain at doses that reduce food intake and body weight, the animals are neither ill nor incapacitated. Rather, they act as if they are maintaining and defending a lower body weight.[123,124] This collective evidence implicates insulin as an adiposity signal to the brain.

Leptin as an Adiposity Signal

Although its existence was inferred from experiments done over 25 years ago on parabiotic mice,[125] leptin was not discovered and described until 1994.[126] Leptin is secreted from adipocytes in direct proportion to the amount of stored fat[127,128] via a mechanism that is sensitive to ongoing metabolic activity of fat cells, in addition to fat content *per se*.[129,130] Hence dissociations can occur between stored fat and leptin release, particularly when there is a rapid decrease of adipocyte glucose metabolism such as occurs in fasting.[131-133] In such instances, plasma leptin decreases more rapidly and to a greater degree than does body fat, but among individuals in neutral energy balance, plasma leptin levels are a reliable indicator of body fat content. As is the case with insulin, circulating leptin is transported through the blood-brain barrier into the brain,[134-138] and leptin receptors are located within the ARC and other nuclei in the ventral hypothalamus (among several other regions).[139,140] Systemic administration of leptin decreases food intake and body weight in rodent models[141-143] and in leptin-deficient humans.[144] The finding that the dose needed to reduce food intake is much lower when leptin is administered into the brain ventricles than into systemic circulation[141,143] implicates the brain as a key target of leptin action (Fig. 10-3). Moreover,

FIGURE 10-3. Rats were administered leptin (3.5 μg) or its vehicle, physiological saline, into the third cerebral ventricle on two separate days. The order of receiving the two substances was random for each rat. When the rats received leptin, food intake was significantly reduced. *(Redrawn from Seeley et al.[143])*

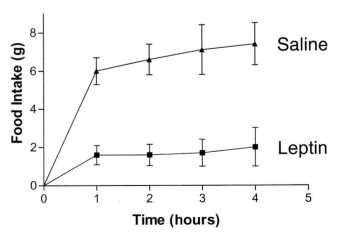

anorexia induced by leptin is dose dependent and is not secondary to illness or incapacitation.[145] Animals with defective leptin signaling (either because they do not synthesize leptin, as in *ob/ob* "obese" mice, or because they have defective leptin receptors, as occurs in *db/db* "diabetic" mice and *fa/fa* "fatty" Zucker rats) are characterized by hyperphagia and extreme obesity, and the same is true for humans with analogous mutations of leptin and its receptor.[146] Hence leptin, like insulin, satisfies the criteria for being an adiposity signal to the brain.

Insulin is secreted in response to minute-to-minute changes in circulating fuels and autonomic activity, and it has a half-life of a few minutes. Thus the rapidly fluctuating titers of insulin reaching the brain reflect instantaneous metabolic needs as well as total body fat. Leptin, on the other hand, has a much longer half-life (around 45 minutes) and therefore provides a more stable signal to the brain regarding body fat stores. Insulin secretion is more highly correlated with visceral fat than with total body fat, and visceral fat is highly associated with insulin resistance. Leptin on the other hand is more highly correlated with subcutaneous than visceral fat. The integration of these different types of signals with central controllers of energy homeostasis is the subject of considerable ongoing research.

CENTRAL CONTROL SYSTEMS

Signals proportional to body adiposity, as well as those that communicate information related to ongoing metabolic processes and what is being eaten and processed in the gut, converge in the central nervous system (CNS). Within the CNS, these signals act on neurochemical systems that influence energy intake and energy expenditure. The best-described CNS systems that regulate energy homeostasis are in the ventral hypothalamus, and they can be roughly divided into those whose activity reduces body fat (catabolic effector systems) and those whose activity increases body fat (anabolic effector systems).[11,97,147] Anabolic effectors are neuronal circuits that elicit increased food intake, decreased energy expenditure and, consequently, increase stored energy in the form of adipose tissue. They become more active when energy stores are low, as indicated by reduced levels of insulin and leptin (i.e., when the body is in negative energy balance). Catabolic effectors are neuronal pathways that do the opposite. Stimulated during times of positive energy balance, they decrease food intake, increase energy expenditure, and result in decreased adiposity. A critical aspect of this negative feedback system is that adiposity signals appear to inhibit anabolic pathways while activating catabolic pathways, and the balance between these two pathways is thought to strongly influence the individual's feeding behavior in response to changes in the level of adiposity.[90,97]

The catabolic and anabolic effector systems are comprised of a number of discrete neurotransmitter systems and axonal pathways within the brain, and many important details of this control system have emerged in recent years. Although receptors for leptin and insulin and binding sites for amylin are located throughout the CNS, all three are concentrated in the ARC in the ventral hypothalamus. Hence, ARC neurons are sensitive to these hormones and consequently to the degree of body adiposity.

Anabolic Effector Systems

The most investigated anabolic effector transmitter is neuropeptide Y (NPY). Although NPY mRNA is made widely throughout the brain, NPY-synthesizing cell bodies in the ARC are implicated as being particularly important in the control of energy homeostasis. Among the many NPYergic projections from these neurons, those to the nearby paraventricular nuclei (PVN) of the hypothalamus and the lateral hypothalamic area (LHA), appear to be major controllers of food intake. ARC NPYergic neurons respond to negative energy balance (i.e., to food deprivation or starvation) by synthesizing more NPY mRNA, and more NPY is consequently released in the PVN[148–150] and presumably the LHA as well. This response is proposed to contribute to increased feeding behavior when food becomes available. Activation of hypothalamic NPY signaling in states of negative energy balance appears to be triggered by reduced levels of adiposity hormones, and the local replacement of either insulin or leptin in the vicinity of the ARC in such individuals attenuates the elevated NPY mRNA in the ARC.[150,151] Hence, the activity of these ARC NPY neurons is directly influenced by at least these two adiposity signals.

Consistent with its proposed role as an anabolic effector peptide, administration of exogenous NPY into the PVN or into the adjacent third cerebral ventricle elicits a rapid and robust increase in food intake[152–156] and decrease of energy expenditure in animals.[157,158] Repeated daily administration of NPY elicits sustained increases of food intake, body weight, and body adiposity,[155] and local administration into the ARC of antisense oligonucleotides to NPY results in reduced NPY synthesis in the ARC and reduced food intake and body weight.[159] Thus NPY satisfies the criteria for being an anabolic effector peptide. Controversy regarding the exact role of NPY stems from experiments on mice with targeted deletion of the NPY gene. These animals do not have differences in food intake or body weight compared to wild-type controls,[160] demonstrating that NPY is not required for normal levels of food intake and body adiposity to be maintained. However, when NPY-deficient mice are crossed with *ob/ob* mice, the hyperphagia and obesity induced by leptin deficiency are partially (but not fully) reversed. Consequently, it would appear that while elevated NPY signaling is an important part of the phenotype of *ob/ob* mice, there must also be other mediators of the response to leptin deficiency.[161]

Hypothalamic Catabolic Effector Systems

At least one catabolic system with effects on energy balance opposite to those of the ARC NPY system also originates within cell bodies in the ARC. Considerable evidence implicates the hypothalamic melanocortin system as an important catabolic effector system. Melanocortins are a family of peptides that includes ACTH and α-melanocyte-stimulating hormone (α-MSH), derived from the precursor molecule proopiomelanocortin (POMC). In the mammalian forebrain, POMC is synthesized only in ARC neurons that are distinct from, but adjacent to, those that synthesize NPY.[162] One of the neuropeptides cleaved from ARC POMC is α-MSH, a peptide transmitter that is an agonist at hypothalamic melanocortin receptors that are concentrated in areas such as the PVN and LHA. When administered into the third ventricle, α-MSH and other melanocortin receptor agonists (including the synthetic drug MTII) reduce food intake and body weight, whereas administration of synthetic melanocortin receptor antagonists (such as SHU-9119) increases food intake and body weight.[163–166] POMC gene expression is reduced during negative energy balance[167] and increased during positive energy balance.[168] Consistent with the hypothesis that the melanocortin system is important in mediating the effects of leptin, leptin receptors are found on POMC neurons in the ARC,[169] leptin stimulates ARC POMC gene expression,[167] and administration of a melanocortin receptor antagonist blocks the effect of leptin to reduce food intake.[164] All of this evidence points to the

hypothalamic POMC-α-MSH-melanocortin receptor system as being a key catabolic effector pathway capable of eliciting robust effects on food intake and body weight that mediates some of the effects of adiposity signals in the CNS. Moreover, it suggests strongly that normal energy homeostasis is dependent on intact melanocortin signaling.

Two melanocortin receptors, termed MC3 and MC4, have been identified within the hypothalamus.[170] Of these, the stronger case can be made for MC4 receptors being involved in the control of energy homeostasis. When administered into the third ventricle of the rat, selective MC4 receptor agonists inhibit and selective MC4 antagonists stimulate food intake.[171] A critical role for MC4 receptor signaling in weight regulation is suggested by the phenotype of MC4 knockout mice. These animals have increased food intake and frank obesity, and they are insensitive to the actions of nonselective MC4 receptor agonists to reduce food intake.[172] MC3 receptor-deficient mice also have increased body fat, but the effect is small and is not driven by increased food intake.[173]

Complexities of the Arcuate Nucleus System

An important interaction that functionally links NPY and POMC neurons in the ARC was recently discovered. Surprisingly, NPY-synthesizing neurons in the ARC make and secrete a second anabolic neuropeptide, agouti-related peptide (AgRP),[174–176] an endogenous antagonist of CNS MC3 and MC4 receptors.[175] Parallel to what occurs following the administration of exogenous NPY, administration of AgRP potently stimulates food intake and body weight gain.[168,177,178] Thus the same ARC neurons release two different orexigenic neuropeptides from their axon terminals. NPY acts at NPY receptors (Y1 and Y5 receptor subtypes) to create an anabolic effect, whereas AgRP acts at MC4 receptors to inhibit α-MSH-mediated catabolic effects (Fig. 10-4). NPY/AgRP neurons of the ARC thereby promote a positive energy balance and weight gain via distinct but complementary mechanisms.

Other Hypothalamic Systems

The model discussed here places ARC anabolic and catabolic neurons at the hub of the system by which input from adiposity signals is transduced into behavioral and autonomic responses. The subsequent downstream neuronal events that control energy homeostasis are complex and diverse. However, as indicated above, two important areas are the nearby PVN and LHA. Each of these pairs of hypothalamic nuclei receives rich inputs from both NPY/AgRP and POMC neurons in the ARC,[179,180] and each synthesizes several neuropeptides that are important in the energy balance equation. The PVN, for example, contains neurons that synthesize corticotropin-releasing hormone (CRH), thyrotropin-releasing hormone (TRH), and oxytocin, and the central administration of any of these has a net catabolic effect.[90,97] Since ablation of the PVN causes a chronic anabolic condition characterized by hyperphagia and obesity (see reference 181), a rough generalization is that the PVN is a key component of the catabolic effector system. Analogously, the LHA, the other major recipient of axons from the ARC, synthesizes melanocyte-concentrating hormone (MCH)[182] and the orexins.[183,184] These neuropeptides, when administered into the CNS, cause a net anabolic response. Thus regulation of activity of ARC neurons by input from adiposity signals may alter feeding behavior in part via changes in the output of catabolic second-order neurons in the PVN and anabolic second-order neurons in the LHA. However, leptin and insulin receptors are present in the PVN and other

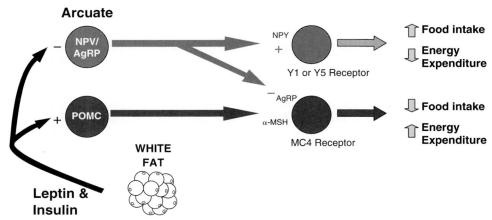

FIGURE 10-4. Model of the initial steps in the hypothalamic control of body fat content. Leptin and insulin are secreted and circulate in direct proportion to body fat, leptin directly from white fat and insulin in direct proportion to white fat. They pass through the blood-brain barrier and interact with two types of cells in the hypothalamic arcuate nucleus. Leptin and insulin inhibit activity in cells that synthesize neuropeptide Y (NPY) and agouti-related peptide (AgRP), and they enhance activity in cells that synthesize proopiomelanocortin (POMC). NPY interacts with Y1 and/or Y5 receptors on neurons in other hypothalamic areas, causing a net anabolic effect by stimulating food intake and decreasing energy expenditure. The peptidergic neurotransmitter cleaved from POMC, α-melanocyte-stimulating hormone (α-MSH), interacts with MC4 receptors on neurons in other hypothalamic areas, causing a net catabolic effect by decreasing food intake and increasing energy expenditure. AgRP is an antagonist at those same MC4 receptors, such that AgRP opposes the actions of α-MSH.

areas, so some neuronal responses to input from these hormones are likely to be independent of the ARC. Moreover, LHA neuronal systems project dense fiber networks to the ARC that may have important effects on the output of NPY/AgRP and POMC neurons. A highly integrated and redundant neurobiological system is thus likely to mediate feeding responses to a change of energy balance.

Interaction of Adiposity Signals with Signals That Control Meal Size

A key question concerns how the various control systems described in this chapter are integrated in the control of food intake. That is, what are the interrelationships among the systems that signal ingested calories and control meal size, those that signal adiposity, and those hypothalamic neuropeptides and other neurotransmitters that receive feeding-pertinent inputs from throughout the brain? Although precise answers are not yet at hand, a model is emerging that is consistent with most of the data, and it is summarized in Fig. 10-5.

When rats have free access to food and can eat whenever they choose, they generally eat 10–12 meals a day, with most intake occurring during the night.[185,186] West and associates observed that when CCK was administered to free-feeding rats at the onset of each meal via an automated delivery system over a 1-week period, the size of each meal was reduced.[187] However, the rats maintained essentially normal total daily caloric intake and body weight, since they increased the number of times they initiated meals each day. This suggests that administration of exogenous CCK alone is an ineffective treatment for losing weight. Nonetheless, rats with a chromosomal deletion that mutates CCK-A receptors[188] gradually become obese over their lifetime,[189] suggesting that an inability to terminate meals appropriately may contribute to a gradual expansion of body fat.[190] Moreover, CCK and adiposity hormones such as insulin or leptin have additive, or even synergistic effects, to reduce food intake. For example, rats treated with very low, sub-threshold doses of either exogenous insulin or leptin manifest a marked increase in the hypophagic response to a low dose of CCK given once a day,[191–194] and they lose weight beyond that achieved by giving these peptides by themselves.[195,196] This observation suggests that the efficacy of CCK (and presumably other signals that reduce meal size as well, such as amylin[84]) is enhanced in the presence of elevated adiposity signaling in the brain. The infusion of a low dose of leptin directly into the brain also increases the sensitivity of the vagus nerve to gastric distension signals that reduce meal size,[197] and leptin-induced anorexia is, in fact, characterized by consumption of smaller meals with no change of meal frequency.[198] The effect of increased adiposity signaling to reduce energy intake may therefore depend largely on an increased response to signals that terminate meals.

These observations have important implications. When an individual goes on a diet and starts losing weight, there is a concomitant reduction of the secretion of adiposity signals (leptin and insulin) and lower titers of these signals enter the brain. In fact, an acute fast, in and of itself, is sufficient to reduce the transport of insulin[199] or leptin[137] into the brain. One consequence of reduced adiposity signaling is a reduced ability of meal-generated peptides such as CCK to terminate a meal, with the result that meals will tend to be larger until adiposity signaling (and body weight) are normalized. Likewise, an individual who overeats and gains weight will have increased adiposity signaling in the brain and will consequently tend to eat smaller meals, providing that they remain sensitive to adiposity signals. Hence, the net action of this control system is to counter long-term changes in body weight, and it does so by changing the average size of meals. Note that individuals are still able to eat according to whatever schedule best meets their

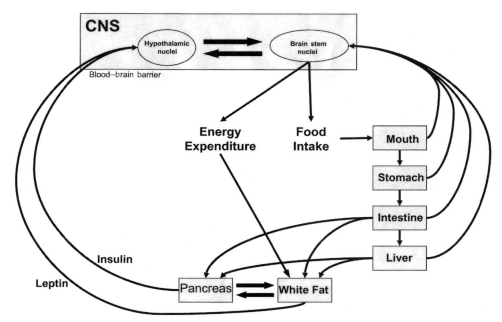

FIGURE 10-5. Model depicting the multiple levels of input and control of energy homeostasis. Body fat content is signaled to the brain via leptin and insulin acting in the hypothalamus. Signals pertinent to food being eaten arise within the gastrointestinal system and reach the brain through sensory nerves converging in the brain stem. The hypothalamic and brain stem areas integrate this information with other factors to determine food intake and energy expenditure.

lifestyle and environmental constraints; it is the meal size rather than the meal pattern that is controlled by this regulatory system.

An important unanswered question relates to what happens to this control system when the diet is changed. A strong case can be made that when individuals habitually consume diets rich in fat, they tend to become obese.[1,4,200–202] This indicates that the normal feedback signaling system must become altered or insensitive on a high-fat diet, and biochemical evidence of leptin resistance in the hypothalamus is beginning to emerge in animals placed on high-fat diets.[203] As the prevalence and associated morbidity of obesity continue to increase in modern society, the importance of understanding the interactions between diet and other environmental factors with the weight-regulatory system increases in parallel. Progress in the prevention and treatment of obesity will likely emerge from an improved understanding of these interactions.

Acknowledgments   Preparation of this review was aided by NIH grants DK 17844, DK 54080, and DK 54890.

REFERENCES

1. Bray GA, Popkin BM: Dietary fat does affect obesity. *J Am Clin Nutr* 1998;68:1157.
2. Flegal KM, Carroll MD, Kuczmarski RJ, *et al*: Overweight and obesity in the United States: prevalence and trends, 1960–1994. *Int J Obes Relat Metab Disord* 1998;22:39.
3. Hill JO, Peters JC: Environmental contributions to the obesity epidemic. *Science* 1998;280:1371.
4. Popkin BM, Doak C: The obesity epidemic is a worldwide phenomenon. *Nutr Rev* 1998;56:106.
5. Mokdad AH, Serdula MK, Dietz WH, *et al*: The continuing epidemic of obesity in the United States. *JAMA* 2000;284:1650.
6. Chinn S, Hughes JM, Rona RJ: Trends in growth and obesity in ethnic groups in Britain. *Arch Dis Child* 2000;78:513.
7. Dwyer JT, Stone EJ, Yang M, *et al*: Prevalence of marked overweight and obesity in a multiethnic pediatric population: findings from the Child and Adolescent Trial for Cardiovascular Health (CATCH) study. *J Am Diet Assoc* 2000;100:1149.
8. Woods SC, Schwartz MW, Baskin DG, *et al*: Food intake and the regulation of body weight. *Ann Rev Psychol* 2000;51:255.
9. Collier G: The dialogue between the house economist and the resident physiologist. *Nutr Behav* 1986;3:9.
10. Bray GA: *The Obese Patient.* Saunders:1976.
11. Schwartz MW, Seeley RJ: The new biology of body weight regulation. *J Am Diet Assoc* 1997;97:54.
12. Stallone DD, Stunkard AJ: The regulation of body weight: evidence and clinical implications. *Ann Behav Med* 1991;13:220.
13. Cannon WB: *The Wisdom of the Body.* Norton:1932.
14. Carlson AJ: *Control of Hunger in Health and Disease.* University of Chicago Press:1916.
15. Mayer J: Regulation of energy intake and the body weight: The glucostatic and lipostatic hypothesis. *Ann NY Acad Sci* 1955;63:14.
16. Mayer J, Thomas DW: Regulation of food intake and obesity. *Science* 1967;156:328.
17. Levin BE, Dunn-Meynell AA, Routh VH: Brain glucose sensing and body energy homeostasis: role in obesity and diabetes. *Am J Physiol* 1999;276:R1223.
18. Hevener AL, Bergman RN, Donovan CM: Portal vein afferents are critical for the sympathoadrenal response to hypoglycemia. *Diabetes* 2000;49:8.
19. Flynn FW: Brain tachykinins and the regulation of salt intake. *Ann NY Acad Sci* 1999;897:432.
20. Stricker EM, Sved AF: Thirst. *Nutrition* 2000;16:821.
21. Grossman SP: The role of glucose, insulin and glucagon in the regulation of food intake and body weight. *Neurosci Biobehav Rev* 1986;10:295.
22. Lotter EC, Woods SC: Injections of insulin and changes of body weight. *Physiol Behav* 1977;18:293.
23. MacKay EM, Calloway JW, Barnes RH: Hyperalimentation in normal animals produced by protamine insulin. *J Nutr* 1940;20:59.
24. Smith GP, Epstein AN: Increased feeding in response to decreased glucose utilization in rat and monkey. *Am J Physiol* 1969;217:1083.
25. Langhans W: Metabolic and glucostatic control of feeding. *Proc Nutr Soc* 1996;55:497515.

26. Langhans W, Scharrer E: Role of fatty acid oxidation in control of meal pattern. *Behav Neural Biol* 1987;47:7.

27. Scharrer E, Langhans W: Control of food intake by fatty acid oxidation. *Am J Physiol* 1986;250:R1003.

28. Langhans W: Role of the liver in the metabolic control of eating: what we know—and what we do not know. *Neurosci Biobehav Rev* 1996;20:145.

29. Virally ML, Guillausseau PJ: Hypoglycemia in adults. *Diabetes Metab* 1999;25:477.

30. Epstein AN, Nicolaidis S, Miselis R: The glucoprivic control of food intake and the glucostatic theory of feeding behavior. In: Mogenson GJ, Calaresci FR, eds. *Neural Integration of Physiological Mechanisms and Behavior.* University Press:1975;148.

31. Campfield LA, Smith FJ: Functional coupling between transient declines in blood glucose and feeding behavior: temporal relationships. *Brain Res Bull* 1986;17:427.

32. Campfield LA, Smith FJ: Transient declines in blood glucose signal meal initiation. *Int J Obes* 1990;14(Suppl. 3):15.

33. Campfield LA, Smith FJ, Rosenbaum M, et al: Human eating: evidence for a physiological basis using a modified paradigm. *Neurosci Biobehav Rev* 1996;20:133.

34. Campfield LA, Brandon P, Smith FJ: On-line continuous measurement of blood glucose and meal pattern in free-feeding rats: the role of glucose in meal initiation. *Brain Res Bull* 1985;14:605.

35. Campfield LA, Smith FJ: Systemic factors in the control of food intake: Evidence for patterns as signals. In: Stricker EM, ed. *Handbook of Behavioral Neurobiology. Neurobiology of Food and Fluid Intake.* Plenum:1990;183.

36. Smith FJ, Campfield LA: Meal initiation occurs after experimental induction of transient declines in blood glucose. *Am J Physiol* 1993;265:R1423.

37. de Vries J, Strubbe JH, Wildering WC, et al: Patterns of body temperature during feeding in rats under varying ambient temperatures. *Physiol Behav* 1993;53:229.

38. Even P, Nicolaidis S: Spontaneous and 2DG-induced metabolic changes and feeding: The ischymetric hypothesis. *Brain Res Bull* 1985;15:429.

39. Nicolaidis S, Even P: Mesure du métabolisme de fond en relation avec la prise alimentaire: Hypothese iscymétrique. *Comptes Rendus Academie de Sciences, Paris* 1984;298:295.

40. Aravich PF, Stanley EZ, Doerries LE: Exercise in food-restricted rats produces 2DG feeding and metabolic abnormalities similar to anorexia nervosa. *Physiol Behav* 1995;57:147.

41. Rieg TS, Aravich PF: Systemic clonidine increases feeding and wheel running but does not affect rate of weight loss in rats subjected to activity-based anorexia. *Pharmacol Biochem Behav* 1994;47:215.

42. Sclafani A, Rendel A: Food deprivation-induced activity in dietary obese, dietary lean, and normal-weight rats. *Behav Biol* 1978;24:220.

43. Stevenson JAF, Rixon RH: Environmental temperature and deprivation of food and water on the spontaneous activity of rats. *Yale J Biol Med* 1957;29:575.

44. Woods SC, Strubbe JH: The psychobiology of meals. *Psychonomic Bull Rev* 1994;1:141.

45. Woods SC, Ramsay DS: Pavlovian influences over food and drug intake. *Behav Brain Res* 2000;110:175.

46. Gibbs J, Young RC, Smith GP: Cholecystokinin decreases food intake in rats. *J Comp Physiol Psychol* 1973;84:488.

47. Smith GP, Gibbs J: The development and proof of the cholecystokinin hypothesis of satiety. In: Dourish CT, Cooper SJ, Iversen SD et al, eds. *Multiple Cholecystokinin Receptors in the CNS.* Oxford University Press,:1992;166.

48. Smith GP, Gibbs J: The satiating effects of cholecystokinin and bombesin-like peptides. In: Smith GP, ed. *Satiation. From Gut to Brain.* Oxford:1998;97.

49. Hewson G, Leighton GE, Hill RG, et al: The cholecystokinin receptor antagonist L364,718 increases food intake in the rat by attenuation of endogenous cholecystokinin. *Br J Pharmacol* 1988;93:79.

50. Reidelberger RD, O'Rourke MF: Potent cholecystokinin antagonist L-364,718 stimulates food intake in rats. *Am J Physiol* 1989;257:R1512.

51. Moran TH, Ameglio PJ, Peyton HJ, et al: Blockade of type A, but not type B, CCK receptors postpones satiety in rhesus monkeys. *Am J Physiol* 1993;265:R620.

52. Schwartz GJ, McHugh PR, Moran TH: Gastric loads and cholecystokinin synergistically stimulate rat gastric vagal afferents. *Am J Physiol* 1993;265:R872.

53. Schwartz GJ, Tougas G, Moran TH: Integration of vagal afferent responses to duodenal loads and exogenous CCK in rats. *Peptides* 1995;16:707.

54. Berthoud HR, Powley TL: Vagal afferent innervation of the rat fundic stomach: Morphological characterization of the gastric tension receptor. *J Comp Neurol* 1992;319:261.

55. Smith GP, Jerome C, Cushin BJ, et al: Abdominal vagotomy blocks the satiety effect of cholecystokinin in the rat. *Science* 1981;213:1036.

56. Smith GP, Jerome C, Norgren R: Afferent axons in abdominal vagus mediate satiety effect of cholecystokinin in rats. *Am J Physiol* 1985;249:R638.

57. Gibbs J, Fauser DJ, Rowe EA, et al: Bombesin suppresses feeding in rats. *Nature* 1979;282:208.

58. Geary N: Glucagon and the control of meal size. In: Smith GP, ed. *Satiation: From Gut to Brain.* Oxford University Press:1998;164.

59. Lotter EC, Krinsky R, McKay JM, et al: Somatostatin decreases food intake of rats and baboons. *J Comp Physiol Psychol* 1981;95:278.

60. Erlanson—Albertsson C, York D: Enterostatin—a peptide regulating fat intake. *Obes Res* 1997;5:360.

61. York DA, Lin L, Smith B, et al: Enterostatin as a regulator of fat intake. In: Berthoud HR, Seeley RJ, eds. *Neural and Metabolic Control of Macronutrient Intake.* CRC Press:2000;295.

62. Fujimoto K, Machidori H, Iwakiri R, et al: Effect of intravenous administration of apolipoprotein A-IV on patterns of feeding, drinking and ambulatory activity in rats. *Brain Res* 1993;608:233.

63. Tso P, Liu M, Kalogeris TJ: The role of apolipoprotein A-IV in food intake regulation. *J Nutr* 1999;129:1503.

64. Smith GP, ed: Satiation: *From Gut to Brain.* Oxford University Press: 1998.

65. Stein LJ, Woods SC: Cholecystokinin and bombesin act independently to decrease food intake in the rat. *Peptides* 1981;2:431.

66. Geary N, Kissileff HR, Pi-Sunyer FX, et al: Individual, but not simultaneous, glucagon and cholecystokinin infusions inhibit feeding in men. *Am J Physiol* 1992;262:R975.

67. Butler PC, Chou J, Carter WB, et al: Effects of meal ingestion on plasma amylin concentration in NIDDM and nondiabetic humans. *Diabetes* 1990;39:752.

68. Lukinius A, Wilander E, Westermark GT, et al: Co-localization of islet amyloid polypeptide and insulin in the B cell secretory granules of the human pancreatic islets. *Diabetologia* 1989;32:240.

69. Pieber TR, Roitelman J, Lee Y, et al: Direct plasma radioimmunoassay for rat amylin-(1–37): concentrations with acquired and genetic obesity. *Am J Physiol* 1994;267:E156.

70. Banks WA, Kastin AJ, Maness LM, et al: Permeability of the blood-brain barrier to amylin. *Life Sci* 1995;57:1993.

71. Banks WA, Kastin AJ: Differential permeability of the blood-brain barrier to two pancreatic peptides: insulin and amylin. *Peptides* 1998;19:883.

72. Beaumont K, Kenney MA, Young AA, et al: High affinity amylin binding sites in rat brain. *Mol Pharmacol* 1993;44:493.

73. Christopoulos G, Paxinos G, Huang XF, et al: Comparative distribution of receptors for amylin and the related peptides calcitonin gene related peptide and calcitonin in rat and monkey brain. *Can J Physiol Pharmacol* 1995;73:1037.

74. Sexton PM, Paxinos G, Kenney MA, et al: In vitro autoradiographic localization of amylin binding sites in rat brain. *Neuroscience* 1994;62:553.

75. Cooper GJ: Amylin compared with calcitonin gene-related peptide: structure, biology, and relevance to metabolic disease. *Endocr Rev* 1994;15:163.

76. Arnelo U, Permert J, Adrian TE, et al: Chronic infusion of islet amyloid polypeptide causes anorexia in rats. *Am J Physiol* 1996;271: R1654.

77. Lutz TA, Del Prete E, Scharrer E: Reduction of food intake in rats by intraperitoneal injection of low doses of amylin. *Physiol Behav* 1994; 55:891.

78. Reidelberger RD, Arnelo U, Granqvist L, et al: Comparative effects of amylin and cholecystokinin on food intake and gastric emptying in rats. *Am J Physiol* 2001;280:R605.

79. Young A: Role of amylin in nutrient intake—animal studies. *Diabet Med* 1997;14(Suppl. 2):S14.

80. Gebre-Medhin S, Mulder H, Pekny M, et al: Increased insulin secretion and glucose tolerance in mice lacking islet amyloid polypeptide (amylin). *Biochem Biophys Res Commun* 1998;250:271.

81. Rushing PA, Hagan MM, Seeley RJ, *et al*: Amylin: A novel action in the brain to reduce body weight. *Endocrinology* 2000;141:850.

82. Chance WT, Balasubramaniam A, Chen X, *et al*: Tests of adipsia and conditioned taste aversion following the intrahypothalamic injection of amylin. *Peptides* 1992;13:961.

83. Lutz TA, Geary N, Szabady MM, *et al*: Amylin decreases meal size in rats. *Physiol Behav* 1995;58:1197.

84. Rushing PA, Lutz TA, Seeley RJ, *et al*: Amylin and insulin interact to reduce food intake in rats. *Horm Metab Res* 2000;32:62.

85. Bhavsar S, Watkins J, Young A: Synergy between amylin and cholecystokinin for inhibition of food intake in mice. *Physiol Behav* 1998; 64:557.

86. Keesey RE: A set-point model of body weight regulation and its implications for obesity. In: Brownell KD, Fairburn CG, eds. *Comprehensive Textbook of Eating Disorders and Obesity.* Guilford Press, NY:1995;46.

87. Keesey RE: Physiological regulation of body weight and the issue of obesity. *Med Clin North Am* 1989;73:15.

88. Pinel JPJ, Assanand S, Lehman DR: Hunger, eating and ill health. *Am Psychol* 2000;55:1105.

89. Schwartz MW, Seeley RJ: Neuroendocrine responses to starvation and weight loss. *N Engl J Med* 1997;336:1802.

90. Woods SC, Seeley RJ, Porte DJ, *et al*: Signals that regulate food intake and energy homeostasis. *Science* 1998;280:1378.

91. Kennedy GC: The role of depot fat in the hypothalamic control of food intake in the rat. *Proc Roy Soc Lond (Biol)* 1953;140:579.

92. Oomura Y: Significance of glucose, insulin, and free fatty acid on the hypothalamic feeding and satiety neurons. In: Novin D, Wyrwicka W, Bray GA, eds. *Hunger. Basic Mechanisms and Clinical Implications.* Raven Press:1976;145.

93. Loftus TM, Jaworsky DE, Frehywot GL, *et al*: Reduced food intake and body weight in mice treated with fatty acid synthase inhibitors. *Science* 2000;288:2299.

94. Friedman MI: Fuel partitioning and food intake. *J Am Clin Nutr* 1998; 67(Suppl. 3):513S.

95. Hervey GR: The effects of lesions in the hypothalamus in parabiotic rats. *J Physiol* 1952;145:336.

96. Schwartz MW, Baskin DG, Kaiyala KJ, *et al*: Model for the regulation of energy balance and adiposity by the central nervous system. *J Am Clin Nutr* 1999;69:584.

97. Schwartz MW, Woods SC, Porte DJ, *et al*: Central nervous system control of food intake. *Nature* 2000;404:661.

98. Woods SC: Insulin and the brain: A mutual dependency. *Prog Psychobiol Physiol Psychol* 1996;16:53.

99. Schwartz MW, Figlewicz DP, Baskin DG, *et al*: Insulin in the brain: a hormonal regulator of energy balance. *Endocrine Rev* 1992; 13:387.

100. Polonsky KS, Given BD, Hirsch L, *et al*: Quantitative study of insulin secretion and clearance in normal and obese subjects. *J Clin Invest* 1988;81:435.

101. Polonsky BD, Given E, Carter V: Twenty-four-hour profiles and pulsatile patterns of insulin secretion in normal and obese subjects. *J Clin Invest* 1988;81:442.

102. Bagdade JD, Bierman EL, Porte D, Jr. The significance of basal insulin levels in the evaluation of the insulin response to glucose in diabetic and nondiabetic subjects. J Clin Invest 1967;46:1549–1557.

103. Schwartz MW, Sipols AJ, Kahn SE, *et al*: Kinetics and specificity of insulin uptake from plasma into cerebrospinal fluid. *Am J Physiol* 1990;259:E378.

104. Schwartz MW, Bergman RN, Kahn SE, *et al*: Evidence for uptake of plasma insulin into cerebrospinal fluid through an intermediate compartment in dogs. *J Clin Invest* 1991;88:1272.

105. Corp ES, Woods SC, Porte D, *et al*: Localization of ^{125}I-insulin binding sites in the rat hypothalamus by quantitative autoradiography. *Neurosci Lett* 1986;70:17.

106. Figlewicz DP, Dorsa DM, Stein LJ, *et al*: Brain and liver insulin binding is decreased in Zucker rats carrying the "fa" gene. *Endocrinology* 1985;117:1537.

107. Baskin DG, Marks JL, Schwartz MW, *et al*: Insulin and insulin receptors in the brain in relation to food intake and body weight. In: Lehnert H, Murison R, Weiner H, *et al*, eds. *Endocrine and Nutritional Control of Basic Biological Functions.* Hogrefe & Huber: 1990;202.

108. LeRoith D, Rojeski M, Roth J: Insulin receptors in brain and other tissues: similarities and differences. *Neurochem Int* 1988;12:419.

109. Woods SC, Lotter EC, McKay LD, *et al*: Chronic intracerebroventricular infusion of insulin reduces food intake and body weight of baboons. *Nature* 1979;282:503.

110. Woods SC, Figlewicz DP, Schwartz MW, *et al*: A re-assessment of the regulation of adiposity and appetite by the brain insulin system. *Int J Obesity* 1990;14(Suppl 3):69.

111. Woods SC, Chavez M, Park CR, *et al*: The evaluation of insulin as a metabolic signal controlling behavior via the brain. *Neurosci Biobehav Rev* 1996;20:139.

112. Schwartz MW, Figlewicz DP, Baskin DG, *et al*: Insulin and the central regulation of energy balance: update 1994. *Endocrine Monogr Rev* 1994;2:109.

113. McGowan MK, Andrews KM, Kelly J, *et al*: Effects of chronic intrahypothalamic infusion of insulin on food intake and diurnal meal patterning in the rat. *Behav Neurosci* 1990;104:373.

114. van Dijk G, de Groote C, Chavez M, *et al*: Insulin in the arcuate nucleus reduces fat consumption in rats. *Brain Res* 1997;777:147.

115. Strubbe JH, Mein CG: Increased feeding in response to bilateral injection of insulin antibodies in the VMH. *Physiol Behav* 1977;19: 309.

116. McGowan MK, Andrews KM, Grossman SP: Chronic intrahypothalamic infusions of insulin or insulin antibodies alter body weight and food intake in the rat. *Physiol Behav* 1992;51:753.

117. Brüning JC, Gautam D, Burks DJ, *et al*: Role of brain insulin receptor in control of body weight and reproduction. *Science* 2000;289:2122.

118. Burks DJ, de Mora JF, Schubert M, *et al*: IRS-2 pathways integrate female reproduction and energy homeostasis. *Nature* 2000;407:377.

119. Stubdal H, Lynch CA, Moriarty A, *et al*: Targeted deletion of the tub mouse obesity gene reveals that tubby is a loss-of-function mutation. *Mol Cell Biol* 2000;20:878.

120. Woods SC, Stein LJ, McKay LD, *et al*: Suppression of food intake by intravenous nutrients and insulin in the baboon. *Am J Physiol* 1984; 247:R393.

121. Vanderweele DA, Haraczkiewicz E, Van Itallie TB: Elevated insulin and satiety in obese and normal weight rats. *Appetite* 1982;3:99.

122. Nicolaidis S, Rowland N: Metering of intravenous versus oral nutrients and regulation of energy balance. *Am J Physiol* 1976;231:661.

123. Chavez M, Kaiyala K, Madden LJ, *et al*: Intraventricular insulin and the level of maintained body weight in rats. *Behav Neurosci* 1995; 109:528.

124. Chavez M, Seeley RJ, Woods SC: A comparison between the effects of intraventricular insulin and intraperitoneal LiCl on three measures sensitive to emetic agents. *Behav Neurosci* 1995;109:547.

125. Coleman DL: Effects of parabiosis of obese with diabetes and normal mice. *Diabetologia* 1973;9:294.

126. Zhang Y, Proenca R, Maffie M, *et al*: Positional cloning of the mouse obese gene and its human homologue. *Nature* 1994;372:425.

127. Considine RV, Sinha MK, Heiman ML, *et al*: Serum immunoreactive-leptin concentrations in normal-weight and obese humans. *N Engl J Med* 1996;334:292.

128. Rosenbaum M, Nicolson M, Hirsch J, *et al*: Effects of gender, body composition, and menopause on plasma concentrations of leptin. *J Clin Endocrinol Metab* 1996;81:3424.

129. Havel PJ, KasimKarakas S, Mueller W, *et al*: Relationship of plasma leptin to plasma insulin and adiposity in normal weight and overweight women: Effects of dietary fat content and sustained weight loss. *J Clin Endocrinol Metab* 1996;81:4406.

130. Havel PJ: Mechanisms regulating leptin production: Implications for control of energy balance. *J Am Clin Nutr* 1999;70:305.

131. Ahren B, Mansson S, Gingerich RL, *et al*: Regulation of plasma leptin in mice: Influence of age, high-fat diet and fasting. *Am J Physiol* 1997;273:R113.

132. Boden G, Chen X, Mozzoli M, *et al*: Effect of fasting on serum leptin in normal human subjects. *J Clin Endocrinol Metab* 1996;81:3419.

133. Wisse BE, Campfield LA, Marliss EB, *et al*: Effect of prolonged moderate and severe energy restriction and refeeding on plasma leptin concentrations in obese women. *J Am Clin Nutr* 1999;70:321.

134. Banks WA, Kastin AJ, Huang W, *et al*: Leptin enters the brain by a saturable system independent of insulin. *Peptides* 1996;17:305.

135. Caro JF, Kolaczynski JW, Nyce MR, *et al*: Decreased cerebrospinalfluid/serum leptin ratio in obesity: a possible mechanism for leptin resistance. *Lancet* 1996;348:159.

136. Golden PL, Maccagnan TJ, Pardridge WM: Human blood-brain barrier leptin receptor: Binding and endocytosis in isolated human brain microvessels. *J Clin Invest* 1997;99:14.

137. Karonen S-L, Koistinen HA, Nikkinen P, *et al*: Is brain uptake of leptin *in vivo* saturable and reduced by fasting? *Eur J Nucl Med* 1998; 25:607.

138. Schwartz MW, Peskind E, Raskind M, *et al*: Cerebrospinal fluid leptin levels: Relationship to plasma levels and to adiposity in humans. *Nat Med* 1996;2:589.

139. Baskin DG, Schwartz MW, Seeley RJ, *et al*: Leptin receptor long form splice variant protein expression in neuron cell bodies of the brain and colocalization with neuropeptide Y mRNA in the arcuate nucleus. *J Histochem Cytochem* 1999;47:353.

140. Baskin DG, Breininger JF, Schwartz MW: Leptin receptor mRNA identifies a subpopulation of neuropeptide Y neurons activated by fasting in rat hypothalamus. *Diabetes* 1999;48:828.

141. Campfield LA, Smith FJ, Gulsez Y, *et al*: Mouse OB protein: Evidence for a peripheral signal linking adiposity and central neural networks. *Science* 1995;269:546.

142. Pelleymounter MA, Cullen MJ, Baker MB, *et al*: Effects of the obese gene product on body weight regulation in ob/ob mice. *Science* 1995; 269:540.

143. Seeley RJ, van Dijk G, Campfield LA, *et al*: The effect of intraventricular administration of leptin on food intake and body weight in the rat. *Horm Metab Res* 1996;28:664.

144. Farooqi IS, Jebb SA, Langmack G, *et al*: Effects of recombinant leptin therapy in a child with congenital leptin deficiency. *N Engl J Med* 1999;341:913.

145. Thiele TE, van Dijk G, Campfield LA, *et al*: Central administration of GLP-1, but not leptin, produce conditioned taste aversions in the rat. *Am J Physiol* 1997;272:R726.

146. Montague CT, Farooqi IS, Whitehead JP, *et al*: Congenital leptin deficiency is associated with severe early-onset obesity in humans. *Nature* 1997;387:903.

147. Kaiyala KJ, Woods SC, Schwartz MW: New model for the regulation of energy balance by the central nervous system. *J Am Clin Nutr* 1995;62(Suppl.):1123S.

148. Kalra SP, Dube MG, Sahu A, *et al*: Neuropeptide Y secretion increases in the paraventricular nucleus in association with increased appetite for food. *Proc Natl Acad Sci USA* 1991;88:10931.

149. Sahu A, Sninsky CA, Kalra PS, *et al*: Neuropeptide Y concentration in microdissected hypothalamic regions and *in vitro* release from the medial basal hypothalamus-preoptic area of streptozotocin-diabetic rats with and without insulin substitution therapy. *Endocrinology* 1990;126:192.

150. Schwartz MW, Sipols AJ, Marks JL, *et al*: Inhibition of hypothalamic neuropeptide Y gene expression by insulin. *Endocrinology* 1992;130: 3608.

151. Schwartz MW, Baskin DG, Bukowski TR, *et al*: Specificity of leptin action on elevated blood glucose levels and hypothalamic neuropeptide Y gene expression in ob/ob mice. *Diabetes* 1996;45:531.

152. Clark JT, Kalra PS, Crowley WR, *et al*: Neuropeptide Y and human pancreatic polypeptide stimulate feeding behavior in rats. *Endocrinology* 1984;115:427.

153. Sahu S, Kalra S: Neuropeptidergic regulation of feeding behavior. *Trends Endocrinol Metab* 1993;4:217.

154. Seeley RJ, Benoit SC, Davidson TL: The discriminative cues produced by NPY administration do not generalize to the interoceptive cues produced by food deprivation. *Physiol Behav* 1995;58:1237.

155. Stanley BG, Kyrkouli SE, Lampert S, *et al*: Neuropeptide Y chronically injected into the hypothalamus: A powerful neurochemical inducer of hyperphagia and obesity. *Peptides* 1986;7:1189.

156. Stanley BG: Neuropeptide Y in multiple hypothalamic sites controls eating behavior, endocrine, and autonomic systems for energy balance. In: Colmers WF, Wahlestedt C, eds. *The Biology of Neuropeptide Y and Related Peptides*. Humana Press:1993;457.

157. Billington CJ, Briggs JE, Grace M, *et al*: Effects of intracerebroventricular injection of neuropeptide Y on energy metabolism. *Am J Physiol* 1991;260:R321.

158. Billington CJ, Briggs JE, Harker S, *et al*: Neuropeptide Y in hypothalamic paraventricular nucleus: a center coordinating energy metabolism. *Am J Physiol* 1994;266:R1765.

159. Akabayashi A, Wahlestedt C, Alexander JT, *et al*: Specific inhibition of endogenous neuropeptide Y synthesis in arcuate nucleus by antisense oligonucleotides suppresses feeding behavior and insulin secretion. *Brain Res* 1994;21:55.

160. Erickson JC, Clegg KE, Palmiter RD: Sensitivity to leptin and susceptibility to seizures of mice lacking neuropeptide Y. *Nature* 1996; 381:415.

161. Erickson JC, Hollopeter G, Palmiter RD: Attenuation of the obesity syndrome of ob/ob mice by the loss of neuropeptide Y. *Science* 1996; 274:1704.

162. Elias CF, Lee C, Kelly J, *et al*: Leptin activates hypothalamic CART neurons projecting to the spinal cord. *Neuron* 1998;21:1375.

163. Fan W, Boston B, Kesterson R, *et al*: Role of melanocortinergic neurons in feeding and the agouti obesity syndrome. *Nature* 1997;385:165.

164. Seeley R, Yagaloff K, Fisher S, *et al*: Melanocortin receptors in leptin effects. *Nature* 1997;390:349.

165. Thiele T, van DG, Yagaloff K, *et al*: Central infusion of melanocortin agonist MTII in rats: assessment of c-Fos expression and taste aversion. *Am J Physiol* 1998;274:R248.

166. Tsujii S, Bray GA: Acetylation alters the feeding response to MSH and beta-endorphin. *Brain Res Bull* 1989;23:165.

167. Schwartz MW, Seeley RJ, Weigle DS, *et al*: Leptin increases hypothalamic proopiomelanocortin (POMC) mRNA expression in the rostral arcuate nucleus. *Diabetes* 1997;46:2119.

168. Hagan M, Rushing P, Schwartz M, *et al*: Role of the CNS melanocortin system in the response to overfeeding. *J Neurosci* 1999; 19:2362.

169. Cheung CC, Clifton DK, Steiner RA: Proopiomelanocortin neurons are direct targets for leptin in the hypothalamus. *Endocrinology* 1997; 138:4489.

170. Mountjoy K, Mortrud M, Low M, *et al*: Localization of the melanocortin-4 receptor (MC4-R) in neuroendocrine and autonomic control circuits in the brain. *Mol Endocrinol* 1994;8:1298.

171. Benoit SC, Schwartz MW, Lachey JL, *et al*: A novel selective melanocortin-4 receptor agonist reduces food intake in rats and mice without producing aversive consequences. *J Neurosci* 2000;20:3442.

172. Huszar D, Lynch CA, Fairchild-Huntress V, *et al*: Targeted disruption of the melanocortin-4 receptor results in obesity in mice. *Cell* 1997; 88:131.

173. Chen AS, Marsh DJ, Trumbauer ME, *et al*: Inactivation of the mouse melanocortin-3 receptor results in increased fat mass and reduced lean body mass [In Process Citation]. *Nat Genet* 2000;26:97.

174. Hahn TM, Breininger JF, Baskin DG, *et al*: Coexpression of Agrp and NPY in fasting-activated hypothalamic neurons. *Nat Neurosci* 1998; 1:271.

175. Ollmann M, Wilson B, Yang Y, *et al*: Antagonism of central melanocortin receptors *in vitro* and *in vivo* by agouti-related protein. *Science* 1997;278:135.

176. Shutter J, Graham M, Kinsey A, *et al*: Hypothalamic expression of ART, a novel gene related to agouti, is up-regulated in obese and diabetic mutant mice. *Genes Dev* 1997;11:593.

177. Rossi M, Kim M, Morgan D, *et al*: A C-terminal fragment of Agouti-related protein increases feeding and antagonizes the effect of alpha-melanocyte stimulating hormone *in vivo*. *Endocrinology* 1998;139: 4428.

178. Hagan MM, Rushing PA, Pritchard LM, *et al*: Long-term orexigenic effects of AgRP-(83–132) involve mechanisms other than melanocortin receptor blockade. *Am J Physiol* 2000;279:R47.

179. Elmquist JK, Maratos-Flier E, Saper CB, *et al*: Unraveling the central nervous system pathways underlying responses to leptin. *Nat Neurosci* 1998;1:445.

180. Elmquist JK, Elias CF, Saper CB: From lesions to leptin: Hypothalamic control of food intake and body weight. *Neuron* 1999;22:221.

181. Bray GA, Fisler J, York DA: Neuroendocrine control of the development of obesity: understanding gained from studies of experimental animal models. *Front Neuroendocrinol* 1990;11:128.

182. Qu D, Ludwig DS, Gammeltoft S, *et al*: A role for melanin-concentrating hormone in the central regulation of feeding behaviour. *Nature* 1996;380:243.

183. de Lecea L, Kilduff TS, Peyron C, *et al*: The hypocretins: hypothalamus-specific peptides with neuroexcitatory activity. *Proc Nat Acad Sci USA* 1998;95:322.

184. Sakurai T, Amemiya A, Ishii M, *et al*: Orexins and orexin receptors: a family of hypothalamic neuropeptides and G protein-coupled receptors that regulate feeding behavior [see comments]. *Cell* 1998;92: 573.

185. Kissileff HR, Van Itallie TB: Physiology of the control of food intake. *Ann Rev Nutr* 1982;2:371.

186. Le Magnen J: Peripheral and systemic actions of food in the caloric regulation of intake. *Ann NY Acad Sci* 1969;157:1126.

187. West DB, Fey D, Woods SC: Cholecystokinin persistently suppresses meal size but not food intake in free-feeding rats. *Am J Physiol* 1984; 246:R776.

188. Miyasaka K, Kanai S, Ohta M, *et al*: Lack of satiety effect of chole-cystokinin (CCK) in a new rat model not expressing the CCK-A receptor gene. *Neurosci Lett* 1994;180:143.

189. Kawano K, Hirashima T, Mori S, *et al*: Spontaneous long-term hyper-glycemic rat with diabetic complications. Otsuka Long-Evans Tokushima Fatty (OLETF) strain. *Diabetes* 1992;41:1422.

190. Schwartz GJ, Whitney A, Skogland C, *et al*: Decreased responsive-ness to dietary fat in Otsuka Long-Evans Tokushima fatty rats lacking CCK-A receptors. *Am J Physiol* 1999;277:R1144.

191. Barrachina MD, Martinez V, Wang L, *et al*: Synergistic interaction be-tween leptin and cholecystokinin to reduce short-term food intake in lean mice. *Proc Natl Acad Sci USA* 1997;94:10455.

192. Figlewicz DP, Sipols AJ, Seeley RJ, *et al*: Intraventricular insulin enhances the meal-suppressive efficacy of intraventricular cholecys-tokinin octapeptide in the baboon. *Behav Neurosci* 1995;109:567.

193. Riedy CA, Chavez M, Figlewicz DP, *et al*: Central insulin enhances sensitivity to cholecystokinin. *Physiol Behav* 1995;58:755.

194. Matson CA, Wiater MF, Kuijper JL, *et al*: Synergy between leptin and cholecystokinin (CCK) to control daily caloric intake. *Peptides* 1997; 18:1275.

195. Matson CA, Ritter RC: Long-term CCK-leptin synergy suggests a role for CCK in the regulation of body weight. *Am J Physiol* 1999; 276:R1038.

196. Matson CA, Reid DF, Cannon TA, *et al*: Cholecystokinin and leptin act synergistically to reduce body weight. *Am J Physiol* 2000;278:R882.

197. Schwartz GJ, Moran TH: Sub-diaphragmatic vagal afferent integra-tion of meal-related gastrointestinal signals. *Neurosci Biobehav Rev* 1996;20:47.

198. Flynn MC, Plata-Salaman CR: Leptin (OB protein) and meal size. *Nutrition* 1999;15:508.

199. Strubbe JH, Porte DJ, Woods SC: Insulin responses and glucose levels in plasma and cerebrospinal fluid during fasting and refeeding in the rat. *Physiol Behav* 1988;44:205.

200. Lichtenstein AH, Kennedy E, Barrier P, *et al*: Dietary fat consumption and health. *Nutr Rev* 1998;56:S3.

201. Poppitt SD: Energy density of diets and obesity. *Int J Obes* 1995; 19(Suppl):S20.

202. Willett WC: Is dietary fat a major determinant of body fat? *J Am Clin Nutr* 1998;67(Suppl):556S.

203. El-Haschimi K, Pierroz DD, Hileman SM, *et al*: Two defects con-tribute to hypothalamic leptin resistance in mice with diet-induced obesity. *J Clin Invest* 2000;105:1827.

204. Bernstein IL, Lotter EC, Kulkosky PJ: Effect of force-feeding upon basal insulin levels in rats. *Proc Soc Exp Biol Med* 1975;150:546.

C H A P T E R 1 1

Diabetes and Atherosclerosis

Daniel Steinberg

Diabetic patients frequently suffer from microvascular disease, but they die more commonly from macrovascular disease. Atherosclerosis affecting the cerebral arteries and the peripheral vasculature takes a toll, but myocardial infarction certainly leads as cause of death. Physicians caring for diabetic patients must be as concerned about the other risk factors for coronary artery disease as they are about the control of glycemia in their patients. Certainly the diabetic patient in poor metabolic control manifests significant derangements of lipoprotein metabolism and this deserves attention. However, diabetic patients who are well controlled do not have significant hypercholesterolemia and only minimal hypertriglyceridemia. Yet they are at significantly higher risk for premature coronary heart disease (CHD). Why? Perhaps due to low high-density lipoprotein (HDL) levels or hypertriglyceridemia. But the blunt answer is that we simply do not know. (The disturbances in lipid metabolism and lipoprotein patterns encountered in diabetes are discussed in detail in Chap. 47). However, there is reason to believe that every effort should be made to correct the acknowledged risk factors for CHD in diabetic patients just as in nondiabetic persons—but even more aggressively, because they are at higher risk. Most of the risk factors, including dyslipidemia, cigarette smoking, hypertension, and obesity, have been shown to apply equally in the presence of diabetes mellitus and, in general, they can be treated in the same ways. Moreover, clinical intervention trials have now shown that diabetic subjects benefit at least as much from lipid-lowering therapy as do nondiabetics.[1–3]

This chapter summarizes recent advances in the understanding of the pathogenesis of atherosclerosis. Over the last two decades a great deal has been learned about the cellular and molecular events in the artery wall that lead to the initiation and progression of lesions. Advances in cell biology and molecular biology have led to the elucidation of a generally agreed-upon sequence of events for lesion initiation in the artery wall and the identification of a number of growth factors and cytokines that influence those events. Particular interest is focused on the role of oxidative modification of LDL in atherogenesis, and some evidence is available to suggest that oxidation of LDL may proceed at a higher rate in diabetic animals. The purpose of this chapter is to briefly review current understanding of atherogenesis and to point out some of the ways that diabetes mellitus may accelerate the process.

CURRENT CONCEPTS OF ATHEROGENESIS

It is probably a mistake to think of atherosclerosis as a single, well-defined disease entity. It is more likely that it has multiple causes

and that the weight of each potential cause varies from individual to individual and possibly even from lesion to lesion. The best established risk factor—and the one most clearly demonstrated to act directly on the vessel wall—is hyperlipoproteinemia. The strikingly low incidence of CHD morbidity and mortality in the Japanese population, where total cholesterol levels have in the past averaged about 165 mg/dL, speaks volumes about the importance of hypercholesterolemia as a risk factor.[4] This is not reflective of a genetic resistance to cholesterol-induced atherosclerosis, because the Japanese who migrate and adopt Western diets in Honolulu or San Francisco acquire higher cholesterol levels and with them a higher incidence of coronary artery disease.[5] The low incidence in Japan is especially remarkable because smoking and hypertension, the two most important additional risk factors, are so prevalent in that population.

There is now general acceptance that an elevated low-density lipoprotein (LDL) or a low HDL level constitutes an important determinant of atherosclerosis, and national programs are in place to deal with dyslipidemia. Many studies have now demonstrated that correction of hypercholesterolemia reduces the rate of progression of atherosclerosis and reduces the incidence of CHD morbidity and mortality.[1–3,6] Only recently, however, have we begun to understand the mechanisms by which a high LDL level in the plasma influences the initiation and progression of the arterial lesion. In the following sections an outline of the current consensus regarding the processes in the artery wall triggered by hypercholesterolemia is presented. A discussion follows of how diabetes mellitus may intersect with and influence the rate at which these processes occur. An overall schema is presented in Fig. 11-1.

Initiation: The Fatty Streak

The fatty streak is the earliest grossly detectable lesion of atherosclerosis. It is a very slightly elevated, yellowish lesion made up predominantly of lipid-laden foam cells. Most of these are derived from circulating monocytes; a smaller number are derived from smooth muscle cells (SMCs). The endothelial lining overlying a fatty streak is intact. The view that loss of endothelial cells might be a necessary first step in the initiation of atherogenesis has been largely discounted. Many carefully conducted studies show no loss of endothelial cells *until later in the course of the disease*. However, the loss of endothelial cells may signal the transition from the first phase of atherosclerosis to the second phase. Thus, the monocyte-derived foam cells represent mostly circulating monocytes that have penetrated between endothelial cells, entered the

ATHEROSCLEROSIS INDUCED BY HYPERCHOLESTEROLEMIA

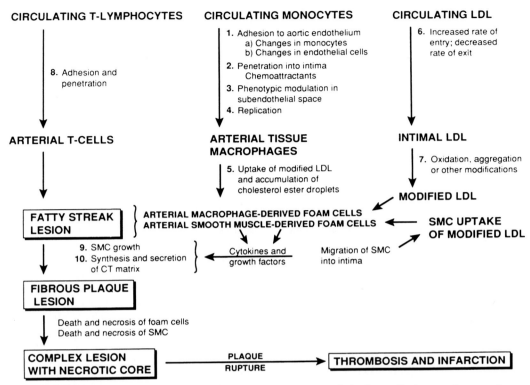

FIGURE 11-1. Schematic summary of the unit processes in the aortic wall contributing to atherogenesis. *(Reprinted with permission from Steinberg* et al.[33]*)*

intima, and taken up lipoproteins with the consequent storage of cholesterol esters in multiple droplets.

One of the earliest observable responses in animals fed a cholesterol-rich diet is an increase in the adherence of circulating monocytes to the arterial endothelium. This was first emphasized by Gerrity[7] and confirmed many times over. Hypercholesterolemia in some way induces the expression of specific adhesion molecules on the endothelial cells, one of which is vascular cell adhesion molecule-1 (VCAM-1) as shown by Li and colleagues.[8] Hypercholesterolemia may also influence the behavior of the circulating monocyte by increasing the probability of its adhesion to endothelium. A large body of literature is developing regarding the selectins and integrins involved in cell–cell interactions, and it seems likely that many additional adhesion molecules will be defined as research progresses. The monocytes that adhere then penetrate in response to chemotactic factors, some of which have been identified. Oxidatively modified LDL can act directly as a chemoattractant.[9] It can also act indirectly by stimulating release of monocyte chemoattractant protein-1 (MCP-1) from endothelial cells.[10] The central importance of monocyte chemoattractant protein 1 (MCP-1) and its receptor on the monocyte CCR2 (CC chemokine receptor 2) has been established by gene targeting. Knocking out either gene in a mouse model of atherosclerosis slows lesion progression by 50–80%.[11,12] Platelet-derived growth factor (PDGF) produced by endothelial cells, macrophages, and SMCs is another candidate chemoattractant.

Once in the subendothelial space, the monocyte undergoes a differentiation process that radically alters the repertoire of genes expressed and the cell acquires the properties of an arterial tissue macrophage. Exactly how this differentiation is accomplished remains uncertain, but it is known that macrophage colony-stimulating factor (MCSF), produced by endothelial cells and macrophages and whose production can be enhanced by oxidized LDL,[13] speeds this differentiation process.

The next step is the accumulation of lipids. It is known that these lipids have their origin in the plasma lipoproteins. The artery wall itself synthesizes almost no cholesterol and the lipid in the foam cells is primarily cholesterol esters. Studies in experimental animals, and some studies in humans, support the conclusion that essentially all of the cholesterol esters that accumulate are derived from circulating lipoproteins. Here a paradox is encountered. In cell culture, neither the circulating monocyte, the tissue macrophage, or the smooth muscle cell can take up native LDL fast enough to build up their cholesterol content significantly.[14,15] This is in part because they take up native LDL by way of the Goldstein-Brown LDL receptor, a receptor that is downregulated as soon as the cholesterol content of the cell begins to increase.[16] This is the normal response that prevents excessive accumulation of cholesterol that can be damaging to cells. How then do we account for the continuing build-up of cholesterol to extremely high levels in macrophages and SMCs in the wall of the artery? These cells can stuff themselves with cholesterol to the point where as much as half of the total dry weight of the cell is represented by lipid.

An even greater paradox is encountered when we consider the lesions in patients with familial hypercholesterolemia. These patients, who totally lack LDL receptors, nevertheless show foam cell accumulation in their lesions much like patients who have normal LDL receptors and very high plasma levels of LDL. Evidently, uptake by way of the LDL receptor, a major route of lipoprotein uptake in most cells of the body, is not the mechanism by which the LDL cholesterol is delivered to these cells (or at least it need not be). These two paradoxes almost forced the conclusion that LDL must be modified in some way prior to its uptake by macrophages. Suffice it to say at this point that oxidation of LDL modifies it into a form not recognized by the native LDL receptor, but recognized by alternative receptors on the macrophage. These presumably are receptors that do not downregulate. In this modified form, LDL can be taken up rapidly enough that there is a progressive build-up of cholesterol esters in the cell.

Fibrous Plaque Formation

The earliest fatty streak lesion consists primarily of monocyte/macrophage-derived foam cells plus some smooth muscle cell-derived foam cells. From the beginning, however, one can find a few T lymphocytes as well. These do not contribute to the foam cell population, but they may play a central role in the transition of the fatty streak to a fibrous plaque. This process shares many of the features seen in chronic inflammatory processes elsewhere in the body. Every one of the major cell types involved—endothelial cells, macrophages, T lymphocytes, and SMCs—is capable of generating and releasing chemotactic factors, mitogenic factors, and cytokines of many kinds. Some are proinflammatory and others anti-inflammatory. The array of factors that *may* be involved has been reviewed extensively elsewhere.[17,18] It is sufficient to note here that the end result is a recruitment of SMCs from the media up through a fragmented internal elastic membrane; the replication of these cells; the secretion of proteoglycans, collagen, elastin, and other connective tissue matrix elements; and the formation of a fibrous cap over the top of the lesion.

Exactly what triggers the transition from fatty streak to fibrous plaque is not certain. There are some populations in which fatty streaks are rather prevalent, but they rarely go on to become fibrous plaques or clinically significant lesions of any kind. Thus the progression is not inevitable, and it would be of great significance if the triggers were identified. One suggestion is that the endothelial cell lining overlying a fully developed fatty streak loses its integrity, exposing the underlying lesion to the bloodstream. This would allow platelet aggregation to occur, with the consequent release of many cytokines, including PDGF, that might then accelerate the progression of the fatty streak to the fibrous plaque. In a sense, this would represent a repair process.

The fibrous cap is not itself a nidus for thrombosis. The fibrous plaque can progress and eventually cause clinically significant stenosis. However, the lesion that is a serious threat is one in which the fibrous cap becomes eroded, culminating in plaque rupture and a terminal thrombosis.

Conversion of the Fibrous Plaque to the Complex Lesion: Plaque Rupture

Over many years the fibrous plaque can build up as a result of SMC replication and deposition of matrix material. There is probably always some continuing lipid accumulation at the growing edges of the lesions that continues to include many macrophages and T lymphocytes. In other words, the lesions extend at their periphery, and at their periphery they retain many of the properties of the original

fatty streak. Eventually, the lesion matures such that there is a fibrous cap and beneath it a pool of lipid. Presumably, the lipid-laden foam cells eventually become necrotic, and it seems likely that the pool in the necrotic core of lesions represents lipid that once was contained within the foam cells. Stenosis as a result of the progressive growth of the lesion can ultimately restrict blood flow to the point that patients will experience angina. They may even have infarction because of disproportion between demand and flow. More commonly, the infarction results from thrombosis that occurs when a plaque ruptures. The pioneering work of Constantinides[19] and the more recent work of Davies[20] make this very clear. What triggers the rupture is not certain, but it could relate to activity of the macrophages at the shoulders of the lesion with release of lytic enzymes, tissue-damaging free radicals, or oxidized lipids. These could erode the thinning fibrous cap, and in concert with hemodynamic forces, bring about the rupture. That in turn exposes the blood to tissue factor and other prothrombogenic factors in the lipid pool, and triggers the potentially fatal thrombosis.

THE OXIDATIVE MODIFICATION HYPOTHESIS

We referred in the section on lesion initiation to the double paradox relating to foam cell formation. Goldstein and coworkers[14] recognized the paradox and attempted to modify LDL into a form that monocytes and macrophages would take up rapidly enough to become foam cells. They demonstrated that chemical acetylation of LDL (treatment with acetic anhydride) converted it into a form that was taken up much more rapidly than native LDL. Moreover, it was taken up by a specific, saturable mechanism. They named the receptor the "acetyl LDL receptor." The key point is that this receptor, unlike the native LDL receptor, does not downregulate as the cholesterol content of the cell increases progressively. The acetyl LDL receptor was subsequently cloned and characterized by Kodama and colleagues. They named it the "scavenger receptor."[21] It now appears that there are several families of scavenger receptors,[22] and the acetyl LDL receptor is now referred to as a class A scavenger receptor.

The work of Goldstein and Brown on macrophage metabolism of lipoproteins was seminal,[14,23] but there was no evidence then (and there is still none) that acetylation of LDL takes place in the body. Henriksen and associates in 1981 were the first to describe a biologically plausible modification of LDL that might account for foam cell formation.[24] They showed that incubation of LDL with cultured endothelial cells led to a modification, later shown to be an oxidative modification,[25,26] that made it a ligand for specific receptors on the macrophage. A part of the uptake, which was saturable, was attributed to the acetyl LDL receptor, but as much as 40% or more could not be via that receptor, but by a different receptor or receptors.

Soon after the discovery that oxidative modification converted LDL to a ligand for specific macrophage receptors, additional biologic properties of oxidized LDL were discovered that could further enhance its atherogenicity. For example, oxidized LDL was shown to be chemotactic for monocytes[9] and later for T lymphocytes.[27] It was shown that oxidized LDL *inhibited* the motility of tissue macrophages and thus might cause a trapping of these cells once they entered the subendothelial space.[28] Work by Morel and coworkers[26,29] showed that oxidized LDL was cytotoxic, which certainly could contribute to its atherogenicity, particularly in the transition from the fatty streak to the fibrous plaque. Studies by

Cushing and associates[10] and by Rajavashisth and coworkers[13] showed that even very mildly oxidized LDL (minimally modified LDL; MM-LDL) has biologic properties that are proatherogenic even before the lipoprotein loses its affinity for the LDL receptor and long before it becomes a ligand for scavenger receptors. They showed that minimally oxidized LDL could stimulate the release of MCP-1 and MCSF from endothelial cells, even though the oxidized LDL used was not a ligand for the scavenger receptor. The list of biologic properties that could in principle make oxidized LDL a more atherogenic lipoprotein than native LDL has grown by leaps and bounds, and at last count there were more than 15 such properties. How many of these properties, demonstrated in cell culture systems, are quantitatively important in the atherogenic process *in vivo* remains to be ascertained. It is sufficient to say here that the conversion of LDL to its oxidized form affects both lipids and protein, and that the oxidized form is significantly more atherogenic than the native form. Consequently, any intervention that inhibits the oxidation of LDL should theoretically be able to slow the progression of atherosclerosis. Conversely, any metabolic error that increases the rate of oxidation of LDL or enhances its proatherogenic properties could speed the progression of atherosclerosis. The next section will identify metabolic abnormalities associated with diabetes that might do this. Before that, an outline of the evidence supporting the oxidative modification hypothesis and some of the uncertainties with regard to its relevance in humans are discussed.

The current status of the oxidative modification hypothesis is summarized in Table 11-1. The theoretical basis for the hypothesis is well supported by an extensive body of work at the experimental level as reviewed in references 30–33. Considerable evidence that oxidative modification does indeed occur *in vivo* has accumulated over the years and includes the following: (1) demonstration of the presence of oxidatively modified LDL in atherosclerotic lesions (but not in normal arteries) and, to a limited extent, in circulating plasma; (2) demonstration by immunohistochemical methods that epitopes of oxidized LDL are represented in lesions but again, not in normal arteries; (3) demonstration of autoantibodies in plasma, signaling the presence *in vivo* of either oxidized LDL itself or a closely related antigen; and (4) demonstration that antioxidants can significantly inhibit the rate of progression of early atherosclerosis in experimental animal models. This last line of evidence is obviously the most critical. The first studies were done by Carew and colleagues[34] and by Kita and coworkers[35] using LDL receptor–deficient rabbits. Both groups showed that probucol, previously shown by Parthasarathy and associates[36] to be a potent antioxidant, inhibited lesion development by 50–80% in young rabbits

TABLE 11-1. Current Status of the Oxidative Modification Hypothesis

- It rests on a well-defined, mechanistically plausible theoretical footing.
- It is consistent with many phenomena demonstrated in cell culture and in experimental animals.
- It is supported by epidemiologic data, both observational and prospective.
- It is strongly supported by positive intervention studies of atherosclerosis in animal models.
- It is supported by the results of the CHAOS trial[47] but not by the three clinical intervention trials with vitamin E so far reported.[46,48,49]
- Only additional appropriately-designed, large double-blind clinical intervention trials will establish the validity of the antioxidant hypothesis in humans. Trials should emphasize stopping the disease in its early stages.

lacking the LDL receptor. Because probucol does have a cholesterol-lowering effect, even in receptor-deficient animals, Carew and coworkers gave a low dose of a 3-hydroxy-3-methylglutaryl coenzyme A (HMG CoA) reductase inhibitor to their control rabbits to keep the cholesterol levels of the two groups matched. Thus it could be concluded that the protective effect of the probucol was not due to cholesterol lowering but to some other property, presumably its antioxidant property. Since these early studies, many additional intervention trials in experimental animals have been reported. These include additional studies in receptor-deficient rabbits, studies in cholesterol-fed rabbits, and studies in cholesterol-fed nonhuman primates (reviewed in reference 37). Recently, antioxidants have also been shown to be effective in mouse models of atherosclerosis.[38–42] All in all, 29 studies have been done, of which 21 are strongly positive. Moreover, different antioxidant compounds have been used by different investigators. These included probucol, butylated hydroxytoluene, N,N′-diphenylphenylenediamine, and vitamin E. The fact that antioxidants, some of them differing quite markedly in their chemical structures and properties, all share the ability to inhibit atherosclerosis strongly supports the interpretation that it is their common antioxidant activity that is operative. However, there is always the possibility that they have additional properties that contribute to or may even account for most of their antiatherogenic potential.

Epidemiologic evidence of several kinds is consistent with the antioxidant hypothesis. Population studies have shown that a high dietary intake or a high plasma concentration of antioxidants (vitamin E, vitamin C, β-carotene, or selenium) is associated with a lower risk of CHD.[43] Prospective within-population studies have also yielded statistically significant associations[44,45]; however, the possibility of confounding factors can never be completely dismissed. Moreover, epidemiologic correlations, no matter how strong, cannot establish a causal relationship. Therefore, large, double-blind, randomized clinical intervention trials are needed to settle the question of whether or not antioxidants can provide significant protection against CHD.

Although a number of clinical intervention trials are underway, only a few have been fully reported as of this writing. A Finnish study of α-tocopherol and β-carotene was designed to test the possible effects of these vitamins against cancer.[46] Administration of 50 mg of vitamin E daily, or 20 mg of β-carotene daily, or both, failed to decrease cancer incidence (and may even have *increased* it). Cardiovascular endpoints, although not a part of the original hypothesis, were also recorded. There was no decrease in CHD deaths and there was a small but significant *increase* in hemorrhagic stroke among the men taking vitamin E. The dose of vitamin E used in this study was probably too small. The results of prospective studies show that only individuals taking vitamin E supplements and having a mean vitamin E intake over 100 mg/d were protected significantly against CHD.[44,45] Moreover, the Finnish study was done in middle-aged men who were heavy smokers and whose lesions must have been far advanced at the time the study was started. Three additional large, double-blind, placebo-controlled vitamin E intervention trials have now been reported. One was strongly positive and two were negative. The Cambridge Heart Antioxidant Study (CHAOS) was a study of 2002 patients with angiographically proved coronary artery disease randomized either to vitamin E (400–800 IU daily) or to placebo.[47] Median follow-up was 1.4 years. The primary endpoint was the combination of cardiovascular death plus nonfatal myocardial infarction. This was reduced by almost 47% ($p = 0.005$). However, there was no decrease in all-cause mortality.[47] The

HOPE trial randomized over 9000 patients in a 2×2 factorial design to evaluate the effects of an angiotensin-converting enzyme inhibitor and vitamin E (400 IU/d). In a 5-year follow-up there was no difference in cardiovascular events between the controls and those on vitamin E.[48] The GISSI trial randomized almost 3000 patients to placebo or vitamin E (300 mg/d). Over a 3.5-year follow-up there was no difference in major cardiovascular endpoints due to vitamin E.[49]

The effectiveness of β-carotene has been tested in three large-scale studies and none has shown any effect on cardiovascular events.[46,50,51] However, whereas the doses of vitamin E used in the intervention trials discussed above are adequate to protect circulating LDL against *ex vivo* oxidation, β-carotene does not do that even at the large doses used in these studies.[52,53] β-carotene does not seem to function as an antioxidant in this context. Consequently, these trials do not constitute tests of the oxidative modification hypothesis.

It should be emphasized that the experimental animal data relate almost exclusively to fatty streaks. In these animal models, lesions seldom go on to more advanced stages during the relatively short course of the study. Thus the experimental evidence is only that antioxidants may inhibit *fatty streak formation*. There is no experimental evidence that antioxidants will have an effect on fibrous plaques or complicated lesions. Eventually, of course, inhibition of fatty streak formation should be reflected by a reduction in the number of fibrous plaques and complicated lesions. However, to see effects on these later lesions may require a longer period of study than the generally accepted 5 years.

It is too early to draw conclusions regarding the effectiveness of antioxidants against human atherosclerosis. However, the strength of the experimental basis for the antioxidant hypothesis justifies continued exploration of its relevance to human disease, and a number of studies are currently in progress.

ATHEROSCLEROSIS IN DIABETIC SUBJECTS

Many studies have been carried out to determine whether the atherosclerosis in diabetic subjects might be qualitatively distinct, which could shed some light on the reason for the excess morbidity from atherosclerosis in persons with diabetes mellitus. None of these studies demonstrates qualitative differences—just more lesions that occur earlier.[54] The histologic appearance of the lesions, their gross appearance, their chemical composition, their sites of predilection, and the clinical expression of the disease are almost exactly the same in diabetic patients and in nondiabetics. One possible exception that calls for special comment is the apparently greater frequency of peripheral vascular disease in diabetic subjects; however, this may be more apparent than real. It is possible that the combination of macrovascular and microvascular disease (or the combination of macrovascular disease and peripheral neuropathy) accounts for the more serious clinical presentation of impaired peripheral circulation in the diabetic. It is of interest that peripheral vascular disease in the diabetic is more closely correlated with the duration of the disease, degree of hyperglycemia, and presence of microvascular disease than is atherosclerosis affecting the coronary or cerebral vessels.[55–57] Janka and associates[57] found that disease below the knee was related to these factors, but that disease above the knee correlated better with hypercholesterolemia, hypertension, and cigarette smoking, the classical risk factors for large-vessel disease. These findings tend to support the conclusion that peripheral vascular disease is more of a clinical problem in diabetics because of interactions between microvascular disease (or neuropathy) and macrovascular disease.

In diabetic subjects, just as in nondiabetic subjects, the risk of clinically evident atherosclerosis increases among cigarette smokers, the obese, hypertensives, those with low HDL values, and those with high LDL values. This concordance with regard to risk factors does not rule out the presence of differences of some kind but is compatible with the premise that the disease is qualitatively no different in diabetic patients.

This conclusion is consonant with the fact that in populations where the general incidence of CHD is low, the incidence in the diabetic population there is also low. For example, in Japan, where the prevalence of CHD in the general population is low, it is also low in the diabetic population and one-sixth the prevalence among Americans with diabetes.[58] Whatever environmental or genetic factors account for the overall lower prevalence of CHD appear to affect its prevalence within the diabetic population in like fashion. A key corollary to this is that interventions that decrease CHD morbidity and mortality in the general population will probably do so also, and to a comparable degree, within the diabetic population. Unfortunately, some physicians tend to regard the development of macrovascular complications as an inevitable accompaniment to diabetes mellitus, not amenable to prevention by intervention. This is not the case. Because the disease process is not qualitatively different, it can be anticipated that the beneficial results already demonstrated in the general population as a result of cholesterol lowering, cessation of smoking, and treatment of hypertension can be expected to be equally impressive within the diabetic population. Once we can identify the reasons the disease progresses more rapidly in diabetic patients, we can hope to intervene more specifically and get even better results.

Some CHD risk factors are found clustered with a high frequency in type 2 diabetes. The constellation of glucose intolerance associated with insulin resistance, hypertension, hypertriglyceridemia with low HDL, and central obesity is variously designated as Syndrome X,[59] the deadly quartet,[60] the insulin resistance syndrome,[61] or the plurimetabolic syndrome. How these elements are related in pathogenetic terms is not clear. Most of these features are associated with obesity,[62,63] even in the absence of frank diabetes. However, some type 2 diabetes patients have most of the elements of the syndrome without obesity.[64] Until the causal relationships are sorted out, one can only treat these abnormalities individually as in nondiabetic patients with these risk factors.

In summary, if there are any differences in the basic nature of the atherosclerotic process in diabetes, they must be subtle. The bulk of the evidence available suggests that the basic nature of the atherosclerotic process in diabetes is the same except that everything moves at a faster rate. If that premise is valid, our goal is to find out what gets speeded up and how and when it happens. The risk factors are the same ones identified in nondiabetic persons. All of them should be treated intensively, even more intensively than in nondiabetic patients. However, the known risk factors simply cannot account for all of the increased risk in diabetic patients.

INTERSECTIONS BETWEEN DIABETES AND ATHEROSCLEROSIS

We should start this section by stating that no one knows with any certainty why diabetic patients suffer premature macrovascular disease. The reader who is interested in knowing what the possibilities are, and which are favored, is invited to read on.

Dyslipidemia

The disturbances in lipoprotein patterns found in diabetes are discussed in Chap. 47, so the discussion here will be brief. Diabetic patients in good control do not have hypercholesterolemia any more frequently than the general population.[65] However, they do have some degree of hypertriglyceridemia as well as low HDL levels (still lower when poorly controlled).[65] Exactly how atherogenic the triglyceride-rich lipoproteins are remains a matter of controversy. They certainly have not been exonerated and the hypertriglyceridemia in diabetes may be highly relevant. A low HDL level is the most powerful predictor of coronary artery disease and could play a significant role in the premature atherosclerosis of diabetes mellitus. Because hypertriglyceridemia and low HDL are closely linked, it has been difficult to assign primacy to one or the other until quite recently. The demonstration that transgenic mice with overexpression of apoA-1 are resistant to atherosclerosis strongly supports a direct effect of low HDL on susceptibility to atherosclerosis.[66] Whether it is the whole story or not is not known. Triglyceride-rich lipoproteins may be directly atherogenic as well. Thus, dyslipidemia may be a contributing factor to the premature atherosclerosis in some diabetic persons. On the other hand, there are many diabetic patients who do not have dyslipidemia but in whom premature atherosclerotic disease is present. Possible contributing factors in these cases are discussed in the following sections.

Lipoprotein Oxidation

Pioneering studies by Sato and associates[67] and by Nishigaki and coworkers[68] showed some years ago that the plasma lipoproteins of patients with diabetes showed higher concentrations of oxidation products. Studies in diabetic animal models, mostly streptozotocin-treated animals, show that there is an increase in oxidized lipids in the plasma lipoproteins and red cell membranes, and that this increase can be prevented by treating the animal with an appropriate antioxidant (see review by Chisolm and coworkers[69]). Thus, to the extent that oxidative modification plays a role in atherogenesis, diabetic subjects might be at a higher risk.

There is a very direct connection between diabetes and oxidative damage: oxidation of LDL proceeds more rapidly in the presence of high levels of glucose, and the rate of generation of glycated proteins is accelerated under pro-oxidant conditions.[69–73] There appears to be a basis for a logarithmic progression: hyperglycemia favoring oxidation of lipids on the one hand, and pro-oxidant conditions and oxidized lipids favoring the formation of advanced glycation end-products on the other. It is of interest that in atherosclerotic lesions one finds both oxidized LDL and advanced glycation end-products,[74–76] compatible with an interaction of the kind just discussed.

Nonenzymatic Glycation

Glucose and other aldoses react nonenzymatically with amino groups to form glucose-protein linkages. The rate of nonenzymatic glycation is proportional to the glucose concentration and it proceeds more rapidly in diabetic patients, especially when their control is poor. All of the plasma proteins, and probably all of the cell surface membrane proteins, are also candidates for glycation. Witztum and coworkers[77] demonstrated that LDL underwent glycation and that this decreased its affinity for the native LDL receptor, consequently prolonging its lifetime in the plasma compartment. Simply prolonging the lifetime of the LDL would increase the proba-

bility of its undergoing oxidative modification with the adverse consequences already discussed. Glycation of connective tissue matrix proteins, particularly when extensive, could increase the probability that LDL will be trapped in the vessel wall and there undergo more extensive oxidative modification and further glycation.[78] The early steps in glycation are reversible, but if it continues, it gives rise to advanced glycation end-products (AGEs). These compounds, heterogeneous in structure and not completely defined chemically, form cross-linkages among macromolecules, are fluorescent, and importantly, are recognized by receptors on the cell surface. A strong case has been made for the possibility that the microvascular complications of diabetes mellitus may be due to the accumulation of AGEs. More recently, evidence has accumulated that the macrovascular complications also may be in part attributable to AGEs. These lines of evidence and the chemistry and pathophysiology of AGEs are explored in detail in Chap. 13. Here we only point to the intersections between AGEs and our current schema for atherogenesis.

Trapping of LDL in the subendothelial space is a critical step in the early stages of atherosclerosis. LDL binds readily to proteoglycans, collagen, elastin, and other matrix proteins, but it binds even more strongly when these matrix proteins carry AGEs.[78] Oxidative modification of such trapped LDL would make it a ligand for uptake by macrophages in the subendothelial space. Also, the additional trapping may encourage the formation of LDL aggregates, also excellent ligands for macrophage phagocytosis.[79]

Another category of interaction, as reviewed by Vlassara,[80] may result from the effects of AGEs on vascular wall cells via specific receptors that recognize them. For example, AGE receptors on the endothelial cell can activate NF-κB, a transcription factor that is also stimulated by oxidized LDL. AGEs in soluble form are chemotactic for monocytes and activate them. They increase the production of PDGF, IGF-1, IL-1, and TNF, all of which have been implicated as contributing to the chronic inflammatory process in an atherosclerotic lesion. As discussed, glycation and lipid oxidation may be reciprocally interactive and synergistic. There is evidence that glycated proteins are more susceptible to oxidative modification and, vice versa, that lipoproteins that have been oxidized are more susceptible to glycation. It is interesting that the complex cross-linking that characterizes AGEs is in a rough way analogous to the cross-linking that characterizes oxidatively modified lipoproteins or oxidatively damaged membranes.

If the mechanisms discussed above were important in the accelerated atherosclerosis of diabetes, it could be anticipated that there would be a good correlation between the level of glycemia and the CHD risk (or other measures of greater progression of atherosclerosis). Some epidemiologic studies show that hyperglycemia is a risk factor for CHD, but the link is not certain. Studies in which glycemia has been carefully controlled, as in the UGDP study, with administration of variable doses of oral agents and insulin in type 2 diabetes,[81] or the Diabetes Control and Complications Trial (DCCT) in type 1 diabetes,[82] have not shown a decrease in CHD mortality, but neither study was designed to test the hypothesis. Both were focused on other complications. There is a need for a large, double-blind test of whether or not close glycemia control reduces the CHD risk in diabetes.

Monocyte/Macrophage Function

Monocytes play a key role in the early stages of fatty streak formation and are the major source of foam cells. It is recognized that diabetic patients have difficulty fighting infections, suggesting the possibility of defects in leukocyte function. Abnormalities in neutrophil function have been described, but the situation with respect to monocyte function is less clear. Recently it has been shown that exposure of cultured endothelial cells to high levels of glucose increases monocyte binding[83] and that endothelial cells in diabetic rabbits overexpress VCAM-1 *in vivo*.[84] Also, monocytes from patients with diabetes show an increased adhesion to normal endothelial cells in culture, and this is attributed to overexpression of β_2 integrins.[85] Monocytes prepared from patients with recent onset of type 1 diabetes showed *less* expression of certain adhesion molecules (LFA-1α, ICAM-1, and HLA-DR). Stewart and coworkers[86] observed a small but statistically significant *decrease* in expression of surface receptors on monocytes from type 1 diabetics with ketoacidosis.

Another mechanism that could link diabetes to atherosclerosis is the chemotactic activity of AGEs.[87] These products of protein glycation exert a chemotactic effect for human blood monocytes and selectively induce monocyte migration across an intact endothelial cell monolayer. When these transmigrating monocytes interact with the AGEs in the matrix, they increase their production of PDGF. Thus the progressive accumulation of glycation products in the subendothelial space could contribute to the progression of the lesion.

Hiramatsu and Aramori[88] reported that monocytes from diabetic patients, especially hypertriglyceridemic diabetic patients, show an increase in the rate of superoxide production. It would be of great interest to extend studies of this kind to determine the enzyme systems responsible for the observed increase in rate of LDL oxidation. The combination of an increase in the ability of cells to oxidize LDL and the greater ease with which LDL is oxidized in the presence of high glucose concentrations could represent a significant driving force for LDL modification in diabetic persons, contributing to their advanced atherosclerosis.

Diabetes may have implications for the later stages of atherogenesis, including the terminal fatal thrombosis. A number of platelet abnormalities have been described, but whether they are causative or reflect underlying vascular disease remains uncertain.[89] The fatal thrombosis is often triggered by erosion of the fibrous cap, exposing blood to tissue factor and other thrombogenic factors in the lipid core of the lesion. This rupture generally occurs at the shoulder of the lesion where there are higher densities of macrophages. On a purely speculative level, if the monocyte/macrophages in diabetic patients were less robust and more inclined to lyse and spill their contents or to release lytic enzymes at a higher rate than macrophages in normal patients, this could explain the higher frequency of clinical events in diabetics. Because there is evidence to suggest that the conversion from a fatty streak to a fibrous plaque is linked to loss of endothelial cells, here might be another way in which the lesions in diabetics advance more rapidly than those in nondiabetic subjects.

Immune Mechanisms

There is mounting evidence that the immune system influences the rate of progression of atherosclerosis. First, autoantibodies against glycated LDL[90] have been demonstrated in both normal subjects and, at higher titers, in diabetic subjects. Autoantibodies against oxidized LDL are also present in the plasma of both diabetic and nondiabetic patients.[75] Immune complexes of oxidized LDL have been demonstrated in atherosclerotic lesions in receptor-deficient

rabbits.[91] Such immune complexes can be recognized by the F_c receptor and provide an additional pathway for rapid uptake and foam cell formation.[92] Immune complexes are potentially cytotoxic and could in this way favor the progression of lesions. Salonen and coworkers[93] reported that in a small series of cases the rate of progression of carotid artery intima/media thickness was closely correlated with the titer of autoantibody against oxidized LDL. Associations of this kind, however, do not necessarily establish a causal relationship and further studies are needed. Palinski and coworkers[94] recently found that deliberately increasing the titer of antibody against oxidized LDL in receptor-deficient rabbits by immunizing them with exogenously oxidized LDL *slowed* rather than *speeded* the progression of early lesions. They suggest that the very high titers reached may have been beneficial by "scavenging" oxidized LDL from the system at early stages and preventing some of the deleterious effects that might otherwise occur. Jonasson and coworkers[95] have shown that T lymphocytes are almost universally present in atherosclerotic lesions. Further studies showed that these include a small percentage of clones that are activated specifically by oxidized LDL.[96] The precise role of T cells in atherogenesis remains uncertain. Hansson and coworkers[97] have shown that a sharp drop in circulating T cells, induced by the injection of a monoclonal antibody against them, actually results in larger proliferative lesions in balloon-catheterized rat aortas. Clearly, additional research needs to be done to resolve this complex problem. Nevertheless, the evidence provided thus far suggests that diabetic patients, because they do have higher titers of antibodies against glycated LDL and other glycated proteins, may be more susceptible.

Abnormalities in Connective Tissue Matrix

We have discussed the possibility that AGEs may contribute. El Khoury and coworkers[98] showed that macrophages do not show calcium-independent binding to native collagen IV but do bind to glycated collagen IV. Interestingly, this binding occurred via the acetyl LDL receptor. Previous studies by Fraser and coworkers[99] showed that this receptor is also the means that macrophages use to attach to plastic dishes in a calcium-independent fashion.

It is possible that the biosynthesis and secretion of proteoglycans, collagen, elastin, or other connective tissue matrix elements may be abnormal in diabetes independently of the nonenzymatic glycation that leads to AGEs. Because trapping of LDL in the artery wall is believed to play an important role in atherogenesis, abnormalities in connective tissue matrix biosynthesis and deposition that enhance such trapping could be proatherogenic.

Relationship between Microvascular and Macrovascular Disease

There has been a tendency to regard microvascular and macrovascular disease as independent and unrelated. However, this is by no means established. We have discussed some of the metabolic links that are emerging as more is learned about the pathogenesis of atherosclerosis. For example, there is now evidence that AGEs may be involved in both the microvascular and macrovascular complications. There is evidence that hyperglycemia may favor the oxidation of LDL and thus could play a role in both macrovascular and microvascular disease. However, intervention trials have yielded negative, or at best borderline, evidence for a decrease in CHD risk with tight control of hyperglycemia.[100,101] A definitive answer must await further large-scale studies to determine whether control of hyperglycemia can decrease the progression of atherosclerosis in diabetic subjects (independent of control of hyperlipidemia or other risk factors).

A unifying hypothesis is always preferable when possible. A possibility that has received little attention is that the vasa vasorum are also subject to microvascular disease, and that this is what enhances the rate of progression of macrovascular disease in the diabetic patient. The oxygen supply and nutrition of the arterial wall in large vessels arise in part from the vasa vasorum. It is well established that even the most mild noxious stimulus on the adventitial side of the artery produces cellular changes in the intima. Certainly the possibility that disease of the vasa vasorum plays a role in atherosclerosis has not been ruled out. However, there are no definitive experiments that assess the relative importance of the vasa vasorum in atherosclerosis either in nondiabetic or diabetic persons. Further research in this area would certainly be warranted.

SUMMARY

Myocardial infarction and other macrovascular diseases are responsible for more deaths in diabetic patients than all of the other causes of death combined. The lesions in diabetic subjects are qualitatively indistinguishable from those in nondiabetic patients, but the rate of progression of the disease is greater and the incidence of fatal outcome higher. The new guidelines on management of hyperlipidemia issued by the National Cholesterol Education Program recommend that diabetic patients should be treated just as aggressively as patients with established coronary heart disease (LDL goal <100 mg/dL).[102] The past decade has seen some remarkable progress in our understanding of vascular pathobiology, such that we can now delineate in some detail the critically important events in atherogenesis. As a result, we can now postulate explicit ways in which diabetes may lead to an acceleration of the atherogenic process. Among the more attractive of these is the interrelationship between glycation and oxidation. Hyperglycemia can promote both the oxidative modification of LDL and the rate of formation of glycated proteins. We still are not in a position to say whether precise control of blood glucose levels will reduce the risk of atherosclerosis and its complications in the diabetic. However, the circumstantial evidence supporting this possibility strengthens the case for rigorous control of hyperglycemia. Most important, management of *all* of the conventional risk factors for atherosclerosis in diabetic patients should rank as high as control of hyperglycemia.

REFERENCES

1. Downs JR, Clearfield M, Weis S, *et al*: Primary prevention of acute coronary events with lovastatin in men and women with average cholesterol levels. *JAMA* 1998;279:1615.
2. Goldberg RB, Mellies MJ, Sacks FM, *et al*: Cardiovascular events and their reduction with pravastatin in diabetic and glucose-intolerant myocardial infarction survivors with average cholesterol levels. *Circulation* 1998;98:2513.
3. The Long-term Intervention with Pravastatin in Ischaemic Disease (LIPID) study group: Prevention of cardiovascular events and death with pravastatin in patients with coronary heart disease and a broad range of initial cholesterol levels. *N Engl J Med* 1998;339:1349.
4. The Inter-Society Commission for Heart Disease Resource Report: Primary prevention of the atherosclerotic diseases. *Circulation* 1984;70:153A.
5. Marmot MG, Syme SL, Kagan A, *et al*: Epidemiologic studies of coronary heart disease and stroke in Japanese men living in Japan, Hawaii and California: Prevalence of coronary and hypertensive heart diseases and associated risk factors. *Am J Epidemiol* 1975;102:514.
6. Tyroler HA: Lowering plasma cholesterol decreases risk of coronary heart disease: An overview of clinical trials. In: Steinberg D, Olefsky JM, eds. *Hypercholesterolemia and Atherosclerosis*. Churchill Livingstone:1987;99.
7. Gerrity RG: The role of the monocyte in atherogenesis. I: Transition of blood-borne monocytes into foam cells in fatty lesions. *Am J Pathol* 1981;103:181.
8. Li H, Cybulsky MI, Gimbrone MA Jr., *et al*: An atherogenic diet rapidly induces VCAM-1, a cytokine-regulatable mononuclear leukocyte adhesion molecule, in rabbit aortic endothelium. *Arterioscler Thromb* 1993;13:197.
9. Quinn MT, Parthasarathy S, Fong LG, *et al*: Oxidatively modified low density lipoproteins: A potential role in recruitment and retention of monocyte/macrophages during atherogenesis. *Proc Natl Acad Sci USA* 1987;84:2995.
10. Cushing SD, Berliner JA, Valente AJ, *et al*: Minimally modified low density lipoprotein induces monocyte chemotactic protein 1 in human endothelial cells and smooth muscle cells. *Nature* 1990;344:254.
11. Gu L, Okada Y, Clinton SK, *et al*: Absence of monocyte chemoattractant protein-1 reduces atherosclerosis in low density lipoprotein receptor-deficient mice. *Mol Cell* 1998;2:275.
12. Boring L, Gosling J, Cleary M, *et al*: Decreased lesion formation in CCR2 −/− mice reveals a role for chemokines in the initiation of atherosclerosis. *Nature* 1998;394:894.
13. Rajavashisth TB, Andalibi A, Territo MC, *et al*: Induction of endothelial cell expression of granulocyte and macrophage colony-stimulating factors by modified low density lipoproteins. *Nature* 1990;344:254.
14. Goldstein JL, Ho YK, Basu SK, *et al*: Binding site on macrophages that mediates uptake and degradation of acetylated low density lipoprotein, producing massive cholesterol deposition. *Proc Natl Acad Sci USA* 1979;76:333.
15. Weinstein DB, Carew TE, Steinberg D: Uptake and degradation of low density lipoprotein by swine arterial smooth muscle cells with inhibition of cholesterol biosynthesis. *Biochim Biophys Acta* 1976;424:404.
16. Brown MS, Goldstein JL: A receptor-mediated pathway for cholesterol homeostasis. *Science* 1986;232:34.
17. Ross R: The pathogenesis of atherosclerosis: A perspective for the 1990s. *Nature* 1993;362:801.
18. Clinton SK, Libby P: Cytokines and growth factors in atherogenesis. *Arch Pathol Lab Med* 1992;116:1292.
19. Constantinides P: Plaque fissures in human coronary thrombosis. *J Athero Res* 1966;6:1.
20. Davies MJ: A macro and micro view of coronary vascular insult in ischemic heart disease. *Circulation* 1990;82(suppl 3):II38.
21. Kodama T, Freeman M, Rohrer L, *et al*: Type I macrophage scavenger receptor contains α-helical and collagen-like coiled coils. *Nature* 1990;343:531.
22. Acton SL, Scherer PE, Lodish HF, *et al*: Expression cloning of SR-BI, a CD36-related class B scavenger receptor. *J Biol Chem* 1994;269:21003.
23. Brown MS, Goldstein JL: Lipoprotein metabolism in the macrophage: Implications for cholesterol deposition in atherosclerosis. *Annu Rev Biochem* 1983;52:223.
24. Henriksen T, Mahoney EM, Steinberg D: Enhanced macrophage degradation of low density lipoprotein previously incubated with cultured endothelial cells: Recognition by receptors for acetylated low density lipoproteins. *Proc Natl Acad Sci USA* 1981;78:6499.
25. Steinbrecher UP, Parthasarathy S, Leake DS, *et al*: Modification of low density lipoprotein by endothelial cells involves lipid peroxidation and degradation of low density lipoprotein phospholipids. *Proc Natl Acad Sci USA* 1984;81:3883.
26. Morel DW, DiCorleto PE, Chisolm GM: Endothelial and smooth muscle cells alter low density lipoprotein in vitro by free radical oxidation. *Arteriosclerosis* 1984;4:357.
27. McMurray HF, Parthasarathy S, Steinberg D: Oxidatively modified low density lipoprotein is a chemoattractant for human T lymphocytes. *J Clin Invest* 1993;92:1004.

28. Quinn MT, Parthasarathy S, Steinberg D: Endothelial cell-derived chemotactic activity for mouse peritoneal macrophages and the effects of modified forms of low density lipoprotein. *Proc Natl Acad Sci USA* 1985;82:5949.

29. Cathcart MK, Morel DW, Chisolm GM III: Monocytes and neutrophils oxidize low density lipoprotein making it cytotoxic. *J Leukocyte Biol* 1985;38:341.

30. Steinberg D, Parthasarathy S, Carew TE, *et al*: Beyond cholesterol: Modifications of low density lipoprotein that increase its atherogenicity. *N Engl J Med* 1989;320:915.

31. Witztum JL, Steinberg D: Role of oxidized LDL in atherogenesis. *J Clin Invest* 1991;88:1785.

32. Esterbauer H, Gebicki J, Puhl H, *et al*: The role of lipid peroxidation and antioxidants in oxidative modification of LDL. *Free Radical Biol Med* 1992;13:341.

33. Steinberg D, Witztum JL: Emerging opportunities for atherosclerosis prevention. In: Rifkind B, ed. *Cholesterol Lowering: Clinical and Population Aspects*. Marcel Dekker:1995;337.

34. Carew TE, Schwenke DC, Steinberg D: Antiatherogenic effect of probucol unrelated to its hypocholesterolemic effect: Evidence that antioxidants in vivo can selectively inhibit low density lipoprotein degradation in macrophage-rich fatty streaks slowing the progression of atherosclerosis in the WHHL rabbit. *Proc Natl Acad Sci USA* 1987;84:7725.

35. Kita T, Nagano Y, Kokode M, *et al*: Probucol prevents the progression of atherosclerosis in Watanabe heritable hyperlipidemic rabbit, an animal model for familial hypercholesterolemia. *Proc Natl Acad Sci USA* 1987;84:5928.

36. Parthasarathy S, Young SG, Witztum JL, *et al*: Probucol inhibits oxidative modification of low density lipoprotein. *J Clin Invest* 1986;77:641.

37. Steinberg D, Witztum JL: Lipoproteins, lipoprotein oxidation and atherogenesis. In: Chien KR, ed. *Molecular Basis of Cardiovascular Disease*. W.B. Saunders:1999;458.

38. Tangirala RK, Casanada F, Miller E, *et al*: Effect of the antioxidant N,N′-diphenyl-phenylenediamine (DPPD) on atherosclerosis in apoE-deficient mice. *Arterioscler Thromb Vasc Biol* 1995;15:1625.

39. Cynshi O, Kawabe Y, Suzuki T, *et al*: Antiatherogenic effects of the antioxidant BO-653 in three different animal models. *Proc Natl Acad Sci USA* 1998;95:10123.

40. Pratico D, Tangirala R, Rader DJ, *et al*: Vitamin E suppresses isoprostane generation *in vivo* and reduces atherosclerosis in apoE-deficient mice. *Nature Medicine* 1998;4:1189.

41. Crawford RS, Kirk EA, Rosenfeld ME, *et al*: Dietary antioxidants inhibit development of fatty streak lesions in the LDL receptor-deficient mouse. *Arterioscler Thromb Vasc Biol* 1998;18:1506.

42. Witting PK, Pettersson K, Ostlund-Lindqvist AM, *et al*: Inhibition by a coantioxidant of aortic lipoprotein lipid peroxidation and atherosclerosis in apolipoprotein E and low density lipoprotein receptor gene double knockout mice. *FASEB J* 1999;13:667.

43. Gey F, Puska P: Plasma vitamins E and A inversely correlated to mortality from ischemic heart disease in cross-cultural epidemiology. *Ann NY Acad Sci* 1989;570:268.

44. Stampfer MJ, Hennekens CH, Manson JE, *et al*: Vitamin E consumption and the risk of coronary disease in men. *N Engl J Med* 1993;328:1444.

45. Rimm EB, Stampfer JM, Ascherio A, *et al*: Vitamin E consumption and the risk of coronary disease in women. *N Engl J Med* 1993;328:1450.

46. Alpha Tocopherol, Beta Carotene Cancer Prevention Study Group: The effects of vitamin E and beta carotene on the incidence of lung cancer and other cancers in male smokers. *N Engl J Med* 1994;330:1029.

47. Stephens NG, Parsons A, Schofield PM, *et al*: Randomised controlled trial of vitamin E in patients with coronary disease: Cambridge Heart Antioxidant Study (CHAOS). *Lancet* 1996;347:781.

48. The Heart Outcomes Prevention Evaluation (HOPE) Study Investigators: Vitamin E supplementation and cardiovascular events in high-risk patients. *N Engl J Med* 2000;342:154.

49. GISSI-Prevenzione Investigators: Dietary supplementation with n-3 polyunsaturated fatty acids and vitamin E after myocardial infarction: Results of the GISSI-Prevenzione trial. *Lancet* 1999;354:447.

50. Hennekens CH, Buring JE, Manson JE, *et al*: Lack of effect of long-term supplementation with beta carotene on the incidence of malignant neoplasms and cardiovascular disease. *N Engl J Med* 1996;334:1145.

51. Omenn GS, Goodman GE, Thornquist MD, *et al*: Effects of a combination of beta carotene and vitamin E on lung cancer and cardiovascular disease. *N Engl J Med* 1996;334:1150.

52. Reaven PD, Khouw A, Beltz WF, *et al*: Effect of dietary antioxidant combinations in humans. *Arterioscler Thromb* 1993;13:590.

53. Reaven PD, Ferguson E, Navab M, *et al*: Susceptibility of human LDL to oxidative modification. Effects of variations in β-carotene concentration and oxygen tension. *Arterioscler Thromb* 1994;14:1162.

54. Sternby NH: Atherosclerosis and diabetes mellitus. *Acta Pathol Microbial Scand* 1968;194(suppl):152.

55. Keen H, Jarrett RJ, Fuller JH, *et al*: Hyperglycemia and arterial disease. *Diabetes* 1981;30(suppl 2):49.

56. Keen H, Jarrett RJ: The WHO multinational study of vascular disease in diabetes, 2. Macrovascular disease prevalence. *Diabetes Care* 1979;2:187.

57. Janka HV, Standl E, Mehnert H: Peripheral vascular disease in diabetes mellitus and its relation to cardiovascular risk factors. *Diabetes Care* 1980;3:207.

58. Goto Y, Sato S, Masuda M: Causes of death in 3151 diabetic autopsy cases. *Tohoku J Exp Med* 1974;112:339.

59. Reaven GM: Role of insulin resistance in human disease. *Diabetes* 1988;37:1595.

60. Kaplan NM: The deadly quartet: Upper body obesity, glucose intolerance, hypertriglyceridemia, and hypertension. *Arch Intern Med* 1989;149:1514.

61. DeFronzo RA, Ferrannini E: Insulin resistance. A multifaceted syndrome responsible for NIDDM, obesity, hypertension, dyslipidemia, and atherosclerotic cardiovascular disease. *Diabetes Care* 1991;14:173.

62. Kissebah AH, Vyelingum N, Murray R, *et al*: Relationship of body fat distribution to metabolic complications of obesity. *Clin Endocrinol Metab* 1982;54:254.

63. Krotkiewski M, Bjorntorp P, Sjostrom L, *et al*: Impact of obesity in metabolism in men and women: Importance of regional adipose tissue distribution. *J Clin Invest* 1983;72:1150.

64. Berntorp K, Lindgard F: Familial aggregation of type 2 diabetes mellitus as an etiological factor in hypertension. *Diabetes Res Clin Pract* 1985;1:307.

65. Reaven P, Picard S, Witztum JL: Low density lipoprotein metabolism in diabetes. In: Draznin B, Eckel RH, eds. *Diabetes and Atherosclerosis*. Elsevier:1993;17.

66. Rubin EM, Krauss RM, Spangler EA, *et al*: Inhibition of early atherogenesis in transgenic mice by human apolipoprotein A1. *Nature* 1991;353:265.

67. Sato Y, Hotta N, Sakamoto N, *et al*: Lipid peroxide level in plasma of diabetic patients. *Biochem Med* 1979;21:104.

68. Nishigaki I, Hagihara M, Tsunekawa HT, *et al*: Lipid peroxides and atherosclerosis. *Biochem Med* 1981;25:373.

69. Chisolm GM, Irwin KC, Penn MS: Lipoprotein oxidation and lipoprotein-induced cell injury in diabetes. *Diabetes* 1992;41(suppl 2):61.

70. Wolff SP, Dean RT: Glucose autoxidation and protein modification. The potential role of autoxidative glycosylation in diabetes. *Biochem J* 1987;245:243.

71. Mullarkey CJ, Edelstein D, Brownlee M: Free radical generation by early glycation products: A mechanism for accelerated atherogenesis in diabetes. *Biochem Biophys Res Comm* 1990;173:932.

72. Hunt JV, Smith CCT, Wolff SP: Autoxidative glycosylation and possible involvement of peroxides and free radicals in LDL modification by glucose. *Diabetes* 1990;39:1420.

73. Hickes M, Delbridge L, Yue DK, *et al*: Catalysis of lipid peroxidation by glucose and glycosylated collagen. *Biochem Biophys Res Commun* 1988;151:649.

74. Haberland ME, Fong D, Cheng L: Malondialdehyde-altered protein occurs in atheroma of Watanabe heritable hyperlipidemic rabbits. *Science* 1988;241:215.

75. Palinski W, Rosenfeld ME, Ylä-Herttuala S, *et al*: Low density lipoprotein undergoes oxidative modification in vivo. *Proc Natl Acad Sci USA* 1989;86:1372.

76. Nakamura Y, Horii Y, Nishino T, *et al*: Immunocytochemical localization of advanced glycosylation endproducts in coronary atheroma and cardiac tissue in diabetes mellitus. *Am J Pathol* 1993;143:1649.

77. Witztum JL, Mahoney EM, Branks MJ, *et al*: Nonenzymatic glycosylation of low density lipoprotein alters its biological activity. *Diabetes* 1981;31:283.

78. Brownlee M, Vlassara H, Cerami A: Nonenzymatic glycosylation products of collagen covalently trap low density lipoprotein. *Diabetes* 1984;34:938.

79. Khoo JC, Miller E, McLoughlin P, *et al*: Enhanced macrophage uptake of low density lipoprotein after self-aggregation. *Arteriosclerosis* 1988;8:348.

80. Vlassara H: Receptor-mediated interactions of advanced glycosylation endproducts with cellular components within diabetic tissues. *Diabetes* 1992;41(suppl 2):52.

81. Knatterud GL, Klimt CR, Levin ME, *et al*: Effects of hypoglycemic agents on vascular complications in patients with adult-onset diabetes, VII. Mortality and selected non-fatal events with insulin treatment. *JAMA* 1978;240:37.

82. The Diabetes Control and Complications Trial Research Group: The effect of intensive treatment of diabetes on the development and progression of long-term complications in insulin-dependent diabetes mellitus. *N Engl J Med* 1993;329:977.

83. Kim JA, Berliner JA, Natarajan RD, *et al*: Evidence that glucose increases monocyte binding to human aortic endothelial cells. *Diabetes* 1994;43:1103.

84. Richardson M, Hadcock SJ, DeReske M, *et al*: Increased expression in vivo of VCAM-1 and E-selectin by the aortic endothelium of normolipidemic and hyperlipidemic diabetic rabbits. *Arterioscler Thromb* 1994;14:760.

85. Dosquet C, Weill D, Wautier JL: Molecular mechanism of blood monocyte adhesion to vascular endothelial cells. *Nouvelle Rev Francaise Hematol* 1992;34(suppl):555.

86. Stewart J, Collier A, Patrick AW, *et al*: Alterations in monocyte receptor function in type 1 diabetic patients with ketoacidosis. *Diabet Med* 1991;8:213.

87. Kirstein M, Britt J, Radoff S, *et al*: Advanced protein glycosylation induces transendothelial human monocyte chemotaxis and secretion of platelet-derived growth factor: Role in vascular disease of diabetes and aging. *Proc Natl Acad Sci USA* 1990;87:9010.

88. Hiramatsu K, Aramori S: Increased superoxide production by mononuclear cells of patients with hypertriglyceridemia and diabetes. *Diabetes* 1988;37:832.

89. Winocour PD: Platelet abnormalities in diabetes mellitus. *Diabetes* 1992;41:26.

90. Witztum JL, Steinbrecher UP, Kesaniemi YA, *et al*: Autoantibodies to glycosylated proteins in the plasma of patients with diabetes mellitus. *Proc Natl Acad Sci USA* 1984;81:3204.

91. Palinski W, Ord V, Plump AS, *et al*: Apoprotein E-deficient mice are a model of lipoprotein oxidation in atherogenesis: Demonstration of oxidation-specific epitopes in lesions and high titers of autoantibodies to malondialdehydelysine in serum. *Arterioscler Thromb* 1994;14:605.

92. Khoo JC, Miller E, Pio F, *et al*: Monoclonal antibodies against LDL further enhance macrophage uptake of LDL aggregates. *Arterioscler Thromb* 1992;12:1258.

93. Salonen JT, Ylä-Herttuala S, Yamamoto R, *et al*: Autoantibody against oxidised LDL and progression of carotid atherosclerosis. *Lancet* 1992;339:883.

94. Palinski W, Miller E, Witztum JL: Immunization of LDL receptor-deficient rabbits with homologous malondialdehyde-modified LDL reduces atherogenesis. *Proc Natl Acad Sci USA* 1995;92:821.

95. Jonasson L, Holm J, Shalli O, *et al*: Regional accumulations of T cells, macrophages, and smooth muscle cells in the human atherosclerotic plaque. *Arteriosclerosis* 1986;6:131.

96. Stemme S, Faber B, Holm J, *et al*: T lymphocytes from human atherosclerotic plaque recognize oxidized LDL. *Proc Natl Acad Sci USA* 1995;92:3893.

97. Hansson GK, Holm J, Holm S, *et al*: T lymphocytes inhibit the vascular response to injury. *Proc Natl Acad Sci USA* 1991;88:10530.

98. El Khoury JE, Thomas CA, Loike JD, *et al*: Macrophages adhere to glucose-modified basement membrane collagen IV via their scavenger receptors. *J Biol Chem* 1994;269:10197.

99. Fraser I, Hughes D, Gordon S: Divalent cation-independent macrophage adhesion inhibited by monoclonal antibody to murine scavenger receptor. *Nature* 1993;364:343.

100. University Group Diabetes Program: A study of the effects of hypoglycemic agents in vascular complications in patients with adult-onset diabetes. *Diabetes* 1970;19(suppl 2):747.

101. UK Prospective Diabetes Study Group: Intensive blood-glucose control with sulfonylureas or insulin compared with conventional treatment and risk of complications in patients with type 2 diabetes (UKPDS 33). *Lancet* 1998;352:837.

102. Expert Panel on Detection, Evaluation, and Treatment of High Blood Cholesterol in Adults: Executive summary of the third report of the National Cholesterol Education Program (NCEP) expert panel on detection, evaluation, and treatment of high blood cholesterol in adults (Adult Treatment Panel III) *JAMA* 2001;285:2486.

Endothelial Dysfunction and Vascular Thrombosis in Diabetes

Douglas E. Vaughan

Patients with diabetes mellitus are at increased risk for a variety of cardiovascular disorders, including myocardial infarction and stroke.[1] The risk for cardiovascular disease is increased up to four-fold among diabetic patients compared with nondiabetic persons. Diabetes is a particularly strong determinant of cardiovascular risk in women. The impact of vascular disease on patients with diabetes mellitus is staggering and accounts for nearly 80 percent of deaths and greater than 70 percent of hospitalizations for patients with this common metabolic disorder. The reasons for this increased risk of atherothrombotic events are widely discussed but only incompletely understood. There is a strong association between the metabolic abnormalities seen in diabetes mellitus and the development of premature atherosclerosis that is reviewed elsewhere in this text. Certainly many of the macrovascular complications of diabetes appear in conjunction with and may reflect the presence of advanced atherosclerosis. In parallel with the development of atherosclerosis, other independent factors coconspire to increase the risk of ischemic cardiovascular events in patients with diabetes. This chapter focuses on the role of endothelial dysfunction and the increased thrombotic tendency found in diabetes.

ENDOTHELIAL DYSFUNCTION IN DIABETES

The vascular endothelium participates in a number of physiologic processes that contribute to vascular health.[2] One of the most important functions involves the production of short-lived vasodilators in response to physiologic stimuli. These vasodilators include nitric oxide, prostacyclin, and endothelial-dependent hyperpolarizing factor (EDHF). The production of nitric oxide (NO) by the vascular endothelium has been the subject of intense investigation for the last two decades. In addition to the important role NO plays in the regulation of vascular tone, NO helps maintain the integrity of the blood vessel wall and blood fluidity by preventing monocyte adhesion and platelet aggregation. NO also retards the growth of vascular lesions by inhibiting cellular proliferation.[3] Taken together, these pleiotropic effects of NO suggest that endothelial NO production may play a pivotal role in the prevention of vascular disease. Although endothelial dysfunction is widely discussed in the context of impaired endothelium-dependent relaxation, impairment of endothelial function also likely impacts on other important physiologic endothelial functions that protect the vasculature from inflammatory processes and thrombosis. Endothelium-dependent

vasodilation and, specifically, the production of NO, is impaired in diabetes. This has been shown in experimental models of chemically induced diabetes[4–7] as well as in genetic models of type 1 diabetes.[8,9] In experimental models, the totality of evidence indicates that the normal vascular relaxation response to nitrates is preserved while agonist-stimulated endothelium-dependent vasodilator function is impaired. The impairment in the endothelial vasodilation can be seen in both conduit and resistance arteries and cannot be explained by physiologic changes in smooth muscle cell responsiveness to NO or by changes in guanylate cyclase reactivity.[10]

There is also substantial clinical evidence that NO-mediated vasodilation is impaired in patients with type 1 diabetes[11,12] and type 2 diabetes mellitus.[13] Abnormalities in vascular reactivity and biochemical markers of endothelial cell activation are present early in individuals at risk of developing type 2 diabetes, even at a stage when normal glucose tolerance exists.[14] Endothelium-dependent vasodilation has also been reported to be impaired in first-degree relatives of patients with type 2 diabetes.[15] The question arises as to the mechanisms through which diabetes impairs endothelial vasodilator function and specifically alters NO production or bioavailability. It has been shown that hyperglycemia *per se* acutely attenuates endothelium-dependent vasodilation in healthy subjects.[16] There are several factors that probably contribute to impaired vasodilation in diabetes over the long term. Diabetes and the metabolic abnormalities that accompany this disorder may reduce endothelial NO production in response to physiologic stimuli. This may be explained by direct effects of advanced glycosylation end products on endothelial NO production[17] or by a relative deficiency of the NO synthase cofactor tetrahydrobiopterin in diabetes.[18] Oxidative degradation of endothelium-derived NO contributes to abnormal endothelium-dependent vasodilation in animal models of diabetes mellitus.[19]

The vascular impairment in NO production seen in diabetes also likely has other important ramifications that impact upon the development of cardiovascular disease. Impairment of NO production enhances the progression in atherosclerosis in animal models.[20,21] Indeed, NO plays an important role in preventing monocyte adhesion to the blood vessel wall, which is one of the initial steps in the development of atherosclerotic lesions. NO possesses other important vasculoprotective properties, and serves as an endogenous inhibitor of smooth cell proliferation and platelet activation.[22] Recently it has been shown that NO also plays a role in enhancing the anticoagulant properties of the vascular endothelium by suppressing the production of plasminogen activator inhibitor type-1 (PAI-1).[23]

Clinical Ramifications

Although this issue has not been selectively examined in diabetes, coronary endothelial vasodilator dysfunction predicts long-term atherosclerotic disease progression and cardiovascular events.[24,25] At present, there is a paucity of data regarding the reversal of endothelial dysfunction in diabetes. Endothelial dysfunction in forearm resistance vessels of patients with type 2 diabetes mellitus can be improved by administration of the antioxidant vitamin C.[19,26] These findings support the hypothesis that NO inactivation by oxygen-derived free radicals contributes to abnormal vascular reactivity in diabetes. In the future, the assessment of forearm and/or coronary endothelial vasoreactivity may gain wider acceptance as both a diagnostic and prognostic tool in patients at risk for coronary heart disease.[27] At present, these measurements remain experimental tools.

DIABETES AND THROMBOSIS

Patients are defined as having a hypercoagulable state if they have laboratory abnormalities or a clinical condition that is associated with increased risk of thrombosis.[28] Certainly patients with diabetes mellitus meet this definition. As noted previously, the vascular endothelium, which is a primary component of the defense against intravascular thrombosis, is dysfunctional in patients with diabetes. The impaired production of NO and prostacyclin seen in diabetes is very likely an important factor in the increased activation of platelets and clotting factors also seen in diabetes. Specifically, with regard to coagulation, there are number of pieces of evidence to indicate that coagulation is enhanced in patients with diabetes mellitus. Several small studies indicate that subclinical evidence of thrombosis can be identified in plasma from diabetic patients by measuring coagulation activation markers such as prothrombin activation fragment 1 + 2 and thrombin/antithrombin complexes.[29–33] With regard to specific coagulation factors, perhaps the strongest epidemiologic evidence indicates that elevated fibrinogen levels are a risk factor for ischemic cardiovascular events.[34] Patients with diabetes generally have elevated plasma fibrinogen levels compared to healthy control subjects, and this may explain some of the increased risk for cardiovascular disease in diabetes.[35] The mechanism for this increase has not been well studied. Fibrinogen is an acute phase reactant, and the increase seen in diabetes may reflect low-level inflammation.[36] Intravascular volume depletion in uncontrolled diabetes may also account for some of the observed increase in plasma fibrinogen. No direct effects of insulin or glucose on fibrinogen production have been described. In addition to fibrinogen, plasma levels of many coagulation factors are modestly increased in diabetes, including factors VII, VIII, XI, and XII and von Willebrand's factor.[32] The significance of these increases is debatable, although in epidemiologic studies, increased levels of factor VII do appear to increase the risk of coronary events.[37] The increased tendency to thrombosis in diabetes may also reflect a failure in circulating anticoagulant mechanisms. Although there is no evidence of important reductions in plasma levels of antithrombin III or heparin cofactor II, it has been reported that the plasma level of activated protein C is reduced in diabetes.[38] However, results from other studies reported increased or unchanged protein C levels in patients with diabetes compared with healthy control subjects.[39–42]

Another system that more likely contributes to the increased thrombotic risk in diabetes is the impairment in endogenous fibrinolytic function seen in patients with type 2 diabetes. The mammalian fibrinolytic system serves as one of the endogenous defense mechanisms against intravascular thrombosis. It functionally complements the effects of endogenous anticoagulants, such as protein C and protein S, and the short-lived endothelium-derived platelet inhibitors NO and prostacyclin. The activity of the fibrinolytic system is ultimately dependent on the generation of the protease plasmin, which is produced from the inactive precursor plasminogen by the action of plasminogen activators. Humans possess two distinct plasminogen activators, tissue-type plasminogen activator (t-PA) and the urokinase-type plasminogen activator (u-PA). Although both of these activators are synthesized in endothelium, t-PA appears to be primary plasminogen activator in the vasculature. It has been proposed that the plasminogen activator system is a critical defender against intravascular thrombosis in the coronary circulation,[43] and the balance between t-PA and its endogenous inhibitor, plasminogen activator inhibitor 1 (PAI-1) is a major determinant of net fibrinolytic activity.

Physiology of PAI-1

PAI-1 is a globular protein comprised of 379 amino acids in a single chain.[44] PAI-1 belongs to the superfamily of serine protease inhibitors (serpins),[45] and as such, it is structurally similar to other serpins including ovalbumin, angiotensinogen, antithrombin III, and α_2-antiplasmin.

Active PAI-1 is readily cleaved by, and forms complexes with, t-PA. The reaction is quite rapid and proceeds with a second-order rate constant of 10^7 M^{-1} s^{-1}.[46] A series of studies involving site-specific mutagenesis have revealed that PAI-1 interacts with t-PA via a two-step mechanism. Replacement of three positively charged amino acids (Lys_{296}, Arg_{298}, and Arg_{299}) in t-PA with negatively charged glutamic residues generates a t-PA mutant that retains its ability to activate plasminogen and is highly resistant to inhibition by PAI-1.[47] The first step in the interaction between t-PA and PAI-1 is reversible and appears to involve an electrostatic interaction between positively charged amino acids in t-PA and negatively charged residues in PAI-1 that are located on a surface loop (residues 350–355). The second step of the interaction of PAI-1 with t-PA is irreversible and involves the cleavage of the PAI-1 reactive site by the active site of t-PA. In addition to its role as the primary inhibitor of t-PA in plasma, PAI-1 also promotes thrombosis by inhibiting activated protein C.

PAI-1 circulates in low but measurable concentrations in plasma, at less than 4:1 molar excess to that of t-PA.[48] The source of plasma PAI-1 is debatable, as it is synthesized in the vascular endothelium and smooth muscle cells, in the liver, and in adipose tissue.[49,50] Platelets also store large quantities of PAI-1 that are secreted following platelet aggregation.[51] Several different fates are possible for PAI-1 after it is secreted. The circulating half-life of PAI-1 is approximately 5 minutes,[52] and the majority of PAI-1 likely circulates briefly in plasma and is removed via a hepatic clearance mechanism. A fraction of secreted, active PAI-1 reacts with plasma t-PA and forms inert, insoluble complexes. There appears to be no endogenous mechanism for recycling t-PA–PAI-1 complexes, which are cleared via receptor-dependent mechanisms.[53] Active PAI-1 can also bind to vitronectin, which actually stabilizes PAI-1 in the active conformation.[54] Binding to vitronectin has also been found to broaden the reactive specificity of PAI-1. Specifically, vitronectin endows PAI-1 with thrombin inhibitory properties.[55]

Endothelial cells also have the capacity to secrete PAI-1 ablumenally.[56] In the extracellular matrix of blood vessels, PAI-1 likely plays a role in vascular remodeling. The relative abundance of vitronectin in the subendothelial matrix provides a mechanism for preserving PAI-1 activity, and, in fact, the PAI-1–vitronectin complex may represent the physiologically relevant form of the inhibitor in the extracellular matrix.

A wide array of cytokines, growth factors, and hormones have been found to stimulate endothelial PAI-1 production. Inflammatory cytokines such as interleukin-1 (IL-1) and tumor neurosis factor α (TNF-α)[57] are potent regulators of PAI-1 production. With acceptance of the concept that atherosclerosis is predominantly an inflammatory process,[58] this functional linkage between PAI-1 and inflammatory cytokines may help explain the increase in PAI-1 reported in atherosclerosis. Transforming growth factor β (TGF-β) is recognized as an important stimulus for the production of PAI-1 in tissues,[57] and this interaction has important ramifications for the understanding of the pathogenesis of vascular fibrosis and nephrosclerosis in diabetes.[59] Thrombin is also a potent stimulus for PAI-1 production in cultured endothelial cells.[60] Angiotensin II[61] and its hexapeptide metabolite angiotensin IV induce dose- and time-dependent increases in endothelial PAI-1 mRNA expression *in vitro*.[62] Angiotensin II is also a potent stimulus of vascular PAI-1 production *in vivo*.[63,64]

The increased production of PAI-1 seen in patients with diabetes has been attributed directly to glucose,[65,66] insulin,[67] and triglycerides. In the upstream regulatory region of the PAI-1 gene, specific sequences have been localized that respond to VLDL[68] and to glucose.[69] Indeed, PAI-1 is one of several genes with transcription that is induced by high glucose concentrations. The glucose-responsive region of the PAI-1 promoter resides in two Sp1 sites located within 90 bases of the transcription start site. Recent studies indicate that hyperglycemia induces mitochondrial superoxide production, which in turn increases hexosamine synthesis and *O*-glycosylation of Sp1.[70] This modification induces a dephosphorylation in Sp1, which has been hypothesized to reduce interactions with transcriptional repressor proteins, thus yielding increased Sp1-dependent gene transcription. Insulin and proinsulin peptides also induce PAI-1 production, which may contribute to increased PAI-1 production in the setting of insulin resistance.

Clinical Consequences of Increased PAI-1

Theoretically, an excess of PAI-1 will reduce the efficiency of the fibrinolytic system, which may create a permissive environment for vascular thrombosis. There is a growing body of evidence that PAI-1 excess (usually measured as PAI-1 activity) may in fact be a risk factor for venous thromboembolic disorders and for ischemic cardiovascular disease.[71] Elevated levels of PAI-1 appear to be a risk factor for recurrent deep vein thrombosis.[72] PAI-1 excess has been identified in youthful survivors of acute myocardial infarction[73] and levels are higher in MI survivors that go on to develop recurrent MI.[74] Low plasma fibrinolytic activity, which may be a reflection of increased PAI-1 activity, appears to be a leading determinant of risk for ischemic heart disease in younger men.[75] There is

compelling evidence that excess PAI-1 is present in atherosclerotic human blood vessels.[76] Vascular PAI-1 content is increased in diabetes and in atherectomy specimens from patients with diabetes compared to healthy control subjects.[77] This finding is relevant to the present discussion in view of the role plasmin plays in "vascular housekeeping." Plasmin activates several different matrix metalloproteinases that are needed to degrade extracellular matrix proteins, including collagen and other glycoproteins.[78] Plasmin itself plays a role in vascular housekeeping by degrading local fibrin deposits, collagen, and fibronectin. Plasmin also plays a role in the activation of the multifaceted cytokine TGF-β, which is felt to have antiatherosclerotic effects related to its antimitogenic properties.[79] Thus, by virtue of these mechanisms and potentially others, an excess of PAI-1 in vascular tissue reduces local plasmin production and diminishes vascular housekeeping capacity. Recent work indicates that PAI-1 deficiency protects against the development of hypertension and perivascular fibrosis in the setting of long-term NO synthase inhibition.[80] Thus, the enhanced production of vascular PAI-1 in clinical conditions associated with a relative NO deficiency may accelerate the development of arteriosclerosis and hypertension.

These local vascular and tissue effects of PAI-1 in retarding vascular defense mechanisms against intravascular clotting and atherosclerotic plaque growth deserve additional emphasis with regard to the understanding of the development of atherothrombotic disease in type 2 diabetes. Plasma levels of PAI-1 are elevated in patients with type 2 diabetes, although the cause of this elevation is likely multifactorial in origin. Patients with type 2 diabetes uniformly exhibit insulin resistance that is associated with several cardiovascular risk factors, including systolic hypertension, hypertriglyceridemia, increased hip–girth ratio, glucose intolerance, hyperinsulinemia, and low HDL levels. Plasma levels of PAI-1 have been found to correlate strongly with insulin resistance.[81] As reviewed previously, insulin, proinsulin-like molecules, glucose, and VLDL have been shown to stimulate PAI-1 production *in vitro*. Similar associations have been reported between plasma PAI-1 activity and plasma insulin and triglyceride levels in obese patients,[82,83] in patients with coronary artery disease,[84] and in patients with type 2 diabetes.[85]

Genetic factors may also impact on the development of thrombosis in diabetes. For example, a common 4/5 guanine-tract (4G-5G) polymorphism in the PAI-1 promoter has been described.[86] The 4G allele has been reported to be associated with high plasma PAI-1 activity. Furthermore, the prevalence of the 4G allele is significantly higher in patients with myocardial infarction before the age of 45 years than in population-based control subjects (allele frequencies of 0.63 versus 0.53).[87] It appears that both alleles are capable of binding a transcriptional activating protein, whereas the normal 5G allele also binds a repressor molecule. Thus, individuals with the 4G polymorphism lose the ability to bind the repressor and exhibit increased plasma levels of PAI-1. Plasma glucose and triglyceride levels also appear to correlate strongly with plasma PAI-1 levels in 4G/4G homozygotes.[88]

Therapeutic Implications

At the present time, thrombolytic agents are the single class of drugs available that are designed to alter fibrinolytic activity directly and acutely. It may be desirable, however, to enhance endogenous fibrinolytic activity for the prevention and treatment of a variety of thrombotic vascular disorders. This is particularly true when considering ways to prevent the development of vascular disease in patients with diabetes mellitus.

Because PAI-1 plays such a major role in regulating fibrinolytic activity, it is a very attractive therapeutic target. Drugs that reduce plasma insulin levels or that attenuate insulin resistance may have secondary benefits in reducing PAI-1 levels. Metformin has been reported to reduce plasma PAI-1 activity in normal subjects and in patients with type 2 diabetes.[89,90] Insulin-sensitizing agents, such as thiazolidinediones, reduced plasma PAI-1 levels by nearly 30% in women with impaired glucose tolerance and polycystic ovary syndrome[91] and in subjects with type 2 diabetes.[92] Because glucose may directly regulate PAI-1 production, especially in individuals with the 4G/4G genotype, improved glycemic control is likely to reduce PAI-1 production over the long term. Other agents may also reduce tissue expression of PAI-1 and may be of benefit in protecting against diabetic complications. ACE inhibitor therapy can significantly reduce plasma PAI-1 levels after MI,[48,93] and in healthy subjects on a low-salt diet.[94] We speculate that this effect may contribute to the beneficial effect of ACE inhibitor therapy in reducing the risk of MI, stroke, and cardiovascular mortality in patients with diabetes.[95] Finally, because NO plays an important role in suppressing vascular PAI-1 production, a unified therapeutic approach to improving vascular health through the restoration and maintenance of endothelial NO production is likely to have compound benefits in the population afflicted with diabetes.

REFERENCES

1. Grundy SM, Balady GJ, Criqui MH, *et al*: Primary prevention of coronary heart disease: Guidance from Framingham: A statement for healthcare professionals from the AHA task force on risk reduction. American Heart Association. *Circulation* 1998;97:1876.
2. Luscher TF, Tanner FC, Tschudi MR, Noll G: Endothelial dysfunction in coronary artery disease. *Annu Rev Med* 1993;44:395.
3. Li H, Forstermann U: Nitric oxide in the pathogenesis of vascular disease. *J Pathol* 2000;190:244.
4. Dai FX, Diederich A, Skopec J, Diederich D: Diabetes-induced endothelial dysfunction in streptozotocin-treated rats: Role of prostaglandin endoperoxides and free radicals. *J Am Soc Nephrol* 1993;4:1327.
5. Chakir M, Plante GE: Endothelial dysfunction in diabetes mellitus. *Prostaglandins Leukot Essen Fatty Acids* 1996;54:45.
6. Vallejo S, Angulo J, Peiro C, *et al*: Prevention of endothelial dysfunction in streptozotocin-induced diabetic rats by gliclazide treatment. *J Diabetes Complications* 2000;14:224.
7. Diederich D, Skopec J, Diederich A, Dai FX: Endothelial dysfunction in mesenteric resistance arteries of diabetic rats: Role of free radicals. *Am J Physiol* 1994;266:H1153.
8. Pieper GM, Moore-Hilton G, Roza AM: Evaluation of the mechanism of endothelial dysfunction in the genetically-diabetic BB rat. *Life Sci* 1996;58:L147.
9. Hink U, Li H, Mollnau H, *et al*: Mechanisms underlying endothelial dysfunction in diabetes mellitus. *Circ Res* 2001;88:E14.
10. Pieper GM: Review of alterations in endothelial nitric oxide production in diabetes: Protective role of arginine on endothelial dysfunction. *Hypertension* 1998;31:1047.
11. Cosentino F, Luscher TF: Endothelial dysfunction in diabetes mellitus. *J Cardiovasc Pharmacol* 1998;32 (suppl 3):S54.
12. Johnstone MT, Creager SJ, Scales KM, *et al*: Impaired endothelium-dependent vasodilation in patients with insulin-dependent diabetes mellitus. *Circulation* 1993;88:2510.
13. Williams SB, Cusco JA, Roddy MA, *et al*: Impaired nitric oxide-mediated vasodilation in patients with non-insulin-dependent diabetes mellitus. *J Am Coll Cardiol* 1996;27:567.
14. Caballero AE, Arora S, Saouaf R, *et al*: Microvascular and macrovascular reactivity is reduced in subjects at risk for type 2 diabetes. *Diabetes* 1999;48:1856.
15. Balletshofer BM, Rittig K, Enderle MD, *et al*: Endothelial dysfunction is detectable in young normotensive first-degree relatives of subjects with type 2 diabetes in association with insulin resistance. *Circulation* 2000;101:1780.
16. Williams SB, Goldfine AB, Timimi FK, *et al*: Acute hyperglycemia attenuates endothelium-dependent vasodilation in humans in vivo. *Circulation* 1998;97:1695.
17. Bucala R, Tracey KJ, Cerami A: Advanced glycosylation products quench nitric oxide and mediate defective endothelium-dependent vasodilatation in experimental diabetes. *J Clin Invest* 1991;87:432.
18. Pieper GM: Acute amelioration of diabetic endothelial dysfunction with a derivative of the nitric oxide synthase cofactor, tetrahydrobiopterin. *J Cardiovasc Pharmacol* 1997;29:8.
19. Timimi FK, Ting HH, Haley EA, *et al*: Vitamin C improves endothelium-dependent vasodilation in patients with insulin-dependent diabetes mellitus. *J Am Coll Cardiol* 1998;31:552.
20. De Meyer GR, Herman AG: Vascular endothelial dysfunction. *Prog Cardiovasc Dis* 1997;39:325.
21. Cooke JP, Dzau VJ: Nitric oxide synthase: Role in the genesis of vascular disease. *Annu Rev Med* 1997;48:489.
22. Cornwell TL, Arnold E, Boerth NJ, Lincoln TM: Inhibition of smooth muscle cell growth by nitric oxide and activation of cAMP-dependent protein kinase by cGMP. *Am J Physiol* 1994;267:C1405.
23. Bouchie JL, Hansen H, Feener EP: Natriuretic factors and nitric oxide suppress plasminogen activator inhibitor-1 expression in vascular smooth muscle cells. Role of cGMP in the regulation of the plasminogen system. *Arterioscler Thromb Vasc Biol* 1998;18:1771.
24. Schachinger V, Britten MB, Zeiher AM: Prognostic impact of coronary vasodilator dysfunction on adverse long-term outcome of coronary heart disease. *Circulation* 2000;101:1899.
25. Suwaidi JA, Hamasaki S, Higano ST, *et al*: Long-term follow-up of patients with mild coronary artery disease and endothelial dysfunction. *Circulation* 2000;101:948.
26. Ting HH, Timimi FK, Boles KS, *et al*: Vitamin C improves endothelium-dependent vasodilation in patients with non-insulin-dependent diabetes mellitus. *J Clin Invest* 1996;97:22.
27. Charbonneau F: Use of measures of endothelial function to stratify risk. *Can J Cardiol* 2001;17 (suppl A):18A.
28. Schafer A: The hypercoagulable states. *Ann Intern Med* 1985;102:814.
29. Matsuda T, Morishita E, Jokaji H, *et al*: Mechanism on disorders of coagulation and fibrinolysis in diabetes. *Diabetes* 1996;45 (suppl 3):S109.
30. Lopez Y, Paloma MJ, Rifon J, *et al*: Measurement of prethrombotic markers in the assessment of acquired hypercoagulable states. *Thromb Res* 1999;93:71.
31. Coccheri S, Palareti G: Pro-thrombotic states and their diagnosis. *Ann Ital Med Int* 1994;9:16.
32. Carr ME: Diabetes mellitus: A hypercoagulable state. *J Diabetes Complications* 2001;15:44.
33. Banga JD, Sixma JJ: Diabetes mellitus, vascular disease and thrombosis. *Clin Haematol* 1986;15:465.
34. Kannel WB, D'Agostino RB, Belanger AJ: Update on fibrinogen as a cardiovascular risk factor. *Ann Epidemiol* 1992;2:457.
35. Kannel WB, D'Agostino RB, Wilson PW, *et al*: Diabetes, fibrinogen, and risk of cardiovascular disease: The Framingham experience. *Am Heart J* 1990;120:672.
36. Sakkinen PA, Wahl P, Cushman M, *et al*: Clustering of procoagulation, inflammation, and fibrinolysis variables with metabolic factors in insulin resistance syndrome. *Am J Epidemiol* 2000;152:897.
37. Meade TW, Ruddock V, Stirling Y, *et al*: Fibrinolytic activity, clotting factors, and long-term incidence of ischaemic heart disease in the Northwick Park heart study. *Lancet* 1993;342:1076.
38. Vukovich TC, Schernthaner G: Decreased protein C levels in patients with insulin-dependent type I diabetes mellitus. *Diabetes* 1986;35:617.
39. Ceriello A, Quatraro A, Dello Russo P, *et al*: Protein C deficiency in insulin-dependent diabetes: A hyperglycemia-related phenomenon. *Thromb Haemost* 1990;64:104.
40. Veglio M, Gruden G, Mormile A, *et al*: Anticoagulant protein C activity in non-insulin-dependent diabetic patients with normoalbuminuria and microalbuminuria. *Acta Diabetol* 1995;32:106.

41. Lee P, Jenkins A, Bourke C, et al: Prothrombotic and antithrombotic factors are elevated in patients with type 1 diabetes complicated by microalbuminuria. Diabet Med 1993;10:122.

42. Gabazza EC, Takeya H, Deguchi H, et al: Protein C activation in NIDDM patients. Diabetologia 1996;39:1455.

43. Rosenberg RD, Aird WC: Vascular-bed–specific hemostasis and hypercoagulable states. N Eng J Med 1999;340:1555.

44. van Mourik JA, Lawrence DA, Loskutoff DJ: Purification of an inhibitor of plasminogen activator (antiactivator) synthesized by endothelial cells. J Biol Chem 1984;259:14914.

45. Pannekoek H, Veerman H, Lambers H, et al: Endothelial plasminogen activator inhibitor (PAI): A new member of the Serpin gene family. EMBO J 1986;5:2539.

46. Wiman B, Chmielewska J, Ranby M: Inactivation of tissue plasminogen activator in plasma. Demonstration of a complex with a new rapid inhibitor. J Biol Chem 1984;259:3644.

47. Madison EL, Goldsmith EJ, Gerard RD, et al: Amino acid residues that affect interaction of tissue-type plasminogen activator with plasminogen activator inhibitor 1. Proc Nat Acad Sci USA 1990;87:3530.

48. Vaughan DE, Rouleau J-L, Ridker PM, et al: Effects of ramipril on plasma fibrinolytic balance in patients with acute anterior myocardial infarction. Circulation 1997;96:442.

49. Sprengers ED, Kluft C: Plasminogen activator inhibitors. Blood 1987;69:381.

50. Loskutoff DJ, Samad F: The adipocyte and hemostatic balance in obesity: Studies of PAI-1. Arterioscl Thromb Vasc Biol 1998;18:1.

51. Erickson LA, Ginsberg MH, Loskutoff DJ: Detection and partial characterization of an inhibitor of plasminogen activator in human platelets. J Clin Invest 1984;74:1465.

52. Vaughan DE, Declerck PJ, Van Houtte E, et al: Studies of recombinant plasminogen activator inhibitor-1 in rabbits. Pharmacokinetics and evidence for reactivation of latent plasminogen activator inhibitor-1 in vivo. Circ Res 1990;67:1281.

53. Andreasen PA, Sottrup-Jensen L, Kjoller L, et al: Receptor-mediated endocytosis of plasminogen activators and activator/inhibitor complexes. FEBS Lett 1994;338:239.

54. Declerck PJ, De Mol M, Alessi MC, et al: Purification and characterization of a plasminogen activator inhibitor 1 binding protein from human plasma. Identification as a multimeric form of S protein (vitronectin). J Biol Chem 1988;263:15454.

55. Ehrlich HJ, Gebbink RK, Keijer J, et al: Alteration of serpin specificity by a protein cofactor. Vitronectin endows plasminogen activator inhibitor 1 with thrombin inhibitory properties. J Biol Chem 1990;265:13029.

56. Mimuro J, Schleef RR, Loskutoff DJ: Extracellular matrix of cultured bovine aortic endothelial cells contains functionally active type 1 plasminogen activator inhibitor. Blood 1987;70:721.

57. Sawdey M, Podor TJ, Loskutoff DJ: Regulation of type 1 plasminogen activator inhibitor gene expression in cultured bovine aortic endothelial cells. Induction by transforming growth factor-beta, lipopolysaccharide, and tumor necrosis factor-alpha. J Biol Chem 1989;264:10396.

58. Ross R: Atherosclerosis—an inflammatory disease. N Eng J Med 1999;340:115.

59. Eddy AA: Molecular basis of renal fibrosis. Pediatr Nephrol 2000;15:290.

60. Dichek D, Quertermous T: Thrombin regulation of mRNA levels of tissue plasminogen activator and plasminogen activator inhibitor-1 in cultured human umbilical vein endothelial cells. Blood 1989;74:222.

61. Vaughan DE, Lazos SA, Tong K: Angiotensin II regulates the expression of plasminogen activator inhibitor-1 in cultured endothelial cells. A potential link between the renin-angiotensin system and thrombosis. J Clin Invest 1995;95:995.

62. Kerins DM, Hao Q, Vaughan DE: Angiotensin induction of PAI-1 expression in endothelial cells is mediated by the hexapeptide angiotensin IV. J Clin Invest 1995;96:2515.

63. Nakamura S, Nakamura I, Ma L, et al: Plasminogen activator inhibitor-1 expression is regulated by the angiotensin type 1 receptor in vivo. Kidney Int 2000;58:251.

64. Chen HC, Bouchie JL, Perez AS, et al: Role of the angiotensin AT(1) receptor in rat aortic and cardiac PAI-1 gene expression. Arterioscler Thromb Vasc Biol 2000;20:2297.

65. Cagliero E, Roth T, Roy S, et al: Expression of genes related to the extracellular matrix in human endothelial cells. Differential modulation by elevated glucose concentrations, phorbol esters, and cAMP. J Biol Chem 1991;266:14244.

66. Nordt TK, Klassen KJ, Schneider DJ, Sobel BE: Augmentation of synthesis of plasminogen activator inhibitor type-1 in arterial endothelial cells by glucose and its implications for local fibrinolysis. Arterioscl Thromb 1993;13:1822.

67. Nordt TK, Sawa H, Fujii S, et al: Augmentation of arterial endothelial cell expression of the plasminogen activator inhibitor type-1 (PAI-1) gene by proinsulin and insulin in vivo. J Mol Cell Cardiol 1998;30:1535.

68. Nilsson L, Gafvels M, Musakka L, et al: VLDL activation of plasminogen activator inhibitor-1 (PAI-1) expression: Involvement of the VLDL receptor. J Lipid Res 1999;40:913.

69. Chen YQ, Su M, Walia RR, et al: Sp1 sites mediate activation of the plasminogen activator inhibitor-1 promoter by glucose in vascular smooth muscle cells. J Biol Chem 1998;273:8225.

70. Du XL, Edelstein D, Rossetti L, et al: Hyperglycemia-induced mitochondrial superoxide overproduction activates the hexosamine pathway and induces plasminogen activator inhibitor-1 expression by increasing Sp1 glycosylation. Proc Natl Acad Sci USA 2000;97:12222.

71. Wiman B, Hamsten A: The fibrinolytic enzyme system and its role in the etiology of thromboembolic disease. Sem Thromb Hemost 1990;16:207.

72. Juhan-Vague I, Valadier J, Alessi MC, et al: Deficient t-PA release and elevated PA inhibitor levels in patients with spontaneous or recurrent deep venous thrombosis. Thromb Haemost 1987;57:67.

73. Hamsten A, Wiman B, de Faire U, Blomback M: Increased plasma levels of a rapid inhibitor of tissue plasminogen activator in young survivors of myocardial infarction. N Engl J Med 1985;313:1557.

74. Hamsten A, de Faire U, Walldius G, et al: Plasminogen activator inhibitor in plasma: Risk factor for recurrent myocardial infarction. Lancet 1987;2:3.

75. Meade TW, Ruddock V, Stirling Y, et al: Fibrinolytic activity, clotting factors, and long-term incidence of ischaemic heart disease in the Northwick Park heart study. Lancet 1993;342:1076.

76. Schneiderman J, Sawdey MS, Keeton MR, et al: Increased type 1 plasminogen activator inhibitor gene expression in atherosclerotic human arteries. Proc Natl Acad Sci USA 1992;89:6998.

77. Sobel BE, Woodcock-Mitchell J, Schneider DJ, et al: Increased plasminogen activator inhibitor type 1 in coronary artery atherectomy specimens from type 2 diabetic compared with nondiabetic patients. Circulation 1998;97:2213.

78. Alexander CM, Werb Z: Proteinases and extracellular matrix remodeling. Curr Opin Cell Biol 1989;1:974.

79. Grainger DJ, Kirschenlohr HL, Metcalfe JC, et al: Proliferation of human smooth muscle cells promoted by lipoprotein(a). Science 1993;260:1655.

80. Kaikita K, Fogo AB, Ma L, Schoenhard AB, Brown NJ, Vaughan DE. Plasminogen activation inhibitor-1 deficiency prevents hypertension and vascular fibrosis in response to long-term nitric oxide inhibition. Circulation 2001;104:839.

81. Potter van Loon BJ, Kluft C, Radder JK, et al: The cardiovascular risk factor plasminogen activator inhibitor type 1 is related to insulin resistance. Metab Clin Exper 1993;42:945.

82. Vague P, Juhan-Vague I, Aillaud MF, et al: Correlation between blood fibrinolytic activity, plasminogen activator inhibitor level, plasma insulin level, and relative body weight in normal and obese subjects. Metab Clin Exp 1986;35:250.

83. Landin K, Stigendal L, Eriksson E, et al: Abdominal obesity is associated with an impaired fibrinolytic activity and elevated plasminogen activator inhibitor-1. Metab Clin Exp 1990;39:1044.

84. Juhan-Vague I, Alessi MC, Joly P, et al: Plasma plasminogen activator inhibitor-1 in angina pectoris. Influence of plasma insulin and acute-phase response. Arteriosclerosis 1989;9:362.

85. Juhan-Vague I, Roul C, Alessi MC, et al: Increased plasminogen activator inhibitor activity in non-insulin dependent diabetic patients—relationship with plasma insulin. Thromb Haemost 1989;61:370.

86. Dawson SJ, Wiman B, Hamsten A, et al: The two allele sequences of a common polymorphism in the promoter of the plasminogen activator inhibitor-1 (PAI-1) gene respond differently to interleukin-1 in HepG2 cells. J Biol Chem 1993;268:10739.

87. Eriksson P, Kallin B, van 't Hooft FM, et al: Allele-specific increase in basal transcription of the plasminogen-activator inhibitor 1 gene

is associated with myocardial infarction. *Proc Nat Acad Sci USA* 1995;92:1851.

88. Mansfield MW, Stickland MH, Grant PI: Plasminogen activator inhibitor-1 (PAI-1) promoter polymorphism and coronary artery disease in non-insulin-dependent diabetes. *Thromb Haemost* 1995;74: 1032.

89. Grant PJ: The effects of metformin on the fibrinolytic system in diabetic and non-diabetic subjects. *Diabet Metab* 1991;17:168.

90. Nagi DK, Yudkin JS: Effects of metformin on insulin resistance, risk factors for cardiovascular disease, and plasminogen activator inhibitor in NIDDM subjects. A study of two ethnic groups. *Diabetes Care* 1993;16:621.

91. Ehrmann DA, Schneider DJ, Sobel BE, *et al*: Troglitazone improves defects in insulin action, insulin secretion, ovarian steroidogenesis, and fibrinolysis in women with polycystic ovary syndrome. *J Clin Endocrinol Metab* 1997;82:2108.

92. Fonseca VA, Reynolds T, Hemphill D, *et al*: Effect of troglitazone on fibrinolysis and activated coagulation in patients with non-insulin-dependent diabetes mellitus. *J Diabetes Complications* 1998;12:181.

93. Soejima H, Ogawa H, Yasue H, *et al*: Effects of imidapril therapy on endogenous fibrinolysis in patients with recent myocardial infarction. *Clin Cardiol* 1997;20:441.

94. Brown NJ, Agirbasli MA, Williams GH, *et al*: Effect of activation and inhibition of the renin-angiotensin system on plasma PAI-1. *Hypertension* 1998;32:965.

95. Yusuf S, Sleight P, Pogue J, *et al*: Effects of an angiotensin-converting-enzyme inhibitor, ramipril, on cardiovascular events in high-risk patients. The Heart Outcomes Prevention Evaluation Study Investigators. *N Engl J Med* 2000;342:145.

Biochemical Mechanisms of Microvascular Disease

Michael Brownlee

James N. Livingston

INTRODUCTION

Diabetes mellitus is by far the most common serious metabolic disorder, with a worldwide prevalence estimated to be between 1% and 5%. All forms of diabetes, both inherited and acquired, are characterized by hyperglycemia, a relative or absolute lack of insulin, and the development of diabetes-specific microvascular pathology in the retina, renal glomerulus, and peripheral nerve. As a consequence of this microvascular pathology, diabetes is now the leading cause of new blindness in people aged 20–74 years, and the leading cause of end-stage renal disease. Diabetics are the fastest growing group of renal dialysis and transplant recipients. The life-expectancy for patients with diabetic end-stage renal failure is only 3 or 4 years. Over 60% of diabetics are affected by neuropathy, which includes distal symmetrical polyneuropathy, mononeuropathies, and a variety of autonomic neuropathies causing erectile dysfunction, urinary incontinence, gastroparesis, and nocturnal diarrhea. Life expectancy is about 7–10 years shorter than for people without diabetes.[1]

Epidemiological studies show a strong relationship between glycemia and diabetic complications in both type 1 (T1DM) and type 2 (T2DM) diabetes mellitus.[2,3] There is a continuous, though not linear, relationship between level of glycemia and the risk of development and progression of complications.[4,5] This chapter integrates the vast amount of data about specific mechanisms by which hyperglycemia may damage diabetic blood vessels into a coherent, unified perspective. The discussion begins with the shared pathophysiologic features of microvascular complications, including the primacy of intracellular hyperglycemia, the development of microvascular complications during posthyperglycemic euglycemia ("hyperglycemic memory") and the influence of genetic factors in determining susceptibility to microvascular complications. After discussing each known major mechanism of hyperglycemia-induced vascular damage, recent data are presented showing that these different pathogenic mechanisms all reflect a single hyperglycemia-induced process. The chapter concludes with a brief consideration of the prospects for mechanism-based pharmacologic intervention.

SHARED PATHOPHYSIOLOGIC FEATURES OF MICROVASCULAR COMPLICATIONS

In the retina, glomerulus, and vasa nervorum, diabetes-specific microvascular disease is characterized by similar pathophysiologic features.

Requirement for Intracellular Hyperglycemia

Clinical and animal model data indicate that chronic hyperglycemia is the central initiating factor for all types of diabetic microvascular disease. Duration and magnitude of hyperglycemia are both strongly correlated with the extent and rate of progression of diabetic microvascular disease. In the Diabetes Control and Complications Trial (DCCT), for example, T1DM patients whose intensive insulin therapy resulted in HbA_{1c} levels 2% lower than those receiving conventional insulin therapy had a 76% lower incidence of retinopathy, a 54% lower incidence of nephropathy, and a 60% reduction in neuropathy.[2,3]

Although all diabetic cells are exposed to elevated levels of plasma glucose, hyperglycemic damage is limited to those cell types, such as endothelial cells, that develop intracellular hyperglycemia. Endothelial cells develop intracellular hyperglycemia because, unlike many other cells, they are unable to downregulate glucose transport when exposed to extracellular hyperglycemia. As illustrated in Fig. 13-1, vascular smooth muscle cells, which are not damaged by hyperglycemia, show an inverse relationship between extracellular glucose concentration and subsequent rate of glucose transport, measured as 2-deoxyglucose uptake. In contrast, vascular endothelial cells show no significant change in subsequent rate of glucose transport after exposure to elevated glucose concentrations.[6] That intracellular hyperglycemia is necessary and sufficient for the development of diabetic pathology is demonstrated by the fact that overexpression of the GLUT-1 glucose transporter in mesangial cells cultured in a normal glucose milieu mimics the diabetic phenotype, inducing the same increases in collagen type IV, collagen type I, and fibronectin gene expression as diabetic hyperglycemia (Fig. 13-2).[7]

Abnormal Endothelial Cell Function

Early in the course of diabetes, before structural changes are evident, hyperglycemia causes abnormalities in blood flow and vascular permeability in the retina, glomerulus, and peripheral nerve vasa nervorum.[8,9] The increase in blood flow and intracapillary pressure is thought to reflect hyperglycemia-induced decreased nitric oxide production on the efferent side of capillary beds, and possibly an increased sensitivity to angiotensin II. As a consequence of increased intracapillary pressure and endothelial cell dysfunction, retinal capillaries exhibit increased leakage of fluorescein and glomerular capillaries have an elevated albumin excretion rate. Comparable changes occur in the vasa vasorum of peripheral

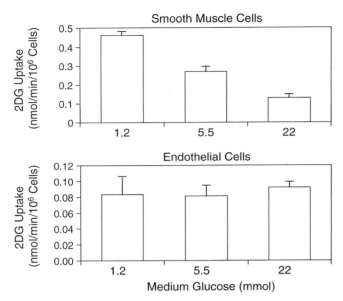

FIGURE 13-1. Lack of downregulation of glucose transport in cells affected by diabetic complications. **Top**: 2-Deoxyglucose uptake in vascular smooth muscle cells pre-exposed to either 1.2, 5.5, or 22 mmol glucose. **Bottom**: 2-Deoxyglucose uptake in vascular smooth muscle cells pre-exposed to either 1.2, 5.5, or 22 mmol glucose. *(Reproduced with permission from Kaiser et al.[6])*

nerve. Early in the course of diabetes, increased permeability is reversible, but as time progresses, it becomes irreversible.

Increased Vessel Wall Protein Accumulation

The common pathophysiologic feature of diabetic microvascular disease is progressive narrowing and eventual occlusion of vascular lumina, which results in inadequate perfusion and function of the affected tissues. Early hyperglycemia-induced microvascular hypertension and increased vascular permeability contribute to irreversible microvessel occlusion by three processes. The first is an abnormal leakage of periodic acid-Schiff (PAS)–positive, carbohydrate-containing plasma proteins, which are deposited in the capillary wall and may stimulate perivascular cells such as pericytes and mesangial cells to elaborate growth factors and extracellular matrix. The second is extravasation of growth factors such as transforming growth factor (TGFβ₁), which directly stimulate overproduction of extracellular matrix components.[10] The third pathologic process is hypertension-induced stimulation of pathologic gene expression by endothelial cells and supporting cells, which include growth factors, growth factor receptors, extracellular matrix components, and adhesion molecules that can activate circulating leukocytes.[11] The observation that unilateral reduction in the severity of diabetic microvascular disease occurs on the side with ophthalmic or renal artery stenosis is consistent with this concept.[12,13]

Microvascular Cell Loss and Vessel Occlusion

The progressive narrowing and occlusion of diabetic microvascular lumina is also accompanied by microvascular cell loss. In the retina, diabetes induces programmed cell death of Muller

cells/ganglion cells,[14] pericytes, and endothelial cells.[15] In the glomerulus, declining renal function is associated with widespread capillary occlusion, but the mechanisms underlying glomerular endothelial cell loss are not yet known. In the vasa nervorum, endothelial cell and pericyte degeneration occur,[16] and these microvascular changes appear to precede the development of diabetic peripheral neuropathy.[17] The multifocal distribution of axonal degeneration in diabetes supports a causal role for microvascular occlusion, but hyperglycemia-induced decreases in neurotrophins may contribute by preventing normal axonal repair and regeneration.[18]

Development of Microvascular Complications During Posthyperglycemic Euglycemia (Hyperglycemic Memory)

Another common feature of diabetic microvascular disease has been termed *hyperglycemic memory*. This refers to the persistence or progression of hyperglycemia-induced microvascular alterations during subsequent periods of normal glucose homeostasis. The most striking example of this phenomenon is the development of severe retinopathy in histologically normal eyes of diabetic dogs, which occurred entirely during a 2.5-year period of normalized blood glucose that followed 2.5 years of hyperglycemia (Fig. 13-3).[19] Normal dogs were compared to diabetic dogs with either poor control for 5 years, good control for 5 years, or poor control for 2.5 years (P→Gₐ) followed by good control for the next 2.5 years (P→G_b). HbA₁c values for both the good control group and the P→G_b group were identical to the normal group. Hyperglycemia-induced increases in selected matrix gene transcription also persist for weeks after restoration of normoglycemia *in vivo*, and a less pronounced, but qualitatively similar, prolongation of hyperglycemia-induced increase in selected matrix gene transcription occurs in cultured endothelial cells.[20]

Data from the DCCT study suggest that hyperglycemic memory occurs in patients. In the secondary intervention cohort, there was no difference in the incidence of sustained progression of retinopathy for the first 3 years, no difference in development of clinical albuminuria for 4 years, and no difference in the rate of change in creatinine clearance during the entire study. For neuropathy, the sural nerve sensory conduction velocity did not differ between the groups for 4 years, and intensive therapy did not slow the rate of decline of autonomic function at all.[2,21–23] Even more strikingly, the effects of former intensive and conventional therapy on the occurrence and severity of retinopathy and nephropathy were shown to persist for 4 years after the DCCT, despite nearly identical glycosylated hemoglobin values during the four-year follow-up (8.2% vs. 7.9%, respectively).[24] Taken together, these observations from animal and clinical studies imply that hyperglycemia induces prolonged and sometimes irreversible changes in long-lived intracellular molecules that persist and cause continued pathologic function in the absence of continued hyperglycemia.

Genetic Determinants of Susceptibility to Microvascular Complications

Clinicians have long observed that different patients with similar duration and degree of hyperglycemia could differ markedly in their susceptibility to microvascular complications. Such observations suggested that genetic differences existed that affected the pathways by which hyperglycemia damaged microvascular cells.

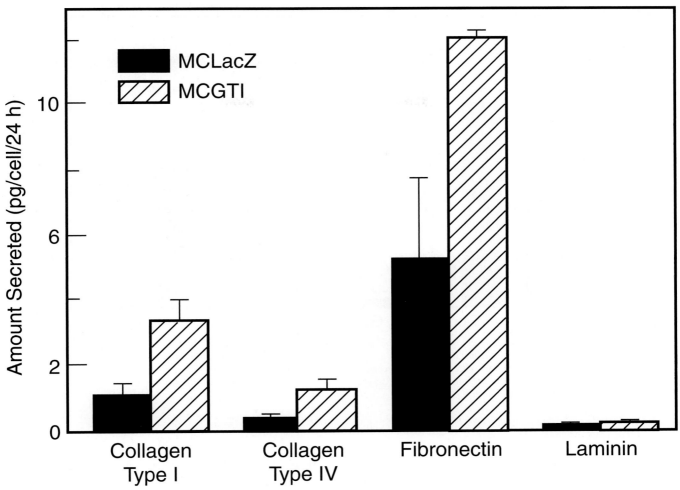

FIGURE 13-2. Overexpression of GLUT-1 in mesangial cells cultured in normal glucose mimics the diabetic phenotype. Mesangial cells transfected with either LacZ (**MCLacZ**) or GLUT-1-expressing constructs (**MCGTI**) were cultured in 5 mmol glucose and the amount of the indicated matrix components secreted was determined. *(Reproduced with permission from Heilig et al.[7])*

The leveling of risk of overt proteinuria after 30 years' duration of type 1 diabetes at 27% is evidence that only a subset of patients are susceptible to developing diabetic nephropathy.[25] A role for genetic determinant of susceptibility to diabetic nephropathy is most strongly supported by the demonstration of familial clustering of diabetic nephropathy. In two studies of families with two or more siblings having type 1 diabetes, if one diabetic sibling has advanced diabetic nephropathy, the other diabetic sibling has a nephropathy risk of 83% or 72%, while the risk is only 17% or 22% if the index case does not have diabetic nephropathy (Fig. 13-4).[26,27] For retinopathy, the DCCT reported familial clustering as well, with an odds ratio of 5.4 for the risk of severe retinopathy in diabetic relatives of positive versus negative subjects from the conventional treatment group.[28] Numerous associations have been made between various genetic polymorphisms and the risk of developing various diabetic complications. Examples include the 5′ insulin gene polymorphism,[29] the G2m (23+) immunoglobulin allotype,[30] angiotensin-converting enzyme insertion/deletion polymorphisms,[31,32] HLA-DQB1*0201/0302 alleles,[33] polymorphisms of the aldose reductase gene,[34] and a polymorphic CCTTT (n) repeat of nitric oxide synthetase 2A.[35] In all of these studies, there is no indication that the polymorphic gene actually plays a functional

role, rather than simply being in linkage disequilibrium with the locus encoding the unidentified relevant gene(s).

MECHANISMS OF HYPERGLYCEMIA-INDUCED DAMAGE

Four major hypotheses about how hyperglycemia causes diabetic complications have generated a large amount of data, as well as several clinical trials based on specific inhibitors of these mechanisms. Until quite recently, there was no unifying hypothesis linking these four mechanisms together, nor was there an obvious connection between any of these mechanisms, each of which responds quickly to normalization of hyperglycemia, and the phenomenon of hyperglycemic memory (discussed above).

Increased Polyol Pathway Flux

Aldose Reductase Function

Aldose reductase [alditol:NAD(P)$^+$ 1-oxidoreductase, EC 1.1.1.21] is a cytosolic, monomeric oxidoreductase that catalyzes the NADPH-dependent reduction of a wide variety of carbonyl

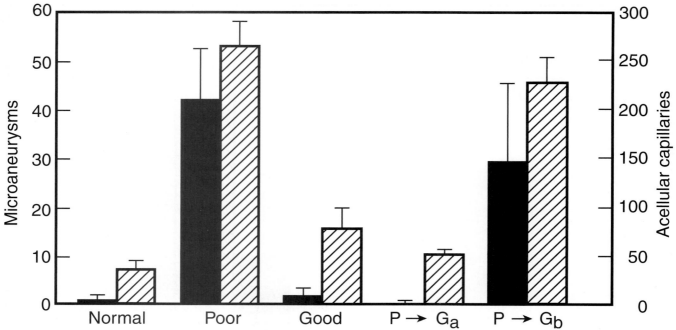

FIGURE 13-3. Development of retinopathy during post-hyperglycemic normoglycemia ("hyperglycemic memory"). Quantitation of retinal microaneurysms and acellular capillaries in normal dogs, dogs with poor glycemic control for 5 years, dogs with good glycemic control for 5 years, dogs with poor glycemic control for 2.5 years (**P→G$_a$**) and the same dogs after a subsequent 2.5 years of good glycemic control (**P→G$_b$**) *(Reproduced with permission from Engerman et al.[19])*

FIGURE 13-4. Familial clustering of diabetic nephropathy. Prevalence of diabetic nephropathy in two studies of diabetic siblings of probands with or without diabetic nephropathy.

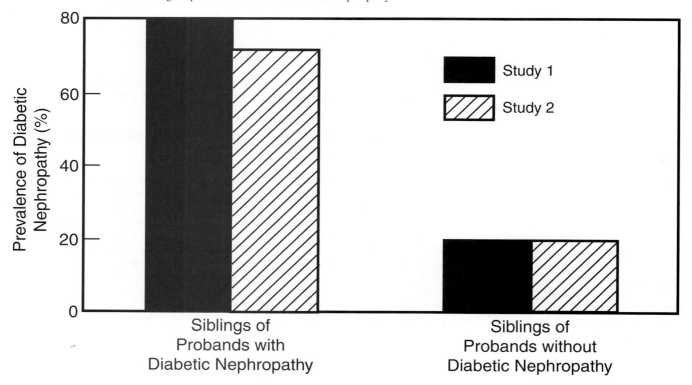

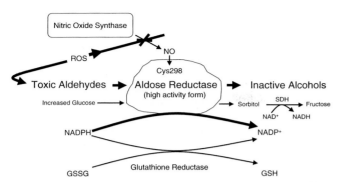

FIGURE 13-5. Aldose reductase function and the polyol pathway. Aldose reductase reduces reactive oxygen species (**ROS**)-generated toxic aldehydes to inactive alcohols, and glucose to sorbitol, using NADPH as a cofactor. Sorbitol dehydrogenase (**SDH**) oxidizes sorbitol to fructose using NAD$^+$ as a cofactor (see text for details). Aldose reductase may be activated by ROS-induced reduction of nitric oxide modification of a cysteine residue in the enzyme's active site *(Reproduced with permission from Brownlee.[175])*

compounds including glucose. Aldose reductase converts a variety of toxic aldehydes (such as 2-oxo-aldehydes and those derived from lipid peroxidation) to inactive alcohols. NADPH is the cofactor in both this reaction and in the regeneration of glutathione by glutathione reductase. Aldose reductase has a low affinity (high K_m) for glucose, and at the normal glucose concentrations found in nondiabetics, metabolism of glucose by this pathway constitutes a very small percentage of total glucose utilization. However, in a hyperglycemic environment, increased intracellular glucose concentration (and possibly oxidant stress-induced aldose reductase activation) results in increased enzymatic conversion to the polyalcohol sorbitol, with concomitant decreases in NADPH. In cells having aldose reductase activity that is sufficient to deplete the endogenous antioxidant glutathione, hyperglycemia-induced oxidative stress would be augmented. In the polyol pathway, sorbitol is oxidized to fructose by the enzyme sorbitol dehydrogenase (SDH), with NAD$^+$ reduced to NADH (Fig. 13-5).

Biochemical Consequences of Increased Polyol Pathway Flux

A number of mechanisms have been proposed to explain the potential detrimental effects of hyperglycemia-induced increases in polyol pathway flux. These include sorbitol-induced osmotic stress, decreased Na$^+$/K$^+$-ATPase activity, increased cytosolic NADH/NAD$^+$, and decreased cytosolic NADPH. Sorbitol does not diffuse easily across cell membranes, and it was originally suggested that this resulted in osmotic damage to microvascular cells. However, sorbitol concentrations measured in diabetic vessels and nerves are far too low to cause osmotic damage.

Another early suggestion was that increased flux through the polyol pathway decreased Na$^+$/K$^+$-ATPase activity. Although this was originally thought to be mediated by polyol-pathway-linked decreases in phosphatidylinositol synthesis, it has recently been shown to result from activation of protein kinase C (PKC; see below). Hyperglycemia-induced activation of PKC increases cytosolic phospholipase A$_2$ activity, which increases the production of two inhibitors of Na$^+$/K$^+$-ATPase, arachidonate and PGE$_2$.[36]

More recently, it has been proposed that oxidation of sorbitol by NAD$^+$ increases the cytosolic ratio of NADH to NAD$^+$, thereby in-

hibiting activity of the enzyme glyceraldehyde-3-phosphate dehydrogenase, and increasing concentrations of triose phosphate.[37] Elevated triose phosphate concentrations could increase formation of both methylglyoxal, a precursor of advanced glycation endproducts, and diacylglycerol (via α-glycerol-3-phosphate), thus activating PKC (discussed in subsequent sections). Although increased NADH production is supported by the observation that hyperglycemia increases both lactate concentration and the lactate:pyruvate ratio, there is no direct evidence that the concentrations of NADH and NAD$^+$, as opposed to NADH and NAD$^+$ flux, are altered. In endothelial cells, where aldose reductase activity is low, increased NADH production may also reflect hyperglycemia-induced increased flux through glycolysis[38] and through the glucuronic acid pathway.[39]

Other evidence presented in support of this hypothesis includes the observation that administration of pyruvate can prevent diabetes-related endothelial dysfunction in some systems. However, the observed effects of pyruvate on microvascular function may reflect its potent antioxidant properties rather than effects on the NADH:NAD$^+$ ratio, since reactive oxygen species also partially inhibit glyceraldehyde-3-phosphate dehydrogenase and increase glyceraldehyde-3-phosphate levels.[40,41] The source of hyperglycemia-induced reactive oxygen species will be discussed later in this chapter.

It has also been proposed that reduction of glucose to sorbitol by NADPH consumes the cofactor NADPH. Since NADPH is required for regenerating reduced glutathione (GSH), this could induce or exacerbate intracellular oxidative stress. Less reduced GSH has in fact been found in the lenses of transgenic mice that overexpress aldose reductase, and this is the most likely mechanism by which increased flux through the polyol pathway has deleterious consequences.[42] Hyperglycemia-induced inhibition of glucose-6-phosphate dehydrogenase, the major source of NADPH regeneration, may further reduce NADPH concentration in some diabetic microvascular cells.[43]

Increased Intracellular AGE Formation

Advanced Glycation Endproducts Form from Intracellular Dicarbonyl Precursors

Advanced glycation endproducts (AGEs) are found in increased amounts in extracellular structures of diabetic retinal vessels[44–46] and renal glomeruli,[47–49] where they can cause damage by mechanisms described later in this section. These AGEs were originally thought to arise from nonenzymatic reactions between extracellular proteins and glucose. However, the rate of AGE formation from glucose is orders of magnitude slower than the rate of AGE formation from glucose-derived dicarbonyl precursors generated intracellularly, and it now seems likely that intracellular hyperglycemia is the primary initiating event in the formation of both intracellular and extracellular AGEs.[50] AGEs can arise from intracellular autoxidation of glucose to glyoxal,[51] decomposition of the Amadori product to 3-deoxyglucosone (perhaps accelerated by an Amadoriase), and fragmentation of glyceraldehyde-3-phosphate to methylglyoxal[52] (Fig. 13-6). These reactive intracellular dicarbonyls react with amino groups of intracellular and extracellular proteins to form AGEs. Methylglyoxal and glyoxal are detoxified by the glyoxalase system.[52] All three AGE precursors are also substrates for other reductases.[53,54]

Intracellular production of AGE precursors damages target cells by three general mechanisms (Fig. 13-7). First, intracellular

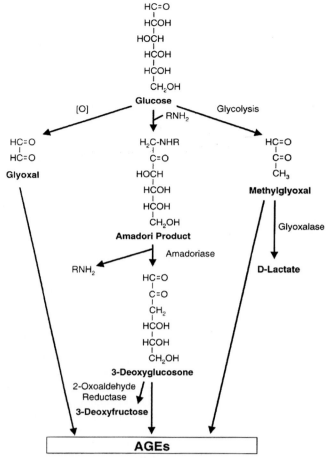

FIGURE 13-6. Intracellular AGE formation. Potential pathways leading to the formation of advanced glycation endproducts (**AGEs**) inside cells (see text for details). (*Reproduced with permission from Shinohara et al.[57]*)

proteins modified by AGEs have altered function. Second, extracellular matrix components modified by AGE precursors interact abnormally with other matrix components and with matrix receptors (integrins) on cells. Third, plasma proteins modified by AGE precursors bind to AGE receptors on cells such as macrophages, inducing receptor-mediated reactive oxygen species production. This AGE receptor ligation activates the pleiotrophic transcription factor NFκB, causing pathologic changes in gene expression.[55]

FIGURE 13-7. Intracellular production of AGE precursors damages cells by three mechanisms. (*Reproduced with permission from Brownlee.[176]*)

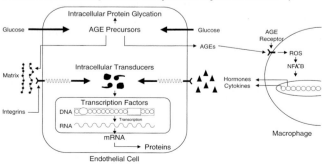

Advanced Glycation Endproducts Alter Intracellular Protein Function

In endothelial cells, intracellular AGE formation occurs very quickly. Within 1 week, AGE content increases 13.8-fold in endothelial cells cultured in media containing high levels of glucose.[56] Basic fibroblast growth factor (bFGF) is one of the major AGE-modified proteins in endothelial cells.[56] Endothelial cell cytosol mitogenic activity is reduced 70% by AGE formation when cytosolic AGE-bFGF is increased 6.1-fold. Proteins involved in macromolecular endocytosis are also modified by AGEs, since the 2.2-fold increase in endocytosis induced by hyperglycemia is also prevented by overexpression of the methylglyoxal-detoxifying glyoxalase I.[57] Glyoxalase-I overexpression also completely prevents the fourfold hyperglycemia-induced increase in Muller cell expression of angiopoietin-2, a factor that has been implicated in both pericyte loss and capillary regression.[58–60] This observation suggests that the α-oxoaldehyde AGE precursors methylglyoxal and glyoxal modify transcriptional complex proteins and thereby activate gene expression.

Advanced Glycation Endproducts Interfere with Normal Matrix-Matrix and Matrix-Cell Interactions

AGE formation alters the functional properties of several important matrix molecules. Collagen was the first matrix protein used to demonstrate that glucose-derived AGEs form covalent, intermolecular bonds. This process is partly mediated by H_2O_2 production.[61,62] On type I collagen, this crosslinking induces an expansion of the molecular packing.[63] These AGE-induced crosslinks alter the function of intact vessels. For example, AGEs decrease elasticity in large vessels from diabetic rats, even after vascular tone is abolished, and increase fluid filtration across the carotid artery.[64] AGE formation on type IV collagen from basement membrane inhibits lateral association of these molecules into a normal network-like structure by interfering with binding of the noncollagenous NC1 domain to the helix-rich domain.[65] AGE formation on laminin causes decreased polymer self-assembly, decreased binding to type IV collagen, and decreased binding of heparan sulfate proteoglycan.[66] *In vitro* AGE formation on intact glomerular basement membrane increases its permeability to albumin in a manner that resembles the abnormal permeability of diabetic nephropathy.[67,68]

AGE formation on extracellular matrix not only interferes with matrix-matrix interactions, it interferes with matrix-cell interactions as well. For example, AGE modification of type IV collagen's cell-binding domains decrease endothelial cell adhesion,[69] and AGE modification of a six-amino-acid growth-promoting sequence in the A chain of the laminin molecule markedly reduces neurite outgrowth.[70] AGE modification of vitronectin reduced cell attachment-promoting activity.[71]

AGE Receptors Mediate Pathologic Changes in Gene Expression

Specific receptors for AGEs were first identified on monocytes and macrophages. Two AGE-binding proteins isolated from rat liver are both present on monocyte/macrophages. Antisera to either the 60-kd or 90-kd protein, recently identified as OST-48 and 80K-H, respectively,[72] block AGE binding.[73] AGE protein binding to this receptor stimulates macrophage production of interleukin-1, insulin-like growth factor IGF-1, tumor necrosis factor α, transforming growth factor-β, macrophage colony-stimulating factor, and granulocyte/macrophage colony-stimulating factor at levels that have been shown to increase glomerular synthesis of type IV collagen and to stimulate proliferation and chemotaxis of both arterial smooth muscle cells and macrophages.[74–82] The macrophage scavenger receptor type 2 and galectin-3 have also been shown to recognize AGEs.[83–86]

AGE receptors have also been identified on glomerular mesangial cells. *In vitro*, AGE protein binding to its receptor on mesangial cells stimulates platelet-derived growth factor secretion, which in turn mediates production of type IV collagen, laminin, and heparan sulfate proteoglycan.[87,88]

Vascular endothelial cells also express AGE-specific receptors (RAGE). A 35-kd and a 46-kd AGE-binding protein have been purified to homogeneity from endothelial cells.[89–91] The N-terminal sequence of the 35-kd protein was identical to lactoferrin, whereas the 46-kd protein was novel. A full-length, 1.5-kb cDNA for the 46-kd protein was cloned and sequenced. This novel AGE-binding protein appears to be a member of the immunoglobulin superfamily, with three disulfide-bonded immunoglobulin homology units. RAGE has been shown to mediate signal transduction via generation of reactive oxygen species, activation of NFκB, and p21 ras.[92–94] AGE signaling is blocked in cells by expression of RAGE antisense cDNA[95] or antiRAGE ribozyme.[96]

In endothelial cells, AGE binding to its receptor induces changes in gene expression that include alterations in thrombomodulin, tissue factor, and vascular cell adhesion molecule 1 (VCAM-1).[97–100] These changes induce procoagulatory changes in the endothelial surface and increase the adhesion of inflammatory cells to the vessel wall. In addition, endothelial AGE receptor binding appears to mediate in part the hyperpermeability induced by diabetes, probably through the induction of vascular endothelial growth factor.[101–103]

Activation of Protein Kinase C

Mechanism of Hyperglycemia-Induced Protein Kinase C Activation

Protein kinase Cs (PKCs) are a family of at least eleven isoforms, nine of which are activated by the lipid second messenger diacylglycerol (DAG). Intracellular hyperglycemia increases DAG content in cultured microvascular cells and in the retina and renal glomeruli of diabetic animals.[104–106] Intracellular hyperglycemia appears to increase DAG content primarily by increasing its *de novo* synthesis from the glycolytic intermediate glyceraldehyde-3-phosphate *via* reduction to glycerol-3-phosphate and stepwise acylation.[105,107] Increased *de novo* synthesis of DAG activates PKC both in cultured vascular cells[106,108–110] and in retina and glomeruli of diabetic animals.[106,108,105] Increased DAG primarily activates the β and δ isoforms of PKC, but increases in other isoforms have also been found, such as PKC-α and -ε isoforms in the retina and PKC-α and -δ in the glomerulus[111,112] of diabetic rats.

Consequences of Hyperglycemia-Induced PKC Activation

In early experimental diabetes, activation of PKC-β isoforms has been shown to mediate retinal and renal blood flow abnormalities,[113] perhaps by depressing nitric oxide production and/or increasing endothelin-1 activity (Fig. 13-8). Abnormal activation of PKC has been implicated in the decreased glomerular production of nitric oxide induced by experimental diabetes,[114] and in the decreased smooth muscle cell nitric oxide production induced by hy-

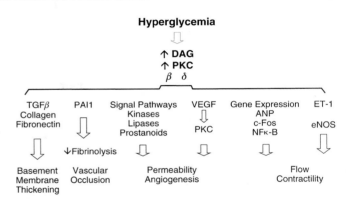

FIGURE 13-8. Potential consequences of hyperglycemia-induced protein kinase C activation. Hyperglycemia increases diacylglycerol (**DAG**) content, which activates PKC, primarily the β and δ isoforms. Activated PKC has a number of pathogenic consequences which are described in the text. (*Reproduced with permission from Koya et al.*[111])

perglycemia.[115] PKC activation also inhibits insulin-stimulated expression of eNOS mRNA in cultured endothelial cells.[116] Hyperglycemia increases endothelin-1-stimulated mitogen-activated protein kinase (MAPK) activity in glomerular mesangial cells by activating PKC isoforms.[117] However, the increased endothelial cell permeability induced by high glucose in cultured cells is mediated by activation of PKCα.[118] Activation of PKC by elevated glucose also induces expression of the permeability-enhancing factor VEGF in smooth muscle cells.[119]

In addition to affecting hyperglycemia-induced abnormalities of blood flow and permeability, activation of PKC contributes to increased microvascular matrix protein accumulation by inducing expression of TGFβ₁, fibronectin, and α1(IV) collagen in both cultured mesangial cells[120,121] and in glomeruli of diabetic rats.[122] This effect appears to be mediated through PKC's inhibition of nitric oxide production.[123] However, hyperglycemia-induced expression of laminin C1 in cultured mesangial cells is independent of PKC activation.[124] Hyperglycemia-induced activation of PKC has also been implicated in the overexpression of the fibrinolytic inhibitor plasminogen activator inhibitor-1,[125] and in the activation of the pleiotrophic transcription factor NFκB in cultured endothelial cells and vascular smooth muscle cells.[126,127]

Increased Hexosamine Pathway Flux

A fourth hypothesis about how hyperglycemia causes diabetic complications has recently been formulated,[128,129] in which glucose is shunted into the hexosamine pathway (Fig. 13–9). In this pathway, fructose-6-phosphate is diverted from glycolysis to provide substrates for reactions that require UDP-N-acetylglucosamine, such as proteoglycan synthesis and the formation of *O*-linked glycoproteins. Inhibition of the rate-limiting enzyme in the conversion of glucose to glucosamine, glutamine:fructose-6-phosphate amidotransferase (GFAT), blocks hyperglycemia-induced increases in the transcription of both transforming growth factor-α[128] and transforming growth factor-β₁ (TGF-β₁).[129] This pathway has previously been shown to play an important role in hyperglycemia-induced and fat-induced insulin resistance.[130–132]

The mechanism by which increased flux through the hexosamine pathway mediates hyperglycemia-induced increases in gene transcription is not clear, but the observation that Sp1 sites reg-

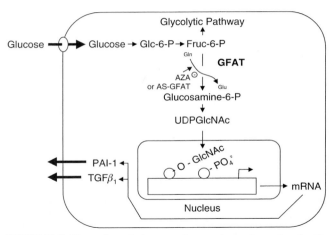

FIGURE 13-9. Hyperglycemia increases hexosamine pathway flux. In this pathway, increased *O*-linked GlcNAc moieties on the transcription factor Sp1 increase its transactivating function and thus increase transcription of genes associated with diabetic complications. *(Reproduced with permission from Kolm-Litty et al.[129])*

ulate hyperglycemia-induced activation of the PAI-1 promoter in vascular smooth muscle cells[133] suggests that covalent modification of Sp1 by N-acetylglucosamine may explain the link between hexosamine pathway activation and hyperglycemia-induced changes in gene transcription. Virtually every RNA polymerase II transcription factor examined has been found to be *O*-GlcNacylated,[134] and the glycosylated form of Sp1 appears to be more transcriptionally active than the deglycosylated form of the protein.[135] A fourfold increase in Sp1 *O*-GlcNacylation caused by inhibition of the enzyme *O*-GlcNac-β-N-acetylglucosaminidase resulted in a reciprocal 30% decrease in its level of serine/threonine phosphorylation, supporting the concept that *O*-GlcNacylation and phosphorylation compete to modify the same sites on this protein.[136]

GlcNac modification of Sp1 may regulate other glucose-responsive genes in addition to TGFβ₁ and PAI-1. Glucose-responsive transcription is regulated by Sp1 sites in the acetyl CoA carboxylase gene, the rate-limiting enzyme for fatty acid synthesis, for example, and it appears that posttranslational modification of Sp1 is responsible for this effect.[137,138] Since virtually every RNA polymerase II transcription factor examined has been found to be *O*-GlcNacylated,[134] it is possible that reciprocal modification by *O*-GlcNacylation and phosphorylation of transcription factors other than Sp1 may function as a more generalized mechanism for regulating glucose-responsive gene transcription.

In addition to transcription factors, many other nuclear and cytoplasmic proteins are dynamically modified by *O*-GlcNAc moieties, and may exhibit reciprocal modification by phosphorylation in a manner analogous to Sp1.[134] Thus, activation of the hexosamine pathway by hyperglycemia may result in many changes in both gene expression and in protein function that together contribute to the pathogenesis of diabetic complications.

DIFFERENT PATHOGENIC MECHANISMS REFLECT A SINGLE HYPERGLYCEMIA-INDUCED PROCESS

Although specific inhibitors of aldose reductase activity, AGE formation, and PKC activation each ameliorate various diabetes-induced abnormalities in animal models, there has been no appar-

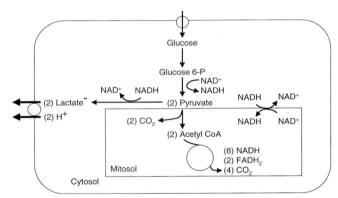

FIGURE 13-10. Glucose oxidation and the production of cytoplasmic and mitochondrial reducing equivalents.

ent common element linking the four mechanisms of hyperglycemia-induced damage discussed in the preceding section.[139–142,113] It has also been conceptually difficult to explain the phenomenon of hyperglycemic memory (discussed in an earlier section) as a consequence of four processes that quickly normalize when euglycemia is restored. These issues may have now been resolved by the recent discovery that each of the four differ... pathogenic mechanisms could reflect a single hyperglycemia-induced process: overproduction of superoxide by the mitochondrial electron transport chain.[38,143]

Hyperglycemia increases reactive oxygen species production inside cultured bovine aortic endothelial cells.[144] To understand how this occurs, a brief overview of glucose metabolism is helpful. Intracellular glucose oxidation begins with glycolysis in the cytoplasm, which generates NADH and pyruvate. Cytoplasmic NADH can donate reducing equivalents to the mitochondrial electron transport chain via two shuttle systems, or it can reduce pyruvate to lactate, which exits the cell to provide substrate for hepatic gluconeogenesis. Pyruvate can also be transported into the mitochondria, where it is oxidized by the tricarboxylic acid (TCA) cycle to produce CO_2, H_2O, four molecules of NADH, and one molecule of $FADH_2$. Mitochondrial NADH and $FADH_2$ provide energy for ATP production via oxidative phosphorylation by the electron transport chain (Fig. 13-10).

Electron flow through the mitochondrial electron transport chain is carried out by four inner membrane-associated enzyme complexes, plus cytochrome *c* and the mobile carrier ubiquinone.[145] NADH derived from both cytosolic glucose oxidation and mitochondrial TCA cycle activity donates electrons to NADH: ubiquinone oxidoreductase (complex I). Complex I ultimately transfers its electrons to ubiquinone. Ubiquinone can also be reduced by electrons donated from several $FADH_2$-containing dehydrogenases, including succinate:ubiquinone oxidoreductase (complex II) and glycerol-3-phosphate dehydrogenase. Electrons from reduced ubiquinone are then transferred to ubiquinol:cytochrome c oxidoreductase (complex III) by the ubisemiquinone radical-generating Q cycle.[146] Electron transport then proceeds through cytochrome *c*, cytochrome c oxidase (complex IV), and finally, molecular oxygen.

Electron transfer through Complexes I, III, and IV generates a proton gradient that drives ATP synthase (Complex V). When the electrochemical potential difference generated by this proton gradient is high, the life of superoxide-generating electron transport intermediates such as ubisemiquinone is prolonged. There appears to be a threshold value above which superoxide production is markedly increased (Fig. 13-11).[147]

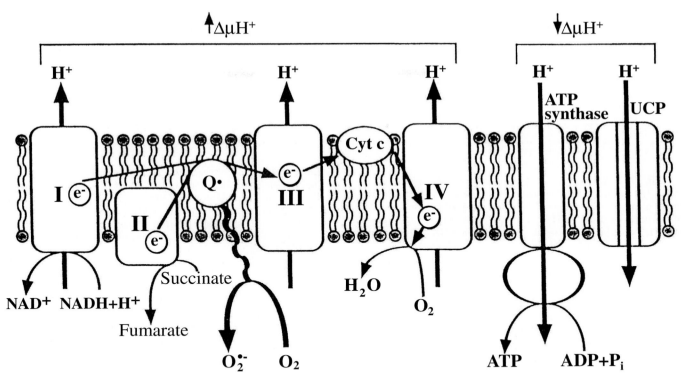

FIGURE 13-11. Production of superoxide by the mitochondrial electron transport chain. Increased hyperglycemia-derived substrate generates a high mitochondrial membrane potential ($\Delta\mu H^+$), which inhibits electron transport and increases the half-life of intermediates capable of reducing O_2 to superoxide (see text for details). *(Reproduced with permission from Boss et al.[177])*

Using inhibitors of both the shuttle that transfers cytosolic NADH into mitochondria, and the transporter that transfers cytosolic pyruvate into the mitochondria, the TCA cycle was shown to be the source of hyperglycemia-induced reactive oxygen species in endothelial cells. To determine the site of hyperglycemia-induced intracellular reactive oxygen species (ROS) production, endothelial cells were first incubated with either rotenone, an inhibitor of complex I, thenoyltrifluoroacetone (TTFA), an inhibitor of complex II, or carbonyl cyanide m-chlorophenylhydrazone (CCCP), an uncoupler of oxidative phosphorylation that abolishes the mitochondrial membrane proton gradient. Compared with baseline conditions (5 mmol glucose), incubation with 30 mmol glucose increased ROS production from 52.08 ± 1.03 (5 mmol glucose) to 154 ± 1.38 nmol/mL (Fig. 13-12). Rotenone did not reduce increased ROS production, while both TTFA and CCCP completely prevented the effect of hyperglycemia (Fig. 13-12).

Since pharmacologic inhibitors are not absolutely specific to one cellular target, experiments were also performed using molecular techniques. Overexpression of uncoupling protein-1 (UCP1), a specific protein uncoupler of oxidative phosphorylation capable of collapsing the proton electrochemical gradient,[148] also prevented the effect of hyperglycemia (Fig. 13-12). Antisense cDNA in the same gene transfer vector did not (Fig. 13-12). These results demonstrate that hyperglycemia-induced intracellular ROS are produced by the proton electrochemical gradient generated by the mitochondrial electron transport chain. Overexpression of manganese superoxide dismutase, the mitochondrial form of this antioxidant enzyme,[149] also prevented the effect of hyperglycemia (Fig. 13-12). This result demonstrates that superoxide is the reactive oxygen radical produced by this mechanism.

The effect of hyperglycemia-induced mitochondrial superoxide overproduction on polyol pathway flux was evaluated after first determining that sorbitol in these cells was exclusively derived from aldose reductase activity. Sorbitol levels were 2.6-fold higher than baseline (5 mmol glucose) when endothelial cells were incubated in 30 mmol glucose (Fig. 13-13). Hyperglycemia-induced sorbitol accumulation was completely prevented by TTFA, UCP1 and Mn-SOD (Fig. 13-13), indicating that mitochondrial superoxide overproduction stimulates aldose reductase activity. This obser-

FIGURE 13-12. Effect of agents that alter mitochondrial metabolism on hyperglycemia-induced reactive oxygen species (**ROS**) formation in bovine aortic endothelial cells. Cells were incubated in 5 mmol glucose, 30 mmol glucose alone, and 30 mmol glucose plus either rotenone, thenoyltrifluoroacetone (**TTFA**), carbonyl cyanide m-chlorophenylhydrazone (**CCCP**), antisense (**AS**), uncoupling protein-1 (**UCP1**), or manganese superoxide dismutase (**Mn-SOD**) HVJ-liposomes, and ROS were quantitated. *(Reproduced with permisison from Nishikawa et al.[38])*

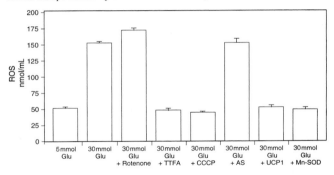

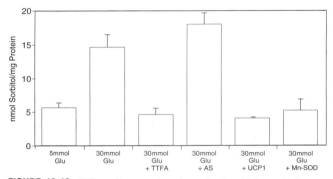

FIGURE 13-13. Effect of agents that alter mitochondrial metabolism on hyperglycemia-induced sorbitol accumulation. Cells were incubated in 5 mmol glucose, 30 mmol glucose alone, and 30 mmol glucose plus either thenoyltrifluoroacetone (**TTFA**), antisense (**AS**), uncoupling protein-1 (**UCP1**), or manganese superoxide dismutase (**Mn-SOD**) HVJ-liposomes, as indicated. (*Reproduced with permission from Nishikawa et al.[38]*)

vation is consistent with recent data suggesting that aldose reductase activity is reversibly downregulated by nitric oxide modification of a cysteine residue in the enzyme's active site,[150] and that reactive oxygen species appear to reduce nitric oxide levels in diabetic endothelium.[151] It may also reflect the well-described reversible inhibition of glyceraldehyde-3-phosphate dehydrogenase by reactive oxygen species,[41,143] which increases glyceraldehyde-3-phosphate levels and the levels of proximal glycolytic metabolites including glucose.

Next, the effect of hyperglycemia-induced mitochondrial superoxide overproduction on intracellular AGE formation was determined. In bovine aortic endothelial cells, hyperglycemia increases intracellular AGEs primarily, if not exclusively, by increasing the formation of AGE-forming methylglyoxal.[57] Therefore, the effect of TTFA, CCCP, UCP1, and Mn-SOD on hyperglycemia-induced formation of intracellular methylglyoxal-derived AGEs was examined (Fig. 13-14). Each of these agents completely prevented hyperglycemia-induced formation of intracellular AGEs (Fig. 13-14), indicating that mitochondrial superoxide initiates intracellular AGE formation. Since methylglyoxal is formed by fragmentation of glyceraldehyde-3-phosphate, this dependency on increased mitochondrial superoxide production also likely reflects increased glyceraldehyde-3-phosphate levels due to inhibition of

FIGURE 13-14. Effect of agents that alter mitochondrial metabolism on hyperglycemia-induced intracellular AGE formation. Cells were incubated in 5 mmol glucose, 30 mmol glucose alone, and 30 mmol glucose plus either thenoyltrifluoroacetone (**TTFA**), uncoupling protein-1 (**UCP1**), or manganese superoxide dismutase (**Mn-SOD**) HVJ-liposomes, as indicated, Age Densitrometry (**AU**). (*Reproduced with permission from Nishikawa et al.[38]*)

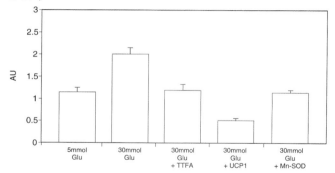

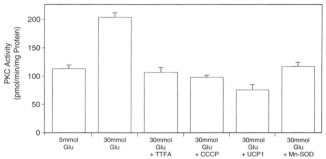

FIGURE 13-15. Effect of agents that alter mitochondrial metabolism on hyperglycemia-induced PKC activation. Cells were incubated in 5 mmol glucose, 30 mmol glucose alone, and 30 mmol glucose plus either thenoyltrifluoroacetone (**TTFA**), carbonyl cyanide m-chlorophenylhydrazone (**CCCP**), uncoupling protein-1 (**UCP1**), or manganese superoxide dismutase (**Mn-SOD**) HVJ-liposomes, as indicated, and PKC activity was determined in the membrane fraction. (*Reproduced with permission from Nishikawa et al.[38]*)

glyceraldehyde-3-phosphate dehydrogenase by reactive oxygen species.[41,143]

The effect of TTFA, CCCP, UCP1, and Mn-SOD on hyperglycemia-induced activation of PKC was also evaluated (Fig. 13-15). Each of these agents completely inhibited PKC activation, suggesting that mitochondrial superoxide overproduction initiates the hyperglycemia-induced *de novo* synthesis of diacylglycerol that activates PKC.[152] Most likely this too reflects increased glyceraldehyde-3-phosphate levels due to inhibition of glyceraldehyde-3-phosphate dehydrogenase by reactive oxygen species.[41,143]

Finally, the effect of hyperglycemia-induced mitochondrial superoxide overproduction on the hexosamine pathway was determined.[143] Hyperglycemia induced an increase in hexosamine pathway activity that was completely prevented by TTFA, CCCP, and by azaserine, an inhibitor of the rate-limiting enzyme in the hexosamine pathway (Fig. 13-16). The increased production of UDP-N-acetyl glucosamine by hyperglycemia-induced mitochondrial superoxide overproduction was shown to increase *O*-glycosylation of the transcription factor Sp1, which activated expression of genes known to contribute to the pathogenesis of diabetic complications.[143]

FIGURE 13-16. Effect of agents that alter mitochondrial metabolism on hyperglycemia-induced hexosamine pathway activity. Cells were incubated in 5 mmol glucose, 30 mmol glucose alone, and 30 mmol glucose plus either thenoyltrifluoroacetone (**TTFA**), carbonyl cyanide m-chlorophenylhydrazone (**CCCP**), manganese (III) tetrakis(4-benzoic acid) porphyrin (**TBAP**), or azaserine as indicated, and UDP-GlcNAc concentration was determined.

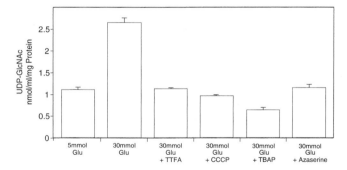

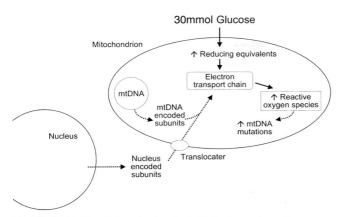

FIGURE 13-17. Potential mechanism for initiating hyperglycemic memory. Hyperglycemia-induced increases in reactive oxygen species are generated as a consequence of increased reducing equivalents entering the mitochondrial electron transport chain. The increased ROS would not only increase aldose reductase activity, AGE formation, PKC activity, and hexosamine pathway activity, but would also induce mutations in mitochondrial DNA. *(Reproduced with permission from Doctrow et al.[174])*

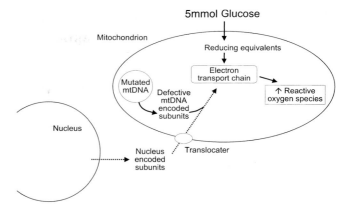

FIGURE 13-18. Potential mechanism for sustaining hyperglycemic memory. Mitochondrial DNA mutated by hyperglycemia-induced ROS would encode defective electron transport chain subunits. These defective subunits would cause increased ROS production by the electron transport chain at physiologic concentrations of glucose and glucose-derived reducing equivalents, thus maintaining the activation of aldose reductase activity, AGE formation, PKC activity, and hexosamine pathway activity. *(Reproduced with permission from Doctrow et al.[174])*

Hyperglycemia-induced activation of the redox-sensitive pleiotrophic transcription factor NfκB was also prevented by inhibition of mitochondrial superoxide overproduction.[38]

A POSSIBLE MOLECULAR BASIS FOR HYPERGLYCEMIC MEMORY

In contrast to the four known hyperglycemia-inducible abnormalities of intracellular metabolism, hyperglycemia-induced mitochondrial superoxide production may provide an explanation for the development of complications during posthyperglycemic normoglycemia (hyperglycemic memory). Hyperglycemia-induced increases in superoxide would not only increase aldose reductase activity, AGE formation, PKC activity, and hexosamine pathway activity, but may also induce mutations in mitochondrial DNA (Fig. 13-17).[153] Mitochondria are more vulnerable to mutation because mtDNA contains virtually no introns, lacks protective histones, and has no effective DNA repair mechanism.[154–156] mtDNA has a 10- to 20-fold higher mutation rate than nuclear DNA.[157,158] Defective electron transport complex subunits encoded by mutated mitochondrial DNA could eventually cause increased superoxide production at physiologic concentrations of glucose, with resultant continued activation of the four pathways despite the absence of hyperglycemia (Fig. 13-18).

PROSPECTS FOR PHARMACOLOGIC INTERVENTION

Aldose Reductase Inhibitors

In vivo studies of polyol pathway inhibition have yielded promising results with neuropathy but disappointing results in other target tissues of diabetic complications. During the course of a 5-year study, nerve conduction velocity progressively decreased in untreated diabetic dogs, while this decrease was prevented by treatment with an aldose reductase inhibitor (ARI).[139] Positive effects of ARIs on human diabetic neuropathy have been reported.[159,160] In

contrast, aldose reductase inhibition failed to prevent retinopathy in a 5-year study in dogs, nor did it prevent capillary basement membrane thickening in the retina, kidney, or muscles.[161] A 3-year human trial also failed to show any effect on diabetic retinopathy.[162]

AGE Inhibitors

The hydrazine compound aminoguanidine was the first AGE inhibitor discovered,[62] and its effect on diabetic pathology has been investigated in the retina, kidney, nerve, and artery. In the rat retina, diabetes causes a 19-fold increase in the number of acellular capillaries. Aminoguanidine treatment of diabetics prevented excess AGE accumulation and reduced the number of acellular capillaries by 80%. Diabetes-induced pericyte dropout also was markedly reduced by aminoguanidine treatments.[44]

Similar results have been obtained in animal models of diabetic kidney disease.[163–165] Diabetes increased AGEs in the renal glomerulus, and aminoguanidine treatment prevented this diabetes-induced increase. Untreated diabetic animals developed albuminuria that averaged 30 mg every 24 hours for 32 weeks. This was more than a 10-fold increase above control levels. In aminoguanidine-treated diabetic rats, the level of albumin excretion was reduced nearly 90%.[36] Untreated diabetic animals also developed the characteristic structural feature of human diabetic nephropathy, increased fractional mesangial volume. When diabetic animals were treated with aminoguanidine, the increase was completely prevented. A structurally unrelated AGE inhibitor, OPB-9195 also prevented the development and progression of experimental diabetic nephropathy by blocking type IV collagen overproduction and normalizing the expression of TGFβ.[166,167]

In the peripheral nerve of diabetic rats, both motor nerve and sensory nerve conduction velocity are decreased after 8 weeks of diabetes.[168] Nerve action-potential amplitude is decreased by 37% and peripheral nerve blood flow is decreased by 57% after 24 weeks of diabetes.[169] Aminoguanidine treatment prevented each of these abnormalities of diabetic peripheral nerve function.[168,169]

In a large randomized, double-blind, placebo-controlled, multicenter trial of aminoguanidine in type 1 diabetic patients with overt nephropathy, aminoguanidine lowered total urinary protein and slowed progression of nephropathy, over and above the effects of existing optimal care. In addition, aminoguanidine reduced the progression of diabetic retinopathy (defined as an increase by three or more steps in the ETDRS scale).[170,171]

PKC Inhibitors

The recent development of a β isoform-specific PKC inhibitor has allowed *in vivo* studies to go forward, since the toxicity of nonselective PKC inhibitors precludes their use. LY333531 inhibits PKCβ$_1$ and PKCβ$_2$ with a half-maximal inhibitory constant (IC$_{50}$) that is at least 50-fold less than for other PKC isoforms.[113] Treatment with LY333531 significantly reduced PKC activity in the retina and renal glomeruli of diabetic animals. Concomitantly, LY333531 treatment significantly reduced diabetes-induced increases in retinal mean circulation time, normalized diabetes-induced increases in glomerular filtration rate, and partially corrected urinary albumin excretion. Treatment of db/db mice with LY333531 for a longer period of time also ameliorated accelerated glomerular mesangial expansion.[172] Clinical trials of LY333531 in human diabetic patients are currently in progress.

Hexosamine Pathway Inhibitors

To date, there have been no *in vivo* trials of hexosamine pathway inhibitors, but the *in vitro* data discussed earlier in this chapter suggest that inhibitors of the rate-limiting enzyme of this pathway, glutamine:fructose-6-phosphate amidotransferase (GFAT), would have beneficial effects.

Future Drug Targets

The recent discovery that each of the four different pathogenic mechanisms discussed in this chapter may reflect a single hyperglycemia-induced process[38,143] suggests that interrupting the overproduction of superoxide by the mitochondrial electron transport chain could normalize polyol pathway flux, AGE formation, PKC activation, and hexosamine pathway flux, as well as a number of other hyperglycemia-induced mechanisms that remain to be discovered.

Novel compounds that act as superoxide dismutase/catalase mimetics already exist,[173,174] and these compounds have been shown to normalize hyperglycemia-induced mitochondrial superoxide overproduction *in vitro*.[143] Compounds that directly prevent hyperglycemia-induced mitochondrial superoxide overproduction may also hold promise. Drugs that normalize superoxide-induced triose phosphate accumulation are another logical therapeutic strategy. These and the other agents described in this section may have unique clinical efficacy in preventing the development and progression of diabetic complications.

REFERENCES

1. Skyler J: Diabetic complications: The importance of glucose control. In: Brownlee MB, King GL, eds. *Endocrinol Metab Clin North Am.* WB Saunders:1996.
2. The Diabetes Control and Complications Trial Research Group: The effect of intensive treatment of diabetes on the development and progression of long-term complications in insulin-dependent diabetes mellitus. *N Engl J Med* 1993;329:977.
3. UK Prospective Diabetes Study (UKPDS) Group: Intensive blood-glucose control with sulphonylureas or insulin compared with conventional treatment and risk of complications in patients with type 2 diabetes (UKPDS 33). *Lancet* 1998;352:837.
4. Krolewski AS, Laffel LM, Krolewski M, et al: Glycosylated hemoglobin and the risk of microalbuminuria in patients with insulin-dependent diabetes mellitus. *N Engl J Med* 1995;332:1251.
5. DCCT Study Group: The absence of a glycemic threshold for the development of long-term complications: the perspective of the Diabetes Control and Complications Trial. *Diabetes* 1996;45:1289.
6. Kaiser N, Feener EP, Boukobza-Vardi N, et al: Differential regulation of glucose transport and transporters by glucose in vascular endothelial and smooth muscle cells. *Diabetes* 1993;42:80.
7. Heilig CW, Concepcion LA, Riser BL, et al: Overexpression of glucose transporters in rat mesangial cells cultured in a normal glucose milieu mimics the diabetic phenotype. *J Clin Invest* 1995;96:1802.
8. Shore AC, Tooke JE: Microvascular function and haemodynamic disturbances in diabetes mellitus and its complications. In: Pickup J, Williams G, eds. *Textbook of Diabetes*, Vol. 1. Blackwell Scientific:1997;43.1.
9. Kihara M, Schmelzer JD, Poduslo JF, et al: Aminoguanidine effects on nerve blood flow, vascular permeability, electrophysiology, and oxygen free radicals. *Proc Natl Acad Sci USA* 1991;88:6107.
10. Kopp JB, Factor VM, Mozes M, et al: Transgenic mice with increased plasma levels of TGF-beta 1 develop progressive renal disease. *Lab Invest* 1996;74:991.
11. Chien S, Li S, Shyy YJ: Effects of mechanical forces on signal transduction and gene expression in endothelial cells. *Hypertension* 1998; (1 Pt 2):162.
12. Walker JD, Viberti GC: Pathophysiology of microvascular disease: an overview. In: Pickup J, Williams G, eds. *Textbook of Diabetes*, Vol. 2. Blackwell Scientific:1991;526.
13. Brownlee M: Advanced products of nonenzymatic glycosylation and the pathogenesis of diabetic complications. In: Rifkin H, Porte D Jr, eds. *Diabetes Mellitus, Theory and Practice.* Elsevier:1990;279.
14. Hammes HP, Federoff HJ, Brownlee M: Nerve growth factor prevents both neuroretinal programmed cell death and capillary pathology in experimental diabetes. *Mol Med* 1995;5:527.
15. Mizutani M, Kern TS, Lorenzi M: Accelerated death of retinal microvascular cells in human and experimental diabetic retinopathy. *J Clin Invest* 1996;97:2883.
16. Giannini C, Dyck PJ: Ultrastructural morphometric features of human sural nerve endoneurial microvessels. *J Neuropathol Exp Neurol* 1993;52:361.
17. Giannini C, Dyck PJ: Basement membrane reduplication and pericyte degeneration precede development of diabetic polyneuropathy and are associated with its severity. *Ann Neurol* 1995;37:498.
18. Tomlinson DR, Fernybough P, Diemel LT: Role of neurotrophins in diabetic neuropathy and treatment with nerve growth factors. *Diabetes* 1997;46(Suppl 2):S43.
19. Engerman RL, Kern TS:. Progression of incipient diabetic retinopathy during good glycemic control. *Diabetes* 1987;36:808.
20. Roy S, Sala R, Cagliero E, et al: Overexpression of fibronectin induced by diabetes or high glucose phenomenon with a memory. *Proc Natl Acad Sci USA* 1990;87:404.
21. The Diabetes Control and Complications Trial Research Group: The effect of intensive treatment of diabetes on the development and progression of long-term complications in insulin-dependent diabetes mellitus. *N Engl J Med* 1993;329:977.
22. The Diabetes Control and Complications Research Group: Effect of intensive therapy on the development and progression of diabetic nephropathy in the Diabetes Control and Complications Trial. *Kidney Int* 1995;47:1703.
23. The Diabetes Control and Complications Research Group: The effect of intensive diabetes therapy on the development and progression of neuropathy. *Ann Intern Med* 1995;122:561.
24. The Diabetes Control and Complications Trial/Epidemiology of Diabetes Interventions and Complications Research Group: Retinopathy and nephropathy in patients with type 1 diabetes four years after a trial of intensive therapy. *N Engl J Med* 2000;342:381.
25. Krolewski AS, Warren JH, Freire MB: Epidemiology of late diabetic complications: A basis for the development and evaluation of preventive programs. In: Brownlee MB, King GL, eds. *Endocrinol Metab Clin North Am.* Saunders:1996.

26. Seaquist ER, Goetz FC, Rich S, *et al*: Familial clustering of diabetic kidney disease. Evidence for genetic susceptibility to diabetic nephropathy. *N Engl J Med* 1989;320:1161.

27. Quinn M, Angelico MC, Warram JH, *et al*: Familial factors determine the development of diabetic nephropathy in patients with IDDM. *Diabetologia* 1996;39:940.

28. The Diabetes Control and Complications Trial Research Group: Clustering of long-term complications in families with diabetes in the Diabetes Control and Complications Trial. *Diabetes* 1997;46:1829.

29. Raffel LJ, Vadheim CM, Roth MP, *et al*: The 5′ insulin gene polymorphism and the genetics of vascular complications in type 1 (insulin-dependent) diabetes mellitus. *Diabetologia* 1991;34:680.

30. Stewart LL, Field LL, Ross S, *et al*: Genetic risk factors in diabetic retinopathy. *Diabetologia* 1993;36:1293.

31. Marre M, Bernadet P, Gallois Y, *et al*: Relationships between angiotensin I converting enzyme gene polymorphism, plasma levels, and diabetic retinal and renal complications. *Diabetes* 1994;43:384.

32. Marre M, Jeunemaitre X, Gallois Y, *et al*: Contribution of genetic polymorphism in the renin-angiotensin system to the development of renal complications in insulin-dependent diabetes: Genetique de la Nephropathie Diabetique (GENEDIAB) study group. *J Clin Invest* 1997;99:1585.

33. Agardh D, Gaur LK, Agardh E, *et al*: LADQB1*0201/0302 is associated with severe retinopathy in patients with IDDM. *Diabetologia* 1996;39:1313.

34. Oates PJ, Mylari BL: Aldose reductase inhibitors: therapeutic implications for diabetic complications. *Exp Opin Invest Drugs* 1999;8:1.

35. Warpeha KM, Xu W, Liu L, *et al*: Genotyping and functional analysis of a polymorphic (CCTTT)(n) repeat of NOS2A in diabetic retinopathy. *FASEB J* 1999;13:1825.

36. Xia P, Kramer RM, King GL: Identification of the mechanism for the inhibition of Na,K-adenosine triphosphatase by hyperglycemia involving activation of protein kinase C and cytosolic phospholipase A2. *J Clin Invest* 1995;96:733.

37. Williamson JR, Chang K, Frangos M, *et al*: Hyperglycemic pseudohypoxia and diabetic complications. *Diabetes* 1993;42:801.

38. Nishikawa T, Edelstein D, Du XL, *et al*: Normalizing mitochondrial superoxide production blocks three pathways of hyperglycemic damage. Nature 2000;404:787.

39. Marano CW, Szwergold BS, Keppler F, *et al*: Human retinal pigment epithelial cells cultured in hyperglycemic media accumulate increased amounts of glycosaminoglycan precursors. *Invest Ophthalmol Vis Sci* 1992;33:2619.

40. Beyer-Mears A, Diecke FP, Mistry K, *et al*: Effect of pyruvate lens myo-inositol transport and polyol formation in diabetic cataract. *Pharmacology* 1997;55:78.

41. Knight RJ, Koefoed KF, Schelbert HR, *et al*: Inhibition of glyceraldehyde-3-phosphate dehydrogenase in post-ischaemic myocardium. *Cardiovasc Res* 1996;32:1016.

42. Lee AY, Chung SS: Contributions of polyol pathway to oxidative stress in diabetic cataract. *FASEB J* 1999;13:23.

43. Zhang Z, Apse K, Pang J, *et al*: High glucose decreases glucose 6 phosphate dehydrogenase (G6PD) activity and impairs G6PD response to oxidative stress, thus predisposing cells to cell death in cultured bovine aortic endothelial cells. *Diabetes* 1999;48(Suppl 1):A127.

44. Hammes H-P, Martin S, Federlin K, *et al*: Aminoguanidine treatment inhibits the development of experimental diabetic retinopathy. *Proc Natl Acad Sci USA* 1991;88:11555.

45. Stitt AW, Moore JE, Sharkey JA, *et al*: Advanced glycation end products in vitreous: Structural and functional implications for diabetic vitreopathy. *Invest Ophthalmol Vis Sci* 1998;39:2517.

46. Stitt AW, Li YM, Gardiner TA, *et al*: Advanced glycation end products (AGEs) co-localize with AGE receptors in the retinal vasculature of diabetic and of AGE-infused rats. *Am J Pathol* 1997;150:523.

47. Nishino T, Horri Y, Shikki H, *et al*: Immunohistochemical detection of advanced glycosylation end products within the vascular lesions and glomeruli in diabetic nephropathy. *Hum Pathol* 1995;26:308.

48. Horie K, Miyata T, Maeda K, *et al*: Immunohistochemical colocalization of glycoxidation products and lipid peroxidation products in diabetic renal glomerular lesions. Implication for glycoxidative stress in the pathogenesis of diabetic nephropathy. *J Clin Invest* 1997;100:2995.

49. Niwa T, Katsuzaki T, Miyazaki S, *et al*: Immunohistochemical detection of imidazolone, a novel advanced glycation end product, in kidneys and aortas of diabetic patients. *J Clin Invest* 1997;99:1272.

50. Degenhardt TP, Thorpe SR, Baynes JW: Chemical modification of proteins by methylglyoxal. *Cell Mol Biol* 1998;44:1139.

51. Wells-Knecht KJ, Zyzak DV, Litchfield JE, *et al*: Mechanism of autoxidative glycosylation: identification of glyoxal and arabinose as intermediates in the autoxidative modification of proteins by glucose. *Biochemistry* 1995;34:3702.

52. Thornalley PJ: The glyoxalase system: new developments towards functional characterization of a metabolic pathway fundamental to biological life. *Biochem J* 1990;269:1.

53. Takahashi M, Fujii J, Teshima T, *et al*: Identity of a major 3-deoxyglucosone reducing enzyme with aldehyde reductase in rat liver established by amino acid sequencing and cDNA expression. *Gene* 1993;127:249.

54. Suzuki K, Koh YH, Mizuno H, *et al*: Overexpression of aldehyde reductase protects PC12 cells from the cytotoxicity of methylglyoxal or 3-deoxyglucosone. *J Biochem* 1998;123:353.

55. Chang EY, Szallasi Z, Acs P, *et al*: Functional effects of overexpression of protein kinase C-alpha, -beta, -delta, -epsilon, and -eta in the mast cell line RBL-2H3. *J Immunol* 1997;1159:2624.

56. Giardino I, Edelstein D, Brownlee M: Nonenzymatic glycosylation *in vitro* and in bovine endothelial cells alters basic fibroblast growth factor activity. A model for intracellular glycosylation in diabetes. *J Clin Invest* 1994;94:110.

57. Shinohara M, Thornalley PJ, Giardino I, *et al*: Overexpression of glyoxalase-I in bovine endothelial cells inhibits intracellular advanced glycation endproduct formation and prevents hyperglycemia-induced increases in macromolecular endocytosis. *J Clin Invest* 1998;101:1142.

58. Maisonpierre PC, Suri C, Jones PF, *et al*: Angiopoietin-2, a natural antagonist for Tie2 that disrupts *in vivo* angiogenesis. *Science* 1997;277:55.

59. Papapetropoulos A, Garcia-Cardena G, Dengler TJ, *et al*: Direct actions of angiopoietin-1 on human endothelium: evidence for network stabilization, cell survival, and interaction with other angiogenic growth factors. *Lab Invest* 1999;79:213.

60. Hanahan D: Signaling vascular morphogenesis and maintenance. *Science* 1997;277:48.

61. Elgawish A, Glomb M, Friedlander M, *et al*: Involvement of hydrogen peroxide in collagen cross-linking by high glucose *in vitro* and *in vivo*. *J Biol Chem* 1996;271:12964.

62. Brownlee M, Vlassara H, Kooney T, *et al*: Aminoguanidine prevents diabetes-induced arterial wall protein cross-linking. *Science* 1986;232:1629.

63. Tanaka S, Avigad G, Brodsky B, *et al*: Glycation induces expansion of the molecular packing of collagen. *J Mol Biol* 1988;203:495.

64. Huijberts MSP, Wolffenbuttel BRH, Struijker Boudier HAJ, *et al*: Aminoguanidine treatment increases elasticity and decreases fluid filtration of large arteries from diabetic rats. *J Clin Invest* 1993;92:1407.

65. Tsilbary EC, Charonis AS, Reger LA, *et al*: The effect of nonenzymatic glucosylation the binding of the main noncollagenous NC1 domain to Type 1V collagen. *J Biol Chem* 1990;263:4302.

66. Charonis AS, Reger LA, Dege JE, *et al*: Laminin alterations after *in vitro* nonenzymatic glucosylation. *Diabetes* 1988;39:807.

67. Cochrane SM, Robinson GB: *In vitro* glycation of a glomerular basement membrane alters its permeability: a possible mechanism in diabetic complications. *FEBS Lett* 1995;375:41.

68. Boyd-White J, Williams JC Jr: Effect of cross-linking on matrix permeability. A model for AGE-modified basement membranes. *Diabetes* 1996;45:348.

69. Haitoglou CS, Tsilibary EC, Brownlee M, *et al*: Altered cellular interactions between endothelial cells and nonenzymatically glucosylated laminin/Type 1V collagen. *J Biol Chem* 1992;267:12404.

70. Federoff HJ, Lawrence D, Brownlee M: Nonenzymatic glycosylation of laminin and the laminin peptide CIKVAVS inhibits neurite outgrowth. *Diabetes* 1993;42:509.

71. Hammes HP, Weiss A, Hess S, *et al*: Modification of vitronectin by advanced glycation 325 alters functional properties *in vitro* and in the diabetic retina. *Lab Invest* 1996;75:325.

72. Li YM, Mitsuhashi T, Wojciechowicz D, *et al*: Molecular identity and cellular distribution of advanced glycation endproduct receptors: relationship of p60 to OST-48 and p90 to 80K-H membrane proteins. *Proc Natl Acad Sci USA* 1996;93:11047.

73. Yang Z, Makita Z, Horii Y, *et al*: Two novel rat liver membrane proteins that bind advanced glycosylation endproducts: Relationship to

macrophage receptor for glucose-modified proteins. *J Exp Med* 1991; 174:515.

74. Vlassara H, Brownlee M, Monogue K, *et al*: Cachectin/TNF and IL-1 induced by glucose-modified proteins: Role in normal tissue remodeling. *Science* 1988;240:1546.

75. Kirstein M, Aston C, Hintz R, *et al*: Receptor-specific induction of insulin-like growth factor I in human monocytes by advanced glycosylation end product-modified proteins. *J Clin Invest* 1992;90:439.

76. Yui S, Sasaki T, Araki N, *et al*: Induction of macrophage growth by advanced glycation end products of the Maillard reaction. *J Immunol* 1994;152:1943.

77. Higashi T, Sano H, Saishoji T, *et al*: The receptor for advanced glycation end products mediates the chemotaxis of rabbit smooth muscle cells. *Diabetes* 1997;46:463.

78. Westwood ME, Thornalley PJ: Induction of synthesis and secretion of interleukin 1 beta in the human monocytic THP-1 cells by human serum albumins modified with methylglyoxal and advanced glycation endproducts. *Immunol Lett* 1996;50:17.

79. Abordo EA, Westwood ME, Thornalley PJ: Synthesis and secretion of macrophage colony stimulating factor by mature human monocytes and human monocytic THP-1 cells induced by human serum albumin derivatives modified with methylglyoxal and glucose-derived advanced glycation endproducts. *Immunol Lett* 1996;53:7.

80. Abordo EA, Thornalley PJ: Synthesis and secretion of tumour necrosis factor-alpha by human monocytic THP-1 cells and chemotaxis induced by human serum albumin derivatives modified with methylglyoxal and glucose-derived advanced glycation endproducts. *Immunol Lett* 1997;58:139.

81. Webster L, Abordo EA, Thornalley PJ, *et al*: Induction of TNF alpha and IL-beta mRNA in monocytes by methylglyoxal- and advanced glycated endproduct-modified human serum albumin. *Biochem Soc Trans* 1997;25:250S.

82. Pugliese G, Pricci F, Romeo G, *et al*: Upregulation of mesangial growth factor and extracellular matrix synthesis by advanced glycation end products via a receptor-mediated mechanism. *Diabetes* 1997;46:1881.

83. Smedsrod B, Melkko J, Araki N, *et al*: Advanced glycation end products are eliminated by scavenger-receptor-mediated endocytosis in hepatic sinusoidal kupffer and endothelial cells. *Biochem J* 1997;322:567.

84. Horiuchi S, Higashi T, Ikeda K, *et al*: Advanced glycation end products and their recognition by macrophage and macrophage-derived cells. *Diabetes* 1996;45:S73.

85. Sano H, Higashi T, Matsumoto K, *et al*: Insulin enhances macrophage scavenger receptor-mediated endocytic uptake of advanced glycation end products. *Biol Chem* 1998;273:8630.

86. Vlassara H, Li YM, Imani F, *et al*: Identification of galectin-3 as a high-affinity binding protein for advanced glycation end products (AGE): a new member of the AGE-receptor complex. *Mol Med* 1995;1:634.

87. Skolnik EY, Yang Z, Makita Z, *et al*: Human and rat mesangial cell receptors for glucose-modified proteins: Potential role in kidney tissue remodeling and diabetic nephropathy. *J Exp Med* 1991;174:931.

88. Doi T, Vlassara H, Kirstein M, *et al*: Receptor specific increase in extracellular matrix productions in mouse mesangial cells by advanced glycosylation end products is mediated via platelet derived growth factor. *Proc Natl Acad Sci USA* 1992;89:2873.

89. Schmidt AM, Vianna M, Gerlach M, *et al*: Isolation and characterization of two binding proteins for advanced glycosylation end products from bovine lung which are present on the endothelial cell surface. *J Biol Chem* 1992;267:14987.

90. Neeper M, Schmidt AM, Brett J, *et al*: Cloning and expression of RAGE: A cell surface receptor for advanced glycosylation end products of proteins. *J Biol Chem* 1992;267:14998.

91. Schmidt AM, Mora R, Cao K, *et al*: The endothelial cell binding site for advanced glycation endproducts consists of A complex: An integral membrane protein and a lactoferrin-like polypeptide. *J Biol Chem* 1994;269:9882.

92. Yan SD, Schmidt AM, Anderson GM, *et al*: Enhanced cellular oxidant stress by the interaction of advanced glycation end products with their receptors/binding proteins. *J Biol Chem* 1994;269:9889.

93. Lander HM, Tauras JM, Ogiste JS, *et al*: Activation of the receptor for advanced glycation end products triggers a p21(ras)-dependent mitogen-activated protein kinase pathway regulated by oxidant stress. *J Biol Chem* 1997;272:17810.

94. Li J, Schmidt AM: Characterization and functional analysis of the promoter of RAGE, the receptor for advanced glycation end products. *J Biol Chem* 1997;272:16498.

95. Yamagishi S, Fujimori H, Yonekura H, *et al*: Advanced glycation endproducts inhibit prostacyclin production and induce plasminogen activator inhibitor-1 in human microvascular endothelial cells. *Diabetologia* 1998;41:1435.

96. Tsuji H, Iehara N, Masegi T, *et al*: Ribozyme targeting of receptor for advanced glycation end products in mouse mesangial cells. *Biochem Biophys Res Commun* 1998;245:583.

97. Vlassara H, Fuh H, Donnelly T, *et al*: Advanced glycation endproducts promote adhesion molecule (VCAM-1, ICAM-1) expression and atheroma formation in normal rabbits. *Mol Med* 1995;1:447.

98. Schmidt AM, Hori O, Chen JX, *et al*: Advanced glycation endproducts interacting with their endothelial receptor induce expression of vascular cell adhesion molecule-1 (VCAM-1) in cultured human endothelial cells and in mice: a potential mechanism for the accelerated vasculopathy of diabetes. *J Clin Invest* 1995;96:1395.

99. Sengoelge G, Fodinger M, Skoupy S, *et al*: Endothelial cell adhesion molecule and PMNL response to inflammatory stimuli and AGE-modified fibronectin. *Kidney Int* 1998;54:1637.

100. Schmidt AM, Crandall J, Hori O, *et al*: Elevated plasma levels of vascular cell adhesion molecule-1 (VCAM-1) in diabetic patients with microalbuminuria: a marker of vascular dysfunction and progressive vascular disease. *Br J Haematol* 1996;92:747.

101. Wautier JL, Zoukourian C, Chappey O, *et al*: Receptor-mediated endothelial cell dysfunction in diabetic vasculopathy: soluble receptor for advanced glycation end products blocks hyperpermeability in diabetic rats. *J Clin Invest* 1996;97:238.

102. Lu M, Kuroki M, Amano S, *et al*: Advanced glycation end products increase retinal vascular endothelial growth factor expression. *J Clin Invest* 1998;101:1219.

103. Hirata C, Nakano K, Nakamura N, *et al*: Advanced glycation end products induce expression of vascular endothelial growth factor by retinal Muller cells. *Biochem Biophys Res Commun* 1997;236:712.

104. Inoguchi T, Battan R, Handler E, *et al*: Preferential elevation of protein kinase C isoform beta II and diacylglycerol levels in the aorta and heart of diabetic rats: Differential reversibility to glycemic control by islet cell transplantation. *Proc Natl Acad Sci USA* 1992;89:11059.

105. Craven PA, Davidson CM, DeRubertis FR: Increase in diacylglycerol mass in isolated glomeruli by glucose from de novo synthesis of glycerolipids. *Diabetes* 1990;39:667.

106. Shiba T, Inoguchi T, Sportsman JR, *et al*: Correlation of diacylglycerol level and protein kinase C activity in rat retina to retinal circulation. *Am J Physiol* 1993;265(5 Pt 1):E783.

107. Inoguchi T, Xia P, Kunisaki M, *et al*: Insulin's effect on protein kinase C and diacylglycerol induced by diabetes and glucose in vascular tissues. *Am J Physiol* 1994;267(3 Pt 1):E369.

108. Derubertis FR, Craven PA: Activation of protein kinase C in glomerular cells in diabetes. Mechanisms and potential links to the pathogenesis of diabetic glomerulopathy. *Diabetes* 1994;43:1.

109. Xia P, Inoguchi T, Kern TS, *et al*: Characterization of the mechanism for the chronic activation of diacylglycerol-protein kinase C pathway in diabetes and hypergalactosemia. *Diabetes* 1994;43:1122.

110. Ayo SH, Radnik R, Garoni JA, *et al*: High glucose increases diacylglycerol mass and activates protein kinase C in mesangial cell cultures. *Am J Physiol* 1991;261(4 Pt 2):F571.

111. Koya D, Jirousek MR, Lin YW, *et al*: Characterization of protein kinase C beta isoform activation on the gene expression of transforming growth factor-beta, extracellular matrix components, and prostanoids in the glomeruli of diabetic rats. *J Clin Invest* 1997;100:115.

112. Kikkawa R, Haneda M, Uzu T, *et al*: Translocation of protein kinase C alpha and zeta in rat glomerular mesangial cells cultured under high glucose conditions. *Diabetologia* 1994;37:838.

113. Ishii H, Jirousek MR, Koya D, *et al*: Amelioration of vascular dysfunctions in diabetic rats by an oral PKC beta inhibitor. *Science* 1996;272:728.

114. Craven PA, Studer RK, DeRubertis FR: Impaired nitric oxide-dependent cyclic guanosine monophosphate generation in glomeruli from diabetic rats. Evidence for protein kinase C-mediated suppression of the cholinergic response. *J Clin Invest* 1994;93:311.

115. Ganz MB, Seftel A: Glucose-induced changes in protein kinase C and nitric oxide are prevented by vitamin E. *Am J Physiol* 2000;278:E146.

116. Kuboki K, Jiang ZY, Takahara N, *et al*: Regulation of endothelial constitutive nitric oxide synthase gene expression in endothelial cells and *in vivo*: a specific vascular action of insulin. *Circulation* 2000;101:676.

117. Glogowski EA, Tsiani E, Zhou X, et al: High glucose alters the response of mesangial cell protein kinase C isoforms to endothelin-1. *Kidney Int* 1999;55:486.

118. Hempel A, Maasch C, Heintze U, et al: High glucose concentrations increase endothelial cell permeability via activation of protein kinase C alpha. *Circ Res* 1997;81:363.

119. Williams B, Gallacher B, Patel H, et al: Glucose-induced protein kinase C activation regulates vascular permeability factor mRNA expression and peptide production by human vascular smooth muscle cells *in vitro*. *Diabetes* 1997;46:1497.

120. Studer RK, Craven PA, DeRubertis FR: Role for protein kinase C in the mediation of increased fibronectin accumulation by mesangial cells grown in high-glucose medium. *Diabetes* 1993;42:118.

121. Pugliese G, Pricci F, Pugliese F, et al: Mechanisms of glucose-enhanced extracellular matrix accumulation in rat glomerular mesangial cells. *Diabetes* 1994;43:478.

122. Koya D, Jirousek MR, Lin YW, et al: Characterization of protein kinase C beta isoform activation on the gene expression of transforming growth factor-beta, extracellular matrix components, and prostanoids in the glomeruli of diabetic rats. *J Clin Invest* 1997;100:115.

123. Craven PA, Studer RK, Felder J, et al: Nitric oxide inhibition of transforming growth factor-beta and collagen synthesis in mesangial cells. *Diabetes* 1997;46:671.

124. Phillips SL, DeRubertis FR, Craven PA: Regulation of the laminin C1 promoter in cultured mesangial cells. *Diabetes* 1999;48:2083.

125. Feener EP, Xia P, Inoguchi T, et al: Role of protein kinase C in glucose- and angiotensin II-induced plasminogen activator inhibitor expression. *Contrib Nephrol* 1996;118:180.

126. Pieper GM, Riaz-ul-Haq J: Activation of nuclear factor-kappaB in cultured endothelial cells by increased glucose concentration: prevention by calphostin C. *Cardiovasc Pharmacol* 1997;30:528.

127. Yerneni KK, Bai W, Khan BV, et al: Hyperglycemia-induced activation of nuclear transcription factor kappaB in vascular smooth muscle cells. *Diabetes* 1999;48:855.

128. Sayeski PP, Kudlow JE: Glucose metabolism to glucosamine is necessary for glucose stimulation of transforming growth factor-alpha gene transcription. *J Biol Chem* 1996;271:15237.

129. Kolm-Litty V, Sauer U, Nerlich A, et al: High glucose-induced transforming growth factor beta1 production is mediated by the hexosamine pathway in porcine glomerular mesangial cells. *J Clin Invest* 1998;101:160.

130. Marshall S, Bacote V, Traxinger RR: Discovery of a metabolic pathway mediating glucose-induced desensitization of the glucose transport system. Role of hexosamine biosynthesis in the induction of insulin resistance. *J Biol Chem* 1991;266:4706.

131. Rossetti L, Hawkins M, Chen W, et al: In vivo glucosamine infusion induces insulin resistance in normoglycemic but not in hyperglycemic conscious rats. *J Clin Invest* 1995;96:132.

132. Hawkins M, Barzilai N, Liu R, et al: Role of the glucosamine pathway in fat-induced insulin resistance. *J Clin Invest* 1997;99:2173.

133. Chen YQ, Su M, Walia RR, et al: Sp1 sites mediate activation of the plasminogen activator inhibitor-1 promoter by glucose in vascular smooth muscle cells. *J Biol Chem* 1998;273:8225.

134. Hart GW: Dynamic O-linked glycosylation of nuclear and cytoskeletal proteins *Annu Rev Biochem* 1997;66:315.

135. Kadonaga JT, Courey AJ, Ladika J, et al: Distinct regions of Sp1 modulate DNA binding and transcriptional activation. *Science* 1988;242:1566.

136. Haltiwanger RS, Grove K, Philipsberg GA: Modulation of O-linked N-acetylglucosamine levels on nuclear and cytoplasmic proteins *in vivo* using the peptide O-GlcNAc-beta-N-acetylglucosaminidase inhibitor O-(2-acetamido-2-deoxy-D-glucopyranosylidene)amino-N-phenylcarbamate. *J Biol Chem* 1998;273:3611.

137. Daniel S, Kim KH: Sp1 mediates glucose activation of the acetyl-CoA carboxylase promoter. *J Biol Chem* 1996;271:1385.

138. Daniel S, Zhang S, DePaoli-Roach AA, et al: Dephosphorylation of Sp1 by protein phosphatase 1 is involved in the glucose-mediated activation of the acetyl-CoA carboxylase gene. *J Biol Chem* 1996;271:14692.

139. Engerman RL, Kern TS, Larson ME: Nerve conduction and aldose reductase inhibition during 5 years of diabetes or galactosaemia in dogs. *Diabetologia* 1994;37:141.

140. Sima AA, Prashar A, Zhang WX, et al: Preventive effect of long-term aldose reductase inhibition (ponalrestat) on nerve conduction and sural nerve structure in the spontaneously diabetic Bio-Breeding rat. *J Clin Invest* 1990;85:1410.

141. Lee AY, Chung SK, Chung SS: Demonstration that polyol accumulation is responsible for diabetic cataract by the use of transgenic mice expressing the aldose reductase gene in the lens. *Proc Natl Acad Sci USA* 1995;92:2780.

142. Brownlee M: Advanced protein glycosylation in diabetes and aging. *Annu Rev Med* 1995;46:223.

143. Du X, Edelstein D, Rossetti L, Fantus IG, Goldberg H, Ziyadeh F, Wu J and Brownlee M. (2000). Hyperglycemia-induced mitochondrial superoxide overproduction activates the hexosamine pathway and induces plasminogen activator inhibitor-1 expression by increasing Sp1 glycosylation. *Proc Natl Acad* Sci USA 97:12222-12226.

144. Giardino I, Edelstein D, Brownlee M: BCL-2 expression or antioxidants prevent hyperglycemia-induced formation of intracellular advanced glycation endproducts in bovine endothelial cells. *J Clin Invest* 1996;97:1422.

145. Wallace DC: Diseases of the mitochondrial DNA. *Annu Rev Biochem* 1992;61:1175.

146. Trumpower BL: The proton motive Q cycle. *J Biol Chem* 1990;265:11409.

147. Korshunov SS, Skulachev VP, Starkov AA: High protonic potential actuates a mechanism of production of reactive oxygen species in mitochondria. *FEBS Lett* 1997;416:15.

148. Casteilla L, Blnodel O, Klaus S, et al: Stable expression of functional mitochondrial uncoupling protein in Chinese hamster ovary cells. *Proc Natl Acad Sci USA* 1990;87:5124.

149. Manna SK, Zhang HJ, Yan T, et al: Overexpression manganese superoxide dismutase suppresses tumor necrosis factor-induced apoptosis and activation of nuclear transcription factor-κB and activated protein-1. *J Biol Chem* 1998;273:13245.

150. Chandra A, Srivastava S, Petrash JM, et al: Active site modification of aldose reductase by nitric oxide donors. *Biochim Biophys Acta* 1997;1341:217.

151. Pieper GM, Langenstroer P, Siebeneich W: Diabetic-induced endothelial dysfunction in rat aorta: role of hydroxyl radicals. *Cardiovasc Res* 1997;34:145.

152. Koya D, King GL: Protein kinase C activation and the development of diabetic complications. *Diabetes* 1998;47:859.

153. Ido Y, McHowat J, Chang KC, et al: Neural dysfunction and metabolic imbalances in diabetic rats. Prevention by acetyl-L-carnitine. *Diabetes* 1994;43:1469.

154. Wallace DC: Diseases of the mitochondrial DNA. *Annu Rev Biochem* 1992;61:1175.

155. Johns DR: The other human genome: mitochondrial DNA and disease. *Nat Med* 1996;2:1065.

156. Yakes FM, Van Houten B: Mitochondrial DNA damage is more extensive and persists longer than nuclear DNA damage in human cells following oxidative stress. *Proc Natl Acad Sci USA* 1997;94:514.

157. Richter C: Reactive oxygen and DNA damage in mitochondria. *Mutat Res* 1992;275:249.

158. Wei YH: Oxidative stress and mitochondrial DNA mutations in human aging. *Proc Soc Exp Biol Med* 1998;217:53.

159. Judzewitsch RG, Jaspan JB, Polonsky KS, et al: Aldose reductase inhibition improves nerve conduction velocity in diabetic patients. *N Engl J Med* 1983;308:119.

160. Greene DA, Arezzo JC, Brown MB: Effect of aldose reductase inhibition on nerve conduction and morphometry in diabetic neuropathy. Zenarestat Study Group. *Neurology* 1999;53:580.

161. Engerman RL, Kem TS, Garment MB: Capillary basement membrane in retina, kidney and muscle of diabetic dogs and galactosemic dogs and its response to 5 years aldose reductase inhibition. *J Diabetes Complications* 1993;7:241.

162. Sorbinil Retinopathy Trial Research Group: A randomized trial of sorbinil, an aldose reductase inhibitor, in diabetic retinopathy. *Arch Ophthalmol* 1990;108:1234.

163. Edelstein D, Brownlee M: Aminoguanidine ameliorates albuminuria in diabetic hypertensive rats. *Diabetologia* 1992;35:96.

164. Ellis EN, Good BH: Prevention of glomerular basement membrane thickening by aminoguanidine in experimental diabetes mellitus. *Metabolism* 1991;40:1016.

165. Soulis-Liparota T, Cooper M, Papazoglou D: et al: Retardation by aminoguanidine of development of albuminuria, mesangial expansion, and tissue fluorescence in streptozocin-induced diabetic rat. *Diabetes* 1991;40:1328.

166. Nakamura S, Makita Z, Ishikawa S, *et al*: Progression of nephropathy in spontaneous diabetic rats is prevented by OPB-9195, a novel inhibitor of advanced glycation. *Diabetes* 1997;46:895.

167. Tsuchida K, Makita Z, Yamagishi S, *et al*: Suppression of transforming growth factor beta and vascular endothelial growth factor in diabetic nephropathy in rats by a novel advanced glycation end product inhibitor, OPB-9195. *Diabetologia* 1999;42:579.

168. Cameron NE, Cotter MA, Dines K, *et al*: Effects of aminoguanidine on peripheral nerve function and polyol pathway metabolites in streptozotocin-diabetic rats. *Diabetologia* 1992;35:946.

169. Kihara M, Schmelzer JD, Poduslo JF, *et al*: Aminoguanidine effects on nerve blood flow, vascular permeability, electrophysiology, and oxygen free radicals. *Proc Natl Acad Sci USA* 1991;88:6107.

170. Appel G, Bolton K, Freedman B, *et al*: Pimagedine (PG) lowers total urinary protein (TUP) and slows progression of overt diabetic nephropathy in patients with type 1 diabetes mellitus (DM). *J Am Soc Nephrol* 1999;10:153.

171. Raskin P, Cattran D, Williams M, *et al*: Pimagedine (PG) reduces progression of retinopathy and lowers lipid levels in patients with type 1 diabetes mellitus (DM). *J Am Soc Nephrol* 1999;10:179.

172. Koya D, Haneda M, Nakagawa H, *et al*: Amelioration of accelerated diabetic mesangial expansion by treatment with a PKC beta inhibitor in diabetic db/db mice, a rodent model for type 2 diabetes. *FASEB J* 2000;14:439.

173. Faulkner KM, Liochev SI, Fridovich J: Stable MN(III) porphyrins mimic superoxide dismutase in vitro and substitute for it in vivo. *J Biol Chem* 1994;269:23471.

174. Doctrow SR, Huffman K, Marcus CB, *et al*: Salen-manganese complexes: combined superoxide dismutase/catalase mimics with broad pharmacological efficacy. *Adv Pharmacol* 1997;38:247.

175. Brownlee M: Mechanisms of hyperglycemic damage in diabetes. In: Kahn CR, ed. *Atlas of Clinical Endocrinology*. Blackwell Science: 1999.

176. Brownlee M: Lilly Lecture 1993. Glycation and diabetic complications. *Diabetes* 1994;43:836.

177. Boss O, Hagen T, Lowell BB: Uncoupling proteins 2 and 3. Potential regulators of mitochondrial energy metabolism. *Diabetes* 2000; 49:143.

Molecular Mechanisms and Genetic Engineering of Insulin-Secreting Cells

Hindrik Mulder

Christopher B. Newgard

In the history of diabetes research, major breakthroughs in understanding of the molecular mechanisms underlying the two predominant forms of the disease have been rare, contributing to the slow development of new therapies. For example, the treatment for type 1 diabetes mellitus (T1DM) is much the same today as it was at the time of the discovery of insulin by Banting and Best in 1922. We also do not yet understand in detail the mechanism by which insulin-containing islet β cells are specifically destroyed by the immune system in T1DM, the mechanisms underlying development of β-cell dysfunction in the majority of patients with type 2 diabetes mellitus (T2DM), or the molecular and biochemical defects that cause insulin resistance.

The tools of molecular biology have been applied to diabetes research with increasing frequency and effectiveness over the past decade. In a preceding edition of this book, we wrote about the various gene transfer methods to help in understanding the mechanics of diabetes, both at the levels of insulin action and insulin secretion.[1] In the ensuing period, tremendous progress has been made, such that it is no longer possible to provide a complete overview of the entire field in a single chapter. For the current volume, we have therefore chosen to focus on new insights gained into the biology of the pancreatic islet β cell via genetic engineering and gene transfer experiments, paying particular attention to mechanisms of fuel-stimulated insulin secretion. We will begin with a brief general overview of gene transfer methods that are applicable to the study of islet β cells, and will close the chapter by discussing the potential use of genetically engineered cells for insulin replacement in diabetes.

OVERVIEW OF GENE TRANSFER METHODS

Strategies for introduction of foreign DNA into animal cells have evolved rapidly in the past two decades, such that today's scientist is confronted with a sometimes bewildering array of options. In our discussion of the application of gene transfer methods to β-cell research, three general approaches will be highlighted. The first is the use of physical or chemical methods to achieve alterations in the properties of cell membranes or of the DNA molecules to be transferred that allow DNA to penetrate an otherwise impermeable barrier. Examples of physicochemical transfection strategies include

(1) Ca_2PO_4 or DEAE-dextran-mediated transfer, in which these carriers form a complex with the DNA that results in efficient endocytosis and deposition of the DNA in the nucleus; (2) electroporation, or the application of brief high-voltage electric pulses to cells to create transient pores in the cell membrane that allow entry of DNA; and (3) lipid-mediated transfection in which liposomes or cationic lipids are mixed with DNA and assist in entry of DNA into the cell by fusion of the lipid complex with the cell membrane. In the field of islet β-cell biology, physical gene transfer methods have been used for transient transfection studies of isolated islets or β-cell lines. Since the efficiency of these methods is generally low, they have been used mainly for evaluation of promoter function, which requires introduction of genetic material into only a small subset of cells in a population. However, physical gene transfer methods can also be used for stable transfection, provided that the DNA to be transferred includes a selectable marker and the cell type under study is capable of sustained growth. By using vectors that contain different antibiotic resistance markers, or by use of single vectors containing multiple genes, it is possible to express multiple transgenes in a given cell. Stable transfection has become an important tool for working with β-cell lines, leading in several instances to creation of new lines with enhanced properties, as described later in this chapter.

The second strategy that will be considered is the creation of transgenic animals. This approach involves microinjection of DNA into the fertilized eggs of animals, usually mice, resulting in integration into the germline DNA. Once integrated, the new gene is replicated along with the chromosomal DNA, allowing for the dissemination of new genetic information in tissues of intact animals. More recently, a variant of this method has emerged, in which embryonic stem cells are transfected with DNA homologous to a chromosomal gene. The transfected DNA integrates into the genome by homologous recombination. This approach can be used for disrupting the chromosomal gene in cases in which the transfected DNA contains an insertion or mutation, or can be used to introduce a variant functional sequence. These methods for genetic manipulation represent powerful tools for modulating the expression of particular genes and assessing impact at the level of whole-organ function and whole-animal fuel homeostasis. In recent years, many examples of specific targeting of transgenes to the pancreatic islet β cell via constructs in which the insulin promoter is used to direct gene expression have come to the fore, and several of these will be highlighted below.

The last approach to be discussed is the use of viral vectors. It has been appreciated for some time that viruses exist by virtue of their capacity to transfer genetic information into host cells. With the advent of recombinant DNA technology, this property of viruses has been exploited in the creation of a wide variety of gene transfer vectors. Much effort has been focused on vectors derived from retroviruses, particularly murine leukemia virus (MuLV), and a variety of packaging systems for propagation of recombinant retroviruses have been developed.[2,3] RNA viruses are generally capable of reverse transcribing their genome to proviral DNA, which must be integrated into genomic DNA of mammalian cells in order to be expressed. This feature of retroviruses ensures permanent transfer of genetic information to target cells, but only under conditions in which cells are able to grow, since integration of the viral genome requires the presence of cellular factors that are only present during periods of DNA replication.[3] Because pancreatic islets do not replicate efficiently *in vitro*, the MuLV class of retroviruses has had very limited application for gene transfer studies in β cells, except in cases in which islet growth is stimulated by culture in the presence of specific cell matrix components or growth factors.[4]

More recently, exciting new vector systems based on lentiviruses, an alternate class of retroviruses that includes human immunodeficiency virus (HIV), have been developed.[5] Of particular importance is the fact that lentiviruses express two genes (*MA* and *Vpr*) that facilitate transport of viral DNA into the nucleus of nondividing cells, allowing viral integration in the absence of cell proliferation. A three-plasmid system for preparing recombinant lentiviruses has been developed, consisting of a modified HIV provirus packaging construct that contains defective genes for envelope proteins, a separate plasmid containing genes encoding MLV or VSV G envelope proteins, and a third plasmid known as a transducing vector that contains *cis*-acting sequences of HIV required for packaging, reverse transcription, and integration, as well as a cloning cassette for insertion of foreign genes.[5] These vectors hold promise for stable gene transfer into cultured cells with low replicative activity, and several reports of lentivirus-mediated gene transfer to cultured pancreatic islets have appeared recently.[6,7] While the use of the three-plasmid system and simian rather than human immunodeficiency virus sequences reduces concerns about safety with these vectors, there is still the potential for generation of replication-competent viruses via recombination with wild-type HIV. Recently, safer vectors have been described, in which just 22% of the HIV genome is included, involving none of the pathogenic sequences.[8,9]

Given the limitations of RNA virus vectors, increasing attention has been paid to DNA viruses for gene transfer studies, in particular herpes simplex virus (HSV), adeno-associated virus (AAV), and adenovirus. HSV has a very large genome, and can accommodate more than 20 kb of insert DNA. However, this vector is largely used for gene transfer to cells of the nervous system, since natural infection by HSV involves invasion of neurons or sensory ganglia and establishment of a state of latency in those cell types.[10]

Recombinant adenovirus has a number of attractive features for metabolic applications. So-called first-generation adenovirus vectors are usually derived from human serotypes 2 or 5, and contain deletions in the E1A region, which controls expression of other early viral genes and is required for viral replication.[11,12] Deletion of just the E1A region allows insert sizes of up to 4.8 kb, but larger inserts can be accommodated by deletion of the nonessential *E3* gene. Adenoviruses can be used to transduce a wide range of mammalian cells, including liver cells, islets of Langerhans, muscle cells, and cells of the central nervous system, independent of cell growth or replication. They can also be grown at remarkably high titers (in excess of 10^{12} plaque-forming units/mL) with minimal effort. Adenoviral vectors are the most efficient of all the viral vectors, with near 100% gene transfer commonly observed in cultured cells. Such high efficiency of gene transfer has been documented for several β-cell lines.[13,14] Furthermore, as shown in Fig. 14-1, exposure of isolated rat islets to recombinant adenoviruses for short time periods (1–2 hours) allows transfer of genes to between 70% and 80% of islet cells.[15] Importantly, insulin secretion is not affected by treatment of islets or insulin-secreting cell lines with recombinant adenoviruses containing irrelevant control genes (e.g., β-galactosidase). Finally, first generation recombinant adenoviruses are easily constructed, and new recombinant viruses can usually be produced in a time frame of 3–6 weeks. Readers interested in detailed methods for preparing first generation adenovirus vectors are referred to reference 16.

While recombinant adenovirus is clearly an excellent tool for high efficiency gene delivery to isolated islets and β-cell lines, it is not useful for gene transfer to islets in living animals. Systemic infusion of adenoviral vectors results in highly efficient and preferential gene transfer to liver.[17–21] The preferential targeting of adenovirus-transferred genes to liver is probably explained by the sinusoidal vasculature of that organ, which allows direct contact of viral particles with hepatocytes, whereas transfer is limited in other tissues by vascular barriers. The pancreatic islets are perifused by an intense network of arterioles and venules, which contain small pores or fenestrations with a diameter of approximately 40 nm.[22] Unfortunately, the adenovirus particle has a diameter of approximately 100 nm, making it too large to pass through the pores of the islet vasculature, even when animals are treated with dilating agents such as mannitol or histamine.[23]

One potential alternative to adenovirus for *in vivo* delivery of genes to pancreatic islets is AAV, which is about one-tenth as large as adenovirus. AAV is also intriguing because it is known to integrate effectively into genomic DNA.[24] Unfortunately, AAV vectors that are currently available are limited to DNA inserts of 4.8 kb or less in size.[25] Furthermore, growth of AAV requires the presence of wild-type adenovirus (which must subsequently be removed from the viral preparation) or the use of packaging cell lines. This means that obtaining AAV stocks of high titer is both laborious and difficult. For all of these reasons, application of AAV to metabolic research in general and islet biology in particular has thus far been limited.

While lentiviral and adenoviral vectors are superb new tools for high efficiency gene delivery to isolated islets and β-cell lines, the only method available today for delivery of genes to the islets of intact animals is microinjection of constructs into fertilized eggs, primarily of mice. Thus an important goal for the field is the continued development of modified adenoviral, lentiviral, and AAV vectors, or other nonviral methods of gene transfer such as peptide/DNA conjugate approaches, for delivery of genes to the pancreatic islets *in vivo*. Development of such methods will be highly useful for studies of islet function in animal models other than mice, including disease models such as the Zucker diabetic fatty (ZDF) rat. The small size of the AAV viral particle relative to either HSV or adenovirus makes this vector potentially attractive for gene delivery to the pancreatic islets of Langerhans *in vivo*, and further work on this system is certainly warranted. Encouragement in this

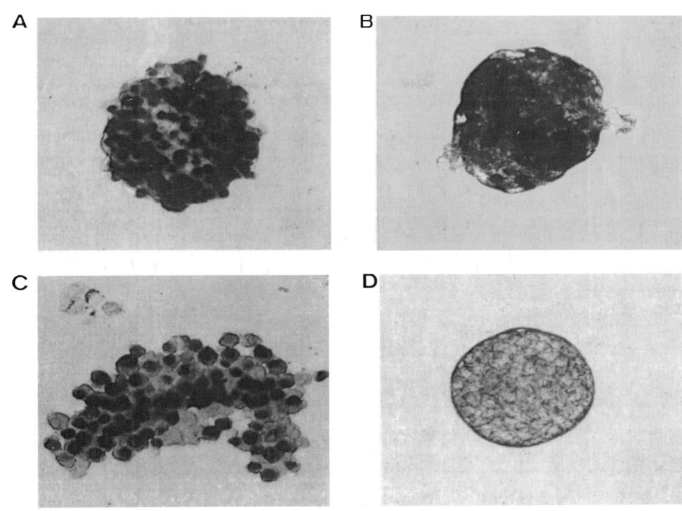

FIGURE 14-1. Recombinant adenovirus is an efficient tool for gene transfer into cultured rat islets of Langerhans. **A**. Rat islet 4 days after treatment with a recombinant adenovirus encoding the β-galactosidase gene (AdCMV-βGAL) and treatment with chromogenic substrate to visualize cells expressing the enzyme. **B**. A similarly treated islet 21 days after AdCMV-βGAL treatment. **C**. Multicell aggregate prepared by trypsin-mediated dispersal of intact AdCMV-βGAL–treated islets to allow quantification of gene transfer efficiency (estimated at 70% of cells in this study). **D**. Control islet not exposed to AdCMV-βGAL and incubated with chromogenic substrate. *(Data are used, with permission, from Becker, et al.[15])*

area comes from a recent article demonstrating efficient AAV-mediated gene transfer to cultured murine islets.[26]

INSIGHTS INTO MECHANISMS OF FUEL-STIMULATED INSULIN SECRETION GAINED FROM GENE TRANSFER STUDIES

General Mechanisms of Fuel-Stimulated Insulin Secretion

Pancreatic islet β cells secrete insulin in response to monomeric fuels such as glucose or fatty acids rather than large polymeric macromolecules such as glycogen or triglycerides. Important nutrient fuels include monosaccharides such as glucose; several L-amino acids such as glutamine, alanine, or leucine; long-chain fatty acids such as palmitate or oleate; or ketone bodies such as β-hydroxybutyrate or acetoacetate.

There is strong evidence in support of the view that nutrient stimulation of insulin secretion requires catabolism of the fuel in question. This is in contrast to the classical mechanism of signal transduction involving recognition of the structure of a stimulant or ligand by a specific receptor, and interaction of the occupied receptor with other molecules to produce second messengers. In the islet β cell, intermediary metabolism integrates the input from multiple fuel molecules to generate specific intermediates known as coupling factors, that link fuel metabolism with hormone secretion. These metabolic signaling systems can interact with classical ligand/receptor pathways. For example, glucose-stimulated insulin secretion is potentiated by glucagon-like peptide-1, which binds to a receptor related to the glucagon receptor, and by neurotransmitters such as acetylcholine, which transduce their signals via muscarinic receptors.[27] Interestingly, these receptor-mediated signaling ligands are ineffective as insulin secretagogues in the absence of a significant threshold of glucose metabolism.

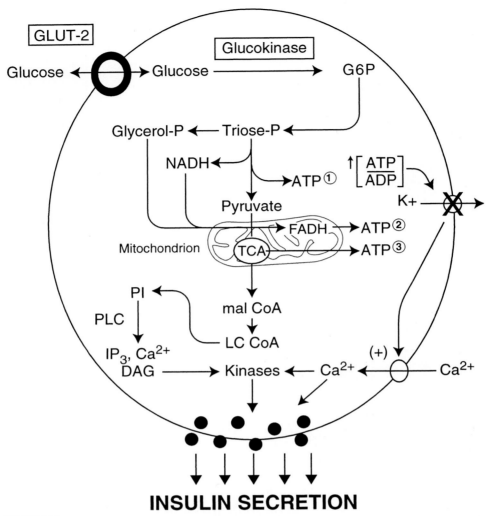

FIGURE 14-2. Schematic summary of basic model of the biochemical mechanism of glucose-stimulated insulin secretion. Insulin secretion is coupled to glucose metabolism in islet β cells. Proposed coupling factors include a rise in the ATP:ADP ratio, with ATP being produced in the distal portion of glycolysis,(1) via NADH shuttles,(2) or via pyruvate oxidation.(3) The potential linkage of glucose and lipid metabolism in regulation of insulin release is also shown.

Among fuel secretagogues, glucose stands out because it is the only one that can stimulate insulin secretion independent of other fuels. In fact, all of the other nutrients mentioned require the presence of physiological glucose levels to be effective. It is therefore not surprising that glucose is the most well-studied β-cell secretagogue. Based on this work, a basic model of the mechanism by which glucose stimulates insulin secretion has evolved, and is shown in Fig. 14-2, although significant questions and areas of disagreement remain to be resolved.

The consensus basic model of the mechanism of glucose-stimulated insulin secretion (GSIS) links glucose metabolism to insulin secretion via modulation in ATP and ADP levels (see Chap. 4). The capacity of glucose to stimulate insulin secretion is directly linked to its transport into β cells and further metabolism to generate coupling factors. Entry of glucose into the β cell is achieved by facilitated glucose transporters known collectively as the GLUTs.[28] GLUT-2 has a higher K_m for glucose and capacity for glucose transport than other members of the family, and is the isoform that

is primarily expressed in rodent islets.[29,30] Human islets also express GLUT-2, but at lower levels than rodent islets, and when isolated from cadaveric pancreata, they also express significant levels of the low-K_m glucose transporters GLUT-1 and GLUT-3.[31,32] Upon entry of glucose into β cells, the sugar is phosphorylated to glucose-6-phosphate (G6P) by glucokinase, also known as hexokinase IV, which contributes more than 90% of the glucose phosphorylating capacity in this cell type.[33] Like GLUT-2, glucokinase is a member of a gene family (the hexokinases), and differs from other members in several functional aspects. Glucokinase has an $S_{0.5}$ for glucose of about 8 mM, sigmoidal substrate dependency (indicated by a Hill coefficient of 1.7), and unlike hexokinases I and II, is not allosterically inhibited by the product of its reaction, G6P.[33,34] Thus, β cells are equipped with specialized proteins that mediate glucose transport and phosphorylation, and both proteins have kinetic features that allow them to regulate glucose metabolism in response to changes in the external glucose concentration.[35] Important new insights into the relative roles of glucose transporters and glucose phosphorylating enzymes in regulation of glycolytic flux and GSIS have come from gene transfer experiments, as summarized below.

At physiological glucose concentrations, most of the G6P produced by the glucokinase reaction in β cells flows efficiently into glycolysis, with little storage in the form of glycogen or entry into the pentose monophosphate shunt.[33] An important coupling factor produced by glucose metabolism in the β cell is ATP, by one of three different pathways. First, a large fraction of the NADH produced in the glyceraldehyde phosphate dehydrogenase reaction can be transferred to the mitochondria for entry into the electron transport chain via the α-glycero-P and aspartate/malate shuttles. In keeping with this idea, the activity level of the mitochondrial glycero-P dehydrogenase is higher in islets than in any other cell type in which it has been measured.[36] Second, ATP is generated in the phosphoglycerokinase and pyruvate kinase reactions of glycolysis. Finally, ATP can be produced in mitochondria from oxidation of pyruvate. Only a small fraction of pyruvate is reduced to lactate in β cells, due to relatively low levels of lactate dehydrogenase.[37–39]

As glucose levels rise and metabolism increases, there is a concomitant increase in the ATP:ADP ratio within β cells that signals that glucose is abundant. The increased ATP:ADP ratio stimulates insulin secretion in part by regulation of the conductance of adenine nucleotide–sensitive K^+ channels (K_{ATP} channels), with ATP serving as an inhibitor and ADP as an activator of the channel.[40–42] Thus, as the ATP:ADP ratio is increased, the open state probability of these channels is decreased and the plasma membrane of the β cell becomes depolarized. Membrane depolarization opens voltage-sensitive Ca^{2+} channels, causing the cytosolic Ca^{2+} level to rise.[43]

However, insulin secretion also seems to be regulated in a K_{ATP} channel–independent fashion. This became clear from experiments of Henquin and coworkers, who incubated islets with diazoxide and 30 mmol K^+ to render K_{ATP} channels insensitive to regulation by cellular ATP.[44] Under these conditions, glucose was still capable of stimulating insulin secretion, albeit not as effectively as in islets with normally-functioning channels. One interpretation of these results is that ATP is required for exocytosis of insulin-containing secretory granules, possibly at the level of providing energy for the movement of granules to the cell surface and fusion with the plasma membrane.

An intriguing and important issue that has emerged in the field of β-cell biology in recent years is the relevance of the interplay between glucose and lipid metabolism in regulation of insulin secretion. The long-chain acyl CoA (LC-CoA) hypothesis of stimulus-secretion coupling holds that part of the signal for insulin secretion that is generated by glucose catabolism is the production of cytosolic malonyl CoA, which is derived from citrate produced in the TCA cycle.[45] Malonyl CoA, in addition to being the proximal precursor of fatty acid biosynthesis, is an important regulatory molecule, in that increases in its levels cause inhibition of the mitochondrial enzyme carnitine palmitoyl transferase I (CPT I), which regulates entry of long-chain acyl CoAs into the mitochondria for oxidation.[46] Thus, increases in malonyl CoA secondary to increased glucose metabolism cause diversion of LC-CoA from oxidation to esterification pathways, and it has been proposed that increases in the levels of cytosolic LC-CoA esters are a key signal in GSIS.[45] Feasible sites at which increased LC-CoA could influence insulin secretion include conversion to bioactive metabolites such as diacylglycerol or inositol trisphosphate (IP_3),[47] contribution to plasma membrane or secretory granule membrane lipid turnover, or direct acylation of proteins involved in secretory granule trafficking.

Biochemical events that mediate insulin secretion distal to the glucose-induced increases in the phosphate potential and intracellular Ca^{2+} are not well understood. Potentially relevant is the activation of two types of protein kinases, protein kinase C (PKC) and Ca^{2+}-calmodulin dependent protein kinase (PKCaCM), during exposure of islets to stimulatory glucose. While it has been speculated that the role of PKCaCM or other Ca^{2+}-calmodulin-regulated kinases such as myosin light chain kinase may be to phosphorylate cytoskeletal or secretory granule proteins, thereby causing movement of granules within cells and exocytosis, definitive evidence for such a process is lacking.

Studies of synaptic vesicle exocytosis from nerve terminals may provide important insights into potential direct actions of Ca^{2+} and ATP on insulin granule exocytosis. Neurotransmitter release from synaptic vesicles involves a cascade of protein-protein interactions that mediate movement of the vesicles to the presynaptic plasma membrane, followed by docking, priming, fusion/exocytosis, and endocytosis of the vesicle.[48] The proteins involved in these processes are well characterized, and several are regulated by Ca^{2+} in either direct or indirect ways. Some of the proteins involved in synaptic vesicle exocytosis and neurotransmitter release have also been identified in insulin-producing cells in the pancreatic islets, including SNAP-25, vesicle-associated protein-2 (VAMP-2), and syntaxins 1A, 4, and 5.[49,50] Others such as synaptobrevin have been localized in a small subset of islet endocrine cells. While it is likely that a subset of the proteins and factors involved in synaptic vesicle exocytosis will also be involved in regulation of insulin secretion, much more work will be required to fully elucidate the specific differences and similarities between the two systems, including islet gene transfer experiments.

To summarize the basic model, increases in circulating glucose concentration are "sensed" by the β cell via a proportional increase in glycolytic rate. Both GLUT-2 and glucokinase participate in translation of changes in glucose concentration to modification in insulin secretion via regulation of entry of glucose into glycolysis, with a dominant role being played by glucokinase, as discussed below. The activation of glycolysis increases the ATP:ADP ratio by generation of ATP at three sites: (1) the distal portion of glycolysis, (2) shuttling of reducing equivalents into the mitochondria and activation of the electron transport chain and oxidative phosphorylation, and (3) glucose oxidation. The increase in ATP:ADP ratio causes inhibition of K_{ATP} channels, resulting in membrane depolarization and Ca^{2+} influx. The rise in intracellular Ca^{2+} triggers insulin secretion by one or some combination of the mechanisms discussed above, or possibly by as yet undiscovered pathways. A fascinating aspect of the glucose signaling pathway is that it can be potentiated by several metabolic fuels, but these potentiating factors are unable to elicit a response in the absence of a minimal level of glucose. This suggests that fuels such as fatty acids, ketone bodies, or amino acids are unable to achieve a threshold of metabolically derived second messengers sufficient to stimulate insulin release.

Within this framework lie a number of fundamental and unanswered questions. First, among the several ways that ATP can be generated during active glucose metabolism, is any one more important or relevant than another? Second, is ATP produced as a result of glucose metabolism the only metabolic coupling signal, or are other events required? Third, what is the overall contribution of the K_{ATP} channel-independent pathway of insulin secretion, and how do specific metabolic fuels regulate this pathway? Finally, in addition to regulating insulin secretion in an acute fashion, glucose also increases insulin gene expression and biosynthesis of the hormone. The effects of glucose on insulin synthesis, like those on secretion, appear to be mediated by glucose metabolism, but a number of lines of evidence suggest that the coupling factors may be different for the two effects. Thus the effects of glucose on insulin secretion are measured on a time scale of seconds, while glucose activation of insulin biosynthesis requires minutes to hours. Also, the threshold glucose concentration required for activation of insulin biosynthesis in islet β cells is considerably lower than that required for stimulation of insulin secretion.[51]

In short, while regulation of insulin secretion has been studied intensively for decades using biochemical and physiological tools, operative mechanisms are not yet fully understood. Recently, however, genetic engineering of islet cells has led to important new insights in this area. Key experiments of this type will now be reviewed.

Regulatory Roles of Glucose Transport and Phosphorylation in β Cells

A large number of gene transfer experiments have focused on the roles of GLUT-2 and glucokinase in regulation of GSIS. Interest in these molecules has been stimulated by the fact that their expression is impaired in diabetes.[35,52] In humans, the important role of glucokinase in glucose sensing has been highlighted by the discovery that a subset of patients with maturity onset diabetes of the young (MODY) are heterozygous for mutations in the glucokinase gene.[53] These mutations render the enzyme less active, diminishing the glucose phosphorylating capacity of the β cells and elevating the threshold for insulin secretion.

Important insights into the role of glucose phosphorylation in regulation of insulin secretion have been gained both from studies in transgenic animals and in experiments on cultured cells *in vitro*. Transgenic methods have been used to investigate the impact of reduced expression of glucokinase in islets of animal models, with results that are generally consistent with findings in MODY patients with glucokinase mutations. Expression of a glucokinase-specific ribozyme under control of the insulin promoter in transgenic mice resulted in a 70% reduction in immunodetectable glucokinase protein and enzyme activity.[54] Insulin secretion was impaired in these animals, with a reduction in total insulin release and an increase in the threshold concentration of glucose required for initiating the response. Unlike MODY patients, however, the transgenic mice were normoglycemic. Somewhat different results were obtained in animals heterozygous for knockout of the glucokinase gene. Animals with specific targeting of exon 1 of the islet isoform of the enzyme exhibited a 52% reduction in islet glucokinase activity, mild fasting hyperglycemia, and an abnormal response to a glucose challenge, despite normal hepatic glucokinase activity.[55] Transgenic mice heterozygous for disruption of a segment of the glucokinase gene that affects gene expression in both the liver and islets of Langerhans had a 30–40% decrease in glucokinase activity in both tissues, significant reduction in GSIS, and mild hyperglycemia.[56,57] Interestingly, animals homozygous for knockout of the glucokinase gene die prior to or shortly after birth.[55–57] Further, homozygous knockout of the β-cell isoform of glucokinase, with retention of normal hepatic expression of the enzyme, is sufficient to cause the neonatal lethality.[57] Also, in animals homozygous for knockout of both hepatic and β-cell glucokinase expression, restoration of β-cell glucokinase restores viability.[56]

The role of glucose phosphorylating enzymes in control of insulin secretion has also been studied by their overexpression in pancreatic islets and β-cell lines. A consistent observation from several laboratories is that overexpression of hexokinases with high affinity for glucose results in a left shift in the glucose dependence of insulin secretion and insulin gene expression. Thus, overexpression of hexokinase I in fetal islets results in a sharp reduction in the concentration threshold for glucose activation of a cotransfected insulin promoter/chloramphenicol acetyl transferase (CAT) plasmid.[58] Similarly, overexpression of low-K_m yeast hexokinase in β cells of transgenic mice results in a left-shifted glucose response and an increase in total insulin output.[59] Treatment of freshly isolated rat islets with a recombinant virus containing the hexokinase I cDNA resulted in a doubling of insulin secretion from islets perifused at a nonstimulatory glucose concentration (3 mM), consistent with a 2.5- to 4-fold increase in 5-^{3}H glucose usage and lactate production at this glucose concentration relative to the control groups.[15] Finally, stable overexpression of hexokinase I in the MIN-6 insulinoma cell line resulted in a threefold enhancement of insulin secretion and glucose usage at low glucose levels.[60]

Surprisingly, in contrast to the results obtained with overexpression of low-K_m hexokinases, overexpression of glucokinase in isolated rat islets or INS-1 insulinoma cells resulted in a substantial increase in glycolytic flux at low but not high glucose concentrations.[39,61] In contrast, overexpression of glucokinase in hepatoma cell lines,[62] isolated hepatocytes,[39,63] or primary human myocytes[64] caused large increases in glycolytic flux and glycogen accumulation, even at glucose concentrations well above 5 mM. A detailed comparison of INS-1 cells and hepatocytes led to the conclusion that a fundamental difference between hepatocytes and islet β cells is the limited capacity of the latter to metabolize glycolytic intermediates beyond the glyceraldehyde-3-phosphate dehydrogenase step.[39]

The foregoing studies may help to explain the finding that culture of GK (+/−) islets at high glucose levels resulted in increased glucokinase expression and near normalization of impaired glucose-stimulated insulin secretion.[65] Culture of GK (+/+) islets at high glucose concentrations also increased glucokinase expression, but in these islets the increased GK activity was accompanied by increased basal insulin secretion and a loss of the normal incremental response to stimulatory glucose. These findings correlate well with the increase in glucose metabolism at low but not high glucose concentrations observed in glucokinase-overexpressing INS-1 cells.[39,61]

In contrast to the consistent experimental support for a critical role for the glucose phosphorylation step in regulation of β-cell glucose sensing, significant controversy exists with regard to the role played by the glucose transporter GLUT-2. To summarize briefly, the following observations have been made that are consistent with the hypothesis:

1. GLUT-2 expression is reduced in concert with the loss of GSIS in a wide variety of rodent models of diabetes (reviewed in references 35 and 52). For example, in diabetes-prone male Zucker diabetic fatty (ZDF) rats, but not in diabetes-resistant female ZDF animals, β-cell GLUT-2 levels decline in inverse proportion to the severity of hyperglycemia. At onset of diabetes, GLUT-2 is detectable in only 60% of the β-cells, and then continues to decline to undetectable levels.[66,67] Similar observations have now been documented in the *db/db* mouse,[68] the GK rat,[69,70] the dexamethasone-treated Wistar and Zucker

fatty female rat,[71] and the streptozocin-treated rat.[72]

2. GLUT-2 expression is lost in concert with loss of glucose-stimulated insulin secretion in islet transplantation experiments.[68] Thus, transplantion of islets from normal animals into diabetic *db/db* mice or animals rendered diabetic by streptozocin injection results in loss of GLUT-2 protein expression and glucose responsivness of the graft, while conversely, transplantation of GLUT-2 deficient islets from diabetic *db/db* mice into normal mice results in restoration of GLUT-2 expression and glucose sensing.[68]

3. Reduced expression of GLUT-2 in β cells of transgenic animals results in impaired glucose sensing.[73,74] Thus, expression of the GLUT-2 cDNA in antisense configuration in islet β cells of transgenic mice under control of the insulin promoter resulted in an 80% depletion of islet GLUT-2 protein.[73] These transgenic animals exhibited an approximate twofold increase in basal glucose concentrations and a markedly impaired response to an intraperitoneal glucose tolerance test. Consistent with these observations, circulating insulin levels were decreased by 32% in the transgenic animals, and GSIS from transgenic islets was also sharply impaired. More recently, homologous recombination techniques have been used to generate GLUT-2 knockout mice.[74] GLUT-2 $-/-$ animals are hyperglycemic, hypoinsulinemic, and die at 3 weeks of age. Analysis of islets isolated from young animals prior to death reveals that the first phase of insulin secretion in response to glucose is abolished, while a modest second phase response remains.[75] Restoration of GLUT-2 expression by lentivirus transduction of cultured islets from GLUT-2 $-/-$ mice restores the first phase of GSIS.[75] Furthermore, expression of GLUT-2 under control of the rat insulin promoter (RIP) restores normal viability and regulation of insulin secretion in GLUT-2 knockout mice.[76]

4. Stable expression of GLUT-2 in neuroendocrine or insulinoma cell lines confers GSIS in cells that are otherwise unresponsive to the sugar,[13,77,78] while GLUT-1, a transporter isoform with higher affinity but lower capacity for glucose uptake than GLUT-2 appears unable to confer responsiveness.[78] Interestingly, in the GLUT-2 $-/-$ mice, GSIS was restored by transgenic expression of either GLUT-1 or GLUT-2.[76] The reasons for the different results obtained with GLUT-1 expression in the transgenic animal versus cell line studies are not known, but could be related to the very high levels of GLUT-1 expression reported in the former.

While the foregoing studies provide support for an important role for GLUT-2 in normal glucose sensing, other work argues that the transporter has little direct influence. Thus depletion of GLUT-2 associated with overexpression of the H-*ras* oncogene,[79] in response to culturing of islets *in vitro*,[80] or as a result of hypoglycemic perfusion of the pancreas[81] does not abrogate GSIS. In addition to these experimental findings, there is an important conceptual issue concerning a rate-determining role for GLUT-2 in glucose sensing, which is that glucose transport capacity has been reported to exceed the rate of glycolytic flux in rodent β cells by as much as two orders of magnitude.[33]

Another observation that seemingly reduces the probability of an important role for GLUT-2 is the finding that human islets express lower levels of the protein than do rat islets, and that human β cells may express other transporter isoforms such as GLUT-1 and GLUT-3 in addition to GLUT-2.[31,32] Thus the ratio of GLUT-2 protein and mRNA in liver and islets is reversed in rats versus humans (rats have higher GLUT-2 expression in islets than in liver, while

humans have less).[32] Consistent with this finding, the rate of 3-O-methyl glucose transport in human islets is only five times higher than the rate of glycolysis, compared to 50–100 times higher in rodent islets.[31] Furthermore, the rate of glucose metabolism in human islets increases by approximately 75% with a change in glucose from 5 to 10 mM, in concert with the increase in glucokinase activity, while glucose uptake increases by only 30%.[31] Nevertheless, the closer relationship of glucose transport capacity and glycolytic rate in human islets compared to rodent islets may suggest that the former cells could be more susceptible to functional impairment in response to decreased GLUT-2 expression. Consistent with this, a single patient with type 2 diabetes has been reported with a point mutation in the GLUT-2 gene (V197L) that renders the expressed mutant protein unable to transport glucose.[82] This finding suggests that reduced GLUT-2 expression may be sufficient to cause diabetes, although the contribution of reduced GLUT-2 expression in β cells relative to other sites of expression of the gene, such as liver or gut, was not determined.

Taken together, the studies performed to date on the role of GLUT-2 and glucokinase in regulation of GSIS are most consistent with a dominant regulatory role of the glucose phosphorylation step, but with an important permissive role played by the glucose transporter. It appears that the functional attribute of GLUT-2 that is most important for its putative role in glucose sensing is its high capacity for glucose transport rather than its low affinity for the sugar. Thus, as a high-capacity glucose transporter, GLUT-2 ensures that the intracellular glucose concentration in the β cell closely mirrors that in the circulation. This function of GLUT-2 allows glucokinase to be the major determinant of the glycolytic rate in β cells in response to changes in the external glucose concentration. Factors that allow glucokinase to fulfill this role include its relatively low level of expression in β cells and its kinetic properties.

Use of Genetic Engineering to Identify Stimulus/Secretion Coupling Factors

There is wide agreement that glucose metabolism generates factors that couple the glucose stimulus to insulin secretion.[33,83,84] In spite of this consensus, the exact nature of these coupling factors remains unresolved. For example, there is conflicting information with regard to the relative importance of discrete pathway segments involved in glucose metabolism. Thus some investigators have reported that inhibitors of glycolytic metabolism, but not enzymes involved in the TCA cycle, abolish GSIS.[85] In contrast, another line of research has shown that the TCA cycle intermediate methyl-succinate or succinate (the latter applied to permeabilized INS-1 cells) evokes insulin secretion.[86] Succinate is an anaplerotic substrate, and its addition to β cells causes both Ca^{2+} influx into mitochondria and hyperpolarization of the mitochondrial membrane. Thus the insulinotropic effect of succinate would appear to be independent of factors generated in the glycolytic pathway. Recently, it has been proposed that glutamate may be the specific coupling factor for insulin secretion derived from mitochondrial metabolism.[87] Data supporting this idea included a measured increase in glutamate content in INS-1 cells exposed to stimulatory glucose and potentiation of GSIS by addition of dimethyl-glutamate to INS-1 cells or glutamate to permeabilized INS-1 cells. It was further proposed that glutamate acts directly on the exocytotic machinery, based on experiments in which inhibitors of vesicular glutamate transporters inhibited insulin secretion. However, another recent paper presents evidence of GSIS independent of changes in

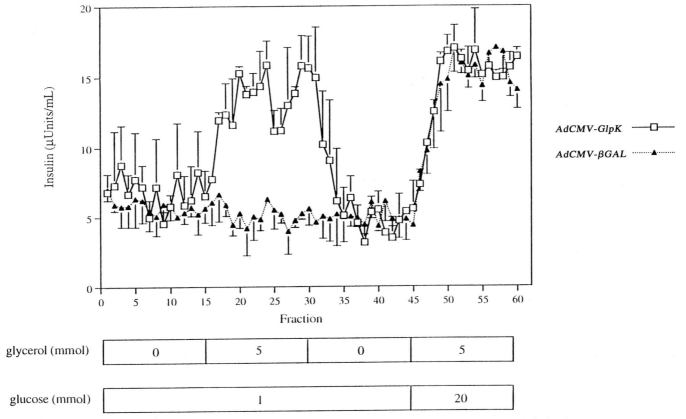

glycerol (mmol)	0	5	0	5

glucose (mmol)	1	20

FIGURE 14-3. Engineering of glycerol-stimulated insulin secretion from perifused rat islets. Freshly isolated rat islets were treated with recombinant adenoviruses containing genes encoding glycerol kinase (AdCMV-GlpK) or, as a control, β-galactosidase (AdCMV-βGAL), and perifusion studies were conducted 48 hours after viral treatment. Islets were perifused at a flow rate of 0.8 mL/min and fractions were collected at 1-minute intervals for measurement of insulin secretion. The perifusate additions are noted at the bottom of the figure. Note that only AdCMV-GlpK–treated islets increased insulin secretion in response to the addition of 5 mM glycerol to the basal perifusate (containing 1 mM glucose), while both groups of islets responded to the combination of 5 mM glycerol and 20 mM glucose. Data represent the mean ± SEM for three independent groups of islets per viral treatment. *(Data used, with permission, from Noel, et al.[14])*

glutamate concentration, leaving open the question of the relevance of this intermediate.[88]

Genetic engineering experiments are helping to resolve the confusion caused by the seemingly conflicting data just summarized. One approach is to compare the metabolic fates of glucose with those of other simple carbohydrates in order to identify those metabolic intermediates that are truly important in regulation of insulin secretion. For example, the triose glycerol is not normally an insulin secretagogue, due to the absence of the first enzyme of its metabolism in the β cell, glycerol kinase. However, as illustrated in Fig. 14-3, adenovirus-mediated expression of glycerol kinase allows INS-1 cells or isolated islets to metabolize glycerol effectively and to respond to glucose as an insulin secretagogue.[14] Comparison of the metabolic fates of glycerol and glucose in glycerol kinase–expressing cells revealed that glucose was oxidized more effectively than glycerol, such that the amount of glycerol oxidized at its maximally stimulatory concentration for insulin secretion was similar to that of glucose at a nonstimulatory concentration (3 mM) of the hexose (Fig. 14-4A). Instead, glycerol was converted effectively to lactate (Fig. 14-4B). These data suggest that oxidation of carbohydrate secretagogues via pyruvate dehydrogenase–catalyzed entry into the TCA cycle is not required

for GSIS, and instead directs attention towards reducing equivalent shuttles, the distal portions of glycolysis, or other metabolic pathways.

Other experiments of this type have been conducted to probe the "pyruvate paradox" of β-cell signaling, which refers to the lack of effect of pyruvate as an insulin secretagogue when applied to pancreatic islets, despite its ability to be oxidized by such cells. This has been investigated by overexpression of the monocarboxylic acid transporter (MCT), which is responsible for transport of lactate and pyruvate across the plasma membrane, and the enzyme lactate dehydrogenase (LDH) in INS-1 cells and isolated rat islets.[89–91] In one study, overexpression of LDH in INS-1 cells had no effect on GSIS, but did confer insulin secretion in response to lactate, while MCT expression had no effect on either variable.[89] The same investigators found that MCT overexpression in isolated islets conferred pyruvate-stimulated insulin secretion, whereas lactate-stimulated insulin secretion required co-overexpression of MCT and LDH. The ability of lactate and pyruvate to stimulate insulin secretion was correlated with their rates of oxidation in the two cell preparations, but was also linked to reducing equivalent shuttles, since aminooxyacetate (AOA) blocked glucose- or lactate-induced insulin secretion in LDH + MCT-overexpressing INS-1

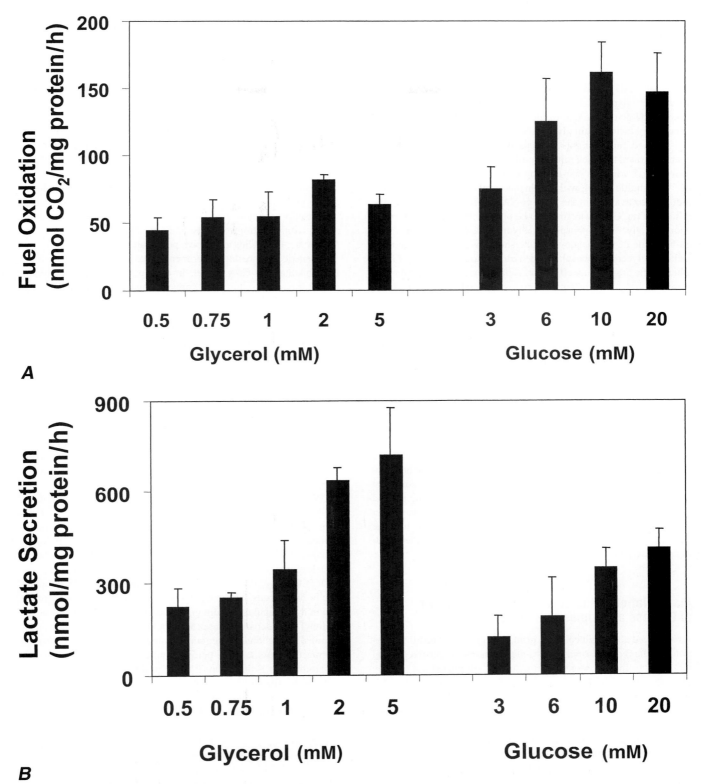

FIGURE 14-4. Comparison of the metabolic fates of glucose and glycerol in INS-1 cells engineered for glycerol kinase expression. **A.** Oxidation of varying concentrations of U-^{14}C glycerol (**left**) and U-^{14}C glucose (**right**) by INS-1 cells treated with a recombinant adenovirus containing the glycerol kinase gene (AdCMV-GlpK). Data are expressed as total nmol CO_2 produced/mg protein/h for each substrate. Note that CO_2 production at concentrations of glycerol that are maximally stimulatory for insulin secretion (2–5 mM) are similar to the CO_2 produced at a concentration of glucose that is nonstimulatory for insulin secretion (3 mM). **B.** Lacate produced at varying concentrations of glycerol (**left**) and glucose (**right**) from the same AdCMV-GlpK–treated INS-1 cells studied in part A. Note that more glycerol is converted to lactate than glucose, the inverse of the oxidation data. For both panels, data represent the mean ± SEM of three independent groups of experiments, each performed in triplicate. *(Data used, with permission, from Noel, et al.[14])*

cells. In contrast to these findings, another group reported that stable expression of LDH in an alternative insulinoma cell line, MIN-6, resulted in significant impairment of GSIS.[90,91] The authors suggested that the LDH-catalyzed conversion of lactate to pyruvate consumes NAD^+, which is required in the glycolytic reaction catalyzed by glyceraldehyde-3-phosphate dehydrogenase. Consequently, the glycolytic rate would be attenuated and the generation of coupling factors from glycolysis abrogated, inhibiting GSIS.

To shed further light on these issues, transgenic mice have been generated that lack mitochondrial glycerol-3-phosphate dehydrogenase,[92] which is rate-limiting in the glycerol phosphate shuttle. This shuttle, along with the malate-aspartate shuttle, transfers reducing equivalents in the form of NADH from the cytosol to the mitochondria. GSIS was found to be normal in mice lacking mitochondrial glycerol-3-phosphate dehydrogenase activity. However, co-blockade of the malate-aspartate shuttle with AOA in the mice lacking glycerol-3-phosphate dehydrogenase abolished GSIS, whereas the drug had no effect on insulin secretion in normal mice. Based on these data, the authors proposed a model in which NADH both from the cytosol, generated by glycolysis, and from the mitochondrion, derived from the TCA cycle, is required for normal stimulus-secretion coupling in β cells. However, a paradoxical finding is that both glucose usage and U-^{14}C-glucose oxidation were unaffected by blockade of the two shuttles, despite an anticipated deficiency in regeneration of NAD for glycolysis.

Taken together, the foregoing studies suggest that oxidation of glucose in the TCA cycle is not the critical event in glucose sensing, since glycerol was a potent secretagogue despite its poor efficiency of oxidation, while glucose failed to stimulate insulin secretion in islets with blockade of shuttle activity, despite normal oxidation of U-^{14}C glucose. These experiments, coupled with the fact that pyruvate and lactate are effective secretagogues when they are transported and metabolized effectively (e.g., when sufficient MCT and LDH are present), instead suggest that signaling is most closely coupled to redox state or to a mitochondrial pathway other than pyruvate dehydrogenase–catalyzed entry of carbon into the TCA cycle. Further studies will be required to gain full understanding of these points.

Manipulation of the Link Between Metabolism of Glucose and Lipids in β Cells

As reviewed above, glucose is a primary regulator of insulin secretion, but the β cell also serves as a more general thermostat for fuel metabolism. Indeed, secretion of insulin is stimulated not only by glucose but also by free fatty acids (FFA) and amino acids. This raises the possibility that some coupling factors that regulate insulin secretion may be common to multiple metabolic pathways. For more than a decade, malonyl CoA has been considered as a potential example of a coupling factor that integrates metabolic pathways for stimulation of insulin secretion.[45] The proposed regulatory role of malonyl CoA originated from the observation that this intermediate rises rapidly in response to stimulatory glucose in HIT-T15 and INS-1 insulinoma cells and in isolated rodent islets.[93] The glucose-induced rise in malonyl CoA coincides with inhibition of fatty acid oxidation and precedes the initiation of insulin secretion. Malonyl CoA is a known allosteric inhibitor of carnitine palmitoyl transferase I (CPT I), the enzyme that transports long-chain acyl CoA (LC-CoA) into the mitochondrion for subsequent β-oxidation.[46] The LC-CoA/malonyl CoA hypothesis also holds that LC-CoA accumulates in the cytosol as a consequence of malonyl CoA–mediated inhibition of CPT I, and that the rise in LC-CoA promotes exocytosis of insulin-containing secretory granules.

A number of observations support this model. For instance, in the perifused rat pancreas, abrogation of the link between glucose and malonyl CoA formation by administration of hydroxycitrate, an inhibitor of citrate lyase, causes an increase in fatty acid oxidation and inhibition of GSIS.[94] Conversely, suppression of fatty acid oxidation with inhibitors of CPT I, such as etomoxir, enhances GSIS. These findings seemingly support a role for malonyl CoA and cytosolic LC-CoA in β-cell stimulus-secretion coupling, but they can also be interpreted differently. Thus, the glucose-induced rise in malonyl CoA is correlated with, but not necessarily causal for, insulin secretion, hydroxycitrate is a potentially toxic compound with pleiotropic effects, and CPT I inhibitors are modified fatty acids; fatty acids are known potentiators of GSIS.

Genetic engineering experiments have been devised to test the LC-CoA/malonyl CoA model. In one such study, a recombinant adenovirus was used to overexpress the goose isoform of malonyl CoA decarboxylase in INS-1 cells.[95] This maneuver significantly attenuated the glucose-induced rise in malonyl CoA and partially reversed glucose-induced inhibition of fatty acid oxidation. The reduction in malonyl CoA levels also impaired the incorporation of glucose and palmitate into cellular lipids. However, despite this perturbation of the link between metabolism of glucose and lipids, GSIS was unaffected. Moreover, addition of an inhibitor of LC-CoA synthetase, triacsin C, to INS-1 cells or intact rat islets impaired glucose incorporation into total cellular lipids and lowered total cellular LC-CoA levels by 50%, but with no effect on GSIS. Finally, in INS-1 cells engineered for glycerol-stimulated insulin secretion by expression of glycerol kinase, incubation of the cells with triacsin C blocked glycerol incorporation into cellular lipids, but did not impair insulin secretion.[14]

While the foregoing study seems to argue against the LC-CoA model of GSIS, it has been criticized at several levels.[96,97] Concerns raised include: (1) The INS-1 cell line used for the work exhibited only a two- to fourfold stimulation of insulin secretion as glucose was raised from 3 to 15 mM, as opposed to freshly isolated rat islets, which can exhibit a 10- to 15-fold response; (2) It is unclear if the K_{ATP} channel–independent pathway of GSIS is operative in INS-1 cells. This pathway has been implicated as the site at which lipids regulate insulin granule exocytosis;[97,98] (3) The goose malonyl CoA decarboxylase (MCD) cDNA used earlier had its N-terminal mitochondrial targeting sequence deleted, but contained an intact C-terminal SKL peroxisomal targeting motif, raising the possibility that a significant fraction of the overexpressed enzyme failed to localize to the cytosol.

These outstanding concerns have been addressed recently. One important advance has been the development of INS-1–derived cell lines (e.g., 832/13) with robust K_{ATP}-channel–dependent and –independent GSIS.[99] The INS-1 cell line was originally derived from radiation-induced rat insulinoma (RIN) cells,[100] and has been popular in the field because it secretes insulin in response to glucose concentrations in the physiological range. However, the magnitude of the response is far less than that seen in freshly isolated rat islets (two- to fourfold in INS-1 cells versus 10- to 15-fold in freshly isolated islets), and even the modest response found in early passage INS-1 cells seems to wane with time in tissue culture. To investigate whether this loss of responsiveness might be due to clonal heterogeneity, parental INS-1 cells were transfected with a plasmid containing the human proinsulin gene, resulting in isolation of more than 60 independent clones.[99] After antibiotic selection and clonal expansion, 67% of the clones were found to be poorly responsive to glucose in terms of insulin secretion ($\leq$ twofold stimulation by 15 mM compared to 3 mM glucose), 17% of the clones were moderately responsive (two- to fivefold stimulation), and 16% were strongly responsive (5- to 13-fold stimulation). The differences in responsiveness among these three groups could not be ascribed to differences in insulin content.[99] More detailed study of one of the strongly responsive lines (832/13) revealed that its responsiveness was stable for prolonged periods of continuous tissue culture, and that the cells exhibit half-maximal stimulation of insulin secretion at 6 mM glucose. Furthermore, insulin secretion was enhanced by known potentiators of islet insulin secretion such as IBMX, FFA, and glucagon-like peptide-1 (GLP-1). GSIS was also potentiated by the sulfonylurea tolbutamide, and abolished by diazoxide, demonstrating the operation of the ATP-sensitive K^+-channel (K_{ATP}) in 832/13 cells. Moreover, when the K_{ATP} channel was bypassed by incubation of cells in depolarizing K^+ (35 mM), insulin secretion was more effectively stimulated by glucose in 832/13 cells than in parental INS-1 cells or the glucose-unresponsive clones.

In addition to the development of new INS-1-derived cell lines, the human MCD cDNA has been cloned,[101] and mutant forms of the cDNA lacking the mitochondrial and peroxisomal localization sequences have been inserted into adenovirus vectors.[102] With this cadre of improved reagents, the effect of MCD overexpression on GSIS has been reexamined, again with the finding of no impairment of robust GSIS in 832/13 cells, despite complete blockade of the glucose-induced rise in malonyl CoA level (Fig. 14-5A).[102] Furthermore, combined treatment of 832/13 cells with an adenovirus containing the modified human MCD cDNA and triacsin C did not impair GSIS (Fig. 14-5B). Interestingly, these maneuvers also did not affect potentiation of GSIS by fatty acids.

The LC-CoA model has also been investigated via modulation of the activity of acetyl CoA carboxylase (ACC), the enzyme that catalyzes malonyl CoA synthesis from acetyl CoA. In one approach, expression of acetyl CoA carboxylase was lowered by stable expression of an ACC-specific antisense construct in parental INS-1 cells.[103] The decrease in acetyl CoA carboxylase activity resulted in decreased malonyl CoA levels and a consequent increase in fatty acid oxidation. GSIS was inhibited over a range of glucose concentrations, as was insulin secretion elicited by other nutrients that require metabolism in β cells, e.g., leucine, glutamine, and ketoisocaproic acid. In contrast, insulin secretion stimulated by KCl was not affected. These results seem to support the LC-CoA model but some caution in interpretation is warranted. A particular concern is that chronic lowering of malonyl CoA levels could result in depletion of stored lipids. Depletion of β-cell lipids in nicotinamide-treated animals or humans[104,105] or in hyperleptinemic rats[106] blocks insulin secretion in response to glucose and many other secretagogues. Interestingly, in both cases GSIS is immediately restored by provision of FFA. These findings clearly support an essential role for lipids in regulation of insulin secretion, possibly at the level of membrane lipid turnover or acylation of regulatory proteins. The latter possibility is also supported by recent studies in which insulin secretion was inhibited by addition of cerulenin, an inhibitor of protein acylation.[98] However, while a minimal pool of lipids may be essential for normal regulation of insulin secretion, the aforementioned studies with malonyl CoA decarboxylase adenoviruses and triacsin C provide strong evidence that glucose sensing can occur in the absence of a rise in malonyl

CoA and despite acute perturbation of lipid metabolism.

Further study will be required to fully understand the role of lipids in regulation of insulin secretion. From the foregoing experiments, it is clear, at least in highly glucose-responsive INS-1–derived cell lines, that perturbation of the normal link between glucose and lipid metabolism and complete blockade of glucose-induced increases in malonyl CoA accumulation have no impact on GSIS. However, it remains possible that an important signal is generated not from changes in the rate of fatty acid oxidation, but rather by flow of LC-CoA into esterification pathways, as has also been suggested by Prentki and associates.[107] This issue remains to be clarified, as does the mechanism by which fatty acids potentiate GSIS.

One possible role for lipids in insulin secretion is their further metabolism to generate by-products with signaling properties. For example, it has been suggested that insulin secretion from pancreatic islets may be mediated in part by activation of phospholipase C (PLC) and phosphoinositide hydrolysis.[47] In freshly isolated rat islets, there is a 15-fold increase in insulin secretion in response to elevated glucose, and this response typically occurs with a biphasic pattern. By contrast, mouse islets lack a sustained second phase of GSIS. It has been proposed that the absence of the second phase response in mouse islets is due to their relatively low capacity for PLC-mediated hydrolysis of phosphoinositides.[108] Indeed, mouse islets have reduced expression of the B and δ isoforms of PLC, while the $\gamma 1$ isoform is expressed at a similar level as in rat islets.[108]

PLC-mediated hydrolysis of phosphoinositides would result in generation of inositol trisphosphate (IP_3) and diacylglycerol, which could link to insulin secretion via mobilization of intracellular Ca^{2+} stores and activation of protein kinase C, respectively. PLC isozyme expression has been characterized in normal rat islets and two insulinoma cell lines, INS-1 and βG 40/110.[109] βG 40/110 is a glucose-responsive cell line derived from RIN 1046-38 insulinoma cells by stable transfection with plasmids encoding human insulin and glucokinase.[110,111] Rat islets contain abundant PLC $\delta 1$ expression, but both cell lines completely lack this isoform. In addition, both lines have similar or slightly reduced levels of expression of PLC $\beta 1$, $\beta 2$, $\beta 3$, $\delta 2$, and γ as found in fresh rat islets. In an attempt to determine whether increases in inositol phosphate (IP) levels enhance insulin secretion, PLC $\delta 1$, $\beta 1$, or $\beta 3$ were overexpressed in INS-1 or βG 40/110 cells using recombinant adenoviruses.[109] In these cell lines, overexpression of PLC isoforms resulted in little or no enhancement in IP accumulation and no improvement in insulin secretion in response to glucose or carbachol, despite the fact that the overexpressed proteins were fully active in cell extracts. Overexpression of the $\beta 1$ or $\beta 3$ isoforms in normal rat islets elicited a larger increase in IP accumulation, but again with no effect on insulin secretion. Since the effect of carbachol on insulin secretion is thought to be mediated through muscarinic receptors that link to the $G_{q/11}$ class of heterotrimeric G proteins, $G_{11\alpha}$ was also overexpressed in INS-1 cells, either alone or in concert with overexpression of PLC $\beta 1$ or $\beta 3$.[112] Overexpression of $G_{11\alpha}$ enhanced IP accumulation, an effect slightly potentiated by co-overexpression of PLC $\beta 1$ or $\beta 3$, but again, these maneuvers were without effect on glucose- or carbachol-stimulated insulin secretion. In sum, these studies showed a lack of correlation between IP accumulation and insulin secretion in INS-1 cells, βG 40/110 cells, or cultured rat islets during stimulation with glucose or carbachol. However, it remains possible that the loss of fuel signaling engendered by complete lipid depletion in islets[104–106] could be due to a requirement for some minimal level of PLC-mediated phosphoinositide metabolism.

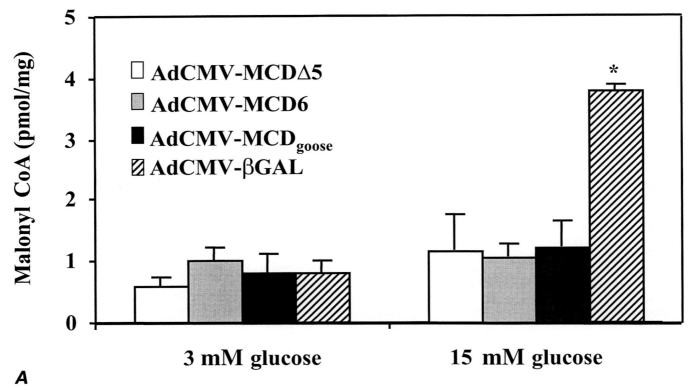

A

FIGURE 14-5A. Adenovirus-mediated expression of malonyl CoA decarboxylase (MCD) in INS-1–derived 832/13 cells blocks glucose-induced malonyl CoA formation, but has no effect on glucose-stimulated insulin secretion. **A.** 832/13 cells were treated with recombinant adenoviruses containing different cDNA constructs encoding MCD (see reference 102 for details) or, as a control, a virus expressing the β-galactosidase gene (AdCMV-βGAL). After viral treatment, cells were cultured in 3 mM glucose for 24 hours, and then switched to buffer containing either 3 or 15 mM glucose for 30 minutes prior to extraction and measurement of malonyl CoA. Data represent the mean ± SEM for three independent measurements. The asterisk (*) indicates that the malonyl CoA level at 15 mM glucose was significantly higher than at 3 mM glucose in the AdCMV-βGAL–treated control cells, with $p < 0.001$.

Insulin Signaling in β Cells

A traditional topic of debate in islet research has been whether insulin controls its own expression and secretion. Recent studies suggest that the insulin receptor and other key components of the insulin signaling cascade are expressed in islet β cells.[113–117] Furthermore, exposure of βTC3 cells to glucose or exogenous insulin results in tyrosine phosphorylation of the insulin receptor and IRS-1, suggesting that the expressed signaling molecules are fully functional in β cells. However, conflicting results have been obtained in insulin-secreting cells with wortmannin, an inhibitor of a key enzyme of insulin signaling, phosphatidylinositol-3-kinase, possibly relating to the different experimental conditions employed.[112,121] In contrast, a role for insulin in regulating its own expression and that of other genes important for β-cell function has been more clearly defined.[122,123]

An important role for signaling molecules implicated in insulin action has also emerged from studies with knockout mice. For example, mice deficient in insulin receptor substrate-2 (IRS-2) become insulin resistant due to impaired insulin signaling in skeletal muscle and liver.[115] Interestingly, while normal mice or mice with IRS-1 knocked out exhibit a compensatory increase in insulin secretion; this does not occur in IRS-2–deficient mice. Instead, they

exhibit a progressive loss of β-cell mass and eventually develop diabetes. These results suggest that IRS-2 plays an important role in regulation of β-cell proliferation and compensation in insulin-resistant states, and implies the existence of signals that balance insulin action and insulin secretion via IRS-2–mediated β-cell expansion.

More recently, mice with specific knockout of the insulin receptor in β cells were created by crossing a strain homozygous for an insulin receptor allele containing loxP sites with one expressing cre recombinase; the latter was under control of the insulin promoter, thereby directing the genetic deletion to pancreatic β cells.[117] The mice developed impaired glucose tolerance, caused by a perturbation of the first phase of insulin secretion in response to a glucose challenge, while the response to arginine remained intact. In addition, insulin content and islet size were slightly decreased in insulin receptor–deficient mice. These findings have led to reexamination of IRS-1–deficient mice with respect to islet function.[124] These animals were initially reported to be highly insulin resistant but normoglycemic due to an effective compensation by islet cell hyperplasia.[125] More recently, it was found that while basal insulin levels are elevated in the IRS-1–deficient mice, glucose- and arginine-stimulated insulin secretion is impaired. Similar findings have been

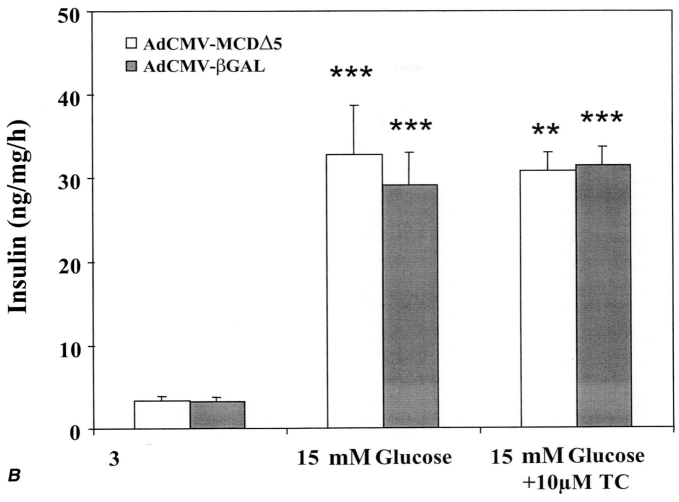

FIGURE 14-5 (continued). B. 832/13 cells were treated with the indicated adenoviruses and cultured for 24 hours in medium containing 3 mM glucose. Insulin secretion was then measured by incubating cells in HBSS containing either 3 or 15 mM glucose for 2 hours. Results represent the mean ± SEM for eight independent experiments.**$p < 0.01$; ***$p < 0.001$. *(Data used, with permission, from Mulder, et al.[102])*

reported in isolated islets and in immortalized cell lines derived from the IRS-1–deficient mice.[124] Insulin content in individual islets of these animals is also decreased, whereas total pancreatic insulin content is not altered due to the increase in total islet mass. Interestingly, morphological examinations showed that the secretory granules are smaller and more condensed in the IRS-1–deficient mice. Also, there is the presence of autophagic vesicles, which are lacking in the wild type β cells.

In a complementary approach to the knockout studies, the effect of stable overexpression of IRS-1 has been studied in clonal mouse β cells, the β-TC-F7 line.[126] This maneuver increased fractional release of insulin, when glucose was raised from 0 to 15 mM, while surprisingly, insulin content was decreased. The glucose-induced increase in intracellular Ca^{2+} was not affected, whereas basal cytoplasmic Ca^{2+} levels were increased. The authors suggest that the mechanism by which basal Ca^{2+} levels are elevated may be inhibition of Ca^{2+} uptake into the endoplasmic reticulum, possibly secondary to an increase in protein kinase C activity. Similar findings were made in single β cells.[120]

At this point, it appears that the insulin receptor is expressed in β cells and that known insulin-stimulated signal transduction pathways are operative. The surprising implication from studies involving genetic manipulation of insulin receptor or insulin signal transduction molecules in β cells is that insulin plays a role in β-cell stimulus–secretion coupling, by augmenting its own secretion. The mechanisms for this are still unclear, particularly in light of the discrepant findings with wortmannin, although Ca^{2+} metabolism may be involved. Another cautionary note about the findings with transgenic animals is that despite the normal appearance of islets in animals with β-cell insulin receptor knockout, the possibility that the altered β-cell function in these animals is due to a developmental impairment has not been rigorously excluded. Further confusion has arisen from the recent finding that transgenic mice carrying a double conditional knockout of the insulin receptor in pancreatic β cells and skeletal muscle unexpectedly exhibited an improvement of their glucose homeostasis compared with the single conditional knockout of the insulin receptor in β cells.[127] This improvement was due in part to an enhancement of GSIS.

GENETIC ENGINEERING APPLIED TO INSULIN REPLACEMENT THERAPY FOR DIABETES

The recently concluded Diabetes Control and Complications Trial (DCCT) has clearly demonstrated the importance of tight glycemic control for limiting onset and progression of the crippling secondary complications of type 1 diabetes mellitus (T1DM). Unfortunately, improvement in glycemic control via self-injection of insulin requires a high level of compliance and discipline, and places the patient at significantly enhanced risk for dangerous hypoglycemic episodes. Transplantation of human pancreatic islets, usually involving instillation of isolated islets via the portal circulation and immunosuppression, has been investigated as an alternative to insulin injection therapy, but historically has had very limited success.[128] Recently, however, in a trial in Edmonton, Alberta, Canada, a combination of mild immunosuppressive agents was used in conjunction with freshly isolated islet tissue to achieve insulin independence in seven successive patients studied for up to 1 year posttransplant.[129]

Two major issues that remain to be overcome in order for cell-based insulin therapy of T1DM to become widely applicable include (1) development of a replenishable source of cells capable of delivering insulin in an appropriately regulated and stable fashion, and (2) development of methods for ensuring immunoprotection of transplanted cells. Because of the difficulty and cost associated with islet isolation and pancreas transplantation, there has been an increasing emphasis on application of the tools of molecular biology for development of novel insulin replacement therapies, including engineering of insulin-secreting cell lines, stem cell development, and expression of insulin in nonislet cells via gene therapy. We will close the chapter by reviewing the current status of these efforts.

Engineering of Cell Lines for Glucose-Stimulated Insulin Secretion

Two basic approaches for engineering of surrogate β cells have emerged. The first involves genetic engineering of preexisting lines to enhance their function. Key goals include overexpression of the human proinsulin cDNA and development of cells that regulate their insulin secretion in response to glucose and its potentiators. Early experiments of this type were carried out in the neuroendocrine cell line AtT-20ins, which is derived from ACTH-secreting corticotrophs of the anterior pituitary. These cells normally do not express the insulin gene, but upon transfection with a plasmid containing the human proinsulin cDNA, are shown to secrete the mature insulin polypeptide.[130,131] Insulin secretion from AtT-20ins cells can be stimulated by agents such as forskolin or 3-isobutyl-1-methylxanthine (IBMX), but not by glucose. Stable expression of GLUT-2 in AtT-20ins cells conferred glucose-stimulated insulin secretion, albeit with a maximal 2.5-fold response occurring at a glucose concentration of approximately 50 μM.[77,78] However, transplantation of engineered AtT-20ins cells into nude rats caused insulin resistance, apparently secondary to ACTH secretion from the cells and resultant adrenal hyperplasia.[132] Thus while these cells served as a proof of principle, they are unlikely to be useful for insulin replacement therapy.

More recent work has instead focused on rodent insulinoma cell lines such as RIN 1046-38 and INS-1. RIN 1046-38 cells respond to glucose, but this response is maximal at subphysiologic glucose concentrations and is lost as a function of time in culture, in concert with loss of expression of GLUT-2 and glucokinase.[13,133] As detailed earlier, INS-1 cells exhibit a modest (two- to fourfold) response to glucose concentrations in the physiologic range, but genetic engineering methods have been applied to procure robustly glucose responsive INS-1–derived subclones.[99]

Using a process of "iterative engineering," or the stepwise stable transfection of cells with plasmids containing different genes and discrete antibiotic resistance markers, RIN 1046-38–derived cell lines have been developed with insulin content comparable to that measured in cultured human islet preparations (2.5–4.0 μg insulin/10^6 cells).[110] Installation of GLUT-2 and glucokinase genes in these cells by stable transfection conferred a large enhancement in glucose-stimulated insulin secretion.[110,111] The multiply engineered lines increase insulin secretion by six-to eightfold in response to glucose, and this response was potentiated by agents that raise cAMP. The engineered cell lines exhibit a maximal response to glucose at low concentrations (0.05–0.25 mM), but when incubated with 5-thioglucose, an inhibitor of low-K_m hexokinase activity, maximal responsiveness occurred at 3–5 mM glucose.[111] These data suggest that further adjustment of glucose sensing to simulate the response threshold of the β cell (4–5 mM) could be achievable by stable suppression of low-K_m hexokinase activity, possibly via gene knockout by homologous recombination.

One advantage of the stable transfection approach outlined above is that it may provide a remarkable genetic and phenotypic stability in the engineered cell lines. Thus transplantation of unencapsulated engineered RIN cell lines into nude rats revealed that stably-integrated transgenes were expressed at constant levels in the *in vivo* environment for up to 48 days, the longest experiment performed.[110] Several endogenous genes expressed in normal β cells, including rat insulin, amylin, sulfonylurea receptor, and glucokinase were also stably expressed in the insulinoma lines during these *in vivo* studies. Endogenous GLUT-2 expression, in contrast, was rapidly extinguished (within 10 days of cell implantation). The loss of GLUT-2 was not observed in engineered cell lines in which GLUT-2 expression was provided by a stably transfected transgene.[110]

The second approach to generation of new cell lines is to direct expression of a transforming gene, generally SV40 T-antigen, to β cells of transgenic mice via the insulin promoter/enhancer. Cell lines derived by transgenic expression of T-antigen in β cells exhibit variable phenotypes.[134–137] In some cases, these differences have been correlated with expression of glucose transporters and glucose phosphorylating enzymes. Some lines such as βTC-6 and βTC-7 were shown to have a glucose response that resembles that of the islet in magnitude and concentration dependence.[135] These cells express GLUT-2 and contained a glucokinase:hexokinase activity ratio similar to that of the normal islet when studied at low passage number, but with time in culture GSIS became maximal at low, subphysiological glucose concentrations. Accompanying this shift in glucose dose-response was a large (approximately sixfold) increase in hexokinase expression. More recently, soft agar techniques have been used to derive new clonal isolates of βTC-6 cells (such as the clone βTC6-F7), which appear to retain differentiated function for longer periods of time in culture.[137] However, the long-term stability of these cell lines is still unclear.[138]

Controlling the growth rate of T-antigen-expressing cell lines by a strategy of conditional immortalization may allow better control of fuel homeostasis. The recently derived βTC-tet insulinoma cell lines express T-antigen under control of a tetracycline-regulatable promoter, such that when tetracycline or its analogues are present, the cells decrease their expression of the transforming gene and stop growing.[139] Syngeneic transplantation of these cells in an unencapsulated state into mice resulted in rapid cell growth and development of hypoglycemia in the absence of tetracycline, but in animals implanted with slow release tetracycline pellets, tumor mass was controlled and normoglycemia was maintained for a period of 150 days. It remains to be determined whether expression of critical glucose-sensing genes is stably maintained in βTC-tet cell lines during tetracycline treatment.

Engineering of Cell Lines for Resistance Against Immunological Attack

As new rodent cell lines with attractive physiological properties are being developed, insights into strategies for immunoprotecting such cell lines are also emerging. As is the case with strategies for engineering of physiological responsiveness, work to date on immunoprotection has been limited to animal cell lines, as appropriate human β cell lines are not yet available. However, it is hoped that emerging approaches will be rapidly transferable to human cells as they are developed.

Immunologic destruction of β cells in type 1 diabetes is thought to be a T-cell-dependent process. Infiltration of pancreatic islets by mononuclear cells of the immune system, mostly macrophages and T lymphocytes, precedes β-cell destruction in human subjects with T1DM and in non-obese diabetic (NOD) mice. Impaired function and destruction of β cells appears to result from direct contact with islet-infiltrating cells and/or exposure to inflammatory cytokines that they produce.[140–143] Since cytotoxic T-cells destroy target cells via docking to MHC class I molecules, resulting in T-cell receptor activation, one approach for protecting unencapsulated islets is MHC class I "masking" by pretreatment with specific antibodies[144] or suppression of MHC class I expression by antisense strategies or by expression of the adenovirus E3 gene.[145,146] These maneuvers have been demonstrated to slow destruction of islet xenografts[144] or cell lines transplanted as allografts.[145] In addition, expression of the entire E3 gene in transgenic mice engineered for virus-induced, β-cell-specific autoimmunity prevents β-cell destruction, although peri-insulitis is still observed.[146] However, it is as yet unclear whether E3 expression will be sufficient to protect transplanted cell lines from immune destruction in all cases. In fact, the protection afforded by E3 expression in transplanted mouse islets is demonstrable in some mouse strains but not in others.[145] Another approach that has been taken is the expression of "protective" or Th2 cytokines such as IL-4 or IL-10 in β cells. Expression of IL-4 in β cells does in fact provide effective protection against β-cell destruction and insulitis in transgenic NOD mice.[147] However, expression of IL-4 fails to protect NOD islets when transplanted into diabetic NOD mice, and also fails to protect islets transplanted from one strain of mouse to another (allografting) in the absence of any autoimmunity.[148] Thus it appears that local production of IL-4 may not be sufficient to provide protection for transplantation of cell lines into animals or humans with diabetes. A final approach that has garnered attention is the engineering of cotransplanted cell lines for expression of Fas ligand (FasL). In one recent study, syngeneic myoblasts engineered for FasL expression provided protection for a cotransplanted islet allograft in mouse experiments.[149] While initially highly encouraging, a subsequent study involving expression of FasL in transplanted islets showed accelerated rather than slowed immunologic destruction of the graft.[150] The reasons for these discrepant results are not yet apparent and further investigation of the FasL approach will be required.

An alternative approach to preventing T-cell/graft interactions is to encapsulate cells in a cell-exclusionary membrane or device. Such an approach obviates the need for suppression or masking of MHC class I expression in the cells to be implanted. Furthermore, implantation of cells in an encapsulated form, particularly when all the cells are within a single device (macroencapsulation), can allow immediate localization or retrieval of cells should problems with cell performance or other complications be encountered. When dealing with cells encapsulated in this fashion, immunoprotective strategies become focused on mechanisms for preventing cell damage in response to small, soluble mediators of the immune response. One approach is to identify and express candidate genes that may interfere with this kind of cell damage. These include the anti-apoptotic gene *bcl-2* and related family members;[7,151] enzymes involved in metabolism of toxic oxygen radicals present at low abundance in β cells such as superoxide dismutase, catalase, or glutathione peroxidase;[152,153] other molecules that interfere with the known signal transduction pathways of inflammatory cytokines, such as dominant-negative FADD domain proteins, which partially block TNF-α signaling;[154,155] or dominant negative forms of the IL-1 receptor interacting protein MyD88.[156] Expression of anti-apoptotic members of the bcl gene family have been reported to confer partial protection against cytokine mixtures,[7,151] but at high levels of expression, these proteins may also impair glucose metabolism and glucose-stimulated insulin secretion.[157]

An alternative, more general approach is to develop cell lines with resistance to inflammatory cytokines. This has been recently achieved by culture of INS-1 cells in incrementally increasing concentrations of IL-1β + IFN-γ, resulting in isolation of clones resistant to the cytotoxic effects of the two cytokines (Fig. 14-6).[158]

The resistance to IL-1β as a result of the selection procedure is permanent, while the resistance to IFN-γ is transient and reinducible.[158] By following the known pathways of IL-1β and IFN-γ signaling, cytokine resistance in the selected cells was shown to be associated with altered activity or expression of transcription factors. Thus the permanent resistance to IL-1β was linked to impaired NF-kB translocation.[158] Selected cells maintained in cytokines were also found to contain very high levels of the transcription factor STAT-1α, whose translocation to the nucleus is mediated by interaction with IFN-γ receptor and its associated Janus kinase (JAK).[159] Furthermore, adenovirus-mediated overexpression of STAT-1α in cytokine-sensitive INS-1 cells confers partial resistance to the cytotoxic effects of IFN-γ or IFN-γ + IL-1β (Fig. 14-7).[159] It remains to be determined whether other factors also participate in the development of complete cytokine resistance. Comparison of gene expression profiles in cytokine-resistant and cytokine-sensitive INS-1–derived cells may allow a more complete understanding of pathways leading to robust resistance to soluble mediators of the immune response.

Approaches to Human Cell Therapy of Diabetes

Important gains have been made in recent years in identifying and developing cell lines that can perform key functions of the normal islet β cell, and in devising strategies that may aid in protecting such cells when transplanted into an immunocompetent host. It is hoped that lessons learned from both transgenic and cellular engineering approaches will be applicable to development of cell lines suitable for treatment of human diabetes. However, it is uncertain if rodent or other xenogeneic cell lines will serve as a useful vehicle

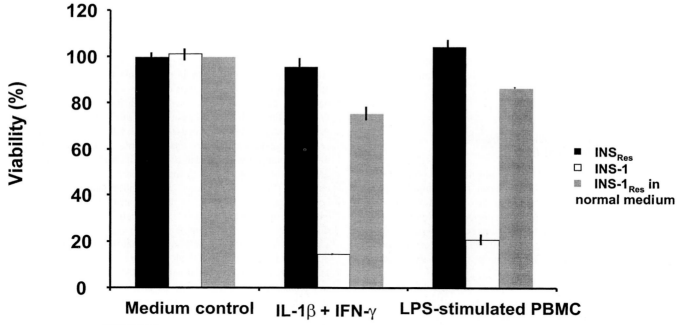

FIGURE 14-6. A selection procedure for isolation of cytokine-resistant INS-1 cells. INS-1 cells were grown in the presence of iterative increases in concentrations of IL-1β + IFN-γ over a period of 8 weeks, as described in Chen, et al.[158] At the end of the 8-week selection procedure, one group of selected cells was cultured for 2 additional months in the continual presence of 10 ng/mL IL-1β + 100 U/mL IFN-γ (INS-1$_{Res}$), while a second group of cells had cytokines withdrawn for the 2-month period (INS-1$_{Res}$ in normal medium). These two cell populations and unselected INS-1 cells (INS-1) were cultured overnight in the absence of cytokines and then subjected to acute treatment (48 hours) with 10 ng/mL IL-1β + 100 U/mL IFN-γ or with conditioned medium from LPS-stimulated rat peripheral blood mononuclear cells (LPS-stimulated PBMC). Viability of the three cell populations was estimated with the MTT viability assay, relative to each group of cells cultured in normal medium without cytokines or PBMC-conditioned medium, which were scored as 100% viable (medium control).

for delivery of insulin to human patients. Problems with such cell lines include their potential transmission of adventitious infectious agents (e.g., retroviruses) and their leak of xenoantigens, resulting in a hyperaggressive immune response that may destroy transplanted cells even if they contain protective genes. It is therefore imperative to develop human cell lines that can serve as functional allografts. The genetic engineering approaches just described are likely to be applicable to the development of such lines. The problem is with the lack of stable human β-cell lines, or alternatively, an expandable population of stem cells that can serve as the starting material for molecular manipulation. We close the chapter by evaluating several approaches for dealing with this problem that have emerged recently.

One approach to procuring an expandable supply of human β cells is to isolate stem cells that can be grown in culture and induced to differentiate to a β-cell phenotype. Two types of stem cells may be suitable for this purpose. First, there is evidence to suggest that the pancreatic ducts contain cells with the capacity to expand and differentiate to normal islet tissue. Thus, islet neogenesis from pancreatic ductal structures has been demonstrated in several models of islet regeneration, including the partially pancreatectomized rat,[160] and in mice transgenic for expression of IFN-γ in islet β cells.[161] More recently, two reports have shown that the portion of the pancreas that remains after islet harvesting can yield islet-like structures when cultured in defined tissue culture media, and that resultant cell clusters express insulin and secrete the hormone in response to known stimulators of secretion.[162,163] These studies provide some encouragement for the idea that the pancreas

contains pluripotent stem cells that can be harnessed to procure functional islets. However, major issues remain to be overcome, including the relatively low and quite variable insulin content achieved in the studies performed to date, and the absence of unequivocal evidence that the insulin-containing cells are derived from stem cells rather than from preexisting β cells. Therefore, a key goal for the future is the isolation and characterization of the putative stem cells from the mixed cellular populations found in the ductal cultures.

The second type of stem cell that may have utility for procurement of functional pancreatic islets is the embryonic stem cell. A recent report has used a cell-trapping system to isolate insulin-producing cells from mouse embryonic stem cells.[164] This involved construction of a vector containing a fragment of the human insulin gene driving expression of a neomycin resistance gene, and a separate transgene consisting of a constitutive promoter (phosphoglycerate kinase) driving expression of a hygromycin resistance gene. This construct was used to transfect mouse embryonic stem cells by electoporation, and transfected cells were selected with hygromycin. Selection of insulin-expressing subpopulations of transfected cells was then achieved by culture of cells in neomycin (G418). Initial populations of insulin-expressing cells procured by culture in the presence of nicotinamide and high (25 mM) glucose had very low insulin content and no response to secretagogues. However, further culture of these cells at low glucose (5.6 mM) resulted in a progressive increase in insulin content and modest glucose-stimulated insulin secretion. Implantation of these cells into streptozocin-induced diabetic mice resulted in partial normaliza-

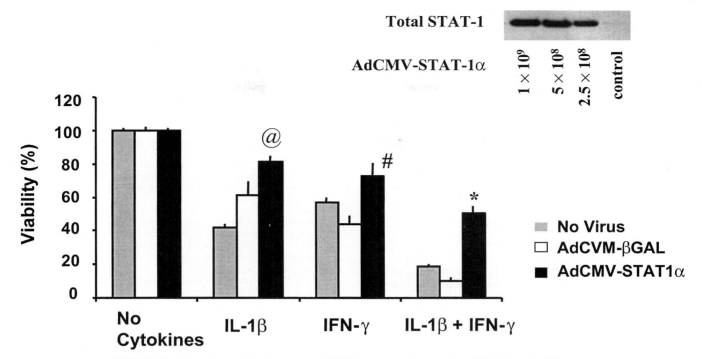

FIGURE 14-7. Adenovirus-mediated expression of STAT-1α in a cytokine-sensitive INS-1–derived cell line confers resistance to cytokine-induced cytotoxicity. **Inset**. INS-1 cells were treated with the indicated concentrations of AdCMV-STAT-1α for 12 hours, and then incubated in fresh medium for 24 hours, prior to cell harvesting and immunoblot analysis with an anti-STAT-1α antibody. Control cells were incubated for the same time period but without virus treatment. The cytokine-sensitive cell line 834/40 was treated with 1×10^9 pfu/mL of AdCMV-STAT1α, the same amount of AdCMV-βGAL virus, or no virus. These cell groups were cultured in normal medium for 24 hours, and then treated with 100 ng/mL IL-1β, 100 U/mL IFN-γ, or both cytokines for 48 hours. Cell viability was then determined with the MTT assay. Data represent the mean ± SEM for four independent experiments. Symbols refer to comparisons of viability of STAT-1α overexpressing cells to other groups, as follows: @, $p < 0.001$ versus untreated control, $p < 0.03$ versus AdCMV-βGAL–treated control; #, $p = 0.05$ versus untreated control, $p < 0.007$ versus AdCMV-βGAL-treated control; *, $p < 0.002$ versus either control group. *(Data used, with permission, from Chen, et al.[159])*

tion of blood glucose levels and improved glucose tolerance during oral glucose or meal challenges. This study provides important proof of principle for the concept that embryonic stem cells can be used to procure cells that resemble pancreatic islets in several important aspects. However, it remains to be determined if the same or related technologies will be applicable to human embryonic stem cells, and whether political considerations will allow such work to progress at an optimal pace. Furthermore, it will also be important to determine whether the insulin-producing cells that are derived by these methods can be induced to become fully differentiated, which could involve application of some of the genetic engineering approaches described earlier.

While human cell line and stem cell development continues, others have investigated the possibility that gene therapy can be used to deliver insulin from extrapancreatic tissues. Three recent publications are notable in this regard.[165–167] In one study, the investigators engineered an insulin molecule containing a short peptide loop connecting the A and B chains of the molecule that allows appropriate folding and interaction of the two chains without a requirement for proteolytic processing.[165] The cDNA encoding this construct was placed under the control of the liver pyruvate kinase promoter and delivered with an AAV vector to liver of streptozocin-induced diabetic mice. Animals that received this vector exhibited near-normalization of blood glucose levels. However, the insulin

secretion response to an oral glucose tolerance test was clearly delayed relative to animals with intact islets, as would be expected given that control of insulin production by glucose in the transgenic mice occurs via activation of the pyruvate kinase promoter, a much slower process than glucose-stimulated insulin exocytosis in normal islets. Transgenic mice were also susceptible to postprandial hypoglycemia, because insulin production persisted beyond the point at which glucose levels began to fall.[165] It must also be noted that further development of viral gene transfer vectors is required to ensure efficacy and patient safety before constructs of this type can be delivered to human diabetic patients. An interesting alternative hepatic engineering strategy that has recently appeared involves adenovirus-mediated expression of a key islet transcription factor, PDX-1.[166] Remarkably, this maneuver results in activation of insulin gene expression in liver of streptozocin-diabetic mice, and partial normalization of their blood glucose levels. While similar concerns can be raised about this approach as for the insulin analogue idea (poor regulation of insulin secretion from liver, concerns about vector efficacy and safety in humans), the PDX-1 study may have broader implications in the context of inducing differentiation of nonislet or stem cells in culture. Finally, a recent study has investigated the expression of human proinsulin under control of the glucose-dependent insulinotropic polypeptide (GIP) promoter in transgenic mice.[167] Initial testing of the construct in gut K cells revealed correct proteolytic processing of proinsulin to insulin, presumably mediated by expression of the proprotein convertases PC1/3 and PC2 in the gut cell line. Furthermore, modest glucose-stimulated insulin secretion (twofold response as glucose was raised from 1 to 10 mM) was demonstrated in the transfected cells. Expression of proinsulin in transgenic mice under control of the GIP promoter resulted in expression of the transgene in gut, normalization of blood glucose levels in streptozocin-induced diabetic mice, and a more normalized response to an oral glucose bolus than observed with the pyruvate kinase/single-chain insulin AAV approach. Whether these intriguing results can be developed into a new strategy for treatment of human diabetes again awaits the development of safe and efficacious gene therapy vectors for gene transfer to the gastrointestinal tract.

REFERENCES

1. Sestak AL, Newgard CB: Gene transfer methods in diabetes research. In: Porte D, Sherwin RS, eds. *Ellenberg and Rifkin's Diabetes Mellitus*, 5th ed. Appleton & Lange:1997; 257.
2. Anderson WF: Human gene therapy. *Nature* 1998;392:25.
3. Varmus H: Retroviruses. *Science* 1988;240:1427.
4. Leibowitz G, Beattie GM, Kafri T, *et al*: Gene transfer to human pancreatic endocrine cells using viral vectors. *Diabetes* 1999;48:745.
5. Naldini L, Blomer U, Gallay P, *et al*: In vivo gene delivery and stable transduction of nondividing cells by a lentiviral vector. *Science* 1996; 272:263.
6. Ju Q, Edelstein D, Brendel MD, *et al*: Transduction of non-dividing adult human pancreatic beta cells by an integrating lentiviral vector. *Diabetologia* 1998;41:736.
7. Dupraz P, Rinsch C, Pralong WF, *et al*: Lentivirus-mediated Bcl-2 expression in beta TC-tet cells improves resistance to hypoxia and cytokine-induced apoptosis while preserving in vitro and in vivo control of insulin secretion. *Gene Therapy* 1999;6:1160.
8. Zufferey R, Nagy D, Mandel RJ, *et al*: Multiply attenuated lentiviral vector achieves efficient gene delivery in vivo. *Nature Biotechnol* 1997;15:871.
9. Kafri T, Blomer U, Peterson DA, *et al*: Sustained expression of genes delivered directly into liver and muscle by lentiviral vectors. *Nature Genet* 1997;17:314.
10. Fink DJ, Glorioso JC: Engineering herpes simplex virus vectors for gene transfer to neurons. *Nature Med* 1997;3:357.
11. Berkner KL: Development of adenovirus vectors for the expression of heterologous genes. *BioTechniques* 1988:6;616.
12. Graham FL, Prevec L: Manipulation of viral vectors. In: Murray EJ, ed. *Methods of Molecular Biology*. Humana Press:1991;109.
13. Ferber S, BeltrandelRio H, Johnson JH, *et al*: GLUT-2 gene transfer into insulinoma cells confers both high and low affinity glucose-stimulated insulin release: Relationship to glucokinase activity. *J Biol Chem* 1994;269:11523.
14. Noel RJ, Antinozzi P, McGarry JD, *et al*: Engineering of glycerol-stimulated insulin secretion in islet β-cells: Differential metabolic fates of glucose and glycerol provide insight into mechanisms of stimulus-secretion coupling. *J Biol Chem* 1997;272:18621.
15. Becker T, BeltrandelRio H, Noel RJ, *et al*: Overexpression of hexokinase I in isolated islets of Langerhans via recombinant adenovirus: Enhancement of glucose metabolism and insulin secretion at basal but not stimulatory glucose levels. *J Biol Chem* 1994;269:21234.
16. Becker T, Noel R, Coats WS, *et al*: Use of recombinant adenovirus for metabolic engineering. *Methods Cell Biol* 1994;43:161.
17. Stratford-Perricaudet LD, Levrero M, Chasse J-F, *et al*: Evaluation of the transfer and expression in mice of an enzyme-encoding gene using a human adenovirus vector. *Hum Gene Ther* 1990;1:241.
18. Herz J, Gerard RD: Adenovirus-mediated transfer of low density lipoprotein receptor gene acutely accelerates cholesterol clearance in normal mice. *Proc Natl Acad Sci USA* 1993;90:2812.
19. Noel RJ, Newgard CB: Prospects for genetic manipulation in diabetes. In: Marshall SM, Home PD, Rizza RA, eds. *The Diabetes Annual*, vol. 10. Elsevier Science:1996;65.
20. Trinh K, O'Doherty R, Anderson P, *et al*: Perturbation of fuel homeostasis caused by overexpression of the glucose-6-phosphatase catalytic subunit in liver of normal rats. *J Biol Chem* 1998;273:31615.
21. O'Doherty RM, Lehman D, Telemaque-Potts S, *et al*: Metabolic impact of glucokinase overexpression in liver: Lowering of blood glucose in fed rats occurs at the expense of hyperlipidemia. *Diabetes* 1999;48:2022.
22. Henderson JR, Moss MC: A morphometric study of the endocrine and exocrine capillaries of the pancreas. *QJ Exp Physiol* 1985;70:347.
23. Noel RJ: Use of recombinant adenovirus for engineering of glucose transport and glycerol metabolism in insulinoma cells and islets of Langerhans. Ph.D. thesis, University of Texas Southwestern Medical Center at Dallas, 1996.
24. Srivastava CH, Samulski RJ, Lu L, *et al*: Construction of a recombinant human parvovirus B19: Adeno-associated virus 2 (AAV) DNA inverted terminal repeats are functional in an AAV-B19 hybrid virus. *Proc Natl Acad Sci USA* 1989;86:8078.
25. Kearns WG, Afione SA, Fulmer SB, *et al*: Recombinant adeno-associated virus (AAV-CFTR) vectors do not integrate in a site-specific fashion in an immortalized epithelial cell line. *Gene Ther* 1996;3:748.
26. Flotte T, Agarwal A, Wang JM, *et al*: Efficient ex vivo transduction of pancreatic islet cells with recombinant adeno-associated virus vectors. *Diabetes* 2001;50:515.
27. Liang Y, Matschinsky FM: Mechanism of action of non-glucose secretagogues. *Ann Rev Nutr* 1994;14:59.
28. Bell GI, Kayano T, Buse JB, *et al*: Molecular biology of mammalian glucose transporters. *Diabetes Care* 1990;13:198.
29. Johnson JH, Newgard CB, Milburn JL, *et al*: The high K_m glucose transporter of islets of Langerhans is functionally similar to the low affinity transporter of liver and has an identical primary sequence. *J Biol Chem* 1990;265:6548.
30. Thorens B, Sarkar HK, Kaback HR, *et al*: Cloning and functional expression in bacteria of a novel glucose transporter in liver, intestine, kidney and beta-pancreatic islet cells. *Cell* 1988;55:281.
31. DeVos A, Heimberg H, Quartier E, *et al*: Human and rat beta cells differ in glucose transporter but not in glucokinase gene expression. *J Clin Invest* 1995;96:2489.
32. Ferrer J, Benito C, Gomis R: Pancreatic islet GLUT-2 glucose transporter mRNA and protein expression in humans with and without NIDDM. *Diabetes* 1995;44:1369.
33. Meglasson MD, Matschinsky FM: Pancreatic islet glucose metabolism and regulation of insulin secretion. *Diabetes Metab Rev* 1986;2:163.
34. Wilson JE: Regulation of mammalian hexokinase activity. In: Beitner R, ed. *Regulation of Carbohydrate Metabolism*. CRC Press:1984;45.
35. Newgard CB: Regulatory role of glucose transport and phosphorylation in pancreatic islet β-cells. *Diabetes Rev* 1996;4:191.
36. MacDonald MJ: Elusive proximal signals of β-cells for insulin secretion. *Diabetes* 1990;29:1461.
37. Sekine N, Cirulli V, Regazzi R, *et al*: Low lactate dehydrogenase and high mitochondrial glycerol phosphate dehydrogenase in pancreatic beta-cells. Potential role in nutrient sensing. *J Biol Chem* 1994;269:4895.
38. Liang Y, Bai G, Doliba N, *et al*: Glucose metabolism and insulin release in mouse βHC9 cells as model for wild-type pancreatic β-cells. *Am J Physiol* 1996;33:E846.
39. Berman HK, Newgard CB: Fundamental metabolic differences between hepatocytes and islet β-cells revealed by glucokinase overexpression. *Biochemistry* 1998;37:4543.
40. Ashcroft FM, Harrison DE, Ashcroft SHJ: Glucose induces closure of single potassium channels in isolated rat pancreatic β-cells. *Nature* 1984;312:446.
41. Cook DL, Hales N: Intracellular ATP directly blocks K^+-channels in pancreatic β-cells. *Nature* 1984;311:269.
42. Misler S, Falke LC, Gillis K, *et al*: A metabolite-regulated potassium channel in rat pancreatic B cells. *Proc Natl Acad Sci USA* 1984;83:7119.
43. Misler S, Pressel DM, Barnett DW: Stimulus transduction in metabolic sensor cells. In: Speralakis N, ed. *Cell Physiology Source Book*. Academic Press:1998;652.
44. Gembal M, Detimary P, Gilon P, *et al*: Mechanisms by which glucose can control insulin release independently from its action on adenosine triphosphate-sensitive K^+ channels in mouse β-cells. *J Clin Invest* 1993;91:871.
45. Prentki M, Corkey BE: Are the β-cell signaling molecules malonyl CoA and cytosolic long-chain-CoA implicated in multiple tissue defects of obesity and NIDDM? *Diabetes* 1996;45:273.

46. McGarry JD, Foster DW: Regulation of hepatic fatty acid oxidation and ketone body production. *Ann Rev Biochem* 1980;49:395.

47. Turk J, Gross RW, Ramanadham S: Amplification of insulin secretion by lipid messengers. *Diabetes* 1993;42:367.

48. Sudhof TC: The synaptic vesicle cycle: A cascade of protein-protein interactions. *Nature* 1995;375:645.

49. Jacobsson G, Bean AJ, Scheller RH, et al: Identification of synaptic proteins and their isoform mRNAs in compartments of pancreatic endocrine cells. *Proc Natl Acad Sci USA* 1994;91:12487.

50. Regazzi R, Sadoul K, Meda P: Mutational analysis of VAMP domains implicated in Ca^{2+}-induced insulin exocytosis. *EMBO J* 1996;15:6951.

51. Skelly RH, Bollheimer LC, Wicksteed BL, et al: A distinct difference in the metabolic stimulus-response coupling pathways for regulating proinsulin biosynthesis and insulin secretion that lies at the level of a requirement for fatty acyl moieties. *Biochem J* 1998;331:553.

52. Unger RH: Diabetic hyperglycemia: Link to impaired glucose transport in pancreatic β-cells. *Science* 1991;251:1200.

53. Frougel P, Zouali H, Vionnet N: Familial hyperglycemia due to mutations in glucokinase. *N Engl J Med* 1993;328:697.

54. Efrat S, Leiser M, Wu Y-J, et al: Ribozyme-mediated attenuation of pancreatic β-cell glucokinase expression in transgenic mice results in impaired glucose-induced insulin secretion. *Proc Natl Acad Sci USA* 1994;91:2051.

55. Terauchi Y, Sakura H, Yasuda K, et al: Pancreatic β-cell-specific targeted disruption of glucokinase gene. *J Biol Chem* 1995;270:30253.

56. Bali D, Svetlanov A, Lee H-W, et al: Animal model for maturity-onset diabetes of the young generated by disruption of the mouse glucokinase gene. *J Biol Chem* 1995;270:21464.

57. Grupe A, Hultgren B, Ryan A: Transgenic knockouts reveal a critical requirement for pancreatic β-cell glucokinase in maintaining glucose homeostasis. *Cell* 1995;83:69.

58. German MS: Glucose sensing in pancreatic islet beta cells: The key role for glucokinase and the glycolytic intermediates. *Proc Natl Acad Sci USA* 1993;90:1781.

59. Epstein PN, Boschero AC, Atwater I, et al: Expression of yeast hexokinase in pancreatic β-cells of transgenic mice reduces blood glucose, enhances insulin secretion and decreases diabetes. *Proc Natl Acad Sci USA* 1992;89:12038.

60. Ishihara H, Asano T, Tsukuda K, et al: Overexpression of hexokinase I but not GLUT 1 glucose transporter alters the concentration dependence of glucose-stimulated insulin secretion in pancreatic beta cells. *J Biol Chem* 1994;269:3081.

61. Wang H, Iynedjian PB: Modulation of glucose responsiveness of insulinoma beta-cells by graded overexpression of glucokinase. *Proc Natl Acad Sci USA* 1997;94:4372.

62. Valera A, Bosch F: Glucokinase expression in rat hepatoma cells induces glucose uptake and is rate limiting in glucose utilization. *Eur J Biochem* 1994;222:533.

63. O'Doherty R, Lehman D, Seoane J, et al: Differential metabolic effects of adenovirus-mediated glucokinase and hexokinase I overexpression in rat primary hepatocytes. *J Biol Chem* 1996;271:20524.

64. Baque S, Montell E, Guinovart JJ, et al: Expression of glucokinase in cultured human muscle cells confers insulin-independent and glucose-concentration dependent glucose disposal and storage. *Diabetes* 1998;47:1392.

65. Sreenan SK, Cockburn BN, Baldwin AC, et al: Adaptation to hyperglycemia enhances insulin secretion in glucokinase mutant mice. *Diabetes* 1998;47:1881.

66. Johnson JH, Ogawa A, Chen L, et al: Underexpression of beta cell high K_m glucose transporters in noninsulin-dependent diabetes. *Science* 1990;250:546.

67. Orci L, Ravazzola M, Baetens D, et al: Evidence that down-regulation of β-cell glucose transporters in non-insulin-dependent diabetes may be the cause of diabetic hyperglycemia. *Proc Natl Acad Sci USA* 1990;87:9953.

68. Thorens B, Wu Y-J, Leahy JL, et al: The loss of GLUT-2 expression by glucose-unresponsive β-cells of db/db mice is reversible and is induced by the diabetic environment. *J Clin Invest* 1992;90:77.

69. Ohneda M, Johnson JH, Inman LR, et al: GLUT-2 expression and function in β-cells of the GK rat with NIDDM: Dissociation between reduction in glucose transport and glucose-stimulated insulin secretion. *Diabetes* 1993;42:1065.

70. Portha B, Serradas D, Bailbe K-I: β-cell insensitivity to glucose in the GK rat, a spontaneous nonobese model for type II diabetes. *Diabetes* 1991;40:227.

71. Ohneda M, Johnson JH, Inman LI, et al: GLUT 2 function in glucose-unresponsive β-cells of dexamethasone-induced diabetes in rats. *J Clin Invest* 1993;92:1950.

72. Thorens B, Weir GC, Leahy JL, et al: Reduced expression of liver/beta cell glucose transporter isoform in glucose-insensitive beta cells of diabetic rats. *Proc Natl Acad Sci USA* 1990;87:6492.

73. Valera A, Solanes G, Fernandez-Alvarez J, et al: Expression of GLUT-2 antisense RNA in β-cells of transgenic mice leads to diabetes. *J Biol Chem* 1994;269:28543.

74. Guillam M-T, Hummler E, Schaerer E: Early diabetes and abnormal postnatal pancreatic islet development in mice lacking GLUT-2. *Nature Genet* 1998;18:88.

75. Guillam M-T, Dupraz P, Thorens B: Glucose uptake, utilization and signaling in GLUT-2 null islets. *Diabetes* 2000;49:1485.

76. Thorens B, Guillam M-T, Beermann F, et al: Transgenic reexpression of GLUT1 or GLUT2 in pancreatic β-cells rescues GLUT2-null mice from early death and restores glucose-stimulated insulin secretion. *J Biol Chem* 2000;275:23751.

77. Hughes SD, Johnson JH, Quaade C, et al: Engineering of glucose-stimulated insulin secretion in non-islet cells. *Proc Natl Acad Sci USA* 1992;89:688.

78. Hughes SD, Quaade C, Johnson JH, et al: Transfection of AtT-20ins cells with GLUT-2 but not GLUT-1 confers glucose-stimulated insulin secretion: Relationship to glucose metabolism. *J Biol Chem* 1993;268:15205.

79. Tal M, Wu Y-J, Leiser M, et al: [Val12] HRAS downregulates GLUT-2 in β-cells of transgenic mice without affecting glucose homeostasis. *Proc Natl Acad Sci USA* 1992;89:5744.

80. Tal M, Liang Y, Najafi H, et al: Expression and function of GLUT-1 and GLUT-2 glucose transporter isoforms in cells of cultured rat pancreatic islets. *J Biol Chem* 1992;267:17241.

81. Chen C, Thorens B, Bonner-Weir S, et al: Recovery of glucose-induced insulin secretion in a rat model of NIDDM is not accompanied by return of the β-cell GLUT-2 glucose transporter. *Diabetes* 1992;41:1320.

82. Mueckler M, Kruse M, Strube M, et al: A mutation in the GLUT2 glucose transporter gene of a diabetic patient abolishes transport activity. *J Biol Chem* 1994;269:17232.

83. Newgard CB, McGarry JD: Metabolic coupling factors in pancreatic beta-cell signal transduction. *Annu Rev Biochem* 1995;64:689.

84. Newgard CB, Matschinsky FM: Substrate control of insulin release. In: Jefferson J, Cherrington A, eds. *Handbook of Physiology.* Oxford University Press:2001;125.

85. Mertz RJ, Worley JF, Spencer B, et al: Activation of stimulus-secretion coupling in pancreatic β-cells by specific products of glucose metabolism: Evidence for privileged signaling by glycolysis. *J Biol Chem* 1996;271:4838.

86. Maechler P, Kennedy ED, Pozzan T, et al: Mitochondrial activation directly triggers the exocytosis of insulin in permeabilized pancreatic beta-cells. *EMBO J* 1997;16:3833.

87. Maechler P, Wollheim CB: Mitochondrial glutamate acts as a messenger in glucose-induced insulin exocytosis. *Nature* 1999;402:685.

88. MacDonald MJ, Fahien LA: Glutamate is not a messenger in insulin secretion. *J Biol Chem* 2000;275:34025.

89. Ishihara H, Wang H, Drewes LR, et al: Overexpression of monocarboxylate transporter and lactate dehydrogenase alters insulin secretory responses to pyruvate and lactate in β-cells. *J Clin Invest* 1999;104:1621.

90. Zhao C, Rutter GA: Overexpression of lactate dehydrogenase A attenuates glucose-induced insulin secretion in stable MIN-6 β-cell lines. *FEBS Lett* 1998;430:213.

91. Ainscow EK, Zhao C, Rutter GA: Acute overexpression of lactate dehydrogenase-A perturbs beta-cell mitochondrial metabolism and insulin secretion. *Diabetes* 2000;49:1149.

92. Eto K, Suga S, Wakui M, et al: Role of NADH shuttle system in glucose-induced activation of mitochondrial metabolism and insulin secretion. *Science* 1999;283:981.

93. Corkey BE, Glennon MC, Chen KS, et al: A role for malonyl-CoA in glucose-stimulated insulin secretion from clonal pancreatic beta-cells. *J Biol Chem* 1989;264:21608.

94. Chen S, Ogawa A, Ohneda M, *et al*: More direct evidence for a malonyl-CoA-carnitine palmitoyltransferase I interaction as a key event in pancreatic beta-cell signalling. *Diabetes* 1994;43:878.

95. Antinozzi P, Segall L, Prentki M, *et al*: Molecular or pharmacologic perturbation of the link between glucose and lipid metabolism is without effect on glucose-stimulated insulin secretion: A re-evaluation of the long-chain acyl CoA hypothesis. *J Biol Chem* 1998;273: 16146.

96. Corkey BE, Deeney JT, Yaney GC, *et al*: The role of long-chain fatty acyl-CoA esters in beta-cell signal transduction. *J Nutr* 2000;130(2S suppl):299S.

97. Komatsu M, Yajima H, Yamada S, *et al*: Augmentation of Ca^{2+}-stimulated insulin release by glucose and long-chain fatty acids in rat pancreatic islets: Free fatty acids mimic ATP-sensitive K^+ channel-independent insulinotropic action of glucose. *Diabetes* 1999;48:1543.

98. Yajima H, Komatsu M, Yamada S, *et al*: Cerulenin, an inhibitor of protein acylation, selectively attenuates nutrient stimulation of insulin release: A study in rat pancreatic islets. *Diabetes* 2000;49:712.

99. Hohmeier HE, Mulder H, Chen G, *et al*: Isolation of INS-1-derived cell lines with robust ATP-sensitive K^+ channel-dependent and -independent glucose-stimulated insulin secretion. *Diabetes* 2000;49:424.

100. Asfari M, Janjic D, Meda P, *et al*: Establishment of 2-mercaptoethanol-dependent differentiated insulin-secreting cell lines. *Endocrinology* 1992;130:167.

101. Gao J, Waber L, Bennett MJ, *et al*: Cloning and mutational analysis of human malonyl-coenzyme A decarboxylase. *J Lipid Res* 1999; 40:178.

102. Mulder H, Lu D, Finley J 4th, *et al*: Overexpression of a modified human malonyl-CoA decarboxylase blocks the glucose-induced increase in malonyl-CoA level but has no impact on insulin secretion in INS-1-derived (832/13) beta-cells. *J Biol Chem* 2001;276:6479.

103. Zhang S, Kim KH: Essential role of acetyl-CoA carboxylase in the glucose-induced insulin secretion in a pancreatic beta-cell line. *Cellular Signalling* 1998;10:35.

104. Stein DT, Esser V, Stevenson BE, *et al*: Essentiality of circulating fatty acids for glucose-stimulated insulin secretion in the fasted rat. *J Clin Invest* 1996;97:2728.

105. Dobbins RL, Chester MW, Daniels MB, *et al*: Circulating fatty acids are essential for efficient glucose-stimulated insulin secretion after prolonged fasting in humans. *Diabetes* 1998;47:1613.

106. Koyama K, Chen G, Wang M *et al*: β-cell function in normal rats made chronically hyperleptinemic by adenovirus-leptin gene therapy. *Diabetes* 1997;46:1276.

107. Segall L, Lameloise N, Assimacopoulos-Jeannet F, *et al*: Lipid rather than glucose metabolism is implicated in altered insulin secretion caused by oleate in INS-1 cells. *Am J Physiol* 1999;277:E521.

108. Zawalich WS, Kelley GG: The pathogenesis of NIDDM: The role of the pancreatic beta cell. *Diabetologia* 1995;38:986.

109. Gasa R, Trinh K, Yu K, *et al*: Overexpression of G11α and isoforms of phospholipase C in islet β-cells reveals a lack of correlation between inositol phosphate accumulation and insulin secretion. *Diabetes* 1999; 48:1035.

110. Clark S, Quaade C, Constandy H, *et al*: Novel insulinoma cell lines produced by iterative engineering of GLUT-2, glucokinase, and human insulin expression. *Diabetes* 1997;46:958.

111. Hohmeier H, BeltrandelRio H, Clark S, *et al*: Regulation of insulin secretion from novel engineered insulinoma cell lines. *Diabetes* 1997; 46:968.

112. Hagiwara S, Sakurai T, Tashiro F, *et al*: An inhibitory role for phosphatidylinositol 3-kinase in insulin secretion from pancreatic B cell line MIN6. *Biochem Biophys Res Comm* 1995;214:51.

113. Rothenberg PL, Willison LD, Simon J, *et al*: Glucose-induced insulin receptor tyrosine phosphorylation in insulin-secreting beta-cells. *Diabetes* 1995;44:802.

114. Harbeck MC, Louie DC, Howland J, *et al*: Expression of insulin receptor mRNA and insulin receptor substrate 1 in pancreatic islet beta-cells. *Diabetes* 1996;45:711.

115. Stenson Holst L, Mulder H, Manganiello V, *et al*: Protein kinase B is expressed in pancreatic beta cells and activated upon stimulation with insulin-like growth factor I. *Biochem Biophys Res Comm* 1998;250:181.

116. Withers DJ, Gutierrez JS, Towery H, *et al*: Disruption of IRS-2 causes type 2 diabetes in mice. *Nature* 1998;391:900.

117. Kulkarni RN, Bruning JC, Winnay JN, *et al*: Tissue-specific knockout of the insulin receptor in pancreatic beta cells creates an insulin secretory defect similar to that in type 2 diabetes. *Cell* 1999;96:329.

118. Gao Z, Konrad RJ, Collins H, *et al*: Wortmannin inhibits insulin secretion in pancreatic islets and beta-TC3 cells independent of its inhibition of phosphatidylinositol 3-kinase. *Diabetes* 1996;45:854.

119. Nunoi K, Yasuda K, Tanaka H, *et al*: Wortmannin, a PI3-kinase inhibitor: Promoting effect on insulin secretion from pancreatic beta cells through a cAMP-dependent pathway. *Biochem Biophys Res Comm* 2000;270:798.

120. Aspinwall CA, Qian WJ, Roper MG, *et al*: Roles of insulin receptor substrate-1, phosphatidylinositol 3-kinase, and release of intracellular Ca^{2+} stores in insulin-stimulated insulin secretion in β-cells. *J Biol Chem* 2000;275:22331.

121. Zawalich WS, Zawalich KC: A link between insulin resistance and hyperinsulinemia: Inhibitors of phosphatidylinositol 3-kinase augment glucose-induced insulin secretion from islets of lean, but not obese, rats. *Endocrinology* 2000;141:3287.

122. Leibiger IB, Leibiger B, Moede T, *et al*: Exocytosis of insulin promotes insulin gene transcription via the insulin receptor/PI-3 kinase/p70 s6 kinase and CaM kinase pathways. *Mol Cell* 1998;1:933.

123. Xu G, Marshall CA, Lin TA: Insulin mediates glucose-stimulated phosphorylation of PHAS-I by pancreatic beta cells. An insulin-receptor mechanism for autoregulation of protein synthesis by translation. *J Biol Chem* 1998;273:4485.

124. Kulkarni RN, Winnay JN, Daniels M, *et al*: Altered function of insulin receptor substrate-1-deficient mouse islets and cultured beta-cell lines. *J Clin Invest* 1999;104:R69.

125. Araki E, Lipes MA, Patti ME, *et al*: Alternative pathway of insulin signalling in mice with targeted disruption of the IRS-1 gene. *Nature* 1994;372:186.

126. Xu GG, Gao ZY, Borge PD, *et al*: Insulin receptor substrate 1-induced inhibition of endoplasmic reticulum Ca^{2+} uptake in beta-cells. Autocrine regulation of intracellular Ca^{2+} homeostasis and insulin secretion. *J Biol Chem* 1999;274:18067.

127. Mauvais-Jarvis F, Virkamaki A, Michael MD, *et al*: A model to explore the interaction between muscle insulin resistance and beta-cell dysfunction in the development of type 2 diabetes. *Diabetes* 2000;49: 2126.

128. Sutherland DER, Gores PF, Hering BJ, *et al*: Islet transplantation: An update. *Diabetes Metab Rev* 1996;12:137.

129. Shapiro AMJ, Lakey JRT, Ryan EA, *et al*: Islet transplantation in seven patients with type 1 diabetes mellitus using a glucocorticoid-free immunosuppressive regimen. *N Engl J Med* 2000;343:230.

130. Moore H-P, Walker MD, Lee F, *et al*: Expressing a human proinsulin cDNA in a mouse ACTH-secreting cell. Intracellular storage, proteolytic processing, and secretion on stimulation. *Cell* 1983;35:531.

131. Hughes SD, Quaade C, Milburn JL, *et al*: Expression of normal and novel glucokinase mRNAs in anterior pituitary and islet cells. *J Biol Chem* 1991;266:4521.

132. BeltrandelRio H, Schnedl WJ, Ferber S, *et al*: Genetic engineering of insulin secreting cell lines. In: Lanza RP, Chick WL, eds. *Pancreatic Islet Transplantation*, vol. 1: *Procurement of Pancreatic Islets*. RG Landes Co.:1994;169.

133. Clark SA, Burnham BL, Chick WL: Modulation of glucose-induced insulin secretion from a rat clonal β-cell line. *Endocrinology* 1990; 127:2779.

134. Miyazaki J-I, Araki K, Yamato E, *et al*: Establishment of a pancreatic β-cell line that retains glucose-inducible insulin secretion: Special reference to expression of glucose transporter isoforms. *Endocrinology* 1990;127:126.

135. Efrat S, Leiser M, Surana M, *et al*: Murine insulinoma cell line with normal glucose-regulated insulin secretion. *Diabetes* 1993;42:901.

136. Efrat S, Linde S, Kofod H, *et al*: Beta-cell lines derived from transgenic mice expressing a hybrid insulin gene-oncogene. *Proc Natl Acad Sci USA* 1988;85:9037.

137. Knaack D, Fiore DM, Surana M, *et al*: Clonal insulinoma cell line that stably maintains correct glucose responsiveness. *Diabetes* 1994;43: 1413.

138. Zhou D, Sun AM, Li X, *et al*: In vitro and in vivo evaluation of insulin-producing βTC6-F7 cells in microcapsules. *Am J Physiol* 1998;43:C1356.

139. Efrat S, Fusco-DeMane D, Lemberg H, *et al*: Conditional transformation of a pancreatic beta-cell line derived from transgenic mice expressing a tetracycline-regulated oncogene. *Proc Natl Acad Sci USA* 1995;92:3576.

140. Mandrup-Poulsen T: The role of interleukin-1 in the pathogenesis of IDDM. *Diabetologia* 1996;39:1005.

141. Rabinovitch A: Roles of cytokines in IDDM pathogenesis and islet β-cell destruction. *Diabetes Rev* 1993;1:215.

142. Corbett JA, McDaniel M: Does nitric oxide mediate autoimmune destruction of β-cells? Possible therapeutic interventions in IDDM. *Diabetes* 1992;41:897.

143. Eizirik DL, Flodstrom M, Karlsen AE, *et al*: The harmony of the spheres: Inducible nitric oxide synthase and related genes in pancreatic beta cells. *Diabetologia* 1996;39:875.

144. Faustman D, Coe C: Prevention of xenograft rejection by masking donor HLA class I antigens. *Science* 1991;252:1700.

145. Efrat S, Fejer G, Brownlee M, *et al*: Prolonged survival of pancreatic islet allografts mediated by adenovirus immunoregulatory transgenes. *Proc Natl Acad Sci USA* 1995;92:6947.

146. von Herrath MG, Efrat S, Oldstone MB: Expression of adenoviral E3 transgenes in beta cells prevents autoimmune diabetes. *Proc Natl Acad Sci USA* 1997;94:9808.

147. Mueller R, Krahl R, Sarvetnick N: Pancreatic expression of interleukin-4 abrogates insulitis and autoimmune diabetes in nonobese diabetic (NOD) mice. *J Exp Med* 1996;184:1093.

148. Mueller R, Davies JD, Krahl T, *et al*: IL-4 expression by grafts from transgenic mice fails to prevent allograft rejection. *J Immunol* 1997;159:1599.

149. Lau HT, Yu M, Fontana A, *et al*: Prevention of allograft rejection with engineered myoblasts expressing FasL in mice. *Science* 1996;273:109.

150. Kang SM, Schneider DB, Lin Z, *et al*: Fas ligand expression in islets of Langerhans does not confer immune privilege and instead targets them for rapid destruction. *Nature Med* 1997;3:738.

151. Rabinovitch A, Suarez-Pinzon W, Strynadka K, *et al*: Transfection of human pancreatic islets with an anti-apoptotic gene (bcl-2) protects beta-cells from cytokine-induced destruction. *Diabetes* 1999;48:1223.

152. Hohmeier H, Thigpen A, Tran V, *et al*: Stable expression of manganese superoxide dismutase (MnSOD) in insulinoma cells prevents IL-1β-induced cytotoxicity and reduces nitric oxide production. *J Clin Invest* 1998;101:1811.

153. Lortz S, Tiedge M, Nachtwey T, *et al*: Protection of insulin-producing RINm5F cells against cytokine-mediated toxicity through overexpression of antioxidant enzymes. *Diabetes* 2000;49:1123.

154. Natoli G, Costanzo A, Ianni A, *et al*: Activation of SAPK/JNK by TNF receptor 1 through a noncytotoxic TRAF2-dependent pathway. *Science* 1997;275:200.

155. Wajant H, Johannes FJ, Haas E, *et al*: Dominant-negative FADD inhibits RNFR60-, FAS/APO1- and TRAIL-R/APO2-mediated cell death but not gene induction. *Curr Biol* 1998;8:113.

156. Dupraz P, Cottet S, Hamburger F, *et al*: Dominant negative MyD88 proteins inhibit interleukin-1 beta/interferon-gamma-mediated induction of nuclear factor kappa B-dependent nitrite production and apoptosis in beta cells. *J Biol Chem* 2000;275:37672.

157. Zhou YP, Pena JC, Roe MW, *et al*: Overexpression of Bcl-x(L) in beta-cells prevents cell death but impairs mitochondrial signal for insulin secretion. *Am J Physiol* 2000;278:E340.

158. Chen G, Hohmeier HE, Gasa R, *et al*: Selection of insulinoma cell lines with resistance to IL-1β- and IFN-γ-induced cytotoxicity. *Diabetes* 2000;49:562.

159. Chen G, Hohmeier HE, Newgard CB: Expression of the transcription factor STAT-1α in insulinoma cells protects against cytotoxicity induced by multiple cytokines. *J Biol Chem* 2001;276:766.

160. Lee HC, Bonner-Weir S, Weir GC, *et al*: Compensatory adaptation to partial pancreatectomy in the rat. *Endocrinology* 1992;124:1571.

161. Sarvetnick N, Liggitt D, Pitts SL, *et al*: Insulin-dependent diabetes mellitus induced in transgenic mice by ectopic expression of class II MHC and interferon-gamma. *Cell* 1988;52:773.

162. Ramiya VK, Maraist M, Arfors KE, *et al*: Reversal of insulin-dependent diabetes using islets generated in vitro from pancreatic stem cells. *Nature Med* 2000;6:278.

163. Bonner-Weir S, Taneja M, Weir GC, *et al*: In vitro cultivation of human islets from expanded ductal tissue. *Proc Natl Acad Sci USA* 2000;97:7999.

164. Soria B, Roche E, Berna G, *et al*: Insulin-secreting cells derived from embryonic stem cells normalize glycemia in streptozotocin-induced diabetic mice. *Diabetes* 2000;49:157.

165. Lee HC, Kim S-J, Kim K-S, *et al*: Remission in models of type 1 diabetes by gene therapy using a single-chain insulin analogue. *Nature* 2000;408:483.

166. Ferber S, Halkin A, Cohen H, *et al*: Pancreatic and duodenal homeobox gene 1 induces expression of insulin genes in liver and ameliorates streptozotocin-induced hyperglycemia. *Nature Med* 2000;6:568.

167. Cheung AT, Dayanandan B, Lewis JT, *et al*: Glucose-dependent insulin release from genetically engineering K cells. *Science* 2000;290:1959.

C H A P T E R   1 5

Immunology Relevant To Diabetes

Charles A. Janeway, Jr.

F. Susan Wong

Type 1 or insulin-dependent diabetes mellitus (T1DM) is widely considered to be an autoimmune disease. This hypothesis is based on a number of independent findings, including the presence of a lymphocytic infiltrate known as insulitis in the islets of recently diabetic individuals, the specificity of pancreatic β-cell destruction, the observation that diabetic patients transplanted with identical twin pancreas grafts rapidly and selectively destroy the β cells in the grafted tissue, the presence of antibodies to islet antigens, and numerous studies in animal models.[1] Thus, to understand the pathogenesis of T1DM, one must have a working knowledge of immunology and of autoimmune diseases.[2,3] In this chapter, relevant features of the immune system will be briefly described, followed by a discussion of the autoimmune pathogenesis of type 1 diabetes in humans as illustrated by studies of experimental animal models. Following that discussion, the possibility of treating, and more importantly of preventing, type 1 diabetes will be discussed. See Chap. 20 for a discussion of the clinical findings and pathophysiology of type 1 diabetes in humans.

ADAPTIVE IMMUNITY: THE CLONAL SELECTION OF ANTIGEN-SPECIFIC LYMPHOCYTES

The immune system has as its primary function the defense of the host against infection. Two discrete classes of immunity exist. Innate immune defense mechanisms such as phagocytosis defend against a broad range of microorganisms but do not provide protection against specific pathogens; these fail to control most pathogens. Adaptive immunity involves immune responses that are specific to individual pathogens and provide long-lasting protection against reinfection with agents previously encountered either naturally or as a result of deliberate immunization. As far as can be determined, innate immune mechanisms have been evolutionarily selected to discriminate self from certain classes of nonself microorganisms. Thus, innate immune mechanisms have no means for recognizing or attacking host cells, and do not participate detectably in autoimmune phenomena. For this reason, this chapter will focus on those aspects of adaptive immune responses that are pertinent to autoimmune disease.

Adaptive immunity operates by clonal selection of individual lymphocytes that recognize specific macromolecular antigens. Clonal selection is the basic operating principle of the adaptive immune response, and is shown schematically in Fig. 15-1. In brief,

the basis of clonal selection is the development within individual lymphocytes of antigen receptors of essentially infinite diversity. During its ontogeny, each lymphocyte generates a unique set of receptor genes that encode a unique cell-surface antigen receptor. As soon as these genes are formed, the receptor is expressed on the surface of the lymphocyte. If the receptor recognizes a ubiquitous self-antigen that is also present in the site of lymphocyte development, this recognition leads to the induction of programmed cell death within the developing lymphocyte. In this way, a repertoire of receptors of random specificity is purged of those receptors that recognize self-antigens.[4] The remaining cells mature functionally and leave the site of lymphocyte development. These cells are now equipped with receptors that recognize all possible antigens other than ubiquitous self-antigens. If a lymphocyte encounters its specific antigen, the binding of antigen to the lymphocyte receptor triggers the lymphocyte's activation, its proliferation to increase the numbers of specific cells, and the differentiation of its expanded progeny into effector cells that can remove the antigen from the body. Some of its progeny also differentiate into long-lived memory lymphocytes that maintain a heightened state of immunity against the initial antigen. In this way, long-lasting protection against a previously encountered pathogen is generated through clonal selection.

In order to fully understand how the adaptive immune response operates through clonal selection, it is necessary to understand the nature of lymphocyte receptors and the genes that encode them, certain aspects of lymphocyte development, and the activation of lymphocytes by antigen. Finally, it is important to understand the effector mechanisms by which lymphocytes rid the body of pathogens, as these same effector mechanisms are used to damage self-tissues.

LYMPHOCYTE RECEPTORS AND THE GENERATION OF LYMPHOCYTE DIVERSITY

There are two main categories of lymphocytes, known as *B lymphocytes* and *T lymphocytes*. B lymphocytes develop in the bursae of Fabricius in birds and the bone marrow in mammals, whereas T lymphocytes develop in the thymus (hence their names). These two classes of lymphocytes have distinct receptors that allow them to recognize antigens displayed in different bodily compartments. B lymphocytes are the precursors of antibody-producing cells, and

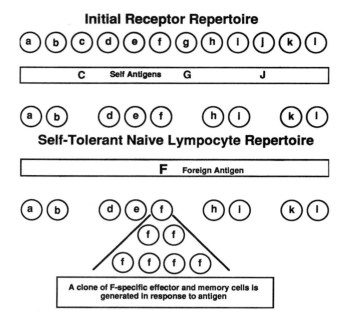

Initial Receptor Repertoire

Self-Tolerant Naive Lymphocyte Repertoire

FIGURE 15-1. Adaptive immunity occurs by clonal selection of lympho-cytes. Each lymphocyte develops bearing a single receptor for antigen. Those lymphocytes whose receptors recognize ubiquitous self-antigens will bind antigen as soon as their receptors are expressed on the cell sur-face, and this induces programmed cell death, purging the initial repertoire of such self-reactive cells. Foreign antigens encountered in the peripheral lymphoid organs induce growth in lymphocytes bearing receptors specific for that antigen; growth is followed by differentiation into effector cells that remove the antigen and generate long-lasting immunologic memory that protects against subsequent encounters with the same antigen.

their cell-surface receptors are identical in specificity to the anti-bodies they will later secrete into the extracellular fluid and are en-coded by the same genes. T lymphocytes, by contrast, have recep-tors that are specialized to recognize antigens actually produced within the cell; this system allows T lymphocytes to detect and act on cells that are sequestering cytoplasmic pathogens. Although performing quite distinct recognition functions, T- and B-lympho-cyte receptors have a great deal in common, having evolved from a common ancestral set of genes and using essentially identical mechanisms to generate the diversity of receptor specificities ne-cessitated by clonal selection.

The diversity of lymphocyte receptors appears to be necessary in order to allow the immune system to recognize all possible pathogens, no matter how recently they arose in evolution. Because microorganisms evolve far more rapidly than their mammalian hosts, the generation of diversity is vested mainly in processes that occur in somatic cells. Thus what evolution has selected for is the ability to generate diverse receptors rather than the genes encoding the receptors themselves.

The antigen recognition sites on antibodies and T-cell recep-tors are formed by the association of two polypeptide chains, each consisting of a series of similarly folded domains of about 110 amino acids. The amino terminal domain is highly variable in se-quence and is called a *variable* or *V domain*. The more C-terminal domains of both B- and T-cell receptor chains have a single amino-acid sequence for all chains of a given type, and are called *constant* or *C domains*. These C domains impart functional capacity to the receptors, whereas the V domains make the extensively varying

antigen-recognition site. Diversity comes from the individual vari-ability of each chain, as well as from the combinatorial diversity produced by pairing two individual variable domains together in all possible combinations to form functional receptors.

There are several distinct sources of diversity that contribute to the variability of variable domains in antibodies and T-cell recep-tors. Each receptor chain is encoded in clusters of gene segments that together encode the finished receptor. The variable domain is encoded in two or three separate gene segments, which must un-dergo recombination in developing lymphocytes before they can be expressed as intact proteins. One chain of each receptor, the light immunoglobulin chain and the α chain of the T-cell receptor, is en-coded in two separate gene segments, a *V-gene segment* that en-codes the first 95 or so amino acids of the domain, and a *J* or *join-ing gene segment* that encodes the last 15 or so amino acids. Any V-gene segment can be joined to any J-gene segment, so the total number of distinct V domains that can be generated is the product of the number of V-gene segments times the number of J-gene seg-ments. In the case of immunoglobulin heavy-chain and T-cell receptor β-chain genes, the complete V domain is assembled from a V-gene segment, a J-gene segment, and a gene segment known as *D* or *diversity* that joins the V- to the J-gene segment. The number of distinct immunoglobulin heavy-chain and T-cell recep-tor β chains that can be formed is the product of the number of V-gene segments, the number of D-gene segments, and the number of J-gene segments. Thus each individual inherits a significant ca-pacity to generate diversity in the form of the different numbers of V-, D-, and J-gene segments for each receptor chain.

A further significant source of receptor diversification occurs at the site of gene segment joining. During the joining process, at least two different processes contribute to diversification at each receptor gene segment junction. First, the precise site at which codons are cleaved and joined is variable. Second, during the formation of gene segment joints, certain nucleotides are removed enzymatically from the site of joining, and more importantly, nucleotides can be added at the site of gene segment joining by two different processes. One of these involves nucleotides of the opposite strand of DNA at the site of gene segment cleavage, forming *palindromic* or *P nucleotides*; the other involves the random addition of *nongenomically encoded* or *N nucleotides* to the ends of the cleaved gene segments by the en-zyme terminal deoxynucleotidyl transferase. These two processes together increase the diversity of lymphocyte receptors very signifi-cantly, adding at least a factor of 100 to the extent of diversity in gene segment junctions. Because there are two junctions of this type in immunoglobulin heavy chains and T-cell receptor β chains, the amplification in diversity in these double junctions is at least 10,000-fold. More importantly, this tremendous diversity is found in the center of the antigen-recognition site in the folded protein. Thus the region of the receptor molecule most involved in antigen recognition is also the site of the greatest somatic diversification (Fig. 15-2).[5]

Finally, for completeness, it is worth mentioning that B-cell re-ceptors and the antibodies produced from them can undergo further diversification upon stimulation by antigen. This diversification oc-curs through a process of *hypermutation* in proliferating B cells. This somatic hypermutation is targeted at the rearranged genes en-coding the antibody variable domains, and acts in such a way that those B cells whose receptors bind antigen most strongly after so-matic hypermutation has occurred are selectively expanded in con-sequence of their improved antigen binding. Because of this, the efficiency of the antibody response increases enormously during the course of the response. This mode of somatic hypermutation

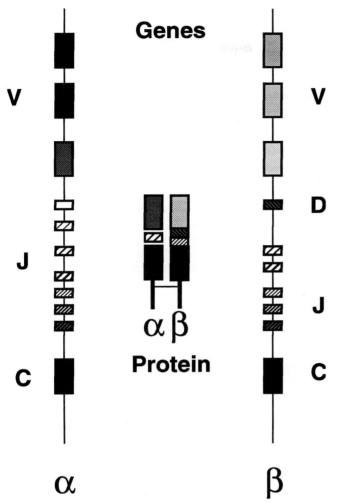

Genes

V

J

C

α β

Protein

V

D

J

C

α   β

FIGURE 15-2. The antigen receptors on T lymphocytes consist of two chains, α and β. Each has a variable (V) domain that is assembled from the somatic recombination of gene segments in developing T cells: V and J in the case of α-chains; V, D, and J in the case of β-chains; and a constant domain. The two chains pair to form a disulfide-bonded heterodimeric protein on the surface of T lymphocytes, with antigen recognition resulting from the pairing of the two variable domains. Diversity comes both from joining different combinations of the multiple V, D, and J gene segments, and from differences in the way in which the gene segments are joined together during lymphocyte development. Immunoglobulin genes that encode B-cell receptors and antibodies are assembled in a very similar fashion in developing B cells.

has not been observed for T cells, so all of the diversity in T-cell receptors is generated prior to the expression of the receptor on the cell surface. This has important consequences for differences in tolerance between T and B lymphocytes.

T-LYMPHOCYTE RECOGNITION OF ANTIGENS AS PEPTIDES BOUND TO MOLECULES ENCODED IN THE MAJOR HISTOCOMPATIBILITY COMPLEX

As mentioned earlier, T lymphocytes are specialized to recognize pathogens that reside in the cytoplasmic compartments of the cell. T cells can detect when a cell is harboring a pathogen because the

receptor on T cells recognizes antigen in the form of peptide fragments of the pathogen bound stably to molecules encoded in the *major histocompatibility complex* (MHC). The sole known function of MHC molecules is to present peptide fragments of antigen to T lymphocytes at the surface of infected cells.[6]

MHC molecules have a novel structure in that the complete molecule expressed at the cell surface consists of three polypeptide chains, only two of which are complete polypeptides shared by all MHC molecules. The third chain in MHC molecules consists of a peptide fragment of a cellular or foreign protein. This third peptidic element is required for the completion of MHC molecular structure; its presence allows MHC molecules to perform their antigen-presenting function.

MHC molecules exist in two distinct forms, known as MHC *class I* and *class II molecules*. MHC class I molecules have a heavy or α chain encoded within the MHC; this heavy chain associates noncovalently with a non-MHC protein known as β_2 microglobulin. The outer two domains of the heavy or α chain, α_1 and α_2, are extensively polymorphic and form a cleft into which an eight- or nine-amino-acid peptide binds during the assembly of the MHC class I molecule. MHC class I molecules that lack this third peptide chain are retained in the endoplasmic reticulum; they are highly unstable at 37°C. When MHC class I molecules are synthesized in the endoplasmic reticulum, they rapidly bind to β_2 microglobulin, but are retained in the endoplasmic reticulum by their association with a specific peptide transporter known as TAP-1/TAP-2. This heterodimeric ATP-binding cassette protein delivers peptides of 8–15 amino acids generated in the cytosolic compartment of the cell to the lumen of the endoplasmic reticulum. If these peptides bind to the associated empty MHC class I molecules, then the MHC class I molecule completes its folding upon binding peptide and is released from the TAP-1/TAP-2 complex. These stable MHC class I molecules are rapidly transported to the cell surface, where they present the peptide to passing T lymphocytes.

The T lymphocytes that recognize MHC class I–associated peptides are a distinct subclass known as *CD8 T cells*, because they express on their surface a molecule known as CD8. CD8 T cells are specialized to kill cells infected with viruses and other pathogens that replicate in the cytosol. CD8 binds to the lateral face of the MHC class I molecule, whereas the T-cell receptor binds over the peptide-binding cleft at the distal end of the MHC class I molecule. Thus, the T-cell receptor discriminates one MHC class I molecule from another on the basis of the peptide bound to it, whereas CD8 can recognize any MHC class I molecule. CD8 not only binds to MHC class I molecules, but when it binds in conjunction with the T-cell receptor, it greatly facilitates antigen recognition by the T-cell receptor. For this reason, CD8 is known as a *coreceptor molecule*.[7,8]

The other type of MHC molecule, the MHC class II, presents peptides at the cell surface that derive from proteins degraded in cellular vesicles. MHC class II molecules consist of two polypeptide chains, both of which are encoded within the MHC. The folded structure of the MHC class II molecule is very similar to that of the MHC class I molecule,[9] but they present peptides derived from different cellular compartments. MHC class II molecules, like class I molecules, are synthesized and assembled in the endoplasmic reticulum. However, MHC class II molecules assemble together with a third, nonpolymorphic chain known as the *invariant chain* or *Ii*, and MHC class II molecules bound to Ii are not able to bind peptide. Moreover, the invariant chain appears to direct MHC class II molecules to a particular cellular vesicle in which the invariant chain is degraded by acidic proteases, and peptides present in this vesicle bind to the now-exposed MHC class II peptide-binding cleft. The invariant chain serves to protect MHC class II molecules from binding peptides in the lumen of the endoplasmic reticulum, and thus avoids the presentation of peptides derived from cytosolic proteins.[6]

MHC class II molecules are recognized at the cell surface by T cells expressing a distinct coreceptor known as *CD4*. Peripheral T cells express either CD4 or CD8 and are specific for MHC class II– or class I–associated peptides, respectively. CD4 T cells have a number of immunologic functions, the most important of which are the activation of infected macrophages to destroy bacteria residing in cellular vesicles and the activation of B lymphocytes to produce antibody. B lymphocytes use their immunoglobulin receptors to convert external antigens into internal ones by binding them and internalizing them into cellular vesicles, and then degrade these proteins into peptides that bind to MHC class II molecules that are expressed on the B-cell surface. Antigen-specific helper T cells recognize those B cells whose surface immunoglobulins effectively bind antigen through the expression of these peptide:MHC class II molecules on the B-cell surface, and selectively activate antigen-binding B cells in this way. In both types of recognition, CD4 binds to the lateral face of the MHC class II molecule and provides coreceptor function to the T-cell receptor in the recognition of peptides bound to MHC class II molecules (Fig. 15-3).[10]

MHC GENE POLYMORPHISM AND ANTIGEN RECOGNITION BY T CELLS

The genes encoding the proteins of the MHC are the most polymorphic genes yet described in the human genome. There are three major loci encoding MHC class I α chains, and four or more encoding MHC class II β chains. At many of these loci,

FIGURE 15-3. T cells come in two distinct types, differentiated by expression of the coreceptor proteins CD4 and CD8. CD8 T cells are specialized to kill cells that present peptide fragments of antigens degraded in cytosol and displayed at the cell surface by MHC class I molecules. The CD8 coreceptor binds the same MHC class I molecule as the T-cell receptor and contributes to signaling for T-cell activation. CD4 T cells are specialized to activate cells, such as macrophages and B cells, that present peptide fragments of antigens degraded in cytoplasmic vesicles, such as endosomes and lysosomes, and displayed at the cell surface by MHC class II molecules. The CD4 coreceptor binds the same MHC class II molecule as the T-cell receptor and contributes to signaling for T-cell activation.

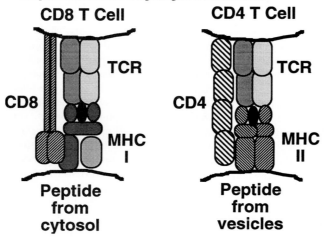

well over 50 alleles are known to exist. Some of this polymorphism is detectable using antibodies, but the remainder must be detected using either T-cell recognition or nucleic acid sequencing. Human MHC proteins are known as *human leukocyte antigens* or *HLAs*, and human MHC class I molecules are known as HLA-A, -B, and -C. Human MHC class II molecules are known as HLA-D proteins, and are subdivided further into DR, DQ, and DP molecules.

The extensive polymorphism of MHC proteins is largely focused on the peptide-binding groove of the MHC molecule. These polymorphic differences alter the peptide-binding characteristics of the MHC molecule, such that different MHC molecules will present different peptides derived from the same protein. Moreover, the polymorphism of MHC molecules also influences the binding of T-cell receptors to MHC:peptide complexes. Precisely how this occurs is not known, but the same exact peptide bound to two different MHC molecules is readily distinguished by T cells. This phenomenon, which is an intrinsic property of T-cell receptors, is known as *MHC restriction*, because genes at the MHC restrict the antigen-recognition capabilities of individual T-cell receptors (Fig. 15-4).[11] In general, MHC restriction is highly MHC specific, such that a given T-cell receptor will recognize its cognate peptide bound only to one or a very few allelic variants of a given MHC molecule. Thus MHC polymorphism affects T-cell recognition in two quite distinct ways: first by altering peptide binding, and second by altering the interaction of the peptide:MHC complex with T-cell receptors. MHC polymorphism is a major genetic factor in determining susceptibility to T1DM and most other autoimmune diseases, and this is likely to reflect the ability of certain MHC allelic variants to present a specific autoantigen to a specific set of T-cell receptors. It also imposes severe constraints on T-cell development, as we will see in the next section.

THE DEVELOPMENT AND SELECTION OF LYMPHOCYTES

We have seen in earlier sections that lymphocyte receptors are assembled from gene segments during the development of individual lymphocytes, and that each lymphocyte assembles different gene segments and makes different junctions that encode its unique receptor, so that the totality of receptors forms a highly diverse repertoire of recognition capabilities. Moreover, we have seen that when ubiquitous self-antigens are now encountered by these receptors, the immature lymphocyte is programmed to die, following an apoptotic pathway. In the case of B lymphocytes, these are the only events about which we have information. However, in the case of T lymphocytes, a further event is necessitated by the nature of antigen recognition by T-cell receptors and by the polymorphism of MHC molecules.

We saw in the preceding section that T-cell receptors will only recognize peptides bound to a particular allelic variant of a MHC molecule, and that a given locus may encode as many as 100 different variants. Because the rearrangement of receptor gene segments is completely random, and because an individual can only express 2 out of the possible 100 alleles at a given MHC locus, it is highly likely that most T-cell receptors that form in an individual will not be able to recognize foreign peptides bound to any of that individual's MHC molecules. If such cells were allowed to differentiate, they would fill the periphery with T lymphocytes that are useless. However, this does not occur because T cells must un-

FIGURE 15-4. Antigen recognition by T cells is governed by polymorphism of MHC molecules. The MHC molecules have a deep cleft in their outer aspect that must be occupied by a peptide in order for the molecule to be displayed at the cell surface. The peptide-binding groove is formed by two α helices overlying a β pleated sheet, and the polymorphic residues in the MHC molecule mainly line the peptide-binding groove. Thus, a T cell is specific for a particular combination of peptide and self-MHC, here MHC IIa (**left**). When this T cell is confronted with a different MHC molecule, here MHC IIb, the nonself-MHC molecules will bind different peptides of a protein (**center**), or will present a different overall conformation of peptide and MHC molecule when binding the peptide (**right**). For this reason, T cells show specificity not only for a particular antigen, but also for a particular allelic form of MHC molecule, a property known as MHC restriction in antigen recognition.

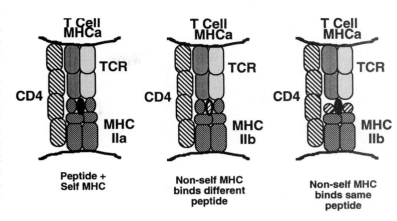

dergo a further selective event during their development within the thymus that circumvents this problem. This process is known as *positive selection* because it selects for further maturation only those T cells whose receptors are capable of recognizing foreign peptides bound to a self-MHC molecule. T cells can only mature if their receptors interact appropriately with MHC molecules binding self-peptide likely that they encounter within the thymus. If the T-cell receptor binds self-MHC/self-peptide sufficiently well to trigger T-cell activation, the result is that the T cell dies, a process called *negative selection*, crucial for preventing the development of autoreactive T cells. The weaker signal that triggers positive selection is not yet understood, but it is clearly essential for T-cell development. The consequence of this process is that all T cells that leave the thymus have receptors able to recognize foreign peptides presented by self-MHC molecules.[12] That is, all of the T cells put into the peripheral repertoire appear to be potentially useful. This positive selection event for self-MHC recognition appears to also involve recognition of self-peptides, but at a level too low to trigger T-cell activation, thus avoiding problems of autorecognition.[13,14]

T-LYMPHOCYTE ACTIVATION, ANTIGEN RECOGNITION, AND COSTIMULATORY SIGNALS

The naïve or unstimulated T cell is a small cell with scanty cytoplasm and condensed nuclear chromatin; it is metabolically very poorly active and cannot carry out any effector function. Moreover, T lymphocytes specific for a given peptide are extremely rare. Thus before a T cell can participate in adaptive immunity, it must recognize antigen and undergo extensive proliferation to increase the number of cells of the relevant specificity, and these must then differentiate into cells capable of mediating effector functions. This occurs over a period of 4–5 days after introducing antigen, and results in an approximately 1000-fold increase in the number of specific cells and their differentiation from resting into active effector cells.

The cells that stimulate T-cell proliferation and differentiation are known as *antigen-presenting cells (APCs)*. For a cell to be able to present antigen to a T cell, it must display the appropriate complex of peptide and MHC on its surface. However, the mere expression of peptide and MHC on the surface of a cell is not sufficient to trigger T-cell proliferation and differentiation into effector

cells. Rather, the T cell needs to receive a signal known as a *costimulatory signal* from the same antigen-presenting cell.[15–17] The major molecules involved in the costimulation of T-cell growth and differentiation are known as B7.1 and B7.2, related molecules that bind to the T-cell molecule CD28 and a related structure known as CTLA4. The simultaneous binding of the T-cell receptor and its coreceptor to specific peptide: MHC and of CD28 to B7.1 or B7.2 triggers the proliferation of T cells and ultimately their differentiation into effector cells. These effector cells can now act on any cell displaying its specific peptide:MHC ligand, allowing effector T cells to act on any cell in the body once activated (Fig. 15-5).

The requirement for costimulation means that only those cells that can express costimulatory molecules can activate naïve T cells. Only a few cell types in the body appear to have this capacity normally, and these are cells that are concentrated in lymphoid organs, the site in which naïve T cells are initially activated by antigen. Tissue cells do not express costimulatory molecules. When a naïve T cell recognizes a peptide:MHC complex on a tissue cell, it tends to be inactivated by that encounter. This is important, because not all tissue antigens are expressed in sites of lymphocyte development, and most specifically in the thymus, the site of T-cell development. These T cells specific for peripheral self-antigens are not eliminated, but they also are not activated when they encounter their specific antigen on a tissue cell, and this is important in avoiding

FIGURE 15-5. T-cell activation requires the expression of antigen and a costimulatory molecule such as B7.1 or B7.2 on the same antigen-presenting cell (**APC**). The simultaneous signaling of the peptide:MHC complex to the T-cell receptor (**TCR**) and of B7.1 or B7.2 to CD28 induces clonal expression of T cells and their differentiation into effector T cells. Effector T cells can be triggered to mediate their function, such as cell killing, in the absence of costimulatory signals on the target cell. Lymphocytes that encounter antigen in the absence of costimulatory signals may be rendered inactive or tolerant by signals received only through the T-cell antigen receptor.

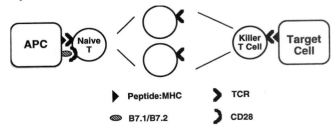

the induction of autoimmunity. Thus T cells may be rendered tolerant either by deletion through recognition of ubiquitous self-antigens in the thymus or through inactivation by recognition of tissue-specific autoantigens in peripheral tissues. The requirement for costimulation also provides a second level of regulation of immune responses, not only through the presence or absence of antigen, but also through the expression or lack of the costimulator on a given cell.

EFFECTOR FUNCTIONS OF ACTIVATED T CELLS

We have already mentioned that CD8 T cells differentiate into cytotoxic effector cells, able to kill any cell expressing specific peptide:MHC class I complexes on the cell surface. The main function of cytotoxic T cells appears to be to eliminate cells that are infected with viruses. Viruses replicate in the cytosolic compartment of host cells, and peptides deriving from the viruses are presented by MHC class I molecules to CD8 T cells. The killing of these infected cells eliminates the site of viral replication, thus contributing to the clearance of viral infections. The cell must be killed, because cells have no internal means for destroying viral genomes they harbor. CD8 T cells also produce interferon-γ, which can inhibit viral replication, and this is also an important mechanism in controlling viral infection.

CD4 T cells, by contrast, are specialized to activate cells expressing peptide associated with MHC class II complexes. MHC class II molecules are expressed mainly by specialized effector cells of the immune system, including macrophages that are infected with vesicular bacteria or have ingested them, and B lymphocytes that bind antigen and can be activated to produce antibody. The CD4 T cells that activate macrophages make small proteins known as *cytokines* that mediate their effector function, and these are distinct from the cytokines made by the CD4 T cells that activate B cells. These two cell types, known respectively as Th1 and Th2, mediate cell-mediated and humoral immunity, respectively.[18,19]

EVIDENCE FOR AUTOIMMUNE DESTRUCTION OF PANCREATIC β CELLS IN TYPE 1 DIABETES

As described at the start of the chapter, there is extensive evidence suggesting immunologically mediated destruction of pancreatic β cells in type 1 diabetes. Inflammatory cell infiltrates have been demonstrated in the islets of patients who have died at the time of clinical diagnosis of diabetes.[20,21] This lymphocytic infiltrate is of mixed lineage, containing macrophages and both CD4 and CD8 T cells.[22] Thus it is assumed that the inflammatory infiltrate is related to the destruction of β cells and is in fact driven by the recognition of β-cell autoantigens, because in the absence of β cells found in long-term diabetic patients, no infiltrate is observed.

This idea was given significant impetus by the results of identical twin hemipancreas grafting.[23] Hemipancreatic grafts from an identical twin who did not have diabetes into a sibling who had been diagnosed with T1DM many years previously led to almost immediate normalization of blood glucose. However, in the absence of immunosuppressive drugs, β-cell function was lost rapidly after grafting as β cells were destroyed. The loss of cells was accompanied by an islet infiltrate dominated by CD8 T cells, and selective β-cell destruction was observed in the grafted tissue.[24] This destructive process could be inhibited by standard immuno-

suppressive drugs such as cyclosporin A. The process was β-cell specific in that other cells in the islet, the exocrine pancreas, and frequently a syngeneic renal graft were all maintained without any sign of inflammation.

Another sign of the involvement of autoimmunity in the pathogenesis of T1DM is the finding of numerous autoantibodies to different proteins found in β cells. The earliest antibodies to be detected were to islet cells,[25,26] although the molecules that these antibodies recognized were not known. Subsequently, detection of specific autoantibodies in prediabetic and newly diagnosed patients with diabetes has given us clues to the nature of the autoantigenic targets. These included proteins such as insulin,[27] glutamic acid decarboxylase (GAD),[28,29] and more recently, the tyrosine phosphatase IA-2/ICA512.[30,31] Others have also been identified, such as bovine serum albumin, insulin receptor, sialoglycolipid, glucose transporter, hsp 65, carboxypeptidase H, 52-kd protein, and 150-kd protein, as reviewed in reference 32.

Because a major role for CD4 cells is to "help" B cells produce antibodies, the production of autoantibodies against proteins found in β cells strongly suggests that helper CD4 T cells specific for peptides contained within these proteins are also activated as part of the diabetic process. Because patients frequently make several different antibodies to distinct proteins, it is likely that the helper CD4 T-cell response in diabetes is quite diverse. However, because the only cells available for study in diabetes in humans are peripheral blood lymphocytes and the quantity of cells likely to be involved in pathogenesis is small, it is difficult to investigate the specificity of potentially pathogenic cells. Nevertheless, it has been possible to clone CD4 T cells to putative autoantigens in humans such as to insulin[33] and IA-2,[34] but the pathogenicity of these cells has not been established. Although much less studied, there is increasing evidence that CD8 T cells may also be equally important, and the presence of cytotoxic CD8 T cells reactive to GAD has also been shown in recently diabetic patients.[35]

The final evidence that diabetes is an autoimmune disease is the linkage of susceptibility to genes in the MHC.[36] The data linking type 1 diabetes to MHC are strong, but in humans there is no conclusive direct evidence that the susceptibility gene is, in fact, an MHC glycoprotein. Much work has concentrated on the HLA-DQ molecules as being crucial for susceptibility to T1DM, but these data are not conclusive. It is interesting, in this context, that certain DQ alleles are highly protective against type 1 diabetes.[37] This further suggests that the pathogenesis of T1DM involves CD4 T cells. However it is clear, in consideration of susceptibility to disease, that larger haplotypes that include the MHC class I molecules are important,[38,39] and although there is no direct evidence, this has implications for the role of CD8 T cells. Nevertheless, the precise roles of MHC molecules and of T cells in β-cell destruction in humans remain to be elucidated. It may ultimately be possible to begin to study the direct role of these molecules in the future with the development of "humanized" animal models, such as those expressing human MHC molecules.[40,41]

EVIDENCE FROM ANIMAL MODELS THAT TYPE 1 DIABETES IS AN AUTOIMMUNE DISEASE

A number of animal models exist for type 1 diabetes. The two that are most extensively studied are the spontaneous type 1 diabetes that occurs in BB/W rats[42] and nonobese diabetic (NOD) mice.[43] Type 1 diabetes in these two animal models is spontaneous. The disease occurs in the majority of individuals, is strongly controlled by genes mapping to the MHC, is transferable with T cells, and is prevented by T cell depletion. T-cell responses in NOD mice of various ages have been shown to a number of putative autoantigens.[44,45] The incidence of disease in NOD mice is also altered by a variety of genetic and immunologic manipulations.[46] The BB rat is rather less susceptible to these manipulations. Autoantibodies are produced in NOD mice to GAD[47] and insulin,[48] although this is not universally found in all NOD mouse colonies. Although much of what we believe about autoimmunity in type 1 diabetes comes from studying animal models, it is clear that no single animal model is a faithful mimic of the human disease, and so all studies with these models must be viewed as possible explanations for the human disease that need to be confirmed by direct study of the disease in humans. More recently, mouse models have been developed in which an antigen is expressed as a transgene in the pancreas and T cells recognizing this antigen are also expressed transgenically in the mouse and these mice have provided important insights.[49,50] As mentioned above, the development of "humanized" animal models expressing human MHC molecules[40,41] may well be important in the future.

Although much of the early information about the autoimmune pathogenesis of T1DM came from studies of the BB/W rat and these data have been available for a longer period of time, more extensive studies have now been carried out using the NOD mouse. Moreover, one of the major contributory factors to type 1 diabetes in the BB/W rat is a gene that creates a lymphopenic state. Although this gene is not essential for diabetes in the BB/W rat, it does contribute to susceptibility. As lymphopenia is not associated with human type 1 diabetes, this particular characteristic may make studies in the BB/W rat less relevant than those in the NOD mouse. Thus this discussion will focus mainly on the NOD mouse.

The NOD mouse was originally produced as part of a genetic experiment that involved crossing several mouse strains to produce an animal with a high degree of susceptibility to cataracts.[51] In the process of this breeding, mice with a high incidence of type 1 diabetes were produced. This line has now been bred to homozygosity and named the nonobese diabetic (NOD) mouse strain. The incidence of diabetes varies from one colony to another, but under excellent conditions of housing, type 1 diabetes begins to appear around 3–4 months of age, and by 6 months over 90% of the females and up to 60% of the males will have developed type 1 diabetes.[52]

The genetics of type 1 diabetes in the NOD mouse are complex, involving many genes.[53] The single genetic factor that appears to be most important is the MHC, although there are at least 17 other regions that have been identified in the genome which may contribute to susceptibility. The MHC genotype of the NOD mouse is denoted $H-2^{g7}$, and mice that are homozygous $H-2^{g7}$ have a high incidence of type 1 diabetes, although this is clearly not the only susceptibility factor. NOD mice expressing even a single haplotype of a different MHC genotype are almost completely protected from developing T1DM. There appear to be a number of components of the unique $H-2^{g7}$ haplotype that contribute to susceptibility to T1DM. First, as in many other mouse strains the I-Eα chain, the mouse equivalent to the human HLA-DR α chain, is mutant, and thus the I-E MHC class II molecule equivalent to HLA-DR is not expressed in NOD mice. NOD mice transgenic for a normal Eα-chain gene are fully protected from type 1 diabetes.[54] This is reminiscent of the protective effect of some HLA haplotypes for

human T1DM, and clearly identifies a single protective gene, Eα. Secondly, the I-A^{g7} molecule, the mouse equivalent of HLA-DQ, is also unique,[55] and it has been shown that changing a single amino acid at either position 56 or 57 of the I-A^{g7}β chain can render NOD mice diabetes-resistant when the gene is inserted as a transgene.[56] Interestingly, position β57, which is aspartic acid in all other mouse I-Aβ chains, is serine in the NOD mouse. This is similar to the finding that DQβ chains with aspartic acid at position 57 tend to be negatively associated with susceptibility to T1DM in Caucasian patients.[57] Biochemically, there is considerable similarity between I-A^{g7} and DQA1*0301/DQB1*0302, the HLA-DQ molecule most strongly associated with diabetes in humans.[58] The fact that alleles at MHC class II loci influence susceptibility to type 1 diabetes also suggests that CD4 T cells play an important role either in the pathogenesis of type 1 diabetes or in protecting against type 1 diabetes. This might be associated with qualitative differences in T-cell responses to putative β-cell autoantigens that may affect insulin-dependent diabetes mellitus by altering the balance of cytokines produced by β-cell autoreactive T cells.[59] More direct evidence for the role of MHC class II molecules is beginning to emerge from the mouse model that has the human MHC class II molecule most closely associated with diabetes, namely, DQA1*0301/DQB1*0302, previously called DQ8, expressed as a transgene instead of mouse MHC class II molecules,[41] in addition to a transgene directing the expression of the costimulatory molecule B7.1 in the pancreas. These mice develop spontaneous diabetes. Although the precise role of the MHC in this process, as in human T1DM, is not yet established, the data from transgenic experiments established that it is the MHC loci themselves that are critical for disease susceptibility.

There is also increasing evidence that MHC class I molecules are important in the NOD mouse. The CTS strain of mice that is related to NOD mice has an identical MHC class II region to NOD mice, but differs at one of the MHC class I loci, D^b in the NOD mouse and D^{dx} in the CTS strain,[60] and these mice have a much lower incidence of diabetes.

Prior to the onset of type 1 diabetes in NOD mice, histopathologic analysis of pancreatic islets of Langerhans reveals an extensive peri-insulitic infiltrate of mononuclear cells, and in some islets an invasion of the islet parenchyma and its apparent destruction by the lymphocytic cells. β-cell destruction is only observed in islets that are invaded by mononuclear cells; islets that are surrounded by lymphocytes but are not invaded do not show destruction. This argues against a diffusible agent being responsible for β-cell destruction, and favors a direct contact mechanism. The infiltrating cells consist of macrophages, dendritic cells, B lymphocytes, CD4 T cells, and CD8 T cells.

There is strong evidence for involvement of T cells in the destruction of pancreatic β cells in type 1 diabetes, and it is likely that both CD4 and CD8 T cells play critical roles. NOD mice carrying a mutation that produces severe combined immunodeficiency (SCID) and that lack lymphocytes, or mice with a mutation such that they do not produce T cells, never develop T1DM, implicating T lymphocytes in the process. Such mice do develop diabetes when they are adoptively reconstituted with lymphocytes. Adoptive transfer can be carried out with bone marrow–derived stem cells, in which case diabetes takes months to develop, or with splenic T cells from recently diabetic syngeneic mice, in which case diabetes develops within 3–4 weeks. The acute adoptive transfer of type 1 diabetes with splenic T cells generally requires both CD4 and CD8 T cells.[61,62] The involvement of MHC class II genes strongly implicates CD4 T cells in the process. In addition, using anti-CD4 antibodies, in the absence of CD4 T cells, insulitis also does not appear to any great extent and diabetes does not develop.[63] However, mice that lack MHC class I molecules due to a mutation in the β_2 microglobulin gene, and that have very few CD8 T cells, do not develop insulitis or diabetes.[64–66] In addition, studies in which anti-CD8 antibodies were injected into young prediabetic NOD mice (before the age of 5 weeks) found that they completely prevented insulitis and diabetes.[67] Thus CD8 T cells also play an early role in the pathogenesis of type 1 diabetes. However, the manner in which cells interact and the CD4 and CD8 T-cell responses required to mediate this complex process in the natural history of disease need still to be determined.

In the effort to characterize the immune response that damages the islets in animal models, isolated cloned T-cell lines from the infiltrate of the islets and from spleen have been useful tools. Cloned CD4 or CD8 T cells, like diabetic spleen cells, have been able to transfer disease.[68,69] In the case of CD4 T cells, it is likely that cells recruited from the recipient provide the required CD8 T cells,[68] although there are clear examples of single populations of both CD8 T cells[69] and CD4 T cells that are able to transfer disease when given alone.[70] Initially, T-cell clones from diabetic spleens that respond to unknown islet antigens, both CD4[68] and CD8,[71] were isolated. More recently, pathogenic CD4 T-cell clones have been isolated that respond to putative autoantigens—insulin[72] and GAD.[73] Highly damaging CD8 T cells isolated from the islets of young NOD mice also recognize insulin,[74] although there are other pathogenic cells present in the islets of young mice that have other specificities,[75] and these differ from those of CD8 T cells isolated from diabetic mice.[71] The cloned T cells from the early infiltrates of NOD mice provide direct evidence that insulin is an important target for both CD4 and CD8 T cells and is the only islet β-cell–specific antigen identified to date. There is also clear evidence for GAD as an autoantigen in this mouse model, although some of it is controversial. There has been much debate about whether a single autoantigen is involved in the initiation of disease, but at present there is no clear evidence, and it is possible that more than one antigen may be a target from the earliest phases of disease.

AUTOIMMUNE PROCESS INITIATION

The normal interaction between the immune system and self-tissues is described as tolerance, the absence of response against self. We have already discussed how tolerance to ubiquitous self-antigens is mediated by deletion of immature T lymphocytes, while tolerance to tissue-specific autoantigens may be mediated by antigen-specific inactivation of T cells that encounter these antigens in the periphery. If autoimmunity represents a failure of self-tolerance mechanisms, which of these mechanisms fails in type 1 diabetes?

There is some suggestion, from the human studies and also from the NOD mouse, that autoreactive cells may be selected rather than deleted in the thymus because there are antigen-presenting cells in the thymus that are able to present peptides of self-antigen such as insulin.[76,77] It has been postulated that one reason for selection of autoreactive T cells by particular MHC class II molecules, such as I-A^{g7} in the mouse, is that these molecules with their peptide ligands are unstable and therefore stimulation of T cells may not be sufficient to induce negative selection.[78] Similarly, this may apply to the MHC class II molecule most closely associated with diabetes: HLA-DQA1*0301/DQB1*0302.[79] In the case of CD8 T cells selected by self-peptides in the context of MHC

class I, autoreactive cells may recognize peptides that bind to the MHC with low affinity, and the concentration of peptide present in the thymus may be insufficient to stimulate deletion. This is one possible mechanism for the selection of autoreactive CD8 T cells that recognize an insulin peptide that binds very poorly to the MHC class I molecule K^d.[74]

Peripheral mechanisms of tolerance that protect against autoreactive T cells are clearly important. It is possible that autoantigens are normally ignored by the immune system. That is to say, the autoantigen is expressed on tissue cells in a form that is recognizable by lymphocytes, and lymphocytes specific for that autoantigen are present but are neither activated nor rendered tolerant. Stimuli that activate T cells specific for these autoantigens can trigger autoimmune processes that then target the tissue itself. A particularly clear example of this is the use of mice transgenic for a viral protein driven by the rat insulin-1 promoter. This leads to expression of the viral protein in pancreatic β cells but does not cause disease. T cells from the transgenic animals are not tolerant to the viral protein. When mice are infected with this virus, the potent antivirus response also causes destruction of pancreatic β cells that express the transgene product.[49,50] Thus the mouse is ignorant of the presence of the transgene-encoded viral antigen and is operationally tolerant until infected by the virus. This suggests that autoantigens may be relatively unique among self-proteins in being expressed too poorly to induce any kind of tolerance, yet expressed well enough to be the target of immune attack.

Most thinking about the induction of autoimmunity has implicated infection as playing a central role. Infection could provoke autoimmune responses in a number of different ways. In the example just cited, the autoantigen is exactly reproduced by a viral antigen. It has been hypothesized that viruses or bacteria could carry peptides sufficiently similar to self-peptides to trigger autoimmune responses. This mechanism is referred to as molecular mimicry.[80] Alternatively, inflammatory responses generated against pathogens could release normally sequestered autoantigens from inside cells or behind tissue barriers, and thus lead to a direct autoimmune attack. It has also been suggested that damage may be caused by a bystander mechanism.[81] A study using transgenic mice had suggested that diabetes induced by Coxsackie virus infection could be a direct result of local infection, leading to inflammation, tissue damage, and the release of sequestered islet antigen resulting in the restimulation of resting autoreactive T cells. Finally, pathogens are known to be able to induce potent costimulatory activity on antigen-presenting cells that are otherwise costimulator negative. Thus the pathogen could trigger expression of costimulatory molecules on tissue cells that do not normally express them. In this regard, the expression of the B7.1 costimulator as a transgene product on pancreatic β cells, together with a permissive genetic background, greatly accelerates autoimmune disease in NOD mice.[82] However, no direct evidence for ectopic expression of costimulator molecules in diabetes has been shown.[83]

Most recently, it has been suggested that normal apoptotic processes involved in the early remodeling of the pancreas may play a role in triggering the development of diabetes.[84] There is a wave of apoptosis occurring 2 weeks after birth, and this is increased in rodent models that are prone to diabetes. Under normal circumstances, it is not thought that apoptosis would trigger immune responses. However, it has recently been shown that the highly specialized antigen-presenting dendritic cells are able to take up antigens released by apoptosis and prime cytotoxic T cells. Perhaps the permissive environment that is encoded by genes other than those in the MHC that are also important in susceptibility may play a role. This mechanism, however, is still speculative.

In conclusion, the autoimmune process in general appears to be triggered by some insult, such as an infection, that upsets a form of tolerance known as immunologic ignorance. The autoimmune response is probably initiated by such an insult.

SUSTAINING AUTOIMMUNE RESPONSES

Most human autoimmune diseases, such as multiple sclerosis, rheumatoid arthritis, and type 1 diabetes, are chronic progressive conditions. Longitudinal studies of individuals at risk of developing type 1 diabetes have suggested that the autoimmune attack takes several years to destroy sufficient β-cell mass to produce overt diabetes.[1] Likewise, in NOD mice, the autoimmune process leading to type 1 diabetes takes at least 3 months to reach completion. These observations suggest that the autoimmune attack must be sustained over long periods of time. Thus, even if a viral infection triggered an initial attack on pancreatic β cells, responses to the autoantigen itself are likely to be required for the production of clinical illness. The tempo of these initial diseases stands in sharp contrast to the tempo of β-cell destruction in human recipients of identical twin hemipancreatic grafts, in which all β cells in the graft can be destroyed within 6 weeks, or to adoptive transfer of T cells from recently diabetic NOD mice into nondiabetic, immunodeficient recipients, in which case all mice become diabetic within 3–4 weeks. Moreover, this adoptive transfer requires only a few percent of the T cells in the diabetic donor for complete penetrance.

These findings suggest that the autoimmune process is normally restrained by mechanisms that protect the target tissue or prevent the development of the autoimmune response. More direct evidence for such restraining cells has been obtained in adoptive transfer experiments using either cell populations or cloned T-cell lines that inhibit the development of type 1 diabetes in NOD mice[85–88] similar results have been reported in several other autoimmune diseases. Some of these cells have been cloned directly from islets[85,86] or from pancreatic lymph nodes,[88] suggesting that their locus of action may be within the islets themselves or locally in the draining nodes. It is not clear how these regulatory populations may be exerting their action. Much interest has centered around the fact that "protective" cells may produce cytokines such as transforming growth factor-β (TGF-β).[88,89] However, there may be other populations producing cytokines that play a protective role such as IL-10, identified as protective in inflammatory bowel disease.[90] In addition, it has been suggested that NOD mice may be deficient in a regulatory population of cells, called natural killer (NK) T cells, that produce large quantities of IL-4.[91–93] This defect has also been reported in BB rats[94] and suggested in the affected twin of identical twins nonconcordant for diabetes.[95] Thus the autoimmune process can be viewed as a balance between effector T cells engaged in β-cell destruction and the protecting T cells that are engaged in restraining the effector cells.

These findings are important because they suggest that the outcome of the autoimmune process is determined by the balance between two sets of activatable lymphocytes. If one could artificially activate a set of protective cells, then type 1 diabetes might be prevented, as outlined in the next section. On the other side, how do the attacking cells sustain their attack on tissue in the face of these regulatory influences? This is still poorly understood.

However, one possibility is that the initial attack on a β cell is focused on a single autoantigen. Such responses are relatively easy to regulate, as few T cells are involved, and the process may be terminated at this point. It has been hypothesized that diversification of the autoimmune process is essential for its progression. If diversification outstrips regulation, then disease results; by contrast, if the protective influences shut the response down prior to its diversification, they may be dominant. These issues are just beginning to be explored.

IMMUNOLOGIC APPROACHES TO PREVENTION OF TYPE 1 DIABETES

If type 1 diabetes indeed represents an autoimmune T-cell attack on the β cells of the pancreatic islets of Langerhans, as all available evidence suggests, and if disease becomes manifest only after the majority of β-cell mass is lost, then it is clearly crucial that we approach this disease with the idea of preventing its occurrence. Numerous strategies have been suggested for doing this. For instance, immunosuppressive drugs had been advocated in the past, but clinical trials had shown only short-term benefit and the toxicity associated with long-term use of drugs such as cyclosporine A make their use untenable. More recently, various other forms of immunomodulation have been suggested. In the NOD mouse, it had been shown that monoclonal antibodies directed at the T-cell receptor complex—nondepleting anti-CD3 antibodies—were able to reverse diabetes when given after the disease had manifested.[96,97] This method has been modified to humanize the antibodies and is currently in clinical trials in patients who have very recently been diagnosed with diabetes.

However, it would be even more attractive to prevent disease at a much earlier stage in pathogenesis, before any significant damage is done to the islets. Many different strategies involving administration of putative autoantigens via a number of different routes have shown the ability to protect against diabetes in the NOD mouse.[46] These are not all applicable in other animal models of diabetes and it is likely that many will not be viable in humans. However, the explanation for the fact that many of these strategies work is the ability to generate cells that have protective qualities. For example, NOD mice have been fed insulin and type 1 diabetes induction was inhibited.[98,99] This was attributed to the induction of cells producing the cytokine TGF-β. Other studies have used insulin administered nasally, and protection is thought to arise through the generation of another subset of protective T cells known as gamma-delta T cells.[100] It may not be possible to generate protective immunity using antigens that are direct targets of the autoimmune attack because there is no way of knowing when autoimmunity has been initiated. While it is clear that we know much about the generation of protective immunity against pathogens—we have considerable ability to vaccinate to generate immune responses against exogenous (non-self) antigens—much less is known in humans about how to alter or turn off immune responses that are already underway. Alternatively, it may be necessary to generate "bystander suppression" to antigens that are not direct targets of the autoimmune response. This has been shown in principle by the ability to protect against diabetes in the mouse model expressing viral protein in the pancreas that develops diabetes on viral infection.[101] In these mice, administration of insulin, but not viral peptides, was able to protect against disease.

One of the major problems associated with all of these approaches is that they require the identification of individuals at risk of developing diabetes. There are two great difficulties associated with this. First, most cases arise sporadically and not in families, making their identification particularly difficult. Second, our ability to predict which individuals will or will not get T1DM is still very imperfect, even using both genetic and immunologic markers.

The ideal approach would be one that could be given to all of the population, as it avoids the problem of identifying individuals at risk. For this approach to work, it must be inexpensive, essentially nontoxic, and highly effective. Based on the preceding description of the autoimmune process as a balance between attacking and protecting cells, the most likely candidate for prevention of T1DM at the present time is a vaccine that selectively immunizes cells that protect the pancreatic β cells from autoimmune attack. Although this may seem a farfetched goal, the results obtained to date in animal models suggest that targeting an immunologic response to a particular tissue can protect that tissue from autoimmune attack. This does not require a sophisticated analysis of the natural means of protection, as protection appears to be tissue- rather than antigen-specific. A far better understanding of the process by which regulatory immune responses protect target tissues is required before this practice can be made more rational. A reliable means of vaccination against autoimmunity that gives sustained protection would be highly desirable, although whether this can be achieved practically remains to be determined. The ability to identify individuals at risk within families will be crucial to the development of such therapies, as ethical testing of these preventive measures will require their use initially on individuals at high risk of developing T1DM.

SUMMARY

Available data suggest that insulin-dependent diabetes mellitus is an autoimmune disease that targets the β cells of the pancreatic islets of Langerhans. The precise mechanism by which β cells are destroyed in type 1 diabetes is not known, but it clearly involves an adaptive immune response by T lymphocytes. We are beginning to understand how the response is initiated, sustained, and regulated. What is particularly encouraging is the finding that type 1 diabetes is not an unrestrained attack on β cells, but rather involves regulatory influences of T lymphocytes, at least in experimental animal studies. This suggests a potential means of preventing T1DM through the selective activation of these restraining or protective T lymphocytes. The major goal in studying the pathogenesis of T1DM is to understand how the β cells are destroyed and how the process might be specifically inhibited. The latter is clearly the more important goal, as it holds the key to prevention of type 1 diabetes. We envision that disease prevention will require the development of a vaccine to stimulate regulatory cells that protect pancreatic β cells from destruction. This is based on the historic success of immunology in vaccinating specific sets of lymphocytes, and its historic failure to restrain specific responses by immunosuppressive drug therapy. To date, little is known about how the immune response regulates itself, and this is even more true in complex processes like autoimmune diseases. Nevertheless, preliminary studies encourage one to hope that such measures may be available in the future.

Acknowledgments The authors' work was supported by the Juvenile Diabetes Foundation International; the National Institutes of Health; the National Institutes of Diabetes, Digestive, and Kidney Diseases; and by the Howard Hughes Medical Institute. The authors thank Eva-Pia Reich, Irene Visintin, Karl Swenson, Jennifer Granata, and Joanne Daugherty for their part in the authors' work in diabetes and Jennifer Boucher-Reid for editorial assistance.

REFERENCES

1. Eisenbarth GS: Type I diabetes mellitus. A chronic autoimmune disease. *N Engl J Med* 1986;314:1360.
2. Janeway C Jr, Travers P, Walport M, Capra JD: *Immunobiology: The Immune System in Health and Disease* 4th Ed. Garland Press: 1999.
3. Paul W: *Fundamental Immunology*, 3rd ed. Raven:1993.
4. Kappler JW, Roehm N, Marrack P: T cell tolerance by clonal elimination in the thymus. *Cell* 1987;49:273.
5. Davis MM, Bjorkman PJ: T-cell antigen receptor genes and T-cell recognition [published erratum appears in *Nature* 1988;335:744]. *Nature* 1988;334:395.
6. Germain RN: MHC-dependent antigen processing and peptide presentation: Providing ligands for T lymphocyte activation. *Cell* 1994;76:287.
7. Janeway CA Jr: T-cell development. Accessories or coreceptors? *Nature* 1988;335:208.
8. Salter RD, Norment AM, Chen BP, et al: Polymorphism in the alpha 3 domain of HLA-A molecules affects binding to CD8. *Nature* 1989;338:345.
9. Brown JH, Jardetzky TS, Gorga JC, et al: Three-dimensional structure of the human class II histocompatibility antigen HLA-DR1. *Nature* 1993;364:33.
10. Janeway CA Jr: The T cell receptor as a multicomponent signalling machine: CD4/CD8 coreceptors and CD45 in T cell activation. *Annu Rev Immunol* 1992;10:645.
11. von Boehmer H: Positive selection of lymphocytes. *Cell* 1994;76:219.
12. von Boehmer H: Developmental biology of T cells in T cell-receptor transgenic mice. *Annu Rev Immunol* 1990;8:531.
13. Hogquist KA, Gavin MA, Bevan MJ: Positive selection of CD8+ T cells induced by major histocompatibility complex binding peptides in fetal thymic organ culture. *J Exp Med* 1993;177:1469.
14. Ashton-Rickardt PG, Van Kaer L, Schumacher TN, et al: Peptide contributes to the specificity of positive selection of CD8+ T cells in the thymus. *Cell* 1993;73:1041.
15. Schwartz RH: Costimulation of T lymphocytes: The role of CD28, CTLA-4, and B7/BB1 in interleukin-2 production and immunotherapy. *Cell* 1992;71:1065.
16. Janeway CA Jr, Bottomly K: Signals and signs for lymphocyte responses. *Cell* 1994;76:275.
17. Liu Y, Janeway CA Jr: Cells that present both specific ligand and costimulatory activity are the most efficient inducers of clonal expansion of normal CD4 T cells. *Proc Natl Acad Sci USA* 1992;89:3845.
18. Janeway CA Jr, Carding S, Jones B, et al: CD4+ T cells: Specificity and function. *Immunol Rev* 1988;101:39.
19. Paul WE, Seder RA: Lymphocyte responses and cytokines. *Cell* 1994;76:241.
20. Gepts W: Pathologic anatomy of the pancreas in juvenile diabetes mellitus. *Diabetes* 1965;14:619.
21. Foulis AK, Liddle CN, Farquharson MA, et al: The histopathology of the pancreas in type 1 (insulin-dependent) diabetes mellitus: A 25-year review of deaths in patients under 20 years of age in the United Kingdom. *Diabetologia* 1986;29:267.
22. Bottazzo GF, Dean BM, McNally JM, et al: In situ characterization of autoimmune phenomena and expression of HLA molecules in the pancreas in diabetic insulitis. *N Engl J Med* 1985;313:353.
23. Sutherland DE, Sibley R, Xu XZ, et al: Twin-to-twin pancreas transplantation: Reversal and reenactment of the pathogenesis of type I diabetes. *Trans Assoc Am Physicians* 1984;97:80.
24. Sibley RK, Sutherland DE, Goetz F, et al: Recurrent diabetes mellitus in the pancreas iso- and allograft. A light and electron microscopic and immunohistochemical analysis of four cases. *Lab Invest* 1985;53:132.
25. Bottazzo GF, Florin-Christensen A, Doniach D: Islet-cell antibodies in diabetes mellitus with autoimmune polyendocrine deficiencies. *Lancet* 1974;2:1279.
26. Lendrum R, Walker G, Gamble DR: Islet-cell antibodies in juvenile diabetes mellitus of recent onset. *Lancet* 1975;1:880.
27. Palmer JP, Asplin CM, Clemons P, et al: Insulin antibodies in insulin-dependent diabetics before insulin treatment. *Science* 1983;222:1337.

28. Baekkeskov S, Nielsen JH, Marner B, *et al*: Autoantibodies in newly diagnosed diabetic children immunoprecipitate human pancreatic islet cell proteins. *Nature* 1982;298:167.

29. Baekkeskov S, Aanstoot HJ, Christgau S, *et al*: Identification of the 64K autoantigen in insulin-dependent diabetes as the GABA-synthesizing enzyme glutamic acid decarboxylase [published erratum appears in *Nature* 1990;347:782]. *Nature* 1990;347:151.

30. Christie MR, Genovese S, Cassidy D, *et al*: Antibodies to islet 37k antigen, but not to glutamate decarboxylase, discriminate rapid progression to IDDM in endocrine autoimmunity. *Diabetes* 1994;43:1254.

31. Solimena M, Dirkx R Jr, Hermel JM, *et al*: ICA 512, an autoantigen of type I diabetes, is an intrinsic membrane protein of neurosecretory granules. *EMBO J* 1996;15:2102.

32. Atkinson MA, Maclaren NK: Islet cell autoantigens in insulin-dependent diabetes. *J Clin Invest* 1993;92:1608.

33. Schloot NC, Willemen S, Duinkerken G, *et al*: Cloned T cells from a recent onset IDDM patient reactive with insulin B-chain. *J Autoimmun* 1998;11:169.

34. Hawkes CJ, Schloot NC, Marks J, *et al*: T-Cell lines reactive to an immunodominant epitope of the tyrosine phosphatase-like autoantigen IA-2 in type 1 diabetes. *Diabetes* 2000;49:356.

35. Panina-Bordignon P, Lang R, van Endert PM, *et al*: Cytotoxic T cells specific for glutamic acid decarboxylase in autoimmune diabetes. *J Exp Med* 1995;181:1923.

36. Davies JL, Kawaguchi Y, Bennett ST, *et al*: A genome-wide search for human type 1 diabetes susceptibility genes. *Nature* 1994;371:130.

37. Nepom GT, Erlich H: MHC class-II molecules and autoimmunity. *Annu Rev Immunol* 1991;9:493.

38. Fennessy M, Metcalfe K, Hitman GA, *et al*: A gene in the HLA class I region contributes to susceptibility to IDDM in the Finnish population. Childhood Diabetes in Finland (DiMe) Study Group. *Diabetologia* 1994;37:937.

39. Reijonen H, Nejentsev S, Tuokko J, *et al*: HLA-DR4 subtype and -B alleles in DQB1*0302-positive haplotypes associated with IDDM. The Childhood Diabetes in Finland Study Group. *Eur J Immunogenet* 1997;24:357.

40. Taneja V, David CS: HLA class II transgenic mice as models of human diseases. *Immunol Rev* 1999;169:67.

41. Wen L, Wong FS, Tang J, *et al*: In vivo evidence for the contribution of human histocompatibility leukocyte antigen (HLA)-DQ molecules to the development of diabetes. *J Exp Med* 2000;191:97.

42. Rossini AA, Mordes JP, Like AA: Immunology of insulin-dependent diabetes mellitus. *Annu Rev Immunol* 1985;3:289.

43. Leiter EH, Serreze DV: The genetics and epidemiology of diabetes in NOD mice. *Immunol Today* 1990;11:147.

44. Kaufman DL, Clare-Salzler M, Tian J, *et al*: Spontaneous loss of T-cell tolerance to glutamic acid decarboxylase in murine insulin-dependent diabetes. *Nature* 1993;366:69.

45. Tisch R, Yang XD, Singer SM, *et al*: Immune response to glutamic acid decarboxylase correlates with insulitis in non-obese diabetic mice. *Nature* 1993;366:72.

46. Atkinson MA, Leiter EH: The NOD mouse model of type 1 diabetes: As good as it gets? *Nat Med* 1999;5:601.

47. De Aizpurua HJ, French MB, Chosich N, *et al*: Natural history of humoral immunity to glutamic acid decarboxylase in non-obese diabetic (NOD) mice. *J Autoimmun* 1994;7:643.

48. Yu L, Robles DT, Abiru N, *et al*: Early expression of antiinsulin autoantibodies of humans and the NOD mouse: Evidence for early determination of subsequent diabetes. *Proc Natl Acad Sci USA* 2000;97:1701.

49. Oldstone MB, Nerenberg M, Southern P, *et al*: Virus infection triggers insulin-dependent diabetes mellitus in a transgenic model: Role of anti-self (virus) immune response. *Cell* 1991;65:319.

50. Ohashi PS, Oehen S, Buerki K, *et al*: Ablation of "tolerance" and induction of diabetes by virus infection in viral antigen transgenic mice. *Cell* 1991;65:305.

51. Makino S, Kunimoto K, Muraoka Y, *et al*: Breeding of a non-obese, diabetic strain of mice. *Jikken Dobutsu* 1980;29:1.

52. Pozzilli P, Signore A, Williams AJ, *et al*: NOD mouse colonies around the world—recent facts and figures. *Immunol Today* 1993;14:193.

53. Wicker LS, Todd JA, Peterson LB: Genetic control of autoimmune diabetes in the NOD mouse. *Annu Rev Immunol* 1995;13:179.

54. Nishimoto H, Kikutani H, Yamamura K, *et al*: Prevention of autoimmune insulitis by expression of I-E molecules in NOD mice. *Nature* 1987;328:432.

55. Acha-Orbea H, McDevitt HO: The first external domain of the nonobese diabetic mouse class II I-A beta chain is unique. *Proc Natl Acad Sci USA* 1987;84:2435.

56. Lund T, O'Reilly L, Hutchings P, *et al*: Prevention of insulin-dependent diabetes mellitus in non-obese diabetic mice by transgenes encoding modified I-A beta-chain or normal I-E alpha-chain. *Nature* 1990;345:727.

57. Todd JA, Bell JI, McDevitt HO: HLA-DQ beta gene contributes to susceptibility and resistance to insulin-dependent diabetes mellitus. *Nature* 1987;329:599.

58. Reizis B, Altmann DM, Cohen IR: Biochemical characterization of the human diabetes-associated HLA-DQ8 allelic product: Similarity to the major histocompatibility complex class II I-A(g)7 protein of non-obese diabetic mice. *Eur J Immunol* 1997;27:2478.

59. Hanson MS, Cetkovic-Cvrlje M, Ramiya VK, *et al*: Quantitative thresholds of MHC class II I-E expressed on hemopoietically derived antigen-presenting cells in transgenic NOD/Lt mice determine level of diabetes resistance and indicate mechanism of protection. *J Immunol* 1996;157:1279.

60. Mathews CE, Graser RT, Serreze DV, *et al*: Reevaluation of the major histocompatibility complex genes of the NOD-progenitor CTS/Shi strain. *Diabetes* 2000;49:131.

61. Miller BJ, Appel MC, O'Neil JJ, *et al*: Both the Lyt-2+ and L3T4+ T cell subsets are required for the transfer of diabetes in nonobese diabetic mice. *J Immunol* 1988;140:52.

62. Bendelac A, Carnaud C, Boitard C, *et al*: Syngeneic transfer of autoimmune diabetes from diabetic NOD mice to healthy neonates. Requirement for both L3T4+ and Lyt-2+ T cells. *J Exp Med* 1987;166:823.

63. Shizuru JA, Taylor-Edwards C, Banks BA, *et al*: Immunotherapy of the nonobese diabetic mouse: Treatment with an antibody to T-helper lymphocytes. *Science* 1988;240:659.

64. Katz J, Benoist C, Mathis D: Major histocompatibility complex class I molecules are required for the development of insulitis in non-obese diabetic mice. *Eur J Immunol* 1993;23:3358.

65. Wicker LS, Leiter EH, Todd JA, *et al*: Beta 2-microglobulin-deficient NOD mice do not develop insulitis or diabetes. *Diabetes* 1994;43:500.

66. Serreze DV, Leiter EH, Christianson GJ, *et al*: Major histocompatibility complex class I-deficient NOD-β2mnull mice are diabetes and insulitis resistant. *Diabetes* 1994;43:505.

67. Wang B, Gonzalez A, Benoist C, *et al*: The role of CD8+ T cells in the initiation of insulin-dependent diabetes mellitus. *Eur J Immunol* 1996;26:1762.

68. Haskins K, McDuffie M: Acceleration of diabetes in young NOD mice with a CD4+ islet-specific T cell clone. *Science* 1990;249:1433.

69. Wong FS, Visintin I, Wen L, *et al*: CD8 T cell clones from young nonobese diabetic (NOD) islets can transfer rapid onset of diabetes in NOD mice in the absence of CD4 cells. *J Exp Med* 1996;183:67.

70. Peterson JD, Haskins K: Transfer of diabetes in the NOD-scid mouse by CD4 T-cell clones. Differential requirement for CD8 T-cells. *Diabetes* 1996;45:328.

71. Nagata M, Santamaria P, Kawamura T, *et al*: Evidence for the role of CD8+ cytotoxic T cells in the destruction of pancreatic beta-cells in nonobese diabetic mice. *J Immunol* 1994;152:2042.

72. Daniel D, Wegmann DR: Protection of nonobese diabetic mice from diabetes by intranasal or subcutaneous administration of insulin peptide B-(9–23). *Proc Natl Acad Sci USA* 1996;93:956.

73. Zekzer D, Wong FS, Ayalon O, *et al*: GAD-reactive CD4+ Th1 cells induce diabetes in NOD/SCID mice. *J Clin Invest* 1998;101:68.

74. Wong FS, Karttunen J, Dumont C, *et al*: Identification of an MHC class I-restricted autoantigen in type 1 diabetes by screening an organ-specific cDNA library. *Nat Med* 1999;5:1026.

75. DiLorenzo TP, Graser RT, Ono T, *et al*: Major histocompatibility complex class I-restricted T cells are required for all but the end stages of diabetes development in nonobese diabetic mice and use a prevalent T cell receptor alpha chain gene rearrangement. *Proc Natl Acad Sci USA* 1998;95:12538.

76. Pugliese A, Zeller M, Fernandez A Jr, *et al*: The insulin gene is transcribed in the human thymus and transcription levels correlated with allelic variation at the INS VNTR-IDDM2 susceptibility locus for type 1 diabetes. *Nat Genet* 1997;15:293.

77. Hanahan D: Peripheral-antigen-expressing cells in thymic medulla: Factors in self-tolerance and autoimmunity. *Curr Opin Immunol* 1998;10:656.

78. Carrasco-Marin E, Shimizu J, Kanagawa O, *et al*: The class II MHC I-Ag7 molecules from non-obese diabetic mice are poor peptide binders. *J Immunol* 1996;156:450.

79. Nepom GT, Kwok WW: Molecular basis for HLA-DQ associations with IDDM. *Diabetes* 1998;47:1177.

80. Fujinami R: Molecular mimicry. In: Rose N, MacKay I, eds. *Book Molecular Mimicry*. Academic Press:1992;153.

81. Horwitz MS, Bradley LM, Harbertson J, *et al*: Diabetes induced by Coxsackie virus: Initiation by bystander damage and not molecular mimicry. *Nat Med* 1998;4:781.

82. Wong S, Guerder S, Visintin I, *et al*: Expression of the co-stimulator molecule B7-1 in pancreatic beta-cells accelerates diabetes in the NOD mouse. *Diabetes* 1995;44:326.

83. Stephens LA, Kay TW: Pancreatic expression of B7 co-stimulatory molecules in the non-obese diabetic mouse. *Int Immunol* 1995;7:1885.

84. Trudeau JD, Dutz JP, Arany E, *et al*: Neonatal beta-cell apoptosis: A trigger for autoimmune diabetes? *Diabetes* 2000;49:1.

85. Reich E-P, Sherwin R, Janeway C Jr: Dissecting insulin-dependent diabetes mellitus in the NOD mouse by preparation of cloned T cell lines from islets. In: Rifkin H, Colwell J, Taylor S, eds. *Diabetes* 1991. Elsevier:1991;9.

86. Utsugi T, Nagata M, Kawamura T, *et al*: Prevention of recurrent diabetes in syngenic islet-transplanted NOD mice by transfusion of autoreactive T lymphocytes. *Transplantation* 1994;57:1799.

87. Akhtar I, Gold JP, Pan LY, *et al*: CD4+ beta islet cell-reactive T cell clones that suppress autoimmune diabetes in nonobese diabetic mice. *J Exp Med* 1995;182:87.

88. Zekzer D, Wong FS, Wen L, *et al*: Inhibition of diabetes by an insulin-reactive CD4 T-cell clone in the nonobese diabetic mouse. *Diabetes* 1997;46:1124.

89. Weiner HL, Friedman A, Miller A, *et al*: Oral tolerance: Immunologic mechanisms and treatment of animal and human organ-specific autoimmune diseases by oral administration of autoantigens. *Annu Rev Immunol* 1994;12:809.

90. Asseman C, Mauze S, Leach MW, *et al*: An essential role for interleukin 10 in the function of regulatory T cells that inhibit intestinal inflammation. *J Exp Med* 1999;190:995.

91. Baxter AG, Kinder SJ, Hammond KJ, *et al*: Association between alphabetaTCR+CD4-CD8-T-cell deficiency and IDDM in NOD/Lt mice. *Diabetes* 1997;46:572.

92. Hammond KJL, Poulton LD, Palmisano LJ, *et al*: Alpha/beta-T cell receptor (TCR)+CD4-CD8-(NKT) thymocytes prevent insulin-dependent diabetes mellitus in nonobese diabetic (NOD)/Lt mice by the influence of interleukin (IL)-4 and/or IL-10. *J Exp Med* 1998;187:1047.

93. Lehuen A, Lantz O, Beaudoin L, *et al*: Overexpression of natural killer T cells protects Valpha14- Jalpha281 transgenic nonobese diabetic mice against diabetes. *J Exp Med* 1998;188:1831.

94. Iwakoshi NN, Greiner DL, Rossini AA, *et al*: Diabetes prone BB rats are severely deficient in natural killer T cells. *Autoimmunity* 1999;31:1.

95. Wilson SB, Kent SC, Patton KT, *et al*: Extreme Th1 bias of invariant Valpha24JalphaQ T cells in type 1 diabetes [published erratum appears in *Nature* 1999;399:84]. *Nature* 1998;391:177.

96. Chatenoud L, Thervet E, Primo J, *et al*: Anti-CD3 antibody induces long-term remission of overt autoimmunity in nonobese diabetic mice. *Proc Natl Acad Sci USA* 1994;91:123.

97. Chatenoud L, Primo J, Bach JF: CD3 antibody-induced dominant self tolerance in overtly diabetic NOD mice. *J Immunol* 1997;158:2947.

98. Zhang ZJ, Davidson L, Eisenbarth G, *et al*: Suppression of diabetes in nonobese diabetic mice by oral administration of porcine insulin. *Proc Natl Acad Sci USA* 1991;88:10252.

99. Hancock WW, Polanski M, Zhang J, *et al*: Suppression of insulitis in non-obese diabetic (NOD) mice by oral insulin administration is associated with selective expression of interleukin-4 and -10, transforming growth factor-beta, and prostaglandin-E. *Am J Pathol* 1995;147:1193.

100. Hanninen A, Harrison LC: Gamma delta T cells as mediators of mucosal tolerance: The autoimmune diabetes model. *Immunol Rev* 2000;173:109.

101. Homann D, Holz A, Bot A, *et al*: Autoreactive CD4+ T cells protect from autoimmune diabetes via bystander suppression using the IL-4/Stat6 pathway. *Immunity* 1999;11:463.

CHAPTER 16

Diabetes in Animals: Contribution to the Understanding of Diabetes by Study of Its Etiopathology in Animal Models

Eleazar Shafrir

Animal models of diabetes, guidelines for their use in investigation, and principles for their classification have been outlined in the fourth and fifth editions of this textbook. In the new sixth edition, the information on various forms of animal diabetes is expanded and updated and new species with diabetes are introduced. In discussing the accrued knowledge, emphasis is placed on its relevance to the pathogenesis of human diabetes. The reader interested in animals extensively investigated in the past should consult Chap. 20 of the fourth edition and Chap. 18 of the fifth edition. During recent years some new books and articles on diabetes in animals have appeared,[1–6] which contain additional information. Table 16-1 summarizes the animals with diabetes in the order that they appear in the text.

DIABETES INDUCED BY CYTOTOXINS SPECIFIC FOR β CELLS

Alloxan, a pyrimidine structurally similar to uric acid and glucose, and streptozocin (STZ), which may be considered glucose with a highly reactive nitrosourea side chain (Fig. 16-1), are selectively toxic to β cells. Their molecular similarity suggests a common site of cytotoxic attack. The elucidation of the mechanism of action of these compounds is important for understanding the destructive processes in β cells in general and for assessing environmental dangers to the endocrine pancreas.

Alloxan

Alloxan is highly unstable in water at neutral pH, but reasonably stable at pH 3. Other uric acid derivatives, dehydrouramil hydrate, 4,5-dihydro-4,5-dihydroxyuric acid, and 5-hydroxypseudouric acid, are also diabetogenic. It has been suggested that alloxan metabolites may be involved in human diabetes; however, no diabetogenic uric acid metabolite has been found in humans except for one report[7] of increased levels of alloxan in blood from children with type 1 diabetes mellitus (T1DM).

Alloxan is rapidly taken up by β cells and has a direct effect on membrane permeability. Morphologic abnormalities suggest disruption of the β-cell membrane. There is evidence that alloxan acts

TABLE 16-1 Animals with Various Forms of Diabetes

Animals with β Cells Destroyed by Chemical Cytotoxins
  Alloxan
  Streptozocin (single dose)
  Streptozocin (multiple subdiabetogenic doses)
Animals with Autoimmune Diabetes with Spontaneous Onset Causing β-Cell Loss
  BB rats
  NOD mice
  LETL rats
  Torri rat
  LEW.1AR1/ZTM-iddm rat
Genetically Altered Animals with Various Forms of Diabetes
Insulin-Resistant Mutant Rodents with Diabesity
  C57BKs *db* mice (*lepr^db^*)
  C57BL6J *ob* mice (*lep^ob^*)
  Yellow A^v and A^{vy} mice
  KK mice
  NZO mice
  Zucker *fa* rats (*lepr^fa^*) and BBZ/Wor rats
  Zdf/Drt-*fa* rats
  Wistar-Kyoto diabetic/fatty rat group
  Corpulent rat group including SHR/N-*cp*, LA/N-*cp*, SHHF/Mcc-*cp*, JCR:LA-*cp* rats
Rodents with Spontaneous Diabetes of Varying Etiology
  NON mice
  WBN/Kob rats
  eSS rats
  BHE/Cdb rats
  OLETF rats
  NSY mice
  Koletzky (SHROB) rats (*fa^K^*)
  Hypertriglyceridemic (HTG) rats
Rodents with Overnutrition-Evoked Diabesity
  Psammomys obesus (sand rats)
  Acomys cahirinus (spiny mice)
  C57BL/6J mice
Diabetic Rodents Isolated by Selective Breeding from Normal Pools
  GK (Goto-Kakizaki) rats
  Cohen sucrose-induced rats
Diabetic Nonrodents
  Primates
  Dogs and cats

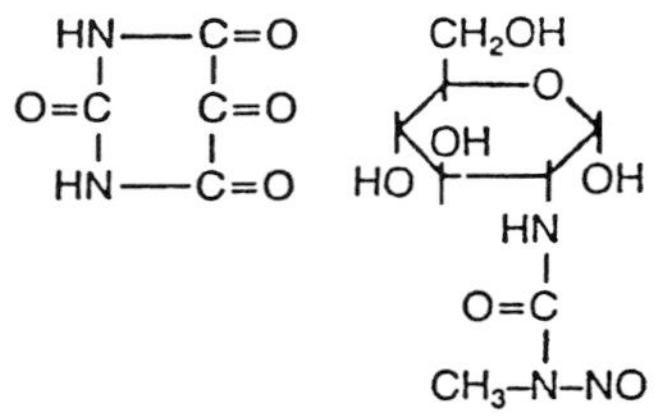

FIGURE 16-1. Molecular structures of alloxan, 2,4-5,6, tetraoxohexahydropyrimidine, and streptozocin, 2-deoxy-2-(3-methyl-nitrosoureido)-D-glucopyranose.

at the site of hexose transport, inhibits glucose-stimulated insulin release, and interferes with the generation of glucose-derived energy by inhibiting glycolytic flux and pyruvate oxidation. Both glucose at high concentration and the nonmetabolizable 2-deoxy- and 3-O-methylglucoses, which share the entry site, block the diabetogenic action and restore insulin production.

Malaisse[8] came to the conclusion that the deleterious effects of alloxan on permeability, transport, intracellular energy generation, and insulin secretion should be attributed to free radical formation. Alloxan is reduced within the cell to dialuric acid, which then autoreoxidizes to alloxan. Superoxide radicals arise from the alloxan–dialuric acid cycle and are decomposed by the enzyme superoxide dismutase (SOD), producing H_2O_2. In the presence of Fe^{2+} ions, extremely reactive OH radicals are formed, which can be visualized by chemiluminescence,[9] and damage various cellular constituents. Pretreatment of cells with SOD, catalase, and a host of nonenzymatic radical scavengers such as NAD or chelators of metal ions protects against alloxan injury.

Boquist[10] provided evidence that alloxan and STZ inhibit enzymes of the tricarboxylic acid cycle and Ca^{2+}-dependent dehydrogenases in β-cell mitochondria, causing ATP deficiency, cessation of insulin production, and cell necrosis. This toxicity mechanism is not an alternative, but rather parallel to that induced by the free radical lesion. This view is supported by Lenzen and coworkers,[11–13] who found that the mitochondrial aconitase and Ca^{2+} transport are inhibited by alloxan, and by the fact that diltiazem, a Ca^{2+} channel blocker, prevents alloxan diabetogenicity. Moreover, pretreatment with verapamil, a Ca^{2+} antagonist, prevents alloxan toxicity and DNA strand breaks by reducing the intracellular influx of Ca^{2+}.[14]

Alloxan is most effective after IV injection in a dose of 40–45 mg/kg, producing irreversible β-cell damage within minutes and structural changes within hours in most rodents, dogs, cats, rabbits, monkeys, sheep, cattle, fish, and birds. The response to alloxan may be divided into three phases: (1) initial hyperglycemia lasting ~2 hours, probably due to liver glycogenolysis; (2) transient hypoglycemia at about 6 hours, due to the release of insulin from damaged cells; and (3) permanent hyperglycemia, due to insulin deficiency, setting on after ~12 hours. The hypoglycemic phase may be quite severe and alloxan should not be given to fasted animals.

Several treatments prevent the alloxan-induced β-cell damage in vivo, apparently by different mechanisms. Metabolic alkalosis induced with sodium bicarbonate or lactate prior to alloxan injection is protective in rats, but when given after alloxan is not. Diethylthiocarbamate and disulfiram, which induce hyperglycemia, are protective when injected prior to alloxan, and so are glucose, mannose, or fructose, whereas leucine is active both before and immediately after alloxan. The mechanism of glucose protection

is thought to be associated with GLUT-2, the β-cell membrane transporter, and intracellular metabolism. Pretreatment with monomethyl, dimethyl, or monoethylurea, scavengers of OH radicals, completely blocks the action of alloxan, in keeping with in vitro observations that inhibition of OH radical formation protects against cellular lesions. Resistance or susceptibility to an alloxaninduced lesion has been observed by Matthews and Leiter[15,16] in β cells of ALR/LT and ALS/LT mice, respectively, due to genes up- or downregulating the antioxidant cell capacity.

Streptozocin

The diabetogenic action of STZ destroys most islet β cells after a single injection. It is effective in different species-specific doses ranging from 25–200 mg/kg in rats, dogs, mice, hamsters, monkeys, miniature pigs, pigs, and rabbits. It is more effective than alloxan in certain species, such as guinea pig and Syrian hamster, which do not develop permanent hyperglycemia after alloxan. Even among different strains of laboratory rats and mice the effective STZ dose may vary. The variation in susceptibility to STZ appears to be related to the pharmacokinetics of the drug rather than to its direct effect on β cells. STZ-treated animals, though insulinopenic, retain some insulin-secretion capacity, are not ketotic, and do not usually require insulin support for survival. In fact, a mild diabetic state, resembling an insulin-poor type 2 diabetes mellitus (T2DM), may be induced in rats by a single low dose of ~35 mg/kg STZ.[17] However, rats tend to recover spontaneously after receiving doses <35 mg/kg.

STZ is unstable in solution even at acid pH, and should be injected promptly after dissolution in citrate buffer at pH 5.0. Its in vivo life span is <15 minutes.[18] As the result of the STZ insult, β cells degranulate but do not completely necrotize, and there is limited proliferation ~4 days after STZ administration to rats. Ductal or acinar cells do not transform into β cells, suggesting that the proliferating cells derive from preexisting precursor β cells.

An impressive body of knowledge on the mechanism of STZ diabetogenicity has been accumulated. Its nitrosourea moiety is responsible for β-cell toxicity, while the deoxyglucose moiety facilitates transport across the cell membrane. The α-anomer of STZ shows higher potency,[19] parallel to the greater effect of the α-glucose anomer on insulin secretion, suggesting the involvement of a membrane glucoreceptor in β-cell penetration. STZ toxicity can be moderated by pretreatment with cortisol, perhaps by augmenting the residual β-cell mass, or by injection of diphenylhydantoin prior to or 60 minutes after STZ. A short-term pretreatment with insulin prevents the STZ diabetogenicity.[20]

STZ reduces the cellular NAD content in several tissues, and this effect is particularly harmful for β cells as their NAD content is lower than in other tissues.[21,22] Nicotinamide, the precursor of NAD, protects against STZ diabetes. The NAD depletion is linked to stimulation of the activity of the nuclear enzyme poly (ADP-ribose) synthase, which is involved in the excision and repair of broken DNA strands and requires NAD as substrate. This enzyme is inhibitable by nicotinamide and picolinamide, which prevent the STZ-induced DNA damage in vivo and help to maintain the NAD content and insulin biosynthesis in vitro. Both STZ and alloxan act by inducing DNA strand breaks first and poly (ADP-ribose) synthase activity subsequently. The profound decline in NAD occurs within minutes after the rise in synthase activity.

A 2-chloroethyl analogue of STZ, chlorotocin, is also diabetogenic and induces DNA strand breaks and DNA–DNA and DNA–

protein crosslinks.[23] Though no islet luminescence can be seen with STZ as with alloxan, the presence of OH radicals can be inferred from the beneficial effect of OH scavengers and/or inhibitors of poly (ADP-ribose) synthase. Nicotinamide exerts considerable protection as late as 2 hours after STZ administration but is effective against alloxan only when given in advance. Poly (ADP-ribose) synthase inhibition alone, without adding OH scavengers, is sufficient to ameliorate STZ diabetogenicity, indicating that the enhanced activity of this enzyme is necessary for the toxic outcome. It is very likely that this action promotes DNA regeneration and the resumption of insulin synthesis. In addition to DNA cleavage by OH radicals, the toxicity of STZ and of its analogue 1-methyl-1-nitrosourea (MNU) also results in alkylation of cell constituents without necessarily being lethal to cells. These nitroso compounds produce highly reactive diazonium and carbonium ions which are able to alkylate and carbamylate, apart from DNA, numerous cytosolic and mitochondrial enzyme proteins vital for energy generation.[24] Because STZ produces a steeper fall in NAD than MNU, it is likely that the acute NAD loss is lethal to cells.

Okamoto[21,22] postulated a uniform mechanism of alloxan and STZ action. This researcher considers fragmentation of β-cell DNA as the crucial event, caused by accumulation of superoxide and OH radicals and DNA alkylation with breaks in DNA strands. This also initiates the processes of excision and repair, involving the activation of poly (ADP-ribose) synthase and the associated NAD depletion. The NAD loss becomes irreplaceable and results in virtual cessation of NAD-dependent energy and protein metabolism, ending in cell necrosis. This unifying concept is supported by preventive effects of nicotinamide and OH scavengers, as mentioned above. Such a mechanism may also apply to other β-cell destructive processes in which there is evidence for generation of free radicals,[25] including autoimmune insulitis due to lymphocyte infiltration.

The likely reasons for the specific β-cell toxicity of alloxan and STZ are: (1) high affinity for the glucose-like moieties related to the exquisite sensitivity of β cells to glucose, raising the concentration of alloxan and STZ to levels higher than in other cells; (2) SH-groups in the β-cell membrane render it especially sensitive to oxidative lesion; (3) β cells have a low capacity for removal of oxidizing radicals due to specific glutathione depletion and low glutathione peroxidase activity[26,27]; and (4) the NAD:DNA ratio in islets is lower than in other tissues, about one-half of that in the liver.

Another phenomenon associated with STZ diabetes is the high frequency of tumors in pancreatic islets, particularly when the STZ toxicity is mitigated by concomitant administration of nicotinamide or poly (ADP-ribose) synthase inhibitors.[28,29] Okamoto[21,22] suggested that the inhibition of DNA repair may cause abnormal DNA recombination, resulting in the formation of tumor-inducing genes. An oncogene was discovered that was expressed in β-cell tumors and was named *rig* for rat insulinoma gene.[30,31] It is of interest that the same gene was expressed in a BK virus–induced hamster insulinoma and in a spontaneous human insulinoma.[21,31]

The discovery of an oncogene that may be unique to β cells appearing subsequent to prevention of cytotoxic assault led to the study of β-cell replication in pancreatectomized rats. This diabetes model is characterized by an exhaustion of insulin production, together with marked hypertrophy of the remaining islets. When these rats receive poly (ADP-ribose) synthase inhibitors starting 7 days before pancreatectomy, the glucosuria and glucose tolerance improve, islet hypertrophy is reduced, and the granulated β-cell

mass increases in the pancreas remnant, compared with pancreatectomized nontreated rats. Okamoto[21,22] constructed from pancreas remnants a poly (A)[1]RNA-derived cDNA library and isolated a *reg* (regeneration) gene. The *reg* gene is expressed only in islets of pancreatectomized, nicotinamide-treated rats, and is not present in control islets or in regenerating liver, brain, kidneys, and insulinoma. The *reg* gene, probably specifically regulating β-cell proliferation, was also isolated from hyperplastic islets of gold thioglucose–treated NON mice (described later) and a *reg* homologue was found in the human pancreas. The *reg* gene has been cloned and shown to induce β-cell replication in cultured islets and in the pancreas remnant of pancreatectomized rats.[32]

METABOLIC AND ENDOCRINE CHANGES IN ALLOXAN- AND STZ-DIABETIC ANIMALS

Glucose Metabolism

Hepatic glucose production and the activity of the rate-limiting enzyme phosphoenolpyruvate carboxykinase (PEPCK) are increased because of lack of control in the virtual absence of insulin. Reduced glucose utilization and lipogenesis are typical outcomes of insulinopenic diabetes induced either by alloxan or STZ. This is due to well-documented inhibition of expression of regulatory enzymes of glycolysis and lipogenesis and not to a direct effect of the toxins. An increased flow of glucogenic precursors, such as lactate alanine or glycerol, from muscle and adipose tissue elevates the hepatic glucose production.

Similarly, changes typical of the absence of insulin are evident in glycogenolysis and glycogenesis through the effects on interconversion of active–inactive forms of glycogen synthase and phosphorylase in the direction favoring glycogen breakdown. A characteristic outcome is the subnormal hepatic glycogen concentration in the fed state and higher than control levels in the fasting state. In several insulin-independent tissues glycogen paradoxically accumulates (kidney, intestine, and placenta).[33,34] This is related to intracellular accumulation of glucose-6-phosphate, an allosteric activator of glycogen synthase in the absence of insulin.

Increased intestinal mass and nutrient absorption are typical of diabetic hyperphagia, evident in STZ- and alloxan-treated rats. There is an elevation in the intestinal brush border membrane hydrolases active in hexose transport. This may result from enhanced specific enzyme synthesis, or intestinal proliferation, or both. There is an overexpression of intestinal GLUT-2 and GLUT-5.[35]

Protein Metabolism

Alloxan- and STZ-diabetic animals have a negative nitrogen balance related to enhanced proteolysis in muscles and other tissues and to reduced protein synthesis. Growth failure is also due to the reduced production of growth factors and increased growth factor–binding protein.[36–38] Proteolysis is effected both by a rapid mechanism and a slow, long-lasting activation of a myofibrillar protease, which is only gradually abolished by insulin.[39,40] The STZ-induced diabetes results in the decrease of collagen synthesis, which exceeds the negative total protein balance in the muscle.[41] Protein catabolism and flow of amino acids to the liver feed the gluconeogenic pathway and accelerate ureagenesis. STZ diabetes is associated with partial loss of hepatic endoplasmic reticulum and of lysosomes, probably related to the enhanced autophagia.[42]

Lipid Metabolism

Alloxan- and STZ-diabetic rats excessively mobilize free fatty acids (FFAs) due to the rise in adipose tissue lipase activity with resultant vigorous muscle and liver FFA oxidation. The activity of carnitine acyl CoA transferase, regulating the transport of fatty acids into the mitochondria, is elevated in rat liver and kidney, whereas the concentration of malonyl CoA, the regulator of acyl CoA entry into mitochondria, is lowered.[43] This is less evident in obese rats. They are also characterized by elevated FFA transport, but their hyperinsulinemia abrogates fat oxidation. In diabetic animals the ratio of FFA oxidation to esterification is double that of nondiabetic animals.[44] Ketosis is present more often in alloxan- than in STZ-diabetic animals, but does not usually progress to ketoacidosis. This is an important distinction from rats and mice with autoimmune type 1-like diabetes, and indicates that insulin secretion from residual or regenerated β cells prevents an unrestrained FFA mobilization with lapse into ketosis. This "spontaneous" amelioration of diabetes limits the period of severe insulin deficiency in STZ- or alloxan-treated animals to a few weeks after the induction of diabetes, and requires scrutiny of β-cell function for long-term experiments.

An elevation in plasma triglycerides, cholesterol, and phospholipids in the VLDL and LDL fractions is evident in diabetic animals, due in part to the hepatic recirculation of inflowing FFAs and other lipids and to the delayed disposal of VLDL and chylomicrons. This is related to decreases in the translation and activity of insulin-dependent lipoprotein lipase (LPL) and in the apoprotein moieties of lipoproteins,[45–48] necessary for the recognition and activation of uptake of the triglyceride-rich particles. It should be emphasized that the HDL fraction is also increased in insulinopenic rodents, in contrast to humans, because HDL functions in both forward and reverse transport of cholesterol in rodents.

Although diabetic animals manifest hypercholesterolemia and atherosclerosis,[48] the hepatic synthesis of cholesterol is either reduced or unchanged.[49] There is evidence for inhibited liver HMG CoA reductase, the rate-limiting enzyme of cholesterol synthesis.[50] Conversely, there is a rise in intestinal synthesis of cholesterol due both to a specific increase and tissue proliferation related to hyperphagia.[49,51] Thus diabetic hypercholesterolemia is mainly of intestinal origin and may be the reason for suppression of hepatic cholesterol production.

Insulin Receptor and Endocrine Derangements

Alloxan- and STZ-diabetic animals excessively secrete somatostatin. Also, arginine- and glucose-induced somatostatin release from isolated rat pancreas is enhanced[52,53] as islet δ cells are not affected. However, the glucose-stimulated islets of STZ-diabetic dogs fail to respond with increased somatostatin and decreased glucagon secretion, whereas the responses to arginine and isoproterenol are normal,[54] suggesting either the blunting of glucose recognition by δ and α cells or compensation by hyperglycemia. Shortly after STZ injection, the basal and stimulated secretion of glucagon is enhanced in rats, but suppressed by exogenous insulin. This suggests that the glucagonemia and somatostatinemia that occur in insulinopenic animals are a consequence of β-cell loss.

With regard to the low fertility of diabetic animals, extensive functional and morphologic neuroendocrine degenerative alterations have been found in the mediobasal hypothalamus of STZ-treated rats.[55] The lesions, affecting luteinizing hormone–releasing hormone synthesis and secretion, were attributed to the direct, local effect of hypoinsulinemia. The reduced neurohormone release from the exhausted pool seems responsible for the wasting of pituitary gonadotrophs and the resulting hypofunction of the pituitary–gonadal hormone axis. There is also evidence of attenuated feedback control of LH release in STZ diabetes[56] and lack of the response of the ovary to FSH in alloxan diabetes, related to atresia shortly after the induction of alloxan diabetes.[57]

Insulin receptors in models of insulinopenic diabetes bind insulin well in adipocytes, hepatocytes, and muscle, in contrast to animals with hyperinsulinemia and insulin resistance, which generally show downregulation of insulin binding and reduced activity of the insulin receptor tyrosine kinase (TK).[58] The increased binding in STZ-treated animals is mainly due to recruitment of receptors and not to higher affinity[59] except in severely diabetic rats.[60] Notwithstanding the increased binding, the activity of hepatic TK per receptor is either reduced or unchanged.[58] However, the TK activity is markedly stimulated after contact with insulin, and total TK receptor autophosphorylation is elevated in muscle and liver, but is not increased per receptor.[61] It is possible that multisite phosphorylation occurs in the presence of added insulin, involving serine/threonine residues on the receptor,[62] which is inhibitory to TK-mediated phosphorylation. It could also be due to increased phosphotyrosine phosphatase activity in diabetic rats.[63] In any case, a relative reduction in phosphorylation in the face of increased insulin binding and receptor number upregulation seems to characterize insulinopenic animals. A similar change was demonstrated in severely insulin-deprived BB rats.[64]

Drug metabolism is altered in insulinopenic diabetes. Microsomal P-450 cytochrome-dependent enzymes (such as aniline hydroxylase and monooxygenase activities) exhibit increased mRNA levels and activity, which may be reversed by insulin treatment.[65] This enhanced capacity of the liver to detoxify xenobiotics may in some cases not be advantageous, as genotoxic intermediates can be formed and the diabetic organism may be susceptible to the toxicity or oncogenicity of such chemicals.[66]

DIABETES ELICITED BY LOW, MULTIPLE DOSES OF STREPTOZOCIN (MD-STZ)

Repeated small doses of STZ, insufficient for immediate diabetogenesis, produce in susceptible species a delayed insulitis-related diabetes. Like and Rossini[67] observed that 200 mg/kg STZ, given to male CD-1 mice in five consecutive daily doses of 40 mg/kg, causes hyperglycemia within 1–2 weeks. A lymphocytic islet infiltration results, preventable by rabbit antiserum against mouse lymphocytes (ALS), suggesting an inflammatory, possibly an autoimmune, reaction. 3-O-methylglucose or nicotinamide, which protects against a single β-cell necrotizing STZ dose, also reduces the MD-STZ syndrome. MD-STZ diabetes is prevented by glucose or 5-thioglucose given before STZ injection or added with STZ to β-cell cultures in vitro.[68] Although the hyperglycemia is fully prevented, attesting to the protection of the insulin-secreting apparatus, the inflammatory response is not. This points to dissociation between insulitis and β-cell destruction. Preservation of β-cell integrity by the above-mentioned and other treatments[69] supports the view that the injury may be due to a combination of cell-mediated autoimmunity and a metabolic, glucose-dependent lesion.

Kolb and associates[69,70] gathered support for a T-cell-mediated mechanism of insulitis. Athymic nude mice, which are less responsive to MD-STZ, fail to show islet lymphocyte infiltration, but when grafted with thymus exhibit the full syndrome. Numerous immunomodulators prevent the syndrome. Silica, a macrophage toxin, also prevents the induction of MD-STZ diabetes, implying a role for cellular immune mechanisms. However, questions remain whether insulitis is causal or only associated with cell death. Treatment of mice with dimethylurea, an OH scavenger, prior to MD-STZ protects against the hyperglycemia but not against insulitis. When dimethylurea is employed to prevent the high-dose STZ diabetes, delayed hyperglycemia and insulitis may occur instead. Evidence has been provided[71] that the type 1 diabetes–like syndrome induced by MD-STZ is not due to the autoimmune T- or B-lymphocyte-mediated mechanisms occurring in NOD mice. When MD-STZ was administered to severely immunodeficient male (*scid/scid*) NOD mice, which are devoid of functional lymphocytes, even low STZ doses of 30 mg/kg induced hyperglycemia without insulitis.

As reviewed by Wilson and Leiter,[72] male C57BKS mice, which are highly sensitive to the induction of both insulitis and hyperglycemia, also show an induction of retroviral genome, such as intracisternal type A and C virus particles in islets, 2 days prior to insulitis. The presence of "silent" viruses in mice islets appears to be frequent, and the possibility that STZ activates some of them, with consequent alteration in islet antigenicity, cannot be ruled out. However, it is certain that MD-STZ mice represent a diabetic condition produced by an exogenous toxin and that this model is distinct from that underlying autoimmune human T1DM. Nevertheless, the MD-STZ model is important for gaining insight into structural and genetic lesions in β cells.

ANIMALS WITH AUTOIMMUNE ETIOLOGY AND INSULIN DEPENDENCE

The discovery of two animal species with spontaneous autoimmune diabetes, BB rats and NOD mice, contributed to the general acceptance of the etiologic role of autoimmunity in T1DM.

The BB Rat

The major features of the syndrome in BB rats in its pathogenic phase are described here. More details on history, husbandry, and complications can be found in special review publications[73–75] (see Chap. 20). The classic symptoms of weight loss, polyuria, polydipsia, glucosuria, and ketoacidosis appear abruptly with marked hyperglycemia, hypoinsulinemia, insulitis, and β-cell loss. The diabetes-prone rats may show IGT a few days before the onset of overt symptoms at 60–120 days of age. Levels of islet insulin become very low, and most diabetic animals are totally insulin dependent for survival within a few days. Several sublines varying in frequency, severity, immunologic characteristics, and time of diabetes onset are available, including three diabetes-resistant lines in which <1% of animals become diabetic.[75]

Breeding of BB rats requires great care because of their lymphopenia, vulnerability to infections, and the need for individual supervision and insulin treatment. As variations in the incidence and expression of diabetes upon exposure to viral or microbial pathogens in various localities occur in BB rats,[76,77] it has been

agreed to denote their derivation by a slash following the BB designation (BB/Wor for the Worcester colony and BB/O for the Ontario colony). Of the inbred BB/Wor rats, the source of several worldwide colonies, 50–80% become diabetic; males and females are equally affected.

The diabetes in BB/Wor rats is probably inherited by autosomal recessive transmission, with about 50% penetrance related to at least two genes. One non-MHC linked gene expresses the T-cell lymphopenia; the second is linked with RT[+], the MHC of the rat.[75] This resembles human T1DM without association with specific HLA types. However, subsequent investigations indicate that the permissive MHC haplotype and the recessive lymphopenic gene[78] are not specifically related to diabetes and are insufficient to produce diabetes susceptibility in the BB rat.[79] Although BB rats share the class II RT1[u] rat MHC, they are not all genetically identical. Genetic heterogeneity of the BB rat has been investigated among 26 distinct lines, analyzing 19 protein markers.[80] Polymorphism in nine markers has been observed and used to define seven distinct haplotypes. Therefore, interpretation of genetic, immune, and metabolic investigations of BB rats should take into account the origin and maintenance of the colonies from which the animals were derived.

Pancreas histology immediately after the outset of hyperglycemia shows a striking lymphocytic islet infiltration (Fig. 16-2). Insulitis precedes the onset of overt diabetes by several days and

FIGURE 16-2. Insulitis in the NOD mouse. **A.** Peripheral accumulation of mononuclear lymphocytes with yet functional β cells. **B.** Penetration of mononuclear lymphocytes into the islet with destruction of β cells. (*Courtesy of Dr. M.C. Appel, Department of Pathology, University of Massachusetts, Worcester, MA.*)

A

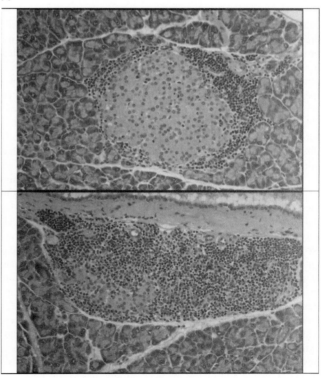

B

disappears after β-cell loss, leaving shrunken end-stage islets composed almost entirely of α, δ, and PP cells. Insulitis to a varying extent is also observed in 50–75% of nonhyperglycemic BB/Wor rats. Nitric oxide is a probable β-cell cytotoxic agent. The inducible NO synthase (iNOS) has been found in the pancreas of BB rats with insulitis by RT-PCR and immunohistochemistry.[81,82] iNOS expression was limited to areas of islet infiltration by macrophages, and produced by macrophages, suggesting iNOS involvement in islet destruction[81] in genetic association with T lymphopenia.[83]

The autoimmune syndrome of BB rats is polyendocrine in nature, as evident from the frequent occurrence of lymphocytic thyroiditis and of autoantibodies against smooth and skeletal muscle, gastric parietal cells, thyroglobulin, and thyroid cells. Islet cell cytoplasmic antibodies (ICAs), thought to arise from cellular constituents after degradation, and islet cell surface antibodies (ICSAs), formed against specific cell membrane components, are often present in the circulation. Although it is known that not all animals with antibodies develop diabetes and not all animals with diabetes carry antibodies, a careful correlation of circulating antibodies with insulitis and diabetes in BB/Wor and BB/O strains reveals that they are more frequent in diabetes-prone than in diabetes-resistant BB rats and are often present at weaning.[84]

Among the features of BB rats resembling human T1DM is the prepubertal onset with a silent prediabetic period, which presents an opportunity for the search for early markers of the disorder. Plasma lymphocyte antibodies[85] and biopterin, released by macrophages upon cytokine activation,[86] have been proposed as predictors. Avoidance of certain wheat- and milk-derived dietary proteins[87–89] was suggested as beneficial for delaying or preventing the expression of diabetes in BB rats and humans. Acividin, the inhibitor of glutamine metabolism, prevents BB rat diabetes, possibly by interacting with the activated insulitis-producing lymphocytes.[90]

The detection of ICSAs 1–2 months before the onset of diabetes in BB rats parallels their early presence in prediabetic children and their association with islet destruction. However, decisive proof of a direct pathogenic role of ICSAs in vivo is still lacking despite correlations between the start of mononuclear islet infiltration and diabetes onset, and between the appearance of complement-fixing ICSAs and β-cell destruction. ICAs have not been conclusively found in BB rats.[74] Moreover, GAD antibodies considered important for the prediction of human T1DM are absent in some lines of BB rats,[91–93] but have been detected in the BB/O line.[94] Also, IA-2 antibodies have been detected in some lines, but not in others.[95]

There is at least one notable difference between the BB rat and human diabetes. The severe generalized lymphopenia occurring in the former, which precedes clinical manifestations of diabetes, involves both primary and secondary lymphoid tissues and affects all subsets of T cells. The T-cell lymphopenia is permissive rather than obligatory for diabetes to occur.[96] It is uniformly present in all diabetes-prone and diabetic BB/Wor rats, and is suggested to originate from a hematopoietic stem cell defect, or from a defective thymic maturation process.[75] All inbred, diabetes-prone BB/Wor rats appear to have reduced phenotypic and functional cytolytic T cells and a lack of RT6+ cells. These defects are absent in diabetes-resistant BB/Wor rats. Although the progression of the lymphocytic infiltration as an intermediate stage of β-cell destruction is now better understood, the initial events remain obscure. The role of lymphopenia and of the involved subsets has yet to be ascertained, as diabetes occurs without lymphopenia in the inbred, re-

sistant BB/Wor lines and in diabetes-prone NOD mice. An alteration of islet β-cell antigenicity is possible, which may result in activation of T lymphocytes, NK cells, and cytotoxic antibodies directed against β cells. The nature and interaction of the humoral antibodies and cell antigens remain to be elucidated. In this respect, it is intriguing that a membrane-bound islet-specific 38-kd autoantigen[97] becomes expressed in diabetes-prone BB rats at 30 days of age, when the immune effectors start to recognize β cells. The delayed expression may be crucial for effecting the breakdown of self-tolerance and for initiating autoimmunity. Another promising aspect of this increasingly immunologic rather than diabetologic discipline is immunomodulation.[75] In BB rats, not only are the various β cell–destroying effectors present at the onset of diabetes, but the regulatory T cells, which control the system, are defective or missing. These may be RT6+ postthymic lymphocytes (carrying the RT6 rat alloantigen), detectable in peripheral lymphocytes of diabetes-resistant BB rats but missing in the diabetes-prone line. Removal of the RT6+ cells in the former with a monoclonal antibody frequently induces insulitis, and renders them diabetic, and their splenocytes are capable of transferring the disease to nondiabetic BB rats. Immunomodulatory interventions may entail changing the balance between subsets of T lymphocytes by cyclophosphamide, or stimulation of lymphopoiesis by blood removal, dietary changes, and immunogenic stimulation.[75]

The Nonobese Diabetic (NOD) Mouse

A large body of information on the development, pathophysiology, immunopathogenesis, and genetics of NOD mice is now available in reviews.[98–102] The NOD mice were raised in Japan in the late 1960s by inbreeding a single female glucosuric mouse from a substrain of ICR mice, and are now distributed worldwide. Their salient feature is the spontaneous lymphocytic islet infiltration, starting at the age of 4–5 weeks, that leads to overt diabetes at 13–30 weeks, with severe hyperglycemia and both plasma and β-cell insulin deficiency. Unlike BB rats they do not become ketoacidotic, but require maintenance on insulin. Insulitis is prevalent both in males and females at 5 weeks, but in the original colony overt diabetes occurs in 80% of females and in only 20% of males at 30 weeks. However, the lines established outside the original colony at Shionogi Laboratories in Japan differ in diabetes incidence, time of onset, and gender ratio.

The lymphocytes infiltrating the islets include CD4+ and CD8+ T cells and B cells. The insulitis differs somewhat from that in the BB rats.[103,104] In the initial invasion stage, the lymphocytes are localized in the periductular capillary spaces with a clear basement membrane boundary without overt contact with the β cells. Later, the lymphocytes invade the islet; β cells are destroyed, but α, δ, and PP cells remain intact. Unlike the pronounced lymphopenia of BB rats, NOD mice exhibit little or no lymphocyte decline. Antibodies directed toward a variety of islet antigens, including GAD, are detectable soon after weaning and ICSAs at 6 weeks, with 50% prevalence between 12 and 18 weeks.

The NOD model is important for the understanding of conditions predisposing to T1DM. Although the contribution of multiple genes on different chromosomes to diabetes susceptibility has been demonstrated,[103–108] the environmental, nutritional, and hormonal impact on the incidence of diabetes, despite the identical genetic background, affects the penetrance of genetic susceptibility. For example, the incidence of diabetes in males may vary from 0–100%. Castration of males increases the incidence of diabetes, whereas implantation of testosterone to young females prevents diabetes, apparently by inhibiting the production or function of autoimmune effectors. This suggests that the gender dimorphism has a genetic background, possibly due to hormonal imprinting early in life, but its expression is amenable to manipulation.

It is striking that the exposure of NOD mice to murine viral pathogens protects against diabetes, probably through general immunostimulation, because several exogenous immunomodulators, such as complete Freund's adjuvant, various cytokines, poly I:C, or gangliosides, also prevent or attenuate the diabetes development, as reviewed by Kolb.[69] These effects are more marked in NOD mice than in BB rats. All these factors are also responsible for the continuing genetic drift in various colonies, which must be considered when analyzing and comparing the experimental results from various sources. To facilitate evaluations, the inbred substrains should be labeled by adding a suffix after a slash (NOD/Shi for the Shionogi colony or NOD/Lt for the Jackson colony).

In contrast to BB rats, the β-cell deterioration in NOD mice is markedly attenuated by nicotinamide, scavengers of free radicals, and inhibitors of poly (ADP-ribose) synthase.[21] Thus, the destructive processes show more similarities to the action of chemical cytotoxins in NOD mice than in BB rats, although these differences may be quantitative in nature. It is of interest that, as in the BB rat, pretreatment with insulin prevents the adoptive transfer of diabetes.[109] The different aspects of human T1DM are compared to those in BB rats and NOD mice in Table 16-2.

Although most investigations of the origin of NOD diabetes have focused on T lymphocytes as effectors, there is strong evidence that functional defects in bone marrow–derived antigen-presenting cells (APCs) may be responsible for the appearance of β-cell autoreactive T lymphocytes. This is based on observations that diabetogenic T lymphocytes become active in diabetes-resistant hybrid NOD strains that are lethally irradiated and transplanted with nonhybrid NOD bone marrow.[110,111] APCs determine the spectrum of the T-cell repertoire by carrying self-antigens into the thymus. Ineffective presentation of antigens by APCs may cause their faulty tolerogenic functions such as the inability to activate functional immunoregulatory T (suppressor) cells in the periphery and to block the thymic development of autoreactive T lymphocytes against islet β cells.

The LETL Rat

The Long Evans Tokushima Lean (LETL) spontaneously diabetic strain of rats was isolated in the 1980s in Japan, from a colony based on a few pairs of outbred Long Evans rats.[112] The diabetes onset in inbred animals occurs at 8–20 weeks of age with an average incidence of 21% in males and 15% in females, influenced by whether one or two parents were diabetic. The incidence of diabetes at 16 weeks of age is doubled by pretreatment with cyclophosphamide, starting at 5–7 weeks.[113] The clinical features of diabetes are typical of type 1 diabetes and the LETL rats require insulin for survival. A control LETO strain which exhibits type 2-like diabetes, was inbred from nondiabetic animals of the same stock.

In contrast to BB rats, the LETL rats are not lymphopenic and the distribution of the thymocyte subsets is similar to that of control rats. A marked lymphocytic infiltration of islets occurs 4–5 days before the onset of clinical diabetes. Insulitis is not observed in nondiabetic siblings and in the LETO control line. Lymphocytic infiltration occurs in other glands, similarly to the polyendocrine character of the disease in BB rats and NOD mice. With regard to genetics, the LETL rats carry the RT1ᵘ haplotype, as does the diabetes-prone BB rat. At least two recessive genes, one closely linked with RT1ᵘ, seem to be involved in the pathogenesis of insulitis.

TABLE 16-2 Characteristics of Autoimmune (Type 1) Diabetes in Humans, NOD Mice, and BB Rats

	Humans	NOD Mice	BB Rats
Hyperglycemia, insulinopenia	+	+	+
Ketoacidosis (if untreated)	+	−	+
Female over male gender bias	−	+	−
Insulitis (T-lymphocyte driven)	+	+	+
Leukocytic infiltrates found in other organs	Sometimes	+	+
Susceptibility of gene penetrance to environmental factors	Probable	Very strong	Strong
Genetic predisposition	+	+	+
Complex polygenic control	+	+	+
Disease transmissible	+	+	+
via bone marrow	Not tested	+	+
via T lymphocytes	Not tested	+	+
Lymphocytopenia	−	−	+
Defective peripheral immunoregulation	−	−	+
Humoral reactivity to β cells			
ICSAs	+	+	+
ICAs	+	+	+
IAAs	+	+	−
Recurrence of aggression against transplanted β cells	+	+	+
Attenuation or prevention by immunomodulation or free radical scavengers	?	+	+
Effective immunotherapy	Possible (safety?)	+	+
Virus induction	Probable	−	+
B lymphocytes required	Not tested	+	Not tested
β Cells required for immune activation	Not tested	+	+

Two new animal with spontaneous autoimmune etiology, which provide new perspective in the clarification of the autoimmune mechanisms, have recently been reported upon. The **Torri rat** of the Sprague Dawley strain manifested an incidence of diabetes of 100% in males and 33% in females at 45 weeks of age.[114] Hyperglycemia, hypoinsulinemia and hyperlipidemia were present at 25 weeks with marked fibrosis of pancreatic islets. Torri rats were characterized by long-term survival without insulin support. The particular characteristics are severe ocular complications, cataract and retinopathy with tractional, retinal detachment, fibrous proliferation and massive hemorrhage at 70–77 weeks of age.

The **LEW.1AR1/Ztm-iddm rat** also exhibits TIDM arising from spontaneous mutation in congenic Lewis rat strain with a defined MHC haplotype.[115] The incidence of TIDM was 20% without sex preference at 8–9 weeks. The proportion of T lymphocytes in the peripheral blood was normal expressing the RT6.1 differentiation antigen. Islets were heavily infiltrated with both T and B lymphocytes, macrophages and NK cells. Apoptotic cell death was evident in the areas of insulitis.

GENETICALLY ALTERED ANIMALS FOR DIABETES RESEARCH

Transgenic and gene-disrupted animals, mainly mice, represent a rapidly expanding technological advance in diabetes research made possible by the ability to introduce transgenes or delete existing genes. These mice are not in a strict sense models of diabetes, but manipulating their genetic expression provides valuable information on the *in vivo* function of a particular gene to assess its role in pathophysiology of diabetes (e.g., glucose transport, insulinogenesis, cell replication, or autoimmunity).

It is beyond the scope of this chapter to overview the plethora of transgenic mice that have been recently investigated. Just a mention of several examples is possible. One of the early studies using transgenic constructs was the implantation of a hybrid insulin oncogene SV40 T antigen (*Tag*) to direct the expression of specific proteins in islet β cells.[116,117] The hybrid-injected eggs were then placed in the oviducts of pseudopregnant female mice, which led to the development of insulinoma. Rat insulin promoter (RIP-Tag) lines have been obtained that vary in their progression to a tumor. These experiments were intended to create insulin-producing cells capable of proliferation at a controlled rate.

Insulin has been overexpressed in β cells with multiple copies of the human insulin gene. These mice manifested a profuse insulin secretion leading to insulin resistance and downregulation of tissue insulin receptors.[118] This illustrates the detrimental effect of insulin excess on receptor number and function typical of type 2-like diabetes. Another transgenic model of a type 2 diabetic condition has been produced by expressing a component of the human insulin receptor with high-affinity insulin binding.[119] In this situation postabsorptive hyperglycemia and hepatic gluconeogenesis ensue despite hyperinsulinemia. Transgenic mice overproducing islet amyloid polypeptide were also prepared, showing an associated insulin storage and increased cosecretion, and eventually amyloid deposits on a high-fat diet.[120]

The glucokinase gene has been overexpressed in the liver to correct the hyperglycemia of type 1 diabetes.[121,122] A phenotype with increased hepatic glycogen content, hypoglycemia, and hypoinsulinemia was obtained. Suppression of the promoter gene driving the insulin-dependent PEPCK in the liver was carried out to reduce the hepatic glucose production in diabetic mice.[123,124]

The selective disruption of the insulin receptor substrate-1 (IRS-1) substrate of the insulin receptor tyrosine kinase has, surprisingly, produced only mild insulin resistance.[125,126] The overexpression of the GLUT-4 gene in several transgenic mouse models resulted in fasting hypoglycemia and hypoinsulinemia due to overutilization of glucose in peripheral tissues.[127,128] The negative result of this hypoinsulinemia was enhanced lipolysis with elevation of plasma triglycerides and ketosis. In general, transgenic animals demonstrated that the GLUT-4 level controls the rate of overall glucose metabolism, particularly in skeletal muscle. Hexokinase II becomes rate limiting only under conditions of hyperglycemia with hypoinsulinemia. Insulin action is correlated with the amount of GLUT-4 protein. Thus the improvement in IGT can be effected by a regulated overexpression of a single protein.[129,130] Severe hyperglycemia and insulin resistance in *db/db* mice were considerably ameliorated by overexpression of GLUT-4.[131] Additional examples of transgenic mice in the study of various aspects of diabetes are listed in reviews.[132,133]

INSULIN-RESISTANT, MUTANT RODENTS WITH DIABESITY

db/db Mice with Hyperinsulinemia, Insulin Resistance, and Hyperglycemia Leading to β-Cell Collapse, Now Labeled as *lepr*[db]

The mutation designated as db occurred spontaneously in the C57BL/Ks inbred strain of mice in Bar Harbor, Maine.[134,135] Diabetes in the *db/db* mice is a recessive, autosomal single-gene mutation on chromosome 4, with complete penetrance. It is now considered to be the homologue of the rat *fa* gene on chromosome 5 and its allele corpulent *cp* (described later). The *db* gene has been linked to the black coat misty gene on chromosome 4, which allows early identification of homozygotes in congenic *mdb* strains. Homozygous *db/db* mice are infertile, so heterozygous db/+ carriers are used to breed the mutants. The *db* gene manifests different expressions on BL/6J and BL/Ks backgrounds. The diabetes is mild and resembles the *ob* mutation on the BL/6J background. In contrast, the Ks background imparts a marked insulin resistance and ketosis and glucose overproduction, associated with marked damage to the insulin secretion apparatus and eventual death in the face of massive glycemia.[134,135] This is a cogent illustration of the impact of deleterious genomic modifiers on the course, severity, and final outcome of the diabesity syndrome (the interrelation of obesity and diabetes, discussed later) caused by a single abnormal gene.

As outlined in Table 16-3, the initial stages of the syndrome are characterized by hyperphagia and hyperinsulinemia at the time of weaning. The mice gain weight and become hyperglycemic [up to 400 mg/dL (33 mmol/L)] between 8 and 12 weeks, in spite of 6- to 10-fold higher than normal insulin levels. At 3–6 months, the insulinemia wanes to subnormal levels, β-cell secretion ceases, and the mice become ketotic with β-cell necrosis and do not survive longer than 10 months. Shifts in the time course of diabetes development may occur in *db/db* mice raised in other colonies, and investigators should establish their own local reference values.

Consistent with hyperglycemia and hyperinsulinemia as the earliest abnormalities in *db/db* mice, the β-cell insulin oversecre-

TABLE 16-3 Genetically Predetermined Time Course of Diabetes Development and Progress in C57BL/KS *db/db* (*lepr ^{db}*) Mice Maintained on Regular Diet*

Stage B <1 month old	Stage C 2–3 months old	Stage D >3 months old	Stage E 8–10 months old
Hyperinsulinemia	Peak insulinemia	Hypoinsulinemia	Severely insulin-deficient, almost complete β-cell loss
Normoglycemia	Hyperglycemia	Marked hyperglycemia	Ketosis
Hyperphagia	Hyperphagia	Hyperphagia	Hyperphagia
Moderate weight gain	Marked weight gain	Weight loss	Leanness
Mild insulin resistance	High gluconeogenesis and lipogenesis	High gluconeogenesis	No survival beyond this age
		Severe β-cell degranulation	

*Because there are no nondiabetic *db/db* mutants, stage A (reference) designation is reserved for the normoinsulinemic-normoglycemic heterozygote siblings.

tion lasts up to 4 months irrespective of the islet content. The reduced β-cell response to glucose, but sustained response to arginine, occurs concurrently with a loss of the β-cell GLUT-2 transporter. This is a reversible phenomenon, because *db* islets transplanted to nondiabetic db/+ controls regain GLUT-2 expression.[136] At the phase of reduced insulin secretion there are ultrastructural changes comprised of dilatation of Golgi apparatus and of rough endoplasmic reticulum.[137] Incorporation of ^{3}H-leucine into insulin indicates first an increased synthesis in young mice, and then a decline concomitant with changes in insulin release. Similar findings were obtained with ^{3}H-thymidine incorporation. β-Cell polyploidy, involving the DNA,[138] enlargement of the islets, and hypertrophy of individual cells, suggests mobilization of β-cell precursors. Although insulin oversecretion initially compensates for the insulin resistance, β cells are unable to sustain the high secretion rate. The end-stage necrosis is drastic, leaving atrophied islets with δ, α, and PP cells only.

Tissue insulin resistance in young *db/db* mice is demonstrated by low response to injected insulin or to implanted islets from isogeneic donors.[134,135] Insulin treatment does not appreciably influence the progression to diabetes. In the young mice, the glycolytic enzymes and glucose oxidation are enhanced by insulin induction, as would be expected. In older, hyperglycemic mice, the activity of glycolytic enzymes declines, while the gluconeogenic pathway escapes control, despite the high concentration of circulating insulin. PEPCK synthesis, assessed by hepatic PEPCK mRNA levels, is normally reduced by physiologic rises in circulating insulin, but suppression of its activity and transcription in *db/db* mice requires enormous amounts of exogenous insulin.[139] Regulatory failure of other liver systems is also evident. Glycogen breakdown proceeds at an accelerated rate and is not inhibited by glucose, as occurs normally. Interestingly, the hepatic insulin resistance does not affect lipogenic enzymes, which remain responsive to insulin and rise in activity, accounting for the prevalent hyperlipidemia in diabetic *db/db* mice. Enhanced lipogenesis is also expressed in the small intestine.[140]

Insulin resistance is evident by reduced insulin binding to receptors and reduced receptor tyrosine kinase activity in muscle, liver, and isolated fibroblasts.[141,142] Adipose tissue of young mice exhibits increased glycolysis and undiminished insulin response. In older mice, an inverse pattern of stimulated FFA outflow reflects insensitivity of adipose tissue lipolysis to insulin.

Dietary restriction does not induce normoinsulinemia in *db/db* mice. Total substitution of protein for carbohydrate has a marked

beneficial effect.[143] The regimen of 83% casein does substantially reduce the insulin resistance and hyperglycemia. It also extends the life span, retards the decrease in islet insulin content,[139] and delays β-cell necrosis, most likely through the alleviation of glucotoxicity. Inclusion of even 8% of carbohydrate in the diet, particularly sucrose, substantially aggravates the diabetes and shortens the life span of these mice. The high-protein diet diminishes the glycemia by making it dependent on endogenously regulated hepatic gluconeogenesis in the absence of intestinally absorbed glucose.

Hypothalamic disturbance is evident in *db/db* mice, manifested by early hyperphagia, insulin secretion, and obesity. The mice fail to respond to satiety signals. Coleman and Hummel impressively demonstrated this by parabiosis with nondiabetic mice.[144] The latter stop eating and starve to death within 2–4 weeks, due to an exaggerated response to the inflow of satiety factors from *db/db* mice now known to be leptin. The *db/db* mice gained weight and did not respond to their own satiety factor or to that of nondiabetic mice because of the defect in the hypothalamic leptin receptor, now known to be a truncation mutation.

Striking results were obtained when *db/db* mice were parabiosed with congenic *ob/ob* partners.[145] The latter stopped eating, became lean, and died from starvation because of the response to the massive inflow of the satiety factor leptin, which they normally lacked. When *ob/ob* mice are parabiosed with normal mice, they lose weight themselves, showing that their own satiety systems react appropriately to leptin.

It took about 20 years to provide the molecular basis for the prescient hypothesis of Coleman about the nature of *db* and *ob* mutations through isolation by Friedman and Halaas of the *ob* gene product leptin[147] and by others of the leptin receptor.[146,148] This discovery provided an explanation for the defects seen in *db* and *ob* mice and revolutionized our view of adipose tissue, not only as a hormonally regulated fat depot, but also as a lipostatic endocrine organ and the source of leptin. Due to the discovery that *db* is a mutation of the leptin receptor gene and *ob* is a mutation of the leptin synthesis gene, the nomenclature of these two mice species has been changed to lepr^{db} and lep^{ob}, respectively. Unfortunately, the early hope that exogenous peripheral injection of leptin would treat obesity in humans has not materialized. However, administration of leptin was highly effective in the rare morbidly obese patients with mutations of the leptin gene that produces an ineffective leptin protein (see Chap. 10). These data suggest an important hitherto unknown role for leptin in human body weight regulation. However, it should be taken into consideration that the mode of action of leptin in mice may not be fully applicable to humans, as discussed by Himms-Hagen.[149]

Leiter[150] proposed to differentiate between the consequences of gene expression and the diabetes susceptibility–conferring effects of the Ks background using the response to estrone. The estrone-treated mice were hyperphagic and obese, but they did not develop hyperglycemia or islet atrophy. He postulated that the estrogen:androgen ratio is critical to glucose homeostasis. In *db/db* mice, this ratio could be regulated by the activity of sulfotransferases, liver enzymes that render steroids receptor-inactive by conjugation with sulfate. At puberty, the sulfotransferases sulfate estrogens but not androgens, thus inducing diabetes. Estrone supplementation is protective, because estrogens appear to prevent the interaction with diabetogenic background modifiers. The hepatic sulfation capacity might then potentiate the diabetogenicity of the *db* mutation,[151] and the development of a diabetic phenotype depends on the strength of interaction between the *db* gene and sulfotransferases. The number of hepatic insulin receptors was reduced in estrone-treated mutants, indicating that this was not a secondary insulin-elicited downregulation. There was no difference in the sensitivity of β cells to glucose. Thus *db* expression appears to be associated with a membrane defect causing scarcity of insulin receptors, independent of obesity and insulinemia.

In addition, the genomic factors inherent in the BLKs background of *db/db* mice facilitate the lesion of β cells. Their influence is harmful by limiting their replication and adversely sensitizing them to hyperglycemia. This is demonstrated by the observation that the growth of islets genetically implanted in the spleens of nondiabetic BL/6J mice far exceeds that of islets implanted in the spleens of nondiabetic BLKs mice.[152,153]

INSULIN-RESISTANT MUTANT RODENTS WITH SUSTAINED INSULIN SECRETION

ob/ob Mice Now Relabeled as *lep^ob*

In contradistinction to *db/db* mice, which lose their β cells in the course of insulin-resistant diabetes, the C57BL/6J-*ob/ob* mice, also originating from the Bar Harbor Jackson Laboratory,[134,135] have been investigated mainly due to their remarkable obesity, reaching up to 90 g body weight. The aspects of hyperinsulinemia and hyperglycemia are mainly discussed here. The autosomal recessive, fully penetrant *ob* mutation is located on chromosome 6 (see Chaps. 10 and 23 for a fuller discussion of obesity).

ob/ob Mice are characterized by hyperphagia, insulin resistance, hyperglycemia, remarkable obesity, and sustained insulin secretion. β-Cell hyperfunction leading to 10- to 50-fold higher than normal hyperinsulinemia persists during their life span, and compensates in large part for resistance, limits the overactive gluconeogenesis to moderate hyperglycemia, and prevents ketosis by promoting lipogenesis despite an increased FFA turnover. Paradoxically, lipogenic enzymes are also highly active, concurrently with those of gluconeogenesis. The close interrelation of obesity and diabetes in this syndrome has led to the definition of this condition as *diabesity*.[5]

Pancreatic insulin content is very high, the highest of any mice mutant with diabesity. In contrast to the *db/db* cells, they exhibit a very pronounced hypertrophy/hyperplasia and a reduced population of α, δ, and PP cells. Islet area doubles by the age of 1 month and increases 30-fold by 6 months.[153] Any degranulation caused by profuse insulin release is offset by regranulation in other islets.

This robust insulin secretion reduces the hyperglycemia by attenuating the hepatic gluconeogenesis on one hand, and pushing glucose carbons into fat synthesis on the other hand. The enhanced lipogenesis leading to obesity actually has an antihyperglycemic effect. By converting the glucose surplus to lipid in the liver and adipose tissue, the hyperglycemia in *ob/ob* mice is moderate. Insulin resistance in *ob/ob* mice, as in other "diabese" animals, appears to be due to diminished insulin binding to receptors, impaired autophosphorylation, and reduced signal transduction.[58]

The genetic defect in *ob/ob* mice is the lack of satiety-controlling factors, as elegantly demonstrated by the parabiosis experiments (see *db/db* mice, above) and confirmed by the discovery that leptin action is missing in *ob/ob* mice by virtue of a mutation in the leptin gene. The role of the associated hypothalamic peptides in neuroendocrine glucoregulation has been recently reviewed.[154–156] Levels of neuropeptide Y (NPY), a potent insulin-suppressible appetite stimulant, are high in diabese animals, possibly as a result of leptin deficiency.

Yellow Obese Mice

The mutation in yellow obese mice was established as an allele at the agouti locus of chromosome 2. It was assigned the gene symbol A^y for yellow, because the yellow skin pigmentation and obesity are interconnected in this dominantly inherited mutation. Homozygosity is lethal and all the obese offspring are heterozygous for the A^y gene. Another dominant allele at the agouti locus, labeled A^vy for viable yellow, arose spontaneously in C3H/HeJ mice at Bar Harbor. Both adiposity and hyperinsulinemia are related to the degree of yellow in the pigmentation.

Two reviews[157,158] supply information on the yellow diabese mice and their response to various pharmacologic interventions. Blood glucose levels are higher in the obese than in nonobese individuals only in the fed state, indicating IGT rather than overt diabetes, but their responses to cortisone are exaggerated. Hypertrophy and hyperplasia of islets appear, especially on a carbohydrate-rich diet, leading to hyperinsulinemia prior to weight gain. Hyperphagia and obesity in the young are more pronounced in males than in females. Fat tissue lipogenesis is enhanced even on fasting. Longevity depends on body weight and fat content of the diet. The adrenal glands of yellow obese mice are enlarged and adrenalectomy prevents islet β-cell hypertrophy and insulin resistance. This may be mediated by the attenuation of hyperphagia that is induced by glucocorticoids, as in other animals with the diabesity syndrome. The underlying abnormality is due to faulty expression of the agouti gene in the hypothalamus, in addition to the hair follicle, due to aberrant splicing of the agouti mRNA coding region.[158]

KK Mice

The history, metabolic-endocrine features, and pharmacologic utility of KK mice have been reviewed by Taketomi and Ikeda,[159] who also listed the trials of antidiabetic modalities in these mice. The KK strains and hybrids differ with respect to the degree of obesity and glucose homeostasis, but obesity seems to be the primary factor precipitating the insulin resistance.

The KK hybrids and the yellow KK mice develop overt diabetes along with weight gain on a regular diet, whereas the Japanese KK mice require a high-energy diet for the diabetes to become expressed. The KK inheritance was suggested to be dominant with 25% penetrance, due to the association with a recessive modifier, but evidence for polygenic inheritance was also provided. Quantitative trait loci analysis was performed by Suto and associates.[160] Nonfasting hyperglycemia is <300 mg/dL (17 mmol/L), and weight reaches a peak of 50 g at 5 months and is more marked in males than females. Nonfasting hyperinsulinemia may reach levels up to 1200 μU/mL. IGT is also more marked in males than in females and improves with age. KK mice have high plasma glucagon levels and deficient suppression of glucagon release by glucose. Treatment with growth hormone or glucagon worsens the hyperglycemia.

The hyperglycemia in all KK strains is associated with high levels of activity of glycolytic and lipogenic enzymes, concordant with the degree of hyperinsulinemia. However, the activity of gluconeogenic enzymes also rises, in spite of hyperinsulinemia. These findings emphasize the failure of insulin to suppress gluconeogenesis, while stimulating glycolysis and lipogenesis, similarly to the metabolic derangements in *db/db* mice. Insulin resistance in KK mice is due to changes in the expression of signal transduction components, among them IRS-1 and phosphatidylinositol-3-kinase (PI-3-kinase).[161]

A prominent feature of the KK mice is β-cell hyperplasia and elevated insulin content, as well as an expanded endoplasmic reticulum, Golgi apparatus, and possible transformation of ductal cells into β cells. Partial β-cell degranulation occurs at high glucose levels, but there is no evidence of necrosis. Like other diabese rodents, yellow KK mice exhibit high corticosterone levels and adrenal hyperplasia. However, obesity, glycemia, and insulinemia precede the adrenal changes, indicating that they are probably secondary rather than causal. Hyperphagia is a common finding in all KK strains, but its onset is not as early as in other diabese mutants. Hyperglycemia, hyperinsulinemia, obesity, the response of hepatic gluconeogenesis to insulin, and sensitivity to exogenous insulin all tend to revert to normal at 1 year of age. Nevertheless, the life span of diabetic KK mice is significantly shorter.

New Zealand Obese (NZO) Mice

The polygenic New Zealand obese (NZO) strain was developed from a mixed colony of mice by selective breeding for heavy weight, until obesity with mild hyperglycemia and hyperinsulinemia became established. Body weight rises rapidly during the first 2 months of life, conforming to the hyperphagia. Later on, weight gain is sluggish, up to a peak of about 90 g at 12–14 months, as in other strains of obese mice. Peak glycemia of ~250 mg/dL (14 mmol/L) occurs at 4–6 months and is more pronounced in males than females. Gluconeogenesis in the liver is increased despite hyperinsulinemia. The features of the NZO diabesity have been reviewed in detail.[162,163]

Hyperfunction of β cells is evident from high insulin secretion, when compared with either Swiss or BL/6 mice as reference, since genetic controls are not available. There is a wide spectrum of plasma insulin values and secretory responses in NZO mice, perhaps due to differences in randomly bred NZO colonies. However, there is definite hyperinsulinemia, though it is less marked than in *ob/ob* or KK mice. Pancreas insulin content is 2–4 times higher in 3-month-old mice and 6–10 times higher in 8-month-old mice. Insulin levels and obesity decline with age.

The insulin secretion pattern in NZO mice is abnormal.[164] The plasma insulin level in fasted mice is similar to that of fed mice and 2–3 times higher than in controls. The islet responses to tolbutamide, cyclic AMP, or glucose are low, and the effects of glucagon or aminophylline are delayed. The calcium ionophore isobutyl-methylxanthine (IBMX) promotes insulin release from islets of fasted mice but does not augment the effect of glucose. Arginine elicits a good response. The refractoriness to glucose may be related to limited islet glucose metabolism in relation to insulin output, with an impediment prior to the triose phosphate step, as glyceraldehyde provokes a potent insulin release. A common denominator in these patterns of insulin secretion is a blunted first phase of release. A single injection of a cyclic AMP elevating "islet activating protein" lowered the blood glucose level for as long as 5 days and improved the secretion of insulin in response to glucose *in vivo* and in isolated islets.

Insulin resistance is remarkable. Large doses of exogenous insulin hardly affect the blood glucose level but intraperitoneally implanted islets from albino mouse donors reverse the hyperglycemia. *In vitro* glucose uptake by muscles is low. Basal and insulin-stimulated 2-deoxyglucose transport is reduced as is glycogen in muscles in young mice.[165] Adipose tissue was also found to be insulin resistant, as evidenced by a defect in insulin-mediated stimulation of the activity of pyruvate dehydrogenase.[166] The activity of glycolytic enzymes, glucokinase, and pyruvate kinase is elevated, and the activity of the gluconeogenic PEPCK and glucose-6-phosphatase is reduced, as would be expected in a hyperinsulinemic state, in contrast to other diabese animals. However, the activity of fructose-1,6-bisphosphatase is not reduced by the hyperinsulinemia, despite high levels of its specific intracellular inhibitor, fructose-2,6-phosphate. It was suggested that the abnormal regulation of this enzyme contributes to the increased hepatic glucose production.[167,168]

Lipogenesis is increased both in the liver and adipose tissue. NZO mice are susceptible to the amount and composition of food, and adipose tissue responds to a fat-rich diet with hypercellularity. The ratio of total to peritoneal adipose tissue is 2.5 in the NZO and 3.5 in the *ob/ob* mice.[169] In NZO mice (as in humans), the peritoneal fat predominance may accentuate the metabolic disturbances.

Of concern is the detection of humoral antibodies to insulin receptors, and possibly also to islets, in NZO mice, suggesting that the tissue insulin resistance may be at least in part of immune origin. However, β-cell autoimmunity in a hyperinsulinemic animal is highly unlikely, and there is no evidence for a β-cell destructive process. The New Zealand strains of mice have, in general, a high incidence of other autoimmune disorders, such as glomerular nephritis with deposition of immune complexes. Therefore, an interaction between general autoimmunity and some aspect of diabesity of NZO mice cannot be completely ruled out.

fa/fa (Zucker) Rats Now Labeled *lepr*^fa

The *fa* gene is a spontaneous autosomal recessive mutation on rat chromosome 5. On the basis of the flanking genetic markers, the *fa* gene is now considered to be the rat homologue of the mouse mutant *db* gene,[170] located on chromosome 4, which has now been shown to produce a mutated leptin receptor.

The pathophysiology of the *fa* mutation has been extensively reviewed.[171,172] Homozygous *fa/fa* rats develop hyperphagia and extreme obesity, recognizable at 1 month of age by the prominent growth of subcutaneous and intraperitoneal fat depots. This is accompanied by mild hyperglycemia, IGT, marked insulin resistance, and hyperinsulinemia. Phenotypically, the *fa/fa* rats appear similar to *ob/ob* mice. They exhibit early and persistent hyperphagia, long-lasting hyperinsulinemia, and obesity without ketosis. However, there are differences in the extent of hyperglycemia in relation to hyperinsulinemia and insulin resistance, and there is a pronounced hyperlipidemia in *fa/fa* rats. No genomic modifiers have been demonstrated, and the nature of primary defect(s) causing the hyperphagia and hyperinsulinemia also appears to differ from those of the obese mice.

Islets of *fa/fa* rats exhibit both hypertrophy and hyperplasia with pronounced microtubule formation, which is sustained throughout most of their life without β-cell exhaustion, despite lasting overstimulation. In these respects *fa/fa* rats resemble *ob/ob* mice. The *fa/fa* rats oversecrete insulin even when fed a diet identical in carbohydrate content to their lean controls. Support for an intrinsic defect causing oversecretion comes from the observation that insulin release from isolated islets is not normalized after culturing for as long as 21 days, and that islets cultured at low glucose concentrations exhibit an exaggerated glucose-stimulated response that is not inhibited by mannoheptulose.[173] The dissociation between hyperphagia and hyperinsulinemia is apparent in long-term experiments. Food restriction throughout life does not preclude the development of hyperinsulinemia, obesity, and the induction of insulin-dependent enzyme systems of hepatic lipogenesis and adipose tissue triglyceride uptake.

The females are sterile and males have also fertility problems, which may be alleviated by adrenalectomy. Lean, heterozygous *fa/+* rats are employed for breeding a progeny with a 25% incidence of obesity, or *fa/fa* males are treated with testosterone. The role of glucocorticoids was discussed in depth by York,[174] stressing that these hormones are required for the development of diabesity in *fa/fa* rats and other mutants by acting both at peripheral and central sites. The diabesity is characterized by increased availability of glucocorticoids from the enlarged adrenal glands. The hyperinsulinemia appears to be caused by CNS signals transmitted to the pancreas via the vagus nerve.[175] Further evidence for the anomalous performance of the hypothalamo-pituitary axis is the dysregulation of NPY mRNA and corticotropin-releasing factor (CRF). Abnormal cerebral glucose utilization has been found by Rohner-Jeanrenaud and colleagues.[176,177] Tissue unresponsiveness to insulin is ameliorated by adrenalectomy, which also lowers food intake, decreases the efficiency of energy use, and depresses lipogenesis.[178]

Insulin resistance is prominent in *fa/fa* rats. A comparison with ventromedial hypothalamus (VMH)–lesioned rats reveals greater tissue insulin resistance in *fa/fa* rats under similar insulin and obesity conditions. Insulin resistance is evident in perfused hindlimb muscle, both with respect to glucose transport and lactate oxidation. However, insulin sensitivity in the heart appears normal, although actual glucose transport and metabolism may be decreased. In a euglycemic insulin clamp study, total glucose use in obese rats was achieved only at 3.5-fold higher insulin concentration, similar to that of lean rats.[179] Muscle insulin resistance was not suggested to be the primary etiologic cause of diabesity, on the basis of 2-deoxyglucose uptake studies in young animals.[180] However, there is a substantial decrease in IRS-1 protein, insulin-stimulated IRS-1 phosphorylation, and the expression of PI-3-kinase,[181] consistent with deficient GLUT-4 translocation,[182,183] which seems to provide the molecular basis for muscle insulin resistance in *fa/fa* diabesity. Oxidative stress has also been implicated in the attenuated glucose transport in skeletal muscle.[184] Hepatic VLDL secretion is increased, giving rise to a marked VLDL hyperlipidemia.[185] The activity of the receptor TK, lipogenic enzymes, and lipoprotein lipase (LPL) was found to be increased in adipose tissue of *fa/fa* rats.[186–188]

The secretion of amylase by the exocrine pancreas is also disturbed. Amylase synthesis is insulin dependent and its activity is reduced in insulinopenic conditions. Interestingly, amylase synthesis was found to be reduced in the hyperinsulinemic, but insulin-resistant *fa/fa* rats and *ob/ob* mice.[189] These observations indicate that insulin resistance is also manifest in proximal acinar cells, preventing the expression of the amylase gene.

In young *fa/fa* rats, adipose tissues grow by hyperplasia and hypertrophy up to week 14, whereas in the older obese rats, adipocyte proliferation continues until at least week 26, in association with striking cell hypertrophy. Early nutritional abundance has a pronounced impact on adipose tissue development, the cellularity increasing in both *fa/fa* and lean rats, while restricted feeding reduces the adipocyte number in lean rats only. Adipose tissue has an increased capacity to take up preformed fat through the insulin-induced LPL. *fa/fa* Rats, compared with normal rats on long-term insulin infusion, had both increased LPL expression and activity, but LPL mRNA was elevated only in the former.

BBZ Rats

Female *fa/fa* rats have been crossed with the autoimmune male BB rats and named BBZ/Wor. As described by Guberski and coworkers,[190,191] when heterozygous *fa/fa* females were mated with diabetic BB/Wor males, the first generation was nondiabetic and lean. When the F_1 females were then backcrossed to BB/Wor diabetic males, 18% of the offspring developed diabetes but remained lean. The third mating was an intercross between the backcross diabetic males and females, of which 74% became diabetic. The fourth cross was between the third-cross progeny and F_1 animals, enabling the selection of carriers of both diabetes and *fa* genes. Of the resultant two groups of lean and obese progeny, about 25% were obese and about half of them became diabetic at around 3 months of age, with a mean blood glucose level near 400 mg/dL (22 mmol/L). Also, slightly more than half of the lean group developed diabetes at around 3 months with a similar blood glucose level.

The BBZ/Wor rat shows surprising differences between the lean and obese offspring. Lean BBZ rats exhibit insulitis with β-cell loss, ketosis, weight loss, and a requirement for exogenous insulin, similarly to the original BB rats. Obese BBZ rats show prominent islet hyperplasia coincident with insulitis and degranulation, are often hyperglycemic but maintain their weight, rarely experience ketosis, and survive without insulin treatment. Apparently the β-cell destructive process is counterbalanced by islet regeneration. Thus the BBZ/Wor rat presents a mixed type 1/type 2 diabetes syndrome, comprising features of both autoimmunity and insulin resistance. They develop hypertension and hyperlipidemia,[192] retinopathy, and neuropathy,[193] and represent a relevant model for exploring the condition of β-cell destruction compensated by β-cell proliferation.

The Diabetic *fa/fa* Rat: ZDF/Drt-*fa*

A substrain of *fa/fa* rats, selectively inbred for hyperglycemia,[194] is useful for the investigation of T2DM. Nonfasting plasma glucose levels exceed 400 mg/dL (22 mmol/L) at 10 weeks of age in males. The hyperlipoproteinemia is similar to that seen in the regular *fa/fa* rats, but the weight gain and insulin levels are lower. These rats also acquire neuropathy and other complications not exhibited in *fa/fa* rats. ZDF/Drt-*fa* rats have a reduced expression of muscle GLUT-4 transporter, most probably as a result of hyperglycemia.[195] In contrast to *fa/fa* rats, the capacity to oversecrete insulin is limited, and they manifest labile, glucose-sensitive β cells that proceed to apoptosis.[196] They also demonstrate downregulation of β-cell GLUT-2 transporters,[197] which may impair insulin synthesis, thus inducing severe type 2-like diabetes. Food restriction in the prediabetic stage in ZDF rats may prevent β-cell deterioration and loss of GLUT-2.[198] A deleterious lipotoxic effect of high plasma FFA and β-cell triglyceride levels on β-cell function has been suggested by Unger and collaborators.[199–201]

Obese-Hyperglycemic Wistar Kyoto Fatty Rat Group

As reviewed by Kava and colleagues[202] and Odaka and associates,[203] this group of rats with polygenic diabetes-hypertension was derived from reciprocal crosses between the *fa/fa* and the glucose-intolerant Wistar Kyoto (WKY) rats in Japan. The original strain, obtained after several crosses and inbreeding, shows both peripheral and hepatic insulin resistance and hyperinsulinemia. Males are hyperglycemic and females become hyperglycemic only on a sucrose-rich regimen. Several variants were developed and referred to as WDF/Ta-*fa* rats,[204] or Wistar diabetic rats, and WKY/N Drt-*fa*,[205] also known as WKY fatty rats.

The outbred males of the WDF/Ta-*fa* substrain exhibit hyperglycemia on a high-sucrose diet; females do not develop hyperglycemia, but both genders are hyperinsulinemic. Castration does not abolish the sexual dimorphism, whereas it does improve insulin sensitivity in *fa/fa* rats. Neonatal ovariectomy did not aggravate the diabesity, indicating no estrogen protection. Males are more hyperphagic than females, which could account in part for the sex difference. High hepatic glucose production with elevated PEPCK activity that was abolished by adrenalectomy was demonstrated. Hypertrophic islets were prominent with pronounced insulin content secretion, but this did not compensate for the hyperglycemia. Insulin resistance in males was associated with downregulation of muscle insulin receptors, leading to decreased insulin binding. TK activity per receptor was also reduced, as compared with *fa/fa* rats, again demonstrating the detrimental effect of hyperinsulinemia on receptor function.[58]

The WKY fatty rats in Japan were reported to be spontaneously hypertensive and nephropathic.[205] Insulin resistance was attributed to enhanced muscle TNFα production, inducing an impairment of postreceptor insulin signaling. The WKY diabetic strain was also raised in the United States by crossing with the WKY/N stock.[204] The colony suffered from infections and had to be maintained in specific-pathogen-free (SPF) condition. The animals delivered by cesarean section were more diabetic than those pre-cesarean derived. It is interesting that the infections reduced the incidence of type 2-like diabetes in these animals, analogously to the effect of pathogens on the diabetes in BB rats and NOD mice, even though the WKY fatty rats were without autoimmune background.

Diabetic Corpulent Rat Group

Rats with type 2-like diabesity and hypertension were developed from two congenic strains, SHR/N and LA/N, at the NIH in Bethesda, Maryland (substrain code N). The SHR/N-*cp* and the LA/N-*cp* rats were obtained by introducing into these backgrounds the *cp* gene of the Koletzky SHR strain, which carries one *fa* allele. The investigators preferred the name "corpulent" and symbol cp^{fa} or fa^{cp}, but the new proposed designation is $lepr^{facp}$. Details on the backcrosses that led to the different substrains have been provided by Greenhouse and associates.[206] The important feature of the *cp* gene is that a small difference in the genomic background leads to substrains that markedly differ in the degree of hyperglycemia, hyperlipidemia, insulin resistance, hypertension, nephropathy, atherosclerosis, and propensity to myocardial lesions.[207] These leptin receptor–abnormal rats are infertile, which requires test mating each generation to identify the individuals for the next cross with the partner strain. Mating the congenic heterozygotes yields a lean to corpulent ratio of 3:1 at 5 weeks of age.

SHR/N-*cp* Rats

SHR/N-*cp* males are moderately hypertensive; manifest hyperlipidemia, hyperinsulinemia, glucosuria, and proteinuria; and become hyperglycemic on a sucrose-rich diet.[208] They show marked and long-lasting β-cell hyperplasia. Insulin receptor malfunction is suggested by decreased insulin binding by liver membranes and by enhanced gluconeogenesis. Muscle GLUT-4 is reduced ~40% in SHR/N-*cp* rats compared with lean controls, whereas the insulin-independent GLUT-1 is increased by ~40%.[209] Corpulence is due to both adipocyte hypertrophy and hyperplasia and pronounced hepatic lipogenesis. Serum concentrations of counterregulatory hormones, glucagon, corticosterone, growth hormone, and somatostatin are elevated. Corpulence and insulin resistance subside after 1 year. SHR/N-*cp* females are smaller and less glucosuric, and rarely exhibit nonfasting hyperglycemia.

Long-term sucrose feeding of SHR/N-*cp* males results in weight gain and accentuates the hyperglycemia, hyperinsulinemia, IGT, and pancreatic islet hyperplasia. SHR/N-*cp* rats are prone to glomerulopathy, which is aggravated by the sucrose diet, as are the hypertension and proteinuria.[210] Renal changes are consistent both with diabetic nephropathy and inflammation, showing segmental, diffuse, and nodular intercapillary mesangial expansion, which may be an outcome of hyperglycemia and concomitant hypertension.

SHHF/Mcc-*cp* Rats

The SHHF/Mcc-*cp* rats maintained by McCune and colleagues[211] evolved on a genomic background conducive to the expression of cardiomyopathy, dramatically presenting as congestive heart failure (CHF). The CHF is expressed in 100% of animals in association with hypertension and diabesity. Renal changes similar to those in the SHR/N-*cp* strain also occur, particularly in females. The mode of inheritance is polygenic, but the presence of the cp^{fa} gene is essential. Sexual dimorphism is seen in the onset of CHF expression, as is the diabesity and hyperlipidemia, which includes also heterozygote littermates. Early death occurs in the following order: males, females, lean males, and lean females. Clinical symptoms resemble those of human CHF: pronounced cardiomegaly, edema, hydrothorax, ascites, dyspnea, and visceral hyperemia, as well as a pattern of changes in atrial natriuretic factor, norepinephrine, aldosterone, and renin. Morphologic observations indicate degeneration of myocytes. Estrone treatment delays but does not prevent CHF. The calcium channel blocker nifedipine reduces body weight, cardiac hypertrophy, and blood pressure, and improves glucose homeostasis, mainly in females.[212]

JCR:LA-*cp* Corpulent Rats

Backcrosses of LA/N-*cp* males with a hooded rat species produced an outbred substrain JCR:LA-*cp* with only about 3% contribution of the SHR gene but the presence of the *fa* allele. As reported by Russell,[213] these rats are not hypertensive, but hyperinsulinemic and insulin resistant, with pronounced hyperlipidemia, diabesity, and hepatic lipogenesis.[214] Their prominent feature is early cardiovascular disease (CVD) with atherosclerotic lesions of major blood vessels. Such lesions do not appear in *fa/fa* or SHR/N-*cp* rats. The lesions were morphologically classified into stages, assumed to represent the progression and repair of the ischemic damage, ranging from inflammatory cell infiltration through myocytolysis to advanced focal infiltration with scavenging and collagen bands, with scars at various stages of maturity.

JCR:LA-*cp* males show a greater incidence of CVD than females, approaching 100% at the age of 9 months. The appearance of occlusive thrombi in coronary arteries indicates that the nature of the lesion is ischemic-atherosclerotic, although not related to plasma cholesterol concentration. Food restriction, strenuous exercise, alcohol intake, or suppression of lipogenesis by a dicarboxylic acid compound (MEDICA 16)[215] delayed the incidence and progression of CVD in association with a decrease in insulin resistance. Castration reduced hypertriglyceridemia, but was without effect on the vascular lesions, indicating that estrogens were not protective. Conversely, nifedipine prevented the formation of advanced lesions without improving insulin resistance. On the other hand, assuming that the hyperinsulinemia is responsible for the frequency and severity of CVD, it was proposed that the susceptibility to CVD is due to hyperinsulinemic stress, which initiates the primary endothelial injury, which in the face of hyperlipidemia, excessive caloric intake, and genetic factors progresses to intimal atheroma and reduces the life span of JCR:LA-*cp* rats.[216,217]

RODENTS WITH SPONTANEOUS DIABETES OF VARYING ETIOLOGY

Nonobese Nondiabetic (NON) Mice

NON mice were bred in Japan from the same CTS line from which the NOD mice were derived, but they do not manifest β-cell targeted autoimmunity. The haplotype of NON mice, H-2[b], is distinct from the H-2[g] of the NOD mice. The derivation, genetics, diabetic features, and complications have been described by various authors in recent reviews.[101,218,219] Male NON mice display IGT at 9 weeks of age. The insulin content and the insulin-mRNA content in the pancreas are low, about one-third that of control ICR mice. The first-phase insulin response is absent in the perfused NON mouse pancreas, and the insulin:glucose ratio after IV glucose injection is low. Insulin-binding studies in muscle do not suggest insulin resistance. However, NON mice show a tendency to obesity on hyper-

caloric diet, islet hyperplasia, and insulin hypersecretion after a hypothalamic gold thioglucose lesion. Thus the NON mice represent a hypoinsulinemic animal, with an "intrinsic" β-cell defect in insulin secretion and synthesis, but retaining the potential for β-cell proliferation when triggered by hyperphagia or hypothalamic stimulation. NON mice are prone to nephropathy, even in the face of only mild hyperglycemia, exhibiting glomerular lesions with lipid deposition and lymphocytic infiltration.

WBN/Kob Rats

WBN/Kob rats have been raised from Wistar specimens originating in Basel, Switzerland, and investigated in Japan by Mori and coworkers.[220,221] Diabetes occurs spontaneously in 40% of males at 9 months and in 90% at 12 months of age. The striking feature of this genetically recessive syndrome is a lesion in both exocrine and endocrine pancreas, involving β and α cells and acini, with decreased insulin, glucagon, and amylase content. The onset of hyperglycemia and glucosuria is gradual and accompanied by weight loss rather than obesity, and is accelerated on a high-energy diet. The animals are not insulin resistant and respond well to exogenous insulin. The insulinopenia is associated with a decrease in the number and size of islets and multifocal fibrosis extending to the exocrine pancreas. An infiltration of the pancreas with inflammatory cells is noted, as well as fibrous exudation around the pancreatic ducts and capillaries, with deposition of hemosiderin by 3 months of age. These changes suggest a slow autoimmune process; however, the morphologic findings are distinct from those of NOD mice and BB rats. Ocular, renal, and neural lesions typical of diabetes have been reported.[222]

eSS Rats

The eSS rats, bred in Argentina, are characterized by a slow onset of IGT and hyperglycemia, more severe in males, which becomes conspicuous at about 1 year of age. The colony development, prolonged inbreeding, and the polygenic inheritance pattern together with metabolic-endocrine and morphologic features have been reviewed in detail.[223] Islets of 6-month-old eSS rats show an interstitial tissue growth, vacuolization, and a disrupted pattern due to separation by fibrous deposits with a compensatory hyperplasia (resembling nesidioblastosis). eSS rats are somewhat overweight, insulin resistant, hyperinsulinemic, and hyperlipidemic. Food restriction slows down the progression to diabetes, whereas a high-energy diet accelerates the onset of metabolic abnormalities and chronic complications in kidneys, nerves, and lenses and shortens the life span of the animals. Aggravation of diabetic symptoms was noted on a high-sucrose diet.[224]

BHE/Cdb Rats

As related by Berdanier,[225] the BHE/Cdb rat strain was developed as a model of type 2 nonobese diabetes, by crossing Osborne-Mendel rats with a Pennsylvania State College strain. Cdb rats, compared with Wistar rats, have a shorter life span, fatty livers, and nephropathy. Females are more susceptible to these changes, whereas males exhibit a moderate hyperglycemia and mild hyperlipidemia prior to insulin elevation. The abnormalities seem to start at the insulin target tissues rather than at the β-cell secretion level; however, at 150 days the pancreatic insulin stores are decreased. As hepatic lipogenesis is enhanced prior to alterations in glucose homeostasis, defects in hepatic metabolism seem to characterize the phenotype. Slow mitochondrial respiratory rates that deteriorate with age were demonstrated, with enhanced lipogenesis linked to lower mitochondrial oxidation. A mutation in the mitochondrial ATPase gene related to the IGT was reported.[226]

OLETF Rats

Male OLETF rats manifest a spontaneous IGT, hyperglycemia, and moderate hyperinsulinemia at about 18 weeks of age and are overweight. This mutation was discovered in the Otsuka Long Evans Tokushima colony of rats, from which the LETL rats with autoimmunity also originated, and was reviewed recently by Kawano and associates.[227,228] β-Cell infiltration with fibrotic tissue and mononuclear cells is seen around the time of onset, followed by β-cell enlargement due to intraislet fibrotic tissue and hemosiderin deposits. Deposition of fat droplets as a consequence of hypertriglyceridemia was also present.

The OLETF rats develop a pronounced nephropathy, with clinical and pathological features resembling human diabetic nephropathy, characterized by marked thickening and rupture of the glomerular basement membrane, focal mesangial lesion, fibrin cap, and aneurysmal dilatations of intraglomerular vessels.

NSY Mice

The Nagoya Shibata Yasuda mice were selectively inbred for glucose intolerance from JcI:JCR mice. They represent a model of T2DM, but are not severely obese, with a cumulative incidence of diabetes of 98% in males and 31% in females. A polygenic inheritance pattern affecting insulin secretion and insulin sensitivity was mapped on four loci on chromosomes 6, 11, and 14. The NSY mouse may serve as a model for studies of the etiology of late onset of T2DM.[229]

Koletzky (SHROB) Rats, Now Labeled *fa*[K]

The SHROB rat exhibits obesity, marked hyperinsulinemia, severe insulin resistance, hypertriglyceridemia, nephropathy, and hypertension.[230] The obese phenotype results from a mutation in the leptin receptor[231] designated *fa*[K] that resides on the same allele as the *fa/fa* rat. Although the SHROB rats have IGT and corticosteronemia, they are normoglycemic in the fasting condition. Because of this property, they may represent a model for investigation of gene modifiers that dissociate obesity from hyperglycemia. The insulin receptor and its IRS-1 substrate are underexpressed. Increased activity of the sympathetic nervous system was proposed to be responsible, by separate pathways, for both hypertension and insulin resistance.

RODENTS WITH OVERNUTRITION-EVOKED INSULIN RESISTANCE AND DIABESITY

Psammomys obesus (Sand Rat)

Although often called sand rats, these animals are gerbils, and their popular nickname stems from the fact that they were trapped on the sandy shores of the Nile Delta. They subsist on a diet of succulent halophilic plants and have no evidence of diabetes in their North African or eastern Mediterranean habitat. Hyperinsulinemia, hyperglycemia, and obesity develop on transfer to *ad libitum* rodent laboratory chow. The history and features of the nutritionally induced diabesity in *Psammomys* have been updated,[232–235] and these reviews should be consulted for details.

Pronounced insulin resistance is evident on a high-energy (HE) diet relative to their native regimen. In the Jerusalem colony, derived from the Dead Sea region, the progression to diabetes was classified into four stages, according to serum insulin and glucose levels.[236] Stage A comprises normoglycemic and normoinsulinemic animals. In stage B the animals gain weight and remain normoglycemic, but become markedly hyperinsulinemic, which compensates for the insulin resistance. In stage C the *Psammomys* animals become hyperglycemic despite extreme hyperinsulinemia. They show a pronounced peripheral insulin resistance, manifested by reduced muscle uptake of 2-deoxyglucose and diminished GLUT-4 protein and mRNA.[235,236] The hepatic resistance is expressed as excessive gluconeogenesis due to nonsuppression of PEPCK; however, the hepatic lipogenesis remains responsive to insulin, with prominent adipose tissue lipid uptake and concomitant obesity. The effectiveness of the augmented insulin secretion is low, as a substantial proportion is secreted as proinsulin and its intermediate conversion products.[237] In stage D, the plasma insulin levels drop and adipose tissue weight decreases, signifying a decline in insulin secretion. Animals at this stage show massive depletion of β-cell insulin granules[238] and apoptosis[152,239] and develop ketoacidosis. They then require exogenous insulin for survival. Longitudinal follow-up[240] demonstrates a characteristic bell-shaped curve (Fig. 16-3). Similar progression to full-fledged diabetes was seen in another colony of *Psammomys* from Algeria that was maintained in France,[241] and in a branch of the Israeli

FIGURE 16-3. Scattergram illustrating the bell-shaped pattern of progression of *Psammomys obesus* to diabesity on a high-energy diet. Stage **A**: Normoglycemia and normoinsulinemia. Stage **B**: Hyperinsulinemia and normoglycemia. Stage **C**: Hyperinsulinemia and hyperglycemia. Stage **D**: Insulin depletion with marked hyperglycemia. Note the clustering of animals in stage B. Longitudinal studies on a group of 37 *Psammomys* for 16 weeks after weaning. The data are from animals that are a branch of the Jerusalem colony maintained at Deakin University in Australia. (*Adapted from Howard.*[270])

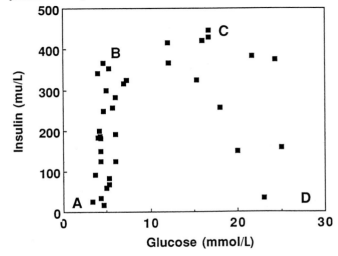

colony maintained in Australia.[242,243] In the latter colony the nutritional obesity and insulin resistance were found to be associated with hyperleptinemia and resistance to exogenous leptin.[244]

The progression of *Psammomys* to diabesity resembles that of *db/db* mice, with an important difference: β-cell loss in *Psammomys* is not solely determined by genetic mutation or by a background genome because the *Psammomys* reverts from stage C or B to A on food restriction alone. Some *Psammomys* were found to remain in stage A even on the HE diet, which led to the isolation of a diabetes-resistant line.[245] The diabetes-prone animals progress on the HE diet to stages C or D within 2–3 weeks, whereas the diabetes-resistant animals stay normoglycemic.

Psammomys represent a model for the β cell loss resulting from massive, continuous insulin resistance imposing compensatory β cell oversecretion. This is evident from fading immunostaining of insulin, of GLUT2 transporter in the plasma membrane and of glucokinase in the cytoplasm of β cells.[246] These changes become apparent only in Stage C with the development of hyperglycemia, with shrinking of β cell volume and content. This is significantly correlated with the level of glycemia. Thus, the increasing glycemia is most likely responsible for the loss of β cell secretory capacity and apoptosis.

Insulin binding by hepatic and muscle insulin receptors is low in stage A *Psammomys*, about one-fifth that in the albino rat, indicating a low receptor density.[247] The activation of TK by insulin on isolated insulin receptors from liver or skeletal muscle at stage A is similar to that of the albino rat per receptor, but it becomes impaired in stages B and C.[247] Hyperinsulinemia is most likely responsible for the reduced TK activation, as it is known to inhibit receptor function in other systems.[58,235,248] By transferring animals to a low-energy diet, it is possible to restore the activation of TK. For complete normalization of TK activity, the return to normoglycemia is not sufficient; the restoration of normoinsulinemia is required. Further studies demonstrated the overexpression of several PKC isoenzymes, particularly of the isoform PKCε.[235] The overexpression and membrane translocation of PKCε appear to contribute to insulin resistance by the inhibition of TK activity through serine/threonine phosphorylation on the receptor and its IRS-1 substrate. In addition, the overexpression of PKCε was associated with attenuation of PKB, an effector of insulin signaling, activating multiple metabolic pathways and partial degradation of the insulin receptor as determined by coincubation in human embryonic kidney (HEK 203) cellls.[249] This finding represents the molecular basis of nutritionally induced insulin resistance in *Psammomys*. It is related to the increase in muscle lipid and diacylglycerol levels, a known activator of several PKC isoforms. This mechanism is supported by findings of an overexpression of PKCε and PKCθ isoenzymes in another model of insulin resistance in the high-fat-fed rat.[250]

These data show that *Psammomys* is a gerbil adapted to subsistence on low-energy food thanks to its endowment with a "thrifty" gene advantageous to survival. Unfortunately, in many diabetes-prone animals this adaptation is not compatible with lavish food provision, and results in hyperinsulinemia, impaired receptor signaling, and diabesity leading to loss of β-cell function. In this sense, the *Psammomys* is a good model for the study of mechanisms evoking hyperinsulinemia and diabesity in human populations emerging into nutritional abundance.

A novel gene that encodes a small protein has recently been discovered by Collier and colleagues[251] in the hypothalamus of *Psammomys* and named "beacon." Beacon mRNA gene expression was positively correlated with percentage of body fat. Intracerebroventricular administration of beacon resulted in a dose-dependent increase in food intake and body weight, and hypothalamic overexpression of neuropeptide Y. Simultaneous infusion of beacon and neuropeptide Y potentiated the orexigenic response and resulted in rapid body weight gain. These novel data suggest a role for beacon and neuropeptide Y in body weight homeostasis.

Acomys cahirinus (Spiny Mice)

These are large mice, with brownish, bristle-like fur, living in semiarid areas of the eastern Mediterranean, that can attain a weight of up to 50 g on rodent chow in captivity. Interest in spiny mice arose when obesity with islet hyperplasia and hypertrophy were discovered in specimens originating from Israel and maintained in Switzerland on fat-rich bird food of sesame, pumpkin, and sunflower seeds. Low insulin secretory capacity was established as a characteristic of spiny mice.[252] The progression of spiny mice to diabesity was characterized by remarkable islet proliferation associated with high insulin content, thought to be compensation for the low capacity of insulin release, with a sudden loss of function at 10–16 months of age, followed by fatal ketosis. Because it took about 40 generations between the transfer to the laboratory and discovery of diabetes, it was suggested by Renold and colleagues[253] that a mutation might have occurred in captivity, causing defective insulin release and compensatory β-cell hypertrophy.

The ultrastructural β-cell features preceding the fulminant diabetes were an overdeveloped Golgi apparatus and gross hypergranulation. This differed from the hypersecretion in other diabese species, because in spiny mice, plasma insulin levels were only marginally increased and hyperglycemia was mild and intermittent. The low sensitivity of β cells to glucose and other secretagogues was attributed to low islet cyclic AMP response to stimulation, low amounts of vincristine-precipitable microtubular material, and scarce autonomic islet innervation.

To investigate the influence of dietary regimens, the diets of Geneva and Jerusalem strains (which did not exhibit marked β-cell hyperplasia) were exchanged for comparison. The Geneva regimen, including *ad libitum* seeds containing 15% fat, appeared to be the cause of obesity and pancreatic insulin overproduction at 8–10 months, whereas on the Jerusalem diet of regular laboratory chow containing 5% fat, the rise in β-cell insulin and insulin resistance was moderate.[254] These studies led to the conclusion that the low insulin response, as well as the obesity, hyperglycemia, and islet hyperplasia seen in spiny mice, is characteristic of a desert species subjected to nutritional stress rather than being due to a monogenic aberration. The low secretory responses of β cells suit the scarce food available in their native habitat, and may be protective against sporadic overstimulation.

On a sucrose-rich diet, spiny mice developed hepatomegaly, hyperactive lipogenesis, and gross hyperlipidemia. Pancreatic insulin content rose, but less so than on the fat-rich seed diet, and no islet disintegration was apparent even at the age of 18 months. The sucrose diet induced an extrathyroidal elevation of triiodothyronine, enhanced thermogenesis, and energy-wasting metabolic reactions.[255] This was thought to be protective against excessive weight gain and a disruptive islet cell lesion.

The difference between spiny mice and other models of nutritionally induced diabesity is that spiny mice do not gradually progress to hyperinsulinemia, hyperglycemia, and ketosis. Overnutrition selectively induces β-cell hypertrophy and proliferation with propensity to disintegration. Perhaps similar mechanisms operate in human low insulin responders when confronted with abundant nutrition.

C57BL/6J Mice

The nonobese, nondiabetic BL/6J mouse, the genomic host of the *ob/ob* mutation, is sensitive to adrenergic stimulation, hypertensive, and insulin resistant, with a weak first-phase insulin release seen at 6 months of age.[256] This indicates that abnormalities in the autonomic nervous system, β-cell function, and adipocyte metabolism are responsible for the IGT, and are expressed in BL/6J mice on a high-energy fat- and sucrose-rich diet. There is no hyperphagia or elevation in corticosterone. Genetic mapping has identified differences in the expression of uncoupling protein UCP2 in adipocytes.[257] Thus inbred laboratory mice without overt metabolic disturbance reveal environmentally induced diabesity and polygenic vulnerabilities on HE nutrition.

Hypertriglyceridemic (HTG) Rats

The nonobese hereditary hypertriglyceridemic rat is also insulin resistant, deficient in muscle GLUT-4, hyperuricemic, and hypertensive.[258] These rats were selected by breeding normal Wistar rats using the hypertriglyceridemic response to a sucrose-rich diet until these symptoms became apparent without nutritional stimulus. The abnormalities were aggravated by continued maintenance on the sucrose-rich diet but were ameliorated by diets rich in ω-3 fatty acids. Enhanced secretion of catecholamines was found.[259] The HTG rats, similarly to the C57BL/6J mice, demonstrate a nutritionally induced genetic predisposition for the insulin resistance syndrome.

SELECTIVE INBREEDING OF DIABETIC RODENTS FROM NORMAL POOLS

Apart from animals with spontaneous alterations that lead to inappropriate hyperglycemia and β-cell loss, lines of animals with diabetes have been selected from normal pools by repeated breeding of individuals with minimal deviation from the mean response to a stressful stimulus. These animal lines manifest the requirement for environmental influences to make the genetic predisposition clinically overt, and emphasize the polygenic basis of diabetes which resides within the "normal" genetic mosaic.

Goto-Kakizaki (GK) Rats

Wistar rats have been bred for over 35 generations in Japan, using relative intolerance to a 2-g/kg glucose load as a selection index.[260] The 10% of rats within the "hyperglycemic zone" were mated in each generation until the offspring had an IGT at F_{10} and fasting hyperglycemia at F_{35}. The GK rats are nonobese, and their diabetes is inheritable and stable with age. Insulin resistance is present and decreased hepatic insulin receptor numbers were noted with normal TK activity per receptor.[261] GK rats aroused interest as a model of nonobese T2DM on a polygenic basis. Neuropathy, glomerulopathy, and retinopathy were observed despite only moderate hyperglycemia.

GK islets are oval or round until 2 months of age, and then become irregular and starfish-shaped, apparently due to the accumulation of fibrous material. Insulin secretion in response to glucose is impaired, lacking the first-phase release. However, the progression to diabetes was also related to the reduced β-cell mass.[262] The response of ATP-sensitive K^+ channels to glucose was impaired[263] as was the action of various secretagogues,[264] pointing to a dysfunction in glycolytic flux before the glyceraldehyde-3-phosphate step or in the glycerol phosphate shuttle. GLUT-2 was also underexpressed in GK rat islets,[265] but not enough to explain the deficient insulin secretion as occurs in *db/db* mice or ZDF rats. The pathogenesis of diabetes in the GK rat has been recently reviewed.[266] It should be pointed out that the GK rats in worldwide colonies maintain IGT and low insulin secretion, but other phenotypic properties may differ between the colonies, suggesting genetic drift.

Cohen Sucrose-Induced Diabetic Rat

Cohen and Rosenmann challenged general-stock rats with a copper-poor, 72% sucrose diet to identify individuals with IGT as related in a monograph describing the pathophysiology, complications and genetics of the strain.[267] A two-way selection was performed by separate mating of those with highest and lowest glucose tolerance values. The offspring were again subjected to sucrose feeding, and the two-way mating continued, producing Cohen diabetes-sensitive (CDs) and Cohen diabetes-resistant (CDr) lines. After 4–5 generations, the CDs rats had a persistent hyperglycemia of ~280 mg/dL (16 mmol/L). The CDr line had normal glucose tolerance even on the sucrose diet. The CDs rats are nonobese, and weigh somewhat less than starch-fed controls even if their food consumption is higher. They are initially hyperinsulinemic, compared with parent rats or the CDr line, which has insulin values lower than the parental stock. The liver enzyme pattern is typical of insulin resistance: The activity of glycolytic enzymes is enhanced, as is that of gluconeogenesis enzymes which are not suppressed by insulin. The insulin response to glucose is low and exogenous insulin produces only a slight effect on blood glucose. With age, the diabetic rats show atrophy of the pancreas with fatty infiltration, and become insulin deficient but not ketotic. The CDs rat was also crossbred with the SHR rat, resulting in a hypertensive, hyperglycemic, and hyperlipidemic hybrid. The Cohen strain was recently newly inbred and the metabolic phenotypes genetically characterized,[268] emphasizing its suitability for studies of the interaction between genetic susceptibility and metabolic-nutritional environment as well as the effect of gender on the development of T2DM.

DIABETIC NONRODENTS

A preference has been expressed for animal models other than rodents in diabetes research. The advantage of using large animals is the possibility of performing catheterizations and clamp studies with multiple sampling across organs, as well as long-term longitudinal follow-up of changes and complications that may be not expressed during the short life of rodents. Rodents have a higher rate of metabolic fuel turnover than humans and differ in patterns of growth, but they have the advantage of enabling performance of statistically reliable observations in large cohorts. Ruminants have metabolic, nutritional, and digestive characteristics dissimilar to humans. Other disadvantages include the necessity for protracted care with considerable expenses for facilities and maintenance. It may take years to document the complications of diabetes in dogs or monkeys because they live much longer than rodents, and their life spans are sometimes nearly equal to that of the investigator.

There is also the difficulty with terminal experiments. Thus both nonrodents and rodents offer a wide range of research opportunities, and the choice of a model depends on the specific aims of the investigator.

Primates with Pancreatic Lesions

Howard[269] found hyperglycemia without hyperinsulinemia with varying degrees of IGT, weight loss, morphologic and functional β-cell defects, total β-cell loss, and amyloidosis among the Celebes black ape (*Macaca nigra*) and other simian species. Amyloidosis was also seen in other monkey species with overt diabetes including *Macaca fascicularis* and *Macaca radiata,* and a baboon, *Papo anubis*.[270] Although amyloid is restricted to islet tissue, it is unknown whether this is the result of a primary reaction or a secondary deposit related to antigen–antibody interaction. However, the islet amyloid content correlates with the intensity of diabetes and the cessation of insulin secretion. Diabetes in these monkeys is severe and associated with hyperlipidemia, xanthomatosis, glucosuria, and ketosis.

The monkey can also develop a type 1 diabetes-like syndrome which progresses over several years. Circulating antibodies to islet cells (ICSAs and ICAs) occur in 80% of macaques with islet dysfunction. Although a correlation between the antibody titers and islet pathology exists, their role in the initiation of insulitis has not been established. The presence of these antibodies may reflect a response to antigens released from β cells disintegrating as the result of damage by other cytotoxins. The overt diabetes stage is similar to human T1DM, requiring insulin treatment.[270]

Primates with Obesity and Pronounced Insulin Resistance

Rhesus monkeys (*Macaca mulatta*) in a colony maintained on an *ad libitum* ration develop a type 2 diabetes-like syndrome. Studies spanning many years performed by Hansen and Bodkin and colleagues[271,272] defined the changes that occur with progression of the disease from leanness to obesity and overt diabetes. Several phases were identified using metabolic and endocrine indices, starting without appreciable elevations of blood glucose and insulin during fasting, but IGT following a glucose load. In phase 4, plasma insulin levels were 161 μU/mL versus 2 μU/mL in phase 1. In phases 5 and 6, body weight peaked at ~19 kg and plasma insulin at ~400 μU/mL. At this stage the monkeys were leptin resistant.[273] Insulin levels dropped in phases 7 and 8, at which time blood glucose levels were two- to threefold higher than in phase 1. Overt diabetes was prevalent in monkeys 10–20 years old, with pronounced weight loss and β-cell malfunction associated with the deposition of amyloid[274] (Fig. 16-4). Hyperinsulinemia in the diabetic obese monkeys was associated with altered muscle insulin receptor mRNA splicing,[275] assumed to be related to the nutritionally induced insulin resistance.

Long-term dietary restriction was beneficial in extending the life span[276] and preventing diabetes.[277] Sedentary lifestyle and obesity in captivity promote the progression to hyperglycemia and β-cell exhaustion. However, IGT with preserved insulin response was found also in 4 out of 30 free-ranging *Macaca fascicularis* in Mauritius, without correlation to age or obesity.[278] The phases of diabetes development in monkeys spanning 10–20 years in captivity are reminiscent of those described in *Psammomys*, occurring during several weeks and representing a common effect of surplus energy intake and low energy expenditure.

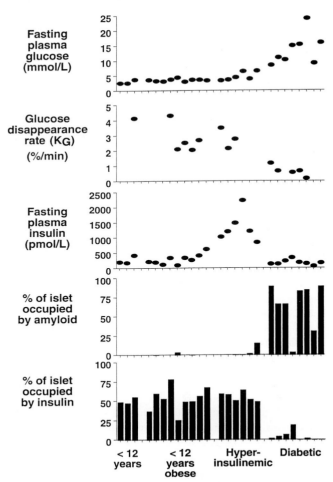

FIGURE 16-4. Progression of rhesus monkeys (*Macaca mulatta*) to diabesity on an *ad libitum* diet over 12 years. The X axis represents individual monkeys arranged left to right from normal to diabetic. Note that the peak plasma insulin concentrations, indicating oversecretion and resistance, occurred prior to the reduction in the peripheral glucose disappearance rate and the onset of fasting hyperglycemia. The exhaustion of β-cell insulin secretion was associated with amyloid deposition. (Personal contribution of Dr. Barbara C. Hansen.)

Dogs and Cats

The frequency of spontaneous, type 1-like diabetes in dogs of various breeds appears to be 1 in 200.[279] Canine diabetes appears to be due to the loss of β cells by a heterogenous autoimmune process,[280] or a result of pancreatitis, which is common in dogs. A general inflammatory reaction with extensive sclerosis and fibrosis was evident in the excised pancreas of diabetic dogs of different breeds transplanted with islets obtained from healthy dogs.[281] An increase in α and δ cells and mononuclear infiltration was seen in the remaining islets, constituting only ~10% of the normal β-cell mass. ICAs, ICSAs, and complement-dependent cytotoxicity were not detected, and no islet immunoglobulin deposits were found. These findings demonstrate characteristics different from those of rodents or monkeys. The pancreata were removed months after the onset of diabetes, by which time any evidence of an immune reaction might have disappeared. A multitargeted immune aggression rather than a specific islet-directed autoimmunity is considered likely. Chronic pancreatitis with an immune defect is also plausible. Extensive studies of retinopathy have been made in spontaneously and experimentally diabetic dogs as well as galactosemic dogs, as reviewed by Kern and colleagues.[282]

A defined genetic disorder in keeshond dogs has been reviewed by Kramer.[283] This type 1-like diabetes in nonobese dogs is a spontaneous autosomal recessive disorder with onset at 2–6 months of age. When not maintained on insulin, these dogs become severely hyperglycemic, hyperlipidemic, and ketotic, and develop cataracts and other complications, as well as becoming infertile. Immunocytochemical investigation of the pancreas revealed a specific absence of β cells, but no basis has been found for an autoimmune etiology of the islet lesion.

The incidence of feline diabetes is estimated to be 1 in 800. Little is known about its pathogenesis or genetics. Morphologic changes in islets are minor, but in some early reports hyaline-amyloid deposits were seen.[279,280,284] Cats exhibit massive deposits of islet amyloid, a product of islet amyloid–associated polypeptide, which is normally coproduced, costored, and most probably co-secreted with insulin, as reviewed by O'Brien and associates[285] (see Chaps. 3, 21, and 17). Amyloid may be involved in the pathogenesis of diabetes by impairing insulin secretion in cats and possibly other species.

Cat insulin's structure differs from that of human insulin at four positions, and appears to be the only insulin with histidine at position A18, close to the receptor-interacting area. This suggests that this histidine position in cat insulin may influence the binding of insulin to its receptor.[286]

CONCLUSION

The animal species with diabetes described in this chapter present an opportunity for investigation of the endocrine, metabolic, and morphologic changes in diverse phenotypic forms of both type 1 and type 2 diabetes. None of the species exhibits the full spectrum of functional or structural lesions associated with diabetes in humans, but each offers an opportunity for investigating certain clusters of derangements that are common in diabetic humans, particularly in their formative stages. A few concluding statements on the lessons learned from the numerous models of type 2 diabetes are appropriate.

A distinction may be made between those endowed with robust β cells with long-lasting secreting capacity that can sustain the huge insulin requirements needed to compensate for the resistance during the entire life span of the animal, and those with labile β cells that fail to compensate for the insulin resistance (Fig. 16-5). The animals of the second group initially oversecrete and present the full picture of typical diabesity. Later their β cells succumb to the pressure of oversecretion and irreversibly necrotize. They are vulnerable to hyperglycemia, either because of the diabetogenic genomic background, or glucotoxicity, or both.

Another feature common to most animal models of T2DM is hyperinsulinemia, which develops early in life, often prior to obesity. This is a result of a hypothalamic aberration that causes hyperphagia by transmitting signals directly to the pancreas through the vagus nerve, or is attributable to the availability of abundant nutrition, or is perhaps due to a low secretion threshold. It should be stressed that the hyperinsulinemia and the hyperglycemia that develop later are the hallmarks of diabesity. When these occur, they signify an advanced stage, with manifest β-cell malfunction. Furthermore, hyperinsulinemia and hyperglycemia are also detrimental by another mechanism. Insulin excess impairs hepatic and mus

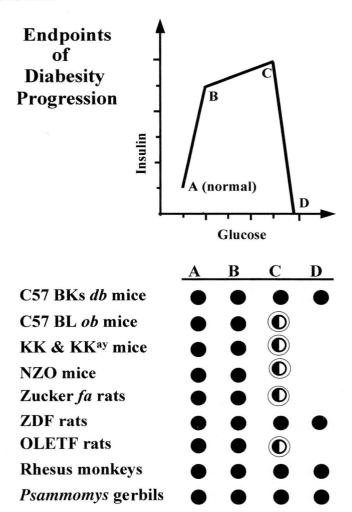

FIGURE 16-5. The inverted U shape of the relation between plasma insulin and glucose levels of several animal species during the development of genetic or nutritionally induced diabesity. The full circles indicate that all listed animals progress to stage B of hyperinsulinemia and obesity. The half-circles in stage C indicate sequential moderate hyperglycemia and remarkable obesity, whereas full circles at stage C indicate pronounced hyperglycemia in *db* mice, male ZDF rats, rhesus monkeys and *Psammomys* gerbils. These four animals progress at varying rates to the endpoint of β-cell loss in stage D, as a result of apoptosis, glucotoxicity, amyloid deposition, or other causes. Other animals continue to oversecrete and compensate for the insulin resistance through the capacity of their β cells to sustain prolonged overstimulation.

cle insulin receptor function by modifying intracellular phosphorylation along the cascade of signaling sequences. One of the most damaging results is the inability to restrain the expression of PEPCK, the rate-limiting enzyme of gluconeogenesis, and this contributes substantially to the hyperglycemia. It is intriguing that in almost all animals with diabesity, the hepatic insulin resistance involves gluconeogenesis, whereas insulin-induced lipogenesis continues to be enhanced, resulting in hyperlipidemia and obesity. By shunting some of the glucose excess to lipids, many of the diabese species are able to maintain moderate hyperglycemia, but the amelioration of glycemia by this mechanism incurs fat deposition that exacerbates obesity.

REFERENCES

1. Shafrir E, ed.: *Lessons from Animal Diabetes, Biennial Review.* Smith-Gordon:1995;5.
2. Shafrir E, ed.: *Lessons from Animal Diabetes.* Birkhauser Press:1996;6.
3. Sima AAF, Shafrir E, eds.: *Primer on Animal Models of Diabetes.* Harwood Academic Press:2000.
4. Sima, AAF, ed.: *Chronic Complications in Diabetes. Animal Models and Chronic Complications.* Harwood Academic Press:1999.
5. Shafrir E: Animal models of non-insulin-dependent diabetes. *Diabetes Metab Rev* 1992;8:179.
6. Bailey CJ, Flatt PR: Islet defects and insulin resistance in models of obese non-insulin-dependent diabetes. *Diabetes Metab Rev* 1993; 9:435.
7. Mrozikiewicz A, Kielczewska-Mrozikiewicz D, Lowick Z, *et al*: Blood levels of alloxan in children with insulin-dependent diabetes mellitus. *Acta Diabetol* 1994;31:236.
8. Malaisse WJ: Alloxan toxicity to the pancreatic B-cell. A new hypothesis. *Biochem Pharmacol* 1982;31:3527.
9. Asayama K, English D, Slonim AE, *et al*: Chemiluminescence as an index of drug-induced free radical production in pancreatic islets. *Diabetes* 1984;33:160.
10. Boquist L: Aspects of the diabetogenicity of alloxan and streptozotocin with special regard to a "mitochondrial hypothesis." In: Shafrir E, ed. *Lessons from Animal Diabetes.* Smith-Gordon:1992;1.
11. Lenzen S, Mirzaie-Petri M: Inhibition of aconitase by alloxan and the differential modes of protection of glucose, 3-O-methylglucose, and mannoheptulose. *Naunyn-Schmiedebergs Arch Pharmacol* 1992; 346:532.
12. Lenzen S, Brunig H, Munster W: Effects of alloxan and ninhydrin on mitochondrial Ca^{2+} transport. *Mol Cell Biochem* 1992;118:141.
13. Flatt P, Lenzen S, eds.: *Frontiers of Insulin Secretion and Pancreatic B-Cell Research.* Smith-Gordon and Nishimura:1994.
14. Kim H-R, Rho H-W, Park H-W, *et al*: Role of Ca^{2+} in alloxan-induced pancreatic β-cell damage. *Biochim Biophys Acta* 1994;1227:87.
15. Mathews CE, Leiter EH: Resistance of ALR/Lt islets to free radical-mediated diabetogenic stress is inherited as a dominant trait. *Diabetes* 1999;48:2189.
16. Mathews CE, Leiter EH: Constitutive differences in antioxidant defense status distinguish alloxan-resistant and alloxan-susceptible mice. *Free Radic Biol Med* 1999;27:449.
17. Ho RS, Aranda CG, Tillery SJ, *et al*: In-vivo and in-vitro glucose metabolism on a low dose streptozotocin rat model on noninsulin-dependent diabetes. In: Shafrir E, Renold AE, eds. *Lessons from Animal Diabetes.* Libbey:1988;202.
18. Agarval MK: Streptozotocin: Mechanism of action. *FEBS Lett* 1980; 120:1.
19. Rossini AA, Like AA, Dulin WE, *et al*: Pancreatic beta toxicity by streptozotocin anomers. *Diabetes* 1977;26:1120.
20. Thulesen J, Orskov C, Holst JJ, *et al*: Short term insulin treatment prevents the diabetogenic action of streptozotocin in rats. *Endocrinology* 1997;138:62.
21. Okamoto H: The molecular basis of experimental diabetes. In: Okamoto H, ed. *Molecular Biology of the Islets of Langerhans.* Cambridge University Press:1990.
22. Okamoto H: The Okamoto model for B-cell damage: Recent advances. In: Shafrir E, ed. *Lessons From Animal Diabetes.* Birkhauser Press:1996;99.
23. Mossman BT, Ireland CM, Filipak M, *et al*: Comparative interactions of streptozotocin and chlorotocin with DNA of an insulin-secreting cell line (RINr). *Diabetologia* 1986;29:186.
24. Wilson GL, Ledoux SP: Interactions of chemicals with pancreatic B-cells. In: Shafrir E, ed. *Lessons From Animal Diabetes.* Smith-Gordon:1992;17.
25. Heller B, Wang ZQ, Wagner EF, *et al*: Inactivation of the poly (ADP-ribose) polymerase gene affects oxygen radical and nitric oxide toxicity in islet cells. *J Biol Chem* 1995;270:11176.
26. Mak DHF, Ip SP, Li PC, *et al*: Alterations in tissue glutathione antioxidant system in streptozotocin-induced diabetic rats. *Mol Cell Biochem* 1996;162:153.
27. Oguzhan B, Yilmaz T, Memisoglu K, *et al*: Tissue glutathione content in streptozotocin diabetes: A proposal to explain the specificity of STZ action. *Mol Sci Med* 1992;21:29.

28. Masiello P, Wollheim CB, Blondel B, *et al*: Studies in vivo and in vitro on chemically-induced primary islet tumours and non-tumour endocrine pancreatic tissue. *Diabetologia* 1983;24:30.
29. Shepherd JG, Chen JR, Tsao MS, *et al*: Neoplastic transformation of propagable cultured rat pancreatic duct epithelial cells by azaserine and streptozotocin. *Carcinogenesis* 1993;14:1027.
30. Takasawa S, Yamamoto H, Terazono K, *et al*: Novel gene activated in rat insulinoma. *Diabetes* 1986;35:178.
31. Inoue C, Shiga K, Takasawa S, *et al*: Evolutionary conservation of the insulinoma gene rig and its possible function. *Proc Natl Acad Sci USA* 1987;84:6659.
32. Watanabe T, Yonemura Y, Yonekura H, *et al*: Pancreatic cell replication and amelioration of surgical diabetes by reg protein. *Proc Natl Acad Sci USA* 1994;9:3589.
33. Debnam ES, Chowrimootoo G: Streptozotocin diabetes and sugar transport by rat ileal enterocytes: Evidence for adaptation caused by an increased luminal nutrient load. *Biochim Biophys Acta* 1992; 1107:86.
34. Shafrir E: Development and consequences of insulin resistance: Lessons from animals with hyperinsulinemia. *Diabetes Metab* 1996;7:122.
35. Burant CF, Flink S, Depaoli FM, *et al*: Small intestine hexose transport in experimental diabetes: Increased transporter mRNA and protein expression in enterocytes. *J Clin Invest* 1994;93:578.
36. Yang H, Scheff AJ, Schalch DS: Effects of streptozotocin induced diabetes mellitus on growth and hepatic insulin-like growth factor I gene expression in the rat. *Metabolism* 1990;39:295.
37. Pao CI, Farmer PK, Begovic S, *et al*: Expression of hepatic insulin-like growth factor I and insulin-like growth factor-binding protein-1 genes is transcriptionally regulated in streptozotocin diabetic rats. *Mol Endocrinol* 1992;6:969.
38. Ooi GT, Tseng LYH, Tren MQ, *et al*: Insulin rapidly decreases insulin-like growth factor-binding protein-1 gene transcription in streptozotocin-diabetic rats. *Mol Endocrinol* 1992;6:2219.
39. Mayer M, Shafrir E: Glucocorticoid and insulin mediated regulation of skeletal muscle protein catabolism. In: Shafrir E, Renold AE, eds. *Lessons from Animal Diabetes.* Libbey:1984;235.
40. Pepato MT, Migliorini RH, Goldberg AL, *et al*: Role of different proteolytic pathways in degradation of muscle protein from streptozotocin-diabetic rats. *Am J Physiol* 1996;34:E340.
41. Han X, Karpakka J, Kainulainen H, *et al*: Effects of streptozotocin-induced diabetes, physical training and their combination on collagen biosynthesis in rat skeletal muscle. *Acta Physiol Scand* 1995;155:9.
42. Lenk SE, Bhat D, Blakeney W, *et al*: Effect of streptozotocin diabetes on rough endoplasmic reticulum and lysosomes in rat liver. *Am J Physiol* 1992;263:E856.
43. McGarry JD: Malonyl-CoA and carnitine palmitoyl transferase I—an expanding partnership. *Biochem Soc Trans* 1995;23:481.
44. Moir AMB, Zammit VA: Effects of insulin treatment of diabetic rats on hepatic partitioning of fatty acids between oxidation and esterification, phospholipid and acylglycerol synthesis, and on the fractional rate of secretion of triacylglycerol *in vivo*. *Biochem J* 1994;304:177.
45. Levy E, Shafrir E, Ziv E, *et al*: Composition, removal and metabolic fate of chylomicrons derived from diabetic rats. *Biochim Biophys Acta* 1985;834:376.
46. Tavangar K, Murata Y, Pedersen ME, *et al*: Regulation of lipoprotein lipase in the diabetic rat. *J Clin Invest* 1992;90:1672.
47. Sparks JD, Zolfghari R, Sparks CE, *et al*: Impaired hepatic apolipoprotein-B and apolipoprotein-E translation in streptozotocin-diabetic rats. *J Clin Invest* 1992;89:1418.
48. Kunjathoor VV, Wilson DL, LeBoeuf RC: Increased atherosclerosis in streptozotocin-induced diabetic mice. *J Clin Invest* 1996;97:1767.
49. Feingold KR, Fulford MH, Zsigmond G, *et al*: Importance of intestinal cholesterol synthesis in diabetic animals. In: Shafrir E, Renold AE, eds. *Lessons from Animal Diabetes.* Libbey:1984;556.
50. Magni F, Cancelleri M, Del Puppo M, *et al*: Diabetes-induced alteration of HMGCoA reductase in rat livers. *Acta Diabetol* 1992;28:211.
51. Feingold KR, Lear SR, Moser SH: De novo cholesterol synthesis in three different animal models of diabetes. *Diabetologia* 1984;26:234.
52. Schauder P, McIntosh C, Herberg L, *et al*: Increased somatostatin secretion from pancreatic islets of streptozotocin-diabetic rats in response to glucose. *Mol Cell Endocrinol* 1980;20:243.
53. Kanatsuka A, Makino H, Matsushima M, *et al*: Effect of glucose on somatostatin secretion from isolated pancreatic islets of normal and streptozotocin diabetic rats. *Endocrinology* 1981;109:652.

54. Grill V, Efendic S: Abnormal D cell secretion in alloxan diabetes: Influence by drug and aberrant metabolism. *Am J Physiol* 1984;246: E483.

55. Bestetti GE, Rossi GL: Neuroendocrine changes in experimentally diabetic rats. In: Shafrir E, Renold AE, eds. *Lessons from Animal Diabetes*. Libbey:1996;444.

56. Foreman D, Kolettios E, Garris D: Diabetes prevents the normal responses of the ovary to FSH. *Endocrinol Res* 1993;19:187.

57. Kienast SG, Fadden C, Steger RW: Streptozotocin induced diabetes blocks the positive feedback release of luteinizing hormone in the female rat. *Brain Res Bull* 1993;32:339.

58. Karasik A, Shafrir E: Function and regulation of insulin receptor in animal models of diabetes and insulin resistance. In: Shafrir E, ed. *Lessons from Animal Diabetes*. Smith-Gordon:1995;161.

59. Sechi LA, Griffin CA, Grady EF, et al: Tissue-specific regulation of insulin receptor mRNA levels in rats with STZ-induced diabetes mellitus. *Diabetes* 1992;41:1113.

60. Tozzo E, Desbuquois B: Effects of STZ-induced diabetes and fasting on insulin receptor mRNA expression and insulin receptor gene transcription in rat liver. *Diabetes* 1992;41:1609.

61. Giorgino F, Chen J, Smith RJ: Changes in tyrosine phosphorylation of insulin receptors and a 170,000 molecular weight nonreceptor protein in vivo in skeletal muscle of streptozotocin induced diabetic rats: Effects of insulin and glucose. *Endocrinology* 1992;130:1433.

62. Iwama N, Watari T, Kajimoto Y, et al: Dephosphorylation of the insulin receptor partially restores the decreased autophosphorylation in streptozotocin-induced diabetic rats. *Diabetes Res* 1991;7:25.

63. Meyerovitch J, Backer M, Kahn CR: Hepatic phosphotyrosine phosphatase activity and its alterations in diabetic rats. *J Clin Invest* 1989; 84:976.

64. Okamoto M, White M, Maron R, et al: Autophosphorylation and kinase activity of insulin receptor in diabetic rats. *Am J Physiol* 1986; 251:E542.

65. Wu D, Cederbaum AI: Combined effects of streptozotocin-induced diabetes plus 4-methypyrazole treatment on rat liver cytochrome P4502E1. *Arch Biochem Biophys* 1993;302:175.

66. Ioannides C, Barnett CR, Ayrton AD, et al: Alterations in chemical toxicity in animal models of insulin-dependent diabetes. In: Shafrir E, ed. *Lessons from Animal Diabetes*. Smith-Gordon:1990;306.

67. Like AA, Rossini AA: Streptozotocin-induced pancreatic insulitis: New model of diabetes mellitus. *Science* 1976;193:415.

68. Wand Z, Dohle C, Friemann J, et al: Prevention of high- and low-dose STZ-induced diabetes with D-glucose and 5-thio-D-glucose. *Diabetes* 1993;42:420.

69. Kolb H: Mouse models of insulin dependent diabetes: Low-dose streptozotocin-induced diabetes and nonobese diabetic (NOD) mice. *Diabetes Metab Rev* 1987;3:751.

70. Kolb H, Oschilewski M, Oschilewski U, et al: Analysis of 22 immunomodulatory substances for efficacy in low-dose streptozotocin-induced diabetes. *Diabetes Res* 1987;6:21.

71. Gerling IC, Friedman H, Greiner DL, et al: Multiple low-dose streptozotocin-induced diabetes in NOD-*scid/scid* mice in absence of functional lymphocytes. *Diabetes* 1994;43:433.

72. Wilson GL, Leiter EH: Streptozotocin interactions with pancreatic β-cells and the induction of insulin-dependent diabetes. In: Dyrberg T, ed. *Topics in Immunology and Microbiology*. Springer:1990;27.

73. Boitard C, Carnaud C: Lessons from animal models regarding pathogenesis of insulin-dependent diabetes mellitus. In: Leslie RDG, ed. *Molecular Pathogenesis of Diabetes Mellitus (Series: Frontiers of Hormone Research)*. Karger:1997;109.

74. Crisa L, Mordes JP, Rossini AA: Autoimmune diabetes in the BB rat. *Diabetes Metab Rev* 1992;8:9.

75. Mordes JP, Bortell R, Groen H, et al: Autoimmune diabetes mellitus in the BB rat. In: Sima AAF, Shafrir E, eds. *Primer on Animal Models of Diabetes*. Harwood Academic Press:2000;1.

76. Ellerman KE, Like AA: Staphylococcal enterotoxin-activated spleen cells passively transfer diabetes in BB/Wor rat. *Diabetes* 1992;41:527.

77. Ellerman KE, Richards CA, Guberski DL, et al: Kilham rat virus triggers T-cell dependent autoimmune diabetes in multiple strains of rat. *Diabetes* 1996;45:557.

78. Jacob HJ, Patterson A, Wilson D, et al: Genetic dissection of autoimmune type I diabetes in the BB rat. *Nat Genet* 1992;2:56.

79. Colle E, Fuks A, Poussier P, et al: Polygenic nature of spontaneous diabetes in the rat. *Diabetes* 1992;41:1617.

80. Prins J-B, Herberg L, Den Bierman M, et al: Genetic characterization and relationship of inbred lines of diabetes-prone and not diabetes-prone BB rats. In: Shafrir E, ed. *Lessons from Animal Diabetes*. Smith-Gordon:1991;19.

81. Kleeman R, Rothe H, Kolb-Bachofen V, et al: Transcription and translation of inducible nitric oxide synthase in the pancreas of prediabetic BB rats. *FEBS Lett* 1993;328:9.

82. Kolb H, Worz-Pagenstert U, Kleeman R, et al: Cytokine gene expression in the BB rat pancreas: Natural course and impact of bacterial vaccines. *Diabetologia* 1996;39:1448.

83. Lau A, Ramanthan S, Poussier P: Excessive production of nitric oxide by macrophages from DP-BB rats is secondary to the T-lymphopenic state of these animals. *Diabetes* 1998;47:197.

84. Dyrberg T, Poussier P, Nakhooda AF, et al: Islet cell surface and lymphocyte antibodies often precede the spontaneous diabetes in the BB rat. *Diabetologia* 1984;26:159.

85. Bertrand S, Vigeant C, Yale JF: Predictive value of lymphocyte antibodies for the appearance of diabetes in BB rats. *Diabetes* 1994;43:137.

86. Davies AJ, Bone AJ, Wilkin TJ, et al: Serum biopterin: A novel marker for immune activation during prediabetes in the BB rat. *Diabetologia* 1994;37:466.

87. Li XB, Scott FW, Park YH, et al: Low incidence of autoimmune type I diabetes in BB rats fed a hydrolysed casein-based diet associated with early inhibition of non-macrophage dependent hyperexpression of MHC class I molecules on beta cells. *Diabetologia* 1995;38:1138.

88. Malkani S, Nompleggi D, Hansen JW, et al: Dietary cow's milk protein does not alter the frequency of diabetes in the BB rat. *Diabetes* 1997;46:1133.

89. Scott FW, Cloutier HE, Kleeman R, et al: Potential mechanisms by which certain foods promote or inhibit the development of spontaneous diabetes in BB rats—dose, timing, early effect on islet area and switch in infiltrate from Th1 to Th2 cells. *Diabetes* 1997;46:589.

90. Misra M, Duguid WP, Marliss EB: Prevention of diabetes in the spontaneously diabetic BB rat by the glutamine antimetabolite acividin. *Can J Physiol Pharmacol* 1996;74:163.

91. Davenport C, Lovell H, James RFL, et al: Brain-reactive antibodies in BB/d rats do not recognize glutamic acid dehydrogenase. *Clin Exp Immunol* 1995;101:127.

92. Mackay IR, Bone A, Tuomi T, et al: Lack of autoimmune serological reactions in rodent models of insulin dependent diabetes mellitus. *J Autoimmun* 1996;9:705.

93. Wilkin T, Kiesel U, Diaz J-L, et al: Autoantibodies to insulin as serum markers for autoimmune insulitis. *Diabetes Res* 1986;3:173.

94. Ziegler M, Schlosser M, Hamann J, et al: Autoantibodies to glutamate dehydrogenase detected in diabetes-prone BB/OK rats do not distinguish onset of diabetes. *Exp Clin Endocrinol* 1994;102:98.

95. Markholst H, Eastman S, Wilson D, et al: Diabetes segregates as a single locus in crosses between inbred BB rats prone or resistant to diabetes. *J Exp Med* 1990;174:297.

96. Like AA, Guberski DL, Butler L: Diabetic Biobreeding/Worcester (BB/Wor) rats need not be lymphopenic. *J Immunol* 1986;136: 3254.

97. Ko IY, Jun HS, Kim GS, et al: Studies on autoimmunity for initiation of beta-cell destruction, 10. Delayed expression of a membrane bound islet cell specific 38 kDa autoantigen that precedes insulitis and diabetes in the diabetes-prone BB rat. *Diabetologia* 1994;37:460.

98. Harada M, Makino S: Biology of the NOD mouse. *Ann Rep Shionogi Res Lab* 1992;42:70.

99. Leiter EH: The nonobese diabetic (NOD) mouse: A model for analyzing the interplay between heredity and environment in development of autoimmune disease. *ILAR News* 1993;35:4.

100. Atkinson MA, Leiter EH: The NOD mouse model of type 1 diabetes; as good as it gets? *Nat-Med* 1999;5:601.

101. Ikegami H, Makino S: The NOD mouse and its related strains. In: Sima AAF, Shafrir E, eds. *Primer on Animal Models of Diabetes*. Harwood Academic Press:2000;43.

102. Baxter AG, Cooke A: The genetics of the NOD mouse. *Diabetes Metab Rev* 1995;11:315.

103. Tisch R, McDevitt H: Insulin-dependent diabetes mellitus. *Cell* 1996; 85:291.

104. Benoist C, Mathis D: Cell death mediators in autoimmune diabetes—no shortage of suspects. *Cell* 1997;89:1.

105. Todd JA: A protective role of the environment in the development of type 1 diabetes? *Diabet Med* 1991;8:906.

106. Ghosh S, Palmer SM, Rodrigues NR, *et al*: Polygenic control of autoimmune diabetes in nonobese diabetic mice. *Nat Genet* 1993;4:404.

107. Wicker L, Todd J, Peterson L: Genetic control of autoimmune diabetes in the NOD mouse. *Annu Rev Immunol* 1995;13:179.

108. Ikegami H, Makino S, Ogihara T: Molecular genetics of insulin-dependent diabetes mellitus: Analysis of congenic strains. In: Shafrir E, ed. *Lessons from Animal Diabetes*. Birkhauser:1996:33.

109. Thivolet CH, Goillot E, Bedosa P, *et al*: Insulin prevents adaptive cell transfer of diabetes in the autoimmune non-obese diabetic mouse. *Diabetologia* 1991;34:314.

110. Wicker LS, Miller BJ, Chai A, *et al*: Expression of genetically determined diabetes and insulitis in the nonobese diabetic (NOD) mouse at the level of bone marrow-derived cells. Transfer of diabetes and insulitis to nondiabetic (NOD × B10)F1 mice with bone marrow cells from NOD mice. *J Exp Med* 1988;167:1801.

111. Serreze DV, Leiter EH: Development of diabetogenic T cells from NOD/Lt marrow is blocked when allo-H-2 haplotype is expressed on cells of hematopoietic origin but not on thymic epithelium. *J Immunol* 1991;147:1222.

112. Natori T, Kawano K: The LETL rat: A model for IDDM without lymphopenia. *ILAR News* 1993;35:15.

113. Mizuno A, Iwami T, Sano T, *et al*: Cyclophosphamide-induced diabetes in Long-Evans Tokushima lean rats: Influence of ovariectomy on the development of diabetes. *Metabolism* 1993;42:865.

114. Shinohara M, Masuyama T, Shoda T, *et al*. A new spontaneously diabetic non-obese Torri rat Strain, with severe ocular complications. *Int J Exp Diab Res* 2000;1:89.

115. Lenzen S, Tiedge M, Elsner M, *et al*. The LEW.1AR1/Ztm-iddm rat: New model of spontaneous insulin-dependent diabetes mellitus. *Diabetologia* 2001;44:1189.

116. Teitelman G, Alpert S, Hanahan D: Proliferation, senescence and neoplastic progression of β-cells in hyperplastic pancreatic islets. *Cell* 1988;52:97.

117. Skowronski J, Alpert S, Hanahan D: Use of transgenic mice to study interactions of novel B-cell antigen with the immune system. In: Shafrir E, Renold AE, eds. *Lessons From Animal Diabetes*. Libbey: 1988;158.

118. Marban SL, Roth J: Transgenic hyperinsulinemia: A mouse model of insulin resistance and glucose intolerance without obesity. In: Shafrir E, ed. *Lessons From Animal Diabetes*. Birkhauser Press: 1996;203.

119. Schaefer EM, Viard V, Morin J, *et al*: A new transgenic mouse model of chronic hyperglycemia. *Diabetes* 1994;43:143.

120. Verschere CB, D'Alessio DA, Palmiter RD, *et al*: Transgenic mice overproducing islet amyloid peptide have increased insulin storage and secretion in vitro. *Diabetologia* 1994;37:725.

121. Ferre T, Pujol A, Riu E, *et al*: Correction of diabetic alterations by glucokinase. *Proc Natl Acad Sci USA* 1996;93:7225.

122. Hariharan N, Farrelly D, Hagan D, *et al*: Expression of human hepatic glucokinase in transgenic mice liver results in decreased glucose levels and reduced body weight. *Diabetes* 1997;46:11.

123. Short MK, Clouthier DE, Schaefer IM, *et al*: Tissue specific developmental, hormonal and dietary regulation of rat phosphoenolpyruvate carboxykinase-human growth hormone fusion genes in transgenic mice. *Mol Cell Biol* 1992;12:1007.

124. Mitanchez D, Chen R, Massias JF, *et al*: Regulated expression of mature human insulin in the liver of transgenic mice. *FEBS Lett* 1988; 421:285.

125. Tamemoto H, Kadowaki T, Tobe K, *et al*: Insulin resistance and growth retardation in mice lacking insulin substrate-1. *Nature* 1994; 372:182.

126. Araki E, Lipes MA, Patti ME, *et al*: Alternative pathway of insulin signaling in mice with targeted disruption of IRS-1 gene. *Nature* 1994;372:186.

127. Liu M-L, Gibbs EM, McCoid SC, *et al*: Transgenic mice expressing the human GLUT4/muscle-fat facilitative glucose transporter protein exhibit efficient glycemic control. *Proc Natl Acad Sci USA* 1993;90: 11346.

128. Deems RO, Evans JL, Deacon RW, *et al*: Expression of GLUT4 in mice results in increased insulin action. *Diabetologia* 1994;37: 1097.

129. Leturque A, Loizeau M, Vaulont S, *et al*: Improvement of insulin action in diabetic transgenic mice selectively overexpressing GLUT4 in skeletal muscle. *Diabetes* 1996;45:23.

130. Zierath JR, Tsao T-S, Stenbit AE, *et al*: Restoration of hypoxia stimulated glucose uptake in GLUT4-deficient muscle by muscle specific GLUT4 transgenic complementation. *J Biol Chem* 1998; 273;20910.

131. von Herrath MG, Efrat S, Oldstone MB, *et al*: Expression of adenoviral E3 transgenes in beta cells prevents autoimmune diabetes. *Proc Natl Acad Sci USA* 1997;94:9808.

132. Miyazaki JI, Tashiro F: Transgenic models of insulin-dependent diabetes mellitus. *ILAR News* 1994;35:37.

133. Mora S, Pessin JE: The use of mouse transgenic and homologous recombination technologies to analyze the physiologic basis of glucose homeostasis. In: Zierath JR, Wallberg-Henricksson H, eds. *Muscle Metabolism in Animal Models of Diabetes*. Taylor and Francis London and New York 2001;227.

134. Coleman DL: Lessons from studies with genetic forms of diabetes in the mouse. *Metabolism* 1983;32:162.

135. Herberg L, Coleman DL: Laboratory animals exhibiting obesity and diabetes syndromes. *Metabolism* 1977;26:59.

136. Thorens B, Wu YJ, Leahy JL, *et al*: The loss of GLUT2 expression by glucose-unresponsive beta-cells of *db/db* mice is reversible and is induced by the diabetic environment. *J Clin Invest* 1992;90:77.

137. Like AA, Chick WL: Studies on the diabetic mutant mouse, 2. Electron microscopy of pancreatic islets. *Diabetologia* 1970;6:216.

138. Pohl MN, Swartz FJ: Development of polyploidy in B-cells of normal and diabetic mice. *Acta Endocrinol* 1979;90:295.

139. Shafrir E: Nonrecognition of insulin as gluconeogenesis suppressant. A manifestation of selective hepatic insulin resistance in several animal species with type II diabetes: Sand rats, spiny mice and *db/db* mice. In: Shafrir E, Renold AE, eds. *Lessons from Animal Diabetes*. Libbey:1988;304.

140. Memon RA, Grunfeld C, Moser AH, *et al*: Fatty acid synthesis in obese insulin resistant diabetic mice. *Horm Metab Res* 1994;26:85.

141. Shargill NS, Tatoyan A, El-Refai MF, *et al*: Impaired insulin receptor phosphorylation in skeletal muscle membranes of db/db mice: The use of a novel skeletal muscle plasma membrane preparation to compare insulin binding and stimulation of receptor phosphorylation. *Biochem Biophys Res Commun* 1986;137:286.

142. Le Marchand-Brustel Y, Tanti JF, Rochet N, *et al*: Insulin receptor alterations in noninsulin-dependent diabetes. In: Shafrir E, Renold AE, eds. *Lessons from Animal Diabetes*. Libbey:1988;362.

143. Leiter EH, Coleman DL, Ingram DK, *et al*: Influence of dietary carbohydrate on the induction of diabetes in C57BL/KsJ-*db/db* diabetes mice. *J Nutr* 1983;113:184.

144. Coleman DL, Hummel KP: Effects of parabiosis of normal with genetically diabetic mice. *Am J Physiol* 1969;217:1298.

145. Coleman DL: Effects of parabiosis of obese with diabetic and normal mice. *Diabetologia* 1973;9:294.

146. Tartaglia LA: The leptin receptor. *J Biol Chem* 1977;272:6093.

147. Friedman JM, Halaas JL: Leptin and the regulation of body weight in mammals. *Nature* 1998;395:763.

148. Maffei M, Fei H, Lee GH, *et al*: Increased expression in adipocytes of Ob RNA in mice with lesions of the hypothalamus and with mutations of the db locus. *Proc Natl Acad Sci USA* 1995;92:6957.

149. Himms-Hagen J: Physiological roles of the leptin endocrine system: Differences between mice and humans. *Crit Rev Clin Lab Sci* 1999; 36:575.

150. Leiter EH: The genetics of diabetes susceptibility in mice. *FASEB J* 1989;3:2231.

151. Leiter EH, Chapman HD, Coleman DL: The influence of genetic background on the expression of mutations at the diabetes locus in the mouse, 5. Interaction between the *db* gene and hepatic sex steroid sulfotransferases correlates with gender-dependent susceptibility to hyperglycemia. *Endocrinology* 1989;124:912.

152. Shafrir E, Ben-Sasson R, Ziv E, *et al*: Insulin resistance, β-cell survival and apoptosis in type 2 diabetes; animal models and human implications. *Diabetes Rev* 1999;7:114.

153. Baetens D, Stefan Y, Ravazolla M, *et al*: Alterations of islet cell populations in spontaneously diabetic mice. *Diabetes* 1978;27:1.

154. Caro JF, Sinha MK, Kolaczynski JW, *et al*: Leptin: The tale of an obesity gene. *Diabetes* 1996;45:1455.

155. Williams G, McCarthy HD, McKibbin PE, *et al*: Neuroendocrine disturbances in diabetes: The role of hypothalamic regulatory peptides. In: Shafrir E, ed. *Lessons from Animal Diabetes*. Smith-Gordon:1992;203.

156. Wang Q, Bing C, Al-Barazanji K, *et al*: Interactions between leptin and hypothalamic neuropeptide Y neurons in the control of food intake and energy homeostasis in the rat. *Diabetes* 1997;46:335.

157. Yen TT, Bue JM, Gill AM: The diabetic obese syndrome of the viable yellow mouse and pharmacological interventions. In: Shafrir E, ed. *Lessons from Animal Diabetes*. Smith-Gordon:1991;293.

158. Yen TT, Gill AM, Frigeri L, *et al*: Obesity, diabetes, and neoplasia in yellow A^vy mice: Ectopic expression of the agouti gene. *FASEB J* 1994;8:479.

159. Taketomi S, Ikeda H: KK and KKA^y mice. In: Sima AAF, Shafrir E, eds. *Primer on Animal Models of Diabetes*. Harwood Academic Press:2000;129.

160. Suto JS, Matsuura S, Imamura K, *et al*: Genetic analysis of non-insulin-dependent diabetes mellitus in KK and yellow KK mice with various diabetic states. *Eur J Endocrinol* 1998;139:654.

161. Bonini JA, Colca JR, Dailey C, *et al*. Compensatory alterations for insulin signal transduction and glucose transport in insulin resistant diabetes. *Am J Physiol* 1995;269:E759.

162. Proietto J, Larkins RG: A perspective on the New Zealand obese mouse. In: Shafrir E, ed. *Lessons from Animal Diabetes*. Smith-Gordon:1992;65.

163. Andrikopoulos S, Thorburn AWE, Proietto J: The New Zealand obese mouse: A polygenic model of type 2 diabetes. In: Sima AAF, Shafrir E, eds. *Primer on Animal Models of Diabetes*. Harwood Academic Press:2000;171.

164. Larkins RG, Simeonova L, Veroni MC: Glucose utilization in relation to insulin secretion in NZO and C57Bl mouse islets. *Endocrinology* 1980;107:1634.

165. Veroni MC, Proietto J, Larkins RG: Evolution of insulin resistance in New Zealand obese mice. *Diabetes* 1991;40:1480.

166. Macaulay SL, Larkins RG: Impaired insulin action in adipocytes of New Zealand obese mice: A role for postbinding defects in pyruvate dehydrogenase and insulin mediator activity. *Metabolism* 1988;37:958.

167. Andrikopoulos S, Proietto J: The biochemical basis of increased hepatic glucose production in a mouse model of type 2 (non-insulin-dependent) diabetes mellitus. *Diabetologia* 1995;38:1389.

168. Andrikopoulos S, Rosella G, Gaskin E, *et al*: Impaired regulation of hepatic fructose-1,6-bisphosphatase in the New Zealand obese mouse model of NIDDM. *Diabetes* 1993;42:1731.

169. Herberg L: Insulin resistance in abdominal and subcutaneous obesity: Comparison of C57BL/6J *ob/ob* with New Zealand obese mice. In: Shafrir E, Renold AE, eds. *Lessons from Animal Diabetes*. Libbey:1988;367.

170. Truett G, Bahary N, Friedman JM, *et al*: The Zucker rat obesity gene fatty (fa) maps to chromosome 5 and is a homolog of the mouse diabetes (db) gene. *Proc Natl Acad Sci USA* 1991;88:7806.

171. Kava R, Greenwood MRC, Johnson PR: Zucker (fa/fa) rat. *ILAR News* 1990;32:4.

172. Bray GA, York DA, Fisler JS: Experimental obesity: A homeostatic failure due to defective nutrient stimulation of the sympathetic nervous system. *Vitam Horm* 1989;45:1.

173. Chan CB, MacPhail RM, Mitton K: Evidence for defective glucose sensing by islets of fa/fa obese Zucker rats. *Can J Physiol Pharmacol* 1993;71:34.

174. York DA: Role of glucocorticoids in the development of obesity and diabetes in experimental animal models. In: Shafrir E, ed. *Lessons from Animal Diabetes*. Smith-Gordon:1992;229.

175. Lee HC, Curry DL, Stern JS: Direct effect of CNS on insulin hypersecretion in obese Zucker rats: Involvement of vagus nerve. *Am J Physiol* 1989;256:E439.

176. Gentil CG, Rohner-Jeanrenaud F, Abramo F, *et al*: Abnormal regulation of the hypothalamo-pituitary adrenal axis in the genetically obese *fa/fa* rat. *Endocrinology* 1990;126:1873.

177. Bchini-Hooft van Huijsduijnen O, Rohner-Jeanrenaud F, Jeanrenaud B: Hypothalamic neuropeptide Y messenger ribonucleic acid levels in preobese and genetically obese (fa/fa) rats; potential regulation thereof by corticotropin-releasing factor. *J Neuroendocrinol* 1993;5:381.

178. Freedman MR, Castonguay TW, Stern JS: Effect of adrenalectomy and corticosterone replacement on meal patterns of Zucker rats. *Am J Physiol* 1985;249:R584.

179. Terretaz J, Assimacopoulos-Jeannet F, Jeanrenaud B: Severe hepatic and peripheral insulin resistance as evidenced by euglycemic clamps in genetically obese *fa/fa* rats. *Endocrinology* 1986;118:674.

180. Zarjevski N, Doyle P, Jeanrenaud B: Muscle insulin resistance may not be a primary etiological factor in the genetically obese fa/fa rat. *Endocrinology* 1993;130:1564.

181. Anai M, Funaki M, Ogihara T, *et al*: Altered expression levels and impaired steps in pathways of phosphatidylinositol-3-kinase activation via insulin receptor substrates. *Diabetes* 1998;47:13.

182. King PA, Horton EO, Hirshman MP, *et al*: Insulin resistance in obese Zucker rat (fa/fa) skeletal muscle is associated with a failure of glucose transporter translocation. *J Clin Invest* 1922;90:1568.

183. Uphues I, Kolter T, Goud B, *et al*: Failure of insulin regulated recruitment of the glucose transporter GLUT4 in cardiac muscle of obese Zucker rats is associated with alterations of small molecular-mass GTP-binding proteins. *Biochem J* 1995;311:161.

184. Henriksen EJ: Oxidative stress and antioxidant treatment: Effects on muscle glucose transport in animal models of type 1 and type 2 diabetes. In: Packer L, Rosen P, Tritscher HJ, *et al*, eds. *Antioxidants in Diabetes Management*. Marcel Decker:2000;303.

185. Bourgeois C, Wiggins D, Hioms R, *et al*: VLDL output by hepatocytes from obese Zucker rats is resistant to the inhibitory effect of insulin. *Am J Physiol* 1995;269:E206.

186. Penicaud L, Ferre P, Assimacopoulos-Jeannet F, *et al*: Increased gene expression of lipogenic enzymes and glucose transporter in white adipose tissue of suckling and weaned obese Zucker rats. *Biochem J* 1991;279:303.

187. Debant A, Guerre-Millo M, Le Marchand-Brustel Y, *et al*: Insulin receptor kinase is hyperresponsive in adipocytes of young obese Zucker rats. *Am J Physiol* 1987;252:E273.

188. Terrettaz J, Cusin I, Etienne J, *et al*: In vivo regulation of adipose tissue lipoprotein lipase in normal rats made hyperinsulinemic and in hyperinsulinemic genetically-obese (fa/fa) rats. *Int J Obes* 1994;18:9.

189. Trimble ER, Bruzzone R, Belin D: Insulin resistance is accompanied by impairment of amylase gene expression in the exocrine pancreas of the obese Zucker rat. *Biochem J* 1986;237:807.

190. Guberski DL, Butler L, Like AA: The BBZ/Wor rat: An obese animal with autoimmune diabetes. In: Shafrir E, Renold AE, eds. *Lessons from Animal Diabetes*. Smith-Gordon:1988;268.

191. Guberski DL, Butler L, Manzi SM, *et al*: The BBZ/Wor rat: Clinical characteristics of the diabetic syndrome. *Diabetologia* 1993;36:912.

192. Murray PT, Wachowski ME, Duiani A, *et al*: Intermediate and long diabetic (type II) complications in the spontaneously BBZ/WOR rat. *Diabetes* 1996;45(suppl 1):272A.

193. Sima AAF, Merry AC, Hall D, *et al*: The BB/Z^DR rat. A model for Type II diabetic neuropathy *Exp Clin Endocrinol Diabetes* 1997;105:63.

194. Peterson RG: The Zucker diabetic fatty (ZDF) rat. In: Sima AAF, Shafrir E, eds. *Primer on Animal Diabetes*. Harwood Academic Press: 2000;109.

195. Friedman JE, Devente JE, Peterson RG, *et al*: Altered expression of muscle glucose transporter GLUT-4 in diabetic fatty Zucker rats (ZDF/Drt-*fa*). *Am J Physiol* 1991;261:E782.

196. Pick A, Clark J, Kubstrup C, *et al*: Role of apoptosis in failure of β-cell mass compensation for insulin resistance and β-cell defects in the male Zucker diabetic rat. *Diabetes* 1998;47:358.

197. Orci L, Ravazzola M, Baetens D, *et al*: Evidence that down-regulation of B-cell glucose transporters in non-insulin-dependent diabetes may be the cause of diabetic hyperglycemia. *Proc Natl Acad Sci USA* 1990;87:9953.

198. Ohneda, M, Inman LR, Unger RH: Caloric restriction in obese prediabetic rats prevents beta-cell depletion, loss of beta-cell GLUT2 and glucose incompetence. *Diabetologia* 1995;38:173.

199. Unger RH: Lipotoxicity in the pathogenesis of obesity-dependent NIDDM. Genetic and clinical implications. *Diabetes* 1995;44:863.

200. Koyama K, Chen GX, Lee Y, *et al*: Tissue triglycerides, insulin resistance and insulin production: Implications for hyperinsulinemia of obesity. *Am J Physiol* 1997;36:E708.

201. Unger RH: How obesity causes diabetes in Zucker Diabetic Fatty rats. *Trends Endocrinol Metab* 1998;7:276.

202. Kava R, Peterson RG, West DB, *et al*: Wistar diabetic fatty rat. *ILAR News* 1990;32:9.

203. Odaka H, Sugiyama Y, Ikeda H: Characteristics of Wistar fatty rat. In: Sima AAF, Shafrir E, eds. *Primer on Animal Diabetes*. Harwood Academic Press:2000;159.

204. Albright AL, Gregoire F, Green S, *et al*: Studies in the Wistar diabetic fatty rat (WDF fa/fa). A model of non-insulin-dependent diabetes

mellitus. In: Shafrir E, eds. *Lessons from Animal Diabetes*. Smith-Gordon:1994;75.

205. Yamakawa T, Tanaka S, Tamura K, *et al*: Wistar fatty rat is obese and spontaneously hypertensive. *Hypertension* 1955;25:146.

206. Greenhouse DD, Hansen CT, Michaelis OE: Development of fatty and corpulent rat strains. *ILAR News* 1990;32:2.

207. Kahle EB, Butz KG, Leibel RL, *et al*: Glucose homeostasis in three interstrains (La/N-BN/Crl *cp/cp*; Zuc13M-BN/Crl *fa/fa*; and Zuc13M-LA/N *fa/cp*) of genetically obese rats. In: Shafrir E, ed. *Lessons from Animal Diabetes*. Birkhauser Press:1996;411.

208. Michaelis OE IV, Hansen CT: The spontaneous hypertensive/NIH corpulent rats: A new rodent model for the study of non-insulin-dependent diabetes mellitus and its complications. *ILAR News* 1990; 32:19.

209. Marette A, Atgie C, Liu Z, *et al*: Differential regulation of GLUT1 and GLUT4 glucose transporters in skeletal muscle of a new model of type II diabetes. The obese SHR/N-cp rat. *Diabetes* 1993;42:1195.

210. Velasquez MT, Kimmel PL, Michaelis OE IV, *et al*: Effect of carbohydrate intake on kidney function and structure in SHR/N-cp rats. *Diabetes* 1989;38:679.

211. McCune SA, Radin MJ, Jenkins JE, *et al*: SHHF/Mcc-fa*cp* rat model: Effects of gender and genotype on age of expression of metabolic complications and congestive heart failure and on response to drug therapy. In: Shafrir E, ed. *Lessons from Animal Diabetes*. Smith-Gordon:1994;255.

212. Radin MJ, Chu YY, Hoepf MM, *et al*: Treatment of obese female and male SHHF/Mcc-*fa^cp* rats with antihypertensive drugs, nifedipine and enalapril: Effects on body weight, fat distribution, insulin resistance and systolic pressure. *Obes Res* 1993;1:433.

213. Russell JC: Insulin resistance and cardiovascular disease: Lessons from the JCR:LA-cp and other strains of obese rat. In: Shafrir E, ed. *Lessons from Animal Diabetes*. Smith-Gordon:1992;137.

214. Shillabeer G, Hornford J, Forden JM, *et al*: Fatty acid synthase and adipsin mRNA levels in obese and lean JCR:LA-cp rats: Effect of diet. *J Lipid Res* 1992;33:31.

215. Russel JC, Shillabeer G, Bar-Tana J, *et al*: Development of insulin resistance in the JCR:LA-*cp* rat. Role of triacylglycerols and effects of Medica 16. *Diabetes* 1998;47:770.

216. Russel JC, Graham SE, Richardson C: Cardiovascular disease in the JCR:LA-*cp* rat. *Mol Cell Biochem* 1988;188:113.

217. Russel JC, Graham SE: The JCR:LA-*cp* rat: An animal model of obesity and insulin resistance with spontaneous cardiovascular disease. In: Sima AAF, Shafrir E, eds. *Primer on Animal Diabetes*. Harwood Academic Press:2000;227.

218. Leiter EH, Prochazka M, Coleman DL, *et al*: Genetic factors predisposing to diabetes susceptibility in mice. In: Jaworski, ed. *The Immunology of Diabetes Mellitus*. Elsevier:1986;29.

219. Sakamoto N, Hotta N, Uchida K, eds.: *Current Concepts of a New Animal Model: The NON Mouse*. Elsevier:1992.

220. Mori Y, Yokoyama J, Nemoto M, *et al*: Expression of diabetes, its genetics and complications in WBN rats with endocrine-exocrine pancreatic lesion. In: Shafrir E, ed. *Lessons from Animal Diabetes*. Smith-Gordon:1992;91.

221. Shimoda I, Koizumi M, Shimosegawa T, *et al*: Physiological characteristics of spontaneously developed diabetes in male WBN/Kob rat and prevention of development of diabetes by chronic oral administration of synthetic trypsin inhibitor (FOY-305). *Pancreas* 1993;8:196.

222. Miyamura N, Amemiya T: Lens and retinal changes in the WBN/Kob rat (spontaneously diabetic strain)—electron microscopic study. *Ophthalmic Res* 1998;30:221.

223. Martinez SM, Tarres MC, Picena JC, *et al*: ESS rat, an animal model for the study of spontaneous non-insulin dependent diabetes. In: Shafrir E, ed. *Lessons from Animal Diabetes*. Smith-Gordon:1992;75.

224. Martinez SM, Tarres MC, Montenegro SM, *et al*: Effects of dietary sucrose option on the diabetic syndrome of the eSS rat. *Isr J Med Sci* 1994;30:761.

225. Berdanier CD: Non-insulin dependent diabetes in the nonobese BHE/cdb rat. In: Shafrir E, ed. *Lessons from Animal Diabetes*. Smith-Gordon:1995;231.

226. Mathews CE, McGraw RA, Dean R, *et al*: Inheritance of a mitochondrial DNA defect and impaired glucose tolerance in BHE/Cdb rats. *Diabetologia* 1999;42:35.

227. Kawano K, Hirashima T, Mori S, *et al*: Spontaneously diabetic rat "OLETF" as a model for NIDDM in humans. In: Shafrir E, ed. *Lessons from Animal Diabetes*. Birkhauser Press:1996;227.

228. Kawano S, Hirashima T, Mori S, *et al*: The OLETF rat. In: Sima AAF, Shafrir E, eds. *Primer on Animal Diabetes*. Harwood Academic Press; 2000;213.

229. Ueda H, Ikegami H, Shibata M, *et al*: The NSY mouse: An animal model of human type 2 diabetes mellitus with polygenic inheritance. In: Sima AAF, Shafrir E, ed. *Primer on Animal Diabetes*. Harwood Academic Press:2000;185.

230. Koletzky RJ, Friedman JE, Ernsberger P: The obese spontaneously hypertensive rat (SHROB, Koletzky rat): A model of metabolic syndrome X. In: Sima AAF, Shafrir E, eds. *Primer on Animal Diabetes*. Harwood Academic Press:2000;143.

231. Ishizuka T, Ernsberger S, Liu D, *et al*: Phenotypic consequences of a nonsense mutation in the leptin receptor gene (*fa^K*) in obese spontaneously hypertensive Koletzky rat (SHROB). *J Nutr* 1998;128:2299.

232. Ziv E, Shafrir E: *Psammomys obesus* (sand rat): Nutritionally induced NIDDM-like syndrome on a "thrifty gene" background. In: Shafrir E, ed. *Lessons from Animal Diabetes*. Smith-Gordon:1995;285.

233. Ziv E, Kalman R: *Psammomys obesus*: Primary insulin resistance leading to nutritionally induced type 2 diabetes. In: Sima AAF, Shafrir E, eds. *Primer on Animal Diabetes*. Harwood Academic Press:2000;321.

234. Shafrir E, Ziv E: Cellular mechanism of nutritionally induced insulin resistance: The desert rodent *Psammomys obesus* and other animals in which insulin resistance leads to detrimental outcome. *J Basic Clin Physiol Pharmacol* 1998;9:347.

235. Shafrir E, Ziv E, Mosthaf L: Nutritionally induced insulin resistance and receptor defect leading to β-cell failure in animal models. *Ann NY Acad Sci* 1999;892:223.

236. Kalderon B, Gutman A, Shafrir E, *et al*: Characterization of stages in the development of obesity-diabetes syndrome in sand rat (*Psammomys obesus*). *Diabetes* 1986;35:717.

237. Gadot M, Leibovitz G, Shafrir E, *et al*: Hyperproinsulinemia and insulin deficiency in the diabetic *Psammomys obesus*. *Endocrinology* 1994;135:610.

238. Like AA, Miki E: Diabetic syndrome in sand rats, 4. Morphologic changes in islet tissue. *Diabetologia* 1967;3:143.

239. Donath MY, Gross DJ, Cerasi E, *et al*: Hyperglycemia-induced β-cell apoptosis in pancreatic islets of *Psammomys obesus* during development of diabetes. *Diabetes* 1999;48:738.

240. Barnett M, Collier GR, Collier FM, *et al*: A cross-sectional and short-term longitudinal characterization of NIDDM in *Psammomys obesus*. *Diabetologia* 1994;37:671.

241. Marquie G, Duhault J, Jacotot B: Diabetes mellitus in sand rats (*Psammomys obesus*). Metabolic pattern during development of the diabetic syndrome. *Diabetes* 1984;33:438.

242. Barnett M, Collier GR, Zimmet P, *et al*: Energy intake with respect to the development of diabetes mellitus in *Psammomys obesus*. *Diabet Nutr Metab* 1995:8:1.

243. Barnett M, Collier GR, Zimmet P, *et al*: The effect of restricting energy intake on diabetes in *Psammomys obesus*. *Int J Obes* 1994;18:789.

244. Collier GR, DeSilva A, Sanigorski A, *et al*: Development of obesity and insulin resistance in the Israeli sand rat (*Psammomys obesus*). Does leptin play a role? *Ann NY Acad Sci* 1997;877:50.

245. Kalman R, Adler H, Lazarovici G, *et al*: The efficiency of sand rat metabolism is responsible for development of obesity and diabetes. *J Basic Clin Physiol Pharmacol* 1993;4:83.

246. Jorns A, Tiedge M, Ziv E, *et al*. Gradual loss of pancreatic beta-cell insulin, glucokinae and GLUT2 glucose transporter immunoreactivities during the time course of nutritionally induced type-2 diabetes in *Psammomys obesus* (sand rat). Virchows Archiv, 2002;440:63.

247. Kanety H, Moshe S, Shafrir E, *et al*: Hyperinsulinemia induces a reversible impairment in receptor function leading to diabetes in the sand rat model of non-insulin-dependent diabetes mellitus. *Proc Natl Acad Sci USA* 1994;91:1853.

248. Miles PD, Li S, Hart M, *et al*: Mechanism of insulin resistance in experimental hyperinsulinemic dogs. *J Clin Invest* 1998;101:202.

249. Ikeda Y, Olsen GS, Ziv E, *et al*: Cellular mechanism of nutrionally induced insulin resistance in *Psammomys obesus*. Overexpression of protein kinase Cε in skeletal muscle precedes the onset of hyperinsulinemia and hyperglycemia. *Diabetes* 2001;50:584.

250. Schmitz-Pfeiffer C, Browne CL, Oakes NJD, *et al*: Alterations in the expression and cellular localization of protein kinase C isozymes ε and θ are associated with insulin resistance in skeletal muscle of the high-fat-fed rat. *Diabetes* 1997;46:169.

251. Collier GR, McMillan JS, Windmill K, *et al*: Beacon: A novel gene involved in the regulation of energy balance. *Diabetes* 2000;49:1766.

252. Cameron DP, Stauffacher W, Orci L, *et al*: Defective immunoreactive insulin secretion in the *Acomys cahirinus*. *Diabetes* 1972;21:1060.

253. Renold AE, Cameron DP, Amherdt M, *et al*: Endocrine-metabolic anomalies in rodents with hyperglycemic syndromes of hereditary and/or environmental origin. *Isr J Med Sci* 1972;8:189.

254. Gutzeit A, Renold AE, Cerasi E, *et al*: Effect of diet-induced obesity on glucose tolerance of a rodent with a low insulin response (*Acomys cahirinus*). *Diabetes* 1979;28:777.

255. Shafrir E: Overnutrition in spiny mice (*Acomys cahirinus*): β-cell expansion leading to rupture and overt diabetes on fat-rich diet and protective energy wasting elevation in thyroid hormone on sucrose-rich diet. *Diabetes Metab Res Rev* 2000;16:94.

256. Surwit RS, Kuhn CM: Diet-induced type 2 diabetes and obesity in the C57BL/6J mouse: A stress-related model of human diabetes. In: Shafrir E, ed. *Lessons from Animal Diabetes*. Smith-Gordon:1992;219.

257. Petro AE, Surwit RS: The C57BL/6J mouse as a model of diet induced type 2 diabetes and obesity. In: Sima AAF, Shafrir E, eds. *Primer on Animal Diabetes*. Harwood Academic Press:2000;337.

258. Klimes I, Sebokova E, Vrana A, *et al*: The hereditary hypertriglyceridemic rat, a new animal model of the insulin resistance syndrome. In: Shafrir E, ed. *Lessons from Animal Diabetes*. Smith-Gordon;:1995;271.

259. Stolba P, Opltova H, Husek P, *et al*: Adrenergic overactivity and insulin resistance in nonobese hereditary hypertriglyceridemic rats. *Ann NY Acad Sci* 1993;683:281.

260. Suzuki KI, Goto Y, Toyota T: Spontaneously diabetic GK (Goto-Kakizaki) rats. In: Shafrir E, ed. *Lessons from Animal Diabetes*. Smith-Gordon:1992;107.

261. Bisbis S, Bailbe D, Tormo MA, *et al*: Insulin resistance in the GK rat: Decreased receptor number but normal kinase activity in liver. *Am J Physiol* 1993;265:E807.

262. Movassat J, Saulnier C, Serradas P, *et al*: Impaired development of pancreatic beta-cell mass is a primary event during the progression of diabetes in the GK rat. *Diabetologia* 1997;40:916.

263. Tsuura Y, Ishida H, Okamoto Y, *et al*: Glucose sensitivity of ATP-sensitive K$^+$ channels is impaired in B-cells of the GK rat. A new genetic model of IDDM. *Diabetes* 1993;41:1446.

264. Sener A, Malaisse-Lagae F, Ostenson CG, *et al*: Metabolism of endogenous nutrients in islets of Goto-Kakizaki (GK) rats. *Biochem J* 1993;296:329.

265. Ohneda M, Johnson JH, Inman LR, *et al*: GLUT2 expression and function in B-cells of GK rats with NIDDM. Dissociation between reductions in glucose transport and glucose-stimulated insulin secretion. *Diabetes* 1993;42:1065.

266. Ostenson CG: The Goto-Kakizaki rat. In: Sima AAF, Shafrir E, eds. *Primer on Animal Diabetes*. Harwood Academic Press:2000;197.

267. Cohen AM, Rosenmann E, eds.: *The Cohen Diabetic Rat*. Karger: 1990.

268. Wexler-Zangen S, Yagil C, Zangen DH, *et al:* The newly inbred Cohen diabetic rat. A nonobese normolipidemic genetic model of diet-induced Type 2 diabetes expressing sex differences. *Diabetes* 2001;50:2521.

269. Howard CF Jr: Use of nonhuman primates to gain insight into diabetes mellitus related hormonal and metabolic controls, and secondary complications. In: Shafrir E, Renold AE, eds. *Lessons from Animal Diabetes*. Libbey:1988;272.

270. Howard CF Jr: Longitudinal studies on the development of diabetes in individual *Macaca nigra*. *Diabetologia* 1986;29:301.

271. Hansen BC, Ortmeyer HK, Bodkin NL: Obesity, insulin resistance, and noninsulin-dependent diabetes mellitus in aging monkeys: Implications for NIDDM in humans. In: Shafrir E, ed. *Lessons from Animal Diabetes*. Smith-Gordon:1994;93.

272. Bodkin NL: The rhesus monkey (*Macaca mulatta*): A unique and valuable model for the study of spontaneous diabetes mellitus and associated conditions. In: Sima AAF, Shafrir E, eds. *Primer on Animal Diabetes*. Harwood Academic Press:2000;303.

273. Bodkin NL, Nicolson M, Ortmeyer HK, *et al*: Hyperleptinemia: Relationship to adiposity and insulin resistance in the spontaneously obese rhesus monkeys. *Hom Metab Res* 1996;28:674.

274. De Koning EJP, Bodkin NL, Hansen BC, *et al*: Diabetes mellitus in *Macaca mulatta* monkeys is characterized by islet amyloidosis and reduction in beta-cell population. *Diabetologia* 1993;36:378.

275. Huang Z, Bodkin NL, Ortmeyer HK, *et al*: Hyperinsulinemia is associated with altered insulin receptor mRNA splicing in muscle of the spontaneously obese diabetic rhesus monkey. *J Clin Invest* 1994;94:1289.

276. Ramsey JJ, Boecker EB, Weinbruch R, *et al*: Energy expenditure of adult male rhesus monkeys during the first 30 mo of dietary restriction. *Am J Physiol* 1997;272:E901.

277. Hansen BC, Bodkin NL: Primary prevention of diabetes mellitus by prevention of obesity in monkeys. *Diabetes* 1993;42:1809.

278. Dunaif A, Tattersall I: Prevalence of glucose intolerance in free-ranging *Macaca fascicularis* of Mauritius. *Am J Perinatol* 1987;13:435.

279. Gepts W, Toussaint D: Spontaneous diabetes in dogs and cats. *Diabetologia* 1967;3:249.

280. Sai P, Debray-Sachs M, Jondet A, *et al*: Anti-B-cell immunity in insulinopenic diabetic dogs. *Diabetes* 1984;33:135.

281. Mintz DH, Alejandro R: Lessons from and for canine diabetes mellitus: Histopathology and islet transplantation. In: Shafrir E, Renold AE, eds. *Lessons from Animal Diabetes*. Libbey:1988;13.

282. Kern TS, Kowluru R, Engerman RL: Dog and rat models of diabetic retinopathy. In: Shafrir E, ed. *Lessons from Animal Diabetes*. Birkhauser:1996;395.

283. Kramer JW: The *dm* diabetic dog with inherited, insulin-dependent diabetes. In: Shafrir E, ed. *Lessons from Animal Diabetes*. Smith-Gordon:1994;217.

284. Schaer M: Feline diabetes mellitus. *Vet Clin North Am* 1976;6:453.

285. O'Brien TD, Westermark P, Betsholtz C, *et al*: Islet amyloid polypeptide: Biology and role in the pathogenesis of islet amyloidosis and diabetes mellitus. In: Shafrir E, ed. *Lessons from Animal Diabetes*. Smith-Gordon:1992;117.

286. Hallden G, Gafvelin G, Mutt V, *et al*: Characterization of cat insulin. *Arch Biochem Biophys* 1986;247:20.

Pathology of the Pancreas in Diabetes Mellitus

Per Westermark

As soon as it became clear that the islets of Langerhans play a central role in the development of diabetes mellitus, pathologists focused their interest on this part of the pancreas. Many of the structural islet lesions that we now know to reflect important pathological events in the pancreas were described at an early date.[1,2] At that time there was no clear distinction between different diabetes mellitus syndromes and although differences between the pathological findings in young and old diabetic individuals were noted, the two diabetes groups were not separated. Only much later was the separation of patients into the syndromes of insulin-dependent or type 1 diabetes mellitus (T1DM) and non-insulin-dependent or type 2 diabetes mellitus (T2DM) performed. We now recognize that the islet pathology in T1DM is very different from the majority of individuals with T2DM. Most recently, distinctive but rare forms of diabetes mellitus have been described, such as familial insulinopathies[3] and maturity onset diabetes of the young (MODY). It should be pointed out that many studies of human islet pathology are based on autopsy materials that may not be completely clean (i.e., they may include cases misinterpreted as either type 1 or type 2). The considerable overlap between T1DM and T2DM concerning islet or β-cell volume may partially depend on this problem.

This chapter deals primarily with the pancreatic pathology of type 1 and type 2 diabetes. Some pathogenetic aspects of these syndromes are also discussed. Comparably little is known about the pancreatic pathology in the rare forms of diabetes.

PANCREAS IN T1DM

General

In recent onset type 1 diabetes, no significant reduction of pancreatic size is found.[4,5] In long-standing T1DM, there is often, but not always, a significant reduction of pancreatic weight[4–7] accompanied by interstitial fibrosis of the exocrine tissue.[6,8] However, the weight reduction only affects the pancreatic peptide (PP)-poor part of the pancreas.[8] Arteriosclerotic and arteriolosclerotic changes are very common in long-standing T1DM and are often pronounced.[5,6] These may lead to secondary changes such as local atrophy and pronounced fibrosis.

Islet Cells and Islet Cell Volume

Even in recent onset T1DM, there is often a reduction in the number of islets[5,6] but in quantitative studies, there is considerable overlap with the normal pancreas.[9] A reduction of β-cell granula-

tion is often conspicuous.[9] Even in islets from individuals with a very brief history of T1DM, the number of β cells is greatly reduced, the majority of islets being devoid of them.[5,10] These so-called pseudoatrophic islets, like islets in long-standing T1DM, consist of α-, δ and PP cells, and thus are devoid of insulin (and islet amyloid polypeptide; IAPP). The islets are composed of cords of small cells (Fig. 17-1). Islets consisting entirely of PP cells increase in frequency with the duration of T1DM,[10] but there is no demonstrable increase of the volume density of PP cells.[8] In long-standing type 1 diabetes, the islets are small[11] and there is a major reduction of islet volume,[4,5,7] which is caused largely by the nearly complete lack of islet β cells.[5] This β-cell atrophy coincides well with the very small amount of extractable insulin in such pancreata.[12] In spite of the pronounced β-cell loss, a few β cells are commonly found in many cases of type 1 diabetes of long duration. A decrease in α-cell volume has been found in one study.[7]

Inflammatory Cell Infiltrate (Insulitis)

Infiltration of the islets with mononuclear inflammatory cells (insulitis or isletitis) (Fig. 17-2) is a common finding in T1DM of recent onset,[4,5,12] especially in children under 10 years of age.[9] In pancreatic material from 16 young persons who had had diabetes for only a few days, Gepts and De Mey found islets with lymphocytic infiltration in 9.[10] However, in specimens of pancreatic biopsies from 17 individuals with recent onset of T1DM, Imagawa and colleagues found insulitis in only 9, and concluded that there may exist at least two mechanisms for β-cell death.[13] Insulitis has also been described rarely in late-onset diabetes in conjunction with islet amyloid.[14] In cases of T1DM of longer duration, insulitis may be absent.[5,10] When present, the inflammatory infiltrate consists mainly of T lymphocytes, B lymphocytes and macrophages.[15] T lymphocytes predominate and there are usually more CD8 T cells than CD4 T cells,[13,16] although the opposite has been found in isolated cases.[17]

Lymphocytic infiltration occurs only in islets with β cells and is seen in at least 80% of pancreata of individuals who have been studied at the clinical onset of T1DM.[16] In type 1 diabetes of recent onset, three main types of islets have been described: apparently normal islets, inflamed islets, and pseudoatrophic islets, which are devoid of β cells but contain all other islet cell types.[5,15] There is reason to believe that these different islet forms reflect a pathologic chain of events and that many islet abnormalities are present long before the clinical onset of diabetes. The end result may be the so-called pseudoatrophic islet.

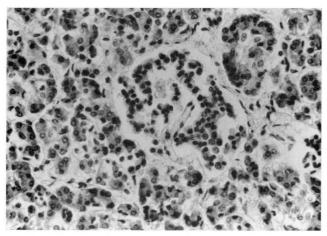

FIGURE 17-1. Islet from the pancreas of a patient with long-standing T1DM. The islet is small and consists of cords of cells, mainly α cells (× 475).

By studying patients that have undergone pancreas transplantation for the treatment of T1DM, evidence has been obtained of the pathogenic importance of the inflammatory infiltrate in β-cell destruction. Some such patients have had recurrence of their diabetes, and in association with this, insulitis similar to that seen in recent onset type 1 diabetes has been found.[18] However, recurrent type 1 diabetes and β-cell loss without signs of insulitis in the transplant has also been recorded.[19]

During recent years it has become evident that some individuals, previously believed to have T2DM in reality are suffering from late onset T1DM. Understandably, few studies of the pancreatic pathology have been performed on such cases. In a pancreatic biopsy from one such individual with "latent autoimmune diabetes in adults," typical insulitis with CD4+ and CD8+ T cells was identified.[17]

Expression of Major Histocompatibility Complex

Like all other cells, islet epithelial cells normally express class I MHC. However, in recent onset type 1 diabetes there is a hyper-

FIGURE 17-2. Heavy infiltration of an islet with lymphocytes from a patient with recently diagnosed T1DM (× 500). (*Reproduced, with permission, from Volk BW: Pathology of the diabetic pancreas. In: Porte D, Sherwin R, eds. Ellenberg & Rifkin's Diabetes Mellitus, 4th ed. Appleton & Lange:1988.*)

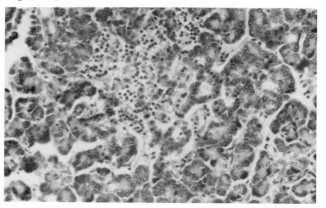

expression of class I MHC in α, δ, and β cells,[13,20,21] which disappears in the pseudoatrophic islets, and which is not seen in other chronic inflammatory pancreatic disorders. There is also an ∝-interferon-like immunostaining of β cells in these islets.[22] Expression of Fas occurs in endocrine cells, mainly β cells, in many islets with insulitis, and inflammatory cells expressing Fas ligand may be found in the same islets, possibly indicating Fas-mediated apoptotic β-cell death.[23] Aberrant expression of class II antigen in some β cells has also been reported in recent onset T1DM.[15,20] The importance of the hyperexpression of class I MHC and aberrant expression of class II MHC in the autoimmune process is not fully understood. However, both events are believed to precede the insulitis and to be involved in its pathogenesis.[21]

Islet Regeneration

Signs of β-cell regeneration are common in recent onset type 1 diabetes. Small new islets appear to differentiate from exocrine ducts and consist of hyperactive β cells.[10] Such islets can also become targets of lymphocytic infiltration.

Other Islet Lesions

Some degree of islet fibrosis is common. Islet amyloidosis is absent in T1DM. In spite of this, there are a few reports of islet amyloidosis in young individuals with diabetes, and this includes Opie's original description.[1] The nature of the amyloid as well as the exact type of diabetes in these patients is not clear.

PANCREAS IN T2DM

General

Since type 2 diabetes is a disease of slow onset, it is difficult to distinguish a definite time of onset of the disease. Therefore very little is known about the early pancreatic pathology of T2DM in humans. Such studies have to be performed in animal models of type 2 diabetes.[24,25]

In contrast to T1DM, the pancreas in T2DM is usually of normal size[7,11,26] but with a tendency toward fatty infiltration,[26] most probably due to the obesity present in many of these patients. Arteriosclerotic changes, often severe, are the rule, and diffuse or focal fibrosis is common.

Islet Cells and Islet Cell Volume

There are several studies showing a moderate reduction of the total islet volume in T2DM.[7,26] This reduction is mainly due to a reduced β-cell mass,[7,27] reflected by a significantly lower relative islet β-cell frequency in type 2 diabetes.[11,28,29] However, there is a significant overlap between nondiabetic and diabetic elderly individuals in both islet volume and percentage of islet β cells,[26,28] and in one study no significant islet volume reduction was found.[11] A pronounced β-cell loss as seen in T1DM does not occur in T2DM. Furthermore, the β cells in type 2 diabetes are rich in granules and not degranulated as in type 1 diabetes. In one study, densitometric studies of insulin immunolabeled sections did not reveal any difference between diabetic and nondiabetic individuals.[30] There are contradictory results concerning the α-cell mass in T2DM, with both reduced α-cell mass,[7,27] and increased α-cell mass[11] reported. In a majority of individuals, many of the islets show pathological alterations, particularly amyloid deposits. The shape of the islets is often more irregular in T2DM[29] and enlarged islets occur in cases with islet amyloidosis.[31] Hyperproinsulinemia is a typical feature of T2DM. In one immunohistochemical study with proinsulin antibody, an increase in β cells with signs of impaired proinsulin processing was found in obese, but not in lean, type 2 diabetic pancreatic islets.[30] Proinsulin gene expression was decreased in β cells in amyloid-containing islets as compared to islets without amyloid.[30]

Islet Hyperplasia

Hyperplasia of islet cells resulting in marked islet hypertrophy has been reported in one study of pancreatic specimens from nondiabetic obese individuals,[32] and in an other study the β-cell volume in obese type 2 diabetic patients was twice that of nonobese diabetic individuals.[33] Obese, nondiabetic individuals had the greatest β-cell volume, which was four times that of nonobese diabetic subjects.

Islet Regeneration

Signs of islet regeneration have sometimes been described in type 2 diabetes. However, the volume distribution of islets is usually normal in T2DM (except for islets with heavy amyloid infiltration), suggesting that there is no significant regeneration of whole islets.[31]

Islet Amyloid

It has sometimes been stated that the pancreas (including the islets) is morphologically normal in T2DM. Nevertheless, the most typical and frequent lesion, deposition of amyloid in the islets of Langerhans, was described independently in two articles at the beginning of the 20th century.[1,2] Although the similarity to amyloid was pointed out early,[34] the deposited material was first described as hyaline, and it was not until the green birefringence under polarization microscopy after Congo red staining was recognized and the fine fibrillar ultrastructure demonstrated that the amyloid nature of the deposits was accepted.[35,36]

Frequency of Islet Amyloid

Some degree of islet amyloidosis is found in a majority of type 2 diabetic patients. The frequency varies among studies. Bell[37] reported some degree of islet amyloidosis in 46% of diabetic patients over 50 years of age. In our own material, 95% of T2DM patients over 60 years old exhibited some degree of islet amyloidosis, but in some modern materials a low frequency (57%) has also been reported.[30] The differences in the frequency of islets with amyloid among studies is probably due to methodological variations; also, the degree of islet amyloidosis is easily underestimated. The frequency of islets with amyloid deposits is higher in the pancreatic tail and body compared to the head,[38] and the distribution of affected islets is often uneven. Sometimes, lobuli with pronounced islet amyloid deposits may be found, while other parts of the pancreas contain no or little amyloid.

Some islet amyloid deposits are also commonly found in nondiabetic individuals.[38,39] In these subjects, the number of affected islets is generally much smaller and the degree of islet amyloidosis is significantly less. There are, however, examples of severe islet amyloidosis in nondiabetic individuals.[38,39] It is possible that these individuals in reality suffered from undiagnosed T2DM.

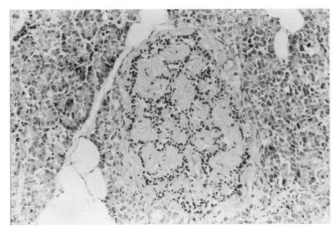

FIGURE 17-3. Islet from a patient with T2DM. The islet is heavily infiltrated with amyloid, which constitutes more than 50% of the islet volume. In this section, residual endocrine cells appear as cords in the amyloid masses ($\times$ 225).

Structure and Topography of Islet Amyloid

Islet amyloid is strictly localized to the endocrine tissue and is not seen in the exocrine tissue (Fig. 17-3). In individuals with slight degrees of islet amyloidosis, the lesion appears as small deposits in the interstitium between islet cells and capillaries, or as a thin amyloid deposit covering the capillary side of the endocrine epithelial cell groups. With more pronounced deposition, islets can become more or less converted into amyloid lumps (Fig. 17-3), although some β, α, and δ cells almost always remain. Ultrastructurally, like all types of amyloid, islet amyloid is composed of thin nonbranched fibrils 7–10 nm in diameter (Fig. 17-4). In the larger deposits, these fibrils form a disorganized network, while in small fibril aggregates and in deposits close to β cells, the amyloid fibrils

FIGURE 17-4. Typical islet amyloid fibrils forming a disorganized network. The section was labeled with antiserum to islet amyloid polypeptide (IAPP) and the reaction visualized with protein A-gold particles. The amyloid fibrils (**A**) react with the antiserum to IAPP, but the collagen (**C**) does not ($\times$ 50,000).

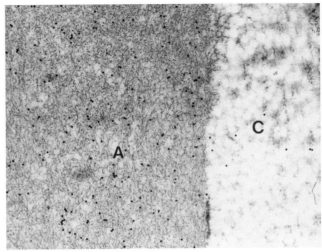

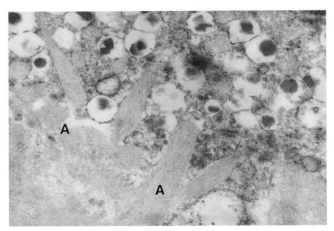

FIGURE 17-5. Electron photomicrograph showing the periphery of β cells containing many typical granules. Amyloid (**A**) is seen extracellularly as parallel bundles in deep plasma membrane-lined pockets of the cells (× 54,000).

tend to form parallel bundles (Fig. 17-5). Such bundles are often seen in deep cytoplasmic membrane-lined pockets in the β cells, but not in other cells.[40] This close relationship between islet amyloid and β cells has been interpreted as a sign of formation of fibrils from a protein produced by these cells.[40]

There is some controversy regarding the exact site of islet amyloid formation. Virtually all islet amyloid is found extracellularly, even in cases with very slight (and therefore probably early) deposits.[40] Formation of the fibrils extracellularly, but in close contact with β cells, has been suggested.[41] However, intracellular formation of the amyloid has also been proposed[42] and studies of amyloid formation in human islets transplanted into nude mice[43] and electron microscopic studies of human insulinomas[44] have supported this supposition. Given the concept that amyloid formation is a nucleation-dependent process, it is possible, but not proven, that the first amyloid forms intracellularly by mechanisms yet to be clarified. The main bulk of amyloid may then be formed extracellularly on the amyloid originally formed, after the death of the cell containing the first amyloid.[45]

Pathogenic Importance of Islet Amyloid

Islet amyloid was long regarded as a characteristic islet lesion of type 2 diabetes, but was thought to be of no pathogenic importance. Study of the phenomenon is difficult in humans, and investigations in the relationship between islet amyloid and diabetes in the primate *Macaca nigra*[46] and the domestic cat[47] were largely disregarded. However, recent experiments with transgenic mice expressing human IAPP have changed this view since a close relationship between glucose intolerance or diabetes and occurrence of islet amyloid deposits has been shown repeatedly in such animals (see Chap. 21).[48–50] Whether islet amyloid is of initial importance in the pathogenesis of type 2 diabetes is thus far uncertain, but there is a growing consensus that islet amyloid is important in the continuing deterioration of β-cell function in type 2 diabetes.[50,51] Beta cells in contact with even small deposits of islet amyloid show signs of degeneration, with parallel bundles of fibrils running through the basement and cell membranes.[40] In islets with more heavy deposition, severe β-cell degeneration occurs. It is rea-

sonable to assume that β-cell function is impaired in such cases, both by direct destruction of the cells and by the barrier formed by the amyloid masses.[26] There is also experimental evidence that IAPP amyloid fibrils, like Aβ-protein fibrils in Alzheimer's disease, exert a cytotoxic effect by a yet unknown mechanism.[52,53] There is also evidence that the most toxic species are not fully developed amyloid fibrils, but the initially formed "protofibrils"[54] (see below). Since severe islet amyloidosis occurs more often in patients who have been treated with insulin,[55,56] it is probable that islet amyloid at least partly explains secondary failure in the treatment of type 2 diabetes with oral hypoglycemic drugs. It should be mentioned, however, that not all investigators believe in the pathophysiologic importance of islet amyloid deposits.[30]

Nature and Pathogenesis of Islet Amyloid

All types of amyloid fibrils are polymers of small proteins, with one specific protein characteristic of each amyloid form.[57] Several polypeptide hormones are known to give rise to local amyloid deposits.[58] Islet amyloid has as a major constituent islet amyloid polypeptide (IAPP; amylin),[59] which is a 37-amino-acid polypeptide related to the neuropeptide calcitonin gene-related peptide (CGRP) (Fig. 17-6).[60,61] IAPP is mainly expressed by islet β cells as a 89-amino-acid prepropolypeptide of which a 22-amino-acid leader sequence is cleaved off initially. The 67-amino-acid proIAPP is converted to mature IAPP by cleavage at two basic amino acid residues flanking the IAPP sequence. IAPP is stored with insulin in the secretory granules[62] and the two peptides are released together. However, on a molar basis, the ratio of IAPP to insulin is less than 1:10 in islets and plasma.

The physicochemical mechanisms by which amyloid fibrils form are likely similar among the different biochemical forms of amyloid, and include adoption of a beta sheet secondary structure

FIGURE 17-6. Human islet amyloid polypeptide is a 37-amino-acid C-terminally amidated peptide. For full biologic activity, IAPP requires a disulfide bond between residues 2 and 7 and the C-terminal amidation.

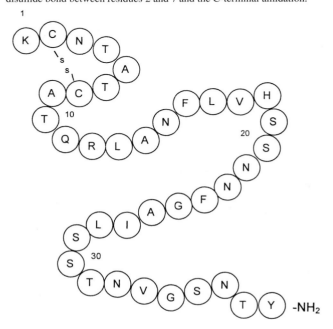

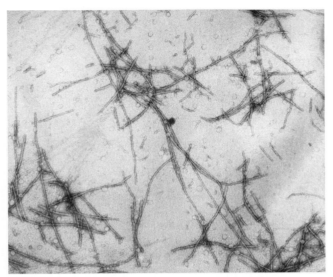

FIGURE 17-7. Fibrils formed from synthetic human IAPP. These fibrils resemble the native islet amyloid fibrils in size and staining properties (× 60,000).

of the protein.[63] The beta strands are arranged perpendicularly to the fibril axis, allowing strong intermolecular noncovalent bonding. There is a growing body of research indicating that very thin "protofibrils" form first and that these subsequently assemble to make up the mature fibrils.[63,64] These protofibrils, which may be the most significant in causing β-cell injury, usually escape detection with ordinary electron microscopic studies and may well be present in islets apparently free of amyloid.

Human IAPP, like IAPP in other primates and in cats, has a strong intrinsic fibril-forming tendency (Fig. 17-7). In contrast, IAPP of most other animal species does not form fibrils due to interspecies amino acid substitutions in the 20-29 segment of the molecule[65–67] (Fig. 17-8).

It is not known why IAPP forms islet amyloid in T2DM, although an overexpression of the peptide may be of importance. However, transgenic mice overexpressing human IAPP do not readily form islet amyloid, indicating that additional factors are of importance. Free fatty acids may induce altered expression, processing, storage or release of IAPP.[51] Beta cells of islets with amyloid contain little or no IAPP immunoreactivity[68,69] in spite of near normal insulin immunoreactivity and the presence of IAPP mRNA

in IAPP-negative islet cells.[70] This lack of immunoreactivity is not due to depletion of (pro)IAPP in the β cells, but IAPP seems to be present in the cells in an abnormal, as yet undefined form.[71]

Islet amyloid contains, like all other types of amyloid, several additional components that are always present. Thus the glycoprotein amyloid P component (SAP), which is a plasma pentraxine protein, is a constituent of islet amyloid. Proteoglycans, especially the heparan sulfate proteoglycan perlecan, is present in islet amyloid[72] and the glycosaminoglycan moiety is the reason why the amyloid can be histologically stained with anionic dyes such as alcian blue.[73] Apolipoprotein E (apo E) has been of considerable interest in the pathogenesis of Aβ-amyloid in Alzheimer's disease, and one allelic form (apoE4) is a risk factor for late-onset Alzheimer's disease. Apo E has also been shown to be a component of human islet amyloid.[51,74] The importance of these additional components in the pathogenesis of the amyloid fibrils is unknown at present, but it has been suggested that they may stabilize a fibrillogenic protein conformation and thereby function as "pathological chaperones."[75]

DIABETES MELLITUS SECONDARY TO PANCREATIC DISEASE AND OTHER RARE FORMS OF DIABETES MELLITUS

Diabetes mellitus commonly occurs in patients with chronic pancreatitis, cystic fibrosis, and hemochromatosis. In all these diseases, the exocrine parenchyma is primarily destroyed, leading to severe fibrosis. Islet atrophy with fibrosis occurs later and is usually not as severe as that of the exocrine parenchyma.[76] The presence of iron in some islet β cells seems to play an important role in the development of diabetes in hemochromatosis.[77] These rare forms of diabetes are not associated with islet amyloidosis. A type of diabetes resembling type 2 diabetes commonly develops in conjunction with pancreatic carcinoma.[78] Although the tumor often causes widespread destruction of pancreatic tissue, loss of islet tissue is not a major cause of the diabetes, since partial pancreatectomy often improves the diabetic state.[79] The pathogenesis of this tumor-associated diabetes form is therefore unknown.

Other rare forms of diabetes mellitus about which little is known of the pancreatic pathology include insulinopathies[3] and maturity onset diabetes of the young (MODY). In patients with diabetes associated with a mutation in mitochondrial DNA, Otabe and colleagues found a reduced number of β cells but no insulitis.[80]

FIGURE 17-8. The 20-29 segment of human CGRP and of IAPP from four species. The sequence differences help to explain why only certain species like humans and cats develop islet amyloid, while others such as mice and hamsters do not. The symbol (−) indicates identity with human IAPP 20-29. Note the complete lack of identity in the 20-29 segments of human CGRP and IAPP.

```
Human IAPP20-29        SNNFGAILSS
Cat IAPP20-29          ---L-----P
Mouse IAPP20-29        ---L-PV-PP
Hamster IAPP20-29      N--L-PV--P
Human CGRP20-29        GGVVKNNFVP
```

REFERENCES

1. Opie EL: On relation of chronic interstitial pancreatitis to the islands of Langerhans and to diabetes mellitus. *J Exp Med* 1901;5:397.
2. Weichselbaum A, Stangl E: Zur Kenntnis der feineren Veränderungen des Pankreas bei Diabetes mellitus. *Wien Klin Wochenshr* 1901;14:968.
3. Nanjo K, Sanke T, Miyano M, *et al*: Diabetes due to secretion of a structurally abnormal insulin (insulin Wakayama). Clinical and functional characteristics of [Leu^A3] insulin. *J Clin Invest* 1986;77:514.
4. Maclean N, Ogilvie RF: Observations on the pancreatic islet tissue of young diabetic subjects. *Diabetes* 1959;8:83.
5. Gepts W: Pathologic anatomy of the pancreas in juvenile diabetes mellitus. *Diabetes* 1965;14:619.
6. Doniach I, Morgan AG: Islets of Langerhans in juvenile diabetes mellitus. *Clin Endocrinol* 1973;2:233.

7. Klöppel G, Drenck CR: Immunzytochemische Morphometrie beim Typ-1- und Typ-2-Diabetes mellitus. *Deutsch Med Wschr* 1983;108:188.

8. Rahier J, Wallon J, Loozen S, *et al*: The pancreatic polypeptide cells in the human pancreas: the effects of age and diabetes. *J Clin Endocrinol Metab* 1983;56:441.

9. Junker K, Egeberg J, Kromann H, *et al*: An autopsy study of the islets of Langerhans in acute-onset juvenile diabetes mellitus. *Acta Path Microbiol Scand A* 1977;85:699.

10. Gepts W, De Mey J: Islet cell survival determined by morphology. An immunocytochemical study of the islets of Langerhans in juvenile diabetes mellitus. *Diabetes* 1978;27(Suppl 1):251.

11. Rahier J, Goebbels RM, Henquin JC: Cellular composition of the human diabetic pancreas. *Diabetologia* 1983;24:366.

12. Warren S, LeCompte PM, Legg MA: *The Pathology of Diabetes Mellitus*, 4th ed. Lea & Febiger:1966.

13. Imagawa A, Hanafusa T, Itoh N, *et al*: Immunological abnormalities in islets at diagnosis paralleled further deterioration of glycaemic control in patients with recent-onset type 1 (insulin-dependent) diabetes mellitus. *Diabetologia* 1999;42:574.

14. LeCompte PH, Legg MA: Insulitis (lymphocytic infiltration of pancreatic islets) in late-onset diabetes. *Diabetes* 1972;21:762.

15. Foulis AK: In type 1 diabetes, does a non-cytopathic viral infection of insulin-secreting B-cells initiate the disease process leading to their autoimmune destruction? *Diabetes Med* 1989;6:666.

16. Foulis AK, Liddle CN, Farquharson MA, *et al*: The histopathology of the pancreas in type 1 (insulin-dependent) diabetes: a 25 year review of deaths in patients under 20 years of age in the United Kingdom. *Diabetologia* 1986;29:267.

17. Shimada A, Imazu Y, Morinaga S, *et al*: T-cell insulitis found in anti-GAD65$^+$ diabetes with residual β-cell function. *Diabetes Care* 1999;22:615.

18. Santamaria P, Lewis C, Jessurun J, *et al*: Skewed T-cell receptor usage and junctional heterogeneity among isletitis αβ and γδ T-cells in human IDDM. *Diabetes* 1994;43:599.

19. Petruzzo P, Andreelli F, McGregor B, *et al*: Evidence of recurrent type I diabetes following HLA-mismatched pancreas transplantation. *Diabetes Metab* 2000;26:215.

20. Bottazzo GF, Dean BM, McNally JM, *et al*: *In situ* characterization of autoimmune phenomena and expression of HLA molecules in the pancreas in diabetic insulitis. *N Engl J Med* 1985;313:353.

21. Foulis AK: The pathology of the endocrine pancreas in type 1 (insulin-dependent) diabetes mellitus. *APMIS* 1996;104:161.

22. Foulis AK, Farquharson MA, Meager A: Immunoreactive α-interferon in insulin-secreting β cells in type 1 diabetes mellitus. *Lancet* 1987;ii:1423.

23. Moriwaki M, Itoh N, Miyagawa J, *et al*: Fas and Fas ligand expression in inflamed islets in pancreas sections of patients with recent-onset type 1 diabetes mellitus. *Diabetologia* 1999;42:1332.

24. Howard CF, van Bueren A: Changes in islet cell composition during development of diabetes in *Macaca nigra*. *Diabetes* 1986;35:165.

25. O'Brien TD, Hayden DW, Johnson KH, *et al*: Immunohistochemical morphometry of pancreatic endocrine cells in diabetic, normoglycaemic glucose-intolerant and normal cats. *J Comp Path* 1986;96:357.

26. Westermark P, Wilander E: The influence of amyloid deposits on the islet volume in maturity onset diabetes mellitus. *Diabetologia* 1978;15:417.

27. Saito K, Yaginuma N, Takahashi T: Differential volumetry of A, B and D cells in the pancreatic islets of diabetic and nondiabetic subjects. *Tohoku J Exp Med* 1979;129:273.

28. Westermark P, Grimelius L: The pancreatic islet cells in insular amyloidosis in human diabetic and non-diabetic adults. *Acta Path Microbiol Scand A* 1973;81:291.

29. Clark A, Wells CA, Buley ID, *et al*: Islet amyloid, increased A-cells, reduced B-cells and exocrine fibrosis: quantitative changes in the pancreas in type 2 diabetes. *Diabetes Res* 1988;9:151.

30. Sempoux C, Guiot Y, Dubois D, *et al*: Human type 2 diabetes: morphological evidence for an abnormal β-cell function. *Diabetes* 2001;50(suppl. 1):172.

31. Hellman B: The frequency distribution of the number and volume of the islets of Langerhans in man. 2. Studies in diabetes of adult onset. *Acta Path Microbiol Scand* 1961;51:95.

32. Ogilvie RF: The islands of Langerhans in 19 cases of obesity. *J Path Bact* 1933;37:473.

33. Klöppel G, Löhr M, Habich K, *et al*: Islet pathology and the pathogenesis of type 1 and type 2 diabetes mellitus revisited. *Surv Synth Path Res* 1985;4:110.

34. Gellerstedt N: Die elektive, insuläre (Para-)Amyloidose der Bauchspeicheldrüse. Zugleich en Beitrag zur Kenntnis der "senilen Amyloidose." *Beitr Path Anat* 1938;101:1.

35. Ehrlich JC, Ratner IM: Amyloidosis of the islets of Langerhans. A restudy of islet hyaline in diabetic and nondiabetic individuals. *Am J Path* 1961;38:49.

36. Lacy PE: The pancreatic beta cell. Structure and function. *N Engl J Med* 1967;276:187.

37. Bell ET: Hyalinization of the islets of Langerhans in diabetes mellitus. *Diabetes* 1952;1:341.

38. Westermark P: Quantitative studies of amyloid in the islets of Langerhans. *Ups J Med Sci* 1972;77:91.

39. Bell ET: Hyalinization of the islets of Langerhans in nondiabetic individuals. *Am J Path* 1959;35:801.

40. Westermark P: Fine structure of islets of Langerhans in insular amyloidosis. *Virchows Arch A* 1973;359:1.

41. Westermark P: Amyloid and polypeptide hormones: What is their inter-relationship? Amyloid: *Int J Exp Clin Invest* 1994;1:47.

42. Clark A, Edwards CA, Ostle LR, *et al*: Localisation of islet amyloid peptide in lipofuscin bodies and secretory granules of human B-cells and in islets of type-2 diabetic subjects. *Cell Tissue Res* 1989;257:179.

43. Westermark P, Eizirik DL, Pipeleers DG, *et al*: Rapid deposition of amyloid in human islets transplanted into nude mice. *Diabetologia* 1995;38:543.

44. O'Brien TD, Butler AE, Roche PC, *et al*: Islet amyloid polypeptide in human insulinomas. Evidence for intracellular amyloidogenesis. *Diabetes* 1994;43:329.

45. Westermark GT, Steiner DF, Gebre-Medhin S, *et al*: Pro islet amyloid polypeptide (proIAPP) immunoreactivity in amyloid formation in the islets of Langerhans. *Ups J Med Sci* 2000;105:97.

46. Howard CF, van Bueren A: Changes in islet cell composition during development of diabetes in *Macaca nigra*. *Diabetes* 1986;35:165.

47. Johnson KH, Hayden DW, O'Brien TD, *et al*: Spontaneous diabetes-islet amyloid complex in adult cats. *Am J Path* 1986;125:416.

48. Verchere CB, D'Alessio DA, Palmiter RD, *et al*: Islet amyloid formation associated with hyperglycemia in transgenic mice with pancreatic beta cell expression of human islet amyloid polypeptide. *Proc Natl Acad Sci USA* 1996;93:3492.

49. Janson J, Soeller WC, Roche PC, *et al*: Spontaneous diabetes mellitus in transgenic mice expressing human islet amyloid polypeptide. *Proc Natl Acad Sci USA* 1996;93:7283.

50. Höppener JWM, Ahrén B, Lips CJM: Islet amyloid and type 2 diabetes mellitus. *N Engl J Med* 2000;343:411.

51. Kahn SE, Andrikopoulos S, Verchere CB: Islet amyloid. A long-recognized but underappreciated pathological feature of type 2 diabetes. *Diabetes* 1999;48:241.

52. May PC, Boggs LN, Fuson KS: Neurotoxicity of human amylin in rat primary hippocampal cultures: similarity to Alzheimer's disease amyloid-β neurotoxicity. *J Neurochem* 1993;61:2330.

53. Lorenzo A, Razzaboni B, Weir GC, *et al*: Pancreatic islet cell toxicity of amylin associated with type-2 diabetes mellitus. *Nature* 1994;368:756.

54. Janson J, Ashley RH, Harrison D, *et al*: The mechanism of islet amyloid polypeptide toxicity is membrane disruption by intermediate-sized toxic amyloid particles. *Diabetes* 1999;48:491.

55. Maloy AL, Longnecker DS, Greenberg ER: The relation of islet amyloid to the clinical type of diabetes. *Hum Path* 1981;12:917.

56. Westermark P: Islet amyloid polypeptide and amyloid in the islets of Langerhans. In: Leslie RGD, Robbins D, eds. *Diabetes: Clinical Science in Practice*. Cambridge Press University:1995;189.

57. Glenner GG: Amyloid deposits and amyloidosis. The β-fibrilloses. *N Engl J Med* 1980;302:1283, 1333.

58. Westermark P, Eriksson L, Engström U, *et al*: Prolactin-derived amyloid in the aging pituitary gland. *Am J Path* 1997;150:67.

59. Westermark P, Wernstedt C, Wilander E, *et al*: A novel peptide in the calcitonin gene related peptide family as an amyloid fibril protein in the endocrine pancreas. *Biochem Biophys Res Commun* 1986;140:827.

60. Westermark P, Wernstedt C, Wilander E, *et al*: Amyloid fibrils in human insulinoma and islets of Langerhans of the diabetic cat are derived from a neuropeptide-like protein also present in normal islet cells. *Proc Natl Acad Sci USA* 1987;84:3881.

61. Cooper GJ, Willis AC, Clark A, *et al*: Purification and characterization of a peptide from amyloid-rich pancreases of type 2 diabetic patients. *Proc Natl Acad Sci USA* 1987;84:8628.

62. Lukinius A, Wilander E, Westermark GT, *et al*: Co-localization of islet amyloid polypeptide and insulin in the B cell secretory granules of the human pancreatic islets. *Diabetologia* 1989;32:240.

63. Rochet J-C, Lansbury PTJ: Amyloid fibrillogenesis: themes and variations. *Curr Opin Struct Biol* 2000;10:60.

64. Goldsbury C, Kistler J, Aebi U, *et al*: Watching amyloid fibrils grow by time-lapse atomic force microscopy. *J Mol Biol* 1999;285:33.

65. Betsholtz C, Svensson V, Rorsman F, *et al*: Islet amyloid polypeptide (IAPP): cDNA cloning and identification of an amyloidogenic region associated with species-specific occurrence of age-related diabetes mellitus. *Exp Cell Res* 1989;183:484.

66. Nishi M, Chan SJ, Nagamatsu S, *et al*: Conservation of the sequence of islet amyloid polypeptide in five mammals is consistent with its putative role as an islet hormone. *Proc Natl Acad Sci USA* 1989;86:5738.

67. Westermark P, Engström U, Johnson KH, *et al*: Islet amyloid polypeptide: pinpointing amino acid residues linked to amyloid fibril formation. *Proc Natl Acad Sci USA* 1990;87:5036.

68. Westermark P, Wilander E, Westermark GT, *et al*: Islet amyloid polypeptide-like immunoreactivity in the islet B cells of type 2 (non-insulin-dependent) diabetic and nondiabetic individuals. *Diabetologia* 1987;30:887.

69. Röcken C, Linke RP, Saeger W: Immunohistology of islet amyloid polypeptide in diabetes mellitus: semi-quantitative studies in a post-mortem series. *Virchows Arch A* 1992;421:339.

70. Westermark GT, Christmanson L, Terenghi G, *et al*: Islet amyloid polypeptide: demonstration of mRNA in human pancreatic islets by *in situ* hybridization in islets with and without amyloid deposits. *Diabetologia* 1993;36:323.

71. Ma Z, Westermark GT, Li Z-C, *et al*: Altered immunoreactivity of islet amyloid polypeptide (IAPP) may reflect major modifications of the IAPP molecule in the amyloidogenesis. *Diabetologia* 1997;40:793.

72. Young ID, Ailles L, Narindrasorasak S, *et al*: Localization of the basement membrane heparan sulfate proteoglycan in islet amyloid deposits in type-II diabetes-mellitus. *Arch Path Lab Med* 1992;116:951.

73. Westermark GT, Johnson KH, Westermark P: Staining methods for identification of amyloid in tissue. *Meth Enzymol* 1999;309:3.

74. Chargé SBP, Esiri MM, Bethune CA, *et al*: Apolipoprotein E is associated with islet amyloid and other amyloidoses: implications for Alzheimer's disease. *J Path* 1996;179:443.

75. Wisniewski T, Frangione B: Apolipoprotein E: a pathological chaperone protein in patients with cerebral and systemic amyloid. *Neurosci Lett* 1992;135:235.

76. Dubin IN: Idiopathic hemochromatosis and transfusion siderosis. *Am J Clin Path* 1955;25:514.

77. Rahier J, Loozen S, Goebbels RM, *et al*: The haemochromatotic human pancreas: a quantitative immunohistochemical and ultrastructural study. *Diabetologia* 1987;30:5.

78. Permert J, Ihse I, Jorfeldt L, *et al*: Pancreatic cancer is associated with impaired glucose metabolism. *Eur J Surg* 1993;159:101.

79. Permert J, Larsson J, Westermark GT, *et al*: Islet amyloid polypeptide in patients with pancreatic cancer and diabetes. *N Engl J Med* 1994;330:313.

80. Otabe S, Yasuda K, Mori Y, *et al*: Molecular and histological evaluation of pancreata from patients with mitochondrial gene mutation associated with impaired insulin secretion. *Biochem Biophys Res Commun* 1999;259:149.

CHAPTER 18

Classification and Diagnosis of Diabetes Mellitus

Silvio E. Inzucchi

Diabetes mellitus is a common metabolic disease characterized by increased circulating glucose concentrations associated with abnormalities in carbohydrate, fat, and protein metabolism, and a variety of microvascular, macrovascular, neurologic, and infectious complications. In stark contrast to the consistency in these cardinal manifestations is a significant variability in its etiopathogenesis. An appreciation of the myriad causes of diabetes is aided by a thorough understanding of the homeostatic mechanisms serving to maintain extracellular glucose concentrations within a specified normal range. These are comprehensively reviewed in Chap. 1. Briefly, in the absence of disease, plasma glucose concentrations during fasting are kept within tight physiologic boundaries through the effects of insulin, the hormone governing intermediary metabolism. During fasting, low circulating insulin concentrations serve to modulate endogenous glucose production, primarily of hepatic origin. This effect is counterbalanced by a variety of other regulatory hormones, chiefly glucagon. In the postprandial setting, ingested carbohydrates are absorbed from the gastrointestinal tract. The resultant tendency for glucose concentrations to rise is blunted by an abrupt increase in pancreatic insulin secretion, shutting off hepatic glucose production and simultaneously augmenting glucose disposal into peripheral tissues, such as muscle and fat as well as the liver. Perturbations in this finely regulated system may result in hyperglycemia.

All diabetic states result from an inadequate supply of insulin or an inadequate tissue response to its actions. The former occurs in, for example, type 1 diabetes, which culminates from the autoimmune destruction of the insulin-producing β cells within the pancreatic islets. The latter occurs when the insulin receptor is defective, or, more commonly, when genetic and/or acquired defects in postreceptor intracellular signaling pathways attenuate the subsequent physiologic response. Such is the case with the more widely prevalent type 2 diabetes, a complex disorder resulting from peripheral insulin resistance, combined with relative insulin deficiency.

In this chapter, the currently accepted clinical classification of diabetes mellitus, the categorization of progressive stages of abnormal glucose homeostasis, and the available diagnostic tests that are commonly used to make these distinctions are reviewed and placed into historical perspective. Distinguishing normality from disease is an ongoing challenge in many areas of endocrinology, and the reader should keep in mind that classification schemas and numerical diagnostic thresholds will always be, in part, artificial constructs emanating from the desire to partition individuals and the conditions that afflict them. Nonetheless, they provide an important framework upon which patients and diseases can be diagnosed, treated, and studied.

ETIOLOGIC CLASSIFICATION OF DIABETES

Not a single disease, diabetes is a heterogenous group of disorders related to each other only because of their primary manifestations: hyperglycemia and resultant vascular complications. In the past, when the understanding of underlying pathophysiologic mechanisms was less mature, its classification was based on either the age groups affected[1] or on conventional treatment paradigms.[2,3] For instance, the currently designated type 1 diabetes mellitus was referred to as "juvenile-onset diabetes mellitus (JODM)" or "insulin-dependent diabetes mellitus (IDDM)," while type 2 diabetes mellitus was labeled "adult-onset diabetes mellitus (AODM)" or "non-insulin-dependent diabetes mellitus (NIDDM)." As knowledge regarding the underlying cellular and even molecular underpinnings of diabetes has matured, a more pathophysiologically based nomenclature has developed. See Table 18–1 for the etiologic classification schema currently accepted by both the American Diabetes Association (ADA)[4] and the World Health Organization (WHO).[5]

Type 1 Diabetes Mellitus

Type 1 diabetes mellitus (T1DM) is responsible for approximately 5–10% of all cases of diabetes in the Western world. It is characterized by severe insulin deficiency resulting from β-cell destruction. Ultimately, circulating insulin concentrations are negligible or completely absent. When the disease is fully expressed (and in the absence of insulin therapy), patients with T1DM exhibit not only hyperglycemia but are also ketosis-prone. Thus, these individuals are "dependent" on insulin for survival. β-Cell destruction in T1DM is autoimmune in nature. Islet inflammation ("insulitis") may be seen in pathologic pancreatic specimens from individuals prior to the development of diabetes. Once hyperglycemia and insulin dependence are well established, however, selective loss of β cells may be the only histologic abnormality (Chap. 20).

As with most autoimmune diseases, T1DM is associated with genes within the major histocompatibility complex (MHC). The prevalence of certain histocompatibility locus antigens (HLAs) is either increased (DR3, DQ2 or DR4, DQ8) or decreased (DR2, DQ6).[6] One or several immune response or other genes are likely to enhance the effect of these HLA antigens, rendering the patient at increased susceptibility to β-cell injury, through the interaction of one or several environmental factors. The presence of islet cell injury in patients with T1DM is reflected in certain circulating antibodies, such as islet cell antibodies (ICAs), insulin autoantibodies (IAAs), and antibodies to glutamic acid decarboxylase (GAD) and

TABLE 18-1. Etiologic Classification of Diabetes Mellitus

Type 1 (formerly insulin-dependent diabetes, IDDM)
Beta-cell destruction, resulting in absolute insulin deficiency.
  Autoimmune
  Idiopathic
Type 2 (formerly non-insulin-dependent diabetes, NIDDM)
Variable disorder ranging from predominately insulin resistance with rela-
    tive insulin deficiency to a predominately insulin secretory defect
    with or without insulin resistance.
Other specific types (secondary diabetes)
  Genetic defects of β-cell function (i.e., MODY)
  Genetic defects of insulin action
  Diseases of the exocrine pancreas
  Other endocrinopathies
  Drug- or chemical-induced
  Infections
  Uncommon forms of immune-mediated diabetes
  Other congenital syndromes associated with diabetes
Gestational diabetes
  Diabetes diagnosed during pregnancy, with usual resolution postpartum.

Source: Adapted with permission from Alberti *et al.*[5]

ICA512 (or IA2).[7] Type 1A diabetes refers to the form that is associated with such immune markers, although it should be noted
that as permanent islet cell destruction is established, antibody
titers may dissipate or disappear entirely. A less common second
subtype, Type 1B, is idiopathic in origin, and may not have an
immune-mediated etiology.[4]

Although the islet autoimmunity can precede clinical manifestations of disease by years or even decades, the presentation
of T1DM is often abrupt and severe because of the eventuation of
a loss of a critical mass of insulin-producing cells. The clinical
onset of T1DM is marked by hyperglycemia developing over
several days to weeks, usually associated with weight loss, fatigue,
polyuria, polydipsia, blurring of vision, and evidence of volume
contraction. The presence of ketoacidosis indicates the severe deficiency of insulin, which leads to both the hyperglycemia as well
as unrestrained lipolysis. In this setting, increased circulating
concentrations of free fatty acids provide substrate to the liver
for the accelerated production of ketones (as well as energy for
gluconeogenesis). Ketone clearance by the kidneys is reduced
due to volume contraction. The result is hyperketonemia, and an
anion-gap metabolic acidosis. If uncorrected, the dehydration
and acid–base disturbance will lead to further electrolyte abnormalities, cardiac dysrhythmias, hemodynamic collapse, and, ultimately,
death.[8]

T1DM is usually diagnosed prior to the age of 30–40 years,
most commonly in childhood or in adolescence. However, T1DM
occurs throughout life and is often misdiagnosed as T2DM when it
appears after the age of 40 years. Individuals with T1DM are typically lean, although the presence of obesity certainly does not preclude the diagnosis. Despite the genetic predisposition for T1DM,
most affected patients, in contrast to type 2 diabetes, have no family
history of diabetes.

T1DM, particularly when poorly controlled, predisposes patients to microvascular diseases, such as retinopathy and nephropathy; atherosclerosis, resulting in cardiovascular, cerebrovascular,
and peripheral vascular disease; neuropathy; complications during
pregnancy; and infection.

Type 2 Diabetes Mellitus

In many ways, type 2 diabetes mellitus (T2DM) is an entirely separate disorder from T1DM. It is a much more common condition,
responsible for more than 90 percent of cases of diabetes worldwide.
The autoimmune markers of type 1 diabetes are typically absent.
While relative beta-cell insufficiency is, by definition, present in all
individuals with T2DM, the disorder in most is characterized by
insulin resistance detected at the level of skeletal muscle, adipose
tissue, and the liver.[9] Insulin resistance at the former site results
in decreased peripheral glucose disposal, while at the latter, in
increased hepatic glucose production. Unlike T1DM, a family history is common, although the inheritance pattern of this disease is
complex and suspected to be polygenic (Chapters 21 to 24).

In many individuals, the natural history of T2DM begins with a
period of insulin resistance with preserved, indeed augmented,
pancreatic insulin secretion, as the insensitivity to insulin action
in peripheral tissues is overcome by hyperinsulinemia.[10] As a result, plasma glucose concentrations remain relatively normal. As
the disease progresses, however, pancreatic islet cell function fal-
ters and is no longer able to meet peripheral demands. As a result,
insulin levels fail to keep up with requirements, and hyperglycemia
ensues. This may be first manifested in the post-prandial setting,
while fasting glucose is preserved early in the disease course. Even
in those with late-stage T2DM, insulin secretion persists to an extent required to suppress lipolysis in most patients, so that ketoacidosis rarely occurs. Ketosis can develop, however, when an intervening medical illness poses a severe metabolic stress, further
heightening insulin resistance and impairing the insulin secretory
response. Because of renal glucose clearance, plasma glucose concentrations in T2DM typically plateau in the 250 to 350 mg/dL
range. However, in the presence of any superimposed deterioration
in renal function or marked dehydration, further elevations may
occur. Hyperosmolar, hyperglycemic nonketotic (HHNK) coma
can result and can be life-threatening.[8]

Compared to patients with T1DM, those with T2DM are typically older, usually over 40 years, and are commonly overweight,
if not frankly obese. Over the past decade, however, a frightening
increase in the prevalence of T2DM has been noted in younger age
groups, even in children.[11] This is felt to result from increasing
rates of obesity and inactivity in populations from certain ethnic
groups predisposed to T2DM, including Native, African, and Hispanic Americans, and Pacific Islanders.

In patients with or at risk for T2DM, a group of other clinical
and biochemical characteristics is frequently encountered. These
include central obesity, hypertension, dyslipidemia (elevated triglycerides, decreased HDL-cholesterol, and increased small dense
LDL-cholesterol), a procoagulant state, endothelial dysfunction,
and an increased risk for premature cardiovascular morbidity. This
constellation of findings is often referred to as the metabolic syndrome (formerly, syndrome X). Insulin resistance is felt by many to
be the root cause of this complex, and, thus, many refer to it as the
"insulin resistance syndrome."[12] The striking predisposition of
patients with T2DM to cardiovascular disease, even prior to their
development of significant hyperglycemia, may result from the
combined effects on the vasculature of these manifestations.

While patients with T2DM can use insulin for blood glucose
control, they rarely require it to avoid the life-threatening complications of ketoacidosis. Importantly, however, when insulin is required for optimal blood glucose control, the designation of disease

type is not changed. It should also be noted that some adult individuals with diabetes mellitus, usually between the ages of 20 and 40 years, share features of both type 1 and type 2 disease and, as a result, escape easy categorization, These individuals are often leaner and more insulin deficient than those with classical T2DM. Frequently, immune markers of T1DM are present, and their hyperglycemia appears to represent a slowly progressive form of autoimmune diabetes. Furthermore, it has recently been discovered that as many as 10 percent of elderly patients classified as T2DM may also have measurable titers of autoantibodies associated with T1DM. Similarly, these patients may also have a slowly evolving form of T1DM, which is now referred to as "latent autoimmune diabetes of adulthood (LADA)"[13] T2DM predisposes patients to the same microvascular, macrovascular, developmental, and infectious complications associated with T1DM.

Other Forms of Diabetes Mellitus (Secondary Diabetes)

Several forms of diabetes result from or are related to another specific disease process or genetic disorder. According to current classifications, these conditions are considered neither T1DM nor T2DM and are grouped together under "other specific types," sometimes referred to as "secondary diabetes."[4,5] This category represents a variety of conditions that are included because of (1) a recognized comprehension of the underlying pathogenesis; (2) the molecular defects governing the hyperglycemia are well defined; or (3) a clear association between the diabetes and an otherwise precisely defined clinical syndrome. These somewhat disparate criteria for inclusion in this category highlight the lack of understanding of the etiologic mechanisms involved in the far more prevalent T1DM and T2DM. It is quite likely, however, that over the next decade, many forms of diabetes currently classified under these broad umbrellas will have their etiologies better defined and be recategorized into this other designation. More likely, as knowledge in the areas of molecular medicine and genetics continues to explode, the classification of diabetes may at some point be completely transformed. At this time, however, this category of diabetes includes genetic disorders of β-cell function and insulin action; inflammatory, infiltrative, and neoplastic diseases of the pancreas; diabetes resulting from other endocrinopathies or infectious diseases, or the use of certain medications or exposure to certain chemical agents; rare forms of immune-mediated diabetes; and a variety of other congenital syndromes frequently associated with hyperglycemia.

Genetic Defects in β-Cell Function

Maturity onset diabetes of the young (MODY) is a clinically heterogeneous group of hyperglycemic disorders with an autosomal dominant mode of inheritance that may account for 1–5% of diabetes cases in the United States. Patients with MODY are usually not obese and may be mildly hyperglycemic. They are generally not predisposed to ketoacidosis. The onset of disease is typically before age 25 years, usually in childhood or adolescence, although the mild nature of the disorder may mask clinical detection for many years. There is a strong family history of diabetes in multiple generations (Chap. 21). Primary defects in β-cell function, which are becoming well defined, appear to be responsible for all cases of MODY. To date, six separate genetic mutations have been characterized and numbered, MODY 1 through MODY 6. The mu-

tated gene in MODY 2 encodes for glucokinase, a glycolytic enzyme. The remaining genes encode for a variety of transcription factors: hepatocyte nuclear factor-4α (HNF-4α) in MODY 1, HNF-1α in MODY 3, insulin promoter factor-1 (IPF-1) in MODY 4, HNF-1β in MODY 5, and neurogenic differentiation factor 1 (NeuroD1) (or beta-cell E-box transactivator 2 (BETA2) in MODY 6.[14] MODY 3 has the highest prevalence rate, and MODY 2 is the next most common form of the disorder. Each of these genes is expressed in islets and their mutations result in abnormal glucorecognition by the β cell, or in insulin secretory dysfunction, or both. Although uncommon, understanding MODY, particularly the mechanisms that attenuate insulin secretion, has led to a better understanding of pancreatic endocrine dysfunction in T2DM.

Genetic Defects in Insulin Action

Abnormalities of the insulin molecule or its receptor can lead to diabetes, but these are extraordinarily rare conditions that are manifested in infancy. Leprechaunism, which results from an inactivating mutation in the insulin receptor, for example, is characterized by severe insulin resistance, dysmorphic features, intrauterine growth retardation, and acanthosis nigricans. Other forms of diabetes in this category include type A insulin resistance with acanthosis nigricans, Rabson-Mendenhall syndrome (dental dysplasia, dystrophic nails, precocious puberty), and lipodystrophic diabetes. More recently, genetic mutations in the nuclear transcription factor known as PPAR-γ (peroxisome proliferator–activated receptor-γ) has been associated with severe insulin resistance and diabetes (Chap. 21).[15]

Exocrine Pancreatic Diseases

Diseases of the nonislet pancreas are also frequently associated with abnormalities of glucose tolerance. Hyperglycemia can be a sequela of both acute and chronic pancreatitis, as well as other diseases that involve the pancreatic parenchyma, such as hemochromatosis and cystic fibrosis. In the tropics, malnutrition-related fibrocalculous pancreatitis has been linked to diabetes.[16] Hyperglycemia is also commonly encountered in patients with carcinoma of the pancreas.

Other Endocrinopathies

Other hormonal disorders are frequently associated with glucose intolerance and sometimes, frank diabetes (Chap. 25). Most of these involve the secretion of counterregulatory factors, leading to a state of decreased insulin sensitivity. Glucose intolerance is seen in 50% of patients with acromegaly, which is usually caused by a growth hormone–secreting pituitary adenoma.[17] In this condition, elevated circulating levels of growth hormone (GH) antagonize insulin action. Circulating concentrations of insulin-like growth factor 1 (IGF-1) are also increased. Although IGF-1 has hypoglycemic properties, its interactions with the insulin and IGF-1 receptors appear to be overwhelmed by the counterregulatory effects of GH. Cushing's syndrome often presents with hyperglycemia, although this condition is notoriously difficult to diagnose until hypercortisolemia leads to other clinical features, such as moon facies, central obesity, hirsutism, hypertension, abdominal striae, emotional lability, and myopathy. Glucocorticoids also antagonize insulin action and augment hepatic gluconeogenesis. Glucose intolerance has been demonstrated in over 80% of patients with Cushing's syndrome.[18] Catecholamines increase hepatic glucose production, decrease and inhibit insulin release. Thus, diabetes can also occur in patients with pheochromocytoma and/or paraganglioma, with up to two-thirds having some degree of glucose intolerance.[19] Diabetes may also occasionally be encountered in patients with hyperthyroidism, presumably due to augmentation of β-adrenergic activity, and primary hyperaldosteronism, possibly related to decreased insulin release from hypokalemia. Finally, several neuroendocrine tumors of the pancreas are also associated with diabetes, including those elaborating primarily glucagon, vasoactive intestinal peptide, and somatostatin. Glucagonoma is rare, but carries the strongest association with diabetes. This tumor is associated with normocytic anemia and a pathognomonic rash involving the groin, genital, and perineal regions, known as necrolytic migratory erythema.[20]

Drug- and Chemical-Induced Diabetes

A number of medications have been implicated in the development of diabetes. In most situations, the use of the drug may simply unmask an underlying tendency toward glucose intolerance.[21] Such drugs include those that contribute to insulin resistance, most notably glucocorticoids, but also growth hormone, levothyroxine (in excess), and niacin.[4,5] Atypical antipsychotics, especially clozapine and olanzapine, are associated with diabetes, at times manifested by severe hyperglycemia or even ketoacidosis.[22] These drugs frequently lead to weight gain but also may directly alter insulin sensitivity. Other diabetogenic medications or chemical agents decrease insulin secretion (β-adrenergic antagonists; calcium channel antagonists; diuretics, especially thiazides; diazoxide; dilantin; and octreotide) or lead to β-cell destruction (pentamidine and the rodenticide, vacor).[4,5] Certain chemotherapeutic agents or immunomodulators, such as mithramycin, L-asparaginase, and α-interferon, have also been associated with new cases of diabetes, although the precise mechanisms involved are not completely understood.

Infections

Certain viral agents have been implicated as the "environmental" factor that triggers the immune response in T1DM, including rubella, CMV, Coxsackie, mumps, and adenovirus. No specific virus appears to be responsible, however, for most cases.

Uncommon Forms of Immune-Mediated Diabetes

Rarely, patients may present with hyperglycemia and/or hypoglycemia due to anti-insulin or anti-insulin receptor antibodies. Stiffman syndrome is an autoimmune neurologic affliction associated with increased circulating titers of anti-GAD antibodies and diabetes.

Other Genetic Syndromes

Diabetes or impaired glucose tolerance is also found with increased frequency in a number of congenital disorders such as Down's syndrome, Turner's syndrome, myotonic dystrophy, Klinefelter's syndrome, Prader-Willi syndrome, Huntington's chorea, Wolfram's syndrome, Werner's syndrome, Alstrom's syndrome, Friedrich's ataxia, porphyria, and the Laurence-Moon-Biedl syndrome.[4,5] In most cases, the diabetes is non-insulin requiring.

Gestational Diabetes Mellitus

Diabetes diagnosed during pregnancy is referred to as gestational diabetes mellitus (GDM), a category that necessarily includes both diabetes first appearing or first being recognized during pregnancy. The diagnosis of GDM is usually made on the basis of a routine oral glucose tolerance test (OGTT) during the late second trimester. It occurs in approximately 2–5% of all pregnancies, with a greater frequency in those populations with a higher incidence for T2DM, such as Native, African-and Hispanic Americans. Treatment usually consists of diet and exercise, although a minority will require insulin. GDM is accompanied by significant risks to both mother and fetus, such as pregnancy-induced hypertension and fetal macrosomia (with resultant increased frequency of obstetric complications and rates of cesarean delivery). Neonatal complications related to fetal hyperinsulinism (hypoglycemia, hypocalcemia, hypomagnesemia, polycythemia, and hyperbilirubinemia) are associated with increased perinatal mortality.[23] The woman with GDM is at high risk for recurrence of hyperglycemia during future pregnancies and for T2DM later in life.[24] Offspring of diabetic pregnancies are themselves at future risk for both T2DM and obesity as adults.[25] GDM and T2DM can be considered two variations of the same general disease process, with insulin resistance and obesity (r 25), decrease playing prominent roles in their pathogeneses.

DIAGNOSTIC CRITERIA AND THE SPECTRUM OF ABNORMALITIES IN GLUCOSE HOMEOSTASIS

Diabetes is characterized by progressive elevations in circulating glucose concentrations. In T2DM, these elevations occur over years to decades. As they pass from the normal into the diabetic range, glucose levels transition through an intermediate and less well-categorized phase referred to as impaired glucose tolerance (IGT). While the hyperglycemia of diabetes is clearly associated with an increased risk of microvascular and macrovascular complications, as well as increased mortality, there has been less agreement on the implications of these earlier and more mild glucose elevations. Over the past decade, however, the risk associated with IGT has become clear, with affected individuals at increased risk not only for progression to diabetes, but also for increased cardiovascular morbidity.[26] IGT, widely recognized to occur in patients destined to develop T2DM, may be seen in individuals prior to the development of T1DM. In the Diabetes Prevention Trial, for example, a group of asymptomatic subjects at risk for T1DM (on the basis of family history and positive islet cell antibody titers and/or abnormal first-phase insulin secretion during an intravenous glucose tolerance test) demonstrated mild elevations of glucose either while fasting or after an oral glucose challenge.[27]

Historical Overview

The modern era of diabetes classification began less than 40 years ago, with the first attempt to not only categorize the various clinical presentations of the disease but also to devise acceptable criteria for its diagnosis. Several revisions of this initial schema have since been undertaken by various international bodies, as knowledge has grown in both epidemiologic and pathophysiologic spheres.

First Report of the WHO Expert Committee on Diabetes Mellitus, 1965

The first attempt to "review the current knowledge on diabetes mellitus and to recommend definitions of the various terms used in application to this disorder in the interests of international uniformity" was performed in 1965 by the WHO.[1] In the manuscript that resulted, patients were divided into several categories:

- *Potential diabetic*: An individual with a normal response to a glucose tolerance test (GTT), but who remains at high risk for the future development of diabetes (because of a strong family history or because of having delivered a macrosomic child).
- *Latent diabetic*: An individual with normal response to a GTT, but in whom a GTT in the past had been abnormal, *or* an abnormal response to a provocative test, such as a cortisone-stimulated GTT.
- *Asymptomatic (subclinical, chemical) diabetic*: An individual with a diabetic response to a GTT but whose fasting venous whole blood glucose is under 125 mg/dL.
- *Clinical diabetic*: An individual with an abnormal GTT response and with symptoms or complications of the disease.

The Committee endorsed the use of some form of oral glucose challenge for the diagnosis of diabetes, although it was not prepared to specify whether the amount of carbohydrate load should be 50 or 100 g. It regarded a normal response 2 hours after a load to be a whole blood venous glucose <110 mg/dL; diabetes was diagnosed if this value reached or exceeded 130 mg/dL. A so-called "borderline state" included those subjects between 110 and 129 mg/dL. While the Committee recognized that the presence of glycosuria with a fasting whole blood glucose of >130 mg/dL likely represented diabetes, their absence in no way ruled out the diagnosis. Each of these parameters was somewhat arbitrary.

Once the diagnosis of diabetes was made, the Committee provided the following recommendations for classifying the various types of this disorder, based solely on age of the patient at the time of disease onset:

- *Infantile or childhood diabetic*: Onset between 0 and 14 years, usually presenting with severe initial symptoms, becoming rapidly insulin-dependent.
- *Young diabetic*: Onset between 15 and 24 years, usually with acute onset of symptoms, with most becoming insulin-dependent.
- *Adult diabetic*: Onset between 25 and 64 years, beginning with variable symptomotology and variable requirements for insulin.
- *Elderly diabetic*: Onset after age 65 years, frequently presenting with symptoms of diabetic complications and often controllable without insulin.

In addition to these types, the Committee also recognized other terminologies, such as *juvenile-type diabetes, brittle diabetes, insulin-resistant diabetes, gestational diabetes, pancreatic diabetes, endocrine diabetes*, and *iatrogenic (drug-induced) diabetes*. It was recommended, however, that such nomenclature, while useful particularly for purposes of research or population reports, not replace the classification based on age of onset. The Committee also recognized that the diagnostic label of "diabetes" was inadequate and that future consideration should be given to a "fuller and more meaningful descriptive classification."

International Workshop of the National Diabetes Data Group, 1979

The decade following the first WHO Expert Committee Report witnessed a significant growth in the understanding of the etiology and pathogenesis of diabetes. This prompted several groups to call for revised international nomenclature, diagnostic criteria, and classification. As a response, the National Institutes of Health convened the National Diabetes Data Group (NDDG).[2] In 1979, the NDDG published a consensus statement, "Classification and Diagnosis of Diabetes Mellitus and Other Categories of Glucose Intolerance." Their proposals were endorsed by multiple bodies, including the ADA and the WHO.

In addition to standardizing the OGTT to a 75-g glucose load for nonpregnant adults, the salient new proposals by the NDDG included the following:

1. The classification of diabetic patients on the basis of age of onset should be eliminated. Instead, diabetes should be divided into several distinct subclasses:
   - *Insulin-dependent diabetes mellitus (IDDM), or Type 1*, describing patients whose clinical presentation was characterized by abrupt onset of symptoms, insulinopenia, dependence on injected insulin to sustain life, and proneness to ketosis.
   - *Non-insulin-dependent diabetes mellitus (NIDDM), or Type 2*, describing those patients frequently presenting with few or no symptoms, in whom insulin levels were variable, and who were not ketosis-prone, and therefore did not depend on insulin to sustain life. Some patients with NIDDM would require insulin, however, for the correction of symptomatic fasting hyperglycemia in the setting of failure of the more conventional therapy, oral agents. Patients in this subclass were further divided into obese NIDDM and nonobese NIDDM.
   - *Diabetes associated with other conditions and syndromes*
   - *Gestational diabetes mellitus*
2. Terminologies previously used, such as "chemical," "latent," "borderline," "subclinical," and "asymptomatic" diabetes should be abandoned. Instead, individuals with plasma glucose (PG) levels intermediate between those considered normal and those considered diabetic should be categorized as "impaired glucose tolerance (IGT)" (see diagnostic criteria below).
3. Individuals with normal glucose tolerance but who had previously experienced transient hyperglycemia, either spontaneously or because of a recognized stimulus, should be categorized as "*previous abnormality of glucose tolerance*."
4. Individuals at significantly higher risk to develop diabetes than the general population, usually due to a strong family or obstetric history, should be categorized as "*potential abnormality of glucose tolerance*."
5. The diagnosis of diabetes (in nonpregnant adults) should be restricted to:
   - Those with classical symptoms of diabetes (polyuria, polydipsia, ketonuria, weight loss) and "gross or unequivocal" hyperglycemia.
   - Those with fasting venous PG (FPG) ≥ 140 mg/dL on more than one occasion.
   - Those who, if FPG < 140 mg/dL, exhibit sustained elevation of PG during a 2-hour OGTT (described as a PG ≥ 200 mg/dL both at 2-hours and at one or more points between 0 and 2 hours).

The NDDG defined normal fasting venous plasma glucose (FPG) as < 115 mg/dL. No category was yet created for those with intermediate FPGs (i.e., 115–139 mg/dL), although the Group did remark that fasting values in this range probably indicated a degree of abnormal glucose tolerance, the implications of which had not yet been fully assessed.

The cutpoints of 140 mg/dL for FPG and 200 mg/dL for 2-hour PG were demarcated for several reasons: (1) These thresholds were found to be the approximate midpoint separating the two components of the bimodal distribution of FPG and 2-hour PG, respectively, in certain population studies, such as Pima Indians; (2) the prevalence of diabetic microvascular complications, as evidenced by epidemiologic data available at the time, appeared to increase sharply beyond an FPG of 140 mg/dL and 2-hour PG of 200 mg/dL; and (3) a large amount of epidemiologic data had already accumulated based upon these thresholds. The new category of IGT was endorsed in order to identify individuals with plasma glucose responses to oral glucose challenge somewhere between normal and diabetic. It was felt that categorizing these persons as "diabetics" was not justified since they appeared to not carry a risk for developing microvascular complications associated with diabetes, they did not reliably progress to frank diabetes, and they often reverted to normal glucose tolerance upon retesting. Thus, the NDDG criteria were more comprehensive and descriptive, although perhaps less stringent than those of the WHO Expert Committee in 1965.

Second Report of the WHO Expert Committee on Diabetes Mellitus, 1980

The WHO adopted the classification and diagnostic criteria of the NDDG in 1980,[3] changing solely the requirements of the OGTT to include only a baseline and 2-hour PG specimen. As a result, IGT could be diagnosed if the 2-hour PG fell between 140 and 199 mg/dL, with the second value $\geq$ 200 mg/dL at 30, 60, or 90 minutes no longer being required. There was continued emphasis by the WHO on the response to oral glucose as a key element in the diagnosis of diabetes.

The WHO Study Group on Diabetes Mellitus, 1985

In 1985, the only changes made to the previous WHO classification and criteria were very minor.[28] The first was the inclusion of "malnutrition-related diabetes mellitus," which was thought to be an important cause of diabetes in tropical developing countries, and included fibrocalculous pancreatic diabetes, as well as protein-deficient pancreatic diabetes. The second was the rounding of SI units for PG values to the nearest tenth of a millimole, instead of to the nearest millimole. Diagnostic criteria were otherwise maintained, with continued emphasis of the plasma glucose response to OGTT.

Report of the Expert Committee on the Diagnosis and Classification of Diabetes Mellitus, 1997

Until 1997, the ADA had endorsed the criteria of the NDDG. In 1995, an international expert committee was invited by the ADA to review the scientific literature since 1979 and to decide if changes to the classification of and diagnostic criteria for diabetes were required.[4] The Committee published its findings in 1997, and these continue to be endorsed by the ADA. The most notable changes recommended by the Committee include the following:

1. The terms "insulin-dependent" and "non-insulin-dependent," as applied to diabetes, should be abandoned, as they were felt to be both confusing and imprecise. Instead, the main subclasses of diabetes would be, simply, "type 1" and "type 2."

TABLE 18-2. Diabetes Mellitus: 1997 ADA Diagnostic Criteria*

1. Symptoms of diabetes plus casual plasma glucose concentration $\geq$ 200 mg/dL (11.1 mmol/L). Casual is defined as any time of day without regard to time since last meal. The classic symptoms of diabetes include polyuria, polydipsia, and unexplained weight loss.

or

2. FPG $\geq$ 126 mg/dL (7.0 mmol/L). Fasting is defined as no caloric intake for at least 8 hours.

or

3. A 2-hour PG $\geq$ 200 mg/dL (11.1 mmol/L) during an OGTT. The test should be performed as described by WHO,[28] using a glucose load containing the equivalent of 75g of anhydrous glucose dissolved in water.

*In the absence of unequivocal hyperglycemia with acute metabolic decompensation, these criteria should be confirmed by repeat testing on a different day. The third measure (OGTT) is not recommended for routine clinical use.

Source: Reprinted with permission from American Diabetes Association.[32]

2. The FPG threshold for the diagnosis of diabetes should be lowered from 140 to 126 mg/dL (Table 18–2).
3. Normal FPG should be < 110 mg/dL; those individuals with FPGs between 110 and 125 mg/dL should be newly categorized as "impaired fasting glucose (IFG)," intended to be the fasting equivalent of IGT.
4. Although the older criteria, using both random (now called "casual") and post-OGTT glucose concentrations, were not changed, FPG was recommended as the preferred screening and diagnostic test due to its wide availability, simplicity, and convenience over OGTT. (See Table 18–3 for the ADA recommended screening guidelines.)

This decision to reduce the diagnostic threshold for FPG was based on epidemiologic data that emerged since the NDDG criteria were developed. It was recognized that only one in four individuals without a prior diagnosis of diabetes but with a 2-hour PG $\geq$ 200 mg/dL during OGTT also had an FPG $\geq$ 140 mg/dL.[29] Thus, the two cutpoints endorsed by the NDDG and WHO did not actually identify equivalent groups of patients. The Committee also had a practical concern. Many individuals who would have a 2-hour PG $\geq$ 200 mg/dL during an OGTT would not necessarily

TABLE 18-3. Criteria for Testing for Diabetes in Asymptomatic, Undiagnosed Individuals

Testing for diabetes should be considered in all individuals at age 45 years and above and, if normal, it should be repeated at 3-year intervals.

Testing should be considered at a younger age or be carried out more frequently in individuals who:

    Are obese ($\geq$ 120% desirable body weight or a BMI $\geq$ 27 kg/m^2).

    Have a first-degree relative with diabetes.

    Are members of a high-risk ethnic population (e.g., African-American, Hispanic American, Native American, Asian American, Pacific Islander).

    Have delivered a baby weighing > 9 lb or have been diagnosed with GDM and are hypertensive ($\geq$ 140/90).

    Have an HDL cholesterol level $\leq$ 35 mg/dL (0.90 mmol/L) and/or a triglyceride level $\geq$ 250 mg/dL (2.82 mmol/L).

    On previous testing, had IGT or IFG.

Source: Reprinted with permission from American Diabetes Association.[32]

undergo such testing, either because they were asymptomatic or because the diagnosis of diabetes had already been confirmed on the basis of an FPG ≥ 140 mg/dL. Since the OGTT identifies more individuals with diabetes than does the FPG, routine use of the OGTT would be necessary for optimal case finding. Yet, in routine practice, the more expensive and inconvenient OGTT was rarely performed. Several studies had also shown that the actual FPG level equivalent to the 2-hour PG cutpoint of 200 mg/dL ranged between 120 and 126 mg/dL. In addition, and perhaps more importantly, the Committee reviewed three studies relating plasma glucose levels to the prevalence of retinopathy, one in Pima Indians,[30] a second in Egyptians,[31] and a third involving participants in the Third National Health and Nutrition Examination Survey (NHANES III).[32] In each of these, the FPG threshold distinguishing those subjects at increased risk for microvascular disease was observed at approximately 120–130 mg/dL (with the 2-hour PG threshold remaining at approximately 200 mg/dL) (Fig. 18–1). Thus, the Committee felt that it was mandatory that the fasting diagnostic criteria for diabetes be revised so that the discrepancy in diagnostic power between the FPG and 2-hour PG would be diminished and in order to facilitate and encourage the use of a simpler test, namely FPG. The cutpoint of 126 mg/dL was chosen.

On the basis of epidemiologic estimates, the Committee expected only slightly fewer individuals would be identified as having diabetes using the new FPG criteria, as compared to the WHO cutpoints using both FPG and 2-hour PG. In the Cardiovascular Health Study, however, Wahl and coworkers reported a significant difference in the prevalence of diabetes as identified by these two sets of criteria. The prevalence of untreated diabetes was found to be 14.8% using the WHO criteria and only 7.7% using the new ADA fasting criteria.[33] Similar conclusions were made by Gabir and colleagues in Pima Indians[34] and Resnick and colleagues, using NHANES III data.[35]

Overall, however, in clinical practice, because of low utilization of OGTTs, the change in the ADA criteria has effectively led to an increase in the number of patients identified as having diabetes. It has been estimated, for example, that the change has resulted in the diagnosis of patients an average of 7 years earlier as compared to the older fasting criteria.[36]

WHO Consultation on the Diagnosis and Classification of Diabetes Mellitus, 1999

In keeping with the new criteria of the ADA, the WHO in 1999[37] similarly reduced their cutpoint for venous FPG to 126 mg/dL and affirmed the new category of IFG (impaired fasting glycemia) for those with FPGs between 110 and 125 mg/dL (Table 18–4). If an OGTT had been performed, however, and if the 2-hour PG reached or exceeded 140 mg/dL, the IGT diagnosis would predominate. The diagnostic glucose ranges for IGT were not changed from the WHO 1985 report, and remained identical to those accepted by the ADA. In contrast to the ADA criteria, however, the WHO continued to recommend use of the OGTT for purposes of clinical research. For clinical practice, unless the FPG was already in the diabetic range, the WHO also recommended an OGTT if a random glucose level was in the "uncertain" range [i.e., between the levels that "establish" (200 mg/dL) or "exclude" (100 mg/dL) diabetes (Fig. 18–2.)] It was also emphasized that IGT and IFG were not diagnostic classes by themselves, but instead stages in the natural history of abnormal carbohydrate metabolism (Fig. 18–3).

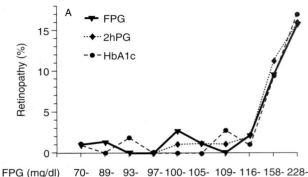

FPG (mg/dl)   70- 89- 93- 97-100-105-109-116-158-228-
2hPG (mg/dl) 88- 94-106-116-126-138-158-185-244-364-
HbA1c (%)   3.4- 4.8- 5.0- 5.2- 5.3- 5.5- 5.7- 6.0- 6.7- 9.5-

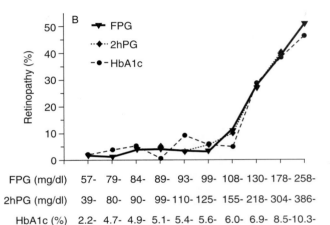

FPG (mg/dl)   57- 79- 84- 89- 93- 99-108-130-178-258-
2hPG (mg/dl) 39- 80- 90- 99-110-125-155-218-304-386-
HbA1c (%)   2.2- 4.7- 4.9- 5.1- 5.4- 5.6- 6.0- 6.9- 8.5-10.3-

FPG (mg/dl)   42- 87- 90- 93- 96- 98-101-104-109-120-
2hPG (mg/dl) 34- 75- 86- 94-102-112-120-133-154-195-
HbA1c (%)   3.3- 4.9- 5.1- 5.2- 5.4- 5.5- 5.6- 5.7- 5.9- 6.2-

FIGURE 18-1.

TABLE 18-4. Diabetes Mellitus: 1999 WHO Diagnostic Criteria

	Venous Plasma Glucose (mg/dL (mmol/L))
Diabetes mellitus	
Fasting	≥126 (≥7.0)
or	
2-hour postglucose load	≥200 (11.1)
or both	
Impaired glucose tolerance (IGT)	
Fasting (if measured)	<126 (<7.0)
and	
2-hour postglucose load	140–199 (7.8–11.0)
Impaired fasting glycemia (IFG)	
Fasting (if measured)	110–125 (6.1–6.9)
and	
2-hour postglucose load (if measured)	<140 (<7.8)

Source: Adapted with permission from Alberti *et al.*[5]

FIGURE 18-2. Random plasmaglucose values in the diagnosis of Diabetes.

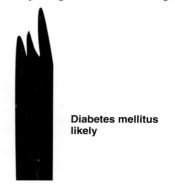
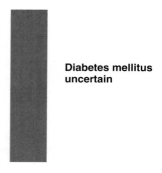
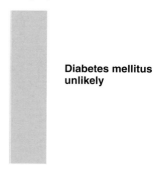

200 (11.1) — Diabetes mellitus likely

100 (5.5) — Diabetes mellitus uncertain

Diabetes mellitus unlikely

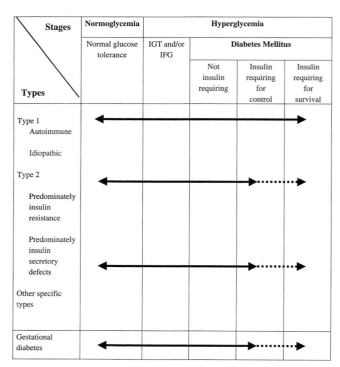

FIGURE 18-3. Disorders of glycemia: etiological types and clinical stages.

Comparison of Current ADA and WHO Criteria

Since the release of the 1997 ADA diagnostic criteria, several studies have compared their performance with those of the WHO. Gabir and colleagues compared the ADA and WHO criteria and their relation to the development of microvascular complications, finding no difference in their predictive value.[38] Others have also affirmed that, although OGTT-driven diagnostic algorithm will find more individuals with diabetes, the current ADA fasting criteria are adequate to identify those persons at risk for microvascular disease resulting from their hyperglycemia.[39]

The DECODE Study Group evaluated the impact of using FPG versus OGTT criteria on the identification of individuals at risk for macrovascular disease. Existing baseline data on glucose concentrations in the fasting state and 2 hours after a 75-g glucose load from 10 prospective European cohort studies including more than 15,000 men and 7000 women were analyzed. Hazard ratios for all-cause mortality and cardiovascular disease end-points were estimated. The investigators concluded that use of 2-hour PG enhanced the predictive value of FPG alone, whereas the converse was not true. Therefore, while both FPG and 2-hour PG appear to perform equivalently in the identification of microvascular risk, FPG alone may fail to sufficiently identify those at increased macrovascular risk, and the 2-hour glucose during an OGTT may provide additional prognostic information.[40] Barzilay and coworkers performed a similar analysis on a separate data set. Not unexpectedly, there was a higher prevalence of cardiovascular disease among individuals with IGT or newly diagnosed diabetes by both ADA and WHO criteria than among those with normal glucose levels. However, since fewer subjects were classified as abnormal by the fasting ADA criteria than by the WHO criteria, the number of cases of cardiovascular disease attributable to abnormal glucose status by ADA criteria was one-third of that attributable by WHO criteria. Conversely, those classified as normal by the ADA fasting criteria had more cardiovascular events during the follow-up period than did those deemed normal by the WHO criteria. The investigator concluded that the current fasting ADA criteria were less predictive than those of the WHO for the burden of cardiovascular disease associated with abnormal glucose metabolism in the elderly.[41] Saydah and colleagues have shown similar trends using NHANES II data.[42]

Comparison of Two Stages of Abnormal Glucose Homeostasis: IGT and IFG

Although IFG was devised to be the fasting equivalent of IGT, studies performed since 1997 demonstrate that these two categories of early abnormal glucose homeostasis are not necessarily interchangeable diagnoses. Based on NHANES III data, for example, 14.9% of Americans between the ages of 40 and 74 have IGT, whereas 8.3% have IFG, and 3.9% carry both diagnoses.[43] That is, only a minority of patients with either IFG or IGT meet criteria for the other diagnosis. Moreover, while almost one-quarter of the U.S. population in this age group has either IFG or IGT, less than 1 in 25 has both conditions simultaneously.[43]

Patients with IFG and those with IGT also appear to have distinct metabolic abnormalities. Investigators studied a large group of Pima Indians using hyperinsulinemic euglycemic clamps, glucose isotope infusions, and intravenous glucose tolerance tests (IVGTTs) to assess insulin sensitivity, insulin secretion, and endogenous glucose production. Subjects with isolated IFG (i.e., IFG, but not IGT) and those with isolated IGT (i.e., IGT, but not IFG) demonstrated equally reduced insulin sensitivity. IFG subjects had worse insulin secretory responses to IVGTTs and increased endogenous glucose production, compared to IGT subjects. Individuals with *both* IFG and IGT had the most severe abnormalities in all metabolic parameters. Thus, Pima Indians with isolated IFG and isolated IGT show similar impairments in insulin action, but those with isolated IFG have a relatively more pronounced defect in early insulin secretion and greater augmentation of endogenous glucose production. The most severe abnormalities are exhibited by those with combined IFG and IGT.[44] The risk of progressing to T2DM appears to be equivalent between those with isolated IFG and isolated IGT, and those who carry both diagnoses progress at the highest rate.[45] From the DECODE study, individuals with IGT seem to have the greater risk for developing cardiovascular disease, which may indicate a greater influence on vascular disease from post-prandial hyperglycemia.[46]

COMMON TESTS USED TO EVALUATE GLUCOSE HOMEOSTASIS

Glucose Concentrations

For *fasting glucose* determinations, blood should be obtained in the morning after an overnight fast of at least 8 hours. It has been recently demonstrated that approximately half of patients with FPG $\geq$ 126 mg/dL in the morning will convert to a nondiabetic FPG if the fast is continued into the afternoon.[47] Although there is a tendency for a gradual climb in FPG with aging, criteria for normal FPG are not age-adjusted.

A "*random*" or "*casual*" *glucose* determination is that which is obtained without regard to meal. Generally, and depending on the amount of time since the most recent consumption of calories, random levels are higher than fasting levels. In the acutely ill or infirm,

or those immobilized or at bed rest, random (and even fasting) plasma glucose may be in an abnormal range, only to normalize when the patient has been returned to proper health. While the implications of such a abnormalities are not entirely clear, it is important to reserve a permanent decision about a patient's glucose tolerance until he or she is back to a baseline health and activity level.

Type and Source of Fluid

Venous plasma or *serum* is considered the standard body fluid for the determination of glucose concentration, being representative of the extracellular glucose content. Serum and plasma glucose values are essentially identical. The latter is measured by most laboratories and has been historically used in most clinical research studies. *Whole blood* determinations are typically 15% lower than plasma or serum[48] and may also be influenced by the hematocrit. Ideally, phlebotomized blood should be collected in test tubes containing sodium fluoride, which will inhibit red blood cell glycolysis. Alternatively, the blood can be chilled immediately, with the plasma or serum expeditiously separated from cellular contents. *Arterial blood* has a glucose content approximately 7% higher than that of venous blood.[5] In the fasting state, this difference is less than in the postprandial setting. *Capillary blood* glucose is similar to that of arterial blood.

The easy availability of capillary blood is taken advantage of by home glucose meters, which are hand-held monitoring devices that provide the patient the ability to test his or her own blood glucose at any time day. Home glucose monitoring has become an integral part of the management of patients with diabetes.[49] A large variety of meters are currently on the market, with many different features, including interfaces with computer software, allowing for intricate forms of data analysis. Many of the newer meters automatically adjust their results to be displayed as standardized to plasma glucose. While extremely useful for the monitoring of established patients, personal glucose monitors are neither accurate nor precise enough for diagnostic purposes.

Urine glucose is a poorly sensitive marker of diabetes, since the renal glucose threshold in most individuals is not reached until the extracellular glucose concentration exceeds 180 mg/dL. In addition, the urine glucose result is in part dependent on the dilutional effects of recent fluid intake. Prior to the availability of home capillary blood glucose meters, urine testing was an acceptable means for the rough assessment of glycemic control. Except for unusual circumstances where capillary glucose monitoring is impractical, urine glucose testing is no longer considered appropriate for either diagnostic or monitoring purposes.

Oral Glucose Tolerance Test

The homeostatic mechanisms serving to maintain normal glucose concentrations can be assessed using the physiologic "stress" of providing the patient a rapidly absorbed carbohydrate load: the oral glucose tolerance test (OGTT). As noted previously, more individuals will be diagnosed with various degrees of abnormal glucose homeostasis on the basis of their performance on OGTT than by the simpler measurement of fasting glucose alone. It is currently recommended by the WHO for use when blood glucose levels are otherwise equivocal, in epidemiologic settings to assess for diabetes and impaired glucose tolerance, and during pregnancy to screen for and diagnose gestational diabetes.[5] Given its relatively cumbersome and time-consuming nature, the ADA recommends that, outside of pregnancy, FPG be used as the routine screening and diagnostic test.[4] However, there is a recent move to expand utilization of the OGTT to detect earlier forms of abnormal carbohydrate metabolism because of recent attention to postchallenge blood glucose being a better prognosticator of cardiovascular morbidity than FPG.[42] In clinical practice, the OGTT is also used in the rare patient who presents with microvascular complications suggesting diabetes (i.e., retinopathy, nephropathy, or neuropathy) but in whom initial glucodiagnostic studies show no abnormalities.

In the standard test, 75 g of anhydrous glucose is dissolved in 250–300 mL of water and administered over 5 minutes.[48] (In children the glucose load should calculate to 1.75 g/kg body weight, up to a maximum of 75 g.) A baseline glucose level is obtained prior to glucose ingestion, and subsequently every 30 minutes for 2 hours. (The WHO standard is for blood to be obtained fasting and then again only at 2 hours.) Variations of the standard OGTT include the 1-hour test using 50 g glucose for GDM screening and the 3-hour 100–g glucose test for formal testing for GDM.[50] The 5-hour OGTT has recently fallen out of favor, having been used in the past for the evaluation of reactive hypoglycemia. The concurrent measurement of plasma insulin concentrations (as a surrogate marker of insulin sensitivity) is used occasionally for the inferential diagnosis of insulin resistance.[51]

Technical Aspects

As in all assessments of glucose metabolism, great care should be taken to ensure that there is no intervening acute illness that might affect the results of the OGTT. The test should be performed in patients who are not bedridden or physically immobilized. In that situation, the test should be postponed until the patient is back to his or her baseline level of activity and health. A variety of host variables that may alter the results of the OGTT have also been identified. Carbohydrate restriction in the days preceding the test may impair insulin secretion to an extent that may render a test abnormal. It is recommended that the daily diet during the 3 days prior to the test contain at least 150 g of carbohydrates. The test should be performed in the morning after an overnight fast of 8–14 hours' duration. Although the patient is allowed to ambulate to the location of the test, he or she should remain seated during the procedure itself. No calories or fluid should be consumed during the test and the patient should refrain from smoking. As with fasting glucose, aging is associated with diminished glucose tolerance, although the diagnostic criteria are the same for all ages.

Glycosylated Hemoglobin, Hemoglobin A$_{1c}$ (HbA$_{1c}$)

Due to wide fluctuations in circulating glucose concentrations in patients with diabetes, random glucose measurements are often not reflective of overall glycemic control. Even fasting determinations, which tend to be more stable, do not provide a complete picture. Like many proteins, erythrocyte hemoglobin is nonezymatically glycosylated at amine residues in the presence of glucose, which passes freely across red blood cell membranes. The percentage of hemoglobin molecules undergoing this reaction is proportional to the average ambient glucose concentrations during the preceding 60–90 days. "Glycohemoglobin" and "hemoglobin A$_{1c}$ (HbA$_{1c}$)" are, therefore, commonly used laboratory tests for assessing long-term diabetic control. HbA$_{1c}$, with a normal range of approximately 4–6% in most laboratories, refers to the percentage of hemoglobin molecules with glucose moieties attached to N-terminal valines of each of the two β-chains.[47] Glycohemoglobin (normal range, approximately 6–8 %) includes HbA$_{1c}$, but also other forms of hemoglobin where glycosylation has occurred at other amino acids.[47] HbA$_{1c}$ is more popular and is primarily used in the ongoing follow-up of diabetic patients. A highly specific test for diabetes, HbA$_{1c}$ is not sensitive enough to be used for screening purposes.[52] That is, patients with mild hyperglycemia, clearly within the diabetic range by FPG or 2-hour PG, may have HbA$_{1c}$ in the high-normal range. This is particularly the case since the lower diagnostic criteria of the ADA have been used. For instance, in one analysis of two large data sets including NHANES III, 87% of individuals with IFG and 61% of those with FPGs in the diabetic range had normal HbA$_{1c}$. In contrast, when the older criteria, FPG $\geq$ 140 mg/dL, were used, only 19% of diabetic patients had normal HbA$_{1c}$.[53] Hemoglobinopathies and states of rapid red cell turnover may make glycohemoglobin and HbA$_{1c}$ values difficult to interpret.

Emerging Technologies

Interstitial sensors are currently available for use in diabetic patients for continuous monitoring of extracellular glucose concentrations. Interstitial glucose approximates plasma glucose, particularly when determining glycemic trends. A current commercially available model is used for a 72-hour period, with the interstitial probe inserted subcutaneously and attached to a computerized unit that can be worn on the belt.[54] The readings are downloaded at the end of the recording period for computerized analysis at the practitioner's office. Several companies are actively pursuing refined versions of sensors that can provide a live display to the patient. Fully implantable sensors are also under investigation, as are units that can communicate directly with insulin delivery pumps to comprise an "artificial pancreas." Recently, a wristwatch-like sensor device was approved by the U.S. Food and Drug Administration (FDA).[55] This unit uses a process known as reverse iontophoresis (applying a gentle electrical current to the skin to express minute amounts of interstitial fluid, which can be analyzed for glucose content) and can measure glucose levels every 20 minutes. The results are provided to the patient on the device's display. Twice–daily calibration with the readings from routine capillary blood glucose monitoring is still required. Others have proposed the direct measure of the glucose content in tears or its indirect measurement, either transcutaneously or through the anterior chamber of the eye using laser technology. At the time of this writing, these and other emerging technologies appear promising for glucose monitoring in diabetic patients, although they will most likely lack the necessary precision for diagnostic purposes. However, if sufficiently sensitive, they may have a role for population screening.

REFERENCES

1. World Health Organization: Diabetes mellitus. Report of a WHO Expert Committee. *World Health Organization Technical Reports Series*, no. 310, 1965.
2. National Diabetes Data Group: Classification and diagnosis of diabetes mellitus and other categories of glucose intolerance. *Diabetes* 1979;28:1039.
3. World Health Organization: Second report of the WHO expert committee on diabetes mellitus. *World Health Organization Technical Reports Series*, no. 646, 1980.
4. American Diabetes Association: Report of the expert committee on the diagnosis and classification of diabetes mellitus. *Diabetes Care* 1997;20:1183.
5. Alberti KGMM, Zimmet PZ: Definition, diagnosis and classification of diabetes mellitus and its complications. Part 1: Diagnosis and classifi-

cation of diabetes mellitus. Provisional report of a WHO consultation. *Diabet Med* 1998;15:553.

6. Atkinson MA, Eisenbarth GS: Type 1 diabetes: New perspectives on disease pathogenesis and treatment. *Lancet* 2001;358:221.
7. Kukreja A, Maclaren NK: Autoimmunity and diabetes. *J Clin Endocrinol Metab* 1999;84:4371.
8. Kitabchi AE, Umpierrez GE, Murphy MB, *et al*: Management of hyperglycemic crises in patients with diabetes. *Diabetes Care* 2001; 24:131.
9. Mahler RJ, Adler ML: Clinical review 102: Type 2 diabetes mellitus: Update on diagnosis, pathophysiology, and treatment. *J Clin Endocrinol Metab* 1999;84:1165.
10. Ferrannini E: Insulin resistance versus insulin deficiency in non-insulin-dependent diabetes mellitus: Problems and prospects. *Endocr Rev* 1998;19:477.
11. Fagot-Campagna A, Pettitt DJ, Engelgau MM, *et al*: Type 2 diabetes among North American children and adolescents: An epidemiologic review and a public health perspective. *J Pediatr* 2000;136:664.
12. Ginsberg HN: Insulin resistance and cardiovascular disease. *J Clin Invest* 2000;106:453.
13. Pozzilli P, Di Mario U: Autoimmune diabetes not requiring insulin at diagnosis (latent autoimmune diabetes of the adult): Definition, characterization, and potential prevention. *Diabetes Care* 2001;24:1460.
14. Fajans SS, Bell GI, Polonsky KS: Molecular mechanisms and clinical pathophysiology of maturity-onset diabetes of the young. *N Engl J Med* 2001;345:971.
15. Barroso I, Gurnell M, Crowley VE, *et al*: Dominant negative mutations in human PPARgamma associated with severe insulin resistance, diabetes mellitus and hypertension. *Nature* 1999;402:880.
16. Mohan V, Nagalotimath SJ, Yajnik CS, Tripathy BB: Fibrocalculous pancreatic diabetes. *Diabetes Metab Rev* 1998;14:153.
17. Kasayama S, Otsuki M, Takagi M, *et al*: Impaired beta-cell function in the presence of reduced insulin sensitivity determines glucose tolerance status in acromegalic patients. *Clin Endocrinol* 2000;52:549.
18. Nestler JE, McClanahan MA: Diabetes and adrenal disease. *Baillieres Clin Endocrinol Metab* 1992;6:829.
19. Stenstrom G, Sjostrom L, Smith U: Diabetes mellitus in phaeochromocytoma. Fasting blood glucose levels before and after surgery in 60 patients with phaeochromocytoma. *Acta Endocrinol* 1984;106:511.
20. Chastain MA: The glucagonoma syndrome: A review of its features and discussion of new perspectives. *Am J Med Sci* 2001;321:306.
21. Bendz H, Aurell M: Drug-induced diabetes insipidus: Incidence, prevention and management. *Drug Safety* 1999;21:449.
22. Mir S, Taylor D: Atypical antipsychotics and hyperglycaemia. *Int Clin Psychopharmacol* 2001;16:63.
23. Ray JG, Vermeulen MJ, Shapiro JL, Kenshole AB: Maternal and neonatal outcomes in pregestational and gestational diabetes mellitus, and the influence of maternal obesity and weight gain: The DEPOSIT study. Diabetes Endocrine Pregnancy Outcome Study in Toronto. *QJM* 2001;94:347.
24. Buchanan TA: Pancreatic beta-cell defects in gestational diabetes: Implications for the pathogenesis and prevention of type 2 diabetes. *J Clin Endocrinol Metab* 2001;86:989.
25. Petry CJ, Hales CN: Long-term effects on offspring of intrauterine exposure to deficits in nutrition. *Hum Reprod Update* 2000;6:578.
26. Shaw JE, Hodge AM, de Courten M, *et al*.: Isolated post-challenge hyperglycaemia confirmed as a risk factor for mortality. *Diabetologia* 1999;42:1050.
27. Greenbaum CJ, Cuthbertson D, Krischer JP: Disease prevention trial of type I diabetes study group. Type I diabetes manifested solely by 2-hour oral glucose tolerance test criteria. *Diabetes* 2001;5:470.
28. World Health Organization: Diabetes mellitus: Report of a WHO study group. *World Health Organization Technical Reports Series*, no. 727, 1985.
29. Harris MI, Hadden WC, Knowler WC, Bennett PH: Prevalence of diabetes and impaired glucose tolerance and plasma glucose levels in the U.S. population aged 20–74 yr. *Diabetes* 1987;36:523.
30. McCance DR, Hanson RL, Charles MA, *et al*: Comparison of tests for glycated hemoglobin and fasting and 2 hour plasma glucose concentrations as diagnostic methods for diabetes. *BMJ* 1994;308:1323.
31. Engelau MM, Thompson TJ, Herman WH, *et al*: Comparison of fasting and 2-hour glucose and HbA1c levels for diagnosing diabetes: Diagnostic criteria and performance revisited. *Diabetes Care* 1997;20: 785.

32. American Diabetes Association. Report of the expert committee on the diagnosis and classification of diabetes mellitus. *Diabetes Care* 2001; 24(suppl1):S5.
33. Wahl PW, Savage PJ, Psaty BM, *et al*: Diabetes in older adults: Comparison of 1997 American Diabetes Association classification of diabetes mellitus with 1985 WHO classification. *Lancet* 1998;352:1012.
34. Gabir MM, Hanson RL, Dabelea D, *et al*: The 1997 American Diabetes Association and 1999 World Health Organization criteria for hyperglycemia in the diagnosis and prediction of diabetes. *Diabetes Care* 2000;23:1108.
35. Resnick H, Harris M, Brock D, Harris T: American Diabetes Association diabetes diagnostic criteria, advancing age, and cardiovascular disease risk profiles. *Diabetes Care* 2000;23:176.
36. Dinneen SF, Maldonado D 3rd, Leibson CL, *et al*: Effects of changing diagnostic criterial on the risk of developing diabetes. *Diabetes Care* 1998;21:1408.
37. World Health Organization: *Definition, Diagnosis and Classification of Diabetes Mellitus and Its Complications: Part 1: Report of a WHO Consultation: Diagnosis and Classification of Diabetes Mellitus.* World Health Organization, 1999.
38. Gabir MM, Hanson RL, Dabelea D, *et al*: Plasma glucose and prediction of microvascular disease and mortality: Evaluation of 1997 American Diabetes Association and 1999 World Health Organization criteria for diagnosis of diabetes. *Diabetes Care* 2000;23:1113.
39. Harris MI, Eastman RC: Early detection of undiagnosed diabetes mellitus: A US perspective. *Diabetes Metab Res Rev* 2000;16:230.
40. DECODE Study Group/European Diabetes Epidemiology Group. Glucose tolerance and cardiovascular mortality: Comparison of fasting and 2 hour diagnostic criteria. *Arch Intern Med* 2001;161:397.
41. Barzilay JI, Spiekerman CF, Wahl PW, *et al*: Cardiovascular disease in older adults with glucose disorders: Comparison of American Diabetes Association criteria for diabetes mellitus with WHO criteria. *Lancet* 1999;354:622.
42. Saydah SH, Miret M, Sung J, *et al*: Postchallenge hyperglycemia and mortality in a national sample of U.S. adults. *Diabetes Care* 2001;24: 1397.
43. Harris M, Eastman R, Cowie C, *et al*: Comparison of diabetes diagnostic categories in the US population according to 1997 American Diabetes Association and 1980–1985 World Health Organization diagnostic criteria. *Diabetes Care* 1997;20:1859.
44. Weyer C, Bogardus C, Pratley RE: Metabolic characteristics of individuals with impaired fasting glucose and/or impaired glucose tolerance. *Diabetes* 1999;48:2197.
45. de Vegt F, Dekker JM, Jager A, *et al*: Relation of impaired fasting and postload glucose with incident type 2 diabetes in a Dutch population: The Hoorn study. *JAMA* 2001;285:2109.
46. DECODE Study Group/European Diabetes Epidemiology Group: Glucose tolerance and mortality: Comparison of WHO and American Diabetes Association diagnostic criteria. *Lancet* 1999;354:617.
47. Troisi RJ, Cowie CC, Harris MI: Diurnal variation in fasting plasma glucose: Implications for diagnosis of diabetes in patients examined in the afternoon. *JAMA* 2000;284:3157.
48. Emancipator K: Laboratory diagnosis and monitoring of diabetes mellitus. *Am J Clin Pathol* 1999;112:665.
49. Karter AJ, Ackerson LM, Darbinian JA, *et al*: Self-monitoring of blood glucose levels and glycemic control: The Northern California Kaiser Permanente diabetes registry. *Am J Med* 2001;111:1.
50. Tam WH, Rogers MS, Yip SK, *et al*: Which screening test is the best for gestational impaired glucose tolerance and gestational diabetes mellitus? *Diabetes Care* 2000;23:1432.
51. Matsuda M, DeFronzo RA: Insulin sensitivity indices obtained from oral glucose tolerance testing: Comparison with the euglycemic insulin clamp. *Diabetes Care* 1999;22:1462.
52. Tanaka Y, Atsumi Y, Matsuoka K, *et al*: Usefulness of stable HbA(1c) for supportive marker to diagnose diabetes mellitus in Japanese subjects. *Diab Res Clin Pract—Suppl* 2001;53:41.
53. Davidson MB, Schriger DL, Peters AL, Lorber B: Relationship between fasting plasma glucose and glycosylated hemoglobin: Potential for false-positive diagnoses of type 2 diabetes using new diagnostic criteria. *JAMA* 1998;281:1222.
54. Chase HP, Kim LM, Owen SL, *et al*: Continuous subcutaneous glucose monitoring in children with type 1 diabetes. *Pediatrics* 2001;107:222.
55. Pitzer KR, Desai S, Dunn T, *et al*: Detection of hypoglycemia with the GlucoWatch biographer. *Diabetes Care* 2001;24:881.

Epidemiology of Diabetes Mellitus

Peter H. Bennett

Marian J. Rewers

William C. Knowler

TYPE 1 DIABETES MELLITUS (T1DM)

According to the current classification of diabetes mellitus,[1,2] type 1 diabetes (T1DM; previously called insulin-dependent or juvenile diabetes) is caused by β-cell destruction, often immune-mediated, that leads to loss of insulin secretion and absolute insulin deficiency. Type 1a (autoimmune form) diabetes (T1aDM) is preceded by a subclinical period of T-cell–mediated autoimmune destruction of β cells, marked by the presence of autoantibodies of variable duration.[3] This is the most common form of diabetes among children and adolescents of European origin. In children, the disease is usually characterized by a rapid onset with acute symptoms and dependence on exogenous insulin for survival. T1aDM is nearly as frequent in adults, but often, less dramatic onset may lead to misclassification as Type 2 (T2DM) and a delayed insulin treatment. In most patients, the etiology of the autoimmune process and β-cell destruction is not known. T1DM also includes cases that are thought not to be immune-mediated, but are characterized by absolute insulin deficiency (T1bDM) (see Chap. 18).[4]

T1DM accounts for 5–10% of all diagnosed diabetes. About 40% of persons with T1DM are younger than 20 years of age at onset, thus making diabetes one of the most common severe chronic diseases of childhood, affecting 0.3% of the general population by the age of 20 years and 0.5–1% during the life span.[5] The incidence of the disease appears to be increasing by 3–5% per year.[6–8] It is estimated that approximately 1.4 million in the United States, and perhaps 10–20 million people globally suffer from the disease.[9,10] The high incidence, associated severe morbidity, mortality (see chapters on complications and mortality), and enormous health care expenditures[11,12] make T1DM a prime target for prevention.

NATURAL HISTORY OF TYPE 1a DIABETES

The natural history of T1aDM (Fig. 19-1) includes four distinct stages that can be observed in a vast majority of the patients: (1) preclinical β-cell autoimmunity with progressive defect of insulin secretion, (2) onset of clinical diabetes, (3) transient remission, and (4) established diabetes associated with acute and chronic complications and premature death. At each stage, a spectrum of clinical manifestations and laboratory measurements helps to define the etiology, severity, prognosis, and prevention goals (Table 19-1).

PRECLINICAL β-CELL AUTOIMMUNITY

T1aDM results from a chronic autoimmune destruction of the pancreatic islet β cells, probably initiated by exposure of a genetically susceptible host to an environmental agent. While the candidate genetic and environmental factors appear to be quite prevalent, β-cell autoimmunity develops in less than 5% and progresses to diabetes in less than 1% of the general population.

The autoimmune process is mediated by macrophages and T lymphocytes with circulating autoantibodies to various β-cell antigens (see Chap. 20). Epidemiologic studies have defined autoimmunity as the presence of autoantibodies,[3] because in contrast to the cellular markers, their measurement is reliable and standardized across laboratories. Earlier studies have described the epidemiology of β-cell autoimmunity by measuring islet cell antibodies (ICAs) in the classical immunoflourescence test using pancreatic tissue.[13] This test has been notoriously difficult to standardize and has been replaced by a combination of assays for antibodies against specific β-cell antigens, such as insulin (IAA)[14–16] glutamic acid decarboxylase (GAD),[17,18] or ICA512 (IA-2).[19] These tests are quite sensitive and predictive in relatives of T1DM patients[20,21] and in the general population.[22]

Prevalence and Incidence

The prevalence data on β-cell autoimmunity in school children from various countries[23] are summarized in Fig. 19-2 and compared with the incidence of T1DM in these countries. The prevalence of ICAs varied from 0.2% in Dutch to 4.4% in Sardinians; however, the rates are not strictly comparable, because of different ICA assays and cut-off values for positivity as well as different age groups screened. The prevalence of β-cell autoimmunity appears to be roughly proportional to the incidence of T1DM in the populations.[24] In contrast, the prevalence of β-cell autoimmunity in first-degree relatives of T1DM persons does not differ as dramatically between high and low T1DM risk countries (Fig. 19-3).

No reliable estimates of the incidence of β-cell autoimmunity in the general population have been published, but appropriate cohort studies are underway in the United States[25] and Finland.[26] In siblings of Finnish T1DM children, the incidence of combined β-cell autoimmunity or T1DM was up to 1.4% per year.[27] In New Zealand, the incidence was 3.7% per year in relatives younger

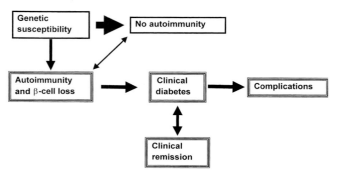

FIGURE 19-1. Natural history of type 1 diabetes.

than 5, compared to 0.5% per year in those 5–9 years old. None of the 356 relatives older than 10 years converted over a period of 5 years.[28] This suggests that relatively few children develop β-cell autoimmunity after the age of 5 and some may recover from autoimmunity.[29,30]

Little data concerning β-cell autoimmunity are available for non-Caucasian populations. Compared with Caucasians, first-degree relatives of African-American T1DM probands had somewhat higher prevalence of ICAs,[31] but at T1DM onset, the proportions were reversed.[32] Among 86,000 relatives of T1DM patients screened for the DPT-1 trial, lower prevalence of ICAs was observed in Asian Americans (2.6%) and in Hispanics (2.7%), compared to African-Americans (3.3%) or non-Hispanic whites (3.9%) (Skyler, unpublished data, 2001). Lower prevalence of GAD antibodies in Asian compared to Caucasian type 1 diabetes patients has also been reported.[33]

No significant gender difference in the prevalence of β-cell autoimmunity, either in first-degree relatives or in the general population, has been published. However, the crude DPT-1 screening data (not adjusted for age, relation to proband of ethnicity) have

suggested higher prevalence of ICAs in males (4.3%) than in females (3.3%). No reliable information is available concerning potential seasonal or annual variation in the incidence of β-cell autoimmunity. Preliminary reports from Finland (Simell, unpublished data, 2001) suggested that the seasonality of autoantibody appearance may mimic that of the clinical onset, indirectly implying that similar infections may trigger autoimmunity and progression to diabetes.

Genetic Factors

Family History

The prevalence of β-cell autoimmunity in first-degree relatives of type 1 diabetic persons is increased 3–5 times, compared to that in school children with no family history of T1DM. This is less than expected, knowing that the risk of T1DM among the relatives is 20 times higher than that in the general population.

Candidate Genes

In contrast to the wealth of data concerning genetic markers associated with clinical diabetes, little is known about the genetic determinants of β-cell autoimmunity. No particular HLA type seems to be associated with β-cell autoimmunity, although inconsistent associations between insulin or GAD autoantibodies and HLA-DR,DQ phenotypes have been reported. The HLA-DR2, DQB1* 0602 haplotype, which almost completely protects from T1DM,[34] is found in about 15% of GAD- and IAA-positive young relatives of T1DM patients.[35–37] However, over 90% of those strongly and/or persistently ICA-positive are HLA-DR3 or 4, similar to T1DM patients.[38] Children with β-cell autoimmunity identified from the general population also show a variety of HLA genotypes, but 90% of those persistently ICA-positive are DRB1*04, DQB1*0302.[39,40] This may suggest that HLA genes are not involved in the initiation of β-cell autoimmunity, but rather deter-

TABLE 19-1. Natural History of Type 1 Diabetes

	Preclinical Autoimmunity	Clinical Onset	Remission	Long-Standing Diabetes

Clinical	—	Polyuria, polydipsia
		Weight loss
		DKA in 20–40%
		Insulin dependence
			Insulin independence
			partial in 20–70%
			Total in 10–30%
				Acute complications:
				  DKA, hypoglycemia, infections
				Chronic complications: retinopathy,
				  nephropathy, neuropathy, hypertension,
				  atherosclerosis, growth impairment
				Premature mortality

Laboratory				
Genetic markers	Initiation: ? Progression: HLA-DR,DQ	IDDM1 ch. 6p21.3 (HLA-DR,DQ,DP) IDDM2 ch.11p15.5 IDDM3-IDDM17?	?	ACE/ApoH—hypertension? Apo E, Apo A-IV—CHD? Others?
Autoantibodies to insulin, GAD$_{65}$, ICA512 (IA-2)	Prevalence 85–100%	Prevalence 85–100%	Prevalence 40–60%	Prevalence ↓ 20–40%
Autoreactive cells	CD4, CD5, CD8	CD4, CD5, CD8	CD4, CD8	Mostly CD8 (?), CD4
Insulin secretion	Normal → low AIR	Low	Partially restored	Progressively lost
Blood glucose	Normal	>200 mg/dL (random)	Mostly <200 mg/dL	Depends on treatment
HbA$_{1c}$	Normal (<6%)	Usually >11%	<7.5%	Depends on treatment
Prevention				
Primary	Of autoimmunity	Of diabetes onset	—	—
Secondary	Of diabetes	Remission induction	Remission extension	—
Tertiary	—	Of onset mortality	Of acute complications	Of complications, mortality

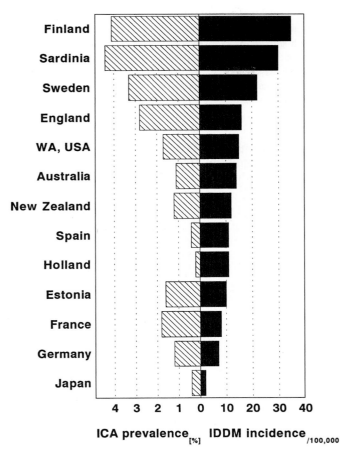

FIGURE 19-2. Geographic differences in the prevalence of islet cell antibodies (ICA) in school children, compared with the incidence of type 1 diabetes (ages 0–14 years) in the area.

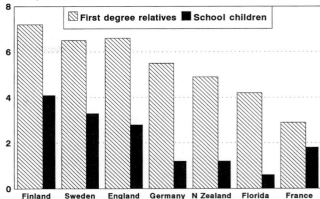

FIGURE 19-3. Prevalence of islet cell antibodies (ICA) in first-degree relatives and in school children in various geographic locations.

mine progression to diabetes. More subjects with β-cell autoimmunity need to be genotyped to precisely determine the role of HLA and additional T1DM candidate genes[41–47] in the initiation of autoimmunity and progression to diabetes.

Environmental Factors

Viruses

Viral infections appear to initiate autoimmunity rather than precipitate diabetes in subjects with autoimmunity. Two infections with similar viruses may be needed. Mice persistently expressing a viral protein in the β cells do not develop β-cell autoimmunity unless exposed to the same virus later in life.[48,49] ICAs or IAAs have been detected after mumps,[50] rubella, measles, chickenpox,[51] Coxsackie,[52] ECHO4,[53] and rotavirus[54] infections. Newborns and infants are particularly likely to develop a persistent infection and among patients with congenital rubella syndrome, 70% have ICAs.[55]

The evidence is strongest for picornaviruses, which include human (enteroviruses and rhinoviruses) and animal pathogens (e.g., mouse EMC virus and Theiler's virus). Picornaviruses induce T1DM in numerous animal models, and their tropism to human β cells has been demonstrated.[56] A molecular mimicry between the P2-C protein of Coxsackie virus and the GAD protein[57] may be responsible for β-cell autoimmunity. Cross-sectional studies of anti-

Coxsackie antibodies in β-cell autoimmunity have been weak and inconclusive[58] and have been recently replaced by studies based on detection of picornaviral RNA in bodily fluids using PCR. Prospective studies of nondiabetic relatives and general population children found a strong relation between enteroviral infections, defined by PCR, and development of islet autoantibodies in Finland[59–61] but not in the United States (Graves, unpublished data, 2000).

Dietary Factors

Exposures to cow's milk bovine serum albumin (BSA) or β-casein prior to gut cellular tight junction closure or during gastroenteritis when the intestinal barrier is compromised are alternative causes of β-cell autoimmunity. Cow's milk or wheat introduced at weaning triggers insulitis and diabetes in animal models,[62] perhaps through a molecular mimicry.[63] Human data are conflicting, but predominantly negative.[64,65–70]

The association between cow's milk and autoimmunity could be due to the effect of β-casein immunostimulating hexapeptide present in enzymatic hydrolysate of milk from *Bos taurus* cows, but not from *Bos indicus* cows.[71] Chemical compounds (streptozocin[72] or dietary nitrates and nitrozamines[73]) induce β-cell autoimmunity in animal models. Multiple hits of dietary β-cell toxins may render genetically resistant individuals susceptible to diabetogenic viruses, leading to T1DM.[74]

Gene–Environment Interactions in β-Cell Autoimmunity

Host–Virus Interactions

Both the susceptibility genes and the environmental risk factors for human β-cell autoimmunity are poorly defined. In mice, the host's genes restrict the diabetogenic effect of picornaviruses in a manner compatible with a recessive trait not related to the MHC (for review see reference 56). In humans, the HLA-DR3 allele is associated with viral persistence. It remains to be established which additional genetic variants interact with infectious agents to promote β-cell autoimmunity in humans.

Host-Diet Interactions

The postulated autoimmune response to cow's milk proteins is likely determined by the host's age and genetic background. The epidemiologic data are extremely limited and suggest that an early

exposure to cow's milk in relatives with HLA-DR3/4,DQB1* 0302,DR3/3 or DRx/4,DQB1*0302 is not associated with the presence of GAAs and/or IAAs at ages 1 to 6 years and may even be protective.[75] It is unclear whether the effect of HLA-DR3 differs from that of HLA-DR4,DQB1*0302, and whether other T1DM-associated genes are involved.

Primary Prevention of β-Cell Autoimmunity

Prevention of Diabetogenic Viral Infection

In mice, it is possible to prevent encephalomyocarditis virus-induced diabetes by immunization with a nondiabetogenic variant of the virus.[76] The interactions between HLA, antigen, and T-cell receptor, as well as the genetic determinants of viral diabetogenecity, are being disentangled. It may become possible to design recombinant vaccines that would provide optimal antigenic stimulus in the context of the host's HLA, providing long-term protection against diabetogenic strains and avoiding adverse effects. Approaches alternative to vaccination include antiviral agents.[77]

Dietary Factors

If early exposure to cow's milk triggers β-cell autoimmunity in humans, a logical primary prevention would include avoidance of cow's milk, especially in those with T1DM-associated HLA alleles. Such an intervention has been piloted in newborn relatives of T1DM patients,[78] and a large multiceneter trial is under way. Current data are insufficient to support cow's milk avoidance for prevention of β-cell autoimmunity and type 1 diabetes.

Progression from β-Cell Autoimmunity to Clinical Diabetes

The duration of preclinical β-cell autoimmunity is variable and precedes the diagnosis of diabetes by up to 9–13 years.[79,80] In most persons with persistent autoantibodies, there is an early loss of spontaneous pulsatile insulin secretion and progressive reduction in the acute insulin response to intravenous glucose load, followed by decreased response to other β-cell secretagogues, impaired oral glucose tolerance, and fasting hyperglycemia.[81] However, a non-progressive β-cell defect can exist for many years in some monozygotic twins and other relatives of T1DM persons.

Studies in first-degree relatives of T1DM patients[80,82,83] and in school children with no family history of T1DM[29,30,39,84,85] have reported ICA "remission" rates between 10 and 78%. It is unclear whether such remissions really occur or are an artifact of low specificity of autoantibody assays. If autoimmunity remits at the reported rates, only 1 in 2–8 of autoimmune children will develop diabetes by the age of 20 years. In those who lose their autoantibodies or remain autoimmune but do not progress to diabetes, it is presumed that the penetrance or number of susceptibility genes or the causative environmental exposures are insufficient. It is possible that β-cell autoimmunity remits spontaneously in genetically resistant persons or when the offending factor is removed, similar to celiac disease. Age also plays a role, because children younger than 10 years have a threefold increased risk of progressing from autoimmunity to T1DM, compared to older relatives.[31]

β-cell autoimmunity may remit and reappear in the course of viral infections or variable exposure to causal dietary factors. The cumulative β-cell damage and increases in insulin resistance with obesity and physical inactivity may eventually cause diabetes at a later age. Those persons in whom the disease process is slow may

present with T1DM as adults, develop diabetes that does not immediately require insulin treatment, or may even fail to develop diabetes altogether. Markers of autoimmunity can be detected in 14–33% of diabetes patients classified on clinical grounds as "type 2"[86,87] and are associated with early failure of oral hypoglycemic drug therapy and insulin dependence in these patients. The term *latent autoimmune diabetes of adults* (LADA)[88] has been coined for this slowly progressing form of T1DM.

Primary Prevention of T1DM in Persons with β-Cell Autoimmunity

ICA-positive relatives of T1DM patients have become the primary target of clinical trials to prevent T1DM.[89–91] Some of the proposed interventions are associated with significant adverse effects.[92–94] The effectiveness of oral nicotinamide[95] is being tested in the ENDIT study[96] (results expected in 2002), but smaller studies[97] have not been promising. Promising results of a pilot trial with parenteral insulin[98] gave impetus to a large randomized unmasked trial of low-dose SC/IV insulin in relatives with confirmed ICA positivity and low acute insulin response to IV glucose (Diabetes Prevention Trial-1[99]). The results of this trial were announced in 2000, but unfortunately showed no efficacy of insulin injections in preventing or delaying diabetes onset. The oral insulin arm of the DPT-1 is in progress, but results of smaller studies in newly diagnosed patients have not been encouraging.[100,101] Trials involving induction of tolerance to insulin or GAD using altered peptide ligands are being tested in phase II clinical studies.

CLINICAL ONSET OF T1DM

In industrialized countries, 20–40% of T1DM patients younger than 20 years present in diabetic ketoacidosis (DKA).[102–105] Younger age, female gender, HLA-DR4 allele,[106] lower socioeconomical status, and lack of family history of diabetes have been associated with more severe presentation. Severe presentation in younger children may result from greater β-cell destruction at diagnosis, an average of 80% of the islets are damaged at diagnosis in children younger than 7 years, 60% in those 7–14 years old, and 40% in those older than 14.[107] Case fatality in industrialized countries ranges between 0.4 and 0.9%,[108] but little is known concerning its predictors.

Both DKA and onset death are largely preventable, because most of the patients have typical symptoms of polyuria, polydipsia, and weight loss 2–4 weeks prior to diagnosis. The diagnosis is straightforward in almost all cases and can be based on the symptoms, random blood glucose over 200 mg/dL, and/or HbA$_{1c}$ higher than 7%.

Traditionally, nearly all children with newly diagnosed T1DM were hospitalized. More recently, an increasing proportion of new-onset children have been managed on an outpatient basis, especially in urban centers with specialized diabetes education and treatment facilities. In Colorado, the proportion of children receiving only outpatient care at diabetes diagnosis increased from 6% in 1978 to 35% in 1988.[109] Hospitalization at onset does not improve short-term outcomes, such as readmission for DKA or severe hypoglycemia.[102,105] Onset hospitalizations and acute complications have similar biologic (younger age, lower endogenous insulin secretion) and psychosocial (lower socioeconomic status, limited access to health care, dysfunctional family) determinants.

Prevalence and Incidence of T1DM

T1DM is one of the most common chronic childhood illnesses, affecting word-wide an estimated 50,000 new cases annually[9] and, in Caucasian populations, 1–3 per 1000 children by the age of 20 years.[5] Prevalence of T1DM, that is, the number of people in the population who have the disease at a given point in time, is determined not only by disease incidence but also by case survival, which may vary markedly in populations. The prevalence of T1DM in the age group 0–15 years ranges from 0.05% to 0.3% in most European and North American populations.[23] Prevalence data are useful in determining the public health impact of T1DM. For example, it is estimated that there are approximately 123,000 persons aged 0–19 years in the United States who currently have T1DM.[10]

Incidence is the rate at which new cases of disease appear in the population and is usually expressed as the annual number of new cases per 100,000 persons. Incidence of T1DM varies by geographic location, ethnicity, age, gender, and time period.

Geographic Location

One of the most striking characteristics of T1DM is the large geographic variability in the incidence (Fig. 19-2).[110–112] Scandinavia and the Mediterranean island of Sardinia have the highest incidence rates in the world. Asian populations have the lowest T1DM incidence rates. A child in Finland is 400 times more likely to develop diabetes than a child in China. The geographic and ethnic variation in T1DM risk may reflect either different pools of susceptibility genes or different prevalence of causative environmental factors or a combination of both.

The clinical picture of the disease is similar in low- and high-risk areas,[113,114] making it unlikely that the interpopulation differences are due to misclassification of different types of diabetes. Since in many populations, T2DM is either increasing[115] or already the predominant form of diabetes in children,[116] it has been suggested that islet autoantibodies should be measured at onset for correct diagnosis and treatment.[117]

Race and Ethnicity

Racial differences in T1DM risk within the same population are striking, although they are not of the same magnitude as the geographic differences (Fig. 19-4). American non-Hispanic whites are about one and a half times as likely to develop T1DM as African-Americans or Hispanics.[110] This is similar to the differences reported from Montreal, where children of British descent had about one and a half times the risk of T1DM as children of French descent.[118]

Age

T1DM incidence peaks at the ages of 2, 4–6, and 10–14 years, perhaps due to alterations in the pattern of infections or increases in insulin resistance. The age distribution of T1DM onset is similar across geographic areas and ethnic groups, as demonstrated by data from Allegheny County, Pennsylvania, and Poland (Fig. 19-5). The incidence decreases in the third decade of life,[119] only to increase again in the fifth to seventh decades of life.[120,121] It is not known whether there are etiologic differences between child- and adult-onset T1DM, but they were not apparent among 3672 adult diabetic participants in the UKPDS. Over 30% of those aged 25–34 were positive for ICA and/or GAD autoantibodies, but the prevalence decreased with age, to less than 10% in those aged 55–65.[122] The presence of the autoantibodies and age of presentation of dia-

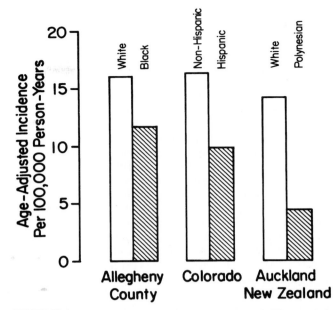

FIGURE 19-4. Incidence of type 1 diabetes in children of different ethnic groups living in the same geographic area.

betes were strongly associated with the presence of the HLA-DRB1*03/DRB1*04-DQB1*0302 genotype.[123]

Gender

In general, males and females have similar risk of T1DM,[124] with the pubertal peak of incidence in females preceding that in males by 1–2 years. In lower-risk populations, such as Japanese or U.S. blacks, there is a female preponderance, whereas in high-risk groups, there is a slight male excess.[5,110,125] T1DM diagnosed in adulthood is associated with male excess.[126–130] These findings contrast with the striking female preponderance in the NOD mouse model of diabetes.[131]

FIGURE 19-5. Age distribution of type 1 diabetes incidence under age 15 years Allegheny County, Pennsylvania and in Wielkopolska, Poland, during 1979–1985. (*Adapted from reference[114]*)

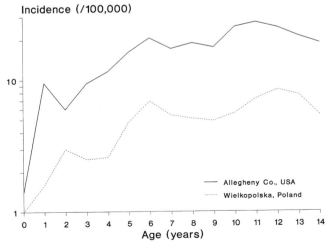

Time

There is evidence for marked variations in the incidence of T1DM over time, both seasonally and annually. In the Northern Hemisphere, the incidence declines during the warm summer months; similarly, in the Southern Hemisphere, the seasonal pattern exhibits a decline during the warm months of December and January, implicating a climatic factor (Fig. 19-6).[132] This seasonal pattern appears to occur only in older children,[133,134] suggesting that factors triggering diabetes may be related to school attendance. The observed seasonality is not an artifact of health care seeking or access, since the seasonality of symptom onset is similar to that of diagnosis and the patterns differ by HLA-DR type.[135,136]

Most population-based registries have shown increasing T1DM incidence over time,[6,137–140] while a few have shown no trend.[133] Some of the inconsistencies may be attributed to insufficient observation time. For example, initial data from Sweden and Allegheny County, Pennsylvania, showed no temporal trend, however, extended data collection showed increase incidence in these locations.[138,141] Most studies have observed periodic outbreaks superimposed on a steady secular increase in incidence. Figure 19-7 displays an example of parallel temporal incidence changes in populations that differ vastly in geographic location and the background risk of T1DM[114] (Allegheny County, Pennsylvania, and Wielkopolska, Poland). Standardized comparisons confirmed that a pandemic of T1DM occurred during 1984–1986.[6] While the increase in T1DM incidence has affected all age groups, several studies reported a particular increase among the youngest children.[142–146]

Genetic models are unable to explain the apparent temporal changes in the incidence.[147] The polio model, where autoimmune diabetes results from delayed exposure to infection that is benign when encountered in early childhood, could explain the recent increase in incidence, but not the shift in diagnosis to earlier ages. An alternative explanation invokes the congenital rubella model.

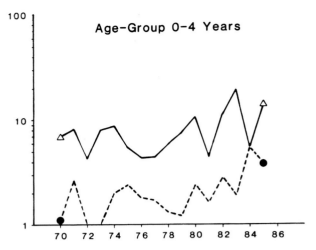
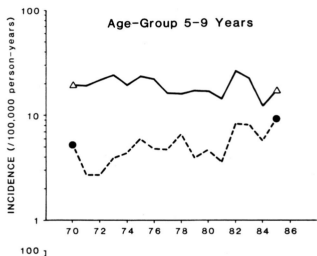
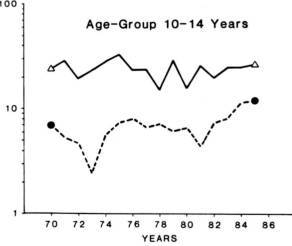

FIGURE 19-7. Annual incidence of type 1 diabetes in Allegheny County, Pennsylvania (Δ) and Wielkopolska, Poland, (◯) by age group, during 1970-1985. (*From reference[114]*)

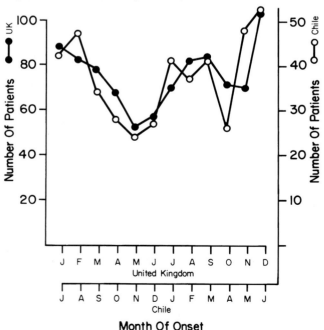

FIGURE 19-6. Seasonal distribution of onset of type 1 diabetes in the United Kingdom and in Chile. (*From reference[132]*)

Briefly, increased hygiene in the Western World has led to a decline in herd immunity to common infections among women of childbearing age. These women are more likely to develop viremia during pregnancy, resulting in congenital persistent infection of β cells and early-onset T1DM in the offspring. This model could explain both the increasing incidence of diabetes and the decreasing age of disease onset.[148]

Genetic Factors

Family History of T1DM

In moderate T1DM risk areas, such as the United States, the risk of T1DM by the age of 15 years is approximately 1/400. The risk is increased to about 1/40 in offspring of type 1 diabetic fathers and to 1/66 in offspring of type 1 diabetic mothers (Dorman and McCarthy, 1993). The risk to siblings of T1DM probands ranges from 1/12–1/35[149,150] and is further increased, to 1/4, in HLA-identical siblings. It is estimated that by the age of 60 years, approximately 10% of the relatives develop T1DM.[151] Family history of T1DM is a surrogate measure of the combination of T1DM genes and environmental exposures shared by family members.

"Familial" cases represent about 10% of T1DM and do not appear to be etiologically different from "sporadic" cases in HLA gene frequencies, seasonality of onset, prevalence of various ICAs, or IgM against Coxsackie B.[152] Familial cases tend to have lower glycated hemoglobin and higher C-peptide levels than sporadic cases, because relatives recognize diabetes symptoms earlier; however, these differences disappear soon after diagnosis.

Candidate Genes

The primary loci of genetic susceptibility to T1DM have been mapped to the HLA-DR and DQ regions[34,153,154], and new candidate genes outside the HLA region are being identified[41–47] (see Chap. 20). While 50% of non-Hispanic whites in the United States have the HLA-DR3 or DR4 allele, at least one of these alleles is present in 95% of patients with T1DM. The estimated risk to HLA-DR3/4 children in the general population ranges from 1/35 to 1/90.[9] The risk is further increased in those with HLA-DR3/4, DQB1*0302 genotype (about 2.2% of the general population versus 30–40% of T1DM patients). For comparison, about 5% of persons in the general population versus 12% of T1DM patients have a first-degree T1DM relative.

Environmental Factors

Twin[155] and family studies indicate that genetic factors alone cannot explain the etiology of T1DM. Seasonality, increasing incidence, and epidemics of T1DM, as well as numerous ecologic, cross-sectional, and retrospective studies, suggest that certain viruses and components of early childhood diet may cause T1DM.

Viruses

Herpesviruses,[156,157] mumps,[50,158] rubella,[55,159] and retroviruses[160,161] have been implicated. An increased incidence of T1DM in patients with congenital rubella syndrome (CRS) is particularly interesting. While CRS is responsible for a minute proportion of T1DM and there is little evidence that postnatal rubella exposure to the wild strain[51] or to the MMR vaccine[162] causes T1DM, CRS provides an example of viral persistence leading to T1DM. The incubation period of T1DM in CRS patients is 5–20 years[159] and persistent rubella virus infection of the pancreas has been demonstrated in some cases. While CRS is not associated with particular HLA-DR alleles, the distribution of the HLA-DR3 and 4 alleles among patients with CRS and diabetes resembles that in non-CRS T1DM patients.[55] Finally, a molecular mimicry has been reported between a rubella virus protein and a 52-kD β-cell autoantigen.[163]

Enteroviruses have been most strongly linked to human T1DM, but convincing proof of causality remains elusive (for review see references 56 and 164). Case and autopsy reports,[165,166] epidemics of T1DM associated with concurrent epidemics of enteroviruses,[167,168] and multiple cross-sectional seroepidemiologic studies[56] have been suggestive, but not entirely convincing. At least 90% of T1DM patients demonstrate a prolonged period of β-cell autoimmunity that is hardly compatible with an acute cytolytic enteroviral infection being a major cause. Enteroviral infection could, however, initiate β-cell autoimmunity through molecular mimicry between CBV P2-C protein and GAD[56,169] or a persistent β-cell infection with impairment of insulin secretion and expression of self-antigens. Alternatively, a combination of acinar cell infection and limited capacity of β cells to neutralize free radicals released in this process could initiate β-cell autoimmunity. Regulating factors could include age of the host, the metabolic activity of the β cell (with the increased demands of puberty or obesity exacerbating the autoimmune process), the HLA-specific restriction of immune responsiveness, and concomitant infection that might cause some degree of immunosuppression or self-tolerance.

Studies from Finland[59] and Sweden[170,171] have suggested *in utero* enteroviral infections can lead to T1DM in a significant proportion of the cases. Additional perinatal factors[171–177] and season of birth[178] have been associated with T1DM. In animal models, viral infection may protect the host from developing T1DM.[179–181] Evidence for such a protective effect in humans is speculative, at best.[182–184]

Routine Childhood Immunization

None of the routine childhood immunization have been shown to increase the risk of diabetes[162,184–188] or prediabetic autoimmunity.[189,190]

Dietary Factors

An ecologic study suggested an association between decrease in breast-feeding and increase in T1DM incidence between 1940 and 1980.[191] Subsequent case-control studies have shown a negative,[192,193] a positive,[194] or no association.[195–197] Certain studies[192,198] but not others[194,196,197] suggested a dose–response relationship between the duration of breastfeeding and protection from T1DM. A meta-analysis found a 50% increase in T1DM risk associated with a breastfeeding duration of less than 3 months, and exposure to breast-milk substitutes prior to 3 months of age.[199] Breastfeeding may be viewed as a surrogate for the delay in the introduction of diabetogenic substances present in formula or early childhood diet. Newly diagnosed T1DM children, compared with age-matched controls, have higher levels of serum antibodies against cow's milk and β-lactoglobulin,[200] as well as against BSA.[201] However, it has been difficult to reproduce some of these reports.[62] More recent cohort studies failed to find an association between infant diet exposures and β-cell autoimmunity.[68,70,190] Interestingly, a study in Finland suggested that current cow's milk consumption was more closely linked to prediabetic autoimmunity and diabetes than infant exposure.[202] Despite these limitations, a dietary intervention trial to prevent T1DM by a short-term elimination of cow's milk from infant diet (TRIGR) is under way.[78]

Circumstantial evidence suggests a connection between T1DM and consumption of foods and water containing nitrates, nitrites, or nitrosamines.[203–205] Anecdotal reports have shown that toxic doses of nitrosamine-containing compounds and generation of free radicals can cause diabetes.[206]

Gene–Environment Interactions

T1DM is likely caused by an interactive effect of genetic and environmental factors within a limited age window. While both the susceptibility genes and the candidate environmental exposures appear to be quite common, the likelihood of these causal components meeting within the susceptibility age window is low.[207] To investigate the environmental causes of T1DM, the study subjects have to be screened for known susceptibility gene markers so that gene–environment interactions can be accounted for.

Interaction Between HLA Class II Alleles and Viral Infection

Susceptibility to diabetogenic enteroviruses in humans appears to be genetically restricted by HLA-DR and DQ alleles.[56] However, the allelic specificity is controversial[106,208–210] and may depend on the viral type and epidemiology. For instance, in Sweden, DR3 was associated with IgM responses to CB4, while DR4 was associated with IgM responses to CB2, CB3, and CB5.[208] Elevated antiviral IgM levels in subjects with a specific HLA phenotype may reflect a greater ability to mount an immune response or a higher susceptibility to infection. This explanation is consistent with no apparent relationship between the presence of enteroviral RNA and HLA phenotypes[189] (Graves, unpublished data, 2001).

Interaction between HLA Class II Alleles and Infant Diet

Very few studies to date have examined a possibility of an interaction between the effects of HLA genes and exposure to cow's milk.[202,211–215] In one of these studies, controlling for birth order, ethnicity, and family income, exposure to whole cow's milk by 3 months of age was associated with T1DM more strongly in children with high-risk HLA than in those with low-risk HLA.[211]

REMISSION ("HONEYMOON PERIOD")

Shortly after clinical onset, most T1DM patients experience a transient fall in insulin requirement due to an improved β-cell function. Total and partial remissions have been reported in, respectively, 2–12% and 18–62%, respectively, of young T1DM patients.[105,212,213] Older age and less severe initial presentation of T1DM[212,215] and low or absent ICA[215–217] or IA-2[218] have been consistently associated with deeper and longer remission. Evidence relating GAD autoantibodies,[215,218,219] non-Caucasian origin, HLA-DR3 allele, female gender, and family history of T1DM to a less severe presentation, greater frequency of remission, and slower deterioration of insulin secretion is inconclusive. Most studies,[212,217] but not all,[213,214] agree that preserved β-cell function is associated with better glycemic control (lower HbA$_{1c}$) and preserved α-cell glucagon response to hypoglycemia.[220] The prevalence of ICA (but not GAD) decreases from 87% at the time of T1DM diagnosis to 38–62% 2–3 years later,[216,221] faster in young boys, subjects lacking HLA-DR3 and 4, and those diagnosed between July and December.[221]

The natural remission is always temporary, ending with a gradual or abrupt increase in exogenous insulin requirements. Destruction of β cells is complete within 3 years of diagnosis in most young children, especially those with the HLA-DR3/4 phenotype.[222] It is much slower and often only partial in older patients,[223] 15% of whom have still some β-cell function preserved 10 years after diagnosis.[224]

Secondary Prevention in New-Onset T1DM Patients

A number of the placebo-controlled randomized trials using azathioprine, cyclosporin A, nicotinamide, prednisone, and other immunosupressive agents attempted to increase the rate and the duration of T1DM remission. Only cyclosporin A treatment has been shown to be partially effective, inducing total remission in 25–40% of patients and sustaining it for 1 year in 18–24% of newly diagnosed patients, compared to 0–10% in the placebo group.[146,225] However, the drug is nephrotoxic, of little value in children, and effective for only as long as it is administered,[226] rendering this approach to secondary prevention of T1DM unacceptable. Trials using intensive insulin treatment,[227,228] oral insulin,[229] or immunomodulation[230] have been even less successful than cyclosporine A trials. Recently completed or ongoing prevention trials are listed in Table 19-2.

ESTABLISHED DIABETES

Complications

Acute complications of T1DM: (diabetic ketoacidosis, hypoglycemia, and infections) are described in detail in Chap 31, 34, and 36. The risk of hospital admission for acute complication is 30/100 patient-years in the first year of the disease and 20/100 in the subsequent 3 years.[105] An estimated 26% of the patients have at least one episode of severe hypoglycemia within the initial 4 years of diagnosis, with little relation to demographic or socioeconomic factors. The incidence of severe hypoglycemic episodes varies between 6 and 20/100 patient-years, depending on age, geographic location, and intensity of insulin treatment.[105]

Diabetes is the leading cause of end-stage renal disease, blindness, and amputation, and a major cause of cardiovascular disease and premature death in the general population.[231] The disease results in over $5 billion in medical care expenditures per year, with costs for patients over 10 times those for nondiabetics.[11] These aspects of diabetes are highlighted in other chapters of this book.

Mortality

Insulin treatment dramatically prolongs survival, but it does not cure diabetes. Although the absolute mortality at onset and within the first 20 years of T1DM is low (3–6%), it is 5 times higher for diabetic males and 12 times higher for diabetic females, compared to the general population.[232] This excess mortality is lowest in Scandinavia, intermediate in the United States, and highest in countries where T1DM is rare, for example, Japan,[233,234] probably due to a combination of the quality of care and access. Even in Finland, at least a half of the deaths are due to currently preventable causes such as acute complications, infections, and suicide.[235] On the other hand, 40% of the patients survive over 40 years and half of these have no major complications. Survival and avoidance of complications have been related to better metabolic control[236]; however, genetic factors also appear to be involved. Inconsistent associations have been reported between diabetic nephropathy and HLA-DR4[237] and several genes involved in blood pressure regulation.[236,238–244] Polymorphisms of apolipoproteins E and A-IV[245] appear to play a role in the development of coronary artery disease in T2DM patients, but have not been extensively studied in persons with T1DM.

TABLE 19-2. Selected Recent or Ongoing Type 1 Diabetes Prevention Trials

Nonantigen Specific	Antigen Specific
Secondary Prevention Trials (in Newly Diagnosed Patients)	
MMF and DZB: P. Gottlieb, Colorado and Seattle	Italy/France[9] Oral Insulin: No effect
Anti-CD3 hOKT3 IV: K. Herold, New York; F. Gorus, The Netherlands	Oral Insulin, N. Maclaren: ↑ C-peptide?
HSP 65 p277 (Peptor) SC: D. Elias, Israel	NBI 6024-003, Neurocrine
Multidose DZB: H. Rodriguez, Indiana	hGAD SC in alum, Diamyd
Oral hIFN-alpha: S. Brod, Texas	
Q fever vaccine SC: K. Lafferty, Australia	
Diazoxide: E. Bjork and A. Karlsson, Sweden	
Lisofylline IV: S. Kirk	
Vitamin E + nicotinamide: P. Pozzilli, Italy	
Primary Prevention Trials (In Nondiabetic Relatives)	
ENDIT: Nicotinamide	Joslin/BDC[9] parenteral insulin: Delay
TRIGR: Casein hydrolysate (cow's milk elimination)	Schwabing[9] parenteral insulin: Delay
	DPT-1[9] parenteral insulin: No effect
	DPT-1[9] oral insulin: ?
	DIPP[9] nasal insulin: ?
	INIT[9] IntraNasal Insulin trial: ?

Tertiary Prevention

The Diabetes Control and Complication Trial[246] and a number of smaller studies have demonstrated that intensive insulin therapy that maintains blood glucose concentrations close to the normal range can delay the onset and slow the progression of diabetic retinopathy, nephropathy, and neuropathy. Additional research is needed to determine the basis for genetic susceptibility to micro- and macrovascular complications[247] and to develop successful tertiary prevention of hypertension and accelerated atherosclerosis in persons with T1DM.

TYPE 2 DIABETES MELLITUS

Type 2 diabetes mellitus (T2DM), formerly known as non-insulin-dependent diabetes, is the most frequent form of diabetes mellitus in all parts of world. The prevalence of the disease is increasing globally.[248] It is estimated that in 2000 there were approximately 150 million individuals with the disease and that this number is likely to double by 2025. In most countries, including those with a high level of medical care, there is typically one undiagnosed case of T2DM for each that is known. Thus, studies that ascertain only previously diagnosed cases are subject to limited interpretation.

As T2DM may remain undetected for many years, investigations of its development, natural history, and complications are compromised when cases are identified only by routine clinical diagnosis. As undiagnosed diabetes represents an important fraction of the population with the disease, most epidemiologic studies are performed by testing all subjects in the population of interest. Without systematic testing, an incomplete and potentially misleading picture of the frequency or distribution of the disease is obtained. Furthermore, because of the differences in criteria, comparisons of rates from recent and earlier studies must be made with caution.

The 1980 internationally accepted WHO criteria for the diagnosis and classification of diabetes led to much greater uniformity of methods used in epidemiologic studies.[231,249] Recently, the diagnostic criteria have been revised, thus complicating comparisons of studies that are analyzed according to the new criteria and those that used the 1980 WHO criteria.[250,251]

Changes in Diagnostic Criteria

The classification and diagnostic criteria for diabetes mellitus were revised by the American Diabetes Association in 1997[250] and by the World Health Organization in 1999 (see Chap. 18).[251] The main changes included the designation of the majority of individuals formerly classified as non-insulin-dependent diabetes mellitus as T2DM mellitus. However, some individuals who fell into this category in earlier classifications were reclassified as Other Specific types of diabetes because the underlying basis for their abnormality of carbohydrate tolerance can now be specifically identified. Several types of non-insulin-dependent diabetes usually presenting in younger adults and widely known as maturity-onset diabetes of the young (MODY) were reclassified because the specific genetic causes of the disease have been identified. Cases of patients with non-insulin-treated diabetes who have circulating autoantibodies, such as islet cell antibodies, glutamic acid dehydrogenase antibodies, or insulin auto-antibodies, or HLA-DR types typically associated with T1DM, are now classified as T1DM. Diabetes of the category formerly known as malnutrition-related diabetes is now subdivided into those with fibrocalculus pancreatopathy, reclassified among Other Specific types of diabetes, whereas the remainder of patients without this specific feature now are considered to have T2DM. Thus, T2DM represents diabetes in the absence of T1DM or Other Specific types of diabetes. Nonetheless, the vast majority of diagnosed and undiagnosed diabetes in most populations falls into the T2DM category.

The revised diagnostic criteria accord greater importance to the fasting plasma glucose concentration (FPG) as a criterion for diagnosis, with the value considered diagnostic of diabetes lowered to greater than or equal to 126 mg/dL or 7.0 mmol/L.[250,251] In addition, a category or clinical stage of diabetes called impaired fasting glycemia (IFG) was introduced to categorize individuals who have fasting plasma glucose levels that are abnormal but fall short of the new diagnostic fasting plasma glucose level for diabetes, that is, FPG = 110 mg/dL (6.1 mmol) −125 mg/dL (<7.0 mmol/L). The category of impaired glucose tolerance (IGT) was retained. These changes in diagnostic criteria have resulted in some individuals being reclassified as having diabetes, that is, individuals with FPG levels at or above 126–139 mg/dL and with postload 2-hour glucose values of less than 200 mg/dL, thereby resulting in an increase in prevalence.[252] Furthermore, some recent papers have reported prevalence of diabetes based solely on fasting glucose values rather than on the 2-hour value based on oral glucose tolerance testing.

While the category of impaired glucose tolerance has been recognized as a risk category for the past 20 years, the category of impaired fasting glucose is new. Furthermore, it is now apparent that less than a majority of individuals with impaired glucose tolerance have impaired fasting glucose, and conversely, less than a majority of those with impaired fasting glucose have impaired glucose tolerance (see Chap. 18).[252,253]

Prevalence

The prevalence of T2DM varies enormously in different countries and among different racial and ethnic groups (Fig. 19-8).[254] Dramatic increases in the prevalence and incidence of T2DM have occurred in many parts of the world, especially in the newly industrialized and developing countries. Indeed, the majority of cases of T2DM in the future will occur in developing countries, with India and China having the highest number of cases in the world.[248]

Estimates have been made of the likely increases in the prevalence of diabetes over the next 20 years. Based on demographic changes, such as the increase and aging of populations, as well as trends in rural to urban migration, it is estimated that the prevalence of diabetes will approximately double in the next 25 years.[248]

T2DM in developed countries most often occurs in the middle to older age groups. In developing countries, because of the younger age distribution of the population, many cases occur in young to middle-aged adults. The disease, however, can develop in childhood or adolescence and its occurrence in these age ranges appears to be increasing rapidly especially in populations that already have a high overall prevalence of T2DM.[255] In Caucasian populations, in the United States and Europe the prevalence of T2DM increases with age at least into the seventies.[256] Prevalence, however, represents the balance between the cumulative rate of development of new cases (cumulative incidence) and the effect of excessive mortality among those with the disease. Furthermore, the patterns seen in prevalence data can be influenced considerably by secular changes in the incidence of the disease.

In the United States, the most complete information on the prevalence of T2DM has been obtained from the U.S. National Health Examination Surveys.[257,258] Surveys carried out in persons age 20–74 years in representative samples of the U.S. population show that the prevalence differs considerably in different ethnic groups.[258,259] The prevalence in Hispanic Americans, particularly Mexican Americans, is higher than in the white or black populations and African-Americans have a greater prevalence than whites.[260] Native American populations have a prevalence of T2DM even higher than Hispanic and African-Americans, although the prevalence does vary from one tribal group to another.[261,262] The exception to this appears to be among Eskimos, who have a prevalence no higher than white Americans.[261]

Data from the health examination surveys (NHANES III) conducted between 1988 and 1994 showed that 5.1% of U.S. adults age 20 years and over already carried a diagnosis of diabetes.[257] The prevalence of undiagnosed diabetes, based on fasting plasma glucose levels of 126 mg/dL or higher, was 2.7%, or based on glucose tolerance tests and the 1985 WHO criteria, was 6.3%.[252] The total prevalence was 7.8% based on diagnosed diabetes and fasting plasma glucose levels only, or 11.4% when based on the 1985 WHO criteria, rates appreciably higher than seen in earlier surveys. Among persons age 40–74 years the prevalence (based on the fasting criteria) had increased from 8.9% in 1976–1980 to 12.3% in 1980–1994—a 38% increase over the course a decade. Data from the Behavioral Risk Factor Surveys, carried out on representative samples of U.S. adults by telephone interviews, indicate that the prevalence of diagnosed diabetes in those aged 18 years and over has continued to increase between 1991 and 1999 from 4.1 to 6.0% in men, and from 5.6 to 7.6% in women, an increase of approximately 40% in less than a decade.[263,264]

Increases in T2DM have been observed in many other populations in the past half-century. For example, among the Pima Indians a 40% increase in the prevalence occurred between 1967 and 1977, primarily due to an increase in the incidence (the rate of development in new cases) of the disease.[262]

Prevalence of Diabetes in Other Countries

The prevalence of T2DM varies considerably among populations of different ethnic origins living in similar environments.[265] For example, in Singapore, the frequency of diabetes in 1992 was 8.5%—7.7% in Chinese men and women aged 18–69 compared to 13.3% and 12.3%, respectively, among the Asian Indians and Malays.[266] High prevalence rates of diabetes have also been found among Asian Indians compared to the indigenous populations in the United Kingdom, Fiji, and the Caribbean.[267] Considerable differences in the prevalence of diabetes have also been described among

FIGURE 19-8. Prevalence of diabetes according to 1980 WHO criteria in men and women aged 30–64 years in different countries and various ethnic groups. (*Adapted from reference*[254])

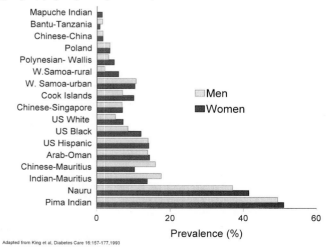

Adapted from King et al, Diabetes Care 16:157-177,1993

the multi-ethnic populations of Hawaii and New Zealand, where the Native Hawaiian and Maori populations, both of Polynesian origin, have higher prevalences than other ethnic groups.[268] Such differences support to the notion that there are racial and ethnic differences in the inherent susceptibility to develop T2DM. Nevertheless, there is also clear evidence that T2DM prevalence varies according to socioeconomic, educational, and other acquired characteristics so that differences in the prevalence of the disease in different ethnic groups living in the same location may be attributable to factors other than genetic predisposition to the disease.

T2DM in Children and Adolescents

T2DM was formerly considered as a disease of adults. In recent years, however, there have been many reports of its occurrence in childhood and adolescence.[255,269,270] As in adults, the disease in children is frequently asymptomatic and is detected mainly by screening. In Japan, a national program for screening school children has been in place since 1992 and the number recognized to have T2DM has increased progressively so that the prevalence and incidence of T2DM greatly exceed those of T1DM.[271] Adolescent T2DM was first described among the Pima Indians[272] and the prevalence has increased steadily over the past 30 years (Fig. 19-9).[269] Reports of T2DM in this age group have appeared from many ethnic groups in recent years, including other Native American tribes, Mexican Americans, African-Americans, Chinese, Polynesians, Asian Indians, and Arabs from the Gulf States. There are few reports among Caucasians, suggesting that the condition is still relatively rare in this ethnic group.

T2DM in childhood and adolescence is associated with obesity and parental diabetes, and in the Pima Indians, about a third of the affected are offspring of mothers who had diabetes during pregnancy.[269] It is also associated with the development of the same vascular complications as are seen in adults, but at an earlier age.[273]

Incidence

Incidence is the rate of development of new cases of disease. Only a few studies of the incidence of T2DM using standardized and comparable methodology have been reported. One method to determine the incidence in a specific population is to test glucose tolerance at two separate points in time and then estimate the cumulative incidence within the interval between the tests. Another method involves multiple tests at regular intervals over a period of time. By this method, the date of onset of disease can be estimated

and the incidence density rate (new cases per person-year at risk) can be calculated.

A less desirable, but easier method of estimating the changes in the incidence of T2DM has been used to examine if there has been a secular increase in the incidence of diabetes in the general U.S. population. In the National Health Interview Survey, the question of whether diabetes has been diagnosed during the past 12 months has been asked on several occasions. The prevalence of diagnosed diabetes and the rate of new diagnoses reported within the previous 12 months, have increased remarkably over time.[256] Some of this increase is undoubtedly attributable to the more frequent and widespread use of blood tests for glucose in routine medical care, but the continuing increase strongly suggests that the incidence of diabetes has risen considerably in the United States since 1940. Incidence studies using standardized glucose tolerance tests have been performed in the Pima Indians of Arizona[274,275] and among Micronesians in the central Pacific island of Nauru.[276] Both groups have very high incidence rates. Among Pima Indians, the age-specific incidence and aged-adjusted incidence rates of diabetes have increased over the course of two decades,[277] whereas in Nauru, the incidence may now be falling.

Mortality

T2DM is associated with excess mortality, mainly attributable to the vascular complications of the disease. In Caucasian populations, much of the excess mortality is attributable to cardiovascular disease, especially ischemic heart disease,[278–280] but in others, such as Asian and American Indian populations, renal disease contributes to a considerable extent.[281,282] In developing nations, an important component of the excess is due to infections.[283]

Age-adjusted mortality rates among persons with diabetes are 1.5–2.5 times higher than in the general population,[278] but the excess is greater in younger age groups and diminishes at older ages. The excess mortality leads to reduced life expectancy among those with T2DM.[284,285] The extent of the reduction of life expectancy is dependent on the age of onset of the disease, but averages approximately 10 years in countries such as the United States. Mortality in women is generally lower than in men, but the relative risk of death in women with diabetes is increased so that the absolute rates approach those seen in men with T2DM.[286,287]

The increased mortality in patients with T2DM is seen mainly among those with complications. Risk factors include proteinuria and retinal disease, and the classic risk factors for heart disease. Hyperlipidemia, hypertension, and smoking, each contribute disproportionately to death rates among those with T2DM.[288] Mortality rates also increase with increasing duration of the disease.[285]

Risk Factors

Familial Aggregation

The empiric risk of having T2DM is increased two- to sixfold if a parent or sibling has the disease.[289] Consequently, a positive family history is a practical, albeit crude, way of estimating if an individual is likely to have inherited susceptibility to the disease. On the other hand, familial aggregation may occur for nongenetic reasons. Family members often share a similar environment, particularly as children and in adolescence thus familial aggregation alone is not definitive evidence of genetic determinants. Furthermore, with a disease as frequent as T2DM two or more family members may well have the disease by chance alone.

FIGURE 19-9. Changes in prevalence of type 2 diabetes in Pima Indian children and adolescents over a 30-year period. *(From reference[269])*

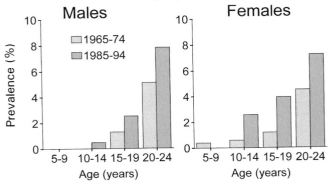

Genetic Factors

Twin Studies

A higher degree of concordance for T2DM in identical twins than in dizygotic twins provides strong evidence that genetic factors are important in determining susceptibility,[290,291] even though twins share the same intrauterine environment and usually grow up in a similar environment. Nevertheless, the high degree of concordance among twins *per se* does not indicate that the majority of individuals who carry genetic susceptibility will develop the disease; thus, among identical twins, there may be pairs who carry the genetic susceptibility and may never manifest the disease.

Further evidence of the importance of genetic factors as predisposing factors for T2DM comes from studies of admixed populations. Differences in prevalence among persons of mixed racial background from that in parent populations with notably different prevalences of the disease are indicative of the importance of genetic determinants. Such relationships have been described among Nauruans and Pima Indians where full-heritage members of these groups have significantly higher rates of diabetes than those of mixed heritage (Fig. 19-9).[292,293] Similarly, among the Mexican American population of San Antonio, the prevalence of T2DM is related to the degree of American Indian admixture, with higher rates associated with greater proportions of American Indian genes.[294]

Genes

Genes that specifically confer risk for the development of T2DM have been identified only to a limited extent. Genes have been identified that determine susceptibility to several rare forms of monogenic diabetes, such as MODY, that were formerly classified as non-insulin-dependent diabetes. Many patients with such forms of diabetes may still be inaccurately diagnosed as T2DM unless specific attempts are made to identify them. These monogenic forms of diabetes, now classified as Other Specific types of diabetes, are discussed in Chap. 21.

T2DM is a complex genetic disorder. Genomic scans have identified several regions in the genome where putative susceptibility genes are located.[295–299] Several genomic scans have indicated the presence of a locus or loci on chromosome 1, but apart from this region, there is limited consensus concerning the likely location of others. These observations suggest that the common forms of T2DM are multigenic and that the relative importance and frequency of the genes determining susceptibility varies from population to population. Certain haplotypes of the calpain 10 gene in the Mexican American population of Starr County, Texas,[300] and polymorphisms of the PPPR1 gene in the Pima Indians[301] have been identified as contributing to susceptibility to T2DM, and polymorphisms in the PPARγ gene have been reported to interact with dietary fat intake to contribute to physiologic characteristics that predispose to the disease (see Chap. 21).[302]

Modest associations of HLA type and T2DM have been reported in the populations of Pima Indians, Nauru, Asiatic Indians in Fiji, and in the Finnish population.[292,303,304] This chromosomal region, however, has shown no definite evidence of linkage in the genomic scans, and in marked contrast to T1DM, seems likely to have only a minor role in contributing to susceptibility in T2DM.

Age and Sex

The prevalence and incidence of T2DM vary to some extent between the sex from one population to another, but these differences are relatively small and appear to be accounted for by differences in other risk factors, such as obesity and physical activity. The prevalence of T2DM increases with age, although these patterns of incidence vary considerably. In populations with high frequencies of the disease, the incidence may be high and the prevalence may increase markedly in the younger adult years (e.g., 20–35 years of age); in others, the incidence and prevalence increase mainly in older individuals (e.g., 55–74 years of age). In most populations a decrease in prevalence is seen in the oldest age groups (e.g., 75+ years) because of higher mortality rates in those with T2DM.

Prevalence rates, however, reflect the balance between the rate of development of new cases (incidence), the duration of disease and mortality. Thus, secular changes in the incidence of the disease can have a marked influence on age-specific patterns of prevalence in different populations and in the same population over different time periods.

Incidence rates provide a much more accurate reflection of changing patterns of disease, but only a limited number of studies have measured age- and sex-specific incidence rates for T2DM. Such rates vary considerably according to other risk factors. Figure 19-10 shows the differences in age-specific incidence rates according to body mass index (BMI) in the Pima Indians.[275] Those with higher BMI have much higher incidence rates of T2DM at earlier ages than those with lower BMI, among whom the incidence rises in the older age groups.

Obesity

Obesity is a frequent concomitant of T2DM. In many longitudinal studies, it has been shown to be a powerful predictor of its development.[275,305] In nonobese individuals, the incidence of T2DM is low, even in populations such as the Pima Indians where the overall risk of the disease is very high. The relationship of incidence of T2DM to obesity also varies with other risk factors. For example, in the Pima Indians, the incidence rises much more steeply with BMI in those whose parents have diabetes than in these who do not (Fig. 19-11). This relationship indicates an interaction between risk factors.

Several studies indicate that waist circumference or waist-to-hip ratio may be a better indicator of the risk of developing diabetes than body mass index.[306–308] Such data suggest that the distribution of body fat is an important determinant of risk as these measures reflect abdominal or visceral obesity. In Japanese American men,

FIGURE 19-10. Incidence of diabetes by age group according to body mass index (BMI) in Pima Indian men and women. *(Updated from reference[262])*

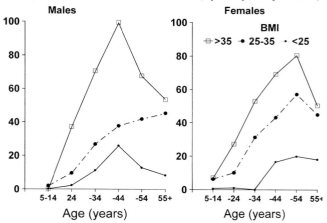

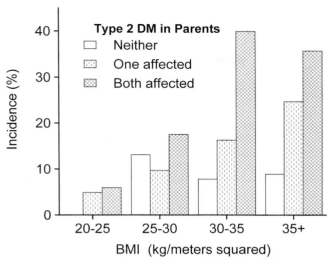

FIGURE 19-11. Age-sex adjusted incidence of diabetes in Pima Indians according to body mass index and whether diabetes was present in both, one or none of their parents. *(Adapted from reference[275])*

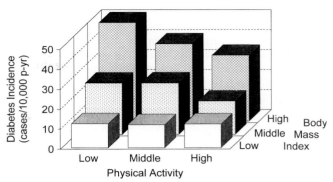

FIGURE 19-12. Incidence of diabetes according to baseline level of physical activity and body mass index (BMI) in men. *(Adapted from reference[312])*

for example, the intraabdominal fat as measured by CAT was the best anthrometric predictor of diabetes incidence.[307]

Obesity has increased rapidly in many populations in recent years. This increase has been accompanied by an increasing prevalence of T2DM. As obesity is such a strong predictor of diabetes incidence, it appears that the rapid increases in the prevalence of T2DM seen in many populations in recent decades are almost certainly related to increasing obesity. Furthermore, interventions directed to reducing obesity reduce the incidence of T2DM in obese individuals with impaired glucose tolerance (*vide infra*).

Physical Activity

Many studies indicate the important role of physical activity in the development of T2DM.[309–312] Nevertheless, its relative importance may be underestimated in most studies because of imprecision in measurement. Several studies do provide evidence of a causal role of physical inactivity in the etiology of T2DM.[309,310,312] The deleterious effect of low levels of physical activity is seen particularly among those subjects who have other risk factors, such as high BMI, hypertension, or parental diabetes. For example, in the Nurses Health Study, women who reported exercising vigorously at least once per week had an age-adjusted incidence rate of self-reported clinically diagnosed diabetes that was two-thirds as high as that of women who exercised less frequently.[309] Similarly, among male physicians, the incidence of self-reported diabetes was negatively related to the frequency of vigorous exercise, and the strength of this relationship was greater in those with higher BMI.[310] For equivalent degrees of obesity, more physically active subjects have a lower incidence of the disease (Fig. 19-12).[312] Intervention studies that have included increased physical activity to prevent diabetes among subjects with impaired glucose tolerance (*vide infra*) demonstrate a reduced incidence of T2DM, but the dose–response relationship of physical activity to diabetes incidence, and the extent that the relationship is confounded by concomitant weight loss, remains unclear.

Gestational Diabetes

Gestational diabetes (diabetes first recognized during pregnancy) is more frequent among women from subgroups of the pop-

ulation who have a high risk of T2DM (e.g., older, overweight or obese women, certain ethnic groups, etc.). In some cases, gestational diabetes represents diabetes that was present, but undiagnosed before pregnancy. In others, it develops during pregnancy, most frequently toward the end of the second trimester. It is in this latter group that glucose tolerance is likely to become normal following delivery, but such women carry a high risk for developing diabetes.[313]

Other Risk Factors

Genes, obesity, and physical inactivity appear to be the most important risk factors for T2DM. There are, however, others that influence the risk of developing T2DM, but their importance on a population level is much less than those of obesity and physical inactivity. These include low birth weight, exposure to a diabetic intrauterine environment, and other metabolic and environmental exposures.

The relative importance of genetics is difficult to assess in the absence of specific knowledge of the genes concerned. The extent to which the effects of obesity and physical activity vary according to the presence or absence of diabetes in parents indicates that genetic factors are important, but not sufficient, for the development of the disease. The strength of the relationship between obesity and physical inactivity suggests that T2DM is, for the most part, a preventable disease.

Low Birth Weight

Studies in many populations indicate that low-birth-weight babies have an increased risk of developing T2DM in adult life.[314–318] This relationship was first described by Hales and Barker,[319] who suggested that low birth weight due to nutritional deprivation *in utero* also resulted in reduced β-cell mass. They suggested that the relationship might represent a "thrifty phenotype"—an acquired rather than inherited defect—that was expressed as T2DM when those with the phenotype were exposed to a more affluent nutritional environment. Low birth weight is also associated with other traits that are associated with the development of diabetes including increased blood pressure, elevated triglycerides, and lower HDL concentrations—all characteristics of the insulin resistance or metabolic syndrome.[320]

Low birth weight (and also high birth weight—see the following discussion) is predictive of diabetes among the Pima Indian population.[315] The fathers, but not the mothers, of low-birth-weight Pima babies have higher rates of diabetes than the fathers of more usual weight babies, suggesting that the low-birth-weight to dia-betes relationship may have a genetic rather than an acquired basis.[321] There are certainly paternally derived genes that are linked to low birth weight, but whether or not these same genes predispose the offspring to T2DM remains to be determined. Low-birth-weight children are relatively insulin-resistant and it has also been suggested that the low-birth-weight to diabetes relationship might represent the selective survival of insulin-resistant babies and that this insulin-resistance would later lead to T2DM.[322] In spite of the importance of this relationship in furthering under-standing of the complex biology of early life events, the proportion of T2DM in most populations that can be accounted for by low birth weight is relatively small.[323]

Intrauterine Environment

The intrauterine environment influences the risk of developing T2DM. Offspring of diabetic pregnancies develop obesity at an early age and also are at high risk of developing T2DM at an early age (Fig. 19-13).[324] Such individuals have lower insulin secretion than similarly aged offspring of nondiabetic pregnancies.[325]

A substantial part of the excess risk of diabetes in the offspring of diabetic pregnancies appears to be the result of exposure to the diabetic intrauterine environment. Among offspring born to moth-ers before and after the development of T2DM, those born after the mother developed diabetes have a three fold higher risk of develop-ing diabetes than those born before.[326] Thus, the enhanced risk among the offspring from diabetic pregnancies among such women is the result of intrauterine programming that has long-term effects on the offspring in later life.

The early appearance of T2DM in female offspring increases the likelihood that their offspring will be exposed to a diabetic in-trauterine environment. This will lead to an increased prevalence of diabetes in subsequent generations.

Inflammation

Several inflammatory markers, such as interleukin 6, C-reactive protein, other cytokines, and acute-phase reactants, such as fibrin-ogen and plasma activator inhibitor-1 (PAI-1), have been associated with T2DM and its metabolic precursor, insulin resistance.[327,328] The extent to which these proteins are involved in the pathogenesis of T2DM is not clear. Nevertheless, it has been suggested that T2DM could be a disease of the innate immune system.[329]

FIGURE 19-13. Prevalence of diabetes in offspring, by age group, accord-ing to whether mother had diabetes at time of pregnancy, developed it later, or remained non-diabetic. *(From reference[324])*

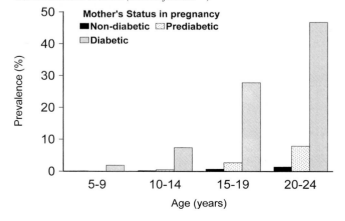

The epidemiologic support for the hypothesis comes from evi-dence that C-reactive protein, interleukin-6, and gamma globulin levels are associated with and also predict the development of T2DM.[327,330] The extent to which these markers are a cause or a consequence of underlying pathogenetic processes is presently uncertain.

Certain infections, such as hepatitis C, have also been associ-ated with T2DM. Patients with hepatitis C infection not infre-quently have glucose intolerance. Furthermore, in the NHANES III survey, anti-HCV antibodies were found 3 times more com-monly in patients with T2DM than those without, but only about one-third of those with T2DM had such antibodies.[331,332] There are no prospective population-based studies to indicate whether hepatitis C infection predicts the development of T2DM or how much of the disease might be attributable to this infection.

Sex Hormones

Low levels of sex hormone binding globulin predict the devel-opment of T2DM in women but not in men.[333,334] Furthermore, men with low testosterone levels and women with high levels of androgens are insulin-resistant.[335] Insulin resistance, or hyperinsu-linemia, and hyperandrogenemia and nulliparity are also character-istic of the polycystic ovarian syndrome. Nulliparity in the Pima Indians is associated with a higher prevalence of T2DM.[336] The significance of these relationships and the importance of sex hor-mones as risk factors for T2DM requires further investigation.

Dietary Factors

Breastfeeding is reported to be associated with a lower preva-lence of T2DM in young adults.[337] This suggests that dietary fac-tors in early life may program the risk of diabetes in later years.

In spite of obesity being such a strong risk factor for T2DM, the role of dietary factors in the development of T2DM is complex. The prevalence of diabetes has risen in many countries as nutrition and caloric intake have increased, for example, Japan. Conversely, marked reductions in T2DM have been recorded in wartime when caloric and nutritional deprivation have been present.[338] Such ob-servations, however, provide no indication of the role of specific effects of diet in the etiology of T2DM.

Many studies have examined nutritional and calorie intake in persons with T2DM and controls. Few consistent differences have emerged from these studies, which are open to the criticism that the purported differences are a result rather than a cause of the dia-betes. There are only a few prospective studies where dietary infor-mation has been obtained in cohorts before the onset of diabetes, who were then followed to ascertain the development of diabetes. Some of these studies have been very small and have lacked power to detect any but large effects,[339–342] but some suggest that total calorie intake and a low polyunsaturated to saturated fat ratio may predispose to the disease. Recently some large studies, such as Nurses Health Study and the Iowa Study, have examined the effects of dietary intake on the incidence of diabetes.[343,344] In each of these studies, however, diabetes has been ascertained by self-report of clinically diagnosed diabetes, which likely underestimates the im-portance of the dietary effects. Furthermore, the lack of precision and poor reproducibility of dietary interviews further reduce the likelihood of detecting important etiologic differences.

The Nurses Health Study involved almost 90,000 women free of diabetes, cardiovascular disease, and cancer at baseline who were followed for 16 years, during which 3300 new cases of T2DM developed.[343] Higher cereal and fiber intake and higher di-etary polyunsaturated to total fat ratios at baseline predicted a significantly lower incidence of T2DM, whereas higher consumption of trans fatty acids and foods with a higher glycemic index was associated with an increased risk of the disease. While each of these relationships was significant, the effects were relatively modest with relative risk for diabetes comparing the first and fifth quintiles, ranging from 0.6 for cereal fiber, 0.8 for polyunsaturated to total fat ratio, and 1.4 for trans fat intake and "glycemic load."[345] The relationships were seen across all strata of body mass index. Similar patterns have been seen in other studies. Neither total fat nor total carbohydrate as a proportion of total energy intake appeared to play a major predictive role in the development of T2DM.[346]

Communities in which there have been rapid changes in the type of diet consumed include many where dramatic changes in the prevalence or incidence of T2DM have been observed (e.g. Pima Indians, Nauru, Japan). In the Pima Indian population, although specific dietary components could not be implicated, individuals stating that they consumed a more traditional "Indian" diet as opposed to a more "Western" or "Anglo" diet experienced less than half the incidence of diabetes over an average 8-year follow-up period.[347] Such an effect, however, may reflect other lifestyle factors, rather than diet alone, that may influence the development of the disease, and these may not be adequately or appropriately considered in the analysis of such data.

Dietary intervention studies designed to delay or prevent the onset of T2DM have been conducted on high-risk individuals with impaired glucose tolerance (*vide infra*). Although these studies have shown that the incidence of T2DM can be reduced and that the reduction is a function of weight loss, they provide no information about whether or not dietary changes *per se* are effective, or if specific dietary constituents alter diabetes risk.

Alcohol Intake

Several studies indicated that moderate alcohol intake is associated with a reduced incidence of T2DM. Among women in the Nurses Health Study, there was a reduced incidence of diabetes in women who consumed alcohol compared to those who did not. There was a strong inverse relation between alcohol consumption and body weight, which could explain much of the apparent protective effect of alcohol consumption.[348] Among 20,000 male physicians, those consuming more than 2–4 drinks per week had a lower incidence of T2DM in the subsequent 12 years compared to nondrinkers, relationships that persisted after adjustment of BMI and other diabetes risk factors.[349,350]

These apparent male to female differences were examined among 12,000 45–64-year-old participants in the Atherosclerosis Risk in Communities Study.[351] After adjustment for other diabetes risk factors, men consuming more than 21 drinks per week had a significant increase in the incidence of diabetes, whereas no significant association with alcohol intake was found among the women. The apparent inconsistencies in the results of these studies suggest that other lifestyle behaviors differ in relation to alcohol consumption in different populations. However, it seems unlikely that moderate alcohol consumption has a deleterious effect on the incidence of T2DM, and may even be associated with a modest degree of protection.

Metabolic Changes During Development of Type 2 Diabetes

The development or worsening of insulin resistance represents a stage in the development of T2DM as reviewed elsewhere (see Chap. 22). Fasting insulin concentrations in subjects with normal glucose tolerance represent a surrogate marker of insulin resistance, and numerous longitudinal studies have shown that higher fasting insulin levels (or other indices of insulin resistance, e.g., HOMA) predict the development of T2DM. The effect of obesity on T2DM risk is probably mediated by its effect to worsen insulin resistance. Insulin resistance is also influenced by physical activity, with lower levels of activity being associated with greater insulin resistance. Consequently, insulin resistance can be considered a mechanism through which many of the risk factors for T2DM exert their pathophysiologic effects (Figure 19-14).[352]

Other factors that increase the risk of T2DM, such as low birth weight, sex-hormone abnormalities, polycystic ovarian syndrome, and inflammatory markers, are all associated with insulin resistance. Component factors of the insulin-resistance or metabolic syndrome also predict the development of T2DM. These include increased blood pressure, raised triglyceride and low high-density lipoprotein concentrations, and obesity and central or visceral adiposity.

Insulin resistance can be identified before any discernable effects on fasting plasma glucose or glucose tolerance can be detected. As insulin resistance worsens, glucose homeostasis may become abnormal and impaired glucose tolerance develops. Marked fasting hyperinsulinemia is characteristic of this stage of the development of T2DM.[353] Impaired or deteriorating β-cell function leads to inadequate insulin secretion to compensate for the insulin resistance and glucose intolerance develops (see Chap. 21).

Impaired glucose tolerance (IGT) and impaired fasting glycemia (IFG) represent clinical stages in the development of T2DM. Both IGT and IFG predict the development of T2DM.[354–356] Data relating to IGT are more numerous, as it was first defined in 1979, whereas IFG was defined only in 1997.

IGT is associated with a high risk of developing T2DM.[357,358] Persons with IGT typically have relatively high BMI, fasting hyperinsulinemia, and various features of the metabolic syndrome. IGT can be considered a further stage in the development of T2DM as a high proportion of those with it progress to T2DM over a period of a few years, although such progression is not inevitable.[358] IGT is associated with a marked degree of insulin resistance and impaired insulin response to the challenge. Progression to T2DM from IGT is most often associated with further worsening of β-cell function and the further inability of insulin secretion to compensate for the insulin resistance.[359] Conversely, improvement in glucose tolerance may occur with weight loss, either

FIGURE 19-14 Stages and risk factors in the development of type 2 diabetes. (*Adapted from reference*[352])

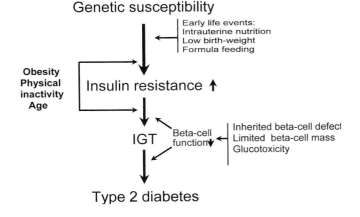

as a result of caloric restriction or increased physical activity, which reduces insulin resistance to the degree that insulin requirements fall so that the existing β-cell function is sufficient to improve glucose tolerance.

Impaired glucose tolerance is associated not only with an increased risk of diabetes, but with increased risks of cardiovascular disease (heart disease and stroke), possibly cancer, and increased total mortality.[360] The risks for cardiovascular disease are intermediate between those seen in persons with diabetes and those with normal glucsose tolerance, but the absolute risks associated with IGT vary from population to population.[361]

Much less is known about the prognostic significance of impaired fasting glucose. A few studies have demonstrated its ability to predict the development of T2DM,[354,356,362] and it is associated with increased risks of cardiovascular disease and mortality, although not to the same extent as IGT.[362,363]

Many persons with IGT do not have IFG and vice versa, and some have both. The dissociation in these two manifestations of impaired glucose regulation suggests that they have somewhat different pathophysiologic bases. Studies in persons with monogenic forms of diabetes suggest that IFG is associated with a greater liver glucose production and a larger β-cell insulin secretory defect than IGT.[359,364] Whether this is true in the general population remains to be established, but may be anticipated in view of the different glucose homeostatic mechanisms that control fasting glycemia and postprandial or post–glucose challenge hyperglycemia.

T2DM Prevention

The prevalence and incidence of T2DM have increased dramatically during the past 50 years in many countries. Countries such as Japan and India that used to have low prevalences now have rates that exceed those found in the United States and Europe. In the United States, the rates have increased considerably in the past 30 years and have continued to do so over the past decade.[256,365]

In 1962, the relatively high frequency of diabetes in populations was proposed to be the result of a "thrifty genotype."[366] As diabetes has a strong genetic basis, it was proposed that the high prevalence was the result of a genotype that had selective advantage at the time when human populations were subject to alternating cycles of feast and famine, but this genotype became deleterious, and gave rise to T2DM, once food supplies become abundant and periodic famines no longer occurred. The rapid increase in T2DM in the past century can only be attributed to changes in lifestyle, primarily increasing obesity and decreasing physical activity. Thus, the thrifty genotype hypothesis provides a plausible explanation of why a disease that has such strong genetic susceptibility determinants has increased markedly in frequency.

As important lifestyle factors have been identified and groups of persons at high risk are identifiable, several recent randomized controlled clinical trials have examined whether or not lifestyle intervention or pharmacologic interventions can reduce the incidence of T2DM.

Studies in DaQing, China, among 530 persons with IGT were the first to show that lifestyle interventions could reduce the rate of progression to diabetes.[367] The effects of diet alone, exercise alone, and both diet and exercise together reduced the incidence of diabetes by about 30% over a 6-year period compared to a control group who received only general lifestyle change recommendations. There was no significant difference among the three intervention groups.

A study from Finland also demonstrated that lifestyle changes reduced the incidence of T2DM among overweight individuals with IGT.[368] Specific dietary goals were given and a target of at least 30 minutes of exercise per day was set. Compared to the control group, who lost 0.8 kg over a 2-year period, the intervention group lost 3.5 kg. After an average of 3.2 years, the incidence of diabetes in the lifestyle intervention group was 58% lower than in the control groups.

A much larger multicenter study, the Diabetes Prevention Program (DPP),[369,370] was conducted in the United States among subjects with IGT and BMI ≥24 kg/m[2] or higher. This study showed a 58% reduction in the incidence of T2DM over a 3-year period in the lifestyle intervention group (Fig. 19-15).[371] One-third of the subjects were randomized to metformin treatment. This therapy resulted in a 31% lower incidence of T2DM, significantly less than in the placebo group, but the lifestyle intervention was significantly more effective overall than the metformin intervention.

Another multicenter study (STOP NIDDM), also among subjects with IGT, examined whether an α-glucosidase inhibitor, acabose, delayed (or prevented) the onset of T2DM.[372] This study reported a 25% reduction in the incidence of T2DM over a 3-year period. However, as the Finnish study, the DPP, and the STOP NIDDM trials were conducted in rather different ways, and the characteristics of the randomized individuals varied to some degree, direct comparisons of effectiveness cannot be made, except in the DPP, where a head-to-head comparison of lifestyle and metformin treatment was made.

Yet another intervention study (TRIPOD; Troglitazone in the Prevention of Diabetes) examined the effect of a thiazolidinedione, troglitazone, on the development of T2DM in women with previous gestational diabetes.[373] Although this trial was stopped prematurely because of the withdrawal of troglitazone from the market, a 50% reduction in the incidence of T2DM was seen compared to the placebo treatment. This trial, therefore, suggests that other thiazolidinedione drugs might also be effective in delaying or preventing the onset of T2DM. Such trials have recently been initiated.

Other pharmacologic agents may also reduce the incidence of T2DM. Secondary analyses of the WOSCOPS (West of Scotland Cardiovascular Disease Prevention Study)[374] and the HOPE (Heart Outcomes Prevention Evaluations) study[375] suggest that the incidence of T2DM may be lower in patients receiving a statin, pravis-

FIGURE 19-15. Results of the Diabetes Prevention Program: diabetes incidence was reduced in persons with impaired glucose tolerance randomized to metformin and to life-style intervention. *(Adapted from reference[371])*

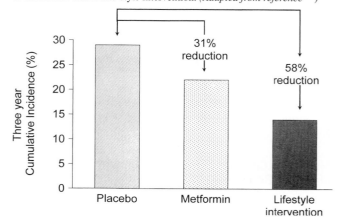

tatin, or ramipril, an angiotensin-converting enzyme inhibitor, than among those receiving placebo. Further trials are required to determine if this is indeed true.

REFERENCES

1. American Diabetes Association: Report of the Expert Committee on the Diagnosis and Classification of Diabetes Mellitus. *Diabetes Care* 1997;20:1183.
2. Alberti KG, Zimmet PZ: Definition, diagnosis and classification of diabetes mellitus and its complications. Part 1: Diagnosis and classification of diabetes mellitus provisional report of a WHO consultation. *Diabet Med* 1998;15:539.
3. Atkinson MA, Eisenbarth GS: Type 1 Diabetes: New perspectives on disease pathogenesis and treatment. *Lancet* 2001;358:221.
4. Imagawa A, Hanafusa T, Miyagawa J, *et al*: A novel subtype of type 1 diabetes mellitus characterized by a rapid onset and an absence of diabetes-related antibodies. Osaka IDDM Study Group. *N Engl J Med* 2000;342:301.
5. Rewers M, LaPorte RE, King H, *et al*: Trends in the prevalence and incidence of diabetes: Insulin-dependent diabetes mellitus in childhood. *World Health Stat Q* 1988;41:179.
6. Diabetes Epidemiology Research International Group: Secular trends in incidence of childhood IDDM in 10 countries. *Diabetes* 1990; 39:858.
7. Onkamo P, Vaananen S, Karvonen M, *et al*: Worldwide increase in incidence of type I diabetes—the analysis of the data on published incidence trends. *Diabetologia* 1999;42:1395.
8. Variation and trends in incidence of childhood diabetes in Europe. EURODIAB ACE Study Group. *Lancet* 2000;355:873.
9. Rewers M: The changing face of the epidemiology of insulin-dependent diabetes mellitus (IDDM): Research designs and models of disease causation. *Ann Med* 1991;23:419.
10. Libman I, Songer T, LaPorte R: How many people in the U.S. have IDDM? *Diabetes Care* 1993;16:841.
11. Songer TJ: Health services and costing in diabetes. *Med J Aust* 1990; 152:115.
12. Songer TJ, LaPorte R, Lave JR, *et al*: Health insurance and the financial impact of IDDM in families with a child with IDDM. *Diabetes Care* 1997;20:577.
13. Bottazzo GF, Florin-Christensen A, Doniach D: Islet-cell antibodies in diabetes mellitus with autoimmune polyendocrine deficiencies. *Lancet* 1974;2:1279.
14. Palmer JP, Asplin CM, Clemons P, *et al*: Insulin antibodies in insulin-dependent diabetics before insulin treatment. *Science* 1983;222:1337.
15. Vardi P, Dib SA, Tuttleman M, *et al*: Competitive insulin autoantibody assay. Prospective evaluation of subjects at high risk for development of type I diabetes mellitus. *Diabetes* 1987;36:1286.
16. Williams AJK, Bingley PJ, Bonifacio E, *et al*: A novel micro-assay for insulin autoantibodies. *J Autoimmun* 1997;10:473.
17. Baekkeskov S, Nielsen JH, Marner B, *et al*: Autoantibodies in newly diagnosed diabetic children immunoprecipitate specific human pancreatic islet cell proteins. *Nature* 1982;298:167.
18. Baekkeskov S, Aanstoot HJ, Christgau S, *et al*: Identification of the 64K autoantigen in insulin-dependent diabetes as the GABA-synthesizing enzyme glutamic acid decarboxylase [published erratum appears in *Nature* 1990 Oct 25;347(6295):782]. *Nature* 1990;347:151.
19. Rabin DU, Pleasic SM, Shapiro JA, *et al*: Islet cell antigen 512 is a diabetes-specific islet autoantigen related to protein tyrosine phosphatases. *J Immunol* 1994;152:3183.
20. Verge CF, Gianani R, Kawasaki E, *et al*: Prediction of type I diabetes in first-degree relatives using a combination of insulin, GAD, and ICA512bdc/IA-2 autoantibodies. *Diabetes* 1996;45:926.
21. Bingley PJ, Christie MR, Bonifacio E, *et al*: Combined analysis of autoantibodies improves prediction of IDDM in islet cell antibody-positive relatives. *Diabetes* 1994;43:1304.
22. Bingley PJ, Bonifacio E, Williams AJ, *et al*: Prediction of IDDM in the general population: Strategies based on combinations of autoantibody markers. *Diabetes* 1997;46:1701.
23. Rewers M, Kostraba JN: *Epidemiology of Type I diabetes*. In: Eisenbarth GS, Lafferty KJ, eds. *Type I Diabetes: Molecular, Cellular, and Clinical Immunology*. London: Oxford University Press; 1995.
24. Adojaan B, Knip M, Vahasalo P, *et al*: Relationship between the incidence of childhood IDDM and the frequency of ICA positivity in non-diabetic children in the general population. *Diabetes Care* 1996; 19:1452.
25. Rewers M, Norris JM, Eisenbarth GS, *et al*: Beta-cell autoantibodies in infants and toddlers without IDDM relatives: Diabetes Autoimmunity Study in the Young (DAISY). *J Autoimmun* 1996;9:405.
26. Kupila A, Muona P, Simell T, *et al*: Feasibility of genetic and immunological prediction of type I diabetes in a population-based birth cohort. *Diabetologia* 2001;44:290.
27. Kulmala P, Savola K, Petersen JS, *et al*: Prediction of insulin-dependent diabetes mellitus in siblings of children with diabetes. A population-based study. The Childhood Diabetes in Finland Study Group. *J Clin Invest* 1998;101:327.
28. Pilcher CC, Dickens K, Elliott RB: ICA only develop in early childhood. *Diabetes Res Clin Pract* 1991;14(suppl. 1):s82.
29. Yu J, Yu L, Bugawan TL, *et al*: Transient anti-islet autoantibodies: Infrequent occurrence and lack of association with genetic risk factors. *J Clin Endocrinol Metab* 2000;85:2421.
30. Lindberg BA, Ericsson UB, Kockum I, *et al*: Prevalence of beta-cell and thyroid autoantibody positivity in schoolchildren during three-year follow-up. *Autoimmunity* 1999;31:175.
31. Riley WJ, Maclaren NK, Krischer J, *et al*: A prospective study of the development of diabetes in relatives of patients with insulin-dependent diabetes. *New Engl J Med* 1990;323:1167.
32. Neufeld M, Maclaren NK, Riley WJ, *et al*: Islet cell and other organ-specific antibodies in U.S. Caucasians and blacks with insulin-dependent diabetes mellitus. *Diabetes* 1980;29:589.
33. Zimmet PZ, Rowley MJ, Mackay IR, *et al*: The ethnic distribution of antibodies to glutamic acid decarboxylase: Presence and levels of insulin-dependent diabetes mellitus in Europid and Asian subjects. *J Diabetes Complications* 1993;7:1.
34. Erlich HA, Griffith RL, Bugawan TL, *et al*: Implications of specific DQB1 alleles in genetic susceptibility and resistance by identification of IDDM siblings with novel HLA-DQB1 allele and unusual DR2 and DR1 haplotypes. *Diabetes* 1991;40:478.
35. Pugliese A, Gianani R, Moromisato R, *et al*: HLA-DQB1*0602 is associated with dominant protection from diabetes even among islet cell antibody-positive first-degree relatives of patients with IDDM. *Diabetes* 1995;44:608.
36. Huang W, She JX, Muir A, *et al*: High risk HLA-DR/DQ genotypes for IDD confer susceptibility to autoantibodies but DQB1*0602 does not prevent them. *J Autoimmun* 1994;7:889.
37. Greenbaum CJ, Cuthbertson D, Eisenbarth GS, *et al*: Islet cell antibody positive relatives with HLA-DQA1*0102, DQB1*0602: Identification by the Diabetes Prevention Trial-1. *J Clin Endocrinol Metab* 2000;85:1255.
38. Chase HP, Voss MA, Butler-Simon N, *et al*: Diagnosis of pre-type J diabetes. *J Pediatr* 1987;111:807.
39. Maclaren N, Horne G, Spillar R, *et al*: The feasibility of using ICA to predict IDDM in US school children. *Diabetes* 1990;39(suppl.1):122A.
40. Levy-Marchal C, Tichet J, Fajardy I, *et al*: Follow-up of children from a background population with high ICA titres. *Diabetologia* 1992: 35(suppl 1):A32.
41. Owerbach D, Gabbay KH: Localization of a type I diabetes susceptibility locus to the variable tandem repeat region flanking the insulin gene. *Diabetes* 1993;42:1708.
42. Davies JL, Kawaguchi Y, Bennett ST, *et al*: A genome-wide search for human type 1 diabetes susceptibility genes. *Nature* 1994;371:130.
43. Hashimoto L, Habita C, Beressi JP, *et al*: Genetic mapping of a susceptibility locus for insulin-dependent diabetes mellitus on chromosome 11q. *Nature* 1994;371:161.
44. Owerbach D, Gabbay KH: The HOXD8 locus (2q31) is linked to type I diabetes: Interaction with chromosome 6 and 11 disease susceptibility genes. *Diabetes* 1995;44:132.
45. Field LL, Tobias R, Magnus T: A locus on chromosome 15q26(IDDM3) produces susceptibility to insulin-dependent diabetes mellitus. *Nat Genet* 1996;8:189.
46. Copeman JB, Cucca F, Hearne CM, *et al*: Linkage disequilibrium mapping of type 1 diabetes susceptibility gene (IDDM7) to chromosome 2q31–q33. *Nat Genet* 1995;9:80.
47. Cox NJ, Wapelhorst B, Morrison VA, *et al*: Seven regions of the genome show evidence of linkage to type 1 diabetes in a consensus analysis of 767 multiplex families. *Am J Hum Genet* 2001;69:820.

48. Oldstone MB, Nerenberg M, Southern P, et al: Virus infection triggers insulin-dependent diabetes mellitus in a transgenic model: Role of anti-self (virus) immune response. Cell 1991;65:319.

49. Ohashi PS, Oehen S, Buerki K, et al: Ablation of "tolerance" and induction of diabetes by virus infection in viral antigen transgenic mice. Cell 1991;65:305.

50. Helmke K, Otten A, Willems WR, et al: Islet cell antibodies and the development of diabetes mellitus in relation to mumps infection and mumps vaccination. Diabetologia 1986;29:30.

51. Bodansky HJ, Dean BM, Bottazzo GF, et al: Islet-cell antibodies and insulin autoantibodies in association with common viral infections. Lancet 1986;Dec 13:1351.

52. Champsaur HF, Bottazzo GF, Bertrams J, et al: Virologic, immunologic, and genetic factors in insulin-dependent diabetes mellitus. J Pediatr 1982;100:15.

53. Uriarte A, Cabrera E, Ventura R, et al: Islet cell antibodies and ECHO-4 virus infection. Diabetologia 1987;30:590A.

54. Honeyman MC, Coulson BS, Stone NL, et al: Association between rotavirus infection and pancreatic islet autoimmunity in children at risk of developing type 1 diabetes. Diabetes 2000;49:1319.

55. Ginsberg-Fellner F, Witt ME, Yagihashi S, et al: Congenital rubella syndrome as a model for type 1 (insulin-dependent) diabetes mellitus: Increased prevalence of islet cell surface antibodies. Diabetologia 1984;27(suppl):87.

56. Kewers M, Atkinson M. The possible role of enteroviruses in diabetes mellitus. In: Rotbart H. ed. Human enterovirus Infections. Washington DC: American Society for Microbiology: 1995:353–385.

57. Kaufmann DL, Erlander MG, Clare-Salzler M, et al: Autoimmunity to two forms of glutamate decarboxylase in insulin-dependent diabetes mellitus. J Clin Invest 1992;89:283.

58. Scherbaum WA, Hampl W, Muir P, et al: No association between islet cell antibodies and Coxsackie B, mumps, rubella and cytomegalovirus antibodies in non-diabetic individuals aged 7–19 years. Diabetologia 1991;34:835.

59. Hyoty H, Hiltunen M, Knip M, et al: A prospective study of the role of Coxsackie B and other enterovirus infections in the pathogenesis of IDDM. Childhood Diabetes in Finland (DiMe) Study Group. Diabetes 1995;44:652.

60. Lonnrot M, Korpela K, Knip M, et al: Enterovirus infection as a risk factor for beta-cell autoimmunity in a prospectively observed birth cohort: The Finnish Diabetes Prediction and Prevention Study. Diabetes 2000;49:1314.

61. Lonnrot M, Salminen K, Knip M, et al: Enterovirus RNA in serum is a risk factor for beta-cell autoimmunity and clinical type 1 diabetes: A prospective study. Childhood Diabetes in Finland (DiMe) Study Group. J Med Virol 2000;61:214.

62. Atkinson MA, Winter WE, Skordis N, et al: Dietary protein restriction reduces the frequency and delays the onset of insulin dependent diabetes in BB rats. Autoimmunity 1988;2:11.

63. Martin JM, Trink B, Daneman D, et al: Milk proteins in the etiology of insulin-dependent diabetes mellitus (IDDM). Ann Med 1991; 23:447.

64. Atkinson MA, Bowman MA, Kuo-Jang K, et al: Lack of immune responsiveness to bovine serum albumin in insulin-dependent diabetes. N Engl J Med 1993;329:1853.

65. Dowse GD, Zimmet PZ, Finch CF, et al: Decline in incidence of epidemic glucose intolerance in Nauruans: Implications for the "thrifty genotype." Am J Epidemiol 1991;133:1093.

66. Martin S, Lampasona V, Dosch M, et al: Islet cell autoantigen 69 antibodies in IDDM. Diabetologia 1996;39:747.

67. Krokowski M, Caillat-Zucman S, Timsit J, et al: Anti-bovine serum albumin antibodies: Genetic heterogeneity and clinical relevance in adult-onset IDDM. Diabetes Care 1995;18:170.

68. Norris JM, Beaty B, Klingensmith G, et al: Lack of association between early exposure to cow's milk protein and beta-cell autoimmunity: Diabetes Autoimmunity Study in the Young (DAISY). JAMA 1996.

69. Virtanen SM, Hypponen E, Laara E, et al: Cow's milk consumption, disease-associated autoantibodies and type 1 diabetes mellitus: A follow-up study in siblings of diabetic children. Childhood Diabetes in Finland Study Group. Diabet Med 1998;15:730.

70. Couper JJ, Steele C, Beresford S, et al: Lack of association between duration of breast-feeding or introduction of cow's milk and development of islet autoimmunity. Diabetes 1999;48:2145.

71. Elliott RB, Harris DP, Hill JP, et al: Type I (insulin-dependent) diabetes mellitus and cow milk: Casein variant consumption. Diabetologia 1999;42:292.

72. Elias D, Prigozin H, Polak N, et al: Autoimmune diabetes induced by the beta-cell toxin STZ. Immunity to the 60-kDa heat shock protein and to insulin. Diabetes 1994;43:992.

73. Rayfield EJ, Ishimura K: Environmental factors and insulin dependent diabetes mellitus. Diabetes Metab Rev 1987;3:925.

74. Toniolo A, Onodera T, Yoon JW, et al: Induction of diabetes by cumulative environmental insults from viruses and chemicals. Nature 1980; 288:383.

75. Norris JM, Beaty B, Klingensmith G, et al: Lack of association between early exposure to cow's milk protein and β-cell autoimmunity: Diabetes Autoimmunity Study in the Young (DAISY). JAMA 1996; 276:609.

76. Notkins AL, Yoon JW: Virus-induced diabetes in mice prevented by a live attenuated vaccine. N Engl J Med 1982;306:486.

77. See DM, Tilles JG: WIN 54954 treatment of mice infected with a diabetogenic strain of group B Coxsackievirus. Antimicrob Agents Chemother 1993;37:1593.

78. Paronen J, Knip M, Savilahti E, et al: Effect of cow's milk exposure and maternal type 1 diabetes on cellular and humoral immunization to dietary insulin in infants at genetic risk for type 1 diabetes. Finnish Trial to Reduce IDDM in the Genetically at Risk Study Group. Diabetes 2000;49:1657.

79. Bonifacio E, Bingley PJ, Shattock M, et al: Quantification of islet-cell antibodies and prediction of insulin-dependent diabetes. Lancet 1990; 335:147.

80. Johnston C, Millward BA, Hoskins P, et al: Islet-cell antibodies as predictors of the later development of type 1 (insulin-dependent) diabetes. A study in identical twins. Diabetologia 1989;32:382.

81. McCulloch DK, Palmer JP: The appropriate use of β-cell function testing in the preclinical period of type 1 diabetes. Diabet Med 1991;8:800.

82. Spinas GA, Matter L, Wilkin T, et al: Islet-cell and insulin antibodies in first-degree relatives of type I diabetics: A 5-year follow-up study in a Swiss population. Adv Exp Med Biol 1988;246:209.

83. Thivolet C, Beaufrere B, Betuel H, et al: Islet cell and insulin autoantibodies in subjects at high risk for development of type 1 (insulin-dependent) diabetes mellitus: The Lyon family study. Diabetologia 1988;31:741.

84. Landin-Olsson M, Palmer JP, Lernmark A, et al: Predictive value of islet cell and insulin autoantibodies for type 1 (insulin-dependent) diabetes mellitus in a population-based study of newly diagnosed diabetic and matched control children. Diabetologia 1992;35:1068.

85. Karjalainen JK: Islet cell antibodies as predictive markers for IDDM in children with high background incidence of disease. Diabetes 1990;39:1144.

86. Groop LC, Bottazzo GF, Doniach D: Islet cell antibodies identify latent type I diabetes in patients aged 35–75 years at diagnosis. Diabetes 1986;35:237.

87. Tuomi T, Groop LC, Zimmet PZ, et al: Antibodies to glutamic acid decarboxylase reveal latent autoimmune diabetes mellitus in adults with a non-insulin-dependent onset of disease. Diabetes 1993;42: 359.

88. Zimmet PZ, Tuomi T, Mackay IR, et al: Latent autoimmune diabetes mellitus in adults (LADA): The role of antibodies to glutamic acid decarboxylase in diagnosis and prediction of insulin dependency. Diabet Med 1994;11:299.

89. Eisenbarth GS, Verge CF, Allen H, et al: The design of trials for prevention of IDDM. Diabetes 1993;42:941.

90. Bingley PJ, Bonifacio E, Ziegler AG, et al: Proposed guidelines on screening for risk of type 1 diabetes. Diabetes Care. 2001;24:398.

91. Schatz DA, Bingley PJ: Update on major trials for the prevention of type 1 diabetes mellitus: The American Diabetes Prevention Trial (DPT-1) and the European Nicotinamide Diabetes Intervention Trial (ENDIT). J Pediatr Endocrinol Metab 2001;14(Suppl 1):619.

92. Silverstein J, Maclaren N, Riley W, et al: Immunosuppression with azathioprine and prednisone in recent-onset insulin-dependent diabetes mellitus. New Engl J Med 1988;319:599.

93. Lipton R, LaPorte RE, Becker DJ, et al: Cyclosporin therapy for prevention and cure of IDDM. Epidemiological perspective of benefits and risks. Diabetes Care 1990;13:776.

94. Mahon JL, Dupre J, Stiller CR, et al: Immunosuppression in IDDM. Rationale, risks, benefits, and strategies. Diabetes Care 1990;13:806.

95. Gale EA: Theory and practice of nicotinamide trials in pre-type 1 diabetes. *J Pediatr Endocrinol Metab* 1996;9:375.

96. Knip M, Douek IF, Moore WP, *et al*: Safety of high-dose nicotinamide: A review. *Diabetologia* 2000;43:1337.

97. Lampeter EF, Klinghammer A, Scherbaum WA, *et al*: The Deutsche Nicotinamide Intervention Study: An attempt to prevent type 1 diabetes. DENIS Group. *Diabetes* 1998;47:980.

98. Keller RJ, Eisenbarth GS, Jackson RA: Insulin prophylaxis in individuals at high risk of type I diabetes. *Lancet* 1993;341:927.

99. The Diabetes Prevention Trial. Type 1 diabetes (DPT-1): Implementation of screening and staging of relatives. DPT-1 Study Group. *Transplant Proc* 1995;27:3377.

100. Pozzilli P, Pitocco D, Visalli N, *et al*: No effect of oral insulin on residual beta-cell function in recent-onset type I diabetes (the IMDIAB VII). IMDIAB Group [in process citation]. *Diabetologia* 2000;43:1000.

101. Chaillous L, Lefevre H, Thivolet C, *et al*: Oral insulin administration and residual beta-cell function in recent-onset type 1 diabetes: A multicentre randomised controlled trial. *Lancet* 2000;356:545.

102. Hamman RF, Cook M, Keefer S, *et al*: Medical care patterns at the onset of insulin-dependent diabetes mellitus: Association with severity and subsequent complications. *Diabetes Care* 1985;8(suppl 1):94.

103. Karjalajnen S, Salema P, Ilonen J.: A comparison of childhood and adult type 1 diabetes mellitus. *N Engl J Med* 1989;320:881.

104. Levy-Marchal C, Papoz L, de Beaufort C, *et al*: Clinical and laboratory features of type I diabetic children at time of diagnosis. *Diabet Med* 1992;9:279.

105. Pinkney JH, Bingley PJ, Sawtell PA, *et al*: Presentation and progress of childhood diabetes mellitus: A prospective population-based study. *Diabetologia* 1994;37:70.

106. Eberhardt MS, Wagener DK, Orchard TJ, *et al*: HLA heterogeneity of insulin-dependent diabetes mellitus at diagnosis. The Pittsburgh IDDM Study. *Diabetes* 1985;34:1247.

107. Foulis AK, Liddle CN, Farquharson MA, *et al*: The histopathology of the pancreas in type I diabetes (insulin dependent) mellitus: A 25-year review of deaths in patients under 20 years of age in the United Kingdom. *Diabetologia* 1986;29:267.

108. Childhood Diabetes Research Committee, Polish Diabetes Research Group, The Netherlands Institute for Preventive Health Care, *et al*: How frequently do children die at the onset of insulin-dependent diabetes? Analyses of registry data from Japan, Poland, the Netherlands, and Allegheny County, Pennsylvania. *Diabetes Nutr Metab* 1990;3:57.

109. Kostraba JN, Gay EC, Rewers M, *et al*: Increasing trend of outpatient management of children with newly diagnosed IDDM. Colorado IDDM registry, 1978–88. *Diabetes Care* 1992;15:95.

110. Diabetes Epidemiology Research International Group: Geographic patterns of childhood insulin-dependent diabetes mellitus. *Diabetes* 1988;37:1113.

111. Green A, Gale EAM, Patterson CC: Incidence of childhood-onset insulin-dependent diabetes mellitus: The EURODIAB ACE Study. *Lancet* 1992;339:905.

112. Karvonen M, Viik-Kajander M, Moltchanova E, *et al*: Incidence of childhood type 1 diabetes worldwide. Diabetes Mondiale (DiaMond) Project Group. *Diabetes Care* 2000;23:1516.

113. Tajima N, LaPorte RE, Hibi I, *et al*: A comparison of the epidemiology of youth-onset insulin-dependent diabetes mellitus between Japan and the United States (Allegheny County, Pennsylvania). *Diabetes Care* 1985;8(suppl 1):17.

114. Rewers M, Stone RA, LaPorte RE, *et al*: Poisson regression modeling of temporal variation in incidence of childhood insulin-dependent diabetes mellitus in Allegheny County, Pennsylvania, and Wielkopolska, Poland, 1970–1985. *Am J Epidemiol* 1989;129:569.

115. Pinhas-Hamiel O, Dolan LM, Daniels SR, *et al*: Increased incidence of non-insulin-dependent diabetes mellitus among adolescents. *J Pediatr* 1996;128:(part 1):608.

116. Dabelea D, Hanson RL, Bennett PH, *et al*: Increasing prevalence of Type II diabetes in American Indian children. *Diabetologia* 1998;41:904.

117. Cornell CN, Stankiewicz W, Asher D, *et al*: Absence of islet autoantibodies at diabetes onset does not rule out type 1a diabetes. *Diabetes* 2000;49(suppl 1):A68.

118. Siemiatycki J, Colle E, Campbell S, *et al*: Case-control study of IDDM. *Diabetes Care* 1989;12:209.

119. Joner G, Sovik O: The incidence of type 1 (insulin-dependent) diabetes mellitus 15–29 years in Norway 1978–1982. *Diabetologia* 1991;34:271.

120. Christau B, Kromann H, Andersen OO, *et al*: Incidence, seasonal and geographic patterns of juvenile-onset insulin-dependent diabetes mellitus is Denmark. *Diabetologia* 1997;13:281.

121. Melton LJ III, Palumbo PJ, Chu CP: Incidence of diabetes mellitus by clinical type. *Diabetes Care* 1983;6:75.

122. Turner R, Stratton I, Horton V, *et al*: UKPDS 25: Autoantibodies to islet-cell cytoplasm and glutamic acid decarboxylase for prediction of insulin requirement in type 2 diabetes. UK Prospective Diabetes Study Group [published erratum appears in *Lancet* 1998;351:376]. *Lancet* 1997;350:1288.

123. Horton V, Stratton I, Bottazzo GF, *et al*: Genetic heterogeneity of autoimmune diabetes: Age of presentation in adults is influenced by HLA DRB1 and DQB1 genotypes (UKPDS 43). UK Prospective Diabetes Study (UKPDS) Group. *Diabetologia* 1999;42:608.

124. Gale EA, Gillespie KM: Diabetes and gender. *Diabetologia* 2001; 44:3.

125. Karvonen M, Pitkaniemi M, Pitkaniemi J, *et al*: Sex difference in the incidence of insulin-dependent diabetes mellitus: An analysis of the recent epidemiological data. World Health Organization DIAMOND Project Group. *Diabetes Metab Rev* 1997;13:275.

126. Green A, Hauge M, Holm NV, *et al*: Epidemiological studies of diabetes mellitus in Denmark. II. A prevalence study based on insulin prescriptions. *Diabetologia* 1981;20:468.

127. Bruno G, Merletti F, Vuolo A, *et al*: Sex differences in incidence of IDDM in age group 15–29 yr. Higher risk in males in Province of Turin, Italy. *Diabetes Care* 1993;16:133.

128. Roglic G, Pavlic-Renar I, Sestan-Crnek S, *et al*: Incidence of IDDM during 1988–1992 in Zagreb, Croatia. *Diabetologia* 1995;38: 550.

129. Vandewalle CL, Coeckelberghs MI, De Leeuw IH, *et al*: Epidemiology, clinical aspects, and biology of IDDM patients under age 40 years. Comparison of data from Antwerp with complete ascertainment with data from Belgium with 40% ascertainment. The Belgian Diabetes Registry. *Diabetes Care* 1997;20:1556.

130. Ustvedt HJ, Olsen E: Incidence of diabetes mellitus in Oslo, Norway 1956–65. *Br J Prev Soc Med* 1977;31:251.

131. Risch N, Ghosh S, Todd JA: Statistical evaluation of multiple-locus linkage data in experimental species and its relevance to human studies: Application to nonobese diabetic (NOD) mouse and human insulin-dependent diabetes mellitus (IDDM). *Am J Hum Genet* 1993; 53:702.

132. Gamble DR: The epidemiology of insulin-dependent diabetes, with particular reference to the relationship of virus infection to its etiology. *Epidemiol Rev* 1980;2:49.

133. Kostraba JN, Gay EC, Cai Y, *et al*: Incidence of insulin-dependent diabetes mellitus in Colorado. *Epidemiology* 1992;3:232.

134. Dahlquist G, Gustavsson KH, Holmgren G, *et al*: The incidence of diabetes mellitus in Swedish children 0–14 years of age. A prospective study 1977–1980. *Acta Paediatr Scand* 1982;71:7.

135. Weinberg CR, Dornan TL, Hansen JA, *et al*: HLA-related heterogeneity in seasonal patterns of diagnosis in type I (insulin-dependent) diabetes. *Diabetologia* 1984;26:199.

136. Ludvigsson J, Afoke AO: Seasonality of type 1 (insulin-dependent) diabetes mellitus: Values of C-peptide, insulin antibodies and haemoglobin A1c show evidence of a more rapid loss of insulin secretion in epidemic patients. *Diabetologia* 1989;32:84.

137. Rewers M, LaPorte R, Walczak M, *et al*: Apparent epidemic of insulin-dependent diabetes mellitus in midwestern Poland. *Diabetes* 1987;36:106.

138. Nystrom L, Dahlquist G, Rewers M, *et al*: The Swedish childhood diabetes study: An analysis of the temporal variation in diabetes incidence, 1978–1987. *Int J Epidemiol* 1990;19:141.

139. Tuomilehto J, Rewers M, Reunanen A, *et al*: Increasing trend in type I (insulin-dependent) diabetes mellitus in childhood in Finland. Analysis of age, calendar time, and birth cohort effects during 1965 to 1984. *Diabetologia* 1991;34:282.

140. Serdula MK, Mokdad AH, Williamson DF, *et al*: Prevalence of attempting weight loss and strategies for controlling weight. *JAMA* 1999;282:1353.

141. Dokheel TM: An epidemic of childhood diabetes in the United States? *Diabetes Care* 1993;16:1606.

142. Karvonen M, Pitkaniemi J, Tuomilehto J: The onset age of type 1 diabetes in Finnish children has become younger. The Finnish Childhood Diabetes Registry Group. *Diabetes Care* 1999;22:1066.

143. Rosenbauer J, Herzig P, von Kries R, et al: Temporal, seasonal, and geographical incidence patterns of type I diabetes mellitus in children under 5 years of age in Germany. *Diabetologia* 1999;42:1055.

144. Cinek O, Lanska V, Kolouskova S, et al: Type 1 diabetes mellitus in Czech children diagnosed in 1990–1997: A significant increase in incidence and male predominance in the age group 0–4 years. Collaborators of the Czech Childhood Diabetes Registry. *Diabet Med* 2000;17:64.

145. Gardner SG, Bingley PJ, Sawtell PA, et al: Rising incidence of insulin dependent diabetes in children aged under 5 years in the Oxford region: Time trend analysis. The Bart's-Oxford Study Group. *BMJ* 1997;315:713.

146. Schoenle EJ, Lang-Muritano M, Gschwend S, et al: Epidemiology of type I diabetes mellitus in Switzerland: Steep rise in incidence in under 5 year old children in the past decade. *Diabetologia* 2001; 44:286.

147. Cordell HJ, Todd JA: Multifactorial inheritance in type 1 diabetes. *Trends Genet* 1995;11:499.

148. Viskari HR, Koskela P, Lonnrot M, et al: Can enterovirus infections explain the increasing incidence of type 1 diabetes? *Diabetes Care* 2000;23:414.

149. Wagener DK, Sacks JM, LaPorte RE, et al: The Pittsburgh study of insulin-dependent diabetes mellitus. Risk for diabetes among relatives of IDDM. *Diabetes* 1982;31:136.

150. Allen C, Palta M, D'Alessio DJ: Risk of diabetes in siblings and other relatives of IDDM subjects. *Diabetes* 1991;40:831.

151. Lorenzen T, Pociot F, Hougaard P, et al: Long-term risk of IDDM in first-degree relatives of patients with IDDM. *Diabetologia* 1994; 37:321.

152. O'Leary LA, Dorman JS, LaPorte RE, et al: Familial and sporadic insulin-dependent diabetes: Evidence for heterogeneous etiologies? *Diabetes Res Clin Pract* 1991;14:183.

153. Bertrams J, Baur MP: Insulin-dependent diabetes mellitus. In: Albert ED, ed. *Histocompatibility Testing 1984*. Springer-Verlag; 1984.

154. Todd JA: The role of MHC class II genes in susceptibility to insulin-dependent diabetes mellitus. *Curr Top Microbiol Immunol* 1990; 164:17.

155. Kaprio J, Tuomilehto J, Koskenvuo M, et al: Concordance for type 1 (insulin-dependent) and type 2 (non-insulin-dependent) diabetes mellitus in a population-based cohort of twins in Finland. *Diabetologia* 1992;35:1060.

156. Pak CY, Hyone-Myong E, McArthur RG, et al: Association of cytomegalovirus infection with autoimmune type 1 diabetes. *Lancet* 1988; 2:1.

157. Sairenji T, Daibata M, Sorli CH: Relating homology between the Epstein-Barr virus BOLF1 and HLA-DQw8 beta chain to recent onset type 1 (insulin-dependent) diabetes mellitus. *Diabetologia* 1991;34:33.

158. Hyoty H, Hiltunen M, Reunanen A, et al: Decline of mumps antibodies in type 1 (insulin-dependent) diabetic children and a plateau in the rising incidence of type 1 diabetes after introduction of the mumps-measles-rubella vaccine in Finland. Childhood Diabetes in Finland Study Group. *Diabetologia* 1993;36:1303.

159. Menser MA, Forrest JM, Bransby RD: Rubella infection and diabetes mellitus. *Lancet* 1978;1:57.

160. Suenaga K, Yoon JW: Association of beta-cell specific expression of endogenous retrovirus with development of insulitis and diabetes in NOD mouse. *Diabetes* 1988;37:1722.

161. Conrad B, Weidmann E, Trucco G, et al: Evidence for superantigen involvement in insulin-dependent diabetes mellitus aetiology. *Nature* 1994;371:351.

162. Blom L, Nystrom L, Dahlquist G: The Swedish childhood diabetes study. Vaccinations and infections as risk determinants for diabetes in childhood. *Diabetologia* 1991;34:176.

163. Karounos DG, Wolinsky JS, Thomas JW: Monoclonal antibody to rubella virus capsid protein recognizes a β-cell antigen. *J Immunol* 1993;150:3080.

164. Graves PM, Norris JM, Pallansch MA, et al: The role of enteroviral infections in the development of IDDM: Limitations of current approaches. *Diabetes* 1997;46:161.

165. Jenson AB, Rosenberg HS, Notkins AL: Pancreatic islet-cell damage in children with fatal viral infections. *Lancet* 1980; Aug 16:354.

166. Yoon JW, Austin M, Onodera T, et al: Virus-induced diabetes mellitus: Isolation of a virus from the pancreas of a child with diabetic ketoacidosis. *N Engl J Med* 1979;300:1173.

167. Donsky J, Massad R: Community medicine in the training of family physicians. *J Fam Pract* 1979;8:965.

168. Wagenknecht LE, Roseman JM, Herman WH: Increased incidence of insulin-dependent diabetes mellitus following an epidemic of Coxsackievirus B5. *Am J Epidemiol* 1991;133:1024.

169. Kaufman DL, Clare-Salzler M, Tian J, et al: Spontaneous loss of T-cell tolerance to glutamic acid decarboxylase in murine insulin-dependent diabetes. *Nature* 1993;366:69.

170. Dahlquist G, Frisk G, Ivarsson SA, et al: Indications that maternal Coxsackie B virus infection during pregnancy is a risk factor for childhood-onset IDDM. *Diabetologia* 1995;38:1371.

171. Dahlquist GG: Viruses and other perinatal exposures as initiating events for beta-cell destruction. *Ann Med* 1997;29:413.

172. McKinney PA, Parslow R, Gurney KA, et al: Perinatal and neonatal determinants of childhood type 1 diabetes. A case-control study in Yorkshire, U.K. *Diabetes Care* 1999;22:928.

173. Dahlquist G, Kallen B: Maternal–child blood group incompatibility and other perinatal events increase the risk of early-onset type 1 (insulin-dependent) diabetes mellitus. *Diabetologia* 1992;35:671.

174. Blom L, Dahlquist G, Nystrom L, et al: The Swedish childhood diabetes study—social and perinatal determinants for diabetes in childhood. *Diabetologia* 1989;32:7.

175. Bache I, Bock T, Volund A, et al: Previous maternal abortion, longer gestation, and younger material age decrease the risk of type 1 diabetes among male offspring. *Diabetes Care* 1999;22:1063.

176. Bock T, Pedersen CR, Volund A, et al: Perinatal determinants among children who later develop IDDM. *Diabetes Care* 1994;17:1154.

177. Patterson CC, Carson DJ, Hadden DR, et al: A case-control investigation of perinatal risk factors for childhood IDDM in northern Ireland and Scotland. *Diabetes Care* 1994;17:376.

178. Rothwell PM, Staines A, Smail P, et al: Seasonality of birth of patients with childhood diabetes in Britain. *Br Med J* 1996;312:1456.

179. Oldstone MB: Viruses as therapeutic agents. I. Treatment of nonobese insulin-dependent diabetes mice with virus prevents insulin-dependent diabetes mellitus while maintaining general immune competence. *J Exp Med* 1990;171:2077.

180. Wilberz S, Partke HJ, Dagnaes-Hansen F, et al: Persistent MHV (mouse hepatitis virus) infection reduces the incidence of diabetes mellitus in non-obese diabetic mice. *Diabetologia* 1991;34:2.

181. Like AA, Guberski DL, Butler L: Influence of environmental viral agents on frequency and tempo of diabetes mellitus in BB/Wor rats. *Diabetes* 1991;40:259.

182. Kolb H, Elliot RB: Increasing incidence of IDDM a consequence of improved hygiene? *Diabetologia* 1994;37:729.

183. McKinney PA, Okasha M, Parslow RC, et al: Early social mixing and childhood type 1 diabetes mellitus: A case-control study in Yorkshire, UK. *Diabet Med* 2000;17:236.

184. EURODIAB Substudy 2 Study Group. Infections and vaccinations as risk factors for childhood type 1 (insulin-dependent) diabetes mellitus: A multicentre case-control investigation. *Diabetologia* 2000; 43:47.

185. Dahlquist G, Gothefors L: The cumulative incidence of childhood diabetes mellitus in Sweden unaffected by BCG-vaccination. *Diabetologia* 1995;38:873.

186. Heijbel H, Chen RT, Dahlquist G: Cumulative incidence of childhood-onset IDDM is unaffected by pertussis immunization. *Diabetes Care* 1997;20:173.

187. Childhood immunization and type 1 diabetes: Summary of an Institute for Vaccine Safety Workshop. The Institute for Vaccine Safety Diabetes Workshop Panel. *Pediatr Infect Dis J* 1999;18:217.

188. Lindberg B, Ahlfors K, Carlsson A, et al: Previous exposure to measles, mumps, and rubella—but not vaccination during adolescence—correlates to the prevalence of pancreatic and thyroid autoantibodies. *Pediatrics* 1999;104:e12.

189. Graves PM, Barriga KJ, Norris JM, et al: Lack of association between early childhood immunizations and beta-cell autoimmunity. *Diabetes Care* 1999;22:1694.

190. Hummel M, Fuchtenbusch M, Schenker M, et al: No major association of breast-feeding, vaccinations, and childhood viral diseases with early islet autoimmunity in the German BABYDIAB Study. *Diabetes Care* 2000;23:969.

191. Borsch-Johnsen K, Joner G, Mandrup-Poulsen T, et al: Relation between breast-feeding and incidence rates of insulin-dependent diabetes mellitus. *Lancet* 1984;2:1083.

192. Mayer EJ, Hamman RF, Gay EC, et al: Reduced risk of IDDM among breast-fed children. The Colorado IDDM Registry. *Diabetes* 1988; 37:1625.

193. Kostraba JN, Dorman JS, LaPorte RE, *et al*: Early infant diet and risk of IDDM in blacks and whites. A matched case-control study. *Diabetes Care* 1992;15:626.

194. Nigro G, Campea L, De Novellis A, *et al*: Breast-feeding and insulin-dependent diabetes mellitus. *Lancet* 1985;1:467.

195. Blom L, Dahlquist G, Nystrom L, *et al*: The Swedish childhood diabetes study—social and perinatal determinants for diabetes in childhood. *Diabetologia* 1989;32:7.

196. Kyvik KO, Green A, Svendsen A, *et al*: Breast feeding and the development of type I diabetes mellitus. *Diabet Med* 1992;9:233.

197. Samuelsson U, Johansson C, Ludvigsson J: Breast-feeding seems to play a marginal role in the prevention of insulin-dependent diabetes mellitus. *Diabetes Res Clin Pract* 1993;19:203.

198. Virtanen SM, Rasanen L, Aro A, *et al*: Feeding in infancy and the risk of type 1 diabetes mellitus in Finnish children. *Diabet Med* 1992;9:815.

199. Gerstein HC: Cow's milk exposure and type I diabetes mellitus—a critical overview of the clinical literature. *Diabetes Care* 1994;17:13.

200. Savilahti E, Akerblom HK, Tainio VM, *et al*: Children with newly diagnosed insulin dependent diabetes mellitus have increased levels of cow's milk antibodies. *Diabetes Res* 1988;7:137.

201. Karjalainen J, Martin JM, Knip M, *et al*: A bovine albumin peptide as a possible trigger of insulin-dependent diabetes mellitus. *N Engl J Med* 1992;327:302.

202. Virtanen SM, Laara E, Hypponen E, *et al*: Cow's milk consumption, HLA-DQB1 genotype, and type 1 diabetes: A nested case-control study of siblings of children with diabetes. Childhood diabetes in Finland study group [in process citation]. *Diabetes* 2000;49:912.

203. Helgason T, Jonasson MR: Evidence for a food additive as a cause of ketosis-prone diabetes. *Lancet* 1981;2:716.

204. Dahlquist GG, Blom LG, Persson LÅ, *et al*: Dietary factors and the risk of developing insulin dependent diabetes in childhood. *Br Med J* 1990;300:1302.

205. Kostraba JN, Gay EC, Rewers M, *et al*: Nitrate levels in community drinking waters and risk of IDDM. *Diabetes Care* 1992;15:1505.

206. Pont A, Rubino JM, Bishop D: Diabetes mellitus and neuropathy following Vacor ingestion in man. *Arch Intern Med* 1979;139:185.

207. Khoury MJ, Flanders WD, Greenland S, *et al*: On the measurement of susceptibility in epidemiologic studies. *Am J Epidemiol* 1989;129:183.

208. Fohlman J, Bohme J, Rask L, *et al*: Matching of host genotype and seotypes of Coxsackie B virus in the development of juvenile diabetes. *Scand J Immunol* 1987;26:105.

209. D'Alessio DJ: A case-control study of group B Coxsackievirus immunoglobulin M antibody prevalence and HLA-DR antigens in newly diagnosed cases of insulin-dependent diabetes mellitus. *Am J Epidemiol* 1992;135:1331.

210. Schernthaner G, Banatvala JE, Scherbaum W, *et al*: Coxsackie-B-virus-specific IgM reponses, complement-fixing islet-cell antibodies, HLA DR antigens, and C-peptide secretion in insulin-dependent diabetes mellitus. *Lancet* 1985;2:630.

211. Kostraba JN, Cruickshanks KJ, Lawler-Heavner J, *et al*: Early exposure to cow's milk and solid foods in infancy, genetic predisposition and risk of IDDM. *Diabetes* 1993;42:288.

212. Knip M, Sakkinen A, Huttunen NP, *et al*: Postinitial remission in diabetic children—an analysis of 178 cases. *Acta Paediatr Scand* 1982;71:901.

213. Agner T, Damm P, Binder C: Remission in IDDM: Prospective study of basal C-peptide and insulin dose in 268 consecutive patients. *Diabetes Care* 1987;10:164.

214. Sochett EB, Daneman D, Clarson C, *et al*: Factors affecting and patterns of residual insulin secretion during the first year of type 1 (insulin-dependent) diabetes mellitus in children. *Diabetologia* 1987;30:453.

215. Ortqvist E, Falorni A, Scheynius A, *et al*: Age governs gender-dependent islet cell autoreactivity and predicts the clinical course in childhood IDDM. *Act Paediatr* 1997;86:1166.

216. Schiffrin A, Suissa S, Possier P, *et al*: Prospective study of predictors of beta-cell survival in type I diabetes. *Diabetes* 1988;37:920.

217. Wallensteen M, Dahlquist G, Persson B, *et al*: Factors influencing the magnitude, duration, and rate of fall of β-cell function in type I (insulin-dependent) diabetic children followed for two years from their clinical diagnosis. *Diabetologia* 1988;31:664.

218. Sabbah E, Savola K, Kulmala P, *et al*: Diabetes-associated autoantibodies in relation to clinical characteristics and natural course in children with newly diagnosed type 1 diabetes. The Childhood Diabetes in Finland Study Group. *J Clin Endocrinol Metab* 1999;84:1534.

219. Petersen JS, Dyrberg T, Karlsen AE, *et al*: Glutamic acid decarboxylase (GAD65) autoantibodies in prediction of β-cell function and remission in recent-onset IDDM after cyclosporin treatment. *Diabetes* 1994;43:1291.

220. Fukuda M, Tanaka A, Tahara Y, *et al*: Correlation between minimal secretory capacity of pancreatic beta-cells and stability of diabetic control. *Diabetes* 1988;37:81.

221. Kolb H, Dannehl K, Gruenklee D, *et al*: Prospective analysis of islet cell antibodies in children with type I (insulin-dependent) diabetes. *Diabetologia* 1988;31:189.

222. Knip M, Llonen J, Mustonen A, *et al*: Evidence of an accelerated β-cell destruction in HLA-Dw3/Dw4 heterozygous children with type I (insulin-dependent) diabetes. *Diabetologia* 1986;29:347.

223. Pipeleers D, Ling Z: Pancreatic beta cell in insulin-dependent diabetes. *Diabetes Metab Rev* 1992;8:209.

224. Madsbad S, Faber OK, Binder C, *et al*: Prevalence of residual beta-cell function in insulin-dependent diabetics in relation to age at onset and duration of diabetes. *Diabetes* 1978;27(suppl 1):262.

225. Feutren G, Assan G, Karsenty G, *et al*: Cyclosporin increases the rate and lengthh of remissions in insulin dependent diabetes of recent onset. Results of a multicentre double-blind trial. *Lancet* 1986;2:119.

226. Martin S, Schernthaner G, Nerup J, *et al*: Follow-up of cyclosporin A treatment in type 1 (insulin-dependent) diabetes mellitus: Lack of long-term effects. *Diabetologia* 1991;34:429.

227. Mirouze J, Selam JL, Pham TC, *et al*: Sustained insulin-induced remissions of juvenile diabetes by means of an external artificial pancreas. *Diabetologia* 1978;14:223.

228. Shah SC, Malone JI, Simpson NE: A randomized trial of intensive insulin therapy in newly diagnosed insulin-dependent diabetes mellitus. *N Engl J Med* 1989;320:550.

229. Pozzilli P, Pitocco D, Visalli N, *et al*: No effect of oral insulin on residual beta-cell function in recent-onset type I diabetes (the IM-DIAB VII). IMDIAB Group [in process citation]. *Diabetologia* 2000;43:1000.

230. Allen HF, Klingensmith GJ, Jensen P, *et al*: Effect of BCG vaccination on new-onset insulin-dependent diabetes mellitus: A randomized clinical study. *Diabetes Care* 1998;22:1703.

231. WHO Study Group: *Diabetes Mellitus—Technical Report Series 727*. World Health Organization; 1985.

232. Dorman JS, LaPorte RE, Kuller LH, *et al*: The Pittsburgh insulin-independent diabetes mellitus (IDDM) morbidity and mortality study. Mortality results. *Diabetes* 1984;33:271.

233. Diabetes Epidemiology Research International Mortality Study Group. Major cross-country differences in risk of dying for people with IDDM. *Diabetes Care* 1991;14:49.

234. Matsushima M, LaPorte RE, Maruyama M, *et al*: Geographic variation in mortality among individuals with youth-onset diabetes mellitus across the world. *Diabetologia* 1997;40:212.

235. Diabetes Epidemiology Research International Mortality Study Group. International evaluation of cause-specific mortality and IDDM. *Diabetes Care* 1991;14:55.

236. Borch-Johnsen K, Nissen H, Henriksen E, *et al*: The natural history of insulin-dependent diabetes mellitus in Denmark: 1. Long-term survival with and without late diabetic complications. *Diabet Med* 1987;4:201.

237. Chowdhury TA, Dyer PH, Mijovic CH, *et al*: Human leucocyte antigen and insulin gene regions and nephropathy in type I diabetes. *Diabetologia* 1999;42:1017.

238. Doria A, Warram JH, Krolewski AS: Genetic predisposition to diabetic nephropathy. Evidence for a role of the angiotensin I-converting enzyme gene. *Diabetes* 1994;43:690.

239. Doria A, Onuma T, Gearin G, *et al*: Angiotensinogen polymorphism M235T, hypertension, and nephropathy in insulin-dependent diabetes. *Hypertension* 1996;27:1134.

240. Fogarty DG, Harron JC, Hughes AE, *et al*: A molecular variant of angiotensinogen is associated with diabetic nephropathy in IDDM. *Diabetes* 1996;45:1204.

241. Nagi DK, Mansfield MW, Stickland MH, *et al*: Angiotensin converting enzyme (ACE) insertion/deletion (I/D) polymorphism, and diabetic retinopathy in subjects with IDDM and NIDDM. *Diabet Med* 1995;12:997.

242. Parving HH, Jacobsen P, Tarnow L, *et al*: Effect of deletion polymorphism of angiotensin converting enzyme gene on progression of dia-

betic nephropathy during inhibition of angiotensin converting enzyme: Observational follow up study. *BMJ* 1996;313:591.

243. Tarnow L, Cambien F, Rossing P, *et al*: Angiotensinogen gene polymorphisms in IDDM patients with diabetic nephropathy. *Diabetes* 1996;45:367.

244. Tarnow L, Cambien F, Rossing P, *et al*: Lack of relationship between an insertion/deletion polymorphism in the angiotensin I-converting enzyme gene and diabetic nephropathy and proliferative retinopathy in IDDM patients. *Diabetes* 1995;44:489.

245. Rewers M, Kamboh MI, Hoag S, *et al*: Apolipoprotein A-IV polymorphism associated with myocardial infarction in obese NIDDM patients. The San Luis Valley Diabetes Study. *Diabetes* 1994;43:1485.

246. The Diabetes Control and Complications Trial Research Group: The effect of intensive treatment of diabetes on the development and progression of long-term complications in insulin-dependent diabetes mellitus. *N Engl J Med* 1993;329:977.

247. Clustering of long-term complications in families with diabetes in the diabetes control and complications trial. The Diabetes Control and Complications Trial Research Group. *Diabetes* 1997;46:1829.

248. King H, Aubert RE, Herman WH: Global burden of diabetes, 1995–2025: Prevalence, numerical estimates, and projections. *Diabetes Care* 1998;21:1414.

249. World Health Organization: *WHO Expert Committee on Diabetes Mellitus*. World Health Organization. Technical Report Series. 1980; 646:1.

250. Gavin JR III, Alberti KGMM, Davidson MB, *et al*: Report of the Expert Committee on the Diagnosis and Classification of Diabetes Mellitus. *Diabetes Care* 1997;20:1183.

251. WHO Consultation Group: *Definition, Diagnosis and Classification of Diabetes Mellitus and its Complications. Part 1: Diagnosis and Classification of Diabetes Mellitus.* World Health Organization; 1999.

252. Harris MI, Eastman RC, Cowie CC, *et al*: Comparison of diabetes diagnostic categories in the U.S. population according to the 1997 American Diabetes Association and 1980–1985 World Health Organization diagnostic criteria. *Diabetes Care* 1997;20:1859.

253. Bennett PH: Impact of the new WHO classification and diagnostic criteria. *Diabetes Obes Metab* 1999;1(suppl 2):S1.

254. King H, Rewers M: Global estimates for prevalence of diabetes mellitus and impaired glucose tolerance in adults. WHO Ad Hoc Diabetes Reporting Group. *Diabetes Care* 1993;16:157.

255. Fagot-Campagna A, Pettitt DJ, Engelgau MM, *et al*: Type 2 diabetes among North American children and adolescents: An epidemiologic review and a public health perspective. *J Pediatr* 2000;136:664.

256. Kenny SJ, Aubert RE, Geiss LS: Prevalence and incidence of non-insulin-dependent diabetes. In: Harris MI, Cowie CC, Stern MP, *et al*, eds. *Diabetes in America*. National Institutes of Health; 1995.

257. Harris MI, Flegal KM, Cowie CC, *et al*: Prevalence of diabetes, impaired fasting glucose, and impaired glucose tolerance in U.S. adults. The Third National Health and Nutrition Examination Survey, 1988–1994. *Diabetes Care* 1998;21:518.

258. Harris MI, Hadden WC, Knowler WC, *et al*: Prevalence of diabetes and impaired glucose tolerance and plasma glucose levels in U.S. population aged 20–74 yr. *Diabetes* 1987;36:523.

259. Harris MI: Noninsulin-dependent diabetes mellitus in black and white Americans. *Diabetes Metab Rev* 1990;6:71.

260. Flegal KM, Ezzati TM, Harris MI, *et al*: Prevalence of diabetes in Mexican Americans, Cubans, and Puerto Ricans from the Hispanic Health and Nutrition Examination Survey, 1982–1984. *Diabetes Care* 1991;14:628.

261. Gohdes D: Diabetes in North American Indians and Alaska Natives. In: Harris MI, Cowie CC, Stern MP, *et al*, eds. *Diabetes in America*. National Institutes of Health; 1995.

262. Knowler WC, Pettitt DJ, Saad MF, *et al*: Diabetes mellitus in the Pima Indians: Incidence, risk factors and pathogenesis. *Diabetes Metab Rev* 1990;61:1.

263. Mokdad AH, Bowman BA, Engelgau MM, *et al*: Diabetes trends among American Indians and Alaska natives: 1990–1998. *Diabetes Care* 2001;24:1508.

264. Mokdad AH, Bowman BA, Ford ES, *et al*: The continuing epidemics of obesity and diabetes in the United States. *JAMA* 2001;286:1195.

265. King H, Rewers M, WHO Reporting Group: Global estimates for prevalence of diabetes mellitus and impaired glucose tolerance in adults. *Diabetes Care* 1993;16:157.

266. Tan CE, Emmanuel SC, Tan BY, *et al*: Prevalence of diabetes and ethnic differences in cardiovascular risk factors. The 1992 Singapore National Health Survey. *Diabetes Care* 1999;22:241.

267. Mather HM, Chaturvedi N, Fuller JH: Mortality and morbidity from diabetes in South Asians and Europeans: 11-year follow-up of the Southall Diabetes Survey, London, UK. *Diabet Med* 1998;15:53.

268. Simmons D: The epidemiology of diabetes and its complications in New Zealand. *Diabet Med* 1996;13:371.

269. Dabelea D, Hanson RL, Bennett PH, *et al*: Increasing prevalence of type II diabetes in American Indian children. *Diabetologia* 1998;41:904.

270. Dean HJ, Mundy RL, Moffatt M: Non-insulin-dependent diabetes mellitus in Indian children in Manitoba. *CMAJ* 1992;147:52.

271. Kitagawa T, Owada M, Urakami T, *et al*: Increased incidence of non-insulin dependent diabetes mellitus among Japanese schoolchildren correlates with an increased intake of animal protein and fat. *Clin Pediatr* 1998;37:111.

272. Savage PJ, Bennett PH, Senter RG, *et al*: High prevalence of diabetes in young Pima Indians: Evidence of phenotypic variation in a genetically isolated population. *Diabetes* 1979;28:937.

273. Krakoff J, Hanson RL, Kobes S, *et al*: Comparison of the effect of plasma glucose concentrations on microvascular disease between Pima Indian youths and adults. *Diabetes Care* 2001;24:1023.

274. Knowler WC, Bennett PH, Hamman RF, *et al*: Diabetes incidence and prevalence in Pima Indians: A 19-fold greater incidence than in Rochester, Minnesota. *Am J Epidemiol* 1978;108:497.

275. Knowler WC, Pettitt DJ, Savage PJ, *et al*: Diabetes incidence in Pima Indians: Contributions of obesity and parental diabetes. *Am J Epidemiol* 1981;113:144.

276. Dowse GD, Zimmet PZ, Finch CF, *et al*: Decline in incidence of epidemic glucose intolerance in Nauruans: Implications for the "thrifty genotype." *Am J Epidemiol* 1991;133:1093.

277. Bennett PH, Knowler WC: Increasing prevalence of diabetes in the Pima (American) Indians over a ten year period. In: Waldhausl WK, ed. *Diabetes 1979*. Excerpta Medica; 1979.

278. Kleinman JC, Donahue RP, Harris MI, *et al*: Mortality among diabetics in a national sample. *Am J Epidemiol* 1988;128:389.

279. Gu K, Cowie CC, Harris MI: Mortality in adults with and without diabetes in a national cohort of the U.S. population, 1971–1993. *Diabetes Care* 1998;21:1138.

280. Roper NA, Bilous RW, Kelly WF, *et al*: Excess mortality in a population with diabetes and the impact of material deprivation: Longitudinal, population based study. *BMJ* 2001;322:1389.

281. Morrish NJ, Wang SL, Stevens LK, *et al*: Mortality and causes of death in the WHO multinational study of vascular disease in diabetes. *Diabetologia* 2001;44:S14.

282. Sievers ML, Nelson RG, Knowler WC, *et al*: Impact of NIDDM on mortality and causes of death in Pima Indians. *Diabetes Care* 1992; 15:1541.

283. McLarty DG, Kinabo L, Swai AB: Diabetes in tropical Africa: A prospective study, 1981–7. II. Course and prognosis. *BMJ* 1990;300:1107.

284. Bale GS, Entmacher PS: Estimated life expectancy of diabetics. *Diabetes* 1977;26:434.

285. Sievers ML, Nelson RG, Knowler WC, *et al*: Impact of NIDDM on mortality and causes of death in Pima Indians. *Diabetes Care* 1992; 15:1541.

286. Barrett-Connor E, Wingard DL: Sex differential in ischemic heart disease mortality in diabetics: A prospective population-based study. *Am J Epidemiol* 1983;118:489.

287. Hu FB, Stampfer MJ, Solomon CG, *et al*: The impact of diabetes mellitus on mortality from all causes and coronary heart disease in women: 20 years of follow-up. *Arch Intern Med* 2001;161:1717.

288. Stamler J, Vaccaro O, Neaton JD, *et al*: Diabetes, other risk factors, and 12-yr cardiovascular mortality for men screened in the Multiple Risk Factor Intervention Trial. *Diabetes Care* 1993;16:434.

289. Everhart JE, Knowler WC, Bennett PH: Incidence and risk factors for noninsulin-dependent diabetes. In: Harris MI, Hamman RF, eds. *Diabetes in America, Diabetes Data Compiled 1984*. J NIH Publication No. 85-1468; 1985.

290. Barnett AH, Eff C, Leslie RD, *et al*: Diabetes in identical twins. A study of 200 pairs. *Diabetologia* 1981;20:87.

291. Newman B, Selby JV, King MC, *et al*: Concordance for type 2 (non-insulin-dependent) diabetes mellitus in male twins. *Diabetologia* 1987; 30:763.

292. Serjeantson SW, Owerbach D, Zimmet P, *et al*: Genetics of diabetes in Nauru: Effects of foreign admixture, HLA antigens and the insulin-gene-linked polymorphism. *Diabetologia* 1983;25:13.

293. Knowler WC, Williams RC, Pettitt DJ, *et al*: Gm3;5,13,14 and type 2 diabetes mellitus: An association in American Indians with genetic admixture. *Am J Hum Genet* 1988;43:520.

294. Gardner LI Jr, Stern MP, Haffner SM, *et al*: Prevalence of diabetes in Mexican Americans. Relationship to percent of gene pool derived from native American sources. *Diabetes* 1984;33:86.

295. Hanis CL, Boerwinkle E, Chakraborty R, *et al*: A genome-wide search for human non-insulin-dependent (type 2) diabetes genes reveals a major susceptibility locus on chromosome 2. *Nat Genet* 1996;13:161.

296. Elbein SC, Hoffman MD, Teng K, *et al*: A genome-wide search for type 2 diabetes susceptibility genes in Utah Caucasians. *Diabetes* 1999;48:1175.

297. Hanson RL, Ehm MG, Pettitt DJ, *et al*: An autosomal genomic scan for loci linked to type II diabetes mellitus and body-mass index in Pima Indians. *Am J Hum Genet* 1998;63:1130.

298. Ghosh S, Watanabe RM, Valle TT, *et al*: The Finland-United States investigation of non-insulin-dependent diabetes mellitus genetics (FUSION) study. I. An autosomal genome scan for genes that predispose to type 2 diabetes. *Am J Hum Genet* 2000;67:1174.

299. Wiltshire S, Hattersley AT, Hitman GA, *et al*: A genomewide scan for loci predisposing to type 2 diabetes in a U.K. population (the Diabetes UK Warren 2 Repository): Analysis of 573 pedigrees provides independent replication of a susceptibility locus on chromosome 1q. *Am J Hum Genet* 2001;69:553.

300. Horikawa Y, Oda N, Cox NJ, *et al*: Genetic variation in the gene encoding calpain-10 is associated with type 2 diabetes mellitus. *Nat Genet* 2000;26:163.

301. Xia J, Scherer SW, Cohen PT, *et al*: A common variant in PPP1R3 associated with insulin resistance and type 2 diabetes. *Diabetes* 1998;47:1519.

302. Luan J, Browne PO, Harding AH, *et al*: Evidence for gene-nutrient interaction at the PPARgamma locus. *Diabetes* 2001;50:686.

303. Williams RC, Knowler WC, Butler WJ, *et al*: HLA-A2 and type 2 (insulin independent) diabetes mellitus in Pima Indians: An association of allele frequency with age. *Diabetologia* 1981;21:460.

304. Tuomilehto-Wolf E, Tuomilehto J, Hitman GA, *et al*: Genetic susceptibility to non-insulin dependent diabetes mellitus and glucose intolerance are located in HLA region. *BMJ* 1993;307:155.

305. Colditz GA, Willett WC, Stampfer MJ, *et al*: Weight as a risk factor for clinical diabetes in women. *Am J Epidemiol* 1990;132:501.

306. Chan JM, Rimm EB, Colditz GA, *et al*: Obesity, fat distribution, and weight gain as risk factors for clinical diabetes in men. *Diabetes Care* 1994;17:961.

307. Boyko EJ, Fujimoto WY, Leonetti DL, *et al*: Visceral adiposity and risk of type 2 diabetes: A prospective study among Japanese Americans. *Diabetes Care* 2000;23:465.

308. Despres JP: Health consequences of visceral obesity. *Ann Med* 2001;33:534.

309. Manson JE, Rimm EB, Stampfer MJ, *et al*: Physical activity and incidence of non-insulin-dependent diabetes mellitus in women. *Lancet* 1991;338:774.

310. Manson JE, Nathan DM, Krolewski AS, *et al*: A prospective study of exercise and incidence of diabetes among U.S. male physicians. *JAMA* 1992;268:63.

311. Kriska AM, LaPorte RE, Pettitt DJ, *et al*: The association of physical activity with obesity, fat distribution and glucose intolerance in Pima Indians. *Diabetologia* 1993;36:863.

312. Helmrich SP, Ragland DR, Leung RW, *et al*: Physical activity and reduced occurrence of non-insulin-dependent diabetes mellitus. *N Engl J Med* 1991;325:147.

313. O'Sullivan JB: Diabetes Mellitus after GDM. *Diabetes* 1991;40(suppl 2):131.

314. Hales CN, Barker DJ, Clark PM, *et al*: Fetal and infant growth and impaired glucose tolerance at age 64. *BMJ* 1991;303:1019.

315. McCance DR, Pettitt DJ, Hanson RL, *et al*: Birth weight and non-insulin dependent diabetes: Thrifty genotype, thrifty phenotype, or surviving small baby genotype? *BMJ* 1994;308:942.

316. Dabelea D, Pettitt DJ, Hanson RL, *et al*: Birth weight, type 2 diabetes, and insulin resistance in Pima Indian children and young adults. *Diabetes Care* 1999;22:944.

317. Hales CN, Desai M, Ozanne SE: The thrifty phenotype hypothesis: How does it look after 5 years? *Diabet Med* 1997;14:189.

318. Lithell HO, McKeigue PM, Berglund L, *et al*: Relation of size at birth to non-insulin dependent diabetes and insulin concentrations in men aged 50–60 years. *BMJ* 1996;312:406.

319. Hales CN, Barker DJ: Type 2 (non-insulin-dependent) diabetes mellitus: The thrifty phenotype hypothesis. *Diabetologia* 1992;35:595.

320. Stern MP, Bartley M, Duggirala R, *et al*: Birth weight and the metabolic syndrome: Thrifty phenotype or thrifty genotype? *Diabetes Metab Res Rev* 2000;16:88.

321. Lindsay RS, Dabelea E, Roumain J, *et al*: Type 2 diabetes and low birth weight: The role of paternal inheritance in the association of low birth weight and diabetes. *Diabetes* 2000;49:445.

322. McCance DR, Pettitt DJ, Hanson RL, *et al*: Birth weight and non-insulin dependent diabetes: Thrifty genotype, thrifty phenotype, or surviving small baby genotype? *BMJ* 1994;308:942.

323. Boyko EJ: Proportion of type 2 diabetes cases resulting from impaired fetal growth. *Diabetes Care* 2000;23:1260.

324. Pettitt DJ, Aleck KA, Baird HR, *et al*: Congenital susceptibility to NIDDM. Role of intrauterine environment. *Diabetes* 1988;37:622.

325. Gautier JF, Wilson C, Weyer C, *et al*: Low acute insulin secretory responses in adult offspring of people with early onset type 2 diabetes. *Diabetes* 2001;50:1828.

326. Dabelea D, Hanson RL, Lindsay RS, *et al*: Intrauterine exposure to diabetes conveys risks for type 2 diabetes and obesity: A study of discordant sibships. *Diabetes* 2000;49:2208.

327. Pradhan AD, Manson JE, Rifai N, *et al*: C-reactive protein, interleukin 6, and risk of developing type 2 diabetes mellitus. *JAMA* 2001;286:327.

328. Festa A, D'Agostino R Jr, Mykkanen L, *et al*: Relative contribution of insulin and its precursors to fibrinogen and PAI-1 in a large population with different states of glucose tolerance. The Insulin Resistance Atherosclerosis Study (IRAS). *Arterioscler Thromb Vasc Biol* 1999;19:562.

329. Pickup JC, Crook MA: Is type II diabetes mellitus a disease of the innate immune system? *Diabetologia* 1998;41:1241.

330. Lindsay RS, Krakoff J, Hanson RL, *et al*: Gamma globulin levels predict type 2 diabetes in the Pima Indian population. *Diabetes* 2001;50:1598.

331. Mason AL, Lau JY, Hoang N, *et al*: Association of diabetes mellitus and chronic hepatitis C virus infection. *Hepatology* 1999;29:328.

332. Mehta SH, Brancati FL, Sulkowski MS, *et al*: Prevalence of type 2 diabetes mellitus among persons with hepatitis C virus infection in the United States. *Ann Intern Med* 2000;133:592.

333. Lindstedt G, Lundberg PA, Lapidus L, *et al*: Low sex hormone-binding globulin as independent risk factor for development of NIDDM: 12-year follow-up of population study in Gothenburg, Sweden. *Diabetes* 1991;40:123.

334. Haffner SM, Valdez RA, Morales PA, *et al*: Decreased sex hormone-binding globulin predicts non-insulin-dependent diabetes mellitus. *J Clin Endocrinol Metab* 1993;76:56.

335. Haffner SM, Karhapää P. Mykkänen L, *et al*: Insulin resistance, body fat distribution and sex hormones in men. *Diabetes* 1994;43:212.

336. Charles MA, Pettitt DJ, McCance DR, *et al*: Gravidity, obesity and non-insulin-dependent diabetes mellitus in Pima Indian women. *Am J Med* 1994;97:250.

337. Pettitt DJ, Forman MR, Hanson RL, *et al*: Breastfeeding and incidence of non-insulin-dependent diabetes mellitus in Pima Indians. *Lancet* 1997;350:166.

338. West KM: *Epidemiology of Diabetes and Its Vascular Complications*. Elsevier; 1978.

339. Bennett PH, Knowler WC, Baird HR, *et al*: Diet and development of noninsulin-dependent diabetes mellitus: An epidemiological perspective. In: Pozza G, Micossi P, Catapano AL, *et al*, eds. *Diet, Diabetes, and Atherosclerosis*. Raven Press; 1984.

340. Marshall JA, Hoag S, Shetterly S, *et al*: Dietary fat predicts conversion from impaired glucose tolerance to NIDDM. *Diabetes Care* 1994;17:50.

341. Williams DE, Wareham NJ, Cox BD, *et al*: Frequent salad vegetable consumption is associated with a reduction in the risk of diabetes mellitus. *J Clin Epidemiol* 1999;52:329.

342. Feskens EJ, Virtanen SM, Rasanen L, *et al*: Dietary factors determining diabetes and impaired glucose tolerance. A 20-year follow-up of the Finnish and Dutch cohorts of the Seven Countries Study. *Diabetes Care* 1995;18:1104.

343. Salmeron J, Hu FB, Manson JE, *et al*: Dietary fat intake and risk of type 2 diabetes in women. *Am J Clin Nutr* 2001;73:1019.

344. Meyer KA, Kushi LH, Jacobs DR, Jr, *et al*: Dietary fat and incidence of type 2 diabetes in older Iowa women. *Diabetes Care* 2001;24:1528.

345. Hu FB, Manson JE, Stampfer MJ, *et al*: Diet, lifestyle, and the risk of type 2 diabetes mellitus in women. *N Engl J Med* 2001;345:790.

346. Hu FB, van Dam RM, Liu S: Diet and risk of type II diabetes: The role of types of fat and carbohydrate. *Diabetologia* 2001;44:805.

347. Williams DE, Knowler WC, Smith CJ, *et al*: The effect of Indian or Anglo dietary preference on the incidence of diabetes in Pima Indians. *Diabetes Care* 2001;24:811.

348. Stampfer MJ, Colditz GA, Willett WC, *et al*: A prospective study of moderate alcohol drinking and risk of diabetes in women. *Am J Epidemiol* 1988;128:549.

349. Rimm EB, Chan J, Stampfer MJ, *et al*: Prospective study of cigarette smoking, alcohol use, and the risk of diabetes in men. *BMJ* 1995;310:555.

350. Ajani UA, Hennekens CH, Spelsberg A, *et al*: Alcohol consumption and risk of type 2 diabetes mellitus among U.S. male physicians. *Arch Intern Med* 2000;160:1025.

351. Kao WH, Puddey IB, Boland LL, *et al*: Alcohol consumption and the risk of type 2 diabetes mellitus: Atherosclerosis risk in communities study. *Am J Epidemiol* 2001;154:748.

352. Saad MF, Knowler WC, Pettitt DJ, *et al*: A two-step model for development of non-insulin-dependent diabetes. *Am J Med* 1991;90:229.

353. Saad MF, Knowler WC, Pettitt DJ, *et al*: Sequential changes in serum insulin concentration during development of non-insulin-dependent diabetes. *Lancet* 1989;i:1356.

354. Shaw JE, Zimmet PZ, de Court, *et al*: Impaired fasting glucose or impaired glucose tolerance. What best predicts future diabetes in Mauritius? *Diabetes Care* 1999;22:399.

355. Gabir MM, Hanson RL, Dabelea D, *et al*: The 1997 American Diabetes Association and 1999 World Health Organization criteria for hyperglycemia in the diagnosis and prediction of diabetes. *Diabetes Care* 2000;23:1108.

356. de Vegt F, Dekker JM, Jager A, *et al*: Relation of impaired fasting and postload glucose with incident type 2 diabetes in a Dutch population: The Hoorn Study. *JAMA* 2001;285:2109.

357. Saad MF, Knowler WC, Pettitt DJ, *et al*: The natural history of impaired glucose tolerance in the Pima Indians. *N Engl J Med* 1988;319:1500.

358. Edelstein SL, Knowler WC, Bain RP, *et al*: Predictors of progression from impaired glucose tolerance to NIDDM: An analysis of six prospective studies. *Diabetes* 1997;46:701.

359. Weyer C, Bogardus C, Mott DM, *et al*: The natural history of insulin secretory dysfunction and insulin resistance in the pathogenesis of type 2 diabetes mellitus. *J Clin Invest* 1999;104:787.

360. Eschwege E, Charles MA, Simon D, *et al*: From policeman to policies: What is the future for 2-h glucose?: The Kelly West Lecture, 2000. *Diabetes Care* 2001;24:1945.

361. Balkau B: The DECODE study. Diabetes epidemiology: Collaborative analysis of diagnostic criteria in Europe. *Diabetes Metab* 2000;26:282.

362. Gabir MM, Hanson RL, Dabelea D, *et al*: Plasma glucose and prediction of microvascular disease and mortality: Evaluation of 1997 American Diabetes Association and 1999 World Health Organization criteria for diagnosis of diabetes. *Diabetes Care* 2000;23:1113.

363. Shaw JE, Hodge AM, de Court, *et al*: Isolated post-challenge hyperglycaemia confirmed as a risk factor for mortality. *Diabetologia* 1999;42:1050.

364. Davies MJ, Raymond NT, Day JL *et al*: Impaired glucose tolerance and fasting hyperglycaemia have different characteristics. *Diabet Med* 2000;17:433.

365. Mokdad AH, Ford ES, Bowman BA, *et al*: Diabetes trends in the United States: 1990–1998. *Diabetes Care* 2000;23:1278.

366. Neel JV: Diabetes Mellitus: A "thrifty" genotype rendered detrimental by "progress"? *Am J Hum Genet* 1962;14:353.

367. Pan XR, Li GW, Hu YH, *et al*: Effects of diet and exercise in preventing NIDDM in people with impaired glucose tolerance. The Da Qing IGT and Diabetes Study. *Diabetes Care* 1997;20:537.

368. Tuomilehto J, Lindstrom J, Eriksson JG, *et al*: Prevention of type 2 diabetes mellitus by changes in lifestyle among subjects with impaired glucose tolerance. *N Engl J Med* 2001;344:1343.

369. The Diabetes Prevention Program Research Group: The Diabetes Prevention Program. Design and methods for a clinical trial in the prevention of type 2 diabetes. *Diabetes Care* 1999;22:623.

370. The Diabetes Prevention Program Research Group. The Diabetes Prevention Program: Baseline characteristic of the randomized cohort. *Diabetes Care* 2000;23:1619.

371. The Diabetes Prevention Program Research Group: Reduction in the incidence of type 2 diabetes with lifestyle intervention or metformin. *New Engl J Med* 2002;346:393–403.

372. Chiasson J-L, Josse RG, Gromis R, et al: Acarbose can prevent the progression of impaired glucose tolerance to type 2 diabetes mellitu: Results of a randomized clinical trial, The Stop-NIDDM Trial Lancet 2002 (in press).

373. Buchanan TA, personal communication, 2002.

374. Freeman DJ, Norrie J, Sattar N, *et al*: Pravastalin and the development of diabetes mellitus: Evidence for a protective treatment effect in the West of Scotland Coronary Prevention Study. *Circulation* 2001;103:357.

375. Yusuf S, Sleight P, Pogue J, *et al*: Effects of an angiotensin-converting-enzyme inhibitor, ramipril, on cardiovascular events in high-risk patients. The Heart Outcomes Prevention Evaluation Study Investigators. *N Engl J Med* 2000;342:145.

CHAPTER 20

The Pathophysiology and Genetics of Type 1 (Insulin-Dependent) Diabetes

Ramachandra G. Naik

Åke Lernmark

Jerry P. Palmer

The term **diabetes** does not denote a single disease entity, but rather a clinical syndrome. Fundamental to all types of diabetes is impairment of insulin secretion by the pancreatic β cells. Except for the β-cell loss that results from known toxins, such as streptozotocin, alloxan, and the rodenticide Vacor™, and from pancreatitis or surgical pancreatectomy, we lack a full understanding of the pathogenic mechanisms leading to diabetes. A major requirement for epidemiologic and clinical research and for the clinical management of diabetes is an appropriate system of classification that provides a framework within which to identify and differentiate the disease's various forms and stages. Although many nomenclatures and diagnostic criteria had been proposed for diabetes, no generally accepted systematic categorization existed until the National Diabetes Data Group (NDDG) classification system was published in 1979.[1] The World Health Organization (WHO) Expert Committee on Diabetes in 1980 and, later, the WHO Study Group on Diabetes Mellitus endorsed the substantive recommendations of the NDDG.[1] These groups recognized two major forms of diabetes, which they termed insulin-dependent diabetes mellitus (IDDM; type 1 diabetes) and non-insulin-dependent diabetes mellitus (NIDDM; type 2 diabetes). However, their classification system went on to include evidence that diabetes mellitus was an etiologically and clinically heterogeneous group of disorders that share hyperglycemia in common.

It is now considered particularly important to move away from a system that appears to base the classification of the disease largely on the type of pharmacologic treatment used in its management and toward a system based on disease etiology. An international Expert Committee, working under the sponsorship of the American Diabetes Association, was established in May 1995 to review the scientific literature since 1979 and to decide whether changes to the classification and diagnosis of diabetes were warranted. The Expert Committee carefully considered the data and rationale for what was accepted in 1979, along with research findings of the last 18 years, and proposed changes to the NDDG/WHO classification scheme.[2]

The main features of these changes are as follows. The terms insulin-dependent diabetes mellitus and non-insulin-dependent diabetes mellitus and their acronyms, IDDM and NIDDM, were eliminated. These terms have been confusing and have frequently resulted in classification of the patient based on treatment rather than etiology. The terms type 1 and type 2 diabetes are retained, with Arabic rather than roman numerals. The class (or form) termed **type 1 diabetes** (T1DM) includes the vast majority of cases that are primarily due to pancreatic islet β-cell destruction and that are prone to ketoacidosis. This form includes those cases currently ascribable to an autoimmune process and those for which an etiology is unknown. It does not include those forms of β-cell destruction or failure for which non-autoimmune-specific causes can be assigned (e.g., cystic fibrosis). Although most type 1 diabetes is characterized by the presence of autoantibodies that identify the autoimmune process leading to β-cell destruction, in some subjects, no evidence of autoimmunity is present; these cases are classified as type 1 idiopathic. The other main class (or form), termed **type 2 diabetes** (T2DM), includes the most prevalent form of diabetes, which results typically from an interaction between insulin resistance and an insulin secretory defect. Although the exact cause(s) of the insulin resistance and the insulin secretory defect are not known, both are strongly genetically determined, and the β-cell defect does not have an autoimmune etiology.

Epidemiologic studies have suggested that the incidence rate of T1DM peaks twice, once close to puberty and again around 40 years of age,[3] and it has been suggested that the overall incidence rate of T1DM is approximately equivalent above and below the age of 20 years.[3] Many of these older patients, especially early in the course of their diabetes, are clinically similar to classical T2DM patients. This relatively high incidence rate of type 1 diabetes in adults is often not appreciated, probably because of the over 10-fold greater frequency of T2DM in this age group. Furthermore, the finding of antibodies characteristic of T1DM such as islet cell antibodies (ICA) and glutamic acid decarboxylase antibodies (GADA) in 10–15% of T2DM patients[4] suggests that in older individuals the type 1 disease process may result in a similar clinical phenotype as the type 2 disease process. This subset has been variously described as latent autoimmune diabetes in adults (LADA),[5,6] slowly progressive T1DM,[7] latent T1DM,[8] late-onset T1DM, antibody-positive T2DM, and type 1½ diabetes.[9,10] It is believed that the autoimmune β-cell destructive process proceeds more slowly than in young patients with T1DM, but this has not been carefully evaluated.[11]

The earliest accounts of diabetes mellitus, written more than a thousand years ago, already took different clinical forms into account, and it was suggested in the preinsulin era that the immune system might be involved in the development of some forms of diabetes mellitus (for review, see ref. 12). The presence of inflammatory cells in the islets of Langerhans was later termed "insulitis."[13] The significance of this insulitis at the clinical onset of insulin-dependent diabetes was first studied in detail by Gepts and LaCompte.[14] Their work is of fundamental importance to our current understanding of T1DM because it showed that the development of T1DM was associated with immunopathologic abnormalities. This chapter deals specifically with T1DM. We discuss what is known and what is controversial about the natural history and the genetic, immunologic, and environmental mechanisms involved in the etiology and pathogenesis of T1DM.

NATURAL HISTORY

Because this chapter deals with the etiology and pathogenesis of T1DM, our discussion of natural history emphasizes events occurring before the development of hyperglycemia or overt clinical T1DM. Because of the acute and dramatic onset of symptoms in most patients, it was previously believed that the disease process underlying T1DM was acute in nature and consequently that individuals were normal or unaffected until shortly before the diagnosis. We now understand that exactly the opposite is usually the case: the T1DM disease process has been active and ongoing for a long period, usually at least several years, before patients develop clinical disease.

Based on data that were mostly obtained by prospective studies of nondiabetic relatives of patients with T1DM, the natural history of T1DM includes the following major components. First, as indicated, there is a long preclinical period. During this time antibodies and T cells reactive with β-cell antigens can be detected, and the immunologic attack on the β cells is occurring. Progressive loss of β-cell function has been observed months to years prior to the onset of clinical T1DM,[15] and hyperglycemia after oral glucose may antedate the diagnosis of clinical T1DM by periods ranging from 3 months to 7 years.[16] Investigators in the ongoing Diabetes Prevention Trial-Type 1 (DPT-1) have recently detected among a cohort of ICA-positive first- and second-degree relatives of T1DM subjects, a group of subjects with T1DM who have a different phenotype. These subjects are asymptomatic, have normal or impaired fasting glucose, but have 2-hour glucose values >11.1 mmol/L on their oral glucose tolerance tests (OGTTs).[17]

Second, at least 80–90% of the functional capacity of the β cells must be lost before hyperglycemia occurs. The normal pancreas has a large reserve capacity and this must be depleted before clinical T1DM becomes manifest. Because even our most sensitive tests of β-cell function remain normal until islet insulin content is very low,[18] the immune markers of T1DM usually antedate evidence of β-cell insulin secretory deficiency by a long period. Until very recently it was believed that β-cell destruction was the primary mechanism responsible for the loss of insulin secretory capacity during the preclinical period of T1DM. We now recognize, as will be discussed in more detail subsequently, that at least some of the impairment in insulin secretion may be functional and due to inhibition of insulin secretion by cytokines and possibly other factors (reviewed in ref. 19).

Third, as implied by the insulitis and the presence of antibodies and T cells directed against islet antigens, the β-cell lesion is autoimmune in nature, and fourth, this autoimmune destructive process specifically occurs in genetically susceptible individuals.

In neonatal rodents, the β-cell mass is believed to undergo a phase of remodeling that includes a wave of apoptosis. Using both mathematical modeling and histochemical detection methods, Trudeau and colleagues[20] have demonstrated that β-cell apoptosis is significantly increased in neonates compared with adult rats, peaking at approximately 2 weeks of age. It was also shown that increased neonatal β-cell apoptosis is also present in animal models of autoimmune diabetes, including both the BB rat and nonobese diabetic (NOD) mouse. Recent studies indicate that apoptotic cells can display autoreactive antigen in their surface blebs, preferentially activate dendritic cells capable of priming tissue-specific cytotoxic T cells, and induce the formation of autoantibodies, thereby challenging the dogma that apoptosis does not elicit an immune response.[20] Initiation of β-cell–directed autoimmunity in murine models appears to be fixed at approximately 15 days of age, even when diabetes onset is dramatically accelerated. Taken together, these observations have led to the hypothesis that the neonatal wave of β-cell apoptosis is a trigger for β-cell–directed autoimmunity.[20]

T1DM is not a disease of unbridled β-cell destruction. The autoimmune attack on pancreatic β cells has two distinct stages (insulitis and diabetes), and progression of the former to the latter appears to be regulated. This has been shown in studies in NOD mice. Starting around 5 weeks of age, NOD mice develop a progressive mononuclear cell infiltration in and around the pancreatic islets. This infiltrate will eventually evolve into a destructive insulitis in those mice progressing to diabetes. By 18–24 weeks of age, most female mice are overtly diabetic. When pancreatic islets with insulitis were isolated from female NOD mice at different ages (5–7, 8–11, or 12–13 weeks), the islets showed a deficient glucose-induced insulin release and defective glucose metabolism that progressively worsened with age.[21,22] The observed β-cell dysfunction showed a close correlation to the severity of the mononuclear cell infiltration and was accompanied by defective glucose metabolism. It is not very clear whether humans have such clear-cut stages as in the NOD mice. Identifying the factors controlling this transition has been difficult because it is a complex process that occurs nonuniversally and asynchronously.[23]

A major question pertaining to the natural history of T1DM centers around whether the diabetogenic process, once initiated, is relentlessly progressive and always culminates in clinical T1DM, or whether it is more variable, waxing and waning, and sometimes remitting without eventual progression to overt T1DM (Fig. 20-1).[24] Whether one or more of the immune markers of T1DM are the direct result of the immune attack and β-cell damage, or possibly are independent of the immune attack, is unknown. In the NOD mouse, for example, although insulitis is usually considered indicative of the T1DM disease process, it is now recognized that insulitis can occur in animals that will not develop clinical T1DM.[25] Therefore, in considering the available human data, it is important to remember that changes in immune markers may not always be reflective of changes in the immune attack on the β cells. ICAs, especially when detected in low titer, may fluctuate over time (26); although it was initially believed that other antibodies such as insulin autoantibodies (IAAs), GADA's, and insulinoma-associated protein-2 antibodies (IA-2A) vary only

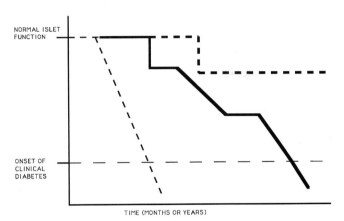

FIGURE 20-1. Hypothetical courses of pancreatic function after islet insult. Inexorable linear decline in function after islet insult leading to rapid onset of clinical disease (- - - -). Multiple islet insults leading to eventual clinical disease (———). Islet insult and recovery, without development of clinical disease (– – –). *(Reproduced with permission from Greenbaum CJ, Brooks-Worrell BM, Palmer JP, Lernmark A: Autoimmunity and prediction of insulin dependent diabetes mellitus. In: Marshall SM, Home PD, eds. The Diabetes Annual/8. Elsevier:1994;21.)*

slightly when measured over several years,[27] more recent data show similar fluctuations as for ICA.[28–35] In nondiabetic individuals with autoantibodies directed against islet antigens, impaired β-cell function is very common. A combination of immune markers with impaired β-cell function is associated with a greater risk of subsequent clinical T1DM than immune markers in combination with normal β-cell function. However, impaired β-cell function is also common in ICA-negative relatives of T1DM patients.[36] Because less than 20% of these individuals would be expected to progress to clinical T1DM, these observations suggest that in many of these individuals the β-cell destructive process has remitted.

In identical twins discordant for diabetes, activated T lymphocytes, ICAs, carbohydrate intolerance, or hyperproinsulinemia are more common in those nondiabetic individuals discordant for a short time vs. those discordant in the long term.[37] Furthermore, β-cell dysfunction is common in long-term discordant identical twins who were ICA-negative at the time of study, but who previously had been ICA-positive.[38] Previous studies suggested that after 6 years of discordance, identical twin pairs rarely become concordant for T1DM.[39] With up to 39 years of follow-up from the onset of diabetes in the index twin, Verge and colleagues[40] have determined how many discordant twins have evidence of β-cell autoimmunity and how many develop overt diabetes. Longitudinal follow-up of 23 pairs of identical twins (or triplets) that were selected from a total group of 30 pairs because they were discordant for T1DM when first ascertained showed that identical twins may develop diabetes after a prolonged period of discordance, and approximately two-thirds of long-term discordant twins have evidence of persistent β-cell autoimmunity and/or β-cell damage. The concordance for β-cell autoimmunity, therefore, is much higher than for overt diabetes.[40]

It should be stressed that the natural history of preclinical T1DM has been described primarily in prospective studies of first-degree relatives of T1DM patients, including the German

BABYDIAB study,[28,30,31] the Diabetes Autoimmunity Study in the Young (DAISY),[41–43] and the Childhood Diabetes in Finland Study.[32–34] This approach has provided a better understanding of the sequence of events preceding the development of hyperglycemia in such individuals.

The temporal development of autoantibodies has been studied in 1353 offspring of parents with T1DM in the German BABY DIAB study.[31] ICA, IAA, GADA, and IA-2A levels were measured at birth, 9 months, 2 years, and 5 years of age. At birth, no offspring had islet autoimmunity other than maternally acquired antibodies. Antibodies detected thereafter were likely to represent a true *de novo* production, since prevalences were the same for offspring from mothers and fathers with diabetes, antibodies detected at 9 months were almost always confirmed in the 2-year sample, and their presence was associated with an increased likelihood of having or developing other antibodies. By 2 years of age, autoantibodies appeared in 11% of offspring, 3.5% having more than one autoantibody. IAAs were detected most frequently, and few had autoantibodies in the absence of IAAs. Development of additional antibodies and changes in levels, including decline of IAAs at older age, was frequent. Overall cumulative risk for disease by 5 years of age was 1.8% (95% CI 0.2–3.4) and was 50% (95% CI 19–81) for offspring with more than one autoantibody in their 2-year sample. It was concluded that autoimmunity associated with childhood diabetes is an early event and a dynamic process, that the presence of IAAs is a consistent feature of this autoimmunity, and that IAA detection can identify children at risk. The group further reported that the humoral autoimmune response to GAD is initially against epitopes within the middle portion of GAD-65 and spreads to epitopes in other regions of GAD-65 and GAD-67[28] (see the Autoantibodies section below).

The Childhood Diabetes in Finland Study Group analyzed 747 children (younger than 15 years of age with newly diagnosed diabetes) for antibodies to GAD, IA-2 protein (IA-2A), insulin (IAA), and islet cells. The aim was to evaluate the influence of positivity for GADA, IA-2A, IAA, or multiple (≥3) autoantibodies at diagnosis on the clinical presentation and natural course of the disease over the first 2 years and to characterize autoantibody-negative patients.[32] At diagnosis, 73.2% of the children tested positive for GADA, 85.7% for IA-2A, 54.2% for IAA, and 72.6% for multiple autoantibodies. The patients testing positive for multiple autoantibodies were younger than the remaining children ($p < 0.001$). A similar age difference was seen when comparing IAA-positive and -negative patients ($p < 0.001$). They further showed that positivity for multiple diabetes-related autoantibodies is associated with accelerated β-cell destruction and an increased requirement for exogenous insulin over the second year of clinical disease, indicating that multiple autoantibodies reflect a more aggressive progression of β-cell destruction. Patients testing negative for diabetes-associated autoantibodies at diagnosis seem to have a milder degree of β-cell destruction, but their metabolic decompensation is similar to that seen in other affected children, suggesting that they do represent classical T1DM.[32–34] Mrena and coworkers[35] studied a total of 801 families taking part in the Childhood Diabetes in Finland Study and observed that it is possible to grade siblings of children with newly diagnosed T1DM into categories with significant differences in the subsequent risk of clinical T1DM and time to diagnosis. Such a classification should become clinically useful as soon as effective measures are available for preventing or delaying the manifestation of overt T1DM.

In the antibody-positive T2DM or the LADA group mentioned earlier, although it is believed that the autoimmune β-cell destructive process proceeds rather slowly or that the destruction stops at a "moderate" stage,[11] it is still not clear from the literature whether the pathophysiologic mechanism(s) of hyperglycemia is more type 1- or type 2-related or a combination of both the diabetes disease processes. A prospective observation on the natural history of the ICA-positive T2DM patients in Japan[7] disclosed the characteristic findings, which included a late onset, a family history of T2DM, a slow progression of β-cell failure over several years with persistently positive low-titer ICA, and incomplete β-cell loss. Similar presentations have been described in various other countries including Australia,[6] Finland,[5] New Zealand,[44] the United States,[45] Hong Kong,[46] Korea,[47] China,[47] Mexico, and Sweden.[4]

The typical patient, however, is generally >35 years old (age at onset 30–50 years) and nonobese (by lower body mass index); the diabetes is often controlled with diet, but within a short period (months to years), metabolic control fails, requiring oral agents, and progression to insulin dependency is more rapid than in antibody-negative, obese patient with T2DM. The eventual clinical features of these patients include weight loss, ketosis proneness, unstable blood glucose levels, and an extremely diminished C-peptide reserve[7,48]; in retrospect, these subjects possess additional classical features of T1DM, i.e., increased frequency of HLA-DR3 and -DR4, and islet-cell antibody positivity.[8]

A number of recent studies have determined ICA, IAA, and GADA levels, usually individually, in patients with phenotypic T2DM.[4,5,49] It has been shown that high GADA levels remain for up to 40 years after diagnosis of T1DM,[50] and there appears to be an ethnic difference in anti-GAD positivity, with higher frequency in Caucasian late-onset T1DM subjects than in adult-onset Asian T1DM patients,[51,52] suggesting that the adult-onset diabetes in the latter groups is less likely to have an autoimmune component to its pathogenesis. Various studies have shown that patients positive for anti-GAD and/or ICA have a more rapid decline in C-peptide, fail oral agents, and require insulin treatment earlier.[45,53–55] A recent study[54] showed that the positive rate for anti-GAD was as high as 23.8% in the nonobese and insulin-deficient patients with sulfonylurea failure, suggesting that autoimmune mechanisms may play an important role in the pathogenesis of secondary failure of sulphonylurea therapy. Thus, loss of β-cell function in approximately two-thirds of phenotypic T2DM subjects can be predicted by anti-GAD and ICA. However, as a result of lower cost and relative ease of performance, and the availability of several simple and robust assays for anti-GAD,[45] GAD antibodies may provide a practical alternative to ICA assay, particularly in population screening. Early detection of these immune markers of β-cell damage creates the potential for immune modulation to limit such damage.

Our current understanding of genetic abnormalities in late-onset T1DM is still not clearly elucidated. The associations between clinical T1DM and HLA genotype appear in part to be determined by age of diagnosis. Patients with onset after age 15 have a higher percentage of non-DR3/non-DR4 genotypes than patients with childhood T1DM, and those with later onset (>20 years) had a lower percentage of DR3/DR4 genotypes and a higher percentage of DQ0602.[56] It appears that the T1DM disease process is more aggressive, resulting in clinical presentation at a younger age in individuals with more susceptibility genes and less protective genes, and *vice versa*, the disease process is less aggressive, resulting in clinical presentation at older ages in individuals with less susceptibility genes and/or more protective genes.

GENETIC ASPECTS

Association with HLA

The association between HLA and T1DM (see Table 20-1 for definitions) was first demonstrated for HLA-B8 and/or B15.[57] Early investigations of these HLA class I molecule specificities were identified by antibodies that were specific for individual alleles or group of alleles. HLA specificities were traditionally defined by serology or by T-lymphocyte proliferation assays such as the mixed lymphocyte culture (MLC) tests. Advancing technologies have allowed a rapid detection of new alleles, and these are now primarily characterized at the genomic level by sequence analysis (see ref. 58 for a detailed review). The HLA molecules have structural similarities to an array of related molecules (Fig. 20-2). The marked polymorphism now explained by gene sequencing is one distinct feature of the HLA complex. Another feature of the HLA class I and II molecule genes encoded on the short arm of chromosome 6 is the phenomenon of linkage disequilibrium. This means that the frequency at which certain alleles are found together on the same haplotype is higher than expected, as calculated from the product of their individual gene frequencies. In other words, certain alleles in a haplotype tend to be inherited together, because the recombination frequency at certain parts of the HLA complex is markedly reduced compared with other parts of the human genome.

The phenomenon of linkage disequilibrium is important when an association between HLA and a disease such as T1DM is analyzed.[59–61] This approach toward estimating susceptibility to a disease differs from that of genetic linkage. The former is based on a comparison between patients and unrelated healthy controls.[62] The latter analysis takes advantage of multiple-generation families in which a disease is inherited through generations together with a given allele. Because of linkage disequilibrium, gene markers in close proximity to such an allele would tend to be inherited with the disease. Analysis of linkage is also used when investigating sib pairs, which is necessary in studying T1DM due to the rarity of large, multigeneration families.[63,64] It is critical to the understanding of T1DM etiology that the majority of new patients do not have a first-degree relative with the disease. It has therefore been extremely complicated to determine the mode of inheritance of T1DM.

Lifetime risks for T1DM (Table 20-2) in first-degree relatives of an individual with T1DM have been calculated to be about 3% for parents, 7% for siblings, and 5% for children.[65] A recent study including patients at an older age at onset and a longer follow-up than in previous studies indicated that 25% of T1DM patients had

TABLE 20-1. Nomenclature and Abbreviations for HLA Molecules

MHC	Major histocompatibility complex
MHC molecules	Proteins encoded on the short arm of chromosome 6; these proteins are involved in various functions of the human immune response
Class I molecules	The heavy chain (M_r 43,000) is encoded in the HLA-A, -B, and -C loci; the light chain is β$_2$-microglobulin, coded for on chromosome 9
Class II molecules	A dimer composed of two transmembrane polypeptide chains (α and β) with M_r 34,000 and 29,000, respectively
Class III molecules	Plasma proteins such as C2 or C4, or cytokines such as tumor necrosis factor (TNF) α and β

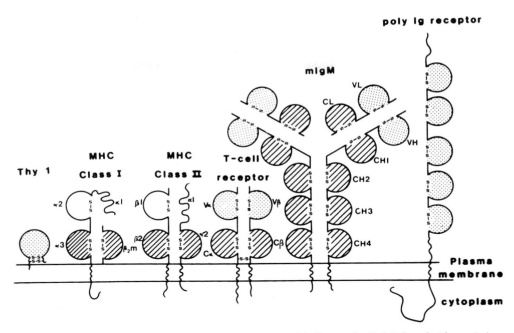

FIGURE 20-2. Schematic structures of proteins in the "immunoglobulin superfamily." *(Adapted with permission from Kaufman JF, Auffray C, Korman AJ, et al: The class II molecules of the human and murine major histocompatibility complex. Cell 1984;28:891.)*

at least one affected sibling. Interestingly, about 50% of the second siblings developed T1DM more than 10 years after the first affected sibling.[66] The lifetime recurrence risk for siblings from time of birth up to 30 years of age was 6%, which increased to 10% at 60 years of age. Studies of families with multiple affected members have shown that the occurrence of T1DM is 16% if the parent or sibling shares both HLA markers with the proband (HLA identical), 5% for one HLA marker (HLA haploidentical), and 1% or less for HLA nonidentical.[59,61] Although these and other studies have failed to clarify the mode of inheritance of T1DM, it is generally held that the HLA types mark genetic susceptibility or risk of developing the disease. This conclusion is based on the calculation of odds ratio or relative risk (RR). This calculation is simply an expression of how often an HLA allele or haplotype occurs in a sample of patients compared with controls. The data may reveal a positive association (interpreted as susceptibility), no association or neutral, or a negative association (interpreted as protection). Certain HLA-DR specificities, such as DR2 (67) or HLA haplotypes such as DQB1*0602-DQA1*0102 (DQ6.2), are rarely found

among young T1DM patients,[68,69] although the frequency of the haplotype among patients increases with age of diagnosis of diabetes.[70] The association with the disease is negative, which is interpreted as protection from T1DM. The mechanisms are not fully understood but may be related to a difference in binding of peptides from autoantigens such as GAD.[71]

Typing sera defined by international workshops for the serologically defined HLA-DR (R for related) specificities showed that the increased frequencies of B8 and B15 were most likely secondary to increased frequencies of DR3 and DR4 because of the linkage disequilibrium between B8 and DR3 and between B15 and DR4, respectively.[67] This concept is important for the discussion that follows. Statistical analyses[67] demonstrate that T1DM patients with HLA-B8 are more often HLA-DR3-positive than healthy HLA-B8 positive controls. These analyses suggested that the DR locus was indeed closer to a putative risk gene for T1DM than the locus coding for the HLA-B specificities. In children or young adults, the overall findings are that >90% of T1DM patients were positive for DR3, DR4, or both compared with 60% of the controls. It was also found that among Caucasians as many as 35–40% of T1DM patients were DR3/4 (heterozygotes).[67] The calculation of RR or absolute RR for the heterozygous combination DR3/4 exceeds the sum of the RR for DR3 and DR4 either as a homozygous specificity or in association with any other DR type. Monozygotic twins concordant for T1DM showed an increased frequency of DR3/4 heterozygosity.[72]

Proliferative responses to cloned T lymphocytes in a primed lymphocyte test (PLT) indicate that DR4 has at least six subtypes—Dw4, Dw10, Dw13, Dw14, Dw15, and a Dw-blank specificity. The DR4 specificity is determined by the DRB1 locus.[73] Although some controversies exist,[74] most investigations have shown the Dw4 subtype to be associated with T1DM.[67] Dw10 was also found to be associated with T1DM, whereas Dw13, Dw14, Dw15, and the blank allele were not.[75] Cellular typing was rapidly super-

TABLE 20-2. Lifetime Recurrence Risk of Type 1 Diabetes

Age-corrected Empirical Risk of Type I Diabetes	Age at Onset of Proband	
	< 25 Years	≥ 25 Years
A. Parents	2.2 ± 0.6%	4.9 ± 1.4%
Siblings	6.9 ± 1.3%	5.8 ± 1.8%
Children	5.6 ± 2.8%	4.3 ± 2.2%
B. HLA-identical siblings	15.5%	ND
HLA-haploidentical siblings	4.9%	ND
HLA-nonidentical siblings	1.2%	ND
C. Identical twins	25–50%	ND

ND, not determined.

seded by molecular techniques after the cloning of DR and DQ A and B genes (for a review, see refs. 60 and 61). Polymerase chain reaction (PCR) analyses with rapid sequencing are widely used.[76] These tools make it possible to relate T-cell responses or antigen presentation to different alleles, haplotypes, or genotypes of DR and DQ and to determine the importance of these cellular responses in the pathogenesis of T1DM.

The HLA class II molecules are central to the human immune response because they present peptide antigens to T-helper (CD4-positive) cells (for review, see ref. 77). It is therefore a reasonable hypothesis that HLA class II molecules associated or linked to T1DM may present peptides that are diabetogenic.[59,61,78] Peptide binding is diverse and variable because there is marked polymorphism of both class I and II molecules. This is of particular importance because class II molecules are dimers composed of one α and one β chain (Fig. 20-2), each coded by a separate gene, and heterodimers can form in heterozygous individuals.[79] For example, the chromosome inherited from the mother (m) would transcribe an α chain (am) and a β chain (bm). The same transcriptions events would take place on the chromosome from the father (p), resulting in ap and bp. The class II molecules that may be formed therefore represent ambm, ambp, apbm, or apbp (Fig. 20-3). It is possible that disease-associated class II molecules are formed because of *trans*-complementation events. These events may be positively associated with the disease, such as in individuals with certain DR2/DQ6.2-containing haplotypes, or negatively associated in individuals heterozygous for DQBI*0302 and DQB1*0602.[68–70,80]

Although DR4 and DR2 are composed of several closely related subtypes, DR3 appears to be more homogeneous.[58] Compiling the results of a large number of studies, the frequency of DR3 among Caucasian T1DM patients amounts to nearly 60% (range, 20–91%), compared with 22% (10–32%) among healthy controls.[59,61] The overall RR was 3.4. It is remarkable that the RRs of DR3 in Japan and China (34% in patients and 17% in controls) and among African Americans (57% in patients and 28% in controls) were similar (3.4 and 3.2, respectively). This was also similar to Caucasians (3.4%), even though the absolute frequency of DR3 varies substantially depending on ethnicity. MLC or PLT failed to reveal additional subtypes of DR3 and/or Dw3.[81] In contrast, a subset of DR3-positive T1DM patients who, in a PLT test, reacted differently from DR3 controls (31% of patients compared with 8% of controls) has been reported.[82] The DR3 specificity is encoded by the DRB1*0301 gene, which is in linkage disequilibrium with the DQA1*050l-B1*0201 (DQ2) haplotype. The role of DQ2 in T1DM is unclear, especially as it has been found that DQ2 is positively associated with T1DM primarily in the presence of DQ8.[56]

Recent advances in molecular genetics have allowed detailed studies of the genes that code for the HLA class II molecules including their precise chromosomal location, nucleotide sequences, and transcriptional regulation. In fact, the entire HLA class II region has been sequenced, and bioinformatic details are available at http://www.anthonynolan.org.uk/HIG/index.html.   PCR-based HLA typing has revolutionized not only HLA typing for transplantation, but also studies of disease associations.[58] Knowledge of the nucleotide sequence permits a derivation of the expected amino acid sequence of the individual class II molecules. A schematic map of the HLA-D region of human chromosome 6 is shown in Fig. 20-4. The reader is referred to refs. 77 and 83 for reviews of the molecular genetics of HLA (Fig. 20-4). The molecular cloning and expression of class II molecules made it possible to determine the structure of these protein complexes,[84,85] and molecular models are shown in Fig. 20-5. The molecular cloning of these genes has also made it possible to define their functions *in vitro* by gene transfection studies or *in vivo* by the production of transgenic mice. The size of the HLA-D region has been estimated to be as large as 1.1×10^6 bp.[86] The DQ and DR subregions are harbored within 450×10^3 bp. The current order of known genes from the centromere toward the telomere is illustrated in Fig. 20-4. Each one of the genes, referred to as A and B genes and coding for the α and β chains, respectively, has been cloned and sequenced. Genomic HLA typing by PCR analyses (Table 20-3) made it possible to test the hypothesis that genetic determinants other than DR explained the association between HLA and T1DM. Evidence that DQ is closer to T1DM than DR was first obtained by restriction fragment length polymorphism (RFLP) analysis,[87] followed by direct cDNA sequence analysis,[88] and was confirmed in numerous investigations by allele-specific PCR analyses.[80,89]

As indicated previously, DR4 is a broad serologic specificity now explained by several DRB1 alleles such as DRB1*0401, DRBI*0402, and DRBI*0403.[58] Due to linkage disequilibrium, these DR4 subtype alleles are commonly inherited with only a limited number of HLA-DQ alleles, as summarized in Tables 20-3 and 20-4. Although DRB1*0401 and DRB1*0405 were strongly associated with T1DM, DRB1*0403 was found to be protective.[56,90] It is therefore possible that antigen presentation by different HLA-DR or DQ molecules may make variable contributions to T1DM risk.

Taken together, the currently available data suggest that certain DQ alleles are more closely associated with T1DM than the associated DR alleles. Data produced by several investigators suggest that among DR4-positive individuals the DQ8 specificity confers the highest risk for T1DM. This risk may, however, be modulated by different DRB1*04 subtypes.[56,90] Comparing the DQ β-chain gene sequences between T1DM patients and controls, Todd and coworkers[88] suggested that susceptibility or resistance to disease is conferred by the amino acid in position 57, as aspartic acid (Asp) in position 57 was rarely seen among diabetic patients. Asp is only one of four polymorphic residues at position 57 of the DQ β chain. The presence of Asp57 in negatively associated HLA-DQ alleles resulted in a simplified view of susceptibility and protection based on this single amino acid.[88,89,91] Several investigations have since

FIGURE 20-3. The location of DQB1 and DQA1 genes on paternal (p) and maternal (m) chromosomes. Possible HLA-DQ class II molecules that may be formed in *cis* and *trans*-complementation are indicated. *(Reproduced with permission from Kockum et al.[68])*

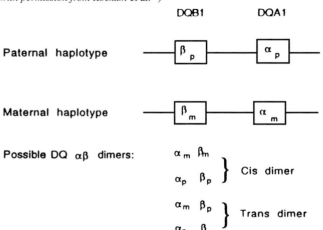

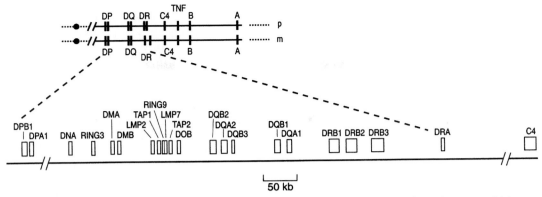

FIGURE 20-4. Schematic map of the HLA region of chromosome 6. The major loci are shown for a paternal (p) and maternal (m) chromosome. The loci between DP and DR are amplified to indicate the location of currently known genetic factors in the HLA class II region.

failed to support this popularized hypothesis. For example, a majority of Chinese[92] and Japanese[93] patients are Asp57-positive on DQ4 and DQ9, which are positively associated with T1DM in these ethnic groups. Other transracial studies[94] indicated that transcomplementation permits the formation of T1DM -permissive DQ heterodimers despite the presence of DQB1Asp 57. Studies in high-incidence countries such as Norway, Sweden, and Finland demonstrate that 2–3% of T1DM children are homozygous Asp57-positive.[79]

The Asp57 hypothesis was subsequently modified to include the DQA1 locus, and Arg52 of DQA1 was suggested to be a critical residue.[89,95] Several investigators have used DQB1 Asp57 and DQA1 Arg52 to calculate RR. These analyses show that DQB1 non-Asp57 and DQA1 Arg52 in homozygous combination only accounted for 47% of Swedish T1DM patients compared with 7% of

controls. All other combinations were neutral or negatively associated with T1DM. Not even combining these two polymorphic amino acids would fully explain susceptibility to T1DM. Position 57 is predicted to be at the far right of the lower α helix in Fig. 20-5. However, about 5% of T1DM patients have been found to be positive for DQw7, which has Asp in position 57.[67,91,96] It is therefore impossible for susceptibility or resistance to T1DM to be conferred solely by this particular amino acid residue.

Large population-based investigations provide sufficient statistical power for the association between HLA and T1DM to be critically analyzed. A genetic factor in the HLA region that totally controlled the development of diabetes would be expected to be present among all (100%) patients. The frequency of this factor in the healthy control population would be expected to be significantly lower, but not necessarily to the level of disease prevalence

FIGURE 20-5. Hypothetical Structure of the HLA Class II Molecule Foreign Antigen Binding Site. *(Reproduced with permission from Bjorkman PJ, Saper MA, Samraou B. Structure of the human class I histocompatibility antigen, HLA A2. Nature 1987;329:506.)*

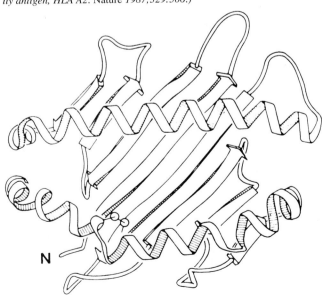

TABLE 20-3. Caucasian HLA Haplotypes

DQB1	DQA1	DRB
0201 (DQ2)	0501	3
0201 (DQ2)	0201	7
0301 (DQ7)	0301	4
0301 (DQ7)	0501	5
0302 (DQ8)	0301	4
0303 (DQ9)	0201	7
0303 (DQ9)	0301	9
0402 (DQ4)	0401	8
0501 (DQ5)	0101	1
0502 (DQ5)	0102	2
0503 (DQ5)	0101	6
0601 (DQ6)	0103	2
0602 (DQ6)	0102	2
0603 (DQ6)	0103	6
0604 (DQ6)	0102	6

TABLE 20-4. Genotypes and Haplotypes Associated with Insulin Dependent Diabetes Mellitus (IDDM)

	Association with IDDM	
	Positive	**Negative**
■ GENOTYPES		
DR	DR4	DR2
	DR3	
DQA1	0301	0102
DQB1	0302	0602
	0501	
■ HETEROZYGOSITY	DQ-DR heterozygotes	
Positive association	DQ 2/8 > DQ 8/8 > DQ8/DQB1*0604-DQA1*0102	
Negative association	DQ 6/6 > DQ 6/8 > DQ6/2	
■ HAPLOTYPES	DQ-DR haplotype	
Positive association	DQB1*0302-DQA1*0301(DQ8)-DR4	
	DQB1*0201-DQA1*0501(DQ2)-DR3	
Negative association	DQB1*0602-DQA1*0102(DQ6)-DR2	
	DQB*0301-DQA1*0301(DQ7)-DR4	

itself. Studies in identical twins[37] and in families[97] suggest that the genetic factors may only account for 30–40% of disease susceptibility, the rest probably being the environment. Among the genetic factors, linkage analysis suggests that HLA contributes 60%.[97]

The major question is whether HLA-DQ is the final answer. To answer this question, studies were conducted on both populations and families including sib-pair analyses[97] using a variety of statistical tests and models to estimate risk.[68] First, individual alleles may be considered, such as DQB1*0302, which is positively associated with T1DM, or DQB1*0602, which is negatively associated with T1DM (Table 20-4). The association between HLA and T1DM with the DQB1 alleles therefore would take into account one-half of the HLA-DQ class II molecule (Fig. 20-2), and a functional consequence that controls T1DM development needs to be identified. The same reasoning is applicable to the many different known alleles of DQA1. It is noted in this respect that most Japanese T1DM patients are DQA1*0301 positive, the same as Caucasians.[95] Second, the Asp-Arg model[89] would represent the other approach in which amino acid polymorphisms in the DQB1 and DQA1 alleles, respectively, are used to estimate risk. As indicated, this approach is not sufficient to explain T1DM susceptibility. Third, disease susceptibility is estimated based on the DQB1-DQA1 haplotype. The hypothesis is that the entire DQ class II molecule is more predictive of susceptibility to T1DM than either DQ chain alone or single amino acids such as DQB1 non-Asp57 and DQA Arg52. Analyses of population-based families suggest that the order of fit is DQB-DQA > DQB1 > DQB1-Asp57/DQA1 Arg52.[68,69] There is no evidence that DQB1*0302 was more strongly associated with T1DM than DQA1*0301. In conclusion, T1DM susceptibility and protection are probably controlled by the expression and function of HLA-DQ class II molecules. The mechanisms may be specific peptide binding to the groove illustrated in Fig. 20-5 and selective initiation of an immune response, perhaps to a T1DM-associated autoantigen such as GAD-65, insulin, or IA-2.

The DQB-DQA molecules that may be formed following either *cis*- or *trans*-complementation are illustrated in Fig. 20-3. Functional studies on peptide loading, binding, and presentation to T lymphocytes are in progress to explain the mechanisms by which

HLA-DQ may control T1DM.[71,99] It has been shown that DQB-DQA heterodimers are able to present peptides of GAD-65 and insulin, the two major autoantigens in T1DM (discussed later). In humans, T-cell responses restricted by HLA-DQ or HLA-DR and dependent on antigen presentation of GAD-65 have been reported.[99,100]

The sequencing of the HLA-DR-DQ-DP region (Fig. 20-4) has identified a number of novel genes. Their products have been shown to fulfill distinct mechanisms in the antigen-presentation pathways for both class I and II molecules. The region between DQ and DR is sufficiently large to harbor yet other genes. It is therefore still possible that the DQ-DR association with T1DM is secondary to yet other genetic factor(s). Sequence analysis of the DQB1*0302 and DQB1*0301 promoter regions has indicated base pair differences that may control rates of transcription of these molecules.[60] Such upstream sequences are important to explore because they often control tissue-specific expression. Sequence analysis combined with functional analyses should make it possible to map the location of putative susceptibility gene loci by comparing absolute RRs with the location on the chromosome. Given the extent or the size of the HLA-D region, it cannot be excluded that genetic elements other than those coding for HLA class II proteins may confer susceptibility to disease. This is exemplified by the observation that congenital severe combined immunodeficiency is linked to flanking sequences that control gene expression.[101]

The HLA class II molecules restrict the immune response to external antigens, and they are thought to control the development of nonresponsiveness or tolerance to self-molecules.[77] Nonresponsiveness to self may primarily be maintained by T-cytotoxic, regulatory, or suppressor cells. These cells are also dependent on antigens presented by class II molecules. It is conceivable that HLA association to disease, including T1DM, is primarily related to mechanisms of protection or nonsusceptibility.[79] Studies on the ability of antigen-presenting cells (APCs) to stimulate T-cell proliferation in response to β cells[102] or specific β-cell autoantigens such as insulin, IA-2, or GAD-65 may help to resolve these issues.

DR3 specificity is most commonly found in association with DR4 because HLA-DR3/4 heterozygotes may comprise as many as 35–45% of T1DM children or young adults.[67,103] As pointed out previously, the DQ locus on DR3-containing chromosomes varies less than the DQ associated with DR4. It is therefore likely that a function of DR3-DQ2 class II molecules influences the pathogenesis of T1DM. In patients with T1DM, DR3 has been associated with low immune responsiveness to insulin,[104] as well as to mumps and coxsackievirus B4, but not to varicella-zoster or purified protein derivative (PPD) of tuberculin.[105,106] In contrast, DR4 was associated with an increased T-cell proliferative response to mumps and coxsackievirus antigens.

These studies need to be confirmed because it is unclear why the two DR types, which are both strongly associated with T1DM, would show opposite effects on antigen-specific T-cell proliferation. One possibility is that DR3, DR4, or both are only in linkage disequilibrium with DQ and that the observations regarding mumps and coxsackievirus are not predictive of T1DM. Another is that DR3 is associated with attenuated immune function, such as removal of immune complexes, which promotes DR4-mediated stimulation of autoreactive T cells and autoantibodies. It is possible that such reactions would either initiate or potentiate an already established immune reaction toward the β cells. It should also be kept in mind that the HLA class II molecules control both T-helper and T-regulatory cell mechanisms.[107] Whether the development of T1DM is dependent on helper cells, regulatory cells, or both is unknown. The former would seem to require an active immunization with an immunogen from the islets directly or a mimicking β-cell antigen to give rise to an immune response toward the β cells. The latter scenario has been invoked based on evidence that there are sequence homologies between GAD-65 and coxsackie B4.[108] GAD-65 has also been used in experiments to test whether HLA class II molecules control the development of T1DM by their ability to present GAD-65 peptides.[109,110] In addition, investigations with GAD-65, coxsackie B4, and peptides of each protein allow a test of the hypothesis that molecular mimicry may initiate autoimmunity but only in certain HLA-susceptible individuals.

The particular proneness to develop T1DM among HLA-DR3/4 DQ-2/8 positive individuals remains to be explained. It has been speculated[111] that the formation of *trans*-complementation HLA class II molecules explains the markedly increased risk of DR3-DQ2 and DR4-DQ8 together (Fig. 20-3). *Trans*-complementation HLA-DQ molecules have been demonstrated in DR3/4-positive IDDM patients.[111] The role of such class II molecules in cell–cell interaction, antigen processing, and presentation is currently not known. The specific amino acid sequence of the α and β chains may determine in part their ability to form such heterodimers.[79] Reagents such as monoclonal antibodies[112] or antibodies against synthetic peptides,[113] which are able to detect α and β chains of defined specificities, should help clarify the presence and functional capacity of *cis*- and *trans*-complementation molecules in the human immune response.

One possible mechanism to explain cell-specific autoimmunity would be if the target cell was able to express HLA class II molecules. It is conceivable that cell-specific self-antigens could be presented by the target cell itself and could thereby induce an immune response by activating appropriate T lymphocytes. Class II molecules are rarely expressed on nonlymphoid cells. The first evidence of aberrant expression was obtained in skin cells of mice with graft-versus-host disease. In organ-specific autoimmunity, thyroid cells may express class II molecules in thyroiditis-affected glands.[114] *In vitro* studies indicated that it was possible to induce class II expression by mitogens[115] or cytokines such as interleukin-1 (IL-1), IL-2, interferon-γ (INF-γ), or tumor necrosis factor (TNF) in both thyroid and islet cells.[116] Studies in the NOD mouse and the BB rat failed to reveal class II expression on β cells, but such expression was found on endothelial cells and on infiltrating mononuclear cells.[117] The detection of class II-positive β cells in a newly diagnosed patient evaluated by immunocytochemistry[118] could not be confirmed in other patients.[12] Aberrant class II expression in human β cells[118] has also been questioned by the observation that at least some of the islet class II-positive cells are macrophages containing insulin granules due to phagocytosis of β cells that have undergone apoptosis.[119,120]

The hypothesis of aberrant expression of class II molecules inducing an autoimmune response was also tested in transgenic mice.[121,122] In these experiments the class II molecule α- and β-chain genes have been inserted into the mouse genome and expressed in the β cell under control of the insulin gene promoter. This aberrant class II expression does not induce insulitis. Hyperglycemia may develop, due presumably to interference with insulin biosynthesis.[121,122] Furthermore, islet β cells expressing class II molecules isolated from the pancreas of transgenic mice were unable to present antigen to induce specific T-lymphocyte responses.[123] These studies suggest that aberrant class II antigen expression on β cells *per se* does not induce an inflammatory response. In contrast, expression of the IFN-γ gene under control of

the insulin gene promoter was associated with the development of both hyperglycemia and insulitis.[121] Similarly, transgenic mice expressing IFN-α in the β cells develop insulitis and diabetes, indicating the possible importance of this cytokine in a pathogenetic immune response.[124] IL-1β transgenic mice did not develop insulitis or diabetes, similar to IL-10-producing transgenic mice.[125] A backcross of the IL-10 transgene onto NOD mice resulted in an acceleration of the T1DM. Therefore, current experimental evidence does not support the hypothesis that aberrant class II expression on target β cells can initiate insulitis, but it does support the possibility that the expression of class I and II molecules within the islet is influenced by the presence of cytokines.

The process of generating endogenous immunogenic peptides is poorly understood. Several genes clustered in the MHC class II region (Fig. 20-4) are thought to be involved in the generation and transport of endogenous immunogenic peptides for MHC class I molecules.[126] The transporter-associated peptide genes TAP 1 and TAP 2, which are located between HLA-DP and HLA-DQ, encode the heterodimeric protein complex responsible for transporting endogenous peptides from the cytosol to the lumen of the endoplasmic reticulum (ER). Two other genes, LMP 2 and LMP 7, also located between HLA-DP and HLA-DQ, interdigitating between the TAP 1 and TAP 2 genes, are believed to be involved in the generation of peptides in the cytosol. These proteosome subunits are present in both cytoplasm and nucleus and generate, through multiple protease specificities, a great diversity of short peptides of different lengths.[127] The gene products of these four genes are members of the adenosine triphosphate (ATP)-binding cassette (ABC) super family. The proteosome subunits LMP 2 and LMP 7 are not essential for the generation of antigenic peptides, because cell lines deficient in these subunits present peptides to T cells.[128]

Each TAP gene encodes an approximately 75-kd IFN-γ-inducible protein. The functional transporter consists of either a heterodimer or some combination of the TAP I and TAP 2 proteins.[129] In TAP 1, two polymorphic residues at position 333 (Ile for Val) and 637 (Asp for Gly), generate four possible alleles. TAP 1A is the most common allele followed by TAP 1B and TAP 1C. In TAP 2, four polymorphic residues at position 379 (Ile for Val), 565 (Ala for Thr), 665 (Ala for Thr), and 687 (stop codon for Gln) allow the formation of eight possible alleles. TAP 2A is the most common followed by TAP 2B and TAP 2C. The TAP-2 allele 0101 was positively associated, and TAP-0201 negatively associated, with T1DM, whereas TAP-1 did not show any significant association.[69] However, the TAP allele association with T1DM was lost when HLA-DR-DQ–matched patients and controls were compared,[130,131] and therefore the effect of the TAP gene was most likely due to linkage disequilibrium.

Association with Other Genes on Chromosome 6

The genes for TNF-α and TNF-β are also located in the MHC region (Fig. 20-4). Both genes have polymorphisms associated with T1DM[132] Although TNF-β alleles differ between HLA-DR–matched Caucasian T1DM patients and controls,[133] this was not found in North Indian Asians, suggesting that TNF-β does not directly predispose to T1DM.[132] The genes for heat shock protein (HSP) are also located in the MHC region. The increased frequency of an HSP70-2 9.5-kb Pst fragment among T1DM patients compared with controls was explained by linkage disequilibrium with DR3.[134] Consistent with this conclusion is the observation that Japanese T1DM patients do not show an association with HSP70.[135]

The properdin factor B (Bf) F1 allele has been reported to be increased among T1DM patients compared with controls, but only among 5–25% of the patients.[136] BfF1 was not increased among DR3/4 T1DM patients compared with DR3/4 controls, suggesting that the Bf association was secondary to the DR association.[137] The two complement genes C4A and C4B also showed associations with T1DM.[138] The data in one study suggested that the association of C4A3 and C4B3 was independent of the HLA-DR association.[137] However, the risk conferred by the C4 genes is lower than that conferred by the DR or DQ class II genes.

Association and Linkage with Chromosome 11

Sequence analysis of the human insulin gene revealed the presence of upstream (5′-flanking) variable-number tandem repeat (VNTR) sequences.[139] Although the function of VNTRs is unknown, numerous studies have been carried out to test whether the large compared with small repeat sequences were associated with T1- or T2DM.[139] Although an association with T2DM was eventually excluded, the T1DM association was reproducible in several ethnic groups.[140] Exploration of other polymorphic sites in and around the insulin gene also revealed an association but no genetic linkage.[139,140] Although the T1DM VNTR was transmitted preferentially to DR4-positive diabetic offspring in multiplex families,[141] there was no difference in frequency among DR4-positive and negative patients, suggesting that the susceptibility conferred by the insulin gene is independent and nonsynergistic with HLA susceptibility.[141] Additional insulin gene polymorphisms have been detected by sequencing patient and control haplotypes.[140,142] Polymorphisms in the 5′-flanking region of the insulin gene[142] were not found to be directly associated with T1DM because these markers were present on haplotypes that were either associated or not with T1DM.[140] It was suggested that the size variation of the VNTR at the 5′ end of the insulin gene could have a direct effect on the insulin gene regulation.[143] The short class I VNTR alleles (26–63 repeats) predispose to T1DM, whereas class III alleles (140–210 repeats) have a dominant protective effect. When expression of insulin in human fetal thymus was examined, it was found that class III VNTR alleles were associated with two- to threefold higher proinsulin mRNA levels than class I.[144,145] It was suggested that higher levels of thymic insulin expression may facilitate immune tolerance induction as a mechanism for the dominant protective effect of class III alleles.

Association with Immunoglobin Genes

The mechanisms by which human immunoglobulins are genetically encoded and synthesized are known.[146] Prior to detailed analyses of the molecular genetics of the immunoglobulin gene heavy and light chains, it was tested whether certain allotypes of the immunoglobulin genes such as Km (light chain) and Gm (heavy chain) were associated with T1DM or linked to the disease in family studies (Table 20-5). The results have been controversial.[147,148] The allotype Glm(l) was reported to be increased among DR3/4 patients compared with controls.[149] An interaction between immunoglobulin allotypes and T-cell receptor genes was also reported,[150] and in a sib-pair analysis there was an HLA-dependent increase in sharing Gm phenotypes,[151] although other studies failed to detect linkage.[152]

Taken together, the data suggest that although Gm and Km allotypes do not provide direct disease susceptibility, they may interact with sex, age, and/or the HLA genes to influence susceptibility.

TABLE 20-5. Candidate Type 1 Diabetes Susceptibility Loci Identified by Linkage Analysis

Locus	Chromosome	Candidate Genes or Microsatellites
IDDM1	6p21.3	HLA (DQA1, DQB1, DRB1)
IDDM2	11p15.5	INS-VNTR, TH
IDDM3	15q26	D15S107
IDDM4	11q13.3	FGF3, D11S1917, MDU1, ZFM1, RT6, ICE, CD3, etc
IDDM5	6q25	ESR, a046Xa9, MnSOD
IDDM6	18q12-q21	D18S487, D18S64, JK (Kidd locus)
IDDM7	2q31-33	D2S152, D2S326, GAD1
IDDM8	6q25-27	D6S281, D6S264, D6S446
IDDM9	3q21-25	D3S1303
IDDM10	10p11-q11	D10S193, D10S208, GAD2
IDDM11	14q24.3-q31	D14S67
IDDM12	2q33	CTLA-4, CD28
IDDM13	2q34	D2S137, D2S164, IGFBP2, IGFBP5
IDDM14	Not assigned	Not assigned
IDDM15	6q21	D6S283, D6S434, D6S1580

It should be kept in mind that the Gm system is a marker for the constant region genes and that variable (V) region gene markers, which are now available as cloned gene probes, may be more likely to detect hypothetical polymorphisms associated with T1DM or other autoimmune disorders. The possible genetic control of antibody formation by HLA also needs to be analyzed, because it was reported that the immunoglobulin allotype association was observed in HLA-DR4 positive individuals only.

Association with T-Cell Receptor Genes

The T-cell receptor (TCR) is a heterodimer composed of an α and a β chain (Fig. 20-2). The genes for these two chains have been cloned and sequenced; the β chain is coded for on chromosome 7. Two additional genes for T-cell receptor chains, δ and γ, have recently been described. The TCR expressed on helper CD4 T lymphocytes recognizes foreign peptides in the context of HLA class II molecules, whereas cytotoxic CD8 T lymphocytes have TCR that recognizes foreign peptides in the context of HLA class I molecules (for review, see ref. 153).

The mechanisms by which TCR is formed or expressed in response to external or internal (autoantigen) antigens are not known. In autoimmunity, is it possible that the TCR involved in activities of the different types of T cells is derived from a limited number of specific variable (V) α- or β-gene sequences? Studies in the spontaneously diabetic NOD mouse and BB rat have so far failed to detect a preferential usage of Vβ or Vα genes.[154] A preferential use of Vβ was reported in experimental autoallergic encephalomyelitis (EAE).[155] This information is of particular interest because monoclonal antibodies against this specific TCR may be used to specifically deplete T lymphocytes expressing this particular TCR and thereby inhibit an immune response and prevent autoimmune disease.[155] Given the complexity of the TCR genes and their transcription and translation to form TCR, it is not surprising that current results on disease association in different ethnic populations are contradictory. Early reports showed that the heterozygotes of the TCR-β Bgl II RFLP were increased among T1DM patients compared with controls.[156] Later studies failed to detect this association.[157] There was no linkage between T1DM and TCR-Cβ.[158] There is one report suggesting that the TCR-Cβ association is dependent on the immunoglobulin heavy-chain region genes, as the distribution of TCR-Cβ differs between patients with G2m(23+) or G2m(23−), as well as between G3m(5+) and G3m(5−).[150] Recently, a polymorphism in the TCR-Cλ but not TCR-Vλ gene was associated with T1DM, in particular among DR3 and DR4 individuals.[159] In further studies to determine the possible role of autoantigen-specific TCR in the development of T1DM, the crystal structure of the NOD mouse I-Ag7 HLA-DQ homolog was determined as a complex with a high-affinity peptide from GAD.[85] I-Ag7 had a wide peptide-binding groove (Fig. 20-5B), which may account for disease-associated peptide binding. Similar results have recently been reported for HLA-DQ8 molecules and may be of importance in understanding the role of peptide binding in T1DM pathogenesis.[160]

Association with Other Genetic Markers from Genome Scanning

Other genetic markers for T1DM (Table 20-5) have been obtained by recent human genome scanning studies to support the previous observation[139] that other genetic factors may contribute to the risk for T1DM. The development of simple sequence repeat (SSR) markers to map the human genome made it possible to identify linkage between SSR markers and T1DM.[63,161,162] These studies required knowledge of the inheritance of T1DM such that genetic linkage was calculated from the simultaneous inheritance of SSR markers in affected siblings. DNA collection available to investigators throughout the world through the Human Biological Data Interchange (HBDI)[163,164] and from the British Diabetic Association (BDA) made it possible to identify several T1DM risk loci.[63,161,165] There may be as many as 14–18 such risk loci, although the number reproducible in all populations is controversial.[63,166]

HLA and insulin VNTR are estimated to contribute to about 40% and 10%, respectively, of familial clustering of T1DM. Other contributing genes are therefore expected. Among these, CTLA-4 on chromosome 2 has been reproduced in several ethnic groups.[167,168] Polymorphisms in the coding as well as noncoding regions of the CTLA-4 gene are associated with autoimmune diseases such as Graves' disease as well as T1DM.[168] The association between CTLA-4 and T1DM in a case-control study indicated that long (AT)n repeats at the 3′ end of the gene are associated with T1DM.[169] The mechanism explaining this association remains to be clarified. One possibility is that the CTLA-4 polymorphism affects the survival of autoreactive regulatory T cells. Although HLA seems necessary, it is clearly not sufficient for the appearance of T1DM; one or several contributing genes may affect the pathogenetic process and age at onset. The possiblity cannot be excluded, however, that other genetic factors important to β-cell function may contribute to T1DM risk. It is predicted that high-throughput genetic typing methods such as analysis of single nucleotide polymorphisms (SNP) will provide novel means by which large numbers of patients and controls can be used to improve the current T1DM genetic map.

IMMUNE ASPECTS

Autoantibodies

Autoantibodies reactive with antigens contained in pancreatic islet cells are common in T1DM (Table 20-6). Antibodies reactive against islet cell antigens (islet cell antibodies [ICAs]) were first

TABLE 20-6. Islet cell autoantigens of Insulin-Dependent Diabetes Mellitus

Autoantigen	Characteristics
Sialoglycolipid	Target of ICA in humans, GM2-1, non-beta-cell specific
Glutamate decarboxylase	Target of 64-kd antigen/GAD antibody in humans and animal models of IDD, two forms (GAD65 and 67), cellular immune antigen, synaptic like microvesicle protein, disease-modifying antigen
Insulin	Target of IAA in humans and non-obese diabetic (NOD) mice, cellular immune antigen, disease-modifying antigen
Insulin receptor	Target of autoantibodies in humans determined by bioassay
38 kd	Target of 38-kd antigen in humans, induced by cytomegalovirus, localized to insulin secretory granules, cellular immune antigen, multiple antigens of this molecular mass?
Bovine serum albumin	Target of BSA antibody, antigen in humans and animal models of IDD, contains ABBOS peptide, has molecular mimic in beta cell p69 protein (PM-1), disease-modifying antigen
Glucose transporter	Target of autoantibodies in humans, inhibit glucose stimulation, Glut-2 directed?
hsp 65	Target of autoantibodies and cellular immunity in NOD mice, disease-modifying antigen, contains p277 peptide.
Carboxypeptidase H	Target of autoantibodies in humans, identified by immunoscreening of islet cDNA, insulin secretory granule protein
52 kd	Target of autoantibodies in humans and NOD mice, molecular mimic with rubella virus
ICA12/ICA512	Target of autoantibodies in humans, identified by immunoscreening of islet cDNA, 5123 homology to CD45
150 kd	Target of autoantibodies in humans, beta-cell specific, membrane associated
RIN polar	Target of autoantibodies in humans and NOD mice, present on insulinoma cells

Reprinted with permission from Atkinson MA, Maclaren NK. Islet cell autoantigens in insulin-dependent diabetes. J Clin Invest. *1993;92:1608–1616.*

described in 1974 and provided strong evidence for an autoimmune etiology and pathogenesis for T1DM. The initial description of ICA has been followed by a large number of reports describing the presence of antibodies reactive with a variety of islet cell components. These include antibodies to insulin, proinsulin, GAD, carboxypeptidase H, a sialoglycolipid, and several other incompletely defined antigens of different molecular weights: 37, 38, 52, 64, 69, and 150 kd.[170] Most of these antibodies occur with high prevalence in newly diagnosed T1DM subjects and prior to clinical appearance of diabetes. Their presence is useful in detecting β-cell autoimmunity and in assessing the risk of subsequent clinical T1DM in genetically susceptible individuals. However, the relationships among the various islet cell autoantibodies, β-cell autoimmunity, and eventual clinical T1DM is very complex and still not fully characterized or understood. Of all the autoantibodies described in T1DM, four are clinically most useful: ICA, IAA, GADA, and IA-2A.

When ICAs were first discovered in 1974, it was felt that all individuals with ICAs would eventually develop clinical T1DM. This is not the case, and recent extensive investigation in this area has revealed considerable complexity. When ICAs are detected in nondiabetic individuals identified because of other autoimmune diseases besides diabetes, the risk of subsequent clinical T1DM is less than when ICAs occur in relatives of T1DM patients.[171] Similarly, ICA-positive individuals from the general population without a family history of T1DM have a much lower risk of T1DM than ICA-positive relatives of T1DM patients.[172,173] In fact, ICAs can occur in people with protective HLA haplotypes, and in these individuals subsequent clinical T1DM is unusual.[174,175] Several subsets of ICAs have been identified with varying risks of T1DM. A subset termed **restrictive**, because the staining pattern is restricted to the β cells and does not stain mouse pancreas, is less predictive of subsequent T1DM than ICAs reactive with all islet endocrine cells and with mouse pancreas.[174] Similarly, ICA binding that is displaceable with GAD or that gives a granular staining pattern is less predictive of subsequent T1DM than conventional ICA.[170,176]

Insulin autoantibodies have become equally complex. In relatives of T1DM patients, the presence of IAAs in addition to ICAs greatly increases the risk of subsequent clinical T1DM compared with ICAs alone, but relatives with IAAs without ICAs have only a minimally increased risk of clinical T1DM.[177] Certain drugs such as methimazole and penicillamine can induce IAAs, but these subjects develop hypoglycemia, not T1DM. Some viral infections can induce IAAs of the IgM subclass, which are also unrelated to T1DM.[178] An international workshop revealed that IAAs measured by fluid-phase assays were predictive of subsequent clinical T1DM, whereas IAAs measured by solid-phase enzyme-linked immunosorbent assay (ELISA) were not.[179] It has not been resolved whether this is due to the two assay formats measuring antibodies of different affinities or to antibodies directed against different epitopes on the insulin molecule, but only fluid-phase IAA assays should be used to assess the risk of T1DM.

In 1990 Baekkeskov and colleagues[180] reported that the 64K autoantigen recognized by antibodies from T1DM patients was GAD. A wealth of data regarding 64K antigens and antibodies to these antigens in T1DM obtained over the last few years has revealed that this area is as complex as for ICAs and IAAs. GAD exists in at least two major isoforms, GAD-65 and GAD-67. Their respective distributions in β cells and neural tissue vary between species, and although antibodies to both isoforms can occur, antibodies to GAD-65 are predominantly associated with T1DM in humans.[181] Several assay formats including fluid-phase, ELISA, and enzymatic assays have been developed, and an international workshop demonstrated, as for IAAs, marked differences related to methodology. In general, fluid-phase measurements of GAD-65 antibodies were most closely correlated with T1DM.[182] GAD autoantibodies are very common in the rare neurologic disorder, stiff-man syndrome, and only a small percentage of these patients develop T1DM. Furthermore, the GAD autoantibodies in T1DM and stiff-man syndrome appear to differ in their ability to inhibit GAD enzymatic activity and in recognizing antigen in Western blot assays.[183] As discussed previously, ICAs that are displaceable with GAD are surprisingly less associated with T1DM than ICAs not recognizing GAD.[170] Recent data have also revealed that antibodies from T1DM subjects binding to 64K islet antigens include antibodies to antigens other than GAD. Some investigators have identified antibodies to HSP65 in T1DM,[184] but others have not,[185] so this remains a controversial area.

The maturation of the humoral response to GAD epitopes sequentially from birth to diabetes onset or current follow-up in GAD antibody (GADA)+ offspring of parents with diabetes was examined recently in the German BABYDIAB Study.[28] Antibodies were measured against GAD-65, GAD-67, and GAD-65/67 chimeras by radiobinding assay. In 28 of 29 offspring, the first GADA contained reactivity against epitopes within GAD-65 residues 96-444, suggesting that the middle GAD-65 region is a primary target of GAD humoral autoimmunity. Subsequent GADA epitope spreading was frequent, and spreading was mostly to NH2-terminal GAD-65 epitopes. In two offspring, spreading to new epitopes was found when antibody titers to GAD-65 and early epitopes were declining, suggesting determinant-specific regulation of the humoral response. None of the GADA reactivities or any changes in reactivity over time were specifically associated with diabetes onset. These findings suggested that the humoral autoimmune response to GAD found in childhood is dynamic, is initially against epitopes within the middle portion of GAD-65, and spreads to epitopes in other regions of GAD-65 and GAD-67. Hampe and colleagues[186] showed that recognition of epitopes by GAD-65 Ab in T1DM is different from that in non-T1DM, GAD-65 Ab-positive individuals. Further studies demonstrated that the N-terminal part is essential for full antibody binding to GAD-65, in particular to the middle epitope. It was suggested that T1DM is associated with restricted GAD-65Ab epitope specificity, and the evolution of GAD-65 autoantibodies in T1DM includes reactivity to a non-human GAD-65 N-terminal end conformation. Progression toward T1DM is, however, associated with a maturation of the immune response toward human GAD-65 autoreactivity.[187–189]

In very elegant experiments, Christie and colleagues[190] have demonstrated antibodies in T1DM to a 64-kd islet protein distinct from known isoforms of HSP or GAD. Antibodies recognizing a 37-kd tryptic fragment of this non-GAD 64-kd antigen were more predictive of T1DM than GAD autoantibodies.[190] These autoantibodies are now known as ICA512 or IA-2 (directed to the neuroendocrine protein insulinoma-associated protein 2, a member of the protein tyrosine phosphatase family).[191,192] Kawasaki and coworkers[193] have examined the overlapping specificities and antigenic epitopes of autoantibodies to IA-2 and phosphatase homolog in granules of insulinoma (phogrin) and determined whether intramolecular epitope spreading occurs during the development of diabetic autoimmunity. IA-2 autoantibodies and phogrin autoantibodies were detected in 65–70% of patients with new-onset T1DM and 60–65% of prediabetic relatives of patients with T1DM. Binding and competition analysis using multiple chimeric IA-2/phogrin constructs demonstrated that a major unique epitope for IA-2 autoantibodies is localized to amino acids 762–887. These studies highlighted the complexity of autoantibody recognition of IA-2/phogrin. Park and colleagues[53] investigated whether alternative splicing could affect humoral autoreactivity to the molecule. Radioimmunoprecipitation assays for IA-2/ICA512 autoantibodies were developed with the widely used ICA512.bdc construct (which has exon 13 deleted) and a series of full-length and modified ICA512/IA-2 molecules. The assays showed that ICA512.bdc and ICA512 604-979 gave the best discrimination between diabetic and control sera. With ICA512 604–979, a somewhat greater proportion of patients expressing antibodies were detected than with ICA512.bdc in the groups studied (70.5% vs. 63.2% of prediabetic/new-onset patients and 25.0% vs. 13.9% of patients with diabetes >20 years). They concluded that important epitopes lie within the exon 13 region and others can be generated by the alternative splicing.

The combinatorial Islet Autoantibody Workshop assessed the ability of individual autoantibody (ab) assays and their use in combination to discriminate between T1DM and control sera.[194] Coded aliquots of sera were measured in a total of 119 assays by 49 participating laboratories in 17 countries. The sera were from 51 patients with new-onset T1DM and 101 healthy control subjects with no family history of diabetes. There were no significant differences in sensitivity among 19 radioimmunoassays (RIAs) for IA-2 autoantibodies (ICA 512) using different constructs that included the intracellular portion of the molecule (mean sensitivity 73%). Among GAD autoantibody assays that achieved sensitivity >70%, 26 were RIAs and 1 was an ELISA. When the sera were ranked according to their autoantibody levels, the concordance for IAAs in different laboratories was markedly less than for IA-2A and GADA. Using a combination of autoantibody assays, several laboratories achieved excellent discrimination between diabetic and control sera (sensitivity up to 80% with a false-positive rate of 0%). A variety of strategies for combining information from different assays were successful (e.g., those including and excluding ICA), and no one strategy emerged as clearly superior.[194]

The relationships between genetic markers and disease-associated autoantibodies were studied in an unselected population of 701 siblings of children with T1DM, and the predictive characteristics of these markers over a period of 9 years were determined.[195] Increased prevalences of all the antibodies were closely associated with HLA identity to the index case, the DR4 and DQB1*0302 alleles, the DR3/4 phenotype, and the DQB1*02/0302 genotype. GADAs were also associated with the DR3 and DQB1*02 alleles, and siblings carrying the protective DR2 and DQB1*0602-3 alleles were characterized by lower frequencies of ICAs, IA-2A, and GADA. A combination of the genetic markers and autoantibodies increased the positive predictive values of all autoantibodies substantially, which may have clinical implications when evaluating the risk of developing T1DM at the individual level or when recruiting high-risk individuals for intervention trials.[195] However, because such combinations also resulted in reduced sensitivity, autoantibodies alone rather than in combination with genetic markers are recommended for first-line screening in siblings. Finally, not all siblings with a broad humoral autoimmune response or high-risk genetic markers present with T1DM, and some with a low genetic risk and weak initial signs of humoral autoimmunity may progress to disease. Lindberg and coworkers[196,197] tested for various islet autoantibodies in cord blood sera from controls and children who developed T1DM between 10 months and 14.9 years of age. An increased frequency of cord blood islet autoantibodies suggested that the T1DM process could already be initiated *in utero*.[196,197]

Although autoantibodies could damage β cells by antibody-dependent complement cytotoxicity or by targeting natural killer cells to β-cell antigens, transfer of T1DM in the animal models requires T cells, and consequently a major direct role for antibodies in causing the β-cell damage of T1DM is unlikely. The findings that intrathymic or intravenous administration of GAD can prevent T1DM in the NOD mouse[198,199] and that T cells reactive with insulin can transfer T1DM in the NOD mouse model[200] suggest important direct roles for GAD and insulin in T1DM. The 9–23-amino acid region of the insulin B chain (B9–23) is a dominant epitope recognized by pathogenic T lymphocytes in NOD mice. Maron and colleagues[201] have shown that oral and nasal administration of insulin or GAD suppresses development of diabetes in the NOD mouse and that this suppression appears secondary to the generation of regulatory T cells that act by secreting anti-inflammatory cytokines such as IL-4 and transforming growth factor (TGF)-β. They analyzed cytokine patterns associated with mucosal administration of insulin B chain, B-chain peptide 10–24, and GAD peptide 524–543, and derived lines and clones from mucosally treated animals. There was significantly less IFN-γ production in mucosally treated mice associated with increased production of IL-10 and TGF-β. The nature of the antigen appeared to determine cytokine production, as the B chain given either orally or nasally primed for TGF-β responses, whereas mucosally administered B-chain peptide 10–24 primed for IL-10.

Their results supported a role for Th2-type cells (see below for discussion on Th1/Th2 cells) in the regulation of diabetes in NOD mice.[201] Their further studies showed that neonatal feeding of human insulin or insulin B-chain peptide (10–24) is effective in inhibiting diabetes when given to the NOD mouse,[202] and this may have applications in preventing diabetes in high-risk human populations. Studies in the BB rat model also demonstrated that immunization with insulin B chain in the presence of adjuvant can reduce diabetes incidence.[203] The absence of any metabolic effect of B chain and the requirement for adjuvant suggested that this effect is mediated via modulation of the autoimmune response. Alleva and coworkers[204] recently described B9–23-specific T-cell responses in peripheral lymphocytes obtained from patients with recent-onset T1DM and from prediabetic subjects at high risk for disease.[204] This is the first demonstration of a cellular response to the B9–23 insulin epitope in human T1DM and suggests that the mouse and human diseases have strikingly similar autoantigenic targets, a feature that should facilitate development of antigen-based therapeutics.

Cellular Immune Response and Cytokines

T1DM is thought to result from a T-cell–mediated destruction of the pancreatic β cells. Antigen-specific T-cell activation requires two signals. One is imparted by interaction of the TCR/CD3 complex with the antigen:MHC class II protein complex expressed by APCs. The second signal is provided by cell-bound and secreted costimulatory molecules, which (although not imparting any antigenic specificity) synergize with TCR/CD3 signals in augmenting T-cell activation.[205,206] Several signal transduction pathways operate as a result of T-cell activation. These include the phospholipase C-1 pathway, the p21^{ras}/RAF kinase (the classical mitogen-activated protein kinase) pathway,[207] and the phosphatidylinositol 3′-hydroxykinase/GDP-Rac (the alternative mitogen-activated protein kinase) signaling pathway.[208]

Coupling to more than one signaling pathway is possible depending on the intensity of the signal generated, the duration of stimulation, and the contribution of costimulatory molecules, which, in turn, affects the duration and outcome of the functional response.[209,210] Insofar as costimulatory signals determine whether TCR recognition of antigen will lead to activation, apoptosis, or anergy, a role for altered costimulation in the pathogenesis of autoimmune diseases including T1DM[211,212] has been proposed. Accordingly, manipulation of costimulatory pathways was proposed as a potential strategy for managing autoimmune diseases, including T1DM.[212]

As part of the insulitis process, a number of cytokines (soluble polypeptide mediators) are released from the immune cells infiltrating the islet. In addition to their immunologic functions of modulating, amplifying, and directing the immune response, several of the cytokines have been found to have direct effects on the pancreatic β cells. The direct effects potentially involved in the pathogenesis of T1DM include inhibition of insulin release, cytotoxicity, and altered antigen expression. The cytokines IL-1, TNF, and IFN have been the most intensively studied. Although there is considerable variability depending on species and possibly other experimental conditions, in general the cytokines mentioned, especially when administered in combination, are cytotoxic to pancreatic β cells.[213,214] In addition to the impairment of insulin secretion resulting from this cytotoxicity, inhibition of insulin secretion, independent of cytotoxicity, is also observed.[19,215]

This distinction is potentially very important because it raises the attractive possibility that, especially early in the preclinical period of T1DM, much of the loss of insulin secretory function may be functional in nature and therefore potentially reversible rather than due to irreversible β-cell destruction. Both *in vitro*[216] and *in vivo*[217] experimental data suggest that β cells are indeed able to repair after damage. Experiments exposing whole rodent islets of Langerhans to various toxic agents showed that the β cells went through an initial phase of suppressed glucose metabolism and decreased glucose-stimulated insulin release.[218,219] After they were cultured for 3–7 days in the absence of toxic agent, the surviving β cells were able to regain their function completely. β-cell repair has also been demonstrated after *in vivo* β-cell damage. When pancreatic islets with insulitis were isolated from female NOD mice at different ages (5–7, 8–11, or 12–13 weeks), the islets showed a deficient glucose-induced insulin release and defective glucose metabolism that progressively worsened with age (Fig. 20-6).[21,22] The observed β-cell dysfunction showed a close correlation to the severity of the mononuclear cell infiltration and was accompanied by defective glucose metabolism. Both abnormal insulin release and glucose oxidation were completely restored after 1 week of culturing, during which the islet mononuclear cell infiltrate was depleted.[21,22] In a subsequent series of experiments, treatment of female 12–13-week-old NOD mice with monoclonal antibodies directed against infiltrating T cells markedly reduced the islet inflammatory reaction and restored islet glucose metabolism, when the islets were isolated after a 10-day period.[21,22,220]

These data suggest that in prediabetic NOD mice, a population of suppressed and/or partially damaged (but still viable) β cells exists. If the immune assault is arrested, either by removing the islets from the *in vivo* environment[21,22] or by eliminating the invading T cells with specific monoclonal antibodies,[220] these β cells can use repair mechanisms and regain normal function. Anti-CD3 monoclonal antibodies suppress immune responses by transient T-cell depletion and antigenic modulation of the CD3/TCR complex, and anti-CD3 treatment of adult NOD mice with recent onset diabetes can restore normoglycemia.[221]

Cytokines also cause alterations in the β-cell expression of many other proteins besides insulin. Some proteins are stimulated, whereas others are inhibited. IFN-γ commonly stimulates MHC class 1 antigen expression in many cell types and may be responsible for the increased class 1 expression on islet β cells in T1DM, as treatment of NOD mice with antibodies to IFN-γ prevents MHC class 1 expression in the insulitis lesion.[222] An important role for IFN-α in T1DM is suggested by transgenic mice expressing IFN-α in their pancreatic β cells; these mice develop insulitis, lymphocyte autoimmune destruction of their islet β cells, and T1DM.[223] Gel electrophoresis has shown that cultured islets exposed to IL-1 decrease the expression of many proteins and increase the expression of others.[224] IL-1 inhibits the expression of GAD (unpublished observations) and stimulates the expression of islet ganglioside,[225] HSP70,[226,227] hemoxygenase,[226] and superoxide dismutase.[228] It has been proposed that some of these proteins, especially HSP70, hemoxygenase, and superoxide dismutase, may be protective to the β cell and/or aid in recovery of the β cell from damage.[229]

Cytokines are recognized to be an important component of the immune mechanism determining whether the immune response of CD4+ T cells to an antigen is primarily cellular (Th1) or humoral (Th2). T-helper cells differentiate into at least two major subtypes, Th1 and Th2, which are functionally distinct and distinguished by different cytokine secretion patterns. Th1 cells produce IL-2, IFN-γ, and TNF-β, whereas Th2 cells produce IL-4, IL-5, and IL-10. Functionally Th1 cells and their respective cytokines are involved in delayed-type hypersensitivity responses, macrophage

FIGURE 20-6. Insulin release (**A**) and glucose oxidation (**B**) from isolated pancreatic islets of 12-week-old female NOD mice or 12-week old NMRI mice. Both insulin release and glucose oxidation rates were measured immediately after islet isolation (day 0) and after 7 days in culture (day 7). (*Reproduced with permission from Eizirik et al.[229]*)

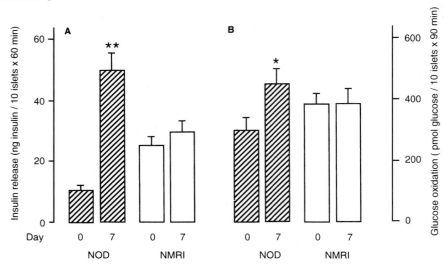

and cytotoxic T-cell activation, and weak B-lymphocyte activation mediating immunoglobulin isotype switching to IgG2a and IgG3.[230] In contrast, Th2 cells and their respective cytokines strongly activate B lymphocytes, stimulate humoral immune responses, and mediate isotype switching to IgG4 and IgE in humans.[231,232] Although Th1 and Th2 lymphocytes can each elicit memory IgG1 responses via different signals,[233] Th1 and Th2 responses are largely mutually inhibitory; Th2 cytokines suppress Th1 responses and *vice versa*. A large number of factors including antigen dose, antigen affinity, route of administration, genetics (including HLA type), and type of APC control differentiation into Th1 vs. Th2 responses.

Considerable data suggest that Th1-type immune responses against islet antigens are associated with progression to clinical T1DM in animals. Transgenic mice expressing the Th1 cytokine IFN-γ in their pancreatic β cells develop insulitis and diabetes,[121] and in both BB rats and NOD mice monoclonal antibodies against IFN-γ prevent T1DM.[234,235] Diabetogenic T-cell clones obtained from the NOD mouse are commonly of the Th1-type phenotype, producing IFN-γ but not IL-4[236]; GAD-reactive T-cells isolated from NOD mice produce IFN-γ[197]; and insulitis developing in transplanted islets in diabetes-prone NOD mice demonstrates a high frequency of IFN-γ-producing cells.[237]

In contrast, a predominantly Th2-type immune response appears to confer protection against T1DM. Thymocytes from NOD mice have markedly reduced IL-4 production when they are stimulated with TCR monoclonal antibodies, anti-CD3, and concanavalin A (Con A), and administration of IL-4 to prediabetic NOD mice prevents diabetes.[237,238] In performing islet transplantation experiments in NOD mice and assessing cytokine production by measuring mRNA, Rabinovitch and colleagues[239] also demonstrated that complete Freund's adjuvant (CFA) resulted in decreased expression of IFN-γ in the islets but increased expression of the Th2-type cytokine IL-10. Autoimmune diabetes and insulitis can be induced in rats by sublethal γ-irradiation and thymectomy and can be prevented by injection of a CD4+ T-cell subset from untreated syngenic rats. These protective cells are of the Th2 phenotype since they produce IL-4 but not IFN-γ when activated *in vitro*.[240]

The Th1/Th2 paradigm may not be as distinct in humans as in the mouse. For example, in humans both Th1 and Th2 clones produce IL-10.[241] Nonetheless, there has been correlation of Th1 vs. Th2 with development of human autoimmune diseases.[242–244] At diagnosis of human T1DM, IL-4 production by peripheral blood mononuclear cells (PBMCs) is markedly reduced[244], and Harrison and coworkers[245] demonstrated that preclinical subjects progressing to clinical diabetes had a predominantly cellular reaction to GAD, whereas subjects at less risk of clinical T1DM had a predominantly humoral response to GAD. However, as an antigen, they used GAD-67, which is not a predominant antigen in human diabetes, and their findings are controversial.[246]

The observations that subjects develop autoantibodies to an increasing number of islet antigens during the preclinical period[247] and that multiple islet autoantibodies are much more predictive of future T1DM than a single antibody[177,248] further support the Th1/Th2 paradigm in humans. Wilson and colleagues[249] investigated a series of at-risk non-progressors and T1DM patients (including five identical twin/triplet sets discordant for disease). The diabetic siblings had lower frequencies of CD4-CD8-Vα24JαQ+ T cells compared with their nondiabetic sibling. All 56 Vα24JαQ+ clones isolated from the diabetic twins/triplets secreted only IFN-γ upon stimulation; in contrast, 76 of 79 clones from the at-risk non-

progressors and normals secreted both IL-4 and IFN-γ. Half of the at-risk non-progressors had high serum levels of IL-4 and IFN-γ. These results support a model for T1DM in which Th1 cell-mediated tissue damage is initially regulated by Vα24JαQ+ T cells producing both cytokines; the loss of the secretion of IL-4 is correlated with T1DM.

Th2-type immune responses are preferentially generated by antigen presentation via the gut, and consequently oral tolerance and the resultant protection against autoimmune disease are in some ways analogous to the Th1/Th2 paradigm. Oral tolerance is a term used to describe the tolerance that can be induced by the exogenous administration of antigen to the peripheral immune system via the gut. It is a form of antigen-driven peripheral immune tolerance and appears to involve two main mechanisms that are in part dependent upon the antigen dose. The tolerance induced by lower doses of orally administered antigen appears to be mediated predominantly by active suppression, whereas higher doses tend to induce clonal anergy and/or deletion.[250] The active suppression by low doses of oral antigen appears to be mediated by the oral antigen: the antigen generates regulatory T cells that migrate to lymphoid and target organs expressing the antigen administered orally, and confers suppression via the secretion of downregulatory cytokines including IL-4, IL-10, and TGF-β.[251] Oral immunization with sheep red blood cells induced predominantly Th2-type cells in Peyer's patches, whereas systemic immunization induced predominantly IFN-γ-producing Th1-type cells.[252] In animals protected against EAE by the oral administration of myelin basic protein (MBP), mesenteric lymph nodes secrete TGF-β, IL-4, and IL-10, but minimal IFN-γ when stimulated *in vitro* with MBP.[253] Immunohistology of brains from animals affected with EAE, and from orally tolerized and therefore protected animals, further supports the Th1 vs. Th2 paradigm. Brains from unprotected animals showed infiltration with activated mononuclear cells secreting IL-1, IL-2, TNF, and IFN-γ, but not IL-4 and TGF-β. In animals orally tolerized with MBP, the inflammatory infiltrate was markedly reduced, IL-1, IL-2, TNF, and IFN-γ were reduced, and TGF-β and IL-4 were increased.[254]

It is fairly well established that T1DM is associated with dysregulated humoral and cellular immunity. There is altered production of and response to macrophage-derived and T-cell–derived cytokines, and a shift in T-helper cell differentiation in favor of a pathogenic Th1 pathway. Th1 cytokines may induce islet β-cell destruction directly by apoptosis and by upregulating the expression of select adhesion molecules, and they may facilitate pancreatic homing of autoreactive leukocytes, hence enhancing β-cell destruction. However, more recently, data are also appearing to suggest that in some cases Th2 cells and their cytokines can accelerate β-cell destruction, arguing against the conventional Th1/Th2 paradigm.[125,255,256] Local production of Th2 cytokines, in particular IL-10, accelerated β-cell destruction by enhancing autoreactive cell infiltration of the pancreas (insulitis) through modulation of the release of other cytokines and by modulating the microvasculature.[255]

Both β-cell antigen-specific and nonspecific immune and inflammatory responses may participate in mediating islet β-cell destruction in T1DM.[257] The β-cell antigen-specific immune response involves binding of CD8+ T cells to β cells. The T cells specifically recognize β-cell antigen or antigens presented by MHC class I molecules on the β cells. This is followed by activation of the T cells (cytotoxic T cells), which may kill the β cells by receptor (Fas/FasL)-mediated mechanisms or by secretion of cytotoxic molecules (granzymes and perforin).[258] The nonspecific immune and inflammatory response that destroys β cells may be mediated by molecules released from activated T cells (both CD4+ and CD8+ T cells) and macrophages, such as proinflammatory cytokines (IL-1, TNF-α, TNF-β, IFN-γ) and free radicals (e.g., superoxide, hydrogen peroxide, the hydroxyl radical, nitric oxide [NO], and peroxynitrite). There is abundant evidence *in vitro* that islet β cells are sensitive to injury mediated by oxygen free radicals[212] and NO.[259] In addition, IL-1, TNF-α, TNF-β, and IFN-γ are cytotoxic to β cells via mechanisms that appear to involve the production of oxygen free radicals or NO (or both) in the β cells themselves.[212,259] NO production has been demonstrated in pancreatic islets *in situ* in conjunction with T1DM development in BB rats[260] and NOD mice.[261] These findings suggest that both oxygen and nitrogen free radicals contribute to β-cell destruction in the insulitis lesion of T1DM. It appears that both β-cell antigen-specific CD8+ T cells and antigen-specific as well as antigen-nonspecific CD4+ T cells and macrophages may contribute to β-cell damage in NOD mice and BB rats; however, the precise cytotoxic mechanisms used by these immunologic cells to kill β cells have not been fully elucidated. Moreover, even less is known regarding the mechanisms of β-cell destruction in human T1DM.

Multiple and sometimes conflicting studies have identified a variety of aberrations in the cellular immune response to autoantigens in persons with the disease. Potential explanations for these discrepancies include different techniques or culture conditions, diversity in the populations of patients or controls tested, and differences in autoantigen preparations. T-cell workshops have been organized by the Immunology of Diabetes Society (IDS) with the aim of evaluating assays for detecting autoreactive T cells associated with T1DM.[262,263]

In the first phase, a series of candidate autoantigens were analyzed by reference laboratories for quality. Subsequently, these preparations, as well as control stimuli, were distributed in a blind fashion to 26 laboratories worldwide, for analysis of T-cell proliferation assays in recent-onset T1DM patients and nondiabetic controls.[262] The results using candidate autoantigens indicated that although a few laboratories could distinguish T1DM patients from nondiabetic controls in proliferative responses to individual islet autoantigens, in general, no consistent differences in T-cell proliferation between type 1 patients and controls were identified. The first T-cell workshop on T-cell autoreactivity in T1DM, although confirming that this was a difficult area for interlaboratory investigations, provided insights for future efforts focused on standardizing autoreactive T-cell measurements. The inability to discriminate normal controls from new-onset T1DM patients suggested that measuring proliferative responses in PBMCs represents an incomplete picture of the immune response, perhaps complicated by difficulties in identifying suitable antigens and assays for standardized use.[262]

Currently, various assays under trial in the second IDS human T-cell workshop (phase II) are those in which peripheral T cells are used without manipulation, are depleted of naïve T cells, or are enriched for activated (HLA DR+) T cells.[263] In each protocol, subjects included are new-onset T1DM subjects, high-risk autoantibody-positive, first-degree relatives, and matched healthy controls. Measurements include proliferation in the presence or absence of added IL-2, cytokine secretion, and cytokine mRNA quantification. Improved assays may provide new mechanistic insights and improved staging of prediabetes and may eventually allow us to measure the effectiveness of intervention therapies well before the onset of overt disease.[264]

ENVIRONMENTAL FACTORS

Epidemiology

Various environmental triggers, e.g., certain viruses and dietary factors, have been proposed as initiators of the autoimmune process, leading to the destruction of the pancreatic β cells and consequent T1DM.[265] Animal models provide solid evidence that environmental factors can, depending on the experimental conditions, both cause and prevent T1DM, but the relevance of these observations to human T1DM is not clear. However, twin studies, major geographic variations in incidence and prevalence rates, temporal seasonal trends in the incidence, and findings in migrant studies suggest that environmental factors play a crucial role in the development of human T1DM.[266] In this section we review the available data dealing with the potential role of environmental factors in the pathogenesis of T1DM.

Perhaps most persuasive are the studies in monozygotic twins. Initial studies had shown that <50% of such twins are concordant for T1DM.[267,268] Concordance can be the result of genetic and/or environmental similarity, but discordance, especially of this degree, suggests that T1DM, at least in part, is due to nongenetic factors. More recent longitudinal twin studies, with up to 39 years of follow-up from the onset of diabetes in index twins have shown that identical twins may develop diabetes after a prolonged period of discordance and that approximately two-thirds of long-term discordant twins have evidence of persistent β-cell autoimmunity and/or β-cell damage.[40] This presence of discordance of age of disease presentation also supports, but does not prove, a role for environmental factors. The diagnosis of T1DM follows a seasonal pattern, with incidence peaks in autumn and winter and a nadir in late spring/early summer. This seasonal pattern was first described in 1926,[269] has been repeatedly observed by numerous other investigators including ourselves,[270] is reversed in the Southern Hemisphere, and is remarkably constant year after year[271] (Fig. 20-7). Such seasonality has suggested a viral connection, because the general incidence pattern of viral infection in children is similar. A single virus is unlikely to be responsible, because in children the autumn peak is primarily enteroviral infections and the winter peak respiratory viruses. Furthermore, because infection usually results in immunity to subsequent infection by similar viruses for several years, most viruses pass through a given community with cycles of 2 or more years. Consequently, if the seasonality were due to viral infections, a number of different viruses would have to be involved to be consistent with the remarkably stable seasonal and yearly incidence of T1DM.[271]

The age pattern of onset of T1DM is in part compatible with an infectious etiology. T1DM is rare in the first 9 months of life. The incidence increases at about 5–6 years of age, peaks at approximately 12 years of age, and has a less well-defined peak at ages 20–35. No known infectious agent has an incidence pattern similar to this, but the low incidence rate of T1DM in the first months of life could be due to protection from infection by maternal antibodies, relative isolation during this period, or both. The increased incidence of T1DM at 5–6 years of age corresponds to the incidence pattern of many viral infections, which is high at this time, probably related to starting school.

Another epidemiologic observation supporting a pathogenetic role for environmental factors is the marked geographic variation in incidence of T1DM. Earlier studies had reported the age-adjusted incidence rates for T1DM with a 30-fold difference be-

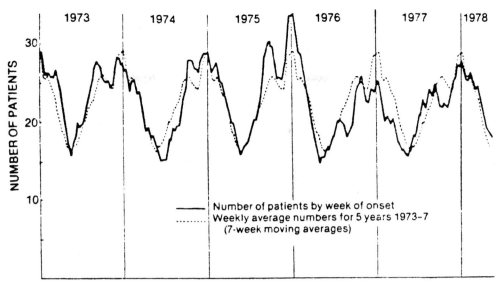

FIGURE 20-7. Seasonal variation in onset of new cases of type 1 diabetes in children reported to the British Diabetic Association Register. *(Reproduced with permission from Gamble.[271])*

tween the population extremes; the highest incidence rate, 29.5/100,000 person-years, was found in Finland and the lowest, 1.6/100,000 person-years, in Hokkaido, Japan.[272] The EURODIAB collaborative group, established in 1988, prospectively analyzed geographically defined registers of new cases diagnosed under 15 years of age in 44 centers representing most European countries and covering a population of about 28 million children[273]; incidence rates ranged from 3.2 cases/100,000/y in the Former Yugoslav Republic of Macedonia to 40.2 cases/100,000/y in two regions of Finland. By pooling over all centers and sexes, the annual rates of increase in incidence were 6.3% for children aged 0–4 years, 3.1% for 5–9 years, and 2.4% for 10–14 years. The very rapid rate of increase in children aged under 5 years has been a matter of particular concern.[273] The Diabetes Mondiale (DiaMond) Project Group recently reported the patterns in incidence of childhood T1DM worldwide[274]; the overall age-adjusted incidence of T1DM varied from 0.1/100,000/y in China and Venezuela to 36.8/100,000/y in Sardinia and 36.5/100,000/y in Finland. This represents a >350-fold variation in incidence among the 100 populations worldwide.[274] This marked difference in incidence is much greater than for most other chronic diseases.[275] Worldwide, a significant correlation was noted between T1DM incidence and average yearly temperature, but this must be interpreted with great caution given the plethora of other factors including diet, gene pool, and ethnicity that also vary geographically in a south to north gradient in the Northern Hemisphere. There are also exceptions to this apparent gradient, with the island of Sardinia being noteworthy. The incidence of T1DM in Sardinia is very similar to Finland.[276] This picture is further complicated by the observation that within the relatively homogeneous Swedish population, T1DM incidence appears to be geographically determined, with high incidence areas only a short distance from areas with consistently lower incidence rates.[276]

Recent findings of time and space clustering of birth dates for later cases of diabetes together with the early observation of a very high prevalence of diabetes in cases with rubella embryopathy suggest that fetal virus exposure may be important.[277] In early perinatal life the immune system is inducible, and exposures in this period may initiate autoimmunity. Findings from Sweden and Finland suggest that enterovirus exposure during fetal life may initiate autoimmunity, leading to diabetes.[277] In addition, food components such as nitrosamine components, cow's milk protein, and gliadin have been proposed to initiate the autoimmune β-cell destruction of T1DM.[277,278] The diversity of determinants that are associated with T1DM risk points at a complex interaction between the genome and environment, and multivariate analyses have disclosed different risk profiles in different age groups.[277] Most of these epidemiologic findings are supported by experimental studies in NOD mice, but their exact mechanisms of action are still unclear. Evidence has been accumulating indicating that perinatal exposures may be important for the initiation of β-cell destruction. Such risk factors may be the targets for primary prevention strategies of T1DM.[277] As discussed earlier, evidence supports the concept that a neonatal wave of β-cell apoptosis precedes insulitis in spontaneous, induced, and accelerated models of autoimmune diabetes, and the wave of apoptosis provides the antigen necessary for priming the β-cell–specific T cells.[20] However, since this neonatal wave of β-cell apoptosis is present in both diabetes-prone and diabetes-resistant animal models, it is believed that other factors (defective APC function, defective clearing of apoptotic debris) determine who goes on to develop autoimmune diabetes.[20]

The precise mechanisms whereby environmental factors contribute to the pathogenesis of human T1DM are not known. Some of the possibilities include the following: (1) the agents may be directly toxic to the β cells and acutely cause sufficient loss of insulin secretory capacity to result in diabetes; (2) the agents, by an effect on the β cells, may trigger an autoimmune response directed against the β cells; (3) the agents, by providing specific peptides that share antigenic epitopes with host-cell protein ("molecular mimicry") may trigger an immune response against β cells; (4) the agents may cause insulin resistance, with resultant increased insulin needs that cannot be met because of prior β-cell damage; and (5) the agents may alter the β cells in a way that increases their susceptibility to damage by other mechanisms (Table 20-7).

TABLE 20-7. Possible Environmental Mechanisms in Type 1 Diabetes

1. Directly toxic to β cells
2. Trigger an autoimmune reaction directed against the β cells
3. Trigger an immune response by "molecular mimicry"
4. Induce increased insulin need that can not be met by damaged β cells
5. Alter β cells to increase susceptibility to damage

Potential environmental factors fall into three main groups: specific drugs or chemicals, nutritional constituents consumed in the diet, and viruses. Even a protective rather than destructive role has also been suggested for specific viral and bacterial antigens.[279] It is also of interest to note that a pathogen-free environment increases diabetes in BB rats and NOD mice and that in NOD mice nonspecific immune stimulation is usually protective.[279,280] As we live in a "cleaner environment," the decreasing chances of natural infection in the general population may contribute to the induction of autoimmunity because the developing immune system is not exposed to the stimulation that may be necessary to generate regulatory cells involved in the modulation and prevention of autoimmunity.[281]

Drugs

Specific drugs or chemicals include alloxan, streptozotocin, pentamidine, and Vacor. Alloxan is directly cytotoxic to β cells, resulting in rapid and selective β-cell destruction, and is frequently used to induce T1DM in experimental animals. Alloxan is a uric acid derivative and is structurally very different from the other drug commonly used to induce diabetes, streptozotocin, which also causes direct β-cell lysis and is used therapeutically in humans to treat malignant insulinomas. In susceptible strains of mice, the β-cell damage induced by multiple subdiabetogenic doses of streptozotocin appears to elicit β-cell autoimmunity, which further contributes to β-cell loss.[282] Consequently, at a mechanistic level, this model provides evidence that a primary β-cell insult can result in secondary β-cell autoimmunity.

Pentamidine (4-4'-diamidino-diphenoxy-pentane) is a drug commonly used in the treatment of *Pneumocystis carinii* and is a recognized cause of drug-induced diabetes.[283] Shortly after receiving the drug, hypoglycemia may be observed, due to release of insulin from damaged β cells, followed subsequently by overt diabetes due to β-cell destruction. Vacor is a rodenticide that, when ingested in large quantities by humans in suicide attempts, causes insulin-dependent diabetes. The major mechanism underlying the diabetes in these patients appears to be direct β-cell toxicity, but these patients also provide evidence that primary β-cell damage can result in secondary autoimmunity, as islet cell antibodies occasionally are found.[284]

Except in rare cases, it is unlikely that drugs or chemicals in the external environment are common and/or major etiologic factors in human T1DM. The observations cited are primarily important because they document that β cells are uniquely sensitive and can be selectively destroyed by certain chemicals and that primary β-cell damage can elicit an immune response directed against the β cells. The latter view is also supported by studies in transgenic mice expressing lymphocytic choriomeningitis virus (LCMV) in their β cells.[285–287] Animals are tolerant to the transgene and remain nondiabetic until infected with the virus exogenously. They then develop an immune response to LCMV, severe insulitis, and T1DM.[288]

Dietary Factors

Among the environmental triggers, exposure to cow's milk in early neonatal life and development of T1DM has received considerable attention.[289–291] The hypothesis was developed more than a decade ago, and the issue is still not settled.[265,292–295] Literature review shows that as many as 19 groups from different parts of the world have implicated exposure to cow's milk protein in early neonatal life in the development of T1DM, whereas 6 other groups have found no such relationship.[265,292–294,296,297] We now review the evidence for and against this hypothesis.

Epidemiologic and experimental evidence has suggested that denial of dietary cow's milk protein early in life may protect genetically susceptible children and animals from T1DM.[298,299] Elimination of intact cow's milk proteins from the diet significantly reduced the incidence of T1DM in the spontaneously diabetic BB rat, the elimination being most effective when it occurred during the preweaning period.[300] Conversely, in newly discovered diabetics (both rats and children), compared with nondiabetic controls, increased levels of antibodies to cow's milk proteins have been reported. Bovine serum albumin (BSA) was proposed as a candidate milk-borne mimicry antigen responsible for the diabetogenic cow's milk effect.[300] Elevated anti-BSA antibodies have been observed in patients and diabetic rodents.[301,302] The anti-BSA antibodies cross-react with a β-cell membrane protein of Mr 69,000 (known as p69 or ICA 69) and precipitate p69 from islet cell lysates. BSA-specific T cells have been detected that recognize a 17-amino acid sequence of BSA, known as ABBOS peptide (pre-BSA position 152–169), previously identified as a possible mimicry epitope.[291–303] ABBOS-sensitized T cells were reported in 28/31 children with recent-onset T1DM but not in nondiabetic controls. Cross-reactive T cells that recognize both Tep69 (dominant NOD T-cell epitope in ICA69) and ABBOS (dominant NOD T-cell epitope in BSA) are routinely generated during human and NOD mouse prediabetes.[304] These findings suggest that bovine milk proteins (mainly BSA) might be an important environmental factor providing specific peptides that share antigenic epitopes with host cell proteins.[305] High titers of antibodies have also been detected against β-lactoglobulin (BLG), in addition to BSA.[298] An enhanced cellular immune response to dietary BLG may reflect a disturbance in the regulation of immune response to oral antigens in T1DM.[306,307] This kind of defect may play a fundamental role in the development of β-cell autoimmunity in T1DM.[306,307]

The clinical evidence relating a short duration of breastfeeding or early cow's milk exposure to T1DM has recently been critically reviewed.[295,308] Ecologic and time-series studies showed a relationship between T1DM and either cow's milk exposure or diminished breastfeeding. In the case-control studies, patients with T1DM were more likely to have been breastfed for <3 months (OR 1.43) and to have been exposed to cow's milk before 4 months (OR 1.63). High dietary intake of cow's milk protein in the 12 months before the onset of diabetes symptoms was also associated with an increased risk (OR 1.84).[299,309]

Results from the Childhood Diabetes in Finland Study Group showed that initially nondiabetic siblings who were ICA-positive also had increased levels of antibodies to cow's milk proteins and suggested that the immune response to cow's milk proteins may be related to progression to clinical T1DM.[310,311] High milk consumption in childhood (≥3 glasses daily) was associated with more frequent emergence of T1DM-associated autoantibodies than low consumption (<3 glasses daily; adjusted OR 3.97), and the estimated RR of childhood milk consumption for progression to T1DM was 5.37 (range: 1.6–18.4) when adjusted for matching and sociodemographic factors, age at introduction of supplementary milk feeding, and genetic susceptibility markers.[312] Moreover, it was shown that children with T1DM have higher levels of cow's milk protein antibodies than their HLA-DQB1–matched sibling controls and that these high levels of antibodies are independent risk markers for T1DM.[313,314] The accumulated evidence provided the basis for recent recommendations by the American Academy of Pediatrics to avoid cow's milk exposure in young infants at risk of T1DM.[315–317]

A recent study examined the composition of milk as well as its consumption together with diabetes incidence in 0–14-year-old children from 10 countries.[318] Total protein consumption did not correlate with diabetes incidence (r = 0.402, level of significance 25%, NS), but the consumption of the β-casein A^1 variant did correlate (r = 0.726, level of significance 2%). Even more pronounced was the relationship between β-casein (A^1+B) consumption and diabetes (r = 0.982, level of significance 0.01%). The ecologic associations shown in this report suggest the necessity to consider not just the role of total milk consumption or its time of introduction into the weaning diet, in the etiology of T1DM, but also the role of individual milk protein variants.

A multicenter trial is being conducted in Finland to test whether avoidance of dietary cow's milk protein (CMP) for at least the first 6 months of life in genetically at-risk infants prevents the subsequent development of T1DM during the first 10 years of life.[296] This Trial to Reduce IDDM in Genetically at Risk" (TRIGR) project is a randomized, prospective trial and involves newborn infants with first-degree relatives who have T1DM. Those genetically determined to be at high risk are randomized to receive a baby formula free of cow's milk (containing a nonantigenic protein hydrolysate) or a conventional cow's milk-based formula. The intervention period is for a 6-month period, with a follow-up of 10 years. This would be a "true" primary prevention strategy.

Generation of insulin-specific T cells in early childhood may provide a pathogenic link between cow's milk and diabetes. Studies among the infants recruited in the TRIGR second pilot study suggested that primary cellular immunization to insulin might occur in infancy by oral exposure to bovine insulin (BI) present in cow's milk. At the T-cell level, this response is first specific for BI but spreads to include reactivity to human insulin (HI) as well.[319,320]

On the other hand, a few other studies including two recent prospective studies found no apparent association between the development of antibodies to islet antigens and feeding patterns in high-risk infants with a first-degree T1DM relative, and there are reports that p69 and BSA are not antigenically cross-reactive.[321–326] It was suggested that studies reporting increased humoral and cellular immunity to cow's milk proteins in children with T1DM often lack appropriate controls and standardization and do not, in themselves, establish a causal connection to disease pathogenesis.[326] Harrison and Honeyman[295] have recently suggested that the cow's milk hypothesis could be productively reframed around mucosal immune function in T1DM. Breast milk contains growth factors, cytokines, and other immunomodulatory agents including cytokines that promote functional maturation of intestinal mucosal tissues. In the NOD mouse model, exposure of the mucosa to in-

sulin (present in breast milk) induces regulatory T cells and decreases diabetes incidence. The mucosa is a major immunoregulatory barrier, and cow's milk happens to be the first dietary protein it encounters. The basic question is whether impaired mucosal immune function predisposes to T1DM.[295] Additional supporting information and further studies are needed to establish a clear role for diet in the pathogenesis of T1DM.

Viruses

Many investigators, employing many different techniques and methodologies, have evaluated whether viruses play an etiologic role in T1DM. Virus-induced diabetes in animal models, *in vitro* studies, epidemiologic investigations, case reports in humans, and research focusing primarily on molecular and cellular mechanisms have all been reported.

Viral infections can cause diabetes in a variety of animal species, frequently with important similarities to human T1DM. Some of these include encephalomyocarditis (EMC) virus, coxsackie B viruses, Mengovirus 2T, and reovirus types 1 and 3.[327] Although EMC virus has not been implicated in human T1DM, elegant studies in mice provide mechanistic information that may be applicable to other viruses and to human T1DM. EMC virus can induce T1DM in genetically susceptible strains of mice, and two antigenically indistinguishable strains of EMC virus have been identified; EMC-D can induce diabetes in >90% of infected animals, whereas EMC-B does not cause diabetes.[328] Genetically these two strains differ by 14 nucleotides, and one amino acid at the 776th position, alanine, is critical for diabetogenicity of the EMC-D variant.[329] This amino acid is located in the attachment site of the virus, and alanine increases the efficiency of viral attachment to pancreatic β cells.[329] Only certain strains of mice are susceptible to EMC-D virus-induced diabetes, and this genetic susceptibility also appears to involve viral attachment. Genetically susceptible mice express more viral receptors on their pancreatic β cells.[330]

Although it is clear that, in certain animal species, viruses can cause diabetes and that sometimes the diabetogenic process is in part immune-mediated, the situation in humans is far more controversial. As a foundation for postulating β-cell viral infection in human T1DM, Yoon, Prince, and coworkers have shown that several human viruses including coxsackie B3, coxsackie B4, reovirus type 3, and mumps can infect human β cells *in vitro* and destroy them.[331,332] Furthermore, in children dying with overwhelming viral infections, histologic examination of their pancreata revealed cytopathology in 5 of 7 cases of coxsackie B infection, 20 of 45 cases of cytomegalovirus infection, and 2 of 45 cases of congenital rubella.[333] Two case reports are also worthy of mention. In the first, a 10-year-old boy died of ketoacidosis, and coxsackie B4 was isolated from his pancreas. This virus produced diabetes when injected into mice.[334] In the second case, diabetes developed a few days after a coxsackie B5 infection, and virus isolated from the feces produced hyperglycemia when injected into mice.

Among the many viruses potentially involved in the etiology of human T1DM, three have received the greatest attention, namely, mumps, coxsackie, and rubella. There has been considerable speculation about the role of wild mumps virus and mumps vaccine in the onset of childhood diabetes. Numerous investigators have noted temporal associations between T1DM and mumps infections, although the proposed time interval between the reported viral infection and T1DM has ranged from several years to weeks or months.[271] Additional support for the possible association of

T1DM with mumps comes from observations that mumps virus can infect human β cells *in vitro*,[335] that altered cytokine and HLA class I and II antigen expression results from mumps-infected human insulinoma cells,[336] and that ICAs are common in nondiabetic children following mumps infection[337]; other reports challenge mumps as an etiologic factor.[338] Available data about mumps and T1DM are incomplete and difficult to interpret.[339] Recent evidence from animal studies has raised the possibility that immunization by vaccines can influence the pathogenesis of T1DM mellitus.[340] The possibility that widespread vaccination against mumps might offer protection against T1DM has also been investigated. A decline in mumps antibodies in T1DM patients and a plateau in the rising incidence of T1DM after introduction of mumps vaccine has been reported from Finland.[341] However, there is no evidence that mumps-measles-rubella (MMR) mass vaccination programs have changed the incidence of diabetes mellitus in any population.[340] Lindberg and associates[342] found no evidence that MMR vaccination during adolescence may trigger autoimmunity.

Several studies have indicated that enterovirus infections, especially with coxsackie B, are frequent at the diagnosis of clinical T1DM or may play a role in the initiation of the β-cell damaging process.[343–346] The first prospective studies were recently published; they suggested that enterovirus infections can also initiate the process several years before clinical T1DM.[347,348] Lonnrot and colleagues[345,349] analyzed the role of enterovirus infections in the initiation of autoimmunity in children who were tested positive for diabetes-associated autoantibodies in a prospective study starting at birth (the Finnish Diabetes Prediction and Prevention Study). Enterovirus infections were detected in 26% of sample intervals in the case subjects and in 18% of the sample intervals in the control children ($p = 0.03$). A temporal relationship between enterovirus infections and the induction of autoimmunity was found; enterovirus infections were detected in 57% of the case subjects during the 6-month period preceding the first appearance of autoantibodies compared with 31% of the matched control children in the same age group (OR 3.7). The frequency of adenovirus infections did not differ between the patient and control groups. Their data implied that enterovirus infections are associated with the development of β-cell autoimmunity and provide evidence for the role of enteroviruses in the initiation of β-cell destruction.

Three other observations support a potential role for coxsackie B in the etiology of T1DM. First, human β cells are susceptible to coxsackie B viral infection, and second, this infection results in decreased insulin production.[350] Third, coxsackie B viral infection of diabetes-susceptible mice results in increased β-cell expression of GAD[351] and GAD antibodies.[352] Finally, a portion of the GAD molecule shares homology to coxsackie B4,[108] and this portion of the GAD molecule appears to contain an immune-dominant epitope stimulatory to T cells from human T1DM patients.[353] However, only some strains of coxsackie B virus are diabetogenic,[354] and exposure to the more common nondiabetic strains probably confers protection against infection with the diabetic strains, similar to the protection afforded against EMC-D virus-induced diabetes by prior EMC-B viral infection.[328]

Molecular mimicry is one mechanism by which infectious agents (or other exogenous substances) may trigger an immune response against autoantigens (Tables 20-8 and 20-9). Structural similarity (molecular mimicry) between viral epitopes and self-peptides can lead to the induction of autoaggressive CD4+ as well as CD8+ T-cell responses.[355] It has been proposed that a self-peptide could replace a viral epitope for T-cell recognition and

TABLE 20-8. Potential Viral Mechanisms in IDDM

1. Direct beta-cell destruction
2. Increased insulin resistance and beta-cell destruction
3. Molecular mimicry
4. Protection from diabetogenic strain by prior infection with nondiabetogenic strain
5. Stimulation of regulatory T cells
6. Stimulation of effector T cells

therefore participate in pathophysiologic processes in which T cells are involved. The tolerance to autoantigens breaks down, and the pathogen-specific immune response that is generated cross-reacts with host structures to cause tissue damage and disease.[356] In patients with T1DM, mimicry related to viral infection has been proposed on the basis of sequence homology between GAD-65, an enzyme concentrated in pancreatic β cells,[357] and coxsackievirus P2-C, an enzyme involved in the replication of coxsackievirus B.[108] Although cross-reactivity between coxsackievirus P2-C and GAD-65 has been demonstrated in mice, and an immune response to the homologous peptides is generated by immunization of mice with full-length P2-C proteins,[358] cross-reactivity between GAD and coxsackievirus P2-C has not been consistently found in studies of T cells or serum antibodies from patients with diabetes.[100,359] Furthermore, a search of databases identified 17 viruses with some homology to various fragments of GAD-65,[360] indicating that cross-reactivity between GAD-65 and coxsackieviruses is not unique.[356]

Poliovirus vaccine, the only currently available enterovirus vaccine, can theoretically modulate the protection against other enteroviruses by inducing cross-reactive T-cell immune responses.[340] Enterovirus-specific cellular immunity was recently studied in Estonian and Finnish children, with the aim of evaluating the level of responsiveness in two neighboring countries that have different poliovirus immunization practices and striking differences in the incidence of T1DM.[343] The results showed that Finnish children have weaker cellular immunity against enteroviruses at the age of 9 months compared with Estonian children at the same age. This was most probably due to the difference in polio vaccination schedules; in Estonia live poliovirus vaccine is used and given at earlier ages than the inactivated vaccines in Finland; the result is stronger T-cell immunity, which cross-reacts with other enterovirus serotypes. This might explain the lower incidence of T1DM in Estonia if live poliovirus vaccine provides effective protection against diabetogenic enterovirus strains in Estonian children. In another study, the cellular immune response to enterovirus antigens was abnormal in children who tested positive for T1DM-associated autoantibodies,[361] and these results showed that the increased responses to virus-infected cell lysates were associated with the early phases of β-cell autoimmunity.

TABLE 20-9. Examples of Molecular Mimicry Potentially Related to Type 1 Diabetes

Pancreatic Antigen	Foreign Antigen
Insulin (IAA)	p73 protein of mouse endogenous retrovirus
GAD	PC2 protein of coxsackie virus
ICA69	ABBOS peptide of bovine serum albumin
38K	Cytomegalovirus
52K	Rubella virus

Lymphocyte proliferation responses to enterovirus antigens were analyzed in 41 children with new-onset T1DM, 23 children with T1DM for 4–72 months, and healthy control children in subgroups matched for HLA-DQB1 risk alleles, sex, and age.[344] Data from this study suggested that T-cell responses to coxsackievirus B4 proteins, particularly to the antigens containing the nonstructural proteins of the virus, are increased in children with T1DM after the onset of the disease. However, in children with new-onset diabetes, responses were normal or even decreased. This phenomenon was specific for enteroviruses and could be caused by trapping of enterovirus-specific T cells in the pancreas. The currently available information supports the assumption that the role of enterovirus infections may be more important than previously estimated. Enterovirus infections are associated with increased risk of T1DM, but whether this association reflects a causal relationship remains to be determined.

In contrast to mumps and coxsackievirus, there is general agreement that congenital rubella infection causes T1DM in later life. The incidence of diabetes in the congenital rubella syndrome has not been definitely determined and may vary between different populations, but it appears to average approximately 10–20%.[362] Most importantly, the diabetes induced by rubella is similar genetically and immunologically to the T1DM occurring spontaneously in the absence of rubella, namely, susceptibility appears to be genetically associated with HLA-B8 and -DR3, and relative protection is associated with HLA-DR2.[363] The viral infection appears to trigger an immune response directed against the β cells because both islet cell antibodies and insulin autoantibodies are commonly found in these patients.[364] These similarities suggest that the diabetes associated with congenital rubella is not etiologically distinct but that rubella virus triggers at least some of the same mechanisms that are operative in most spontaneous cases of T1DM.

Rubella virus has also been demonstrated to infect human β cells and to result in impaired insulin production,[365] and there is antigen homology between a rubella virus capsid protein and an epitope in an unidentified 52-kd islet protein.[366] The similarity between these findings and those previously summarized for coxsackievirus make it tempting to speculate that molecular mimicry may be applicable to both viruses. Ou and coworkers[367] examined cross-reaction between virus antigens and β-cell protein determinants to understand further the potential role of this mechanism in T1DM. Cellular immune responses to a panel of human β-cell protein peptides (GAD-65, GAD-67, and a 38-kd protein) and to a panel of peptides of viral proteins (rubella virus E1, E2 and C, coxsackie B4 virus P2-C) were studied in 60 T1DM subjects. Amino acids (252–266) induced responses of patients with recent-onset diabetes in proliferation assays at the highest frequency (77%), whereas GAD-67 (212–226) stimulated cellular responses at the highest rate (61%) in patients with late-onset diabetes. Rubella virus E1 (RVE1; 157–176) was recognized by all groups of patients at the highest frequency and with the largest amplitude among the viral peptides tested. T-cell clones specific to GAD-65 (252–266), GAD-65 (274–286), or GAD-67 (212–226) were tested in cytotoxicity assays for their responses to rubella virus peptides. Each of these T-cell clones cross-reacted with two to four rubella virus peptides, including RVE1 (157–176) and rubella virus E2 (RVE2; [87–107), again supporting a potential role for molecular mimicry.

Recent data have reported an association of rotavirus infection and T1DM.[368,369] Rotavirus, the most common cause of childhood gastroenteritis, contains peptide sequences highly similar to T-cell epitopes in the islet autoantigens GAD and tyrosine phosphatase IA-2 (IA-2), suggesting that rotavirus could also trigger islet autoimmunity by molecular mimicry. Honeyman and colleagues[368,369] sought an association between rotavirus infection and islet autoantibody markers in children at risk for diabetes who were followed from birth. There was a specific and highly significant association between rotavirus seroconversion and increases in three antibodies: 86% of antibodies to IA-2, 62% to insulin, and 50% to GAD first appeared or increased with increases in rotavirus IgG or IgA. It appears that rotavirus infection may trigger or exacerbate islet autoimmunity in genetically susceptible children. However, rotavirus infection is ubiquitous, occurring in all children, and hence the specific role in the small percentage that develop T1DM, usually many years later, is not clear.

With the exception of diabetes associated with congenital rubella infection, the large amount of research investigating a viral component to the etiology of human T1DM has raised as many questions as have been answered. Several different mechanisms have been suggested (Table 20-8), and these may not be mutually exclusive. Viral infections can directly damage β cells. Massive and sudden β-cell destruction may occasionally cause T1DM, whereas a smaller degree of injury may provide the initial insult that activates dormant autoimmune responses or the final insult to β cells previously damaged by a long autoimmune attack. It is also very likely that viral infections can act as a nonspecific, precipitating factor by causing insulin resistance and increased insulin needs. If prior β-cell damage and destruction make it impossible to meet the increased insulin demand, clinical diabetes would ensue.

Molecular mimicry, as discussed earlier, is considered the most attractive mechanism: viral infections might trigger subsequent immune-mediated β-cell destruction. The process of molecular mimicry and the use of transgenic models in which viral and host genes can be manipulated to analyze their effects in causing autoimmunity have been particular objects of research.[370] For example, there is a transgenic murine model of virus-induced autoimmune disease, in which a known viral gene is selectively expressed as a self-antigen in β cells of the pancreas. In these mice, insulin-dependent diabetes develops after either a viral infection, the release of a cytokine such as IFN-γ, or the expression of the costimulatory molecule B7.1 in the islets of Langerhans. Recent studies using this model have contributed to the understanding of the pathogenesis of virus-induced autoimmune disease and have furthered the design and testing of novel immunotherapeutic approaches.[370,371] Perhaps the most convincing evidence supporting this mechanism comes from transgenic mice expressing LCMV in their β cells.[286,287] Animals are tolerant to the transgene and remain nondiabetic until infected with the virus exogenously. They then develop an immune response to LCMV, severe insulitis, and T1DM.[288]

Viral infections may also protect against T1DM. Infection with a nondiabetogenic strain of a virus can elicit an immune response that protects against subsequent infection with a diabetogenic strain, as demonstrated for EMC virus.[328] Viral infections can also directly affect the immune system and result in resistance to T1DM. In both the NOD mouse and BB rat, infection with a lymphotropic virus confers protection against the development of diabetes. In the BB rat, Kilham's rat virus appears to affect the immune system directly and to increase the population of immune cells mediating the T1DM.[372] von Herrath and colleagues[373] have recently described an intriguing approach to the prevention of autoimmune disease, in which a DNA vaccine encoding a self-antigen is used to abrogate autoimmune diabetes. The success of this strategy relies on the nature of the immune response induced by the DNA vaccine. Finally, environmental factors that alter β-cell activity may alter the β-cell susceptibility to injury and/or alter the β cells' repair mechanisms. It has been demonstrated that stimulated β-cells are more susceptible to cytokine-induced inhibition of insulin secretion and cytotoxicity,[214,374] and recovery from a brief exposure to streptozotocin is improved by culturing islet cells in a high glucose-containing medium.[375]

SUMMARY

Dramatic advances have been made in recent years in our understanding of the pathogenesis of T1DM. Using this information plus genetic and immunologic measurements, nondiabetic individuals can now be identified who are at high risk of subsequent clinical T1DM. In turn, this ability to identify high-risk subjects and to predict subsequent clinical T1DM plus knowledge of pathogenic mechanisms has set the stage for large-scale intervention trials to test whether T1DM can be prevented (the Diabetes Prevention Trial-Type 1 [DPT-1]; the European Nicotinamide Diabetes Intervention Trial [ENDIT]; the Finnish Diabetes Type 1 Prediction and Prevention Project [DIPP]; and the Trial to Reduce IDDM in Genetically at Risk [TRIGR]). The long-term goal of researchers working in this field may soon be realized; the T1DM disease process may be susceptible to interruption, and some people may be prevented from developing clinical T1DM.

Acknowledgments This work was supported in part by the Medical Research Service of the Department of Veterans Affairs and by grants from the National Institutes of Health (P01 DK53004 and P30 DK17047).

REFERENCES

1. World Health Organization (WHO) Study Group: *Diabetes Mellitus.* WHO Technical Report Series. WHO:1985;727.
2. The Expert Committee on the Diagnosis and Classification of Diabetes Mellitus. Diagnosis and classification of diabetes mellitus. *Diabetes Care* 2000;23(Suppl 1):S4.
3. Karjalainen J, Salmela P, Ilonen J, et al: A comparison of childhood and adult type I diabetes mellitus. *N Engl J Med* 1989;320:881.
4. Hagopian WA, Karlsen AE, Gottsater A, et al: Quantitative assay using recombinant human islet glutamic acid decarboxylase (GAD65) shows that 64K autoantibody positivity at onset predicts diabetes type. *J Clin Invest* 1993;91:368.
5. Tuomi T, Groop LC, Zimmet PZ, et al: Antibodies to glutamic acid decarboxylase reveal latent autoimmune diabetes mellitus in adults with a non-insulin-dependent onset of disease. *Diabetes* 1993;42:359.
6. Zimmet PZ, Tuomi T, Mackay IR, et al: Latent autoimmune diabetes mellitus in adults (LADA): the role of antibodies to glutamic acid decarboxylase in diagnosis and prediction of insulin dependency. *Diabetes Med* 1994;11:299.
7. Kobayashi T: Subtype of insulin-dependent diabetes mellitus (IDDM) in Japan: slowly progressive IDDM—the clinical characteristics and pathogenesis of the syndrome. *Diabetes Res Clin Pract* 1994;24 (Suppl 2):S95.
8. Groop LC, Bottazzo GF, Doniach D: Islet cell antibodies identify latent type 1 diabetes in patients aged 35–75 years at diagnosis. *Diabetes* 1986;17:1214.
9. Anonymous: Insulin-dependent? *Lancet* 1985;2:809.
10. Harris MI, Zimmet P: Classification of diabetes mellitus and other categories of glucose intolerance. In: Keen H, DeFronzo R, Alberti KGMM, et al, eds. *International Textbook of Diabetes Mellitus.* John Wiley:1992;3.
11. Kuzuya T, Matsuda A: Classification of diabetes on the basis of etiologies versus degree of insulin deficiency. *Diabetes Care* 1997;20:219.
12. Pipeleers D, Ling Z: Pancreatic beta cells in insulin dependent diabetes. *Diabetes Metabol Rev* 1992;8:209.
13. Von Meyenburg H: Uber "Insulitis" bei Diabetes. *Schweitz Med Wochenschr* 1940;21:554.
14. Gepts W, LaCompte PM: The pancreatic islets in diabetes. *Am J Med* 1981;70:105.
15. Srikanta S, Ganda OP, Eisenbarth GS, et al: Islet cell antibodies and beta-cell function in monozygotic triplets and twins initially discordant for type I diabetes mellitus. *N Engl J Med* 1983;308:321.
16. Rosenbloom AL, Hunt SS, Rosenbloom EK, et al: Ten year prognosis of impaired glucose tolerance in siblings of patients with insulin-dependent diabetes. *Diabetes* 1982;31:385.
17. Greenbaum CJ, Cuthbertson D, Krischer JP: Type I diabetes manifested solely by 2-h oral glucose tolerance test criteria. *Diabetes* 2001; 50:470.
18. McCulloch DK, Raghu PK, Johnston C: Defects in B-cell function and insulin sensitivity in normoglycemic streptozotocin-treated baboons: a model of preclinical insulin dependent diabetes. *J Clin Endocrinol Metab* 1988;67:785.
19. Mehta VK, Hao W, Brooks-Worrell BM, et al: Low dose interleukin 1 and tumor necrosis factor individually stimulate insulin release but in combination cause suppression. *Eur J Endocrinol* 1994;130:208.
20. Trudeau JD, Dutz JP, Arany E, et al: Neonatal beta-cell apoptosis: a trigger for autoimmune diabetes? *Diabetes* 2000;49:1.
21. Strandell E, Eizirik DL, Sandler S: Reversal of beta cell suppression in vitro in pancreatic islets isolated in nonobese diabetic mice during the phase preceding insulin-dependent diabetes mellitus. *J Clin Invest* 1990;85:1944.
22. Eizirik DL, Strandell E, Sandler S: Prolonged exposure of islets isolated from prediabetic nonobese diabetic mice to a high glucose concentration does not impair B cell function. *Diabetologia* 1991;34:6.
23. Luhder F, Chambers C, Allison JP, et al: Pinpointing when T cell costimulatory receptor CTLA-4 must be engaged to dampen diabetogenic T cells. *Proc Natl Acad Sci USA* 2000;97:12204.
24. Barmeier H, McCulloch DK, Neifing JL, et al: Risk for developing type 1 (insulin-dependent) diabetes mellitus and the presence of islet 64K antibodies. *Diabetologia* 1991;34:727.
25. Garchon HJ, Bedossa P, Eloy L, et al: Identification and mapping to chromosome 1 of a susceptibility locus for periinsulitis in non-obese diabetic mice. *Nature* 1991;353:260.
26. Spencer KM, Tarn A, Dean BM, et al: Fluctuating islet cell autoimmunity in unaffected relatives of patients with insulin-dependent diabetes. *Lancet* 1984;1:764.
27. Palmer JP: Predicting IDDM. The use of humoral immune markers. *Diabetes Rev* 1993;1:104.
28. Bonifacio E, Lampasona V, Bernasconi L, et al: Maturation of the humoral autoimmune response to epitopes of GAD in preclinical childhood type 1 diabetes. *Diabetes* 2000;49:202.
29. Schenker M, Hummel M, Ferber K, et al: Early expression and high prevalence of islet autoantibodies for DR3/4 heterozygous and DR4/4 homozygous offspring of parents with type I diabetes: the German BABYDIAB study. *Diabetologia* 1999;42:671.
30. Naserke HE, Bonifacio E, Ziegler AG: Immunoglobulin G insulin autoantibodies in BABYDIAB offspring appear postnatally: sensitive early detection using a protein A/G-based radiobinding assay. *J Clin Endocrinol Metab* 1999;84:1239.
31. Ziegler AG, Hummel M, Schenker M, et al: Autoantibody appearance and risk for development of childhood diabetes in offspring of parents with type 1 diabetes: the 2-year analysis of the German BABYDIAB Study. *Diabetes* 1999;48:460.
32. Sabbah E, Savola K, Kulmala P, et al: Diabetes-associated autoantibodies in relation to clinical characteristics and natural course in children with newly diagnosed type 1 diabetes. The Childhood Diabetes in Finland Study Group. *J Clin Endocrinol Metab* 1999;84:1534.
33. Sabbah E, Savola K, Ebeling T, et al: Genetic, autoimmune, and clinical characteristics of childhood- and adult-onset type 1 diabetes. *Diabetes Care* 2000;23:1326.
34. Komulainen J, Kulmala P, Savola K, et al: Clinical, autoimmune, and genetic characteristics of very young children with type 1 diabetes. Childhood Diabetes in Finland (DiMe) Study Group. *Diabetes Care* 1999;22:1950.

35. Mrena S, Savola K, Kulmala P, et al: Staging of preclinical type 1 diabetes in siblings of affected children. Childhood Diabetes in Finland Study Group. *Pediatrics* 1999;104:925.

36. Carel JC, Boitard C, Bougneres PF: Decreased insulin response to glucose in islet cell antibody-negative siblings of type 1 diabetic children. *J Clin Invest* 1993;92:509.

37. Leslie RDG, Heaton DA, Millward BA: Identical co-twins of type I (insulin-dependent) diabetic patients can show evidence of B-cell dysfunction which does not lead to diabetes. *Diabetologia* 1986;29:564A.

38. Heaton DA, Millward BA, Gray P, et al: Evidence of B-cell dysfunction which does not lead on to diabetes: a study of identical twins of insulin dependent diabetic. *BMJ* 1987;294:145.

39. Gottlieb PA, Eisenbarth GS: Mouse and man: multiple genes and multiple autoantigens in the etiology of type I DM and related autoimmune disorders. *J Autoimmun* 1996;9:277.

40. Verge CF, Gianani R, Yu L, et al: Late progression to diabetes and evidence for chronic beta-cell autoimmunity in identical twins of patients with type I diabetes. *Diabetes* 1995;44:1176.

41. Norris JM, Beaty B, Klingensmith G, et al: Lack of association between early exposure to cow's milk protein and beta-cell autoimmunity. Diabetes Autoimmunity Study in the Young (DAISY). *JAMA* 1996;276:609.

42. Rewers M, Bugawan TL, Norris JM, et al: Newborn screening for HLA markers associated with IDDM: diabetes autoimmunity study in the young (DAISY). *Diabetologia* 1996;39:807.

43. Rewers M, Norris JM, Eisenbarth GS, et al: Beta-cell autoantibodies in infants and toddlers without IDDM relatives: diabetes autoimmunity study in the young (DAISY). *J Autoimmun* 1996;9:405.

44. Scott R, Willis J, Brown L, et al: Antibodies to glutamic acid decarboxylase (GAD) predict insulin deficiency in adult-onset diabetes mellitus. *Diabetes* 1993;42(Suppl):220A.

45. Zimmet PZ, Shaten BJ, Kuller LH, et al: Antibodies to glutamic acid decarboxylase and diabetes mellitus in the Multiple Risk Factor Intervention Trial. *Am J Epidemiol* 1994;140:683.

46. Yeung V, Chan JCN, Chow CC, et al: Antibodies to glutamic acid decarboxylase (anti-GAD) in Chinese IDDM patients. 15th International Diabetes Federation Congress Proceedings. Kobe, Japan, 1994;432.

47. Zimmet PZ: The pathogenesis and prevention of diabetes in adults: genes, autoimmunity, and demography. *Diabetes Care* 18:1050, 1995.

48. Kobayashi T, Tamemoto K, Nakanishi K, et al: Immunogenetic and clinical characterization of slowly progressive IDDM. *Diabetes Care* 1993;16:780.

49. Gottsater A, Landin Olsson M, Fernlund P, et al: Beta-cell function in relation to islet cell antibodies during the first 3 yr. after clinical diagnosis of diabetes in type II diabetic patients. *Diabetes Care* 1993;16:902.

50. Rowley MJ, Mackay IR, Chen QY, et al: Antibodies to glutamic acid decarboxylase discriminate major types of diabetes mellitus. *Diabetes* 1992;41:548.

51. Min HK: Non-insulin-dependent diabetes mellitus (NIDDM) in Korea. *Diabetic Med* 1996;13:S13.

52. Park Y, Lee HK, Koh CS, et al: The low prevalence of immunogenetic markers in Korean adult-onset IDDM patients. *Diabetes Care* 1996;19:241.

53. Park YS, Kawasaki E, Kelemen K, et al: Humoral autoreactivity to an alternatively spliced variant of ICA512/IA-2 in type I diabetes. *Diabetologia* 2000;43:1293.

54. Fukui M, Nakano K, Shigeta H, et al: Antibodies to glutamic acid decarboxylase in Japanese diabetic patients with secondary failure of oral hypoglycaemic therapy. *Diabetic Med* 1997;14:148.

55. Kasuga A, Maruyama T, Ozawa Y, et al: Antibody to the Mr 65,000 isoform of glutamic acid decarboxylase are detected in non-insulin-dependent diabetes in Japanese. *J Autoimmun* 1996;9:105.

56. Kockum I, Sanjeevi CB, Eastman S, et al: Complex interaction between HLA DR and DQ in conferring risk for childhood type 1 diabetes. *Eur J immunogenet* 1999;26:361.

57. Nerup J, Platz P, Anderssen OO: HLA antigens and diabetes mellitus. *Lancet* 1974;2:864.

58. Bodmer JG, Marsh SG, Albert ED, et al: Nomenclature for factors of the HLA system, 1998. *Hum Immunol* 1999;77:60.

59. Wassmuth R, Lernmark A: The genetics of susceptibility to diabetes. *Clin Immunol Immunopathol* 1989;53:358.

60. Nepom GT: Immunogenetics and IDDM. *Diabetes Reviews* 1:93, 1993.

61. Wassmuth R, Kockum I, Karlsen A, et al: Etiology of type 1 diabetes: genetic aspects. In: Ashcroft FM, Ashcroft SJH, eds. *Insulin: Molecular Biology to Pathology*. Oxford University Press:1992;285.

62. Cardon LR, Bell JI: Association study designs for complex diseases. *Nat Rev Genet* 2001;2:91.

63. Concannon P, Gogolin E-KJ, Hinds DA, et al: A second-generation screen of the human genome for susceptibility to insulin-dependent diabetes mellitus. *Nat Genet* 1998;19:292.

64. Herr M, Dudbridge F, Zavattari P, et al: Evaluation of fine mapping strategies for a multifactorial disease locus: systematic linkage and association analysis of IDDM1 in the HLA region on chromosome 6p21. *Hum Mol Genet* 2000;9:1291.

65. Tillil H, Kobberling J: Age-corrected empirical genetic risk estimates for first-degree relatives of IDDM patients. *Diabetes* 1987;36:93.

66. Lorenzen T, Pociot F, Hougaard P, et al: Long-term risk of IDDM in first-degree relatives of patients with IDDM. *Diabetologia* 1994;37:321.

67. Platz P, Jakobsen BK, Morling M, et al: HLA-D and DR antigens in genetic analysis of insulin-dependent diabetes mellitus. *Diabetologia* 1981;21:108.

68. Kockum I, Wassmuth R, Holmberg E, et al: HLA-DQ primarily confers protection and HAL-DR susceptibility in type I (insulin-dependent) diabetes studied in population-based affected families and controls. *Am J Human Genet* 1993;53:150.

69. Caillat-Zucman S, Bertin E, Timsit J, et al: Protection from insulin-dependent diabetes mellitus is linked to a peptide transporter gene. *Eur J Immunol* 1993;23:1784.

70. Graham J, Kockum I, Sanjeevi CB, et al: Negative association between type 1 diabetes and HLA DQB1*0602- DQA1*0102 is attenuated with age at onset. Swedish Childhood Diabetes Study Group. *Eur J Immunogenet* 1999;26:117.

71. Kwok WW, Domeier ML, Raymond FC, et al: Allele-specific motifs characterize HLA-DQ interactions with a diabetes-associated peptide derived from glutamic acid decarboxylase. *J Immunol* 1996;156:2171.

72. Johnston C, Pyke DA, Cudworth AG, et al: HLA-DR typing in identical twins with insulin-dependent diabetes: difference between concordant and discordant pairs. *BMJ* 1983;286:253.

73. Korman AJ, Boss JM, Spies T: Genetic complexity and expression of human class II histocompatibility antigens. *Immunol Rev* 1985;85:45.

74. Suciu-Foca N, Rubenstein P, Nicholson J. Juvenile diabetes mellitus and the HLA system. *Transplant Proc* 1979;11:1309.

75. Rowe JR, Mickelson EM, Hansen JA: T cell-defined DR4 subtypes as markers for type I diabetes. *Hum Immunol* 1988;22:51.

76. Erlich H, Bugawan T, Begovich AB, et al: HLA-DR, DQ and DP typing using PCR amplification and immobilized probes. *Eur J Immunogenet* 1991;18:33.

77. Castellino F, Zhong G, Germain RN, et al: Antigen presentation by MHC class II molecules: invariant chain function, protein trafficking, and the molecular basis of diverse determinant capture. *Hum Immunol* 1997;54:159.

78. Nepom GT: A unified hypothesis for the complex genetics of HLA, associations. *Diabetes* 1990;39:1153.

79. Thorsby E, Ronningen KS: Particular HAL-DQ molecules play a dominant role in determining susceptibility or resistance to type I (insulin-dependent) diabetes mellitus. *Diabetologia* 1993;36:371.

80. Sanjeevi CB, Lybrand TP, Landin-Olsson M, et al: Analysis of antibody markers, DRB1, DRB5, DQA1 and DQB1 genes and modeling of DR2 molecules in DR2 positive patients with insulin-dependent diabetes. *Tissue Antigens* 1994;44:110.

81. Segall M, Bach FH: HLA and diabetes from a T-cell perspective. *Diabetes Metab Rev* 1987;3:803.

82. Sheehy MJ, Rowe JR, Fuller TC, et al: A minor subset of HAL-DR3 haplotypes is preferentially increased in type I (insulin-dependent) diabetes. *Diabetologia* 1985;28:891.

83. Nepom GT, Kwok WW: Molecular basis for HLA-DQ associations with IDDM. *Diabetes* 1998;47:1177.

84. Brown J, Jardetsky T, Saper M, et al: A hypothetical model of the foreign antigen binding site of class II histocompatibility molecules. *Nature* 1988;332:845.

85. Corper AL, Stratmann T, Apostolopoulos V, et al: A structural framework for deciphering the link between I-Ag7 and autoimmune diabetes. *Science* 2000;288:505.

86. Hardy DA, Bell JI, Lona EO, *et al*: Mapping of the class II region of the human major histocompatibility complex by pulsed-field gel electrophoresis. *Nature* 1986;323:453.

87. Owerbach D, Lernmark A, Platz P, *et al*: HLA-D region B-chain DNA endonuclease fragments differ between HLA-DR identical healthy and insulin-dependent diabetic individuals. *Nature* 1983;303:815.

88. Todd JA, Bell JI, McDevitt HO: HLA DQ B gene contributes to susceptibility and resistance to insulin dependent diabetes mellitus. *Nature* 1987;329:599.

89. Khalil I, d'Auriol L, Gobet M, *et al*: A combination of HLA-DQβ Asp57-negative and HLA-DQα Arg52 confers susceptibility to insulin-dependent diabetes mellitus. *J Clin Invest* 1990;85:1315.

90. Undlien DE, Friede T, Rammensee HG, *et al*: HLA-encoded genetic predisposition in IDDM: DR4 subtypes may be associated with different degrees of protection. *Diabetes* 1997;46:143.

91. Baisch JM, Weeks T, Giles R, *et al*: Analysis of HLA-DQ genotypes and susceptibility in insulin-dependent diabetes mellitus. *N Engl J Med* 1990;322:1836.

92. Bao MZ, Wang JX, Dorman JS, *et al*: HLA-DQβ non-asp-57 allele and incidence of diabetes in China and the USA. *Lancet* 1989;2:497.

93. Yamagata K, Nakajima H, Hanafusa T, *et al*: Aspartic acid in position 57 of DQβ chain does not protect against type 1 (insulin-dependent) diabetes mellitus in Japanese subjects. *Diabetologia* 1989;32:762.

94. Todd JA, Mijovic C, Fletcher J, *et al*: Identification of susceptibility loci for insulin-dependent diabetes mellitus by trans-racial gene mapping. *Nature* 1989;338:587.

95. Todd JA, Fukui Y, Kitagawa T, *et al*: The A3 allele of the HLA DQA1 locus is associated with susceptibility to type I diabetes in Japanese. *Proc Natl Acad Med Sci USA* 1990;87:1094.

96. Aparicio JMR, Wakisaka A, Takada A, *et al*: HLA-DQ system and insulin-dependent diabetes mellitus in Japanese: does it contribute to the development of IDDM as it does in Caucasians? *Immunogenetics* 1998;28:240.

97. Risch N: Genetics of IDDM: evidence for complex inheritance with HLA. *Genet Epidemiol* 1989;6:143.

98. Graham J, Kockum I, Breslow N, *et al*: A comparison of three statistical models for IDDM associations with HLA. *Tissue Antigens* 1996; 48:1.

99. Nepom GT, Lippolis JD, White FM, *et al*: Identification and modulation of a naturally processed T cell epitope from the diabetes-associated autoantigen human glutamic acid decarboxylase 65 (hGAD65). *Proc Natl Acad Sci USA* 2001;98:1763.

100. Endl J, Otto H, Jung G, *et al*: Identification of naturally processed T cell epitopes from glutamic acid decarboxylase presented in the context of HLA-DR alleles by T lymphocytes of recent onset IDDM patients. *J Clin Invest* 1997;99:2405.

101. Reith W, Satola S, Herrero-Sanchez C: Congenital immunodeficiency with a regulatory defect in MHC class II gene expression lacks a specific HLA-DR promoter binding protein, RF-X. *Cell* 1988;53:897.

102. De Berardinis P, James RFL, Wise PH, *et al*: Do CD4-positive cytotoxic T cells damage islet B-cells in type I diabetes? *Lancet* 1988; 1:823.

103. Michelsen B, Wassmuth R, Ludvigsson J, *et al*: HLA heterozygosity in insulin-dependent diabetes is most frequent at the DQ locus. *Scand J Immunol* 1990;31:405.

104. Reeves WG, Barr D, Douglas CA: Factors governing the human immune response to injected insulin. *Diabetologia* 1984;26:266.

105. Bruserud O, Thorsby E: HLA control of the proliferative T lymphocyte response to antigenic determinants on mumps virus: studies of healthy individuals and patients with type I diabetes. *Scand J Immunol* 1985;22:509.

106. Bruserud O, Stenersen M, Thorsby E: T lymphocyte responses to coxsackie B4 and mumps virus, 2. Immunoregulation by HLA-DR3 and -DR4 associated restriction elements. *Tissue Antigens* 1985;26:179.

107. Sasazuki T, Nishimura Y, Muto M, *et al*: HLA-linked genes controlling immune response and disease susceptibility. *Immunol Rev* 1983; 70:51.

108. Kaufman DL, Erlander MG, Clare-Salzler M, *et al*: Autoimmunity to two forms of glutamate decarboxylase in insulin-dependent diabetes mellitus. *J Clin Invest* 1992;89:283.

109. Lohmann T, Leslie RDG, Hawa M, *et al*: Immunodominant epitopes of glutamic acid decarboxylase 65 and 67 in insulin-dependent diabetes mellitus. *Lancet* 1994;343:1607.

110. Rharbaoui F, Mayer A, Granier C, *et al*: T cell response pattern to glutamic acid decarboxylase 65 (GAD65) peptides of newly diagnosed

111. Nepom BS, Schwarz D, Palmer JP, *et al*: Transcomplementation of HLA genes in IDDM: HLA DQα- and β-chains produce hybrid molecules in DR3/ 4 heterozygotes. *Diabetes* 1987;36:114.

112. Radka SF, Scott RG, Stewart SJ: Molecular complexity of HLA-DQw3: the TA10 determinant is located on a subset of DQw3 b chains. *Hum Immunol* 1987;18:287.

113. Atar D, Dyrberg T, Michelsen B, *et al*: Site-specific antibodies distinguish single amino acid substitutions in position 57 in HLA-DQ b-chain alleles associated with insulin-dependent diabetes. *J Immunol* 1989;143:533.

114. Hanafusa I, Chiovato L, Doniach D, *et al*: Aberrant expression of HLA-DR antigen on thyrocytes in Graves' diseases: relevance for autoimmunity. *Lancet* 1983;2:1111.

115. Pujoll-Borrell R, Hanafusa T, Chiovato L, *et al*: Lectin-induced expression of DR antigen on human cultured follicular thyroid cells. *Nature* 1983;303:71.

116. Pujoll-Borrell R, Doshi M: HLA class II induction in human islet cells by interferon-gamma plus tumor necrosis factor or lymphotoxin. *Nature* 1987;326:304.

117. Ono SJ, Badia IC, Colk E, *et al*: Enhanced MHC class I heavy-chain gene expression in pancreatic islets. *Diabetes* 1988;37:1411.

118. Bottazzo GF, Dean BM, McNally JM, *et al*: In situ characterization of autoimmune phenomena and expression of HLA molecules in the pancreas in diabetic insulitis. *N Engl J Med* 1985;313:353.

119. Pipeleers DG, In't Veld PA, Pipeleers-Marichal MA, *et al*: Presence of pancreatic hormones in islet cells with MHC-class II antigen expression. *Diabetes* 1987;36:872.

120. In't Veld PA, Pipeleers DG: In situ analysis of pancreatic islets in rats developing diabetes: appearance of nonendocrine cells with surface MHC class II antigens and cytoplasmic insulin immunoreactivity. *J Clin Invest* 1988;82:1123.

121. Sarvetnick N, Liggitt D, Pitts SL, *et al*: Insulin dependent diabetes mellitus induced in transgenic mice by ectopic expression of class II MHC and interferon-gamma. *Cell* 1988;52:773.

122. Lo D, Burkly LC, Widera G: Diabetes and tolerance in transgenic mice expressing class II MHC molecules in pancreatic beta cells. *Cell* 1988;53:159.

123. Markmann J, Lo D, Naji A, *et al*: Antigen presenting function of class II MHC expressing pancreatic beta cells. *Nature* 1988;336:476.

124. Stewart TA, Hultaren B, Huang X, *et al*: Induction of type I diabetes by interferon-alpha in transgenic mice. *Science* 1994;199:1942.

125. Wogensen L, Lee M-S, Sarvetnick N: Production of interleukin 10 by islet cells accelerates immune-mediated destruction of β cells in nonobese diabetic mice. *J Exp Med* 1994;179:1379.

126. Trowsdale J, Hanson I, Mockridge I, *et al*: Sequences encoded in the class II region of the MHC related to 'ABC' superfamily of transporters. *Nature* 1990;348:741.

127. Dick LR, Moomaw CR, Dematino GN, *et al*: Degradation of oxidized insulin B chain by the multiproteinase complex macroplain (proteosome). *Biochemistry* 1991;30:2725.

128. Arnold D, Driscoll J, Androlewicz M, *et al*: Proteasome subunits encoded in the MHC are not generally required for the processing of peptides bound by MHC class I molecules. *Nature* 1992;360:171.

129. Colonna M, Bresnahan M, Bahram S, *et al*: Allelic variants of the human putative peptide transporter involved in antigen processing. *Proc Natl Acad Sci USA* 1992;89:3932.

130. Ronningen KS, Undlien DE, Ploski R, *et al*: Linkage disequilibrium between TAP2 variants and HLA class II alleles; no primary association between TAP2 variants and insulin-dependent diabetes mellitus. *Eur J Immunol* 1993;22:1050.

131. Rau H, Nicolay A, Donner H, *et al*: Polymorphisms of TAP1 and TAP2 genes in German patients with type 1 diabetes mellitus. *Eur J Immunogenet* 1997;24:229.

132. Jenkins D, Penny MA, Mijovic CH, *et al*: Tumour necrosis factor-beta polymorphism is unlikely to determine susceptibility to type I (insulin-dependent). diabetes mellitus. *Diabetologia* 1991;34:576.

133. Badenhoop K, Schwarz G, Trownsdale J, *et al*: TNF-alpha gene polymorphisms in type I (insulin-dependent). diabetes mellitus. *Diabetologia* 1989;32:445.

134. Pociot F, Ronningen KS, Nerup J: Polymorphic analysis of the human MHC-linked heat shock protein 70 (HSP70-2) and HSP70-Hom genes in insulin-dependent diabetes mellitus (IDDM). *Scand J Immunol* 1993;38:491.

type 1 diabetic patients sharing susceptible HLA haplotypes. *Clin Exp Immunol* 1999;117:30.

135. Kawaguchi Y, Ikegami H, Fukuda M, et al: Polymorphism of HSP70 gene is not associated with type I (insulin-dependent) diabetes mellitus in Japanese. Diabetes Res Clin Pract 1993;21:103.

136. Bertrams J, Baur MP, Gruneklee D, et al: Age-related association of insulin-dependent diabetes mellitus with BfF1 and the HLA-B18, BfFl haplotype. Diabetologia 1981;21:47.

137. Thomsen M, Molvig J, Zerbib A, et al: The susceptibility to insulin-dependent diabetes mellitus is associated with C4 allotypes independently of the association with HLADQ alleles in HLA-DR3, 4 heterozygotes. Immunogenetics 1988;28:320.

138. Partanen J, Koskimies S, Ilonen J, et al: HLA antigens and haplotypes in insulin-dependent diabetes mellitus. Tissue Antigens 1986;27:291.

139. Bell GI, Aorita S, Koran JH: A polymorphic locus near the human insulin gene is associated with insulin-dependent diabetes mellitus. Diabetes 1984;33:176.

140. Owerbach D, Gabbay KH: Localization of a type I diabetes susceptibility locus to the variable tandem repeat region flanking the insulin gene. Diabetes 1993;42:1708.

141. Julier C, Hyer RN, Davies J, et al: Insulin-IgF2 region on chromosome 11p encodes a gene implicated HLA-DR4 dependent diabetes susceptibility. Nature 1991;354:155.

142. Lucassen AM, Julier C, Beressi JP, et al: Susceptibility to insulin dependent diabetes mellitus maps to a 4.1 kb segment of DNA spanning the insulin gene and associated VNTR. Nat Genet 1993;4:305.

143. Permutt MA, Rotwein P, Andreone T, et al: Islet beta-cell function and polymorphism in the 5'-flanking region of the human insulin gene. Diabetes 1986;34:311.

144. Pugliese A, Zeller M, Fernandez JA, et al: The insulin gene transcribed in the human thymus and transcription level correlate with allelic variation at the INS VNTR-IDDM2 susceptibility locus for type 1 diabetes. Nat Genet 1997;15:293.

145. Vafidias P, Bennett STJAT, Nadeau J, et al: Insulin expression in human thymus is modulated by INS VNTR alleles at the IDDM2 locus. Nat Genet 1997;15:289.

146. Honjo T, Habu S: Origin of immune diversity: genetic variation and selection. Annu Rev Biochem 1985;54:803.

147. Rich SS, Weitkamp LR, Guttormsen S, et al: Gm, Km, and HLA in insulin-dependent type I diabetes. Diabetes 1986;35:927.

148. Bertrams J, Baur MP: No interaction between HLA and immunoglobulin IgG heavy chain allotypes in early onset type I diabetes. J Immunogenet 1985;12:81.

149. Schernthaner G, Mayr WR: Immunoglobulin allotype markers and HLA-DR genes in type I diabetes mellitus. Metab Clin Exp 1984; 33:833.

150. Field LL, Stephure DK, McArthur RG: Interaction between T cell receptor beta chain and immunoglobulin heavy chain region genes in susceptibility to insulin dependent diabetes mellitus. Am J Hum Genet 1991;49:627.

151. Dizier MH, Deschamps I, Hors J, et al: Interactive effect of HLA and Gm tested in a study of 135 juvenile insulin-dependent diabetic families. Tissue Antigens 1986;27:269.

152. Field L, Dugoujon JM: Immunoglobulin allotyping (Gm, Km) of GAW5 families. Genet Epidemiol 1989;6:31.

153. Garcia KC, Teyton L, Wilson IA: Structural basis of T cell recognition. Annu Rev Immunol 1999;17:369.

154. Leiter E: The genetics of diabetes susceptibility in mice. FASEB J 1989;3:2231.

155. Acha-Orbea H, Mitchell DJ, Timmermann L: Limited heterogeneity of T cell receptors from lymphocytes mediating autoimmune encephalomyelitis allows specific immune intervention. Cell 1998; 54:263.

156. Hoover ML, Capra JD: HLA and T-cell receptor genes in insulin-dependent diabetes mellitus. Diabetes Metab Rev 1987;3:835.

157. Martinez-Naves E, Coto E, Gutierrez V, et al: Germ line repertoire of T-cell receptor beta-chain genes in patients with insulin-dependent diabetes mellitus. Hum Immunol 1991;27:77.

158. Sheehy MJ, Meske LM, Emler CA, et al: Allelic T-cell receptor alpha complexes have little or no influence on susceptibility to type I diabetes. Hum Immunol 1989;26:261.

159. Martinez-Naves E, Pena M, Lopez-Larrea C: T-cell receptor alpha, delta, and gamma chain genes in insulin-dependent diabetes mellitus. Eur J Immunogenet 1993;20:317.

160. Lee KH, Wucherpfennig KW, Wiley DC: Structure of a human insulin peptide-HLA-DQ8 complex and susceptibility to type 1 diabetes. Nat Immunol 2001;2:501.

161. Davies JL, Kawaguchi Y, Bennett ST, et al: A genome-wide search for human type 1 diabetes susceptibility genes. Nature 1994;371: 130.

162. Mein CA, Esposito L, Dunn MG, et al: A search for type 1 diabetes susceptibility genes in families from the United Kingdom. Nature Genetics 1998;19:297.

163. Lernmark Å, Ducat L, Eisenbarth GE, et al: Family cell lines available for research. Am J Hum Genet 1990;47:1028.

164. Lernmark A, Eisenbarth G, Ducat L, et al: Family cell lines available for research—an endangered resource? [letter]. Am J Hum Genet 1997;61:778.

165. Luo DF, Buzzetti R, Rotter JI, et al: Confirmation of three susceptibility genes to insulin-dependent diabetes mellitus: IDDM4, IDDM5 and IDDM8. Hum Mol Genet 1996;5:693.

166. Schranz DB, Lernmark A: Immunology in diabetes: an update. Diabetes Metab Rev 1998;14:3.

167. Buzzetti R, Quattrocchi CC, Nistico L: Dissecting the genetics of type 1 diabetes: relevance for familial clustering and differences in incidence. Diabetes Metab Rev 1998;14:111.

168. Nisticó L, Buzzetti R, Pritchard LE, et al: The CTLA-4 gene region on chromosome 2q33 is linked to, and associated with type 1 diabetes. Belgian-Diabetes Registry. Hum Mol Genet 1996;5:1075.

169. Lowe RM, Graham J, Sund G, et al: The length of the CTLA-4 microsatellite (AT)N-repeat affects the risk for type 1 diabetes. Autoimmunity 2000;32:173.

170. Atkinson MA, Maclaren NK: Islet cell autoantigens in insulin-dependent diabetes. J Clin Invest 1993;92:1608.

171. Bosi E, Becker F, Bonifacio E, et al: Progression to type I diabetes in autoimmune endocrine patients with islet cell antibodies. Diabetes 1991;40:977.

172. Bingley PJ, Bonifacio E, Gale EAM: Can we really predict IDDM? Diabetes 1993;42:213.

173. Knip M, Karjalainen J, Akerblom HK: Islet cell antibodies are less predictive of IDDM among unaffected children in the general population than in sibs of children with diabetes. The Childhood Diabetes in Finland Study Group. Diabetes Care 1998;21:1670.

174. Gianani R, Pugliese A, Bonner-Weir S, et al: Prognostically significant heterogeneity of cytoplasmic islet cell antibodies in relatives of patients with type I diabetes. Diabetes 1992;41:347.

175. Landin-Olsson M, Arnqvist HJ, Blohme G, et al: Appearance of islet cell autoantibodies after clinical diagnosis of diabetes mellitus. Autoimmunity 1999;29:57.

176. Timsit J, Caillat-Zucman S, Blondel H, et al: Islet cell antibody heterogeneity among type I (insulin-dependent) diabetes patients. Diabetologia 1992;35:792.

177. Krischer JP, Schatz D, Riley WJ, et al: Insulin and islet cell antibodies as time-dependent covariates in the development of insulin-dependent diabetes: a prospective study in relatives. J Clin Endocrinol Metab 1993;77:743.

178. Palmer JP: Insulin autoantibodies: their role in the pathogenesis of IDDM. Diabetes Metab Rev 1987;3:1005.

179. Greenbaum CJ, Palmer JP: Insulin antibodies and insulin autoantibodies. Diabete Med 1991;8:97.

180. Baekkeskov S, Aanstoot HJ, Christgau S, et al: Identification of the 64K autoantigen in insulin-dependent diabetes as the GABA-synthesizing enzyme glutamic acid decarboxylase. Nature 1990;347: 151.

181. Hagopian WA, Michelsen B, Karlsen AE, et al: Autoantibodies in IDDM primarily recognize the 65,000-Mr rather than the 67,000-Mr isoform of glutamic acid decarboxylase. Diabetes 1993;42:631.

182. Colman PG: IDW GAD Antibody Workshop. 13th International Immunology and Diabetes Workshop, Montvillargenne, France, 1994.

183. Bjork E, Velloso LA, Kampe O, et al: GAD autoantibodies in IDDM, stiff-man syndrome, and autoimmune polyendocrine syndrome type I recognize different epitopes. Diabetes 1994;43:161.

184. Jones DB, Hunter NR, Duff GW: Heat-shock protein 65 as a B-cell antigen of insulin-dependent diabetes. Lancet 1990;336:583.

185. Atkinson MA, Holmes LA, Scharp DW, et al: No evidence for serological autoimmunity to islet cell heat shock proteins in insulin-dependent diabetes. J Clin Invest 1991;87:721.

186. Hampe CS, Ortqvist E, Rolandsson O, et al: Species-specific autoantibodies in type 1 diabetes. J Clin Endocrinol Metab 1999;84:643.

187. Hampe CS, Ortqvist E, Persson B, et al: Glutamate decarboxylase (GAD) autoantibody epitope shift during the first year of type 1 diabetes. Horm Metab Res 1999;31:553.

188. Hampe CS, Hammerle LP, Bekris L, *et al*: Recognition of glutamic acid decarboxylase (GAD) by autoantibodies from different GAD antibody-positive phenotypes. *J Clin Endocrinol Metab* 200085:4671.

189. Hampe CS, Lundgren P, Daniels TL, *et al*: A novel monoclonal antibody specific for the N-terminal end of GAD65. *J Neuroimmunol* 2001113:63.

190. Christie MR, Hollands JA, Brown TJ, *et al*: Detection of pancreatic islet 64,000 Mr autoantigens in insulin dependent diabetes distinct from glutamate decarboxylase. *J Clin Invest* 1993;92:240.

191. Schmidli RS, Colman PG, Cui L, *et al*: Antibodies to the protein tyrosine phosphatases IAR and IA-2 are associated with progression to insulin-dependent diabetes (IDDM) in first-degree relatives at-risk for IDDM. *Autoimmunity* 1998;28:15.

192. Ellis TM, Schatz DA, Ottendorfer EW, *et al*: The relationship between humoral and cellular immunity to IA-2 in IDDM. *Diabetes* 1998; 47:566.

193. Kawasaki E, Yu L, Rewers MJ, *et al*: Definition of multiple ICA512/phogrin autoantibody epitopes and detection of intramolecular epitope spreading in relatives of patients with type 1 diabetes. *Diabetes* 1998;47:733.

194. Verge CF, Stenger D, Bonifacio E, *et al*: Combined use of autoantibodies (IA-2 autoantibody, GAD autoantibody, insulin autoantibody, cytoplasmic islet cell antibodies) in type 1 diabetes: Combinatorial Islet Autoantibody Workshop. *Diabetes* 1998;47:1857.

195. Kulmala P, Savola K, Reijonen H, *et al*: Genetic markers, humoral autoimmunity, and prediction of type 1 diabetes in siblings of affected children. Childhood Diabetes in Finland Study Group. *Diabetes* 2000; 49:48.

196. Lindberg B, Ivarsson SA, Landin-Olsson M, *et al*: Islet autoantibodies in cord blood from children who developed type I (insulin-dependent) diabetes mellitus before 15 years of age. *Diabetologia* 1999;42:181.

197. Lindberg B, Ivarsson SA, Lernmark A: Islet autoantibodies in cord blood could be a risk factor for future diabetes. *Diabetologia* 1999; 42:1375.

198. Kaufman DL, Clare-Salzler MC, Tian J, *et al*: Spontaneous loss of T-cell tolerance to glutamic acid decarboxylase in murine insulin dependent diabetes. *Nature* 1993;366:69.

199. Tisch R, Yang XD, Singer SM, *et al*: Immune response to glutamic acid decarboxylase correlates with insulitis in non-obese diabetic mice. *Nature* 1993;366:72.

200. Wegmann DR, Gill RG, Daniel D: The role of insulin-specific T cells in IDDM in NOD mice. 13th Immunology of Diabetes Workshop. Montvillargenne, France, 1994.

201. Maron R, Melican NS, Weiner HL: Regulatory Th2-type T cell lines against insulin and GAD peptides derived from orally- and nasally-treated NOD mice suppress diabetes. *J Autoimmun* 1999;12:251.

202. Maron R, Guerau-De-Arellano M, Zhang X, *et al*: Oral administration of insulin to neonates suppresses spontaneous and cyclophosphamide induced diabetes in the nod mouse. *J Autoimmun* 2001;16:21.

203. Song HY, Abad MM, Mahoney CP, *et al*: Human insulin B chain but not A chain decreases the rate of diabetes in BB rats. *Diabetes Res Clin Pract* 1999;46:109.

204. Alleva DG, Crowe PD, Jin L, *et al*: A disease-associated cellular immune response in type 1 diabetics to an immunodominant epitope of insulin. *J Clin Invest* 2001;107:173.

205. Garcia K, Scott C, Brunmark A, *et al*: CD8 enhances formation of a stable T-cell receptor/MHC class I molecule complexes. *Nature* 1996; 384:577.

206. Hampl J, Chien T-H, David MM: CD4 augments the response of a T-cell to agonist but not to antagonist ligands. *Immunity* 1997;7:379.

207. Izquierdo Pastor M, Reif K, Cantrell D: The regulation and function of p21ras during T-cell activation and growth. *Immunol Today* 1995; 16:159.

208. Cantrell D: T cell antigen receptor signal transduction pathways. *Annu Rev Immunol* 1996;14:259.

209. Constant S, Pfeifer C, Woodard A, *et al*: Extent of T cell receptor ligation can determine the functional differentiation of naive CD4+ T-cells. *J Exp Med* 1996;182:1591.

210. Kundig TM, Shahinian A, Kawai K, *et al*: Duration of TCR stimulation determines co-stimulatory requirements of T cells. *Immunity* 1996;5:41.

211. Kuchroo VK, Das MP, Brown JA, *et al*: B7-1 and B7-2 costimulatory molecules differentially activate the Th1/Th2 developmental pathways: application to autoimmune disease therapy. *Cell* 1995;80:707.

212. Tivol EA, Schweitzer NA, Sharpe AH: Costimulation and autoimmunity. *Curr Opin Immunol* 1996;8:822.

213. Rabinovitch A: Roles of cytokines in IDDM pathogenesis and islet beta-cell destruction. *Diabetes Rev* 1993;1:215.

214. Mehta V, Hao W, Brooks-Worrell M, *et al*: The functional state of the B cell modulates IL-1 and TNF-induced cytotoxicity. *Lymphokine Cytokine Res* 1993;12:255.

215. Ling Z, In't Veld PA, Pipeleers DG: Interaction of interleukin-1 with islet B-cells. Distinction between indirect specific functional suppression. *Diabetes* 1993;42:56.

216. Eizirik DL, Sandler S: Function and metabolism of pancreatic beta-cells maintained in culture following experimentally induced damage. *Pharmacol Toxicol* 1989;65:163.

217. Tochino Y: The NOD mouse as a model of type I diabetes. *Crit Rev Immunol* 1987;8:49.

218. Eizirik DL, Sandler S, Ahnström G, *et al*: Exposure of pancreatic islets to different alkylating agents decreases mitochondrial DNA content but only streptozotocin induces long-lasting functional impairment of B-cells. *Biochem Pharmacol* 1991;42:2275.

219. Rabinovitch A, Pukel C, Baquerizo H: Interleukin-1 inhibits glucose-modulated insulin and glucagon secretion in rat islet monolayer cultures. *Endocrinology* 1988;122:2393.

220. Strandell E, Sandler S, Boitard C, *et al*: Role of infiltrating T cells for impaired glucose metabolism in pancreatic islets isolated from nonobese diabetic mice. *Diabetologia* 1992;35:924.

221. Chatenoud L, Primo J, Bach JF: CD3 antibody-induced dominant self tolerance in overtly diabetic NOD mice. *J Immunol* 1997;158: 2947.

222. Kay TWH, Campbell IL, Oxbrow L, *et al*: Overexpression of class I major histocompatibility complex accompanies insulitis in the nonobese diabetic mouse and is prevented by anti-interferon-1 antibody. *Diabetologia* 1991;34:779.

223. Sarvetnick N, Shizuru J, Liggitt D, *et al*: Loss of pancreatic islet tolerance induced by B-cell expression of interferon-gamma. *Nature* 1990; 346:844.

224. Welsh N, Welsh M, Lindquist S, *et al*: Interleukin-I-beta increases the biosynthesis of the heat shock protein hsp70 and selectively decreases the biosynthesis of five proteins in rat pancreatic islets. *Autoimmununity* 1991;9:33.

225. Kjaer TW, Rygaard J, Bendtzen K, *et al*: Interleukins increase surface ganglioside expression of pancreatic islet cells in vitro. *APMIS* 1992; 100:509.

226. Helqvist S, Sehested Hansen BS, *et al*: Interleukin 1 induces new protein formation in isolated rat islets of Langerhans. *Acta Endocrinol (Copenh)* 1989;121:136.

227. Eizirik DL, Welsh M, Strandell E, *et al*: Interleukin-1-beta depletes insulin messenger ribonucleic acid and increases the heat shock protein HSP70 in mouse pancreatic islets without impairing the glucose metabolism. *Endocrinology* 1990;127:2290.

228. Borg LAH, Cagliero E, Sandler S, *et al*: Interleukin-l-beta increases the activity of superoxide dismutase in rat pancreatic islets. *Endocrinology* 1992;130:2851.

229. Eizirik DL, Sandler S, Palmer JP: Repair of pancreatic B-cells. A relevant phenomenon in early IDDM? *Diabetes* 1993;42:1383.

230. DeKruyff R, Rizzo L, Umetsu D: Induction of immunoglobulin synthesis by CD4+ T cell clones. *Semin Immunol* 1993;5:421.

231. Field E, Noelle R, Rouse T, *et al*: Evidence for excessive Th2 CD4+ subset activity in vivo. *J Immunol* 1993;151:48.

232. King C, Mahanty S, Kumaraswami V, *et al*: Cytokine control of parasite-specific anergy in human lymphatic filariasis—preferential induction of a regulatory T helper type 2 lymphocyte subset. *J Clin Invest* 1993;92:1667.

233. Abbas A, Burstein H, Bogen S: Determinants of helper T-cell dependent antibody production. *Semin Immunol* 1993;5:441.

234. Debray-Sachs M, Carnaud C, Boitard C, *et al*: Prevention of diabetes in NOD mice treated with antibody to murine IFN. *J Autoimmun* 1991;4:237.

235. Nicoletti F, Meroni PL, Landolfo S, *et al*: Prevention of diabetes in BB/Wor rats treated with monoclonal antibodies to interferon. (Abstract). *Lancet* 1990;336:319.

236. Bergman B, Haskins K: Islet-specific T-cell clones from NOD mouse respond to B-granule antigen. *Diabetes* 1994;43:197.

237. Shehadeh NN, LaRosa F, Lafferty KJ: Altered cytokine activity in adjuvant inhibition of autoimmune diabetes. *J Autoimmun* 1993;6:291.

238. Rapoport MJ, Jaramillo A, Zipris D, *et al*: Interleukin 4 reverses T cell proliferative unresponsiveness and prevents the onset of diabetes in nonobese diabetic mice. *J Exp Med* 1993;178:87.

239. Rabinovitch A, Sorensen O, Suarez-Pinzon WL, *et al*: Analysis of cytokine mRNA expression in syngenic islet grafts of NOD mice: interleukin 2 and interferon gamma mRNA expression correlate with graft rejection and interleukin 10 with graft survival. *Diabetologia* 1994;37:833.

240. Fowell D, Mason D: Evidence that the T cell repertoire of normal rats contains cells with the potential to cause diabetes. Characterization of the CD4+ T cell subset that inhibits this autoimmune potential. *J Exp Med* 1993;177:627.

241. Del Prete G, DeCarli FM, Almerigogna F, *et al*: Human IL-10 is produced by both type 1 helper (Th1) and type 2 helper (Th2) T cell clones and inhibits their antigen-specific proliferation and cytokine production. *J Immunol* 1993;150:353.

242. Del Prete G, Maggi E, Romagnani S: Human Th1 and Th2 cells: functional properties, mechanism of regulation, and role in disease. *Lab Invest* 1994;70:299.

243. Correale J, Gilmore W, McMillan M, *et al*: Patterns of cytokine secretion by autoreactive proteolipid protein-specific T cell clones during the course of multiple sclerosis. *J Immunol* 1995;154:2959.

244. Berman MA, Sandborg CI, Wang Z, *et al*: Decreased IL-4 production in new onset type1 insulin-dependent diabetes mellitus. *J Immunol* 1996;157:4690.

245. Harrison LC, Honeyman MC, DeAizpurua HJ, *et al*: Inverse relation between humoral and cellular immunity to glutamic acid decarboxylase in subjects at risk of insulin-dependent diabetes. *Lancet* 1993;341:1365.

246. Atkinson M, Leslie DR: Inverse relation between humoral and cellular immunity to glutamic acid decarboxylase in subjects at risk of insulin-dependent diabetes. *J Endocrinol Invest* 1994;17:581.

247. Yu L, Rewers M, Gianani R, *et al*: Antiislet autoantibodies usually develop sequentially rather than simultaneously. *J Clin Endocrinol Metab* 1996;77:743.

248. Bingley PJ, Christie MR, Bonifacio E, *et al*: Combined analysis of autoantibodies improves prediction of IDDM in islet cell antibody-positive relatives. *Diabetes* 1994;43:1304.

249. Wilson SB, Kent SC, Patton KT, *et al*: Extreme Th1 bias of invariant Valpha24JalphaQ T cells in type 1 diabetes. *Nature* 1998;391:177.

250. Friedman A, Weiner HL: Induction of anergy or active suppression following oral tolerance is determined by antigen dosage. *Proc Natl Acad Sci USA* 1994;91:6688.

251. Miller A, Lider O, Roberts AB, *et al*: Suppressor T cells generated by oral tolerization to myelin basic protein suppress both in vitro and in vivo immune responses by the release of TGF-beta following antigen-specific triggering. *Proc Natl Acad Sci USA* 1992;89:421.

252. Ku-Amano J, Aicher WK, Taguchi T, *et al*: Selective induction of Th2 cells in murine Peyer's patches by oral immunization. *Int Immunol* 1992;4:433.

253. Chen Y, Kuchroo VK, Inobe JI, *et al*: Regulatory T cell clones induced by oral tolerance: suppression of autoimmune encephalomyelitis. *Science* 1994;265:1237.

254. Khoury SJ, Hancock WW, Weiner HL: Oral tolerance to myelin basic protein and natural recovery from experimental autoimmune encephalomyelitis are associated with downregulation of inflammatory cytokines and differential upregulation of transforming growth factor-beta, interleukin 4, and prostaglandin E expression in the brain. *J Exp Med* 1992;176:1355.

255. Almawi WY, Tamim H, Azar ST: T helper type 1 and 2 cytokines mediate the onset and progression of type I (insulin-dependent) diabetes. *J Clin Endocrinol Metab* 1999;84:1497.

256. Shimada A, Charlton B, Rohane P, *et al*: Immune regulation in type 1 diabetes. *J Autoimmun* 1996;9:263.

257. Rabinovitch A, Skyler JS: Prevention of type 1 diabetes. *Med Clin North Am* 1998;82:739.

258. Benoist C, Mathis D: Cell death mediators in autoimmune diabetes—no shortage of suspects. *Cell* 1997;89:1.

259. Corbett JA, McDaniel ML: Does nitric oxide mediate autoimmune destruction of beta-cells? Possible therapeutic interventions in IDDM. *Diabetes* 1992;41:897.

260. Kleemann R, Rothe H, Kolb-Bachofen V, *et al*: Transcription and translation of inducible nitric oxide synthase in the pancreas of prediabetic BB rats. *FEBS Lett* 1993;328:9.

261. Rothe H, Faust A, Schade U, *et al*: Cyclophosphamide treatment of female non-obese diabetic mice causes enhanced expression of inducible nitric oxide synthase and interferon-gamma, but not of interleukin-4. *Diabetologia* 1994;37:1154.

262. Roep BO, Atkinson MA, van Endert PM, *et al*: Autoreactive T cell responses in insulin-dependent (type 1) diabetes mellitus. Report of the First International Workshop for Standardization of T Cell Assays. *J Autoimmun* 1999;13:267.

263. Peakman M, Atkinson M, Roep BO, *et al*: The Second IDS Human T-Cell Workshop-Phase II: Distribution of high quality islet autoantigen preparations for novel T cell assays. *Diabetes Metab* 2001;17 (Suppl 1):S12.

264. Dosch HM, Becker DJ: Measurement of T-cell autoreactivity in autoimmune diabetes. *Diabetologia* 2000;43:386.

265. Akerblom HK, Knip M: Putative environmental factors in type 1 diabetes. *Diabetes Metab Rev* 1998;14:31.

266. Verge CF, Howard NJ, Irwig L, *et al*: Environmental factors in childhood IDDM. A population-based, case-control study. *Diabetes Care* 1994;17:1381.

267. Romagnani S: Human TH1 and TH2 subsets: regulation of differentiation and role in protection and immunopathology. *Int Arch Allergy Immunol* 1992;98:279.

268. Kaprio J, Tuomilehto J, Koskenvuo M, *et al*: Concordance for type I (insulin-dependent) and type 2 (noninsulin-dependent) diabetes mellitus in a population-based cohort of twins in Finland. *Diabetologia* 1992;35:1060.

269. Adams SF: The seasonal variation in the onset of acute diabetes. *Arch Intern Med* 1926;37:861.

270. Weinberg CR, Dornan TL, Hansen JA, *et al*: HAL-related heterogeneity in seasonal patterns of diagnosis of type I (insulin-dependent) diabetes. *Diabetologia* 1984;26:199.

271. Gamble DR: The epidemiology of insulin-dependent diabetes, with particular reference to the relationship of virus infection to its etiology. *Epidemiol Rev* 1980;2:49.

272. Tajima N, LaPorte RE, Hibi I, *et al*: A comparison of the epidemiology of youth-onset insulin-dependent diabetes mellitus between Japan and the United States. *Diabetes Care* 1985;8(Suppl 1):17.

273. Anonymous: Variation and trends in incidence of childhood diabetes in Europe. EURODIAB ACE Study Group. *Lancet* 2000;355:873.

274. Karvonen M, Viik-Kajander M, Moltchanova E, *et al*: Incidence of childhood type 1 diabetes worldwide. Diabetes Mondiale (DiaMond) Project Group. *Diabetes Care* 2000;23:1516.

275. Akerblom HK, Ballard DJ, Bauman B: Geographic patterns of childhood insulin-dependent diabetes mellitus. *Diabetes* 1988;37:1113.

276. Muntoni S, Songini M, IDDM S: High incidence rate of IDDM in Sardinia. *Diabetes Care* 1992;15:1317.

277. Dahlquist GG: Viruses and other perinatal exposures as initiating events for beta-cell destruction. *Ann Med* 1997;29:413.

278. Ahmed T, Kamota T, Sumazaki R, *et al*: Circulating antibodies to common food antigens in Japanese children with IDDM. *Diabetes Care* 1997;20:74.

279. Singh B, Rabinovitch A: Influence of microbial agents on the development and prevention of autoimmune diabetes. *Autoimmunity* 1993;15:209.

280. Yoon J-W: Environmental factors: viruses. In: Palmer JP, ed. *Prediction, Prevention, and Genetic Counseling in IDDM*. John Wiley & Sons:1996;145.

281. Singh B: Stimulation of the developing immune system can prevent autoimmunity. *J Autoimmun* 2000;14:15.

282. Nederaaard M, Egeberg J, Kromann H: Irradiation protects against pancreatic islet degeneration and hyperglycemia following streptozotocin treatment of mice. *Diabetologia* 1983;24:392.

283. Bouchard PH, Sai P, Reach G, *et al*: Diabetes mellitus following pentamidine-induced hypoglycemia in humans. *Diabetes* 1982;31:40.

284. Karam JH, Lewitt PA, Young CW, *et al*: Insulinopenic diabetes after rodenticide (Vactor) ingestion. A unique model of acquired diabetes in man. *Diabetes* 1980;29:971.

285. von Herrath MG, Evans CF, Horwitz MS, *et al*: Using transgenic mouse models to dissect the pathogenesis of virus-induced autoimmune disorders of the islets of Langerhans and the central nervous system. *Immunol Rev* 1996;152:111.

286. von Herrath MG, Homann D, Gairin JE, *et al*: Pathogenesis and treatment of virus-induced autoimmune diabetes: novel insights gained

from the RIP-LCMV transgenic mouse model. *Biochem Soc Trans* 1997;25:630.

287. von Herrath MG: Selective immunotherapy of IDDM: a discussion based on new findings from the RIP-LCMV model for autoimmune diabetes. *Transplant Proc* 1998;30:4115.

288. Ohashi PS, Oehen S, Buerki K, *et al*: Ablation of "tolerance" and induction of diabetes by virus infection in viral antigen transgenic mice. *Cell* 1991;65:305.

289. Holmes W: Association of exposure to cow's milk protein and beta-cell autoimmunity. *JAMA* 1996;276:1799.

290. Johnston CS, Spear SE: Association of exposure to cow's milk protein and beta- cell autoimmunity. *JAMA* 1996;276:1800.

291. Karjalainen J, Martin JM, Knip M, *et al*: Cow's milk and IDDM. *Lancet* 1996;348:905.

292. Bodington MJ, McNally PG, Burden AC: Cow's milk and type 1 childhood diabetes: no increase in risk. *Diabete Med* 1994;11:663.

293. Dosch HM: Cow's milk and the diabetes debate. *Pediatrics* 1995; 96:541.

294. Hammond McKibben D, Dosch HM: Cow's milk, bovine serum albumin, and IDDM: can we settle the controversies? *Diabetes Care* 1997; 20:897.

295. Harrison LC, Honeyman MC: Cow's milk and type 1 diabetes: the real debate is about mucosal immune function. *Diabetes* 1999; 48:1501.

296. Akerblom HK, Savilahti E, Saukkonen TT, *et al*: The case for elimination of cow's milk in early infancy in the prevention of type 1 diabetes: the Finnish experience. *Diabetes Metab Rev* 1993;9:269.

297. Akerblom HK, Vaarala O: Cow milk proteins, autoimmunity and type 1 diabetes. *Exp Clin Endocrinol Diabetes* 1997;105:83.

298. Atkinson MA, Bowman MA, Kao KJ, *et al*: Increased levels of cow's milk and beta-lactoglobulin antibodies in young children with newly diagnosed IDDM. The Childhood Diabetes in Finland Study Group. *Diabetes Care* 1993;16:984.

299. Gerstein HC: Cow's milk exposure and type I diabetes mellitus. A critical overview of the clinical literature. *Diabetes Care* 1994;17:13.

300. Dahlquist G, Savilahti E, Landin-Olsson M: An increased level of antibodies to beta-lactoglobulin is a risk determinant for early-onset type 1 (insulin-dependent) diabetes mellitus independent of islet cell antibodies and early introduction of cow's milk. *Diabetologia* 1992; 35:980.

301. Füchtenbusch M, Karges W, Standl E, *et al*: Antibodies to bovine serum albumin (BSA) in type 1 diabetes and other autoimmune disorders. *Exp Clin Endocrinol Diabetes* 1997;105:86.

302. Lévy Marchal C, Karjalainen J, Dubois F, *et al*: Antibodies against bovine albumin and other diabetes markers in French children. *Diabetes Care* 1995;18:1089.

303. Cheung R, Karjalainen J, Vandermeulen J, *et al*: T cells from children with IDDM are sensitized to bovine serum albumin. *Scand J Immunol* 1994;40:623.

304. Winer S, Gunaratnam L, Astsatourov I, *et al*: Peptide dose, MHC affinity, and target self-antigen expression are critical for effective immunotherapy of nonobese diabetic mouse prediabetes. *J Immunol* 2000;165:4086.

305. Dahlquist G: Milk proteins in the etiology of insulin-dependent diabetes mellitus (IDDM). *Ann Med* 1991;23:447.

306. Vaarala O, Kaste J, Klemetti P, *et al*: Development of immune response to orally administered cow milk protein in young children. *Ann N Y Acad Sci* 1996;778:429.

307. Vaarala O, Klemetti P, Savilahti E, *et al*: Cellular immune response to cow's milk beta-lactoglobulin in patients with newly diagnosed IDDM. *Diabetes* 1996;45:178.

308. Gerstein HC, VanderMeulen J: The relationship between cow's milk exposure and type 1 diabetes. *Diabetic Med* 1996;13:23.

309. Gimeno SG, de Souza JM: IDDM and milk consumption. A case-control study in São Paulo, Brazil. *Diabetes Care* 1997;20:1256.

310. Vähäsalo P, Petäys T, Knip M, *et al*: Relation between antibodies to islet cell antigens, other autoantigens and cow's milk proteins in diabetic children and unaffected siblings at the clinical manifestation of IDDM. The Childhood Diabetes in Finland Study Group. *Autoimmunity* 1996;23:165.

311. Virtanen SM, Hypponen E, Laara E, *et al*: Cow's milk consumption, disease-associated autoantibodies and type 1 diabetes mellitus: a follow-up study in siblings of diabetic children. Childhood Diabetes in Finland Study Group. *Diabetic Med* 1998;15:730.

312. Virtanen SM, Laara E, Hypponen E, *et al*: Cow's milk consumption, HLA-DQB1 genotype, and type 1 diabetes: a nested case-control study of siblings of children with diabetes. Childhood Diabetes in Finland Study Group. *Diabetes* 2000;49:912.

313. Saukkonen T, Virtanen SM, Karppinen M, *et al*: Significance of cow's milk protein antibodies as risk factor for childhood IDDM: interactions with dietary cow's milk intake and HLA-DQB1 genotype. Childhood Diabetes in Finland Study Group. *Diabetologia* 1998;41:72.

314. Vaarala O, Knip M, Paronen J, *et al*: Cow's milk formula feeding induces primary immunization to insulin in infants at genetic risk for type 1 diabetes. *Diabetes* 1999;48:1389.

315. American Academy of Pediatrics, Work Group on Cow's Milk Protein and Diabetes: Infant feeding practices and their possible relationship to the etiology of diabetes mellitus. *Pediatrics* 1994;94:752.

316. Harrison LC: AAP recommendations on cow milk, soy, and early infant feeding. *Pediatrics* 1995;96:515.

317. Gerstein HC, Simpson JR, Atkinson S, *et al*: Feasibility and acceptability of a proposed infant feeding intervention trial for the prevention of type I diabetes. *Diabetes Care* 1995;18:940.

318. Elliott RB, Harris DP, Hill JP, *et al*: Type I (insulin-dependent) diabetes mellitus and cow's milk: casein variant consumption. *Diabetologia* 1999;42:292.

319. Paronen JM, Akerblom HK, Vaarala O: Cow milk insulin as a trigger of cellular and humoral immunity to infants with genetic risk for IDDM. *Diabetes* 1999;48(Suppl 1):A207.

320. Paronen J, Knip M, Savilahti E, *et al*: Effect of cow's milk exposure and maternal type 1 diabetes on cellular and humoral immunization to dietary insulin in infants at genetic risk for type 1 diabetes. Finnish Trial to Reduce IDDM in the Genetically at Risk Study Group. *Diabetes* 2000;49:1657.

321. Couper JJ, Steele C, Beresford S, *et al*: Lack of association between duration of breast-feeding or introduction of cow's milk and development of islet autoimmunity. *Diabetes* 1999;48:2145.

322. Ivarsson SA, Mu MÄ, Jakobsson IL: IgG antibodies to bovine serum albumin are not increased in children with IDDM. *Diabetes* 1995; 44:1349.

323. Ronningen KS, Atrazhev A, Smith D, *et al*: The 69kD islet cell autoantigen (ICA69) and bovine serum albumin are not antigenically cross-reactive. *Diabetes* 1995;44(Suppl 1):78A.

324. Atkinson MA, Bowman MA, Kao KJ, *et al*: Lack of immune responsiveness to bovine serum albumin in insulin-dependent diabetes. *N Engl J Med* 1993;329:1853.

325. Atkinson MA, Ellis TM: Infants' diets and insulin-dependent diabetes: evaluating the "cows' milk hypothesis" and a role for anti-bovine serum albumin immunity. *J Am Coll Nutr* 1997;16:334.

326. Norris JM, Scott FW: A meta-analysis of infant diet and insulin-dependent diabetes mellitus: do biases play a role? *Epidemiology* 1996;7:87.

327. Yoon JW: Viral pathogenesis of insulin-dependent diabetes mellitus, In: Ginsbera-Fellner FM, ed. *Autoimmunity and the Pathogenesis of Diabetes.* Springer-Verlag:1990;206.

328. Yoon JW, McClintock PR, Onodera T, *et al*: Virus-induced diabetes mellitus. Inhibition by a non-diabetogenic variant of encephalomyocarditis virus. *J Exp Med* 1980;152:878.

329. Bae YS, Yoon JW: Determination of diabetogenecity attributable to a single amino acid Ala-776, on the polyprotein of encephalomyocarditis virus. *Diabetes* 1993;42:435.

330. Kang Y, Yoon JNNI: A genetically determined host factor controlling susceptibility to encephalomyocarditis virus-induced diabetes in mice. *J Genet Virol* 1993;74:1203.

331. Yoon JW, Silvaggio S, Onodera T, *et al*: Infection of cultured human pancreatic B cells with reovirus type 3. *Diabetologia* 1981;20:462.

332. Heurtier AH, Boitard C: T-cell regulation in murine and human autoimmune diabetes: the role of TH1 and TH2 cells. *Diabetes Metab* 1997;23:377.

333. Jenson A-B, Rosenberg HS, Notkins AL: Pancreatic islet cell damage in children with fatal viral infections. *Lancet* 1980;2:354.

334. Yoon JW, Austin M, Onodera T, *et al*: Virus induced diabetes mellitus. Isolation of a virus from the pancreas of a child with diabetic ketoacidosis. *N Engl J Med* 1979;300:1173.

335. Prince GA, Jenson AB, Billups LC, *et al*: Infection of human pancreatic beta cell cultures with mumps virus. *Nature* 1978;271:158.

336. Cavallo MG, Baroni MG, Toto A, *et al*: Viral infection induces cytokine release in beta islet cells. *Immunology* 1992;75:664.

337. Helmke K, Otten A, Willems W: Islet cell antibodies in children with mumps infection. *Lancet* 1980;9:211.

338. Banatvala JE, Schernthaner G, Schober E, *et al*: Coxsackie B, mumps, rubella and cytomegalovirus specific IgM response in patients with juvenile-onset diabetes mellitus in Britain, Austria and Australia. *Lancet* 1985;2:1409.

339. Milne LM: Difficulties in assessing the relationship, if any, between mumps vaccination and diabetes mellitus in childhood. *Vaccine* 2000; 19:1018.

340. Hiltunen M, Lonnrot M, Hyoty H: Immunisation and type 1 diabetes mellitus: is there a link? *Drug Saf* 1999;20:207.

341. Hyoty H, Hiltunen M, Reunanen A, *et al*: Decline of mumps antibodies in type I (insulin-dependent) diabetic children and a plateau in the rising incidence of type I diabetes after introduction of the mumps-measles-rubella vaccine in Finland. *Diabetologia* 1993;36:1303.

342. Lindberg B, Ahlfors K, Carlsson A, *et al*: Previous exposure to measles, mumps, and rubella—but not vaccination during adolescence—correlates to the prevalence of pancreatic and thyroid autoantibodies. *Pediatrics* 1999;104:12.

343. Juhela S, Hyoty H, Uibo R, *et al*: Comparison of enterovirus-specific cellular immunity in two populations of young children vaccinated with inactivated or live poliovirus vaccines. *Clin Exp Immunol* 1999; 117:100.

344. Juhela S, Hyoty H, Roivainen M, *et al*: T-cell responses to enterovirus antigens in children with type 1 diabetes. *Diabetes* 2000;49:1308.

345. Lonnrot M, Korpela K, Knip M, *et al*: Enterovirus infection as a risk factor for beta-cell autoimmunity in a prospectively observed birth cohort: the Finnish Diabetes Prediction and Prevention Study. *Diabetes* 2000;49:1314.

346. Serreze DV, Ottendorfer EW, Ellis TM, *et al*: Acceleration of type 1 diabetes by a coxsackievirus infection requires a preexisting critical mass of autoreactive T-cells in pancreatic islets. *Diabetes* 2000; 49:708.

347. Roivainen M, Knip M, Hyoty H, *et al*: Several different enterovirus serotypes can be associated with prediabetic autoimmune episodes and onset of overt IDDM. Childhood Diabetes in Finland (DiMe) Study Group. *J Med Virol* 1998;56:74.

348. Hyoty H, Hiltunen M, Lonnrot M: Enterovirus infections and insulin dependent diabetes mellitus—evidence for causality. *Clin Diagn Virol* 1998;9:77.

349. Lonnrot M, Knip M, Roivainen M, *et al*: Onset of type 1 diabetes mellitus in infancy after enterovirus infections. *Diabete Med* 1998; 15:431.

350. Szopa TM, Ward T, Taylor KW: Impaired metabolic functions in human pancreatic islets following infection with coxsackie B4 virus in vitro. *Diabetologia* 1986;30:587A.

351. Hou J, Sheikh S, Martin DL, *et al*: Coxsackie virus B4 alters pancreatic glutamate decarboxylase expression in mice soon after infection. *J Autoimmun* 1993;6:529.

352. Gerling I, Chatterjee NK, Nejman C: Coxsackie virus B4-induced development of antibodies to 64,000 Mr islet autoantigen and hyperglycemia in mice. *Autoimmunity* 1991;6:49.

353. Atkinson M, Bowman M, Darrow B, *et al*: Cellular immunity to an epitope common to glutamate decarboxylase (GAD) and coxsackie virus in insulin dependent diabetes (IDD). *Diabetes* 1994;43 (Suppl 1):93A.

354. Prabhakar BS, Haspel MV, McClintock PR, *et al*: High frequency of antigenic variants among naturally occurring human coxsackie B4 virus isolated identified by monoclonal antibodies. *Nature* 1982;300: 374.

355. Hudrisier D, Riond J, Burlet-Schiltz O, *et al*: Structural and functional identification of major histocompatibility complex class I-restricted self-peptides as naturally occurring molecular mimics of viral antigens: implication in CD8+ T cell-mediated, virus-induced autoimmune disease. *J Biol Chem* 2001;8:8.

356. Albert LJ, Inman RD: Molecular mimicry and autoimmunity. *N Engl J Med* 1999;341:2068.

357. Solimena M, Folli F, Aparisi R, *et al*: Autoantibodies to GABA-ergic neurons and pancreatic beta cells in stiff-man syndrome. *N Engl J Med* 1990;322:1555.

358. Tian J, Lehmann PV, Kaufman DL: T cell cross-reactivity between coxsackievirus and glutamate decarboxylase is associated with a murine diabetes susceptibility allele. *J Exp Med* 1994;180:1979.

359. Atkinson MA, Bowman MA, Campbell L, *et al*: Cellular immunity to a determinant common to glutamate decarboxylase and coxsackie virus in insulin-dependent diabetes. *J Clin Invest* 1994;94:2125.

360. Jones DB, Armstrong NW. Coxsackie virus and diabetes revisited. *Nat Med* 1995;1:284.

361. Juhela S, Hyoty H, Hinkkanen A, *et al*: T cell responses to enterovirus antigens and to beta-cell autoantigens in unaffected children positive for IDDM-associated autoantibodies. *J Autoimmun* 1999;12:269.

362. McIntosh EDG, Menser MA: A fifty-year follow-up of congenital rubella. *Lancet* 1992;340:414.

363. Rubinstein P, Walker ME, Fedun B, *et al*: The HLA system in congenital rubella patients with and without diabetes. *Diabetes* 1982; 31:1088.

364. Ginsberg-Fellner F, Fedun B, Cooper LZ: Interrelationships of congenital rubella and type I insulin-dependent diabetes mellitus. In: Ma J, ed. *The Immunology of Diabetes Mellitus*. Elsevier:1986;279.

365. Numazaki K, Goldman H, Seemayer TA, *et al*: Infection by human cytomegalovirus and rubella virus of cultured human fetal islets of Langerhans. *In Vivo* 1990;4:49.

366. Karounos DG, Wolinsky JS, Thomas JW: Monoclonal antibody to rubella virus capsid protein recognizes a B-cell antigen. *J Immunol* 1993;150:3080.

367. Ou D, Mitchell LA, Metzger DL, *et al*: Cross-reactive rubella virus and glutamic acid decarboxylase (65 and 67) protein determinants recognised by T cells of patients with type I diabetes mellitus. *Diabetologia* 2000;43:750.

368. Honeyman MC, Stone NL, Harrison LC: T-cell epitopes in type 1 diabetes autoantigen tyrosine phosphatase IA-2: potential for mimicry with rotavirus and other environmental agents. *Mol Med* 1998;4:231.

369. Honeyman MC, Coulson BS, Stone NL, *et al*: Association between rotavirus infection and pancreatic islet autoimmunity in children at risk of developing type 1 diabetes. *Diabetes* 2000;49:1319.

370. von Herrath MG, Oldstone MB: Virus-induced autoimmune disease. *Curr Opin Immunol* 1996;8:878.

371. von Herrath MG, Holz A, Homann D, *et al*: Role of viruses in type I diabetes. *Semin Immunol* 1998;10:87.

372. Brown DW, Welsh RM, Like AA: Infection of peripancreatic lymph nodes but not islets precedes Kilham's rat virus-induced diabetes in BB/Wor rats. *J Virol* 1993;67:5873.

373. von Herrath MG, Whitton JL: DNA vaccination to treat autoimmune diabetes. *Ann Med* 2000;32:285.

374. Palmer JP, Helqvist S, Spinas GA, *et al*: Interaction of B-cell activity and IL-1 concentration and exposure time in isolated rat islets of Langerhans. *Diabetes* 1989;38:1211.

375. Pipeleers D, Van de Winkel M: Pancreatic B cells possess defense mechanisms against cell-specific toxicity. *Proc Natl Acad Sci USA* 1986;83:5267.

The Pathophysiology and Genetics of Type 2 Diabetes Mellitus

Steven E. Kahn

Daniel Porte, Jr.

Both fasting hyperglycemia and excessive increases in glucose concentration following oral glucose loading are criteria for the diagnosis of type 2 diabetes mellitus (T2DM). In both the post-absorptive and fed states, three important defects have been demonstrated in subjects with T2DM: (1) impaired basal and stimulated insulin secretion, (2) an increased rate of endogenous hepatic glucose release, and (3) inefficient peripheral tissue glucose use. In this chapter we will review the closed feedback loop comprising the pancreatic islet, liver, and peripheral tissues, which together are responsible for the regulation of plasma glucose. Then we will describe the nature of the three major defects observed in T2DM and how they interact in the pathophysiology of hyperglycemia. We will use this same feedback loop to provide a perspective of how the different therapeutic interventions act to alter the steady-state glucose level. Finally, we will discuss studies of the genetic basis for hyperglycemic syndromes including type 2 diabetes, maturity-onset diabetes of the young (MODY), and other rare genetic forms of T2DM.

NORMAL PHYSIOLOGY OF GLUCOSE REGULATION

The maintenance of a stable fasting plasma glucose level is dependent on a closed feedback loop relationship between the circulating glucose level and the pancreatic islet hormones (Fig. 21-1). After an overnight fast, glucose is produced largely in the liver by glycogen breakdown and gluconeogenesis, and the rate of production is dependent on the availability of hepatic glycogen and gluconeogenic precursors. About 80% of this glucose released by the liver is metabolized independent of insulin by the brain and other insulin-insensitive tissues, such as the gut and red blood cells. Insulin-sensitive tissues, such as muscle and fat, use only small quantities. A number of neural and hormonal influences regulate hepatic glucose production, and in the presence of adequate amounts of insulin, the glucose level itself can regulate hepatic glucose release.[1,2] Short-term hormonal regulators of physiologic importance include insulin, glucagon, and the catecholamines; a more long-term influence on hepatic glucose production is provided by growth hormone, thyroid hormone, and glucocorticoids.

The liver is exquisitely sensitive to changes in insulin and glucagon levels, which, due to the fact that these hormones drain directly into the liver, are ideally suited to regulate moment-to-moment changes in hepatic glucose output. A reduction in insulin concentration removes the inhibitory effect of insulin on the liver and permits a slow rise in hepatic glucose production and the development of hyperglycemia.[3] On the other hand, a decrease in the glucagon level reduces glucose production by the liver and is associated with a concomitant fall in plasma glucose level.[4,5] Restoration of the original plasma glucose level will occur if the feedback loop is intact due to the effect of the glucose level to in turn regulate pancreatic insulin and glucagon secretion. In situations in which peripheral insulin sensitivity changes, this will also be reflected by a change in plasma glucose level. For example, if peripheral glucose use decreases, a rise in the fasting plasma glucose level will occur, to which the pancreatic islet will appropriately modify its secretion by reducing glucagon output by the α cell and increasing insulin secretion by the β cell. These secretory changes will reduce the rate of hepatic glucose output so that the glucose level will tend to be restored to near normal. In instances in which peripheral glucose use rises, the opposite will occur, so that hepatic glucose production will increase and glucose level will once again return toward normal. It is important to realize that complete islet adaptation cannot occur; otherwise no stimulus for the changes in insulin and glucagon secretion would be present. Thus, when tissue insulin sensitivity changes, a new steady-state glucose level results, at a value somewhere between that expected for the change in insulin action and that expected for the change in pancreatic hormone secretion, with the exact level depending on islet α- and β-cell responsiveness and sensitivity to glucose.

Following food ingestion, plasma glucose excursions are minimized by the islet. This is accomplished by a reduction in hepatic glucose production and an increase in peripheral glucose uptake. These changes in glucose metabolism arise as a result of alterations in insulin and glucagon secretion, which are regulated on a minute-to-minute basis by an interaction between glucose, amino acids, and the gut hormones. Glucose is the key regulator of the islet in this system since it not only regulates insulin and glucagon secretion directly, but it also modulates responses to the other substrates as well as gut hormones and neural factors released during nutrient ingestion (see Chap. 4).

From this description it is clear that when the feedback loop is functional, interpretation of any isolated aspect of this glucose homeostatic mechanism cannot be meaningfully performed without

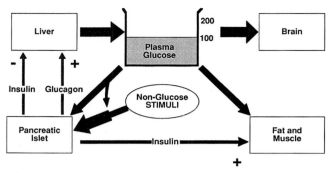

FIGURE 21-1. A model for the normal steady-state regulation of plasma glucose level. Plasma glucose has direct effects on the pancreas to modulate insulin and glucagon secretion as well as interacting with nonglucose stimuli to modify α- and β-cell responses to these stimuli. During hyperglycemia, insulin secretion is increased and glucagon secretion reduced. When hypoglycemia prevails, glucagon secretion is enhanced and insulin secretion is diminished. Glucagon stimulates hepatic glucose production. Insulin inhibits glucose release by the liver and stimulates glucose use in insulin-sensitive tissues. Glucose uptake by the brain is insulin independent, but in the periphery glucose uptake by fat and muscle is enhanced by insulin. Any change in hormone or substrate concentration or glucose use will be modulated by the loop in order that glucose use and production remain balanced. The plasma glucose level at which this occurs is determined by the efficiency with which the peripheral tissues take up glucose, the rate of hepatic glucose production, and islet α- and β-cell responsiveness to glucose. *(Adapted, with permission, from Porte.[92])*

taking into account all of the participating variables. Thus it is vitally important that comparisons of islet secretory function, hepatic glucose output, or peripheral tissue glucose uptake between different groups of individuals be performed at similar hormonal and substrate levels or that differences in these levels be taken into account. Failure to do so could lead to a gross misinterpretation of the status of these various components of the feedback loop.

PATHOPHYSIOLOGY OF ISLET DYSFUNCTION IN T2DM

Basal Insulin Secretion

Fasting plasma insulin levels in patients with T2DM, as compared with nondiabetic controls, have been reported as low, normal, and elevated.[6–10] However, as is evident from the closed feedback loop relationship just described, it is important that type 2 diabetic patients be adiposity (insulin resistance)-matched and have their insulin levels evaluated at matched plasma glucose concentrations. Such evaluations have been performed in two ways. Glucose has been infused into normal subjects to match their glucose levels with those of diabetic subjects, and diabetic individuals have had their glucose levels lowered to achieve normoglycemia by means of an insulin infusion followed by an insulin washout period. Under these conditions the resulting steady-state insulin levels in diabetic patients are lower than those of weight-matched and presumably insulin sensitivity–matched controls.[11,12] Use of such methods has unmasked a deficiency of basal insulin secretion in patients with T2DM.[13] It appears, therefore, that in T2DM there is a fundamental decrease in β-cell responsiveness to the prevailing plasma glucose level, but that the effect of the resultant hyperglycemia is to stimulate basal insulin output to the point where the

insulin levels will often appear normal or, if insulin resistance is present, may even be higher than those of normal lean subjects.

Insulin release is not simply a continuous process, but rather it has both pulsatile and oscillatory characteristics. Pulsatile insulin secretion has been demonstrated in healthy subjects, with distinct pulses occurring approximately every 10–15 minutes (Fig. 21-2A).[14] These pulses occur on a background of longer oscilla-

FIGURE 21-2. **A.** Two-hour plasma insulin profile in a healthy nondiabetic subject. From samples drawn every minute, it is apparent that insulin is released in regular pulses every 12–15 min. **B.** Twenty-four-hour insulin secretion profile in a healthy nondiabetic subject. Meals were eaten at 0900, 1300, and 1800 hours. The arrows indicate statistically significant pulses of secretion occurring approximately every 105–120 minutes during the waking hours (0900–2300 hours) and approximately every 180 minutes in the subsequent 10 hours during sleep. *(A. Reprinted with permission from O'Rahilly et al.[14] B. Reprinted with permission from Polonsky et al.[15])*

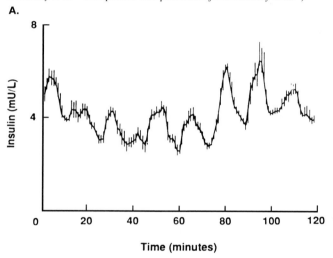

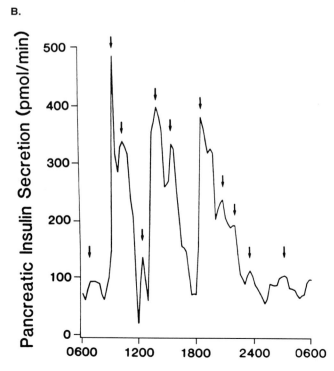

tions with cycles approximately every 120 minutes (Fig. 21-2B).[15] Examination of these patterns reveals both to be abnormal in subjects with T2DM and in individuals at high risk for developing the disease.[14,16–18] Although the exact cause of these abnormalities has not been determined, it would appear that the derangement in pulsatile secretion is likely to be intrinsic to the pancreatic β cell, since isolated islets have been found to have an intrinsic pacemaker that stimulates pulsatile insulin release *in vitro* with a periodicity similar to that observed *in vivo*.[19]

Comparisons of basal insulin secretion in type 2 diabetic subjects and normal individuals may be confounded by the fact that proinsulin cross-reacts in conventional insulin radioimmunoassays. Using a radioimmunoassay specific for insulin, it has been shown that proinsulin and proinsulin intermediates contribute an average of twice as much to basal insulin immunoreactivity (approximately 30%) in subjects with T2DM as in healthy subjects (approximately 15%).[20–24] Thus depending on the assay the true insulin levels in these patients may be actually lower than those measured as immunoreactive insulin.

Glucose-Stimulated Insulin Secretion

Although measurement of plasma glucose levels during the oral glucose tolerance test provides a method for the diagnosis of T2DM, the use of this test as a means of assessing β-cell function in patients with this disorder is somewhat problematic. This is because it is difficult to control factors such as gastric emptying time, gut hormone secretion rates, and the differences in glucose levels, which are important variables during the test. Thus, although some patients with T2DM will demonstrate an exaggerated insulin response late in the oral test,[6,7] this seems to be the result of an early deficient response leading to the markedly increased glucose levels that provide both a prolonged and exaggerated stimulus to the β cell.[25,26] However, the magnitude of the insulin response over the first 30 minutes following oral glucose administration is reduced in both T2DM and impaired glucose tolerance (Fig. 21-3A).[26] In fact, in subjects with reduced glucose tolerance, small changes in the magnitude of this response can have dramatic effects on glucose tolerance (Fig. 21-3B).[26]

Use of an intravenous glucose challenge avoids many of the complicating variables associated with oral glucose tolerance testing. Using this test, T2DM has been shown to be characterized by total absence of the acute or first-phase insulin response measured during the first 10 minutes following intravenous glucose administration (Fig. 21-4). Loss of this response can be documented at a fasting plasma glucose level above 115 mg/dL (6.4 mmol/L; Fig. 21-4).[27,28] Some individuals with the highest fasting plasma glucose levels have even been observed to have an absolute decrease below basal insulin levels following the administration of an intravenous glucose challenge.[29] The insulin response after the first 10 minutes is called the second phase. Like the fasting insulin level, it is a function of the prevailing fasting glucose level. Thus, in subjects whose fasting plasma glucose levels are less than 200 mg/dL (11.1 mmol/L), second-phase insulin responses may appear normal or even increased in some patients with obesity and insulin resistance (Fig. 21-5).[13] However, when comparisons are made to adiposity-matched normal subjects at equal plasma glucose levels, it is apparent that second-phase insulin secretion is also decreased in type 2 diabetic patients. Once plasma glucose levels rise above 200–250 mg/dL (11.1–13.9 mmol/L), glycosuria ensues, thus preventing a sufficient rise in glucose level to compensate for the

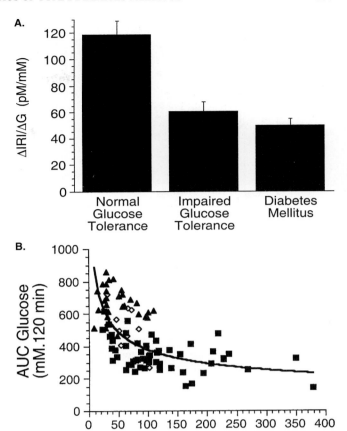

FIGURE 21-3. Ratio of the incremental responses of immunoreactive insulin (ΔIRI) and glucose (ΔG) over the first 30 minutes following oral glucose ingestion in 94 Japanese-American subjects with varying glucose tolerance. **A.** Of the 94 subjects, 56 had normal glucose tolerance, 10 impaired glucose tolerance, and 28 T2DM. Significant decreases in the ΔIRI/ΔG (*p* <0.0001) occurred with decreasing glucose tolerance. **B.** Relationship between the ratio of the incremental immunoreactive insulin and glucose responses (ΔIRI/ΔG) over the first 30 minutes following oral glucose ingestion and glucose tolerance, the latter determined as the incremental glucose area (AUC G) during the oral glucose tolerance test. Subjects with normal glucose tolerance (□), impaired glucose tolerance (□), and T2DM (▲) are indicated. The relationship between these variables is nonlinear with an r² value of 0.38 (*p* <0.0001). *(Reprinted with permission from Kahn et al.*[26]*)*

impaired insulin secretion. Therefore, patients with fasting plasma glucose levels above 250 mg/dL (13.9 mmol/L) are usually absolutely insulin deficient and their second-phase responses are characterized by absolute reductions in insulin release.[13] These individuals have been termed as having *decompensated type 2 diabetes*.

The regulation of insulin secretion by glucose can also be studied during an oscillating glucose infusion. When the periodicity of the glucose oscillations is varied, the β cell can be stimulated to oscillate in concert with these exogenous glucose cycles.[18] An inability to entrain is another marker of β-cell dysfunction present in subjects with T2DM. This lack of stimulation has also been demonstrated in subjects with impaired glucose tolerance, consistent with an early abnormality of β-cell function in these individuals (Fig. 21-6).[18]

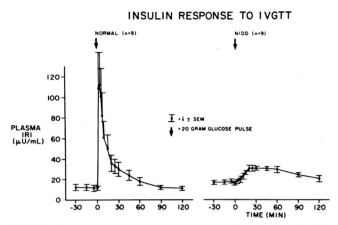

FIGURE 21-4. Relation between incremental acute (3- to 5-minute) insulin response and fasting glucose level in normal and type 2 diabetic subjects. *(Reprinted with permission from Bounzell et al.[13])*

Non-Glucose-Stimulated Insulin Secretion

Administration of one of a variety of nonglucose stimuli, such as the amino acid arginine,[13] the gastrointestinal hormones secretin[30] or glucagon-like peptide 1 (GLP-1),[31] the β-adrenergic agent isoproterenol,[30] or the sulfonlyurea tolbutamide,[32] is also followed by an acute insulin response.[20] In type 2 diabetic patients with a fasting plasma glucose level less than 200 mg/dL (11.1 mmol/L), the acute insulin response to any of these secretagogues is of normal magnitude when subjects are matched for body adiposity

(Fig. 21-7).[13,30,32] However, as is the case for basal and second-phase insulin secretion, the elevated plasma glucose level appears to be responsible for the maintenance of these apparently normal insulin responses to nonglucose stimuli. When plasma glucose levels are matched by either a glucose infusion in normal subjects or an insulin infusion in type 2 diabetic subjects, the acute insulin response to a nonglucose stimulus is also found to be reduced in diabetic subjects (Fig. 21-8).[11,33] This regulatory effect of glucose, termed *glucose potentiation*, can be expressed as the slope of the line relating the acute insulin response to a nonglucose secretagogue as a function of plasma glucose level between 100 and 250 mg/dL (5.6 and 13.9 mmol/L). Type 2 diabetic subjects with fasting hyperglycemia have been shown to have a much flatter slope of potentiation than normal individuals.[11]

At a glucose level above 450 mg/dL (25.0 mmol/L) both normal and diabetic subjects reach their maximal acute insulin responses, termed AIRmax (Fig. 21-8).[33] The observed reduction in maximal responsiveness in diabetic subjects denotes a decrease in insulin secretory capacity. The similarity of the glucose level giving a half-maximal response (PG_{50}) in both diabetic and healthy individuals indicates an equivalent β-cell sensitivity to glucose.[33] However, AIRmax has a curvilinear relationship to the fasting plasma glucose level (Fig. 21-9).[34] Thus there is already a reduction of 50–75% in secretory capacity by the time the diagnostic level of hyperglycemia is reached.

Basal and Stimulated Glucagon Secretion

Abnormalities of glucagon secretion have also been demonstrated in T2DM. The normal regulation of glucagon release is not en-

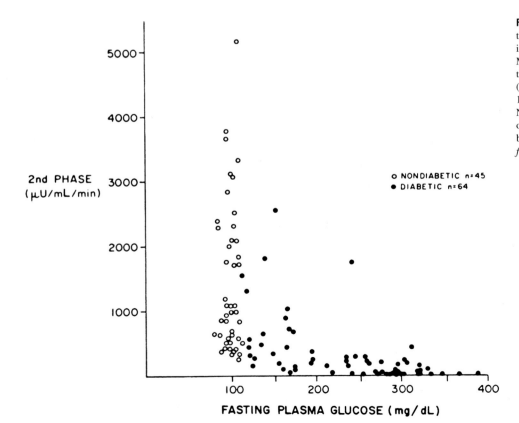

FIGURE 21-5. Insulin release in response to intravenous administration of glucose in normal and type 2 diabetic subjects. Mean fasting plasma glucose concentrations: normal subjects, 85 ± 3 mg/dL (4.7±0.2 mmol/L); diabetic subjects, 160±(10 mg/dL (5.9 ± 0.6 mmol/L). Note the relative preservation of the second-phase insulin response in type 2 diabetic subjects. *(Reprinted with permission from Pfeifer et al.[13])*

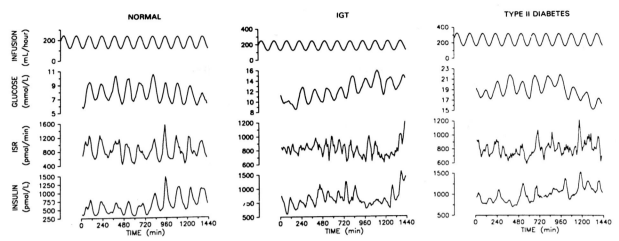

FIGURE 21-6. Entrainment of insulin secretion by glucose in subjects with normal glucose tolerance (**left panel**), impaired glucose tolerance (**middle panel**), and T2DM (**right panel**). Profiles of the glucose infusion rate, glucose and insulin concentrations, and the derived insulin secretory rates are illustrated for a typical subject from each group. Studies for each individual are shown during a slow oscillatory infusion with periods of 144 minutes. In the control subject, the increase in amplitude of the glucose oscillations is accompanied by an increase in insulin secretory rate oscillations, while in the subjects with impaired glucose tolerance and T2DM, the amplitude of the insulin secretory rate oscillations did not increase with the increase in amplitude of the glucose oscillations. (*Reprinted with permission from O'Meara et al.*[18])

tirely understood but appears to be dependent on inhibition of the α cell by glucose or insulin alone or by insulin and glucose together (see Chap. 7).[35] Bearing this in mind, type 2 diabetic patients with plasma glucose levels below 250 mg/dL (13.9 mmol/L) have been shown to have apparently normal basal plasma glucagon levels.[36] Though matching of plasma glucose levels does not pro-

vide evidence as to whether glucose or insulin regulation of the α cell is impaired, it has demonstrated that these normal glucagon levels are inappropriately elevated for the prevailing hyperglycemia.[33,36]

The glucagon response to an intravenous glucose challenge is also abnormal in type 2 diabetic patients. Although bolus admin-

FIGURE 21-7. Insulin responses to the nonglucose stimulant arginine in normal and type 2 diabetic subjects. Mean fasting plasma glucose concentrations: normal subjects, 85 ± 3 mg/dL (4.7 ± 0.2 mmol/L); diabetic subjects, 172 ± 9 mg/dL (9.6 ± 0.5 mmol/L). The insulin responses to arginine were not statistically different in the two groups. (*Reprinted with permission from Pfeifer et al.*[13])

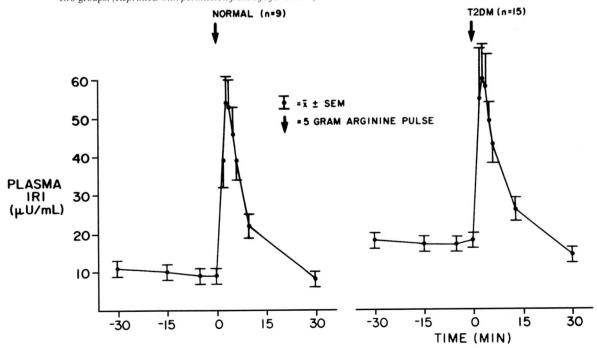

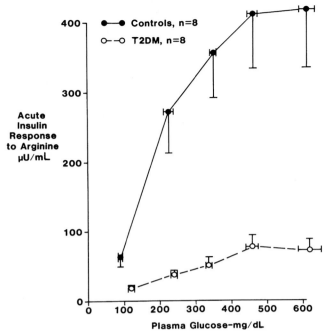

FIGURE 21-8. A comparison of acute insulin responses to 5 g IV arginine (mean 2- to 5-minute insulin increment) at five matched plasma glucose levels in eight patients with T2DM and in eight controls of similar age and body weight. The slope of potentiation is the linear portion of the relation between plasma glucose (100–250 mg/dL, 5.5–13.9 mmol/L) and the acute insulin response. It is much flatter in the diabetic group. The maximal insulin response, a measure of β-cell secretory capacity, is the response at a glucose concentration greater than 450 mg/dL (25 mmol/L). It is also much lower in the diabetic group. The half-maximal glucose level, a measure of glucose sensitivity of the β cell, is between 150 mg/dL (8.3 mmol/L) and 200 mg/dL (11.1 mmol/L) and is unchanged in the diabetic group. *(Reprinted with permission from Ward et al.[33])*

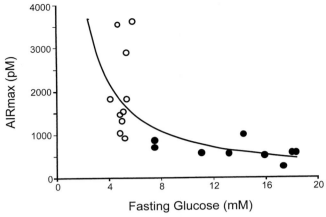

FIGURE 21-9. Curvilinear relationship between β-cell secretory capacity (AIRmax) and fasting plasma glucose in nine subjects with T2DM (●) and ten subjects with normal glucose tolerance (○). There is a broad range of β-cell secretory capacity in the healthy subjects due to large differences in insulin sensitivity while in the subjects with T2DM, the range is narrower as a manifestation of the impaired islet function. The nonlinear relationship between these two parameters ($r = -0.76$; $p < 0.0001$) demonstrates that the degree of β-cell function is a determinant of the fasting glucose level. This relation predicts that a relatively large initial loss of β-cell function should result in only a small increase of fasting plasma glucose level. However, further small declines in β-cell function would lead to much larger increases of glucose level. *(Adapted from Røder et al.[34])*

glucagon response in type 2 diabetic patients regardless of whether their fasting glucose levels are normal or elevated.[38]

Thus it appears that an abnormality in α-cell function is present in most patients with T2DM. At the present time, however, it is unclear whether this abnormality results from reduced insulin regulation of the α cell, diminished glucose sensing, or a combination.

FIGURE 21-10. A comparison of acute glucagon responses to arginine as a function of glucose level in eight normal subjects and in eight patients with T2DM. *(Reprinted with permission from Ward et al.[33])*

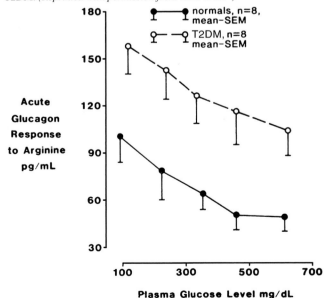

istration of intravenous glucose results in normal suppression of glucagon release, this suppression is a slow phenomenon. Although there may be less insulin present, glucose disposal rates are lower and therefore a higher glucose level prevails, causing only what appears to be a normal suppressive response. That this is indeed the case is demonstrated by the fact that during a glucose infusion, glucagon levels are elevated at a variety of matched glucose levels in type 2 diabetic subjects as compared to controls.[33] In addition, the magnitude of the acute glucagon response to amino acid stimulation is greater at all glucose levels in type 2 diabetic subjects (Fig. 21-10).[33] This is consistent with an abnormality in glucose and/or insulin regulation of α-cell secretory function.

Assessment of α-cell secretory function by oral glucose tolerance testing is, as in β-cell evaluation, confounded by the inability to control the plasma glucose level, the rate of gastric emptying, and gut peptide secretion. Despite these caveats, when oral testing is performed, defects in α-cell function are often more apparent than β-cell defects. Following carbohydrate ingestion, a gross abnormality in glucagon secretion is apparent in type 2 diabetic subjects, who may even demonstrate a paradoxical increase rather than the usual suppression observed with hyperglycemia.[37] Furthermore, ingestion of a pure protein meal produces an exaggerated

Nature of the Islet Lesion in T2DM

Although it is clear that islet dysfunction is present in T2DM, it is still not certain whether the defects in insulin secretion are the result of a reduction of β-cell mass, dysfunction of a normal number of β cells, or some combination. In addition, as the normal physiologic regulation of glucagon secretion is incompletely understood, the contribution of the β-cell defect to α-cell dysfunction is also not entirely clear.

Examination of β-cell mass, islet size, and islet characteristics in postmortem studies of type 2 diabetics have been performed by a number of investigators. Direct quantification of β-cell mass is difficult due to postmortem changes, but most studies have demonstrated that the islets in affected individuals are smaller and that β-cell mass is decreased by 40–60% compared to appropriately matched nondiabetic subjects.[39] Although islet size is reduced, it appears that this loss of volume is due purely to the change in β-cell mass since no significant reduction in α, δ, and PP cells has been documented in T2DM. Although the precise etiology of this β-cell mass reduction is unknown, changes in islet morphology, including islet fibrosis and amyloid deposition, have been demonstrated,[39] the latter evidently due to deposition of a second β-cell–specific peptide called islet amyloid polypeptide (IAPP) or amylin.[40,41] IAPP may be a significant factor in the pathogenesis of the β-cell loss of T2DM in that the amyloid deposits appear to replace the β cells specifically (see Chap. 17). Although the human peptide has a predilection to form amyloid at high concentrations *in vitro*,[42] the mechanism underlying its propensity to deposit in the islets of individuals with T2DM is not understood. The peptide is normally cosecreted with insulin,[43] but it does not appear that simple overproduction under conditions of increased β-cell secretory demand can explain amyloid formation, as obese individuals without diabetes are no more likely to have amyloid than lean subjects. Furthermore, studies in transgenic mice overproducing human IAPP failed to demonstrate amyloid[44] until they were treated with a high-fat diet[45] or were made markedly insulin resistant by crossbreeding them with lines of genetically modified insulin-resistant mice.[46,47] Perhaps the demonstration in neonatal rat islet cultures[48] and isolated human islets[49] of a dissociation of insulin and IAPP secretion due to the isolated release of IAPP through the constitutive secretory pathway,[48] the finding of amyloid fibrils in transgenic islets expressing human IAPP exposed to severe hyperglycemia *in vitro*,[50] the toxic effect of amyloid fibrils,[42,51] and the presence of other components such as the heparan sulfate proteoglycan perlecan[52,53] may be important clues to the mechanism(s) underlying islet amyloid formation.

Although it is difficult to evaluate the effect of a 50% reduction of β-cell mass in humans; an animal study suggests that this amount of cell loss alone is insufficient to result in fasting hyperglycemia and the insulin secretion abnormalities observed in T2DM.[54] Therefore, it appears that the development of fasting hyperglycemia and defective secretory responses requires either a greater loss of β-cell mass or a 50% reduction in mass along with dysfunction of the remaining cells or insulin resistance.

In an attempt to clarify whether larger degrees of β-cell loss can reproduce the features of T2DM, animal models have been created by either pancreatectomy or neonatal administration of streptozocin. Removal of two-thirds of a canine pancreas does not result in fasting hyperglycemia, nor is the classic loss of first-phase insulin release observed.[54] Although the insulin response to non-

glucose secretagogues is present, at matched glucose levels the magnitude of this response is reduced, as is the slope of glucose potentiation, indicating that this measure is a sensitive indicator of β-cell mass reduction. In rodents, a 60% pancreatectomy had similar effects, with an unchanged fasting glucose level and a reduced glucose potentiation slope.[55] Only when islet mass was reduced by 90% were hyperglycemia and insulin secretory responses similar to those observed in T2DM seen.[56,57] However, α-cell function could not be tested due to the marked reduction in glucagon secretion, implying that this model does not precisely replicate the islet lesion of T2DM. With neonatal streptozocin administration, abnormal glucose-regulated α-cell secretion has been demonstrated, but the glucagon response to arginine is unlike that of T2DM in that the magnitude of the response is reduced, rather than increased, when compared to controls.[58] This same model of β-cell mass loss is associated with a loss of first-phase insulin secretion, but the response to arginine administration does not simulate that observed in type 2 diabetes,[59] in that it is increased at low glucose concentrations and reduced at high glucose levels. Thus, neither surgical reduction of β- and α-cell mass nor cytotoxic β-cell destruction can produce an exact model of the insulin- and glucagon secretory abnormalities found in human T2DM.

Models of islet dysfunction have been created in normal human subjects by the prolonged administration of cyclic somatostatin or an analogue of this peptide. When normal human subjects received a cyclic somatostatin infusion together with glucagon replacement for 2 days, the observed metabolic derangements were fairly similar to those in type 2 diabetic subjects: fasting hyperglycemia with near-normal basal insulin levels, markedly diminished first- and second-phase insulin responses to glucose, a preserved insulin response to a nonglucose secretagogue, and increased glucose turnover.[3,59] Healthy individuals who were treated for 8 days with a somatostatin analogue without glucagon replacement also developed fasting hyperglycemia, markedly impaired first- and second-phase responses to glucose, and a preserved insulin response to arginine.[60] However, this latter study demonstrated that although the β-cell dysfunction produced by somatostatin closely mimics many of the features of T2DM, the mechanism by which it does this is different. β-Cell secretory capacity (AIRmax) remains unchanged while the sensitivity to glucose (PG_{50}) is impaired—the reverse of T2DM. Whether some combination of the type of islet dysfunction produced by somatostatin together with a reduction in islet mass can duplicate the α- and β-cell defects of T2DM is as yet unknown.

The theory that overactivity of the α-adrenergic component of pancreatic sympathetic innervation could also contribute to the pathogenesis of T2DM has been suggested by the finding that phentolamine, which blocks the α-adrenergic system, can partially restore the acute insulin response to glucose and the ability of glucose to potentiate insulin secretion in these patients.[61,62] However, similarly to somatostatin, elevated catecholamines do not change β-cell secretory capacity (AIRmax) but impair β-cell sensitivity to glucose (PG_{50}).[63] Furthermore, the mildly elevated catecholamine levels documented in some diabetic subjects offer additional support for enhanced activity of the α-adrenergic nervous system under some conditions (see Chap. 8).[61] Two other inhibitory peptides, galanin and pancreastatin, have been isolated in pancreatic tissue.[64,65] Galanin has been demonstrated in pancreatic sympathetic nerves in dogs.[64] Intravenous administration of these peptides increases glucose levels, inhibits insulin secretion, and stimulates glucagon release.[64,65] Because these peptides can simulate the islet secretory changes that characterize T2DM, it was proposed that increased intrapancreatic concentrations or islet sensitivity to either of these peptides may be present in T2DM. However, evidence suggests that galanin is not effective in primates or humans.[66] Thus, some other peptide would need to be involved for this mechanism to be operative. IAPP has been suggested as an alternate peptide with this function, and some studies suggest that IAPP impairs insulin release.[67] This impairment has not been a universal finding, and at present it appears unlikely that physiologic levels of IAPP modulate β-cell function.[67] Enhanced endogenous prostaglandin effects may also contribute to diminished β-cell function, as suggested by the increase in first- and second-phase insulin responses to intravenous glucose and the increase in glucose potentiation slope observed in type 2 diabetic subjects who received an intravenous infusion of the prostaglandin synthesis inhibitor sodium salicylate.[68,69]

A number of studies have demonstrated that hyperglycemia not only may induce structural damage to the islet, but also can reproduce some of the secretory findings of T2DM. Following partial pancreatectomy in rats, the islet remnant often regenerates with new islet tissue also developing from pancreatic ductal tissue.[70] However, the new tissue comprises not only normal-appearing islets but also islets that are disorganized and fibrotic.[56] These changes in islet structure appear to be the result of hyperglycemia, because the development of these histologic abnormalities can be prevented by insulin treatment.[71] Mild chronic hyperglycemia produced by a continuous glucose infusion is capable of altering islet function, resulting in a loss of glucose-stimulated insulin release, and when hyperglycemia becomes more severe, a loss of the potentiating effect of glucose.[72] The combination of a 60% pancreatectomy and 6 weeks of mild chronic hyperglycemia produces not only a loss of glucose potentiation as is seen after β-cell mass reduction alone, but also an impairment of glucose-stimulated insulin secretion.[55] Although these studies addressed the effects of mild prolonged increases in plasma glucose concentrations, more recent animal studies have demonstrated that marked hyperglycemia produced by intravenous glucose administration to healthy animals results in changes in β-cell function as early as 14 hours after commencing the infusion.[73] In addition, animals given phlorizin, an agent capable of lowering the glucose level by inhibiting renal tubular cell reabsorption of glucose, demonstrate a decline in plasma glucose levels and a restoration of β-cell function toward normal.[57] These studies add credence to the idea that hyperglycemia is a cellular toxin or leads to suppression of islet function and may therefore contribute to the pancreatic defect observed in T2DM.

Recently, work has focused on the potential adverse effects of dietary fat and free fatty acids on islet function. Consumption of a high-fat diet is associated with an increased risk of developing diabetes that is related in part to the obesity and associated insulin resistance that develops with the increased caloric intake, but may also be the result of alterations in β-cell function that occur.[74,75] It is unclear what period of time is required for these changes to occur but it is clear that altering the balance of the diet to more carbohydrate results in an improvement in glucose tolerance within a period as short as 3 days.[76–78] Free fatty acids have also been shown to have a negative impact on islet function because prolonged incubation of islets with free fatty acids *in vitro* results in a reduction in insulin secretion, with changes in proinsulin mRNA levels and insulin biosynthesis also having been demonstrated.[79–81]

Furthermore, in the presence of both glucose and free fatty acids, neutral lipid accumulation occurs within islets,[82] with increased quantities of this morphologic change being observed with aging.[83] Whether this change is even greater in type 2 diabetes and whether it impacts islet function or is simply a marker of such are presently unknown.

As mentioned, other evidence for β-cell dysfunction in T2DM is a change in the proportion of circulating proinsulin, the circulating insulin precursor. Under basal conditions, about 15% of insulin-like immunoreactivity measured by conventional insulin radioimmunoassays is comprised of proinsulin and its conversion intermediates des 31,32 and des 64,65 proinsulin.[84] This proportion is doubled in subjects with T2DM,[21–23,84] with the vast majority of circulating proinsulin-like molecules being intact proinsulin and the conversion intermediate des 31,32 proinsulin.[24] This increase in type 2 diabetic subjects appears to represent a fundamental change in the production of insulin from its precursor proinsulin. Although no single study has been able to identify the mechanism(s), a number of studies suggest that defective processing of proinsulin to insulin may be the underlying basis for the observed differences. Administration of glucocorticoids and growth hormone to humans,[84,85] as well as the induction of a subclinical defect in β-cell function in nonhuman primates with streptozocin,[86] has resulted in disproportionate proinsulinemia. Although it is possible that the ability of the β cell to normally process proinsulin may be limited and that an increase in secretory demand may result in the release of a granular pool that has not had sufficient time to cleave proinsulin to insulin, data from studies in healthy insulin-resistant humans would not support this concept. Thus, neither obesity[22,23,87] nor insulin resistance induced experimentally with nicotinic acid[88] induces disproportionate proinsulinemia. Furthermore, women with a history of gestational diabetes have been demonstrated to have disproportionate proinsulinemia following pregnancy even though their glucose tolerance has returned to normal.[89] Japanese-American men with normal or impaired glucose tolerance who developed T2DM after 5 years of observation have disproportionately increased proinsulin levels at baseline when compared to subjects who do not progress to T2DM,[90] suggesting that this defect is present early in the course of the development of T2DM. A similar observation has been made in older Finnish subjects.[91]

From the foregoing discussion it is apparent that although many different perturbations can reproduce some features of the β-cell secretory abnormalities observed in T2DM, no single experimental approach has been able to fully replicate the findings of this disorder. This suggests the possibility that the abnormalities of islet function characteristic of T2DM are the result of a combination of a variety of lesions and supports the concept that considerable heterogeneity is probably involved in the pathogenesis of the β-cell defects of this disorder.[92]

PATHOPHYSIOLOGY OF INSULIN RESISTANCE AND GLUCOSE RESISTANCE IN T2DM

Tissue resistance to insulin is an important component of the glucose intolerance of T2DM (see Chap. 22). Rare syndromes of extreme insulin resistance associated with diabetes mellitus and acanthosis nigricans have been described in which genetic defects in insulin receptor function are present,[93] as has a syndrome of extreme insulin resistance with diabetes as a result of a dominant negative mutation in the peroxisome proliferator activated receptor gamma (PPAR-γ).[94] The etiology of defects in insulin action observed in the liver and peripheral tissues of the more common forms of type 2 diabetes is much less clear. However, it does appear that a major component of this abnormality may be related to obesity, with central fat distribution, and particularly intra-abdominal fat, being important.[95–97] The recent elucidation of the importance of glucose-mediated glucose disposal to glucose tolerance requires that its role in the pathophysiology of T2DM also be considered.

Hepatic Insulin Resistance

Basal rates of hepatic glucose production in patients with T2DM have been documented as normal or increased.[98–100] As with measurements of insulin secretion, it is important that these production rates be evaluated in the context of the glucose concentration at which they were measured. When this is done, it is apparent that even the "normal" values are inappropriately elevated for the ambient glucose level. In many studies, the degree of the abnormality in hepatic glucose output is positively correlated with the degree of fasting hyperglycemia, suggesting that the rate of hepatic glucose production is an important determinant of the fasting plasma glucose level (Fig. 21-11).

The increased rate of hepatic glucose production results from an impairment of the effects of insulin and glucose to normally suppress glucose release by the hepatocyte. A shift to the right in the insulin dose–response curve with no reduction in the maximal suppressive response at supraphysiologic insulin levels has been demonstrated in diabetic subjects studied at euglycemia.[101] This type of change is compatible with a reduction in hepatic sensitivity to insulin produced by a decrease in insulin receptor number. However, when similar studies are performed in type 2 diabetic subjects at basal hyperglycemia, maximal suppression of hepatic glucose

production occurs at lower insulin levels, but the dose–response relation still demonstrates a defect in insulin action when compared to control subjects studied at normoglycemia.[100] Thus hyperglycemia appears capable of exerting a suppressive effect on hepatic glucose output independent of insulin, but is unable to fully compensate for the reduction in insulin sensitivity found in T2DM. This suggests that a defect in the ability of glucose to inhibit its own release from the liver is also contributing to the observed glucose overproduction in the basal state. Glucagon, of major importance in the maintenance of postabsorptive hepatic glucose release,[4,5] appears to be capable of maintaining more than half of the hepatic glucose production observed in T2DM.[102] As a result, the abnormal regulation of glucagon secretion in these subjects may help explain the observed hepatic resistance of type 2 diabetics to the suppressive effects of both insulin and glucose.

During oral intake the liver plays a critical role in the maintenance of glucose homeostasis. The meal-induced alterations in the concentrations of glucose, insulin, and glucagon entering the liver through the portal circulation contribute to the liver changing from its status in the fasted condition as an organ responsible solely for glucose production to one that, during refeeding, restores its glycogen content by increasing its uptake and/or synthesis of glucose. Therefore, considering the defects in hepatic sensitivity to glucose and insulin, it is not surprising that following an oral glucose load a delayed reduction in hepatic glucose production can be demonstrated in T2DM.[8,103] This failure of the liver to adequately suppress its glucose production accounts for a considerable proportion of the observed rise in plasma glucose concentrations following meal ingestion. Although a large proportion of this defect in suppression of hepatic glucose release may result from the deficient insulin response, neither the contribution of the increased glucagon response during meals nor the potential for variability in hepatic sensitivity to other neurohormonal responses following oral intake has yet been defined.

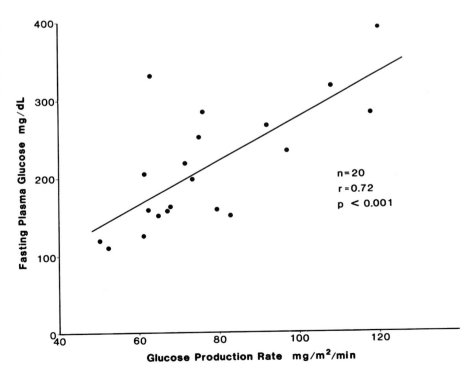

FIGURE 21-11. Correlation between fasting plasma glucose levels and glucose production rate in 20 patients with untreated T2DM. Despite the suppressive effect of hyperglycemia on glucose production, those patients with the highest glucose levels had the highest production rates. *(Reprinted with permission from Best et al.[98])*

Peripheral Insulin Resistance

Using the euglycemic insulin clamp technique, it has been conclusively demonstrated that a reduction of more than 55% in the mean glucose disposal rate exists in subjects with T2DM.[101] Further analysis of the *in vivo* dose–response relation suggests that this reduction in insulin responsiveness is the result of two abnormalities (Fig. 21-12A). First, the rightward shift in the curve is compatible with a reduction in cellular insulin receptor number. A decrease in receptor number has been reported in *in vitro* studies using monocytes,[104] erythrocytes,[105] and adipocytes.[101] Despite the presence of spare or unoccupied receptors, the marked decrease in the maximal rate of glucose disposal suggests the existence of a second defect in peripheral insulin action, namely, a postbinding (intracellular) defect.[101] Insulin-binding studies on isolated adipocytes from individuals with T2DM have shown that the predominant determinant of the severity of the peripheral insulin resistance in untreated patients is this reduction in postbinding insulin action.[101] Initial analysis suggested that part of this defect in intracellular insulin action resulted from a reduction in the number of glucose transporters.[106] However, it appears that the total amount of GLUT-4 mRNA and protein is normal although the function or the intracellular movement to the cell membrane of this insulin-dependent glucose transporter may be diminished (see Chap. 22).[107] Assessments of a number of the key molecules involved in intracellular transmission of the insulin signal following insulin binding to its receptor (e.g., insulin receptor substrate-1 [IRS-1] and phosphoinositol 3

kinase [PI3 kinase]) have demonstrated defects in the action of some of these molecules, but these changes are not distinct from those observed in obesity.[108,109]

These preceding observations of reduced insulin effectiveness were all made under euglycemic conditions and thus do not take into account the ability of glucose, by virtue of mass action, to augment its own disposal into the peripheral tissues.[110,111] When incremental insulin dose–response studies are performed at the basal level of hyperglycemia in type 2 diabetic subjects, the relation of insulin's effect on peripheral glucose disposal is essentially identical to that observed in matched control subjects studied at euglycemia (Fig. 21-12B).[100] These findings suggest that in the presence of hyperglycemia, any impairment of peripheral insulin action is overcome by a mass action increase of glucose uptake. Therefore, as glucose levels rise due to the increase in hepatic glucose production, peripheral glucose uptake increases by mass action so that a new steady state is created in which the increased glucose levels are associated with increased glucose use despite the impairment of insulin action.

The efficiency of glucose uptake following oral glucose ingestion is also defective in type 2 diabetic subjects. In the peripheral tissues, ingested glucose normally undergoes oxidative and nonoxidative metabolism, with the rate of these processes being controlled by the enzymes pyruvate dehydrogenase and glycogen synthase, respectively. At low insulin concentrations the major route of peripheral glucose disposal is via glucose oxidation, while at higher levels disposal occurs predominantly by glycogen synthesis.[112] In

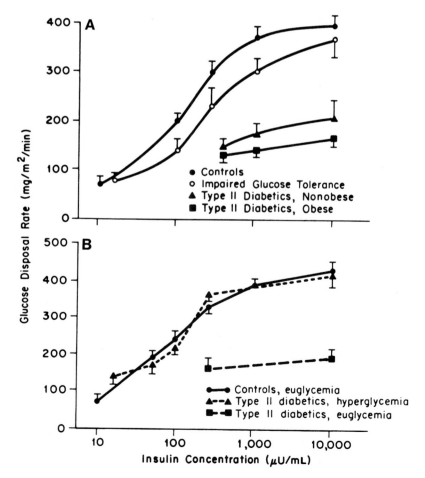

FIGURE 21-12. A. Mean dose–response curves for insulin-stimulated peripheral glucose disposal in control subjects (●), subjects with impaired glucose tolerance (○), and nonobese (▲) and obese (■) type 2 diabetic subjects. Note the large reduction in maximum glucose disposal in the diabetic subjects. **B.** The effect of hyperglycemia on the dose–response relation for insulin-stimulated peripheral glucose disposal: normal subjects at euglycemia (●), type 2 diabetic subjects at hyperglycemia (▲), and type 2 diabetic subjects at euglycemia (■). Note the similarity of glucose uptake at spontaneous levels of glycemia. *(A. Reprinted with permission from Kolterman et al.[101] B. Reprinted with permission from Revers et al.[100])*

T2DM, the efficiency of glucose uptake by both processes is reduced, with the predominant abnormality being a defect in nonoxidative glucose storage.[113] As glycogen synthase activity is stimulated by insulin, the diminished insulin sensitivity compounded by the reduced insulin secretory response to meals leads to a failure to stimulate normal enzyme activity.[114]

Glucose Resistance

Besides insulin resistance and islet dysfunction as causes of decreased glucose tolerance, insulin-independent glucose uptake or glucose-mediated glucose uptake is an important factor determining glucose use. In fact, about 80% of tissue glucose uptake in the fasting state occurs by insulin-independent mechanisms, primarily into the brain, but glucose uptake also takes place in muscle, fat, and other tissues.[115] During intravenous glucose tolerance testing, glucose-mediated glucose uptake, also known as glucose effectiveness, is important in determining the rate of glucose disappearance.[116]

Glucose-mediated glucose uptake has been quantified using a number of methods,[115,116] and has been shown to be regulated in normal subjects[31,60] and abnormal in patients with type 2 diabetes.[117] As suggested in the foregoing discussions of hepatic and peripheral insulin resistance, glucose-mediated glucose disposal is important in decreasing glucose production by the liver and increasing glucose uptake in muscle. Thus it could be envisaged that in type 2 diabetes, glucose resistance would result in a reduced ability of the liver to suppress glucose production and/or a decrease in the effectiveness of peripheral tissues to take up glucose by mass action, thereby contributing to hyperglycemia.

The cellular processes underlying alterations in glucose effectiveness have not been fully elucidated. This function could be dependent on glucose transporter number and/or activity as well as processes involving glucose metabolism after its entry into the cell. These posttransport processes could include regulation of enzymes responsible for glucose use, as well as others that may regulate glucose transporter function such as the enzyme glucosamine fructose amino transferase (GFAT), which metabolizes glucose through a shunt from the glycolytic breakdown process.[118] Although glucose effectiveness is independent of a sudden change in insulin level, this process can apparently be regulated by changes in circulating insulin over time. Up until now, all conditions in which glucose effectiveness has been shown to be reduced have been associated with impaired islet function and therefore associated with reduced circulating basal and stimulated insulin levels.[60,117,119] This finding suggests that improvements in insulin secretion should be associated with an increase in glucose effectiveness, a hypothesis that has yet to be tested. Based on the demonstration that a short infusion of GLP-1 results in an enhancement of glucose effectiveness without a change in basal plasma insulin concentrations,[31] it would appear that other hormones may also be important in regulating this function.

Role of Obesity, Counterregulatory Hormone Secretion, and Insulin Deficiency

It has long been recognized that obesity is associated with insulin resistance. In the absence of carbohydrate intolerance, dramatic compensatory hyperinsulinemia is present.[120,121] Though this adaptive response effectively maintains normoglycemia in more than 85% of obese individuals, these elevated plasma insulin levels may contribute to the alterations in insulin action that are a feature of obesity. With mild degrees of obesity, the predominant change is a reduction in tissue insulin binding.[122] As body weight and fat cell size increase further, a proportional increase in basal insulin secretion occurs.[123] These changes are associated with the development of a postreceptor defect, the severity of which is related to the change in body weight and plasma insulin concentration.[124] Because central adiposity rather than lower body adiposity is the major determinant of the insulin resistance of obesity,[123,125] and intra-abdominal fat appears to be an important determinant of insulin sensitivity,[95–97] there are also great difficulties in estimating the role of obesity in the insulin resistance of any particular type 2 diabetic person (see Chap. 23). The differences in estimations of adiposity and the corrections applied by some investigators for age differences probably contribute to the controversy in the literature regarding obesity and its role in the insulin resistance of T2DM. Nevertheless, because more than 80% of type 2 diabetic subjects are obese, their elevated basal insulin levels are a manifestation of their diminished insulin sensitivity, which is at least partly the result of their obesity.

Secretion of counterregulatory hormones has been shown to be altered in some patients with T2DM. Increased diurnal fluctuations of plasma growth hormone concentration[126] and enhanced responses to exercise[127] have been reported. Basal growth hormone levels, on the other hand, are usually normal except in those patients who are severely hyperglycemic.[128] Marked hyperglycemia by inducing glycosuria and resultant volume depletion leads to baroreceptor stimulation and increased sympathetic nervous system activation, which would explain the increased levels of catecholamines observed in type 2 diabetic subjects.[61] This effect is more marked as hyperglycemia becomes more severe due to greater urinary glucose losses. Thus, hyperglycemia acts as a stimulus for a neuroendocrine stress response, which leads to counterregulatory hormone secretion. This excessive catecholamine release in turn impairs islet function, and reduces both insulin-mediated and glucose-mediated glucose disposal,[129–131] thus producing more hyperglycemia (see Chap. 8). Although treatment to lower plasma glucose can return these levels toward or even to normal, more subtle abnormalities of many of these counterregulatory hormones have been reported in subjects with relatively mild hyperglycemia in whom a neuroendocrine stress response as a result of baroreceptor stimulation seems unlikely.[132] Since counterregulatory hormones are all capable of producing insulin resistance, it appears that even the mild increase in plasma concentrations of such hormones observed in type 2 diabetes patients could contribute to their insulin resistance. With severe hyperglycemia it is likely that the more pronounced neuroendocrine abnormalities contribute to the greater degrees of insulin and glucose resistance observed with poorer glycemic control.

A variety of studies suggest that insulin deficiency, or the metabolic derangements arising from it, is involved in the development of insulin and glucose resistance. Animal studies in which insulin deficiency has been created using agents toxic to the β cell, such as streptozocin, have demonstrated the existence of an abnormality in insulin action. This defect is apparent in *in vitro* studies using adipocytes[133] and in the intact animal in the presence of high concentrations of plasma insulin and only trivial elevations in the glucose level.[134] Although it could be argued that this effect is a result of a direct action of the agent on insulin-sensitive tissues, a similar degree of insulin resistance has been observed in animals following a 90% pancreatectomy.[135] Demonstration of this relation in type 2 diabetic individuals is more difficult in view of the complicating effects of obesity and residual insulin secretion. However, indirect support for this concept can be obtained from other human studies. First, type 1 diabetic subjects who are totally insulin deficient are insulin resistant.[136] Second, both type 1 and type 2 diabetic subjects increase their rates of glucose disposal with an amelioration of the postreceptor defect in insulin action when treated with insulin.[137–139] Third, states of glucose resistance have been associated with an absolute or relative reduction of β-cell function. For example, type 1 diabetic subjects who have absent insulin responses have reduced glucose effectiveness.[140] In addition, impaired insulin responses produced by somatostatin or epinephrine administration are associated with reduced glucose effectiveness in humans and animals,[60,141] and β-cell mass reduction with streptozocin in dogs has also been associated with reduced efficiency of glucose-mediated glucose disposal.[119] Thus, even though integrated 24-hour plasma insulin levels may be within the normal range in type 2 diabetics, for their degree of hyperglycemia they are relatively insulin deficient and it is this relative hypoinsulinemia that may at least in part be responsible for the observed changes in the efficiency of tissue glucose uptake. From the foregoing discussion it is apparent that the simultaneous presence and interaction of obesity, excessive counterregulatory hormone effects, and the metabolic events related to hypoinsulinemia contribute significantly to the diminished insulin and glucose sensitivity of T2DM. The inability to control for all these factors makes it difficult to discern whether a primary alteration in insulin or glucose action exists in this disease. However, by virtue of its relation with islet function, it is clear that insulin and glucose resistance are of major importance in determining the degree of the metabolic derangement present in T2DM.

THE INTERACTION BETWEEN INSULIN RESISTANCE AND INSULIN SECRETION IN T2DM

The feedback loop comprising the liver, pancreas, and peripheral tissues requires that islet function be an important determinant of the basal glucose level. If islet responsiveness to glucose is high,

then changes in insulin action will not perturb the plasma glucose level very much. Thus in the presence of normal islet function, isolated insulin resistance does not usually result in the development of fasting hyperglycemia. A common condition that exemplifies this is obesity in which the majority of subjects are insulin resistant, but do not have impaired glucose tolerance or diabetes. This lack of change in fasting glycemia is because there is a reciprocal and proportionate increase in insulin secretion, representing an adaptive phenomenon by the normal β cell to insulin resistance (Figs. 21-13 and 21-14A).[142] From percentile charts based on data from healthy subjects, it is possible to determine the adequacy of insulin secretion for the degree of insulin sensitivity (Fig. 21-14B–D). Where the relationship places an individual in a low percentile, this would be predicted to be associated with reduced glucose tolerance.

Further support for the capability of normal islets to adapt their responsiveness is the finding that normal-weight individuals made insulin resistant with nicotinic acid for a period of 2 weeks demonstrate an increase in basal as well as glucose- and non-glucose-stimulated insulin secretion,[88] and that a decrease in these same measures of β-cell function in individuals who have had an improvement in insulin sensitivity following a 6-month endurance exercise training program.[143] The enhanced insulin secretion observed under conditions of natural and experimental insulin resistance results from an increase in β-cell secretory capacity without any change in β-cell sensitivity to glucose, while the decreased insulin release that occurs with the exercise-induced improvement in insulin sensitivity results from a decrease in β-cell secretory capacity and no change in β-cell sensitivity to glucose. Furthermore, with experimental insulin resistance basal and stimulated glucagon levels are reduced, providing evidence for α-cell adaptation to prolonged insulin resistance in normal subjects. Although the exact mediator responsible for this alteration in α- and β-cell function has not been identified, evidence in normal subjects suggests that glucose may be responsible for this change. When healthy individuals are given glucose infusions for 2–3 hours, they demonstrate enhanced insulin-secretory responses to a later intravenous glucose challenge despite the fact that glucose levels under both the basal and postinfusion conditions are similar at the time of the test.[144]

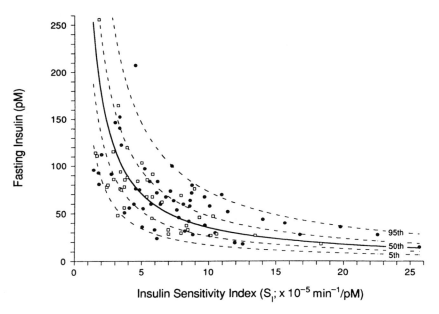

FIGURE 21-13. Relationship between insulin sensitivity and fasting insulin in 93 healthy subjects (55 males [●] and 38 females [□]). The best fit of the relationship is described by a hyperbolic function (i.e., insulin sensitivity times fasting insulin is a constant). The 5th, 25th, 50th, 75th, and 95th percentiles for the relationship are illustrated. *(Reprinted with permission from Kahn et al.[142])*

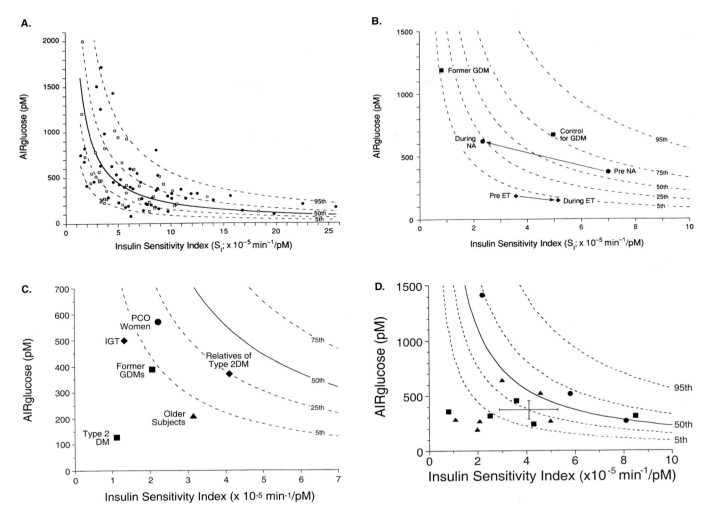

FIGURE 21-14. **A**. Relationship between insulin sensitivity and the first-phase insulin response (AIRglucose) in 93 healthy subjects (55 males [●] and 38 females [□]). The best fit of the relationship is described by a hyperbolic function (i.e., insulin sensitivity times first-phase insulin response is a constant). The 5th, 25th, 50th, 75th, and 95th percentiles for the relationship are illustrated. **B**. Percentile lines for the relationship between insulin sensitivity and the first-phase insulin response (AIRglucose). Data from three studies[69,145,146] are plotted. Individual data for a former gestational diabetic (**former GDM**) and a control individual (**control for GDM**)[141] demonstrate that although β-cell function may be greater in absolute terms, when evaluated relative to the degree of insulin sensitivity, the response is inappropriately low in the former GDM, compatible with β-cell dysfunction. Mean data show that exercise training (**ET**) in older males[146] does not alter the relationship between insulin sensitivity and the first-phase insulin response, and thus glucose tolerance does not change. In contrast, nicotinic acid (**NA**)–induced insulin resistance in young males[109] results in a change in the relationship between insulin sensitivity and the first-phase insulin response, which is associated with a reduction in glucose tolerance. **C**. Percentile lines for the relationship between insulin sensitivity and the first-phase insulin response (AIRglucose) based on data from 93 normal subjects.[142] Mean data from six other studies are plotted. The 10 subjects with type 2 diabetes are insulin resistant and have markedly impaired insulin secretion.[117] Thirteen healthy older subjects demonstrate that aging is associated with insulin resistance and a reduction in β-cell function.[143] Reduced β-cell function is also manifest in 8 women with a history of gestational diabetes (GDM),[312] 11 women with polycystic ovarian disease (PCO) and a family history of T2DM,[313] 21 subjects with impaired glucose tolerance (IGT),[170] and 14 subjects with a first-degree relative with T2DM.[314] The reduction in β-cell function in these latter three groups is compatible with their high risk of subsequently developing T2DM. **D**. Individual measurements of insulin sensitivity and the first-phase insulin response (AIRglucose) in a group of first-degree relatives of subjects with T2DM from three different families indicated by different symbols. These individuals, studied when their fasting glucose levels were normal, exhibit broad ranges of both insulin sensitivity and first-phase insulin response. When these two parameters are assessed together, it is apparent that some individuals have well-preserved β-cell function while others have markedly deficient responses and thus would be predicted to be at very high risk of developing hyperglycemia. *(A and B. Reprinted with permission from Kahn et al.[142] C. Reprinted with permission from Vidal J, Kahn SE: Regulation of insulin secretion in vivo. In: Lowe WL Jr, ed.* Genetics of Diabetes Mellitus. *Kluwer:2001;109. D. Reprinted with permission from Kahn SE: Regulation of beta-cell function in vivo: From health to disease.* Diabetes Rev *1996;4: 372.*

When studies of islet secretory function are performed following a 20-hour glucose infusion, consistent increases in the slope of glucose potentiation provide evidence of β-cell adaptation, while consistent decreases in the acute glucagon responses suggest adaptation of α-cell function.[145] Thus it appears that the normal pancreatic islets possess an adaptive capability involving both the α and β cells, and that this adaptation, which may be mediated by changes in glucose level, prevents the development of marked hyperglycemia in individuals with insulin resistance and normal islet function (Fig. 21-15). However, when β-cell dysfunction is present, hyperglycemia will be the expected compensatory response.

When insulin sensitivity is normal, it is unclear what degree of β-cell mass reduction is necessary before fasting hyperglycemia occurs. Some individuals do not develop diabetes mellitus after 70–90% pancreatectomies.[146,147] Whether this or lesser degrees of β-cell loss are associated with clinically significant hyperglycemia if insulin resistance develops is as yet undetermined. Because this question cannot be easily addressed in humans, mathematical modeling has been utilized to predict the various degrees of β-cell loss and insulin resistance required to produce fasting hyperglycemia.[148] Such modeling predicts that in the presence of marked insulin resistance a 50% decrease in β-cell function would result in significant hyperglycemia. From this type of analysis it is predicted that tissue insensitivity to insulin will become a more important determinant of plasma glucose concentration as the loss of β-cell function becomes greater.

The observations in normal-weight and obese subjects cited previously, as well as the application of mathematical models, are consistent with observations in T2DM. Whereas a decrease in insulin sensitivity such as that induced by the development of adiposity will cause only a small change in glucose level in a person with a normal pancreas, in the patient with reduced islet function a much larger rise in glucose concentration will be observed (Fig. 21-16). This is due to the curvilinear relation between islet β-cell function and glucose.[34] As shown in Fig. 21-16, it requires more than a 75% loss of islet function for plasma glucose to rise above 126 mg/dL (7.0 mmol/L), but there is an increasingly greater glucose rise as islet function deteriorates further. Insulin resistance shifts the curve to the right, amplifying this effect. When tissue insulin sensitivity is improved by weight loss, again only small changes in fasting plasma glucose levels will be observed in sub-

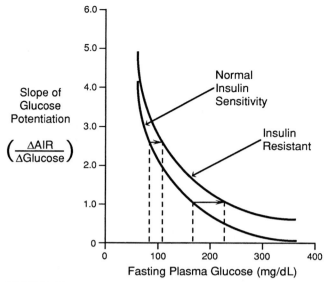

FIGURE 21-16. Relationship of β-cell function to plasma glucose concentration and the impact of insulin resistance. The curvilinear relationship between β-cell function and fasting plasma glucose concentration dictates that in an individual with normal insulin sensitivity, the fasting glucose concentration will only reach the diagnostic level for T2DM (126 mg/dL; 7.0 mmol/L) when approximately 75% of β-cell function has been lost. When insulin resistance coexists in an individual with intact islet function and normal fasting plasma glucose, the compensatory enhancement in insulin output will prevent a marked change in plasma glucose concentration. Alternatively, in an individual with islet dysfunction sufficient to produce an elevation in the fasting glucose concentration, the additive effect of insulin resistance will produce a large increase in fasting glucose. A therapeutic intervention that reduces insulin resistance will reverse this change, resulting in a reduction in the glucose concentration.

jects with normal α- and β-cell function, but a marked lowering of the glucose concentration will occur in the hyperglycemic obese individual with impaired islet β-cell function. Taken together, these observations imply that a change in the degree of insulin sensitivity will have a greater effect on the fasting glucose level as islet function deteriorates.

A PATHOPHYSIOLOGIC MODEL OF T2DM

Figure 21-17A illustrates how the basal glucose concentration is regulated by a feedback loop in which the pancreatic islet acts as a glucose sensor to balance hepatic glucose delivery to the rate of insulin-dependent and insulin-independent glucose use. The occurrence of any change in glucose production by the liver or glucose use by the peripheral tissues is sensed by the islet and leads to changes in insulin and glucagon secretion to achieve a new steady state, which minimizes the overall change in glucose level. This new steady state returns the glucose concentration toward normal, but complete compensation cannot occur because this would result in the loss of the stimulus responsible for this adaptive change. The development of a β-cell lesion in T2DM would reduce plasma insulin levels. Because glucagon secretion is either wholly or partially regulated by the neighboring β-cell, an abnormal rise in α-cell release of glucagon would also occur (Fig. 21-17B). This reduction in insulin and increase in glucagon draining into the liver

FIGURE 21-15. Impact of insulin resistance on basal glucose regulation. The impairment of insulin action in the liver and insulin-sensitive peripheral tissues increases the glucose level, but as the islet compensates by increasing its insulin output and decreasing its glucagon release, hepatic glucose output and glucose disposal are modulated. The net effect is a small rise in glucose concentration and a large increase in insulin secretion. *(Adapted with permission from Porte.[92])*

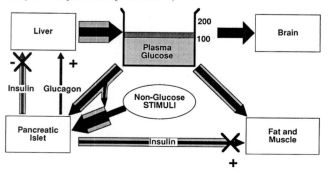

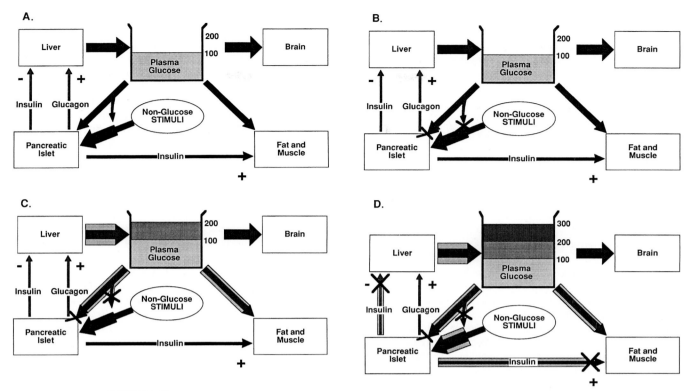

FIGURE 21-17. Model for the development of hyperglycemia in T2DM. **A.** Normal basal glucose regulation. Insulin and glucagon, through their effects on the liver, fat, and muscle, modulate the plasma glucose level. Plasma glucose, by its direct interaction with the endocrine pancreas and by its modulation of the secretory response to nonglucose stimuli, feeds back to the islet to regulate insulin and glucagon output. **B.** Hypothetical initial islet lesion of T2DM. The impairment of islet function would be expected to reduce insulin and increase glucagon output, which would result in overproduction of glucose by the liver and underuse of glucose in the periphery, with a resultant increase in the glucose level. **C.** Hyperglycemia's effect to compensate for the islet lesion of T2DM. The increased glucose concentration that develops as a result of the deficient insulin and enhanced glucagon secretion in turn modulates the islet by increasing insulin secretion and decreasing glucagon release. As a result of these secretory changes, glucose production and use return toward normal but still remain elevated. **D.** Interaction of islet dysfunction and insulin resistance on basal glucose regulation in T2DM. The impairment of insulin action in the liver and peripheral tissues requires a marked additional increase in glucose concentration so that, in the presence of an impaired islet, a new steady state is achieved. Under these conditions, the islet may secrete "normal" or even "supranormal" quantities of insulin while secreting "normal" or "subnormal" amounts of glucagon, despite the presence of islet α- and β-cell dysfunction. The net result is a further increase in glucose production by the liver and glucose use by the peripheral tissues, until the renal threshold is exceeded when decompensation occurs. *(Adapted with permission from Porte.[92])*

would be expected to produce an increase in hepatic glucose production. Further, the reduced peripheral insulin level would impair glucose use by both fat and muscle, while glucose use in the non-insulin-dependent tissues proceeds normally. Due to the reduction in insulin secretion, insulin-mediated glucose uptake cannot increase sufficiently to compensate for the increased rate of hepatic glucose release, and the fasting glucose level tends to rise. This situation is only transient, because the elevation in the fasting plasma glucose level would lead to increased β-cell stimulation, thereby producing a more "normal" plasma insulin level, as depicted in Fig. 21-17C. In addition, the increase in glucose and insulin concentrations results in a reduction in glucagon secretion, but at the new steady state the glucagon level is not appropriately reduced for the degree of glycemia. Concurrent with these changes in islet hormone secretion, glucose production and use are moderated. However, at the new steady state, the rate of hepatic glucose

release will remain elevated and total glucose uptake will be increased due to the hyperglycemia. When hepatic and peripheral insulin resistance develops, the impairment of glucose uptake leads to a further increase in plasma glucose level. This additional hyperglycemia leads to further stimulation of the β cell with resultant normal or even supranormal insulin levels as well as further increase in hepatic glucose delivery and peripheral glucose uptake (Fig. 21-17D). Although a further reduction in the glucagon level occurs, the resultant level is still inappropriately elevated for the degree of hyperglycemia.

From this model it is apparent that islet dysfunction may be present regardless of whether basal insulin and glucagon levels are normal, high, or low in T2DM. Hyperglycemia is a compensatory mechanism that occurs in an attempt to overcome the islet secretory defect and insulin resistance. These adaptive changes result in a reregulated steady-state hyperglycemia, but complete compensation can occur only at glucose levels below the renal threshold. Once the renal threshold is exceeded, glycosuria occurs and the plasma glucose level cannot rise sufficiently to compensate for the islet defect. This then results in the development of a state of absolute insulin deficiency and glucagon excess with metabolic decompensation.

TREATMENT OF T2DM

At the present time, three major therapeutic modalities are used in type 2 diabetic subjects: diet, oral agents, and insulin administration. These interventions produce alterations in hepatic glucose production, insulin sensitivity, and/or insulin secretion and, as is apparent from the previously described closed feedback loop, any change in these variables should result in a reregulated steady state at a new level of glycemia.

Body weight reduction comprises two distinct phases: a period of weight loss, during which time there is a marked reduction in caloric intake, and weight maintenance at a new lower level, during which time more calories are being consumed, albeit less than the quantity taken prior to the initiation of weight loss. While a decline in glucose level occurs during both these phases, the mechanism by which glucose decreases is different. For an individual to lose weight, a reduction in caloric intake is required so that a state of negative caloric balance exists. Although it has been claimed that caloric restriction is associated with an improvement in insulin sensitivity, this does not occur during the period of weight loss. In fact, during periods of severe caloric restriction, the opposite is true and a state of insulin resistance exists.[149] Therefore, the initial decrease in fasting plasma glucose level that is observed during caloric restriction results from a reduction in hepatic glycogen stores with a resultant decline in glycogenolysis and a reduced rate of hepatic glucose release. As glycogen stores become progressively depleted, the liver tends to produce glucose predominantly by gluconeogenesis, with the rate of hepatic glucose production remaining low as the body attempts to maintain energy stores and minimize the loss of protein. Thus, after a period of fasting as short as 3 days, type 2 diabetes patients will demonstrate a significant reduction in their glucose levels, but these levels, while approximating those of healthy individuals, never reach the same low levels as normal subjects during a similar fast.[150] However, as soon as caloric intake increases, and weight maintenance is achieved, hepatic glycogen is replaced, glucose release is enhanced, and glucose levels tend to rise once again. Thus although improved insulin action is not a factor in the lowering of glucose levels during a hypocaloric diet, once body adiposity is reduced and weight is stabilized at a new lower level, any lowering of plasma glucose is due to improved hepatic and peripheral insulin sensitivity. The magnitude of the glucose level reduction will in large part be related to this enhancement of insulin sensitivity and is of most benefit to those individuals with poor islet function and marked hyperglycemia, in whom even a small improvement in insulin action can lower glucose concentrations (Fig. 21-16). This improvement in peripheral insulin sensitivity is largely due to an enhancement of postreceptor insulin action,[151] with some increase in insulin receptor number also occurring.[152] Some of these improvements in hepatic and peripheral glucose metabolism may also be the result of an increase in insulin secretion. Enhanced insulin release has been demonstrated in type 2 diabetes patients given an oral glucose challenge following weight reduction[151–153] and in a group of severely hyperglycemic subjects in whom the plasma glucose level was halved to approximately 150 mg/dL (8.3 mmol/L) following 4–12 weeks of severe caloric restriction, with a resultant increase of about 65% in the insulin response to tolbutamide.[154]

A number of oral agents are now available that are capable of stimulating insulin secretion (see Chap. 32). All these agents can effectively lower plasma glucose levels, but this effect is dependent on the presence of a responsive endocrine pancreas. Long-term administration of sulfonylureas is associated with reduced plasma glucose levels, but basal and stimulated insulin levels are often unchanged.[155,156] This similarity of insulin levels is misleading, however, because when glucose is administered to match the glucose levels to those present prior to initiation of treatment, marked increases in basal and stimulated insulin levels are apparent.[157,158] This observed increase in the slope of glucose potentiation suggests that sulfonylureas improve β-cell responsiveness to glucose.[158] Sulfonylureas are also capable of reducing basal hepatic glucose production, and this reduction has been maintained for periods of up to 18 months.[98,99] The magnitude of this reduction appears to be a major determinant of the hypoglycemic effectiveness of these compounds. This decrease in the rate of hepatic glucose output is related to the change in basal insulin secretion. This relation between hepatic glucose release and basal insulin secretion, coupled with a marked enhancement of β-cell responsiveness to glucose, clearly links a major proportion of the decline in hepatic glucose production and the resultant glucose-lowering effect of these agents to the improved insulin secretion. Although it has been suggested that these compounds have a direct effect on hepatic sensitivity, the variability of findings preclude the drawing of a definite conclusion regarding this possibility. However, in many patients, sulfonylurea administration does appear to improve peripheral insulin sensitivity measured *in vivo*, resulting in an increase in insulin binding and an enhancement of postreceptor function, the latter being the predominant improvement.[99] This change in intracellular insulin action results in an increase of nearly 40% in the maximal response to insulin in some type 2 diabetics.[99] This ability of sulfonylureas to improve peripheral insulin sensitivity also appears to be a function of their capacity to enhance insulin secretion. This is suggested by the fact that type 1 diabetic subjects who are insulin resistant and incapable of enhancing their insulin output do not exhibit an improvement of insulin sensitivity when treated with these agents.[159] Therefore, we conclude that sulfonylureas result in a steady-state reregulation of plasma glucose at a lower level largely due to their direct and persistent effects on the pancreatic islet. More recently, two new classes of β-cell secretagogues have been developed and introduced into clinical practice. The first is the meglitinide repaglinide and the second the D-phenylalanine analogue nateglinide. As with the sulfonylureas, they appear to bind to the ATP-sensitive potassium channel.[160,161] However, due to the fact that these newer classes of agents have a more rapid onset of action and a shorter half-life, they tend to have a greater effect on early postprandial insulin release compared to basal insulin, thereby being more efficient in suppressing meal-related hepatic glucose production.[162]

The biguanide metformin has long been available for the treatment of type 2 diabetes. Its predominant effect appears to be on the liver, where it primarily reduces basal hepatic glucose production.[163] This effect may be mediated by an enhancement of the action of insulin in the liver or perhaps by an alteration in substrate flow, primarily from the splanchnic bed.[164] It has been postulated that a portion of the effect of this agent to improve glucose metabolism may also be mediated by an improvement in peripheral insulin sensitivity.[165] However, this effect does not appear to be consistent, although it is clear that the major beneficial effect is mediated through the liver.

Another recent addition to the classes of oral medications available for treating hyperglycemia are the PPAR-γ–agonist thiazolidinediones. These agents work primarily by enhancing insulin sensitivity in the peripheral insulin-sensitive tissues, namely, the muscle and adipose tissue, while having a much smaller effect on the liver.[166,167] The mechanism by which enhancement of signaling via PPAR-γ improves glucose uptake has not been determined. It has been suggested that the effect of these agents to enhance insulin action may be mediated in part by a change in free fatty acid flux from the adipocyte.[168] In this context, it is also of interest that in small studies it has been demonstrated that administration of these compounds has been associated with a redistribution of central adiposity from the intra-abdominal to the subcutaneous fat depot.[169] It also appears that these agents may improve β-cell function as the relationship between insulin sensitivity and insulin levels is improved and disproportionate proinsulinemia is partially ameliorated.[170,171] The recent suggestion that PPAR-γ receptors may be present on islets raises the interesting possibility that this effect of thiazolidinediones to improve β-cell function may be in part occurring via a direct effect on the β cell.[172]

Exogenous insulin serves to substitute for the β-cell defect of type 2 diabetes, and if sufficient insulin is administered, normoglycemia can be achieved.[138,139] This reduction in glucose level is a function of insulin's ability to suppress hepatic glucose release and enhance peripheral glucose uptake. Intensive insulin treatment is capable of reducing hepatic glucose production so that after only 3 weeks of therapy, the rate of glucose output approximates that observed in normal subjects.[139] Using this same treatment regimen, near normalization of fasting glucose levels is associated with a 74% improvement in the maximal glucose disposal rate without any improvement in adipocyte insulin binding.[139] This improvement in postreceptor function with insulin administration suggests that a reversible component of the postbinding abnormality is the result of hypoinsulinemia or some other metabolic factor, such as hyperglycemia. Improved glucose utilization has been demonstrated for periods of up to 2 weeks following withdrawal of insulin therapy.[139] Although this lower plasma glucose level may provide less stimulation to the β cell, resulting in reduced basal insulin secretion, it has been demonstrated that intensive glucose control may improve the insulin response to glucose and nonglucose stimuli.[138,139,173] Although the first-phase insulin response to glucose, long considered a marker of T2DM, does not improve, the second-phase insulin response is enhanced. Furthermore, the improved glucose control results in a nearly threefold increase in the insulin response to glucagon[138] and an improvement in the C-peptide response to arginine.[173] However, once intensive insulin therapy is discontinued, the subsequent rise in glucose levels is again associated with steadily deteriorating β-cell function.[173] As noted, even though β-cell function may improve when glucose levels decline as a result of insulin treatment, islet stimulation is reduced, and usually the endocrine pancreas is suppressed. Therefore, the total insulin requirement will need to be met by exogenous insulin administration and the treatment program for an insulin-treated type 2 diabetic subject becomes very similar to the regimen of a type 1 diabetes patient. Thus the treatment program will require well-spaced meals and multiple doses of insulin. When complete replacement is required, the amount of insulin needed is not related to the degree of hyperglycemia, but rather relates to body adiposity and other factors that determine insulin resistance. Thus in lean individuals a daily dose of 40–50 U may suffice, while in grossly obese subjects the requirement may be as great as 150–200 U/d.

GENETIC FACTORS IN T2DM

The advancement in our knowledge related to the pathogenesis of type 2 diabetes and the improved effectiveness of therapy that is based on this information have been matched in part by progress in our understanding and ability to identify genetic causes of disease. It now appears that type 2 diabetes is a polygenic disease that in most instances probably requires the interaction of at least two genetic factors: one related to β-cell dysfunction and one related to insulin resistance. In the process of searching for the genetic causes of type 2 diabetes, several rare forms of disordered glucose metabolism have been shown to be caused by gene defects involving the β cell and the insulin receptor.

Two groups of patients with type 2 diabetes and identified gene defects associated with β-cell dysfunction have been described. The first group consists of the maternally inherited mitochondrial syndromes with diabetes originally described as being associated with various neuromuscular disorders, but recently found to present at any age independently of or prior to neuromuscular disease with glucose intolerance or type 2 diabetes.[174,175] The second group also presents as glucose intolerance or type 2 diabetes with a different inheritance pattern and has been called maturity-onset diabetes of the young (MODY) since it was first described clinically on the basis of its presentation under age 40 with a dominant inheritance pattern.[36,176] For a comprehensive description see the reviews by Fajans and associates[177] and Kahn and Porte.[178]

Similarly, molecular studies have found relatively rare defects associated with insulin resistance that are associated with T2DM and mutations in the insulin receptor gene.[179–181] Two clinical features commonly observed in these syndromes are acanthosis nigricans and hyperandrogenism (in female patients). However, each set of defects is defined by the presence or absence of specific clinical features. One, called *type A insulin resistance,* is defined by the triad of insulin resistance, acanthosis nigricans, and hyperandrogenism in the absence of obesity or lipoatrophy.[93] Another consists of patients with the clinical diagnosis of *leprechaunism* with multiple abnormal features presenting during gestation or soon after birth, including intrauterine growth restriction and impaired glucose tolerance (IGT) with intermittent fasting hypoglycemia.[182,183] These patients usually die within the first year of life. A third syndrome is the *Rabson-Mendenhall syndrome* that is associated with short stature, abnormalities of teeth and nails, and pineal hyperplasia.[184] For a comprehensive description see the review by Taylor.[93]

These known β-cell and insulin receptor genetic syndromes and the high concordance of T2DM in identical twins compared with fraternal twins have stimulated a major search for predisposing gene defects in the more typical older-onset T2DM patients, but the likely heterogeneity of defects has made their identification difficult, and despite many promising associations between gene polymorphisms and hyperglycemia, there is no genetic defect that has yet been unequivocally identified to cause the disease more commonly affecting T2DM patients. Before describing in greater detail the known rarer causes of diabetes mentioned above, some discussion of the status of genetic studies on the more common form of type 2 diabetes is warranted.

Genetic Studies of T2DM

A variety of metabolic studies have demonstrated impaired β-cell function and insulin resistance in family members of subjects with type 2 diabetes[185,186] and in identical twins of type 2 diabetic patients with normal glucose tolerance who have a high likelihood of developing the syndrome.[187] It is still not clear in any individual patient which of these two disorders began first, how much is related to the environment and to genetic dysfunction, and how much of the full-blown syndrome is secondary to the hyperglycemia. There is evidence that both β-cell function[188,189] and insulin sensitivity[190] are familial traits in certain populations, and abnormalities of insulin secretion and sensitivity have been reported to predate the onset of glucose intolerance.[185,186] Nevertheless, there remain many uncertainties regarding progression from normal to impaired glucose tolerance and eventually to fasting hyperglycemia and clinical T2DM. For this reason it has been difficult to identify the genetic defects that are presumed to underlie much of the risk of T2DM. The most convincing evidence of a genetic factor is derived from twin studies.[191–195] Although there is some variation in reported risk when comparing monozygotic and dizygotic twins, concordance is always higher for monozygotic twins than dizygotic twins. Initial studies reported almost 100% concordance in monozygotic twins and roughly 50% in dizygotic twins, but ascertainment bias was believed to be a serious problem in the generation of these data. More recent studies suggest that concordance is more likely to be in the 60–70% range in monozygotic twins and roughly 10–20% in dizygotic twins. Thus the relative risk of development of T2DM in the sibling of an identical twin with the disease was increased 2- to 3.4-fold compared with nonidentical twins, and this increases with age. Further evidence for genetic factors is the familial aggregation of type 2 diabetes in a variety of ethnic groups, and a variation of prevalence among these groups, ranging from as high as 80% in subjects such as the Pima Indians whose parents both had early onset diabetes to the estimates of approximately 5% in Caucasian Americans, 10% in African Americans, 25% in Mexican Americans, and 35% in Pima Indians overall.[196]

Positional cloning has been attempted after locating susceptibility genes from either a genome scan using random markers or discrete regions of a chromosome which are strongly associated with the rare genetic forms of the disease, or one of the physiological markers believed to contribute to the etiology of the disease. The generally disappointing results have now led to the common belief that T2DM is a polygenic disorder which probably results from several combined gene defects that interact with environmental factors to produce the eventual clinical syndrome. This being the case, it is perhaps not surprising that none of these genetic approaches has been particularly successful so far in unraveling the important, underlying etiological factors in late-onset T2DM. Nevertheless, success using the MODY phenotype has encouraged continuing efforts using more powerful techniques. To date, the study of candidate genes has been by far the most commonly used approach. However, a high degree of heterozygosity is required to optimize sib-pair analysis, and identification of affected subjects is arbitrary, being based on a continuous physiological variable. Identity by descent or identity by state can be utilized, but considering the age of onset of T2DM, identity by state is by far the most frequent method. Unfortunately, this requires determination of the frequency of the alleles in an appropriately matched population and may require a large number of pairs. Until recently, candidate genes have usually been evaluated in populations of unrelated individuals. Avoiding errors in conclusions in these studies requires careful clinical and metabolic phenotyping using well-matched case and control populations, with particular regard to avoiding differences in ethnicity and genetic background. Since many genes have now been cloned and sequenced using molecular scanning methods designed to detect changes in nucleotide sequence in fragments of DNA, such as single-strand confirmation polymorphism (SSCP) or heteroduplex analysis, it is possible to test a very large number of potential associations. While an association between a mutation or polymorphism with β-cell dysfunction, insulin resistance, impaired glucose tolerance, or diabetes can then be analyzed, care must be taken to confirm positive findings using some other method to eliminate a chance occurrence or an unknown difference in the background of the affected and control subjects.

Candidate Genes for T2DM

Glucokinase

All of the known MODY genes have been considered as possible candidates for gene defects in late-onset T2DM. Positive associations between T2DM and particular glucokinase polymorphisms were originally observed in American Blacks and Mauritian Creoles,[197] suggesting that the glucokinase locus might be implicated in diabetes in these populations. However, mutations in the coding region were not found. Variants were observed in the liver promoter at −258 and the islet β-cell promoter at −30. A block transversion mutation near this latter region in the rat promoter resulted in a 22% reduction in promoter activity in vitro,[198] and the region of the −30 base is known to be completely homologous between the rat and the human. However, the functional importance of this region in humans is not known for certain. This variant promoter was associated with an increased frequency of impaired glucose tolerance in a group of Japanese middle-aged men who were surveyed in a population under study in Seattle, and when this population was resurveyed 5 years later, this was confirmed.[199] Further analysis of the population demonstrated an association between this variant and a 30% reduction in early insulin responses to oral glucose challenge. This was true whether or not the individual had normal or impaired glucose tolerance. Thus it was concluded that the −30 promoter variant may be an example of a common genetic variation which increases the risk of impaired glucose tolerance and contributes to the increased frequency of T2DM in this population. However, the pathophysiology of impaired glucose tolerance is heterogeneous even in this population, and therefore multiple factors are probably interacting to produce clinical hyperglycemia. Furthermore, as discussed earlier, for this phenotyping it is necessary to recognize that insulin sensitivity modulates β-cell responses to glucose, and therefore the assessment of β-cell function can be complex. This may explain why populations do not show linkage between the glucokinase locus when clinical diabetes is used as the phenotype,[188,200–203] but may show association with glucose intolerance.[199,204]

The High-Affinity β-Cell Sulfonylurea Receptor (SUR-1)

This molecule couples with an inwardly rectifying potassium channel (Kir6.2) and acts as a regulatory subunit for coupling glucose metabolism through its nucleotide binding sites for ATP and ADP to regulate the potassium channel and membrane conductance for control of calcium influx and insulin secretion.[205] A number of variants of this receptor have been described.

A silent variant in exon 22, ACC → ACT at nucleotide 761 was more common in patients than in controls with an odds ratio of 3, while an intronic T → C change at position −3 of the exon 24 splice acceptor site was also more common, with an odds ratio of 1.9. The combination occurred in 8.9% of patients and 0.5% of control subjects. Therefore, it was suggested that this locus may be a contributor to T2DM in Northern European Caucasians.[206]

Sixty-three T2DM patients were completely screened from a Danish population.[207] One variant, a C/T in the silent exon 18 at position 775 and an intron 3c/−3t were found together more frequently in T2DM patients than control subjects. Ten of 300 unrelated, healthy, young Danish Caucasians had the combined at-risk genotype associated with a 50% reduction in serum C peptide and a 40% reduction in serum insulin responses to tolbutamide, but not to glucose injection. Therefore, there is only a possible association with T2DM and SUR-1 in some populations.

GLUT-2

GLUT-2 is a high-K_m (low affinity) glucose transporter expressed in liver, islet β cells, kidney, and intestine. Coupled with glucokinase, GLUT-2 has been proposed to act as part of the glucose-sensing mechanism in β cells.[208] A sib-pair analysis in Pima Indians demonstrated significant linkage between GLUT-2 and the acute insulin response to glucose, but no linkage with T2DM.[188] Studies in a Japanese group of pedigrees with affected members showed a possible association between a polymorphic marker near the GLUT-2 locus, but follow-up in 60 subjects with complete gene scans found three Thr110Ile mutations and one Pro68Leu mutation that were not associated with disease.[209] In summary, association with disease has not been found.

Glucagon Receptor

A screening study of the glucagon receptor gene was reported in 1995 in a population of Sardinian and French families.[210] Eighty multiplex, French type 2 diabetic families were investigated first. In exon 2 a single heterozygous missense mutation GGT 40 → AGT 40 (Gly40Ser) was identified in 5 of the 80 tested. Subsequently, a further 136 unrelated patients from additional families and 96 unrelated patients from Sardinia were screened. The overall frequency was 4.6% in the French and 8.3% in the Sardinians. Three control groups were also tested. The trend of the two populations was similar. When tested together, there was a highly significant association with T2DM. Linkage was tested using the transmission/dysequilibrium (TD) test and the estimated transmission frequency of .727 was significantly higher than the expected value of .5. This required subjects with impaired glucose tolerance, impaired fasting glucose, or T2DM to be considered affected, although impaired glucose tolerance and impaired fasting glucose combined were also significant. Overt T2DM assessed alone was not. This receptor variant was expressed in BHK cells and transfected clones tested for binding. Compared to wild-type receptor, labeled glucagon had a threefold lower affinity for the mutant.

Unfortunately, subsequent studies were quite variable and not confirmatory.[211–219] Similar association data have been reported with the −30 β-cell glucokinase promoter (see above), and suggest the possibility that there may be genetic factors which predispose to impaired glucose tolerance, but whose impact on blood glucose is so modest that because they are common variants, the effect does not become noticeable when surveying the entire population and comparing overt diabetes as the affected with a group including impaired glucose tolerance and impaired fasting glucose among the nonaffected populations. Thus detailed phenotypic characterization may be critical if such a variation is a significant contributor to the eventual development of risk for T2DM in a population.

Other Candidate Genes

Many other candidate genes have been screened, but none has been consistently associated with type 2 diabetes. Total genome scans have been almost as equally disappointing to date, although not nearly as extensive.[220–224]

Genome-Wide Scanning for Type 2 Diabetes

There are five groups that have assembled the necessary resources, including identification of a suitable population, clinical phenotyping, metabolic studies, and genetic analytic techniques, that are enabling them to pursue this approach. However, since the populations vary and the selection criteria are different, it is likely that the outcomes will be different.

The first group reported on a population of 217 individuals from 26 families screened from 4000 individuals in a population isolated in western Finland (Botnia), an area where Swedes are living.[220] The total population of the region is 60,000. Over a 5-year period, families with a positive history of diabetes at four health centers were recruited to participate in clinical characterization studies with an overall participation rate of 90%. In total, 1180 type 2 diabetes patients and 3005 family members were phenotyped. Families containing three or more affected individuals, with at least one subject having disease onset before age 60 years and another before age 65 years, were selected for analysis. A 10-cM sequence length polymorphic map was made of the 217 individuals and a nonparametric method used for evaluation. This analysis revealed no significant or even suggestive evidence for susceptibility loci predisposing to T2DM. However, to further phenotype individuals, they selected the early insulin response during the oral glucose tolerance test (30-minute insulin level) among affected individuals as an indicator of insulin secretion to rank families. Families were partitioned into four quartiles and the data reanalyzed. In the quartile with the lowest insulin levels, a region near D12S366 on chromosome 12q was highly significant, and with additional markers in this region, evidence for linkage was observed with an approximate LOD score of 3.65. This is the region of the *MODY-3* gene, but the lowest quartile families do not fit the usual phenotypic definition of *MODY-3* families. Subsequent screening of 86 of these subjects failed to demonstrate a mutation in the HNF1α gene, suggesting that a nearby gene is possibly involved.

Hanis and colleagues performed a sib-pair analysis on a group of Mexican American families from Starr County, Texas.[225] This group consisted of 408 Mexican American individuals with 330 affected sib-pairs from 170 sibships. One marker at D2S125 showed evidence for linkage with an LOD score >2.6. Follow-up studies were made in another group of Mexican-Americans consisting of 166 individuals from 76 sibships for a total of 110 affected sib-pairs, and were compared with a group of Japanese affected sib-pairs consisting of 213 individuals from 97 sibships for a total of 140 affected sib-pairs. An oral glucose tolerance test using WHO criteria, current oral hypoglycemic agent, or insulin use was used to determine the affected. Several markers showed some evidence for linkage with type 2 diabetes in this second sample. When combined, only D2S125 met the genome-wide criteria with significant evidence for linkage with IBS X_2 and MLS values in the combined sample of 30.25 and 4.10. There was no evidence for linkage in the Japanese population or in a group of heterogeneous non-Hispanic whites who were also screened. Subsequently, positional cloning at this location on chromosome 2 demonstrated a common (G/A) variation in an intron of the gene encoding calpain-10.[226] A homozygous polymorphism (G/G) of UCSNP-43 was the at-risk genotype in this Mexican-American population. Recently, three biallelic polymorphisms UCSNP-43 (G/A), −19 (32 bp ins/del), and −63 (C/T) have been found to have the greatest association with T2DM in this population.[227] In Pima Indians this genotype was not associated with type 2 diabetes, but in normal glucose-tolerant relatives, GG homozygotes were found to be relatively insulin resistant and to have reduced calpain-10 mRNA expression in skeletal muscle.[228] A northern European population from Botnia, Finland was also tested and the G/G polymorphism was again associated with T2DM.[226] Therefore, it appears to be a risk factor in some populations despite being in a noncoding region of the gene without any clear-cut function. The message is expressed in many tissues and therefore its physiologic impact is not yet known.

In summary, whole genome searches using the affected sib-pair method have been undertaken by a variety of groups to complement the ongoing work on candidate genes for T2DM. The results to date have been modest, largely because of the difficulties of the effort. The FUSION group has pointed out that 400 pairs typed on a 10-cM map will require a 1.8-fold excess risk to siblings of affected individuals at an LOD score of 3.0 with 82% power. However, this drops to an LOD score of 1.0 for a 1.4-fold excess risk. It is also pointed out that it would require 800 such pairs to have 70% power to detect a locus with an impact estimated by the Starr County investigators for their chromosome 2 finding to produce an LOD score of 3.0, and even this would be reduced to an LOD score of 1.59 if the locus only confers a 1.2-fold excess risk. Thus it is becoming obvious that detection of genes for type 2 diabetes is going to be extremely complex and difficult if the impact of these genes is relatively modest and their frequencies either relatively low or very high or if they interact in some way, which is likely. This probably explains why even the results of the initial efforts have not replicated one another, and only one potential gene has been identified. Thus identification of genes for type 2 diabetes will almost certainly require pooling of data among investigative groups. Fortunately, such efforts have begun, and with the recent success of the human, mouse, and rat genome sequencing efforts, should lead to rapid progress.

GENETIC STUDIES OF RARER FORMS OF ALTERED GLUCOSE METABOLISM ASSOCIATED WITH DEFECTS IN β-CELL GENES

Mitochondrial Diabetes

The first case of mitochondrial disease with diabetes without muscle or nerve dysfunction except for sensorineural hearing loss was reported a decade ago,[174] with an increasing number of cases seen since. The general characteristic appears to be an early, selective impairment of insulin secretion and a later global metabolic dysfunction similar to classical T2DM with insulin resistance and fasting hyperglycemia.[229–231] However, the diabetes often progresses to absolute insulin deficiency and the need for insulin treatment. In some cases an autoantibody to glutamic acid decarboxylase (GAD)[232] or islet cells (ICAs)[233] is present. Since these markers are

used to assist in the diagnosis of T1DM, there can be confusion regarding classification. In a detailed analysis of subjects with a known mitochondrial defect from families with associated diabetes, those with normal glucose tolerance or impaired glucose tolerance appear to have either a failure to prime the insulin secretory response by a prolonged glucose infusion or an inability to stimulate ultradian insulin secretory-oscillations.[231,233] As the disease progresses, clear-cut impaired insulin secretion in response to a standard glycemic challenge becomes obvious, and insulin resistance may develop.[175,234] Since it has been shown that islet β cells are dependent on mitochondrial metabolism for function,[235,236] with associated high rates of blood flow to the organ and relatively high rates of oxygen consumption, it is assumed that islets are a critical tissue, along with nerve and muscle, that depend on mitochondrial oxidative phosphorylation. Despite the general similarities that have been described, there are great differences among individuals in clinical presentation, age of onset, rate of progression, and eventual dependence on insulin. Furthermore, individuals with the same molecular lesion may have vastly different clinical manifestations, and/or several quite different clinical syndromes may have the same underlying genetic defect. Some of the heterogeneity can be explained by the tissue variability or cellular heterogeneic (i.e., heteroplasmic) nature of the mitochondrial basis for the disease and some by varying genetic backgrounds of the subjects. However, from the studies that have been performed it is clear that there is not always a correlation between molecular and clinical findings.

Maternally Inherited Diabetes and Deafness (MIDD)

The first single large pedigree with MIDD associated with a 10.4-kb deletion of mitochondrial DNA was described in 1992 by Ballinger and associates.[174] Further studies of this pedigree have shown the presence of a variety of mitochondrial rearrangements, and it is likely that the primary defect is mitochondrial DNA duplication.[230] Shortly afterward, van den Ouweland and colleagues described a pedigree with maternally inherited diabetes and deafness with a heteroplasmic A → G mutation at 3243 in the tRNA[leu(UUR)] portion of the mitochondrial genome.[237] This was rather surprising since the same mutation had been previously reported to be associated with the MELAS syndrome (mitochondrial encephalopathy, lactic acidosis, and stroke-like episodes).[238] The reasons why the phenotype varies are unknown, but may be because of differences in the degree of heteroplasmy. The clinical diagnosis of diabetes usually, but not always, precedes the detection of clinical sensorineural hearing loss, but the age of presentation in a rather large Japanese population has varied from 11 to 68 years.[239] The identical clinical picture has also been associated with several other less common mitochondrial mutations. The most common of these, the tRNA[(lys)] 8296 A → G mutation, was estimated to explain 1% of Japanese T2DM cases,[240] and the 3271 T → C tRNA[leu(UUR)] mutation to explain one-tenth as many.[241] An explanation for the poor correlation between the degree of heteroplasmy in peripheral tissues and the severity of the diabetes mellitus suggests that other genes or environmental factors are probably important to the clinical picture.

Other Mitochondrial Syndromes

Several neuromuscular mitochondrial syndromes are also associated with diabetes. The most common one is the MELAS syndrome, and it is usually also associated with the same 3243 A → G mutation that can lead to MIDD. The explanation for the variation is not known, but presumably it results from heteroplasmy which can result in a variable phenotype, or from the interaction with other unknown genetic defects or polymorphisms. Furthermore, other mutations[238,241] have been reported to be associated with this syndrome. Another rare mitochondrial syndrome is the Kearns-Sayre syndrome (KS syndrome), which is usually associated with a mitochondrial DNA deletion on muscle biopsy and is frequently associated with diabetes mellitus.[229,242]

Maturity-Onset Diabetes of the Young (MODY)

In the great majority of patients with T2DM, a diagnosis is made in middle age. However, a subclass of this syndrome includes families in whom diabetes can be recognized in children, adolescents, and young adults, and has been clinically termed MODY.[176] Autosomal dominant inheritance has been established in these families, and at least five specific mutations have been described. However, this does not include all of the families in whom a dominant genetic pattern with young family members has been observed, so more mutations are yet to be discovered. At times these patients have been confused with T1DM patients because they are young, some variants lead to relatively severe forms of insulin-deficient diabetes, and by and large most patients with this syndrome are lean. However, most of the patients are ketosis resistant, and even those who need insulin for control of glycemia are not usually ketosis prone. Since the more common variety of T2DM can also be present among these families, it is possible for an individual family member to have both syndromes, and therefore relative insulin deficiency may become more evident in the presence of insulin resistance and obesity and during periods of stress, infection or trauma. In some MODY patients, there may be easily diagnosable clinical hyperglycemia, but in other members of the family with the same mutation, much milder degrees of hyperglycemia or glucose intolerance may be present. In the younger members diagnosed by genetic screening, some may have normal glucose tolerance although, when studied carefully, subtle abnormalities of insulin secretion may be detectable. MODY can be suspected and recognized if T2DM occurs in three or more generations and the pattern of inheritance conforms to an autosomal dominant type. Families have been diagnosed in Europe and the United States, as well as Japan and other Asian countries. Progression of hyperglycemia depends on the specific genetic defect. Glucose tolerance may fluctuate depending on other factors, and variability among family members is assumed to be related to other genetic and environmental factors that can fluctuate over time. The true prevalence of MODY is unknown, but estimates have varied from 2–5% of patients with T2DM to 10–20% of families with T2DM in multiple family members. Studies of the insulin secretory defects early in the course of the disease can distinguish among the various genetic mutations.

MODY-1 (Hepatocyte Nuclear Factor-4α [HNF-4α])

In 1996, mutations in the HNF-4α gene were shown to be the cause of MODY-1.[243] In this early large pedigree, there was a C → T substitution in codon 130 leading to a threonine-to-isoleucine substitution and a C → T substitution in codon 268 which generated a nonsense mutation CAG (Gln) → TAG (AM) (Q268X). Both the isoleucine 130 and the amber mutation at codon 268 were present on the same allele.[243]

There are some affected subjects that have normal glucose tolerance and some that have impaired glucose tolerance, but most have clinical hyperglycemia, although the age of diabetes onset is variable.[244] Study of marker-positive family members with normal or slightly impaired fasting glucose shows reduced insulin secretory rates above 7 mmol/L glucose at steady state and an impaired ability to prime β-cell function after a 42-hour intravenous glucose infusion (Fig. 21-18).[244,245] This pattern is different from MODY-2 and MODY-3. Approximately one-third of affected individuals will require insulin treatment, and patients with this form of diabetes may have microvascular complications. Homozygous loss of functional protein in mice leads to embryonic lethality and defects in gastrulation.[246] However, there are no obvious hepatic, renal, or gastrointestinal defects in family members.

Several other families in the UK, Japan, and Scandinavia have been reported (Fig. 21-19), but this mutation is still a relatively infrequent cause of MODY. By 2001 only 13 families had been identified.[177]

MODY-2 (Glucokinase)

The first candidate gene linkage in the MODY syndrome was described from a study of 16 French families with three or more generations of IGT or type 2 diabetes, and was found to link to a polymorphic marker adjacent to glucokinase at chromosomal

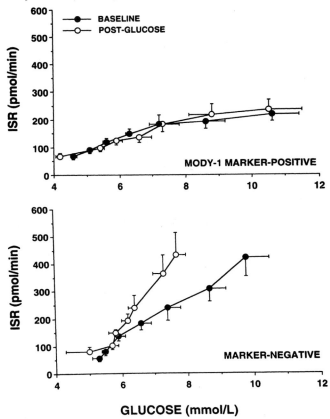

FIGURE 21-18. Insulin secretion rates during graded intravenous glucose infusions administered to 6 marker-negative and 10 marker-positive subjects from the R-W MODY-1 family after an overnight fast (**baseline**) and after a 42-hour intravenous infusion of glucose (**postglucose**) at a rate of 4–6 mg · kg^{-1} · minute^{-1}. Data expressed as means ± SE. (*Reproduced with permission from Froguel et al.[244,245]*)

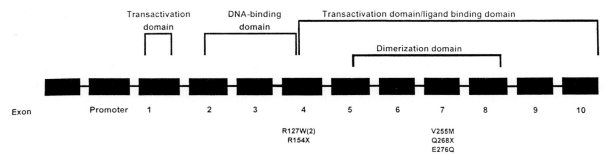

FIGURE 21-19. The distribution of HNF-4α gene mutations in MODY-1 families. When there is more than one family with a mutation, the number of families is shown in parentheses. *(Reproduced with permission from Hattersley.[261])*

locus 7p.[247] By 2001, a large number of families with more than 130 different mutations involving all 10 exons, in populations distributed worldwide of all racial types (Caucasian, black, and Asian) were described (Fig. 21-20).[177,244] Twenty-eight of these mutations alter the protein sequence by changing one amino acid; six transform the sequence at the site of RNA splicing of an intron-exon or exon-intron junction, resulting in the expression of an abnormal species of messenger RNA; and eight are responsible for the synthesis of a truncated protein by creating a premature termination codon by point mutation or deletion. Most are only present in single families.

Glucokinase is present at critical levels in the liver and the pancreas, playing an important role in hepatic glucose storage by phosphorylation of glucose after absorption and in the endocrine pancreas by coupling the first step of glucose metabolism to insulin secretion through the generation of ATP and regulation of β-cell potassium conductance and calcium levels.[248] The degree of hyperglycemia is relatively mild, although it can be usually detected in children. Long-term complications are relatively unusual with this form of diabetes. Hyperglycemia remains stable for many years whether treated or not and progresses very little, in contrast to typical T2DM. Treatment with oral agents is usually satisfactory, and can lead to reasonable control for many years (Fig. 21-21).[176,244,249,250]

The major functional defect that has been observed is impaired insulin secretion; however, this may not be evident unless sophisticated testing is performed. Twenty-four-hour profiles of affected subjects show persistent, round-the-clock hyperglycemia, but insulin levels are only slightly reduced after meals and are no different at baseline and between meals. However, when glucose levels are matched during continuous infusions, they are reduced by at least 50%. As glycemia is increased, they are markedly reduced compared to healthy controls (Fig. 21-22).[250–252] Islet priming by a 42-hour glucose infusion shows a response, but one of smaller magnitude than controls, and it is quite different from that observed in MODY-1 or MODY-3.[244,245,253] After an overnight fast, the entire curve is shifted down and to the right, whereas in MODY-1 the curve rises normally until approximately 8 mmol/L and is then essentially flat throughout as it is in MODY-3. In MODY-2, glucose potentiation of arginine-induced insulin secretion is reduced, and glucose suppression of arginine-induced glucagon secretion is impaired.[254] The average fasting hepatic glycogen content has been shown to be similar in glucokinase-deficient and control subjects, but it is increased in both groups after meals, following a normal pattern throughout the day. However, the net increment in hepatic glycogen content after each meal was 30–60% lower in glucokinase-deficient subjects.[255] Occasional cases of late-onset T2DM have been reported with muta-

FIGURE 21-20. The exon-intron organization of the human glucokinase gene and mutations found in subjects with MODY-2. Amino acid residues are numbered as in the β-cell form of human glucokinase. The two amino acid polymorphisms in the unique NH$_2$-terminal portion of β-cell glucokinase that is encoded by exon 1a are indicated (Asn/Gln-4 [D/N4] and Ala/Thr-11). *(Reproduced with permission from Froguel et al.[244])*

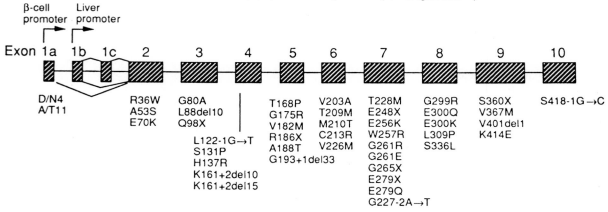

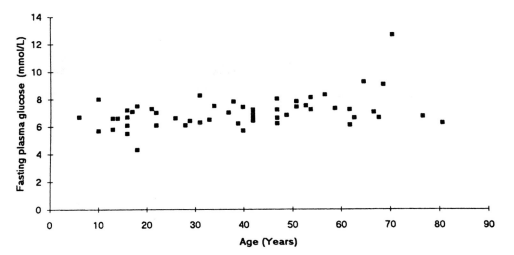

FIGURE 21-21. The relationship between age and fasting plasma glucose values in MODY-2 patients with glucokinase mutations. The fasting plasma glucose values increase very gradually with age (r = 0.41; p = 0.002). *(Reproduced with permission from Tanizawa, Y, Chiu KC: Role of glucokinase in the defective insulin secretion of diabetes. In: Flatt PR, Lenzen S, eds.* Insulin Secretion and Pancreatic β-Cell Research. *Smith-Gordon:1994; 437.)*

tions in glucokinase,[256] and the pattern of inheritance could not be differentiated from that of MODY. It is likely that some mutations produce a syndrome so mild that only obesity in middle age or aging-associated insulin resistance is associated with clinical hyperglycemia.

FIGURE 21-22. Insulin secretion rates during graded intravenous glucose infusions administered to six MODY-2 subjects with glucokinase (**GCK**) mutations and six control subjects after an overnight fast (**BASELINE**) and a 42-hour intravenous infusion of glucose (**POSTGLUCOSE**) at a rate of 4–6 mg · kg^{-1} · min^{-1}. Administration of the glucose infusion enhanced the insulin secretory response to glucose in both control and glucokinase-deficient subjects. Data are expressed as means ± SE. *(Reproduced with permission from Froguel et al.[244])*

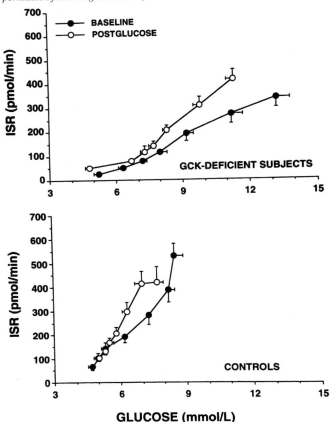

MODY-3 (Hepatocyte Nuclear Factor-1α [HNF-1α])

In 1995, a genome-wide segregation analysis of highly informative microsatellite markers in 12 French families with MODY reported the localization of a gene to the long arm of chromosome 12 in 6 of 12 families.[257] In 1996, Yamagata and associates showed that MODY-3 was the gene encoding HNF-1α, a transcription factor involved in tissue-specific regulation of liver genes which is also expressed in pancreatic islets and other tissues.[243] Seven different mutations in HNF-1α were found to cosegregate with MODY-3 diabetes. More than 120 different mutations have now been identified in MODY-3 families of various populations (Fig. 21-23).[243,258–261] HNF-4α is a transcription factor for HNF-1α. There is a mutation in one family with MODY-3 diabetes in the conserved region of the promoter that disrupts the binding site for the transcription factor HNF-4α.[262] This finding suggests that a 50% reduction in HNF-1α activity can lead to β-cell dysfunction and hyperglycemia. The true frequency of genetic variation in HNF-1α remains to be determined.

An insulin secretory defect in the absence of insulin resistance was observed in diabetic and nondiabetic carriers of MODY-3 mutations with a pattern that during sequential glucose infusions is distinct from MODY-1 and MODY-2.[244,253] In marker-positive normal glucose tolerance (NGT) subjects, the defect was not observed at glucose levels lower than 8 mmol/L, but became evident as glucose rose above this level (Fig. 21-24). Priming was still present in nondiabetic marker-positive subjects, but not in those with clinical hyperglycemia (Fig. 21-25). This type of MODY resembles late-onset type 2 diabetes in its natural history, with patients progressing rapidly from impaired glucose tolerance to overt hyperglycemia with severe deterioration of insulin secretion. Thus it is frequently treated with oral hypoglycemic agents for a time, but often later requires insulin therapy.[263] Complications, such as proliferative retinopathy, have been observed frequently and at rates comparable to those seen in late-onset type 2 diabetics. However, there is a low prevalence of obesity, dyslipidemia, and arterial hypertension, and unlike MODY-2, clinical disease with hyperglycemia usually develops after puberty.[263]

MODY-4 (Insulin Promoter Factor-1 [IPF-1])

One family with a mutation in the IPF-1 gene has been reported.[264] IPF-1, also known as IDX-1, STF-1, and PDX-1, regulates both early pancreatic development and the expression of key

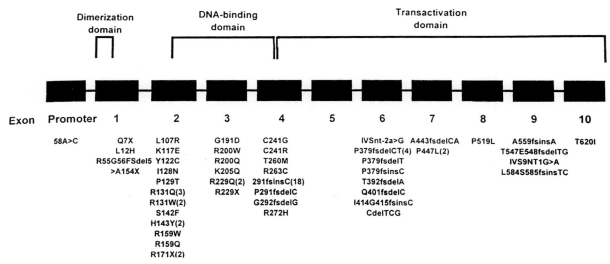

FIGURE 21-23. The distribution of HNF-1α gene mutations in MODY-3 diabetes. When there is more than one family with a mutation, the number of families is shown in parentheses. *(Reproduced with permission from Hattersley.[261])*

endocrine β-cell–specific genes, most notably insulin. Targeted homozygous destruction in mice results in pancreatic agenesis.[265] Family studies simulated by a case with homozygous mutations in exon 1 of the coding sequence with pancreatic agenesis and neonatal diabetes[266] found a high prevalence of diabetes mellitus with age-dependent autosomal dominant transmission in six generations.[264] The average age of onset of hyperglycemia is 35 years (range, 17–67 years) with the hyperglycemia clinically resembling MODY diabetes in that it is mild and treated with diet or oral hypoglycemic agents. The association between the mutation and the clinical syndrome was so significantly strong that the authors suggested the term MODY-4. Further screening in type 2 diabetic families in the UK uncovered several mutations associated with reduced function *in vitro* and an increased risk of

impaired glucose tolerance or type 2 diabetes, but not MODY. It thus appears that these mutations are risk factors for type 2 diabetes.[267,268]

MODY-5 (Hepatocyte Nuclear Factor-1β [HNF-1β])

HNF-1β is a member of a complex transcriptional regulatory network that includes HNF-1α and HNF-4α. It is a homeodomain-containing factor that is structurally related to HNF-1α, and functions as a homodimer or a heterodimer with HNF-1α. Fifty-seven unrelated Japanese subjects with MODY were screened for mutations in these genes, and one family with a nonsense mutation in codon 177 (R177X) of HNF-1β was found, which in this family was associated with diabetes.[269] This family is complex in that one parent has what appears to be late-onset T2DM with no mutations identified. Further screening has been reported in additional families with early-onset T2DM and a frameshift mutation with a GG insert in exon 3 of HNF-β for Ala 263 designated A263fsinsGG has been found.[270] This MODY family has diabetes in three generations with renal dysfunction consisting of renal cysts, proteinuria, and/or elevated creatinine. Additional families screened for MODY or renal disease in the UK uncovered additional mutations segregating with hyperglycemia and renal disease.[267,271–273]

More MODY mutants presumably will be found as only 60% of clinically dominant families with T2DM had an identified defect in 2001.

GENETIC STUDIES OF RARER FORMS OF ALTERED GLUCOSE METABOLISM ASSOCIATED WITH MUTATIONS IN THE INSULIN RECEPTOR GENE

Although insulin resistance plays a key role in the pathogenesis of type 2 diabetes, the molecular mechanisms that cause insulin resistance have not been elucidated in the majority of patients. However, there has been considerable success in identifying the cause of diabetes in several uncommon syndromes of insulin resistance due to mutations in the insulin receptor gene (see review by Taylor[93]).

FIGURE 21-24. Relationship between average plasma glucose concentrations and insulin secretion rates during the stepped glucose infusion studies in seven diabetic MODY-3 subjects (□), six nondiabetic MODY-3 subjects (▲), and six control subjects (○). The lowest glucose levels and insulin secretion rates were measured under basal conditions, and subsequent levels were obtained during glucose infusion rates of 1, 2, 3, 4, 6 and 8 mg · kg^{-1} · min^{-1}. *(Reproduced with permission from Byrne et al.[253])*

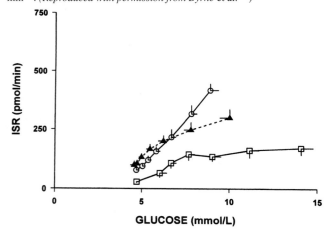

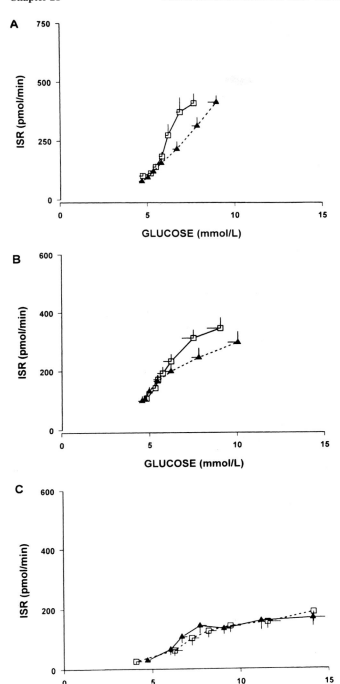

FIGURE 21-25. Graded intravenous glucose infusions were administered to six control subjects (**A**), six nondiabetic MODY-3 subjects (**B**), and seven diabetic MODY-3 subjects (**C**) after an overnight fast (baseline, ▲) and after a 42-hour intravenous infusion of glucose (postglucose, □) at a rate of 4–6 mg · kg⁻¹ · min⁻¹. *(Reproduced with permission from Byrne et al.[253])*

Clinical Syndromes

Leprechaunism

Leprechaunism is the most severe clinical syndrome caused by mutations in the insulin receptor gene.[179–181,274] These patients have glucose intolerance despite having extremely high insulin levels (100-fold above the normal range). In addition to insulin

resistance, patients have multiple abnormalities (e.g., intrauterine growth restriction and fasting hypoglycemia) and usually die within the first year of life. These patients have inactivating mutations in both alleles of the insulin receptor gene. In inbred pedigrees, the patients are usually homozygous for a single mutant allele.[274,275] In the absence of consanguinity, they are usually compound heterozygotes with two different mutant alleles.[276,277]

Type A Insulin Resistance

Type A insulin resistance is defined by the triad of insulin resistance, acanthosis nigricans, and hyperandrogenism (in female patients) in the absence of obesity or lipoatrophy.[93,181,278] Acanthosis nigricans and hyperandrogenism correlate with hyperinsulinemia, and it is believed that they are caused by "toxic" effects of insulin upon the skin and the ovaries, respectively.[279] Because these patients have defects in the function of their insulin receptors, it is unlikely that the toxic effects of insulin are mediated by insulin receptors, but more likely by receptors for homologous peptides such as insulin-like growth factor 1.

Most patients with type A insulin resistance are heterozygous for a single mutant allele, most often a mutation in the tyrosine kinase domain of the receptor.[93,180,181,280,281] Although some heterozygotes have abnormal glucose tolerance, most do not exhibit fasting hyperglycemia. These patients are usually less insulin resistant than patients with two mutant alleles. Patients with type A insulin resistance with two mutant alleles of the insulin receptor gene can develop overt diabetes with fasting hyperglycemia during childhood or adolescence, but usually do not have fasting hyperglycemia as infants.[93,180,181,274,282,283]

Rabson-Mendenhall Syndrome

The Rabson-Mendenhall syndrome is defined by the presence of several clinical features, including extreme insulin resistance, acanthosis nigricans, short stature due to growth retardation, abnormalities of teeth and nails, and pineal hyperplasia.[179–181,184] This syndrome is intermediate in clinical severity between leprechaunism and type A insulin resistance. Although the distinction between leprechaunism and the Rabson-Mendenhall syndrome may not be clear at the time of birth, it has been suggested that diagnosis of Rabson-Mendenhall syndrome only be made in patients who survive beyond 2 years of age. As in leprechaunism, patients with the Rabson-Mendenhall syndrome have inactivating mutations in both alleles of the insulin receptor gene.[274,284,285]

Specific Mutations

Many different mutations have been identified in the insulin receptor. However, there are insufficient data to provide a reliable estimate of the prevalence of mutations in the insulin receptor gene, although currently available data are consistent with estimates that about 1% of patients with T2DM may have such mutations in their receptor gene.[180,181] In several instances the same mutation has been identified in two apparently unrelated patients. However, most of the published mutations have only been identified in single kindreds. The mutations have been separated into five classes based on the mechanisms that impair insulin receptor function (Fig. 21-26). This approach is a modification of the scheme proposed by Brown and Goldstein for the LDL receptor.[286]

Class 1: Impaired Receptor Biosynthesis

Several types of premature chain termination mutations have been identified in the insulin receptor gene (Fig. 21-27): nonsense

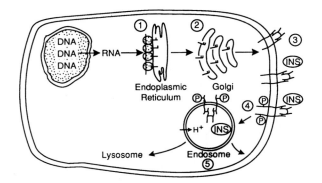

Class of Mutation	Synthesis	Transport to Plasma Membrane	Insulin Binding	Trans-membrane Signalling	Endocytosis, Recycling, Degradation
①	→✗				
②		→✗			
③			→✗		
④				→✗	
⑤					→✗

FIGURE 21-26. Classification of mutations in the insulin receptor gene. This drawing illustrates the major steps in the life of an insulin receptor. First, the gene is transcribed, and the RNA is spliced. The mature mRNA is transported from the nucleus to the cytosol where it is translated by ribosomes on the rough endoplasmic reticulum. The receptor is transported through the endoplasmic reticulum and Golgi complex, the organelles that cause it to undergo multiple posttranslational modifications. Eventually the mature receptor is inserted in the plasma membrane. Insulin binds to the receptor on the cell surface. As a result, the receptor undergoes autophosphorylation and becomes activated as a tyrosine kinase. The interaction of insulin with its receptor initiates the various responses of the target cell to insulin. In addition, insulin binding triggers receptor endocytosis. The acid pH in the endosome dissociates insulin from its receptor. Subsequent to receptor internalization, the receptor is either transported to lysosomes for degradation or recycled back to the plasma membrane for reutilization. The five major classes of genetic defects in receptor function are summarized in the table at the bottom of the figure. This classification scheme is based on the classification for genetic defects in the function of the low-density lipoprotein receptor originally proposed by Brown and Goldstein.[286] *(Reproduced with permission from Taylor.[181])*

mutations,[274,276,277] mutations at intron-exon junctions that impair splicing of mRNA,[287] and deletion mutations that shift the reading frame.[281,288] Premature chain termination mutations interfere with receptor biosynthesis, and lead to the synthesis of truncated receptor fragments. In addition, most premature chain termination mutations exert a *cis*-acting effect to decrease the level of mRNA transcribed from the mutant allele.[274,277] In some patients, mutant alleles have been demonstrated to decrease the level of insulin receptor mRNA, but the mutations map outside the protein coding regions, most likely in regions of the gene that regulate its level of expression.[277,289] At least one patient with leprechaunism has been reported who was homozygous for a total deletion of both insulin receptor genes,[275] and several patients were homozygous for other null alleles.[290–293]

Class 2: Impaired Transport of Receptors to the Cell Surface

The insulin receptor precursor undergoes multiple posttranslational processing steps within the endoplasmic reticulum and Golgi complex. Some mutations impair transport through the endoplasmic reticulum and Golgi to the plasma membrane, thereby reducing the number of receptors on the cell surface.[93,180,181,281,283, 294–297] Because these mutations prevent the receptor from folding into its normal conformation, some class 2 mutations also impair receptor function, e.g., decreasing the affinity of insulin binding[296] or inhibiting activation of the receptor tyrosine kinase.[294] Most of the published mutations in this class are located in the N-terminal half of the α subunit. However, at least one mutation that inhibited posttranslational processing of the proreceptor and transport of the receptor to the plasma membrane was located in the intracellular domain and inhibited receptor tyrosine kinase activity.[298]

Class 3: Decreased Affinity of Insulin Binding

Some mutations decrease the affinity with which the receptor binds insulin.[180,181] This is predicted to cause a rightward shift in the dose–response curve for insulin action, i.e., to decrease the sensitivity with which the target cell responds to insulin. A mutation substituting serine for arginine (R735S) was the first mutation reported to decrease the affinity of insulin binding.[282,299] Arg735 is the last amino acid in the Arg-Lys-Arg-Arg motif at the proteolytic cleavage site between the α and β subunits. In addition to decreasing the affinity of insulin binding, the R735S mutation inhibits cleavage of the precursor into two subunits.

Two mutations in the N-terminal half of the α subunit have also been reported to decrease the affinity of insulin binding, consistent with the hypothesis that the insulin binds to this region of the receptor.[93,180,181] The N15K mutation causes a fivefold reduction of affinity, and the S323L mutation essentially abolishes insulin binding.[284,300,301]

Class 4: Impaired Tyrosine Kinase Activity

Many mutations have been identified in the tyrosine kinase domain that inhibit receptor tyrosine kinase activity. The G1008V mutation was among the first mutations to be identified in this domain.[302] Valine is substituted for Gly1008, the third glycine in the highly conserved Gly-X-Gly-X-X-Gly motif in the ATP binding site. Because ATP is the phosphate donor for the tyrosine kinase reaction, it is not surprising that a mutation in the ATP binding site inactivates the tyrosine kinase. Unlike most mutations in the extracellular domain of the insulin receptor, mutations in the tyrosine kinase domain cause insulin resistance in a dominant fashion.[93,180,181]

Class 5: Accelerated Receptor Degradation

Insulin binding triggers endocytosis of the insulin-receptor complex.[303] Internalized receptors are located in endosomes with the insulin-binding site oriented on the inside of the vesicle.[304] Endosomal proton pumps acidify the interior of the endosome (pH 5.5), and the acidic pH promotes dissociation of insulin from the receptor.[305] Subsequent to internalization, there are at least two pathways available to the receptor: recycling back to the plasma membrane for reutilization and degradation within the lysosome. Some mutations (i.e., K460E and N462S) impair the ability of acidic pH to dissociate insulin from the receptor.[276,305,306] Both mutations are associated with an impaired recycling pathway and preferential targeting of mutant receptors toward lysosomal degradation, thereby accelerating receptor degradation and decreasing the number of receptors on the cell surface.[276,305,307] Receptor missense mutations from classes 2–5 are shown in Fig. 21-28.

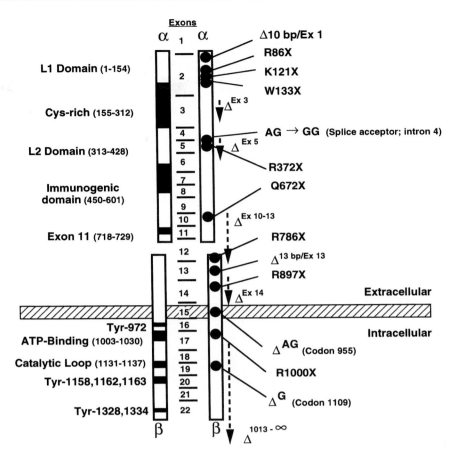

FIGURE 21-27. Mutations that impair receptor biosynthesis (class 1). In this drawing of the receptor, the structural landmarks are indicated on the left side of the figure. Examples of class 1 mutations are indicated on the right side of the figure. These include nonsense mutations, as well as frameshifts and splicing mutations. (In the right half of the drawing, the tetrapeptide connecting the two subunits has not been removed in order to illustrate the sequence of the uncleaved prereceptor.) *(Modified from and based on Taylor SI, Arioglu E: Syndromes associated with insulin resistance and acanthosis nigricans. J Basic Clin Physiol Pharmacol 1998;9:419. Used with permission.)*

Correlation of Molecular Defects with Clinical Syndromes

At least three different theories have been considered to explain the fact that mutations in the insulin receptor gene cause several distinct clinical syndromes.[179–181]

Severity of Insulin Resistance

According to this hypothesis, the severity of insulin resistance determines the clinical manifestations. Patients with leprechaunism have mutations in both alleles of the insulin receptor gene,[180,181] and exhibit the most extreme degree of insulin resistance. In contrast, heterozygosity for a single mutant allele causes the less severe syndrome of type A insulin resistance. Furthermore, even among patients with type A insulin resistance, the patients with two mutant alleles have a more severe form of the syndrome, characterized by fasting hyperglycemia.

Existence of Branched Pathways

Insulin is a hormone that has multiple biologic actions. The pathways for insulin action diverge in the biochemical steps distal to the receptor. According to this hypothesis, the effect of a mutation would depend on which biologic actions are impaired and which are preserved.[308] For example, a mutation that impairs both the metabolic actions and the growth-promoting effects of insulin might cause leprechaunism (a syndrome with growth retardation as well as abnormal glucose tolerance). If a mutation selectively impairs only the ability of the receptor to mediate the metabolic actions of insulin, this might cause type A insulin resistance (a syndrome with abnormal glucose tolerance but normal growth).

Genetic Variation at Different Loci

According to this theory, the insulin receptor locus is the major disease gene responsible for the insulin resistance, but other genetic loci modulate the clinical syndrome. For example, defects in various growth factor receptors have been reported in patients with leprechaunism, and these defects may contribute to the growth retardation associated with the syndrome.[309] However, if the difference between type A insulin resistance and leprechaunism were due to mutations at another genetic locus, then one would predict that mutations at the two genetic loci would segregate independently. If a child inherited the insulin receptor mutations in the absence of the mutations at the other locus, the patient would manifest type A insulin resistance. If another child in the same pedigree inherited mutations in both the insulin receptor and the other locus, then that child would develop leprechaunism. This pattern of inheritance has not been reported, although many kindreds have been reported with two or more siblings having the same clinical syndrome (i.e., either leprechaunism or type A insulin resistance).

Nevertheless, it is likely that polygenic influences may explain some clinical variation between individuals with the same genotype at the insulin receptor locus. Two sisters with type A insulin resistance (both homozygous for the F382V mutation) illustrate this clinical variability in the syndrome.[283,310,311] Although the

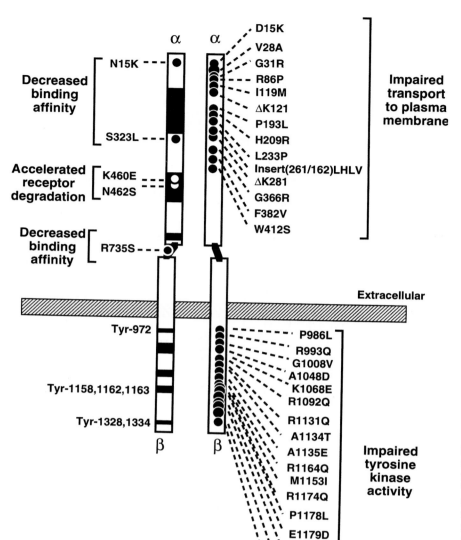

FIGURE 21-28. Missense mutations in the insulin receptor gene. Examples of missense mutations in the insulin receptor gene are indicated in the figure. These mutations either impair the transport of receptors to the plasma membrane (class 2), decrease the affinity of insulin binding (class 3), impair tyrosine kinase activity (class 4), or accelerate the rate at which receptors are degraded (class 5). *(Modified from and based on Taylor SI, Arioglu E: Syndromes associated with insulin resistance and acanthosis nigricans.* J Basic Clin Physiol Pharmacol *1998;9: 419. Used with permission.)*

younger sister required treatment with several thousand units of insulin per day, the older sister responded to dietary management. The younger sister had such severe hyperandrogenism that she had never menstruated spontaneously and did not experience withdrawal bleeding when treated with estrogen-progestin, while the older sister twice became pregnant.

Acknowledgements This work was supported in part by NIH grants DK-02654, DK-17047, DK-50703, and RR-37, and grants from the Medical Research Service of the Department of Veterans Affairs, and the American Diabetes Association.

REFERENCES

1. Sacca L, Hendler R, Sherwin RS: Hyperglycemia inhibits glucose production in man independent of changes in glucoregulatory hormones. *J Clin Endocrinol Metab* 1978;47:1160.

2. Liljenquist JE, Mueller GL, Cherrington AD, *et al*: Hyperglycemia per se (insulin and glucagon withdrawn) can inhibit hepatic glucose production in man. *J Clin Endocrinol Metab* 1979;48:171.

3. Ward WK, Best JD, Halter JB, *et al*: Prolonged infusion of somatostatin with glucagon replacement increases plasma glucose and glucose turnover in man. *J Clin Endocrinol Metab* 1984;58:449.

4. Liljenquist JE, Mueller GL, Cherrington AD, *et al*: Evidence for an important role of glucagon in the regulation of hepatic glucose production in normal man. *J Clin Invest* 1977;59:369.

5. Wahren J, Efendic S, Luft R, *et al*: Influence of somatostatin on splanchnic glucose metabolism in postabsorptive and 60-hour fasted humans. *J Clin Invest* 1977;59:299.

6. Bagdade JD, Bierman EL, Porte D Jr: The significance of basal insulin levels in the evaluation of the insulin response to glucose in diabetic and nondiabetic subjects. *J Clin Invest* 1967;46:1549.

7. Perley MJ, Kipnis DM: Plasma insulin responses to oral and intravenous glucose: Studies in normal and diabetic subjects. *J Clin Invest* 1967;46:1954.

8. Felig P, Wahren J, Hendler R: Influence of maturity-onset diabetes on splanchnic glucose balance after oral glucose ingestion. *Diabetes* 1978;27:121.

9. Hollenbeck CB, Chen YD, Reaven GM: A comparison of the relative effects of obesity and non-insulin-dependent diabetes mellitus on in vivo insulin-stimulated glucose utilization. *Diabetes* 1984;33:622.

10. Holman RR, Turner RC: Maintenance of basal plasma glucose and insulin concentrations in maturity-onset diabetes. *Diabetes* 1979;28:227.

11. Halter JB, Graf RJ, Porte D Jr: Potentiation of insulin secretory responses by plasma glucose levels in man: Evidence that hyperglycemia in diabetes compensates for impaired glucose potentiation. *J Clin Endocrinol Metab* 1979;48:946.

12. Turner RC, McCarthy ST, Holman RR, et al: Beta-cell function improved by supplementing basal insulin secretion in mild diabetes. *Br Med J* 1976;1:1252.

13. Pfeifer MA, Halter JB, Porte D Jr: Insulin secretion in diabetes mellitus. *Am J Med* 1981;70:579.

14. O'Rahilly S, Turner RC, Matthews DR: Impaired pulsatile secretion of insulin in relatives of patients with non-insulin-dependent diabetes. *N Engl J Med* 1988;318:1225.

15. Polonsky KS, Given BD, Cauter EV: Twenty-four-hour profiles and patterns of insulin secretion in normal and obese subjects. *J Clin Invest* 1988;81:442.

16. Lang DA, Matthews DR, Burnett M, et al: Brief, irregular oscillations of basal plasma insulin and glucose concentrations in diabetic man. *Diabetes* 1981;30:435.

17. Polonsky KS, Given BD, Hirsch LJ, et al: Abnormal patterns of insulin secretion in non-insulin-dependent diabetes mellitus. *N Engl J Med* 1988;318:1231.

18. O'Meara NM, Sturis J, Van Cauter E, et al: Lack of control by glucose of ultradian insulin secretory oscillations in impaired glucose tolerance and in non-insulin-dependent diabetes mellitus. *J Clin Invest* 1993;92:262.

19. Bergstrom RW, Fujimoto WY, Teller DC, et al: Oscillatory insulin secretion in perifused isolated rat islets. *Am J Physiol* 1989;257:E479.

20. Ward WK, LaCava EC, Paquette TL, et al: Disproportionate elevation of immunoreactive proinsulin in type 2 diabetes and insulin resistance. *Diabetologia* 1987;30:698.

21. Yoshioka N, Kuzuya T, Matsuda A, et al: Serum proinsulin levels at fasting and after oral glucose load in patients with type 2 (non-insulin-dependent) diabetes mellitus. *Diabetologia* 1988;31:355.

22. Saad MF, Kahn SE, Nelson RG, et al: Disproportionately elevated proinsulin in Pima Indians with non-insulin-dependent diabetes mellitus. *J Clin Endocrinol Metab* 1990;70:1247.

23. Kahn SE, Leonetti DL, Prigeon RL, et al: Relationship of proinsulin and insulin with noninsulin-dependent diabetes mellitus and coronary heart disease in Japanese American men: impact of obesity. *J Clin Endocrinol Metab* 1995;80:1399.

24. Kahn SE, Halban PA: Release of incompletely processed proinsulin is the cause of the disproportionate proinsulinemia of NIDDM. *Diabetes* 1997;46:1725.

25. Mitrakou A, Kelley D, Mokan M, et al: Role of reduced suppression of glucose production and diminished early insulin release in impaired glucose tolerance. *N Engl J Med* 1992;326:22.

26. Kahn SE, Verchere CB, Andrikopoulos S, et al: Reduced amylin release is a characteristic of impaired glucose tolerance and type 2 diabetes in Japanese Americans. *Diabetes* 1998;47:640.

27. Cerasi E, Luft R, Efendic S: Decreased sensitivity of the pancreatic beta cells to glucose in prediabetic and diabetic subjects. A glucose dose-response study. *Diabetes* 1972;21:224.

28. Brunzell JD, Robertson RP, Lerner RL, et al: Relationships between fasting plasma glucose levels and insulin secretion during intravenous glucose tolerance tests. *J Clin Endocrinol Metab* 1976;42:222.

29. Metz SA, Halter JB, Robertson RP: Paradoxical inhibition of insulin secretion by glucose in human diabetes mellitus. *J Clin Endocrinol Metab* 1979;48:827.

30. Halter JB, Porte D Jr: Mechanisms of impaired acute insulin release in adult onset diabetes: Studies with isoproterenol and secretin. *J Clin Endocrinol Metab* 1978;46:952.

31. D'Alessio DA, Kahn SE, Leusner C, et al: Glucagon-like peptide 1 enhances glucose tolerance both by stimulation of insulin release and by increasing insulin-independent glucose disposal. *J Clin Invest* 1994;93:2263.

32. Varsano-Aharon N, Echemendia E, Yalow RS, et al: Early insulin responses to glucose and to tolbutamide in maturity-onset diabetes. *Metabolism* 1970;19:409.

33. Ward WK, Bolgiano DC, McKnight B, et al: Diminished B-cell secretory capacity in patients with non-insulin-dependent diabetes mellitus. *J Clin Invest* 1984;74:1318.

34. Røder ME, Porte D Jr, Kahn SE: Disproportionately elevated proinsulin levels reflect the degree of impaired B-cell secretory capacity in patients with non-insulin dependent diabetes mellitus. *J Clin Endocrinol Metab* 1988;83:604.

35. Gerich JE, Charles MA, Grodsky GM: Regulation of pancreatic insulin and glucagon secretion. *Annu Rev Physiol* 1976;38:353.

36. Unger RH, Aguilar-Parada E, Muller WA, et al: Studies of pancreatic alpha cell function in normal and diabetic subjects. *J Clin Invest* 1970;49:837.

37. Muller WA, Faloona GR, Aguilar-Parada E, et al: Abnormal alpha-cell function in diabetes. Response to carbohydrate and protein ingestion. *N Engl J Med* 1970;283:109.

38. Raskin P, Aydin I, Yamamoto T, et al: Abnormal alpha cell function in human diabetes: The response to oral protein. *Am J Med* 1978;64:988.

39. Westermark P, Wilander E: The influence of amyloid deposits on the islet volume in maturity onset diabetes mellitus. *Diabetologia* 1978;15:417.

40. Cooper GJS, Willis AC, Clark A, et al: Purification and characterization of a peptide from amyloid-rich pancreases of type 2 diabetic patients. *Proc Natl Acad Sci USA* 1987;84:8628.

41. Westermark P, Wernstedt C, Wilander E, et al: Amyloid fibrils in human insulinoma and islets of Langerhans of the diabetic cat are derived from a neuropeptide-like protein also present in normal islets. *Proc Natl Acad Sci USA* 1987;84:3881.

42. Lorenzo A, Razzaboni B, Weir GC, et al: Pancreatic islet cell toxicity of amylin associated with type-2 diabetes mellitus. *Nature* 1994;368:756.

43. Kahn SE, D'Alessio DA, Schwartz MW, et al: Evidence of cosecretion of islet amyloid polypeptide and insulin by β-cells. *Diabetes* 1990;39:634.

44. D'Alessio DA, Verchere CB, Kahn SE, et al: Pancreatic expression and secretion of human islet amyloid polypeptide in a transgenic mouse. *Diabetes* 1994;43:1457.

45. Verchere CB, D'Alessio DA, Palmiter RD, et al: Islet amyloid formation associated with hyperglycemia in transgenic mice with pancreatic beta cell expression of human islet amyloid polypeptide. *Proc Natl Acad Sci USA* 1996;93:3492.

46. Soeller WC, Janson J, Hart SE, et al: Islet amyloid-associated diabetes in obese Avy/a mice expressing human islet amyloid polypeptide. *Diabetes* 1998;47:743.

47. Höppener JW, Oosterwijk C, Nieuwenhuis MG, et al: Extensive islet amyloid formation is induced by development of Type II diabetes mellitus and contributes to its progression: Pathogenesis of diabetes in a mouse model. *Diabetologia* 1999;42:427.

48. Kahn SE, Verchere CB, D'Alessio DA, et al: Evidence for selective release of rodent islet amyloid polypeptide through the constitutive secretory pathway. *Diabetologia* 1993;36:570.

49. Gasa R, Gomis R, Casamitjana R, et al: High glucose concentration favors the selective secretion of islet amyloid polypeptide through a constitutive secretory pathway in human pancreatic islets. *Pancreas* 2001;22:307.

50. de Koning EJP, Morris ER, Hofhuis FM, et al: Intra- and extracellular amyloid fibrils are formed in cultured pancreatic islets of transgenic mice expressing human islet amyloid polypeptide. *Proc Natl Acad Sci USA* 1994;91:8467.

51. Janson J, Ashley RH, Harrison D, et al: The mechanism of islet amyloid polypeptide toxicity is membrane disruption by intermediate-sized toxic amyloid particles. *Diabetes* 1999;48:491.

52. Young ID, Ailles L, Narindrasorasak S, et al: Localization of the basement membrane heparan sulfate proteoglycan in islet amyloid deposits in type II diabetes mellitus. *Arch Pathol Lab Med* 1992;116:951.

53. Kahn SE, Andrikopoulos S, Verchere CB: Islet amyloid: A long-recognized but underappreciated pathological feature of type 2 diabetes. *Diabetes* 1999;48:241.

54. Ward WK, Wallum BJ, Beard JC, et al: Reduction of glycemic potentiation: A sensitive indicator of β-cell loss in partially pancreatectomized dogs. *Diabetes* 1988;37:723.

55. Leahy JL, Bonner-Weir S, Weir GC: Minimal chronic hyperglycemia is a critical determinant of impaired insulin secretion after an incomplete pancreatectomy. *J Clin Invest* 1988;81:1407.

56. Bonner-Weir S, Trent DF, Weir GC: Partial pancreatectomy in the rat and subsequent defect in glucose-induced insulin release. *J Clin Invest* 1983;71:1544.

57. Rossetti L, Shulman GI, Zawalich W, et al: Effect of hyperglycemia on in vivo insulin secretion in partially pancreatectomized rats. *J Clin Invest* 1987;80:1037.

58. Leahy JL, Bonner-Weir S, Weir GC: Abnormal insulin secretion in a streptozocin model of diabetes. Effects of insulin treatment. *Diabetes* 1985;34:660.

59. Giroix MH, Portha B, Kergoat M, et al: Glucose insensitivity and amino-acid hypersensitivity of insulin release in rats with non-insulin-dependent diabetes. A study with the perfused pancreas. *Diabetes* 1983;32:445.

60. Kahn SE, Klaff LJ, Schwartz MW, et al: Treatment with a somatostatin analog decreases pancreatic B-cell and whole body sensitivity to glucose. *J Clin Endocrinol Metab* 1990;71:994.

61. Robertson RP, Halter JB, Porte D Jr: A role for alpha-adrenergic receptors in abnormal insulin secretion in diabetes mellitus. *J Clin Invest* 1976;57:791.

62. Broadstone VL, Pfeifer MA, Bajaj V, et al: α-Adrenergic blockade improves glucose-potentiated insulin secretion in non-insulin-dependent diabetes mellitus. *Diabetes* 1987;36:932.

63. Ortiz-Alonso FJ, Herman WH, Zobel DL, et al: Effect of epinephrine on pancreatic β-cell and α-cell function in patients with NIDDM. *Diabetes* 1991;40:1194.

64. Dunning BE, Ahren B, Veith RC, et al: Galanin: A novel pancreatic neuropeptide. *Am J Physiol* 1986;251:E127.

65. Ahren B, Lindskog S, Tatemoto K, et al: Pancreastatin inhibits insulin secretion and stimulates glucagon secretion in mice. *Diabetes* 1988;37:281.

66. Holst JJ, Bersani M, Hvidberg A, et al: On the effects of human galanin in man. *Diabetologia* 1993;36:653.

67. Cooper GJS: Amylin compared with calcitonin gene-related peptide: Structure, biology, and relevance to metabolic disease. *Endocr Rev* 1994;15:163.

68. Robertson RP, Chen M: A role for prostaglandin E in defective insulin secretion and carbohydrate intolerance in diabetes mellitus. *J Clin Invest* 1977;60:747.

69. McRae JR, Metz SA, Robertson RP: A role for endogenous prostaglandins in defective glucose potentiation of nonglucose insulin secretagogues in diabetics. *Metabolism* 1981;30:1065.

70. Bonner-Weir S, Baxter LA, Schuppin GT, et al: A second pathway for regeneration of adult exocrine and endocrine pancreas. A possible recapitulation of embryonic development. *Diabetes* 1993;42:1715.

71. Clark A, Bown E, King T, et al: Islet changes induced by hyperglycemia in rats. Effect of insulin or chlorpropamide therapy. *Diabetes* 1982;31:319.

72. Leahy JL, Cooper HE, Weir GC: Impaired insulin secretion associated with near normoglycemia. *Diabetes* 1987;36:459.

73. Leahy JL, Weir GC: Evolution of abnormal insulin secretory responses during 48-h in vivo hyperglycemia. *Diabetes* 1988;37:217.

74. Kaiyala KJ, Prigeon RL, Kahn SE, et al: Reduced beta-cell function contributes to impaired glucose tolerance in dogs made obese by high-fat feeding. *Am J Physiol* 1999;277:E659.

75. Mittelman SD, Van Citters GW, Kim SP, et al: Longitudinal compensation for fat-induced insulin resistance includes reduced insulin clearance and enhanced β-cell response. *Diabetes* 2000;49:2116.

76. Brunzell JD, Lerner RL, Hazzard WR, et al: Improved glucose tolerance with high carbohydrate feeding in mild diabetes. *N Engl J Med* 1971;284:521.

77. Chen M, Bergman RN, Pacini G, et al: Pathogenesis of age-related glucose intolerance in man: Insulin resistance and decreased β-cell function. *J Clin Endocrinol Metab* 1985;60:13.

78. Chen M, Halter JB, Porte D Jr: The role of dietary carbohydrate in the decreased glucose tolerance of the elderly. *J Am Geriatr Soc* 1987;35:417.

79. Zhou YP, Grill VE: Long-term exposure of rat pancreatic islets to fatty acids inhibits glucose-induced insulin secretion and biosynthesis through a glucose fatty acid cycle. *J Clin Invest* 1994;93:870.

80. Zhou YP, Grill V: Long term exposure to fatty acids and ketones inhibits B-cell functions in human pancreatic islets of Langerhans. *J Clin Endocrinol Metab* 1995;80:1584.

81. Bollheimer LC, Skelly RH, Chester MW, et al: Chronic exposure to free fatty acid reduces pancreatic beta cell insulin content by increas-ing basal insulin secretion that is not compensated for by a corresponding increase in proinsulin biosynthesis translation. *J Clin Invest* 1998;101:1094.

82. Briaud I, Harmon JS, Kelpe CL, et al: Lipotoxicity of the pancreatic beta-cell is associated with glucose-dependent esterification of fatty acids into neutral lipids. *Diabetes* 2001;50:315.

83. Cnop M, Grupping A, Hoorens A, et al: Endocytosis of low-density lipoprotein by human pancreatic beta cells and uptake in lipid-storing vesicles, which increase with age. *Am J Pathol* 2000;156:237.

84. Ward WK, LaCava EC, Paquette TL, et al: Disproportionate elevation of immunoreactive proinsulin in type 2 (non-insulin-dependent) diabetes mellitus and experimental insulin resistance. *Diabetologia* 1987;30:698.

85. Kahn SE, Horber FF, Prigeon RL, et al: Effect of glucocorticoid and growth hormone treatment on proinsulin levels in humans. *Diabetes* 1993;42:1082.

86. Kahn SE, McCulloch DK, Schwartz MW, et al: Effect of insulin resistance and hyperglycemia on proinsulin release in a primate model of diabetes mellitus. *J Clin Endocrinol Metab* 1992;74:192.

87. Shiraishi I, Iwamoto Y, Kuzuya T, et al: Hyperinsulinaemia in obesity is not accompanied by an increase in serum proinsulin/insulin ratio in groups of human subjects with and without glucose intolerance. *Diabetologia* 1991;34:737.

88. Kahn SE, Beard JC, Schwartz MW, et al: Increased β-cell secretory capacity as mechanism for islet adaptation to nicotinic acid-induced insulin resistance. *Diabetes* 1989;38:562.

89. Persson B, Hanson U, Hartling SG, et al: Follow-up of women with previous GDM: insulin, C-peptide, and proinsulin responses to oral glucose load. *Diabetes* 1991;40(Suppl 2):136.

90. Kahn SE, Leonetti DL, Prigeon RL, et al: Proinsulin as a marker for the development of NIDDM in Japanese-American men. *Diabetes* 1995;44:173.

91. Mykkanen L, Haffner SM, Kuusisto J, et al: Serum proinsulin levels are disproportionately increased in elderly prediabetic subjects. *Diabetologia* 1995;38:1176.

92. Porte D Jr: β-Cells in type II diabetes mellitus. *Diabetes* 1991;40:166.

93. Taylor SI: Insulin action, insulin resistance, and type 2 diabetes mellitus. In: Scriver CR, Beaudet AL, Sly WS et al, eds. *The Metabolic and Molecular Bases of Inherited Disease.* McGraw-Hill:2001;1433.

94. Barroso I, Gurnell M, Crowley VE, et al: Dominant negative mutations in human PPARgamma associated with severe insulin resistance, diabetes mellitus and hypertension. *Nature* 1999;402:880.

95. Peiris AN, Sothmann MS, Hoffmann RG, et al: Adiposity, fat distribution, and cardiovascular risk. *Ann Intern Med* 1989;110:867.

96. Goodpaster BH, Kelley DE, Wing RR, et al: Effects of weight loss on regional fat distribution and insulin sensitivity in obesity. *Diabetes* 1999;48:839.

97. Cnop M, Landchild M, Vidal J, Havel PJ, Knowles NG, Carr DR, Wang F, Hull RL, Boyko EJ, Retzlaff BM, Walden CE, Knopp RH, Kahn SE: The concurrent accumulation of intra-abdominal and subcutaneous fat explains the association between insulin resistance and plasma leptin concentrations: Distinct metabolic effects of two fat compartments. *Diabetes* 2002;51:1005.

98. Best JD, Judzewitsch RG, Pfeifer MA, et al: The effect of chronic sulfonylurea therapy on hepatic glucose production in non-insulin-dependent diabetes. *Diabetes* 1982;31:333.

99. Kolterman OG, Gray RS, Shapiro G, et al: The acute and chronic effects of sulfonylurea therapy in type II diabetic subjects. *Diabetes* 1984;33:346.

100. Revers RR, Fink R, Griffin J, et al: Influence of hyperglycemia on insulin's in vivo effects in type II diabetes. *J Clin Invest* 1984;73:664.

101. Kolterman OG, Gray RS, Griffin J, et al: Receptor and postreceptor defects contribute to the insulin resistance in noninsulin-dependent diabetes mellitus. *J Clin Invest* 1981;68:957.

102. Baron AD, Schaeffer L, Shragg P, et al: Role of hyperglucagonemia in maintenance of increased rates of hepatic glucose output in Type II diabetics. *Diabetes* 1987;36:274.

103. Kelley D, Mokan M, Veneman T: Impaired postprandial glucose utilization in non-insulin-dependent diabetes mellitus. *Metabolism* 1994;43:1549.

104. Olefsky JM, Reaven GM: Insulin binding in diabetes. Relationships with plasma insulin levels and insulin sensitivity. *Diabetes* 1977;26:680.

105. DePirro R, Fusco A, Lauro R, *et al*: Erythrocyte insulin receptors in non-insulin-dependent diabetes mellitus. *Diabetes* 1980;29:96.

106. Garvey WT, Huecksteadt TP, Matthaei S, *et al*: Role of glucose transporters in the cellular insulin resistance of Type II non-insulin-dependent diabetes mellitus. *J Clin Invest* 1988;81:1528.

107. Pedersen O, Bak JF, Andersen PH, *et al*: Evidence against altered expression of GLUT1 or GLUT4 in skeletal muscle of patients with obesity or NIDDM. *Diabetes* 1990;39:865.

108. Kim YB, Nikoulina SE, Ciaraldi TP, *et al*: Normal insulin-dependent activation of Akt/protein kinase B, with diminished activation of phosphoinositide 3-kinase, in muscle in type 2 diabetes. *J Clin Invest* 1999;104:733.

109. Cusi K, Maezono K, Osman A, *et al*: Insulin resistance differentially affects the PI 3-kinase- and MAP kinase-mediated signaling in human muscle. *J Clin Invest* 2000;105:311.

110. Verdonk CA, Rizza RA, Gerich JE: Effects of plasma glucose concentration on glucose utilization and glucose clearance in normal man. *Diabetes* 1981;30:535.

111. Best JD, Taborsky GJ Jr, Halter JB, *et al*: Glucose disposal is not proportional to plasma glucose level in man. *Diabetes* 1981;30:847.

112. Mandarino LJ, Wright KS, Verity LS, *et al*: Effects of insulin infusion on human skeletal muscle pyruvate dehydrogenase, phosphofructokinase, and glycogen synthase. Evidence for their role in oxidative and nonoxidative glucose metabolism. *J Clin Invest* 1987;80:655.

113. Boden G, Ray TK, Smith RH, *et al*: Carbohydrate oxidation and storage in obese non-insulin-dependent diabetic patients. Effects of improving glycemic control. *Diabetes* 1983;32:982.

114. Wright KS, Beck-Nielsen H, Kolterman OG, *et al*: Decreased activation of skeletal muscle glycogen synthase by mixed-meal ingestion in NIDDM. *Diabetes* 1988;37:436.

115. Baron AD, Brechtel G, Wallace P, *et al*: Rates and tissue sites of non-insulin and insulin-mediated glucose uptake in humans. *Am J Physiol* 1988;255:E769.

116. Kahn SE, Prigeon RL, McCulloch DK, *et al*: The contribution of insulin-dependent and insulin-independent glucose uptake to intravenous glucose tolerance. *Diabetes* 1994;43:587.

117. Welch S, Gebhart SSP, Bergman RN, *et al*: Minimal model analysis of intravenous glucose tolerance test-derived insulin sensitivity in diabetic subjects. *J Clin Endocrinol Metab* 1990;71:1508.

118. Marshall S, Bacote V, Traxinger RR: Discovery of a metabolic pathway mediating glucose-induced desensitization of the glucose transport system. Role of hexosamine biosynthesis in the induction of insulin resistance. *J Biol Chem* 1991;266:4706.

119. Tobin BL, Finegood DT: Reduced insulin secretion by repeated low doses of STZ impairs glucose effectiveness but does not induce insulin resistance in dogs. *Diabetes* 1993;42:474.

120. Rabinowitz D, Zieler KL: Forearm metabolism in obesity and its response to intraarterial insulin: Characterization of insulin resistance and evidence for adaptive hyperinsulinism. *J Clin Invest* 1962;41:2173.

121. Kreisberg RA, Boshell BR, DiPlacido J, *et al*: Insulin secretion in obesity. *N Engl J Med* 1967;276:314.

122. Kashiwagi A, Bogardus C, Lillioja S, *et al*: In vitro insensitivity of glucose transport and antilipolysis to insulin due to receptor and postreceptor abnormalities in obese Pima Indians with normal glucose tolerance. *Metabolism* 1984;33:772.

123. Krotkiewski M, Björntorp P, Sjöstrom L, *et al*: Impact of obesity on metabolism in men and women. Importance of regional adipose tissue distribution. *J Clin Invest* 1983;72:1150.

124. Kolterman OG, Insel J, Saekow M, *et al*: Mechanisms of insulin resistance in human obesity: Evidence for receptor and post-receptor defects. *J Clin Invest* 1980;65:1272.

125. Evans DJ, Hoffmann RG, Kalkhoff RK, *et al*: Relationship of body fat topography to insulin sensitivity and metabolic profiles in premenopausal women. *Metabolism* 1984;33:68.

126. Kjeldsen H, Hansen AP, Lundbaek K: Twenty-four-hour serum growth hormone levels in maturity-onset diabetics. *Diabetes* 1975;24:977.

127. Hansen AP: Abnormal serum growth hormone response to exercise in maturity-onset diabetics. *Diabetes* 1973;22:619.

128. Vigneri R, Squatrito S, Pezzino V, *et al*: Growth hormone levels in diabetes: Correlation with the clinical control of the disease. *Diabetes* 1976;25:167.

129. Beard JC, Weinberg C, Pfeifer MA, *et al*: Interaction of glucose and epinephrine in the regulation of insulin secretion. *Diabetes* 1982;31:802.

130. Rizza RA, Cryer PE, Haymond MW, *et al*: Adrenergic mechanisms for the effects of epinephrine on glucose production and clearance in man. *J Clin Invest* 1980;65:682.

131. Deibert D, DeFronzo R: Epinephrine-induced insulin resistance in man. *J Clin Invest* 1980;65:717.

132. Linde J, Deckert T: Increase of insulin concentration in maturity-onset diabetics by phentolamine (Regitine) infusion. *Horm Metab Res* 1973;5:391.

133. Kobayashi M, Olefsky JM: Effects of streptozotocin-induced diabetes on insulin binding, glucose transport, and intracellular glucose metabolism in isolated rat adipocytes. *Diabetes* 1979;28:87.

134. Levy J, Gavin JR, Fausto A, *et al*: Impaired insulin action in rats with non-insulin-dependent diabetes. *Diabetes* 1984;33:901.

135. Rossetti L, Smith D, Shulman GI, *et al*: Correction of hyperglycemia with phlorizin normalizes tissue sensitivity to insulin in diabetic rats. *J Clin Invest* 1987;79:1510.

136. DeFronzo RA, Simonson D, Ferrannini E: Hepatic and peripheral insulin resistance: A common feature of type 2 (non-insulin-dependent) and type 1 (insulin-dependent) diabetes mellitus. *Diabetologia* 1982;23:313.

137. Lager I, Lonnroth P, von Schenck H, *et al*: Reversal of insulin resistance in type I diabetes after treatment with continuous subcutaneous insulin infusion. *Br Med J Clin Res Ed* 1983;287:1661.

138. Garvey WT, Olefsky JM, Griffen J, *et al*: The effect of insulin treatment on insulin secretion and insulin action in type II diabetes mellitus. *Diabetes* 1985;34:222.

139. Andrews WJ, Vasquez B, Nagulesparen M, *et al*: Insulin therapy in obese, non-insulin dependent diabetes induces improvements in insulin action and secretion that are maintained for two weeks after insulin withdrawal. *Diabetes* 1984;33:634.

140. Finegood DT, Hramiak IM, Dupre J: A modified protocol for estimation of insulin sensitivity with the minimal-model of glucose kinetics in patients with insulin-dependent diabetes. *J Clin Endocrinol Metab* 1990;70:1538.

141. Martin IK, Weber KM, Boston RC, *et al*: Effects of epinephrine infusion on determinants of intravenous glucose tolerance in dogs. *Am J Physiol* 1988;255:E668.

142. Kahn SE, Prigeon RL, McCulloch DK, *et al*: Quantification of the relationship between insulin sensitivity and B-cell function in human subjects. Evidence for a hyperbolic function. *Diabetes* 1993;42:1663.

143. Kahn SE, Larson VG, Beard JC, *et al*: Effect of exercise on insulin action, glucose tolerance and insulin secretion in aging. *Am J Physiol* 1990;258:E937.

144. Cerasi E: Potentiation of insulin release by glucose in man. I. Quantitative analysis of the enhancement of glucose-induced insulin secretion by pretreatment with glucose in normal subjects. *Acta Endocrinol* 1975;79:483.

145. Ward WK, Halter JB, Beard JC, *et al*: Adaptation of B and A cell function during prolonged glucose infusion in human subjects. *Am J Physiol* 1984;246:E405.

146. Warren K, Braasch J, Thurn C: Diagnosis and surgical treatment of carcinoma of the pancreas. *Curr Prob Surg* 1968;132:3.

147. Brooks JR: Operative approach to pancreatic carcinoma. *Semin Oncol* 1979;6:357.

148. Turner RC, Holman RR, Matthews D, *et al*: Insulin deficiency and insulin resistance interaction in diabetes: Estimation of their relative contribution by feedback analysis from basal plasma insulin and glucose concentrations. *Metabolism* 1979;28:1086.

149. Bjorkman O, Eriksson LS: Influence of a 60-hour fast on insulin-mediated splanchnic and peripheral glucose metabolism in humans. *J Clin Invest* 1985;76:87.

150. Bagdade JD, Bierman EL, Porte D Jr: Counter-regulation of basal insulin secretion during alcohol hypoglycemia in diabetic and normal subjects. *Diabetes* 1972;21:65.

151. Henry RR, Wallace P, Olefsky JM: Effects of weight loss on mechanisms of hyperglycemia in obese non-insulin-dependent diabetes mellitus. *Diabetes* 1986;35:990.

152. Savage PJ, Bennion LJ, Flock EV, *et al*: Diet-induced improvement of abnormalities in insulin and glucagon secretion and in insulin receptor binding in diabetes mellitus. *J Clin Endocrinol Metab* 1979;48:999.

153. Kosaka K, Kuzuya T, Akanuma Y, *et al*: Increase in insulin response after treatment of overt maturity-onset diabetes is independent of the mode of treatment. *Diabetologia* 1980;18:23.

154. Stanik S, Marcus R: Insulin secretion improves following dietary control of plasma glucose in severely hyperglycemic obese patients. *Metabolism* 1980;29:346.

155. Seltzer HS, Allen EW, Brennan MT: Failure of prolonged sulfonylurea administration to enhance insulogenic response to glycemic stimulus. *Diabetes* 1965;14:392.

156. Reaven G, Dray J: Effect of chlorpropamide on serum glucose and immunoreactive insulin concentration in patients with maturity onset diabetes mellitus. *Diabetes* 1967;16:487.

157. Pfeifer MA, Halter JB, Beard JC, et al: Insulin responses to nonglucose stimuli in non-insulin-dependent diabetes mellitus during a tolbutamide infusion. *Diabetes* 1982;31:154.

158. Judzewitsch RG, Pfeifer MA, Best JD, et al: Chronic chlorpropamide therapy of noninsulin-dependent diabetes augments basal and stimulated insulin secretion by increasing islet sensitivity to glucose. *J Clin Endocrinol Metab* 1982;55:321.

159. Grunberger G, Ryan J, Gorden P: Sulfonylureas do not affect insulin binding or glycemic control in insulin-dependent diabetes. *Diabetes* 1982;31:890.

160. Akiyoshi M, Kakei M, Nakazaki M, et al: A new hypoglycemic agent, A-4166, inhibits ATP-sensitive potassium channels in rat pancreatic beta-cells. *Am J Physiol* 1995;268:E185.

161. Gromada J, Dissing S, Kofod H, et al: Effects of the hypoglycaemic drugs repaglinide and glibenclamide on ATP-sensitive potassium-channels and cytosolic calcium levels in beta TC3 cells and rat pancreatic beta cells. *Diabetologia* 1995;38:1025.

162. Landgraf R, Bilo HJ, Muller PG: A comparison of repaglinide and glibenclamide in the treatment of type 2 diabetic patients previously treated with sulphonylureas. *Eur J Clin Pharmacol* 1999;55:165.

163. DeFronzo RA, Barzilai N, Simonson DC: Mechanism of metformin action in obese and lean noninsulin-dependent diabetic subjects. *J Clin Endocrinol Metab* 1991;73:1294.

164. Bailey CJ, Wilcock C, Day C: Effect of metformin on glucose metabolism in the splanchnic bed. *Br J Pharmacol* 1992;105:1009.

165. Prager R, Schernthaner G, Graf H: Effect of metformin on peripheral insulin sensitivity in non insulin dependent diabetes mellitus. *Diabetes Metab* 1986;12:346.

166. Frias JP, Yu JG, Kruszynska YT, et al: Metabolic effects of troglitazone therapy in type 2 diabetic, obese, and lean normal subjects. *Diabetes Care* 2000;23:64.

167. Mudaliar S, Henry RR: New oral therapies for type 2 diabetes mellitus: The glitazones or insulin sensitizers. *Annu Rev Med* 2001;52:239.

168. Oakes ND, Thalen PG, Jacinto SM, et al: Thiazolidinediones increase plasma-adipose tissue FFA exchange capacity and enhance insulin-mediated control of systemic FFA availability. *Diabetes* 2001;50:1158.

169. Kelly IE, Han TS, Walsh K, et al: Effects of a thiazolidinedione compound on body fat and fat distribution of patients with type 2 diabetes. *Diabetes Care* 1999;22:288.

170. Cavaghan MK, Ehrmann DA, Byrne MM, et al: Treatment with the oral antidiabetic agent troglitazone improves beta cell responses to glucose in subjects with impaired glucose tolerance. *J Clin Invest* 1997;100:530.

171. Prigeon RL, Kahn SE, Porte D Jr: Effect of troglitazone on B cell function, insulin sensitivity, and glycemic control in subjects with type 2 diabetes mellitus. *J Clin Endocrinol Metab* 1998;83:819.

172. Dubois M, Pattou F, Kerr-Conte J, et al: Expression of peroxisome proliferator-activated receptor gamma (PPARgamma) in normal human pancreatic islet cells. *Diabetologia* 2000;43:1165.

173. Herman WH, Morrow LA, Halter JB: Maladaptation of beta cell function to hyperglycemia in noninsulin-dependent diabetes mellitus. *Diabetes* 1988;37(suppl 1):5A.

174. Ballinger S, Shoffner J, Hedaya E, et al: Maternally transmitted diabetes and deafness associated with a 10.4 kb mitochondrial DNA deletion. *Nat Genet* 1992;1:11.

175. Kadowaki T, Kadowaki H, Mori Y, et al: A subtype of diabetes mellitus associated with a mutation of mitochondrial DNA. *N Engl J Med* 1994;330:962.

176. Tattersall R: Maturity-onset diabetes of the young: A clinical history. *Diabet Med* 1998;15:11.

177. Fajans SS, Bell GI, Polonsky KS: Molecular mechanisms and clinical pathophysiology of maturity-onset diabetes of the young. *N Engl J Med* 2001;345:971.

178. Kahn SE, Porte D Jr: B-cell dysfunction in type 2 diabetes: Pathophysiologic and genetic bases. In: Scriver CR, Beaudet AL, Sly WS, et al, eds. *The Metabolic and Molecular Bases of Inherited Disease.* McGraw-Hill:1999;1407.

179. Taylor SI, Accili D, Cama A, et al: Unusual forms of insulin resistance. *Annu Rev Med* 1991;42:373.

180. Taylor SI, Cama A, Accili D, et al: Mutations in the insulin receptor gene. *Endocr Rev* 1992;13:566.

181. Taylor SI: Lilly Lecture: Molecular mechanisms of insulin resistance. Lessons from patients with mutations in the insulin-receptor gene. *Diabetes* 1992;41:1473.

182. Donohue WL, Uchida I: Leprechaunism: A euphemism for a rare familial disorder. *J Pediatr* 1954;45:505.

183. Rosenberg AM, Haworth JC, Degroot GW, et al: A case of leprechaun-ism with severe hyperinsulinemia. *Am J Dis Child* 1980;134:170.

184. Rabson SM, Mendenhall EN: Familial hypertrophy of pineal body, hyperplasia of adrenal cortex and diabetes mellitus. *Am J Clin Pathol* 1956;26:283.

185. Gerich JE: The genetic basis of type 2 diabetes mellitus: Impaired insulin secretion versus impaired insulin sensitivity. *Endocr Rev* 1998;19:491.

186. Ferrannini E: Insulin resistance versus insulin deficiency in non-insulin-dependent diabetes mellitus: Problems and prospects. *Endocr Rev* 1998;19:477.

187. Vaag A, Henriksen J, Madsbad S, et al: Insulin secretion, insulin action, and hepatic glucose production in identical twins discordant for non-insulin-dependent diabetes mellitus. *J Clin Invest* 95:690.

188. Janssen RC, Bogardus C, Takeda J, et al: Linkage analysis of acute insulin secretion with GLUT2 and glucokinase in Pima Indians and the identification of a missense mutation in GLUT2. *Diabetes* 1994;43:558.

189. Elbein SC, Hasstedt SJ, Wegner K, et al: Heritability of pancreatic beta-cell function among nondiabetic members of Caucasian familial type 2 diabetic kindreds. *J Clin Endocrinol Metab* 1999;84:1398.

190. Lillioja S, Mott DM, Zawadzki JK, et al: In vivo insulin action is a familial characteristic in nondiabetic Pima Indians. *Diabetes* 1987;36:1329.

191. Gottlieb MS, Root HF: Diabetes mellitus in twins. *Diabetes* 1968;17:693.

192. Barnett AH, Eff C, Leslie RDG, et al: Diabetes in identical twins: A study of 200 pairs. *Diabetologia* 1981;20:87.

193. Newman B, Selby JV, King M-C, et al: Concordance for type 2 (non-insulin-dependent) diabetes mellitus in male twins. *Diabetologia* 1987;30:763.

194. Society JD: Diabetes mellitus in twins: A cooperative study in Japan. *Diabetes Res Clin Pract* 1988;5:271.

195. Kaprio J, Tuomilehto J, Koshenvuo M, et al: Concordance for type 1 (insulin-dependent) and type 2 (non-insulin-dependent) diabetes mellitus in a population-based cohort of twins in Finland. *Diabetologia* 1992;35:1060.

196. Harris MI, Hadden WC, Knowler WC, et al: Prevalence of diabetes and impaired glucose tolerance and plasma glucose levels in U.S. population aged 20–74 yr. *Diabetes* 1987;36:523.

197. Chiu KC, Province MA, Permutt MA: Glucokinase gene is genetic marker for NIDDM in American blacks. *Diabetes* 1992;41:843.

198. Shelton KD, Franklin AJ, Khoor A, et al: Multiple elements in the upstream glucokinase promoter contribute to transcription in insulinoma cells. *Mol Cell Biol* 1992;12:4578.

199. Stone LM, Kahn SE, Fujimoto WY, et al: A variation at position −30 of the B-cell glucokinase gene promoter is associated with reduced B-cell function. *Diabetes* 1996;45:422.

200. Elbein SC, Hoffman M, Chiu D, et al: Linkage analysis of the glucokinase locus in familial Type 2 diabetic pedigrees. *Diabetologia* 1993;36:141.

201. Zouali H, Vaxillaire M, Lesage S, et al: Linkage analysis and molecular scanning of glucokinase gene in NIDDM families. *Diabetes* 1993;42:1238.

202. Cook JTE, Hattersley AT, Christopher P, et al: Linkage analysis of glucokinase gene with NIDDM in caucasian pedigrees. *Diabetes* 1992;41:1496.

203. McCarthy MI, Hitchins M, Hitman GA, et al: Absence of linkage suggests a minor role for the glucokinase gene in the pathogenesis of Type 2 diabetes in South Indians. *Diabetologia* 1993;36:633.

204. McCarthy MI, Hitman GA, Hitchins M, *et al*: Glucokinase gene polymorphisms: A genetic marker for glucose intolerance in a cohort of elderly Finnish men. *Diabet Med* 1994;11:198.

205. Cook DL, Taborsky GJ Jr: B-cell function and insulin secretion. In: Porte D Jr, Sherwin RS, eds. *Diabetes Mellitus*. Appleton & Lange: 1997;49.

206. Inoue H, Ferrer J, Welling C, *et al*: Sequence variants in the sulfonylurea receptor (SUR) gene are associated with NIDDM in Caucasians. *Diabetes* 1996;45:825.

207. Hansen T, Echwald S, Hansen L, *et al*: Decreased tolbutamide-stimulated insulin secretion in healthy subjects with sequence variants in the high-affinity sulfonylurea receptor gene. *Diabetes* 1998; 47:598.

208. Matschinsky F: A lesson in metabolic regulation inspired by the glucokinase glucose sensor paradigm. *Diabetes* 1996;45:223.

209. Matsubara A, Tanizawa Y, Matsutani A, *et al*: Sequence variations of the pancreatic islet/liver glucose transporter (GLUTZ) gene in Japanese subjects with non-insulin-dependent diabetes mellitus. *J Clin Endocrinol Metab* 1995;80:3131.

210. Hager J, Hansen L, Vaisse C, *et al*: A missense mutation in the glucagon receptor gene is associated with non-insulin-dependent diabetes mellitus. *Nat Genet* 1995;9:299.

211. Fujisawa T, Ikegami H, Yamato E, *et al*: A mutation in the glucagon receptor gene (Gly40Ser): Heterogeneity in the association with diabetes mellitus. *Diabetologia* 1995;38:983.

212. Hart L, Stolk R, Jansen J, *et al*: Absence of the Gly40-Ser mutation in the glucagon receptor among diabetic patients in the Netherlands. *Diabetes Care* 1995;18:1400.

213. Gough S, Saker P, Pritchard L, *et al*: Mutation of the glucagon receptor gene and diabetes mellitus in the UK: Association or founder effect. *Hum Mol Genet* 1995;4:1609.

214. Ristow M, Busch K, Schatz H, *et al*: Restricted geographical extension of the association of a glucagon receptor gene mutation (Gly40Ser) with non-insulin-dependent diabetes mellitus. *Diabetes Res Clin Pract* 1996;32:183.

215. Odawara M, Tachi Y, Yamashita K: Absence of association between the Gly(40)Ser mutation in the human glucagon receptor and Japanese patients with non-insulin-dependent diabetes mellitus or impaired glucose tolerance. *Hum Genet* 1996;98:636.

216. Ogata M, Iwasaki N, Ohgawara H, *et al*: Absence of the Gly(40)Ser mutation in the glucagon receptor gene in Japanese subjects with NIDDM. *Diabetes Res Clin Pract* 1996;33:71.

217. Fujisawa T, Ikegami H, Babaya N, *et al*: Gly40Ser mutation of glucagon receptor gene and essential hypertension in Japanese. *Hypertension* 1996;28:1100.

218. Morris B, Chambers S: Hypothesis: Glucagon receptor glycine to serine missense mutation contributes to one in 20 cases of essential hypertension. *Clin Exp Pharmacol Physiol* 1996;23:1035.

219. Tonolo G, Melis M, Ciccarese M, *et al*: Glucagon receptor Gly40Ser amino acid variant in Sardinian hypertensive non-insulin-dependent diabetic patients. *Acta Diabetologica* 1997;34:75.

220. Mahtani M, Widen E, Lehto M, *et al*: Mapping of a gene for type 2 diabetes associated with an insulin secretion defect by a genome scan in Finnish families. *Nat Genet* 1996;14:90.

221. Ghosh S, Hauser ER, Magnuson VL, *et al*: A large sample of Finnish diabetic sib-pairs reveals no evidence for a non-insulin-dependent diabetes mellitus susceptibility locus at 2qter. *J Clin Invest* 1998;102:704.

222. Stern M, Duggirala R, Mitchell B, *et al*: Evidence for linkage of regions on chromosomes 6 and 11 to plasma glucose concentrations in Mexican Americans. *Genome Res* 1996;6:724.

223. Pratley R, Thompson D, Prochazka M, *et al*: An autosomal genomic scan for loci linked to prediabetic phenotypes in Pima Indians. *J Clin Invest* 1998;101:1757.

224. Valle T, Tumomilehto J, Bergman R, *et al*: Mapping genes for NIDDM. *Diabetes Care* 1998;21:949.

225. Hanis C, Boerwinkle E, Chakraborty R, *et al*: A genome-wide search for human non-insulin-dependent (type 2) diabetes genes reveals a major susceptibility locus on chromosome 2. *Nat Genet* 1996;13:161.

226. Horikawa Y, Oda N, Cox NJ, *et al*: Genetic variation in the gene encoding calpain-10 is associated with type 2 diabetes mellitus. *Nat Genet* 2000;26:163.

227. Cox NJ, Horikawa Y, Oda N, *et al*: Genetic variations in the calpain 10 gene affects susceptibility to type 2 diabetes in Mexican Americans. *Diabetes* 2000;40:A7.

228. Baier LJ, Permana PA, Yang X, *et al*: A calpain-10 gene polymorphism is associated with reduced muscle mRNA levels and insulin resistance. *J Clin Invest* 2000;106:R69.

229. Sherratt E, Thomas A, Alcolado J: Mitochondrial DNA defects: A widening clinical spectrum of disorders. *Clin Sci* 1997;92:225.

230. Ballinger S, Wallace D: Maternally transmitted diabetes and deafness. *Endocrinologist* 1995;5:104.

231. Velho G, Byrne M, Clement K, *et al*: Clinical phenotypes, insulin secretion, and insulin sensitivity in kindreds with maternally inherited diabetes and deafness due to mitochondrial tRNA Leu(UUR) gene mutation. *Diabetes* 1996;45:478.

232. Suzuki Y, Hata T, Miyaoka H, *et al*: Diabetes with the 3243 mitochondrial tRNA Leu(UUR) mutation. *Diabetes Care* 1996;19:739.

233. Oka Y, Katagiri H, Yazaki Y, *et al*: Mitochondrial gene mutation in islet cell antibody positive patients who were initially non-insulin-dependent diabetes. *Lancet* 1993;342:527.

234. Gebhart S, Shoffner J, Koontz D, *et al*: Insulin resistance associated with maternally inherited diabetes and deafness. *Metabolism* 1996; 45:526.

235. Kennedy ED, Maechler P, Wollheim CB: Effects of depletion of mitochondrial DNA in metabolism secretion coupling in INS-1 cells. *Diabetes* 1998;47:374.

236. Maechler P, Wollheim CB: Mitochondrial signals in glucose-stimulated insulin secretion in the beta cell. *J Physiol* 2000;529:49.

237. van den Ouweland J, Lemkes H, Ruitenbeek W, *et al*: Mutation in mitochondrial tRNA(Leu)(UUR) gene in a large pedigree with maternally transmitted type 2 diabetes mellitus and deafness. *Nat Genet* 1992;1:368.

238. Ciafaloni E, Ricci E, Shanske S, *et al*: MELAS: Clinical features, biochemistry, and molecular genetics. *Ann Neurol* 1992;31:391.

239. Katagiri H, Asano T, Ishihara H, *et al*: Mitochondrial diabetes mellitus: Prevalence and clinical characterization of diabetes due to mitochondrial tRNA Leu(UUR) gene mutation in Japanese patients. *Diabetologia* 1994;37:504.

240. Kameoka K, Isotani H, Tanaka K, *et al*: Novel mitochondrial DNA mutation in tRNA(Lys) (88296A-G) associated with diabetes. *Biochem Biophys Res Commun* 1998;245:523.

241. Tsukuda K, Suzuki Y, Kameoka K, *et al*: Screening of patients with maternally transmitted diabetes for mitochondrial gene mutations in the tRNA Leu(UUR) region. *Diabet Med* 1997;14:1032.

242. Harvey J, Barnett D: Endocrine dysfunction in Kearns-Sayre syndrome. *Clin Endocrinol* 1992;37:97.

243. Yamagata K, Furuta H, Oda N, *et al*: Mutations in the hepatocyte nuclear factor-4alpha gene in maturity-onset diabetes of the young (MODY1). *Nature* 1996;384:458.

244. Froguel P, Vaxillaire M, Velho G: Genetic and metabolic heterogeneity of maturity-onset diabetes of the young. *Diabetes Rev* 1997;5:123.

245. Byrne MM, Sturis J, Fajans SS, *et al*: Altered insulin secretory response to glucose in subjects with a mutation in the MODY 1 gene on chromosome 20. *Diabetes* 1995;44:699.

246. Chen WS, Manova K, Weinstein C, *et al*: Disruption of the HNF-4 gene, expressed in visceral endoderm, leads to cell death in embryonic ectoderm and impaired gastrulation of mouse embryos. *Genes Dev* 1994;8:2466.

247. Froguel P, Vaxillaire M, Sun F, *et al*: Close linkage of glucokinase locus on chromosome 7p to early-onset non-insulin-dependent diabetes mellitus. *Nature* 1992;356:162.

248. Matchinsky FM: Glucokinase as glucose sensor and metabolic signal generator in pancreatic beta-cells and hepatocytes. *Diabetes* 1990; 39:647.

249. Velho G, Blanche H, Vaxillaire M, *et al*: Identification of 14 new glucokinase mutations and description of the clinical profile of 42 MODY-2 families. *Diabetologia* 1997;40:217.

250. Bell G, Pilkis S, Weber I, *et al*: Glucokinase mutations, insulin secretion, and diabetes mellitus. *Annu Rev Physiol* 1996;58:171.

251. Byrne MM, Sturis J, Clement K, *et al*: Insulin secretory abnormalities in subjects with hyperglycemia due to glucokinase mutations. *J Clin Invest* 1994;93:1120.

252. Polonsky KS: The B-cell in diabetes: From molecular genetics to clinical research. *Diabetes* 1995;44:705.

253. Byrne M, Sturis J, Menzel S, *et al*: Altered insulin secretory responses to glucose in diabetic and nondiabetic subjects with mutations in the diabetes susceptibility gene MODY3 chromosome 12. *Diabetes* 1996; 45:1503.

254. Wajngot A, Alvarsson M, Glaser A, *et al*: Glucose potentiation of arginine-induced insulin secretion in subjects with a glucokinase Glu256Lys. *Diabetes* 1994;43:1402.

255. Tappy L, Dussoix P, Iynedjian P, *et al*: Abnormal regulation of hepatic glucose output in maturity-onset diabetes of the young caused by a specific mutation of the glucokinase gene. *Diabetes* 1997;46:204.

256. Katagiri H, Asano T, Ishihara H, *et al*: Nonsense mutation of glucokinase gene in late-onset non-insulin-dependent diabetes mellitus. *Lancet* 1992;340:1316.

257. Vaxillaire M, Boccio V, Philippi A, *et al*: A gene for maturity onset diabetes of the young (MODY) maps to chromosome 12q. *Nat Genet* 1995;9:418.

258. Frayling T, Bulman M, Ellard S, *et al*: Mutations in the hepatocyte nuclear factor-1alpha gene are a common cause of maturity-onset diabetes of the young in the U.K. *Diabetes* 1997;46:720.

259. Glucksmann M, Lehto M, Tayber O, *et al*: Novel mutations and a mutational hotspot in the MODY3 gene. *Diabetes* 1997;46:1081.

260. Velho G, Froguel P: Genetic, metabolic and clinical characteristics of maturity onset diabetes of the young. *Eur J Endocrinol* 1998;138:233.

261. Hattersley A: Maturity-onset diabetes of the young: Clinical heterogeneity explained by genetic heterogeneity. *Diabet Med* 1998;15:15.

262. Gragnoli C, Lindner T, Cockburn BN, *et al*: Maturity-onset diabetes of the young due to a mutation in the hepatocyte nuclear factor-4 α binding site in the promoter of the hepatocyte nuclear factor 1-α gene. *Diabetes* 1997;46:1648.

263. Velho G, Vaxillaire M, Boccio V, *et al*: Diabetes complications in NIDDM kindreds linked to the MODY3 locus on chromosome 12q. *Diabetes Care* 1996;19:915.

264. Stoffers DA, Ferrer J, Clarke WL, *et al*: Early-onset type-II diabetes mellitus (MODY 4) linked to IPF1. *Nat Genet* 1997;17:138.

265. Jonsson J, Carlsson L, Edlund T, *et al*: Insulin-promoter-factor 1 is required for pancreas development in mice. *Nature* 1994;371:606.

266. Stoffers DA, Zinkin NT, Stanojevic V, *et al*: Pancreatic agenesis attributable to a single nucleotide deletion in the human IPF-1 gene coding sequence. *Nat Genet* 1997;15:106.

267. Frayling TM, Evans JC, Bulman MP, *et al*: Beta-cell genes and diabetes: Molecular and clinical characterization of mutations in transcription factors. *Diabetes* 2001;50(suppl 1):S94.

268. Weng J, Macfarlane WM, Lehto M, *et al*: Functional consequences of mutations in the MODY4 gene (IPF1) and coexistence with MODY3 mutations. *Diabetologia* 2001;44:249.

269. Horikawa Y, Iwasaki N, Hara M, *et al*: Mutation in hepatocyte nuclear factor-1β gene (TCF2) associated with MODY. *Nat Genet* 1997; 17:384.

270. Nishigori H, Yamada S, Kohama T, *et al*: Frameshift mutation, A263fsinsGG, in the hepatocyte nuclear factor-1β gene associated with diabetes and renal dysfunction. *Diabetes* 1998;7:1354.

271. Lindner TH, Njolstad PR, Horikawa Y, *et al*: A novel syndrome of diabetes mellitus, renal dysfunction and genital malformation associated with a partial deletion of the pseudo-POU domain of hepatocyte nuclear factor-1beta. *Hum Mol Genet* 1999;8:2001.

272. Iwasaki N, Okabe I, Momoi MY, *et al*: Splice site mutation in the hepatocyte nuclear factor-1 beta gene, IVS2nt + 1G > A, associated with maturity-onset diabetes of the young, renal dysplasia and bicornuate uterus. *Diabetologia* 2001;44:387.

273. Betsholtz C, Christmansson L, Engstrom U, *et al*: Sequence divergence in a specific region of islet amyloid polypeptide (IAPP) explains differences in islet amyloid formation between species. *FEBS Lett* 1989;251:261.

274. Kadowaki T, Kadowaki H, Rechler MM, *et al*: Five mutant alleles of the insulin receptor gene in patients with genetic forms of insulin resistance. *J Clin Invest* 1990;86:254.

275. Wertheimer E, Lu SP, Backeljauw PF, *et al*: Homozygous deletion of the human insulin receptor gene. *Nat Genet* 1993;5:71.

276. Kadowaki T, Bevins CL, Cama A, *et al*: Two mutant alleles of the insulin receptor gene in a patient with extreme insulin resistance. *Science* 1988;240:787.

277. Kadowaki T, Kadowaki H, Taylor SI: A nonsense mutation causing decreased levels of insulin receptor mRNA: Detection by a simplified technique for direct sequencing of genomic DNA amplified by the polymerase chain reaction. *Proc Natl Acad Sci USA* 1990;87:658.

278. Kahn CR, Flier JS, Bar RS, *et al*: The syndromes of insulin resistance and acanthosis nigricans. Insulin-receptor disorders in man. *N Engl J Med* 1976;294:739.

279. De Fea K, Roth RA: Modulation of insulin receptor substrate-1 tyrosine phosphorylation and function by mitogen-activated protein kinase. *J Biol Chem* 1997;272:31400.

280. Moller DE, Flier J: Detection of an alteration in the insulin-receptor gene in a patient with insulin resistance, acanthosis nigricans, and the polycystic ovary syndrome (type A insulin resistance). *N Engl J Med* 1988;319:1526.

281. Wertheimer E, Litvin Y, Ebstein RP, *et al*: Deletion of exon 3 of the insulin receptor gene in a kindred with a familial form of insulin resistance. *J Clin Endocrinol Metab* 1994;78:1153.

282. Yoshimasa Y, Seino S, Whittaker J, *et al*: Insulin-resistant diabetes due to a point mutation that prevents insulin proreceptor processing. *Science* 1988;240:784.

283. Accili D, Frapier C, Mosthaf L, *et al*: A mutation in the insulin receptor gene that impairs transport of the receptor to the plasma membrane and causes insulin-resistant diabetes. *EMBO J* 1989;8:2509.

284. Roach P, Zick Y, Formisano P, *et al*: A novel human insulin receptor gene mutation uniquely inhibits insulin binding without impairing posttranslational processing. *Diabetes* 1994;43:1096.

285. Wertheimer E, Barbetti F, Muggeo M, *et al*: Two mutations in a conserved structural motif in the insulin receptor inhibit normal folding and intracellular transport of the receptor. *J Biol Chem* 1994;269:7587.

286. Brown MS, Goldstein JL: A receptor-mediated pathway for cholesterol homeostasis. *Science* 1986;232:34.

287. Kadowaki H, Takahashi Y, Ando A, *et al*: Four mutant alleles of the insulin receptor gene associated with genetic syndromes of extreme insulin resistance. *Biochem Biophys Res Commun* 1997;237:516.

288. Taira M, Hashimoto N, Shimada F, *et al*: Human diabetes associated with a deletion of the tyrosine kinase domain of the insulin receptor. *Science* 1989;245:63.

289. Imano E, Kadowaki H, Kadowaki T, *et al*: Two patients with insulin resistance due to decreased levels of insulin-receptor mRNA. *Diabetes* 1991;40:548.

290. Krook A, Brueton L, O'Rahilly S: Homozygous nonsense mutation in the insulin receptor gene in infant with leprechaunism. *Lancet* 1993; 342:277.

291. Psiachou H, Mitton S, Alaghband-Zadeh J, *et al*: Leprechaunism and homozygous nonsense mutation in the insulin receptor gene. *Lancet* 1993;342:924.

292. Hone J, Accili D, Psiachou H, *et al*: Homozygosity for a null allele of the insulin receptor gene in a patient with leprechaunism. *Hum Mutat* 1995;6:17.

293. Jospe N, Kaplowitz PB, Furlanetto RW: Homozygous nonsense mutation in the insulin receptor gene of a patient with severe congenital insulin resistance: Leprechaunism and the role of the insulin-like growth factor receptor. *Clin Endocrinol (Oxf)* 1996;45:229.

294. Accili D, Mosthaf L, Ullrich A, *et al*: A mutation in the extracellular domain of the insulin receptor impairs the ability of insulin to stimulate receptor autophosphorylation. *J Biol Chem* 1991;266:434.

295. Accili D, Kadowaki T, Kadowaki H, *et al*: Immunoglobulin heavy chain-binding protein binds to misfolded mutant insulin receptors with mutations in the extracellular domain. *J Biol Chem* 1992; 267:586.

296. Kadowaki T, Kadowaki H, Accili D, *et al*: Substitution of lysine for asparagine at position 15 in the alpha-subunit of the human insulin receptor. A mutation that impairs transport of receptors to the cell surface and decreases the affinity of insulin binding. *J Biol Chem* 1990; 265:19143.

297. Kadowaki T, Kadowaki H, Accili D, *et al*: Substitution of arginine for histidine at position 209 in the alpha-subunit of the human insulin receptor. A mutation that impairs receptor dimerization and transport of receptors to the cell surface. *J Biol Chem* 1991;266:21224.

298. Cama A, de la Luz Sierra M, Quon MJ, *et al*: Substitution of glutamic acid for alanine 1135 in the putative "catalytic loop" of the tyrosine kinase domain of the human insulin receptor. A mutation that impairs proteolytic processing into subunits and inhibits receptor tyrosine kinase activity. *J Biol Chem* 1993;268:8060.

299. Yoshimasa Y, Paul JI, Whittaker J, *et al*: Effects of amino acid replacements within the tetrabasic cleavage site on the processing of the human insulin receptor precursor expressed in Chinese hamster ovary cells. *J Biol Chem* 1990;265:17230.

300. Taouis M, Levy-Toledano R, Roach P, *et al*: Rescue and activation of a binding-deficient insulin receptor. Evidence for intermolecular transphosphorylation. *J Biol Chem* 1994;269:27762.

301. Taouis M, Levy-Toledano R, Roach P, *et al*: Structural basis by which a recessive mutation in the alpha-subunit of the insulin receptor affects insulin binding. *J Biol Chem* 1994;269:14912.

302. Odawara M, Kadowaki T, Yamamoto R, *et al*: Human diabetes associated with a mutation in the tyrosine kinase domain of the insulin receptor. *Science* 1989;245:66.

303. Carpentier JL, Paccaud JP, Gorden P, *et al*: Insulin-induced surface redistribution regulates internalization of the insulin receptor and requires its autophosphorylation. *Proc Natl Acad Sci USA* 1992;89:162.

304. Hedo JA, Simpson IA: Internalization of insulin receptors in the isolated rat adipose cell. Demonstration of the vectorial disposition of receptor subunits. *J Biol Chem* 1984;259:11083.

305. Kadowaki H, Kadowaki T, Cama A, *et al*: Mutagenesis of lysine 460 in the human insulin receptor. Effects upon receptor recycling and cooperative interactions among binding sites. *J Biol Chem* 1990;265:21285.

306. Cama A, Sierra ML, Kadowaki T, *et al*: Two mutant alleles of the insulin receptor gene in a family with a genetic form of insulin resistance: A 10 base pair deletion in exon 1 and a mutation substituting serine for asparagine-462. *Hum Genet* 1995;95:174.

307. McElduff A, Hedo JA, Taylor SI, *et al*: Insulin receptor degradation is accelerated in cultured lymphocytes from patients with genetic syndromes of extreme insulin resistance. *J Clin Invest* 1984;74:1366.

308. Flier JS: Lilly Lecture: Syndromes of insulin resistance. From patient to gene and back again. *Diabetes* 1992;41:1207.

309. Reddy SS, Kahn CR: Epidermal growth factor receptor defects in leprechaunism. A multiple growth factor-resistant syndrome. *J Clin Invest* 1989;84:1569.

310. Barnes ND, Palumbo PJ, Hayles AB, *et al*: Insulin resistance, skin changes, and virilization: A recessively inherited syndrome possibly due to pineal gland dysfunction. *Diabetologia* 1974;10:285.

311. Taylor SI, Accili D, Imai Y: Insulin resistance or insulin deficiency. Which is the primary cause of NIDDM? *Diabetes* 1994;43:735.

312. Ward WK, Johnston CL, Beard JC, *et al*: Abnormalities of islet B-cell function, insulin action, and fat distribution in women with histories of gestational diabetes: Relationship to obesity. *J Clin Endocrinol Metab* 1985;61:1039.

313. Ehrmann DA, Sturis J, Byrne MM, *et al*: Insulin secretory defects in polycystic ovary syndrome. Relationship to insulin sensitivity and family history of non-insulin-dependent diabetes mellitus. *J Clin Invest* 1995;96:520.

314. Kahn SE: Regulation of B-cell function in vivo: From health to disease. *Diabetes Rev* 1996;4:372.

Insulin Resistance

Jerrold M. Olefsky

Yolanta T. Kruszynska

In 1889 Mering and Minkowski[1] demonstrated that total pancreatectomy in dogs was followed by hyperglycemia, glycosuria, ketosis, and death. The similarity between this syndrome and diabetes mellitus was noted, and this suggested that diabetes mellitus was due to pancreatic deficiency. Following this, Banting and Best[2,3] published their classic studies in which they showed that the sequelae of total pancreatectomy could be controlled if dogs were treated with parenteral injections of a pancreatic extract obtained following ligation of the pancreatic ducts. Because of the enormous importance of these studies, most scientists in the field came to the conclusion that all human diabetes was entirely due to insulin deficiency. Despite this apparent consensus, it is important to realize that 27 years after the discovery of insulin, Himsworth[4] pointed out "that in the diabetic patient insulin appears to vary in efficiency at different times." He suggested that diabetes could be differentiated into "insulin sensitive" and "insulin insensitive" types on the basis of the blood glucose response to insulin administered immediately following an oral glucose load.

Continuing this line of investigation, Himsworth published the accumulated evidence in support of his notion that insulin insensitivity, and not insulin deficiency, was present in many patients with diabetes. He further suggested that the classification of patients with diabetes into two groups corresponded to the clinical forms of diabetes: patients who are insulin-sensitive tended to be ketosis-prone, while the middle-aged, nonketotic diabetic tended to be insulin-insensitive. In 1960 Yalow and Berson published their study of the immunoassay of endogenous plasma insulin in humans.[5] These results demonstrated that plasma insulin was indeed measurable in diabetic patients, and that on average, higher levels existed in the subjects with the adult-onset form of the disease. This term generally corresponds to the new classification of non-insulin-dependent (NIDDM) or type 2 diabetes mellitus (T2DM). On the basis of these results, they concluded "that the tissues of the maturity onset diabetic do not respond to insulin as well as the tissues of the non-diabetic subjects respond to insulin."

Since that time, plasma insulin levels have been measured many times under a variety of circumstances in diabetic patients. Rabinowitz and Zierler[6] provided the first direct evidence of insulin resistance in man when they demonstrated that intra-arterial administration of insulin produced significantly less glucose uptake by forearm muscle in obese subjects than in normal individuals. In addition, newer techniques have been devised to directly estimate *in vivo* insulin action in a number of clinical and pathophysiologic states. From these studies it is now clear that resistance to the action of insulin is a characteristic feature of human obesity and non-insulin-dependent, or type 2, diabetes mellitus. In addition to these common clinical conditions, insulin resistance is also present in several unusual but well-defined syndromes such as acromegaly and lipodystrophy. In this chapter, the general problem of insulin resistance and its mechanisms will be discussed, and then we will turn to specific issues related to obesity and diabetes mellitus. Relatively less attention will be paid to the unusual syndromes of insulin resistance.

GENERAL CONSIDERATIONS

Insulin is produced in the pancreatic β cell as the primary biosynthetic product preproinsulin. Preproinsulin is rapidly converted to proinsulin (MW $\sim$ 9000), most of which is cleaved into insulin (MW $\sim$ 6000) and C peptide with only about 5% remaining as proinsulin. Insulin is secreted in response to a number of stimuli with glucose being the most important. After a brief circulating time ($t_{1/2}$, 5–10 minutes), the hormone interacts with a specific receptor on target tissues to exert its biologic effects.

Insulin resistance is a state in which a given concentration of insulin produces a less than normal biologic response. Because one of insulin's major effects is to promote overall glucose metabolism, abnormalities of this action of insulin can lead to a number of important clinical and pathophysiologic states. Because insulin travels from the β cell through the circulation to the target tissue, events at any one of these loci can influence the ultimate action of the hormone. Therefore, it is useful to categorize insulin resistance according to known etiologic mechanisms (Table 22-1). In general, insulin resistance can be due to (1) an abnormal β-cell secretory product, (2) circulating insulin antagonists, or (3) a target tissue defect in insulin action. Subclassifications exist within each of these categories.

CAUSES OF INSULIN RESISTANCE

Abnormal β-Cell Secretory Product

Several patients have been described who secrete a structurally abnormal, biologically defective insulin molecule as a result of a mutation in the structural gene for insulin.[7–9] Others have been

TABLE 22-1. Causes of Insulin Resistance

Abnormal β-cell secretory product
   Abnormal insulin molecule
   Incomplete conversion of proinsulin to insulin
Circulating insulin antagonists
   Elevated levels of counterregulatory hormones,
     (e.g., growth hormone, cortisol, glucagon, or catecholamines)
   Elevated free fatty acid levels
   Anti-insulin antibodies
   Anti-insulin receptor antibodies
   Resistin
   Cytokines (TNF-α, interleukin 6)
Target tissue defects
   Insulin receptor defects
   Postreceptor defects

described with familial hyperproinsulinemia, caused by incomplete conversion of proinsulin to insulin within the β-cell secretory granule as a result of structural abnormalities at the proteolytic cleavage sites of the proinsulin molecule.[10,11] These syndromes are dealt with in more detail in Chaps. 3 and 21 and will not be discussed further here, except to note that they do not represent insulin-resistant states in the most common usage of the term. Thus in these syndromes it is the hormone that is abnormal and the patients are only resistant to their endogenous insulin and not to exogenous insulin.

Circulating Insulin Antagonists

Circulating antagonists may be hormonal or nonhormonal.

Hormonal Antagonists

Hormonal antagonists include all of the known counterregulatory hormones such as cortisol, growth hormone, glucagon, and catecholamines. Well-known clinical syndromes exist (Cushing's disease, pheochromocytoma, glucagonoma, acromegaly) in which elevated levels of these hormones can induce an insulin-resistant diabetic state (see Chap. 25). However, in the usual case of obesity or T2DM, excessive levels of counterregulatory hormones are not an important contributory factor to insulin resistance.

Glucocorticoids

It is well known that excess endogenous or exogenous glucocorticoids impair carbohydrate metabolism, and this is often referred to as *steroid diabetes*. This effect is perhaps best exemplified in patients with Cushing's syndrome. In these patients, carbohydrate tolerance is often impaired. However, fasting hyperglycemia and overt symptomatic diabetes occur in less than 20% of patients, and the abnormalities of carbohydrate tolerance are generally limited to those that can be elicited only through the stress of a glucose challenge. Analogous results are seen in patients who receive exogenous glucocorticoids. In a patient with normal baseline carbohydrate tolerance, the usual effect of glucocorticoid administration will be some degree of deterioration of the ability to respond to a glucose load. Analysis of glucose tolerance tests after treatment with glucocorticoids reveals increased plasma insulin values accompanied by only mild to moderate increases in glucose concentration.[12] This pattern of glucose intolerance—increased glucose concentrations in the face of increased insulin concentrations—is characteristic of an insulin-resistant state.

A number of mechanisms cause this decrease in insulin action, since glucocorticoids counteract the effects of insulin at several steps in glucose homeostasis. Hepatic glucose output increases in some patients with Cushing's syndrome,[13] as well as after infusion of cortisol,[14] and the liver becomes resistant to the normal suppressive effect of insulin on hepatic glucose output.[14] Glucocorticoids increase the activity of key hepatic gluconeogenic enzymes[15] and the release of gluconeogenic substrates (amino acids, lactate, and glycerol) from peripheral tissues.[16–18] Both increased substrate availability and increased hepatic ability to produce glucose from substrates are involved in the glucocorticoid-induced increase in hepatic glucose production. Furthermore, glucocorticoid treatment raises plasma glucagon levels,[16,19] which also augments hepatic glucose production. Glucocorticoids can also decrease peripheral glucose utilization.[14] Again, this effect is mediated through several mechanisms. Corticosteroids decrease the activity of the plasma membrane glucose transport system by decreasing the transport V_{max}.[20] They appear to do this by inhibiting the ability of insulin to mediate the recruitment, or translocation, of glucose transport proteins from the cell interior to the cell surface.[21] Additionally, some glucocorticoids can cause a decrease in insulin binding to receptors, both *in vivo* and *in vitro*; this is mediated through a decrease in both receptor affinity[22,23] and number.[22] *In vivo*, the effects of glucocorticoids that cause insulin resistance have been well documented using the glucose clamp technique; they reduce the effect of insulin at all insulin concentrations[14] and also markedly slow the rate of activation of insulin's *in vivo* biologic effects.[24] Insulin secretory abnormalities have also been reported after steroid treatment (see Chaps. 21 and 25).

Growth Hormone

Growth hormone is a well-recognized circulating insulin antagonist. In chronic excess it can lead to carbohydrate intolerance.[25] Acromegaly can be associated with hyperinsulinemia, glucose intolerance, and decreased effectiveness of exogenous insulin. In most cases of acromegaly, compensatory hyperinsulinemia is sufficient to prevent gross deterioration of glucose homeostasis. Thus mild abnormalities of glucose tolerance are the rule, and less than 20% of patients develop fasting hyperglycemia.[25] The mechanism underlying the anti-insulin effects of growth hormone has not been clearly elucidated, in part due to the multiplicity of cellular effects of growth hormone and the heterogeneity of circulating forms of the hormone. Although excess growth hormone clearly leads to an insulin-resistant state in the chronic situation, the acute effects of growth hormone on insulin action are less clear. For example, *in vitro* the acute effects of growth hormone can be anabolic and insulin-like. Early *in vivo* studies showed that infusion of growth hormone leads to hyperinsulinemia and higher plasma glucose levels after an oral glucose load, suggesting insulin resistance;[26] fasting plasma free fatty acid and ketone body levels are also increased despite the hyperinsulinemia.[26] Most studies have shown that growth hormone leads to an impairment of insulin-stimulated glucose uptake and may also impair insulin's ability to suppress hepatic glucose output.[25,27,28] These effects develop 2–12 hours after exposure to high growth hormone levels and are most marked at submaximally stimulating insulin concentrations.[27] An additional major effect of this hormone is to induce the production of insulin-like growth factor 1 (IGF-1), and IGF-1 has its own cellular effects. Finally, insulin secretory abnormalities have also been reported. For a more detailed discussion of this subject the reader is referred to Chaps. 21 and 25.

Catecholamines

Excessive levels of circulating catecholamines can also antagonize the effects of insulin, and several mechanisms are involved. Catecholamines can stimulate glucagon secretion (β-effect) and increase hepatic glucose production by direct stimulation of glycogenolysis and gluconeogenesis (α- and β₂-effect). In combination, these effects tend to cause hyperglycemia and are opposite to the actions of insulin. Additionally, catecholamines directly inhibit peripheral glucose uptake (β-effect), and this has been demonstrated both *in vitro* in isolated adipocytes[29] and *in vivo* using the glucose clamp technique.[30,31] It is also possible that in addition to direct insulin antagonistic effects, the β-adrenergic–induced augmentation of lipolysis[31] leads to a secondary fatty acid–induced decrease in glucose uptake, at least *in vivo*. Catecholamines also impair β-cell insulin secretion by an α-adrenergic effect (see Chaps. 9, 21, and 25)

Placental Lactogen

Lactogen is a placental-derived hormone that may be causally involved in the insulin resistance that develops during the late second and third trimesters of normal pregnancy. Other than its potential role in the development of gestational diabetes, this hormone has little relevance to obesity or T2DM. Its mechanisms of action are not understood.

Glucagon

Glucagon influences glucose metabolism by augmenting hepatic glycogenolysis and gluconeogenesis, and in this sense, glucagon can counteract some of insulin's effects. However, glucagon has no influence on insulin's ability to promote peripheral glucose metabolism and does not lead to a true state of insulin resistance. For a detailed discussion of glucagon action, the reader is referred to Chap. 7.

Nonhormonal Antagonists

Free Fatty Acids

Fasting plasma free fatty acid (FFA) levels tend to be higher in type 2 diabetic patients than in lean normal subjects, and suppression of FFA levels after meals is impaired. These abnormalities are more marked in type 2 diabetic patients with significantly impaired insulin secretion and in obese patients. Elevated FFA levels are also found in other insulin-resistant states such as cirrhosis, uremia, and sepsis. A number of years ago Randle and coworkers[32] showed that FFAs could compete with glucose for oxidative metabolism in skeletal muscle and heart muscle. They hypothesized that elevated circulating levels of FFAs could impair peripheral glucose use. Studies using the glucose clamp technique have confirmed that elevated FFAs can induce mild insulin resistance.[33–36] However, the intracellular mechanism may differ from that originally proposed.[32] Thus, according to Randle's hypothesis, the inhibition of glucose oxidation and glycolysis as a result of enhanced cellular FFA uptake would lead to increased intracellular glucose-6-phosphate levels, which in turn would inhibit the phosphorylation of incoming glucose and hence glucose uptake. It now appears that the decreased glucose uptake that develops after several hours of raised plasma FFA levels must involve additional direct effects of FFAs on insulin-stimulated glucose transport. Evidence for this comes from the finding that when plasma FFA levels were elevated during a hyperinsulinemic glucose clamp in normal subjects, gastrocnemius muscle glucose-6-phosphate levels progressively decreased instead of

increasing,[35] as did intracellular free glucose levels.[36] These findings strongly suggest that prolonged elevation of FFA levels impairs insulin-stimulated muscle glucose transport. Recent data indicate that the mechanism may involve FFA-induced defects at several early steps in the insulin signaling pathway, including decreased activation of phosphatidylinositol-3-kinase (PI-3-kinase), which is thought to be important for insulin's enhancement of glucose transport.[36,37] These effects of FFAs may be mediated by accumulation of long-chain fatty acyl coenzyme A.

Skeletal muscle also uses FFAs from intramuscular triglyceride depots. Increased circulating FFA levels might be expected to promote the accumulation of triglycerides within the muscle if their supply exceeds immediate energy needs. Skeletal muscle triglyceride levels in nondiabetic subjects correlate inversely with whole-body insulin sensitivity and are a better predictor of insulin sensitivity than either body mass index or percentage of body fat.[38,39] Muscle triglyceride levels are increased in type 2 diabetic patients.[40] Moreover, insulin-resistant offspring of type 2 diabetic patients have a much higher intramyocyte lipid content than do insulin-sensitive offspring matched for age, body mass index, physical activity, and percentage of body fat.[39,41]

Support for the hypothesis that increased availability of FFAs may contribute to insulin resistance and glucose intolerance also comes from studies using acipimox, a long-acting nicotinic acid analogue that potently inhibits lipolysis. When obese type 2 diabetic and nondiabetic subjects were treated with this drug, FFA levels were reduced well into the normal range, and this was associated with an improvement in oxidative and nonoxidative glucose metabolism. However, these were not normalized and the improvement in oral glucose tolerance was rather modest. Whether further improvements in glucose metabolism might be seen with prolonged treatment that normalizes hepatic and muscle fat levels as well as circulating FFA levels remains to be seen. FFAs also play an important role in the regulation of hepatic glucose output and may contribute to hepatic insulin insensitivity in obesity and T2DM. This is discussed later in this chapter. Available evidence indicates that increased FFAs may contribute to both hepatic and peripheral tissue insulin insensitivity, but that FFAs probably explain only a portion of the defect in carbohydrate metabolism that exists in T2DM.

Anti-Insulin Antibodies

Essentially all patients who receive animal-derived insulin for a long enough period of time eventually develop anti-insulin antibodies. In past years, insulin preparations were commonly a mixture of beef and pork insulins, and the antigenicity of these preparations has been related to the insulin as well as the impurities within the mixture. In more recent years, highly purified insulins have been available and these have proven to be much less antigenic. With the use of these newer preparations, the development of anti-insulin antibodies is much less of a problem than in the past. However, even with completely pure beef or pork insulin, some antigenicity would still exist, since there are structural differences between human and pork or beef insulin. Pork insulin differs from human insulin only at a single residue: B 30 is threonine in human and alanine in pork insulin. Beef insulin differs from human insulin at three amino acid residues, including the region of the intra-A-chain disulfide bridge, and this has a significant effect on the tertiary structure of beef insulin. This explains the reduced antigenicity of pork insulin versus beef, and most anti-insulin sera have a lower affinity for pork insulin compared with beef. With the more recent use of highly purified human insulin made by either recombinant or chemical methods, the problem of insulin antibodies has become even less of an issue, although low titers of insulin antibodies have been noted even in patients treated only with pure human insulin. The immunogenicity of an insulin preparation may be influenced by the route of insulin delivery. Thus insulin infused intraperitoneally appears to be more immunogenic than subcutaneously infused insulin.[42]

Although anti-insulin antibodies do not usually lead to a clinically significant insulin-resistant state, the presence of these antibodies alters the pharmacokinetics of insulin.[43,44] High titers of high-affinity antibodies can act as a reservoir for insulin by binding the hormone when it initially enters the circulation and later releasing it. This increases the half-life of circulating insulin[43,44] and prolongs the time course of insulin action.[45]

Anti-Insulin Receptor Antibodies

In a few well-documented cases, circulating endogenous immunoglobulins directed against the insulin receptor have been described in insulin-resistant diabetic patients.[46,47] This syndrome is extremely rare and is discussed in more detail later in this chapter. Possibly, patients will be discovered with antibodies against other critical proteins in the insulin action scheme, such as the glucose transporter.

Resistin

Resistin is a novel protein secreted by adipocytes that circulates in plasma and has been shown to antagonize some of the metabolic actions of insulin.[48] Levels decrease with prolonged fasting and increase with refeeding. Acute administration of resistin to normal mice resulted in higher blood glucose and insulin responses to an oral glucose load and a blunted hypoglycemic response to exogenous insulin. Conversely, administration of antiresistin antibody to mice that became insulin resistant and glucose intolerant on a high-fat diet resulted in improved insulin sensitivity and glucose tolerance. These findings, and the observation that plasma resistin levels were increased in the genetically obese *db/db* and *ob/ob* mice, and in mice that developed obesity and insulin resistance after 8 weeks on a high-fat diet,[48] suggest that resistin could provide a link between obesity, insulin resistance, and T2DM.

Other Insulin Antagonists

Over the years a variety of antagonist activities have been reported in plasma of type 2 diabetic subjects. However, none of these earlier "insulin resistance factors" have been isolated and chemically identified, and thus cannot be substantiated, although reports continue to appear.[49] One such factor is islet amyloid polypeptide (IAPP). IAPP has a high degree of homology to calcitonin gene–related peptide (CGRP), and is cosecreted with insulin from the islet β cell (see Chaps. 17 and 21). It can inhibit insulin-stimulated glucose uptake when pharmacologic doses are infused.[50,51] However, subsequent studies have shown no anti-insulin actions of IAPP at high physiologic doses.[52] Furthermore, transgenic mice have been produced that overexpress the human IAPP gene, leading to markedly elevated circulating concentrations of IAPP. These animals were not hyperglycemic, nor were they hyperinsulinemic or insulin resistant.[53] Based on these studies, it seems unlikely that circulating IAPP plays a significant role in causing insulin resistance in human disease. In fact, IAPP may have a beneficial role in glucose homeostasis because it inhibits postprandial glucagon secretion and gastric emptying.[51,54]

Cytokines

Cytokines such as tumor necrosis factor-α (TNF-α) and interleukin-6 (IL-6) may contribute to the insulin resistance associated with sepsis, cirrhosis, or other severe illness. Recent studies have raised the provocative idea that they may also play a role in the insulin resistance of obesity and T2DM.[55–57] TNF-α is produced in adipose tissue, and elevated amounts of TNF-α are produced in a variety of genetic forms of obesity in animal models.[55,57] *In vitro* studies have shown that TNF-α can impair insulin receptor signaling.[58] Furthermore, neutralization of TNF-α by *in vivo* administration of soluble TNF-α receptors or TNF-α antibodies greatly ameliorated the insulin resistance in obese animals.[55–57] However, in obese type 2 diabetic patients, intravenous infusion of an antibody that neutralizes TNF-α had no effect on insulin resistance.[56,59] Thus if excess adipocyte production of TNF-α in obesity contributes to insulin resistance, it probably does so not in an endocrine fashion, but in a local autocrine or paracrine fashion. This is an interesting hypothesis, but one which will require considerable future experimentation before the role of TNF-α in human pathophysiologic states characterized by insulin resistance will be fully understood.

IL-6 is another cytokine that has recently been suggested to play a role in the insulin resistance of obesity and type 2 diabetes.[60,61] IL-6 is produced by adipocytes as well as immune cells and circulating levels are increased in obesity and T2DM. As well as stimulating the hypothalamic-pituitary-adrenal axis, it also has direct effects on adipocyte metabolism. A C → G polymorphism at −174 in the IL-6 gene was found to be associated with higher IL-6 gene transcription and IL-6 secretion rates from adipocytes, and healthy carriers of this polymorphism had a twofold increase in fasting triglyceride and FFA levels. Postprandial FFA levels were also elevated.[62] Thus IL-6 could contribute to insulin resistance through its effects on adrenal steroid production or as discussed above through a chronic elevation of plasma FFA levels.

GENERAL CONSIDERATIONS OF INSULIN ACTION

Before considering cellular causes of insulin resistance, it is useful to review some of the general concepts concerning normal and abnormal insulin action. Figure 22-1 presents a schematic diagram of cellular insulin action. The first step involves binding of insulin to specific cell surface receptors. The amino acid sequence of the receptor has been deduced from the cloned insulin receptor cDNA and consists of two identical α subunits and two β subunits, all linked together by disulfide bonds to form the full heterotetrameric structure.[63–66] The α subunits are entirely extracellular, whereas the β subunits have an extracellular, transmembrane, and cytoplasmic domain. The α subunit contains the insulin binding site, and after the hormone binds, a transmembrane signal is generated which initiates the insulin action program. The first known event following binding of insulin to its receptor is stimulation of a tyrosine kinase enzymatic activity intrinsic to the β subunit. Once activated, the β subunit undergoes an autocatalytic reaction (autophosphorylation) in which specific tyrosine residues within the subunit are phosphorylated.[64–67] As a result of autophosphorylation the tyrosine kinase activity of the receptor β subunit is enhanced[64–67] such that it can now phosphorylate tyrosine residues on endogenous phosphoprotein substrates, such as insulin receptor substrate-1 (IRS-1) (see below). A substantial body of evidence has accumulated indicating

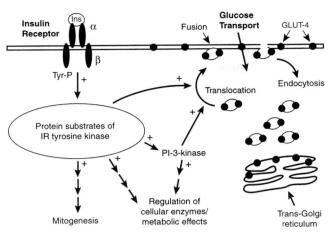

FIGURE 22-1. Model of insulin action. Abnormalities can occur at the pre-receptor phase, involving biosynthesis and secretion of abnormal β-cell products; at the receptor binding phase, involving decreased insulin binding to receptors due to decreased receptor number or affinity; or at the postreceptor binding phase, involving any defect in the insulin action cascade distal to the initial binding event.

that the receptor kinase is a critical initial step in a variety of insulin's biologic effects. For example, it has been shown by site-directed mutagenesis of the insulin receptor cDNA that a kinase-defective mutant insulin receptor can be made which, after transfection into host cells, is incapable of mediating insulin's bioeffects.[66,68,69] Additionally, intracellular injection of antiphosphotyefrosine antibodies effectively blocks insulin action.[70]

Activation of the receptor initiates a signaling cascade which culminates in the metabolic and growth effects of insulin. Considerable progress has been made in elucidating the mechanisms by which the insulin signal is transmitted downstream from the activated insulin receptor to the various insulin-regulated enzymes, transporters, and insulin-responsive genes (Fig. 22-1). This complex and rapidly evolving field is discussed only briefly as it is covered in detail in Chap. 5. A number of cytosolic protein substrates of the insulin receptor kinase have been reported. The first of these to be identified as a key player in the insulin signaling pathway was insulin receptor substrate-1 (IRS-1).[66,67] It belongs to a growing family of proteins that also includes IRS-2, IRS-3, IRS-4, and a protein called shc. All of these are immediate substrates of the insulin receptor kinase and are involved in insulin signaling in different cells. A shared characteristic of these proteins is that they have no enzymatic activity, but instead act as docking proteins. Thus when tyrosine phosphorylates, they can associate with other proteins that contain src homology-2 (SH2) domains.[66,67] The latter are sequences of approximately 100 amino acids that can bind to specific short sequences that encompass a phosphotyrosine moiety. When specific SH2 domain–containing downstream signaling proteins bind to tyrosine phosphorylated IRS proteins or shc, a large multicomponent signaling complex is formed, leading ultimately to the modulation of the activities of lipid kinases, serine and threonine kinases, and phosphatases that act on insulin-regulated enzymes and transcription factors. Recent evidence indicates that insulin receptors can phosphorylate Gαq/11, which would provide a mechanism for modulation of G protein signaling to glucose transport.[71] It is now clear that a number of signaling pathways diverge at different points in the insulin action cascade. For example, the

mitogenic and metabolic actions of insulin are mediated by distinct pathways downstream of the insulin receptor kinase, and even a single action of insulin, such as activation of glucose transport, may involve more than one signaling pathway.[72] Although tyrosine phosphorylation is a critical early step in insulin action, other signaling processes may either modulate the phosphorylation mechanism or separately mediate specific insulin effects. These may include the generation of various second messengers such as diacylglycerol, phosphoinositide-glycans, or changes in ion flux, G proteins, and the like.[73]

Regardless of the precise nature of the signaling mechanism, it eventually interacts with a variety of effector units, which mediate the entire host of biological actions attributable to insulin. In many instances the effector unit consists of a series of steps such as a sequentially linked enzyme system (the glycogen synthase/phosphorylase system) or a series of enzymes involved in the degradation of a particular substrate (glucose). Clearly, insulin action involves a cascade of events, and abnormalities anywhere along this sequence can lead to insulin resistance. For convenience, cellular abnormalities in insulin action can be categorized under the headings of binding and postbinding defects.

Decreased cellular insulin receptors have been described in a variety of pathophysiologic situations. The most common of these are obesity[74–76] and T2DM.[75–79] Decreased insulin receptors have also been described in acromegaly,[80] following glucocorticoid[81] or oral contraceptive therapy,[82] and in several other less common conditions.[83,84] Since the first step in insulin action involves binding to the receptor, it is apparent that a decrease in cellular insulin receptors could lead to insulin resistance. However, this potential relationship is not as clear as it would seem because insulin target tissues possess "spare" receptors.[85,86]

The spare receptor concept is based on the observation that a maximal insulin effect is achieved at a concentration of insulin at which less than the total number of cellular receptors are occupied. For example, for glucose transport in adipocytes and muscle, maximal response is achieved with only 10–20% of the receptors occupied. Thus 80–90% of the normal complement of receptors are "spare." All of these spare receptors are potentially fully functional, but which receptors are occupied at any given time is purely a random event; any group of occupied receptors amounting to 10–20% of the total would lead to the same metabolic response. Therefore, the cellular response to increasing insulin concentration is a continuous increase in receptor occupancy and biologic action until the critical number of occupied receptors needed to generate a maximal response is reached. Further increases in the prevailing insulin concentration beyond this point lead to a continued increase in receptor occupancy with no further increase in biological response, since a step distal to the receptor is now rate-limiting. The predicted functional consequence of a decrease in the number of receptors is a rightward shift in the dose–response curve for insulin action (i.e., a decreased response at lower insulin concentrations, but a normal response at maximally effective hormone concentrations).[76,85,87] This is illustrated in Fig. 22-2. The degree of rightward shift of the insulin dose–response curve is proportional to the decrease in the number of receptors. The only time a decrease in the number of insulin receptors can lead to a decrease in maximal insulin action is when less than 10–20% of the original receptor complement is present (Fig. 22-2). The proportion of spare receptors varies according to cell type and is also dependent upon which action of insulin is measured.

EFFECT OF RECEPTOR LOSS ON INSULIN DOSE–RESPONSE CURVE

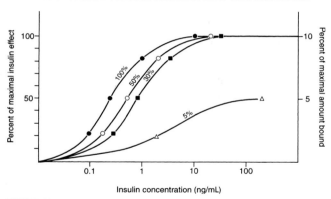

FIGURE 22-2. Predicted functional consequence of a progressive loss of insulin receptors on the insulin biologic function dose–response curve. Results represent theoretical dose–response curves in which the percentage of the maximal insulin effect (**left axis**) and the percentage of the normal maximal amount bound (**right axis**) are plotted as a function of insulin concentration. With progressive receptor loss, the dose–response curves are increasingly shifted to the right with no change in maximal insulin action, although more insulin is necessary to elicit a maximal insulin response. If enough receptors are lost (95%) so that 5% of the original receptor complement is present, both a rightward shift in the dose–response curve and a decrease in maximal insulin response occur.

It is apparent that the overall scheme of insulin action represents a multistep sequence in which the binding of insulin to receptors is only the initial event. A defect in any of the effector systems distal to receptor binding can also lead to impaired insulin action and insulin resistance. These defects can involve abnormal coupling between insulin-receptor complexes and the effector system (e.g., glucose transport), decreased activity of the effector system *per se*, or a variety of intracellular enzymatic defects. In this context the term *postbinding defect* refers to any abnormality in the insulin action sequence following the initial insulin-receptor binding event. This defect could include an abnormality of the insulin receptor that does not affect insulin binding but does affect the transmembrane signaling function of the receptor (e.g., β-subunit kinase activity), or any defect in the insulin action sequence distal to the receptor. The latter can be termed a *postreceptor defect* and generally refers to abnormalities in effector proteins such as the glucose transporter or target enzymes. The most common type of postreceptor defect leads to a proportionate decrease in insulin action at all insulin concentrations, including maximally effective hormone levels.[76,87] Thus a decrease in the capacity of a rate-limiting step in the insulin action–glucose metabolism scheme leads to a reduction in the maximal insulin effect, and this defect cannot be overcome by the addition of more insulin.

On the basis of our understanding of normal insulin action, the effects of binding versus postbinding defects on the *in vivo* insulin biologic function dose–response curve can be predicted, and by studying the insulin dose–response curve in insulin-resistant states the following distinctions, which are summarized in Fig. 22-3, can be made.

1. An isolated decrease in the number of insulin receptors leads to a rightward shift in the insulin dose–response curve with no

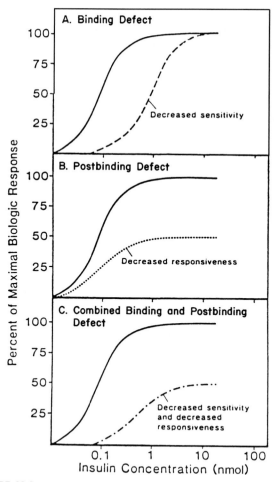

FIGURE 22-3. Theoretical insulin biologic action dose–response curves. **A.** Binding defect (this includes decreased insulin binding and/or decreased coupling of insulin binding to biologic responses). **B.** Isolated postbinding defects. **C.** A combined binding and postbinding defect.

change in maximal insulin action, and this is termed *a decrease in insulin sensitivity* (Fig. 22-3A). Certain kinds of postbinding defects involving the coupling mechanisms can also lead to rightward-shifted dose–response curves, leading to decreased insulin sensitivity.

2. A pure postreceptor defect in insulin action usually leads to a proportionate reduction in biological effects at all insulin concentrations. This is termed *a decrease in insulin responsiveness* (Fig. 22-3B).

3. If both a receptor and a postreceptor defect coexist, the dose–response curve shifts to the right and maximal insulin responsiveness decreases (Fig. 22-3C).

Hereafter, the terms *decreased insulin sensitivity* and *decreased insulin responsiveness* will be used in relation to the concepts depicted in Fig. 22-3.[87] One caveat when applying these concepts to *in vivo* insulin action is important to keep in mind: the heterogeneous nature of the system under study *in vivo*.

IN VIVO INSULIN RESISTANCE IN T2DM AND OBESITY

Type 2 Diabetes

Pathogenesis and Etiology

Before beginning a detailed discussion of the insulin resistance in T2DM, it is useful to put this metabolic defect into perspective by examining the overall pathophysiology of this disease. Figure 22-4 summarizes the physiologic abnormalities commonly seen in patients with T2DM. Although this is a genetically heterogeneous disease, once the diabetic syndrome is fully manifest, there is a final common metabolic pathway for the pathogenesis of hyperglycemia which involves defects in the liver, in the pancreatic islets, and in peripheral target tissues, particularly skeletal muscle.[88–91] As shown in Fig. 22-4, increased basal hepatic glucose production is characteristic of essentially all type 2 diabetic patients with fasting hyperglycemia.[88,92–94] Skeletal muscle is depicted as the prototypical peripheral insulin target tissue, because in the *in vivo* insulin-stimulated state, 70–80% of all glucose uptake is into skeletal muscle. Target tissues are insulin resistant in T2DM, and this is a characteristic feature of this disease, seen in essentially all population groups studied. Lastly, abnormal islet cell function plays a central role in the eventual development of hyperglycemia in T2DM; decreased β-cell function and increased glucagon secretion are also frequently present in the diabetic state. Taken together, abnormalities in these three organ systems account for the full-blown syndrome of T2DM.

Figure 22-4 represents a pathophysiologic view at a single point in time after overt type 2 diabetes has developed. However, such a description does not provide insight into the natural history of the disease. The disorder is progressive, evolving in stages, as depicted in Fig. 22-5. Whether or not the insulin resistance of T2DM is a primary or a secondary phenomenon has been the subject of intense study in recent years. To answer this question, various prediabetic populations have been examined prospectively.[95–98] In these studies, conducted in a wide variety of ethnic populations, it has been reported that insulin resistance and hyperinsulinemia exist in the prediabetic state, many years before T2DM supervenes. At this stage, insulin secretion in response to intravenous glucose is also often increased.[95,97–99] Thus, while acquired factors, such as obesity and a sedentary lifestyle, may be additive, insulin resistance is likely to be a primary inherited component of the disease in most patients. In the presence of primary insulin resistance, if β-cell function is normal, hyperinsulinemia ensues with maintenance of relatively normal glucose homeostasis. Impaired glucose tolerance (IGT) eventually develops in a subpopulation of individuals with compensated insulin resistance. Those with IGT also typically have fasting and postprandial hyperinsulinemia, but this is not sufficient to fully compensate for insulin resistance. This may be because they have a more profound degree of insulin resistance or because of a limited ability to augment their insulin secretion rates.[100] Although some subjects with IGT may revert to normal glucose tolerance, many will progress to overt T2DM. The proportion of insulin-resistant subjects who progress to T2DM depends on the particular ethnic group studied. In most populations the rate of progression of IGT to type 2 diabetes is 2–6% per year over 10 years.[101] Those who progress to T2DM display a marked decline in insulin secretion. The etiology of this decrease in β-cell function is not known. It may result from preprogrammed genetic abnormalities and/or from acquired insults such as that caused by the chronic effects of mild hyperglycemia or elevated FFA levels, commonly referred to as glucotoxicity and lipotoxicity,

FIGURE 22-4. Summary of the metabolic abnormalities in type 2 diabetes mellitus (T2DM) that contribute to hyperglycemia. Increased hepatic glucose production, impaired insulin secretion, and insulin resistance due to receptor and postreceptor defects all combine to generate the hyperglycemic state.

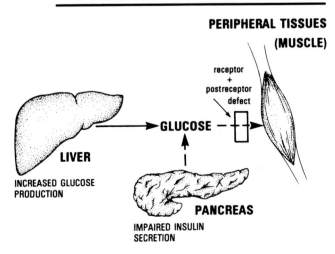

CAUSES OF HYPERGLYCEMIA IN NIDDM

FIGURE 22-5. Proposed etiology for the development of type 2 diabetes mellitus. HGO = hepatic glucose output.

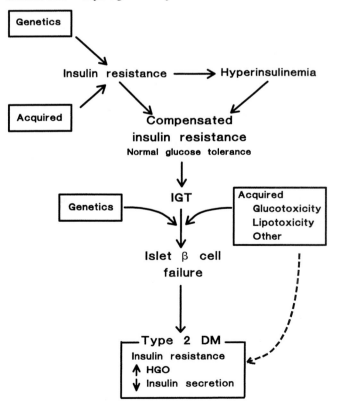

respectively. It could also result from an inherited susceptibility to the effects of chronic hyperglycemia or elevated FFA levels. Regardless of the etiology, this decrease in insulin secretion is a major contributor to the development of the overt type 2 diabetic state.

The contribution of genetics to the etiology of T2DM is well accepted,[102] and is demonstrated by studies showing a greater than 90% concordance rate for T2DM in identical twins.[103] In addition, the incidence of T2DM is much higher in individuals with first-degree relatives with the disease.[104] Given this strong genetic component to T2DM and that insulin resistance predates the development of T2DM in most populations, it is likely that insulin resistance is an inherited initial lesion in most patients. However, considerable data also exist that indicate that the magnitude of the insulin resistance is greater in T2DM than it is in the prediabetic IGT state. Although not all reports agree with this conclusion, most do. For example, Eriksson and colleagues showed that offspring of type 2 diabetic parents are insulin resistant.[96] When they divided the cohort of offspring into weight- and age-matched groups with normal glucose tolerance (NGT), IGT, and T2DM, they found that the hyperglycemic diabetic offspring were more insulin resistant than the NGT or IGT groups. Perhaps more compelling is the work by Vaag and associates, who studied monozygotic twins in which only one twin had T2DM.[105] They found that the nondiabetic twins were insulin resistant compared to matched controls, but that the diabetic twins were considerably more insulin resistant. Obviously, these subjects were well matched for genetic influences as well as other factors. These studies are quite consistent with population-based results showing that type 2 diabetic subjects are more insulin resistant than those with IGT.[93] Thus one can propose that once T2DM develops, some factor creates a secondary component of insulin resistance that is additive to the component that existed in the prediabetic state. There is strong evidence that hyperglycemia *per se* plays a role and that elevated glucose levels can cause insulin resistance or exacerbate an underlying insulin-resistant state.[106,107]

For example, poorly controlled type 1 diabetic patients are insulin resistant,[106,108] as are alloxan diabetic dogs[109] and pancreatectomized diabetic rats.[110] The insulin resistance in recently diagnosed type 1 diabetic patients is completely reversed by intensive insulin therapy,[106,108] and in pancreatectomized diabetic rats it is normalized by controlling the hyperglycemia via phlorhizin-mediated renal glycosuria.[110] In more direct experiments, when well-controlled type 1 diabetic patients were infused with glucose, whole-body insulin sensitivity, forearm glucose uptake, and muscle glycogen deposition were all reduced by approximately 35% after blood glucose had been maintained at 20 mmol/L (360 mg/dL) for a period of 24 hours.[111] In specific regard to T2DM, it has been shown that tight glycemic control achieved by intensive insulin therapy improves peripheral tissue insulin sensitivity by 17–75% in various studies.[107,112,113] Other forms of treatment which improve glycemia are also associated with partial restoration of insulin sensitivity in T2DM.[78,107,114–116] The most likely cause of this reversible component of insulin resistance is hyperglycemia-mediated glucotoxicity, although other factors associated with the poorly controlled hyperglycemic state such as elevated FFA levels may also play a role.

From the foregoing it can be concluded that in established T2DM there are two components to insulin resistance. The first is a primary, probably inherited abnormality, and the second is an acquired component, most likely due to hyperglycemia-related toxicity. In this way, a vicious cycle is created in which hyperglycemia begets more hyperglycemia.

As discussed above, insulin resistance is also a characteristic feature of subjects with IGT.[76,88–90] In general, subjects with IGT have less severe insulin resistance than patients with overt T2DM.[76,77,96,105] Furthermore, as the degree of carbohydrate intolerance worsens, the frequency of insulin resistance increases.[77] Thus many, but not all, subjects with IGT are insulin resistant, while essentially every type 2 diabetic patient with significant fasting hyperglycemia displays this abnormality. Obesity, particularly when it is centrally distributed, is a well-known condition also associated with insulin resistance. Since most adult type 2 diabetic patients are overweight, obesity-induced insulin resistance is thought to be a contributing factor in the hyperglycemia of these patients. However, obesity does not account for all of the insulin resistance in this type of diabetic patient, since the insulin resistance exceeds that caused by obesity alone, and nonobese type 2 diabetic patients are also insulin resistant.[88–90,117]

In Vivo Studies of Insulin Sensitivity

All methods of assessing insulin action *in vivo* rely, in one way or another, on measurement of the ability of a fixed dose or concentration of insulin to promote glucose disposal. Thus a blunted decline in the plasma glucose concentration following intravenous insulin in T2DM has been demonstrated.[117,118] One approach to quantifying insulin sensitivity has been to infuse insulin and glucose at fixed rates while endogenous insulin secretion is inhibited by either a combination of epinephrine and propranolol, or by somatostatin.[117,119,120] With this method, the resulting steady-state plasma glucose level reflects the action of the concomitantly infused insulin; the higher the steady-state plasma glucose, the greater the degree of insulin resistance.[117] Another method of assessing insulin sensitivity is the "minimal model" developed by Bergman and colleagues,[117] in which the plasma glucose and insulin levels following an intravenous glucose bolus are fed into a mathematical model to generate an index of insulin sensitivity (S_i). The test was adapted for type 2 diabetic patients with poor insulin secretion by giving an injection of insulin 20 minutes after the glucose bolus. With all these methods, significant insulin resistance has been demonstrated in the overwhelming majority of type 2 diabetic patients.

The site of this resistance to insulin-stimulated glucose disposal is primarily at the level of skeletal muscle. Thus, forearm and leg glucose balance studies have shown that 80–85% of overall *in vivo* insulin-mediated glucose uptake is accounted for by skeletal muscle, and that skeletal muscle is markedly resistant to insulin's ability to stimulate glucose uptake in T2DM.[121–123]

More detailed *in vivo* studies of insulin sensitivity have been carried out using the euglycemic glucose clamp method developed by Andres and colleagues.[117,124] With this approach, insulin is infused at a constant rate to maintain a given steady-state plasma insulin level. At the same time, the plasma glucose level is frequently monitored and hypoglycemia is prevented by infusing glucose at a variable rate, which is periodically adjusted to maintain a constant plasma glucose level. The amount of glucose that has to be infused to keep plasma glucose constant increases gradually until a steady state is reached. If a radioactive or stable isotope of glucose is also infused during the study, the rate of hepatic glucose output during the clamp can be quantified. At steady state, the isotopically measured rate of glucose disposal provides an excellent quantitative assessment of the biological effect of a particular steady-state insulin concentration. If several studies at different insulin levels are performed in a given subject, the dose–response curve for insulin-

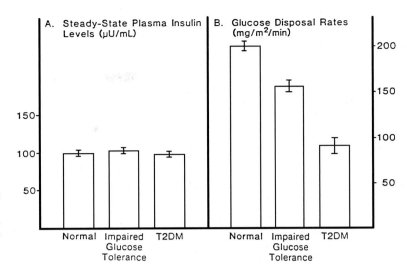

FIGURE 22-6. Mean steady-state glucose disposal rates (**right panel**) and plasma insulin levels (**left panel**) for control subjects, nonobese subjects with impaired glucose tolerance, and type 2 diabetic patients (T2DM) during euglycemic glucose clamp studies performed at an insulin infusion rate of 40 mU/m^2/min. Results are plotted as means ± SEM.

stimulated glucose disposal and suppression of hepatic glucose output can be constructed. The steady-state glucose disposal data from such a glucose clamp study, in which a submaximally stimulating insulin infusion rate was used in normal, nonobese IGT subjects and obese or nonobese type 2 diabetic subjects, are shown in Fig. 22-6.[93] As can be seen, steady-state insulin levels were comparable in all subjects, but the glucose disposal rates were decreased in the patient groups and the magnitude of this defect was greatest in the patients with the worst carbohydrate intolerance.

To further explore the mechanisms of this insulin resistance, the *in vivo* dose–response relationship was examined by performing additional euglycemic glucose clamp studies at insulin infusion rates of 40, 120, 240, or 1200 mU/m^2/min.[93] As seen in Fig. 22-7, the subjects with IGT had a rightward shift in their dose–response curves (diminished sensitivity), but their maximal rate of glucose disposal was not significantly different from that of the control sub-

jects, indicating normal insulin responsiveness. The patients with T2DM (obese and nonobese) exhibited both a rightward shift in their dose–response curves and a marked decrease in the maximal rate of glucose disposal. These changes tended to be more pronounced in the obese diabetic patients, especially at the highest insulin concentration. Clearly, the predominant lesion responsible for the insulin-resistant state in the patients with fasting hyperglycemia appears to be a postbinding defect in insulin action, leading to a marked decrease in maximal insulin responsiveness. This abnormality is present in both nonobese and obese T2DM patients, showing that this postbinding defect in insulin action is not simply a result of obesity.

Inspection of the individual data in the type 2 diabetic patients showed that the patients with the lower fasting glucose levels were less insulin resistant and had the smallest reductions in maximal glucose disposal rates (Fig. 22-8), which suggests that the degree of the postbinding defect is greater as the severity of the diabetic state increases. Clearly, this is consistent with the concept discussed earlier that there is a primary and an acquired component to the insulin resistance in T2DM, and that the acquired component may be secondary to the development of chronic hyperglycemia.

Hepatic Glucose Metabolism

The liver is capable of extracting glucose from the blood delivered via portal vein and hepatic artery as well as releasing glucose derived from glycogenolysis or gluconeogenesis into the hepatic vein.

Hepatic Glucose Production

After an overnight fast, about 90% of the glucose released into the circulation comes from the liver. In normal subjects, basal glucose production rates are around 1.8–2.2 mg/kg/min. After carbohydrate ingestion, hepatic glucose output (HGO) falls and this helps to limit the rise in plasma glucose levels. As intestinal delivery of glucose wanes, basal HGO rates must be restored to prevent hypoglycemia. These changes in HGO are largely mediated by changes in insulin and other hormones that oppose insulin's effects on hepatic gluconeogenesis and glycogenolysis through alterations in the supply of gluconeogenic substrate, and by the effects of the hepatic plasma glucose concentration *per se*.

FIGURE 22-7. Mean insulin dose–response curves for glucose disposal in control subjects (●), subjects with impaired glucose tolerance (○), and nonobese (△) and obese (▲) type 2 diabetic subjects.

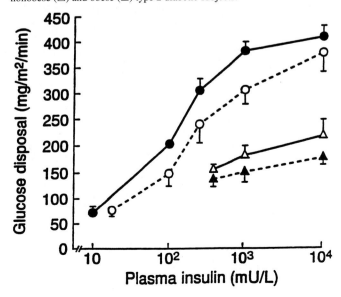

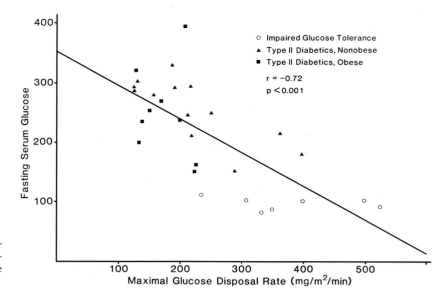

FIGURE 22-8. Relationship between fasting serum glucose level and maximal glucose disposal rate in individual subjects with IGT (○) and nonobese (▲) and obese (■) type 2 diabetes.

HGO is abnormal in T2DM.[92–94,112,115] The basal rate of HGO is increased, whether or not the diabetic patients are obese, but is normal in subjects with IGT (Fig. 22-9A). The importance of this abnormality in sustaining the hyperglycemic state is best illustrated by examining the relationship between HGO and the fasting plasma glucose level in individual subjects. Figure 22-9B illustrates the very close correlation between these two variables, indicating that it is the rate of glucose production by the liver that appears to be most directly responsible for the level of fasting hyperglycemia in T2DM.

Most studies suggest that gluconeogenesis is increased in T2DM and that this is the proximate cause of their increased HGO.[125–127] However, the exact mechanisms remain unclear, and it is likely that the abnormalities of gluconeogenesis and HGO are multifactorial in origin. Glucagon levels are elevated in T2DM (see Chap. 7), and the effect of glucagon to stimulate the synthesis and release of glucose by the liver is well known. Hyperglycemia normally exerts a potent suppressive effect on α-cell glucagon secretion, and the presence of hyperglucagonemia in the face of hyperglycemia is consistent with the view that pancreatic α cells are resistant to the inhibitory effects of glucose in type 2 diabetic subjects. Insulin also normally suppresses glucagon secretion, and this may reflect an intraislet paracrine function of β-cell insulin secretion inhibiting α-cell glucagon release.[128] This effect is also possibly impaired in T2DM. Other factors could be at work, but regardless of the mechanisms, increased α-cell function in T2DM is an important and consistent abnormality. If somatostatin is infused to induce isolated glucagonopenia, it can be demonstrated that about two-thirds of basal HGO is glucagon dependent in normal and type 2 diabetic subjects.[129,130]

Hepatic glucose production can be completely suppressed by high physiologic or supraphysiologic insulin levels in T2DM, but there is resistance to suppression of HGO at lower insulin concentrations.[131,132] This hepatic insulin resistance also likely contributes to exaggerated glucose production rates in this condition. Because insulin's effect on HGO may in part be indirect and mediated by suppression of adipose tissue lipolysis and plasma FFA levels,[133] it is possible that the defect of HGO suppression in T2DM may in part be secondary to impaired suppression of plasma FFA levels by

FIGURE 22-9. A. Rates of hepatic glucose output (HGO) in the basal state (7 to 9 AM following an overnight fast) in normal subjects, subjects with IGT, and obese or nonobese subjects with type 2 diabetes. HGO is normal in patients with IGT but is increased in type 2 diabetes. **B**. Relationship between hepatic glucose production rates and fasting serum glucose levels in type 2 diabetic subjects.

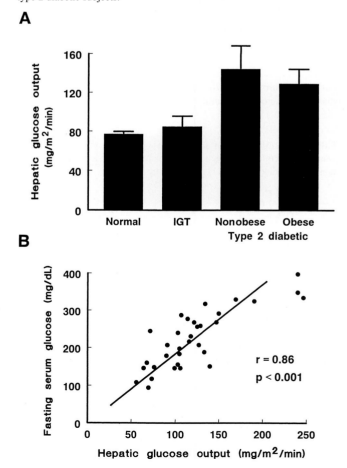

insulin.[131,133–135] However, resistance to insulin's direct effects on HGO is undoubtedly also present in T2DM.[136]

Finally, the increased flux of the gluconeogenic precursors lactate, alanine, and glycerol from peripheral tissues to the liver may participate in the maintenance of the increased rate of HGO in T2DM[137] The finding that plasma alanine levels are usually normal in T2DM despite increased entry of alanine into the circulation[126] is consistent with an increased uptake of alanine by the liver. The substrate-induced increase in HGO could be at least partly related to differences in intracellular disposition of glucose in peripheral target tissues in normal versus insulin-resistant type 2 diabetic subjects. In the basal state, Ra (the rate of glucose appearance) is increased in hyperglycemic type 2 diabetic patients because of increased HGO, and under the near steady-state conditions that exist in the basal state this means that total glucose disposal (Rd) is also elevated. When basal tissue glucose uptake is enhanced by hyperglycemia in diabetes, the proportion of glucose metabolized by glycolysis to lactate and pyruvate tends to be increased.[138] Some of the pyruvate is converted to alanine by transamination and these three-carbon compounds can be recycled to the liver (Cori cycle) to be reconverted to glucose, facilitating increased HGO. Consistent with this formulation, increased flow of three-carbon precursors from muscle in the basal state and their reincorporation into glucose has been described in T2DM.[126,127] The increased FFA levels generally observed in hyperglycemic diabetic subjects could provide the energy, via fatty acid oxidation, to drive the increased rate of hepatic gluconeogenesis.

Hepatic Glucose Uptake

Although earlier data held that the majority of orally ingested glucose was extracted by the liver and largely converted to glycogen,[139] more recent studies suggest that only 20–35% of oral glucose is directly taken up (as glucose) by the liver, and even less (about 10%) of the glucose absorbed from the gut is taken up on first pass.[140] Thus the majority of the incoming glucose load enters the peripheral circulation and skeletal muscle is quantitatively the predominant site of glucose disposal.[141] Taylor and colleagues, using ^{13}CNMR spectroscopy to quantitate liver glycogen in normal subjects, estimated that only 19% of the carbohydrate content of a liquid meal consumed after an overnight fast was incorporated into liver glycogen.[142] Furthermore, much of the liver glycogen is derived through the indirect pathway from incoming amino acids, lactate, and pyruvate via gluconeogenesis (more properly glyconeogenesis) rather than directly from glucose.[141–143] Insulin does not directly stimulate hepatic glucose uptake; it plays a permissive role. An increase in the portal venous glucose concentration and the establishment of a positive portal–arterial glucose gradient is a prerequisite for net hepatic glucose uptake;[144,145] under these circumstances insulin will augment the net uptake of glucose by the liver.[145] After glucose ingestion, uptake of glucose by the liver (newly absorbed and recirculating) is impaired in T2DM.[146] A recent study found that in patients with T2DM, splanchnic glucose uptake during combined hyperinsulinemia and hyperglycemia was impaired, as was the incorporation of glucose into hepatic glycogen by the direct pathway, whereas hepatic glycogen synthesis via the indirect pathway from three-carbon intermediates was not significantly decreased.[132]

In summary, in T2DM the liver overproduces glucose in the basal state and the metabolic milieu is ideal to sustain this ability. Exaggerated hormonal stimulation is provided by the increased glucagon levels in combination with hepatic insulin resistance, and

augmented gluconeogenic precursor flow ensures adequate substrate availability. Finally, elevated FFA levels could provide the necessary source of intracellular energy, via fatty acid oxidation, to drive the gluconeogenic process. Postprandially, suppression of HGO and uptake of glucose by the liver are impaired in T2DM and these defects contribute to postprandial hyperglycemia.

Insulin-Mediated versus Non-Insulin-Mediated Glucose Uptake and the Pathogenesis of Hyperglycemia

Overall glucose uptake can be conveniently divided into non-insulin-mediated glucose uptake (NIMGU) and insulin-mediated glucose uptake (IMGU) (Fig. 22-10). Because of the differences in the relative proportions of insulin-mediated and non-insulin-mediated glucose uptake with fasting and feeding, the cause of fasting hyperglycemia is different from the cause of postprandial hyperglycemia. By definition, IMGU occurs only in insulin target tissues under the influence of insulin. NIMGU comprises glucose uptake not under the influence of insulin and has two components. NIMGU occurs in tissues (primarily the central nervous system) that are not targets for insulin action; it also involves insulin target cells and consists of the basal rate (non-insulin-mediated) of glucose disposal (Rd) by these tissues. Total glucose Rd equals the sum of NIMGU plus IMGU (Fig. 22-10). NIMGU can be assessed *in vivo* by measuring glucose Rd under conditions of severe insulinopenia induced by an infusion of somatostatin.[147,148] Following measurement of basal glucose Rd (at basal or fasting insulin and glucose levels), somatostatin is administered to inhibit insulin secretion to negligible levels. Glucose Rd gradually falls to a new steady state that equals NIMGU, because insulin action is nearly absent under these conditions. Using this method, approximately 70% of basal glucose Rd is non-insulin-mediated in normal euglycemic subjects and in type 2 diabetic subjects studied at their basal level of hyperglycemia.[147] This means that in the basal state, at all levels of glycemia, most of the glucose is disposed of by non-insulin-mediated mechanisms, and that the elevated rates of basal glucose Rd (due to an increased HGO) that prevail in T2DM are associated with increased rates of NIMGU.

How does this consideration of non-insulin-mediated and insulin-mediated glucose uptake relate to the cause of fasting hyperglycemia? This is summarized in Table 22-2. Because IMGU comprises only 30% of basal glucose Rd, it follows that an impairment of IMGU due to insulin resistance and/or decreased insulin secretion will have little effect on overall basal glucose Rd or

FIGURE 22-10. Overall basal glucose uptake divided into its constituent parts. Most non-insulin-mediated glucose uptake occurs in the central nervous system.

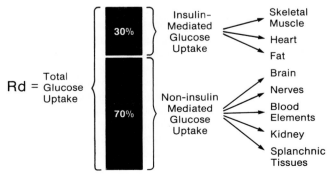

TABLE 22-2. Etiology of Fasting versus Postprandial Hyperglycemia

Basal State

1. Non-insulin-mediated glucose uptake predominantes (70% of basal glucose disposal)
2. Glucose output (hepatic glucose production) equals glucose disposal (insulin-mediated glucose uptake plus non-insulin-mediated glucose uptake) equals 2 mg/kg/min
3. Non-insulin-mediated glucose uptake equals 1.4, and insulin-mediated glucose uptake equals 0.6 mg/kg/min
4. A 50% decrease in insulin-mediated glucose uptake equals a 15% decrease in glucose disposal to 1.7 mg/kg/min
5. Fasting blood glucose (85 mg/dL) increases to about 100 mg/dL, and glucose disposal increases 15%, back to 2.0 mg/kg/min
6. If glucose output increases from 2.0 to 2.6 mg/kg/min, then insulin-mediated glucose uptake must increase from 0.6 to 1.2 mg/kg/min to prevent hyperglycemia
7. This requires a five- to sixfold increase in insulin level, which cannot be readily achieved in type 2 diabetes mellitus
8. Fasting hyperglycemia is largely secondary to increased glucose output (hepatic glucose production)

Postprandial State

1. Insulin-mediated glucose uptake predominates (80–90% of glucose disposal)
2. Postprandial glucose disposal increases to 7 mg/kg/min
3. Non-insulin-mediated glucose uptake then equals 1.4, and insulin-mediated glucose uptake equals 5.6 mg/kg/min
4. A 50% decrease in insulin-mediated glucose uptake leads to a 40% decrease in glucose disposal
5. Postprandial hyperglycemia is largely secondary to a restricted rise in insulin-mediated glucose uptake

fasting glucose levels. For example, if a normal basal rate of glucose Rd is 2 mg/kg/min and IMGU is equal to 0.6 mg/kg/min (30%), then a 50% decrease in IMGU will lower glucose Rd by 0.3 mg/kg/min, a 15% reduction. A slight (about 15%) rise in plasma glucose level is all that is necessary to provide a sufficient mass action effect of glucose to restore glucose Rd back to the original level. Thus the restriction of IMGU in type 2 diabetes is not the proximate cause of fasting hyperglycemia. Because the fasting glucose level reflects the balance between glucose output and glucose Rd, then if reduced glucose Rd does not lead to significant fasting hyperglycemia, it follows that increased glucose entry into the circulation (essentially HGO) is the factor most directly responsible for fasting hyperglycemia. This is because in the setting of peripheral insulin resistance and impaired insulin secretion, the ability of IMGU to rise and accommodate an increase in glucose output is severely curtailed. Thus, using the above example (Table 22-2), if basal HGO and glucose Rd are 2 mg/kg/min at euglycemia, with IMGU accounting for only 30% of glucose Rd, then a modest increase in HGO to 2.6 mg/kg/min would require a doubling of IMGU (from 0.6 to 1.2 mg/kg/min) to maintain glucose Rd equal to the new HGO with no change in basal glucose level.

A normal subject can increase basal IMGU twofold with less than a twofold increase in plasma insulin above the basal concentration. Thus, with a normal ability to secrete insulin and a normal capacity of peripheral tissues to respond to insulin, a control subject can easily accommodate a rise in glucose output from 2.0 to 2.6 mg/kg/min with little if any change in fasting glucose level. In T2DM, the situation is quite different; a five- to sixfold increase in plasma insulin is necessary to increase IMGU twofold over the basal value. Thus, because of insulin resistance, type 2 diabetic

subjects need much larger increases in plasma insulin to increase IMGU, and in view of their impaired insulin secretion, this is unlikely to be achieved. Therefore, the fasting glucose level must rise until the mass action effect of glucose raises glucose Rd sufficiently to match the increased glucose output and thus bring the system back into balance. At this point increased glucose output is matched by increased glucose Rd in the presence of fasting hyperglycemia. Thus, in T2DM, the inability to augment IMGU due to the presence of insulin resistance and restricted insulin secretion provides the metabolic foundation that allows relatively small increases in glucose output (HGO) to cause direct and proportionate increases in the fasting glucose level.[92]

The cause of postprandial hyperglycemia is quite different (Table 22-2). The majority of ingested glucose bypasses the liver and enters the peripheral circulation.[140] This is accompanied by rapid suppression (60-90%) of HGO for 2–3 hours after carbohydrate ingestion.[138,140,142] Therefore, in the postprandial state, the main source of glucose appearing in the circulation is the ingested carbohydrate. Glucose absorbed from the gut largely enters the systemic circulation to be disposed of mostly by skeletal muscle through a severalfold increase in IMGU. Since IMGU can make up 80–90% of overall glucose disposal, decreases in IMGU due to insulin resistance and insulin deficiency will markedly reduce glucose disposal at any given glucose level. In T2DM, systemic delivery of ingested glucose appears to be normal, but suppression of HGO is impaired as a result of insulin resistance and impaired insulin secretion,[138] which means that the total quantity of glucose appearing in the circulation is somewhat higher. In addition, the efficiency of peripheral glucose removal is greatly reduced because of insulin resistance and impaired insulin secretion. Hepatic uptake of glucose (newly absorbed plus recirculating) is also impaired in T2DM.[138,146] Thus, postprandial hyperglycemia in T2DM is primarily due to impaired IMGU by peripheral tissues, with impaired suppression of HGO and impaired hepatic glucose uptake compounding the problem. Because of the very limited capacity for an acute increase in IMGU, postprandial glucose levels must rise markedly until the mass action effect of glucose raises glucose Rd to match glucose input and allow disposal of the incoming glucose load.

In summary, in the basal state, NIMGU predominates, and decreased IMGU will raise fasting blood glucose levels only modestly. Fasting hyperglycemia is primarily due to increased hepatic glucose production. In the postprandial state, IMGU normally predominates, and the limited ability of type 2 diabetic subjects to increase IMGU allows the marked postprandial glucose excursions. Postprandial hyperglycemia is thus primarily due to glucose underutilization by peripheral tissues (primarily muscle).

Obesity

Insulin resistance has been widely described in human obesity, and this has been documented by observing an attenuated ability of exogenous insulin to promote glucose disposal using a variety of techniques. These range from measurements of hypoglycemic responses to bolus insulin injections,[149] forearm perfusions,[6] and glucose clamp studies.[88,124,150] Using the euglycemic clamp technique over a range of insulin infusion rates to construct individual insulin dose–response curves for *in vivo* glucose disposal and HGO (as discussed earlier), a rightward shift in the dose–response curve for insulin-stimulated glucose disposal is a consistent finding in obese subjects. However, the response to a maximally stimulating insulin concentration is quite variable, covering the whole spectrum from normal to markedly reduced.[150] Figure 22-11 shows the mean insulin dose–response curves obtained in a group of normal and obese subjects. Some of the obese subjects achieved a normal or near-normal maximal insulin stimulated glucose disposal rate, whereas others displayed a markedly decreased maximal glucose disposal rate. In the figure, the obese subjects have been arbitrarily divided into two groups: (1) those showing a normal maximal rate of insulin-stimulated glucose disposal (group I obese) and (2) those displaying a markedly decreased maximal glucose disposal rate (group II obese). With this analysis, the insulin resistance associated with obesity is heterogeneous; some patients display only a rightward shift in the dose–response curve, consistent with decreased insulin binding as the sole abnormality (decreased insulin sensitivity), while others show a decreased maximal response, consistent with a postbinding defect in insulin action (decreased insulin responsiveness). Indeed, there are several reports of postbinding defects in insulin signaling in muscle and adipocytes from obese subjects.

It is apparent that the patients with normal maximal rates of glucose disposal are less insulin resistant. They also are less hyperinsulinemic and have a smaller reduction in insulin receptors than the subjects with reduced maximal responsiveness (Fig. 22-12). Although all of the subjects were hyperinsulinemic and insulin resistant, the data suggest that no postbinding defect exists in the least affected subjects. The findings indicate a continuum of insulin resistance in human obesity such that in the mildly hyperinsulinemic,

insulin-resistant state, only a binding defect exists; however, as the hyperinsulinemic, insulin-resistant state worsens, a postbinding defect appears.

Hepatic glucose output (HGO) was measured during all studies and these results are plotted in Fig. 22-13. Basal HGO was comparable for all groups when expressed as mg/m^2/min (66 ± 5, 63 ± 4, and 67 ± 5 mg/m^2/min for control, group I obese, and group II obese, respectively), but was significantly higher for the normal subjects when expressed on a per kilogram basis (2.0 ± 0.2 mg/kg/min versus 1.4 ± 0.1 and 1.3 ± 0.1 mg/kg/min for the group I obese and group II obese, respectively). Several conclusions can be drawn from the data in Fig. 22-13. First, HGO can be totally suppressed in all subjects, provided high enough insulin concentrations are employed. Thus, in contrast to insulin's effects on peripheral glucose disposal, the liver of obese subjects does not appear to exhibit a postbinding defect in this insulin effect. Second, the dose–response curves for HGO are shifted to the right in the obese groups, and the half-maximally effective insulin levels were 33, 75, and 130 mU/L in normal, group I obese, and group II obese subjects, respectively. This parallels the results for peripheral glucose disposal.

A number of factors, including the habitual physical activity level[151] and the regional distribution of body fat,[152–155] could contribute to the heterogeneity of insulin resistance in human obesity. Overweight individuals tend to be sedentary. Bogardus and associates[151] found that the level of habitual physical activity (estimated by measurement of maximal oxygen consumption) accounted for about 25% of the variance in insulin-mediated glucose disposal in normal subjects over a wide range of body mass indices. It follows that the habitual physical activity level of obese subjects participating in studies of insulin action could be one determinant of whether they have a decrease in maximal responsiveness or only a rightward shift in their insulin dose–response curve.

Several studies suggest that obese subjects with a predominantly central (abdominal/truncal) distribution of body fat are more insulin resistant and have higher circulating insulin levels than those with peripheral obesity, independent of the overall degree of

FIGURE 22-11. Dose–response curves for *in vivo* glucose disposal in control subjects (●), and obese subjects separated into two groups on the basis of their maximal response: group I (○) and group II (▲) (see text for details). Results were obtained by performing euglycemic clamp studies in each subject with insulin infusion rates of 15, 40, 120, 240, or 1200 mU/m^2/min. The initial point on the curve represents glucose disposal in the basal state as measured by a primed continuous infusion of 3-3H-glucose. Data are presented as mean ± SEM.

FIGURE 22-12. Insulin binding by isolated adipocytes from control (●), group I (○), and group II (▲) obese subjects. All data are corrected for nonspecific binding and represent the mean (± SEM) percentage of ^{125}I-insulin specifically bound/2 × 10^5 cells.

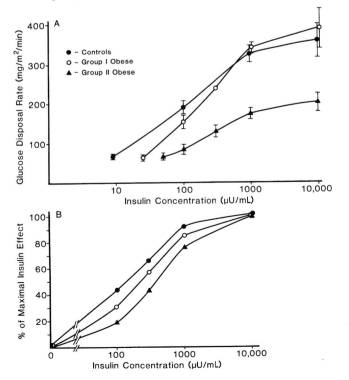

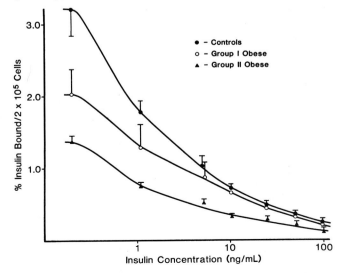

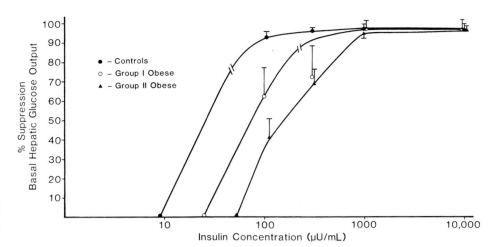

FIGURE 22-13. Mean dose–response curves for insulin-mediated suppression of basal hepatic glucose output for control (●), group I (○), and group II (▲) obese subjects.

obesity.[152–155] In contrast, total body fat content rather than its distribution is an important determinant of insulin sensitivity in mildly obese subjects. Once an individual exceeds 25–30% of ideal body weight (BMI > 27 kg/m^2), further increases in total fat mass have relatively little additional influence on insulin sensitivity, and the distribution of fat (i.e., central versus peripheral) assumes greater importance as a determinant of insulin action and circulating insulin levels.[153,155,156] Therefore, a more central distribution of body fat could be a determinant of whether obese subjects exhibit a decrease in maximal insulin responsiveness.

The prevailing view is that the adverse metabolic effects associated with central obesity are due to the accumulation of visceral fat, which is lipolytically more active.[157,158] FFAs may impair hepatocyte insulin receptor function,[159] and if so, this would cause decreased hepatic insulin clearance in subjects with central obesity.[160] High circulating insulin levels may desensitize the target tissues at several steps in the insulin action sequence. This raises the possibility that the hyperinsulinemia in subjects with central abdominal obesity may cause a decrease in maximal insulin responsiveness. This formulation fits with the observation that a decrease in maximal insulin responsiveness is seen in the most hyperinsulinemic obese subjects, and that the magnitude of the defect is directly related to the degree of hyperinsulinemia.

CELLULAR DEFECTS IN INSULIN ACTION

From the foregoing discussion, it is likely that in obese or type 2 diabetic patients with mild degrees of insulin resistance, the defect is characterized by decreased insulin sensitivity, which may be attributable, at least in part, to a decreased number of insulin receptors. In those subjects with more severe insulin resistance, a postbinding defect in cellular insulin action is the predominant abnormality. A great deal of recent attention has been paid to elucidating potential postbinding abnormalities in insulin action in tissues from type 2 diabetic and obese subjects.

Insulin Binding

As discussed earlier, a large number of studies have found that insulin binding to a variety of tissues is decreased in type 2 diabetic patients relative to controls, and many studies, but not all, have also

shown a decrement in obese patients.[74–79,93,150,161,162] Using partially purified adipocyte insulin receptors, it was found that at all concentrations of added insulin, the amount of insulin bound was 20% lower in obese subjects and nearly 50% less per milligram of protein in the obese diabetics relative to lean controls.[150]

Insulin-Stimulated Autophosphorylation

The first known event following insulin binding to its receptor is activation of the tyrosine kinase property intrinsic to the cytoplasmic domain of the β subunit. For functional studies of receptor kinase activity, receptors can be partially purified from cells by affinity chromatography using the lectin wheat germ agglutinin to adsorb the receptors from solubilized cells. When wheat germ–purified receptors were preincubated with increasing concentrations of insulin, and then exposed to [γ-^{32}P]ATP, there was an insulin-dependent increase in the amount of ^{32}P incorporated into the ~92,000 MW β subunit, as shown in Fig. 22-14A for a control subject. When the bands corresponding to the β subunit were excised and counted, a dose–response curve for insulin stimulation of autophosphorylation was constructed for subjects, as shown in Fig. 22-14B.

Figure 22-15 illustrates the dose–response curves for autophosphorylation of adipocyte insulin receptors in control, obese, and type 2 diabetic subjects.[162] In the absence of insulin, basal autophosphorylation was not significantly different among the three groups (control, 1.73 ± 0.24; obese, 1.65 ± 0.28; type 2 diabetic, 1.47 ± 0.37 fmol phosphate/76 fmol insulin-binding activity), and the basal level was subtracted from all corresponding values measured in the presence of different concentrations of insulin. Analyzed in this manner, the results displayed in Fig. 22-16 reflect only insulin-stimulated autophosphorylation. When equal amounts of insulin receptors were allowed to autophosphorylate, the amount of phosphate incorporated into the β subunit of the receptor was similar in the lean controls and nondiabetic obese subjects at all insulin concentrations. In contrast, the amount of autophosphorylation was markedly reduced (p <0.01) in the type 2 diabetic subjects relative to the two other groups.

As previously discussed, skeletal muscle represents the major insulin target tissue with respect to insulin-stimulated glucose disposal, and therefore it is important to examine insulin receptor kinase activity in this tissue. To accomplish this, the kinase activity

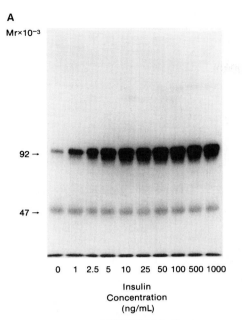

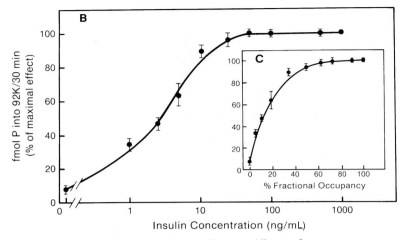

FIGURE 22-14. Dose–response of autophosphorylation of insulin receptors from human adipocytes. Aliquots of wheat germ–purified receptors from three lean nondiabetic subjects were preincubated in the presence and absence of increasing concentrations of unlabeled insulin, with or without 0.5 ng/mL ^{125}I-insulin. After 18 hours at 4°C, autokinase and insulin-binding assays were performed. **A.** Representative autoradiograph of insulin-stimulated autophosphorylation from a control subject. **B.** The phosphorylated proteins corresponding to 92,000 MW were located by autoradiography, excised, and counted. The amount of phosphate incorporated into the 92-kd band, expressed as the percentage of the maximal effect achieved at 1000 ng/mL insulin, is plotted as a function of increasing concentrations of added insulin. **C.** Kinase data from **B** redrafted as a function of the fraction of total receptors occupied with insulin at each concentration of added insulin, as determined by Scatchard plots of the binding data.

of insulin receptors was measured during glucose clamp studies using a technique which determines the magnitude of receptor kinase activity as it existed in the *in vivo* situation stimulated by the exogenous insulin infusion.[163] With this approach, glucose clamp studies were performed at different insulin infusion rates, and skeletal muscle biopsies were performed 3 hours after each insulin infusion. Kinase activity is then assessed using receptors purified

from these biopsies, and this provides a measure of the ability of circulating insulin to stimulate skeletal muscle insulin receptor kinase activity *in vivo*. As shown in Fig. 22-16, the results are comparable to those observed in adipocytes, with decreased kinase activity in type 2 diabetic patients compared to lean and obese nondiabetic subjects.[163] Similar findings have been reported using insulin receptors from liver[164] and erythrocytes.[165]

FIGURE 22-15. Insulin dose–response of autophosphorylation. Aliquots of receptor preparations (76 fmol of insulin-binding capacity/80 μL) were preincubated with 0, 2, 5, or 500 ng/mL insulin, after which autokinase reactions were conducted for 30 minutes at 4°C. For each subject, the amount of ^{32}P incorporated into the 92-kd band in the absence (basal) of insulin was subtracted from all corresponding values measured in the presence of insulin. The results are graphed as the mean (± SEM) increase over basal from 10 control (●), 13 obese (△), and 13 type 2 diabetic (○) subjects.

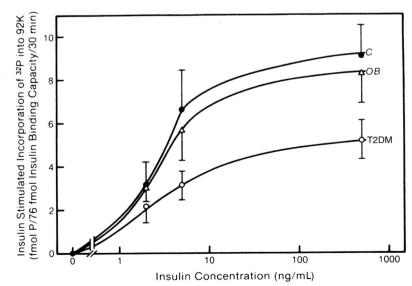

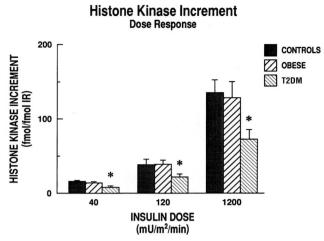

FIGURE 22-16. Dose–response stimulation of skeletal muscle insulin receptor phosphorylation of histone-2B *in vivo* during euglycemic clamp studies. The results represent the kinase activity (mean ± SEM) expressed as increment over the basal values for lean nondiabetics (■), obese nondiabetics (▨), and type 2 diabetic subjects (▧). Type 2 diabetic versus lean controls, $p = 0.01$; type 2 diabetic versus obese, $p < 0.05$; obese versus lean controls, $p =$ NS (by ANOVA).

The impaired receptor kinase activity seen in the type 2 diabetic subjects appears to be relatively specific for the hyperglycemic diabetic state since no decrease in kinase activity was observed in adipocyte-,[162] erythrocyte-,[165] and skeletal muscle-derived[163] receptors prepared from insulin–resistant nondiabetic obese subjects compared to lean nondiabetic controls. This suggests that the insulin receptor kinase defect is a consequence of the diabetic state rather than a primary inherited cause of insulin–resistance, and several lines of evidence support this idea. First, molecular studies have shown that the sequence of the insulin receptor gene is normal in >99% of subjects with "garden variety" T2DM, demonstrating that the insulin receptor does not represent a diabetes susceptibility gene, except in a small fraction of patients.[166,167] Second, when obese type 2 diabetic patients lose weight, hyperglycemia is markedly improved and this is associated with partial amelioration of insulin resistance and normalization of receptor kinase activity.[78] One can speculate that hyperglycemia, or some closely related factor, causes the receptor kinase defect, and ample *in vitro* evidence exists to support this contention.[168] In summary, evidence exists to indicate that glucotoxicity causes the acquired secondary component of insulin resistance in T2DM at least in part by reversibly decreasing the autophosphorylation/kinase activity of target tissue insulin receptors. With this analysis, the cellular mechanism underlying the primary inherited component of insulin resistance in T2DM remains to be elucidated. With regard to simple obesity, since these subjects are insulin resistant with normal receptor kinase activity, it would appear that the cause of impaired insulin action in those subjects with a reduced V_{max} involves some other postreceptor defect.

Insulin Receptor Subpopulations

This decrease in kinase activity in T2DM could be due to (1) a decrease in the intrinsic kinase activity of each individual receptor within the total receptor preparation, or (2) the existence of two

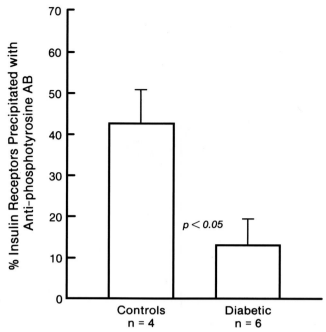

FIGURE 22-17. Percentage of receptors immunoprecipitable with anti-phosphotyrosine antibody. Receptors were labeled with ^{125}I-NAPA-DP-insulin, autophosphorylated, and immunoprecipitated. Washed receptor-antibody complexes were boiled in Laemmli's buffer and analyzed by SDS-polyacrylamide gel electrophoresis (7.5% resolving gel). Areas of the gel containing the ^{125}I-NAPA-DP-insulin–labeled β subunit were excised and counted in a gamma counter. Equal areas of the dried gel free of any ^{125}I activity were counted and subtracted as background. The graph shows the amount of ^{125}I-labeled insulin receptors immunoprecipitated by anti-phosphotyrosine antibody as a percentage of the total amount of receptors immunoprecipitated by the anti-insulin receptor antibody.

populations of receptors that bind insulin, one subpopulation having normal kinase activity and the other subpopulation having no kinase activity, with a relative increase in the kinase-defective population in T2DM. To discriminate between these two possibilities, phosphorylated ^{125}I-NAPA-DP-labeled receptors were immunoprecipitated using a monoclonal antireceptor antibody and an antiphosphotyrosine antibody.[169] ^{125}I-NAPA-DP-insulin is a photoactive insulin derivative which binds to the receptor α subunit; when exposed to UV light, the ^{125}I-NAPA-DP-insulin becomes activated and photoaffinity labels the insulin receptor by forming covalent bonds with the α subunit. The monoclonal anti-insulin receptor antibody immunoprecipitates all of the ^{125}I-NAPA-DP-labeled insulin receptors. In order to determine the proportion of insulin receptors that contain phosphotyrosine in the type 2 diabetic subjects compared to those of control subjects, an anti-phosphotyrosine antibody was used to immunoprecipitate only those insulin receptors containing phosphorylated tyrosine residues. Control studies showed that the monoclonal antireceptor antibody quantitatively immunoprecipitates the total receptor pool, whereas the phosphotyrosine antibody quantitatively immunoprecipitates only the autophosphorylated receptors. Therefore, a comparison of the ^{125}I counts immunoprecipitated by the antiphosphotyrosine antibody indicates the percentage of the total insulin receptors that are autophosphorylated and contain phosphotyrosine.

Figure 22-17 illustrates, for both control and type 2 diabetic subjects, the percentage of the insulin receptors, after maximal *in vitro* insulin-stimulated autophosphorylation, that contain phosphotyrosine. Forty-three percent of the insulin receptors derived from control subjects contained phosphotyrosine residues, while only 14% of the type 2 diabetic subjects' insulin receptors were phosphorylated.[169] A much smaller fraction of the total receptors from type 2 diabetic subjects were able to undergo insulin-stimulated autophosphorylation compared to the normals. Additional studies have shown that the insulin receptors not precipitated by the antiphosphotyrosine antibody were completely devoid of kinase activity, and thus the kinase activity found in the total receptor preparations was attributable to those receptors precipitated by the antiphosphotyrosine antibody. These studies demonstrate the existence of at least two distinct populations of receptors—one containing phosphotyrosine residues and one apparently incapable of insulin-stimulated tyrosine phosphorylation. The results show that 43% of the receptors from nondiabetic subjects were capable of autophosphorylation, indicating that 50–60% of the receptors do not undergo tyrosine phosphorylation and presumably do not contribute to the kinase activity of the normal cell's complement of insulin receptors. Interestingly, since about 90% of the adipocyte insulin receptors are at the cell surface in the basal state,[170] most of these kinase-negative receptors must be at the cell surface, where they apparently bind insulin in a physiologic manner. In the type 2 diabetic group, only 14% of the receptors were capable of tyrosine autophosphorylation, and this decrease in the proportion of receptors that were phosphorylated appears to largely explain the defect in receptor kinase activity which has been observed in T2DM.[75,162–165,171]

Glucose Transport

In vivo, insulin resistance is usually defined as an impaired ability of insulin to stimulate overall glucose disposal, and any cellular mechanism of insulin resistance must account for decreased glucose disposal. In the insulin action sequence, abnormalities in insulin receptor binding and receptor kinase activity *per se* do not account for all of the decreased glucose uptake. Decreased numbers of insulin receptors do not explain decrements in maximal insulin responsiveness in T2DM, since receptor downregulation does not commonly proceed below the level of spare insulin receptors. In addition, insulin concentrations that elicit maximal insulin bioeffects (1–5 ng/mL) produce only a submaximal degree of insulin receptor phosphorylation (see Fig. 22-16). This indicates, in a sense, that there is also "spare" insulin receptor kinase activity. Therefore, postreceptor defects may account for a large portion of insulin resistance. One potential cellular locus for such a postreceptor defect is the glucose transport effector system. In humans there are at least five known glucose transporter species (GLUT-1 to GLUT-5), each the product of a separate gene, with a distinct pattern of tissue expression for each transporter isoform. The insulin-regulatable glucose transporter is termed GLUT-4, and is almost exclusively expressed in skeletal muscle, cardiac muscle, and adipose tissue. As discussed in detail in Chap. 5, insulin stimulates glucose transport primarily by causing translocation of GLUT-4 proteins from an intracellular vesicular compartment to the plasma membrane. Once inserted into the plasma membrane, cellular glucose uptake is initiated. Consequently, insulin stimulation of glucose transport in target tissues reflects GLUT-4 activity. In this regard, decreased insulin-stimulated glucose transport has been observed in isolated adipocytes[161,172–175] and skeletal muscle strips[176–178] from obese and/or type 2 diabetic subjects. Decreased

insulin-stimulated glucose transport has also been found in cultured skeletal muscle cells derived from the insulin-resistant nondiabetic relatives of type 2 diabetic patients.[179]

Although adipose tissue accounts for only a small amount of *in vivo* glucose metabolism, whereas over 85% of insulin-stimulated glucose disposal occurs in skeletal muscle, for technical reasons most studies of glucose transport have been performed in isolated adipocytes. Figure 22-18 displays glucose transport dose–response curves using isolated adipocytes from normal, IGT, and type 2 diabetic subjects. In the IGT subjects, there is a rightward shift in the glucose transport dose–response curve with no change in the maximal response. This decrease in insulin sensitivity (rightward-shifted curve) is largely accounted for by the decreased number of insulin receptors in cells from subjects with IGT. In the type 2 diabetic groups, however, a marked decrease in glucose transport rates is observed at all insulin concentrations. Thus there is a major decrease in glucose transport activity even at maximally effective insulin concentrations, and this *in vitro* reduction in glucose transport correlates quite well with the decrease in maximal overall glucose disposal rates observed *in vivo*. Similar results are seen in nondiabetic obese subjects, with a marked decrease in adipocyte glucose transport activity compared to controls (Fig. 22-19).

In extrapolating from *in vitro* adipocyte transport data to *in vivo* glucose disposal, several assumptions are made. First, it is assumed that adipose tissue glucose transport is reflective of muscle glucose transport, since muscle is the major site of insulin-stimulated glucose uptake. Available data strongly support this contention. Thus an excellent correlation has been found between adipocyte glucose transport activity and *in vivo* glucose disposal in individual type 2 diabetic or obese subjects both before[161,175] and after[180–182] therapy. Additionally, a number of more direct studies have shown that changes in adipocyte transport are paralleled by quantitatively similar changes in skeletal muscle glucose transport in a number of different pathophysiologic conditions in rodents.[183,184] Most importantly, the few studies that have been conducted on muscle fiber strips from normal, obese, and type 2 diabetic subjects have found that glucose transport is decreased in

FIGURE 22-18. Dose–response curve for insulin's ability to stimulate glucose transport (3-0-methylglucose uptake) in isolated adipocytes prepared from normal subjects, subjects with IGT, and obese or nonobese subjects with type 2 diabetes. The functional form of these dose–response curves is quite comparable to the shape of the dose–response curves for *in vivo* insulin-stimulated overall glucose disposal (Fig. 22-7).

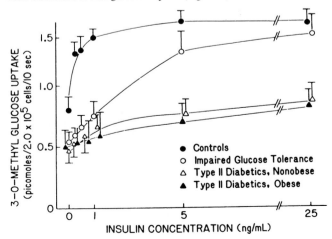

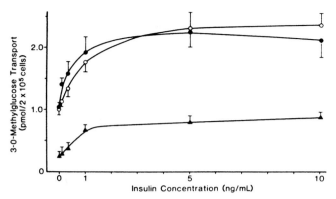

FIGURE 22-19. Dose–response curves for insulin's ability to simulate 3-0-methylglucose transport in isolated adipocytes from normal subjects (●), group I (○), and group II (▲) obese subjects.

the insulin-resistant groups[176–178] (Fig. 22-20), and that, as in the adipocyte studies, insulin-stimulated glucose transport in isolated muscle fiber strips correlates with whole-body insulin sensitivity in normal and type 2 diabetic subjects.[177]

The second assumption inherent in relating glucose transport to *in vivo* glucose disposal is that the transport step is rate-determining for glucose metabolism *in vivo*. Available data indicate that this is the case. For example, if intracellular metabolism, rather that transport, were limiting the rate of glucose disposal, one would expect an accumulation of free intracellular glucose. However, a build-up of intracellular glucose is not observed in skeletal muscle, even at brisk rates of glucose uptake.[185–187] Additionally, apparent K_m values reported for *in vivo* glucose disposal[188] are similar to measured values of muscle glucose transport *in vitro*,[189] consistent with the view that transport governs glucose disposal. Furthermore, the insulin-induced increases in *in vitro* glucose transport are quite comparable to insulin-mediated increases in in vivo glucose disposal.

FIGURE 22-20. 3-0-Methylglucose transport in muscle fiber strips from nonobese subjects, morbidly obese subjects with normal glucose tolerance, and morbidly obese subjects with type 2 diabetes. (*Significantly different [$p < 0.05$] from nonobese group + insulin.) *(Reprinted with permission from Dohm et al.[176])*

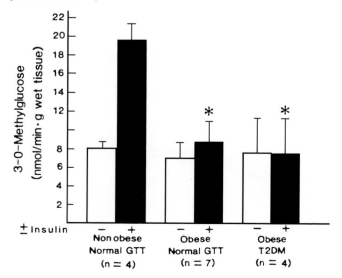

Bonadonna and coworkers[190] used the forearm glucose balance technique in humans, combined with a simultaneous infusion of 3-0-methylglucose, to assess concomitant rates of glucose transport and *in vivo* muscle glucose uptake. They found that insulin-stimulated forearm glucose transport was very well correlated with overall muscle glucose disposal.[190] Studies with transgenic mice also support this concept. Thus, when GLUT-4 is overexpressed in skeletal muscle, enhanced insulin sensitivity and increased glucose disposal occur,[191] pointing to the importance of glucose transport in regulating overall glucose metabolism.

Cline and colleagues,[187] using nuclear magnetic resonance spectroscopy to measure skeletal muscle glucose-6-phosphate levels and intracellular free glucose levels during a hyperinsulinemic, hyperglycemic clamp, have produced compelling *in vivo* evidence that glucose transport is also the rate-controlling step in insulin-stimulated muscle glucose uptake in T2DM. They found that the reduction in muscle glucose uptake and glycogen synthesis in patients with T2DM was associated with lower steady-state muscle glucose-6-phosphate levels and very low intracellular free glucose levels, implying a defect at the level of glucose transport. Of course, it is possible that the additional postglucose transport intracellular defects in glucose metabolism which have been reported[123,135,192–197] alter the intracellular pathways for glucose metabolism, and contribute to abnormal glucose homeostasis.

Because decreased glucose transport is such a prominent defect in T2DM, a number of mechanistic studies have been conducted. Several groups have examined skeletal muscle GLUT-4 content at both the protein and mRNA levels, with uniform agreement. Skeletal muscle GLUT-4 mRNA and protein levels are normal in type 2 diabetic subjects.[198–200] Since total skeletal muscle GLUT-4 protein is not decreased in T2DM, the explanation for the decreased glucose transport activity is related to either decreased insulin-mediated translocation of GLUT-4 to the plasma membrane, decreased GLUT-4 intrinsic activity, or both. Evidence that insulin-stimulated translocation of GLUT-4 is impaired in skeletal muscle of obese and type 2 diabetic patients comes from the study of Kelley and associates.[201] These investigators used quantitative confocal laser scanning microscopy to study insulin-stimulated recruitment of GLUT-4 to the sarcolemma in muscle biopsies from normal, obese, and type 2 diabetic subjects. In the basal state, sarcolemmal GLUT-4 labeling was similar in the three groups, but in response to a 3-hour hyperinsulinemic euglycemic clamp (plasma insulin ~500–600 pmol/L), the increase in sarcolemmal GLUT-4 labeling in type 2 diabetic subjects and in obese nondiabetic subjects was only 25% of that in the controls. This defect in GLUT-4 translocation in the type 2 diabetic and obese subjects was associated with a marked impairment of insulin-stimulated muscle glucose transport as determined by positron emission tomography. Others using biochemical muscle subfractionation techniques have also suggested a defect in GLUT-4 translocation in patients with T2DM.[202]

A decrease in GLUT-4 intrinsic activity in T2DM is also a possibility. Such a defect could be a result of an alteration in the primary structure of the GLUT-4 protein due to genetic variation in the GLUT-4 gene. An answer to this question was made possible by the studies of Buse and associates, who elucidated the intron-exon structure of the human GLUT-4 gene.[203] A determination of the coding sequences of GLUT-4 was conducted in seven typical type 2 diabetic patients.[166] In six patients, no abnormalities in the amino acid sequence were seen. Two patients were heterozygous and one homozygous for a silent polymorphism at nucleotide position 535, but this polymorphism is commonly seen in nondiabetic individuals.[204] Interestingly, one of the six patients had a substitution at codon 383, leading to an isoleucine-for-valine substitution at this position. The biological significance of this substitution is unclear, but larger-scale molecular scanning studies have verified that this mutation exists in only a small percentage (1–2%) of type 2 diabetic subjects, and it also exists in low frequency in nondiabetic subjects.[204] Since no other mutations in the GLUT-4 gene have been identified in T2DM, it would appear that abnormalities in the GLUT-4 gene are rare in T2DM and that the coding sequence of GLUT-4 is not a diabetes gene locus.

Translocation of GLUT-4 involves a complex system, and an expanding list of proteins involved in GLUT-4 vesicle trafficking, regulation of membrane fusion, and endocytotic events are being identified.[72] Thus it is quite possible that decreased GLUT-4 translocation could be due to altered expression or a functional defect of one or more of the GLUT-4 vesicle-trafficking proteins. An impairment of insulin signaling downstream of the receptor is also a likely cause of the decreased insulin-stimulated GLUT-4 translocation, and these are areas of intensive investigation.

Postreceptor Signaling Defects

After insulin binding and receptor autophosphorylation, a number of endogenous protein substrates are phosphorylated on tyrosine residues by the insulin receptor kinase. Insulin receptor substrate-1 (IRS-1) is the most thoroughly studied of these substrates. The ability of insulin to stimulate IRS-1 phosphorylation is decreased in both adipocytes[205] and skeletal muscle[206,207] from type 2 diabetic subjects. Rondinone and associates found that the IRS-1 protein content of adipose tissue was reduced by 70% in type 2 diabetic patients.[208] Clearly, this reduction in IRS-1 protein content could contribute to the decrease in IRS-1 phosphorylation observed in adipocytes.[205] However, this cannot be a factor in muscle because skeletal muscle IRS-1 levels are no different in type 2 diabetic patients than in lean or obese normal subjects.[206,207,209] Insulin-stimulated phosphorylation of IRS-2 is also impaired in skeletal muscle from type 2 diabetic subjects.[210] Thus IRS-2 does not compensate for the defect of IRS-1 phosphorylation in skeletal muscle from diabetic patients.

Studies in adipocytes from control, obese, and type 2 diabetic subjects showed that the insulin dose–response curves for stimulation of tyrosine phosphorylation of IRS-1 and of the insulin receptor β subunit were almost identical and that the ability of phosphorylated insulin receptors to phosphorylate IRS-1 was normal.[205] Because of this normal coupling between autophosphorylated β subunits and IRS-1 in adipocytes from type 2 diabetic patients, it is likely that the reduction in IRS-1 phosphorylation in adipocytes from these patients is essentially secondary to the insulin receptor kinase defect. Although similar detailed studies have not been performed in skeletal muscle, the finding that the abnormalities of the insulin receptor kinase and of IRS-1 phosphorylation in muscle parallel those in adipocytes suggests that the impairment of IRS-1 phosphorylation in muscle is also largely a consequence of the insulin receptor kinase defect.[207]

The enzyme PI-3-kinase is essential for insulin's effects on GLUT-4 translocation and glycogen synthase activation. As outlined earlier, this enzyme is activated by the binding of its regulatory subunit to tyrosine phosphorylated IRS-1 and IRS-2. Thus, tyrosine phosphorylation of IRS-1 and IRS-2 in response to insulin allows the regulatory subunit of PI-3-kinase to bind, leading to activation of the catalytic subunit of the enzyme. Several studies have shown that association of the p85 regulatory subunit with IRS-1 and IRS-2 in response to insulin is impaired in muscle of type 2 diabetic patients and there is a corresponding defect of PI-3-kinase activation.[207,210] Some[207,211] but not all[210] studies have found that activation of muscle PI-3-kinase by insulin is also impaired in obese nondiabetic subjects.

Glycogen Synthesis

Glycogen synthase, the rate-controlling enzyme of glycogen synthesis, is another potential locus for acquired or inherited insulin resistance in T2DM. Glycogen synthase activity has been measured in muscle biopsy samples, and the level of enzyme activity correlates with the magnitude of nonoxidative glucose disposal, as measured by indirect calorimetry during glucose clamp studies. Diminished activation of glycogen synthase, decreased insulin-stimulated muscle glycogen deposition, impaired insulin-mediated glucose disposal, and defective nonoxidative glucose disposal all exist in type 2 diabetic subjects.[194–197,212,213]

Glycogen synthase activity is reduced in T2DM by 35–50% as compared to controls at submaximal insulin levels, but the defect can be normalized by increasing insulin levels fourfold.[194] The glucose-6-phosphate activation constant was also increased, demonstrating a decreased sensitivity of muscle glycogen synthase in type 2 diabetes to allosteric activation by glucose-6-phosphate.[194] Importantly, the reduction in glycogen synthase activity in T2DM patients persists even when glucose uptake rates are normalized, indicating that the effect of insulin on glycogen synthesis is separate from its effect on glucose transport and that the defect in glycogen synthase activity is not simply due to a decline in glucose flux into the cell.[194]

The defect in glycogen synthase activity can be partially reversed by an 8-week course of sulfonylurea therapy,[196] raising the possibility that the irreversible component may be genetic in nature. This is also suggested by a study of 16 type 2 diabetic subjects, 18 first-degree relatives of type 2 diabetic patients, and 16 nondiabetic subjects. Activation of muscle glycogen synthase was impaired in the relatives with a high known genetic risk of developing T2DM, indicating that this may represent an early defect in the evolution of T2DM.[214]

To complement the cellular and biochemical studies cited above, the gene for glycogen synthase has been examined in T2DM. Groop and colleagues[215] reported an association between a rare polymorphism located in intronic sequences of the glycogen synthase gene and the type 2 diabetic phenotype in Finnish subjects. However, this association was not found in subsequent studies of French or American Caucasian subjects.[216,217] Molecular scanning of the entire glycogen synthase gene in Finnish subjects identified a missense mutation at position 464 in exon 11 in only 2 of 228 type 2 diabetic patients but none of 154 controls.[218] Clearly, glycogen synthase gene mutations are uncommon in T2DM. A Danish study failed to detect any abnormalities in the coding sequence of the glycogen synthase gene in eight subjects with T2DM.[219] These authors did, however, find a 39% reduction in the steady-state level of glycogen synthase mRNA per microgram of muscle DNA, which correlated with the reduced total glycogen synthase activity of vastus lateralis muscle of type 2 diabetic subjects as compared to matched controls. Recent studies of twin pairs discordant for T2DM suggest that this reduction in muscle glycogen synthase mRNA and protein levels found in some diabetic patients may be an acquired defect, perhaps secondary to hyperglycemia.[220]

FUNCTIONAL ASPECTS OF INSULIN RESISTANCE

From the earlier discussion, it is apparent that insulin resistance may be due to changes in insulin sensitivity, responsiveness, or both. This analysis relies on *in vivo* measures of the biologic effectiveness of a given concentration of insulin under steady-state conditions. However, steady-state analysis does not take into account potential alterations in the rate of insulin action. The kinetics of insulin action may be thought of as having two components: activation, and its opposite process, deactivation. The rate of activation of insulin's effects can be measured *in vivo* by assessing the time course of the increase in glucose disposal after starting an insulin infusion. Conversely, when insulin is removed from the system, deactivation of glucose disposal ensues. Early studies on the kinetics of insulin action were performed by Zierler and Rabinowitz.[221] These investigators infused insulin into the brachial artery and measured forearm glucose uptake. They found that when the insulin infusion was stopped, glucose uptake by the forearm persisted for up to an hour. They dubbed this the "memory effect" of insulin. Later, Sherwin and coworkers[222] and Insel and associates[124] confirmed that insulin's *in vivo* biologic effects dissipated slowly compared to the rapid decay of insulin from plasma. Finally, studies performed with isolated rat adipocytes have shown that deactivation of insulin's effect on glucose transport *in vitro* is slower than dissociation of insulin from its receptor. The glucose clamp technique is excellent for studying insulin's *in vivo* effects, and has generated much valuable information. However, it takes several hours before steady-state biologic effects of constant insulin infusions are reached, and this clearly does not reproduce the phasic way in which insulin is delivered into the circulation under physiologic conditions of meal ingestion. Furthermore, assessments confined to steady-state measurements of insulin action will not detect kinetic alterations in the onset (activation) or offset (deactivation) of insulin's biologic effects. Indeed, in view of the fact that in response to food, insulin is secreted in a phasic rather than a constant manner, a defect in the dynamics of insulin action might be a physiologically more important manifestation of insulin resistance than reduced steady-state hormonal effects. To evaluate the above ideas, a modification of the euglycemic glucose clamp technique was used to test the hypothesis that a common human insulin-resistant state (obesity) is characterized by abnormally slow activation and rapid deactivation of insulin's effects to stimulate peripheral glucose uptake.[223]

In these studies, insulin was given as a constant infusion and the time course of activation of insulin-stimulated glucose disposal was measured. To study deactivation, the insulin infusion was stopped and the rate of fall in glucose disposal rate was observed. Insulin was infused intravenously at rates of 15, 40, 120, and 1200 mU/m²/min in a group of obese, nondiabetic patients compared to a group of lean normal control subjects. Comparable plasma insulin levels were attained in the two groups at each insulin infusion rate (Fig. 22-21). The time course of glucose disposal during and after the termination of the insulin infusions is shown in Fig. 22-22A. It can be seen from this figure that at each insulin infusion the normals achieved higher maximal insulin-stimulated glucose disposal rates. Additionally, the rate of activation of insulin-stimulated glucose disposal was slower in the obese subjects (Fig. 22-22B); in each case, the normal subjects had a steeper initial rise in insulin-stimulated glucose disposal. In addition, the rate of deactivation of insulin-stimulated glucose disposal occurred more quickly in the obese subjects. The apparent $t_{1/2}$

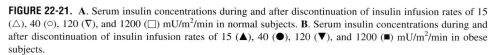

FIGURE 22-21. **A**. Serum insulin concentrations during and after discontinuation of insulin infusion rates of 15 (△), 40 (○), 120 (▽), and 1200 (□) mU/m²/min in normal subjects. **B**. Serum insulin concentrations during and after discontinuation of insulin infusion rates of 15 (▲), 40 (●), 120 (▼), and 1200 (■) mU/m²/min in obese subjects.

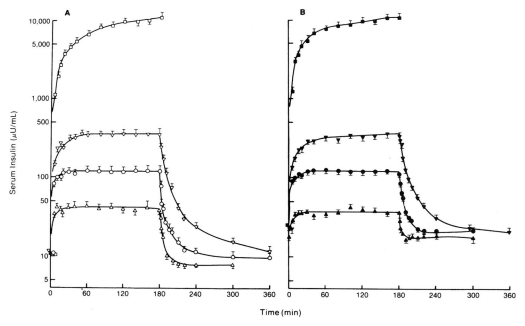

Time (min)

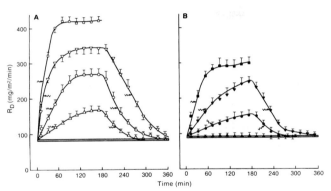

FIGURE 22-22A. A. Time course of total glucose Rd during and after termination of insulin infusion rates of 15 ($\triangle$), 40 ($\circ$), 120 ($\triangledown$), and 1200 ($\square$) mU/m^2/min in normal subjects. **B.** Time course of glucose Rd during and after termination of insulin infusion rates of 15 ($\blacktriangle$), 40 ($\bullet$), 120 ($\blacktriangledown$), and 1200 ($\blacksquare$) mU/m^2/min in obese subjects.

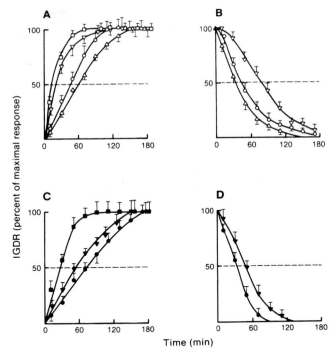

FIGURE 22-22B. Time course of activation (**A, C**) and deactivation (**B, D**) of insulin-stimulated glucose disposal. Data are expressed as a percentage of the maximal response, observed at the end of the infusion, and the insulin-stimulated glucose disposal rate (**IGDR**) is defined as the difference between the initial basal Rd value and the Rd values during and after cessation of the insulin infusion. Controls at insulin infusion rates of 15 ($\triangle$), 40 ($\circ$), 120 ($\triangledown$), and 1200 ($\square$) mU/m^2/min. Obese subjects at insulin infusion rates of 15 ($\blacktriangle$), 40 ($\bullet$), 120 ($\blacktriangledown$), and 1200 ($\blacksquare$) mU/m^2/min.

values for activation and deactivation are provided in Table 22-3. Since the insulin levels achieved in these studies were identical in obese and normal controls, the differences in glucose disposal must reflect differences in insulin action in normal and insulin-resistant subjects.

Thus, in insulin-resistant subjects the rate of activation of insulin-stimulated glucose disposal was two- to threefold slower compared to controls at every insulin level, and the rate of deactivation of insulin's effects was faster at all insulin levels. Therefore, one can postulate that the abnormal kinetics of insulin action in insulin-resistant obese subjects represent a functionally important manifestation of the insulin resistance in this condition. This concept is depicted in Fig. 22-23, which shows a theoretical time course of insulin action under conditions in which there is a 30% decrease in maximal steady-state insulin effects combined with a twofold slower rate of activation. At early points during the time course, the magnitude of the deficit in insulin's effects is far greater than that achieved at steady state. Considering that insulin rises and falls after meals, coupled with the kinetic defects in insulin action shown in Figs. 22-22 and 22-23, one can hypothesize that insulin's effects never reach steady state in the physiologic situation in obesity, and that the decrease in the rate of onset of insulin action and rapid deactivation serves to greatly minimize the biologic effects of the insulin secreted after oral glucose or meals in obesity, despite the fact that obese subjects are hyperinsulinemic.

To test this hypothesis, glucose disposal was measured in normal versus insulin-resistant obese subjects during phasic, rather than steady-state, insulin infusions. First, oral glucose tolerance

tests (OGTTs) with measurement of the plasma insulin profile were performed in a series of normal and obese subjects. The subjects then underwent two separate glucose clamp–type studies in each of which insulin was infused in a phasic stepped manner that reproduced the OGTT insulin profiles observed initially (Fig. 22-24). Each subject received an insulin infusion which reproduced the "normal" insulin profile as well as the "obese" insulin profile. Figure 22-25 demonstrates that this stepped insulin infusion method faithfully reproduced the insulin secretory profiles observed during the OGTTs. During these "insulin rate clamp" studies, stimulation of Rd and suppression of hepatic glucose production were measured. The results demonstrated that at comparable phasic, stepped insulin infusion rates, insulin-stimulated glucose disposal was reduced by 80–90% in the obese compared to

TABLE 22-3. Half-Maximal Activation (A$_{50}$IGRD) and Deactivation (D$_{50}$IGDR) Values in Normal and Obese Subjects

Insulin Infusion Rate	A$_{50}$IGDR		D$_{50}$IGDR	
	Normal (min)	Obese (min)	Normal (min)	Obese (min)
15 mU/m^2/min	52 ± 4	—	34 ± 3	—
40 mU/m^2/min	44 ± 2	74 ± 6†	43 ± 2	31 ± 6*
120 mU/m^2/min	29 ± 3	64 ± 8†	78 ± 5	46 ± 2*
1200 mU/m^2/min	21 ± 2	28 ± 3*		

*$p < 0.01$.

†$p < 0.001$; obese vs. nonobese.

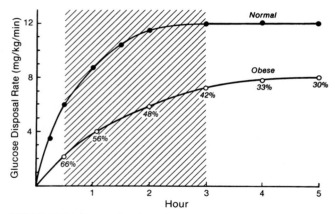

FIGURE 22-23. Effect of a theoretical defect in activation of the time course of glucose disposal. The lower curve depicts the results of a twofold slower rate of activation combined with a 30% decrease in maximal steady-state glucose disposal. As can be seen, this leads to a far greater decrease in the magnitude of the insulin effect at early time points than would be predicted based on the steady-state defect alone. Given the fact that insulin levels rise and fall relatively quickly (2–3 hours) after a meal, this kinetic defect is functionally important during the time interval over which post-prandial insulin is normally secreted.

FIGURE 22-24. Glucose and insulin levels during oral glucose tolerance tests (OGTTs) in normal (○) and obese (●) subjects (*$p < 0.01$).

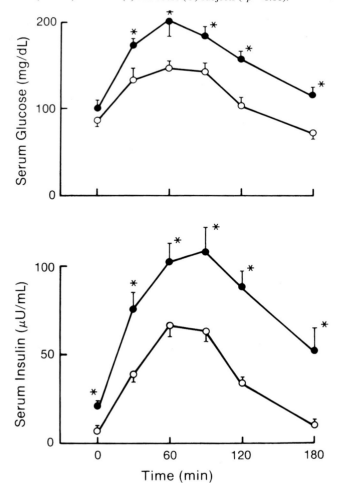

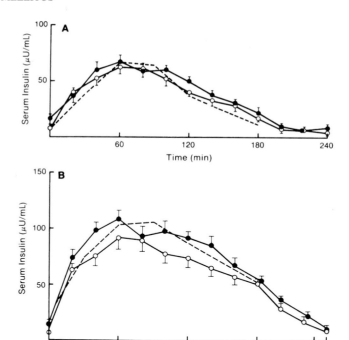

FIGURE 22-25. **A.** Insulin levels during the low-dose stepped insulin infusion in normal (○) and obese (●) subjects. **Dotted line**, mean OGTT insulin levels observed during OGTTs in normal subjects. **B.** Insulin levels during the high-dose stepped insulin infusion in normal (○) and obese (●) subjects. **Dotted line**, mean OGTT insulin levels observed during OGTTs in obese subjects.

control subjects (Fig. 22-26). More importantly, however, when the obese subjects were compared during the "hyperinsulinemic" infusion to the normal subjects at the "normoinsulinemic" infusion, a 60% reduction in glucose disposal was still observed in the obese group (Fig. 22-26C). Therefore, one can conclude that the post-prandial hyperinsulinemia of obesity is unable to fully compensate for the insulin resistance, primarily due to the kinetic defects of insulin action, and that *in vivo* in the physiologic setting, insulin-stimulated glucose disposal is still markedly reduced in obesity.[224] This conclusion was confirmed by carrying out glucose clamp studies in which insulin was infused at a constant rate to reach steady state at the same peak insulin levels as achieved during the phasic infusions. During these latter studies, the obese subjects achieved glucose disposal rates at hyperinsulinemia which were identical to the glucose disposal rates achieved in normal subjects at euinsulinemia [224] (Fig. 22-27). Thus, the differences between phasic insulin infusions versus constant insulin infusions bring out the marked kinetic abnormalities of insulin action in obesity. Doeden and Rizza have obtained similar results using a modification of the glucose clamp technique.[225]

Because hyperinsulinemia does not fully compensate for insulin resistance in obesity, what does? Upon analysis of the oral glucose tolerance profile, it is clear that obese subjects, while not diabetic or glucose intolerant, are somewhat hyperglycemic compared to controls, and it is the hyperglycemia, by virtue of mass action, that helps compensate for the insulin resistance to restore glucose disposal to normal during meals. Thus, following a meal, insulin-resistant obese subjects achieve relatively normal rates of

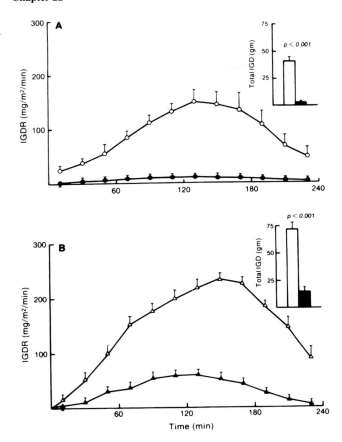

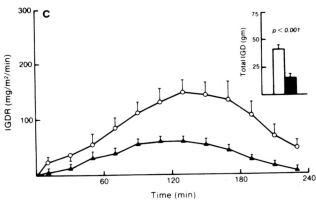

FIGURE 22-26. **A**. Insulin-stimulated glucose disposal rate (**IGDR**) in normal (○) and obese (●) subjects at the low-dose insulin infusion. **Inset**, Total absolute incremental glucose disposal (**IGD**) over 4 hours in normal (**open bars**) and obese (**solid bars**) subjects. **B**. IGDR (**solid**) in normal (○) and obese (●) subjects at the high-dose insulin infusion. **Inset**, total absolute incremental glucose disposal (**IGD**) over 4 hours in normal (**open bars**) and obese (**solid bars**) subjects. **C**. IGDR in normal subjects (○) at the low-dose insulin infusion compared with IGDR in obese subjects (●) at the high-dose insulin infusion. **Inset**, total absolute incremental glucose disposal (**IGD**) over 4 hours in normal (**open bars**) and obese (**solid bars**) subjects.

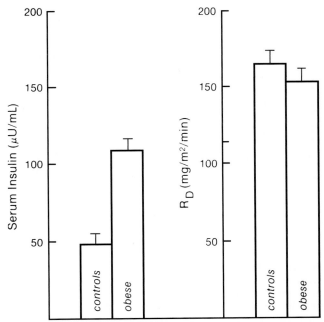

FIGURE 22-27. Steady-state plasma insulin levels and total glucose disposal rates (Rd) during 15-mU/m²/min insulin infusions in control subjects compared to 40-mU/m²/min insulin infusions in obese subjects.

glucose disposal (and therefore can accommodate an incoming glucose load), but only at the expense of hyperinsulinemia and relative hyperglycemia.

In confirmation of this notion, studies have shown[226] that when glucose disposal is measured during infusions in which both the OGTT insulin plus glucose profiles are reproduced in obese subjects, glucose disposal rates can be normalized. Thus, the mass action effects of postprandial glycemia contribute importantly to the maintenance of normal absolute rates of postprandial glucose disposal in obesity. Insulin resistance leads to a defect in postprandial glucose disposal in obesity. Hyperinsulinemia is an attempt to compensate for this defect by enhancing IMGU. When this compensatory effect is insufficient, absolute rates of glucose disposal remain impaired and the postprandial glucose level rises, so that by the mass action effect of glucose, glucose disposal rates are further augmented to a normal level (but at the expense of hyperinsulinemia and relative hyperglycemia). The obese patients depicted in Fig. 22-24 have substantial insulin resistance, and it can be roughly estimated that the hyperinsulinemia and postprandial glycemia each compensate ~50% for the deficit in glucose disposal induced by the insulin resistance. It seems likely that in subjects with milder states of insulin resistance, and/or in those obese subjects with particularly exuberant insulin secretion patterns, the hyperinsulinemia will be more effective as a compensatory mechanism.

Functional studies of adipocyte glucose transport in obesity have indicated that the kinetic abnormalities observed *in vivo* are most likely related to cellular defects in insulin action.[173] Thus, when the time course of insulin's ability to activate glucose transport was measured, a slower activation rate was observed in cells from obese subjects (Fig. 22-28); it took 15 ± 2 minutes to achieve half-maximal activation of insulin-stimulated glucose transport in cells from obese subjects compared to 9.4 ± 1.2 minutes ($p < 0.05$) in controls (Fig. 22-28). This decrease in the *in vitro* rate of

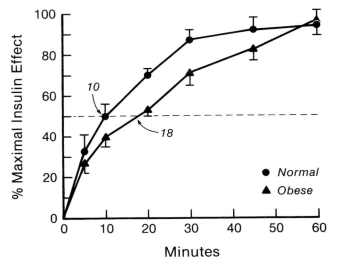

FIGURE 22-28. Time course of insulin-stimulated glucose transport. Adipocytes from lean (●) or obese (▲) subjects were exposed to a maximally effective concentration of insulin (25 ng/mL) at time 0, and 3-0-methylglucose uptake was measured at the indicated time points. Data are expressed as a percentage of the maximal effect for each subject and represent the mean (± SEM).

activation of glucose transport correlates quite well with the slower rates of activation of glucose disposal *in vivo*.

Comparable findings have been reported in T2DM.[174] Thus, marked kinetic defects in activation and deactivation of insulin's *in vivo* effects on glucose disposal are found. Nolan and colleagues[227] showed that the kinetic defect in insulin's ability to stimulate leg glucose uptake in type 2 diabetic patients was not accompanied by any delay in the activation of leg muscle insulin receptors by insulin. This suggests that the kinetic defect is distal to the insulin receptor. As in obesity, delayed activation of glucose transport is demonstrable in isolated adipocytes from type 2 diabetic patients. In general, the magnitude of the kinetic defects is greater in T2DM than in simple obesity. The presence of insulin resistance in T2DM, coupled with the impaired insulin secretion, explains the marked postprandial hyperglycemia in this condition. With this formulation it is evident that hyperglycemia is the major factor driving glucose disposal in T2DM, allowing these subjects to eventually dispose of an incoming meal or glucose load. These concepts may have implications regarding the treatment of type 2 diabetic patients. For example, intensive insulin therapy relies on algorithms for insulin delivery that were largely developed in type 1 diabetic patients. Clearly, such algorithms do not account for the kinetic defects present in insulin-resistant type 2 diabetic subjects. As such, these kinetic defects provide part of the explanation of why such large daily doses of insulin are needed to achieve ideal control in type 2 diabetic patients.

MOLECULAR GENETICS OF INSULIN RESISTANCE AND T2DM

Heredity plays a key role in the etiology of T2DM. Thus, although acquired factors such as obesity may be necessary for the phenotypic manifestation of T2DM, acquired factors alone are insufficient in most patients without preexisting genetic determinants.

Because insulin resistance predates the development of T2DM in most populations, it seems likely that some of the diabetogenic genes involve some aspect of insulin action. Available evidence indicates that T2DM is a genetically heterogeneous, polygenic disease. In other words, more than one diabetes gene occurs within a population, and it is possible that an individual must carry more than one abnormal gene in order to develop T2DM. For example, one or more genes involved in insulin action could be affected, along with a separately inherited defect responsible for the loss of β-cell function that occurs late in the course of T2DM.

Two basic strategies have been employed to identify potential diabetes genes. First is the candidate gene approach, in which it is hypothesized that a certain gene that has already been cloned and sequenced may be involved in the pathogenesis of T2DM. This hypothesis is then tested by comparing the sequence of this candidate gene in normal and type 2 diabetic subjects, looking for abnormalities in the disease state. The second approach makes use of polymorphic genetic markers or single nucleotide polymorphisms (SNPs), which are distributed throughout the genome, to map the location of the disease phenotype to a particular locus. This is done by determining whether the DNA markers cosegregate with the type 2 diabetic phenotype in a pedigree or population.

The insulin receptor glycogen synthase and GLUT-4 have been examined as potential candidate genes in insulin resistance and T2DM. As discussed earlier, the primary sequences of these proteins are normal in T2DM, eliminating them as diabetes gene loci, except in rare individuals. In some populations, polymorphisms of IRS-1 may be two to three times more common in type 2 diabetic patients than in normal subjects, and in some studies an association between polymorphisms affecting the region of IRS-1 thought to be important for PI-3-kinase binding and a reduction in insulin sensitivity has been found.[67] The most common IRS-1 variant involves a substitution of arginine for glycine at codon 972. Expression of this Arg[972] IRS-1 variant in a skeletal muscle cell line resulted in decreased activation of PI-3-kinase, decreased insulin-stimulated GLUT-4 translocation, and activation of glycogen synthase compared to cells expressing wild-type IRS-1.[228] Clearly, further studies are needed to assess the importance of these IRS-1 variants because they could contribute to the genetic basis of T2DM in a small subset of subjects. Very little information is available on other downstream insulin-signaling molecules. Several polymorphisms have been described in IRS-2, but there is general agreement that these are not associated with either insulin resistance or T2DM.[229,230] A polymorphism of the p85α subunit of PI-3-kinase in which isoleucine is substituted for methionine at codon 326 is common. In one study 2% of Danish Caucasians were found to be homozygous for the Met[326]Ile mutation, and this was associated with a reduction in insulin sensitivity, glucose effectiveness, and intravenous glucose tolerance.[231] However, subsequent studies do not support a role for this p85α variant in the etiology of insulin resistance or T2DM.[232,233]

The thiazolidinedione class of oral hypoglycemic agents act by increasing peripheral tissue insulin sensitivity. Because these agents work by binding to the nuclear peroxisome proliferator–activated receptor γ (PPAR-γ),[234] it follows that this receptor may play a role in modulating insulin sensitivity. Because PPAR-γ is also an important regulator of adipogenesis, it could influence whole-body insulin sensitivity indirectly through an effect on fat mass and lipid metabolism.[234] Several studies have therefore examined PPAR-γ as a potential candidate gene for insulin resistance and obesity in T2DM. The PPAR-γ gene gives rise to two alternate transcripts, PPAR-γ1 and PPAR-γ2, with PPAR-γ2 being expressed only in fat tissue. Molecular scanning of the PPAR-γ gene in diabetic Caucasians identified a Pro12Ala missense mutation in PPAR-γ2.[235] This mutation was associated with decreased PPAR-γ2 receptor activity and is found in about 10% of Caucasians and Mexican-Americans. The Pro12Ala variant was associated with lower BMI and improved insulin sensitivity in Finnish subjects,[236] but with a higher BMI and waist:hip ratio in Mexican-Americans.[237] These contrasting findings may be due to the different populations studied. However, two other large studies of European Caucasians concluded that the Pro12Ala mutation is not associated with either obesity or T2DM.[238,239] Another very rare inactivating mutation of PPAR-γ was found in three severely insulin resistant subjects characterized by marked hyperinsulinemia, acanthosis nigricans, and early-onset diabetes in the absence of obesity.[240] Thus, inactivating PPAR-γ mutations may account for a small number of subjects with very unusual forms of insulin resistance, but PPAR-γ does not appear to be an insulin-resistance gene locus in patients predisposed to typical T2DM.

Given the importance of obesity in most type 2 diabetic patients, genes that predispose to obesity, and in particular a more central distribution of body fat, could also underlie the genetic predisposition. The discovery that the genetic syndromes of obesity and diabetes in the ob/ob mouse and db/db mouse were due, respectively, to failure of leptin production and an abnormality of the leptin receptor suggested that similar defects may play a role in human obesity. However, leptin levels are generally increased in human obesity, and leptin-receptor gene mutations do not appear to cosegregate with common obesity in humans.[241,242] A polymorphism in the β$_2$-adrenergic receptor was found to be associated with obesity; replacement of glutamine by glutamate at codon 27 (Gln27Glu) was found in 24% of obese women but only 3% of nonobese women.[243] Homozygotes for Glu27 had on average 20 kg more adipose tissue, larger fat cells, higher fasting insulin levels, and a more central distribution of body fat. Although this particular polymorphism does not alter β-adrenoreceptor function, it is in strong linkage disequilibrium with another polymorphism (Arg16Gly) that is associated with increased sensitivity to agonist-induced downregulation.[243]

Gene mapping studies have generally sought linkage with the established type 2 diabetic phenotype rather than the underlying pathophysiological traits of insulin resistance and insulin secretory abnormalities (see Chap. 21). The few studies that have specifically looked for linkage between chromosomal loci and *in vivo* insulin action or fasting insulin levels (an index of insulin sensitivity) have been conducted in populations with a high prevalence of T2DM, such as the Pima Indians or Mexican-Americans. In Mexican-Americans, linkage was found between fasting insulin levels and markers on chromosome 3p.[244] This region contains two possible candidate genes for insulin resistance, namely, a glycogen branching enzyme involved in glycogen synthesis and a peroxisomal branched-chain acyl-CoA oxidase that is involved in the degradation of long-branched fatty acids.[244] Family studies in Pima Indians[245] and Mexican-Americans[246] have also suggested linkage between *in vivo* insulin resistance and a locus on chromosome 4q that encodes the intestinal fatty acid binding protein-2 (FABP-2). However, in three different European populations, no differences in allelic frequency at this locus were found between diabetic and nondiabetic individuals.[247]

A major development has been the positional cloning by Horikawa and colleagues of the gene for calpain 10 in the poly-

morphic "NIDDM1" region of chromosome 2 that shows linkage with T2DM in Mexican-Americans.[248] Horikawa and colleagues found that an SNP (UCSNP-43) in intron 3 of the calpain 10 gene showed an increased frequency of the common G allele in type 2 diabetic patients compared to controls, and evidence for linkage with T2DM. Interestingly, subjects homozygous for the putative at-risk G/G genotype were not at increased risk of T2DM, and it appears that other variations in the calpain 10 gene, in combination with the G allele at UCSNP-43, contribute to disease susceptibility. These investigators identified a number of high-risk calpain 10 gene haplotypes and found that the heterozygous 112/121 haplotype was the most common combination in Mexican-Americans with T2DM. They estimated that the 112/121 haplotype combination played a role in 14% of cases of T2DM in Mexican-Americans, but only 4% of Europeans participating in the study, in whom the combination was less common.[248] Calpain 10 is a member of the family of cysteine proteases that have a ubiquitous tissue distribution. Its involvement in the mechanisms of insulin action or secretion is unknown and will be the focus of much research in light of these genetic findings. In one study, Pima Indians homozygous for the UCSNP-43 G allele had lower skeletal muscle calpain 10 mRNA levels, higher insulin levels 2 hours after an oral glucose load, and a marginally lower (~5%) glucose disposal rate during a glucose clamp.[249]

A major advance in our understanding of potential genetic mechanisms of insulin resistance leading to the development of the type 2 diabetic phenotype has come from transgenic mouse models in which a specific gene thought to play a key role in insulin action has been disrupted either at the whole-body level or in a specific tissue. Mice with targeted disruption of the insulin receptor die a few days after birth, while heterozygous animals have a virtually normal phenotype.[250] These results in the heterozygous animals were perhaps not unexpected given the presence of spare insulin receptors on insulin target tissues. However, animals heterozygous for the IRS-1 null allele also do not develop diabetes, even though they display mild insulin resistance, hyperinsulinemia, and mildly impaired glucose tolerance as they age.[251,252] Mice homozygous for the IRS-1 null allele show growth retardation, but again only mild insulin resistance, because IRS-2 appears to provide an alternative signaling pathway, particularly in liver.[251] IRS-1 and IRS-2 are not, however, simply interchangeable proteins. Thus IRS-2 is critical for certain actions of insulin. For example, in the liver it plays an important role in the activation of PI-3-kinase by insulin and regulation of gluconeogenic enzyme levels.[253,254] Insulin signaling to PI-3-kinase in livers of IRS-2 −/− mice is markedly impaired, and this is associated with impaired suppression of glucose production despite normal IRS-1 levels.[253,255] Thus in hepatocytes IRS-1 does not compensate for IRS-2 deficiency, whereas IRS-2 is able to fully compensate for loss of IRS-1 in liver. Distinct roles of IRS-1 and IRS-2 have also been demonstrated in adipocytes. In brown adipocytes from IRS-2 knockout mice, insulin-stimulated glucose uptake is decreased by 50%. This defect is partially corrected by reexpression of IRS-2, but not by overexpression of IRS-1.[256]

Because severe deficiencies of insulin-signaling molecules are extremely rare in T2DM, and because T2DM is thought to be a polygenic disease, Bruning and colleagues[252] generated mice heterozygous for the null allele of more than one of the key signaling molecules. They found that mice heterozygous for the null alleles of both the insulin receptor and IRS-1 developed insulin resistance, hyperinsulinemia, and a progressive impairment of glucose tolerance, with overt diabetes developing in approximately 40% of these mice by the age of 6 months.[252] Mice heterozygous for deficiencies of the insulin receptor, IRS-1, and IRS-2 had an even more profound degree of insulin resistance in muscle and liver, and a higher percentage went on to develop overt diabetes.

Taken together, these studies indicate that combinations of relatively minor defects, which in isolation may not cause significant phenotypic abnormalities, can act synergistically to cause insulin resistance and glucose intolerance. The particular mix of defects is likely to differ between different populations. Clearly, some defects may be acquired (e.g., the downregulation of insulin receptors by high circulating insulin levels), and act in concert with inherited genetic defects to produce significant insulin resistance and impairment of insulin secretion.

Another key finding from studies of mouse genetics is that insulin receptor signaling in islet β cells is essential for normal function. Thus, mice in which the insulin receptor gene has been specifically ablated in islet β cells, but not in other tissues, have smaller islet β cells, and no first-phase insulin secretion in response to glucose, reminiscent of the β-cell defect in T2DM.[257] Second-phase glucose-induced insulin secretion is also blunted in these mice, and as they age, their glucose tolerance deteriorates, although they do not develop overt diabetes. IRS-2 rather than IRS-1 appears to be important for post-insulin-receptor signaling in islet β cells.[253] IRS-2 also mediates IGF-1 receptor signaling in the β cells.[258] IRS-2 thus plays a role in proliferative and neogenic responses. Thus IRS-2–deficient mice have a smaller β-cell mass than wild-type animals, whereas IRS-1–deficient mice develop β-cell hyperplasia to compensate for insulin resistance. IRS-2–deficient mice have hepatic, adipocyte, and muscle insulin resistance. Initially, they display fasting hyperinsulinemia and normal glucose-induced insulin secretion, but unlike IRS-1 deficient mice, their insulin secretion subsequently declines. They then become progressively hyperglycemic and overtly diabetic at several weeks of age.[253] These studies indicate that functional insulin receptors and postreceptor signaling are essential for normal β-cell function, and raise the possibility that insulin resistance at the level of the β cell may contribute to the decline in insulin secretion that supervenes during the natural history of T2DM.

INSULIN-DEPENDENT (TYPE 1) DIABETES MELLITUS

When applied to the patient with type 1 diabetes mellitus (T1DM), the term "insulin resistance" is more difficult to evaluate. It usually denotes a patient who requires a large amount of insulin (>100 U/d) to maintain an acceptable level of diabetic control. These patients are unusual and sometimes have high titers of anti-insulin antibodies. However, the great majority of T1DM patients do not require more than 100 U/d for control. In fact, daily insulin dose requirements of C-peptide–negative type 1 diabetic patients are similar to endogenous 24-hour insulin secretion rates in normal subjects matched for age, sex, and BMI.[259] Thus the question of whether the typical T1DM patient responds normally to insulin must be asked. No clear-cut answer emerges from the literature. One reason for this is that an insulin-dependent diabetic subject's insulin sensitivity is at least partially dependent on the degree of diabetic control, with resulting changes in the metabolic milieu, and these patients hardly represent a homogeneous population. By definition, subjects in poor control are more hyperglycemic, and the effect of hyperglycemia *per se* to induce a secondary state of

insulin resistance has already been discussed. In addition to hyperglycemia, changes in pH, counterregulatory hormones, and FFA concentrations can all influence insulin action, and as the degree of metabolic control deteriorates, these factors can change in such a way as to impair insulin action. Certainly, patients in ketoacidosis are insulin resistant.[260] In a longitudinal study of 15 type 1 diabetic patients, Yki-Jarvinen and Koivisto[261] found a 32% decrease in *in vivo* insulin action 2 weeks from diagnosis. However, 3 months after starting insulin therapy, sensitivity was restored to normal. Other studies also suggest that insulin sensitivity may be normal if a T1DM patient is maintained in euglycemic control.[108,262,263] Most T1DM patients have relatively poor glycemic control and lie somewhere between these extremes, so the status of insulin sensitivity is difficult to evaluate.

Studies using the forearm perfusion technique to assess insulin sensitivity have found that T1DM patients take up less glucose than normal, suggesting that peripheral tissues do not respond normally to insulin.[264] Hepatic sensitivity to insulin, however, appears to be normal in most conventionally treated type 1 diabetic patients. Thus, although glucagon levels are often increased in T1DM patients, the ability of insulin to inhibit glucose production is normal or even increased;[265] this might be explained by reduced hepatic sensitivity to glucagon.[266,267] Studies in which whole-body insulin-stimulated glucose disposal in type 1 diabetes has been assessed using the glucose clamp technique at several insulin infusion rates have generally shown a decrease in the maximal response without any rightward shift in the insulin dose–response curve.[262,263,268] This is thought to indicate that the abnormality is primarily distal to the insulin binding step. *In vitro* studies in isolated adipocytes from untreated type 1 diabetic patients showing a marked decrease in glucose transport at maximally stimulating insulin concentrations with no displacement of the insulin dose–response curve for this action of insulin, as well as unchanged insulin binding, support this view.[269]

When interpreting studies of insulin action in T1DM, it is important to bear in mind that in addition to the problem of variable diabetic control, the study populations may be heterogeneous. For example, a Danish study found that about 10% of patients originally classified as having type 1 diabetes, but without a high-risk HLA haplotype for the disease, carried mutations in the HNF-1α gene and were thus MODY-3 patients.[270] Furthermore, some studies may well have included some type 2 diabetic patients with very poor residual β-cell function. While the exact mechanism of insulin resistance in type 1 diabetic patients is unknown, since good metabolic control can reverse the insulin resistance, the defect must be acquired.[261–263,268,269] Most likely, hyperglycemia is the major factor causing this secondary state of insulin resistance, although other acquired factors may be contributory. In a sense, this aspect of glucotoxicity represents another complication of chronic hyperglycemia, and provides additional rationale for attempts to achieve the best possible glycemic control in patients with diabetes.

UNUSUAL FORMS OF INSULIN RESISTANCE

Syndromes of Insulin Resistance and Acanthosis Nigricans

In a series of well-documented reports Flier, Kahn, Roth, and their colleagues have described a group of patients with extreme insulin resistance and marked acanthosis nigricans, in the absence of any other diseases associated with insulin resistance such as lipodystrophy, Cushing's disease, or acromegaly.[271–273] Patients with these syndromes are classified into two general groups.[271,274] Type A patients tend to be young females with hirsutism, polycystic ovaries, mild virilism, coarse features, early accelerated growth, and, of course, acanthosis nigricans. Type B patients tend to be middle-aged females, although two males with this entity have now been reported. The syndrome in these patients is suggestive of an autoimmune disease with features such as hypergammaglobulinemia, proteinuria, hypocomplementemic nephritis, leukopenia, arthralgia, alopecia, enlarged salivary glands, and positive nuclear and anti-DNA antibodies. Patients with either of these subtypes have carbohydrate intolerance ranging from mild abnormalities of the oral glucose tolerance test to severe fasting hyperglycemia requiring enormous amounts of exogenous insulin. All of these patients are extremely hyperinsulinemic and respond poorly to the administration of exogenous insulin.

The mechanisms of this insulin resistance have been well studied, and in addition to learning about the cause of insulin resistance in a rare form of diabetes, these studies have provided important insights into overall insulin action. In type B patients, the mechanisms for the insulin resistance are fairly clear-cut. These patients have a severe defect in insulin binding to circulating monocytes, which is due primarily to an apparent reduction in binding affinity.[271,272] These patients have circulating antibodies directed against some portion of the insulin receptor, which impairs insulin binding to the patients' cells.[272,274] When immunoglobulins from these patients' sera are isolated and incubated *in vitro* with various cell types, subsequent measurements of insulin binding are also decreased. Furthermore, when the patients' freshly isolated circulating monocytes are "stripped" of adherent immunoglobulins, insulin binding returns to normal. Thus the role of the antireceptor antibody to directly interfere with the ability of insulin to bind to receptors *in vivo* is undisputed in these patients.

The insulin resistance of these patients can be quite severe, and one subject received as much as 177,000 U of insulin per day. The metabolic abnormalities in this syndrome can wax and wane, and a few patients have been described who have experienced complete remission of the insulin-resistant diabetic state with disappearance of antireceptor antibodies from the plasma. In a few patients remission occurred during immunosuppressive therapy;[275] however, the documented occurrence of spontaneous remissions makes the potential causal relationship between drug therapy and remission unclear.

In other patients with genetic forms of severe insulin resistance (such as type A patients), various defects in insulin action have been described.[274,276,277] Some of these patients show marked decreases in insulin binding affinity, whereas others show reduced levels of receptor expression. Intrinsic defects in receptor kinase activity or postreceptor abnormalities have also been reported. Many of these patients have been studied using molecular biologic approaches, and this has led to the identification of a large number of different mutations in the insulin receptor gene. These mutations can lead to abnormal insulin binding, decreased receptor kinase activity, impaired processing of the receptor polypeptide, or abnormal receptor gene transcription, and the reader is referred to Chap. 5 for a full discussion of this subject.

Generalized Lipodystrophy and Lipoatrophy

Many patients have been described as having generalized loss of subcutaneous and deep adipose tissue, hepatosplenomegaly, hyperlipoproteinemia, and diabetes mellitus. Frequently, these patients also have acanthosis nigricans. Diabetes associated with this syndrome is of the insulin-resistant type. Thus these patients have highly elevated circulating plasma insulin levels and respond poorly to the administration of exogenous insulin. Similar findings can be observed in patients with partial lipodystrophy, in whom adipose tissue loss can occur exclusively above the waist, or less frequently, only below the waist. Both genetic and acquired forms of these lipodystrophic syndromes are recognized. A number of missense mutations in the gene for lamin A/C, a component of the nuclear envelope, have recently been identified in kindreds with the familial form of partial lipodystrophy.[278,279] Presumably these mutations interfere with adipocyte differentiation. The gene for congenital generalized lipodystrophy has been mapped to a region of chromosome 9 that encodes the retinoid X receptor alpha gene.[280] The latter would be a plausible candidate gene given its critical role in adipocyte differentiation.

The mechanism of the insulin resistance in the lipodystrophies is poorly understood and only a few conflicting reports exist. Oseid and colleagues[281] found that patients with generalized lipodystrophy have decreased insulin binding to circulating monocytes due to a slight decrease in receptor number and a large decrease in receptor affinity. However, upon fasting, the ability of cells from these patients to bind insulin increased normally, suggesting that this defect was secondary to the existing hyperinsulinemia rather than a primary abnormality. On the other hand, Kriauciunas and coworkers[282] found decreased insulin binding and decreased tyrosine kinase activity of receptors in cultured fibroblasts from patients with this syndrome, suggesting that the defect may be genetic and primary. However, others found normal insulin binding to cultured fibroblasts and to circulating monocytes from these patients.[283,284] Possibly, these disparate findings indicate that different defects exist in different patients. The insulin resistance may well be secondary to the lipoatrophy and not due to any primary genetic defect in the insulin action pathway. A characteristic finding in patients with lipodystrophy is muscle hypertrophy associated with accumulation of triglyceride and glycogen within muscle fibers.[276] The link between intramuscular fat and insulin resistance was discussed earlier. In two patients studied using the hyperinsulinemic euglycemic clamp, an impairment of HGO suppression by insulin was found together with a decrease in insulin-stimulated glucose disposal and a marked impairment of suppression of lipid oxidation.[285] These findings could all be explained by the high circulating FFA and triglyceride levels and accumulation of fat in the liver and skeletal muscles of these patients.

Ataxia Telangiectasia

Ataxia telangiectasia is a rare recessive syndrome caused by inactivating mutations in a gene on chromosome 11 that encodes a protein that plays an important role in the cellular response to DNA damage.[286] Homozygous patients develop progressive cerebellar ataxia, oculocutaneous telangiectasia, recurrent sinopulmonary infections, and a number of diverse abnormalities of the immune system. Frequently, this syndrome is accompanied by glucose intolerance and insulin resistance. Schalch and associates[287] reported that about 60% of patients with this syndrome displayed glucose intolerance, hyperinsulinemia, and an attenuated hypoglycemic response to exogenously injected insulin. In the patients who have been well studied, secondary causes of insulin resistance such as circulating insulin antibodies, obesity, lipoatrophy, and excessive growth hormone or corticosteroid secretion have been ruled out. Thus the insulin resistance that may occur in ataxia telangiectasia appears to be an intrinsic component of this syndrome.

In general, the degree of glucose intolerance has been mild, rarely requiring insulin therapy. Furthermore, a tendency toward exacerbation and remission of the insulin-resistant state has been noted. Earlier researchers[287] recognized the resistance to the hypoglycemic effects of exogenous insulin and suggested an unknown circulating insulin antagonist might be a causative factor. Bar and associates[83] published detailed studies in two patients with ataxia telangiectasia and insulin resistance. A marked decrease in the binding affinity of insulin receptors on freshly isolated circulating monocytes was noted, while the insulin receptors of fibroblasts cultured from skin biopsies were normal. The fact that the insulin receptor abnormality did not persist in cell culture indicated that this defect was not genetic and was likely to be secondary to some aspect of the *in vivo* environment. In confirmation of this idea, these workers were able to demonstrate a circulating inhibitor of insulin binding, most likely an immunoglobulin, in the plasma of these patients. On the basis of these studies, it would appear that the insulin resistance in ataxia telangiectasia is due to the production of an antibody that inhibits insulin binding. Serial studies in one patient demonstrated the disappearance of this circulating inhibitor, coincident with the remission of the insulin resistance,[83] and this greatly strengthens the argument for a cause-and-effect relationship between these variables.

Leprechaunism

Leprechaunism is a very rare autosomal recessive disease characterized by an unusual facial appearance, hirsutism, clitorimegaly, acanthosis nigricans, sparse subcutaneous fat stores, and a number of other somatic abnormalities. This syndrome is almost always fatal. Most patients die during the first 1–2 years of life, with hyperglycemia and the histologic findings of β-cell hyperplasia. Several children with this syndrome have now been studied.[276,277,288] In those patients in whom *in vivo* data are available, hyperinsulinemia and severe insulin resistance are present.[277,288] The immunoreactive material in the plasma of these patients has been shown to be genuine insulin of normal biologic activity.[288] Circulating insulin antagonists have not been detected, and this points to a cellular defect in insulin action.[277,288] This concept is supported by molecular studies that have revealed the presence of insulin-receptor gene mutations in these patients. Interestingly, the mutations thus far described have been different, indicating that more than one genotype can lead to a common phenotype. It is important to eventually unravel the relationship between the receptor mutations and the multiple congenital anomalies displayed by these subjects, and this is discussed more thoroughly in Chap. 5.

Common Features of Severe Insulin-Resistant States

There are several somatic features that many of these unusual insulin-resistant states share (acanthosis nigricans, hirsutism, and mild virilism). Certainly, not every patient with one of these syndromes has these characteristics, but many do. Additionally, it is well known that severely obese insulin-resistant women often have acanthosis nigricans, hirsutism, and mild virilism. These frequent associations suggest some basic relationship between these phenomena, and it seems possible that some metabolic feature of hyperinsulinemia and insulin resistance leads to the associated so-

matic characteristics described. Although no mechanism is known, it is interesting to note that insulin is able to bind to IGF-1 receptors and can exert growth-like properties through this mechanism. Although insulin binds with a much higher affinity to the insulin receptor than to the IGF-1 receptor, it is possible to speculate that at very high circulating insulin levels (as seen in severe insulin-resistant states) insulin is capable of binding (or overlapping) into IGF-1 receptors, stimulating growth and proliferation of various cell types. With this formulation, high levels of circulating insulin could cross-react with other hormone receptors, possibly leading to some of the somatic features associated with a variety of insulin-resistant states.

REFERENCES

1. Major RH: Diseases of metabolism. Diabetes mellitus. In: Major RH, Thomas CC, eds. *Classic Descriptions of Disease,* with biographical sketches of the authors. Springfield, Ill., CC Thomas 1945;245.
2. Banting FG, Best CH: The internal secretion of the pancreas. *J Lab Clin Med* 1922;7:251.
3. Banting FG, Best CH: Pancreatic extracts. *J Lab Clin Med* 1922;7:464.
4. Himsworth H: The syndrome of diabetes mellitus and its cause. *Lancet* 1949;1:465.
5. Yalow RS, Berson SA: Immunoassay of endogenous plasma insulin in man. *J Clin Invest* 1960;39:1157.
6. Rabinowitz D, Zierler KL: Forearm metabolism in obesity and its response to intraarterial insulin. *J Clin Invest* 1962;41:2173.
7. Given BD, Mako ME, Tager H, *et al*: Circulating insulin with reduced biological activity in a patient with diabetes. *N Engl J Med* 1980;302:129.
8. Olefsky JM, Saekow M, Tager H, *et al*: Characterization of a mutant human insulin species. *J Biol Chem* 1980;255:6098.
9. Tager H, Given B, Baldwin D, *et al*: A structurally abnormal insulin causing human diabetes. *Nature* 1979;281:122.
10. Gabbay KH, De Luca K, Fisher JN, *et al*: Familial hyperproinsulinemia: An autosomal dominant defect. *N Engl J Med* 1976;294:911.
11. Warren-Perry MG, Manley SE, Ostrega D, *et al*: A novel point mutation in the insulin gene giving rise to hyperproinsulinemia. *J Clin Endocrinol Metab* 1997;82:1629.
12. Perley M, Kipnis DM: Effect of glucocorticoids on plasma insulin. *N Engl J Med* 1966;274:1237.
13. Nosadini R, Del Prato S, Tiengo A, *et al*: Insulin resistance in Cushing's syndrome. *J Clin Endocrinol Metab* 1983;57:529.
14. Rizza R, Mandarino LJ, Gerich JF: Cortisol-induced insulin resistance in man: Impaired suppression of glucose production and stimulation of glucose utilization due to a postreceptor defect of insulin action. *J Clin Endocrinol Metab* 1982;54:131.
15. Pilkis SJ, Granner DK: Molecular physiology of the regulation of hepatic gluconeogenesis and glycolysis. *Annu Rev Physiol* 1992;54:885.
16. Wise JK, Hendler R, Felig P: Influence of glucocorticoids on glucagon secretion and plasma amino acid concentrations in man. *J Clin Invest* 1973;52:2774.
17. Simmons PS, Miles JM, Gerich JE, *et al*: Increased proteolysis: An effect of increases in plasma cortisol within the physiologic range. *J Clin Invest* 1984;73:412.
18. Divertie GD, Jensen MD, Miles JM: Stimulation of lipolysis in humans by physiological hypercortisolemia. *Diabetes* 1991;40:1228.
19. Marco J, Calle C, Roman D, *et al*: Hyperglucagonism induced by glucocorticoid treatment in man. *N Engl J Med* 1973;288:128.
20. Olefsky JM: Effect of dexamethasone on insulin binding glucose transport, and glucose oxidation of isolated rat adipocytes. *J Clin Invest* 1975;56:1499.
21. Dimitriadis G, Leighton B, Parry-Billings M, *et al*: Effects of glucocorticoid excess on the sensitivity of glucose transport and metabolism to insulin in rat skeletal muscle. *Biochem J* 1997;321:707.
22. Olefsky JM, Johnson J, Liu F, *et al*: The effects of acute and chronic dexamethasone administration on insulin binding to isolated rat hepatocytes and adipocytes. *Metabolism* 1975;24:517.

23. Kahn CR, Goldfine ID, Neville DM Jr, *et al*: Alterations in insulin binding induced by changes in vivo in the levels of glucocorticoids and growth hormone. *Endocrinology* 1978;103:1054.

24. Baron AD, Wallace P, Brechtel G: *In vivo* regulation of non-insulin mediated glucose uptake and insulin mediated glucose uptake by cortisol. *Diabetes* 1987;36:1230.

25. Sharp PS, Beshyah SA, Johnston DG: Growth hormone disorders and secondary diabetes. In: Alberti KGMM, Johnston DG, eds. *Baillieres Clin Endocrinol Metab* 1992;6:819.

26. Sherwin RS, Schulman GA, Hendler R, *et al*: Effect of growth hormone on oral glucose tolerance and circulating metabolic fuels in man. *Diabetologia* 1983;24:155.

27. Rizza RA, Mandarino LJ, Gerich JE. Effects of growth hormone on insulin action in man: Mechanisms of insulin resistance, impaired suppression of glucose production, and impaired stimulation of glucose utilization. *Diabetes* 1982;31:663.

28. Moller N: The role of growth hormone in the regulation of human fuel metabolism. In: Flyvberg A, Orskov H, Alberti KGMM, eds. *Growth Hormone and Insulin-Like Growth Factor I in Human and Experimental Diabetes*. Wiley:1993;77.

29. Ferrara CM, Cushman SW: GLUT4 trafficking in insulin-stimulated rat adipose cells: Evidence that heterotrimeric GTP-binding proteins regulate the fusion of docked GLUT4- containing vesicles. *Biochem J* 1999;343:571.

30. Baron AD, Wallace P, Olefsky JM: In vivo regulation of non-insulin-mediated and insulin-mediated glucose uptake by epinephrine. *J Clin Endocrinol Metab* 1987;64:889.

31. Kruszynska YT, Frias JP: The role of β-adrenergic signalling in the regulation of fat and energy metabolism. In: Marshall SM, Home PD, Rizza RA, eds. *The Diabetes Annual*. Elsevier Science:1999;12:181.

32. Randle PJ, Hales CN, Garland PB, *et al*: The glucose fatty-acid cycle. Its role in insulin sensitivity and the metabolic disturbances of diabetes mellitus. *Lancet* 1963;2:785.

33. Boden G: Free fatty acids, insulin resistance, and type 2 diabetes mellitus. *Proc Assoc Am Physicians* 1999;111:241.

34. Bonadonna RC, Zych K, Boni C, *et al*: Time dependence of the interaction between lipid and glucose in humans. *Am J Physiol* 1989;257:E49.

35. Roden M, Price TB, Perseghin G, *et al*: Mechanism of free fatty acid induced insulin resistance in humans. *J Clin Invest* 1996;97:2859.

36. Dresner A, Laurent D, Marcucci M, *et al*: Effects of free fatty acids on glucose transport and IRS-1 associated phosphatidylinositol 3-kinase activity. *J Clin Invest* 1999;103:253.

37. Griffin ME, Marcucci MJ, Cline GW, *et al*: Free fatty acid induced insulin resistance is associated with activation of protein kinase C theta and alterations in the insulin signaling cascade. *Diabetes* 1999;48:1270.

38. Krssak M, Falk Petersen K, Dresner A, *et al*: Intramyocellular lipid concentrations are correlated with insulin sensitivity in humans: A ^{1}H NMR spectroscopy study. *Diabetologia* 1999;42:113.

39. Perseghin G, Scifo P, De Cobelli F, *et al*: Intramyocellular triglyceride content is a determinant of in vivo insulin resistance in humans: A ^{1}H-^{13}C nuclear magnetic resonance spectroscopy assessment in offspring of type 2 diabetic parents. *Diabetes* 1999;48:1600.

40. Falholt K, Jensen I, Lindkaer-Jensen S, *et al*: Carbohydrate and lipid metabolism of skeletal muscle in type 2 diabetic patients. *Diabet Med* 1988;5:27.

41. Jacob S, Machann J, Rett K, *et al*: Association of increased intramyocellular lipid content with insulin resistance in lean nondiabetic offspring of type 2 diabetic subjects. *Diabetes* 1999;48:1113.

42. Jeandidier N, Boivin S, Sapin R, *et al*: Immunogenicity of intraperitoneal insulin infusion using programmable implantable devices. *Diabetologia* 1995;38:577.

43. Kurtz AB, Nabarro JDN: Circulating insulin-binding antibodies. *Diabetologia* 1980;19:329.

44. Waldhausl WK, Bratusch-Marrain P, Kruse V, *et al*: Effect of insulin antibodies on insulin pharmacokinetics and glucose utilization in insulin-dependent diabetic patients. *Diabetes* 1985;34:166.

45. Roy B, Chou MCY, Field JB: Time-action characteristics of regular and NPH insulin in insulin-treated diabetics. *J Clin Endocrinol Metab* 1980;50:475.

46. Flier JS, Kahn CR, Roth J, *et al*: Antibodies that impair insulin receptor binding in an unusual diabetic syndrome with severe insulin resistance. *Science* 1975;190:63.

47. Kahn CR, Baird KL, Flier JS, *et al*: Effects of autoantibodies to the insulin receptor on isolated adipocytes: Studies of insulin binding and insulin action. *J Clin Invest* 1977;60:1094.

48. Steppan CM, Bailey ST, Bhat S, *et al*: The hormone resistin links obesity to diabetes. *Nature* 2001;409:307.

49. Misbin RI, Green A, Alvarez IM, *et al*: Inhibition of insulin-stimulated glucose transport by factor extracted from serum of insulin-resistant patient. *Diabetes* 1988;37:1217.

50. Molina JM, Cooper G, Leighton B, Olefsky JM: Induction of insulin resistance in vivo by amylin and calcitonin gene-related peptide. *Diabetes* 1990;39:260.

51. Ludvik B, Kautzky-Willer A, Prager R, *et al*: Amylin: History and overview. *Diabet Med* 1997;14(suppl):9.

52. Kassir AA, Upadhyay AK, Lim TJ, *et al*: IAPP does not cause peripheral or hepatic insulin resistance in conscious dogs, but does have a hypocalcemic effect. *Diabetes* 1991;40:998.

53. Hoppener JWM, Verbeek JS, de Koning EJP, *et al*: Chronic overproduction of islet amyloid polypeptide/amylin in transgenic mice: Lysosomal localization of human islet amyloid polypeptide and lack of marked hyperglycaemia or hyperinsulinaemia. *Diabetologia* 1993;36:1258.

54. Schmitz O: The amylin analogue pramlintide: Mechanisms of actions and possible therapeutic implications. In: Marshall SM, Home PD, Rizza RA, eds. *The Diabetes Annual*. Elsevier Science:1999;12:181.

55. Hotamisligil GS, Spiegelman BM: Tumor necrosis factor-α: A key component of the obesity-diabetes link. *Diabetes* 1994;43:1271.

56. Ledgerwood E, Prins JB: Tumour necrosis factor alpha. In: Marshall SM, Home PD, Rizza RA, eds. *The Diabetes Annual*. Elsevier Science:1999;12:161.

57. Spiegelman BM, Choy L, Hotamisligil GS, *et al*: Regulation of adipocyte gene expression in differentiation and syndromes of obesity/diabetes. *J Biol Chem* 1993;268:6823.

58. Hotamisligil GS, Peraldi P, Budavari A, *et al*: IRS-1 mediated inhibition of insulin receptor tyrosine kinase activity in TNF-α and obesity induced insulin resistance. *Science* 1996;271:665.

59. Ofei F, Hurel S, Newkirk J, *et al*: Effects of an engineered human anti TNF-α antibody (CDP571) on insulin sensitivity and glycemic control in patients with NIDDM. *Diabetes* 1996;45:881.

60. Yudkin JS, Kumari M, Humphries SE, *et al*: Inflammation, obesity, stress and coronary heart disease: Is interleukin-6 the link? *Atherosclerosis* 1999;148:209.

61. Kern PA, Ranganathan S, Li C, *et al*: Adipose TNF and IL-6 expression in human obesity-associated insulin resistance. *Diabetes* 2000;(suppl 1)49:A24.

62. Fernandez-Real JM, Broch M, Vendrell J, *et al*: Interleukin-6 gene polymorphism and lipid abnormalities in healthy subjects. *J Clin Endocrinol Metab* 2000;85:1334.

63. Ullrich A, Bell JR, Chen EY, *et al*: Human insulin receptor and its relationship to the tyrosine kinase family of oncogenes. *Nature* 1985;313:756.

64. Kahn CR, White MF: The insulin receptor and the molecular mechanisms of insulin action. *J Clin Invest* 1988;82:1151.

65. Wilden PA, Siddle K, Haring H, *et al*: The role of insulin receptor kinase domain autophosphorylation in receptor mediated activities. *J Biol Chem* 1992;267:13719.

66. White MF: The IRS-signalling system and the IRS proteins. *Diabetologia* 1997;40(suppl 2):S2.

67. Virkamaki A, Ueki K, Kahn RC: Protein-protein interaction in insulin signaling and the molecular mechanisms of insulin resistance. *J Clin Invest* 1999;103:931.

68. McClain DA, Maegawa H, Lee J, *et al*: A mutant insulin receptor with defective tyrosine kinase displays no biologic activity and does not undergo endocytosis. *J Biol Chem* 1987;262:14663.

69. Ebina Y, Araki E, Taira M, *et al*: Replacement of lysine residue 1030 in the putative ATP-binding region of the insulin receptor abolishes insulin- and antibody-stimulated glucose uptake and receptor kinase activity. *Proc Natl Acad Sci USA* 1987;84:704.

70. Morgan DO, Ho L, Korn LJ, *et al*: Insulin action is blocked by a monoclonal antibody that inhibits the insulin receptor kinase. *Proc Natl Acad Sci USA* 1986;83:328.

71. Imamura T, Vollenweider P, Egawa K, *et al*: G alpha-q/11 protein plays a key role in insulin-induced glucose transport in 3T3-L1 adipocytes. *Mol Cell Biol* 1999;19:6765.

72. Elmendorf JS, Pessin JE: Insulin signaling regulating the trafficking and plasma membrane fusion of Glut 4-containing intracellular vesicles. *Exp Cell Res* 1999;253:55.

73. Saltiel AR: Diverse signaling pathways in the cellular actions of insulin. *Am J Physiol* 1996;270:E375.

74. Bar RS, Gorden P, Roth J, et al: Fluctuations in the affinity and concentration of insulin receptors on circulating monocytes of obese patients: Effects of starvation, refeeding and dieting. *J Clin Invest* 1976;58:1123.

75. Caro JF, Sinha MK, Raju SJ, et al: Insulin receptor kinase in human skeletal muscle from obese subjects with and without non-insulin dependent diabetes. *J Clin Invest* 1987;79:1330.

76. Olefsky JM: Insulin resistance and insulin action: An in vitro and in vivo perspective. *Diabetes* 1981;20:148.

77. Olefsky JM, Reaven GM: Insulin binding in diabetes: Relationships with plasma insulin levels and insulin sensitivity. *Diabetes* 1977;26:680.

78. Freidenberg GR, Reichart D, Olefsky JM, et al: Reversibility of defective adipocyte insulin receptor kinase activity in non-insulin dependent diabetes mellitus: Effect of weight loss. *J Clin Invest* 1990;82:1398.

79. Maegawa H, Shigeta Y, Egawa K, et al: Impaired autophosphorylation of insulin receptors from abdominal skeletal muscles in nonobese subjects with NIDDM. *Diabetes* 1991;40:815.

80. Muggeo M, Bar RS, Roth J, et al: The insulin resistance of acromegaly: Evidence for two alterations in the insulin receptor on circulating monocytes. *J Clin Endocrinol Metab* 1977;48:17.

81. Kahn CR, Goldfine ID, Neville DM Jr, et al: Alterations in insulin binding induced by changes in vivo in the levels of glucocorticoids and growth hormone. *Endocrinology* 1978;103:1054.

82. Bertoli A, De Pirro R, Fusco A, et al: Differences in insulin receptors between men and menstruating women and influence of sex hormones on insulin binding during the menstrual cycle. *J Clin Endocrinol Metab* 1980;50:246.

83. Bar RS, Lewis WR, Rechler MM, et al: Extreme insulin resistance in ataxia telangiectasia. Defect in affinity of insulin receptors. *N Engl J Med* 1978;298:1164.

84. Oseid S, Beck-Nielsen H, Pedersen O: Decreased binding of insulin to its receptor in patients with congenital generalized lipodystrophy. *N Engl J Med* 1977;296:245.

85. Gliemann J, Gammeltoft S, Vinten J: Time course of insulin-receptor binding and insulin-induced lipogenesis in isolated rat fat cells. *J Biol Chem* 1975;250:3368.

86. Kono T, Barham FW: The relationship between the insulin-binding capacity of fat cells and the cellular response to insulin: Studies with intact and trypsin-treated fat cells. *J Biol Chem* 1971;246:6210.

87. Kahn CR: Insulin resistance, insulin insensitivity, and insulin unresponsiveness: A necessary distinction. *Metab Clin Exp* 1978;27:1893.

88. Seely BL, Olefsky JM: Potential cellular and genetic mechanisms for insulin resistance in common disorders of obesity and diabetes. In: Moller D, ed. *Insulin Resistance and Its Clinical Disorders*. Wiley: 1993;187.

89. Reaven GM: Role of insulin resistance in human disease. *Diabetes* 1988;37:1595.

90. Granner DK, O'Brien RM: Molecular physiology and genetics of NIDDM. Importance of metabolic staging. *Diabetes Care* 1992;15:369.

91. Kruszynska YT, Olefsky JM: Cellular and molecular mechanisms of non-insulin dependent diabetes mellitus. *J Invest Med* 1996;44:413.

92. Ferrannini E, Groop LC: Hepatic glucose production in insulin resistant states. *Diabetes Metab Rev* 1989;5:711.

93. Kolterman OG, Gray RE, Griffin J, et al: Receptor and post-receptor defects contribute to the insulin resistance in non-insulin dependent diabetes mellitus. *J Clin Invest* 1981;68:957.

94. Dinneen S, Gerich J, Rizza R: Carbohydrate metabolism in non-insulin-dependent diabetes mellitus. *N Engl J Med* 1992;327:707.

95. Warram JH, Martin BC, Krolewski AS, et al: Slow glucose removal rate and hyperinsulinemia precede the development of Type II diabetes in the offspring of diabetic parents. *Ann Int Med* 1990;13:909.

96. Eriksson J, Franssila-Kallunki A, Ekstrand A, et al: Early metabolic defects in persons at increased risk for non-insulin-dependent diabetes mellitus. *N Engl J Med* 1989;321:337.

97. Zimmet PZ: Kelly West Lecture 1991. Challenges in diabetes epidemiology from West to East. *Diabetes Care* 1991;15:232.

98. Pershegin G, Ghosh S, Gerow K, et al: Metabolic defects in lean non-diabetic offspring of NIDDM parents: A cross sectional study. *Diabetes* 1997;46:1010.

99. Taylor SI, Accili D, Imai Y: Insulin resistance or insulin deficiency. Which is the primary cause of NIDDM? *Diabetes* 1994;43:735.

100. Polonsky KS, Sturis J, Bell GI: Non-insulin-dependent diabetes mellitus—a genetically programmed failure of the beta cell to compensate for insulin resistance. *N Engl J Med* 1996;334:777.

101. Alberti KGMM: The clinical implications of impaired glucose tolerance. *Diabet Med* 1996;13:927.

102. Kahn CR, Vicent D, Doria A: Genetics of non-insulin-dependent (type II) diabetes mellitus. *Annu Rev Med* 1996;47:509.

103. O'Rahilly S, Wainscoat JS, Turner RC: Type 2 (non-insulin-dependent) diabetes mellitus. New genetics for old nightmares. *Diabetologia* 1988;31:407.

104. Permutt MA: Genetics of NIDDM. *Diabetes Care* 1990;13:1150.

105. Vaag A, Henriksen JE, Madsbad S, et al: Insulin secretion, insulin action, and hepatic glucose production in identical twins discordant for non-insulin-dependent diabetes mellitus. *J Clin Invest* 1995;95:690.

106. Yki-Jarvinen H: Glucose toxicity. *Endocr Rev* 1992;13:415.

107. Yki-Jarvinen H: Toxicity of hyperglycaemia in type 2 diabetes. *Diabetes Metab Rev* 1998;14(suppl 1):S45.

108. Kruszynska YT, Home PD: Insulin insensitivity in type 1 diabetes. *Diabet Med* 1987;4:414.

109. Reaven GM, Sageman WS, Swenson RS: Development of insulin resistance in normal dogs following alloxan-induced insulin deficiency. *Diabetologia* 1997;13:459.

110. Rossetti L, Lauglin MR: Correction of chronic hyperglycemia with vanadate, but not with phlorizin, normalizes in vivo glycogen repletion and in vitro glycogen synthase activity in diabetic skeletal muscle. *J Clin Invest* 1989;84:892.

111. Vuorinen-Markkola H, Koivisto VA, Yki-Jarvinen H: Mechanisms of hyperglycemia-induced insulin resistance in whole body and skeletal muscle of type 1 diabetic patients. *Diabetes* 1992;41:571.

112. Garvey WT, Olefsky JM, Griffin J, et al: The effects of inulin treatment on insulin secretion and action in type II diabetes mellitus. *Diabetes* 1985;34:222.

113. Olefsky JM, Kruszynska YT: Type 2 diabetes mellitus: Etiology, pathogenesis, and natural history. In: DeGroot LJ, Jameson JL, eds. *Endocrinology*, 4th ed. Philadelphia Saunders: 2001; vol 1:776-797.

114. Henry RR, Wallace P, Olefsky JM: The effects of weight loss on the mechanisms of hyperglycemia in obese noninsulin-dependent diabetes mellitus. *Diabetes* 1986;35:990.

115. Kolterman OG, Gray RS, Shapiro G, et al: The acute and chronic effects of sulfonylurea therapy in type II diabetics. *Diabetes* 1984;33:346.

116. Vestergaard H, Weinreb JE, Rosen AS, et al: Sulfonylurea therapy improves glucose disposal without changing skeletal muscle Glut 4 levels in non-insulin-dependent diabetes mellitus: A longitudinal study. *J Clin Endocrinol Metab* 1995;80:270.

117. Bergman RN, Finegood DT, Ader M: Assessment of insulin sensitivity *in vivo*. *Endocr Rev* 1985;1:45.

118. Himsworth HP, Kerr RB: Insulin-sensitive and insulin-insensitive types of diabetes mellitus. *Clin Sci* 1939;4:119.

119. Ginsberg H, Kimmerling G, Olefsky JM, et al: Demonstration of insulin resistance in maturity-onset diabetic patients with fasting hyperglycemia. *J Clin Invest* 1975;55:454.

120. Harano Y, Ohgaku S, Hidaka H, et al: Glucose, insulin and somatostatin infusion for the determination of insulin sensitivity. *J Clin Endocrinol Metab* 1977;45:1124.

121. Bonadonnna RC, Del Prato S, Saccomani MP, et al: Transmembrane glucose transport in skeletal muscle of patients with non-insulin-dependent diabetes. *J Clin Invest* 1993;92:486.

122. Baron AD, Laakso M, Brechtel G, et al: Reduced capacity and affinity of skeletal muscle for insulin mediated glucose uptake in non-insulin dependent diabetic subjects. Effects of insulin therapy. *J Clin Invest* 1991;87:1186.

123. Kelley DE, Mokan M, Mandarino LJ: Intracellular defects in glucose metabolism in obese patients with NIDDM. *Diabetes* 1992;41:698.

124. Insel PA, Liljenquist JE, Tobin JD, et al: Insulin control of glucose metabolism in man. *J Clin Invest* 1975;55:1057.

125. Magnusson I, Rothman DL, Katz LD, et al: Increased rate of gluconeogenesis in type II diabetes mellitus: A ^{13}C nuclear magnetic resonance study. *J Clin Invest* 1992;90:1323.

126. Consoli A, Nurjhan N, Reilly JJ, et al: Mechanism of increased gluco-neogenesis in non-insulin-dependent diabetes mellitus: Role of alter-ations in systemic, hepatic, and muscle lactate and alanine metabo-lism. *J Clin Invest* 1990;86:2038.

127. Tayek JA, Katz J: Glucose production, recycling, and gluconeogene-sis in normals and diabetics: A mass isotopomer [U-^{13}C] glucose study. *Am J Physiol* 1996;270:E709.

128. Orci L: The insulin cell: Its cellular environment and how it processes (pro)insulin. *Diabetes Metab Rev* 1986;2:71.

129. Liljenquist JE, Mueller GL, Cherrington AD, et al: Evidence for an important role of glucagon in the regulation of hepatic glucose pro-duction in normal man. *J Clin Invest* 1977;59:369.

130. Baron AD, Schaeffer L, Shragg P, Kolterman OG: Role of hyper-glucagonemia in maintenance of increased rates of hepatic glucose output in type II diabetics. *Diabetes* 1987;36:274.

131. Groop LC, Bonadonna RC, Del Prato S, et al: Glucose and free fatty acid metabolism in non-insulin dependent diabetes mellitus: Evidence for multiple sites of insulin resistance. *J Clin Invest* 1989;84:205.

132. Basu A, Basu R, Shah P, et al: Effects of type 2 diabetes on the ability of insulin and glucose to regulate splanchnic and muscle glucose me-tabolism: Evidence for a defect in hepatic glucokinase activity. *Dia-betes* 2000;49:272.

133. Rebrin K, Steil GM, Getty L, et al: Free fatty acid as a link in the reg-ulation of hepatic glucose output by peripheral insulin. *Diabetes* 1995;44:1038.

134. Kruszynska YT: The role of fatty acid metabolism in the hypertriglyc-eridaemia and insulin resistance of type 2 (non-insulin dependent) di-abetes. In: Marshall SM, Home PD, Rizza RA, eds. *The Diabetes An-nual*. Elsevier:1995;9:107.

135. Boden G, Ray TK, Smith RH, Owen OE: Carbohydrate oxidation and storage in obese non-insulin-dependent diabetic patients. Effect of im-proving glycemic control. *Diabetes* 1983;32:982.

136. Lewis GF, Carpentier A, Vranic M, et al: Resistance to insulin's acute direct hepatic effect in suppressing steady-state glucose production in individuals with type 2 diabetes. *Diabetes* 1999;48:570.

137. McGuiness OP, Ejiofor J, Audoly LP, et al: Regulation of glucose pro-duction by NEFA and gluconeogenic precursors during chronic glucagon infusion. *Am J Physiol* 1998;275:E432.

138. Mitrakou A, Kelley D, Veneman T, et al: Contribution of abnormal muscle and liver glucose metabolism to postprandial hyperglycemia in NIDDM. *Diabetes* 1990;39:1381.

139. Felig P, Wahren J, Hendler R: Influence of oral glucose ingestion on splanchnic glucose and gluconeogenic substrate metabolism in man. *Diabetes* 1975;24:468.

140. Ferrannini E, Bjorkman O, Reichard GA, et al: The disposal of an oral glucose load in healthy subjects: A quantitative study. *Diabetes* 1985; 34:580.

141. Katz J, McGarry JD: The glucose paradox: Is glucose a substrate for liver metabolism? *J Clin Invest* 1984;74:1901.

142. Taylor R, Magnusson I, Rothman DL, et al: Direct assessment of liver glycogen storage by ^{13}C nuclear magnetic resonance spectroscopy and regulation of glucose homeostasis after a mixed meal in normal subjects. *J Clin Invest* 1996;97:126.

143. Shulman GI, Cline G, Schumann WC, et al: Quantitative comparison of pathways of hepatic glycogen repletion in fed and fasted humans. *Am J Physiol* 1990;259:E335.

144. Niewoehner CB, Nuttall FQ: Relationship of hepatic glucose uptake to intrahepatic glucose concentration in fasted rats after glucose load. *Diabetes* 1988;37:1559.

145. Cherrington AD: Banting Lecture 1997. Control of glucose uptake and release by the liver in vivo. *Diabetes* 1999;48:1198.

146. Ludvik B, Nolan JJ, Roberts A, et al: Evidence for decreased splanch-nic glucose uptake after oral glucose administration in non-insulin-dependent diabetes mellitus. *J Clin Invest* 1997;100:2354.

147. Baron AD, Kolterman OG, Bell J, et al: Rates of non-insulin mediated glucose uptake are elevated in type II diabetic subjects. *J Clin Invest* 1986;76:1782.

148. Felber JP, Thiebaud D, Maeder E, et al: Effect of somatostatin-induced insulinopenia on glucose oxidation in man. *Diabetologia* 1983;25:325.

149. Frankson JRM, Malaise W, Arnould Y, et al: Glucose kinetics in human obesity. *Diabetologia* 1966;2:96.

150. Kolterman OG, Insel J, Saekow M, et al: Mechanisms of insulin re-sistance in human obesity: Evidence for receptor and post-receptor defects. *J Clin Invest* 1980;65:1272.

151. Bogardus C, Lillioja S, Mott DM, et al: Relationship between degree of obesity and in vivo insulin action in man. *Am J Physiol* 1985;248:E286.

152. Abate N, Garg A, Peshock RM, et al: Relationship of generalized and regional adiposity to insulin sensitivity in men. *J Clin Invest* 1995;96:88.

153. Bonora E, Prato SD, Bonadonna RC, et al: Total body fat content and fat topography are associated differently with in vivo glucose metabo-lism in nonobese and obese nondiabetic women. *Diabetes* 1992;41:1151.

154. Peiris AN, Mueller RA, Smith GA, et al: Splanchnic insulin metabo-lism in obesity: Influence of body fat distribution. *J Clin Invest* 1986;78:1648.

155. Pouliot MC, Despres J-P, Nadeau A, et al: Visceral obesity in men: Associations with glucose tolerance, plasma insulin, and lipoprotein levels. *Diabetes* 1992;41:826.

156. Golay A, Felber JP, Jequier E, et al: Metabolic basis of obesity and non-insulin dependent diabetes mellitus. *Diabetes Metab Rev* 1988;4:727.

157. Wahrenberg H, Lonnqvist F, Arner P: Mechanisms underlying re-gional differences in lipolysis in human adipose tissue. *J Clin Invest* 1989;84:458.

158. Lonnqvist F, Thorne A, Nilsell K, et al: A pathogenetic role of visceral fat β_3-adrenoceptors in obesity. *J Clin Invest* 1995;95:1109.

159. Svedberg J, Bjontorp P, Smith U, et al: Free fatty acid inhibition of in-sulin binding, degradation, and action in isolated rat hepatocytes. *Di-abetes* 1990;39:570.

160. Peiris AN, Mueller RA, Smith GA, et al: Splanchnic insulin metabo-lism in obesity. Influence of body fat distribution. *J Clin Invest* 1986;78:1648.

161. Kashiwagi A, Verso MA, Andrews J, et al: In vitro insulin resistance of human adipocytes isolated from subjects with noninsulin-dependent diabetes mellitus. *J Clin Invest* 1983;72:1246.

162. Freidenberg GR, Henry RR, Klein HH, et al: Decreased kinase activ-ity of insulin receptors from adipocytes of non-insulin dependent dia-betic (NIDDM) subjects. *J Clin Invest* 1987;79:240.

163. Nolan JJ, Freidenberg G, Henry R, et al: Role of human skeletal mus-cle insulin receptor kinase in the in vivo insulin resistance of NIDDM and obesity. *J Clin Endocrinol Metab* 1994;78:471.

164. Caro JF, Hoop IO, Pories WJ, et al: Studies on the mechanism of in-sulin resistance in the liver from humans with non-insulin dependent diabetes. *J Clin Invest* 1986;78:249.

165. Comi RJ, Grunberger G, Gorden P: Relationship of insulin binding and insulin-stimulated tyrosine kinase activity is altered in type II dia-betes. *J Clin Invest* 1987;79:453.

166. Kusari J, Verma US, Buse JB, et al: Analysis of the gene sequences of the insulin receptor and the insulin sensitive glucose transporter (Glut-4) in patients with common type non-insulin dependent diabetes mel-litus. *J Clin Invest* 1991;88:1323.

167. Rich SS: Mapping genes in diabetes: Genetic epidemiological per-spective. *Diabetes* 1990;39:1315.

168. Muller HK, Kellerer M, Ermel B, et al: Prevention by protein kinase C inhibitors of glucose-induced insulin-receptor tyrosine kinase re-sistance in rat fat cells. *Diabetes* 1991;40:1440.

169. Brillon DJ, Freidenberg GR, Henry RR, et al: Mechanism of defective insulin-receptor kinase activity in NIDDM: Evidence for two receptor populations. *Diabetes* 1989;38:397.

170. Heidenreich K, Brandenburg D, Berhanu P: Metabolism of pho-toaffinity-labeled insulin receptors by adipocytes: Role of inter-nalization, degradation, and recycling. *J Biol Chem* 1984;259:6511.

171. Arner P, Pollare T, Lithell H, et al: Defective insulin receptor tyrosine kinase in human skeletal muscle in obesity and Type II (non-insulin-dependent) diabetes mellitus. *Diabetologia* 1987;30:437.

172. Ciaraldi TP, Kolterman OG, Scarlett JA, et al: Role of the glucose transport system in the postreceptor defect of non-insulin dependent diabetes mellitus. *Diabetes* 1982;31:1016.

173. Molina JM, Ciaraldi TP, Brady D, et al: Decreased activation rate of insulin-stimulated glucose transport in adipocytes from obese sub-jects. *Diabetes* 1989;38:991.

174. Ciaraldi TP, Molina JM, Olefsky JM: Insulin action kinetics in adipocytes from obese and noninsulin-dependent diabetes mellitus subjects: Identification of multiple cellular defects in glucose trans-port. *J Clin Endocrinol Metab* 1991;72:872.

175. Ciaraldi TP, Kolterman OG, Olefsky JM: Mechanism of the postre-ceptor defect in insulin action in human obesity. *J Clin Invest* 1981; 68:875.

176. Dohm GL, Tapscott EB, Pories WJ, *et al*: An in vitro human muscle preparation suitable for metabolic studies: Decreased insulin stimula-tion of glucose transport in muscle from morbidly obese and diabetic subjects. *J Clin Invest* 1988;82:486.

177. Zierath JR, He L, Guma A, *et al*: Insulin action on glucose transport and plasma membrane Glut 4 content in skeletal muscle from patients with NIDDM. *Diabetologia* 1996;39:1180.

178. Krook A, Bjornholm M, Galuska D, *et al*: Characterization of signal transduction and glucose transport in skeletal muscle from type 2 dia-betic patients. *Diabetes* 2000;49:284.

179. Jackson S, Bagstaff SM, Lynn S, *et al*: Decreased insulin responsive-ness of glucose uptake in cultured human skeletal muscle cells from insulin-resistant nondiabetic relatives of type 2 diabetic families. *Dia-betes* 2000;49:1169.

180. Henry RR, Wallace P, Olefsky JM: The effects of weight loss on the mechanisms of hyperglycemia in obese noninsulin-dependent dia-betes mellitus. *Diabetes* 1986;35:990.

181. Scarlett JA, Kolterman OG, Ciaraldi TP, *et al*: Insulin treatment re-verses the post-receptor defect in adipocyte 3-0-methyl glucose trans-port in Type II diabetes mellitus. *J Clin Endocrinol Metab* 1983;56: 1195.

182. Olefsky JM, Ciaraldi TP, Scarlett JA, *et al*: Role of the glucose trans-port system in the post-receptor defect of non-insulin dependent dia-betes mellitus and reversibility of this abnormality with insulin treat-ment. In: Angel A, Hollenberg CH, Roncari DAK, eds. *Proceedings of International Conference on the Adipocyte and Obesity: Cellular and Molecular Mechanisms.* Raven:1983;85.

183. Storlien LH, James DE, Burleigh KM, *et al*: Fat feeding causes wide-spread in vivo insulin resistance, decreased energy expenditure, and obesity in rats. *Am J Physiol* 1986;251:E576.

184. Goodman MN, Berger M, Ruderman ND: Glucose metabolism in rat skeletal muscle at rest. Effects of starvation, diabetes, ketone bodies and free fatty acid. *Diabetes* 1974;23:881.

185. Katz A, Nyomba BL, Bogardus C: No accumulation of glucose in human skeletal muscle during euglycemic hyperinsulinemia. *Am J Physiol* 1988;255:E942.

186. Ziel FH, Venkatesan N, Davidson MB: Glucose transport is rate-limiting for skeletal muscle glucose metabolism in normal and streptozotocin-induced diabetic rats. *Diabetes* 1988;37:885.

187. Cline GW, Petersen KF, Krssak M, *et al*: Impaired glucose transport as a cause of decreased insulin-stimulated muscle glycogen synthesis in type 2 diabetes. *N Engl J Med* 1999;341:240.

188. Gottesman I, Mandarino L, Verdonk C, *et al*: Insulin increases the maximum velocity of glucose uptake without altering the Michaelis constant in man. Evidence that insulin increases glucose uptake merely by providing additional transport sites. *J Clin Invest* 1982;70: 1310.

189. Rennie MJ, Edstrom JP, Mann GE, *et al*: A paired-tracer dilution method for characterizing membrane transport in the perfused rat hindlimb. Effects of insulin, refeeding and fasting on the kinetics of sugar transport. *Biochem J* 1983;214:737.

190. Bonadonna RC, Saccomani MP, Seely L, *et al*: Glucose transport in human skeletal muscle: The in vivo response to insulin. *Diabetes* 1993;42:191.

191. Ren JM, Marshall BA, Mueckler MM, *et al*: Overexpression of Glut4 protein in muscle increases basal and insulin-stimulated whole body glucose disposal in conscious mice. *J. Clin Invest* 1995;95:429.

192. Bonadonna RC, Del Prato S, Bonora E, *et al*: Roles of glucose trans-port and glucose phosphorylation in muscle insulin resistance of NIDDM. *Diabetes* 1996;45:915.

193. Kruszynska YT, Mulford MI, Baloga J, *et al*: Regulation of skeletal muscle hexokinase II by insulin in non-diabetic and NIDDM subjects. *Diabetes* 1998;47:1107.

194. Thorburn AW, Gumbiner B, Bulacan F, *et al*: Multiple defects in mus-cle glycogen synthase activity contribute to reduced glycogen synthe-sis in non-insulin dependent diabetes mellitus. *J Clin Invest* 1991;87: 489.

195. Damsbo P, Vaag A, Hother-Nielsen O, *et al*: Reduced glycogen syn-thase activity in skeletal muscle from obese patients with and without type 2 (non-insulin-dependent) diabetes mellitus. *Diabetologia* 1991; 34:239.

196. Bak JF, Schmitz O, Schwartz N, *et al*: Postreceptor effects of sulfony-lurea on skeletal muscle glycogen synthase activity in type II diabetic patients. *Diabetes* 1989;38:1343.

197. Bogardus C, Lillioja S, Stone K, *et al*: Correlations between muscle glycogen synthase activity and in vivo insulin action in man. *J Clin Invest* 1984;73:1185.

198. Pedersen O, Bak JF, Andersen PH, *et al*: Evidence against altered ex-pression of Glut 1 or Glut 4 in skeletal muscle of patients with obesity or NIDDM. *Diabetes* 1990;39:865.

199. Eriksson J, Koranyi L, Bourey R, *et al*: Insulin resistance in type 2 (non-insulin dependent) diabetic patients and their relatives is not as-sociated with a defect in the expression of the insulin-responsive glu-cose transporter (GLUT-4) gene in human skeletal muscle. *Diabetolo-gia* 1992;35:143.

200. Garvey WT, Maianu L, Hancock JA, *et al*: Gene expression of Glut4 in skeletal muscle from insulin-resistant patients with obesity, IGT, GDM, and NIDDM. *Diabetes* 1992;41:465.

201. Kelley DE, Mintun MA, Watkins SC, *et al*: The effect of non-insulin-dependent diabetes mellitus and obesity on glucose transport and phosphorylation in skeletal muscle. *J Clin Invest* 1996;97:2705.

202. Garvey WT, Maianu L, Zhu J-H, *et al*: Evidence for defects in the traf-ficking and translocation of Glut 4 glucose transporters in skeletal muscle as a cause of human insulin resistance. *J Clin Invest* 1998;101: 2377.

203. Buse JB, Yasuda K, Lay TP, *et al*: Human Glut4/muscle fat glucose transporter gene: Characterization and genetic variation. *Diabetes* 1992;41:1436.

204. Choi WH, O'Rahilly S, Buse JB, *et al*: Molecular scanning of insulin-responsive glucose transporter (Glut 4) gene in NIDDM subjects. *Di-abetes* 1991;40:1712.

205. Thies RS, Molina JM, Ciaraldi TP, *et al*: Insulin receptor autophos-phorylation and endogenous substrate phosphorylation in human adipocytes from control, obese, and non- insulin dependent diabetic subjects. *Diabetes* 1990;39:250.

206. Bjornjolm M, Kawano Y, Lehtihet M, *et al*: Insulin receptor substrate-1 phosphorylation and phosphatidylinositol 3-kinase activity in skele-tal muscle from NIDDM subjects after in vivo insulin stimulation. *Di-abetes* 1997;46:524.

207. Cusi K, Katsumi M, Osman A, *et al*: Insulin resistance differentially affects the PI-3-kinase- and MAP kinase-mediated signaling in human muscle. *J Clin Invest* 2000;105:311.

208. Rondinone CM, Wang LM, Lonnroth P, *et al*: Insulin receptor sub-strate (IRS)-1 is reduced and IRS-2 is the main docking protein for phosphatidylinositol 3-kinase in adipocytes from subjects with non-insulin-dependent diabetes mellitus. *Proc Natl Acad Sci USA* 1997; 94:4171.

209. Krook A, Bjornholm M, Galuska D, *et al*: Characterization of signal transduction and glucose transport in skeletal muscle from type 2 dia-betic patients. *Diabetes* 2000;49:284.

210. Kim Y-B, Nikoulina SE, Ciaraldi TP, *et al*: Normal insulin-dependent activation of Akt/protein kinase B, with diminished activation of phosphoinositide 3-kinase, in muscle in type 2 diabetes. *J Clin Invest* 1999;104:733.

211. Goodyear LJ, Giorgino F, Sherman LA, *et al*: Insulin receptor phos-phorylation, insulin receptor substrate-1 phosphorylation and phos-phatidylinositol 3-kinase activity are decreased in skeletal muscle strips from obese subjects. *J Clin Invest* 1995;95:2195.

212. Freymond D, Bogardus C, Okubo M, *et al*: Impaired insulin-stimulated muscle glycogen synthase activation in vivo in man is re-lated to low fasting glycogen synthase phosphatase activity. *J Clin Invest* 1988;82:1503.

213. Wright KS, Beck-Nielsen H, Kolterman OG, *et al*: Decreased activa-tion of skeletal muscle glycogen synthase by mixed-meal ingestion in NIDDM. *Diabetes* 1988;37:436.

214. Schalin-Jantti C, Harkonen M, Groop LC: Impaired activation of glycogen synthase in people at increased risk for developing NIDDM. *Diabetes* 1992;41:598.

215. Groop LC, Kankuri M, Schalin-Jantti C, *et al*: Association between polymorphism of the glycogen synthase gene and non-insulin-dependent diabetes mellitus (published erratum appears in *N Engl J Med* 1993;328:1136, see comments). *N Engl J Med* 1993;328:10.

216. Zouali H, Velho G, Froguel P: Polymorphism of the glycogen syn-thase gene and non- insulin-dependent diabetes mellitus (letter, com-ment). *N Engl J Med* 1993;328:1569.

217. Elbein SC, Hoffman M, Ridinger D, *et al*: Description of a second microsatellite marker and linkage analysis of the muscle glycogen synthase locus in familial NIDDM. *Diabetes* 1994;43:1061.

218. Orho M, Nikula-Ijas P, Schalin-Jantti C, *et al*: Isolation and characterization of the human muscle glycogen synthase gene. *Diabetes* 1995; 44:1099.

219. Vestergaard H, Bjorbaeck C, Andersen PH, *et al*: Impaired expression of glycogen synthase mRNA in skeletal muscle of NIDDM patients. *Diabetes* 1991;40:1740.

220. Huang X, Vaag A, Hansson M, *et al*: Impaired insulin-stimulated expression of the glycogen synthase gene in skeletal muscle of type 2 diabetic patients is acquired rather than inherited. *J Clin Endocrinol Metab* 2000;85:1584.

221. Zierler K, Rabinowitz D: Roles of insulin and growth hormone, based on studies of forearm metabolism in man. *Medicine* 1963;42:385.

222. Sherwin RS, Kramer KJ, Tobin JD, *et al*: A model of the kinetics of insulin in man. *J Clin Invest* 1974;53:1481.

223. Prager R, Wallace P, Olefsky JM: In vivo kinetics of insulin action on peripheral glucose disposal and hepatic glucose output in normal and obese subjects. *J Clin Invest* 1986;78:472.

224. Prager R, Wallace P, Olefsky JM: Hyperinsulinemia does not compensate for the peripheral insulin resistance in obesity. *Diabetes* 1987;36:327.

225. Doeden B, Rizza R: Use of a variable insulin infusion to assess insulin action in obesity: Defects in both the kinetics and amplitude of response. *J Clin Endocrinol Metab* 1987;64:902.

226. Klauser R, Prager R, Schernthaner G, *et al*: Contribution of postprandial insulin and glucose levels to the stimulation of glucose disposal and suppression of hepatic glucose production in normal and insulin resistant obese subjects. *J Clin Endocrinol Metab* 1991;73:758.

227. Nolan JJ, Ludvik B, Baloga J, *et al*: Mechanisms of the kinetic defect in insulin action in obesity and NIDDM. *Diabetes* 1997;46:994.

228. Hribal ML, Federici M, Porzio O, *et al*: The Gly → Arg^{972} amino acid polymorphism in insulin receptor substrate-1 affects glucose metabolism in skeletal muscle cells. *J Clin Endocrinol Metab* 2000;85:2004.

229. Bernal D, Almind K, Yenush L, *et al*: Insulin receptor substrate-2 amino acid polymorphisms are not associated with random type 2 diabetes among Caucasians. *Diabetes* 1998;47:976.

230. Almind K, Fredriksen SK, Bernal D, *et al*: Search for variants of the gene-promoter and the potential phosphotyrosine encoding sequence of the insulin receptor substrate-2 gene: Evaluation of their relation with alterations in insulin secretion and insulin sensitivity. *Diabetologia* 1999;42:1244.

231. Hansen T, Andersen CB, Echwald SM, *et al*: Identification of a common amino acid polymorphism in the p85α regulatory subunit of phosphatidylinositol 3-kinase. *Diabetes* 1997;46:494.

232. Baier LJ, Wiedrich C, Hanson RL, Bogardus C: Variant in the regulatory subunit of phosphatidylinositol 3-kinase (p85α): Preliminary evidence indicates a potential role of this variant in the acute insulin response and type 2 diabetes in Pima women. *Diabetes* 1998;47:973.

233. Baynes KCR, Beeton CA, Panayatou G, *et al*: Natural variants of human p85α phosphoinositide 3-kinase in severe insulin resistance: A novel variant with impaired insulin-stimulated lipid kinase activity. *Diabetologia* 2000;43:321.

234. Saltiel AR, Olefsky JM: Thiazolidinediones in the treatment of insulin resistance and type 2 diabetes. *Diabetes* 1996;45:1661.

235. Yen CJ, Beamer BA, Negri C, *et al*: Molecular scanning of the human peroxisome proliferator activated receptor gamma (hPPAR gamma) gene in diabetic Caucasians: Identification of a Pro12Ala PPAR gamma 2 missense mutation. *Biochem Biophys Res Commun* 1997; 241:270.

236. Deeb SS, Fajas L, Nemoto M, *et al*: A Pro12Ala substitution in PPARgamma2 associated with decreased receptor activity, lower body mass index and improved insulin sensitivity. *Nat Genet* 1998;20:284.

237. Cole SA, Mitchell BD, Hsueh WC, *et al*: The Pro12Ala variant of peroxisome proliferator-activated receptor-gamma2 (PPAR-gamma2) is associated with measures of obesity in Mexican Americans. *Int J Obes Relat Metab Disord* 2000;24:522.

238. Clement K, Hercberg S, Passinge B, *et al*: The Pro115Gln and Pro12Ala PPAR gamma gene mutations in obesity and type 2 diabetes. *Int J Obes Relat Metab Disord* 2000;24:391.

239. Haddad L, Saker P, Gharani N, *et al*: Evaluation, using family-based association methods, of the role of the Pro12Ala variant in PPARG in

240. Barroso I, Gurnell M, Crowley VEF, *et al*: Dominant negative mutations in human PPARγ associated with severe insulin resistance, diabetes mellitus and hypertension. *Nature* 1999;402:880.

241. Matsuoka N, Ogawa Y, Hosoda K, *et al*: Human leptin receptor gene in obese Japanese subjects: Evidence against either obesity-causing mutations or association of sequence variants with obesity. *Diabetologia* 1997;40:1204.

242. Rolland V, Clement K, Dugail I, *et al*: Leptin receptor gene in a large cohort of massively obese subjects: No indication of the fa/fa rat mutation. Detection of an intronic variant with no association with obesity. *Obes Res* 1998;6:122.

243. Large V, Hellstrom L, Reynisdottir S, *et al*: Human beta-2 adrenoceptor gene polymorphisms are highly frequent in obesity and associate with altered adipocyte beta-2 adrenoceptor function. *J Clin Invest* 1997;100;3005.

244. Mitchell BD, Cole SA, Hsueh W-C, *et al*: Linkage of serum insulin concentrations to chromosome 3p in Mexican Americans. *Diabetes* 2000;49:513.

245. Pratley RE, Thompson DB, Prochazka M, *et al*: An autosomal genomic scan for loci linked to prediabetic phenotypes in Pima Indians. *J Clin Invest* 1998;101:1757.

246. Mitchell BD, Kammerer CM, O'Connell P, *et al*: Evidence for linkage of postchallenge insulin levels with intestinal fatty acid-binding protein (FABP2) in Mexican-Americans. *Diabetes* 1995;44:1046.

247. Humphreys P, McCarthy M, Tuomilehto J, *et al*: Chromosome 4q locus associated with insulin resistance in Pima Indians: Studies in three European NIDDM populations. *Diabetes* 1994;43:800.

248. Horikawa Y, Oda N, Cox NJ, *et al*: Genetic variation in the gene encoding calpain-10 is associated with type 2 diabetes mellitus. *Nat Genet* 2000;26:163.

249. Baier LJ, Permana PA, Yang X, *et al*: A calpain-10 gene polymorphism is associated with reduced muscle mRNA levels and insulin resistance. *J Clin Invest* 2000;106:R69.

250. Joshi RL, Lamothe B, Cordonnier N, *et al*: Targeted disruption of the insulin receptor gene in the mouse results in neonatal lethality. *EMBO J* 1996;15:1542.

251. Araki E, Lipes MA, Patti M-E, *et al*: Alternative pathway of insulin signalling in mice with targeted disruption of the IRS-1 gene. *Nature* 1994;372:186.

252. Bruning JC, Winnay J, Bonner-Weir S, *et al*: Development of a novel polygenic model of NIDDM in mice heterozygous for IR and IRS-1 null alleles. *Cell* 1997;88:561.

253. Withers DJ, Gutierrez JS, Towery H, *et al*: Disruption of IRS-2 causes type 2 diabetes in mice. *Nature* 1998;391:900.

254. Shimomura I, Matsuda M, Hammer RE, *et al*: Decreased IRS-2 and increased SREBP-1c lead to mixed insulin resistance and sensitivity in livers of lipodystrophic and ob/ob mice. *Mol Cell* 2000;6:77.

255. Kubota N, Tobe K, Teranchi Y, *et al*: Disruption of insulin receptor substrate-2 causes type 2 diabetes due to liver insulin resistance and lack of compensatory β-cell hyperplasia. *Diabetes* 2000;49:1880.

256. Fasshauer M, Klein J, Ueki K, *et al*: Essential role of IRS-2 in insulin stimulation of Glut 4 translocation and glucose uptake in brown adipocytes. *J Biol Chem* 2000;275:25494.

257. Kulkarni RN, Bruning JC, Winnay JN, *et al*: Tissue-specific knockout of the insulin receptor in pancreatic β cells creates an insulin secretory defect similar to that in type 2 diabetes. *Cell* 1999;96:329.

258. Withers DJ, Burks DJ, Towery HH, *et al*: Irs-2 coordinates Igf-1 receptor mediated beta-cell development and peripheral insulin signalling. *Nat Genet* 1999;23:32.

259. Kruszynska YT, Home PD, Hanning I, *et al*: Basal and 24 hour C-peptide and insulin secretion rate in normal man. *Diabetologia* 1987;30:16.

260. Barrett EJ, DeFronzo RA, Bevilacqua S, *et al*: Insulin resistance in diabetic ketoacidosis. *Diabetes* 1982;31:923.

261. Yki-Jarvinen H, Koivisto VA: Natural course of insulin resistance in type I diabetes. *N Engl J Med* 1986;315:224.

262. Revers RR, Kolterman OG, Scarlett JA, *et al*: Lack of in vivo insulin resistance in controlled insulin dependent, Type I, diabetic patients. *J Clin Endocrinol Metab* 1984;58:353.

263. Lager I, Lonnroth P, Von Schenck H, *et al*: Reversal of insulin resistance in Type 1 diabetes after treatment with continuous subcutaneous insulin infusion. *Br Med J* 1983;287:1661.

264. Makimattila S, Virkamaki A, Malmstrom R, *et al*: Insulin resistance in type 1 diabetes mellitus: A major role for reduced glucose extraction. *J Clin Endocrinol Metab* 1996;81:707.

265. Hother-Nielsen O, Schmitz O, Bak J, *et al*: Enhanced hepatic sensitivity, but peripheral insulin resistance in patients with Type 1 (insulin-dependent) diabetes. *Diabetologia* 1987;30:834.

266. Orskov L, Alberti KGMM, Mengel A, *et al*: Decreased hepatic glucagon responses in Type 1 (insulin-dependent) diabetes mellitus. *Diabetologia* 1991;34:521.

267. Launay B, Zinman B, Tildesley HD, *et al*: Effect of subcutaneous insulin infusion with lispro on hepatic responsiveness to glucagon in type 1 diabetes. *Diabetes Care* 1998;21:1627.

268. Del Prato S, Nosadini R, Tiengo A, *et al*: Insulin-mediated glucose disposal in Type 1 diabetes: Evidence for insulin resistance. *J Clin Endocrinol Metab* 1983;57:904.

269. Hjollund E, Pedersen O, Richelsen B, *et al*: Glucose transport and metabolism in adipocytes from newly diagnosed untreated insulin-dependent diabetics. Severely impaired basal and postinsulin binding activities. *J Clin Invest* 1985;76:2091.

270. Moller AM, Dalgaard LT, Pociot F, *et al*: Mutations in the hepatocyte nuclear factor-1 alpha gene in Caucasian families originally classified as having Type 1 diabetes. *Diabetologia* 1998;41:1528.

271. Kahn CR, Flier JS, Bar RS, *et al*: The syndromes of insulin resistance and acanthosis nigricans. Insulin-receptor disorders in man. *N Engl J Med* 1976;294:739.

272. Flier JS, Kahn CR, Roth J, *et al*: Antibodies that impair insulin receptor binding in an unusual diabetic syndrome with severe insulin resistance. *Science* 1975;190:63.

273. Kahn CR, Baird KL, Flier JS, *et al*: Effects of autoantibodies to the insulin receptor on isolated adipocytes: Studies of insulin binding and insulin action. *J Clin Invest* 1977;60:1094.

274. Tritos N, Mantzoros CS: Syndromes of severe insulin resistance. *J Clin Endocrinol Metab* 1998;83:3025.

275. Auclair M, Vigouroux C, Desbois-Mouthon C, *et al*: Antiinsulin receptor autoantibodies induce insulin receptors to constitutively associate with insulin receptor substrate-1 and -2 and cause severe cell resistance to both insulin and insulin-like growth factor I. *J Clin Endocrinol Metab* 1999;84:3197.

276. Taylor SI, Arioglu E: Genetically defined forms of diabetes in children. *J Clin Endocrinol Metab* 1999;84:4390.

277. Krook A, O'Rahilly S: Mutant insulin receptors in syndromes of insulin resistance. *Baillieres Clin Endocrinol Metab* 1996;10:97.

278. Speckman RA, Garg A, Du F, *et al*: Mutational and haplotype analyses of families with familial partial lipodystrophy (Dunnigan variety) reveal recurrent missense mutations in the globular C-terminal domain of lamin A/C. *Am J Hum Genet* 2000;66:1192.

279. Shackleton S, Lloyd DJ, Jackson SN, *et al*: LMNA, encoding lamin A/C, is mutated in partial lipodystrophy. *Nat Genet* 2000;24:153.

280. Garg A, Wilson R, Barnes R, *et al*: A gene for congenital generalized lipodystrophy maps to human chromosome 9q34. *J Clin Endocrinol Metab* 1999;84:3390.

281. Oseid S, Beck-Nielsen H, Pedersen O, *et al*: Decreased binding of insulin to its receptor in patients with congenital generalized lipodystrophy. *N Engl J Med* 1977;296:245.

282. Kriauciunas KM, Kahn CR, Muller-Wieland D, *et al*: Altered expression and function of the insulin receptor in a family with lipoatrophic diabetes. *J Clin Endocrinol Metab* 1988;67:1284.

283. Whittaker J, Zick Y, Roth J, *et al*: Insulin stimulated receptor phosphorylation appears normal in cultured Epstein-Barr virus transformed cell lines derived from patients with extreme insulin resistance. *J Clin Endocrinol Metab* 1985;60:381.

284. Wachslicht-Rodbard H, Muggeo M, Kahn CR, *et al*: Heterogeneity of the insulin receptor interaction in lipoatrophic diabetes. *J Clin Endocrinol Metab* 1981;52:416.

285. Sovik O, Vestergaard H, Trygstad O, *et al*: Studies of insulin resistance in congenital generalized lipodystrophy. *Acta Paediatr Suppl* 1996;13:29.

286. Li A, Swift M: Mutations at the ataxia-telangiectasia locus and clinical phenotypes of A-T patients. *Am J Med Genet* 2000;92:170.

287. Schalch DS, McFarlin DE, Barlow MH: An unusual form of diabetes mellitus in ataxia telangiectasia. *N Engl J Med* 1970;282:1396.

288. Taylor SI, Moller DE: Mutations of the insulin receptor. In: Moller DE, ed. *Insulin Resistance*. Wiley:1993;83.

Obesity and Diabetes Mellitus

P. Antonio Tataranni

Clifton Bogardus

OBESITY

Throughout evolution, animals and humans have developed redundant mechanisms promoting accumulation of fat tissue during periods of abundance to survive periods of famine. However, what once was an asset has become a liability in the current obesogenic environment of readily available high-fat foods and reduced physical activity.[1] As a consequence, obesity has reached epidemic proportions in both industrialized countries and in urbanized populations around the world.[2]

Obesity is clinically defined as a body mass index (BMI) of ≥ 30 kg/m^2 [a BMI of 30 represents an excess of weight of approximately 30 lb (14 kg) for any given height] (Table 23-1).[3] In the United States during the late 1990s one out of two adults was overweight and one of four were obese.[4] More alarming, the prevalence of obesity has been increasing drastically among children.[5] The World Health Organization has identified obesity as one of the major emerging chronic diseases.[2] Obesity increases the risk for a number of noncommunicable diseases (i.e., type 2 diabetes, hypertension, dyslipidemias) and reduces life expectancy.[6] In the U.S. the annual cost of obesity to the public health system is estimated to be nearly $100 billion. This represents between 5% and 10% of the U.S. health care budget.[7]

The exact cause of obesity in the majority of humans is not known. It is, however, widely accepted that it results from a chronic imbalance between energy intake and energy expenditure (Fig. 23-1). Studies in twins,[8] adoptees,[9] and family members[10] indicate that obesity is a heritable disease and that 70% of the interindividual variability in BMI is genetically determined.[9] Because only 30% of BMI's heritable components can be attributable to familial traits such as daily energy expenditure (10–15%), respiratory quotient (5%), and spontaneous physical activity (10%),[11–13] one has to conclude that a large proportion of the genetic variance in BMI may be due to the effect of genes on eating behavior and/or habitual daily physical activity (Fig. 23-2).

Recent research has provided an unprecedented expansion of our knowledge of the molecular mechanisms regulating food intake. Perhaps the greatest impact has resulted from cloning the genes corresponding to several mouse monogenic obesity syndromes and the subsequent characterization of the pathways involved.[14] Many of these gene discoveries (*ob, db,* and *Ay*) have already led to potential anorexigenic drugs (leptin) or drug targets

(agonists for the leptin receptor and the melanocortin stimulating hormone receptor 4 [MC4-R], and antagonists for the neuropeptide Y receptors 1 and 5 [NPY1-R, NPY5-R] and others) currently in pharmaceutical development (see Chap. 10).

In contrast to animal models, the study of the molecular mechanisms and resulting behaviors that underlie excessive energy intake in humans has been very difficult. Nevertheless, the identification of severe hyperphagia in individuals with mutations of the leptin, leptin receptor, and MC4-receptor genes leaves little doubt that energy intake is as tightly regulated in humans as it is in animals, and suggests that these are highly conserved pathways[15] (Table 23-2). Furthermore, based on the results that have emerged from the recent use of new imaging techniques (such as positron emission tomography and functional MRI), it seems likely that brain responses to a meal may be substantially different between lean and obese subjects.[16,17] Such techniques applied to postobese subjects as well as subjects suffering from eating disorders may help identify the neurological pathways responsible for hyperphagia and obesity in humans.

Past difficulties in measuring habitual physical activity in humans have largely been alleviated by the advent of the doubly labeled water technique.[18] Thus in the near future it should be possible to better understand the interaction between the energy expended in daily physical activities and the development of obesity in children and adults.

A greater knowledge of the pathophysiology of obesity will ultimately come from the current efforts to isolate all of the genes related to weight gain. Over the past 5 years, genetic linkage studies have increasingly focused on complex traits such as obesity. Genome-wide scans have been completed in Mexican-Americans,[19] in Pima Indians,[20,21] in a diverse population of whites and blacks,[22] in French-Canadian families,[23] and in French families.[24] From these studies major loci linked to obesity have been found on chromosomes 2, 5, 10, 11, and 20. Those areas of the genome are currently under intense investigation as they may lead to the cloning of obesity susceptibility genes.

While obesity is likely a disease with multiple genetic and molecular causes, the impact of an obesogenic environment on this disease is substantial.[25] Therefore research should be conducted to uncover the major environmental determinants of obesity, and most importantly, to understand which are realistically modifiable.

TABLE 23-1. Classification of Overweight and Obesity by Body Mass Index (BMI) According to the 1998 National Institutes of Health Guidelines

	Obesity Class	BMI kg/m^2
Underweight		<18.5
Normal		18.5–24.9
Overweight		25.0–29.9
Obesity	I	30.0–34.9
	II	35.0–39.9
Extreme obesity	III	≥40

TABLE 23-2. Some Forms of Human Obesity Caused by Single Gene Mutations

Gene	Mutation	Location
LEP	G deletion @ codon 133 C → T codon 105 exon 3	7q31
LEPR	G → A exon 16	1p31
MC4-R	CTCT deletion @ codon 211 GATT insertion @nt732	18q21.3

LEP, leptin gene; LEPR, leptin receptor gene; MC4-R melanocortin = stimulating hormone receptor-4 gene.

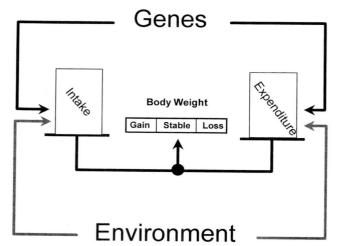

FIGURE 23-1. Obesity is the result of a chronic imbalance between energy intake and energy expenditure. Obesity susceptibility genes and their interaction with the obesogenic environment are likely to control both sides of the energy balance equation (i.e., energy intake and energy expenditure).

FIGURE 23-2. Studies in twins, adoptees, and family members indicate that approximately 70% of the interindividual variability in BMI is attributable to genetic factors. From prospective studies in Pima Indians, we can ascribe 10% of the variability in BMI to resting metabolic rate (RMR), 5% to fat oxidation (estimated from the respiratory quotient, RQ), and another 10% is likely due to the level of spontaneous physical activity (SPA)/fidgeting. Based on these data we estimate that at least 40% of the variability in BMI is related to genetic factors involved in the regulation of food intake (hyperphagia) and/or volitional activity (inactivity). Future studies are warranted to confirm these theoretical estimates.

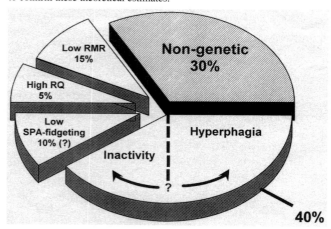

ASSOCIATION BETWEEN OBESITY AND T2DM

Individuals with type 2 diabetes mellitus (T2DM) are so commonly obese that Ethan Sims coined the term *diabesity* to describe this increasingly common syndrome. The association between obesity and T2DM has been observed in comparisons of different populations and within populations. In 10 different populations from divergent areas of the world, West and Kalbfleish discovered a strong correlation between prevalence of mean percentage standard weight and prevalence of T2DM.[26] Similar associations were found within populations, starting as early as 1921 in a study by Joslin.[27] Epidemiologic data indicates that both obesity and T2DM are more prevalent in affluent than in poor countries, suggesting that differences in life style and nutrition account for some of the differences observed between populations. However, within the same environment, certain ethnic groups have a markedly increased prevalence of obesity and T2DM. This has been interpreted by some to indicate that a common genetic predisposition may underlie the increased propensity for obesity and T2DM.

In addition to being more obese than nondiabetic people, people with T2DM have a more central distribution of body fat. As early as 1956, Vague suggested that central obesity was more common in people with T2DM.[28] Using different measures of body fat distribution, Feldman and colleagues confirmed these findings.[29] In a survey of over 30,000 women, Hartz and associates reported a higher prevalence of T2DM in women with a greater proportion of body fat at the waist relative to the hips, even at comparable degrees of obesity.[30] In a addition to these intrapopulation surveys, West reported that the Plains Indians of Oklahoma, a population with a high prevalence of T2DM, had a more central distribution of body fat when compared with whites in the U.S. population, a group with a lower prevalence of T2DM.[31]

Despite the overwhelming evidence showing the association between obesity and diabetes, a closer look at these cross-sectional data indicates that obesity is neither necessary nor sufficient for the development of T2DM. First, a number of lean people have diabetes.[32] Second, in some populations a high prevalence of obesity is associated with a low prevalence of T2DM[33] and pairs of diabetic monozygotic twins who are discordant for body weight have been described.[34] Third, in most populations obesity is more prevalent in females than in males, whereas the prevalence of T2DM is no different between genders. Finally and most importantly, in all populations a vast majority of the individuals who are obese do not

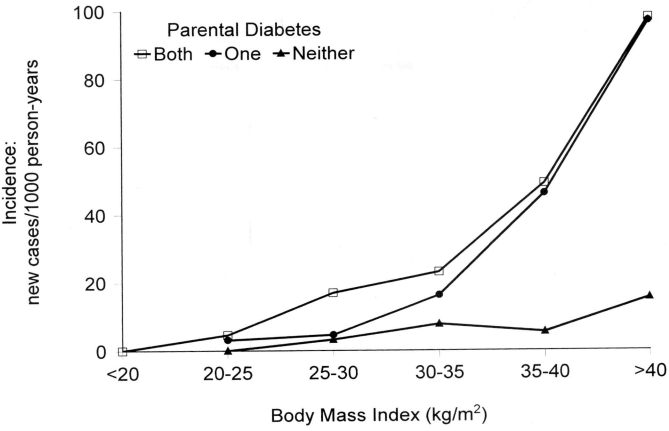

FIGURE 23-3. Incidence of T2DM correlated with BMI and parental diabetes in Pima Indians. This and other evidence (see text) indicates that obesity in neither sufficient nor necessary for the development of T2DM. *(Adapted from Knowler et al.[36])*

have T2DM. Although more than 50% of U.S. individuals are overweight, less than 10% of the population has T2DM (see Chap. 19 for a complete review). Among Caucasians[35] and Pima Indians[36] the latter, a population with one of the highest reported prevalence rates of obesity and diabetes in the world, the association between obesity and diabetes is strongly influenced by parental diabetes (Fig. 23-3). This seems to suggest that obesity may be more harmful in subjects who are genetically predisposed to develop T2DM. Cross-sectional studies do not establish whether obesity and T2DM are causally related, or if there is a third factor that causes both. However, prospective and longitudinal studies strongly support a direct role of obesity in the pathogenesis of diabetes.

OBESITY IS A RISK FACTOR FOR T2DM

Prospective studies on Caucasians in Norway,[37] Sweden,[38] Israel,[39] and the United States,[35,40,41] as well as Mexican-Americans in Texas[42] and Pima Indians in Arizona[43] have shown conclusively that obesity is a major risk factor for T2DM. Furthermore, studies of Israelis[39] and Pima Indians[44] have indicated that duration of obesity, in addition to degree of obesity, is a risk factor for T2DM. The risk of T2DM in Pima Indians is twice as high in those who have been obese for 10 years or more compared with those obese for less than 5 years.[44] A central distribution of body fat is also a major risk factor for T2DM, independently of the degree of obesity. This was demonstrated in prospective studies of Swedish, Pima Indian, and

Japanese populations, irrespective of the methodology used to assess body fat distribution.[43,45,46]

Obesity and visceral fat are neither the only nor the strongest predictors of T2DM. The relative role of obesity, body fat distribution, insulin sensitivity, insulin secretion, and hepatic glucose production was assessed in a prospective study of nondiabetic Pima Indians followed annually to detect the development of T2DM and to compare baseline measurements of those who developed the disease and those who did not.[43] Consistent with studies in other populations, univariate analyses revealed that insulin resistance is the single strongest predictor of T2DM (Table 23-3). In multivariate analyses, insulin resistance and insulin secretory dysfunction had an independent and cumulative effect on the development of diabetes, while hepatic glucose production did not (Fig. 23-4). The degree of obesity had little or no effect in predicting diabetes when insulin resistance was taken into account, suggesting that insulin resistance may be the major mechanism behind the association of obesity with increased risk of diabetes. In contrast, insulin resistance remained a strong predictor of T2DM when obesity (and insulin secretory function) was taken into account, indicating that in this population, insulin resistance predisposes to T2DM as a result of factors other than obesity alone. Central obesity, which predicts diabetes in other populations, was also predictive in Pima Indians and remained a significant risk factor when percentage of body fat and insulin resistance were taken into account. A reduced acute insulin response to glucose was also a significant independent risk factor.[43]

TABLE 23-3. Risk Factors for the Development Type 2 Diabetes in 200 Pima Indians

Factor	Values at 10th or 90th percentile*	Relative Hazard	95 % CI
Body fat (%)	22, 52	7.8	2.3–26.8
Ratio of waist to thigh circumference	1.4, 1.8	12.2	4.0–36.8
M_{130} (mg glucose/kg MBS · min)	4.4, 2.0	31.1	4.9–197.1
Hepatic glucose production (mg/kg MBS · min)	1.79, 2.47	1.3	0.3–1.9
Acute insulin response (μU/mL)	402, 104	2.2	0.9–5.9

M_{130} represents glucose uptake at a mean plasma insulin concentration of 130 μU/mL during euglycemia. MBS, metabolic body size (fat-free mass + 17 kg). Relative hazards were computed by proportional hazard analysis. *The first value in this column is the value associated with a lower risk of diabetes.

Together, prospective studies in Pimas and other populations indicate that obesity and defects in both insulin action and insulin secretion predispose to diabetes, but they give little information about the time course of these abnormalities and how they interact with one another. Longitudinal data in a group of Pima Indians followed for 5 years indicate that the transition from normal glucose tolerance to impaired glucose tolerance was associated with increased body weight, a decline in insulin action, and a decline in insulin secretion, but no changes in hepatic glucose production.[47] Further increase in body weight and further decrease in both insulin action and insulin secretion, but an increase in hepatic glucose production, characterized progression from IGT to diabetes. By comparison, in Pimas who remained NGT over the same period

of time, a twofold smaller increase in body weight was associated with a decline in insulin action and an increase in insulin secretion[47,48] (Fig. 23-5). These data are consistent with a pathogenic role of obesity and longer duration in the progressive impairment of insulin action and insulin secretion that lead to diabetes.

OBESITY AND INSULIN RESISTANCE

Experimental weight gain causes hyperinsulinemia and insulin resistance in animals and humans.[49–53] The effect of short-term overnutrition on insulin action is thought to be mediated by a decrease in muscle glycogen synthase activity and glycogenesis.[51]

FIGURE 23-4. Seven-year cumulative incidence of T2DM in Pima Indians. This analysis shows the independent and additive effect of insulin resistance and insulin secretory dysfunction on the development of T2DM in this population.

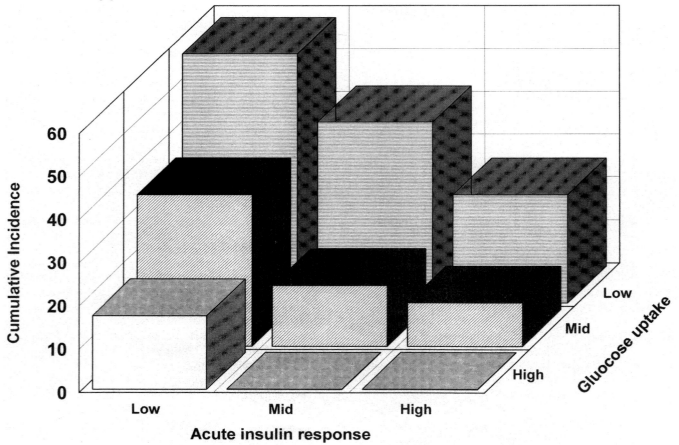

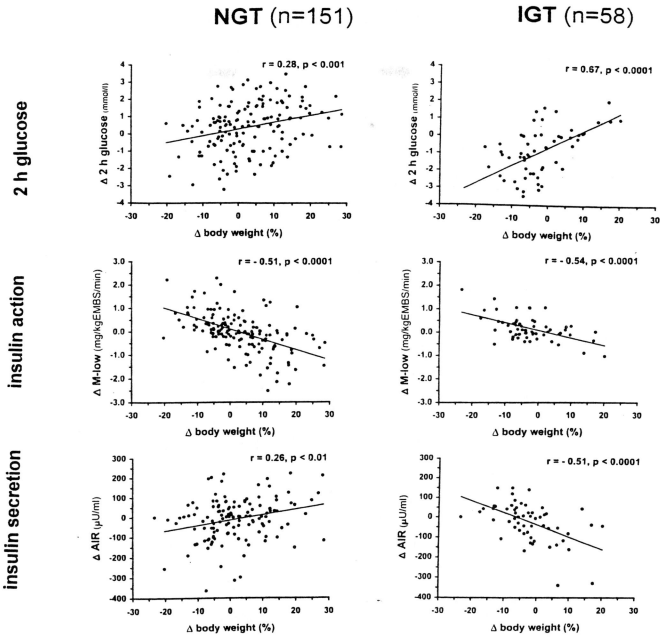

FIGURE 23-5. Relation of changes in 2-hour glucose concentration, insulin action (Δ**M-low**), and insulin secretion (Δ**AIR**) to change in body weight in 209 Pima Indians with normal (**NGT**) or impaired (**IGT**) glucose tolerance at baseline, who were studied a second time while still free of diabetes after either losing or gaining weight over an average of 2.5 years. While weight gain was associated with a similar decline in insulin action in individuals with NGT and IGT (**middle panels**), the effect of weight gain on insulin secretory function was opposite in the two groups (**lower panels**). Thus, weight gain seems to have more detrimental effects in subjects with IGT than in subjects with NGT, since in the former insulin secretion fails to increase to compensate for the decreased insulin action. Consequently, the raise in 2-hour glucose in response to the same degree of weight gain is greater in people with IGT compared to people with NGT (**upper panels**). *(Adapted from Weyer et al.[48])*

Recent data suggest that this may be due to activation of the intracellular hexosamine pathway in response to excessive availability of nutrients.[54]

The relationship between degree of obesity and *in vivo* insulin action has been investigated extensively. In nondiabetic Pima Indians the relationship between obesity and insulin action was studied using a two-step euglycemic-hyperinsulinemic clamp technique.[55] In combination with indirect calorimetry, this technique allows the assessment of whole body (reflecting mostly skeletal muscle glucose metabolism) insulin-mediated glucose disposal and its two major components, oxidative and nonoxidative (glycogen storage) glucose disposal. A negative, nonlinear relationship

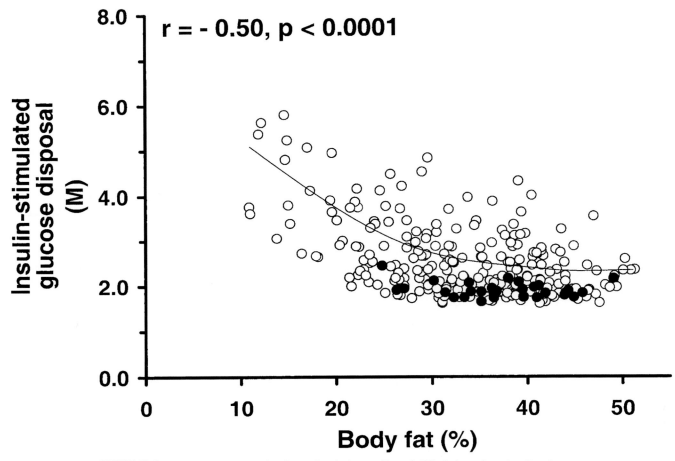

FIGURE 23-6. The relation between insulin-mediated glucose disposal (**M**) during a hyperinsulinemic eug-lycemic clamp and percentage of body fat study in 280 Pima Indians with either NGT (n = 179, **open circles**), IGT (n = 79, **gray circles**), or T2DM (n = 29, **dark circles**). At each level of adiposity, individuals with a rela-tively high, normal, or low M can be identified.

between the degree of obesity and *in vivo* insulin action at physio-logic insulin concentrations was observed[55–57] (Fig. 23-6). At maximally-stimulating plasma insulin concentrations there was a significant, negative linear relationship between degree of obesity and insulin action. It is important to point out that in Pima Indians, adiposity only accounts for approximately 36% of the variance in insulin action at physiologic insulin concentration, and even less, approximately 15%, at maximally-stimulating insulin concentra-tions.[55–57] While some of this variance can be explained by differ-ences in body fat distribution, this indicates that some very obese individuals can have a normal peripheral tissue sensitivity to the effect of insulin on glucose uptake (Fig. 23-6).

Many studies have indicated that over a wide range of insulin action, from the greatest *in vivo* insulin resistance to the greatest insulin sensitivity, glucose storage, not glucose oxidation, makes a progressively greater contribution to glucose uptake.[58–62] Together with the evidence that during a hyperinsulinemic euglycemic clamp there is little hepatic glucose uptake[63–65] but significant pe-ripheral glucose uptake, these studies emphasize the role of skele-tal muscle glucose storage in determining insulin resistance. In 1989, Shulman and associates demonstrated directly that the rate of insulin-mediated glycogenesis, measured by nuclear magnetic resonance, was reduced in people with T2DM compared with non-diabetic subjects.[66] Despite the many theories proposed to explain

the etiologic link between obesity and insulin resistance, a con-vincing explanation of how excess adiposity and/or its metabolic and hormonal consequences impair glucose uptake and storage in the muscle remains elusive.

Role of Free Fatty Acids (FFA)

After years of controversy, there is now very strong evidence that acute elevation of plasma FFA levels, such as can be generated by intralipid/heparin infusion, can result in insulin resistance.[67] Furthermore, acute[68,69] and chronic[70] lowering of FFA improves insulin sensitivity.

The question as to how an increased fatty acid supply from fat depots, especially visceral adipose tissue, induces insulin resis-tance in peripheral tissues has been difficult to resolve. Lipolytic activity in abdominal adipocytes is considerably higher than in subcutaneous adipocytes.[71] Because FFA released from the ab-dominal fat deposits are delivered directly to the liver through the portal vein, hepatic insulin resistance, accompanied by increased gluconeogenesis and increased lipoprotein and triglyceride export to other tissues, has been invoked as a possible mechanism. How-ever, it has been difficult to directly demonstrate an increase in FFA flux to the muscle in obese subjects and in subjects with increased visceral obesity, and in fact the reverse has been reported.[72] Nevertheless, insulin sensitivity in animals and humans has been found to be inversely related to total muscle triglyceride content as measured in muscle biopsies.[73–75] In humans, this correlation is much stronger when intramyocellular fat is the measured variable.[76] While there appears to be increasing evidence for an accumulation of muscle lipid in insulin resistance states in humans, the causal mechanism that links tissue accumulation of fat and reduced glucose uptake remains to be established.

It has been proposed that increased availability of FFA or ketones for oxidation may be responsible for an inhibition of carbohydrate metabolism in muscle, thus producing a reduction in glucose tolerance. The concept has been extended to suggest that one role of insulin is to control glucose uptake by controlling the rate of release of FFA from adipose tissue.[77,78–80] However, in both humans and rodents the effect of intralipid/heparin infusion on insulin resistance takes several hours to occur.[67,81] Thus the prompt effect of FFA to reduce glucose oxidation/glycolysis at the mitochondrial level by competing for the same oxidative pathways as first described by Randle and colleagues[77] is at best an incomplete explanation for a direct effect of FFA on insulin resistance.

While there is substantial evidence of a primary role of skeletal muscle glucose storage (not oxidation) in determining insulin resistance, an unequivocal biochemical explanation for a role for FFA in regulating glycogen synthesis is lacking. Some possible mechanisms have been proposed. Long-chain acyl CoA (LCACs, the activated form of FFA that can be transported across the mitochondrial membrane for oxidation) and especially palmitoyl CoA have been shown to inhibit the activity of liver glycogen synthase,[82] but there are no reports of this effect in muscle. The effect of FFA on glucose storage may be indirectly mediated via an inhibitory effect on insulin signaling and/or glucose transport. Some evidence points to the possible modulatory effect of LCACs on PKC activity[83] and its inhibition of insulin-mediated glycogen synthesis. In animal and human studies, a significant correlation has been found between FFA composition of muscle membranes and insulin action.[84,85] The mechanisms by which lipid composition of the membrane influences insulin action are not clear but may involve changing membrane fluidity, which could affect insulin and other membrane receptor action.[86] FFA may directly affect glucose transport, and there is substantial evidence that LCACs are intimately involved in the regulation of the normal translocation of GLUT-4–containing vesicles.[87–89] UDP-N-acetyl-glucosamine (UDP-N-GlcNAc) is the end product of the hexosamine pathway and stimulation of this pathway by hyperglycemia, infusion of glucosamine, or increased availability of FFA causes insulin resistance in the muscle.[90] By glycosylation and stabilization of transcription factors, UDP-N-GlcNAc may regulate expression of genes involved in the control of glycogen synthesis.

Role of Adipocyte Secreted Hormones

While the response of adipocytes to sex steroids and glucocorticoids has been known for a long time,[91] it is only recently that the adipose tissue has been recognized as an endocrine and paracrine organ from which a number of signals emanate. These include leptin, tumor necrosis factor-α (TNF-α), interleukin-6 (IL-6), complement C3 and its cleavage product acylation stimulating protein (ASP), enzymes of lipoprotein metabolism (LPL, CETP, and Apo-E), growth factors (TGFβ and IGF-1), angiotensinogen, and PAI-1.[92] It has been proposed that the role of adipose tissue in regulating glucose metabolism may in part be explained through the action of leptin and the other adipocyte-secreted cytokines TNF-α and IL-6 on peripheral tissues (Fig. 23-7).

Leptin levels are usually elevated in proportion to the degree of obesity in animals and humans.[93,94] Leptin has been shown to have both central and peripheral effects.[95–97] Experimental studies have suggested that leptin may impair insulin signaling both in the skeletal muscle and the adipose tissue. Leptin impairs insulin-mediated glucose uptake in mouse myotubules by inhibiting phosphorylation of IRS-1.[98] The same type of mechanism was reported for the insulin-mediated glucose uptake inhibition induced by leptin in Hep-G2 cells.[99] In rat adipocytes, leptin has been found to inhibit insulin-mediated glucose uptake, possibly via PKA activation.[100] These in vitro data contrast sharply with the data from experiments in several animal models of obesity and diabetes that show improvement in glucose/insulin metabolism in response to peripheral administration of leptin.[101–104] Leptin administration in humans is not associated with the development of diabetes in the short-term.[105] Thus the role of leptin as a mediator of the insulin resistance observed in obese individuals remains largely unsubstantiated and the balance of data suggest that leptin improves insulin sensitivity.

Adipose tissue is a significant source of endogenous TNF-α production and its expression is elevated in association with obesity in both animals and humans.[106,107] Adipocytes are also responsible for the expression of the soluble form of both type 1 and type 2 TNF-α receptors.[108] Release from subcutaneous adipose tissue of both forms of TNF-α receptors into the circulation has been observed, but not release of TNF-α itself.[108,109] The exact role of the soluble receptors in modulating the effects of TNF-α in target tissues in not well understood. In vitro studies suggest that TNF-α impairs insulin signaling, but the exact mechanism is still under investigation. TNF-α has been reported to decrease phosphorylation of IR/IRS-1,[110] decrease IRS-1 and GLUT-4 expression,[111] and increase intracellular calcium concentration.[112] However, whether TNF-α is an endocrine or paracrine signal from distant or local adipocytes to the muscle remains the subject of some debate. Therefore, the in vivo significance of these data is as yet unclear.[92]

Like TNF-α, IL-6 is a proinflammatory cytokine with potent actions in host defense. IL-6 is also expressed in and released by adipose tissue and its circulating concentration increases with obesity.[113,114] In animals, IL-6 has been shown to stimulate insulin secretion.[115] In humans, IL-6 was found to increase hepatic glucose release and to induce the release of glucagon and cortisol.[115] Thus, a direct role of IL-6 in causing insulin-resistance in the obese state is currently only based on circumstantial evidence.

Human adipocytes also synthesize and secrete the three proteins of the alternative complement pathway: complement C3, factor B, and factor D (adipsin). The interaction of these three factors results in the generation of C3a, which is rapidly converted to C3adesarg, also termed acylation stimulating protein (ASP).[116] In vitro studies indicate that ASP stimulates glucose uptake in adipocytes,[117] fibroblasts,[118] and myotubules.[119] Experimental data indicate that ASP stimulates the translocation of glucose transporters to the cell surface and that this effect is independent of insulin.[118,119] Elevated C3 levels have been reported in association with obesity and other conditions associated with insulin resistance.[120–122] A negative correlation between insulin action and C3, but not ASP, plasma concentration has been reported in Pima Indians.[123] The exact biological mechanism underlying this association remains obscure, especially in view of the positive effects of ASP on glucose metabolism.

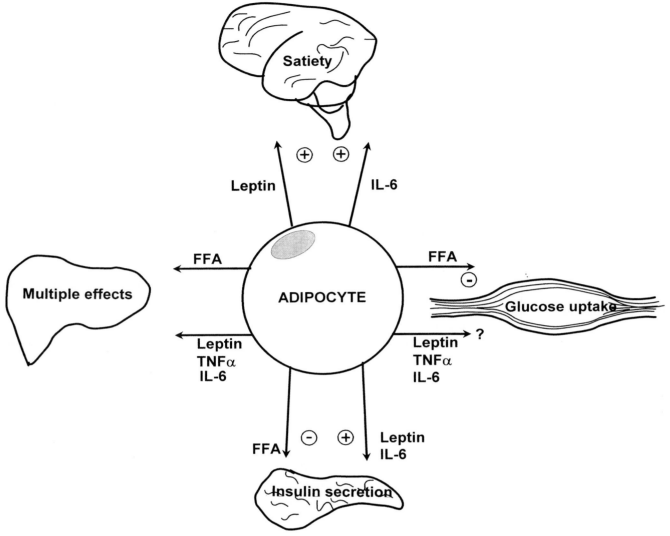

FIGURE 23-7. The adipose tissue is an endocrine organ. Several signals (endocrine, paracrine, and metabolic) emanate from adipocytes and are believed to affect several organs including brain, liver, skeletal muscle, and pancreas. The strength and direction of the effect of the signals emanating from the adipose tissue to other organs are the object of intense investigation.

Role of Obesity-Induced Changes in Skeletal Muscle

Obesity is associated with an increase in both fat mass and fat-free mass.[124] A role for the increase in fat-free tissue in producing insulin resistance has been studied in the past. With an increase in fat-free mass, muscle cells are hypertrophied and capillaries in the muscle are more widely spaced. Several human studies have indicated that muscle cell size and muscle capillary supply are associated with changes in fasting insulin concentration and glucose tolerance.[125–127] It has been proposed that the association between obesity-induced changes in skeletal muscle morphology and insulin action may be explained by the fact that lower capillary density results in reduced access of insulin to muscle of obese subjects.[128] Studies of insulin kinetics have indicated that insulin penetrates the capillary wall slowly and equilibrates slowly in a nonvascular compartment.[129] If muscle cell membranes are able to take up and degrade insulin more rapidly than the diffusion of insulin from capillary to interstitial space and down to fibers, then physiologic effects would be important. Theoretical models based on the principles that insulin diffuses from the capillary and is taken up and degraded by muscle cell membrane, predict that the average insulin concentration around a hypertrophied muscle cell with a poor capillary supply will be reduced even at steady state.[57] In support of this theory, a reduced capillary density,[128] a delayed onset of insulin action in the muscle,[130,131] and a 26% lower tissue insulin concentration at the same plasma concentration have been observed in obese compared with lean individuals.[132]

OBESITY AND INSULIN SECRETION

FFA serve as an important energy source for most body tissues, but they have a broader function in whole-body fuel homeostasis by virtue of their ability to act as signals in a variety of cellular processes. One such role of FFA is to enhance the responsiveness of the pancreas to a variety of insulin secretagogues. However, recent studies indicate that chronic exposure of the pancreas to excessive FFA concentration may have deleterious effects on the β cells.[133]

Studies in animals indicate that FFA are indispensable to the β cells for stimulus-secretion coupling during fasting. In fasted rats, β cells are virtually unresponsive if FFA are lowered by an infusion of nicotinic acid before a glucose load, and the insulinotropic efficiency of FFA increases with their degree of saturation.[134,135] The situation appears to be similar in humans during prolonged food deprivation.[136] Thus it has been proposed that at any given time, insulin secretion will be governed not only by the blood glucose concentration, but also by the prevailing concentration and nature of the circulating fatty acids. The exact mechanism by which FFA (or an active form like LCACs) modulate insulin secretory function is not known, but the site of action appears to be at a late step of the insulin secretory process, since it is common to a variety of insulin-secretory stimuli.[137]

The ability of circulating FFA to sustain basal β-cell function in the fasted state and to assure efficient nutrient-stimulated insulin secretion when the fast is terminated must be considered a physiologic phenomenon. In prediabetic obese individuals, basal hyperinsulinemia and exaggerated postprandial insulin secretion are widely accepted as compensatory responses to the preexisting muscle insulin resistance. However, because at this early stage only a small increase in plasma glucose concentration is observed in association with insulin resistance and hyperinsulinemia, it is not clear how the β cells sense peripheral insulin resistance and become hyperresponsive to glucose. An attractive hypothesis is that tissue accumulation of fat plays a role in inducing both muscle insulin resistance and pancreatic glucose hyperresponsiveness.

Both experimental and circumstantial evidence is mounting, however, that chronic exposure to FFA has deleterious effects on insulin secretion. Long-term intravenous infusions of FFA impair insulin secretion in both animals and humans.[138,139] Elevated FFA plasma concentrations have been found to predict diabetes.[140,141] In Pima Indians, a high fasting plasma FFA concentration predicted the development of diabetes independently of insulin resistance, but not independently of insulin secretion.[141] Results from this prospective study are consistent with the hypothesis of a deleterious effect of chronically elevated FFA concentrations on insulin secretion. Possible mechanisms underlying the "lipotoxic" effects of FFA on the β cell include overproduction of NO,[142] interleukin-1β,[143] and/or ceramide,[144] the latter possibly being responsible for the accelerated apoptosis observed in fat-laden β cells.

OBESITY, T2DM, AND THE AUTONOMIC NERVOUS SYSTEM

Fasting hyperinsulinemia and exaggerated insulin response to glucose are typical characteristics of various animal models of genetic or hypothalamic obesity and diabetes. They include the *ob/ob* mouse, the *fa/fa* rat, and rodents with lesions of the ventromedial hypothalamus.[145–153] The metabolic abnormalities observed in these animals are thought to be due to an abnormal function of the autonomic nervous system, namely low sympathetic nervous system activity and an exaggerated parasympathetic drive to the pancreas. In humans, the autonomic nervous system is also thought to be involved in the regulation of energy[154] and glucose/insulin metabolism.[155]

Studies in Caucasians indicate that the activity of the sympathetic nervous system is related to the three major components of energy expenditure: resting metabolic rate,[156] the thermic effect of food,[157] and spontaneous physical activity.[158] We have recently shown that sympathetic nervous system (SNS) activity is also correlated with daily fat oxidation rates.[159] Further indications of the possible role of SNS activity in the regulation of energy balance in humans comes from a study showing that low SNS activity was associated with poor weight loss outcome in obese subjects treated with diet.[160] Furthermore, Pima Indians, who are prone to obesity, have low rates of muscle sympathetic nerve activity compared to weight-matched Caucasians.[156] In a prospective study, baseline urinary excretion rate of norepinephrine, a global index of SNS activity, was negatively correlated with body weight gain in male Pima Indians.[161] Thus low activity of the SNS is associated with the development of obesity, which in turn is a risk factor for T2DM.

Parasympathetic, sympathetic, and sensory nerves richly innervate the pancreatic islets. Experimental evidence indicates that insulin secretion is stimulated by parasympathetic nerves and their neurotransmitters and inhibited by sympathetic nerves and their neurotransmitters.[155,162] The autonomic innervation of the pancreas seems to be of physiologic importance in mediating the cephalic phase of insulin secretion.[155,163] However, the autonomic nerves could also be involved in the islet adaptation to insulin resistance with possible implications for the development of T2DM[155] (see Chap. 9).

At the opposite extremes of the relationship between autonomic nervous system activity and insulin secretion, are patients with Prader-Willi syndrome and the Pima Indians of Arizona.[164,165] Patients with Prader-Willi syndrome, a relatively common form of genetic obesity, who are hypoinsulinemic and have a delayed insulin response to a meal, have a very low parasympathetic drive to the pancreas.[164] Pima Indians seem to have a complex disturbance of the autonomic function, including not only lower sympathetic nervous system activity,[156] but also an increased parasympathetic drive to the pancreas, which is detectable in childhood.[165] This is thought to contribute, at least in part, to the high prevalence of hyperinsulinemia in this population.[166] Of note, fasting hyperinsulinemia has recently been reported to be an independent risk factor for T2DM in the Pimas.[167]

OBESITY AND T2DM IN CHILDREN AND ADOLESCENTS

Childhood obesity is a very serious problem because obese children tend to grow into obese adults.[168] Furthermore, duration of obesity is an independent predictor of poor health outcomes.[169] The risk of developing obesity seems to be especially elevated during early infancy, the adiposity rebound period during prepubertal growth, and the adolescent growth phase.[170]

The observation that obesity occurs more frequently in children of obese parents has led to a variety of studies to determine how much of the genetic predisposition to obesity is related to energy metabolism. As in adults, some but not all studies have reported that excessive energy intake and/or a low energy expenditure in early childhood increase the risk of obesity later in life.[171–176] Despite large inconsistencies in the literature and because low levels of aerobic fitness,[177] excessive TV viewing,[178] and limited playing time[179] have all been associated with increased risk of weight gain, it seems reasonable to conclude that a sedentary lifestyle in early childhood should be discouraged.

One of the most troubling aspects of the current epidemic of obesity is the increasing prevalence of T2DM among children and adolescents.[4] Until recently, immune-mediated type 1 diabetes was the only type of diabetes considered prevalent among children. Recent reports indicate that 8–45% of children with newly diagnosed diabetes have non-immune-mediated diabetes. While percentages vary greatly depending on ethnicity and sampling strategies, the majority of these children have T2DM.[180]

Because the emergence of T2DM in children and adolescents is a relatively recent phenomenon, there is only a limited amount of data on the epidemiology of the disease in the general U.S. population, but it seems that certain ethnic minorities are disproportionately affected.[181] Among the Pima Indians of Arizona an analysis performed from 1992 to 1996 revealed a prevalence of T2DM of 2.2% in the 10- to 14-year-old age group and 5% in children 15–19 years of age.[182]

Obesity is the hallmark of T2DM in youth, with up to 85% of affected children being either overweight or obese at diagnosis.[180] Usually a family history of diabetes is also present, with up to 80% of patients having at least one parent and close to 100% of the patients having a first- or second-degree relative with diabetes.[180,182] Female sex and puberty are other possible risk factors for developing T2DM at an early age.[180] Studies in Pima Indians indicate that offspring of women who had diabetes during pregnancy are especially at risk of T2DM at an early age.[183] Exposure to the diabetic intrauterine environment was responsible for about 40% of the T2DM seen in children aged 5–19 between 1987 and 1994, approximately twice the attributable risk found between 1967 and 1976.[183] It remains to be seen whether gestational diabetes is a factor in the alarming rise of T2DM seen in youth nationally.

SUMMARY AND CONCLUSION

Obesity is a chronic disease that is quickly reaching epidemic proportions, and one that increases the risk for other noncommunicable diseases, and thus reduces life expectancy. Obesity is heritable and it results from a chronic imbalance between energy intake and energy expenditure. However, its exact etiology is unknown.

While it is often observed in association with T2DM, obesity is neither necessary nor sufficient alone to cause T2DM. In some predisposed individuals and populations, obesity substantially increases the risk of developing T2DM by lowering insulin sensitivity, and possibly by increasing insulin secretory dysfunction. The precise links between obesity and T2DM have yet to be unequivocally identified.

In conclusion, further research is needed to understand the etiology of obesity and how obesity precipitates the development of T2DM in predisposed individuals.

REFERENCES

1. Swinburn B, Egger G, Raza F: Dissecting obesogenic environments: the development and application of a framework for identifying and prioritizing environmental interventions for obesity. *Prev Med* 1999; 29:563.
2. WHO Report: *Obesity, Preventing and Managing the Global Epidemic.* WHO/NUT/NCD/98.1. WHO:1997.
3. NIH, NHLBI: Clinical guidelines on the identification, evaluation and treatment of overweight and obesity in adults—The Evidence Report. *Obes Res* 1998;6:(Suppl 2).
4. Mokdad AH, Serdula MK, Dietz WH, *et al*: The spread of the obesity epidemic in the United States, 1991–1998. *JAMA* 1999;282:1519.
5. Ogden CL, Troiano RP, Briefel RR, *et al*: Prevalence of overweight among preschool children in the United States, 1971 through 1994. *Pediatrics* 1997;99:E1.
6. Must A, Spadano J, Coakley EH, *et al*: The disease burden associated with overweight and obesity. *JAMA* 1999;282:1523.
7. Wolf AM, Colditz GA: Current estimates of the economic cost of obesity in the United States [see comments]. *Obes Res* 1998;6:97.
8. Bouchard C, Perusse L: Heredity and body fat. *Annu Rev Nutr* 1988; 8:259.
9. Allison DB, Kaprio J, Korkeila M, *et al*: The heritability of body mass index among an international sample of monozygotic twins reared apart. *Int J Obes Relat Metab Disord* 1996;20:501.
10. Sakul H, Pratley R, Cardon L, *et al*: Familiality of physical and metabolic characteristics that predict the development of non-insulin-dependent diabetes mellitus in Pima Indians. *Am J Hum Genet* 1997; 60:651.
11. Ravussin E, Lillioja S, Knowler WC, *et al*: Reduced rate of energy expenditure as a risk factor for body-weight gain. *N Engl J Med* 1988; 318:467.
12. Zurlo F, Lillioja S, Esposito-Del PA, *et al*: Low ratio of fat to carbohydrate oxidation as predictor of weight gain: study of 24-h RQ. *Am J Physiol* 1990;259:E650.
13. Zurlo F, Ferraro RT, Fontvielle AM, *et al*: Spontaneous physical activity and obesity: cross-sectional and longitudinal studies in Pima Indians. *Am J Physiol* 1992;263:E296.
14. Yanovski JA, Yanovski SZ: Recent advances in basic obesity research. *JAMA* 1999;282:1504.
15. Barsh GS, Farooqi IS, O'Rahilly S: Genetics of body-weight regulation. *Nature* 2000;404:644.
16. Tataranni PA, Gautier JF, Chen K, *et al*: Neuroanatomical correlates of hunger and satiation in humans using positron emission tomography. *Proc Natl Acad Sci USA* 1999;96:4569.
17. Matsuda M, Liu Y, Mahankali S, *et al*: Altered hypothalamic function in response to glucose ingestion in obese humans. *Diabetes* 1999; 48:1801.
18. Schoeller DA, Taylor PB: Precision of the doubly labelled water method using the two-point calculation. *Hum Nutr Clin Nutr* 1987; 41:215.
19. Comuzzie AG, Hixson JE, Almasy L, *et al*: A major quantitative trait locus determining serum leptin levels and fat mass is located on human chromosome 2. *Nat Genet* 1997;15:273.
20. Hanson RL, Ehm MG, Pettitt DJ, *et al*: An autosomal genomic scan for loci linked to type II diabetes mellitus and body-mass index in Pima Indians. *Am J Hum Genet* 1998;63:1130.
21. Norman RA, Tataranni PA, Pratley R, *et al*: Autosomal genomic scan for loci linked to obesity and energy metabolism in Pima Indians. *Am J Hum Genet* 1998;62:659.
22. Lee JH, Reed DR, Li WD, *et al*: Genome scan for human obesity and linkage to markers in 20q13. *Am J Hum Genet* 1999;64:196.
23. Chagnon YC, Perusse L, Weisnagel SJ, *et al*: The human obesity gene map: the 1999 update. *Obes Res* 2000;8:89.
24. Hager J, Dina C, Francke S, *et al*: A genome-wide scan for human obesity genes reveals a major susceptibility locus on chromosome 10. *Nat Genet* 1998;20:304.
25. Hill JO, Peters JC: Environmental contributions to the obesity epidemic. *Science* 1998;280:1371.
26. West KM, Kalbfleish JM: Influence of nutritional factors on prevalence of diabetes. *Diabetes* 1971;20:99.
27. Joslin EP: The prevention of diabetes mellitus. *JAMA* 1921;76:79.
28. Vague J: The degree of masculine differentiation of obesities: a factor determining predisposition to diabetes, atherosclerosis, gout, and uric calculus disease. *Am J Clin Nutr* 1956;4:20.
29. Feldman R, Sender AJ, Siegelaub AB: Difference in diabetic and non-diabetic fat distribution patterns by skinfold measurements. *Diabetes* 1969;18:478.
30. Hartz AJ, Rupley DC, Rimm AA: The association of girth measurements with disease in 32,856 women. *Am J Epidemiol* 1984;119:71.
31. West KM: Diabetes in American Indians and other native populations of the New World. *Diabetes* 1974;23:841.

32. Amner P, Pollare T, Lithell H: Different aetiologies of type 2 (non-insulin-dependent) diabetes mellitus in obese and non-obese subjects. *Diabetologia* 1991;34:483.
33. Jackson WPU: Epidemiology of diabetes in South Africa. *Adv Metab Disord* 1978;9:111.
34. Barnett AH, Eff C, Leslie RD, et al: Diabetes in identical twins. A study of 200 pairs. *Diabetologia* 1981;20:87.
35. O'Sullivan JB, Mahan CM: Blood sugar levels, glycosuria, and body weight related to development of diabetes mellitus. The Oxford epidemiologic study 17 years later. *JAMA* 1965;194:587.
36. Knowler WC, Pettitt DJ, Saad MF, et al: Diabetes mellitus in the Pima Indians: incidence, risk factors and pathogenesis. *Diabetes Metab Rev* 1990;6:1.
37. Westlund K, Nicolaysen R: Ten-year mortality and morbidity related to serum cholesterol. A follow-up of 3,751 men aged 40–49. *Scand J Clin Lab Invest Suppl* 1972;127:1.
38. Ohlson LO, Larsson B, Eriksson H, et al: Diabetes mellitus in Swedish middle-aged men. The study of men born in 1913 and 1923. *Diabetologia* 1987;30:386.
39. Modan M, Karasik A, Halkin H, et al: Effect of past and concurrent body mass index on prevalence of glucose intolerance and type 2 (non-insulin-dependent) diabetes and on insulin response. The Israel study of glucose intolerance, obesity and hypertension. *Diabetologia* 1986;29:82.
40. Dunn JP, Ipsen J, Elsom KO, et al: Risk factors in coronary artery disease, hypertension and diabetes. *Am J Med Sci* 1970;259:309.
41. Wilson PW, McGee DL, Kannel WB: Obesity, very low density lipoproteins, and glucose intolerance over fourteen years: The Framingham Study. *Am J Epidemiol* 1981;114:697.
42. Haffner SM, Stern MP, Mitchell BD, et al: Incidence of type II diabetes in Mexican Americans predicted by fasting insulin and glucose levels, obesity, and fatty-fat distribution. *Diabetes* 1990;39:283.
43. Lillioja S, Mott DM, Spraul M, et al: Insulin resistance and insulin secretory dysfunction as precursors of non-insulin-dependent diabetes mellitus. Prospective studies of Pima Indians. *N Engl J Med* 1993;329:1988.
44. Everhart JE, Pettitt DJ, Bennett PH, et al: Duration of obesity increases the incidence of NIDDM. *Diabetes* 1992;41:235.
45. Ohlson LO, Larsson B, Svardsudd K, et al: The influence of body fat distribution on the incidence of diabetes mellitus. 13.5 years of follow-up of the participants in the study of men born in 1913. *Diabetes* 1985;34:1055.
46. Bergstrom RW, Newell-Morris LL, Leonetti DL, et al: Association of elevated fasting C-peptide level and increased intra-abdominal fat distribution with development of NIDDM in Japanese-American men. *Diabetes* 1990;39:104.
47. Weyer C, Bogardus C, Mott DM, et al: The natural history of insulin secretory dysfunction and insulin resistance in the pathogenesis of type 2 diabetes mellitus. *J Clin Invest* 1999;104:787.
48. Weyer C, Hanson K, Bogardus C, et al: Long-term changes in insulin action and insulin secretion associated with gain, loss, regain and maintenance of body weight. *Diabetologia* 2000;43:36.
49. Sims EA, Danforth EJ, Horton ES, et al: Endocrine and metabolic effects of experimental obesity in man. *Recent Prog Horm Res* 1973;29:457.
50. Kashiwagi A, Mott D, Bogardus C, et al: The effects of short-term overfeeding on adipocyte metabolism in Pima Indians. *Metabolism* 1985;34:364.
51. Mott DM, Lillioja S, Bogardus C: Overnutrition induced decrease in insulin action for glucose storage: *in vivo* and *in vitro* in man. *Metabolism* 1986;35:160.
52. Oppert JM, Nadeau A, Tremblay A, et al: Plasma glucose, insulin, and glucagon before and after long-term overfeeding in identical twins. *Metabolism* 1995;44:96.
53. Kolaczynski JW, Ohannesian JP, Considine RV, et al: Response of leptin to short-term and prolonged overfeeding in humans. *J Clin Endocrinol Metab* 1996;81:4162.
54. Rossetti L: Perspective: Hexosamines and nutrient sensing. *Endocrinology* 2000;141:1922.
55. Bogardus C, Lillioja S, Mott D, et al: Relationship between obesity and maximal insulin-stimulated glucose uptake *in vivo* and *in vitro* in Pima Indians. *J Clin Invest* 1984;73:800.
56. Bogardus C, Lillioja S, Mott DM, et al: Relationship between degree of obesity and *in vivo* insulin action in man. *Am J Physiol* 1985;248:E286.
57. Lillioja S, Bogardus C: Obesity and insulin resistance: lessons learned from the Pima Indians. *Diabetes Metab Rev* 1988;4:517.
58. Felber JP, Meyer HU, Curchod B, et al: Glucose storage and oxidation in different degrees of human obesity measured by continuous indirect calorimetry. *Diabetologia* 1981;20:39.
59. Jacot E, DeFronzo RA, Jequier E, et al: The effect of hyperglycemia, hyperinsulinemia, and route of glucose administration on glucose oxidation and glucose storage. *Metabolism* 1982;31:922.
60. Lillioja S, Mott DM, Zawadzki JK, et al: Glucose storage is a major determinant of *in vivo* "insulin resistance" in subjects with normal glucose tolerance. *J Clin Endocrinol Metab* 1986;62:922.
61. Thiebaud D, Jacot E, DeFronzo RA, et al: The effect of graded doses of insulin on total glucose uptake, glucose oxidation, and glucose storage in man. *Diabetes* 1982;31:957.
62. Boden G, Ray TK, Smith RH, et al: Carbohydrate oxidation and storage in obese non-insulin-dependent diabetic patients. Effects of improving glycemic control. *Diabetes* 1983;32:982.
63. DeFronzo RA, Jacot E, Jequier E, et al: The effect of insulin on the disposal of intravenous glucose. Results from indirect calorimetry and hepatic and femoral venous catheterization. *Diabetes* 1981;30:1000.
64. DeFronzo RA, Ferrannini E, Hendler R, et al: Regulation of splanchnic and peripheral glucose uptake by insulin and hyperglycemia in man. *Diabetes* 1983;32:35.
65. DeFronzo RA, Gunnarsson R, Bjorkman O, et al: Effects of insulin on peripheral and splanchnic glucose metabolism in noninsulin-dependent (type II) diabetes mellitus. *J Clin Invest* 1985;76:149.
66. Shulman GI, Rothman DL, Jue T, et al: Quantitation of muscle glycogen synthesis in normal subjects and subjects with non-insulin-dependent diabetes by 13C nuclear magnetic resonance spectroscopy [see comments]. *N Engl J Med* 1990;322:223.
67. Boden G: Role of fatty acids in the pathogenesis of insulin resistance and NIDDM. *Diabetes* 1997;46:3.
68. Balasse EO, Neef MA: Influence of nicotinic acid on the rates of turnover and oxidation of plasma glucose in man. *Metabolism* 1973;22:1193.
69. Gomez F, Jequier E, Chabot V, et al: Carbohydrate and lipid oxidation in normal human subjects: its influence on glucose tolerance and insulin response to glucose. *Metabolism* 1972;21:381.
70. Kumar S, Boulton AJ, Beck-Nielsen H, et al: Troglitazone, an insulin action enhancer, improves metabolic control in NIDDM patients. Troglitazone Study Group [published erratum appears in *Diabetologia* 1996;39:1245] *Diabetologia* 1996;39:701.
71. Hoffstedt J, Arner P, Hellers G, et al: Variation in adrenergic regulation of lipolysis between omental and subcutaneous adipocytes from obese and non-obese men. *J Lipid Res* 1997;38:795.
72. Colberg SR, Simoneau JA, Thaete FL, et al: Skeletal muscle utilization of free fatty acids in women with visceral obesity [see comments]. *J Clin Invest* 1995;95:1846.
73. Pan DA, Lillioja S, Kriketos AD, et al: Skeletal muscle triglyceride levels are inversely related to insulin action. *Diabetes* 1997;46:983.
74. Phillips DI, Caddy S, Ilic V, et al: Intramuscular triglyceride and muscle insulin sensitivity: evidence for a relationship in nondiabetic subjects. *Metabolism* 1996;45:947.
75. Oakes ND, Cooney GJ, Camilleri S, et al: Mechanisms of liver and muscle insulin resistance induced by chronic high-fat feeding. *Diabetes* 1997;46:1768.
76. Stein DT, Dobbins R, Szczepaniak L, et al: Skeletal muscle triglycerides stores are increased in insulin resistance. *Diabetes* 1997;46(Suppl 1):A206.
77. Randle PJ, Hales CN, Garland PB, et al: The glucose-fatty acid cycle. Its role in insulin insensitivity and the metabolic disturbances of diabetes mellitus. *Lancet* 1963;1:785.
78. Randle PJ, Garland PB, Hales CN, et al: Interactions of metabolism and the physiological role of insulin. *Recent Prog Horm Res* 1966;22:1.
79. Newsholme EA: Carbohydrate metabolism *in vivo*: regulation of the blood glucose level. *Clin Endocrinol Metab* 1976;5:543.
80. Lillioja S, Bogardus C, Mott DM, et al: Relationship between insulin-mediated glucose disposal and lipid metabolism in man. *J Clin Invest* 1985;75:1106.
81. Jenkins AB, Storlien LH, Chisholm DJ, et al: Effects of nonesterified fatty acid availability on tissue-specific glucose utilization in rats *in vivo*. *J Clin Invest* 1988;82:293.

82. Wititsuwannakul D, Kim KH: Mechanism of palmityl coenzyme A inhibition of liver glycogen synthase. *J Biol Chem* 1977;252:7812.

83. Brindley DN: Intracellular translocation of phosphatidate phosphohydrolase and its possible role in the control of glycerolipid synthesis. *Prog Lipid Res* 1984;23:115.

84. Pan DA, Hulbert AJ, Storlien LH: Dietary fats, membrane phospholipids and obesity. *J Nutr* 1994;124:1555.

85. Borkman M, Storlien LH, Pan DA, *et al*: The relation between insulin sensitivity and the fatty-acid composition of skeletal-muscle phospholipids. *N Engl J Med* 1993;328:238.

86. Storlien LH, Kriketos AD, Calvert GD, *et al*: Fatty acids, triglycerides and syndromes of insulin resistance. *Prostaglandins Leukot Essent Fatty Acids* 1997;57:379.

87. Glick BS, Rothman JE: Possible role for fatty acyl-coenzyme A in intracellular protein transport. *Nature* 1987;326:309.

88. Pfanner N, Glick BS, Arden SR, *et al*: Fatty acylation promotes fusion of transport vesicles with Golgi cisternae. *J Cell Biol* 1990;110:955.

89. Pfanner N, Orci L, Glick BS, *et al*: Fatty acyl-coenzyme A is required for budding of transport vesicles from Golgi cisternae. *Cell* 1989;59:95.

90. Rossetti L, Hawkins M, Chen W, *et al*: *In vivo* glucosamine infusion induces insulin resistance in normoglycemic but not in hyperglycemic conscious rats. *J Clin Invest* 1995;96:132.

91. Bjorntorp P: Endocrine abnormalities of obesity. *Metabolism* 1995;44:21.

92. Mohamed-Ali V, Pinkney JH, Coppack SW: Adipose tissue as an endocrine and paracrine organ. *Int J Obes Relat Metab Disord* 1998;22:1145.

93. Zhang Y, Proenca R, Maffei M, *et al*: Positional cloning of the mouse obese gene and its human homologue [published erratum appears in *Nature* 1995;374:479] *Nature* 1994;372:425.

94. Maffei M, Halaas J, Ravussin E, *et al*: Leptin levels in humans and rodents: measurement of plasma leptin and ob RNA in obese and weight-reduced subjects. *Nat Med* 1995;1:1155.

95. Caro JF, Sinha MK, Kolaczynski JW, *et al*: Leptin: the tale of an obesity gene. *Diabetes* 1996;45:1455.

96. Unger RH, Zhou YT, Orci L: Regulation of fatty acid homeostasis in cells: novel role of leptin. *Proc Natl Acad Sci USA* 1999;96:2327.

97. Wang MY, Lee Y, Unger RH: Novel form of lipolysis induced by leptin. *J Biol Chem* 1999;274:17541.

98. Berti L, Gammeltoft S: Leptin stimulates glucose uptake in C2C12 muscle cells by activation of ERK2. *Mol Cell Endocrinol* 1999;157:121.

99. Wang Y, Kuropatwinski KK, White DW, *et al*: Leptin receptor action in hepatic cells. *J Biol Chem* 1997;272:16216.

100. Muller G, Ertl J, Gerl M, *et al*: Leptin impairs metabolic actions of insulin in isolated rat adipocytes. *J Biol Chem* 1997;272:10585.

101. Gavrilova O, Marcus-Samuels B, Leon LR, *et al*: Leptin and diabetes in lipoatrophic mice. *Nature* 2000;403:850.

102. Shimomura I, Hammer RE, Ikemoto S, *et al*: Leptin reverses insulin resistance and diabetes mellitus in mice with congenital lipodystrophy. *Nature* 1999;401:73.

103. Ogawa Y, Masuzaki H, Hosoda K, *et al*: Increased glucose metabolism and insulin sensitivity in transgenic skinny mice overexpressing leptin. *Diabetes* 1999;48:1822.

104. Chinookoswong N, Wang JL, Shi ZQ: Leptin restores euglycemia and normalizes glucose turnover in insulin-deficient diabetes in the rat. *Diabetes* 1999;48:1487.

105. Heymsfield SB, Greenberg AS, Fujioka K, *et al*: Recombinant leptin for weight loss in obese and lean adults: a randomized, controlled, dose-escalation trial [see comments]. *JAMA* 1999;282:1568.

106. Hotamisligil GS, Shargill NS, Spiegelman BM: Adipose expression of tumor necrosis factor-alpha: direct role in obesity-linked insulin resistance. *Science* 1993;259:87.

107. Kern PA, Saghizadeh M, Ong JM, *et al*: The expression of tumor necrosis factor in human adipose tissue. Regulation by obesity, weight loss, and relationship to lipoprotein lipase. *J Clin Invest* 1995;95:2111.

108. Mohamed-Ali V, Goodrick S, Bulmer K, *et al*: Production of soluble tumor necrosis factor receptors by human subcutaneous adipose tissue *in vivo*. *Am J Physiol* 1999;277:E971.

109. Mohamed-Ali V, Goodrick S, Rawesh A, *et al*: Subcutaneous adipose tissue releases interleukin-6, but not tumor necrosis factor-alpha, *in vivo*. *J Clin Endocrinol Metab* 1997;82:4196.

110. Stephens JM, Lee J, Pilch PF: Tumor necrosis factor-alpha-induced insulin resistance in 3T3-L1 adipocytes is accompanied by a loss of insulin receptor substrate-1 and GLUT4 expression without a loss of insulin receptor-mediated signal transduction. *J Biol Chem* 1997;272:971.

111. Guo D, Donner DB: Tumor necrosis factor promotes phosphorylation and binding of insulin receptor substrate 1 to phosphatidylinositol 3-kinase in 3T3-L1 adipocytes. *J Biol Chem* 1996;271:615.

112. Sayeed MM: Alterations in calcium signaling and cellular responses in septic injury. *New Horiz* 1996;4:72.

113. Hotamisligil GS, Arner P, Caro JF, *et al*: Increased adipose tissue expression of tumor necrosis factor-alpha in human obesity and insulin resistance. *J Clin Invest* 1995;95:2409.

114. Purohit A, Ghilchik MW, Duncan L, *et al*: Aromatase activity and interleukin-6 production by normal and malignant breast tissues. *J Clin Endocrinol Metab* 1995;80:3052.

115. Yudkin JS, Kumari M, Humphries SE, *et al*: Inflammation, obesity, stress and coronary heart disease: is interleukin-6 the link? *Atherosclerosis* 1999;148:209.

116. Cianflone K: Acylation stimulating protein and the adipocyte. *J Endocrinol* 1997;155:203.

117. Maslowska M, Sniderman AD, Germinario R, *et al*: ASP stimulates glucose transport in cultured human adipocytes. *Int J Obes Relat Metab Disord* 1997;21:261.

118. Germinario R, Sniderman AD, Manuel S, *et al*: Coordinate regulation of triacylglycerol synthesis and glucose transport by acylation-stimulating protein. *Metabolism* 1993;42:574.

119. Tao Y, Cianflone K, Sniderman AD, *et al*: Acylation-stimulating protein (ASP) regulates glucose transport in the rat L6 muscle cell line. *Biochim Biophys Acta* 1997;1344:221.

120. Pomeroy C, Mitchell J, Eckert E, *et al*: Effect of body weight and caloric restriction on serum complement proteins, including factor D/adipsin: studies in anorexia nervosa and obesity. *Clin Exp Immunol* 1997;108:507.

121. Figueredo A, Ibarra JL, Bagazgoitia J, *et al*: Plasma C3d levels and ischemic heart disease in type II diabetes. *Diabetes Care* 1993;16:445.

122. Ylitalo K, Porkka KV, Meri S, *et al*: Serum complement and familial combined hyperlipidemia [see comments]. *Atherosclerosis* 1997;129:271.

123. Weyer C, Tataranni PA, Pratley RE: Insulin action and insulinemia are closely related to the fasting complement C3, but not acylation stimulating protein concentration. *Diabetes Care* 2000;23:779.

124. Tataranni PA, Ravussin E: Use of dual-energy X-ray absorptiometry in obese individuals. *Am J Clin Nutr* 1995;62:730.

125. Lithell H, Lindgarde F, Hellsing K, *et al*: Body weight, skeletal muscle morphology, and enzyme activities in relation to fasting serum insulin concentration and glucose tolerance in 48-year-old men. *Diabetes* 1981;30:19.

126. Lindgarde F, Eriksson KF, Lithell H, *et al*: Coupling between dietary changes, reduced body weight, muscle fibre size and improved glucose tolerance in middle-aged men with impaired glucose tolerance. *Acta Med Scand* 1982;212:99.

127. Krotkiewski M, Bylund-Fallenius AC, Holm J, *et al*: Relationship between muscle morphology and metabolism in obese women: the effects of long-term physical training. *Eur J Clin Invest* 1983;13:5.

128. Lillioja S, Young AA, Culter CL, *et al*: Skeletal muscle capillary density and fiber type are possible determinants of *in vivo* insulin resistance in man. *J Clin Invest* 1987;80:415.

129. King GL, Johnson SM: Receptor-mediated transport of insulin across endothelial cells. *Science* 1985;227:1583.

130. Prager R, Wallace P, Olefsky JM: *In vivo* kinetics of insulin action on peripheral glucose disposal and hepatic glucose output in normal and obese subjects. *J Clin Invest* 1986;78:472.

131. Doeden B, Rizza R: Use of a variable insulin infusion to assess insulin action in obesity: defects in both the kinetics and amplitude of response. *J Clin Endocrinol Metab* 1987;64:902.

132. McGuire EA, Tobin JD, Berman M, *et al*: Kinetics of native insulin in diabetic, obese, and aged men. *Diabetes* 1979;28:110.

133. McGarry JD, Dobbins RL: Fatty acids, lipotoxicity and insulin secretion. *Diabetologia* 1999;42:128.

134. Stein DT, Esser V, Stevenson BE, *et al*: Essentiality of circulating fatty acids for glucose-stimulated insulin secretion in the fasted rat. *J Clin Invest* 1996;97:2728.

135. Stein DT, Stevenson BE, Chester MW, *et al*: The insulinotropic potency of fatty acids is influenced profoundly by their chain length and degree of saturation. *J Clin Invest* 1997;100:398.

136. Dobbins RL, Chester MW, Daniels MB, *et al*: Circulating fatty acids are essential for efficient glucose-stimulated insulin secretion after prolonged fasting in humans. *Diabetes* 1998;47:1613.

137. Liu YQ, Tornheim K, Leahy JL: Fatty acid-induced beta cell hypersensitivity to glucose. Increased phosphofructokinase activity and lowered glucose-6-phosphate content. *J Clin Invest* 1998;101:1870.

138. Bollheimer LC, Skelly RH, Chester MW, *et al*: Chronic exposure to free fatty acid reduces pancreatic beta cell insulin content by increasing basal insulin secretion that is not compensated for by a corresponding increase in proinsulin biosynthesis translation. *J Clin Invest* 1998;101:1094.

139. Paolisso G, Gambardella A, Amato L, *et al*: Opposite effects of short- and long-term fatty acid infusion on insulin secretion in healthy subjects. *Diabetologia* 1995;38:1295.

140. Tataranni PA, Baier LJ, Paolisso G, *et al*: Role of lipids in development of noninsulin-dependent diabetes mellitus: lessons learned from Pima Indians. *Lipids* 1996;31(Suppl):S267.

141. Paolisso G, Tataranni PA, Foley JE, *et al*: A high concentration of fasting plasma non-esterified fatty acids is a risk factor for the development of NIDDM. *Diabetologia* 1995;38:1213.

142. Shimabukuro M, Ohneda M, Lee Y, *et al*: Role of nitric oxide in obesity-induced beta cell disease. *J Clin Invest* 1997;100:290.

143. Shimabukuro M, Koyama K, Lee Y, *et al*: Leptin- or troglitazone-induced lipopenia protects islets from interleukin 1beta cytotoxicity. *J Clin Invest* 1997;100:1750.

144. Shimabukuro M, Zhou YT, Levi M, *et al*: Fatty acid-induced beta cell apoptosis: a link between obesity and diabetes. *Proc Natl Acad Sci USA* 1998;95:2498.

145. Rohner-Jeanrenaud F, Jeanrenaud B: A role for the vagus nerve in the etiology and maintenance of the hyperinsulinemia of genetically obese fa/fa rats. *Int J Obes* 1985;9(Suppl 1):71.

146. Penicaud L, Rohner-Jeanrenaud F, Jeanrenaud B. *In vivo* metabolic changes as studied longitudinally after ventromedial hypothalamic lesions. *Am J Physiol* 1986;250:E662.

147. Rohner-Jeanrenaud F, Jeanrenaud B: Involvement of the cholinergic system in insulin and glucagon oversecretion of genetic preobesity. *Endocrinology* 1985;116:830.

148. Inoue S, Mullen YS, Bray GA: Hyperinsulinemia in rats with hypothalamic obesity: effects of autonomic drugs and glucose. *Am J Physiol* 1983;245:R372.

149. Rohner-Jeanrenaud F, Ionescu E, Jeanrenaud B: The origins and role of efferent vagal nuclei in hyperinsulinemia in hypothalamic and genetically obese rodents. *J Auton Nerv Syst* 1983;9:173.

150. Berthoud HR, Jeanrenaud B: Acute hyperinsulinemia and its reversal by vagotomy after lesions of the ventromedial hypothalamus in anesthetized rats. *Endocrinology* 1979;105:146.

151. Tokunaga K, Fukushima M, Kemnitz JW, *et al*: Effect of vagotomy on serum insulin in rats with paraventricular or ventromedial hypothalamic lesions. *Endocrinology* 1986;119:1708.

152. Inoue S, Bray GA: The effects of subdiaphragmatic vagotomy in rats with ventromedial hypothalamic obesity. *Endocrinology* 1977;100:108.

153. Inoue S, Bray GA, Mullen YS: Transplantation of pancreatic beta-cells prevents development of hypothalamic obesity in rats. *Am J Physiol* 1978;235:E266.

154. Ravussin E, Tataranni PA: The role of altered sympathetic nervous system activity in the pathogenesis of obesity. *Proc Nutr Soc* 1996;55:793.

155. Ahren B: Autonomic regulation of islet hormone secretion—implications for health and disease. *Diabetologia* 2000;43:393.

156. Spraul M, Ravussin E, Fontvieille AM, *et al*: Reduced sympathetic nervous activity. A potential mechanism predisposing to body weight gain. *J Clin Invest* 1993;92:1730.

157. Schwartz RS, Jaeger LF, Veith RC: Effect of clonidine on the thermic effect of feeding in humans. *Am J Physiol* 1988;254:R90.

158. Christin L, O'Connell M, Bogardus C, *et al*: Norepinephrine turnover and energy expenditure in Pima Indian and white men. *Metabolism* 1993;42:723.

159. Snitker S, Tataranni PA, Ravussin E: Respiratory quotient is inversely associated with muscle sympathetic nerve activity. *J Clin Endocrinol Metab* 1998;83:3977.

160. Astrup A, Buemann B, Gluud C, *et al*: Prognostic markers for diet-induced weight loss in obese women. *Int J Obes Relat Metab Disord* 1995;19:275.

161. Tataranni PA, Young JB, Bogardus C, *et al*: A low sympathoadrenal activity is associated with body weight gain and development of central adiposity in Pima Indian men. *Obes Res* 1997;5:341.

162. Ahren B, Taborsky GJJ, Porte DJ: Neuropeptidergic versus cholinergic and adrenergic regulation of islet hormone secretion. *Diabetologia* 1986;29:827.

163. Berthoud HR, Bereiter DA, Trimble ER, *et al*: Cephalic phase, reflex insulin secretion. Neuroanatomical and physiological characterization. *Diabetologia* 1981;20(Suppl):393.

164. Tomita T, Greeley GJ, Watt L, *et al*: Protein meal-stimulated pancreatic polypeptide secretion in Prader-Willi syndrome of adults. *Pancreas* 1989;4:395.

165. Weyer C, Salbe A, Lindsay R, *et al*: Exaggerated pancreatic polypeptide secretion in Pima Indians: can an increased parasympathetic drive to the pancreas contribute to hyperinsulinemia and diabetes in humans? *Metabolism* 2001;50:223.

166. Lillioja S, Nyomba BL, Saad MF, *et al*: Exaggerated early insulin release and insulin resistance in a diabetes-prone population: a metabolic comparison of Pima Indians and Caucasians. *J Clin Endocrinol Metab* 1991;73:866.

167. Weyer C, Hanson R, Tataranni PA, *et al*: A high fasting insulin concentration predicts type 2 diabetes independent of insulin resistance: evidence for a pathogenic role of "relative" hyperinsulinemia. *Diabetes* 2000;49:2094.

168. Serdula MK, Ivery D, Coates RJ, *et al*: Do obese children become obese adults? A review of the literature. *Prev Med* 1993;22:167.

169. McCance DR, Pettitt DJ, Hanson RL, *et al*: Glucose, insulin concentrations and obesity in childhood and adolescence as predictors of NIDDM. *Diabetologia* 1994;37:617.

170. Dietz WH: Critical periods in childhood for the development of obesity. *Am J Clin Nutr* 1994;59:955.

171. Stunkard AJ, Berkowitz RI, Stallings VA, *et al*: Energy intake, not energy output, is a determinant of body size in infants [see comments]. *Am J Clin Nutr* 1999;69:524.

172. Griffiths M, Payne PR, Stunkard AJ, *et al*: Metabolic rate and physical development in children at risk of obesity. *Lancet* 1990;336:76.

173. Roberts SB, Savage J, Coward WA, *et al*: Energy expenditure and intake in infants born to lean and overweight mothers. *N Engl J Med* 1988;318:461.

174. Goran MI, Gower BA, Nagy TR, *et al*: Developmental changes in energy expenditure and physical activity in children: evidence for a decline in physical activity in girls before puberty. *Pediatrics* 1998;101:887.

175. Goran MI, Shewchuk R, Gower BA, *et al*: Longitudinal changes in fatness in white children: no effect of childhood energy expenditure [see comments]. *Am J Clin Nutr* 1998;67:309.

176. Goran MI, Hunter G, Nagy TR, *et al*: Physical activity related energy expenditure and fat mass in young children. *Int J Obes Relat Metab Disord* 1997;21:171.

177. Johnson MS, Figueroa-Colon R, Herd S, *et al*: Does fitness or energy expenditure predict increasing adiposity in African-American and Caucasian children? *Pediatrics* 2000;106:E50.

178. Robinson TN: Reducing children's television viewing to prevent obesity: a randomized controlled trial. *JAMA* 1999;282:1561.

179. Salbe AD, Weyer C, Fontvielle AM, *et al*: Low levels of physical activity and time spent viewing television at 9 years of age predict weight gain 8 years later in Pima Indian children. *Int J Obes* 1998;22(Suppl 4):S10.

180. Anonymous: Type 2 diabetes in children and adolescents. American Diabetes Association. *Pediatrics* 2000;105(3 Pt 1):671.

181. Fagot-Campagna A, Pettitt DJ, Engelgau MM, *et al*: Type 2 diabetes among North American children and adolescents: An epidemiologic review and a public health perspective. *J Pediatr* 2000;136:664.

182. Dabelea D, Hanson RL, Bennett PH, *et al*: Increasing prevalence of type II diabetes in American Indian children. *Diabetologia* 1998;41:904.

183. Dabelea D, Knowler WC, Pettitt DJ: Effect of diabetes in pregnancy on offspring: follow-up research in the Pima Indians. *J Matern Fetal Med* 2000;9:83.

CHAPTER 24

Aging and Diabetes

Robert V. Hogikyan

Jeffrey B. Halter

CLASSIFICATION AND DEFINITION

The American Diabetes Association (ADA) criteria for diabetes and impaired glucose tolerance, provided in Chap. 8, are currently applied to adults of any age, despite the fact that glucose tolerance is known to deteriorate with age. However, as discussed later in this chapter, the increased likelihood of intercurrent illness and medication use in an older adult needs to be taken into account when interpreting any serum glucose level in an older person.

Older persons with diabetes are a heterogeneous group. While 90% have type 2 diabetes mellitus (T2DM), these individuals may vary from lean to obese, from good general health to having multiple comorbid conditions, and from being fully functional to having major functional disabilities. They may be treated with diet, oral hypoglycemic agents, insulin, or a combination of these approaches. Some older adults may initially appear to have typical T2DM and have significant residual β-cell function at the time of diagnosis, but then progress with time to insulin dependency. This progression may take months to years before an insulin-deficient state develops. Rarely, an older person may present with classical autoimmune type 1 diabetes. Others with type 1 diabetes mellitus (T1DM) survive until old age and become part of the heterogeneous population of elderly diabetic patients. This heterogeneity must be taken into account when deciding about treatment goals and interventions for a given elderly patient.

EPIDEMIOLOGY

Diabetes mellitus is a very common health problem among older adults. Nearly half of all patients with T2DM are aged 65 years or older.[1,2] The proportion of the U.S. population meeting current ADA criteria increases dramatically with advancing age through at least the mid-70s (Fig. 24-1), but many are undiagnosed.[3] Some older diabetes patients are first identified by screening fasting plasma glucose (FPG) levels. Oral glucose tolerance tests (OGTTs) identify others who do not have elevated FPG but meet the diabetes criterion of a 2-hour OGTT glucose level ≥200 mg/dL, a situation known as isolated postchallenge hyperglycemia (IPH). IPH increases dramatically with advancing age[1–3] and has raised problems due to the recent focus on use of fasting glucose levels to make the diagnosis. The overall total prevalence of diabetes in people aged 60–74 years is 26%, a rate ten times greater than that seen in people under age 40.[1] The high prevalence rate of diabetes persists in populations 70 years of age and older. In addition to the high prevalence of diabetes in older adults, 14% of the U.S. population over age 60 meet the ADA criteria for impaired fasting glucose (IFG) and 20% meet the criteria for impaired glucose tolerance (IGT). Ethnic differences in rates of diabetes appear to apply to elderly populations as well, with higher rates in older Hispanic and African-American adults than in Caucasians.[4]

While identifying individuals with diabetes in order to initiate treatment early is clearly a priority, to be able to protect individuals from developing diabetes could also be worthwhile. Total expenditure of energy during leisure time appears to protect against the development of type 2 diabetes independent of age, obesity, history of hypertension, or parental history of diabetes.[5,6] This protective effect was not limited to intensive exercise, which may be less sustainable into older age. Recent findings indicate that lifestyle intervention including diet and exercise can delay progression from IGT to diabetes in middle-aged and older adults.[7]

Given that people over age 85 are the fastest growing segment of the population, there is significant growth expected in the population living in institutional long-term care settings. Those living in an institutional long-term care setting may carry a diagnosis of diabetes, and there may be special considerations in the treatment of diabetes in this population. However, the epidemiology of diabetes in this population has not been adequately studied.

Older adults with T2DM are at increased risk for all of the long-term diabetes complications,[8] as summarized in Table 24-1. Observational studies suggest that poor glycemic control in older people with diabetes contributes to excessive risk of stroke and cardiovascular events.[9,10] Atherosclerotic macrovascular disease accounts for 75% of the mortality among people with diabetes in the U.S.[11] Increased risk for cardiovascular disease is also associated with IGT, in the absence of overt diabetes.[12,13] Diabetes is the major cause of renal failure and dialysis in people over 65 in the U.S.[14] The risks of end-stage renal disease, loss of vision, myocardial infarction, stroke, and peripheral vascular disease increase with age in the absence of diabetes, but these risks in elderly patients with diabetes are even greater (Table 24-1). Because diabetes complications are generally viewed as long term, it could be argued that such complications are not of concern in someone who is already very old. However, even a new diagnosis of diabetes in an older person may be preceded by an unknown period of undetected hyperglycemia. In addition, the average remaining life expectancy for a 65-year-old person is nearly 20 years, and for a 75-year-old person over 10 years.[15]

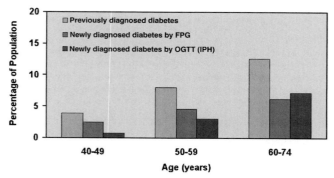

FIGURE 24-1. Prevalence of type 2 diabetes among elderly people according to age and ADA diagnostic criteria (NHANES III). FPG, fasting plasma glucose; OGTT, oral glucose tolerance test; IPH, isolated postchallenge hyperglycemia. *(Adapted from Harris* et al[1] *and Resnick* et al.[2])

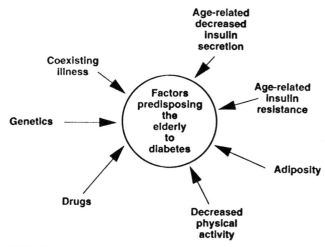

FIGURE 24-2. A summary of factors that may contribute to the high rate of diabetes mellitus and impaired glucose tolerance among older adults. *(Reproduced with permission from* Diabetes Update: Elderly Patients with Non-Insulin Dependent Diabetes Mellitus. *The Upjohn Company, 1990.)*

Diabetic retinopathy is a major cause of visual loss in older adults, and even if it does not lead to blindness is associated with disability and depression.[16,17] Peripheral neuropathy, due both to micro- and macrovascular disease, and peripheral vascular disease are particularly prevalent in older age groups. Amputations increase with age, as do balance problems, mobility impairment, and chronic pain related to diabetic nerve disorders.[18] Diabetic neuropathy is common in this population, but the epidemiology is not yet sufficiently defined to establish the degree of increased risk.

MECHANISMS FOR AGE-RELATED CHANGES OF CARBOHYDRATE METABOLISM

Studies of the effects of aging on carbohydrate metabolism have been reviewed.[19] A major challenge to the interpretation of age-related differences in measures of glucose metabolism is that glucose metabolism is sensitive to a wide range of factors. Thus it may be very difficult to specifically define effects of aging that are independent of other factors. As summarized in Fig. 24-2, it is likely that there are primary changes in pancreatic β-cell function and possibly changes in insulin action with aging that contribute to age-related changes in glucose metabolism. It is also likely that there are specific genetic factors that may influence the expression of glucose intolerance with aging, although such genetic factors have yet to be defined. Several studies have attempted to control for the other variables that may affect glucose metabolism in studies of human aging. Although there are exceptions, these studies suggest

TABLE 24-1. Important Long-Term Complications of Diabetes in Older Adults and Their Relative Risk*

Complication	Relative Risk
Macrovascular disease	
Coronary heart disease	2
Stroke	2
Amputation	10
Capillary microangiopathy	
Retinopathy/macular edema	1.4†
Renal disease	2
Neuropathy	?

*Risk compared to people of the same age who do not have diabetes (see reference 8).

†Relative risk for blindness.

that there is a gradual decline in glucose tolerance with age, both in healthy men and women, but that this age effect is relatively modest in magnitude. Glucose intolerance occurs in older people accompanied by delayed absorption of oral glucose and delayed posthepatic glucose delivery. Greater hyperglycemia in older people results from delayed suppression of hepatic glucose output and a decreased rate of peripheral glucose uptake following oral glucose ingestion.[20]

Many studies have been carried out to assess the effects of aging on insulin secretion in experimental animals and in humans. A delayed insulin response during an OGTT has been observed in some studies. OGTT and hyperglycemic glucose clamp studies suggest that gross impairment of pancreatic β-cell function is not characteristic of normal human aging.[19,21] However, clear age-related pancreatic β-cell functional deficits have been demonstrated in pulsatile insulin secretion[22] and with quantitation of the potentiating effect of glucose on insulin secretory responses to a nonglucose stimulus such as the amino acid arginine.[19,23]

A problem in the interpretation of studies of pancreatic β-cell function in aging is the confounding effect of coexistent obesity and insulin resistance in elderly people. As described below, a number of studies have provided evidence for the presence of insulin resistance in elderly humans.[19] The normal physiologic feedback control mechanism for regulation of glucose homeostasis should result in hyperinsulinemia to compensate for the presence of insulin resistance if pancreatic β-cell function is completely normal. Thus the finding of similar pancreatic β-cell responses to glucose challenge in old and young subjects may in fact represent a relative impairment in β-cell function among the older subjects if they are also insulin resistant. When the confounding effects of obesity, insulin resistance, and age-related declines in insulin clearance have been taken into account, diminished pancreatic β-cell function is observed in older humans.[23–26]

Many studies have demonstrated resistance to the metabolic effects of insulin in aging animals and humans (see reference 19 for review). Age-related deficits in postreceptor insulin signaling have been observed in fat, muscle, and liver. Increased adiposity is one factor that contributes to age-related alterations in insulin action. Several studies of age group differences in humans have attempted to control for the influence of adiposity by including a large sample size and multiple measurements of various aspects of body fat mass and distribution. Although all of these studies are not in full agreement, overall they suggest that there is a persistent effect of age on both glucose tolerance and insulin action that is independent of body fat mass and distribution in humans.[27–29] However, there is heterogeneity among the elderly population. Older people who have been selected to meet criteria for normal glucose tolerance are less obese with less central adiposity, and did not have a detectable decrease of insulin sensitivity[30,31] independent of obesity.

Aging-associated decreased mobility and diminished physical activity may also contribute to age-related changes in glucose homeostasis. Healthy older men with greater degrees of physical fitness, usually as assessed by measurement of maximal oxygen uptake during exercise, have better glucose tolerance and less evidence of insulin resistance than less active older adults.[19,28] More physically fit elderly people also tend to have less body fat and less central adiposity. While some glucose intolerance appears to persist with age even when controlling for these factors, the age-related change is modest.

A significant improvement in insulin action has been demonstrated in older adults following exercise training.[32–34] The reduction of insulin resistance accompanying exercise training under these circumstances is associated with diminished pancreatic β-cell responses to stimulation,[32] as would be expected from the physiology of the feedback control system affecting glucose and insulin. This compensation may explain why the improvement of insulin action associated with exercise training has generally not affected overall glucose tolerance.

Some groups of people with essential hypertension have associated insulin resistance and glucose intolerance.[35] Given the high prevalence of hypertension among the elderly population, blood pressure may be an important variable when trying to understand age-related glucose intolerance. However, the degree of association between insulin resistance or hyperinsulinemia and hypertension has varied considerably in different studies, perhaps related to the degree of obesity and the pathophysiology of hypertension in the populations.[36,37] In the predominantly Caucasian population of the Baltimore Longitudinal Study of Aging, little if any relationship between hyperinsulinemia and blood pressure was found after adjusting for other variables.[38]

A number of pharmacologic agents in common use have known effects on glucose metabolism. Since older adults are frequent users of pharmacologic agents, interpretation of alterations of glucose metabolism in such individuals must take into account drugs that they are using. Table 24-2 includes a list of some of the drugs that are known to affect glucose metabolism. Because of the association of hypertension with insulin resistance and glucose intolerance as described previously, effects of antihypertensive agents on glucose metabolism have been of particular interest. Though none of the drug effects on glucose metabolism seem to be of large magnitude, a variety of adverse effects have been documented.[39]

INITIAL PRESENTATION OF THE OLDER PATIENT WITH DIABETES

Type 2 diabetes is frequently asymptomatic in older adults. When signs or symptoms are present, they may be difficult to interpret in

TABLE 24-2. Drugs That May Contribute to Hyperglycemia

Antihypertensives
  Diuretics
  β-Adrenergic blockers
  α$_2$-Agonists
  ? Calcium channel blockers
Antinflammatory agents
  Glucocorticoids
  NSAIDS (nonsteroid anti-inflammatory drugs)
Others
  Estrogen and progesterone
  Phenytoin
  Pentamidine
  Nicotinic acid

older people. The atypical presenting symptom or sign may be misinterpreted as the consequence of an illness other than diabetes, or may be fully attributed to a condition other than diabetes, when in fact diabetes is in part responsible for the sign or symptom. One such presenting sign may be unexplained weight loss. While a number of etiologies such as malignancy need to be considered, substantial weight loss can occur in an older person with marginal oral intake in the setting of poorly controlled diabetes. Other atypical symptoms in an older person with poorly controlled hyperglycemia include generalized weakness or malaise, anorexia, and confusion.

With the expanded use of blood chemistry screening, the presence of hyperglycemia is readily established. More challenging is the interpretation of an elevated random serum glucose in an older person. One example is the acutely ill hospitalized older person who is physiologically stressed. Known interactions between stress hormones, insulin secretion, and insulin sensitivity will acutely elevate the serum glucose, which may return to a normal range upon resolution of the acute stress.[40] As summarized in Table 24-2, medication use may also complicate the interpretation of hyperglycemia in an older person, as there is an increased likelihood of use of multiple medications.

Urinary incontinence may be confused with hyperglycemia-related polyuria. The insensate neuropathic bladder with overflow incontinence may be a sign indicating diabetes presenting as neuropathy. Urinary frequency may be attributed to prostatic hypertrophy, urinary tract infection, or diuretic therapy, when in fact these problems are only contributing causes and hyperglycemia is a major problem for the patient.

Since thirst perception may be altered in older people, polydipsia may not occur in response to the increase of osmolality associated with hyperglycemia. Even when thirst is appreciated by the patient, access to water or other fluids may be limited, especially for the older patient with functional dependence on others. Intravascular fluid depletion and orthostatic hypotension may result, and the patient may present with a history of falling or hyperosmolar coma.

COMPREHENSIVE ASSESSMENT OF THE OLDER ADULT WITH DIABETES

Medical care of a geriatric patient should begin with a comprehensive geriatric assessment. A comprehensive geriatric assessment is a multidisciplinary evaluation in which the multiple problems of older persons are uncovered, described, and explained, if possible, and in which the resources and strengths of the person are catalogued, need for services assessed, and a coordinated care plan developed.[41] In this section, consideration will be given to some of the physical, mental, social, economic, functional, and environmental domains requiring special attention.[41]

Functional Status

The functional assessment of geriatric patients is a critical component of a comprehensive geriatric assessment, and is recommended for all older patients.[42] Older adults with diabetes are about two to three times more likely to have physical limitations[43] and 1.5 times more likely to have decrements in activities of daily living (ADL) than those without. Much of this excess disability is a direct result of complications of diabetes, such as eye disease, increased strokes and cardiovascular disease, and increased neuropathy and peripheral vascular disease.[43] The assessment of functional status can begin prior to the physician-patient encounter with a self- or family-completed questionnaire. ADL can be further assessed during the history and physical examination. It is important that the patient's family or caregiver assist in completing this assessment.

Cognitive Function

The older patient with diabetes, like all patients with diabetes, will need to maintain control over a variety of aspects of day-to-day life that may affect glucose regulation. Maintaining a proper diet, medication administration, and skin care, for example, require cognitive skills and reliable memory function. A number of age-related deficits in cognition and memory function have been identified, but there is a great deal of variability in how an individual's memory and cognition may change. Older individuals will perform tasks requiring retrieval of newly-learned material from secondary memory less well than younger individuals. Older persons will also perform less well when the process requires carrying out two tasks concurrently. However, these changes have little effect on ADL.

When compared with age-matched controls, older subjects with T2DM who do not have evidence of a coexisting cognitive disorder perform more slowly and less well on complex tasks.[44] No differences were observed between type 2 diabetics and controls in the areas of basic attentional processes, short-term memory, and semantic memory.[45] However, these deficits are relatively minor in older people who do not have central nervous system (CNS) pathology. Of much greater potential impact in an older person with diabetes is coexistence of a major cognitive disorder. The prevalence rate of cerebrovascular disease is high in the diabetic older population. Alzheimer's disease is common and may coexist, although it is uncertain whether the prevalence is higher or lower in people with diabetes.[44,46] Therefore cognition and memory function need evaluation in the comprehensive assessment of an older patient with diabetes. The possible presence of deficits in the performance of complex tasks, speed and memory tasks, serial learning tasks, and primary CNS pathology need to be assessed. Speed of processing and memory function may have implications for activities such as driving, where a problem may not otherwise be brought to light until there is an accident. There are a number of good screening instruments which have been shown to be valid and reproducible in older adults.[47] These can be administered quickly and highlight deficits. When the deficits are less clear, the performance of more complete neuropsychological testing may be indicated.

Psychosocial Situation

With the growing complexity of our day-to-day lives, there may be less availability of the extended family, putting many elderly people with diabetes at risk for psychosocial difficulties. The older individual's health can affect their self-esteem, recreational activities, social contacts, and family relationships, including contact with younger family members. Since the older patient with diabetes and no informal system of support may be at high risk for functional decline, delivering quality care can be a substantial challenge. When health care is compromised by the home situation, entry into an assisted living situation or other institutionalization must be considered.

Diet Maintenance and Access to Food

One of the cornerstones of working with a patient with diabetes is assuring that the patient maintains a proper diet. Specific recommendations with regard to nutrition and diet for patients with diabetes are presented in Chap. 26. In the older patient with diabetes there are some areas of special concern which need to be considered, as summarized in Table 24-3. Nutritional needs of elderly patients may differ due to a number of factors. Physiologic alterations include a decrease in energy needs due to decreased activity. Some may experience declining health status, including increased prevalence of chronic disease with poor nutrition, depression, dementia, medication-induced anorexia, or feeding dependency. In addition, some may be socially isolated, possibly due to the loss of a spouse, and find eating alone a problem.

Although there is little research in the area, no specific modifications in the diet currently recommended by the ADA are suggested for older adults with diabetes. Functional ability and financial considerations are important areas that need assessment in the older patient with diabetes. In those patients with reduced food access, a network of formal and/or informal support services may be available to assist them and needs to be explored. For those community-dwelling older adults with diabetes and limited access to food, home delivered meals may enhance the likelihood of following a diabetic diet and reduce "food insecurity" (concern about obtaining and preparing food), as well as decrease the frequency of being hospitalized for hyper- or hypoglycemia.[48] A program of home delivered meals is available in many communities and should be considered a valuable resource. This problem of access to proper diet may exist among residents of long-term care facilities. Thus residents who are dependent on staff for feeding are at significant risk for inadequate dietary intake.

TABLE 24-3. Dietary Therapy: Special Considerations for Older Adults with Diabetes

Access to food
  Functional disability
    Poor meal preparation skills
    Lack of formal and/or informal support to obtain food
  Limited financial resources
Food intake
  Decline in taste and smell appreciation
  Poor dentition and/or xerostomia
Ingrained dietary habits
  Past experience and ethnic food preferences
Impaired cognitive function

Assuming food is available, intake may be reduced because of an age-associated decrease in the ability to appreciate taste and smell. To the extent that taste influences dietary intake, decreased taste may be a contributor to the decreased caloric intake which has been reported among older humans. A decline in physical activity, particularly common among older people with diabetes,[49,50] may also play a role in this decreased caloric intake.

In the institutional long-term care setting, inappropriate or absent dietary prescriptions are sometimes found.[51] Particularly in an institutional long-term care setting, weight maintenance as a goal of therapy may be more important for older patients than weight reduction, since low body weight and undernutrition may be more prevalent than obesity in this setting. A careful nutritional assessment on a regular basis of the institutionalized older adult with diabetes is very important in guiding the dietary prescription.

Adequacy of food intake may also be affected by oral health problems in older patients. Tooth loss is common in the older adult population, and severe tooth loss limits the foods that are considered acceptable. Thus for geriatric patients with diabetes who may already be struggling to identify foods that meet their dietary needs, tooth loss may further limit their choices. Another concern of many older patients with diabetes is dry mouth. It is not clear if diabetes *per se* increases the likelihood of xerostomia, but xerostomia is common in this population and associated with use of multiple medications.

Vision Problems Including Cataracts and Retinopathy

For the older patient with diabetes who may already have functional deficits, loss of sight may be devastating. Thus proliferative retinopathy with possible hemorrhage into the vitreous or macular edema are manifestations with potentially disastrous results. Many older people with diabetes do not comply with the ADA recommendation that patients with diabetes have a yearly dilated ophthalmoscopic examination.[52] Some of the responsibility for not having annual examinations rests with health care providers who fail to refer patients for examination. The percentage of patients who do not undergo annual dilated examinations may be even higher among institutionalized elderly people with diabetes.

Cataracts, macular degeneration, and glaucoma also place the older patient with diabetes at increased risk of blindness. Cataracts are the most common age-related ocular disorder, and subjects with diabetes have a higher rate than those without diabetes. Performance of regular ophthalmologic examinations in the older patient with diabetes, given the potential for other functional deficits, is at least as important as in a younger patient with diabetes.

Urinary Continence

Urinary incontinence is common both among community-dwelling elderly people (10–43%) and among those living in institutional long-term care settings (36–62%).[53] Changes in bladder function are very common in patients with diabetes and are characterized by some as "diabetic cystopathy." The noteworthy clinical feature of bladder involvement in diabetes is the insidious onset and progression of bladder paresis, eventually leading to retention. Urinary retention with overflow incontinence represents one of the major causes of urinary incontinence in geriatric patients.

In one study in an institutional long-term care setting, involuntary bladder contractions were the presumed contributor to urinary incontinence among 61% of the older patients with diabetes. All patients with urinary retention had poor or no bladder contractions.[53] While diabetic cystopathy is one factor contributing to urinary incontinence in this population, older patients with diabetes are at risk for the other common causes of urinary incontinence: detrusor overactivity, outlet incompetence, outlet obstruction, and detrusor underactivity. In the patient who is functionally dependent on others for assistance in transferring from bed to wheelchair or wheelchair to toilet, urinary incontinence may be termed environmental when the necessary assistance is not available. The evaluation of an older adult with diabetes for urinary incontinence should follow guidelines for the evaluation of any older adult with urinary incontinence.[54] These guidelines differ for community-dwelling elderly as compared with those living in an institutional long-term care setting.

Sexual Function and Dysfunction

Sexual activity can persist well into older adulthood, although there is a general decrease with age. In a survey of 225 elderly male veterans in a geriatric ambulatory care clinic 47% of those aged >75 years reported absent libido.[55] Overall this study found sexual dysfunction to be related to subjective poor health, diabetes, and incontinence. At present little information is available about sexual function in older women with diabetes.

By virtue of age, older men and women are at risk for social factors contributing to decreased sexuality. Three social factors contribute to whether an older patient remains sexually active. First, a patient must feel the desire to do so; second, they must have access to a sexually functional partner; and third, they must have access to an environment with privacy. Chronic diseases, simple demographics, and living with children or in an institutional long-term care setting contribute to these social factors.

Polypharmacy and Drug Interactions

The older patient with diabetes is likely to have a number of other chronic medical conditions which are treated with medications. The number of medications prescribed for older patients increases with increasing age, both in inpatient and outpatient settings. One of the major concerns with the increased number of prescriptions per patient is the risk of adverse drug reactions, since the percentage of patients with adverse drug reactions increases exponentially with the number of medications taken. Elderly patients with diabetes are at increased risk for adverse drug reactions for a variety of reasons: age-related alterations of pharmacokinetics and in some cases pharmacodynamics; decreased vision and cognition; peripheral diabetic neuropathy and coexisting arthritis making childproof lids unusable; and as mentioned above, the greater likelihood that elderly patients are taking multiple medications. Effective methods for reducing polypharmacy and improving prescription of medications have been demonstrated in both the outpatient and institutional long-term care settings,[56,57] and explicit criteria have been developed to identify inappropriate medication use in the institutional long-term care setting.[58]

APPROACHES TO THERAPY

The comprehensive geriatric assessment should provide the information needed to decide upon a therapeutic approach to the older patient with diabetes. Such information includes current general health, remaining life expectancy, motivation and commitment of the patient and family, finances, and support services. All of these factors can have a significant impact on the treatment approach.

Management of Atherosclerotic Risks and Complications

Reduction in risk factors for atherosclerotic disease is a major goal of diabetes management in older adults. A high proportion of older diabetes patients have associated hypertension, hyperlipidemia, and atherosclerotic arterial disease.[59–62] Although fewer older people smoke cigarettes, smoking cessation programs should be encouraged for those who do. Older diabetes patients have been shown to benefit as much or more than nondiabetes patients from hypertension treatment.[63,64] Aspirin use is beneficial in older patients with diabetes and atherosclerosis risk or atherosclerosis.[65] Treatment of hyperlipidemia in diabetes patients with cardiovascular disease has been shown to be beneficial and may decrease mortality in those who may develop cardiovascular disease; no age limit has been defined, although there are limited data available for people over age 75. Peripheral vascular occlusive disease and amputations increase with age, so monitoring and evaluation for circulatory problems is indicated. Preventative treatment and monitoring for complications is not just for those older patients who are seriously ill or have advanced dementia. Most older people, even those with comorbidities and disability, will benefit from interventions shown to prevent or slow an increasing burden of illness over a period of several years.

Management of Microvascular Risks and Complications

Treatment with an ACE inhibitor and aggressive management of hypertension and hyperglycemia are the major recommended interventions for preventing end-stage renal disease due to diabetes.[14] These interventions are appropriate for the majority of older diabetes patients. Peripheral neuropathy leading to pain, neuropathic joints, wounds, mobility problems, and amputations contribute to disability and poor quality of life in older patients. The little evidence that is available suggests that foot care and monitoring may be associated with better outcomes.

Yearly retinal examinations and intervention as appropriate are recommended for older people with diabetes. Although simulations have suggested that few older persons with late-onset diabetes are likely to go blind due to diabetes,[66] it is important to remember that most older people do not have late-onset diabetes; many have had diabetes for 10 years or more and the true duration of diabetes is not known for many others.

Treatment of Hyperglycemia

There are two general approaches to treatment of hyperglycemia in this group of patients: basic care and intensive care. When the goal is primarily the prevention of symptoms of hyperglycemia, a basic care approach is sufficient. The alternative is intensive care when treatment is aimed at achieving ADA guidelines for glucose levels as close to euglycemia as possible with the goal of preventing the long-term complications of diabetes. Unfortunately, as in other patient groups, only a minority of older people with diabetes achieve recommended goals for treatment of hyperglycemia,[3,67,68] as illustrated in Fig. 24-3. Nonpharmacologic treatment, oral hypoglycemic agents, and insulin therapy can each play a role in the

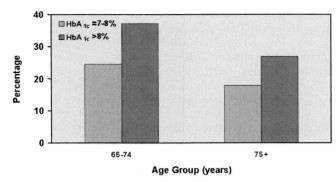

FIGURE 24-3. Percentage of patients in NHANES III who did not achieve the level of hemoglobin A_{1c} (HbA_{1c}) recommended by the American Diabetes Association ($HbA_{1c} < 7\%$). Patients were analyzed by age group and according to whether their HbA_{1c} was in the range at which the ADA recommends therapeutic action ($>8\%$) or not ($7–8\%$). *(Adapted from Shorr RI, et al., 2000[67]).*

management of the older adult with diabetes, whether the treatment goal is control of symptoms of hyperglycemia or achievement of euglycemia.

The prevention of symptomatic hyperglycemia by delivering basic care includes the prevention of glycosuria and associated intravascular volume depletion. Glycosuria may result in urinary incontinence, and intravascular depletion may result in hyperglycemic hyperosmolar nonketotic coma, the most severe acute complication of diabetes in an older adult. Glycosuria may also result in weight loss due to calorie loss in the urine. The resultant catabolic state can lead to excess protein breakdown and the loss of lean body tissue. The goal of prevention of symptoms of hyperglycemia can be accomplished and glycosuria minimized by maintaining a serum glucose averaging about 200 mg/dL.

The decision about goals of treatment in the older adult with diabetes is critical to planning the management of hyperglycemia in an individual patient. This decision may be made with the patient alone. However, when comprehensive geriatric assessment indicates that the patient may need assistance, others may need to be involved in the decisionmaking process. A primary caregiver or other responsible party along with consultants may be needed to clarify the patient's condition.

Education

Education is an important component in the management of an older patient with diabetes. Short-term diabetes education program sessions can increase patient knowledge, reduce stress, improve diet, and enhance quality of life. When a spouse is involved there is greater improvement in knowledge, less patient stress and better glycemic control.[69] The Colorado Diabetes Control Program was able to document an improved level of patient care and a significantly reduced length of hospital stay for patients with diabetes who were admitted to an acute care hospital following a 2-year educational intervention. Care of the older adult with diabetes in an institutional long-term care setting can be made easier and may be more effective with an educational intervention aimed at the patient care staff.

Diet

Dietary therapy is a basic building block of therapy for the older adult with diabetes. There is no evidence to suggest that dietary therapy is more or less effective in older adults with diabetes than younger ones. Dietary restriction and weight loss should help the older adult with diabetes achieve better control of the hyperglycemia, but caution is indicated. If functional restrictions prevent the older adult with diabetes from increasing caloric expenditure during dietary restriction, weight loss may be more difficult to achieve. In this situation, caloric restriction sufficient to cause weight reduction may be severe enough to put the patient at risk for nutrient or vitamin deficiencies, thereby potentially exacerbating functional limitations by reducing muscle strength.

The general dietary recommendations for patients with diabetes are discussed in Chap. 26. There are no specific alterations to the recommended diet for treatment of older adults, but there is a lack of studies in the area. The ability of an older adult with diabetes to follow a therapeutic diet may be limited by circumstances discussed earlier, such as physical limitations in obtaining food, financial limitations, alterations in taste and smell, and ingrained lifelong dietary habits which may be further complicated by ethnic food preferences. A dietician experienced in working with older adults can be of great help.

Exercise

The beneficial effect of progressive resistance exercise on muscle strength and function is clear even among the elderly.[70] Exercise would be expected to result in improved physical functioning in resistance-trained older adults with type 2 diabetes. As summarized in Table 24-4, in addition to improved physical functioning, benefits of exercise may be in two areas: direct effects on glucose metabolism, and effects on other common comorbidities in patients with T2DM. Although large-scale studies in older adults with T2DM are not yet available, lower fasting plasma glucose and glycosylated hemoglobin, improved oral and intravenous glucose tolerance, and enhancement of insulin action may be seen in older adults with T2DM on a regular exercise program.[71]

Exercise may also offer substantial reduction of risk for the development of cardiovascular disease. However, there are also some potential problems and risks in prescribing exercise for an older adult with diabetes. One study found that 81% of a population of older men with newly diagnosed diabetes were unable to participate in an exercise program due to medical treatment or comorbid diseases.[72] Despite the potential benefits of exercise in the older adult with diabetes, it may not be prescribed by health care providers. For example, highly experienced nurse providers of

health care to older adults with diabetes reported not teaching clients about exercise. This was due to lack of resources, lack of specific knowledge about exercise, and a negative perception about their patients' ability to exercise.[73] The general approach to the use of exercise in patients with diabetes is discussed in Chap. 27.

Pharmacologic Intervention

There are some special considerations in the older adult with diabetes when nonpharmacologic treatment has been unsuccessful in controlling glucose levels and the addition of an oral hypoglycemic agent or insulin is being considered. Of these the risk of hypoglycemia is the most serious.

Oral Hypoglycemic Agents

The efficacy and mechanism of action of oral hypoglycemic agents are discussed in detail in Chap. 32. There are no data to suggest that the efficacy or mechanism of action of these drugs are different in the older adult with diabetes than in younger patients. Safety and efficacy studies of all the newer agents have included older adults. Studies of combination oral agent therapy have also included older patients and have demonstrated both safety and efficacy.[74–76] Although the rate of severe hypoglycemia appears to be low in older people with diabetes, age is an independent risk factor for hypoglycemia during oral agent therapy.[77] This may be related in part to an age-associated decrease in hepatic oxidative metabolism. Combined with the apparent decrease in hepatic blood flow with age, the metabolism of some oral agents may decline in older patients with diabetes, requiring use of lower dosages. The decline of renal function with age may prolong the duration of action of oral hypoglycemic agents excreted by the kidneys.

The presence of coexisting disease may decrease serum albumin in an older patient, thereby influencing bioavailability of drugs that are protein-bound. Polypharmacy and the potential for drug-drug interactions need to be taken into account when prescribing oral hypoglycemic agents for the older adult with diabetes. Though each medication should be reviewed for potential interaction with the oral hypoglycemic agent being used, there are some general classes of medications that may increase the risk for hypoglycemia: β-adrenergic blockers, salicylates, warfarin, sulfonamides, and alcohol. The longer acting sulfonylureas are reported to cause the greatest number of hypoglycemic episodes in older adults, including prolonged hypoglycemia.[78]

Insulin

The use of insulin therapy can be as appropriate in the older adult with diabetes as in a younger individual. Failure of maximal oral hypoglycemic therapy to achieve the treatment goal is the most common reason to consider insulin therapy in the older adult with diabetes. No studies have shown that insulin therapy is any less effective or more risky in older adults with diabetes than in the young. When the treatment goal is control of symptomatic hyperglycemia, a single daily dose of insulin may be adequate. However, when the goal is euglycemia, a split regimen of mixed insulin will likely be necessary and is tolerated well by older adults.[79] No special insulin regimens have been identified as more or less efficacious in treating older adults (see Chap. 30 for intensive insulin therapy recommendations in T2DM).

There are some special considerations when prescribing insulin therapy for an older adult with diabetes. A comprehensive geriatric assessment of the older adult with diabetes as discussed earlier in this chapter should identify which, if any, of these special

TABLE 24-4. Potential Benefits and Risks of Exercise for Older Adults with Diabetes

Benefits	Risks
Diabetes-Related	*Diabetes-Related*
Improved glucose tolerance and increased insulin sensitivity	Hypoglycemia, exercise-induced and delayed
Decreased central and overall adiposity	
General Health	*General Health*
Increased maximal oxygen consumption	Sudden cardiac death
Decreased blood pressure	Musculoskeletal injuries
Improved physical function and increased muscle strength	
Improved lipid profile	
Increased bone mineral content	
Improved self-image	

considerations apply to each patient. Coexisting conditions commonly found in older adults combined with complications secondary to diabetes may impair the visual, fine motor, cognitive and/or sensory skills necessary for the delivery of insulin therapy and home blood glucose monitoring. Home blood glucose monitoring is important for any older patient treated with insulin.

Hypoglycemia

Since older people with diabetes mellitus receiving pharmacologic treatment are at risk for hypoglycemia, information about hypoglycemia recognition, prevention, and management should be part of their diabetes education program. Studies of hypoglycemia counterregulation under controlled conditions in carefully defined populations of normal older adults and older adults with T2DM have demonstrated some subtle alterations of neuroendocrine function,[80–82] but these are unlikely to be of sufficient magnitude to limit the ability to counterregulate hypoglycemia. Effects of hypoglycemia on autonomic symptoms and cognitive function are also minimal in such patients, although a mild impairment of reaction times during hypoglycemia has been observed in older type 2 diabetes patients.[81]

Thus otherwise healthy older adults can tolerate hypoglycemia reasonably well and mount an appropriate counterregulatory response. However, older patients with coexisting conditions may have greater risk. Older diabetic patients with autonomic neuropathy or with other neurologic disorders that affect autonomic nervous system function may be less able to counterregulate appropriately, or may develop symptoms requiring corrective action. While many antihypertensive drugs affect autonomic nervous system function and could therefore interfere with counterregulation of hypoglycemia, no increased risk of severe hypoglycemia was observed with antihypertensive drug use in a population study.[83]

Older individuals with a significant cognitive disorder, poor or irregular nutrition, or those who are prescribed sedating agents or frequently use alcohol may be unable to recognize symptoms of hypoglycemia, or may have an impaired ability to initiate the feeding response to hypoglycemia. The presence of coexisting kidney or liver dysfunction in an older person contributes to the risk of hypoglycemia by reducing the clearance of insulin or oral hypoglycemic agents. The concomitant use of other medications may contribute to increased risk for hypoglycemia or impaired counterregulation in such individuals. The social setting of the patient may also increase the risk for severe hypoglycemia or its sequelae. Thus the identification of risk factors for hypoglycemia should be part of the comprehensive geriatric evaluation.

Older Patients in Institutionalized Long-Term Care

Diabetes is prevalent among the institutionalized long-term care population. Since life expectancy is limited for many patients admitted to long-term care institutions, basic diabetes care aimed at controlling symptoms of hyperglycemia is often the appropriate goal. Maintenance of good nutrition is important for institutionalized patients. Each patient should be assessed by a dietician at the time of admission and on a regular basis thereafter, because aggressive nutritional support may be needed to treat or avoid malnutrition. For the minority of institutionalized patients who are overweight, it may be necessary to decrease their caloric intake. For patients receiving pharmacologic therapy, dosage reduction at the time of admission should be considered to prevent hypoglycemia, because the resident may receive all scheduled medications and a tightly controlled institutional diet. Thus a regimen which may

have appeared inadequate at home due to poor patient compliance may be more effective in the institutional setting.

A frail institutionalized older adult with diabetes may benefit from an exercise program that reduces physical disability,[84] even if the exercise program is not sufficient to affect glucose levels. Consideration should be given for an exercise program for each patient and the final decision based on information from all appropriate practitioners of the institution's multidisciplinary assessment team.

With regard to pharmacologic treatment, oral hypoglycemic agents or a single dose of mixed insulin will often be adequate to achieve the basic treatment goal of preventing symptomatic hyperglycemia. Insulin will be required in some patients when there is an intolerance or contraindication to oral hypoglycemics, such as acute medical illness or renal or hepatic insufficiency. The monitoring of fingerstick glucose levels by staff in this setting can be a significant aid to the treating physician.

Older Patients in the Acute Care Hospital

The management of diabetes in the hospitalized older adult is, with a few precautions, not very different from managing diabetes in a hospitalized younger adult. The major precautions include an awareness that functional, cognitive, and pharmacokinetic or pharmacodynamic changes may place older patients at increased risk for complications. Therapy for the older patient with diabetes during an acute care hospital admission should emphasize delivering an adequate amount of insulin to prevent the patient from becoming catabolic. To maintain adequate glucose control, some hospitalized older patients with diabetes may need to have insulin added temporarily, despite being adequately controlled at home on diet or oral agents. Therapy needs to be monitored closely to avoid hypoglycemia. Management of hyperosmolar, hyperglycemic nonketotic coma, which occurs primarily in older adults, is discussed in Chap. 35. It emphasizes the importance of fluid and electrolyte replacement, provision of insulin, and treatment of the underlying major illness which is usually present.

REFERENCES

1. Harris MI, Flegal KM, Cowie CC, *et al*: Prevalence of diabetes, impaired fasting glucose, and impaired glucose tolerance in U.S. adults. The Third National Health and Nutrition Examination Survey, 1988–1994. *Diabetes Care* 1998;21(4):518–524.
2. Resnick HE, Harris MI, Brock DB, *et al*: American Diabetes Association diabetes diagnostic criteria, advancing age, and cardiovascular disease risk profiles: results from the Third National Health and Nutrition Examination Survey. *Diabetes Care* 2000;23:176.
3. Halter J B: Diabetes mellitus in older adults: underdiagnosis and undertreatment. *J Am Geriatr Soc* 2000;48:340.
4. Lindeman RD, Romero LJ, Hundley R: Prevalences of type 2 diabetes, the insulin resistance syndrome, and coronary heart disease in an elderly, biethnic population. *Diabetes Care* 1998;21:959.
5. Helmrich SP, Ragland DR, Leung RW, *et al*: Physical activity and reduced occurrence of non-insulin-dependent diabetes mellitus. *N Engl J Med* 1991;325:147.
6. Tuomilehto J, Lindstrom J, Eriksson J, *et al*: Prevention of type 2 diabetes mellitus by changes in lifestyle among subjects with impaired glucose tolerance. *N Engl J Med* 2001;344:1343.
7. Diabetes Prevention Program Research Group. Reduction in the incidence of type 2 diabetes with lifestyle intervention or metformin. *N Engl J Med* 2002;346:393.
8. Carter Center of Emory University: Closing the gap: the problem of diabetes mellitus in the United States. *Diabetes Care* 1985;8:391.
9. Kuusisto J, Mykkanen L, Pyorala K, *et al*: Non-insulin-dependent diabetes and its metabolic control are important predictors of stroke in elderly subjects. *Stroke* 1994;25:1157.

10. Kuusisto J, Mykkanen L, Pyorala K, *et al*: Non-insulin-dependent diabetes and its metabolic control predict coronary heart disease in elderly subjects. *Diabetes* 1994;43:960.

11. Geiss LS, Herman WH, Smith PJ: Mortality in non-insulin-dependent diabetes. In: Harris MI, ed. *Diabetes in America*. National Institute of Diabetes and Digestive and Kidney Diseases:1995;233.

12. Rodriguez BL, Curb JD, Burchfiel CM, *et al*: Impaired glucose tolerance, diabetes, and cardiovascular disease risk factor profiles in the elderly. *Diabetes Care* 1996;19:587.

13. Barzilay JI, Spiekeman CF, Wahl PW, *et al*: Cardiovascular disease in older adults with glucose disorders: comparison of American Diabetes Association criteria for diabetes mellitus with WHO criteria. *Lancet* 1999;354:622.

14. American Diabetes Association: Position statement: diabetic nephropathy. *Diabetes Care* 2000;23(Suppl 1):69.

15. National Center for Health Statistics: *National Vital Statistics Report*. 1999;47:12.

16. Klein R, Klein BEK: Vision disorders in diabetes. In: Harris MI, ed. *Diabetes in America*. National Institute of Diabetes and Digestive and Kidney Diseases:1995;293.

17. American Diabetes Association: Position statement: diabetic retinopathy. *Diabetes Care* 2000;23(Suppl. 1):S73.

18. Vinik AI, Park TS, Stansberry KB, *et al*: Diabetic neuropathies. *Diabetologia* 2000;43:957.

19. Halter JB: Aging and carbohydrate metabolism. In: Masoro EJ, ed. *Handbook of Physiology, Volume on Aging*. Oxford University Press: 1995;119.

20. Jackson RA: Mechanisms of age-related glucose intolerance. *Diabetes Care* 1990;13:9.

21. Chen M, Halter JB, Porte D Jr: The role of dietary carbohydrate in the decreased glucose tolerance of the elderly. *J Am Geriatr Soc* 1987;35:417.

22. Meneilly GS, Veldhuis JD, Elahi D: Disruption of the pulsatile and entropic modes of insulin release during an unvarying glucose stimulus in elderly individuals. *J Clin Endocrinol Metab* 1999;84:1938.

23. Kahn SE, Larson VG, Schwartz RS, *et al*: Exercise training delineates the importance of B-cell dysfunction to the glucose intolerance of human aging. *J Clin Endocrinol Metab* 1992;74:1336.

24. Iozzo P, Beck-Nielsen B, Laakso M, *et al*: Independent influence of age on basal insulin secretion in nondiabetic humans. *J Clin Endocrinol Metab* 1999;84:863.

25. Dechenes CJ, Verchere CB, Andrikopoulos S, *et al*: Human aging is associated with parallel reductions in insulin and amylin release. *Am J Physiol* 1998;275(Pt. 1):E785.

26. Roder ME, Schwartz RS, Prigeon RL, *et al*: Reduced pancreatic B cell compensation to the insulin resistance of aging: impact on proinsulin and insulin levels. *J Clin Endocrinol Metab* 2000;85:2275.

27. Busby MJ, Bellantoni MF, Tobin JD, *et al*: Glucose tolerance in women: the effects of age, body composition, and sex hormones. *J Am Geriatr Soc* 1992;40:497.

28. Meyers DA, Goldberg AP, Bleecker ML, *et al*: Relationship of obesity and physical fitness to cardiopulmonary and metabolic function in healthy older men. *J Gerontol Med Sci* 1991;46:M57.

29. Shimokata H, Muller DC, Fleg JL, *et al*: Age as independent determinant of glucose tolerance. *Diabetes* 1991;40:44.

30. Coon PJ, Rogus EM, Drinkwater D, *et al*: Role of body fat distribution in the decline in insulin sensitivity and glucose tolerance with age. *J Clin Endocrinol Metab* 1992;75:1125.

31. Kohrt WM, Kirwan JP, Staten MA, *et al*: Insulin resistance in aging is related to abdominal obesity. *Diabetes* 1993;42:273.

32. Kahn SE, Larson VG, Beard JC, *et al*: Effect of exercise on insulin action, glucose tolerance, and insulin secretion in aging. *Am J Physiol* 1990;258:E937–E943.

33. Ryan AS, Pratley RE, Goldberg AP, *et al*: Resistive training increases insulin action in postmenopausal women. *J Gerontol Med Sci* 1996; 51A:M199.

34. Dela F, Mikines KJ, Larsen JJ, *et al*: Training-induced enhancement of insulin action in human skeletal muscle: the influence of aging. *J Gerontol Biol Sci* 1996;51A:B247.

35. Reaven PD, Barrett-Connor EL, Browner DK: Abnormal glucose tolerance and hypertension. *Diabetes Care* 1990;13:119.

36. Haffner SM: Insulin and blood pressure: fact or fantasy? *J Clin Endocrinol Metab* 1993;76:541.

37. Dengel DR, Hogikyan RV, Brown MD, *et al*: Insulin sensitivity is associated with blood pressure response to sodium in older hypertensives. *Am J Physiol* 1998;274:E403.

38. Muller DC, Elahi D, Pratley RE, *et al*: An epidemiological test of the hyperinsulinemia-hypertension hypothesis. *J Clin Endocrinol Metab* 1993;76:544.

39. Lithell HOL: Effect of antihypertensive drugs on insulin, glucose, and lipid metabolism. *Diabetes Care* 1991;14:203.

40. Morrow LA, Morganroth GS, Herman WH, *et al*: Effects of epinephrine on insulin secretion and action in humans. *Diabetes* 1993;42:307.

41. Brown AS, Brummel-Smith K, Burgess L, *et al*: National Institutes of Health consensus development conference statement: geriatric assessment methods for clinical decision-making. *J Am Geriatr Soc* 1988; 36:342.

42. Rubenstein LV, Calkins DR, Greenfield S, *et al*: Health status assessment for elderly patients. Report of the Society of General Internal Medicine task force on health assessment. *J Am Geriatr Soc* 1988;37:562.

43. Gregg EW, Beckles GLA, Williamson DE, *et al*: Diabetes and physical disability among older U.S. adults. *Diabetes Care* 2000;23:1272.

44. Kumari M, Brunner E, Fuhrer R: Minireview: mechanisms by which the metabolic syndrome and diabetes impair memory. *J Gerontol Biol Sci* 2000;55A:B228.

45. Tun PA, Nathan DM, Perlmuter LC: Cognitive and affective disorders in elderly diabetics. *Clin Geriatr Med* 1990;6:731.

46. Halter JB: Alzheimer's disease and non-insulin dependent diabetes mellitus: common features do not make common bedfellows. *J Am Geriatr Soc* 1996;44:992.

47. White H, Davis PB: Cognitive screening tests: an aid in the care of elderly outpatients. *J Gen Int Med* 1990;5:438.

48. Edwards DL, Frongillo EA, Fauschenback B, *et al*: Home-delivered meals benefit the diabetic elderly. *J Am Diet Assoc* 1993;93:585.

49. Hays LM, Clark DO: Correlates of physical activity in a sample of older adults with type 2 diabetes. *Diabetes Care* 1999;22:706.

50. Caruso LB, Silliman RA, Demissie S, *et al*: What can we do to improve physical function in older persons with type 2 diabetes? *J Gerontol Med Sci* 2000;55A:M372.

51. Lan S-JJ, Justice CL: Use of modified diets in nursing homes. *J Am Diet Assoc* 1991;91:46.

52. Brechner RJ, Cowie CC, Howie LJ, *et al*: Ophthalmic examination among adults with diagnosed diabetes mellitus. *JAMA* 1993;270:1714.

53. Starer P, Libow L: Cystometric evaluation of bladder dysfunction in elderly diabetic patients. *Arch Intern Med* 1990;150:810.

54. Resnick NM: Urinary incontinence in older adults. *Hosp Pract* 1992;27:139.

55. Mulligan T, Retchin SM, Chinchilli VM, *et al*: The role of aging and chronic disease in sexual dysfunction. *J Am Geriatr Soc* 1988;36:520.

56. Kroenke KK, Pinholt EM: Reducing polypharmacy in the elderly. A controlled trial of physician feedback. *J Am Geriatr Soc* 1990;38:31.

57. Gurwitz JH, Soumerai SB, Avorn J: Improving medication prescribing and utilization in the nursing home. *J Am Geriatr Soc* 1990;38:542.

58. Beers MH, Rollingher I, Reuben DB, *et al*: Explicit criteria for determining inappropriate medication use in nursing home residents. *Arch Intern Med* 1991;151:1825.

59. Moritz DJ, Ostfeld AM, Blazer DI, *et al*: The health burden of diabetes for the elderly in four communities. *Public Health Reps* 1994;109:782.

60. Fillenbaum GG, Pieper CF, Cohen HJ, *et al*: Comorbidity of five chronic health conditions in elderly community residents: determinants and impact on mortality. *J Gerontol Med Sci* 2000;55A:M84.

61. Wingard DL, Barrett-Connor E: Heart disease and diabetes. In: Harris MI, ed. *Diabetes in America*. National Institute of Diabetes and Digestive and Kidney Diseases:1995;429.

62. Kuller LH: Stroke and diabetes. In: Harris MI, ed. *Diabetes in America*. National Institute of Diabetes and Digestive and Kidney Diseases:1995;449.

63. Curb JD, Pressel SL, Cutler JA, *et al*: Effect of diuretic-based antihypertensive treatment on cardiovascular disease risk in older diabetic patients with isolated systolic hypertension. *JAMA* 1996;276;1886.

64. Tuomilehto J, Rastenyte D, Birkenhager WH, *et al*: Effects of calcium-channel blockade in older patients with diabetes and systemic hypertension. *N Engl J Med* 1999;340:677.

65. Antiplatelet Trialists' Collaboration: Collaborative overview of randomised trials of antiplatelet therapy. Prevention of death, myocardial infarction, and stroke by prolonged antiplatelet therapy in various categories of patients. *Br Med J* 1994;308:81.

66. Vijan S, Hofer TP, Hayward RA: Cost-utility analysis of screening intervals for diabetic retinopathy in patients with type 2 diabetes mellitus. *JAMA* 2000;283:889.

67. Shorr RI, Franse LV, Resnick HE, *et al*: Glycemic control of older adults with type 2 diabetes: findings from the Third National Health and Nutrition Examination Survey, 1988–1994. *J Am Geriatr Soc* 2000;48:264.

68. Smith NL, Heckbert SR, Bittner VA, *et al*: Antidiabetic treatment trends in a cohort of elderly people with diabetes, The Cardiovascular Health Study, 1989–1997. *Diabetes Care* 1999;22:736.

69. Gilden JL, Hendryx MS, Clar S, *et al*: Diabetes support groups improve health care of older diabetic patients. *J Am Geriatr Soc* 1992; 40:147.

70. Fiatarone MA, O'Neill RF, Ryan ND, *et al*: Exercise training and nutritional supplementation for physical frailty in very elderly people. *N Engl J Med* 1994;330:1769.

71. Schwartz RS: Exercise training in treatment of diabetes mellitus in elderly patients. *Diabetes Care* 1990;13:77.

72. Skarfors ET, Wegener TA, Lithell H: Physical training as treatment for type 2 (non-insulin-dependent) diabetes in elderly men. A feasibility study over 2 years. *Diabetologia* 1987;30:930.

73. Ruby KL, Blainey CA, Haas LB, *et al*: The knowledge and practices of registered nurse, certified diabetes educators: teaching elderly clients about exercise. *Diabetes Educator* 1993;19:299.

74. Gregorio F, Ambrosit F, Manfrini S, *et al*: Poorly controlled elderly type 2 diabetic patients: the effects of increasing sulphonylurea dosages or adding metformin. *Diabet Med* 1999;16:1016.

75. Fonseca V, Rosenstock J, Patwardhan R, *et al*: Effect of metformin and rosiglitazone combination therapy in patients with type 2 diabetes mellitus. A randomized controlled trial. *JAMA* 2000;283:1695.

76. Horton ES, Clinkingbeard C, Gatlin M, *et al*: Nateglinide alone and in combination with metformin improves glycemic control by reducing mealtime glucose levels in type 2 diabetes. *Diabetes Care* 2000;23: 1660.

77. Shorr RI, Ray WA, Daugherty JR, *et al*: Incidence and risk factors for serious hypoglycemia in older persons using insulin or sulfonylureas. *Arch Intern Med* 1997;157:1681.

78. Shorr RI, Ray WA, Daugherty JR, *et al*: Individual sulfonylureas and serious hypoglycemia in older people. *J Am Geriatr Soc* 1996;44:751.

79. Wolffenbuttel BHR, Sels J-PJE, Rondas-Colbers GJWM, *et al*: Comparison of different insulin regimens in elderly patients with NIDDM. *Diabetes Care* 1996;19:1326.

80. Ortiz-Alonso FJ, Galecki A, Herman WH, *et al*: Hypoglycemia counterregulation in elderly humans: relationship to glucose levels. *Am J Physiol* 1994;267:E497.

81. Meneilly GS, Cheung E, Tuokko H: Counterregulatory hormone responses to hypoglycemia in the elderly patient with diabetes. *Diabetes* 1994;43:403.

82. Matyka K, Evans M, Lomas J, *et al*: Altered hierarchy of protective responses against severe hypoglycemia in normal aging in healthy men. *Diabetes Care* 1997;20:135.

83. Shorr RI, Ray WA, Daugherty JR, *et al*: Antihypertensives and the risk of serious hypoglycemia in older persons using insulin or sulfonylureas. *JAMA* 1997;278:40.

84. Mulrow CD, Gerety MB, Kanten D, *et al*: A randomized trial of physical rehabilitation for very frail nursing home residents. *JAMA* 1994; 271:519.

Diabetes Secondary to Endocrinopathies

Om P. Ganda

Eric S. Bachman

A number of endocrine disorders are associated with varying degrees of glucose intolerance (Table 25-1). In most instances, the excess of a counterregulatory hormone (such as growth hormone, cortisol, epinephrine, or glucagon) is manifested by a distinct clinical syndrome associated with hyperglycemia or glucose intolerance. However, overt diabetes with symptomatic hyperglycemia, glycosuria, and ketosis secondary to an endocrinopathy is a relatively uncommon event, unless an underlying genetic diabetic diathesis is also present. Because of various beta-cell regulatory mechanisms,[1] endocrine factors potentially capable of disrupting glucose homeostasis in normal humans are offset primarily by appropriate increments and other adjustments of insulin secretion. The net outcome of the metabolic effects of an endocrinopathy in producing glucose intolerance is, therefore, usually dependent on its direct or indirect impact on one or more of the following: (1) insulin sensitivity (hepatic glucose production and/or peripheral glucose utilization); (2) insulin secretion (direct inhibition or compensatory hyperinsulinism); (3) unmasking of genetic diabetes; or (4) a familial polyendocrine disorder with a common underlying mechanism, such as a genetic mechanism (multiple endocrine neoplasia syndromes) and/or autoimmune factors. This chapter deals with the pathophysiology of glucose intolerance and related metabolic derangements associated with various types of endocrine disorders. The role of counterregulatory hormones in the pathogenesis and complications of genetic diabetes has been presented elsewhere.

DISORDERS OF GROWTH HORMONE SECRETION

A relation between the anterior pituitary gland and diabetes mellitus was first shown in the classic experiments by Houssay[2] and by Young[3] using crude pituitary extracts. Subsequently, it was demonstrated that the administration of human growth hormone resulted in a marked deterioration of metabolic control in patients with diabetes.[4]

Secretion and Actions of Growth Hormone

Human growth hormone (GH) is secreted as a single strand of 191 amino acids sharing marked structural homology with placental lactogen and prolactin. A number of physiologic factors affect the secretion of GH in a healthy person.[5,6] The stimuli for the release of GH include sleep, muscular exercise, stress, hypoglycemia, and amino acids, whereas hyperglycemia is a potent suppressor of its release under normal circumstances.

GH has diverse metabolic effects on carbohydrate, protein, and lipid metabolism.[5,7] Evidence indicates that GH contains multiple domains that determine its growth-promoting, diabetogenic, and insulin-like activities. For example, the carboxy-terminal sequences 44 to 191 and 182 to 191 were shown to induce hyperglycemia and insulin resistance in animal models,[8,9] whereas the amino-terminal sequences 32 to 46 and 8 to 13 within the parent molecule have insulin-like actions.[8,10] Employing a human forearm technique in a series of elegant experiments, Zierler and Rabinowitz showed the diabetogenic effects of acute increments of GH to occur via (1) an inhibition of glucose uptake by the skeletal muscle and the adipose tissue and (2) an augmentation of lipolysis.[11] Whether a significant lipolytic effect is seen during physiologic circumstances in normal individuals has not always been confirmed.[5,12] With regard to in vivo glucose tolerance, supraphysiologic increments in circulating GH (30 to 40 ng/mL) were shown to result in an early but transient insulin-like effect consisting of a diminished glucose production and an enhanced peripheral glucose clearance; however, this was subsequently followed by a delayed insulin-antagonistic effect leading to hyperglycemia.[13] In normal human subjects, several studies employing human pituitary growth hormone[14,15] or recombinant DNA-derived human growth hormone administration,[16] over a period of hours to days, reported the development of insulin resistance. In none of these studies was the degree of insulin resistance explained by changes in insulin receptor binding on monocytes, suggesting a postreceptor mechanism. Chronic administration of GH resulting in permanent diabetes in dogs is accompanied by eventual exhaustion of pancreatic beta cells.[17]

Up to 50% of GH is bound to growth hormone binding proteins (GHBP).[18,19] The high-affinity GHBP has been found to correspond to the extracellular domain of the GH receptor. Although GHBP thus provides an indirect estimate of tissue GH responsiveness in general, there may be some exceptions to this relationship.[19] Considerable evidence exists that many of the metabolic and growth-promoting effects of GH are mediated via the generation of a family of growth factors or somatomedins, produced by the liver in response to this hormone.[5,7,20] The most prominent among these is insulin-like growth factor I (IGF-I). In contrast, there is also evidence that at least some of the effects of GH may be elicited by the physiologic concentrations of GH directly and

TABLE 25-1. Certain Endocrinopathies Associated with Glucose Intolerance

Disorders of growth hormone secretion
Growth hormone excess (acromegaly)
Growth hormone deficiency (sexual ateliotic dwarfism)
Hyperprolactinemic states
Glucocorticoid excess (Cushing's syndrome)
Catecholamine excess (pheochromocytoma)
Primary hyperaldosteronism
Hyperthyroidism
Disorders of calcium and/or phosphorus metabolism
Tumors of endocrine pancreas or gut
Glucagonoma
Somatostatinoma
Gastrinoma (Zollinger–Ellison syndrome)
Pancreatic cholera syndrome (Verner–Morrison syndrome)
Carcinoid syndrome
Multiple endocrine neoplasia (MEN)

independent of somatomedin generation.[21] This view is further supported by the demonstration of the receptors for growth hormone in a variety of cell types including cultured human lymphocytes.

Acromegaly

The prevalence of glucose intolerance in acromegaly is about 50 to 60 percent, although symptomatic diabetes requiring treatment has been observed only in 10 to 30% of all patients.[22–26] Even more frequent than glucose intolerance is a striking increase in serum insulin concentrations and decrease in insulin sensitivity to both endogenous and exogenous insulin that accompanies the GH excess in acromegaly. Defects in both hepatic and peripheral insulin action have been described, using insulin clamp studies.[27] GH levels correlate poorly with both the degree of glucose intolerance and the hyperinsulinemia; a better correlation of disease activity, including glucose intolerance, is found with the serum concentrations of IGF-I or IGF-binding protein 3 (IGFBP-3) levels.[28,29] Muggeo and associates[30] showed a decreased concentration of insulin receptors on circulating monocytes and an inverse correlation of receptor concentration with the basal plasma insulin level in acromegaly. However, in most studies, there was no significant alteration in insulin receptor binding, probably explained by reciprocal changes in receptor affinity.[26] In some patients with acromegaly, the failure of the compensatory increase in receptor affinity may explain the development of hyperglycemia,[31] although insulin dose–response studies in such patients suggest a postreceptor defect in insulin action.[27] The precise nature of the GH-induced postreceptor defect leading to inhibition of glucose transport across cell membrane remains unknown.

In contrast to the majority of patients with acromegaly who have hyperinsulinemia and impaired glucose tolerance, those with overt diabetes with or without ketosis clearly have a subnormal insulin reserve, suggesting an underlying genetic diabetic trait. Studies with somatostatin infusions in the human have provided evidence that growth hormone has significant effects on lipolysis or ketogenesis mainly in the presence of significant insulin deficiency.[32,33]

Successful treatment of acromegaly is accompanied by striking improvement in glucose tolerance and restoration of normal serum insulin levels and normalization of insulin sensitivity in the majority of patients with impaired glucose tolerance but infrequently so in those with overt, symptomatic diabetes.[24–26,34] Lack of a complete remission in many patients may be due to incomplete cure of acromegaly, defined as suppression of GH to less than 2.5 ng/mL or to less than 1 ng/mL after oral glucose, using newer, ultra-sensitive assays.[35] The increase in mortality rate in acromegaly may persist unless GH levels are suppressed to near-normal range.[36,37] Moreover, glucose intolerance and hypertension are independent determinants of acromegalic cardiomyopathy.[38]

The long-acting somatostatin analog, octreotide, has been shown to be a useful adjunct in the treatment of acromegaly. In large, multicenter trials of 58 and 103 patients, lasting up to 30 months,[39,40] most of whom had been previously treated with surgery or radiotherapy, treatment with octreotide for more than 6 months resulted in substantial improvement in about 65% of patients. However, biochemical cure, defined by GH less than 5 ng/mL and normal IGF-I occurred in about 50 percent of patients, and only 20 to 40 percent of patients fulfilled the more stringent criterion of GH suppression to less than 2ng/mL in both of these large series of patients.[39,40]

Regarding the effects of octreotide therapy on glucose tolerance, the results from various reports indicate a mixed outcome, depending on the baseline metabolic status.[26] On the one hand, in patients with overt diabetes or IGT, significant improvement in glucose tolerance or normalization of diabetes may result after several weeks of treatment. Impressive decreases in insulin requirements among the diabetic subjects within the largest, randomized, multicenter trial were observed.[40] Normalization of GH and IGF-I were associated with improvements in insulin sensitivity and greater suppression of hepatic glucose output (HGO) as determined by the euglycemic-hyperinsulinemic clamp technique, whereas peripheral glucose disposal was not affected.[41] On the other hand, in patients with normal or minimally impaired glucose tolerance, treatment with octreotide resulted in either slight improvement, no change, or even a worsening of glucose tolerance, despite improvements in GH and IGF-I levels.[26,39,42] Thus, an adverse outcome in glucose homeostasis may be seen in some nondiabetic acromegalic patients following treatment with octreotide, depending on baseline characteristics such as β-cell reserve and degree of insulin resistance. Finally, long-term octreotide therapy may result in other side affects, the most important of which is the 40 to 50 percent incidence of cholelithiasis and/or biliary sludge.[40]

Recently, results with longer-acting somatostatin analogs (Octreotide LAR and Lanreotide) have shown comparable decreases in GH and IGF-I levels but the long-term effects on glucose homeostasis with these agents are awaited. Similarly, impressive short-term clinical outcome data with a growth hormone receptor antagonist, Pegvisomant, in a large series of patients with acromegaly were reported recently.[43] The effects of this novel approach on glucose intolerance will also be of interest.

Diabetes Associated with Growth Hormone Deficiency

The presence of diabetes in the setting of GH-deficient dwarfs presents an interesting paradox. However, it has been known for a number of years that exogenous administration of GH to both normal and hypopituitary subjects augments the insulin response to a variety of secretagogues before a significant change in blood glucose occurs.[44] Martin and Gagliardino[45] showed a β-cytotropic effect of GH on isolated pancreatic islets of rat in vitro. Similarly, some workers have shown direct effects of GH on islet β-cell replication in neonatal rat islet monolayer cultures.[46]

The majority of adult sexual ateliotic dwarfs with monotropic GH deficiency studied by Merimee and coworkers, showed evidence of a mild to moderately severe glucose intolerance and insulin deficiency.[47] In addition, GH deficiency may promote visceral obesity, and in turn reduce insulin action as well (see Chapter xxxxxxx). Interestingly, after 10 years of follow-up, there was no evidence of diabetic microangiopathy in these dwarfs, despite worsening of glucose intolerance.[48] On the one hand, these observations support the concept of a permissive role of GH in the pathogenesis of diabetic vascular disease. On the other hand, the incidence and severity of microangiopathy in patients with acromegaly with a striking increase of ambient GH concentrations does not appear to be increased and may indeed be significantly lower than in patients with genetic diabetes. Further studies on groups of patients well matched for the degree and duration of hyperglycemia are required to settle this question.

A number of long-term follow-up studies in adult patients with hypopituitarism have suggested an increased cardiovascular mortality even after replacement of other hormones.[49] This has been partly ascribed to an atherogenic lipid profile, visceral adiposity, and insulin resistance in such patients. Administration of GH in such patients may restore, although not normalize the cardiovascular risk profile.[50] Short-term studies with GH therapy over 12 to 30 months have also reported adverse effects on glucose tolerance and insulin sensitivity in hypopituitary adults.[51,52] Retinal changes, mimicking diabetic retinopathy, were reported in two non-diabetic patients after 14 to 17 months of treatment with GH.[53] However, only 12 cases of overt diabetes were reported among 8136 GH-treated children.[54]

GH is currently being proposed by some as therapeutic agent for several indications (e.g., preservation of lean body mass during aging, HIV-related disorders, prolonged illness, osteoporosis, enhancing tissue repair following surgery or trauma, and stimulation of muscle mass in athletes). Besides its potential for diabetogenic effects, other long-term risks of GH therapy need to be studied before specific recommendations can be made.[55]

Hyperprolactinemia

GH and prolactin share considerable structural homology. A role of prolactin in the pathogenesis of a human diabetogenic syndrome was suggested by the studies of Landgraf and colleagues.[56] These investigators studied the blood glucose and insulin levels during oral glucose tolerance tests in 26 patients with prolactin-secreting pituitary tumors. The basal glucose and insulin levels were similar to control subjects despite chronic, endogenous hyperprolactinemia; however, glucose tolerance was significantly impaired and was accompanied by a relative peripheral insulin insensitivity as reflected by the associated hyperinsulinemia. Both glucose intolerance and hyperinsulinism improved after suppression of prolactin release following treatment with bromocriptine. In a study of nine patients with amenorrhea-galactorrhea syndrome and hyperprolactinemia, mildly abnormal glucose tolerance and elevated insulin levels were found.[57] On the other hand, the 24-hour plasma prolactin pattern in a group of relatively stable, insulin-dependent (juvenile) diabetics was found to be identical to that in normal controls,[58] suggesting a normal regulation of prolactin secretion in such diabetics. In contrast, elevated plasma concentrations of prolactin have been reported in diabetics in ketoacidosis,[59] a finding not confirmed by oth-

ers,[60] even after stimulation with TRH. Further studies are clearly required in the delineation of metabolic aberrations, if any, associated with the syndrome of prolactin excess.

Cushing's Syndrome

It has been known for a long time that glucocorticoids antagonize the actions of insulin. The spectrum of insulin insensitivity in patients with Cushing's syndrome and the insulin hypersensitivity in Addison's disease is clinically well recognized. Cahill[61] has reviewed extensive evidence for the diverse metabolic actions of glucocorticoids on liver, adipose tissue, and muscle.

In the liver, glucocorticoids appear to accelerate the biochemical actions at every rate-limiting step in the sequence of events leading to gluconeogenesis.[61,62] Some of these crucial loci are (1) hepatic uptake of amino acids, (2) activation of pyruvate carboxylase in generating pyruvate from amino acid precursors, and (3) activation of phosphoenolpyruvate carboxykinase, the unidirectional rate-limiting enzyme in the initiation of the cascade of glucogenesis from pyruvate. Glucocorticoids, paradoxically, stimulate glycogen deposition and in this respect resemble the action of insulin; in fact, some evidence suggests that the glycogen-synthesizing effect of glucocorticoids may be mediated via insulin, rather than a direct steroid effect. At the level of adipose tissue and muscle, the main effect of glucocorticoids involves an antagonism of insulin-induced glucose transport by multiple mechanisms including a decrease in insulin-receptor affinity, as well as a defect in insulin-receptor signaling.[62–64] In addition, glucocorticoids appear to exert a permissive effect on lipolysis by promoting the activation of cAMP-dependent, hormone-sensitive lipase in the adipose tissue of several species. However, the net clinical effect of glucocorticoid excess in humans is generally not fat mobilization but a relocation of fat depots, resulting in typical truncal obesity. Recent studies have suggested differential effects of glucocorticoids on adipose tissue of omental versus subcutaneous regions.[65] In these studies, both the glucocorticoid receptor binding and the LPL activity were two- to fourfold higher in the omental adipose tissue. Several in vitro studies have shown an augmentation of proteolysis in skeletal muscle and perhaps a decreased incorporation of amino acids in the muscle protein. A shift in muscle fiber composition from type I to type IIb has been described in patients with Cushing's syndrome.[66] Finally, glucocorticoids may have a direct effect on insulin release by inhibition of Ca^{++}-induced exocytosis.[67]

In normal humans, short-term increments of plasma cortisol within the ranges up to those seen in moderate stress situations result in a mild increase of glucose levels secondary to both hepatic and extrahepatic effects, as well as in a significant increase in blood ketone and branched-chain amino acid levels.[62,63] These changes were accompanied by no significant alterations in insulin receptors, supporting a role for postreceptor mechanisms underlying the decrease in insulin sensitivity. However, the hyperglycemic effects of chronic administration of glucocorticoids in normal subjects with an intact islet reserve are partially compensated for by secondary changes in insulin release, so that the net effects observed on glucose levels may be minimal or moderate. The spectrum of glucose intolerance in a patient with Cushing's syndrome is therefore largely dependent upon the endogenous beta-cell reserve, similar to the situation in acromegaly. Glucose intolerance in Cushing's syndrome has been reported to be present in 75 to 80 percent of patients, although overt diabetes occurs in about 10 to 15 percent of all patients.[68] Nearly all patients manifest basal and stimulated hyperinsulinemia and insulin insensitivity. The diabetogenic effect in glucocorticoid-excess states also involves a stimulation of glucagon secretin. Glucocorticoid administration in normal volunteers over 3 to 4 days[69,70] was shown to induce an augmented alpha-cell responsiveness both in the basal state and following protein ingestion or amino acid infusion. This effect may be mediated indirectly via hyperaminoacidemia brought about by augmented proteolysis and, perhaps by other factors, such as decreased islet glucose utilization, or a direct effect of the steroid upon the alpha cell.

Pheochromocytoma

Catecholamines, acting via adrenergic receptors, produce their effects on islet secretion and in several loci of intermediary metabolism.[71] The classical effect of epinephrine (E) in enhancing hepatic glucose output via glycogenolysis results primarily via β_{-2} adrenergic stimulation of adenylcyclase and cAMP release. In addition, E stimulates glycogenolysis also by an α-adrenergic, Ca^{++}-dependent but cAMP-independent mechanism.[72] On the other hand, stimulation of adipose tissue lipolysis and muscle glycogenolysis is mediated by β-adrenergic mechanisms.[71] In vitro studies performed by Garber and associates[73] have revealed a significant inhibition of the release of gluconeogenic amino acids (alanine and glutamine) in response to β-adrenergic agonists. Moreover, recent studies with E infusions in normal humans achieving physiologic concentrations in the range of 350 to 400 pg/mL revealed a significant decline in circulating amino acids (particularly branched-chain), which was preventable by the β-adrenergic antagonist propranolol. The significance of these effects of catecholamines on muscle protein balance requires further elucidation.

Studies in normal subjects receiving physiologic infusions of E have shown only a transient stimulation of hepatic glucose output and a sustained inhibition of peripheral glucose uptake.[74] The latter effect is mediated via a β-adrenergic stimulation in muscle. Norepinephrine was found to have much less pronounced direct hyperglycemic effects, and the effects of epinephrine were not mediated via glucagon hypersecretion.[74]

A number of studies have been performed to study the adrenergic regulation of islet hormone secretion. Robertson and co-workers[75] provided evidence for inhibition of basal insulin secretion by α-adrenergic stimulation or by β-adrenergic blockade. In addition, they postulated that an excessive endogenous α-adrenergic activity may contribute to the defective glucose-stimulated insulin secretion in type 2 diabetes. However, the role of catecholamines in the physiologic regulation of insulin secretion and in the pathogenesis of diabetes remains controversial. Recently, a 29-amino-acid polypeptide, galanin, was proposed as an important mediator of sympathetic neural activation in the endocrine pancreas.[76] However, its effects may be restricted to nonprimates. Regarding the pancreatic α cell, both α- and β-adrenergic stimulation have been shown to augment glucagon secretion, although the relative importance of α- and β-sympathetic versus the parasympathetic tone in maintaining basal glucagon release remains uncertain.[71,77]

In patients with pheochromocytoma, fasting glucose at or higher than 126 mg/dL was reported in about 30% of patients[78] from multiple mechanisms, including (1) an inhibition of insulin secretion, (2) stimulation of hepatic and muscle glycogenolysis and hepatic glucose output, and (3) enhanced lipolysis. In animals epinephrine has been shown to decrease the transcription of the glucose transporter 4 (GLUT-4) gene.[79] Administration of α-adrenergic blocking agents, such as phenoxybenzamine, characteristically improves β-cell secretory response and glucose tolerance.[71] Glucagon levels were found to be within the normal range in the basal state, and suppressed in response to arginine[80] or hypoglycemia[81] in patients with confirmed pheochromocytoma. As a rule, surgical removal of the tumor restores or improves glucose tolerance[78,80] within several weeks postoperatively. However, others have reported a normal increase with arginine.[71,82]

Table 25-2 summarizes the major sites of action of various counterregulatory hormones at the levels of target organs and the principal mechanisms of diabetogenic effects. In addition, the net outcome of these effects is dependent upon the direct or indirect influences on the secretion or actions of insulin (Table 25-3), as discussed previously.

Primary Hyperaldosteronism

The triad of hypertension, hypokalemia, and glucose intolerance was first described by Conn.[83] Contrary to previous expectations, it has been estimated that this syndrome accounts for certainly no more than 1–2% of the hypertensive population.

Glucose intolerance was earlier reported to be present in about 50% of the patients with this syndrome,[83] but a more accurate incidence would be considerably lower in view of a relatively mild abnormality in most patients even with the current criteria for the diagnosis of diabetes. The metabolic abnormality linked to glucose intolerance is generally thought to be secondary to potassium depletion, which may be responsible for the reported blunted insulin secretion[83,84] and perhaps accelerated glycogenolysis. Sagild and associates[85] were able to induce glucose intolerance in normal men commensurate with the induction of a potassium depletion to the extent of 200–500 mEq during a 5-day period, while the insulin

TABLE 25-2. Major Metabolic Sites of Action of Counterregulatory Hormones*

Hormone	Liver		Muscle		Adipose Tissue	
	Glycogen[†]	Gluconeogenesis	Glucose Uptake	Amino Acid Release	Glucose Uptake	Lipolysis
Growth hormone	1	1	2	?	2	1
Glucocorticoids	1	1	2	1	2	1[‡]
Epinephrine	2	1	2	2[§]	?	1
Glucagon	2	1	0	?	0	?

* 1, Stimulation or increase; 2, inhibition or decrease; 0, no effect; ?, uncertain.

[†] Net effect on glycogen content via glycogen synthesis or glycogenolysis.

[‡] A permissive role.

[§] A β-adrenergic effect, common to several β-adrenergic agonists.

TABLE 25-3. Summary of Hormonal Effects on Insulin Secretion and Action*

Hormone	Insulin Secretion	Insulin Action[†]
Growth hormone	1	2
Prolactin	?	2
Glucocorticoids	1[‡]	2
Catecholamines	2	2
Aldosterone[§]	?2	?
Glucagon	1[¶]	2
Thyroid hormones (T$_4$, T$_3$)	?	2
Somatostatin	2	?
Parathyroid hormone[#]	0	2

* 1, Stimulation; 2, inhibition or antagonism; 0, no effect; ?, uncertain.

[†] Via receptor, postreceptor, or both mechanisms.

[‡] Indirectly via insulin resistance. The direct effect appears to be a decrease in insulin secretion.

[§] Indirectly via potassium depletion.

[¶] A pharmacologic effect.

[#] Probably via an effect on phosphorus metabolism as a major mechanism.

sensitivity remained unchanged. However, potassium depletion may not be the only explanation for the glucose intolerance in primary aldosteronism.[86]

THYROID DISORDERS

Hyperthyroidism

Mild to moderately severe degrees of glucose intolerance have been documented in 30–50% of patients with hyperthyroidism.[87,88] Several effects of thyroid hormone excess have been related with aberrations of intermediary metabolism of carbohydrate, lipid, and protein.[88] Induction of hyperthyroidism in subjects with and without diabetes has been found to augment hepatic glucose production and perhaps renal gluconeogenesis. A rapid gastric emptying rate itself may contribute to postprandial hyperglycemia in some thyrotoxic patients. The data on insulin secretion and insulin sensitivity in hyperthyroid patients are controversial.[68,89,90] Several studies have shown subnormal insulin responsiveness to oral glucose, IV glucagon, and IV arginine; however, others have reported normal or increased β-cell responsiveness, but a decreased C-peptide to insulin molar ratio. The significance of the latter finding is uncertain in view of reports of a significantly increased metabolic clearance rate of insulin in such patients.[91] The elevated free fatty acid levels seen in hyperthyroid patients[88] might also contribute to glucose intolerance. Beylot and associates have found evidence for augmented ketogenesis, probably mediated in part by a β-adrenergic mechanism.[92] Along with the evidence from isolated liver perfusion experiments in which thyroxine was shown to enhance gluconeogenesis from alanine,[88] these observations would support the clinical observation of worsening glycemic control and recurrent ketoacidosis in patients with preexisting diabetes mellitus who develop thyrotoxicosis.[93] Glucose intolerance persisted in 32% (7 of 22) of patients studied by Maxon and coworkers[87] after 12 years of follow-up after treatment. Because both Graves' disease and type I diabetes share similar autoimmune mechanisms, an increased coexistence of these two disorders may be at least partly explained on this basis.[94]

DISORDERS OF CALCIUM AND/OR PHOSPHORUS METABOLISM

Disorders of calcium and phosphorus metabolism produce significant alterations in insulin secretion and/or insulin sensitivity, although the extent of these alterations and their precise mechanisms remain uncertain. In primary hyperparathyroidism, elevated serum calcium levels are associated with hyperinsulinism.[95,96] and the insulin hypersecretion pattern has been found to correlate with the serum calcium level.[95] The presence of glucose intolerance in up to 40% of such patients[97] suggests a state of tissue insensitivity to insulin due to the raised intracellular free calcium in primary hyperparathyroidism. However, studies in dogs[98] and humans[99] also point to an important role of hypophosphatemia in inhibiting glucose disposal and an impairment of tissue sensitivity to insulin. This could be, therefore, an important contributory mechanism underlying the insulin resistance of primary hyperparathyroidism. That parathyroid hormone has little direct effect on glucose disposal or insulin secretion is suggested by the studies in dogs with diet-induced secondary hyperparathyroidism[94] and in patients with renal insufficiency who showed no significant effect of parathyroidectomy on any of these parameters.[100] Patients with idiopathic hypoparathyroidism or pseudohypoparathyroidism may have impaired insulin secretion associated with hypocalcemia.[95]

The α-cell responses to arginine or to a protein meal and glucose were studied in a series of patients with primary hyperparathyroidism before and after removal of parathyroid adenoma and were found to be intact.[96] In several, but not all, patients with preexisting diabetes mellitus who underwent parathyroidectomy for primary hyperparathyroidism, evidence for significant improvement in glucose tolerance and for increased sensitivity to exogenous or endogenous insulin was reported.[97,101] These observations further indicate potential consequences of the disorders of calcium and/or phosphorus metabolism on glucose tolerance, insulin secretion, and insulin sensitivity.

TUMORS OF THE ENDOCRINE PANCREAS OR GUT

Non-β-cell tumors of the endocrine pancreas associated with glucose intolerance include particularly those characterized by glucagon and somatostatin hypersecretion. Subtle abnormalities of carbohydrate metabolism have also been encountered in some patients with gastrinoma, vasoactive inhibitory polypeptide tumor (VIP-oma), and carcinoid syndrome. Additionally, diabetes or glucose intolerance may be a component of the multiple endocrine neoplasia (MEN) syndromes.

GLUCAGONOMA

Clinical Features

Since the first well-described patient with a glucagon-secreting tumor in 1966 and a clear definition of the glucagonoma syndrome in 1974, there are now more than 130 definite, well-documented cases in the literature.[102–104] The salient clinical features are summarized in Table 25-4. The syndrome is most prevalent in postmenopausal women, and the tumor is found to be malignant in the majority of patients, usually originating in the body or tail of the

TABLE 25-4. Salient Features of the Glucagonoma Syndrome

Incidence: women > men
Clinical features:
    Glucose intolerance
    Skin rash: necrolytic migratory erythema
    Anemia: normochromic, normocytic
    Atrophic glossitis or stomatitis
    Thromboembolic disease
    Weight loss
Biochemical features:
    Hyperglucagonemia, usually > 1000 pg/mL
    Hypoaminoacidemia
Associated hormonal secretion:
    Insulin, ACTH, parathyroid hormone, or PTH-like substance, pancreatic
    polypeptide, gastrin, serotonin, vasoactive intestinal polypeptide,
    melanocyte-stimulating hormone
Pathology: malignant >> benign

pancreas. Glucose intolerance, a characteristic skin rash, and anemia, the clinical triad of this syndrome, are present in 70–80% of patients. The less common features include unexplained severe weight loss, atrophic glossitis or stomatitis, thromboembolic phenomena, diarrhea, and psychiatric disturbances. Rarely, glucagonoma has been described as part of the MEN I syndrome. More commonly, in about 20–30% of patients, the pancreatic tumor itself was documented to secrete one or more of several other polypeptide hormones, including insulin, ACTH, PTH, or PTH-like substances, pancreatic polypeptide (PP), gastrin, VIP, MSH, and, rarely, serotonin.

The necrolytic migratory erythema[105] is characterized as a disabling, chronic, intermittent, bullous dermopathy presenting as single or confluent areas of desquamating, maculopapular, exudative lesions. The areas most commonly involved include groin, perineum, and buttocks, but almost any other area may be involved. Healing of several lesions is followed by hyperpigmentation; recurrence in the areas of trauma or friction is frequent.

Biochemical Features

The circulating glucagon levels in most patients are very high, ranging between 1000 and 7000 pg/mL, two orders of magnitude higher than those seen in other states of marked glucagon excess such as uncontrolled diabetes, stress, trauma, hepatic or renal insufficiency, and hypercortisolism. However, in a rare syndrome of familial hyperglucagonemia, probably inherited as an autosomal dominant trait,[106,107] striking hyperglucagonemia may sometimes be observed at levels indistinguishable from those usually seen in glucagonoma syndrome. Interestingly, in one study[106] elevated basal glucagon levels were observed in several relatives of a patient with glucagonoma. Most patients with glucagonoma secrete variable proportions of both 3500- and 9000-d (proglucagon) fractions, whereas the major fraction of glucagon in patients with familial hyperglucagonemia elutes in the 9000- and 30,000-d range.[107]

Hypoproteinemia and, more consistently, marked hypoaminoacidemia have been frequently reported in patients with glucagonoma. In some patients, concentrations of several gluconeogenic amino acids including threonine, proline, arginine, and alanine were decreased to 10% of normal but returned to normal range after successful resection of the tumor.[108] The markedly decreased amino acid levels probably reflect enhanced hepatic ex-

traction. Regardless of the exact mechanism of hypoaminoacidemia, it has been suggested that the amino acid deficiency may be causally related to the dermopathy of the syndrome, because parenteral supplementation with amino acids may result in marked amelioration in skin rash, commensurate with the restoration of amino acid levels.[109]

GLUCOSE INTOLERANCE

Despite striking elevations of circulating glucagon levels, the glucose intolerance in this syndrome is usually only mild to moderately severe, reflecting the key role of pancreatic insulin reserve in determining the diabetic status. In some patients, hyperglycemia may worsen simply because of the infiltration of the normal pancreatic tissue by the tumor mass, spuriously suggesting a correlation between the rising glucagon levels and the glucose intolerance.[102] In patients in whom the tumor mass is not overwhelming, the peripheral insulin levels have been found to be normal or appropriately increased, in keeping with hyperglycemia. Development of ketoacidosis has been a rare occurrence[110]; when demonstrable, it probably reflects an insulin-deficient state due to an underlying true genetic diabetic trait.

Therapy

The skin lesions of the glucagonoma syndrome have been treated with various modalities including tropical corticosteroids, antifungal agents, oral tetracyclines, or zinc, with variable success rates. Rapid improvement of skin lesions was noted in two patients following prolonged infusions of somatostatin.[111] and in some patients after parental amino acid infusions or total parenteral nutrition.[109] The occasional spontaneous remissions of the dermopathy in the natural history present some difficulty in assessing the response to any of the therapeutic maneuvers.

The definitive treatment of glucagonoma syndrome consists of total excision of tumor, although this is feasible in only a minority of patients. When complete, a dramatic remission of the dermopathy and all the other manifestations of the syndrome has been reported. For the nonresectable tumors, most of which are accompanied by hepatic metastases, streptozocin has been the most frequently employed chemotherapy. The results have not been uniformly good. A combination of streptozocin and doxorubicin was found to be significantly more efficacious than streptozocin alone or streptozocin plus fluorouracil for the treatment of all forms of islet-cell carcinoma,[112] although enough experience with this regimen in glucagonoma is yet to be established. Encouraging results have also been obtained with dimethyltriazenoimidazole carboxamide (DTIC) in several patients with glucagonoma. In patients with hepatic-dominant metastases, hepatic artery occlusion by surgery or embolization, followed by chemotherapy, may be more effective than chemotherapy alone.[113] The effectiveness of a long-acting somatostatin analogue, octreotide, in suppressing glucagon release from inoperable tumors and associated clinical benefits were demonstrated in some patients.[114]

SOMATOSTATINOMA

The association of diabetes in patients with somatostatin-containing pancreatic tumors is part of a fascinating, although rare, clinical syndrome. The somatostatinoma syndrome also provides an opportunity to study the diverse pathophysiologic effects of chronic endogenous somatostatin excess resulting from such tumors.

Since the initial reports in 1977,[115,116] more than 20 patients with somatostatinoma-secreting pancreatic tumors have been well documented.[117] Occasionally, variable amounts of somatostatin may be an incidental finding in a variety of neuroendocrine tumors, reflecting the multihormonal heterogeneity of such tumors. In addition, there are more than 50 recorded cases of duodenal carcinoids containing somatostatin, frequently in association with neurofibromatosis type I.[117,118] Interestingly, almost all of the patients with pancreatic somatostatinoma had diabetes, whereas those with extrapancreatic somatostatinoma lacked diabetes, suggesting that a paracrine action of somatostatin in inhibiting islet hormone secretion, particularly insulin, might be the predominant diabetogenic mechanism in these patients. However, the presence of a number of other clinical manifestations, such as gallbladder disease (most common), diarrhea (with or without steatorrhea), hypo- or achlorhydria, weight loss, and anemia, in many of the patients would suggest that the markedly raised circulating somatostatin concentrations do produce expected multiple biologic effects in patients with this syndrome.[117] Table 25-5 presents a clinicopathologic classification of somatostatin-secreting tumors.

The diabetes in the patients with pancreatic somatostatinoma has generally been of mild to moderate severity, although in a few patients, significant ketosis and even ketoacidosis were present.[119,120] The immunoreactive insulin, glucagon, pancreatic polypeptide, and growth hormone levels were often blunted when measured. In all except a few of the patients, there was evidence of significant metastases by the time of diagnosis, culminating in fatal outcome or necessitating chemotherapy. In only one patient, successful excision of the pancreatic tumor resulted in complete disappearance of diabetes,[121] and she remains asymptomatic after 25 years. A follow-up arginine stimulation test in this patient revealed restoration of insulin, glucagon, and growth hormone responses, suggesting a causal relation between the patient's tumor and the induced metabolic aberrations. Another patient was free of symptoms, including remission of diabetes, 2 years after successful resection.[122]

The characterization of circulating and tissue somatostatin-like immunoreactivity (SLI) carried out in some of the patients revealed predominantly large-molecular-weight SLI, suggesting precursor secretory proteins.[117,123,124] In one patient, there was evidence of a greater release of precursor proteins from the metastatic than from the primary tumor tissue,[123] and in one patient the tumor cells could be grown in monolayer cultures and released somatostatin into the culture medium.[117] The ultrastructural and immunohistochemical studies in most of the reported patients revealed the presence of typical D cells as the predominant cell form in these tumors. However, multiple hormone production due to mixed cellularity of malignant islet cell tumors is not an uncommon occurrence. In some patients, the clinical symptoms from the secretion of a second or even third major hormone may result months to years following the initial diagnosis.[125] This may also explain the seemingly unrelated symptoms in certain patients thought to have "somatostatinoma" on a morphologic basis in whom the clinical presentation may be due to a different major hormonal secretion, such as insulin.[126,127] In several other patients, there was evidence of overproduction of calcitonin from the pancreatic tumor as seen by the immunohistochemical studies as well as by the markedly elevated plasma calcitonin levels in the absence of evidence for coexisting medullary carcinoma of thyroid. Of additional interest in this regard are the findings[117] of ectopic somatostatin-secreting cells in some patients with medullary carcinoma of thyroid, and in oat-cell tumors of lung. These findings support the theory of a common derivation of these three types of tumors among those from the amine precursor uptake decarboxylation (APUD) cellular origin.

The experience with chemotherapy in patients with metastatic somatostatinoma is limited. Several patients underwent treatment with streptozocin, 5-fluorouracil, or both, but long-term follow-up was generally disappointing. Newer regimens including doxorubicin in combination with streptozocin may hold promise, as shown for other forms of islet cell malignancies.[113]

GLUCOSE INTOLERANCE IN PATIENTS WITH OTHER TYPES OF ENDOCRINE TUMORS

Gastrinoma (Zollinger–Ellison) Syndrome

Glucose intolerance has occasionally been reported in patients with the Zollinger–Ellison (ZE) syndrome, chiefly characterized by (1) hypersecretion of gastric acid, (2) recurrent peptic ulcers, and

TABLE 25-5. Classification of Somatostatin-Producing Tumors

Type	Common Site(s) of Origin	Mode of Clinical Presentation	Associated Diseases or Syndromes	Cases Reported (n)
A	Pancreas	Somastatinoma syndrome (diabetes, cholelithiasis, diarrhea, anemia, hypochlorhydria)	—	20–25
B	Duodenal, ampullary, or periampullary mucosa	Abdominal pain, GI bleeding, biliary obstruction, incidental finding	Von Recklinghausen's neurofibromatosis, MEN type IIb syndrome, pheochromocytomas, paragangliomas, carcinoids elsewhere, carcinoma of pancreas	50–55
C	Pancreas, GI tract, paraganglia, thyroid, lung, etc.	Very variable: Cushing's syndrome, ZE syndrome, carcinoid syndrome, hypoglycemia	Celiac disease (one case)	15–20

Modified with permission from Ganda OP, Dayal Y. Somatostatin-producing tumors. In: Dayal Y, ed. *Endocrine Pathology of the Gut and Pancreas*. Boca Raton: CRC Press; 1991:241–277.

(3) a gastrin-producing tumor. The tumors of this type originate from the pancreas or, not infrequently, from the duodenum or from both sites. The cell of origin in pancreas is probably from a subset of D cells, and some evidence indicates that both gastrin and somatostatin may be secreted by the same D cells,[128] although others have been unable to detect gastrin in normal islets.[129]

The effect of hypergastrinemia associated with the ZE syndrome on pancreatic islet hormone secretion has not been studied in detail. It is, therefore, not clear if the glucose intolerance seen in some patients with ZE syndrome is causally related to gastrin overproduction. Moreover, in about 20–60% of patients with ZE syndrome,[130] other endocrine tumors coexist as part of the multiple endocrine neoplasia (MEN) syndrome, one or more of which may have diabetogenic effects (as is discussed later).

Pancreatic Cholera Syndrome

In 1958, Verner and Morrison described a syndrome characterized by severe watery, cholera-like diarrhea, hypokalemia, and achlorhydria (WDHA syndrome or Verner–Morrison syndrome) in association with an islet cell tumor and subsequently reviewed 55 patients with this entity.[131] Other clinical features of the syndrome include episodic flushing of skin, hypercalcemia, and hyperglycemia, the latter being found in about one-third of patients.[132] The possibility exists that glucose intolerance, at least in some patients, is related to the severe hypokalemia, an integral component of this syndrome.

Many, but not all, patients with this syndrome have elevated concentrations of vasoactive intestinal peptide (VIP). Several investigators have reported patients with classical pancreatic cholera syndrome with normal concentrations of VIP (pseudo-Verner–Morrison syndrome). In this latter situation, the nature of the causative agent(s) mediating the syndrome remains uncertain although a number of likely candidates have been proposed, including calcitonin, pancreatic polypeptide, prostaglandins, substance P, neurotensin, and peptide histidine-methionine (PHM), a peptide that shares a common precursor with VIP.[133]

Carcinoid Syndrome

Glucose intolerance is occasionally seen in patients with carcinoid syndrome, an endocrine disorder with protean manifestations.[134] Feldman and coworkers[135] showed an inhibitory effect of serotonin on insulin secretion in several experimental animals, and reported a potentiation of insulin secretion *in vitro* by a serotonin antagonist, methysergide maleate. These observations supported the concept of biogenic amines modulating insulin secretion. Subsequently, the same investigators studied a series of patients with carcinoid syndrome.[136] Glucose intolerance (by intravenous glucose tolerance testing) was documented in 8 of 10 patients with metastatic carcinoid tumors, presenting with the carcinoid syndrome and elevated serum serotonin levels. In contrast, all seven patients with metastatic carcinoid tumors but without the carcinoid syndrome (normal serotonin levels) had a normal IV glucose tolerance. Administration of a serotonin antagonist, cyproheptadine, or *p*-chlorophenylalanine, which blocks serotonin synthesis, resulted in enhanced insulin secretion and, in the latter instance, some improvement in glucose disposal rates. None of the patients in this series had evidence of overt diabetes, although oral glucose tolerance tests were not performed. Thus, subtle aberrations of carbohydrate metabolism may exist in patients with carcinoid syndrome.

Multiple Endocrine Neoplasia

As discussed previously, it is important to recognize that the clinical picture and differential diagnosis of several endocrine tumor syndromes are sometimes complicated by the fact that multiple hormones might be produced by one "specific" type of tumor, as reported in some patients with glucagonoma or somatostatinoma. Perhaps more commonly, the pathologic hypersecretion of several hormones occurs in an individual patient simply on the basis of multiple endocrine neoplasia. Three such constellations of multiple endocrine neoplasia (MEN) syndromes have been described, each as a familial syndrome with autosomal dominant inheritance.[137] MEN type I (Wermer's syndrome) most frequently consists of the involvement of the pituitary gland, pancreatic islets, and parathyroids, sometimes in association with tumors of the adrenal cortex or thyroid, or with carcinoid tumors, lipomas, or thymomas. Of the pancreatic tumors present in 60–80% of patients with MEN I, gastrinomas and insulinomas are the ones most frequently observed. MEN type IIA (Sipple's syndrome) is characterized by pheochromocytoma, hyperparathyroidism, and medullary carcinoma of the thyroid. A variant of the syndrome, MEN type IIB, consists of pheochromocytoma, medullary carcinoma of the thyroid, mucosal neuromas, hyperplastic corneal nerves, and marfanoid habitus. However, overlap between these MEN categories does occur, so that it is not certain if these are distinct genetic syndromes and discrete classification types.[137] Recently, a MEN type II gene was identified on chromosome 10 and a MEN I gene on chromosome 11q13.[138,139] Mutations in the RET protooncogene have been identified in MEN IIA and IIB syndromes, but the role of this gene product in the pathogenesis of diabetes remains uncertain. The RET protooncogene is a transmembrane tyrosine kinase receptor whose overexpression in transgenic mice results in medullary thyroid cancer but not glucose intolerance syndromes.[140]

POEMS Syndrome

POEMS syndrome (polyneuropathy, organomegaly, endocrinopathy, monoclonal gammopathy, and skin changes), also known as Krow–Fukasi syndrome, is a rare form of plasma cell disorder associated with osteosclerotic myeloma. About 100 cases have been reported.[141] The endocrine components of this syndrome include diabetes, hypogonadism with or without hyperprolactinemia, hypothyroidism, and adrenal insufficiency. Polyneuropathy is almost always a clinically manifested feature along with IgG or IgA type M protein and lambda-type light chain. Glucose intolerance, sometimes requiring insulin, has been reported in 30–50% of cases.[142]

REFERENCES

1. Porte D Jr: Banting lecture 1990. Beta-cells in type II diabetes mellitus. *Diabetes* 1991;40:166.
2. Houssay B: The hypophysis and metabolism. *N Engl J Med* 1936; 214:961.
3. Young FG: The relationship of the anterior pituitary gland to carbohydrate metabolism. *Br Med J* 1939;2:393.
4. Luft R, Guillemin R: Growth hormone and diabetes in man. Old concepts—new implications. *Diabetes* 1974;23:783.
5. Press M: Growth hormone and metabolism. *Diabetes Metab Rev* 1988;4:391.
6. Casanueva FF: Physiology of growth hormone secretion and action. *Endocrinol Metab Clin North Am* 1992;21:483.

7. Davidson MB: Effect of growth hormone on carbohydrate and lipid metabolism. *Endocr Rev* 1987;8:115.
8. Lewis UJ: Variants of growth hormone and prolactin and their post-translational modifications. *Annu Rev Physiol* 1984;46:33.
9. Sinha YN, Jacobsen BP: Human growth hormone (hGH)-(44-191), a reportedly diabetogenic fragment of hGH, circulates in human blood: measurement by radioimmunoassay. *J Clin Endocrinol Metab* 1994; 78:1411.
10. Ng FM, *et al*: The minimal amino acid sequence of the insulin-potentiating fragments of human growth hormone: Its mechanism of action. *Diabetes* 1980;29:782.
11. Zierler KL, Rabinowitz D: Roles of insulin and growth-hormone on studies of forearm metabolism in man. *Medicine* 1863;42:385.
12. Harant I, *et al*: Response of fat cells to growth hormone (GH): Effect of long term treatment with recombinant human GH in GH-deficient adults. *J Clin Endocrinol Metab* 1994;78:1392.
13. McGorman LR, Rizza RA, Gerich JE: Physiological concentrations of growth-hormone exert insulin-like and insulin antagonistic effects on both hepatic and extrahepatic tissues in man. *J Clin Endocrinol Metab* 1981;53:556.
14. Brautsch-Marrain PR, Smith D, Defronzo RA: The effect of growth hormone on glucose metabolism and insulin secretion in man. *J Clin Endocrinol Metab* 1982;55:973.
15. Rizza RA, Mandarino LJ, Gerich JE: Effects of growth hormone on insulin action in man. Mechanisms of insulin resistance, impaired suppression of glucose production, and impaired stimulation of glucose utilization. *Diabetes* 1982;31:663.
16. Rosenfeld RG, *et al*: Both human pituitary growth hormone and recombinant DNA-derived human growth hormone cause insulin resistance at a postreceptor site. *J Clin Endocrinol Metab* 1982;54:1033.
17. Pierluissi J, Campbell J: Metasomatotrophic diabetes and its induction: basal insulin secretion and insulin release responses to glucose, glucagon, arginine and meals. *Diabetologia* 1980;18:223.
18. Baumann G: Growth hormone-binding proteins: State of the art. *J Endocrinol* 1994;141:1.
19. Amit T, Youdim MB, Hochberg Z: Clinical review 112: Does serum growth hormone (GH) binding protein reflect human GH receptor function? *J Clin Endocrinol Metab* 2000;85:927.
20. Van Wyk JJ, Underwood LE: Relation between growth hormone and somatomedin. *Ann Intern Med* 1975;26:426.
21. Golde DW, *et al*: Growth factors. *Ann Intern Med* 1980;92:650.
22. Wass JA, *et al*: An assessment of glucose intolerance in acromegaly and its response to medical treatment. *Clin Endocrinol* 1980;12:53.
23. Nabarro JD: Acromegaly. *Clin Endocrinol* 1987;26:481.
24. Molitch ME: Clinical manifestations of acromegaly. *Endocrinol Metab Clin North Am* 1992;21:597.
25. Ezzat S, *et al*: Acromegaly. Clinical and biochemical features in 500 patients. *Medicine* 1994;73:233.
26. Ganda OP, Simonson DS: Growth-hormone, acromegaly and diabetes. *Diabet Rev* 1993;1:286.
27. Hansen I, *et al*: Insulin resistance in acromegaly: Defects in both hepatic and extrahepatic insulin action. *Am J Physiol* 1986;250:E269.
28. Rieu M, *et al*: The importance of insulin-like growth factor (somatomedin) measurements in the diagnosis and surveillance of acromegaly. *J Clin Endocrinol Metab* 1982;55:147.
29. Grinspoon S, *et al*: Serum insulin-like growth factor-binding protein-3 levels in the diagnosis of acromegaly. *J Clin Endocrinol Metab* 1995;80:927.
30. Muggeo M, *et al*: The insulin resistance of acromegaly: Evidence for two alterations in the insulin receptor on circulating monocytes. *J Clin Endocrinol Metab* 1979;48:17.
31. Muggeo M, *et al*: Insulin receptor on moncytes from patients with acromegaly and fasting hyperglycemia. *J Clin Endocrinol Metab* 1983;56:733.
32. Gerich JE, *et al*: Effects of physiologic levels of glucagon and growth hormone on human carbohydrate and lipid metabolism. Studies involving administration of exogenous hormone during suppression of endogenous hormone secretion with somatostatin. *J Clin Invest* 1976; 57:875.
33. Metcalfe P, *et al*: Metabolic effects of acute and prolonged growth hormone excess in normal and insulin-deficient man. *Diabetologia* 1981;20:123.
34. Moller N, *et al*: Basal- and insulin-stimulated substrate metabolism in patients with active acromegaly before and after adenomectomy. *J Clin Endocrinol Metab* 1992;74:1012.
35. Giustina A, *et al*: Criteria for cure of acromegaly: A consensus statement. *J Clin Endocrinol Metab* 2000;85:526.
36. Bates AS, *et al*: An audit of outcome of treatment in acromegaly. *Q J Med* 1993;86:293.
37. Rajasoorya C, *et al*: Determinants of clinical outcome and survival in acromegaly. *Clin Endocrinol* 1994;41:95.
38. Colao A, *et al*: Systemic hypertension and impaired glucose tolerance are independently correlated to the severity of the acromegalic cardiomyopathy. *J Clin Endocrinol Metab* 2000;85:193.
39. Sassolas G, Harris AG, James-Deidier A: Long term effect of incremental doses of the somatostatin analog SMS 201-995 in 58 acromegalic patients. French SMS 201-995 approximately equal to Acromegaly Study Group. *J Clin Endocrinol Metab* 1990;71:391.
40. Newman CB, *et al*: Safety and efficacy of long-term octreotide therapy of acromegaly: Results of a multicenter trial in 103 patients—a clinical research center study. *J Clin Endocrinol Metab* 1995;80:2768.
41. Ho KK, *et al*: Impact of octreotide, a long-acting somatostatin analogue, on glucose tolerance and insulin sensitivity in acromegaly. *Clin Endocrinol* 1992;36:271.
42. Breidert M, *et al*: Long-term effect of octreotide in acromegaly on insulin resistance. *Horm Metab Res* 1995;27:226.
43. Trainer PJ, *et al*: Treatment of acromegaly with the growth hormone-receptor antagonist pegvisomant. *N Engl J Med* 2000;342:1171.
44. Daughaday WH, Kipnis DM: The growth-promoting and anti-insulin actions of somatotropin. *Recent Prog Horm Res* 1966;22:49.
45. Martin JM, Gagliardino JJ: Effect of growth hormone on the isolated pancreatic islets of rat in vitro. *Nature* 1967;213:630.
46. Rabinovitch A, Quigley C, Rechler MM: Growth hormone stimulates islet β-cell replication in neonatal rat pancreatic monolayer cultures. *Diabetes* 1983;32:307.
47. Merimee TJ, *et al*: Diabetes mellitus and sexual ateliotic dwarfism: A comparative study. *J Clin Invest* 1970;49:1096.
48. Merimee TJ: A follow-up study of vascular disease in growth-hormone-deficient dwarfs with diabetes. *N Engl J Med* 1978; 298:1217.
49. Thomas AM, Berglund L: Growth hormone and cardiovascular disease: An area in rapid growth. *J Clin Endocrinol Metab* 2001; 86:1871.
50. Colao A, *et al*: Improved cardiovascular risk factors and cardiac performance after 12 months of growth hormone (GH) replacement in young adult patients with GH deficiency. *J Clin Endocrinol Metab* 2001;86:1874.
51. Beshyah SA, *et al*: The effects of short and long-term growth hormone replacement therapy in hypopituitary adults on lipid metabolism and carbohydrate tolerance. *J Clin Endocrinol Metab* 1995;80: 356.
52. Rosenfalck AM, *et al*: The effect of 30 months of low-dose replacement therapy with recombinant human growth hormone (rhGH) on insulin and C-peptide kinetics, insulin secretion, insulin sensitivity, glucose effectiveness, and body composition in GH-deficient adults. *J Clin Endocrinol Metab* 2000;85:4173.
53. Koller EA, *et al*: Retinal changes mimicking diabetic retinopathy in two nondiabetic, growth hormone-treated patients. *J Clin Endocrinol Metab* 1998;83:2380.
54. Czernichow P, *et al*: Growth hormone treatment and diabetes: Survey of the Kabi Pharmacia international growth study. *Acta Paediatr Scand Suppl* 1991;379:104.
55. Thorner MO: Critical evaluation of the safety of recombinant human growth hormone administration: Statement from the Growth Hormone Research Society. *J Clin Endocrinol Metab* 2001;86:1868.
56. Landgraf R, *et al*: Prolactin: A diabetogenic hormone. *Diabetologia* 1977;13:99.
57. Gustafson AB, *et al*: Correlation of hyperprolactinemia with altered plasma insulin and glucagon: Similarity to effects of late human pregnancy. *J Clin Endocrinol Metab* 1980;51:242.
58. Hanssen KF, *et al*: Plasma prolactin in juvenile diabetics. 24-h studies with somatostatin. *Diabetologia* 1978;15:369.
59. Hanssen KF, Torjesen PA: Increased serum prolactin in diabetic ketoacidosis: Correlation between serum sodium and serum prolacting concentration. *Acta Endocrinol* 1977;85:372.
60. Naejie R, *et al*: Prolactin response to TRH in diabetic ketoacidosis. *Diabetologia* 1979;16:381.
61. Cahill GFJ: Actions of adrenal corical steroids on carbohydrate metabolism. In: Christy NP, ed. *The Human Adrenal Cortex*. New York: Harper and Row; 1971.

62. Boyle PJ: Cushing's disease. *Diabetes Rev* 1993;1:301.
63. Rizza RA, Mandarino LJ, Gerich JE, Cortisol-induced insulin resistance in man: Impaired suppression of glucose production and stimulation of glucose utilization due to a postreceptor defect of insulin action. *J Clin Endocrinol Metab* 1982;54:131.
64. Dimitriadis G, *et al*: Effects of glucocorticoid excess on the sensitivity of glucose transport and metabolism to insulin in rat skeletal muscle. *Biochem J* 1997;321:707.
65. Pedersen SB, Jonler M, Richelsen B: Characterization of regional and gender differences in glucocorticoid receptors and lipoprotein lipase activity in human adipose tissue. *J Clin Endocrinol Metab* 1994; 78:1354.
66. Rebuffe-Scrive J, *et al*: Muscle and adipose tissue morphology and metabolism in Cushing's syndrome. *J Clin Endocrinol Metab.* 1988; 67:1122.
67. Lambillotte C, Gilon P, Henquin JC: Direct glucocorticoid inhibition of insulin secretion. An in vitro study of dexamethasone effects in mouse islets. *J Clin Invest* 1997;99:414.
68. Ganda OP: Secondary forms of diabetes. In: Kahn CR, Weir, GC, eds. *Joslin's Diabetes Mellitus.* Philadelphia: Lea & Febiger; 1994.
69. Marco J, *et al*: Hyperglucagonism induced by glucocorticoid treatment in man. *N Engl J Med* 1973;288:128.
70. Wise JK, Hendler R, Felig P: Influence of glucocorticoids on glucagon secretion and plasma amino acid concentrations in man. *J Clin Invest* 1973;52:2774.
71. Cryer PE: Catecholamines, pheochromocytoma, and diabetes. *Diabetes Rev* 1993;1:309.
72. Strickland WG, Blackmore PF, Exton JH: The role of calcium in alpha-adrenergic inactivation of glycogen synthase in rat hepatocytes and its inhibition by insulin. *Diabetes* 1980;29:617.
73. Garber AJ, Karl IE, Kipnis DM: Alanine and glutamine synthesis and release from skeletal muscle. IV. Beta-adrenergic inhibition of amino acid release. *J Biol Chem* 1976;251:851.
74. Sacca L, *et al*: Influence of epinephrine, norepinephrine, and isoproterenol on glucose homeostasis in normal man. *J Clin Endocrinol Metab* 1980;50:680.
75. Robertson RP, Halter JB, Porte D Jr: A role for alpha-adrenergic receptors in abnormal insulin secretion in diabetes mellitus. *J Clin Invest* 1976;57:791.
76. Dunning BE, Taborsky GJ Jr: Galanin—sympathetic neurotransmitter in endocrine pancreas? *Diabetes* 1988;37:1157.
77. Palmer JP, Porte DJ: Neural control of glucagon secretion. In: Lefebvre PJ, ed. *Glucagon II.* New York: Springer-Verlag; 1983.
78. Stenstrom G, Sjostrom L, Smith U: Diabetes mellitus in phaeochromocytoma. Fasting blood glucose levels before and after surgery in 60 patients with phaeochromocytoma. *Acta Endocrinol* 1984;106:511.
79. Jones I, Dohm G: Regulation of glucose transporter GLUT-4 and hexokinase II gene transcription by insulin and epinephrine. *AJP Endocrinol Metab* 1997;273;E682.
80. Hamaji M: Pancreatic alpha- and beta-cell function in pheochromocytoma. *J Clin Endocrinol Metab* 1979;49:322.
81. Bolli G, *et al*: Circulating catecholamine and glucagon responses to insulin-induced blood glucose decrement in a patient with pheochromocytoma. *J Clin Endocrinol Metab* 1982;54:447.
82. Sicolo N, *et al*: Endocrine pancreatic function in pheochromocytoma. *J Endocrinol Invest* 1991;14:225.
83. Conn JW: Hypertension, the potassium ion and impaired carbohydrate tolerance. *N Engl J Med* 1965;273:1135.
84. Podolsky S, Melby JC: Improvement of growth hormone response to stimulation in primary aldosteronism with correction of potassium deficiency. *Metabolism* 1976;25:1027.
85. Sagild U, Anderson V, Andreasen PB: Glucose tolerance and insulin responsiveness in experimental potassium depletion. *Acta Med Scand* 1961;169:243.
86. Grunfeld C, Chappell DA: Hypokalemia and diabetes mellitus. *Am J Med* 1983;75:553.
87. Maxon HR, Kreines KW, Goldsmith RE: Long-term observations of glucose tolerance in thyrotoxic patients. *Arch Intern Med* 1975; 135:1477.
88. Loeb JN: Metabolic changes in thyrotoxicosis. In: Braverman LE, Utiger RD, eds. *Werner and Inbar's the Thyroid.* Philadelphia: Lipincott; 1996.
89. O'Meara NM, *et al*: Alterations in the kinetics of C-peptide and insulin secretion in hyperthyroidism. *J Clin Endocrinol Metab* 1993; 76:79.
90. Gonzalo MA, *et al*: Glucose tolerance, insulin secretion, insulin sensitivity and glucose effectiveness in normal and overweight hyperthyroid women. *Clin Endocrinol* 1996;45:689.
91. Randin JP, *et al*: Insulin sensitivity and exogenous insulin clearance in Graves' disease. Measurement by the glucose clamp technique and continuous indirect calorimetry. *Diabetes* 1986;35:178.
92. Beylot M, *et al*: Increased ketonaemia in hyperthyroidism. Evidence for a beta-adrenergic mechanism. *Diabetologia* 1980;19:505.
93. Cooppan R, Kozak GP: Hyperthyroidism and diabetes mellitus. An analysis of 70 patients. *Arch Intern Med* 1980;140:370.
94. Payami H, Joe S, Thomson, G. Autoimmune thyroid disease in type I diabetic families. *Genet Epidemiol* 1989;6:137.
95. Yasuda K, *et al*: Glucose tolerance and insulin secretion in patients with parathyroid disorders. Effect of serum calcium on insulin release. *N Engl J Med* 1975;292:501.
96. Kalkhoff RK, *et al*: Plasma alpha-cell glucagon in primary hyperparathyroidism. *Metabolism* 1976;25:769.
97. Taylor WH, Khaleeli AA: Coincident diabetes mellitus and primary hyperparathyroidism. *Diabetes Metab Res Rev* 2001;17:175.
98. Harter HR, *et al*: The relative roles of calcium, phosphorus, and parathyroid hormone in glucose- and tolbutamide-mediated insulin release. *J Clin Invest* 1976;58:359.
99. DeFronzo RA, Lang R: Hypophosphatemia and glucose intolerance: Evidence for tissue insentivity to insulin. *N Engl J Med* 1980; 303:1259.
100. Amend WJ Jr, *et al*: The influence of serum calcium and parathyroid hormone upon glucose metabolism in uremia. *J Lab Clin Med* 1975; 86:435.
101. Akgun S, Ertel NH: Hyperparathyroidism and coexisting diabetes mellitus. Altered carbohydrate metabolism. *Arch Intern Med* 1978; 138:1500.
102. Leichter SB: Clinical and metabolic aspects of glucagonoma. *Medicine* 1980;59:100.
103. Stapoole PW: The glucagonoma syndrome: Clinical features, diagnosis and treatment. *Endocr Rev* 1980;2:347.
104. Polak JM, Bloom SR: Glucagon-producing tumors and the glucagonoma syndrome. In: Dayal Y, ed. *Endocrine Pathology of the Gut and Pancreas.* Boca Raton: CRC Press; 1991.
105. Sweet RD: A dermatosis specifically associated with a tumour of pancreatic alpha cells. *Br J Dermatol* 1974;90:301.
106. Ensinck JW, Palmer JP: Dominant inheritance of large molecular weight species of glucagon. *Metabolism* 1976;25:1409.
107. Boden G, Owen OE: Familial hyperglucagonemia—an autosomal dominant disorder. *N Engl J Med* 1977;296:534.
108. Boden G, *et al*: An islet cell carcinoma containing glucagon and insulin. Chronic glucagon excess and glucose homeostasis. *Diabetes* 1977;26:128.
109. Norton JA, *et al*: Amino acid deficiency and the skin rash associated with glucagonoma. *Ann Intern Med* 1979;91:213.
110. Domen RE, *et al*: The glucagonoma syndrome. Report of a case. *Arch Intern Med* 1980;140:262.
111. Sohier J, *et al*: Rapid improvement of skin lesions in glucagonomas with intravenous somatostatin infusions. *Lancet* 1980;1:40.
112. Moertel CG, *et al*: Streptozocin-doxorubicin, streptozocin-fluorouracil or chlorozotocin in the treatment of advanced islet-cell carcinoma. *N Engl J Med* 1992;326:519.
113. Moertel CG, *et al*: The management of patients with advanced carcinoid tumors and islet cell carcinomas. *Ann Intern Med* 1994; 1204:302.
114. Boden G, *et al*: Treatment of inoperable glucagonoma with the long-acting somatostatin analogue SMS 201-995. *N Engl J Med* 1986; 314:1686.
115. Ganda OP, *et al.*: "Somatostatinoma": A somatostatin-containing tumor of the endocrine pancreas. *N Engl J Med* 1977;296:963.
116. Larsson LI, *et al*: Pancreatic somatostatinoma. Clinical features and physiological implications. *Lancet* 1977;1:666.
117. Ganda OM, Dayal, Y: Somatostatin-producing tumors. In Dayal Y, ed. *Endocrine Pathology of the Gut and Pancreas.* Boca Raton: CRC Press; 1991.
118. Erbe RW: A 52-year-old man with neurofibromatosis and jaundice. *N Engl J Med* 1989;320:996.
119. Axelrod L, *et al*: Malignant somatostatinoma: Clinical features and metabolic studies. *J Clin Endocrinol Metab* 1981;52:886.
120. Jackson JA, *et al*: Malignant somatostatinoma presenting with diabetic ketoacidosis. *Clin Endocrinol* 1987;26:609.

121. Ganda OP, Soeldner JS: "Somatostatinoma": Follow-up studies. *N Engl J Med* 1977;297:1352.

122. Kelly TR: Pancreatic somatostatinoma. *Am J Surg* 1983;146:671.

123. Conlon JM, *et al*: Characterization of somatostatin-like components in the tumors and plasma of a patient with a somatostatinoma. *J Clin Endocrinol Metab* 1981;52:66.

124. Patel YC, Ganda OP, Benoit R: Pancreatic somatostatinoma: Abundance of somatostatin-28(1-12)-like immunoreactivity in tumor and plasma. *J Clin Endocrinol Metab* 1983;57:1048.

125. Wynick D, Williams SJ, Bloom SR: Symptomatic secondary hormone syndromes in patients with established malignant pancreatic endocrine tumors. *N Engl J Med* 1989;319:605.

126. Wright J, *et al*: Pancreatic somatostatinoma presenting with hypoglycaemia. *Clin Endocrinol* 1980;12:603.

127. Pipeleers D, *et al*: Five cases of somatostatinoma: Clinical heterogeneity and diagnostic usefulness of basal and tolbutamide-induced hypersomatostatinemia. *J Clin Endocrinol Metab* 1983;56:1236.

128. Erlandsen SL, *et al*: Pancreatic islet cell hormones distribution of cell types in the islet and evidence for the presence of somatostatin and gastrin within the D cell. *J Histochem Cytochem* 1976;24:883.

129. Lotrstra F, Vanderloo W, Gepts W: Are gastrin cells present in mammalian pancreatic islets? *Diabetologia* 1974;10:291.

130. Pipeleers-Marichal M, *et al*: Gastrinomas in the duodenums of patients with multiple endocrine neoplasia type 1 and the Zollinger-Ellison syndrome. *N Engl J Med* 1990;322:723.

131. Verner JV, Morrison AB: Endocrine pancreatic islet disease with diarrhea. Report of a case due to diffuse hyperplasia of nonbeta islet tissue with a review of 54 additional cases. *Arch Intern Med* 1974;133:492.

132. Walsh JH, *et al*: Gastrointestinal hormones in clinical disease: Recent developments. *Ann Intern Med* 1979;90:817.

133. Yiangou Y, *et al*: Peptide histidine-methionine immunoreactivity in plasma and tissue from patients with vasoactive intestinal peptide-secreting tumors and watery diarrhea syndrome. *J Clin Endocrinol Metab* 1987;64:131.

134. Creutzfeldt W, Stockmann F: Carcinoids and carcinoid syndrome. *Am J Med* 1987;82:4.

135. Feldman JM, Quickel KE Jr, Lebovitz HE: Potentiation of insulin secretion in vitro by serotonin antagonists. *Diabetes* 1972;21:779.

136. Feldman JM: Glucose intolerance in the carcinoid syndrome. *Diabetes* 1975;24:664.

137. DeLillis RA: The multiple endocrine neoplasia syndromes. In: Dayal Y, ed. *Endocrine Pathology of the Gut and Pancreas*. Boca Raton: CRC Press; 1991.

138. Ponder BA: The gene causing multiple endocrine neoplasia type 2 (MEN 2). *Ann Med* 1994;26:199.

139. Larsson C, Friedman E: Localization and identification of the multiple endocrine neoplasia type 1 disease gene. *Endocrinol Metab Clin North Am* 1994;23:67.

140. Kawai K, *et al*: Tissue-specific carcinogenesis in transgenic mice expressing the RET protooncogene with a multiple endocrine neoplasia type 2A mutation. *Cancer Res* 2000;60:5254.

141. Miralles GD, O'Fallon JR, Talley NJ: Plasma-cell dyscrasia with polyneuropathy. The spectrum of POEMS syndrome. *N Engl J Med* 1992;327:1919.

142. Soubrier MJ, Dubost JJ, Sauvezie BJ: POEMS syndrome: A study of 25 cases and a review of the literature. French study group on POEMS syndrome. *Am J Med* 1994;97:543.

Nutritional Management of the Person with Diabetes

Abhimanyu Garg

Joyce P. Barnett

INTRODUCTION

Nutritional guidelines for patients with diabetes mellitus have been changing over the past century based on new scientific knowledge. The American Diabetes Association (ADA) Task Force on Nutritional Guidelines made major revisions compared to the previous guidelines of 1994.[1] Most recently, evidence-based nutrional guidelines have been proposed.[2] These guidelines address the importance of optimizing plasma glucose and lipid levels, as well as issues related to growth and development, pregnancy and lactation, aging, prevention of short- and long-term complications, and overall optimal health through good nutrition. Nutritional management, or medical nutrition therapy, is an integral component of overall management of diabetes, but is extremely challenging to implement successfully. The goal of nutrition therapy "is to assist individuals with diabetes in making changes in nutrition and exercise habits leading to improved metabolic control."[1,3] Specific goals of therapy are outlined in Table 26-1. The purpose of this chapter is to review the scientific rationale for nutritional management and provide practical insight on how to implement nutrition therapy to optimize diabetes management.

HISTORICAL PERSPECTIVE

The earliest known recommendations for treatment of diabetes included references to what we now consider to be carbohydrate-containing foods. Even then the debate was whether a high-carbohydrate or a low-carbohydrate diet was most beneficial for someone with diabetes. In the 1600s and 1700s this controversy continued. In the 1800s attention was given for the first time to specific amounts of foods, when it was recognized that amino acids could yield glucose in the body via gluconeogenesis.[4] Prior to the discovery of insulin in 1921, the primary treatment for diabetes mellitus was an extremely low-energy, low-carbohydrate diet (Table 26-2).[3] Although the ADA guidelines somewhat liberalized carbohydrate intake in the 1950s, the focus continued to be primarily on restriction of carbohydrate until the 1970s. The longer survival of people with diabetes that resulted from improved treatment then shifted attention to long-term complications. The increased risk for cardiovascular disease in individuals with diabetes shifted the focus toward restriction of dietary fats, particularly saturated fats, and cholesterol, which received increasing emphasis through the 1980s and into the 1990s. This led to further liberalization of carbohydrate intake. The recommendations issued in 1994 and 2002 are based to a greater degree on scientific evidence and less on clinical practice than previously issued recommendations. Recent studies have emphasized the importance of rigorous glycemic control in the prevention of long-term diabetic complications, and therefore greater emphasis on nutritional management should help achieve normoglycemia.[5,6]

The most recent ADA guidelines emphasize the importance of individualizing the nutrition prescription to meet specific goals of therapy for each patient, and allow for more variation in proportion of energy from carbohydrate and fat and limited variation in protein intake (10–20%), depending on individual needs. The focus for carbohydrate intake shifted away from restriction of sugar, or sucrose, to the total amount of carbohydrate included in the diet. Based on scientific evidence, sucrose can be incorporated into the meal plan as a part of an overall healthful diet.[1] In recognition of the difficulty of the task of nutritional management of patients with diabetes, the concept of a coordinated team approach was expanded to include an active role for the patient.

NUTRITION RECOMMENDATIONS

Energy Needs

The most important decision for nutrition management in patients with diabetes involves deciding the appropriate total energy intake, which may differ from patient to patient (Tables 26-3 and 26-4).[7] During childhood and adolescence, patients with type 1 diabetes mellitus (T1DM) need extra energy for normal growth and development. Pregnant and lactating women also have increased energy demands, and total energy intake should be appropriately increased in such patients. Because most patients with type 2 diabetes mellitus (T2DM) are obese, usually total energy intake should be less than that needed for weight maintenance. After achieving reasonable body weight, it can be adjusted to maintain body weight and prevent future weight gain. However, in some instances, when patients with T2DM have lost considerable weight, such as at the time of diagnosis of diabetes mellitus or during chronic infections, severe illness, a postoperative period, or chronic severe hyperglycemia, they may in fact need extra energy beyond that needed for weight maintenance. Such patients lose not only body fat but also lean body mass that needs to be recovered.

TABLE 26-1 Goals of Medical Nutrition Therapy

- Maintenance of as near-normal blood glucose levels as possible by balancing food intake with insulin (either endogenous or exogenous) or oral glucose-lowering medications and physical activity levels
- Achievement of optimal serum lipid levels
- Provision of adequate calories for maintaining or attaining reasonable weights for adults, normal growth and development rates in children and adolescents, increased metabolic needs during pregnancy and lactation, or recovery from catabolic illnesses
- Prevention and treatment of the acute complications of insulin-treated diabetes such as hypoglycemia, short-term illnesses, and exercise-related problems, and of the long-term complications of diabetes such as renal disease, autonomic neuropathy, hypertension, and cardiovascular disease
- Improvement of overall health through optimal nutrition

Source: Modified with permission from American Diabetes Association.[3]

TABLE 26-2 Historical Perspective of Nutrition Recommendations

| Year | Distribution of Calories (%) | | |
	Carbohydrate	Protein	Fat
Before 1921		Starvation diets	
1921	20	10	70
1950	40	20	40
1971	45	20	35
1986	≤60	12–20	<30
1994, 2002	*	10–20	<30[†]

* Amount of carbohydrate and cis-monounsaturated fat is based on nutritional assessment and treatment goals.

†Less than 10% of calories from saturated fats.

Source: Reprinted with permission from American Diabetes Association.[3]

TABLE 26-3 Estimating Energy Requirements for Adults

Basal energy requirements:	20–25 kcal/kg (80–100 kJ/kg) of desirable body weight
*Adjustment of additional energy required for activity level:	
Sedentary	30% of estimated basal energy requirements
Moderate	50% of estimated basal energy requirements
Strenuous	100% of estimated basal energy requirements
*Adjustments:	
During pregnancy (2nd and 3rd trimester)	Add 300 kcal (1250 kJ) per day
During lactation	Add 500 kcal (2100 kJ) per day
For weight gain (0.5 kg/wk)	Add 500 kcal (2100 kJ) per day
For weight loss (0.5 kg/wk)	Subtract 500 kcal (2100 kJ) per day

*Adjustments are approximate; weight changes should be monitored and compared to energy intake.

TABLE 26-4 Estimating Energy Requirements for Children and Adolescents

Age in Years	kcal(kJ)/kg body weight*
≤3	~100 (~400)
4–6	90 (375)
7–10	70 (300)
11–14 Males	55 (230)
15–18 Males	45 (190)
11–14 Females	47 (200)
15–18 Females	40 (165)

*Adjustments may be needed for activity level and other individuals variations.

Source: National Research Council.[7]

Obesity is a major predisposing factor for T2DM; thus reduced energy intake is an important aspect of management for these patients as well as for prevention of diabetes in susceptible individuals. Some patients with T2DM are prone to truncal obesity as well as generalized excess body fat.[8,9] Beyond the detrimental effects of overall adiposity, distribution of body fat, particularly in the truncal region, further predisposes subjects to insulin resistance. In addition, the threshold for developing insulin resistance in response to adiposity may vary in different ethnic groups as well among individuals belonging to the same ethnic group.[8,10,11] Therefore, even mild increases in truncal subcutaneous fat and intra-abdominal fat can lead to insulin resistance in susceptible subjects. Patients who are not considered overweight by weight-for-height standards may have excess adiposity, and thus could also benefit from reduction of body fat. Interestingly, even small amounts of weight loss (5–10%) can markedly improve glycemic control and serum lipid levels.[12–15]

Controversy exists over whether high-carbohydrate or high-fat diets are more effective in causing weight loss. Studies show that if reduction of total energy intake is similar, the diets cause equal loss of body weight.[16] On the other hand, studies conducted in the United States revealed that total energy consumption was higher on a high-fat diet compared to a high-carbohydrate diet.[17,18] However, whether this excess energy intake on high-fat diets continues for the long term remains unclear. Since people in the United States tend to consume high-fat diets, whether other groups such as Asians or Africans who are habituated to high-carbohydrate diets will also tend to consume extra energy when given high-fat diets remains unclear. Therefore, the major emphasis should be on reduction of total energy intake.

Two approaches may be considered for reduction of total energy intake: a very-low-calorie diet (VLCD) or a low-calorie diet (LCD). The very-low-calorie diet (less than 800 kcal or 3350 kJ per day) will promote rapid weight loss and lead to reduction of blood pressure and serum glucose and lipid levels. The VLCD may be either a food-based plan or a liquid formula. To safely implement the VLCD, close medical supervision is required. Care must be taken to include adequate protein (1.0–1.4 g/kg of ideal body weight per day), vitamins, electrolytes, and fluids. Side effects of VLCDs include rapid loss of lean body mass, electrolyte imbalance, cardiac arrhythmias, gout, and gallstones. Less serious side effects include hair loss, anemia, cold intolerance, constipation, fatigue, and menstrual irregularities. VLCDs should only be used for those with body mass index (BMI) greater than 30 kg/m², not for mildly overweight individuals.[19] There is some evidence that VLCDs may produce disordered binge eating in some people.[20] Even though short-term weight loss is greater on VLCDs, the long-term results (i.e., producing weight loss after 1 year) are no more effective than a low-calorie diet.[21] The preferred approach to energy reduction is the LCD (800–1500 kcal or 3350–6300 kJ per day). This approach represents a reduction of 500–1000 kcal (2100–4200 kJ) per day to produce weight loss of 0.5–1 kg per week.[22] However, reduction in energy intake of 1000 kcal (4200 kJ) per day, a significant change in food habits for most individuals, can be difficult to sustain for an extended period of time.

An alternative approach is to reduce energy intake by 250–500 kcal (1050–2100 kJ) per day to promote gradual weight loss of approximately 0.25–0.5 kg per week.[1] Gradual changes in types of foods and moderate reduction in portion size can lead to gradual weight loss that is more likely to be sustained over the extended period most obese individuals will need to achieve their goal weight.

Some people claim that high-protein, low-carbohydrate diets promote weight loss. They suggest that carbohydrate intake, by stimulating insulin secretion, contributes to insulin resistance, obesity, and other metabolic abnormalities, and therefore should be reduced. However, such diets have not been investigated clinically. Proposed benefits of the low-carbohydrate diet are initial rapid weight loss and short-term improvements in serum lipids. The low-carbohydrate intake of some of these diets leads to induction of ketosis. Studies of ketogenic diets used to control seizures in children have reported adverse effects such as an increased risk of kidney stones, as well as constipation and dehydration. Other relevant but less common side effects associated with use of ketogenic diets include hyperlipidemia, impaired neutrophil function, osteoporosis, and optic neuropathy.[23,24] Very-low-energy ketogenic diets have also been reported to have a negative effect on cognitive function.[25]

High protein intake can lead to hypercalciuria, hyperuricemia, and hypocitraturia that can contribute to kidney stone formation, gout, and possible reduction in bone density.[26–29] Most individuals can tolerate unlimited intake of high-protein, high-fat foods for only a short time, leading to decreased total energy intake and thus weight loss. The limited variety of food allowed also contributes to decreased energy intake. In addition, decreased intake of vitamins and minerals may be deleterious.

Macronutrients

After deciding total energy intake, the patient and the dietitian should consider the choice of macro- and micronutrients.

Dietary Carbohydrates

Traditionally, intake of complex carbohydrates has been recommended for patients with diabetes, and intake of simple carbohydrates (mono- and disaccharides) such as glucose, fructose, and sucrose is discouraged. This is based on the notion that simple sugars are more rapidly absorbed and therefore can cause wide fluctuations in blood glucose. Equal energy intake from complex carbohydrates such as starch or naturally occurring simple carbohydrates causes similar increases in plasma glucose concentrations.[2,30–34] Fructose causes a reduced glycemic excursion.[35–37] However, sucrose or fructose intake may increase serum triglyceride and cholesterol concentrations compared to starch intake, although results have been inconsistent.[38–41] Therefore, while small amounts of simple sugars can be ingested as part of a healthful diet, overall intake should be limited.[42]

Nutritive sweeteners, including honey and fructose, may not have any advantage or disadvantage over sucrose.[1,2] While sucrose and other refined sugars can be substituted for other carbohydrates in the meal plan, caution is still needed. Foods containing sugars are also often high in fat as well as energy. Fruit as a source of fructose is not of concern as long as total carbohydrate intake is controlled; however, high-fructose corn syrup, which is added to many foods and beverages today, should be limited.[35,43]

Sucrose can increase palatability and thus interfere with weight loss efforts. It can also contribute to the development of dental caries. The amount of carbohydrate in the meal plan should be based on an assessment of current intake and must be individualized. Patients who are using oral antidiabetes agents or insulin need to maintain day-to-day consistency and meal-to-meal consistency in the amount of carbohydrate consumed to maintain good glycemic control. Some experts advise dietary carbohydrate-based calculation of insulin dose in patients with T1DM. Complex carbohydrates should be encouraged and simple sugars from fruits and vegetables are preferred because of the vitamins, minerals, and other nutrients in those foods.

The glycemic index of foods has been proposed as a criterion to select carbohydrate-containing foods.[44] The glycemic index is a ranking of foods based on their immediate effect on an individual's blood glucose levels. Following ingestion of a 50-g carbohydrate portion of a food, the blood glucose concentration area under the curve above the fasting glucose concentration is compared with the blood glucose area obtained with 50-g carbohydrate portion of white bread or glucose.[45] Interestingly, bread, some cereals, and potatoes have a higher glycemic index than simple sugars. Lower-glycemic foods include pasta, unprocessed grain products, legumes, dairy products, and some fruits. Several factors, including differences in cooking methods and processing, molecular and physical characteristics of the starch in the product, and individual variations in blood glucose response, can affect glycemic index.[46] Further, long-term intake of low-glycemic-index foods has not shown consistent improvement in plasma glucose or lipid concentrations in patients with diabetes.[47,48] Therefore, many experts, including the ADA, do not recommend the use of the glycemic index in nutritional management of patients with diabetes.

Sweeteners

Sugar alcohols (or polyols) such as sorbitol, mannitol, lactitol, and isomalt provide 2–3 kcal (8–12 kJ) per gram (Table 26-5). Hydrogenated starch hydrolysates and polyols are often used in sugar-free candies and cough drops. All of the polyols can cause significant gastrointestinal distress (cramping and diarrhea) if consumed in large amounts (20–50 grams, depending on the product). Small children may be particularly susceptible to developing diarrhea resulting from ingestion of as little as 0.5 g/kg body weight of polyols.[49] Sugar alcohols should not be used to treat hypoglycemia.

Non-nutritive sweeteners include saccharin, aspartame, acesulfame K, and sucralose. Both saccharin and acesulfame K are excreted unchanged from the body and provide no energy. Saccharin has been found to cross the placenta and is cleared slowly by the fetus; therefore, its use in pregnancy is not recommended.[50] Although aspartame contains 4 kcal (17 kJ) per gram, it is consumed in very small amounts, and thus contributes a negligible amount of energy. Aspartame cannot be used in cooking due to heat instability. People with phenylketonuria should not use aspartame because its metabolism yields phenylalanine. Sucralose (trichlorogalacto-sucrose) is being used in certain products such as fruit juice and pie fillings, with a substantial reduction in energy in those items. Sucralose provides no energy, is heat stable, and can be used in desserts, confections, and beverages.[43] The commercial version of sucralose (Splenda®) is packaged with a small amount of dextrose, thus contributing a minimal amount of energy.

Protein

Adequate protein intake is necessary for maintenance of lean body mass in adults. Children have higher protein needs to support growth, as well as for maintenance. Protein needs are also increased during pregnancy, lactation, catabolic illness or stress, and during vigorous exercise. Typical intake of protein in the United States ranges from 15–20% of total energy, while the recommended dietary allowance (RDA) for protein is approximately 10% of total energy (0.8 g/kg).[7] Protein intake of 10–20% of total energy is recommended by the ADA, and this will meet protein needs in most situations.[3] When using reduced energy diets, it is especially important to include adequate protein.

Reduction of protein intake to 0.8 g/kg is recommended for patients with chronic renal insufficiency and diabetic renal disease; however, protein malnutrition can occur on lower intakes.[51] Although studies suggest that decreasing protein intake in people with T1DM may delay the progression of nephropathy, it is not clear if all patients with diabetes would benefit from reduced protein intake.[52,53] In addition, it is unclear whether protein from different sources, e.g., from meat, vegetables, eggs, or milk, has variable effects on renal function.[54–56]

Good sources of protein include meat, poultry, fish, dairy products, legumes such as soybeans, chickpeas, other seeds and nuts, grain products, and vegetables. Because meat, poultry, and dairy products tend to be major sources of saturated fat and cholesterol, lower-fat selections should be made. Besides supplying protein, dairy products are excellent sources of calcium, and red meats are good sources of iron and zinc. Consumption of 500 mL (~2 cups) of milk and 140–170 g of meat, poultry, or fish per day can provide approximately 20% of total daily energy requirements from protein in adults. In contrast, a lacto-ovo vegetarian diet provides about 12–14% of energy from protein, while vegan diets provide about 10–12% energy from protein.[57] Although soy protein has some serum cholesterol–lowering effects, the mechanisms remain unclear. Whether protein from other legumes will have similar cholesterol-reducing potential has not been established.

Dietary Fats

Dietary fats, or triglycerides, usually contain a mixture of saturated (no double bonds), monounsaturated (one double bond), and polyunsaturated (two or more double bonds) fatty acids. Mono-

TABLE 26-5 Comparison of Sweeteners

Compound	Energy (kcal/kg)	Relative Sweetness Compared to Sucrose
Sucrose	4.0	1.0
Fructose	4.0	1.2–1.8
Sugar alcohols (polyols)		
Erythritol	0.2	0.7
Hydrogenated starch hydrolysates	3.0	0.25–0.5
Isomalt	2.0	0.45–0.65
Lactitol	2.0	0.3–0.4
Mannitol	1.6	0.5
Sorbitol	2.6	0.5–0.7
Xylitol	2.4	1.0
Non-Nutritive Sweeteners		
Acesulfame K	0	200
Alitame*	1.4	2000
Aspartame†	4.0	160–220
Cyclamate*	0	30
Saccharin	0	200–700
Sucralose	0	600

*Not approved for use in the United States.

†Negligible energy contribution due to intense sweetening capability.

Source: American Dietetic Association.[43]

and polyunsaturated fatty acids can be further classified as *cis* or *trans* depending on the geometric configuration of the double bonds. Approximately 90% of total fat intake in the United States comes from fats and oils, red meat, poultry, fish, and dairy products. Two-thirds of the saturated fat in the diet comes from animal fats, emphasizing the need to limit the quantity of animal products eaten. Invisible or hidden fats and oils are often overlooked. The importance of reducing cholesterol-raising fatty acids (mainly the saturated and *trans* variety) in the diet to achieve maximum reduction in serum low-density lipoprotein (LDL) cholesterol is well established. The goals for serum lipid and glycemic control may be used as the basis for individualization of the amount of fat included in the diet.

Saturated Fatty Acids

Saturated fatty acids should be limited to <10% and preferably to <7% of total energy.[3,58] The saturated fatty acids with the most potent serum cholesterol–raising effect are lauric (C12:0; 12-carbon chain length and no double bonds), myristic (C14:0), and palmitic (C16:0) acids.[59] Stearic acid (C18:0) does not raise serum LDL-cholesterol.[60,61] Recent studies have found that the medium-chain fatty acids caprylic (C8:0) and capric (C:10) acids, as well as the long-chain fatty acid behenic acid (C22:0), also raise serum LDL-cholesterol.[62,63]

Polyunsaturated Fatty Acids

Polyunsaturated fatty acids should also be limited to 10% or less of total energy intake.[3,58] Polyunsaturated fatty acids are classified as n-6 (ω-6) or n-3 (ω-3), depending on the location of the first double bond counting from the methyl end of the carbon chain. Consumption of approximately 2–3% of total energy intake from n-6 polyunsaturated fatty acids supplies adequate amounts of essential fatty acids. The essential fatty acids are linoleic acid (n-6, C18:2) and α-linolenic acid (n-3, C18:3). Arachidonic and γ-linolenic acids can be formed from linoleic acid. Linoleic acid, when substituted for saturated fatty acids, lowers LDL-cholesterol, but does not decrease triglycerides. Large intakes of linoleic acid, however, may decrease HDL-cholesterol concentrations.[64]

Omega-3 (n-3) fatty acids have been shown to reduce serum triglycerides by competitively inhibiting hepatic triglyceride synthesis. Fish oils are the major sources of eicosapentaenoic acid (C20:5) and docosahexaenoic acid (C22:6). Fish oil intake in large quantities (up to 5–10 g of n-3 polyunsaturated fatty acids per day) can cause hyperglycemia by increasing hepatic glucose output.[65] Such adverse effects, however, have not been noted with small doses of fish oil and when energy intake is adequately controlled.[66] Fish oils can also raise serum LDL-cholesterol concentrations, particularly in patients with hypertriglyceridemia.[67,68] Reduced risk of

acute myocardial infarction as a result of decreased platelet aggregation could be another potential benefit of n-3 fatty acids. For all patients with diabetes, the increase in consumption of n-3 fatty acids should be via increased intake of fish, except in those with hypertriglyceridemia, who need moderate to large doses of fish oils for reduction of serum triglycerides.

cis-Monounsaturated Fatty Acids

The *cis*-monounsaturated fatty acids are abundant in nature. People from Mediterranean countries who consume diets rich in *cis*-monounsaturated fats have lower mortality rates, particularly from coronary heart disease. Recent studies have shown that when oleic acid (C18:1) is substituted for saturated fatty acids, serum LDL-cholesterol declines just as much as with polyunsaturated fatty acids.[69–74] A preliminary study showed that erucic acid (C22:1) may also have cholesterol-lowering properties similar to those of oleic acid, but little is known about the effects of other *cis*-monounsaturated fatty acids such as palmitoleic (C16:1) and gadoleic (C20:1) acid.[75] This led us to explore potential beneficial effects of *cis*-monounsaturated fatty acids for patients with T2DM.

In a randomized, crossover study in patients with T2DM, in comparison to a high-carbohydrate diet, a diet high in *cis*-monounsaturated fatty acids, with reduced plasma triglycerides and very-low-density-lipoprotein (VLDL) cholesterol levels, raised high-density lipoprotein (HDL) cholesterol and apolipoprotein A-I concentrations, but caused no changes in plasma total cholesterol, LDL-cholesterol, and apolipoprotein B. The high-*cis*-monounsaturated-fat diet also lowered plasma glucose and insulin concentrations.[76] A recent meta-analysis of nine randomized, crossover trials showed that compared to high-carbohydrate diets, the high-*cis*-monounsaturated-fat diets reduced fasting plasma triacylglycerol by 19% and VLDL-cholesterol concentrations by 22%. A modest increase in HDL-cholesterol was noted with no adverse effect on LDL-cholesterol concentrations (Table 26-6).[77]

Besides beneficial effects of diets rich in *cis*-monounsaturated fatty acids on serum lipids and glycemic control, such diets may increase compliance for some individuals used to a high-fat diet. When weight loss is a goal, attention should be given to overall energy intake. Good sources of *cis*-monounsaturated fatty acids include canola, olive, mustard, and peanut oils, avocados, olives, and some nuts (Table 26-7).[78] Certain genetically modified varieties of safflower and sunflower oils are also rich in *cis*-monounsaturated fatty acids.

trans-Fatty Acids

Partial hydrogenation of oils yields a firmer and more stable product than the original oil, but the process also leads to formation

TABLE 26-6 Net Change in Lipids and Lipoprotein Concentrations in Type 2 Diabetic Patients with the High Monounsaturated Fat Diet, as Compared with the High Carbohydrate Diet*

Parameter	Total Cholesterol	Triglycerides	VLDL Cholesterol	LDL Cholesterol	HDL Cholesterol
No. of studies	9	9	4	6	9
No. of subjects	133	133	68	105	133
Change in mmol/L*	−0.15	−0.36	−0.20	−0.01	+0.05
(95% CI)	(−0.24 to −0.06)	(−0.43 to −0.29)	(−0.24 to −0.15)	(−0.10 to +0.08)	(+0.03 to +0.07)
Percent change*	−3.0	−19.0	−22.5	0.0	+4.0

*Results of a meta-analysis of nine studies. Net or percent change is expressed as the concentration during the high monounsaturated fat diet minus that during the high carbohydrate diet.[77]

CI, confidence interval; VLDL, very-low-density lipoprotein; LDL, low-density lipoprotein; HDL, high-density lipoprotein.

Modified with permission from Gang.[77]

TABLE 26-7 Various *cis*-Monounsaturated Fatty Acids and Their Dietary Sources

Common Name	Notation	Sources
Lauroleic	C12:1	Fish oils
Myristoleic	C14:1	Fish oils, beef fat
Palmitoleic	C16:1	Fish oils, beef and pork fat
Oleic	C18:1	*Oils:* olive, canola, ground nut (peanuts), high-oleic safflower and sunflower, avocado, aceituno, shea nut, rice bran, sesame, *Jessenia bataua*, tea seed
		Nuts: filberts, almonds, pistachios, pecans, macadamias, cashews
		Others: mowrah butter; illipe butter; *fat of cattle, pigs, goats, chicken, and sheep; *cocoa butter
Gadoleic	C20:1	Fish oils (such as herring, sardines, mackerel), jojoba oil
Erucic	C22:1	Mustard seed oil, rape seed oil, nasturtium seed oil

*Although a source of oleic acid, these fats should be used sparingly because they are high in cholesterol-raising saturated fatty acids.

Source: Padley, *et al.*[78]

of *trans*-monounsaturated or *trans*-polyunsaturated fatty acids. Partially hydrogenated oils are often used as a substitute for saturated fats in foods such as spreads, shortenings, and baked goods. Approximately 3% of the total daily energy is provided by *trans*-fatty acids in the United States.[79] In other western countries 0.5–2.1% of the total energy consumption is from *trans*-fatty acids.[80] Dietary *trans*-fatty acids should be limited as much as possible because they have been shown to raise serum LDL-cholesterol and apolipoprotein B levels and may lower serum HDL-cholesterol and apolipoprotein A-I.[81,82] Furthermore, intake of *trans*-fatty acids has also been associated with higher risk of coronary heart disease.[83]

Fat Replacers

Fat replacers can help to lower overall fat intake; however, these products cannot counteract the effects of a diet high in fat and cholesterol. Patients may need education in label reading to understand the difference between reduced-fat, low-fat, and fat-free products. Fat replacers are of questionable benefit in weight management, as many have only slightly reduced energy than the regular product. In addition, satiety value may be less for the reduced-fat product, leading to increased overall intake.

Fat replacers can be made from carbohydrates, proteins, or fat.[84] Carbohydrate-based fat replacements are gums, gels, and maltodextrins that add creaminess and texture to foods such as salad dressings. A significant amount of carbohydrate may be consumed in a low-fat product made with a carbohydrate-based fat replacement, especially if the serving size listed on the label is small. Protein-based fat replacers are made of microparticulated egg white or milk protein. They can be used in cheese, salad dressings, and some baked products. Most protein-based fat replacers lose their desired effect due to coagulation when subjected to high temperatures, thus limiting the types of products in which they can be used. Protein-based fat replacers add 1–4 kcal (4–16 kJ) per gram.[84] Fat-based substitutes are either synthetic or modified fats. Olestra, a sucrose polyester, is a synthetic fat that is not digested or absorbed and thus contributes no energy. Large amounts of olestra can cause gastrointestinal distress and may reduce absorption of fat-soluble vitamins.[85] Salatrim® and caprenin are examples of fats altered to decrease absorption. Salatrim provides ~20 kJ (5 kcal) per gram and is a modified triglyceride containing acetic, propionic, and stearic acids. Caprenin also provides ~20 kJ per gram and contains caprylic (C8:0), capric (C:10), and behenic (C22:0) acids. Even though absorption of caprenin and Salatrim is decreased, caprylic, capric, and behenic acids can raise serum cholesterol concentration.[59]

Dietary Cholesterol

Both serum LDL- and total cholesterol are increased by high intake of dietary cholesterol. Limiting dietary cholesterol to 300 mg or less per day is recommended, while further reduction to 200 mg or less may be necessary to achieve maximal lowering of LDL-cholesterol. Animal products are the sole sources of dietary cholesterol, and their intake should be limited.[1,58] Consumption of 140–170 grams per day of lean meat, poultry, or fish and 500–750 mL (2–3 cups) of nonfat or low-fat dairy products is recommended. Certain high-cholesterol foods, such as egg yolks and organ meats, should be limited. Egg yolks should be limited to 2–4 per week, including those used in cooking. Egg whites may be used in place of whole eggs. Certain shellfish (i.e., shrimp) have higher cholesterol content than other meats or fish, but may be consumed in moderation because of their lower saturated fat content.[58]

Dietary Fiber

The recommended intake for dietary fiber for patients with diabetes is 20–35 grams per day, a significant increase over the usual intake of 16 to 17 grams per day in the United States.[86] In other Western countries fiber intake is also quite low, approximately 22 grams per day.[87] Dietary fiber can be classified as soluble or insoluble. Insoluble fibers such as cellulose, lignin, and some hemicelluloses increase stool volume and shorten intestinal transit time, but do not affect serum cholesterol levels. Soluble fibers such as pectin, gums, mucilages, and some hemicelluloses reduce serum cholesterol by approximately 5%.[88] A recent study in subjects with T2DM, comparing a diet high in total fiber (50 grams total fiber, 25 grams each of soluble and insoluble fiber) from foods unfortified with fiber supplements to a moderate-fiber diet (24 grams total, 8 grams soluble and 16 grams insoluble), reported a 10% reduction in 24-hour plasma glucose and a 12% reduction in plasma insulin levels, as well as decreased daily urinary glucose excretion (Fig. 26-1).[89] The high-fiber diet also reduced plasma cholesterol by 7%, triglycerides by 10%, and VLDL-cholesterol by 12.5%. Selection of such fruits, vegetables, and grains with a high proportion of soluble to insoluble fiber is recommended (Table 26-8).[90]

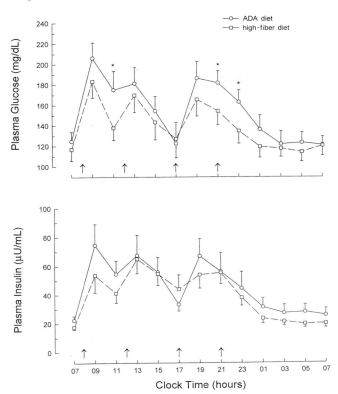

FIGURE 26-1. Profile of 24-hour plasma glucose and insulin levels (means ± SEM) obtained on the last day of each diet period. The **circles** represent mean values on the American Diabetes Association (ADA) diet and the **squares** represent mean values on the high-fiber diet. The **arrows** indicate the times at which the major meals and a snack were consumed during the day. An **asterisk** denotes $p < 0.05$ for the ADA diet versus the high-fiber diet values. To convert values of plasma insulin to picomoles per liter, multiply by 6. (*Modified with permission from Chandalia et al.*[89])

Alcohol

The ADA recommends the same guidelines for alcohol consumption for patients with diabetes as those for the general population; however, there are some additional concerns.[91–94] Pregnant women and people with a history of alcohol abuse, pancreatitis, gastritis, and certain other conditions should abstain from alcohol intake. One recent study reported increased risk for developing T2DM in men who abstain or drink large amounts of alcohol when compared with those who are moderate drinkers.[95] Low to moderate alcohol intake on a regular basis in nondiabetic subjects can increase serum HDL-cholesterol and apolipoprotein A-I levels, thus contributing to lower cardiovascular risk; however, these effects are somewhat negated by an accompanying increase in blood pressure and decrease in concentration of antithrombin III.[96] In large amounts, alcohol causes peripheral insulin resistance, and may lead to hyperglycemia, hypertriglyceridemia, and hypertension.[97–99] Alcohol may also contribute to development of truncal obesity and fatty liver.[100–102] Because alcohol ingestion may enhance glucose-stimulated insulin secretion and reduce gluconeogenesis, binge drinking and/or failing to consume food with alcohol increases the likelihood of hypoglycemic events. The likelihood of hypoglycemic unawareness also increases with alcohol ingestion. To reduce the risk of hypoglycemia when insulin is required, food should never be omitted to compensate for the alcohol consumed

and meals must be eaten at the scheduled times.[1,103,104] People with T2DM, particularly elderly individuals, who drink alcohol and require oral antidiabetes agents are also at increased risk for hypoglycemia, but their risk is less than that for T1DM.[105] With good glycemic control, moderate ingestion of alcohol (two drinks for men and one for women) has limited acute effect on blood glucose levels. Alcohol provides 7 kcal (30 kJ) per gram and in T2DM where weight management is usually a concern, energy from alcohol should be substituted for fat energy.

Micronutrients

Vitamins

There is little need for vitamin and mineral supplementation in patients who eat a variety of foods and consume adequate energy to maintain body weight.[106] Patients following reduced-energy diets for long periods of time, however, can be at risk for consuming less than the recommended intake of some nutrients. In addition, those individuals who consume meals or snacks prepared away from home are more likely to have diets lower in vitamin and mineral content than those who consume more conventional meals prepared in the home. During pregnancy and in times of illness and stress, nutrient needs are increased. A thorough assessment of the patient's current diet by a dietitian can be helpful to determine if supplementation may be indicated.

Because of increased risk for coronary heart disease in people with diabetes, the antioxidant vitamins such as vitamins C and E are of particular interest. They may protect LDL-cholesterol particles from oxidation or modification, but clinical trials that support the benefits from the effects are lacking.[107,108] In fact, a recent large clinical trial evaluating cardiovascular outcomes found no positive effect for vitamin E supplementation.[109] Earlier enthusiasm for the antioxidant beta-carotene has declined after reports of either no beneficial effect or slightly increased risk for lung cancer in subjects who took beta-carotene supplements.[110,111]

Minerals

Chromium

Chromium is often touted as a mineral that needs to be supplemented in diabetes because it is a component of glucose tolerance factor. However, unless the diet is deficient in chromium, its supplementation does not improve glucose tolerance.[112,113]

Magnesium

Magnesium serves many important functions in the body. Patients with diabetes tend to have low blood magnesium levels, most likely due to urinary loss of magnesium associated with chronic glycosuria.[114–116] However, repletion with oral magnesium chloride is recommended only for those who have documented hypomagnesemia. Good food sources of magnesium include liver, leafy green vegetables, legumes, and nuts. Those who follow a nutritionally balanced meal plan and consume adequate energy should be able to obtain adequate magnesium from their food.[117]

Sodium

Scientific evidence strongly supports the effectiveness of good blood pressure control to prevent complications of diabetes, and reduction of sodium intake has been found to be effective in lowering blood pressure in subjects with hypertension.[118–120] Older individuals, especially those with diabetes, appear to be more sensitive to

TABLE 26-8 Fiber Content of Some Foods Particularly Rich in Soluble Fiber

Food Item	Amount	Weight (g)	Total Dietary Fiber (g)	Insoluble Fiber (g)	Soluble Fiber (g)
Legumes and Grains					
Beans, lima	1 c	188	13.6	6.2	7.4
Beans, navy	1 c	182	15.4	6.6	5.2
Chickpeas	1 c	164	9.5	5.7	3.8
Peas, split	1 c	196	6.3	4.1	2.2
Oatmeal, cooked	1 c	234	3.6	1.7	1.9
Fruits					
Apple with skin	1 med	138	2.8	1.8	1.0
Banana	1 med	114	2.2	1.6	0.6
Cantaloupe	½ med	461	3.7	1.5	2.2
Grapefruit	½ med	145	1.8	0.7	1.1
Mango	1 med	207	4.1	2.2	1.9
Nectarine	1 med	136	2.2	1.1	1.1
Orange	1 med	131	3.1	1.2	1.9
Papaya	1 c	140	3.5	1.3	2.2
Peach	1 med	87	1.4	0.5	0.9
Plums	1 med	66	1.0	0.3	0.7
Vegetables					
Artichokes	1 c	168	5.6	2.5	3.1
Broccoli	1 c	184	5.2	2.8	2.3
Cabbage	1 c	150	3.0	1.9	1.1
Corn, whole kernel	1 c	164	6.1	3.4	2.6
Kohlrabi	1 c	165	4.4	1.4	3.0
Okra	1 c	185	5.9	2.4	3.5
Squash, winter	1 c	245	6.9	2.9	3.9
Sweet potatoes	1 c	255	7.7	4.6	3.1
Zucchini	1 c	130	2.0	0.7	1.3

Source: Schakel *et al.*[90]

sodium than others.[121] For individuals with hypertension, moderate restriction of sodium (2400 mg/d) is usually recommended.[122] Patients with diabetic nephropathy should limit intake of sodium to ≤2000 mg per day.[3] Acute severe sodium restriction (<500 mg/d) has been shown to adversely affect serum total and LDL-cholesterol and to increase resistance to the vasodilating effects of insulin.[123–125] For older individuals who are thin or at normal body weight, severe sodium restriction may adversely affect energy intake due to decreased palatability of food and thus could contribute to malnutrition. Dietary intake of sodium usually greatly exceeds the minimum needed for normal body function due to its frequent use in foods such as canned soups, salty snacks, and processed meats. Meals and snacks purchased in restaurants are also likely to have a higher sodium content than meals prepared from fresh foods at home. Reduction of sodium intake can be difficult to achieve unless the diet is based primarily on fresh rather than processed foods.

Phytochemicals and Supplements

Evidence is growing in support of increased intake of fruits and vegetables in the diet as more is learned about potential health benefits of newly identified substances in those foods. Isoflavones are an example of phytoestrogens found in vegetables, fruits, and legumes. Some potential beneficial effects of isoflavones, such as genistein and daidzein from soy products, include antioxidant properties, weak estrogenic effects, and action as modulators of intestinal glucose transport.

Sitostanol, a plant sterol incorporated into margarine, lowers serum LDL-cholesterol by 10–15% in mildly hypercholesterolemic subjects by competitive inhibition of gastrointestinal absorption of cholesterol.[126–128] It may be a useful dietary adjunct for patients with diabetes.[129,130]

Other substances in plants, such as lutein, lycopene, lignans, and saponins, are currently being investigated and may eventually play a role in enhancing health. As studies are conducted using these substances, foods are emerging as the preferred source. The isolated individual components taken in the form of a supplement do not always have the same effect as the substance when consumed in a whole food along with all the other elements present in the food.

Use of botanical (herbal) supplements is widespread and growing among the general population and is especially prevalent among patients with chronic diseases.[131] Clinical evidence to support the efficacy and safety of use of many of these products is very limited. Because of the potential for harmful effects and possible interaction with prescription medications, patients should be asked about their use of all types of supplements.

Meal Frequency and Timing

For patients with T1DM, consistency in timing of meals in relation to insulin action is important to prevent wide fluctuations in blood glucose levels. Adjustments should be made in the timing of insulin injections to match peak glucose excursion after meals and snacks.

As discussed earlier, consistency in the amount of carbohydrate eaten is of greatest importance, as dietary protein and fat have a lesser effect than carbohydrates on blood glucose levels. If there are more than 5 hours between meals, a snack may be needed to prevent a hypoglycemic event. Multiple daily injections or use of an insulin pump provides greater flexibility in timing of meals for the person with T1DM.

For patients whose diabetes is controlled by diet alone or with oral agents, eating 3–5 small meals per day may be beneficial. Although frequency of feeding does not appear to affect rate of weight loss when energy intake is constant, more frequent eating may lead to less fluctuation in satiety level, thus curbing the tendency to consume excessive energy.[132,133] Patients taking oral agents to lower blood glucose levels should be advised to avoid skipping meals to prevent hypoglycemic events. Multiple small meals have been shown to have a positive effect on serum lipids and lipoproteins, insulin, and postprandial glucose when compared to a pattern of less frequent meals.[133–135] In addition, less impulsive eating and a reduced dietary fat intake have been noted when breakfast is eaten.[136]

SPECIAL ISSUES

Type 1 Diabetes Mellitus

Infants and Young Children

Providing adequate nutrition for normal growth and development and prevention of hypoglycemic events are two major goals in management of diabetes in infants and children. Children with poor glycemic control may grow at a slower rate. Growth should be monitored every 3–6 months so that appropriate intervention can be made if growth is not optimal. To help prevent hypoglycemia, blood glucose target goals for infants and children are higher than for adults. Preprandial target blood glucose ranges for infants and toddlers are 120–220 mg/dL, for preschool children, 100–200 mg/dL, and for school-age children, 70–150 mg/dL.[137] Because the risks of hypoglycemia are greater for infants and young children due to ineffective communication and brain growth, blood glucose should be monitored frequently. For infants, a flexible 3- to 4-hour feeding schedule of breast milk or iron-fortified formula can help to maintain normoglycemia. Other foods can be added to the diet at the usual recommended age (4–6 months) to help maintain glucose levels and provide other sources of carbohydrate. Careful blood glucose monitoring is needed due to the fluctuating activity level in infants.

Toddlers present special challenges, because their physical activity and eating habits are sporadic and spontaneous. Toddlers need three meals and three snacks, and usually are good judges of how much they need to eat. The focus of food intake should be the overall picture over a period of time, rather than concern over limited food choices on a day-to-day basis. The dosage and timing of insulin administration should be adjusted to match the amount of carbohydrate that has been consumed.

Adolescents

The adolescent years also present challenges in diabetes management from a physiologic as well as developmental perspective. Rapid growth and hormonal changes influence insulin needs. From a meal planning perspective, the importance of eating a consistent amount of carbohydrate on a regular schedule requires creativity. The use of the carbohydrate counting method for meal planning can provide flexibility.[138] Since this method focuses on a single nutrient, it gives more options and allows the adolescent to include foods his or her peers are eating, but still maintain consistent carbohydrate intake for good glycemic control.

For children of normal weight, usual intake is a good baseline to determine nutrition needs and establish a meal plan. Extra energy intake may be needed for catch-up growth if the child has lost weight or experienced growth faltering prior to the time of diagnosis. If intensive glycemic control is implemented for adolescents, excessive weight gain may become a problem. While children with T1DM are typically thin or even underweight at the time of diagnosis, with the increased prevalence of childhood obesity in the United States, approximately 25% of children diagnosed with T1DM are now obese.[139]

Age-appropriate physical activity should be encouraged to help establish lifelong habits early and emphasize the benefits for overall good health as well as diabetes management. As children begin to participate in organized sports and other physical activities, periodic guidance by nutritionists is needed to adjust the meal plan so that additional carbohydrate and energy are planned to maintain good glycemic control.

Type 2 Diabetes Mellitus

Adults

When the focus of management for T2DM is on improved serum glucose, hypertension, and lipid levels rather than on weight loss, there is greater incentive for continued and long-term changes. However, long-term maintenance of reduced weight is problematic for many individuals. Studies of those who have successfully maintained reduced weight reveal that continued self-monitoring by keeping food records and weighing themselves regularly is important.[140–142] Increased physical activity, however, seems to be a key factor in maintenance of reduced weight.[143–145] In addition to increased energy expenditure, physical activity seems to provide a sense of self-efficacy in overall weight management efforts.[146,147] For lifelong adherence to a physical activity regimen, a person needs to find something enjoyable to do in order to increase the likelihood of continued activity.

Coronary heart disease, peripheral vascular disease, foot problems or amputation, osteoarthritis of hip or knee, and cerebrovascular accidents may limit patients' physical activity. A number of medications can adversely affect weight loss efforts. Tricyclic antidepressants and antihistamines may increase appetite. Nonsteroidal anti-inflammatory drugs as well as aspirin (even at prophylactic doses used for coronary heart disease and cerebrovascular disease) can cause gastritis. Energy balance can be affected by beta-blockers that can cause a slight decrease in metabolic rate.[148]

Children and Adolescents

The prevalence of T2DM in children and adolescents is growing at an alarming rate, up from 1–2% in the past to recent reports of 8–25% of diabetes cases in children.[139] The increasing prevalence of obesity among children in the United States is likely a contributing factor to the increase in T2DM in this group. Except when life-threatening comorbidities exist, the goal for weight management in younger children is to maintain weight while providing adequate energy for continued linear growth. Modest energy restriction to promote weight loss in adolescents who are past the growth spurt is appropriate. When weight loss is indicated, energy intake should be reduced as discussed previously; however, increased physical activity should be stressed. Decreased physical activity has been implicated as a major factor in development of obesity in children. As for adults, it is equally important that children find an activity they like and will continue to do over the long term. Family involvement is extremely important in promoting healthy weight in children.

Pregnancy and Lactation

Good diabetes management is essential for successful pregnancy outcome for a woman with diabetes. Nutritional planning 3–6 months prior to conception is essential to achieve near-normal glycemic control before and during pregnancy. Increased energy should be provided during pregnancy and lactation. The increased energy intake needed for development of the fetus and maternal tissue is approximately 300 additional kcal (1250 kJ) per day during the second and third trimesters of pregnancy.[149] Women with a body mass index of >26 to 29.0 kg/m^2 should gain 7–11.5 kg, while women with BMI >29.0 kg/m^2 should gain ~7 kg. Protein intake should be increased by 10 grams per day. Folic acid, calcium, and iron should be increased appropriately.

Approximately 4% of women develop gestational diabetes. They are often overweight and are at increased risk for future development of T2DM. Energy restriction during pregnancy is controversial. Severe energy restriction can result in ketosis and can adversely affect the fetus. However, energy consumption of 1600–1800 kcal (6700–7500 kJ) per day can improve hyperglycemia without causing ketosis.[150,151] Some experts recommend 30 kcal/kg of present pregnant weight for normal-weight women, 24 kcal/kg for overweight women, and 12 kcal/kg for morbidly obese women.[152] To control postprandial glucose response, carbohydrates are limited to 40% of total energy intake and are distributed into three meals and three snacks. If an energy-restricted diet is used during pregnancy, adequate protein must be provided because pregnant women with diabetes may be more susceptible to protein malnutrition than those without diabetes.[153–155] Weight loss efforts should continue during the postpartum period with a long-term goal of gradual weight reduction.

Consistent patterns of food intake and physical activity are important during pregnancy to avoid ketonemia and maintain stable blood glucose levels. Frequent meals and snacks may be eaten. Blood glucose levels in nondiabetic women are generally lower during pregnancy. Morning sickness can increase the likelihood of hypoglycemia. As the pregnancy progresses, increasing insulin resistance affects blood glucose levels and insulin needs. Carbohydrate intake should be adjusted to approximately 40–45% of total energy to maintain glycemic goals.[156]

Breastfeeding should be encouraged, particularly for obese women with T2DM, as it can assist in their efforts to lose weight. Approximately 500 kcal (2100 kJ) per day are needed to provide the extra energy required for lactation. Because breastfeeding lowers blood glucose levels, the dose of insulin may be reduced appropriately and additional energy may be consumed, particularly during the night. Moderate weight loss can occur on energy consumption of approximately 35 kcal/kg of body weight as the maternal stores laid down during the pregnancy are used to support lactation. Weight loss of 0.5–1.0 kg per month is acceptable and up to 2 kg weight loss per month does not appear to compromise milk volume.[157,158]

Eating Disorders

The prevalence of eating disorders, clinical and subclinical, among people with diabetes is at least as great as in the general population,

and some studies report higher rates.[159–161] Eating disorders can significantly complicate short- and long-term diabetes management. Mostly young females, who tend to have greater concern about body weight and shape, are affected. Omission or reduction of insulin to control weight may be practiced by up to 30% of females with diabetes.[159,162] Those who omit insulin are more likely to exhibit disordered eating, have a greater fear of hypoglycemia, report more psychological distress, and have poorer adherence to diabetes management protocols, leading to increased diabetes-related hospitalizations.[162] Most studies report poorer glycemic control when disordered eating is present. Binge eating and purging are the most commonly reported types of disordered eating among patients with diabetes.[161,163] Women who intentionally omit or reduce insulin dosage tend to have elevated plasma triglycerides, cholesterol, and hemoglobin A$_{1c}$ concentrations, which may increase the risk for long-term complications of diabetes such as retinopathy and neuropathy.[164] Those who report bulimic behavior have an increased intake of energy, dietary fat, and cholesterol compared with those who do not.[165] In a German study that included subjects with T2DM, binge eating disorder often preceded the diagnosis of diabetes, possibly contributing to the obesity associated with T2DM.[160]

Acute and Chronic Illnesses

Sick Day Guidelines

Nutritional management during acute illnesses requires adequate fluids (orally or intravenously) to avoid dehydration and at least 150 grams of carbohydrates to avoid ketosis. When solid food is not tolerated, energy can be provided in the form of liquids, such as juice, lemonade, sodas, gelatin, soup, ice cream, or sherbet.

Metabolic stress and pain during surgery or trauma increases circulating counterregulatory hormones and can lead to hyperglycemia. During such periods, it is extremely important to monitor and maintain appropriate fluid and electrolyte balance, metabolic control, and body weight. The nutritional goal during periods of stress is to avoid over- and underfeeding. Overfeeding further exaggerates the hyperglycemia caused by metabolic stress. Maintenance of blood glucose levels between 100 and 200 mg/dL is recommended to limit extremes of hypo- and hyperglycemia.[166] Impaired wound healing has been observed when blood glucose exceeds 200 mg/dL.[167] Adequate pain management is important, but the sedating effects of pain medication can increase risk of hypoglycemia.

Enteral and Parenteral Nutrition Support

The indications for such nutritional support for patients with diabetes are similar to those without diabetes. Energy and protein needs should be determined based on thorough nutrition assessment. Unintentional weight loss of 10–20% in a 6-month period suggests moderate malnutrition and >20% weight loss indicates severe malnutrition. Protein catabolism is often a consequence of the metabolic stress of severe illness or injury. Protein needs can usually be met with 1.0–1.5 g protein/kg body weight, but some patients may require higher protein intake. Monitoring of blood glucose and urine ketones is recommended every 6 hours during enteral nutrition and every 4 hours during parenteral nutrition.[168]

Enteral Nutrition

Enteral nutrition is preferred if the gut is functioning because of less expense and fewer complications, and because it is more physiologic and may have beneficial trophic effects on the gastrointestinal cells. Enteral nutrition is best supplied by commercially prepared formulas to limit risk of contamination; however, with careful attention to sanitation, nutritionally adequate formulas can be prepared by blending together milk and other foods. If the patient is lactose intolerant, cooked, pureed meat can provide the protein needed. Adequate liquid must be added to provide the proper consistency to avoid clogging of the feeding tube. Reduced fluid intake and high-carbohydrate formulas may increase risk of hyperosmolar nonketotic coma.

Total Parenteral Nutrition

Total parenteral nutrition (TPN) is recommended when oral intake is not adequate and enteral nutrition is not feasible. Accurate intake and output records are essential. Excess administration of glucose (>5 mg/kg body weight/min) may cause hyperglycemia and require a higher dose of insulin for good glycemic control. Continuous infusion of fat emulsion is recommended to maintain approximately 30% of energy intake (not greater than 2.5 g/kg body weight).[168] Use of lipid emulsions may need to be reduced or discontinued if serum triglyceride concentrations exceed 400 mg/dL.[166]

Other Complications

Chronic Pancreatitis

Chronic severe pancreatitis can lead to destruction of the pancreas and subsequent development of diabetes. In addition, loss of exocrine function due to pancreatitis or pancreatectomy causes malabsorption. With adequate enzyme replacement therapy, greater intake of fat can be allowed with alleviation of fat and protein malabsorption.[169]

Diabetic Nephropathy

Adjustments in dietary protein intake may help to slow the progression of diabetic nephropathy. In chronic renal insufficiency, a reduction in dietary protein to 0.8 g/kg is recommended.[2] The recommendation for protein intake in patients with nephrotic syndrome is also 0.8 g/kg. When protein intake is less than 0.8 g/kg, patients are at greater risk for malnutrition.[170] Adequate energy intake in the range of 35–40 kcal/kg may be needed in some instances to maintain body weight.[171] Increased use of simple carbohydrates and unsaturated fats may be needed to achieve the desired level of energy intake. Hyperphosphatemia in chronic renal failure requires reduction of phosphorus intake to prevent metabolic bone disease. Intake of sodium and potassium must be monitored and adjusted as needed to maintain appropriate serum concentrations. Fluid intake must also be adjusted as renal failure progresses. As much as 80% of the dextrose in the dialysate used for peritoneal dialysis is absorbed and thus can contribute a significant amount of energy. Supplementation of certain vitamins and minerals may be needed due to the metabolic alterations of renal failure as well as poor dietary intake.

Autonomic Neuropathy

Gastroparesis

Gastroparesis is a complication of diabetes with significant nutrition and diabetes management implications. The symptoms of bloating, fullness, early satiety, nausea and vomiting, and abdominal pain can lead to decreased intake and weight loss. At the same time the patient may experience postprandial hypoglycemia and fluctuating plasma glucose levels. Optimal glycemic control is important because hyperglycemia can slow gastric emptying. Nutritional management for gastroparesis includes (1) small frequent meals, (2) a low-fat, low-fiber diet, (3) use of foods of soft consistency, and (4) replacement of solid foods with liquid meals.[172] Eating meals with more solid foods earlier in the day, then switching to liquids later in the day seems to help some patients. While fat usually slows gastric emptying, many patients can tolerate fat in a liquid form, such as milkshakes. Patients should be instructed to sit up during and after meals. If enteral feeding is necessary, a jejunostomy feeding route is recommended.[173]

Diarrhea and Constipation

Diabetic diarrhea occurs in approximately 10–20% of patients with poorly controlled diabetes. Before diagnosis of diabetic diarrhea can be definitively established, pancreatic insufficiency, bacterial overgrowth, lactose intolerance, or gluten-induced enteropathy must be considered as possible causes of persistent diarrhea. Constipation is another common complaint that occurs in patients with diabetes. Adjustments in diet have not been very effective in management of diarrhea or constipation that results from diabetic autonomic neuropathy; therefore, good glycemic control for prevention of development of neuropathy is essential.[174]

Gluten-Induced Enteropathy

Celiac disease, or gluten-induced enteropathy, is a disease with a reported higher incidence (estimated at 1–8%) among patients with T1DM.[175–177] Patients with celiac disease usually present with abdominal distention, diarrhea, weight loss (or failure to thrive in children), lactose intolerance, fatigue, and irritability. Depending on the severity of the gluten sensitivity and length of time prior to diagnosis, the patient may be at significant nutritional risk. The treatment requires avoidance of the protein gliadin and several other prolamins from the diet, which means elimination of wheat, rye, oats, and barley. Strict adherence to the diet results in significant improvement in symptoms but is difficult to achieve. The offending grains can be found in many products and are often hidden, making careful label reading essential. Nutrition advice should be obtained to plan nutritionally balanced meals for overall health.[178]

OVERCOMING BARRIERS TO CHANGE

Barriers

Numerous obstacles to dietary compliance have been cited: a sense of isolation, time pressures and competing priorities, lack of support from friends and family, social events, negative emotions, and feelings of deprivation.[179] In a recent survey of dietitians who work with patients with diabetes, the greatest barrier to change identified was the complication of lifestyle and competing demands.[180] Included in this barrier category are (1) time constraints, (2) eating out, (3) lack of finances, (4) portion control, and (5) denial or unwillingness to make changes. The primary factors needed to overcome these barriers were individualization and simplification of meal plans and help with time management (scheduling). Medical nutrition therapy that involves assessment and individualized intervention has been shown to be effective in improving metabolic control in other studies as well.[181,182] Physician referral for medical nutrition therapy in diabetes management is extremely important due the difficulty in achieving dietary change. For approximately half of the patients with T2DM in one study, lack of physician referral was the reason for not consulting a dietitian.[183] Infrequent referral for dietary counseling was found to be as ineffective in facilitating dietary change as no referral.[184] The importance of following a meal plan for improved glycemic control in T1DM was recognized in The Diabetes Control and Complication Trial (DCCT).[185,186] Increased adherence to meal plans occurs when patients attend follow-up nutrition counseling sessions.[187] Additional education about the complications of diabetes was identified as a means to overcome the barrier of denial or the perception that diabetes is not serious. Increased emphasis on blood glucose monitoring, more follow-up sessions, use of support groups, and further individualized education were recommended by dietitians involved in diabetes education.

Tools and Techniques

Practice guidelines have been developed to provide a systematic approach for provision of medical nutrition therapy for patients with diabetes mellitus. The major components of medical nutrition therapy are assessment, intervention, and evaluation. Intervention includes the nutrition prescription, education, and goal setting. For the intervention to be effective, the patient must be an active participant in this process.[188] Improved fasting plasma glucose, glycosylated hemoglobin, serum lipids, and body weight have demonstrated effectiveness of medical nutrition therapy. Use of cognitive motivational techniques, as well as programs of longer duration with greater simplicity and repetition, has been found to improve outcome.[189] Patients with diabetes of long duration, with poor metabolic control, and with major obstacles to lifestyle changes are most likely to benefit from intensive nutrition therapy.[190]

A wide range of tools is available to facilitate meal planning for patients with diabetes.[191] Which meal planning approach to use depends on the assessment of the individual patient's needs. *The Exchange Lists for Meal Planning*, long used to help patients select appropriate foods and portion sizes, may be too complex for some situations. A simplified version of the exchange system was found to be an effective meal planning tool during the DCCT. The carbohydrate counting method, which focuses on the nutrient with greatest influence on glycemic control, provides flexibility and can be implemented with varying degrees of complexity.[138]

SUMMARY

The goals of nutritional management for diabetes mellitus can be achieved in a number of ways to meet patient needs. Provision of adequate energy intake to meet needs during periods of growth and development, pregnancy and lactation, and times of stress, injury, or illness are of primary importance. For patients with T2DM, reduction of total energy intake and an increase in physical activity consistent with the patient's physical capabilities should be recommended in order to reduce body fat, decrease insulin resistance, and improve glycemic and lipid control. Either a high-carbohydrate diet or a diet rich in *cis*-monounsaturated fats can be used as long as intake of dietary cholesterol and cholesterol-raising fats is limited. Intake of added sugars should be limited and carbohydrates rich in soluble fiber should be preferentially consumed. Recommendations for protein, vitamins, minerals, and fluids are similar to those for the nondiabetics. Emphasis should be on a healthy lifestyle with a diet low in saturated and *trans*-unsaturated fats and rich in whole grains, fresh fruits, and vegetables. Referral to a qualified dietitian to assist the patient in establishing an individualized, realistic meal plan is essential. Because changing dietary habits is difficult, frequent follow-up will increase the likelihood of long-term positive outcomes of good glycemic control and prevention of short- and long-term complications.

REFERENCES

1. American Diabetes Association: Nutrition recommendations and principles for people with diabetes mellitus. *Diabetes Care* 1994;17: 519.
2a. American Diabetes Association Position Statement: Evidence-based nutrition principles and recommendations for the treatment and prevention of diabetes and related complications. *Diabetes Care* 2002; 25:202.
2b. Franz MJ, Bantle JP, Beebe CA, et al: Evidence-based nutrition principles and recommendations for the treatment and prevention of diabetes and related complications, Technical Review. *Diabetes Care* 2002;25:148.
3. American Diabetes Association: Nutrition recommendations and principles for people with diabetes mellitus. *Diabetes Care* 2000;23: S43.
4. Vinik AI, Wing RR, Lauterio TJ: Nutritional management of the person with diabetes. In: Porte D Jr, Sherwin RS, eds. *Diabetes Mellitus*, 5th ed. Appleton & Lange:1997;610.
5. UK Prospective Diabetes Study Group (UKPDS): Intensive blood-glucose control with sulphonylureas or insulin compared with conventional treatment and risk of complications in patients with type 2 diabetes (UKPDS 33). *Lancet* 1998;352:837.
6. UK Prospective Diabetes Study Group (UKPDS): Effect of intensive blood-glucose control with metformin on complications in overweight patients with type 2 diabetes (UKPDS 34). *Lancet* 1998;352: 854.
7. National Research Council: *Recommended Dietary Allowances*, 10th ed. National Academy Press:1989.
8. Abate N, Garg A, Peshock RM, et al: Relationship of generalized and regional adiposity to insulin sensitivity in men with NIDDM. *Diabetes* 1996;45:1684.
9. Abate N, Garg A: Heterogeneity in adipose tissue metabolism: Causes, implications and management of regional adiposity. *Prog Lipid Res* 1995;34:53.
10. Abate N, Garg A, Peshock RM, et al: Relationships of generalized and regional adiposity to insulin sensitivity. *J Clin Invest* 1995; 96:88.
11. Chandalia M, Abate N, Garg A, et al: Regional adiposity and insulin resistance in Asian Indian migrant men to the United States. *J Invest Med* 1995;43(suppl 2):303A.
12. Markovic TP, Jenkins AB, Campbell LV, et al: The determinants of glycemic responses to diet restriction and weight loss in obesity and NIDDM. *Diabetes Care* 1998;21:687.
13. Bosello O, Armellini F, Zamboni M, et al: The benefits of modest weight loss in type II diabetes. *Int J Obesity* 1997;21(suppl 1):S10
14. Van Gaal LF, Wauters MA, De Leeuw IH: The beneficial effects of modest weight loss on cardiovascular risk factors. *Int J Obes* 1997; 21(suppl 1):S5.
15. Wing RR, Koeske R, Epstein LH, et al: Long-term effects of modest weight loss in type II diabetic patients. *Arch Intern Med* 1987;147: 1749.
16. Shah M, Garg A: High-fat and high-carbohydrate diets and energy balance. *Diabetes Care* 1996;19:1142.
17. Gazzaniga JM, Burns TL: Relationship between diet composition and body fatness, with adjustment for resting energy expenditure and physical activity in preadolescent children. *Am J Clin Nutr* 1993; 58:21.
18. Romieu I, Willett WC, Stampfer MJ, et al: Energy intake and other determinants of relative weight. *Am J Clin Nutr* 1988;47:406.
19. National Task Force on Prevention and Treatment of Obesity: Very low-calorie diets. *JAMA* 1993;270:967.

20. Telch CF, Agras WS: The effects of a very low calorie diet on binge eating. *Behav Ther* 1993;24:177.

21. Wadden TA, Foster GD, Letizia KA: One-year behavioral treatment of obesity: Comparison of moderate and severe caloric restriction and the effects of weight maintenance therapy. *J Consult Clin Psychol* 1994;62:165.

22. National Heart, Lung & Blood Institute Obesity Education Initiative Expert Panel: Clinical guidelines on the identification, evaluation, and treatment of overweight and obesity in adults, The evidence report. *Obes Res* 1998;6(suppl 2):92S.

23. Freeman JM, Vining EP, Pillas DJ, et al: The efficacy of the ketogenic diet—1998: A prospective evaluation of intervention in 150 children. *Pediatrics* 1998;102:1358.

24. Tallian K, Nahata M, Tsao CY: Role of ketogenic diet in children with intractable seizures. *Ann Pharmacother* 1998;32:349.

25. Wing RR, Vazquez JA, Ryan CM: Cognitive effects of ketogenic weight reducing diets. *Int J Obes Relat Metab Disord* 1995;19:811.

26. Kerstetter JE, Mitnick ME, Gundberg CM, et al: Changes in bone turnover in young women consuming different levels of dietary protein. *J Clin Endocrinol Metab* 1999;84:1052.

27. Barzel US, Massey LK: Excess dietary protein can adversely affect bone. *J Nutr* 1998;128:1051.

28. Robertson WG, Heyburn PJ, Peacock M: The effect of high animal protein intake on the risk of calcium stone-formation in the urinary tract. *Clin Sci* 1979;57:285.

29. Sakhaee K, Williams RH, Oh MS, et al: Alkali absorption and citrate excretion in calcium nephrolithiasis. *J Bone Miner Res* 1993;8:789.

30. Jeppesen J, Chen Y-DI, Zhou M-Y, et al: Effect of variations in oral fat and carbohydrate load on postprandial lipemia. *Am J Clin Nutr* 1995; 62:1201.

31. Bantle JP, Swanson JE, Thomas W, et al: Metabolic effects of dietary sucrose in type II diabetic subjects. *Diabetes Care* 1993;16:1301.

32. Peters AL, Davidson MB, Eisenberg K: Effect of isocaloric substitution of chocolate cake for potato in type I diabetic patients. *Diabetes Care* 1990;13:888.

33. Hollenbeck CB, Coulston A, Donner CC, et al: The effects of variations in percent of naturally occurring complex and simple carbohydrates on plasma glucose and insulin response in individuals with non-insulin-dependent diabetes mellitus. *Diabetes* 1985;34:151.

34. Coulston AM, Hollenbeck CB, Donner CC, et al: Metabolic effects of added dietary sucrose in individuals with non-insulin-dependent diabetes mellitus (NIDDM). *Metabolism* 1985;34:962.

35. Jeppesen J, Chen Y-DI, Zhou M-Y, et al: Postprandial triglyceride and retinyl ester responses to oral fat: Effects of fructose. *Am J Clin Nutr* 1994;61:787.

36. Bantle JP, Swanson JE, Thomas W, et al: Metabolic effects of dietary fructose in diabetic subjects. *Diabetes Care* 1992;15:1468.

37. Crapo PA, Kolterman OG, Henry RR: Metabolic consequence of two-week fructose feeding in diabetic subjects. *Diabetes Care* 1986; 9:111.

38. Malerbi DA, Paiva ESA, Duarte AL, et al: Metabolic effects of dietary sucrose and fructose in type II diabetic subjects. *Diabetes Care* 1996; 19:1249.

39. Grant KI, Marais MP, Dhansay MA: Sucrose in a lipid-rich meal amplifies the postprandial excursion of serum and lipoprotein triglyceride and cholesterol concentrations by decreasing triglyceride clearance. *Am J Clin Nutr* 1994;59:853.

40. Abraira C, Derler J: Large variations of sucrose in constant carbohydrate diets in type II diabetes. *Am J Med* 1988;84:193.

41. Bantle JP, Laine DC, Thomas JW: Metabolic effects of dietary fructose and sucrose in types I and II diabetic subjects. *JAMA* 1986;256: 3241.

42. Bantle JP: Current recommendations regarding the dietary treatment of diabetes mellitus. *Endocrinologist* 1994;4:189.

43. American Dietetic Association: Position paper: Use of nutritive and nonnutritive sweeteners. *J Am Diet Assoc* 1998;98:580.

44. Joint FAO/WHO Expert Consultation, April 14–18, 1997. Carbohydrates in Human Nutrition. Food and Agriculture Organization Food and Nutrition, Paper 66. FAO:1998.

45. Wolever TMS, Jenkins DJA, Jenkins AL, et al: The glycemic index: Methodology and clinical implications. *Am J Clin Nutr* 1991;54: 846.

46. Foster-Powell K, Miller JB: International tables of glycemic index. *Am J Clin Nutr* 1995;62:871S.

47. Luscombe ND, Noakes M, Clifton PM: Diets high and low in glycemic index versus high monounsaturated fat diets: Effects on glucose and lipid metabolism in NIDDM. *Eur J Clin Nutr* 1999;53: 473.

48. Jarvi AE, Karlstrom BE, Granfeldt YE, et al: Improved glycemic control and lipid profile and normalized fibrinolytic activity on a low glycemic index diet in type 2 diabetic patients. *Diabetes Care* 1999; 22:10.

49. Payne ML, Craig WJ, Williams AC: Sorbitol is a possible risk factor for diarrhea in young children. *J Am Diet Assoc* 1997;97:532.

50. Pitkin RM, Reynolds WA, Filer LJ, et al: Placental transmission and fetal distribution of saccharin. *Am J Obstet Gynecol* 1971;111:280.

51. Brodsky IG, Robbins DC, Hiser E, et al: Effects of low-protein diets on protein metabolism in insulin-dependent diabetes mellitus patients with early nephropathy. *J Clin Endocrinol Metab* 1992;75:351.

52. Zeller KR: Low-protein diets in renal disease. *Diabetes Care* 1991; 14:856.

53. Brenner BM, Meyer TW, Hostetter TH: Dietary protein intake and the progressive nature of kidney disease: The role of hemodynamically mediated glomerular injury in the pathogenesis of progressive glomerular sclerosis in aging, renal ablation and intrinsic renal disease. *N Engl J Med* 1982;307:652.

54. Nakamura H, Ito S, Ebe N, et al: Renal effects of different types of protein in healthy volunteer subjects and diabetic patients. *Diabetes Care* 1993;16:1071.

55. Jibani MM, Bloodworth LL, Foden E, et al: Predominantly vegetarian diet in patients with incipient and early clinical diabetic nephropathy: Effects on albumin excretion rate and nutritional status. *Diabetic Med* 1991;8:949.

56. Kontessis P, Jones S, Dodds R, et al: Renal, metabolic and hormonal responses to ingestion of animal and vegetable proteins. *Kidney Int* 1990;38:136.

57. Messina M, Messina V: *The Dietitian's Guide to Vegetarian Diets: Issues and Applications.* Aspen Publishers, Inc.:1996.

58. National Cholesterol Education Program: *Second Report of the Expert Panel on Detection, Evaluation, and Treatment of High Blood Cholesterol in Adults.* National Institutes of Health:1993.

59. Cater NB, Garg A: Serum low-density lipoprotein cholesterol response to modification of saturated fat intake: Recent insights. *Curr Opin Lipidol* 1997;8:332.

60. Kris-Etherton PM, Yu S: Individual fatty acid effects on plasma lipids and lipoproteins: Human studies. *Am J Clin Nutr* 1997;65:(suppl) 1628S.

61. Bonanome A, Grundy SM: Effect of dietary stearic acid on plasma cholesterol and lipoprotein levels. *N Engl J Med* 1988;318:1244.

62. Cater NB, Heller HJ, Denke MA: Comparison of the effects of medium-chain triacylglycerols, palm oil, and high oleic acid sunflower oil on plasma triacylglycerol fatty acids and lipid and lipoprotein concentrations in humans. *Am J Clin Nutr* 1997;65:41.

63. Cater NB, Denke MA: Comparison of effects of behenate oil, high oleic acid sunflower oil, and palm oil on lipids and lipoproteins in humans [Abstract]. *Circulation* 1996;94:I–97.

64. Mattson FH, Grundy SM: Comparison of effects of dietary saturated, monounsaturated, and polyunsaturated fatty acids on plasma lipids and lipoproteins in man. *J Lipid Res* 1985;26:194.

65. Glauber H, Wallace P, Griver K, et al: Adverse metabolic effect of omega-3 fatty acids in non-insulin-dependent diabetes mellitus. *Ann Intern Med* 1988;108:663.

66. Prince MJ, Deeg MA: Do n-3 fatty acids improve glucose tolerance and lipemia in diabetics? *Curr Opin Lipidol* 1997;8:7.

67. Connor WE, Prince MJ, Ullman D, et al: The hypotriglyceridemic effect of fish oil in adult-onset diabetes without adverse glucose control. *Ann NY Acad Sci* 1993;683:337.

68. Rivellese AA, Mafettone A, Iovine C, et al: Long-term effects of fish oil on insulin resistance and plasma lipoproteins in NIDDM patients with hypertriglyceridemia. *Diabetes Care* 1996;19:1207.

69. Mensink RP, Katan MB: Effects of dietary fatty acids on serum lipids and lipoproteins: A meta-analysis of 27 trials. *Arterioscler Thromb* 1992;12:911.

70. Valsta LM, Jauhiainen M, Aro A, et al: Effects of a monounsaturated rapeseed oil and a polyunsaturated sunflower oil diet on lipoprotein levels in humans. *Arterioscler Thromb* 1992;12:50.

71. Berry EM, Eisenberg S, Haratz D, et al: Effects of diets rich in monounsaturated fatty acids on plasma lipoproteins—the Jerusalem Nu-

trition Study: High MUFAs vs high PUFAs. *Am J Clin Nutr* 1991;53: 899.

72. Dreon DM, Vranizan KM, Krauss RM, *et al*: The effects of polyunsaturated fat vs. monounsaturated fat on plasma lipoproteins. *JAMA* 1990;263:2462.

73. McDonald BE, Gerrard JM, Bruce VM, *et al*: Comparison of the effect of canola oil and sunflower oil on plasma lipids and lipoproteins and on *in vivo* thromboxane A$_2$ and prostacyclin production in healthy young men. *Am J Clin Nutr* 1989;50:1382.

74. Mensink RP, Katan MB: Effect of a diet enriched with monounsaturated or polyunsaturated fatty acids on levels of low-density and high-density lipoprotein cholesterol in healthy women and men. *N Engl J Med* 1989;321:436.

75. Grande FY, Matsumoto Y, Anderson JT, *et al*: Effect of dietary rapeseed oil on man's serum lipids. *Circulation* 1962;26:653.

76. Garg A, Bonanome A, Grundy SM, *et al*: Comparison of a high-carbohydrate diet with a high-monounsaturated-fat diet in patients with non-insulin-dependent diabetes mellitus. *N Engl J Med* 1988; 319:829.

77. Garg A: High-monounsaturated-fat diets for patients with diabetes mellitus: A meta-analysis. *Am J Clin Nutr* 1998;67(suppl):577S.

78. Padley FB, Gunstone FD, Harwood JL: Occurrence and characteristics of oils and fats. In: Gunstone FD, Harwood JL, Padley FB, eds. *The Lipid Handbook*, 2nd ed. Chapman & Hall:1994;49.

79. Allison DB, Egan SK, Barraj LM, *et al*: Estimated intakes of *trans* fatty and other fatty acids in the US population. *J Am Diet Assoc* 1999;99:166.

80. Hulshof KF, van Erp-Baart MA, Anttolainen M, *et al*: Intake of fatty acids in western Europe with emphasis on trans fatty acids: The TRANSFAIR Study. *Eur J Clin Nutr* 1999;53:143.

81. Nestel P, Noakes M, Belling B, *et al*: Plasma lipoprotein lipid and Lp[a] changes with substitution of elaidic acid for oleic acid in the diet. *J Lipid Res* 1992;33:1029.

82. Mensink RP, Katan MB: Effect of dietary *trans* fatty acids on high-density and low-density lipoprotein cholesterol levels in healthy subjects. *N Engl J Med* 1990;323:439.

83. Hu FB, Stampfer MJ, Manson JE, *et al*: Dietary fat intake and the risk of coronary heart disease in women. *N Engl J Med* 1997;337:1491.

84. The American Dietetic Association: Position paper on fat replacers. *J Am Diet Assoc* 1998;98:463.

85. Prince DM, Welschenbach MA: Olestra: A new food additive. *J Am Diet Assoc* 1998;98:565.

86. National Health and Nutrition Examination Survey III, 1988–1994. NCHS CD-ROM series 11. No. 2A. ASCII version. National Center for Health Statistics:April 1998.

87. Eeley EA, Stratton IM, Hadden DR, *et al*: UKPDS 18: Estimated dietary intake in type 2 diabetic patients randomly allocated to diet, sulphonylurea or insulin therapy. UK Prospective Diabetes Study Group. *Diabet Med* 1996;13:656.

88. Hunninghake DB, Miller VT, LaRosa JC, *et al*: Hypocholesterolemic effects of a dietary fiber supplement. *Am J Clin Nutri* 1994;59: 1050.

89. Chandalia M, Garg A, Lutjohann D, *et al*: Beneficial effects of high dietary fiber intake in patients with type 2 diabetes mellitus. *N Engl J Med* 2000;342:1392.

90. Schakel SF, Sievert YA, Buzzard IM: Dietary fiber values for common foods (Appendix I). In: Spiller GA, ed. *CRC Handbook of Dietary Fiber in Human Nutrition*, 2nd ed. CRC Press:1993;567.

91. Dietary Guidelines Committee: *Dietary Guidelines for Americans, 2000*. U.S. Department of Agriculture, U.S. Department of Health and Human Services:2000.

92. Suh I, Shaten BJ, Cutler JA, *et al*: Alcohol use and mortality from coronary heart disease: The role of high-density lipoprotein cholesterol. *Ann Intern Med* 1992;116:881.

93. Steinberg D, Pearson TA, Kuller LH: Alcohol and atherosclerosis. *Ann Intern Med* 1991;114:967.

94. Burr ML, Fehily AM, Butland BK, *et al*: Alcohol and high-density lipoprotein cholesterol: A randomized controlled trial. *Br J Nutr* 1986;56:81.

95. Wei M, Gibbons LW, Mitchell TL, *et al*: Alcohol intake and incidence of type 2 diabetes in men. *Diabetes Care* 2000;23:18.

96. Kiechl S, Willeit J, Poewe W, *et al*: Insulin sensitivity and regular alcohol consumption: Large, prospective, cross sectional population study (Bruneck study). *Br Med J* 1996;313:1040.

97. Ben G, Gnudi L, Maran A, *et al*: Effects of chronic alcohol intake on carbohydrate and lipid metabolism in subjects with type II (non-insulin-dependent) diabetes. *Am J Med* 1991;90:70.

98. Puhakainen I, Koivisto VA, Yki-Jarvinen H: No reduction in total hepatic glucose output by inhibition of gluconeogenesis with ethanol in NIDDM patients. *Diabetes* 1991;40:1319.

99. Yki-Jarvinen H, Koivisto VA, Ylikahri R, *et al*: Acute effects of ethanol and acetate on glucose kinetics in normal subjects. *Am J Physiol* 1988;254:E175.

100. Bjorntorp P, Rosmond R: Visceral obesity and diabetes. *Drugs* 1999; 58(suppl 1):13.

101. Naveau S, Giraud V, Borotto E, *et al*: Excess weight risk factor for alcoholic liver disease. *Hepatology* 1997;25:108.

102. Leiber CS: Alcohol and the liver, 1994 update. *Gastroenterology* 1994;106:1085.

103. Menzel R, Mentel DC, Brunstein U, *et al*: Effect of moderate ethanol ingestion on overnight diabetes control and hormone secretion in type I diabetic patients [Abstract]. *Diabetologia* 1991;34:A188.

104. Kerr D, Macdonald IA, Heller SR, *et al*: Alcohol causes hypoglycaemic unawareness in healthy volunteers and patients with type 1 (insulin-dependent) diabetes. *Diabetologia* 1990;33:216.

105. Burge MR, Zeise T-M, Sobhy TA, *et al*: Low-dose ethanol predisposes elderly fasted patients with type 2 diabetes to sulfonylurea-induced low blood glucose. *Diabetes Care* 1999;22:2037.

106. Mooradian AD, Failla M, Hoogwerf B, *et al*: Selected vitamins and minerals in diabetes. *Diabetes Care* 1994;17:464.

107. Jialal I, Grundy SM: Effect of combined supplementation with α-tocopherol, ascorbate, and β-carotene on low-density lipoprotein oxidation. *Circulation* 1993;88:2780.

108. Steinberg D, Parthasarathy S, Carew TE, *et al*: Beyond cholesterol: Modifications of low-density lipoproteins that increase its atherogenicity. *N Engl J Med* 1989;320:915.

109. Yusuf S, Dagenais G, Pogue J, *et al*: Vitamin E supplementation and cardiovascular events in high-risk patients. The Heart Outcomes Prevention Evaluation Study Investigators. *N Engl J Med* 2000;342: 154.

110. Hennekens CH, Buring JE, Manson JE, *et al*: Lack of effect of long-term supplementation with beta carotene on the incidence of malignant neoplasms and cardiovascular disease. *N Engl J Med* 1996;334: 1145.

111. Albanes D, Heinonen OP, Taylor PR, *et al*: Alpha-tocopherol and beta-carotene supplements and lung cancer incidence in the alpha-tocopherol, beta-carotene cancer prevention study: Effects of baseline characteristics and study compliance. *J Natl Cancer Inst* 1996;88: 1560.

112. Abraham AS, Brooks BA, Eylate U: The effects of chromium supplementation on serum glucose and lipids in patients with and without non-insulin-dependent diabetes. *Metabolism* 1992;41:768.

113. Anderson RA, Polansky MM, Bryden NA, *et al*: Supplemental-chromium effects on glucose, insulin, glucagon, and urinary chromium losses in subjects consuming controlled low-chromium diets. *Am J Clin Nutr* 1991;54:909.

114. Lima JDL, Cruz T, Pousada JC, *et al*: The effect of magnesium supplementation in increasing doses on the control of type 2 diabetes. *Diabetes Care* 1998;21:682.

115. Nadler JL, Malayan S, Luong H, *et al*: Intracellular free magnesium deficiency plays a key role in increased platelet reactivity in type II diabetes mellitus. *Diabetes Care* 1992;15:835.

116. Sjogren A, Floren CH, Nilsson A: Magnesium, potassium, zinc deficiency in subjects with type II diabetes mellitus. *Acta Med Scand* 1988;224:461.

117. American Diabetes Association: Magnesium supplementation in the treatment of diabetes (Consensus Statement). *Diabetes Care* 1992;15: 1065.

118. UK Prospective Diabetes Study Group (UKPDS): Tight blood pressure control and risk of macrovascular and microvascular complications in type 2 diabetes (UKPDS 38). *Br Med J* 1998;317:703.

119. UK Prospective Diabetes Study Group (UKPDS): Efficacy of atenolol and captopril in reducing risk of macrovascular and microvascular complications in type 2 diabetes (UKPDS 39). *Br Med J* 1998;317: 713.

120. Midgley JP, Matthew AG, Greenwood CM, *et al*: Effect of reduced dietary sodium on blood pressure: A meta-analysis of randomized controlled trials. *JAMA* 1996;275:1590.

121. Overlack A, Ruppert M, Lkolloch R, *et al*: Age is a major determinant of the divergent blood pressure responses to varying salt intake in essential hypertension. *Am J Hypertens* 1995;8:829.

122. The Sixth Report of the Joint National Committee on Prevention, Detection, Evaluation, and Treatment of High Blood Pressure. *Arch Intern Med* 1997;157:2413.

123. McCarron DA, Weder AB, Egan BM, *et al*: Blood pressure and metabolic responses to moderate sodium restriction in israpidine-treated hypertensive patients. *Am J Hypertens* 1997;10:68.

124. Feldman RD, Logan AG, Schmidt ND: Dietary salt increased vascular insulin resistance. *Clin Pharm Ther* 1996;60:444.

125. Fliser D, Nowack R, Allendorf-Ostwald N, *et al*: Serum lipid changes on low salt diet. Effects of alpha 1-adrenergic blockade. *Am J Hypertens* 1993;6:320.

126. Cater NB, Grundy SM: Lowering serum cholesterol with plant sterol and stanols. Historical perspectives. A *Postgraduate Med* Special Report. Nov. 1998:6.

127. Mensink RP, Plat J: Efficacy of dietary plant stanols. A *Postgraduate Med* Special Report. Nov. 1998:27.

128. Miettinen TA, Puska P, Gylling H, *et al*: Reduction of serum cholesterol with sitostanol ester margarine in a mildly hypercholesterolemic population. *N Engl J Med* 1995;333:1308.

129. Gylling H, Miettinen TA: Cholesterol absorption, synthesis and LDL metabolism in NIDDM. *Diabetes Care* 1997;20:90.

130. Gylling H, Miettinen TA: Serum cholesterol and cholesterol and lipoprotein metabolism in hypercholesterolaemic NIDDM patients before and during sitostanol ester-margarine treatment. *Diabetologia* 1994;37:773.

131. Eisenberg DM, Davis RB, Ettner SL, *et al*: Trends in alternative medicine use in the United States, 1990–1997: Results of a follow-up national survey. *JAMA* 1998;280:1569.

132. Verboeket-van den Venne WPHG, Westerterp KR: Frequency of feeding, weight reduction and energy metabolism. *Int J Obes* 1993; 17:31.

133. Jenkins DJA, Ocana A, Jenkins AL, *et al*: Metabolic advantages of spreading the nutrient load: Effects of increased meal frequency in non-insulin-dependent diabetes. *Am J Clin Nutr* 1992;55:461.

134. Bertelsen J, Christiansen C, Thomsen C, *et al*: Effect of meal frequency on blood glucose, insulin, and free fatty acids in NIDDM subjects. *Diabetes Care* 1993;16:4.

135. Jenkins DJA, Wolever TMS, Vuksan V, *et al*: Nibbling versus gorging: Metabolic advantages of increased meal frequency. *N Engl J Med* 1989;321:929.

136. Schlundt DG, Hill JO, Sbrocco T, *et al*: The role of breakfast in the treatment of obesity: A randomized clinical trial. *Am J Clin Nutr* 1992;55:645.

137. Kaufman FR: Diabetes mellitus. *Pediatrics in Review* 1997;18:383.

138. Gillespie SJ, Kulkarni KD, Daly AE: Using carbohydrate counting in diabetes clinical practice. *J Am Diet Assoc* 1998;98:897.

139. American Diabetes Association: Type 2 diabetes in children and adolescents. *Diabetes Care* 2000;23:381.

140. Shick SM, Wing RR, Klem ML, *et al*: Persons successful at long-term weight loss and maintenance continue to consume a low-energy, low-fat diet. *J Am Diet Assoc* 1998;98:408.

141. French SA, Jeffery RW: Current dieting, weight loss history, and weight suppression: Behavioral correlates of three dimensions of dieting. *Addict Behav* 1997;22:31.

142. Klem ML, Wing RR, McGuire MT, *et al*: A descriptive study of individuals successful at long-term maintenance of substantial weight loss. *Am J Clin Nutr* 1997;66:239.

143. Harris JK, French SA, Jeffery RW, *et al*: Dietary and physical activity correlates of long-term weight loss. *Obesity Res* 1994;2:307.

144. Pronk NP, Wing RR: Physical activity and long-term maintenance of weight loss. *Obes Res* 1994;2:587.

145. Kayman S, Bruvold W, Stern JS: Maintenance and relapse after weight loss in women: behavioral aspects. *Am J Clin Nutr* 1990;52: 800.

146. Perri MG, McAllister DA, Gange JJ, *et al*: Effects of four maintenance programs on the long-term management of obesity. *J Consult Clin Psychol* 1988;56:529.

147. Perri MG, McAdoo WG, McAllister DA, *et al*: Enhancing the efficacy of behavior therapy for obesity: Effects of aerobic exercise and a multicomponent maintenance program. *J Consult Clin Psychol* 1986;54: 670.

148. Lamont LS: Beta-blockers and their effects on protein metabolism and resting energy expenditure. *J Cardiopulm Rehabil* 1995;15:183.

149. Institute of Medicine, Food and Nutrition Board, Committee on Nutritional Status During Pregnancy and Lactation, Subcommittee on Dietary Intake and Nutrient Supplements During Pregnancy, Subcommittee on Nutrition Status and Weight Gain During Pregnancy: *Nutrition During Pregnancy*. National Academy Press:1990;1.

150. Knopp RH, Magee MS, Raisys V, *et al*: Hypocaloric diets and ketogenesis in the management of obese gestational diabetic women. *J Am Coll Nutr* 1991;10:649.

151. Magee MS, Knopp RH, Benedetti TJ: Metabolic effects of 1200 kcal diet in obese pregnant women with gestational diabetes. *Diabetes* 1990;39:234.

152. Jovanovic L: American Diabetes Association's Fourth International Workshop-Conference on Gestational Diabetes Mellitus: Summary and Discussion. Therapeutic interventions. *Diabetes Care* 1998;21: B131.

153. Eriksson UJ, Swenne I: Diabetes in pregnancy: Fetal macrosomia, hyperinsulinism, and islet hyperplasia in the offspring of rats subjects to temporary protein-energy malnutrition early in life. *Pediatr Res* 1993; 34:791.

154. Barbosa FB, Gravena C, Mathias P, *et al*: Blockade of the 32P phosphate flush of pancreatic β-cells from adult rats who received a low-protein diet during early lactation. *Braz J Med Biol Res* 1993;26: 1355.

155. Giavini E, Broccia ML, Prati M, *et al*: Diet composition modifies embryotoxic effects induced by experimental diabetes in rats. *Biol Neonate* 1991;59:278.

156. Major CA, Henry MJ, De Veciana M, *et al*: The effects of carbohydrate restriction in patients with diet-controlled gestational diabetes. *Obstet Gynecol* 1998;91:600.

157. Lovelady CA, Garner KE, Moreno KL, *et al*: The effect of weight loss in overweight, lactating women on the growth of their infants. *N Engl J Med* 2000;342:449.

158. Murtaugh MA, Ferris AM, Capacchione CM, *et al*: Energy intake and glycemia in lactating women with type 1 diabetes. *J Am Diet Assoc* 1998;98:642.

159. Bryden KS, Neil A, Mayou RA, *et al*: Eating habits, body weight, and insulin misuse. *Diabetes Care* 1999;22:1956.

160. Herpetz S, Albus C, Wagener R, *et al*: Comorbidity of diabetes and eating disorders. Does diabetes control reflect disturbed eating behavior? *Diabetes Care* 1998;21:1110.

161. Neumark-Sztainer D, Story M, Toporoff E, *et al*: Psychosocial predictors of binge eating and purging behaviors among adolescents with and without diabetes mellitus. *J Adolesc Health* 1996;19:289.

162. Polonsky WH, Anderson BJ, Lohrer PA, *et al*: Insulin omission in women with IDDM. *Diabetes Care* 1994;17:1178.

163. Engstrom I, Kroon M, Arvidson CG, *et al*: Eating disorders in adolescent girls with insulin-dependent diabetes mellitus: A population-based case-control study. *Acta Paediatr* 1999;88:175.

164. Rydall AC, Rodin GM, Olmsted MP, *et al*: Disordered eating behavior and microvascular complications in young women with insulin-dependent diabetes mellitus. *N Engl J Med* 1997;336:1849.

165. Affenito SG, Lammi-Keefe CJ, Vogel S, *et al*: Women with insulin-dependent diabetes mellitus (IDDM) complicated by eating disorders are at risk for exacerbated alterations in lipid metabolism. *Eur J Clin Nutr* 1997;51:462.

166. McMahon MM: Nutrition support and diabetes. In: Franz MJ, Bantle JP, eds. *American Diabetes Association Guide to Medical Nutrition Therapy for Diabetes*. ADA:1999;335.

167. Boswell E, Lipps J: Diabetes management during illness and surgery. In: Funnell MM, Hunt C, Kulkarni K, *et al*, eds. *A Core Curriculum for Diabetes Education*, 3rd ed. American Association of Diabetes Educators:1998;475.

168. Gaare-Porcari JM, O'Sullivan J: Care for persons with diabetes during surgery. In: Powers MA, ed. *Handbook of Diabetes Medical Nutrition Therapy*, 2nd ed. Aspen Publishers, Inc.:1996;602.

169. Parrish CR: Gastrointestinal issues in persons with diabetes. In: Powers MA, ed. *Handbook of Diabetes Medical Nutrition Therapy*, 2nd ed. Aspen Publishers, Inc.:1996;618.

170. American Diabetes Association: Diabetic nephropathy. *Diabetes Care* 2000;23:S69.

171. Dallas-Fort Worth Hospital Council: Nutritional therapy in renal disease and transplantation. *Manual of Medical Nutrition Therapy*. 1998.

172. Wheeler ML: Diabetic gastropathy and medical nutrition therapy. In: Franz MJ, Bantle JP, eds. *American Diabetes Association Guide to Medical Nutrition Therapy for Diabetes*. ADA:1999;330.

173. Fontana RJ, Barnett JL: Jejunostomy tube placement in refractory diabetic gastroparesis: A retrospective review. *Am J Gastroenterol* 1996;91:2174.

174. Ogbonnaya KI, Arem R: Diabetic diarrhea. Pathophysiology, diagnosis, and management. *Arch Intern Med* 1990;150:262.

175. Sjoberg K, Eriksson KF, Bredberg A, *et al*: Screening for coeliac disease in adult insulin-dependent diabetes mellitus. *J Intern Med* 1998;243:133.

176. Cronin CC, Feighery A, Ferriss JB, *et al*: High prevalence of celiac disease among patients with insulin-dependent (type I) diabetes mellitus. *Am J Gastroenterol* 1997;92:2210.

177. Rensch MJ, Merenich JA, Lieberman M, *et al*: Gluten-sensitive enteropathy in patients with insulin-dependent diabetes mellitus. *Ann Intern Med* 1996;124:564.

178. Inman-Felton AE: Overview of gluten-sensitive enteropathy (celiac sprue). *J Am Diet Assoc* 1999;99:352.

179. Schlundt DG, Rea MR, Kline SS, *et al*: Situational obstacles to dietary adherence for adults with diabetes. *J Am Diet Assoc* 1994;94:874, 879.

180. Williamson AR, Hunt AE, Pope JF, *et al*: Recommendations of dietitians for overcoming barriers to dietary adherence in individuals with diabetes. *Diabetes Educ* 2000;26:272.

181. Johnson EQ, Valera S: Medical nutrition therapy in non-insulin-dependent diabetes mellitus improves clinical outcome. *J Am Diet Assoc* 1995;95:700.

182. Laitinen JH, Ahola IE, Sarkkinen ES, *et al*: Impact of intensified dietary therapy on energy and nutrient intakes and fatty acid consumption on serum lipids in patients with recently diagnosed non-insulin-dependent diabetes mellitus. *J Am Diet Assoc* 1993;93:1423.

183. Arnold MS, Stepien CJ, Hess GE, *et al*: Guidelines vs. practice in the delivery of diabetes nutrition care. *J Am Diet Assoc* 1993;93:34.

184. Close EJ, Wiles PG, Lockton JA, *et al*: The degree of day-to-day variation in food intake in diabetic patients. *Diabet Med* 1993;10:514.

185. The Diabetes Control and Complication Trial (DCCT) Research Group: Nutrition interventions for intensive therapy in The Diabetes Control and Complications Trial. *J Am Diet Assoc* 1993;93:768.

186. Delahanty LM, Halford BN: The role of diet behaviors in achieving improved glycemic control in intensively treated patients in the diabetes control and complications trial. *Diabetes Care* 1993;16:1453.

187. Travis T: Patient perceptions of factors that affect adherence to dietary regimens for diabetes mellitus. *Diabetes Educ* 1997;23:152.

188. Warshaw HS: Nutrition management of diabetes must be individualized. *Diabetes Care* 1993;16:843.

189. Campbell LV, Barth R, Gosper JK, *et al*: Impact of intensive educational approach to dietary change in NIDDM. *Diabetes Care* 1990;13:841.

190. Franz MJ, Monk A, Barry B, *et al*: Effectiveness of medical nutrition therapy provided by dietitians in the management of non-insulin-dependent diabetes mellitus: A randomized, controlled clinical trial. *J Am Diet Assoc* 1995;95:1009.

191. Diabetes Care and Education Dietetic Practice Group: *Meal Planning Approaches for Diabetes Management*, 2nd ed. American Dietetic Association:1994.

CHAPTER 27

Metabolic Implications of Exercise and Physical Fitness in Physiology and Diabetes

David H. Wasserman

Zhi-Qing Shi

Mladen Vranic

Exercise has long been considered beneficial in the treatment of diabetes mellitus. Its therapeutic usefulness was widely recognized by physicians in the nineteenth and early twentieth centuries. Following the discovery of insulin, Joslin and coworkers[1] and others recommended exercise as one of three basic principles in the management of diabetes. In the last two decades, many studies employing modern technology have investigated the relationship between fitness and metabolic control in diabetes. The rationale for the use of exercise as part of the treatment program is much clearer in type 2 diabetes mellitus (T2DM) than in type 1 diabetes mellitus (T1DM).[2] Thus, exercise is not currently regarded as a necessary management component for every diabetic individual, as it was in the past. Because physical exercise is related to improved quality of life, an assumption that has been made since classical Greek civilization, and has beneficial effects on the cardiovascular system, metabolic control should not be the only criterion by which to judge the benefits of a training program for diabetic patients.

A distinction must be made between the effects of acute exercise and those of physical training. For the body to meet the acute oxygen and fuel requirements of physical work and still minimize the deviations from homeostasis, metabolic, circulatory, and temperature-controlling adaptations are necessary. These short-lived regulations vary with the type, intensity, and duration of exercise; the muscles used; and a variety of environmental factors, such as physical condition and nutritional state. In contrast, the changes induced by physical training are long-term adaptations resulting from regularly performed exercise. In addition to improvements in work capacity, these chronic adaptations may also change the metabolic parameters during both rest and exercise. By nature, both local (muscular) and systemic effects of physical training are chronic and continue to be demonstrable for variable periods after physical exercise has stopped. Significant advances have been made in understanding the hormonal and substrate regulation of glucose fluxes during exercise in physiology and diabetes. This chapter highlights recent progress.

PHYSIOLOGY OF FUEL METABOLISM DURING EXERCISE

The increase in energy demand during exercise necessitates an accelerated flow of carbohydrate and fat from their storage sites to the energy-transducing machinery in the working muscle. To a lesser extent, amino acids may be used as fuel, particularly when the availability of other substrates becomes limited. During the transition from rest to moderate-intensity exercise, the muscle shifts from using primarily free fatty acids (FFAs) to using a blend of FFAs, glucose, and muscle glycogen. During the early stages of exercise, muscle glycogen is the chief source of energy. With prolonged duration of exercise, the contributions of circulating glucose and, particularly, of FFAs, become increasingly important, as muscle glycogen gradually depletes. In addition, the origin of circulating glucose shifts from hepatic glycogenolysis to gluconeogenesis, as intrahepatic mechanisms channel a greater portion of the three-carbon molecules taken up by the liver into glucose.[3] With increasing exercise intensity, the balance of substrate usage shifts to a greater oxidation of carbohydrates.[4] Although the metabolic response to exercise will be influenced by such factors as nutritional state, age, type of exercise, and physical condition, the contribution of each specific substrate will always depend on work intensity and duration. Specific aspects of substrate metabolism can be defined in terms of three functional aims discussed as follows.

Preserving Glucose Homeostasis

Endogenous glucose production (GP) is so closely coupled to the exercise-induced increase in muscle glucose uptake that circulating glucose levels are generally not perturbed even though large increments in glucose usage may be present. Under certain conditions, however, blood glucose concentration may deviate from resting levels even in normal subjects. During prolonged exercise, gradually diminishing carbohydrate stores often result in a fall in blood glucose levels, whereas during heavy exercise, a rise in glycemia can ensue, as GP may exceed glucose metabolism.

Metabolizing the Most Efficient Substrate

Metabolic Efficiency

During high-intensity work when adenosine triphosphate (ATP) hydrolysis is accelerated and O_2 availability may be limited, carbohydrates are the preferred substrate. Generation of ATP from glucose oxidation in the cytoplasm occurs more rapidly than from fat oxidation in the mitochondria. Furthermore, since glucose carbon atoms are already partially oxidized compared to the highly saturated carbon skeleton of fats, they require less oxygen for complete metabolism. Hence, when oxygen availability is limited, such as during heavy exercise, glucose is the most efficient fuel.

Storage Efficiency

Low-intensity exercise that can potentially be sustained for long intervals is characterized by a preference for fat oxidation. Under these circumstances, speed and efficiency of energy transduction become secondary to fuel storage efficiency. Differences in the degree of saturation of FFAs and glucose carbons predict that twice as much energy can be gained from the oxidation of triglycerides than an equal quantity of glycogen. In addition, while glycogen is stored with water, fats are immiscible with water and are stored in pure form. Hence, the economy of fat storage makes this fuel the most efficient for muscular activity of long duration.

Delaying Exhaustion

Fatigue during exercise that is not limited by the cardiopulmonary system is probably due to muscle glycogen depletion.[5] To preserve muscle glycogen, a number of processes are accelerated. Glycerol, lactate, pyruvate, alanine, and other amino acids are channeled into the gluconeogenic pathway at an increased rate, thereby conserving carbon-based compounds. The contribution of FFA oxidation to total energy needs increases, thus sparing muscle glycogen. To a far lesser extent, branched-chain amino acid and ketone body oxidation will also increase. Prolonged exercise necessitates that extramuscular substrates be mobilized and made available to the working muscle with the goal of delaying muscle glycogen depletion. The rate at which these alternate substrates are used, however, must also preserve glucose homeostasis and allow for optimal metabolic efficiency.

REGULATION OF SUBSTRATE METABOLISM DURING EXERCISE

Control of the optimal substrate balance during exercise is achieved largely by the combined actions of insulin, glucagon, and the catecholamines (Fig. 27-1). In general, decreased insulin secretion and increased glucagon, catecholamine and cortisol secretion, among other hormones, characterize exercise. The signal for these hormonal and neural changes has been postulated to be increased afferent nerve activity originating at the working limb and splanchnic bed, a deficit in fuel availability, and/or neural feed-forward. In addition to hormonal factors, it is likely that other parameters, such as neural outflow originating in the central nervous system, blood flow shifts, and subtle changes in glycemia or the metabolic state, play a role in control of fuel metabolism during exercise.

Regulation of Endogenous Glucose Production

The interaction of increased glucagon and decreased insulin is the primary mechanism by which increases in hepatic glycogenolysis and gluconeogenesis are coordinated with the increase in glucose uptake during moderate-intensity exercise.[6–8] For reasons that are discussed, it is possible that endogenous GP is regulated differently during high-intensity exercise.

Studies in humans using the pancreatic clamp technique show that simultaneously preventing the increase in glucagon and de-

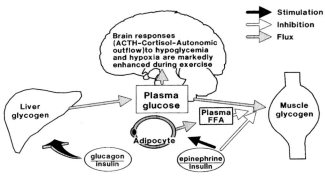

FIGURE 27-1. Hormonal control and the interaction between the brain, liver, muscle, and fat cell in control of glucose homeostasis. It is indicated that glucagon/insulin interaction mainly controls hepatic glucose production, while epinephrine/insulin interaction controls peripheral glucose uptake, but the main role of the latter could be indirect through control of lipolysis in adipocytes (FFA–glucose cycle.)

crease in insulin leads to a fall in glucose ranging from about 25–50 mg/dL over the course of 1 hour.[9–11] This fall in blood glucose can occur despite a large compensatory increase in catecholamines. From these studies, it is apparent that changes in glucagon and/or insulin are essential to the maintenance of glucose homeostasis during exercise. These studies were extended by work in exercising dogs, and later in humans, that assessed the specific role of changes in insulin and glucagon.[6,11] To selectively determine the role of the glucagon increment during moderate exercise in the dog, somatostatin was infused to suppress endogenous pancreatic hormone release, and insulin was replaced intraportally at basal rates at rest and with the normal fall in this hormone simulated during exercise.[12] Circulating glucose levels were clamped to prevent the confounding influence of hypoglycemic counterregulation. These studies showed that about 60% of the exercise-induced increment in GP is controlled by glucagon. This was consistent with findings in humans, showing that the rise in glucagon is necessary for glucose homeostasis during moderate exercise.[11] Studies in the dog also showed that the rise in glucagon is necessary for the full increment in both hepatic glycogenolysis and gluconeogenesis (Fig. 27-2).[6] This stimulatory effect of glucagon on gluconeogenesis was due to an accelerated rate of gluconeogenic precursor extraction by the liver and enhanced channeling of precursor to glucose within the liver.

The role of the decrease in insulin level during moderate exercise was first ascertained in the dog by infusing insulin in the portal vein at a rate that prevented the fall in this hormone.[13] Glucose levels were clamped throughout the exercise period in these studies. When the fall in insulin was selectively eliminated, the increase in hepatic GP was impaired due to an attenuation of hepatic glycogenolysis. The fall in insulin was calculated to control 55% of the increase in hepatic GP. The importance of the fall in insulin was subsequently confirmed by a study in human subjects showing that selectively preventing the exercise-induced fall in insulin using the pancreatic clamp technique led to a more expeditious fall in blood glucose.[11] In the dog, when the fall in insulin was prevented and glucose levels were not clamped, counterregulation (i.e., excessive catecholamine, glucagon, and cortisol increases) prevented

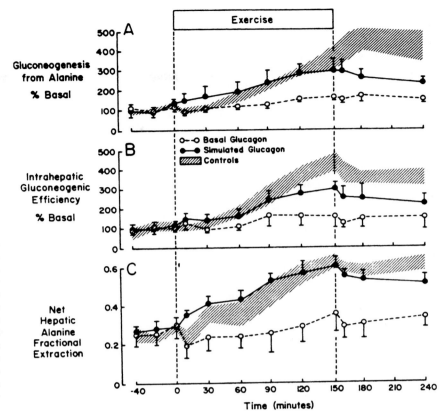

FIGURE 27-2. Role of the exercise-induced increase in glucagon in gluconeogenic regulation. Effect of exercise alone (**shaded area**), exercise with somatostatin plus simulated glucagon and insulin (**solid line**), and somatostatin plus basal glucagon and simulated insulin (**dashed line**) on (**A**) gluconeogenic conversion from alanine, (**B**) intrahepatic gluconeogenic efficiency from alanine, and (**C**) hepatic fractional alanine extraction. The exercise-induced increment in glucagon enhances gluconeogenesis by stimulating the gluconeogenic precursor extraction by the liver and channelling into glucose within the liver. Data are mean ± SE. (*Reprinted with permission from Wasserman DH, Williams PE, Lacy DB, et al: Exercise-induced fall in insulin and hepatic carbohydrate metabolism during muscular work. Am J Physiol 1989; 256:E500.*)

severe hypoglycemia by stimulating hepatic glycogenolysis and gluconeogenesis.[6] Thus, while the fall in insulin plays an important physiologic role in the liver, effective counterregulation can partially compensate for the absence of the exercise-induced decrease in this hormone, and minimize the fall in glucose.

From the previous discussion, it is evident that coordinated and reciprocal changes in glucagon and insulin play important physiologic roles in accounting for virtually the entire increments in hepatic glycogenolysis and gluconeogenesis during moderate-intensity exercise. While changes in glucagon and insulin are individually very important, several lines of evidence indicate that it is the interaction of these changes that is the most critical. First, although changes in glucagon and insulin are both well correlated to the increase in endogenous GP, the ratio between glucagon and insulin exhibits the strongest correlation to this variable.[7,8] Second, the glucagon increment controls about fourfold more of the increment in GP when insulin is allowed to fall, compared to when it is maintained at basal levels. Hence, during exercise, as is the case at rest, a fall in insulin sensitizes the liver to the effects of glucagon. Third, the fall in insulin has no effect on endogenous GP when biologically active glucagon levels are suppressed using somatostatin.[6]

It seems that epinephrine is unimportant in controlling endogenous GP during moderate-intensity exercise.[6] Human subjects who were adrenalectomized for treatment of Cushing's disease or bilateral pheochromocytoma had a normal increase in GP during 60 minutes of moderate-intensity exercise, even though the changes in pancreatic hormone levels were similar to those in normal controls.[14] Moreover, the increase in epinephrine plays only a minor

role in stimulating the increase in GP with moderate-intensity exercise in the dog and appears to occur only during the later stage of prolonged exercise (>120 minutes).[6] Because of this, and the fact that it coincides with a diminished arterial lactate response, one can speculate that the effect of epinephrine is to facilitate gluconeogenic substrate mobilization from peripheral sites. This hypothesis is supported by the increased importance of epinephrine to glucoregulation in fasted rats, who are far more reliant on gluconeogenesis.[15]

A role for hepatic nerves in the stimulation of endogenous GP during exercise has been proposed based on two premises. First, an increase in hepatic glycogenolysis is evident during stimulation of the anterior hepatic nerve plexus, presumably caused by activation of sympathetic nerves.[16] Second, the increase in endogenous GP that occurs with exercise is more rapid than changes in arterial glucagon, insulin, and epinephrine levels.[16] Despite circumstantial evidence that seems to implicate the sympathetic nerves, a role during moderate exercise remains to be established. Combined α- and β-adrenergic blockade does not impair the increase in hepatic GP during moderate exercise in humans,[17] implying that sympathetic drive is unimportant in this process. In addition, surgical hepatic denervation does not affect the increment in endogenous GP in rats,[18] dogs,[19] or humans.[20] It has recently been shown that sympathetic nerve blockade to the liver and adrenal medulla using local anesthesia of celiac ganglion in humans has no effect on the increase in hepatic GP.[10]

In humans, the hepatic response to high-intensity exercise and the regulation of this response are different from exercise of lesser intensity. The main difference in glucoregulation is that the increase in GP is maximal, and no longer matches, but exceeds the rise in glucose utilization.[21,22] This results in an increase in arterial glucose levels that extends into the postexercise state. In addition, insulin secretion is not suppressed and it is markedly increased in the postexercise period, facilitating recovery of muscle glycogen. Since a single bout of high-intensity exercise can only be sustained for a short interval, it is likely that the additional glucose released by the liver originates from liver glycogen. It has been hypothesized by Marliss and associates that during exercise of high intensity, there may be a shift in the control of GP away from the pancreatic hormones to the catecholamines.[22] Most research indicates that catecholamines are unimportant in controlling hepatic GP during moderate-intensity exercise. However, during strenuous exercise, norepinephrine and epinephrine can increase by 10- to 20-fold, whereas the increase in the glucagon to insulin ratio is very small.[22]

Using octreotide (a somatostatin analogue), the endogenous secretions of insulin, glucagon, and growth hormone were suppressed and replaced by infusion of the three hormones (islet and growth hormone clamp). Despite prevention of increases in growth hormone and glucagon and decrease of insulin, increments of glucose production were not affected. This strongly supports the notion that catecholamines are the primary regulators of glucose production during exercise in normal humans.[23] During moderate exercise glucose infusions inhibit GP, presumably by stimulating insulin release and suppressing glucagon secretion. In contrast, during strenuous exercise endogenous GP is partially preserved, despite glucose infusions or the postprandial state, supporting the role of catecholamines rather than the glucagon/insulin ratio.[24,25] An additional argument is that epinephrine and norepinephrine infusions during moderate exercise can substantially increase GP, thus mimicking the effects of strenuous exercise.[26] Nevertheless, human studies that have attempted directly to assess the role of catecholamines in stimulating hepatic GP during heavy exercise (> 80% maximum O_2 uptake) have been negative.[10] A recent study in dogs showed that complete blockade of α- and β-adrenergic receptors, specifically at the liver, had no effect on high-intensity exercise that resulted in a twofold increase in hepatic norepinephrine spillover.[27] However, the exercise was much less intense in these human and dog studies than in those reported by Marliss.[22] It remains to be explored whether nonadrenergic or noncholinergic mechanisms could also be involved.

The question of whether the GP increment in humans during strenuous exercise is regulated by α- and β-catecholamine receptors was studied by Marliss's group in healthy subjects in whom a complete β-blockade was achieved during exercise at 87% V_{max}.[28] The GP increment was not suppressed by β-blockade, but actually rose twofold more than controls, attributed to an excessive and "unmasked" α-adrenergic effect that can also stimulate hepatic GP.[29] It is unknown whether GP might be increased in strenuous exercise through an additive effect of both catecholamine receptors, although this is feasible since α-effects can increase glycogenolysis through Ca^{2+} and protein kinase C, whereas β-effects work through cAMP and protein kinase A signaling mechanisms. Blockade of α-receptors also does not decrease GP, suggesting that enhanced β-effects maintain GP unchanged.[29]

Regulation of Fat Metabolism

Moderate exercise is typically associated with an approximate 10-fold increase in fat oxidation due to increased energy expenditure coupled with greater FFA availability. Lipolysis, assessed by the increase in arterial glycerol concentration and isotopic techniques, increases with the onset of moderate exercise.[30] Arterial FFA levels increase gradually. The slower time course for the rise in plasma FFA levels reflects an increase in clearance of this fuel by the working muscle.[30] The increase in FFA availability is largely due to an increase in lipolysis from adipose tissue triglycerides. In addition, the percentage of released fatty acids that are reesterified is decreased by 50%,[30] presumably because of alterations in blood flow that facilitate the delivery of fatty acids from adipose tissue to working muscles.

FFA release from adipose tissue is regulated primarily by the actions of insulin and the catecholamines. When the exercise-induced fall in insulin is prevented in dogs[6] and humans,[11] the increase in FFA levels is prevented. In the dog, this effect is accompanied by an attenuated rise in arterial glycerol. Adipocytes taken from human subjects following exercise have an increased lipolytic responsiveness to catecholamines, which is mediated through β-adrenergic mechanisms and occurs without an increase in the binding of the β-receptor–specific catecholamine, ^{125}I-cyanopindolol.[31]

In contrast to the role of FFA mobilization from adipose tissue during moderate-intensity exercise, its role during high-intensity exercise is considerably less important. Despite the increased adrenergic drive that is present during high-intensity work, the arterial FFA level in plasma decreases. A diminished lipolytic response and increased rate of reesterification to the diminished increase in FFA mobilization could lead to a decrease in FFA availability. Stimulation of adipocytes' β-adrenergic receptors is negatively coupled to adenylate cyclase and decreases lipolysis. The decrease in FFA mobilization during high-intensity exercise may be due to stimulation of β-adrenergic receptors by the high epinephrine concentrations that occur under these conditions.[32] Increased reesterification of FFAs due to excessive lactate levels during high-intensity exercise has been proposed as a possible reason for the decrease in FFA availability. This is consistent with the observation that blood glycerol levels may still rise during heavy exercise even when FFAs are not increased. It is also possible that increased blood glycerol levels are due to release from triglycerides within the working muscle. FFAs that are liberated in the process are oxidized locally, within the muscle.

With regard to the possible role of intramuscular triglycerides stores during exercise, there is a large body of evidence suggesting that they may represent an important metabolic substrate.[33] Estimates of the oxidation of intramuscular fat stores that were calculated indirectly using whole-body isotopic methods suggest that intramuscular fats provide more than 50% of the total fat oxidized during exercise[34] and muscle contraction.[35] Results obtained using muscle biopsies or arteriovenous differences, however, generally cannot account for such a large contribution of muscle fat stores during exercise.[36]

The increase in ketogenesis that occurs with prolonged exercise seems to be in large part due to the increased lipolytic rate and consequent increase in FFA delivery to the liver. When the increase in FFA levels is abolished either by preventing the fall in insulin[6] or by β-blockade,[17] ketone body levels do not rise. In addition to hepatic FFA delivery, the exercise-induced rise in glucagon appears to be necessary for the full increase in ketogenesis.[6] The ketogenic effect of glucagon that occurs without altering net hepatic FFA uptake indicates that glucagon stimulates this process at a site within the liver.

Control of Muscle Glycogenolysis

Muscle glycogen is an important local fuel during the early stages of exercise. With prolonged duration of exercise, glycogen stores decline in working muscle and glycogenolysis is stimulated in inactive muscle fibers.[6] In these muscles, glycogen is metabolized to lactate, where it is released and then delivered to the liver to be used in the gluconeogenic pathway. Increasing work intensities accelerate the rate of glycogen breakdown in contracting muscle. Glycogen breakdown is regulated by the rate-limiting enzyme glycogen phosphorylase. Phosphorylase is phosphorylated by phosphorylase kinase, creating the active form of the enzyme, phosphorylase *a*. The enzyme is dephosphorylated to its inactive form, phosphorylase *b*, by phosphorylase phosphatase. It is interesting, however, that although muscle glycogenolysis increases with increasing workload, there is no increase in phosphorylase transformation to its active form.[37] This suggests that allosteric regulators, such as AMP and inorganic phosphate, allow for glycogen phosphorylase to be matched to energy demands. Studies using β-adrenergic blockade indicate that catecholamines play a major role in mobilization of muscle glycogen during exercise.[6] Studies in the isolated rat hindlimb indicate that in addition to epinephrine, contraction *per se* can stimulate muscle glycogenolysis even in the complete absence of catecholamines.[38] Intracellular cAMP levels mediate the activation of phosphorylase *a* and the stimulation of muscle glycogenolysis by catecholamines. It appears that contraction causes the events by releasing calcium from the muscle sarcoplasmic reticulum.

Exercise-Induced Muscle Glucose Uptake

Muscle glucose uptake is closely regulated by hormonal and nonhormonal mechanisms (Fig. 27-3). Kinetic analyses of glucose uptake conducted *in vivo*[6] and *in vitro*[39–41] generally indicate that the maximal velocity (V_{max}) for this process is increased by exercise without affecting the Michaelis–Menten constant (K_m) (Fig. 27-4). The K_m for glucose oxidation by the working limb is the same as for glucose uptake, implying that both processes are controlled at the same step.[6] Stimulation of muscle glucose uptake by exercise depends, as it does for insulin and other regulators of glucose uptake, on the muscle interstitial to intracellular glucose gradient (transport gradient) and the permeability of the sarcolemma to glucose. Exercise increases muscle glucose transport dramatically while maintaining the transport gradient. Both effects of exercise are obviously critical for muscle glucose uptake and are described below.

Glucose Transport Gradient

The glucose transport gradient is determined by the rate that glucose is delivered to the muscle and the rate that free glucose transported across the sarcolemma is cleared once it is inside the cell. It is important to recognize that muscle interstitial glucose would fall precipitously and the glucose transport gradient would be insufficient to sustain glucose uptake if it were not for a marked increase in muscle blood flow that replenishes the interstitial glucose as it enters the working muscle. The increase in muscle blood flow is due to an increase in cardiac output and local vasodilation of the arterioles to the working muscle and is directly related to work rate.[42] The capillary endothelium is permeable to glucose and is not a limiting factor in supplying glucose to the working muscle. The diffusion distance to the sarcolemma, once glucose exits the

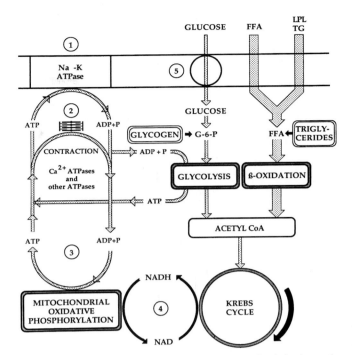

FIGURE 27-3. Pathways regulating glucose transport in skeletal muscle during exercise. Pathways of glycolysis, glycogenolysis, lipolysis, β-oxidation, and oxidative phosphorylation are shown in outline. The circled numbers refer to the following sequence of metabolic events: (1) the release of acetylcholine from motor neurons, (2) the activation of muscle contractile activity, (3) the increase in ATP turnover leading to a decrease in the molar ratio of ATP/ADP × Pi, and (4) the increased mitochondrial oxidation of reduced coenzymes. This leads to an increased oxidation of acetyl-CoA deriving from glucose or fatty acids. A decrease in the levels of glucose-6-phosphate might enhance extracellular glucose uptake mediated via cytochalosin β-inhibitable glucose transporters. Thus, in the absence of extracellular insulin, contraction triggers extracellular glucose uptake via insulin-independent pathways. Note that there are at least three sources for endogenous FFAs in muscle: plasma FFAs, plasma triglycerides associated with lipoproteins (**LPL, TG**), and endogenous triglycerides. The thick arrows delineating the pathways of FFA oxidation emphasize the fact that fatty acids are the principal substrates oxidized by muscles at rest and during prolonged exercise. If FFAs are present in excess (such as in diabetes), they retro-inhibit glucose oxidation. Likewise, if fatty acid oxidation is inhibited (by drugs such as methylpalmoxirate or by anaerobic conditions), then glucose oxidation is increased. Although the detailed biochemical mechanism of the FFA–glucose cycle remains to be determined, it is hypothesized that this cycle is more important for the regulation of glucose metabolism in red oxidative muscle than in white glycolytic muscles. *(This scheme is kindly provided by Dr. L. Bukowiecki of Laval University School of Medicine, Quebec.)*

capillary, however, may be critical. Fast-twitch fibers have a low capillary density and are poorly perfused; therefore, the diffusion distance is greater in fast-twitch than slow-twitch fibers that are well perfused. One would predict that at equivalent rates of muscle glucose transport, glucose concentration at the sarcolemma of fast-twitch muscle, and therefore the glucose transport gradient, would be lower than it is in slow-twitch fibers. It may, in part, be for this reason that fast-twitch muscle fibers are not able to sustain rates of glucose uptake as high as slow-twitch fibers.[43]

The importance of glucose supply to working muscle is supported by several observations. First, there is a close correlation of

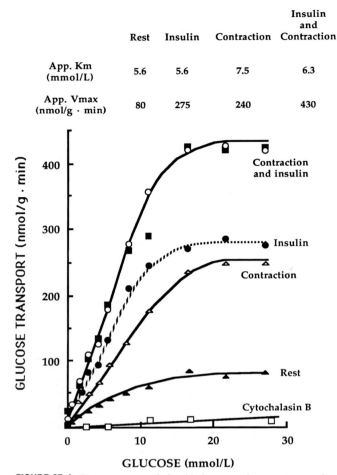

	Rest	Insulin	Contraction	Insulin and Contraction
App. Km (mmol/L)	5.6	5.6	7.5	6.3
App. Vmax (nmol/g · min)	80	275	240	430

FIGURE 27-4. Dose–response relationship between glucose concentration and glucose transport in apilrochlearis muscle at rest, during contractions (48 twitches/min), incubated in the presence and absence of insulin (10 mU/mL). Also shown are the rates of nonfacilitated glucose diffusion abtained by incubating the muscle in the presence of cytochalasin 8 (50 uM). Note that both insulin and contractile activity increase the apparent V_{max} without significantly changing the apparent K_m (5–8 mmol). (*Reprinted with permission from Nesher R, Korl IE, Kipris KM. Dissociation of the effect(s) of insulin and contraction on glucose transport in rat epitrochlearis muscle. Am J. Physiol. 1985;249:C226*)

muscle blood flow to glucose uptake by the working human limb.[44,45] Second, an increase in perfusion of the isolated rat hindlimb is necessary for the full contraction-induced glucose uptake in this preparation.[46] Finally, increasing blood glucose supply by creating hyperglycemia with an intravenous glucose infusion resulted in a marked increase in limb glucose uptake in the exercising dog, even when hyperinsulinemia was prevented using somatostatin.[6] The exercise-induced increase in glucose delivery is so effective at maintaining interstitial glucose that an increase in muscle fractional glucose extraction is not required for the increase in muscle glucose uptake.[6]

The muscle intracellular free glucose concentration determines the "downward" slope of the glucose transport gradient. As a consequence, the ability to metabolize glucose critically determines the glucose flux across the sarcolemma. The first step in glucose metabolism is phosphorylation by hexokinase II. In addition to maintaining intracellular glucose concentration low, glucose phos-

phorylation is important because the product, G6P, cannot exit the cell and is the substrate for subsequent glucose metabolism. Although glucose uptake is probably rate-limited by glucose transport at rest, there is evidence that glucose phosphorylation becomes limiting if glucose transport is stimulated to a critically high level of G6P, which inhibits hexokinase II.[47–50] Not only are muscle glucose delivery and transport elevated during exercise, but glycogenolysis is high, flooding the G6P pool. The consequence is a greater role for glucose phosphorylation in control of muscle glucose uptake during exercise.[51,52] Figure 27-5 illustrates how overexpression of hexokinase II improves the ability to consume the 2-deoxyglucose in mice and how a glycogen-depleting fast can enhance the uptake of this glucose analog even further, presumably by reducing the size of the G6P pool.[51] Conversely, the importance of muscle glycogenolysis as a factor controlling muscle glucose uptake is reflected by the high G6P concentration and attenuated increase in contraction-stimulated glucose transport in perfused rat hindlimb muscle with a high initial glycogen mass.[53] This concept is further supported by results from human subjects' cycling after a single leg has been glycogen-depleted by prior exercise.[54] The limb with glycogen-depleted muscle has a higher net rate of glucose uptake and lower muscle G6P levels than the contralateral control limb.

FIGURE 27-5. [2-³H]DGP content in soleus, gastrocnemius (gastroc), vastus lateralis (vastus), and diaphragm normalized to brain [2-³H]DGP content after a 30-minute sedentary period (**A**), or a 30-minute treadmill exercise period in 5-hour fasted (**B**) or 18-hour fasted (**C**) mice overexpressing hexokinase II or wild-type litter mates. Data shown are mean ± SE; n = 8 and 6 for sedentary wild-type and transgenic, n = 8 and 12 for 5-hour fasted exercise wild-type and transgenic, and n = 6 and 6 for 18-hour fasted wild-type and transgenic. *Indicates significantly greater [2-³H]DGP content in transgenic than wildtype ($p < 0.05$–0.005).

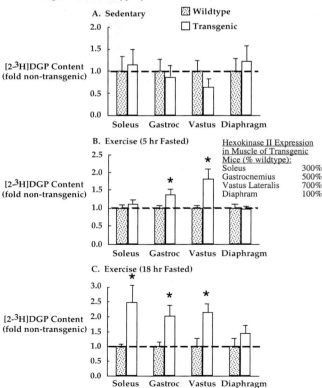

In contrast to the extensive work assessing exercise and glucose transport, very little is known regarding the effects of exercise on hexokinase II and glucose phosphorylation. There have been no positive allosteric regulators of hexokinase II identified. Therefore, enzyme compartmentation and mass are likely to be key regulatory factors. It has been shown in this regard that prolonged, moderate exercise to exhaustion in the rat results in a small increase in the percentage of muscle hexokinase activity associated with mitochondria.[55] Consistent with this is the observation that chronic, low-frequency stimulation can lead to a redistribution of muscle hexokinase activity so that more of the enzyme is in an insoluble fraction.[56] In marked contrast, however, is the demonstration that the percentage of hexokinase activity bound to mitochondria fell by about 80% in skeletal muscles of horses run to exhaustion at 100% of their maximum oxygen uptake.[57] Based on the latter results, it was hypothesized that the reduction in bound hexokinase during high-intensity exercise was a result of the increase in muscle G6P that induced the release of hexokinase from mitochondria.

Acute exercise has been shown to stimulate skeletal muscle hexokinase II gene transcription.[58] Interestingly, increases in gene transcription,[58,59] mRNA,[60–62] and protein synthesis[61,62] with exercise or electrical stimulation of the nerve to a muscle precede and are larger for hexokinase II than GLUT-4. The increase in hexokinase activity lags behind the increase in hexokinase II mRNA[60,61] and may, therefore, be more significant to the persistent increase in insulin action following exercise or the adaptations that occur with training.

Because G6P is such a potent inhibitor of hexokinase II activity, the capacity to metabolize it is necessary for the accelerated rate of glucose phosphorylation required by the working muscle. In contrast to insulin-stimulated glucose utilization where glycogen formation is the primary fate of G6P, the muscle G6P formed during exercise is, at least in a net sense, metabolized entirely glycolytically.[6,63–65] Consequently, the capacity for muscle glycolysis and glucose oxidation is a determinant of muscle G6P concentration and, as a result, glucose uptake.

Sarcolemma Glucose Transport

Exercise is associated with an increase in glucose transporter number in sarcolemma[40,66–68] and specifically at T tubules[66] isolated from rat skeletal muscle. It has been proposed that the intrinsic activity of the glucose transporter is also increased in sarcolemma from exercised rats.[67] The finding of increased intrinsic activity, however, is probably a consequence of measuring glucose transporters that are both accessible and inaccessible to extracellular glucose.[69] Studies using a photo-label that identifies only GLUT-4 accessible to extracellular glucose has shown that the exercise-induced increase in glucose transport can be explained entirely by an increase in sarcolemma GLUT-4 number.[70,71] The increased transporter number is due specifically to an increase in plasma membrane GLUT-4, as plasma membrane GLUT-1, the other isoform found in muscle, is unaffected by exercise.[72,73] The increase in plasma membrane GLUT-4 in response to exercise is, like that due to insulin stimulation, a result of an increase in translocation from an intracellular pool.

The studies just described show that an increase in glucose transport is clearly important to muscle glucose uptake and metabolism during exercise and that GLUT-4 is the protein responsible for the increase in glucose transport. The importance of other regulatory factors, however, is clearly exemplified during submaximal

work by the negative correlation between rate of whole body glucose utilization and muscle total GLUT-4 in humans.[74] This seemingly paradoxical relationship can exist since muscles rich in GLUT-4 also have metabolic properties that make them better able to derive energy from fats and therefore require less glucose. The higher muscle total GLUT-4 levels better enable an individual to meet the challenges of maximal exercise. However, "glucose-sparing" mechanisms take precedence at submaximal work rates. As a consequence, there is less muscle glucose uptake even though the key glucose transport protein is more abundant.

Important advances in how contraction triggers the increases in GLUT-4 translocation and muscle glucose uptake have been made over the last several years. As discussed as follows, the mechanism for the increase is clearly different from that of insulin. A hypothesis that is gaining growing support is that the exercise-induced increase in muscle AMP stimulates AMP kinase, which then causes an increase in muscle glucose uptake.[75] This is supported by the demonstration that the pharmacological agent 5-aminoimadazole-4-carboxamide 1-□-D-ribfuranoside (AICAR) activates AMP kinase and has a stimulatory effect to increase uptake in perfused rat hindlimb[76] and isolated muscle.[77] As is the case with muscle contraction, AICAR appears to activate muscle glucose uptake by GLUT-4 translocation.[77]

In addition to the stimulation of AMP kinase by AMP, Ca^{2+} and nitric oxide (NO) have also been proposed to mediate the exercise-induced increase in muscle glucose uptake. Because increased cytoplasmic Ca^{2+} is an essential part of the contraction process and is involved in many aspects of intracellular metabolic regulation, it has been proposed that deficient depancreatized dogs is increased by only 25–50% of the response seen when insulin is replaced.[82] The reason for the difference between studies in isolated muscle and studies in the whole organism is that insulin acts indirectly to maintain a metabolic state that is conducive to exercise-stimulated glucose uptake in vivo. This is exemplified by studies that show that if characteristics of chronic insulin deficiency (e.g., enhanced nonesterified fatty acid levels, elevated catecholamines) are minimized, insulin-independent mechanisms are sufficient to stimulate glucose utilization in vivo. Consistent with this hypothesis, β-adrenergic blockade during exercise suppresses FFA levels and increases the impaired rise in glucose utilization present in diabetes.[83,84] Somatostatin has been used to create an acute insulin deficiency in dogs, since in combined insulin and glucagon deficiency, a time period exists when the animal is not hyperglycemic or hyperlipidemic.[64] Under these conditions, the contribution of insulin-independent mechanisms to the exercise-induced increase in whole-body glucose utilization, limb glucose uptake, and limb glucose oxidation in dogs ranges from 50–70%. The contribution of insulin-independent mechanisms has also been estimated in humans by the extrapolation of data obtained in humans during insulin clamps to a theoretical insulin value of zero.[85] These estimates suggest that virtually all of the exercise-induced increases in glucose uptake and carbohydrate oxidation are insulin-independent. Taken together, in vivo and in vitro experiments consistently show that muscular work is a potent stimulus for insulin-independent glucose uptake and metabolism when severe insulin deficiency is not present.

The cell-signaling pathway of contraction-stimulated glucose transport is distinct from that for insulin-stimulated glucose transport. Although the increase in plasma membrane transporters in response to both insulin and exercise results from an increase in translocation of GLUT-4, these stimuli recruit GLUT-4 from different intracellular pools.[66,78,86] Evidence that cell signaling for glucose uptake is different for exercise and insulin is supported by the demonstration that these two stimuli are functionally additive,[70,71] as are the corresponding increases in GLUT-4 translocation.[70,71,87] Moreover, electric stimulation of rat skeletal muscle *in situ* does not lead to the phosphorylation of proteins involved in insulin signaling, such as insulin receptor substrate-1,[88] PI 3-kinase,[88] Akt2 kinase,[89] Akt3 kinase,[89] and p70^{s6k}.[90] In addition, wortmannin, an inhibitor an insulin of PI 3-kinase, eliminates insulin-stimulated glucose transport but does not impair[71,91,92] contraction-stimulated glucose transport in isolated rat skeletal muscle.

In further support of unique mechanisms for insulin- and contraction-stimulated glucose transport is the demonstration that physiologic and pathologic factors can affect them differently. High-fat feeding[93] and maturation[94] both decrease insulin-stimulated skeletal muscle glucose uptake, without diminishing contraction-stimulated glucose uptake. Furthermore, muscles isolated from the obese Zucker rat have diminished glucose transport and sarcolemma GLUT-4 with insulin stimulation, but respond normally to contraction.[43,70] The differential effects of these conditions on insulin emphasize that the insulin signaling pathway is different from that stimulated by contraction.

Modulation of Glucose Uptake by the Working Muscle by the Internal Milieu

The preceding discussion describes the basic mechanisms that control muscle glucose uptake during exercise. Hormones and substrates in the circulation can further regulate this response. The following are some of the means by which humoral factors influence the exercise response.

Insulin Sensitivity of the Working Muscle

In addition to the increase in insulin-independent glucose utilization during exercise, insulin sensitivity is also increased.[6,39,44,95,96] Studies conducted in humans show that exercise and insulin stimulate glucose utilization and carbohydrate oxidation synergistically over a range of insulin doses by affecting both the K_m of insulin and V_{max} of these pathways.[85] The effects of this increase in insulin action are probably most important in the postprandial state and in the intensively treated diabetic state when insulin levels can be higher than those that normally accompany exercise. There is, nevertheless, an increased sensitivity of glucose uptake to the subbasal insulin levels present during exercise in the postabsorptive state.[97] Exercise also has a potent effect on the intracellular pathway for insulin-stimulated muscle glucose metabolism. The primary route of insulin-mediated glucose metabolism at rest[98] and in the postexercise state[99] is nonoxidative metabolism. Acute exercise, however, shifts the route of insulin-stimulated glucose disposal so that all the glucose consumed by the muscle is oxidized.[85]

Several mechanisms have been proposed to explain how exercise enhances insulin action. These mechanisms can be classified as those that exert their effect on muscle indirectly through the hormone's action at another site and those that act directly at the muscle. The increased blood flow to the working muscle increases the exposure of this tissue to circulating insulin and may reflect one mechanism for increasing insulin action on muscle indirectly.[44,100] The relationship between the exercise-induced increase in muscle blood flow and the increase in insulin sensitivity has been illus-

trated by studies in the perfused rat hindlimb.[46] Increasing the perfusate flow augmented the effect of insulin on glucose uptake when the hindlimb muscles were stimulated to contract. If trans-endothelial insulin transport determines the kinetics of insulin action, as discussed elsewhere,[101] then the hemodynamic adjustments result in increased capillary surface area in the working muscle, which may enhance insulin action by increasing insulin transport across the endothelium.

Exercise may also increase insulin-stimulated glucose utilization by a mechanism secondary to insulin's suppressive effect on nonesterified FFA availability. The absolute magnitude of the insulin-induced suppression of plasma FFA levels and fat oxidation is greater during exercise. This may represent a second indirect mechanism by which exercise increases insulin action. The K_m's for total carbohydrate and fat oxidation occur at similar insulin levels during exercise, suggesting that the greater stimulation of carbohydrate oxidation may be an essential response to a primary suppression of lipolysis.[85] The interaction of circulating FFA concentrations and muscle glucose uptake during exercise is described in a subsequent section.

Studies in humans[102] and rats[102–105] generally indicate that insulin binding affinity to skeletal muscle is unaffected by acute moderate exercise. Since insulin binding affinity is unaltered, it has been concluded that a step distal to binding must be altered.[105] It has been proposed that a postreceptor modification may be linked to the glycogen-depleting effect of exercise. One recent study showed that the ability of muscle contraction to enhance insulin-stimulated glucose uptake and transport in the perfused rat hindquarter was eliminated by adenosine receptor blockade.[96] Adenosine receptor blockade had no effect during contraction in the absence of insulin. This suggests that the increased adenosine production that occurs in response to muscular work[106] plays a role in facilitating insulin action.

Effect of Circulating FFA Concentrations on the Working Muscle

Insulin-stimulated muscle glucose uptake can be attenuated by elevated circulating FFAs concentrations.[107,108] A similar link between elevated FFA and depressed muscle glucose uptake during exercise has also been shown in studies using arteriovenous difference methods across the working human leg.[109] A twofold increase in FFA concentrations elicited by infusion of a lipid emulsion reduced leg glucose uptake from 30–60% during 60 minutes of knee extension in human subjects. This finding was supported by a study in the exercising dog that showed that reducing FFA levels by about 70% by suppressing lipolysis with nicotinic acid leads to an increase in whole-body glucose utilization and an approximately 70% increase in limb glucose oxidation.[110] The mechanism for the high FFA-induced impairment in glucose uptake by working muscle may be different than the one originally proposed by Randle and coworkers.[111] Randle and colleagues proposed that fats impaired muscle glucose uptake by metabolic feedback resulting from accumulation of metabolic intermediates involved in fat oxidation. During lipid infusion, glucose uptake by the working human limb was impaired during lipid infusion even though G6P was not increased.[109] Moreover, increasing fat availability to working human muscle by diet, triglyceride infusion[112] does not decrease pyruvate dehydrogenase activity or lead to an accumulation of citrate or acetyl-CoA in muscle biopsies. Taken together, these studies suggest that an increase in fat availability impairs glucose uptake in working muscle by a different mechanism. Since the inhibition of glucose uptake does not necessitate the buildup of G6P or metabolic intermediates downstream from this metabolite, the conclusion may be that elevated FFA levels inhibit muscle glucose uptake at either the glucose transport or glucose phosphorylation step. These findings are in agreement with studies that show that high FFA levels decrease whole-body glucose utilization during hyperinsulinemic euglycemic clamps without increasing G6P in resting human subjects.[113,114]

Effect of Decreased Oxygen Availability on the Working Muscle

Excessive increments in muscle glucose uptake occur when O_2 availability is limited, such as exercise under anemic conditions,[115] when breathing a hypoxic gas mixture,[116] or at high altitude.[117] This occurs even when energy expenditure is no greater. Moreover, elevated rates of glucose uptake occur under these circumstances even though insulin levels are no higher and catecholamines, which may be antagonistic to glucose uptake, are greater. These findings are consistent with studies, conducted in perfused[118] rat skeletal muscle, that show the close relationship of hypoxia, and the consequent metabolic state, to glucose uptake. The mechanism that links muscle metabolism to glucose uptake remains to be identified. It is noteworthy, however, that hypoxia-stimulated and contraction-stimulated skeletal muscle glucose transport share common features and may, in fact, involve the same signaling steps.

Effect of Adrenergic Stimulation on the Working Muscle

Glucose uptake by working muscle may also be impaired when adrenergic stimulation is excessive. Epinephrine infusion inhibits tracer-determined whole-body glucose clearance in the exercising dog,[119] and a local infusion of epinephrine into an artery of one leg led to a reduction in leg glucose uptake compared to the contralateral leg during cycle exercise in humans.[120] Conversely, β-adrenergic receptor blockade increased whole-body glucose utilization[117,121] and oxidation[117,121] and leg glucose uptake[117] in humans during cycling. One mechanism for the inhibitory effect of the catecholamines on muscle glucose uptake is the inhibition of hexokinase due to the increase in muscle G6P resulting from stimulation of glycogenolysis. The potential importance of this mechanism is illustrated by the 50% reduction in G6P that occured during β-adrenergic receptor blockade in the working muscle of humans.[122] In addition, metabolic effects due to catecholamine-stimulated lipolysis (as discussed) may also be a factor.[111]

Effect of Carbohydrate Ingestion on Glucose Metabolism During Exercise

An important factor limiting exercise endurance is the depletion of endogenous carbohydrate stores. Many studies have indicated that glucose feeding during exercise was shown to improve exercise endurance or allow resumption of exercise after exhaustion. The principal underlying mechanism for this improvement is probably related to increased glucose availability to the working muscle. The prevention of neuroglycopenia is not likely to be the mechanism by which carbohydrate ingestion prevents fatigue since severe hypoglycemia is not necessarily present at exhaustion. During exercise, moderate levels of hypoglycemia (consequent to liver glycogen depletion) induce marked glucagon and catecholamine responses,

further increasing the stimuli for muscle and liver glycogen breakdown and expediting glycogen depletion. This cycle can be broken by carbohydrate ingestion. The amount, form, and timing of an oral carbohydrate load, along with the duration and intensity of exercise, will determine how effectively glucose enters the bloodstream, thus becoming available to the working muscle.

Multiple factors determine the metabolic availability of ingested carbohydrates. Two components are involved in the absorption of an oral carbohydrate load: transit time through the small intestine and intestinal sugar absorption. Transit time through the intestine is determined by gastric emptying and intestinal motility. Gastric emptying is influenced by the volume, osmolality, temperature, energy content, acidity, and presence of specific nutrients in the ingested meal. Of these, volume is the most potent activator of gastric emptying, whereas high carbohydrate concentrations slow the emptying rate. The question of whether moderate exercise changes gastric emptying is controversial. The discrepant results may pertain to methodology or study design. Exercise at greater than 70% of the maximum oxygen uptake has consistently been shown to slow gastric emptying.[123] It is clear that specific conditions that accompany intense exercise, such as dehydration and sympathetic nervous activity, may inhibit gastric emptying. Generally, experiments show that small intestine transit time is increased by exercise.

The direct effect of exercise on intestinal absorption has received very little attention. Moderate-intensity cycling (around 45% maximum oxygen uptake) has been shown to lead to a reduction in water and electrolyte absorption as determined using jejunal perfusion.[124] This finding is consistent with other work that showed that the vascular appearance of ingested deuterium oxide was reduced by high-intensity exercise.[125] High intensity exercise reduces splanchnic blood flow in humans by as much as 70% during high-intensity exercise.[126] This hemodynamic change may, therefore, impair the absorption of ingested glucose.

The metabolic availability of ingested carbohydrates has been assessed in numerous studies by spiking the oral load with sugar labeled with isotopic carbon and measuring the appearance of the isotope in expired CO_2. Initial studies were done using ^{14}C-glucose to trace the oxidation rate of ingested glucose. However, these studies underestimated exogenous glucose oxidation due to technical problems that arise from the extensive interval required for the $H_{14}CO_3$ to equilibrate with the endogenous HCO_3 stores. In subsequent years, the metabolic availability of ingested glucose was measured using ^{13}C-labeled sugars. Use of this label, on the other hand, has given rise to overestimates due to the presence of naturally occuring ^{13}C label. Since the ^{13}C enrichment of glucose is greater than fats, an increased contribution of carbohydrate to total fuel oxidation (as is seen during exercise) will result in an increase in $^{13}CO_2$ production. Early work that did not consider the contribution of endogenous carbohydrates overestimated the rate of ingested carbohydrate oxidation. More recent work determined that the exact metabolic availability of ingested carbohydrate depends on many factors related to the composition and quantity of the substrate load. In addition, exercise parameters (i.e., work intensity, duration, modality) will also be an important determinant of how readily ingested glucose will be made available. As a consequence, it is difficult to ascribe an exact efficiency for metabolism of ingested glucose. A reasonable estimate might be that approximately 40% of a 50-g oral glucose load ingested at the start of moderate-intensity exercise is metabolized during the first hour.[127]

During light work rates, there is probably little difficulty in delivering adequate amounts of ingested glucose to the working muscle. As glucose oxidation by the working muscle increases at higher work rates, it may no longer be possible to absorb adequate amounts of ingested glucose from the gastrointestinal tract. Thus, what limits ingested oxidation may shift at different work intensities—low muscle demand limits glucose oxidation at light work rates, whereas absorption from the gastrointestinal tract limits it at high work rates. One study showed that as exercise intensity increased from 22 to 51% of the maximum oxygen uptake, the oxidation of ingested glucose (100 g) increased proportionally.[128] With further increases in work rate, total carbohydrate oxidation continued to rise, but the oxidation of ingested glucose increased no further, suggesting that the rate at which glucose is made available from the gastrointestinal tract had become limiting.

Several approaches have been used to increase the rate of ingested carbohydrate availability to the working muscle. Some of these are described as follows:

1. *Increasing the mass of ingested carbohydrates*. One approach for increasing the amount of carbohydrate that is absorbed is simply to increase the mass of ingested glucose. This is an effective approach even though the fraction of the ingested glucose that is made available for metabolism is actually decreased with a greater oral glucose load. In one study, a 400% increase in the carbohydrate ingested mass induced only a 25% increase in exogenous glucose oxidation; as a result, a large increase (from 45% to 81%) of ingested carbohydrates remained in the gastrointestinal tract.[129] The decreased percentage of ingested glucose oxidized when larger quantities of ingested glucose are consumed suggests one or more steps involved in the intestinal absorption or delivery of glucose to the working muscle have become saturated.

2. *Ingestion of different carbohydrate types*. Sucrose ingestion has been used as a source of substrate during exercise, with the goal of decreasing ingestant osmolarity with similar effectiveness as ingested glucose.[130] This is not surprising because the hydrolysis of this sugar leads to the entry of glucose into the circulation. More sugar can be made metabolically available by using different sugar types. A greater percentage of ingested sugar is oxidized during exercise if 50 g of glucose and 50 g of fructose are ingested than if 100 g of glucose alone is consumed.[127] Studies examining the effectiveness of fructose[127] alone suggest that it is less effective than glucose at sparing endogenous carbohydrate stores. Due to a smaller insulin response with nonglucose sugars, FFA levels are higher than following glucose ingestion, but this does not seem to improve exercise tolerance.[130]

3. *Timing of ingested glucose*. The beneficial effect of carbohydrate ingestion on exercise endurance seems to be equal whether the meal is fed prior to, at the onset of, or during exercise, provided that the onset of exercise does not coincide with the postingestion insulin peak (about 45 minutes after ingestion)[131] and signs of fatigue are not already present.[132]

At least two important endocrine changes accompany the increase in glucose availability. The exercise-induced fall in insulin and rise in glucagon are attenuated or eliminated altogether.[133] The absence of the fall in insulin will attenuate the increases in lipolysis and GP,[6,11] whereas a reduction in glucagon will reduce the latter.[6,11] The suppression of lipolysis will result in a reduction in

circulating FFA levels, which has been shown to stimulate tracer-determined glucose utilization and glucose oxidation by the working limb.[110] Although insulin acts to suppress net muscle glycogen breakdown, multiple signals are present in the working muscle and these counterbalance the antiglycogenolytic effects of insulin more often than not.

Because of the difficulties in studying liver metabolism directly in humans, very little direct information as to the effects of carbohydrate ingestion on hepatic GP is available. The available data, however, all uniformly show that exogenous glucose reduces the demands on the liver. Glucose infusion reduces hepatic GP during low- and moderate-intensity exercise in humans.[6,134] Furthermore, glucose ingestion inhibits the uptake of gluconeogenic precursors by the splanchnic bed during prolonged low-intensity exercise.[133] The potent effect of glucose infusion and carbohydrate ingestion at the liver is probably mediated, in large part, by a highly sensitive pancreatic hormone response.[6]

Postexercise Glucose Metabolism

Stimulatory effects of exercise on muscle glucose uptake can persist well after cessation of exercise. In contrast to moderate exercise, where all the glucose taken up by muscle is oxidized, the added glucose taken up after exercise is channeled into glycogen.[6,85,99,135,136] The repletion of muscle glycogen after exercise occurs in two phases, which can be distinguished by their reliance on insulin and kinetics.[137,138] In phase one, the sarcolemma permeability to glucose is elevated,[138] glycogen synthase activity is elevated,[138] and muscle glycogen is rapidly restored.[137,138] This phase occurs immediately after exercise and is notable in that it does not require insulin.[137,138] In the second phase, muscle glycogen has returned to near-normal levels and glucose uptake is no longer elevated in the absence of insulin. Phase two is characterized by a marked and persistent increase in insulin action.[138] Estimates of the duration of this second phase are highly variable. The increase in insulin sensitivity is probably more persistent after more extensive glycogen depletion and can be protracted by an absence of dietary carbohydrate.[139] It has been shown that glycogen repletion to preexercise levels requires approximately 24 hours in humans maintained on a high-carbohydrate diet, but may take as long as 8–10 days in the absence of dietary carbohydrate.[139] It has also been shown, using ^{13}C-NMR spectroscopy, that muscle glycogen resynthesis can be slowed if the ingested medium is high in lipid content even if glucose content is equivalent.[140]

As is the case during exercise, an increase in insulin binding to muscle insulin receptor is not necessary for the increase in insulin action following exercise,[138] indicating that post receptor events are responsible. Prior exercise enhances insulin-stimulated glucose uptake and glycogen synthase activity, but does not result in a greater increase in insulin receptor tyrosine kinase, Akt phosphorylation, or glycogen synthase kinase-3 phosphorylation.[141] Muscle glycogen depletion, such as that which occurs with exercise, is a potent stimulant of muscle glycogen synthesis. The presence of the muscle insulin receptor may not even be necessary for the increased effects of insulin on muscle glucose uptake and glycogen synthase after exercise, implying that the effects of prior exercise are mediated by nonmuscle cells or by downstream signaling.[142] It has been proposed that a postreceptor modification may be linked to the glycogen-depleting effect of exercise.[99] Nevertheless, the improved effect of insulin on glucose uptake can persist after exercise even when preexercise glycogen levels have been restored.[138]

GLUT-4 is the primary means by which glucose enters the cell in the postexercise state. While GLUT-4 null mice have normal fed, fasted, and postexercise muscle glycogen content, the restoration of glycogen following a glucose load after exercise was markedly slowed.[143] It is possible that overexpression of GLUT-1 could compensate for any shortage of GLUT-4 in the plasma membrane as mice overexpressing this protein have increased muscle glycogenesis in the postexercise state.[144]

The increase in muscle insulin sensitivity following exercise is reliant on a local factor since glucose uptake during one-legged cycling was increased across the exercised limb, but not the contralateral rested limb.[135] When extramuscular influences were eliminated by isolating and directly stimulating the muscle, however, insulin sensitivity was not increased.[145] The exercise-induced increase in insulin sensitivity seems, therefore, to require a local extracellular factor.[146] It is possible that a neurotrophic or paracrine factor released at or near the working muscle is required.

The cellular basis for the persistent increase in insulin sensitivity may, at least in part, relate to the demonstrations that skeletal muscle GLUT-4 protein,[147] glycogenin,[148] and hexokinase II activity[60] can be increased during recovery from acute exercise. Both these adaptations are accompanied by increases in the respective mRNA pools for these proteins.[60,147] The increases in GLUT-4[59] and hexokinase II[60] mRNA levels appear to be due primarily to increases in the nuclear transcription rate of the genes for these proteins. Other posttranscriptional[60] and posttranslational[59] mechanisms may also be involved. One difference in the regulation of these proteins by exercise is that hexokinase II induction occurs more rapidly, and is initially more pronounced, than the induction of GLUT-4. Skeletal muscle GLUT-4 mRNA in the rat is unchanged immediately after 2 hours of electrical stimulation[149] or 90 minutes of treadmill exercise.[60] An increase in hexokinase II mRNA, on the other hand, is already present in rat muscle after 90 minutes of running.[60] Increases in skeletal muscle GLUT-4 mRNA and protein do occur but require a more strenuous exercise protocol or a longer exercise recovery period.[147] The more sensitive induction of hexokinase II as compared to GLUT-4 mRNA in muscle is reflected by differences in the transcription of their respective genes. An increase in hexokinase II gene transcription of almost threefold is seen immediately after 45 minutes of treadmill exercise in nuclei isolated from rat hindlimb muscles.[60] The transcription rate for the GLUT-4 gene is increased by only about 80% over basal rates and does not occur until 3 hours after exercise.[59]

There can be a paradoxical decrease in glucose tolerance immediately following exhaustive or extremely intense exercise.[150–152] This has been shown to correspond to elevated catecholamine and FFA levels[151,152] and muscle damage,[150] as evidenced by elevated plasma creatine kinase and myoglobin.

In addition to the well-known adaptations in skeletal muscle, prior exercise can lead to persistent effects on splanchnic tissue. Studies in a dog model that provided access to gut and liver *in vivo* showed that prior exercise increased the intestinal absorption of an intraduodenal glucose load[136] and increased the intrinsic capacity of the liver to consume glucose (Fig. 27-6).[153] The increase in the ability of the liver to consume glucose is not due to a sensitization to the stimulatory effects of the arterial to portal vein glucose gradient.[154] Whether the effect on liver glucose uptake, like the effect on muscle glucose uptake, is related to an increase in insulin action is unknown. Studies using ^{13}C magnetic resonance spectroscopy showed that ingestion of 1 g/kg of glucose or sucrose immediately after completion of prolonged moderate exercise caused liver

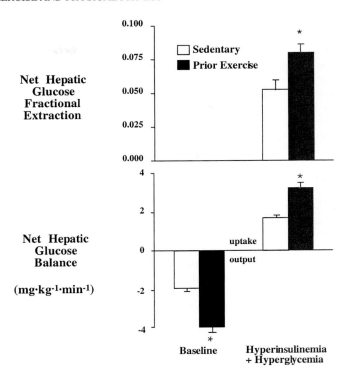

FIGURE 27-6. Net hepatic glucose fractional extraction (**top**) and balance (**bottom**) following 150 minutes of moderate treadmill exercise or an equivalent period of rest. Data are mean ± SE; n = 6 in each group. Insulin levels were fixed at ~30 μU/mL using somatostatin with intraportal insulin replacement and arterial blood glucose was clamped at ~130 mg/dL. The portal to arterial glucose gradient was ~19 mg/dL during hyperinsulinemic, hyperglycemic periods in both groups. The measurements made in the presence of a hyperglycemic, insulin-stimulated state were taken after a 60-minute equilibration period, during which time a steady state was achieved. *Indicates significantly greater values than corresponding sedentary period ($p < .05$). (*Reprinted with permission from Helmrich SP, et al.*[210])

glycogen resynthesis to increase by 0.7 and 1.3 mg/kg^{-1}/min^{-1}, respectively, over a period of 4 hours of postexercise recovery.[155] There was no liver glycogen resynthesis over the same period when a placebo was ingested. The ability to replenish liver glycogen after exercise may be functionally important in performance of subsequent exercise as there was a significant positive correlation between liver glycogen content and exercise endurance.[155]

EFFECTS AND MEDICAL BENEFITS OF EXERCISE IN DIABETES

The rationale and benefits of physical training in the general population were extensively reviewed in 1994 at the International Conference on Exercise, Fitness and Health.[156] The first conference on exercise and diabetes was organized in 1978 in Santa Ynes Valley, California.[157] We believe that this conference greatly stimulated this area of basic and clinical research, eventually demonstrating that exercise not only improves but can also prevent or delay the onset of diabetes, as described later in this chapter. This initial conference was followed by symposia in Olympia, Greece (1980); Burlington, Vermont (1983); Dusseldorf, Germany (1990); and at frequent intervals thereafter. The 2000 American Diabetes Association Position Statement on "Diabetes Mellitus and Exercise" unequivocally states that "with the publication of new clinical reviews, it is becoming increasingly clear that exercise may be a therapeutic tool in a variety of patients with, or at risk for diabetes," and that "all patients with diabetes" should be able to "benefit from the many valuable effects of exercise."[158] The founding of the International Diabetes Athlete Association (IDAA) in 1985 greatly stimulated the interest in exercise among diabetic populations around the world, and has established an information-, experience-, and knowledge-sharing system for diabetic people who are active in sports.[159] In 1988, diabetologists from 14 European countries, representing the European NIDDM Policy Group, met and prepared a consensus view of management of type 2 diabetes.[160] With respect to exercise, this document indicates overall benefits, improved glucose tolerance, decreased hyperinsulinemia, improved plasma lipoprotein profiles, and reduction of body weight and hypertension. Exercising muscle has been shown to increase glucose utilization by 7- to 20-fold compared to the resting muscle. In addition to the many general benefits of exercise enjoyed by nondiabetic individuals, exercise in type 2 diabetic individuals can potentially bring about medical improvements. These include better glycemic control, increased insulin sensitivity, reduced insulin requirement, improved plasma lipid profile and blood pressure, reduction in fat mass, preservation of lean body mass, and strengthened cardiovascular fitness.[161] Persistent and well-controlled exercise programs are expected to help lower glycated hemoglobin levels, which is the key to prevention of many chronic diabetic complications. In recent years, the traditional bias against diabetic individuals to engage in high-intensity, competitive sports has been challenged by a growing number of successful athletes, including Olympic gold medalists and world champions, who had type 1 diabetes.[162] However, the majority of diabetic individuals who are not professional athletes will benefit most by engaging in regular, aerobic exercise of moderate intensity. Due to the many pathologic, hormonal, and biochemical disparities, type 1 and type 2 diabetic individuals respond to and benefit from exercise with different clinical patterns as discussed below.

Exercise in Individuals with Type 1 Diabetes

The American Diabetes Association recommends that "all levels of exercise, including leisure activities, recreational sports, and competitive professional performance, can be performed by people with type 1 diabetes who do not have complications and are in good blood glucose control."[158]

In type 1 diabetes, exercise should not be used for the sole purpose of improving unsatisfactory glycemic control. All efforts should be made to advise and support those type 1 diabetic patients who are motivated to exercise to do so under optimal conditions for performance and enjoyment and with minimal risk of causing acute complications. A number of studies have found that physical training can increase Vo_2max,[163] decrease insulin dose,[163] and reduce levels of HbA_1. It is noteworthy that each of these studies achieved improvement of some, but not all parameters, which may be related to the differences in patient selection and training protocols. Small sample size and lack of adequate controls may also account for the discrepancy in results. Given the importance of diet and insulin therapy as determinants of glycemic control in type 1 diabetes, it is not surprising that glycosylated hemoglobin is little affected by increased physical activity. The importance of the general benefits of exercise, especially on the cardiovascular system, lends strong support to the promotion of physical training in type 1 diabetes.

Whether exercise improves insulin sensitivity in this particular population is still unresolved, but aerobic exercise in type 1 diabetic patients has been shown to substantially improve cardiorespiratory endurance, muscle strength, lipid profile, blood pressure, and glucose regulation.[164] Exercise training also reduces insulin requirement in these patients.[165] In general, exercise is safe and can be well tolerated in most patients even with 24–40 years of type 1 diabetes.[164,166] The peak oxygen consumption, respiratory exchange ratio, heart rate, and cardiac output in these exercising diabetic people are not significantly different from those of nondiabetic subjects.[166] Exercise in type 1 diabetic patients needs to be properly prescribed and closely monitored while their insulin dosages are adjusted. Without these precautions, exercise in type 1 diabetic subjects may provoke excessive glucose counterregulation, impaired glucose disposal, and even severe clinical complications, such as life-threatening hypoglycemia.

It is well accepted that exercise enhances glucose uptake and reduces insulin requirement for the working muscle. This fact, however, should be construed by no means as a diminished importance of insulin during exercise. On the contrary, adjustment of proper insulin dosage becomes even more critical during exercise than in the resting state. In general, diabetics are able to meet the energy needs of exercise; however, it is often with less than the optimal balance of fuel usage. Both insulin sensitivity (SI) and glucose effectiveness (SG) are impaired in type 1 diabetes, even when glycemia is under apparent control.[167] Exercise stimulates release of catecholamines, among other counterregulatory factors, which can decrease SI in type 1 diabetes.[168] The metabolic response to exercise in type 1 diabetic subjects varies with age, fitness, type of exercise, and nutritional status. The metabolic abnormalities and complications accompanying the disease often render exercise difficult for some patients. Due to a left-shifted oxygen dissociation curve as a result of high levels of glycosylated hemoglobin and the high frequency of vasculopathy, oxygen delivery to the muscle may be impaired. Furthermore, the development of neuropathies in patients with long-standing diabetes may hinder work tolerance.

Individuals with type 1 diabetes rely on gluconeogenesis substantially more than nondiabetic individuals for glucose fuel to feed the exercising muscle. The exercise-induced increments in glucose utilization are, by and large, similar in individuals with and without diabetes. Nevertheless, a few differences exist. First, in healthy individuals, this increase is associated with a higher rate of metabolic clearance. In patients with poorly-controlled diabetes, it is a result of an increased mass action of exaggerated hyperglycemia coupled with a small increment in metabolic clearance.[82] Second, a smaller percentage of the glucose utilized is completely oxidized in patients with diabetes, probably due to an impaired pyruvate dehydrogenase activity. This leads to an accelerated Cori cycle featuring augmented lactate release from muscle and augmented lactate-derived hepatic gluconeogenesis. Third, underinsulinization and exaggerated counterregulation result in increased mobilization and utilization of noncarbohydrate fuels, such as FFAs, especially in subjects with severe diabetes. Type 1 diabetes is also associated with a greater availability of ketone bodies for energy metabolism due to an increased splanchnic fractional extraction and a greater intrahepatic conversion of FFAs to ketone bodies as assessed by ^{14}C-oleic acid infusion.[169] The effects of insulin on muscle glucose utilization can be partly mediated by insulin's effects on fat metabolism.[170,171] Exercise-induced increases in glucose uptake and clearance were markedly enhanced by suppression of FFA oxidation in alloxan-diabetic dogs[83] or suppression of both FFA oxidation and lipolysis in depancreatized dogs.[170] Suppression of lipolysis using acipimox reduced fat oxidation and increased carbohydrate oxidation during and after moderate exercise in patients with T2DM. Respiratory quotient (RQ) was elevated by acipimox during exercise. In contrast, heparin treatment increased plasma FFA levels by 150%, increased fat oxidation by 7%, and reduced carbohydrate oxidation by 29%. Insulin-deficient diabetes may also exhibit differences in intramuscular substrate metabolism in response to exercise.

Patients with diabetes deprived of insulin for 24 hours have decreased intramuscular glycogen storage and increased intramuscular fat storage. This shift in fuel storage leads to a greater metabolism of intramuscular fat and a diminished breakdown of intramuscular glycogen. By using ratio-labeled palmitate and glucose in combination with gas-exchange measurements, it was calculated that in the insulin-deficient depancreatized dog more than twice as much intramuscular fat, but only about 60% of the muscle glycogen, are used. Thus, glucose and fatty acids, as fuels for exercising muscle, are utilized in a reciprocal and complementary fashion. An important issue is that decreased fatty acid oxidation may facilitate glucose utilization and improve hyperglycemia in exercising diabetic people.[83,170] Resistance exertions should be conducted under professional guidance. In patients with physical limitations, graded walking may be preferred. In those with low back pain, lower extremity arthritis, sensory loss, and other medical conditions, moderate-intensity swimming may be a good choice. When initiating a physical training program, all patients with type 1 diabetes should seek professional guidance from physicians, nurses, and/or diabetes educators.[172]

Inadequate Insulinization

Individuals with type 1 diabetes require adequate insulinization for improvement of metabolic control. Insulin deficiency can cause serious metabolic decompensation in diabetic patients during exercise, which is manifested by aggravated hyperglycemia and ketosis. When type 1 diabetic patients deprived from insulin treatment for a prolonged period (18–48 hours) underwent a 3-hour bout of exercise, blood glucose rose further.[173] The worsening in hyperglycemia is due to an attenuated increase in glucose metabolic clearance in the face of rising GP that is generally similar or excessive when compared to nondiabetic subjects. Underinsulinization during exercise may also lead to further increases in FFA and ketone body levels.

Exercise as a form of physical stress invokes a surge of counterregulatory hormones, glucagon,[83,173–175] epinephrine and norepinephrine,[83] and cortisol,[83,173] all of which can exacerbate the diabetic state in an underinsulinized individual. The magnitude of increase in these hormones depends not only on the extent of insulinization and the physical fitness of the subject, but also on the intensity and duration of the exercise. Owing to the overresponsiveness of the counterregulatory system in diabetes, high-intensity exercise can be more deleterious to the diabetic state than moderate exercise of similar duration, as is described later.

Excessive counterregulation does not occur only during exercise, but is a general characteristic of stress response in diabetes. For example, a stress model induced by injecting carbachol into the third cerebral ventricle in normal dogs caused a surge of counterregulatory hormones and stimulated glucose utilization. The stress-mediated increase in glucose uptake was independent of insulin release and not mediated by adrenergic pathways. However, the same type of stress in diabetic dogs failed to increase glucose utilization,

resulting in markedly worsened hyperglycemia.[176,177] This resistance of glucose uptake to exercise could not be improved by acute normalization with basal or high insulin infusion rates, indicating that stress can offset glucose homeostasis even in the presence of hyperinsulinemia. However, similarly to exercise,[83] β-blockade improved glucose uptake and prevented hypoglycemia. This indicates that during severe stress, transient treatment with β-blockade could improve glucose homeostasis.[178] An unresolved, intriguing question is whether there are similarities in the mechanisms of stimulating glucose utilization in stress and exercise, because under both conditions, glucose utilization increases despite release of counterregulatory hormones and without a concurrent increase in insulin release. Finding the mechanism for this intriguing observation may help improve glucose homeostasis in diabetics during stress.

When hypoinsulinemic, the diabetic liver becomes more sensitive to glucagon while the glucagon response to exercise is exaggerated.[175] Catecholamines clearly have potent peripheral effects in type 1 diabetic humans and dogs.[82] In the total absence of insulin, catecholamines play an even more important role than glucagon in control of GP. The effects of catecholamines are related to the mobilization of FFAs to sustain gluconeogenesis and to the stimulation of glycogenolysis. These effects are minimized by β-blockade in insulin-infused type 1 diabetic subjects, and in insulin-deficient diabetic dogs.[82,83] Adequate insulin therapy is critical in improving metabolic control and normalizing the excessive counterregulatory response to exercise in people with type 1 diabetes.

Overinsulinization

The most feared acute complication of exercise in patients with type 1 diabetes is hypoglycemia caused by relative overinsulinization, that is, an otherwise moderate dose of insulin becoming excessive during exercise. In normal individuals, physical exercise is associated with a physiologically regulated reduction in endogeneous insulin release. This low rate of insulin secretion carries a number of physiologic benefits. One such benefit is the protection against overinsulinization and excessive glucose utilization, because muscle glucose uptake is increased by both insulin-dependent and insulin-independent mechanisms. Another physiologic benefit lies in the unleashing of the glucagon stimulation of hepatic GP. In spite of reduced secretion, insulin delivery to the exercising muscle is not compromised because of accelerated blood circulation. Therefore, a moderate dose of insulin under nonexercising conditions can cause overinsulinization during exercise in the insulin-treated, exercising diabetic person. Relative or absolute overinsulinization may take place, due to the following factors:

1. Absorption of subcutaneously injected insulin accelerates during exercise.[179,180]
2. Unlike endogenous insulin secretion, insulinemia due to exogenous injections does not fall during muscular work.
3. Exercise enhances insulin sensitivity in the skeletal muscle.[181]

Whatever the cause, overinsulinization diminishes hepatic GP while further increasing glucose utilization. Consequently, hypoglycemia ensues during or after exercise. It is also noteworthy that individuals with antecedent hypoglycemia may be at an increased risk for subsequent hypoglycemic attacks during exercise due to blunted neuroendocrine defense and impaired metabolic response with insufficient endogenous GP.[182]

The time of day exercise is performed and the prevailing levels of insulin are of importance when considering appropriate measures to prevent hypoglycemia. The risk of exercise-induced hypoglycemia is lowest in the morning before insulin injection when low insulin levels usually prevail. However, this may be achieved at the cost of hyperglycemia. Exercise in the evening or afternoon carries a higher risk of nocturnal hypoglycemia due to enhanced insulin sensitivity extended beyond the exercise period when the muscle glycogen store continues to be replenished.[183]

A reduction in insulin dosage in anticipation of exercise helps prevent hypoglycemia. Patients with diabetes undergoing intensive insulin therapy were able to avoid hypoglycemia during 45 minutes of postprandial exercise at 55% maximum oxygen uptake by reducing insulin treatment from 30–50%.[184] Patients with diabetes with 80% reduction in insulin dosage were able to exercise for nearly 3 hours without hypoglycemia, whereas a 50% reduction in insulin dosage allowed exercise for only 90 minutes.[185] In contrast to patients with tightly controlled diabetes, those with fasting hypoglycemia were able to perform sustained exercise with a less substantial reduction in insulin.[185] High-intensity exercise elicits a greater glucose-lowering effect than moderate-intensity exercise. The exercise intensity should be taken into consideration when adjusting preexercise insulin dosage. *In vivo* insulin sensitivity was increased in patients with type 1 diabetes up to 2 hours after one bout of exercise at 50% of maximal oxygen uptake for 30 minutes.

Instant ingestion of extra carbohydrate can effectively prevent and/or treat hypoglycemia, as glucose derived from exogenous sources is readily utilizable by the working muscle.[183,186] The choice of carbohydrate supplements should exclude bulky food and include only rapidly absorbable carbohydrates ingested in small amounts to avoid exercising on a full stomach.[183] Injection of insulin into a nonexercising part of the body can help prevent an acceleration in insulin absorption.[183] In addition to insulin dose adjustments, the use of lispro insulin, a rapid- and short-acting formulation of insulin, may also be used to minimize the risk of hypoglycemia during and after exercise.[187]

It is well known that the responses of glucagon and epinephrine to insulin-induced hypoglycemia are impaired in resting patients with type 1 diabetes and in alloxan-diabetic dogs.[188] However, the secretion of counterregulatory hormones was found to be adequate in the face of hypoglycemia during a long-distance run in reasonably well-controlled, well-trained subjects with diabetes, but without long-term complications.[189] It appears that the degree of diabetic control and state of physical fitness may influence the difference in counterregulatory response to hypoglycemia.

Although a fall in insulin is essential for the normal metabolic response to exercise, it is not clear whether this is the case in subjects with type 1 diabetes receiving a peripheral insulin infusion (Fig. 27-7).[180,190] When patients with type 1 diabetes were exercised during a constant insulin infusion that maintained normoglycemia, the response of GP was either insufficient or adequate[180,190] to prevent a fall in glycemia. The actions and mechanisms of peripheral insulin infusion on hepatic GP in these patients during exercise are not clear. It should be noted that in diabetic dogs and humans, at least during rest, insulin exerts its inhibition of hepatic GP primarily through a peripheral mechanism.[191,192] The responses seen in diabetes, therefore, cannot always be extrapolated to normal physiology.

The three panels of Fig. 27-8 summarize the interactions of insulin and glucagon in regulating glucose turnover in exer-

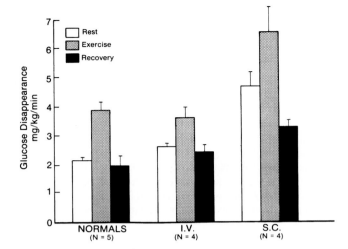

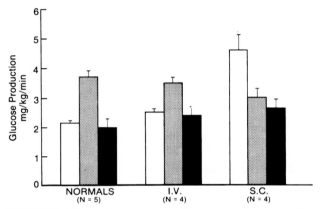

FIGURE 27-7. Glucose turnover: glucose disappearance (**upper panel**) and glucose production (**lower panel**) at rest, at 45 minutes of exercise, and 60 minutes recovery for the normal controls. Insulin-infused (**IV**), and subcutaneous (**SC**) insulin-treated diabetics. *(Reprinted with permission from Zinman B, et al.[180])*

cising patients with type 1 diabetes and in depancreatized dogs[82,170,174,175,179,180]:

1. During constant intravenous infusion of insulin, glucose homeostasis is preserved because GP and utilization are balanced as in nondiabetic subjects.
2. Due to the direct or indirect (FFA-glucose cycle) effects of insulin deficiency,[170,174] exercise does not stimulate glucose utilization adequately, and hence, the exercise-induced increase in hepatic GP leads to or enhances hyperglycemia, a key factor restraining metabolic glucose clearance during exercise.[174]
3. Absolute or relative overinsulinization, due to absorption of subcutaneous insulin injected before exercise, results in inhibition of hepatic GP, enhanced peripheral glucose uptake, and a fall in blood glucose levels.[185]

Intense Exercise in Type 1 Diabetes

The effect of intense exercise was examined in patients with type 1 diabetes whose glycemia was normalized or kept moderately elevated by constant insulin infusions maintained overnight and during the experimental period. As in normal subjects, it ap-

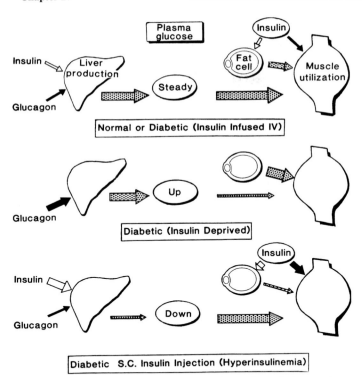

FIGURE 27-8. Scheme indicating changes in glucose fluxes during exercise in insulin-treated diabetes.

pears that catecholamines are the main regulators of GP during intense exercise and that they induce a relative inhibition of glucose utilization. The main difference in glucose homeostasis between normal subjects and those with diabetes was that the elevation in glycemia induced by exercise was sustained throughout the postexercise period in both normoglycemic and hyperglycemic individuals with type 1 diabetes. During this prolonged period of hyperglycemia, the metabolic clearance rate (MCR) of glucose was reduced. However, hyperglycemia during intense exercise in both groups of patients with type 1 diabetes fully compensated for the low MCR (decreased efficiency of glucose extraction) such that overall glucose utilization was the same as in control subjects (Fig. 27-9).[28] Thus, hyperglycemia appears to be an adaptive phenomenon to reduced MCR, which ensures that during strenuous exercise, glucose delivery to the muscle is kept constant. This corresponds to similar observations in diabetic dogs subjected to moderate exercise.[170,174] On a cellular level, the efficiency of glucose uptake is related to the number of glucose transporters in the plasma membrane.[193] The observation that hyperglycemia decreases the number of glucose transporters in the plasma membrane also supports the notion of an adaptive effect of hyperglycemia.[193]

This postexercise hyperglycemia can be normalized by an additional postexercise administration of insulin. Postexercise hyperinsulinemia was required to further increase MCR and gradually return plasma glucose concentrations to preexercise levels.[28,194] Therefore, special strategies, differing from those for less strenuous exercise, are required for management of insulin therapy in type 1 diabetes during and after intense exercise.

The difference from moderate exercise is largely accounted for by the difference in catecholamine responses. As noted, the stimu-

lation of muscle glycogenolysis increases the glucose-6-phosphate, which in intense exercise is likely to be sufficient to restrain the uptake of circulating glucose and account for the hyperglycemia. Consistent with this explanation is the effect of β-adrenergic receptor blockade during stress[178] or moderate exercise in dogs,[83] and intensely exercised normal[195] and type 1 diabetic subjects[196] in whom β-blockade increased metabolic clearance.

Effect of Hyperglycemia: Possible Protection of Muscle Against Excessive Glucose

The effect of hyperglycemia on metabolic glucose clearance (MCR) is of pivotal importance during exercise in diabetes. This section summarizes the effects during both rest and exercise. Decreased MCR in hyperglycemia may reflect a protective mechanism against excessive glucose in the muscle. It is tempting to speculate that this is the reason that muscle does not have the diabetic complications seen in so many other tissues. Restoration of normal glycemia by phlorizin treatment normalizes glucose transporters in plasma membrane. Importantly, this effect of normalization of plasma glucose occurs without any changes in plasma insulin. In the same experiments, hyperglycemia also suppressed GLUT-4 mRNA and normoglycemia brought about partial restoration. The conclusion is that hyperglycemia itself suppresses both gene expression and translocation of the GLUT-4 protein (Fig. 27-10).[193] This adaptive mechanism of glucose uptake could also be demonstrated in the absence of insulin in glucose-perfused rat hindquarter. Glucose uptake was maintained both during hyper- and hypoinsulinemia due to decreased or increased GLUT-4 transporter and glucose clearance, respectively.[197]

Similarly, normalization of glycemia with phlorizin in alloxandiabetic dogs increases MCR, while glucose uptake is unchanged. This applies both to resting conditions[188,198] and to exercise (Fig. 27-11).[199,200] This mechanism of self-regulation also explains observations in streptozocin-diabetic rats where endogenous pH and energy stores measured with nuclear magnetic resonance (NMR) techniques and the activity of pyruvate dehydrogenase during rest and muscular contraction were normal, not only in insulin-treated rats but also in rats with insulin treatment discontinued for 3 days (Fig. 27-12).[201]

Exercise in Individuals with Type 2 Diabetes

It is well documented that chronic exercise is particularly important in type 2 diabetes, since it can prevent the onset of the disease and improve glycemia and other metabolic parameters. Glucoregulation, which has been extensively studied in type 1 diabetes, has scarcely been studied in type 2 diabetes. During exercise in type 2 diabetes, plasma glucose declines. In studies in which insulin levels failed to decrease during exercise, perhaps due to neuropathy, the decline in plasma glucose was due to a blunted increase in GP.[202] However, in a study in which insulin levels decreased, greater than normal rates of glucose utilization were found due to residual mild hyperglycemia, because glucose clearance increased similarly to control subjects.[203,204]

There is a close association between the metabolic syndrome, or syndrome X, and type 2 diabetes. Indeed, many individuals with obesity, dyslipidemia, hyperinsulinemia, and hypertension eventually develop type 2 diabetes. Most patients with type 2 diabetes lead a sedentary lifestyle and have a low Vo₂max.[165] Therefore, physical exercise is one of the three principal therapeutic measures

HYPERGLYCEMIA FULLY COMPENSATES FOR DEFECTIVE MCR IN INSULIN INFUSED HYPERGLYCEMIC IDDM'S

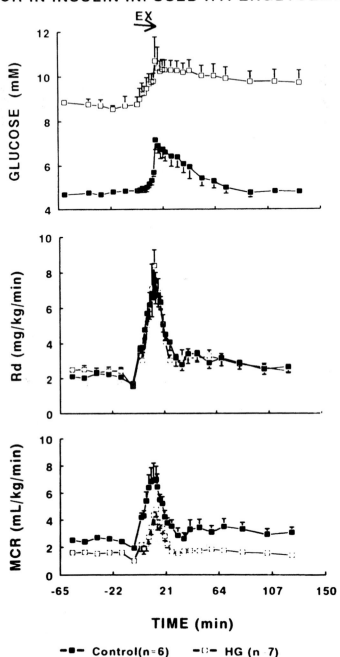

FIGURE 27-9. Effect of intense exercise in IDDM subjects whose glycemia was normalized (■) or kept moderately elevated (□) by constant insulin infusions maintained overnight and during the experiment.

recommended, along with diet and weight control and hypoglycemic medicines, for type 2 diabetic patients.[156,165]

DIABETES PREVENTION

Historically, a number of factors have shifted emphasis from the use of physical activity for diabetes treatment to its use for diabetes prevention. They include difficulty in obtaining compliance with an exercise program in middle-aged and elderly individuals,

the variable response of patients with established type 2 diabetes, and the fact that vascular complications of diabetes are present in many patients at the time of diagnosis. For these reasons, it was suggested that an optimum target population for an exercise program might be people at increased risk for type 2 diabetes such as individuals with impaired glucose tolerance and/or insulin resistance.[205,206] In keeping with this hypothesis, cross-sectional studies in Melanesian and Indian Fijian men[207] by Taylor and colleagues, other populations,[208] and in college alumni,[209] demonstrated an

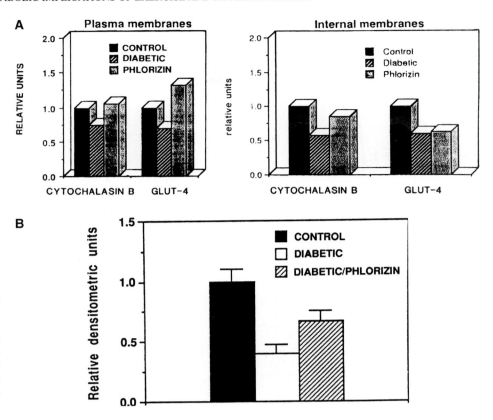

FIGURE 27-10. **A**. Effect of normalization of glycemia on cytochalasin B binding and GLUT-4 glucose transporters in hyperglycemic normainsulinemic diabetic rats. The isolated fractions were isolated for protein and 5-nucleotidase activity. Forty micrograms of protein-isolated membrane fractions were analyzed by Western blot using an anti–GLUT-4 antibody. The blots were quantified by laser densitometry and the results were plotted in arbitrary units relative to the values in the plasma membrane of control animals. Plasma membrane glucose transporters were suppressed by diabetes and restored by normalization of glucose with phlorizin. Normalization of glucose with phlorizin restores cytochalasin B binding but not the GLUT-4 transporters in internal membranes. **B**. GLUT-4 mRNA is suppressed by diabetes and partially restored by normalization of glucose with phlorizin. *(Reprinted with permission from Dimitrakoudis D, Vranic M, Klip A: Effects of hyperglycemia on glucose transporters of the muscle: Use of the renal glucose reabsorption inhibitor phlorizin to control glycemia.* J Am Soc Nephrol *1992;3:1078.)*

inverse relationship between physical activity and risk of type 2 diabetes, as did later studies of male college alumni by Helmrich and coworkers[210] (Fig. 27-13) and in nurses[211] and male physicians[212] by Manson and coworkers. In the college alumni and male physicians, the risk reduction was particularly pronounced among obese men.

Further proof of the benefit of exercise in diabetes prevention came from two later studies, in which the effect of 5–6 years of increased physical activity was examined prospectively in several hundred patients with impaired glucose tolerance in China (DaQuing)[213] (Table 27-1) and Sweden (Malmo).[214] In Malmo, therapy consisted of dietary advice during the first 6 months and exercise throughout. In DaQuing, the effects of exercise, diet, and the two in combination were independently evaluated. In both studies, progression to diabetes over 5–6 years was diminished by 30–50% in all intervention groups, with no additive effect of exercise plus diet observed.[213] Plasma triglycerides and insulin levels were also reduced in the Malmo exercising subjects.[214] A critical finding in the Malmo study was that after 12 years, overall mortality due to ischemic heart disease and other causes was diminished in the exercise group to levels similar to those of nondiabetic control subjects.[215] Thus, an emerging body of evidence suggests that in people with impaired glucose tolerance, exercise can be efficacious in preventing, or at least retarding progression to, diabetes, and in diminishing overall mortality. Of particular note is that lifestyle changes that include exercise or exercise and diet, which also increase insulin sensitivity, prevent or at least substantially delay the progression of individuals with impaired glucose tolerance to overt type 2 diabetes.[216] The Diabetes Prevention Program (DPP) also showed this. In a randomized clinical trial of diabetes prevention in 3234 overweight men and women aged 25–85 years

with impaired glucose tolerance, who exercised 150 minutes per week (corresponding to a brisk walk) and reduced their weight by 7%, there was a 58% reduced risk of developing type 2 diabetes. Logic suggests that this is somehow related to exercise's effect of enhancing insulin action and reversing some of the risk factors associated with the metabolic syndrome, or of lowering blood glucose levels independent of insulin (e.g., by directly simulating glucose utilization by muscle). This, however, remains to be proven.

Insulin resistance is a common clinical feature of type 2 diabetes that can be related to receptor and/or postreceptor defects. Intriguingly, many individuals with type 2 diabetes exhibit normal or even slightly above normal rates of glucose utilization and normal splanchnic glucose output during exercise.[204] However, muscle lactate output during exercise was elevated twofold and muscle glycogen store was one-third lower in these patients in comparison to the nondiabetic control subjects, indicating higher rates of glycolysis and glycogenolysis.[204] This suggests that muscle insulin resistance in at least part of the type 2 diabetic population involves defects in glucose oxidative metabolism, the steps downstream to those of glucose transport and glycolysis. Therefore, to understand the effects of exercise in type 2 diabetes, the severity of the disease and the specific treatments the patient receives must be taken into account. Bicycle ergometer exercise for 30 minutes stimulated sympathetic hypersensitivity in patients with type 2 diabetes and fasting hyperglycemia and hyperketonemia, but not in those who were well controlled.[216] Some individuals with type 2 diabetes with postabsorptive hyperglycemia and near-normal basal insulin secretion display a significant fall in glycemia following exercise due to a failure of insulin to decrease during exercise. These patients have a defect in control of insulin secretion when challenged

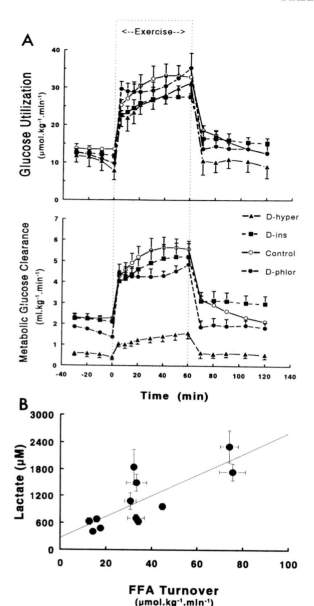

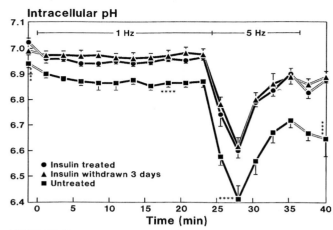

FIGURE 27-12. Changes in intracellular pH in gastrocnemius muscle during stimulation at 1 and 5 Hz and during the initial recovery period for insulin-treated diabetic (•), untreated diabetic (■), and diabetic animals from which insulin therapy was withdrawn for 72 hours prior to study (▲). Values are shown as mean ± SE for six experiments in each study group. *(Reprinted with permission from Challis RAJ, et al.[201])*

FIGURE 27-11. A. Glucose utilization and metabolic clearance rates of plasma glucose in dogs before, during, and after 60-minute treadmill exercise (100 m/min, 5% slope). Experiments were conducted in four dog protocols consisting of one protocol with normal control dogs (C, O) and three protocols with alloxan-diabetic dogs studied under conditions of hyperglycemia (DH, γ), and during acutely induced normoglycemia (<160 minutes) with either insulin (2.6 ± 0.6 pmol.kg$_{-1}$/min$_{-1}$, DI (■) or phlorizin (50 kg$_{-1}$/min$_{-1}$, DP). Values are presented as mean ± SE from six experiments in each protocol. During hyperglycemia metabolic clearance of glucose was markedly suppressed during rest and exercise. It was normalized with normoglycemia and independently of insulin or FFA levels—glucose utilization was only slightly decreased in hyperglycemic dogs, reflecting the balance between mass effect of hyperglycemia and suppressed clearance. **B.** Correlation between rates of FFA turnover and lactate concentrations in all four dog protocols consisting of normal control dogs and alloxan-diabetic dogs studied under conditions of hyperglycemia and during acutely induced normoglycemia (<160 minutes) with either insulin or phlorizin. Plotted data indicate the mean ± SE during the basal period, exercise period, and recovery period for each protocol (r = 0.72, p < .001). Increased FFA turnover did not affect glucose uptake, but it decreased glucose oxidation—a reflection of lactate release.

both with glucose (inadequate increase) and exercise (inadequate decrease). The latter could be a consequence of hyperglycemia prevailing over the adrenergic stimulation, or part of the intrinsic abnormality of islet β-cell function, or of neuropathy. In addition, hyperglycemia, acting synergistically with insulin, can suppress GP and sustain a normal rate of peripheral glucose uptake.

In general, exercise is associated with improvements in insulin action and glucose metabolism. Twelve to 16 hours after a single bout of glycogen-depleting exercise, hepatic insulin sensitivity was enhanced in patients with type 2 diabetes.[181] The prior exercise reduced basal hepatic GP by 25%, while a low-dose insulin infusion suppressed it by 85%. Peripheral insulin sensitivity was also enhanced, which was reflected by an increased rate of nonoxidative glucose disposal.[191] In a 10-year lifestyle modification program, persistent physical exercise has resulted in a significant improvement in glycated hemoglobin, blood pressure, and plasma triglycerides profile.[165] In a recent study, patients with type 2 diabetes with a mean body mass index of 30.2 underwent a 2-month exercise program that consisted of a twice weekly supervised 45-minute cycling at 75% VO$_2$ peak. This resulted in a 41% increase in VO$_2$ peak and 61% increase in glucose disappearance during an intravenous glucose tolerance test (IVGTT). The improvement was associated with a reduction of visceral adipose tissue (VAT) that was greater than the loss of subcutaneous fat (Fig. 27-14).[218] Thus, in obese individuals with type 2 diabetes, regular- and moderate-intensity exercise can lead to improvements in both obesity and insulin sensitivity.[218] These studies emphasize the significance of exercise in improving energy fuel metabolism, and its importance as an adjuvant therapy for type 2 diabetes.

Patient participation may be affected by length and severity of the illness that in turn affect the medical benefits of exercise. For example, a high incidence of complications can preclude participation for some patients, but in some studies, no complications or dropouts were reported with exercise training in type 2 diabetic patients for 3 months.[219,220]

Type 2 diabetic patients who have no major vascular complication should be able to exercise as normal people. Single bouts of

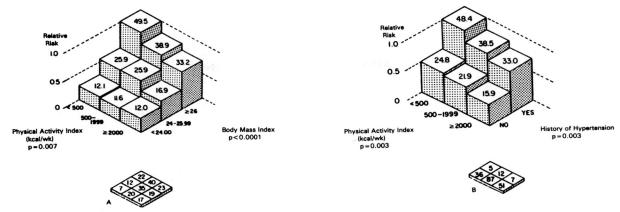

FIGURE 27-13. Age-adjusted incidence rates and relative risks of T2DM among 5990 men, based on 1962 data for the physical activity index in relation to the body mass index (**A**) and any history of hypertension (**B**). Each block represents the relative risk based on the rate of T2DM per 10,000 person-years of follow-up, with the risk for the tallest block set at 1.0. The numbers on the blocks are the incidence rates of T2DM, and the numbers of patients with T2DM are shown below in the corresponding grid. *(Reprinted with permission from Helmrich SP, et al.[210])*

exercise in type 2 diabetic men have been shown to enhance peripheral and splanchnic insulin sensitivity for up to 16 hours.[181] Although the incidence of hypoglycemia is much lower in the type 2 than in the type 1 diabetic population, the use of sulfonylurea and insulin in patients with type 2 diabetes increases the susceptibility to this complication, especially among those who exercise after taking the drugs.[221] It is interesting that in the majority of patients with type 2 diabetes, exercise-induced glucose utilization was not impaired but actually greater than in the nondiabetic individuals. In the meantime, the exercise-induced rise in hepatic GP can be restrained by the prior use of hypoglycemic drugs, including sulfonylureas, insulin, and inhibitors of FFA oxidation. The actions of sulfonylurea drugs and exercise can potentiate each other and the hypoglycemic responses are further enhanced by sulfonylurea-induced insulin secretion, which restrains hepatic GP and reduces glucose supply to the working muscle.[222] When glyburide was given to normal subjects before exercise, insulin levels increased about twofold and blood glucose levels fell to about 50 mg/dL.[223] The nadir in blood glucose levels was deeper and occurred more promptly than when glyburide was administered to resting subjects.

Thus, normoglycemic patients with type 2 diabetes may be at increased risk of developing hypoglycemia if they exercise 1–2 hours after ingesting sulfonylureas. In general, however, type 2 diabetic individuals should avoid high-intensity exercise, which induces an exaggerated rise in counterregulatory hormones. Excessive hyperglycemia can be triggered or worsened by a greater increase in GP than glucose utilization.

An appropriate exercise program should be a powerful adjunct to the diet and drug therapies to improve glycemic control, reduce cardiovascular risk factors, and increase psychological well-being in individuals with type 2 diabetes. It has been clearly demonstrated that leisure-time physical activity, expressed in kilocalories expended per week in walking, stair climbing, and sports, was inversely related to the development of type 2 diabetes (Fig. 27-14).[210] The incidence rates declined as energy expenditure increased from less than 500 kcal to 3500 kcal. For each 500-kcal increment in energy expenditure, the age-adjusted risk of type 2 diabetes was reduced by 6%.[210] In most patients, the benefits of exercise substantially outweigh the risks. However, attention must be paid to minimizing potential exercise complications.

TABLE 27-1. Effects of 6 Years of Diet and Exercise Therapy on Progression to Type II Diabetes in Lean and Overweight Patients with Impaired Glucose Tolerance (DaQuing Study)

	Control	Diet	Exercise	Diet and Exercise
Lean				
n	50	55	57	46
Initial BMI (kg/m^2)	22.4	21.8	21.7	22.3
Percent diabetic (6 yrs)	30	21	15*	16*
Overweight				
n	83	75	84	80
Initial BMI (kg/m^2)	28.5	28.3	27.9	28.6
Percent diabetic (6 yrs)	60	36*	43*	42*

*Significantly different from control group, $p < 0.05$.

Roughly equal numbers of men and women, ages 44–46 at the onset of the study, were followed in each group. Results are means for indicated number of subjects. Diet consisted of a decrease in ethanol and refined sugar intake and an increase in vegetables in the lean young group and a similar diet with reduced calories in the overweight subjects. Exercise consisted of an increase in daily leisure physical activity of varying intensity. Lean and overweight groups experienced small increases and decreases in body mass index, respectively, over 6 years. Body fat and its distribution were not measured, or plasma insulin or triglyceride levels. Blood pressure was measured but not reported.

Adapted from Pan *et al.*[213]

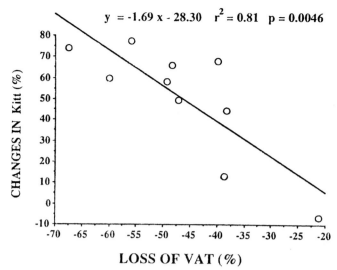

$$y = -1.69 x - 28.30 \quad r^2 = 0.81 \quad p = 0.0046$$

FIGURE 27-14. In overweight, type 2 diabetic patients (BMI: 30.2 ± 0.9 kg/m²), physical training with 45 minutes of cycling at 75% of V_{O_2} peak twice weekly for 2 months resulted in a marked (48%) loss of visceral adipose tissue (VAT). The loss of VAT was associated with a significant improvement in insulin sensitivity indicated by the glucose disposal during an intravenous glucose tolerance test (Kitt). *(Reprinted with permission from Mourier A, et al.[218])*

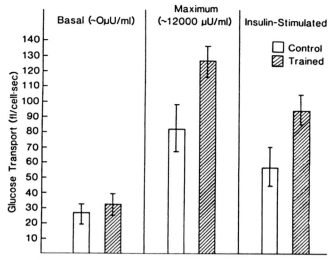

FIGURE 27-15. Mean ± SE values for basal, maximum, and insulin-stimulated glucose transport in adipocytes isolated from control (**open bars**) and trained (**hatched bars**) individuals. *(Reprinted with permission from Rodnick KJ, et al.[224])*

Effect on Insulin Sensitivity in Nondiabetics

The general effects of exercise on improvement of glucose tolerance and insulin sensitivity have been well documented.[224] Insulin action in trained nondiabetic distance runners was enhanced in muscle, liver, and adipose tissue (Fig. 27-15).[224] These effects of training are probably specific for aerobic exercise. Interestingly, no difference in specific binding of insulin to its receptor on monocytes was noted between the two groups. The increased insulin effect is primarily mediated by postrecepter events, such as increased glucose transport and intracellular metabolism. Enzyme activities for both glycogen synthesis and glucose oxidation are stimulated by physical training. Decreased adiposity and increased muscle mass, due to long-term training, can also contribute to improvement in insulin sensitivity. Insulin levels are lowered as a result of enhanced insulin sensitivity. Single bouts of exercise in untrained nondiabetic subjects are also associated with increased insulin sensitivity, presumably due to depletion of muscle and liver glycogen stores. Single bouts of exercise can also decrease insulin resistance in obese normoglycemic and obese type 2 diabetic subjects, probably related to improvements at both insulin receptor and postreceptor levels.

The effect of exercise on insulin sensitivity may be dependent on specific types of physical work. Strength training, for example, results in a net increase in submaximal insulin-stimulated glucose disposal and glucose tolerance that is proportional to the increased muscle mass and probably does not represent an increase in insulin sensitivity *per se*. Cycling at 70% V_{O_2}max and 4 hours per week for 12 weeks did not significantly affect insulin-stimulated glucose disposal in either lean and obese nondiabetic men, or diet-controlled type 2 diabetic patients.[225] There are many other effects of training that can directly or indirectly affect carbohydrate metabolism during rest and exercise. One study[226] showed that ath-

letes have a larger capacity to secrete epinephrine in response to a variety of stimuli during rest.

The metabolic benefits of physical training can also be appreciated from observing the effects of cessation of training or bed rest. It is known that exercise-trained people have a reduced insulin response to a glucose load. As rapidly as 14 days after cessation of exercise training, this insulin response increased. However, rates of whole-body glucose disposal were not different between exercising and inactive states, indicating a large increase in insulin resistance due to inactivity.[227] A 7-day bed rest also affected insulin responsiveness of protein metabolism in humans.[228] After bed rest, subjects exhibited decreased glucose tolerance, increased endogenous insulin secretion, and a negative nitrogen balance compared with the control period. Because negative nitrogen balance and skeletal muscle atrophy occurred in the six rested subjects in the absence of changes in the two indices of protein breakdown used in this study, it seems likely that muscle protein synthesis was inhibited when compared with the period before bed rest.

Studies also suggest that exercise can positively impact a population of insulin-resistant, normal-weight individuals.[220] These individuals are not obese on the basis of weight and height, but are hyperinsulinemic, insulin resistant, and predisposed to type 2 diabetes, hypertriglyceridemia, and coronary heart disease. The specific factors associated with insulin resistance in this population are central fat distribution, inactivity, and a low V_{O_2}max Long-term exercise and diet can significantly diminish their incidence of diabetes.[220]

Effect on Insulin Sensitivity in Patients with Diabetes

Insulin binding to skeletal muscle in type 2 diabetic subjects was unaffected, but glycogen synthase activity was increased by training.[163] However, hepatic insulin sensitivity, as judged by suppression of hepatic GP, was not affected by training.[229] When type 1 diabetic patients undergo exercise training that significantly increases their maximum oxygen consumption, glucose uptake in response to a hyperinsulinemic euglycemic clamp is increased markedly.[229] Studies in streptozocin-diabetic rats indicate that the ability to adapt to chronic exercise in insulin-deficient states may depend on the severity of the condition. Mildly diabetic rats increase insulin sensitivity in response to exercise training, whereas severely diabetic rats do not show this change.[230]

Studies in patients with type 2 diabetes have shown that an exercise training program that is feasible for most individuals can cause an improvement in glucose tolerance[219] and lower glucose-stimulated insulin levels.[219] Insulin sensitivity, as assessed by glucose disposal during hyperinsulinemic euglycemic clamps, improves with exercise training.[219] By combining euglycemic clamps, infusion of radioactive glucose, and measurement of glucose metabolic rate, it is possible to differentiate between glucose oxidation and glucose storage, because the latter is a nonoxidative pathway. A combined exercise training and diet program increased the total glucose disposal rate during an insulin clamp in type 2 diabetes by approximately 27%, due primarily to an accelerated rate of nonoxidative carbohydrate disposal (storage) (Fig. 27-16).[231] In contrast, diet alone did not affect glucose storage. Exercise alone does not appear to normalize muscular insulin sensitivity in insulin-resistant states. However, diet and exercise together may correct this condition.[232] In the perfused hindlimb of trained and sedentary insulin-resistant obese Zucker rats, training and a high-carbohydrate diet independently increased glucose uptake above that in sedentary, obese Zucker rats (on a high-fat diet) but still below that in lean control rats. A combination of high-carbohydrate diet and training had a synergistic effect. Thus, it appears that the combination of diet and exercise has a more physiologic metabolic effect than diet alone. Basal and insulin-suppressed hepatic glucose output was also reduced by diet and training, but no more than by the diet program alone. Training programs lead to an improvement in insulin sensitivity in obese subjects even without concurrent weight loss or change in body composition (Fig. 27-17).[219] Nevertheless, since weight reduction by itself can also improve insulin sensitivity, it is likely that exercise training that results in loss of body fat will yield optimal results on carbohydrate metabolism.

Although insulin sensitivity is improved and muscular metabolic capacity is increased, it is unresolved whether glycemic control is effectively improved in trained individuals with type 1 diabetes. Indeed, there was no improvement in glycosylated hemoglobin levels, glycosuria, or fasting plasma glucose levels following training programs that resulted in significant increments in maximal oxidative capacity.[233] In contrast, training can improve glycemic control in type 2 diabetes. It is important to note that individuals with different degrees of insulin resistance do not adapt to training in the same way. For example, training in insulin-resistant conditions characterized by high rates of insulin secretion can lead to a decrease in the release of this hormone.[219] On the other hand, training in subjects with insulin resistance and low insulin secretion has been shown to increase the rate of insulin secretion.[219] Finally, an improvement in insulin action in trained diabetic and nondiabetic subjects could be due to the cumulative effects of single exercise bouts rather than to long-term adaptations to exercise training.[234] This is based on two lines of evidence. First, the effects of training on insulin action are rapidly reversed by inactivity, whereas the effects of training on oxygen uptake and lean

FIGURE 27-16. Carbohydrate disposal by nonoxidative processes, "storage." The single asterisk indicates the significant increase in estimated storage within the group in the dietary therapy plus physical training group ($p < .05$), and the double asterisk shows the significant reduction in the group given dietary therapy alone. *(Reprinted with permission from Bogardus C, et al.[231])*

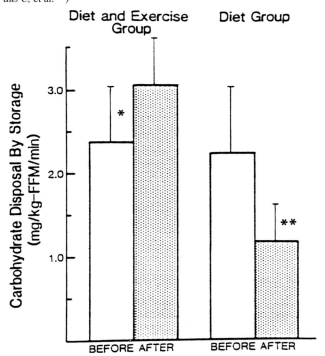

FIGURE 27-17. Glucose disposal in diabetic subjects (n = 10) and controls (n = 13) during euglycemic clamp before (**hatched bars**) and after (**open bars**) physical training for 3 months, 3× weekly 50-minute alternate heavy (80%–90% Vo₂max) and light periods. There was no change in BW, cell mass, or adipose cellularity. *(Reprinted with permission from Kratkiewski M, et al.[219])*

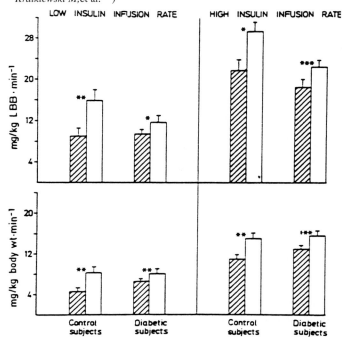

body mass are more sustained.[234] Second, an acute bout of exercise and exercise training share similar effects.[181]

Effects on Muscle and Adipose Tissues

The skeletal muscle is the major site of the increase in insulin action that occurs with training, due to its large mass of insulin-sensitive tissue and its fundamental role during physical work. Skeletal muscle in trained rats is more insulin sensitive than in sedentary control animals, due mainly to increased glucose oxidation.[80] Hyperinsulinemic euglycemic clamps combined with the 2-deoxy-glucose technique demonstrated an increase in maximal insulin-stimulated glucose metabolism in soleus and red gastrocnemius, and an increased insulin sensitivity in soleus, gastrocnemius, extensor digitorum longus, and diaphragm in exercise-trained rats compared with sedentary control rats.[80,156] The increase in insulin action in skeletal muscle during habitual exercise may be due in part to an increase in insulin binding to its skeletal muscle receptor. It is surprising, however, that for similar amounts of bound insulin, trained rats had a decrease in the activity of the tyrosine kinase activity.[235,236] Skeletal muscle adapts to aerobic exercise training so that it more readily uses fuel and oxygen. Physical training greatly enhanced mitochondrial oxidative enzyme activities, which last 4–6 weeks following the cessation of training in both type 1 and type 2 diabetic individuals.[237] Streptozocin-diabetic rats have deficits in cytoplasmic and mitochondrial enzyme in muscle fibers, which are increased by training. In type 1 diabetic patients, training programs can lead to increases in skeletal muscle citrate synthase and succinate dehydrogenase that parallel an increase in insulin sensitivity.[238] Improvement in insulin sensitivity with exercise training is associated with upregulated enzymes responsible for the phosphorylation, storage, and oxidation of glucose, and also with conversion of fast-twitch glycolytic IIb fibers to fast-twitch oxidative IIa fibers that are more insulin sensitive.[239]

It is well documented that both insulin and exercise translocate GLUT-4 from intracellular sites to the plasma membrane. The effect of insulin is more pronounced in red than in white muscle.[240] The translocation from internal membranes to the muscle transverse tubules is at lest least as important as the transfer to plasma membrane[241] because the area of transverse tubules that penetrates the various muscle structures is much larger than that of plasma membrane. Swimming or free-wheel running induces rapid increases in the expression of the insulin-sensitive GLUT-4 protein and enhancement of glucose transport capacity and insulin-induced glycogen storage in the muscle in the normal rat.[242] In male patients with type 1 diabetes, acute exercise (3 hours at cycling) decreased cellular GLUT-4 mRNA content, while GLUT-4 protein content remained unchanged in the quadriceps femoris.[243] In type 2 diabetic patients, physical training increased both muscle GLUT-4 protein and mRNA.[244] However, human studies thus far could only measure total GLUT-4 content but not translocation of GLUT-4. Since glucose transport does not depend on the total cellular amount of GLUT-4 but on plasma membrane abundance of this protein, the human studies are not conclusive.

A recent study provided compelling evidence that regular exercise results in a marked preferential reduction (48%) in central obesity and a significant increase (23%) in thigh muscle tissue area, both of which help improve insulin resistance in type 2 diabetes.[218] Another new role of insulin is to induce vasodilation in skeletal muscle and increase muscle blood flow, leading to an increase in blood glucose extraction by the muscle.[239] It is known that a re-duced ability of insulin to vasodilate skeletal muscle contributes to insulin resistance in type 2 diabetes. Exercise training has been found to improve both muscle blood flow and glucose extraction in response to insulin.[239]

Changes in muscle capillary density can also affect insulin sensitivity by altering the exposure of muscle to insulin and glucose. In the rat, muscles with highest blood flow are the most insulin sensitive.[245] In humans, muscle capillary density is strongly correlated to the total glucose disposal rate during a hyperinsulinemic euglycemic glucose clamp.[246] However, postexercise muscle blood flow was 40.1 mL/min/100 g of tissue in the nondiabetic subjects and was significantly reduced in 10 type 1 diabetic (25.7 mL/min/100 g) and 11 type 2 diabetic patients (14 mL/min/100 g).[247] Muscle capillary density was not improved by exercise training in the diabetic patients,[248] although it increased significantly (50%) in nondiabetic athletes.

In addition to skeletal muscle, adipose tissue represents another site of adaptation to training. Regular physical activity increases insulin-stimulated glucose uptake,[80,249] oxidation,[80] and incorporation into fatty acids[80] in rat adipocytes. The improvement of insulin action may relate to the reduced fat cell size after physical training. One such study demonstrated that insulin-stimulated 2-deoxyglucose uptake and 1-^{14}C-glucose oxidation in adipocytes were highly correlated to fat cell size in exercise-trained, sedentary, and calorie-restricted sedentary rats. The increase in insulin action in adipocytes of trained rats occurs in the absence of any changes in insulin binding, indicating a modification in a postbinding event.

Exercise and Cardiovascular Health in Diabetes

Regular aerobic exercise results in significant improvements in lipid profile, blood pressure, and body fat distribution in type 2 diabetes.[250] Regular exercise can potentially diminish the risk for atherosclerotic macrovascular disease in type 2 diabetic patients, as it does in the general population. Hyperinsulinemia, insulin resistance, and/or increases in intra-abdominal adipose mass (central obesity) are related to a high risk of atherosclerosis in type 2 diabetes. The basis for the effect of exercise may be its ability to diminish or prevent these risk factors.[251] Cardiovascular benefits of exercise are best achieved by aerobic exercise that improves maximal aerobic work capacity, (Vo_2max) by both enhanced cardiopulmonary function and increased oxidative metabolism in the muscle.[172]

Atherosclerotic vascular complications, affecting arteries in the heart, brain, and extremities, account for most morbidity and mortality in type 2 diabetic patients. Epidemiologic data and animal studies all indicate that physical training might retard atherosclerotic vascular disease in the general population although hard epidemiologic data are still lacking.[251] The incidence of fatal myocardial infarction among persons who exercised regularly for more than 10 years could be reduced by one-half in comparison with the sedentary controls, independent of other known risk factors including hypertension, cigarette smoking, and hypercholesterolemia.

It was shown that in type 2 diabetes, training can affect a number of parameters related to blood coagulation, but it is too early to indicate whether or not this represents an antiatherogenic effect of exercise. In the untrained state, fibrinolytic activity was impaired in diabetics and resting levels of plasma fibrinogen and the prothrombin time (PT) were increased. Activation of fibrinolysis occurred following exercise in both groups but the increment was less in patients with diabetes. Physical training could improve the resting and postexercise activated partial thromplastin time (APTT), Vo₂max, and resting fibrinolytic activity in diabetics, in association with improved glycemic control.[252] Hyperlipidemia and disorders in lipoprotein metabolism are major risk factors for cardiovascular disease and occur with higher frequency in both type 1 and 2 diabetes. There is an increased prevalence of hyperlipidemia and diminished high-density lipoprotein (HDL) cholesterol in diabetics, presumably a function of metabolic control. Recent studies in type 1 diabetes[233] show that intensive training increases the ratio of HDL cholesterol to total cholesterol. Training can reduce triglyceride levels in type 2 diabetes, an effect that appears to be rapidly reversed by inactivity. Hypertension markedly increases the frequency of vascular disease and occurs with greater frequency in patients with diabetes than in normal subjects. It is now recognized that essential hypertension is associated with insulin resistance and hyperinsulinemia, even in the absence of diabetes and obesity. In general, active individuals have lower systolic and diastolic blood pressure than sedentary control individuals matched for age.[251]

SUMMARY AND SOME PRACTICAL RECOMMENDATIONS

The sedentary and over nourished lifestyle in nearly two-thirds of the population in modern society plays a critical part in the twentieth century "epidemic" of coronary heart disease. Physical activity and fitness are key determinants of whole-body or total health, that is, physical, social, cultural, and spiritual well-being. Inspired by the desire of diabetic patients to participate in various physical activities, sports, and games, there is a drastic increase in the number of publications related to sports activities for people with diabetes.[161,172,251]

With the discovery of insulin, Joslin recommended that diet, insulin, and exercise represent the management triad in diabetes. The importance of exercise and general considerations with respect to exercise and diabetes have been reviewed and detailed plans for specific exercise prescriptions have been discussed.[251]

Exercise cannot be regarded as an isolated, separate therapy but must be incorporated into the total program of treatment, including medication and diet. While most experts recommend aerobic exercise for improving insulin sensitivity and carbohydrate metabolism, some researchers suggest that some patients might benefit from resistance training. Some very general guidelines are recommended:

1. Before prescribing an exercise program, perform a complete history and physical examination. Evaluate diabetes control and complications.
2. Prescribe a moderate work load that is enjoyable and can increase slowly. Lifting and strong resistance training should be avoided.
3. Encourage self-managed blood glucose monitoring to document glycemic responses to various exercise modalities.
4. Encourage patients to schedule exercise to reduce postprandial hyperglycemia and discourage exercise during insulin action peak.
5. Exercising extremities should not be used as insulin injection sites.
6. Alert patients about the possibility of delayed exercise-induced hypoglycemia. Always have carbohydrate liquid handy.

7. Individuals who have been sedentary for years should begin exercising with a warm-up and proceed gradually to vigorous, preferably aerobic activity and conclude with a cool-down period.
8. Patients with evidence of peripheral neuropathy should shy away from running and sports involving pounding of the lower extremities that are likely to produce chafing and blisters. Bicycling and swimming are ideal for most patients with diabetes.
9. Be aware of the potential problems of combining exercise with a diet that is deficient in calories or essential nutrients. Diets containing low calories and low carbohydrates can increase risks of cardiac arrhythmia, ketosis, and sudden death.

In conclusion, significant medical, physical, and psychological benefits of exercise can and should be achieved in most patients with diabetes. Appropriate planning will optimize these benefits and minimize potential complications and risks.

REFERENCES

1. Joslin EP, Root HF, White P, et al: *The treatment of Diabetes Mellitus.* Philadelphia: Lea & Febiger: 1935; 299.
2. American Diabetes Association: Diabetes mellitus and exercise: Position statement. *Diabetes Care* 1990;13:804.
3. Wasserman DH, Williams PE, Lacy DB, et al: Importance of intrahepatic mechanisms to gluconeogenesis from alanine during prolonged exercise and recovery. *Am J Physiol* 1988; 254:E518.
4. Wahren J, Felig P, Ahlborg G, et al: Glucose metabolism during leg exercise in man. *J Clin Invest* 1971;50:2715.
5. Bergstrom J, Hermansen L, Hultman E, et al: Diet, muscle glycogen and physical performance. *Acta Physiol Scand* 1967;71:140.
6. Wasserman D: Control of glucose fluxes during exercise in the postabsorptive state. *Annu Rev Physiol* 1995; 191.
7. Issekutz B, Vranic M: Role of glucagon in regulation of GP in exercising dogs. *Am J Physiol* 1980;238:E13.
8. Wasserman DH, Lickley HLA, Vranic M: Interactions between glucagon and other counterregulatory hormones during normoglycemic and hypoglycemic exercise. *J Clin Invest* 1984;74:1404.
9. Wolfe RR, Nadel ER, Shaw JHF, et al: Role of changes in insulin and glucagon in glucose homeostasis in exercise. *J Clin Invest* 1986;77:900.
10. Kjaer M, Engfred K, Fernandez A, et al: Regulation of hepatic GP during exercise in humans: Role of sympathoadrenergic activity. *Am J Physiol* 1993;265:E275.
11. Hirsch IB, Marker JC, Smith LJ, et al: Insulin and glucagon in prevention of hypoglycemia during exercise in humans. *Am J Physiol* 1991;260:E695.
12. Wasserman DH, Spalding JS, Lacy DB, et al: Glucagon is a primary controller of hepatic glycogenolysis and gluconeogenesis during muscular work. *Am J Physiol* 1989;257:E108.
13. Wasserman DH, Lacy DB, Goldstein RE, et al: Exercise-induced fall in insulin and increase in fat metabolism during prolonged muscular work. *Diabetes* 1989;38:484.
14. Howlett K, Galbo H, Lorentsen J, et al: Effect of adrenaline on glucose kinetics during exercise in adrenalectomised humans. *J Physiol* 1999;519:911.
15. Winder WW, Terry ML, Mitchell VM, et al: Role of plasma epinephrine in fasted exercising rats. *Am J Physiol* 1985;248:R302.
16. Garceau D, Yamaguchi N, Goyer R, et al: Correlation between endogenous noradrenaline and glucose released from the liver upon hepatic sympathetic nerve stimulation in anesthetized dogs. *Can J Physiol Pharmacol* 1984;62:1086.
17. Hoelzer D, Dalsky G, Clutter W, et al: Glucoregulation during exercise: Hypoglycemia is prevented by redundant glucoregulatory systems during exercise: Sympathochromaffin activation and changes in hormone secretion. *J Clin Invest* 1986;77:212.
18. Sonne B, Mikines KL, Richter EA, et al: Role of liver nerves and adrenal medulla in glucose turnover in running rats. *J Appl Physiol* 1985; 59:1640.

19. Wasserman DH, Williams PE, Lacy DB, *et al:* Hepatic nerves are not essential to the increase in hepatic GP during muscular work. *Am J Physiol* 1990;259:E195.

20. Kjaer M, Keiding S, Engfred K, *et al:* Glucose homeostasis during exercise in humans with a liver or kidney transplant. *Am J Physiol* 1995; 268:E636.

21. Calles J, Cunningham JJ, Nelson L, *et al:* Glucose turnover during recovery from intense exercise. *Diabetes* 1983;32:734.

22. Marliss EB, Simantirakis E, Miles PDG, *et al:* Glucoregulatory and hormonal responses to repeated bouts of intense exercise in normal male subjects. *J Appl Physiol* 1991;71:924.

23. Sigal RJ, Fisher S, Halter JB, *et al:* The roles of catecholamines in glucoregulation in intense exercise as defined by the islet cell clamp technique. *Diabetes* 1996;45:148.

24. Manzon A, Fisher S, Morais J, *et al:* Glucose infusion partially attenuates glucose production and increases glucose uptake during intense exercise. *J Applied Physiol* 1998;85:514.

25. Kreisman SH, Manzon A, Nessim SJ, *et al:* Glucoregulatory responses to intense exercise performed in the postprandial state. *Am J Physiol* 2000;278:E786.

26. Kreisman SH, Mew NA, Arsenault M, *et al:* Epinephrine infusion during moderate exercise mimics intense exercise increments in GP and utilization. *Am J Physiol* 2000;278:E949.

27. Coker RH, Krishna MG, Lacy DB, *et al:* Role of hepatic alpha- and beta-adrenergic receptor stimulation on hepatic GP during heavy exercise. *Am J Physiol* 1997; Nov, 273:E831–8.

28. Sigal R, Purdon C, Bilinski D, *et al:* Glucoregulation during and after intense exercise: Effects of beta-blockade. *J Clin Endocrinol Metab* 1994;78:359.

29. Sigal RJ, Fisher SJ, Manzon M *et al:* Glucoregulation during and after intense exercise: Effects of alpha-adrenergic blockade. *Metabolism* 2000;49:386.

30. Wolfe RR, Klein S, Carraro F, *et al:* The role of the triglycerides-fatty acid cycle in controlling fat metabolism in humans during and after exercise. *Am J Physiol* 1990;258:E382.

31. Wahrenberg H, Engfeldt P, Bolinder J, *et al:* Acute adaptation in adrenergic control of lipolysis during physical exercise in humans. *Am J Physiol* 1987;253:E383.

32. Stich V, DeGliesezinski I, Crampes F, *et al:* Activation of antilipolytic alpha₂-adrenergic receptors by epinephrine during exercise in human adipose tissue. *Am J Physiol* 1999;277:R1076.

33. Horowitz JF, Klein S: Lipid metabolism during endurance exercise. *Am J Clin Nutr* 2000;72:558S.

34. Salvadori A, Fanari P, Mazza P, *et al:* Metabolic aspects and sympathetic effects in the obese subject undergoing exercise testing. *Minerva Med* 1993;84:171.

35. Dyck DJ, Bonen A: Muscle contraction increases palmitate esterification and oxidation and triacylglycerol oxidation. *Am J Physiol* 1998; 275:E888.

36. Bergman BC, Butterfield GE, Wolfe EE, *et al:* Evaluation of exercise and training on muscle lipid metabolism. *Am J Physiol* 1999;276:E106.

37. Howlett RA, Parolin ML, Dyck DJ, *et al:* Regulation of skeletal muscle glycogen phosphorylase and PDH at varying exercise power outputs. *Am J Physiol* 1998;275:R418.

38. Richter EA, Ruderman NB, Gavras H, *et al:* Muscle glycogenolysis during exercise: Dual control by epinephrine and contractions. *Am J Physiol* 1982;242:E25.

39. Nesher R, Karl IE, Kipnis KM: Dissociation of the effect(s) of insulin and contraction on glucose transport in rat epitrochlearis muscle. *Am J Physiol* 1985;249:C226.

40. Ploug T, Wojtaszewski J, Kristiansen S, *et al:* Glucose transport and transporters in muscle giant vesicles: Differential effects of insulin and contractions. *Am J Physiol* 1993;264:E270.

41. Hilsted J, Madsbad S, Hvidberg A, *et al:* Intranasal insulin therapy: The clinical realities. *Diabetologia* 1995;38:680.

42. Andersen PH, Saltin B: Maximal perfusion of skeletal muscle in man. *J Physiol* 1985;366:233.

43. Brozinick JT Jr, Etgen GJ, Yaspelkis BBI, *et al:* Contraction-activated glucose uptake is normal in insulin-resistant muscle of the obese Zucker rat. *J Appl Physiol* 1992;73:382.

44. DeFronzo RA, Ferrannini E, Sato Y, *et al:* Synergistic interaction between exercise and insulin on peripheral glucose uptake. *J Clin Invest* 1981;68:1468.

45. Ahlborg G: Metabolism in exercising arm vs leg muscle. *Clin Physiol* 1991;11459.

46. Hespel P, Vergauwen L, Vandenberghe K, *et al:* Important role of insulin and flow in stimulating glucose uptake in contracting skeletal muscle. *Diabetes* 1995;44:210.

47. Furler S, Jenkins AB, Storlien LH, *et al:* In vivo location of the rate-limiting step of hexose uptake in muscle and brain tissue of rats. *Am J Physiol* 1991;261:E337.

48. Kubo K, Foley JE: Rate-limiting steps for insulin-mediated glucose uptake into perfused rat hindlimb. *Am J Physiol* 1986; 250:E100.

49. Ren JM, Adkins-Marshall B, Gulve EA, *et al:* Evidence from transgenic mice that glucose transport is rate-limiting for glycogen deposition and glycolysis in skeletal muscle. *J Biol Chem* 1993;268:16113.

50. Katz A, Sahlin K, Broberg S: Regulation of glucose utilization in human skeletal muscle during moderate dynamic exercise. *Am J Physiol* 1991;260:E411.

51. Halseth A, Bracy D, Wasserman D: Overexpression of hexokinase II increases insulin- and exercise-stimulated muscle glucose uptake in vivo. *Am J Physiol* 1999;276:E70.

52. Halseth AE, Bracy DP, Wasserman DH: Limitations to exercise- and maximal insulin-stimulated muscle glucose uptake in vivo. *J Appl Physiol* 1998;85:2305.

53. Hespel P, Richter EA: Glucose uptake and transport in contracting, perfused rat muscle with different pre-contraction glycogen concentrations. *J Physiol (Lond)* 1990;427:347.

54. Gollnick P, Pernow B, Essen B, *et al:* Availability of glycogen and plasma FFA for substrate utilization in let muscle of man during exercise. *Clin Physiol* 1981;1:27.

55. VanHouten DR, Davis JM, Meyers DM, *et al:* Altered cellular distribution of hexokinse in skeletal muscle after exercise. *Int J Sports Med* 1992;13:436.

56. Weber FE, Pette D: Changes in free and bound forms and total amount of hexokinase isozyme II of rat muscle in repsonse to contractile activity. *Eur J Biochem* 1990;191:85.

57. Chen J, Gollnick PD: Effect of exercise on hexokinase distribution and mitochondrial respiration in skeletal muscle. *Pflugers Arch* 1994; 427:527.

58. Halseth AE, Bracy DP, O'Doherty RM, *et al:* Analysis of basal and insulin-stimulated skeletal muscle glucose uptake in vivo. *Diabetes* 1996;45:20A.

59. Neufer PD, Dohm GL: Exercise induces a transient increase in transcription of the GLUT-4 gene in skeletal muscle. *Am J Physiol* 1993; 265:C1597.

60. O'Doherty RM, Bracy DP, Osawa H, Wasserman DH, Granner DK: Rat skeletal muscle hexokinase II mRNA and activity are increased by a single bout of acute exercise. *Am J Physiol* 1994;266:E171.

61. Hofmann S, Pette D: Low frequency stimulation of rat fast-twitch muscle enhances the expression of hexokinase II and both the translocation and expression of glucose transporter 4 (GLUT4). *Eur J Biochem* 1994;219:307.

62. Koval JA, DeFronzo RA, O'Doherty RM, *et al:* Regulation of hexokinase II activity and expression in human muscle by moderate exercise. *Am J Physiol* 1998;274:E304.

63. Coggan AR, Kohrt WM, Spina RJ, *et al:* Endurance training decreases plasma glucose turnover and oxidation during moderate intensity exercise in men. *J Appl Physiol* 1990;68:990.

64. Wasserman DH, Mohr T, Kelly P, *et al:* Impact of insulin deficiency on glucose fluxes and muscle glucose metabolism during exercise. *Diabetes* 1992;41:1229.

65. Williams BD, Plag I, Troup J, *et al:* Isotopic determination of glycolytic flux during intense exercise in humans. *J Appl Physiol* 1995;78:483.

66. Roy D, Marette A: Exercise induces the translocation of GLUT4 to transverse tubules from an intracellular pool in rat skeletal muscle. *Biochem Biophys Res Comm* 1996;223:147.

67. Kristiansen S, Hargreaves M, Richter EA: Exercise-induced increase in glucose transport, GLUT4 and VAMP2 in plasma membrane from human muscle. *Am J Physiol* 1996;270:E197.

68. Kennedy JW, Hirshman MF, Gervino EV, *et al:* Acute exercise induces GLUT4 translocation in skeletal muscle of normal human subjects and subjects with type 2 diabetes. *Diabetes* 1999;48:1192.

69. Lund S, Vestergaard H, Andersen PH, *et al:* GLUT4 content in plasma membrane of muscle from patients with non-insulin-dependent diabetes mellitus. *Am J Physiol* 1993;265:E889.

70. Etgen GJ, Wilson CM, Jensen J, *et al:* Glucose transport and cell surface GLUT4 protein in skeletal muscle of the obese Zucker rat. *Am J Physiol* 1996;271:E294.

71. Lund S, Holman GD, Schmitz O, *et al:* Contraction stimulates translocation of glucose transporter GLUT4 in skeletal muscle through a mechanism distinct from that of insulin. *Proc Natl Acad Sci USA* 1995;92:5817.

72. Goodyear LJ, Hirshman MF, Horton ES: Exercise-induced translocation of skeletal muscle glucose transporters. *Am J Physiol* 1991;261: E795.

73. Douen AG, Ramlal T, Rastogi S, *et al:* Exercise induces recruitment of the "insulin-responsive glucose transporter." Evidence for distinct intracellular insulin- and exercise-recruitable transporter pools in skeletal muscle. *J Biol Chem* 1990;265:13427.

74. McConnell G, McCoy M, Proietto J, *et al:* Skeletal muscle GLUT-4 and glucose uptake during exercise in humans. *J Appl Physiol* 1994; 77:1565.

75. Winder WW, Hardie DG: Inactivation of acetyl-CoA carboxylase and activation of AMP-activated protein kinase in muscle during exercise. *Am J Physiol* 1996;270:E299.

76. Merrill GF, Kurth EJ, Hardie DG, *et al:* AICA riboside increases AMP-activated protein kinase, fatty acid oxidation, and glucose uptake in rat muscle. *Am J Physiol* 1997;273:E1107.

77. Hayashi T, Hirshman MF, Kurth EJ, *et al:* Evidence for 5'AMP-activated protein kinase mediation of the effect of muscle contraction on glucose transport. *Diabetes* 1998;47:1369.

78. Balon TW, Nadler JL: Nitric oxide release is present from incubated skeletal muscle preparations. *J Appl Physiol* 1994;77:2519.

79. Bradley SJ, Kingwell BA, McConnell GK: Nitric oxide synthase inhibition reduces let glucose uptake but not blood flow during dynamic exercise. *Diabetes* 1999;48:1815.

80. James DE, Kraegen EW, Chisholm DJ: Effects of exercise training on in vivo insulin action in individual tissues of the rat. *J Clin Invest* 1985;76:657.

81. Ploug T, Galbo H, Vinten J, *et al:* Kinetics of glucose transport in rat muscle: Effects of insulin and contractions. *Am J Physiol* 1987;253: E12.

82. Bjorkman O, Miles P, Wasserman D, *et al:* Regulation of glucose turnover during exercise in pancreatectomized, totally insulin deficient dogs: Effects of beta-adrenergic blockade. *J Clin Invest* 1988;81: 1759.

83. Wasserman DH, Lickley HLA, Vranic M: Role of beta-adrenergic mechanisms during exercise in poorly-controlled insulin deficient diabetes. *J Appl Physiol* 1985;59:1282.

84. Benn JJ, Brown PM, Beckwith LJ, *et al:* Glucose turnover in type I diabetic subjects during exercise. *Diabetes Care* 1992;15:1721.

85. Wasserman DH, Geer RJ, Rice DE, *et al:* Interaction of exercise and insulin action in humans. *Am J Physiol* 1991;260:E37.

86. Coderre L, Kandror KV, Vallega G, *et al:* Identification and characterization of an exercise-sensitive pool of glucose transporters in skeletal muscle. *J Biol Chem* 1995;270:27584.

87. Gao J, Ren J, Gulve EA, *et al:* Additive effect of contractions and insulin on GLUT-4 translocation into the sarcolemma. *J Appl Physiol* 1994;77:1597.

88. Goodyear LJ, Giorgino F, Balon TW, *et al:* Effects of contractile activity on tyrosine phosphoproteins and PI 3-kinase activity in rat skeletal muscle. *Am J Physiol* 1995;268:E987.

89. Turinsky J, Damrau-Abney A: Akt kinases and 2-deoxyglucose uptake in rat skeletal muscles in vivo: Study with insulin and exercise. *Am J Physiol* 1999;276:R277.

90. Sherwood DJ, Dufresne SD, Markus JF, *et al:* Differential regulation of MAP kinase, p709(s6k) and akt by contraction and insulin in rat skeletal muscles. *Am J Physiol* 1999;276:E870.

91. Lee AD, Hansen PA, Holloszy JO: Wortmannin inhibits insulin-stimulated but not contraction-stimulated glucose transport activity in skeletal muscle. *FEBS Lett* 1995;361:51.

92. Yeh J, Culve EA, Rameh L, *et al:* The effects of wortmannin on rat skeletal muscle. Dissociation of signaling pathways for insulin- and contraction-activated hexist transport. *J Biol Chem* 1995;270: 2107.

93. Kusunoki M, Storlien LH, MacDessi J, *et al:* Muscle glucose uptake during and after exercise is normal in insulin-resistant rats. *Am J Physiol* 1993;264:E167.

94. Houmard JA, Weidner MD, Dolan PL, *et al:* Skeletal muscle GLUT4 protein concentration and aging in humans. *Diabetes* 1995;44:555.

95. Richter EA, Garetto LP, Goodman MN, *et al:* Muscle glucose metabolism following exercise in the rat. Increased sensitivity to insulin. *J Clin Invest* 1982;69:785.

96. Vergauwen L, Hespel P, Richter EA: Adenosine receptors mediate synergistic stimulation of glucose uptake and transport by insulin and by contractions in rat skeletal muscle. *Clin Invest* 1994;93:974.

97. Wasserman DH, Bupp JL, Johnson JL, *et al:* Glucoregulation during rest and exercise in depancreatized dogs: Role of the acute presence of insulin. *Am J Physiol* 1992;262:E574.

98. Young AA, Bogardus C, Stone K, *et al:* Insulin response of components of whole-body and muscle carbohydrate metabolism in humans. *Am J Physiol* 1988;254:E231.

99. Bogardus C, Thuillez P, Ravussin E, *et al:* Effect of muscle glycogen depletion on in vivo insulin action in man. *J Clin Invest* 1983;72: 1605.

100. Baron AD, Steinberg H, Brechtel G, *et al:* Skeletal muscle blood flow independently modulates insulin-mediated glucose uptake. *Am J Physiol* 1994;266:E248.

101. Mandarino LJ, Bonadonna RC, McGuinness OP, *et al:* Regulation of muscle glucose uptake in vivo. In: Jefferson LS, Cherrington AD, eds. *The American Physiological Society Handbook of Physiology-Endocrine Pancreas.* Waverly Press; 2000.

102. Bonen A, Tan MH, Clune P, *et al:* Effects of exercise on insulin binding to human muscle. *Am J Physiol* 1985;248:E403.

103. Treadway JL, James DE, Burcel E, *et al:* Effect of exercise on insulin receptor binding and kinase activity in skeletal muscle. *Am J Physiol* 1989;256:E138.

104. Michel G, Vocke T, Fiehn W, *et al:* Bidirectional alteration on insulin receptor affinity by different forms of physical exercise. *Am J Physiol* 1984;246:E153.

105. Zorzano A, Balon TW, Garetto LP, *et al:* Muscle alpha-aminoisobutyric acid transport after exercise: Enhanced stimulation by insulin. *Am J Physiol* 1985;248:E546.

106. Achike FI, Ballard HJ: Influence of stimulation parameters on the release of adenosine, lactate, and CO_2 from contracting dog gracilis muscle. *J Physiol (Lond)* 1993;463:107.

107. Nuutila P, Koivisto VA, Knuuti J, *et al:* Glucose-free fatty acid cycle operates in human heart and skeletal muscle in vivo. *J Clin Invest* 1992;89:1767.

108. Boden G, Jadali F, White J, *et al:* Effects of fat on insulin-stimulated carbohydrate metabolism in normal men. *J Clin Invest* 1991;88:960.

109. Hargreaves M, Kiens B, Richter EA: Effect of increased plasma free fatty acid concentrations on muscle metabolism in exercising men. *J Appl Physiol* 1991;70:194.

110. Bracy DP, Zinker BA, Jacobs JC, *et al:* Carbohydrate metabolism during exercise:influence of circulating fat availability. *J Appl Physiol* 1995;79.

111. Randle PJ, Garland PB, Hales CN, *et al:* The glucose-fatty acid cycle: Its role in insulin sensitivity and the metabolic disturbances of diabetes mellitus. *Lancet* 1963;1:785.

112. Dyck DJ, Putman CT, Heigenhauser GJF, *et al:* Regulation of fat-carbohydrate interaction in skeletal muscle during intense aerobic cycling. *Am J Physiol* 1993;265:E852.

113. Boden G, Chen X, Ruiz J, *et al:* Mechanisms of fatty acid-induced inhibition of glucose uptake. *J Clin Invest* 1994;93:2438.

114. Roden M, Price TB, Perseghin G, *et al:* Mechanism of free fatty acid-induced insulin resistance in humans. *J Clin Invest* 1996;97: 2859.

115. Wasserman DH, Lickley HLA, Vranic M: Effect of hematocrit reduction on hormonal and metabolic responses to exercise. *J Appl Physiol* 1985;58:1257.

116. Cooper DM, Wasserman DH, Vranic M, *et al:* Glucose turnover in response to exercise during high- and low-FIo_2 in humans. *Am J Physiol* 1986;251:E209.

117. Kang J, Robertson RJ, Hagberg JM, *et al:* Effect of exercise intensity on glucose and insulin metabolism in obese individuals and obese NIDDM patients. *Diabetes Care* 1996;19:341.

118. Idstrom JP, Subramanian VH, Chance B, *et al:* Oxygen dependence of energy metabolism in contracting and recovering rat skeletal muscle. *Am J Physiol* 1985;248:H40.

119. Issekutz B: Effect of epinephrine on carbohydrate metabolism in exercising dogs. *Metabolism* 1985;34:457.

120. Jansson E, Hjemdahl P, Kaijser L: Epinephrine-induced changes in muscle carbohydrate metabolism during exercise in male subjects. *J Appl Physiol* 1986;60:1466.

121. Issekutz B: Role of beta-adrenergic receptors in mobilization of energy sources in exercising dogs. *J Appl Physiol* 1978;44:869.

122. Broberg S, Katz A, Sahlin K: Propranolol enhances adenine nucleotide degradation in human muscle during exercise. *J Appl Physiol* 1988;65:2478.

123. Rehrer NJ, Beckers E, Brouns F, *et al:* Effects of dehydration on gastric emptying and gastrointestinal distress while running. *Med Sci Sports Exerc* 1990;22:790.

124. Barclay GR, Turnberg LA: Effect of moderate exercise on salt and water transport in the human jejunum. *Gut* 1988;29:816.

125. Maughan RJ, Leiper JB, McGraw A: Effects of exercise intensity on absorption of ingested fluids in man. *Exp Physiol* 1990;75:419.

126. Rowell LB, Blackmon JR, Bruce RA: Indocyanine green clearance and estimated blood flow during mild to maximal exercise in upright man. *J Clin Invest* 1964;43:1677.

127. Adopo E, Peronnet F, Massicotte D, *et al:* Respective of oxidation of exogenous glucose and fructose given in the same drink during exercise. *J Appl Physiol* 1994;76:1014.

128. Pirnay F, Crielaard JM, Pallikarakis N, *et al:* Fate of exogenous glucose during exercise of different intensities in humans. *J Appl Physiol* 1982;43:258.

129. Rehrer NJ, Wagenmakers AJ, Beckers EJ, *et al:* Gastric emptying, absorption, and carbohydrate oxidation during prolonged exercise. *J Appl Physiol* 1992;72:468.

130. Murray R, Paul GL, Siefert JG, *et al:* The effects of glucose, fructose, and sucrose ingestion during exercise. *Med Sci Sports Exerc* 1989;21:275.

131. Costill D, Coyle E, Dalsky G, *et al:* Effects of elevated plasma FFA and insulin on muscle glycogen usage during exercise. *J Appl Physiol* 1997;43:695.

132. Coggan AR, Coyle EF: Reversal of fatigue during prolonged exercise by carbohydrate infusion or ingestion. *J Appl Physiol* 1987;63:2388.

133. Ahlborg G, Felig P: Influence of glucose ingestion on fuel-hormone response during prolonged exercise. *J Appl Physiol* 1976;41:683.

134. Jenkins AB, Chisholm DJ, James DE, *et al:* Exercise induced hepatic glucose output is precisely sensitive to the rate of systemic glucose supply. *Metabolism* 1985;34:431.

135. Goke R, Trautmann ME, Haus E, *et al:* Signal trnsmission after GLP-1-(7-36)amide binding in RINm5F cells. *Am J Physiol* 1989;257:G397.

136. Hamilton-Wessler M, Donovan CM, Bergman R: Role of the liver as a glucose sensor in the integrated response to hypoglycemia. In *Glucose Fluxes, Exercise and Diabetes.* Smith-Gordon: 1996.

137. Price TB, Rothman DL, Taylor R, *et al:* Human muscle glycogen after exercise: Insulin-dependent and independent phases. *J Appl Physiol* 1994;76:104.

138. Garetto LP, Richter EA, Goodman MN, *et al:* Enhanced muscle glucose metabolism after exercise in the rat: The two phases. *Am J Physiol* 1984;246:E471.

139. Hultman E, Nilsson LH: Liver glycogen in man. Effect of different diets and muscular exercise. In: Pernow B, Saltin B, eds. *Metabolism During Exercise.* Plenum Press: 1971.

140. Delmas-Deauvieu MD, Quesson B, Thiaudiere E, *et al:* 13C nuclear magnetic resonance study of glycogen resynthesis in muscle after glycogen-depleting exercise in healthy men receiving an infusion of lipid emulsion. *Diabetes* 1999;48:327.

141. Wojtaszewski JF, Hansen BF, Kien B, *et al:* Insulin signaling and insulin sensitivity after exercise in human skeletal muscle. *Diabetes* 2000;49:325.

142. Wojtaszewski JF, Higaki Y, Hirshman MF, *et al:* Exercise modulates postreceptor insulin signaling and glucose transport in muscle-insulin receptor knockout mice. *J Clin Invest* 1999;104:1257.

143. Ryder JW, Kawano Y, Galuska D, *et al:* Postexercise glucose uptake from glycogen synthesis in skeletal muscle from GLUT4-deficient mice. *FASEB J* 1999;13:2246.

144. Ren JM, Barucci N, Marshall BA, *et al:* Transgenic mice overexpressing GLUT1 protein in muscle exhibit increased muscle glycogenesis after exercise. *Am J Physiol* 2000;278:E588.

145. Cartee GD, Holloszy JO: Exercise increases susceptibility of muscle glucose transport to activation by various stimuli. *Am J Physiol* 1990;258:E390.

146. Gao J, Gulve EA, Holloszy JO: Contraction-induced increase in muscle insulin sensitivity: Requirement for a serum factor. *Am J Physiol* 1994;266:E186.

147. Ren J-M, Semenkovich CF, Gulve EA, *et al:* Exercise induces rapid increases in GLUT4 expression, glucose transport capacity, and insulin-stimulated glycogen storage in muscle. *J Biol Chem* 1994;269:14396.

148. Kraniou Y, Cameron-Smith D, Misso M, Collier G, Hargreaves M: Effects of exercise on GLUT4 and glycogenin gene expression in human skeletal muscle. *J Appl Physiol* 2000;88:794.

149. Han XX, Handberg A, Petersen LN, *et al:* Stability of GLUT1 and GLUT4 expression in perfused rat muscle stimulated by insulin and exercise. *J Appl Physiol* 1995;78:46.

150. Higaki Y, Kagawa T, Fujitani J, *et al:* Effects of a single bout of exercise on glucose effectiveness. *Am J Physiol* 1996;80:754.

151. Pestell RG, Ward GM, Galvin P, *et al:* Impaired glucose tolerance after endurance exercise is associated with reduced insulin secretion rather than altered insulin sensitivity. *Metabolism* 1993;42:277.

152. Yale J, Leiter L, Marliss E: Metabolic responses to intense exercise in lean and obese subjects. *J Clin Endocrinol Metab* 1989;68:438.

153. Galassetti P, Coker RH, Lacy DB, *et al:* Prior exercise increases net hepatic glucose uptake during a glucose load. *Am J Physiol* 1999;276:E1022.

154. Galassetti P, Koyama Y, Coker RH, *et al:* Role of a negative arterial-portal venous glucose gradient in the post-exercise state. *Am J Physiol* 1999;277:E1038.

155. Casey A, Mann R, Banister K, *et al:* Effect of carbohydrate ingestion on glycogen resynthesis in human liver and skeletal muscle, measured by 13C MRS. *Am J Physiol* 2000;2778:E65.

156. Bouchard C, Shepard RJ, Stevens T, *Physical Activity, Fitness, and Health.* Human Kinetics Publishers: 1994.

157. Vranic M, Horvath S, Wahren J: Proceedings of a Conference on Diabetes and Exercise. Sponsored by the Kroc Foundation, Santa Ynez Valley, California. *Diabetes* 1979;28:1.

158. American Diabetes Association: Diabetes mellitus and exercise. *Diabetes Care* 2000;23:S50.

159. Thurm U, Harper PN: I'm running on insulin. *Diabetes Care* 1992;15:1811.

160. Alberti KGMM, Gries FA: Management of non-insulin-dependent diabetes mellitus in Europe: A care for diabetes worldwide. 1988; 13.

161. Horton E: Exercise. In: Lebovitz HE, ed. *Therapy for Diabetes Mellitus and Related Disorders.* American Diabetes Association: 1998.

162. Peirce NS: Diabetes and exercise. *Br J Sports Med* 1999;33:161.

163. Bak JF, Jacobsen UK, Jorgensen FS, *et al:* Insulin receptor function and glycogen synthase activity in skeletal muscle biopsies from patients with insulin-dependent diabetes mellitus: Effects of physical training. *J Clin Endocrinol Metab* 1989;69:158.

164. Lehman R, Kaplan V, Bingisser R, *et al:* Impact of physical activity on cardiovascular risk factor in IDDM. *Diabetes Care* 1997;20:1603.

165. Schneider SH, Khachadurian AK, Amorosa LF, *et al:* Ten-year experience with an exercise-based outpatient life-style modification program in the treatment of diabetes mellitus. *Diabetes Care* 1992;15:1800.

166. Nugent AM, Steele IC, AlModaris F, *et al:* Exercise responses in patients with IDDM. *Diabetes Care* 1997;20:1814.

167. Ward GM, Weber KM, Walters JM: A modified minimal model analysis of insulin sensitivity and glucose-mediated glucose disposal in insulin-dependent diabetes. *Metabolism* 1991;40:4.

168. Walters JM, Ward GM, Kalfas A, *et al:* The effect of epinephrine on glucose-mediated and insulin-mediated glucose disposal in insulin-dependent diabetes. *Metabolism* 1992;41:671.

169. Wahren J, Sato Y, Ostman J, *et al:* Turnover and splanchnic metabolism of FFA and ketones in insulin-dependent diabetics during exercise. *J Clin Invest* 1984;73:1367.

170. Yamatani K, Shi Z, Giacca A, *et al:* Role of FFA-glucose cycle in glucoregulation during exercise in total absence of insulin. *Am J Physiol* 1992;263:E646.

171. Akanji AO, Osifo E, Kirk M, *et al:* The effects of changes in plasma nonesterified fatty acid levels on oxidative metabolism during moderate exercise in patients with non-insulin-dependent mellitus. *Metabolism* 1993;42:426.

172. Devlin J: Exercise in the management of type 1 diabetes mellitus. In: DeFronzo RA, ed. *Current Therapy of Diabetes Mellitus.* Mosby-Year Book: 1998.

173. Berger M, Berchtold P, Cuppers HJ, *et al:* Metabolic and hormonal effects of muscular exercise in juvenile type diabetics. *Diabetologia* 1977;13:355.

174. Shi ZQ, Giacca A, Yamatani K, *et al:* Effects of subbasal insulin infusion on resting and exercise-induced glucose uptake in depancreatized dogs. *Am J Physiol* 1993;264:E334.

175. Vranic M, Kawamori R, Pek S, *et al:* The essentiality of insulin and the role of glucagon in regulating glucose turnover during strenuous exercise. *J Clin Invest* 1975;57:245.

176. Miles PDG, Yamatani K, Brown MR, *et al:* Intracerebroventicular administration of somatostatin octapeptide counteracts the hormonal and metabolic responses to stress in normal and diabetic dogs. *Metabolism* 1994;43:1134.

177. Miles PDG, Yamatani K, Lickley HLA, *et al:* Mechanism of glucoregulatory responses to stress and their deficiency in diabetes. *Proc Natl Acad Sci USA* 1991;88:1296.

178. Rashid S, Shi ZQ, Niwa M, *et al:* Beta-blockade but not normoglycemia nor hyperinsulinemia markedly diminished stress-induced hyperglycemia in diabetic dogs. *Diabetes* 2000;49:253.

179. Kawamori R, Vranic M: Mechanism of exercise-induced hypoglycemia in depancreatized dogs maintained on long-acting insulin. *J Clin Invest* 1977;59:331.

180. Zinman B, Murray FT, Vranic M *et al:* Glucoregulation during moderate exercise in insulin treated diabetics. *J Clin Endocrinol Metab* 1977;45:641.

181. Devlin JT, Hirshman M, Horton ED, *et al:* Enhanced peripheral and splanchnic insulin sensitivity in NIDDM men after single bout of exercise. *Diabetes* 1987;36:434.

182. Davis SN, Galassetti P, Wasserman DH, *et al:* Effects of antecedent hypoglycemia on subsequent counterregulatory responses to exercise. *Diabetes* 2000;49:73.

183. Kemmer FW: Prevention of hypoglycemia during exercise in type I diabetes. *Diabetes Care* 1992;15:1732.

184. Schiffrin A, Parikh S: Accomodating planned exercise in type I diabetic patients on intensive treatment. *Diabetes Care* 1985;8:337.

185. Kemmer FW, Berger M: Therapy and better quality of life: The dichotomous role of exercise in diabetes mellitus. *Diabetes Metab Rev* 1986;2:53.

186. Ramires PR, Forjza CLM, Strunz CMC, *et al.:* Oral glucose ingestion increases endurance capacity in normal and diabetic (type 1) humans. *J Appl Physiol* 1997;83:608.

187. Puttagunta AL, Toth EL: Insulin lispro (Humalog), the first marketed insulin analogue: Indications, contraindications and need for further study. *Can Med Assoc J* 1998;158:506.

188. Hetenyi G Jr, Gauthier C, Byers M, Vranic M: Phlorizin induced normoglycemia partially restores glucoregulation in diabetic dogs. *Am J Physiol* 1989;256:E277.

189. Meinders AE, Willekens FLA, Heere LP: Metabolic and hormonal change in IDDM during long-distance run. *Diabetes Care* 1988;11:1.

190. Tuttle K, Marker J, Dalsky G, *et al:* Glucagon, not insulin, may play a secondary role in defense against hypoglycemia during exercise. *Am J Physiol* 1988;17:E713.

191. Lewis GH, Carpentier A, Vranic M, *et al:* Resistance to insulin's direct hepatic effect in suppressing steady state GP in individuals with type 2 diabetes mellitus. *Diabetes* 1999;48:570.

192. Giacca A, Fisher S, Shi ZQ, *et al:* Importance of peripheral insulin levels for insulin-induced suppression of GP in depancreatized dogs. *J Clin Invest* 1992;90:1769.

193. Dimitrakoudis D, Ramlal T, Rastogi S, *et al:* Glycemia regulates the glucose transporter number in the plasma membrane of rat skeletal muscle. *Biochem J* 1992;284:341.

194. Purdon C, Brousson M, Nyveen SL, *et al:* The roles of insulin and catecholamines in the glucoregulatory response during intense exercise and early recovery in insulin-dependent diabetic and control subjects. *J Clin Endocrinol Metab* 1993;76:566.

195. Sigal RJ, Purdon C, Bilinski D, *et al:* Glucoregulation during and after intense exercise: Effects of beta-blockade in subjects with type 1 diabetes mellitus. *J Clin Endocrinol Metab* 1999;84:3961.

196. Marliss EB, Vranic M. Intense exercise has unique effects on both insulin release and its role in glucoregulation. Implications for diabetes. Diabetes 51 (suppl 1); 271, 2002.

197. Mathoo J, Shi Q, Klip A, *et al:* Opposite effects of acute hypoglycemia and acute hyperglycemia on glucose transport and glucose transporters in perfused rat skeletal muscle. *Diabetes* 1999;48:1281.

198. Lussier B, Vranic M, Kovacevic N, *et al:* Glucoregulation in alloxan diabetic dogs. *Metabolism* 1986;35:18.

199. Fisher SJ, Lekas M, Shi ZQ, *et al:* Glycemia acutely regulates glucose clearance during exercise in diabetic dogs. *Diabetes* 1997;46:1805.

200. Klip A, Marette A, Dimitrakoudis D, *et al:* Effect of diabetes on glucoregulation. From glucose transporters to glucose metabolism in vivo. *Diabetes Care* 1992;15:1747.

201. Challis RAJ, Vranic M, Radda GK: Bioenergetic changes during contraction and recovery in diabetic rat skeletal muscle. *Am J Physiol* 1989;256:E129.

202. Minuk HL, Vranic M, Marliss EB, *et al:* Glucoregulatory and metabolic response to exercise in obese noninsulin-dependent diabetes. *Am J Physiol* 1981;240:E458.

203. Giacca A, Groenewoud Y, Tsui E, *et al:* GP, utilization, and cycling in response to moderate exercise in obese subjects with type 2 diabetes and mild hyperglycemia. *Diabetes* 1998;47:1763.

204. Martin IK, Katz A, Wahren J: Splanchnic and muscle metabolism during exercise in NIDDM patients. *Am J Physiol* 1995;269:E583.

205. Ruderman NB, Apelian AZ, Schneider SH: Exercise in therapy and prevention of type II diabetes. Implications for blacks. *Diabetes Care* 1990;13:1163.

206. Ruderman NB, Schneider SJ, Berchtold P: The "metabolically obese," normal-weight individual. *Am J Clin Nutr* 1981;34:1617.

207. Taylor R, Ram P, Zimmet P, *et al:* Physical activity and prevalence of DM in Melanesian and Indian man in Fiji. *Diabetologia* 1984;27:578.

208. Dowse GK, Zunnet OZ, Gareeboo H, *et al:* Abdominal obesity and physical inactivity as risk factors for NIDDM and impaired glucose tolerance in Indian, Creole and Chinese Mauritians. *Diabetes Care* 1991;14:271.

209. Frisch RE, Wyshak G, Albright TE, *et al:* Lower prevalence of diabetes in female former college athletes compared with nonathletes. *Diabetes* 1986;35:1101.

210. Helmrich SP, Ragland DR, Leung RW, *et al:* Physical activity and reduced occurrence of non-insulin-dependent diabetes mellitus. *N Engl J Med* 1991;325:147.

211. Manson JE, Rimm EB, Stampfer MJ, *et al:* Physical activity and incidence of non-insulin-dependent diabetes mellitus in women. *Lancet* 1991;338:774.

212. Manson JE, Nathan DM, Krolewski AS, *et al:* A prospective study of exercise and incidence of diabetes among US male physicians. *JAMA* 1992;268:63.

213. Pan XR, *et al:* Effects of diet and exercisein preventing NIDDM in people with impaired glucose tolerance. The Da Qing IGT and Diabetes Study. *Diabetes Care* 1997;20:537.

214. Eriksson KF, Lindgarde F: Prevention of type 2 (non-insulin-dependent) diabetes mellitus by diet and physical exercise. *Diabetologia* 1991;34:891.

215. Eriksson KF, Lindgarde F: No excess 12-year mortality in men with impaired glucose tolerance who participated in the Malmo preventive trial with diet and exercise. *Diabetologia* 1998;41:1010.

216. Tuomilehto J, Lindstrom J, Eriksson JG, *et al:* Prevention of type 2 diabetes mellitus by changes in lifestyle among subjects with impaired glucose tolerance. *N Engl J Med* 2001;344:1343.

217. Ohoshi T, Sasaki H, Bessho H, *et al:* Sympathetic hypersensitivity to exercise in NIDDM patients with fasting hyperketonemia. In: Shigeta Y, Lebovitz HE, Gerich JE, *et al:* eds. *Best Approach to the Ideal Theraphy of Diabetes Mellitus.* Elsevier Science Publishers: 1987.

218. Mourier A, Gautier JM, DeKerviler R, *et al:* Mobilization of visceral adipose tissue related to the improvement in insulin sensitivity in response to physical training in NIDDM. *Diabetes Care* 1997;20:385.

219. Krotkiewski M, Lonroth P, Mandroukas K, *et al:* The effects of physical training on insulin secretion and effectiveness and on glucose metabolism in obesity and type II (non-insulin dependent) diabetes mellitus. *Diabetologia* 1985;28:881.

220. Ruderman NB, Chisholm D, Pi-Sunyer FX, *et al:* The metabolically obese, normal weight individual: Revisited. *Diabetes* 1998;47:699.

221. Evans A, Krentz AJ: Benefits and risks of transfer from oral agents to insulin in type 2 diabetes melliuts. *Drug Saf* 1999;21:7.

222. Larsen JJ, Dela F, Madsbad S, *et al:* Interaction of sulfonylureas and exercise on glucose homeostasis in type 2 diabetes. *Diabetes Care* 1999;22:1647.

223. Kemmer FW, Tacken M, Berger M: Mechanism of exercise-induced hypoglycemia during sulfonylurea treatment. *Diabetes* 1987;36:1178.

224. Rodnick KJ, Haskell WL, Swislocki ALM, *et al:* Improved insulin action in muscle, liver and adipose tissue in physically trained human subjects. *Am J Physiol* 1987;253:E489.

225. Segal KR, Edano A, Abalos A, *et al:* Effect of exercise training on insulin sensitivity and glucose metabolism in lean, obese, and diabetic men. *J Appl Physiol* 1991;71:2401.

226. Kjaer M, Galbo H: Effect of physical training on the capacity to secrete epinephrine. *J Appl Physiol* 1988;64:11.

227. King DS, Dalsky GP, Clutter WE, *et al:* Effects of lack of exercise on insulin secretion and action in trained subjects. *Am J Physiol* 1988;254:E537.

228. Shangraw RE, Stuart CA, Prince MJ, *et al:* Insulin responsiveness of protein metabolism in vivo following bedrest in humans. *Am J Physiol* 1988;255:E548.

229. Yki-Jarvinen H, DeFronzo R, Koivisto V: Normalization of insulin sensitivity in type I diabetic subjects by physical training during insulin pump therapy. *Diabetes Care* 1984;7:520.

230. Goodyear LJ, Hirshman MF, Knutson SM, *et al:* Effect of exercise training on glucose homeostasis in normal and insulin-deficient diabetic rats. *J Appl Physiol* 1988;65:844.

231. Bogardus C, Ravussin E, Robbins DC, *et al:* Effects of physical training and diet therapy on carbohydrate metabolism in patients with glucose intolerance and non-insulin dependent diabetes mellitus. *Diabetes* 1984;33:311.

232. Vallerand AL, Lupien J, Bukowiecki LJ: Synergistic improvement of glucose tolerance by sucrose feeding and exercise training. *Am J Physiol* 1986;250:E607.

233. Wallberg-Henriksson H, Gunnarsson R, Rossner S, Wahren J: Long-term physical training in female type I (insulin dependent) diabetic patients: Absence of significant effect on glycemic control and lipoprotein levels. *Diabetologia* 1986;29:53.

234. Burstein R, Polychronakos C, Toews CJ, *et al:* Acute reversal of the enhanced insulin action in trained athletes associated with insulin receptor changes. *Diabetes* 1985;34:756.

235. Bonen A, Clune PA, Tan MH: Chronic exercise increases insulin binding in muscles but not liver. *Am J Physiol* 1986;251:E196.

236. Dohm GL, Sinha MK, Caro JF: Insulin receptor binding and protein kinase activity in muscles of trained rats. *Am J Physiol* 1987;252:E170.

237. Henriksson J: Effects of physical training on the metabolism of skeletal muscle. *Diabetes Care* 1992;15:1701.

238. Katz A, Sahlin K: Regulation of lactic acid production during exercise. *J Appl Physiol* 1988;65:509.

239. Ivy JL: Role of exercise training in the prevention and treatment of insulin resistance and non-insulin-dependent diabetes mellitus. *Sports Med* 1997;24:323.

240. Marette A, Richardson JM, Ramlal T, *et al:* Abundance, localization and insulin-induced translocation of glucose transporters in red and white muscle of the rat hindlimb. *Am J Physiol* 1992;263:C443.

241. Klip A, Ramlal T, Bilan PJ, *et al:* Recruitment of GLUT-4 glucose transporter by insulin in diabetic rat skeletal muscle. *Biochem Biophys Res Comm* 1990;172:728.

242. Rodnick KJ, Henriksen EJ, James DE, *et al:* Exercise training, glucose transporters, and glucose transport in rat skeletal muscles. *Am J Physiol* 1992;262:C9.

243. Koivisto VA, Bourey RE, Vuorinen-Markkola H, *et al:* Exercise reduces muscle glucose transport protein (GLUT-4) mRNA in type I diabetic patients. *J Appl Physiol* 1993;74:1755.

244. Dela F, Ploug T, Handberg A, *et al:* Physical training increases muscle GLT4 protein and mRNA in patients with NIDDM. *Diabetes* 1994;43:862.

245. James DE, Jenkins AB, Kraegen EW: Heterogeneity of insulin action in individual muscles in vivo: Euglycemic clamp studies in rats. *Am J Physiol* 1985;248:E567.

246. Lilloja S, Young AA, Cutler CL, *et al:* Skeletal muscle capillary density and fiber type are possible determinants of in vivo insulin resistance in man. *J Clin Invest* 1987;80:415.

247. Menon RK, Grace AA, Burgoyne W, *et al:* Muscle blood flow in diabetes mellitus. *Diabetes Care* 1992;15:693.

248. Lithell H, Krotkiewski M, Kiens B: Non-response of muscle capillary density and lipoprotein-lipase activity to regular training in diabetic patients. *Diabetes Res* 1985;2:17.

249. Craig BW, Garthwaite SM, Holloszy JO: Adipocyte insulin resistance: Effects of aging, obesity exercise and food restriction. *J Appl Physiol* 1987;62:95.

250. Lehmann R, Vokac A, Niedermann K, *et al:* Loss of abdominal fat and the improvement of the cardiovascular risk profile by regular moderate exercise training in patients with NIDDM. *Diabetologia* 1995;38:1313.

251. Ruderman NB, Schneider SH: Diabetes, exercise and atherosclerosis [review]. *Diabetes Care* 1992;15:1787.

252. Schneider SH, Vitug A, Ruderman NB: Atherosclerosis and physical activity. *Diabetes Metab Rev* 1986;1:513.

CHAPTER 28

Insulin Chemistry and Pharmacokinetics

Michael R. DeFelippis

Bruce H. Frank

Ronald E. Chance

INTRODUCTION

In the early 1920s, Banting and Best[1] demonstrated the blood glucose lowering effect of pancreatic extracts and discovered a method for treating diabetes mellitus using an exogenous source of insulin. Since this breakthrough discovery, the intense focus on insulin research has produced extensive knowledge about the hormone's three-dimensional structural properties (see Chaps. 3 and 5),[2] its biosynthesis at the molecular and cellular level,[3,4] and its biologic and physiologic effects.[5] Despite the current understanding of insulin biochemistry, subcutaneous injection therapy remains the predominant method for effectively treating the more severe type 1 form of diabetes mellitus (T1DM). Therefore additional research efforts have been directed toward improving the overall effectiveness of insulin treatment, the goal being to mimic as closely as possible insulin secretion patterns in normal individuals. Frequently, this more practical emphasis on enhancing drug therapy has been directly influenced by discoveries made from more fundamental scientific explorations.

The chronology of the major achievements forming the basis of modern diabetes treatment have been discussed in previous reviews.[6,7] In the area of pharmaceutical formulation, significant developments have been made involving the optimization of excipients, improvements in insulin purity, and the nearly total replacement of animal insulins with both recombinant human insulin and recombinant human insulin analogs. Consequently, insulin therapy has evolved from the early crude solutions of pancreatic insulin to a series of pharmaceutical preparations with short-, intermediate-, and long-acting profiles. Although the invention of the longer-acting, insoluble depot insulin preparations in the 1930s (protamine zinc insulin), the 1940s (NPH insulin), and the 1950s (zinc insulins) gave patients some reprieve from multiple daily injections of soluble insulin, for the most part these insulin formulations have not adequately mimicked normal insulin secretion, and thus have not provided optimal glycemic control.[8] The large intra- and intersubject variability of absorption from the subcutaneous injection site is another major problem associated with current insulin preparations. Various approaches have been proposed in an effort to optimize insulin therapy using the available insulin preparations, involving multiple injection regimens,[9] continuous subcutaneous insulin infusion (CSII),[10] and delivery devices.[11] Alternative modes and routes of delivery for insulin and other therapeutic agents have also been investigated.[12]

Large-scale, controlled multicenter clinical trials such as the Diabetes Control and Complications Trial (DCCT)[13] have recently provided conclusive evidence that effective blood glucose control using intensive insulin therapy reduces the development and progression of long-term microvascular and neurologic complications of T1DM. Normalization of plasma glucose concentration requires duplication of the physiologic plasma insulin secretion profile, with elevations associated with meal consumption and a low basal concentration during fasting. The intensive injection therapy required to achieve normoglycemia is very demanding and imposes rigid constraints on the life style of the patient, and also presents an increased risk of severe hypoglycemia. There is optimism that the new human insulin analogs recently approved will at least partially overcome the many inadequacies of older, traditional insulins. Clinical experience to date suggests these new analogs (insulin lispro and insulin aspart, both very rapid-acting, soluble, mealtime insulins; and insulin glargine, a soluble, basal insulin) display more desirable pharmacokinetic and glucodynamic behavior than the older insulins.[14]

The previous approaches to optimize insulin preparations were not directed towards the intrinsic physicochemical properties of the insulin molecule. In particular, the potential role of insulin self-association on absorption was not considered, largely because detailed molecular information was lacking and conventional methodology to manipulate the primary structure was limited. Two achievements derived from basic biochemical research on insulin changed the current thinking about the nature of insulin preparations. High-resolution x-ray crystallographic data[2] and advances in molecular biology[15] provided both the insight and ability to explore the impact of insulin self-association on pharmacologic properties. The crystal structure of insulin provided a detailed understanding of the amino acids and molecular interactions involved in insulin self-association. Recombinant DNA technology made it possible to specifically modify any amino acid in the native sequence of insulin without having to rely on chemical modification or semisynthetic methods that are generally site-restricted.[16] Thus optimization approaches based on a rational design of the insulin molecule became possible.

In this chapter, the various molecular modifications resulting in insulin analogs displaying altered pharmacological properties are reviewed. Specific emphasis is placed on analogs with amino acid modifications that disrupt insulin self-association. Research in this area has resulted in the creation of "monomeric" insulin analogs that are formulated as solution preparations and display more desirable pharmacokinetic profiles to cover meal-related insulin requirements. Efforts to modify the self-association of insulin to produce basal therapies have been more challenging. In this case, other design strategies to manipulate the properties of insulin have been employed.

For example, insulin glargine's basal action results from low solubility at physiologic pH due to a shift of the isoelectric point to near neutrality. The physicochemical properties of insulin and the formulation and pharmacologic aspects of conventional insulin preparations are also discussed to provide the necessary background information and the basis for application of rational design-based drug regimens for modern insulin treatment.

PHYSICOCHEMICAL PROPERTIES OF NATIVE INSULIN

The primary structure of insulin was determined by the pioneering work of Sanger and colleagues at Cambridge University beginning in the late 1940s and culminating with the elucidation of amino acid sequences for several mammalian insulins in the 1950s.[17] Insulin is a 5800-Dalton-molecular-weight protein having 51 amino acids and consisting of two polypeptide chains designated the A chain and the B chain (Fig. 28-1). The A chain contains 21 amino acids, while the longer B chain is composed of 30 residues. Two intermolecular disulfide bonds involving cysteine residues A7,B7 and A20,B19 connect the individual chains. There is one additional intramolecular disulfide bond in the A-chain sequence between cysteine residues at positions A6 and A11. Putative residues involved with receptor interactions have been deduced from studies involving modification of selected residues.[18]

Much of the structural knowledge of insulin has been derived from studies conducted on bovine and porcine insulins. Bovine insulin differs from the human sequence at two positions in the A chain, in which alanine replaces threonine at position A8 and valine substitutes for isoleucine at residue A10. The B chain of bovine insulin additionally differs at position B30, where threonine is replaced by alanine. A similar alanine substitution at position B30 occurs in porcine insulin, and is the only difference relative to the human sequence. These sequence differences are not thought to affect the structural aspects or ligand binding properties of the three wild-type insulins. Today, the primary structures for more than 100 species of insulin and related molecules are known. Considering all the species of insulin and the various insulin analogs synthesized for structure and activity studies, more than 1000 molecules have likely been studied in insulin chemistry laboratories throughout the world [personal communication with J.E. Shields].

Structure of the Monomer

At dilute solution concentrations (<0.1 μM, $\sim$0.6 μg/mL), insulin exists as a monomer. Insulin circulates in plasma as a monomer,[19] and it is this form that interacts with the receptor.[4] X-ray crystallographic studies suggest that the three-dimensional structure of the monomer is not substantially altered upon self-association to the dimer and the hexamer.[20] The tertiary structure of the insulin monomer derived from x-ray crystallography[2] (Fig. 28-2A) indicates that the A chain consists of two α-helical segments involving residues A1–A8 and A13–A19, that are connected by a short loop from A9 to A12. The remaining two C-terminal residues are in an extended conformation. Structural elements of the B chain consist of a straight chain at the N-terminus (B1–B8) followed by an α helix (B9–B19) and ending with a long β strand (B20–B30) at the C terminal end. There is extensive conformational flexibility in the N-terminal region of the B chain, such that binding of certain ligands to insulin hexamers can induce an α-helix structure involv-

FIGURE 28-1. Primary structure of human insulin with amino acid residues involved in dimer formation shown in black and those involved in assembly of the Zn^{2+}-insulin hexamer in gray. The arrows indicate putative sites involved in receptor interactions. *(Reproduced with permission from Brange et al.[80])*

A chain

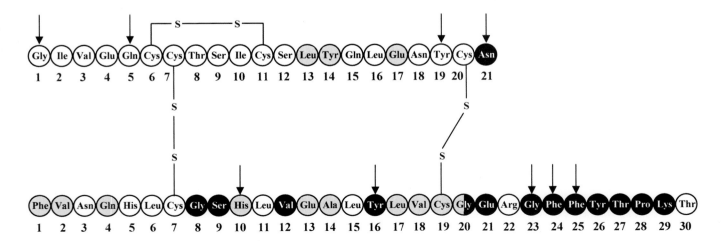

B chain

ing residues B1–B8 in the monomer subunits.[21] This structural transition is discussed further in the section on self-association and ligand binding.

The solution state conformation of the insulin monomer has been examined by several experimental and theoretical techniques including NMR,[22] circular dichroism,[23] competitive labeling of functional groups,[24] and molecular dynamics simulations.[25] In contrast to x-ray crystallography data, the results of some of these studies suggest that there are conformational differences between the free and associated insulin monomer. While the significance of the purported differences is still not entirely understood, the results of other studies suggest that conformational flexibility in the insulin monomer is necessary for receptor interactions.[26]

High-resolution (500 MHz), [1]H Fourier transform nuclear magnetic resonance (NMR) imaging conducted on dilute solutions of insulin at pH 8.0 (pH electrode reading) and higher has allowed the spectrum of the native insulin monomer to be obtained.[22] Spectral changes observed under conditions at which the dimer predominates were interpreted as differences between the monomer conformation in the free and associated states. A vacuum ultraviolet (UV) circular dichroism study exploring the changes in secondary structure associated with the dissociation of insulin hexamers also revealed structural differences between the free and associated monomers.[23]

Insulin Self-Association and Ligand Binding

The self-association of insulin has important implications in *in vivo* processes[4] and in pharmaceutical formulation.[27] Insulin association has been studied in solution with several elegant physical chemistry methods as reviewed recently by DeFelippis and colleagues.[28] These include ultracentrifugation, light scattering, equilibrium dialysis, difference UV absorbance spectroscopy, stopped-flow kinetics, osmometry, circular dichroism spectroscopy, and NMR. In the absence of divalent metal ions, insulin exhibits a complex association pattern consisting of monomer, dimer, tetramer, hexamer, and higher-order species, all in dynamic equilibrium and further influenced by protein concentration, pH, ionic strength, and temperature. Multiple models have been used to describe insulin self-assembly; however, it is clear that dimer formation is a necessary prerequisite for higher order aggregation.[29] Metal ions such as zinc will shift the equilibrium towards the formation of insulin hexamers.[30]

X-ray crystallography has provided the most detailed information concerning the interactions involved in insulin self-association.[2] The predominant forces resulting in dimer formation are nonpolar interactions and hydrogen bonds. With the exception of the asparagine residue at position A21 (a highly conserved amino acid among insulin species), the amino acids involved in dimer formation are all located in the B chain (Fig. 28-1). Most of the nonpolar interactions occur in the extended, C-terminal region of the B chain involving residues B23–26 and B28. A short, antiparallel β sheet with hydrogen bonds involving residues B24 and B26 also secures the C-terminal B chains of adjoining monomers (Fig. 28-2B). The importance of the C-terminal B chain residues in monomer-monomer association is demonstrated by despentapeptide insulin (lacking residues B26–B30).[20,31]

The divalent metal ion binding capacity of insulin was first demonstrated by Scott,[32] and the presence of zinc is known to cause specific aggregation to hexamers. Hexamer formation is strongly pH-dependent, occurring when the molar ratio of zinc to

insulin is between 0.33 and 1.0 and the protein concentration is above 0.5 mg/mL.[30,33] Note that these conditions are achieved in commercial solution preparations of insulin. A value of 10^{11} M^{-2} has been reported for the dimer-hexamer association constant of zinc-containing porcine insulin.[33,34] Two classes of zinc binding sites have been identified in the insulin hexamer. The stronger zinc binding site has an apparent association constant of 10^5–10^6 M^{-1} while the weaker one is in the range of 10^3–10^4 M^{-1}.[29] The insulin hexamer is capable of binding additional zinc ions.[35] Multiple, weak zinc-binding sites involving interactions with carboxylate groups have also been observed by x-ray crystallography studies on zinc-soaked crystals.[36]

X-ray crystallography studies have led to the identification of three hexameric insulin structures designated 2-Zn, 4-Zn, and the phenol-induced species.[2,21,37] The naming convention originally based on analytically-determined zinc content[35] leads to confusion since the 2-Zn form can bind more than two zinc ions[36] and the 4-Zn hexamer does not bind four zinc ions in all examples studied.[37] Therefore, the three structures are more appropriately defined in accordance with allosteric nomenclature as T_6, T_3R_3, and R_6, respectively.[38] The T and R designations refer to the conformational transitions associated with the B1–B8 residues in the insulin monomer subunits of the hexamers (Fig. 28-2D). Regardless of these structural differences, all three hexamer forms are oblate spheroidal assemblies having a diameter of ~5 nm and a height of ~3.5 nm.

Evidence for the existence of the various hexamer forms in solution has been obtained using circular dichroism,[39] UV-visible absorption spectroscopy,[38,40,41] and NMR.[42] Direct evidence for the existence of a solution state R6 hexamer structure has been recently obtained by ^{1}H-NMR.[42] The exceptional thermal stability of this hexamer form allowed high-resolution NMR spectra to be obtained, demonstrating an overall similarity between the secondary, tertiary, and quaternary structure between solution and crystal structures. Furthermore, the distinctive secondary structural features of the N terminus of the B chain were observed. Of the three hexamer structures, the R_6 species is particularly relevant to pharmaceutical solution preparations of insulin, since phenolic excipients are added as antimicrobial agents. The other structures, specifically the T_6 form, may be associated with the events controlling hexamer dissociation at the subcutaneous injection depot.

In the T_6 insulin structure, three dimers are assembled around two centrally-located zinc ions positioned in a solvent-filled cavity running through the hexamer (Fig. 28-2C). Each of the zinc ions is coordinated to three histidine B10 side chains, one from each dimer and three water molecules in an octahedral arrangement.[2] At the center of the hexamer, six glutamic acid B13 residues are arranged in a circular pattern, and the charge repulsion caused by the close proximity of the normally ionized carboxyl side chains necessitates zinc binding to stabilize hexamers. This fact is emphasized by substitution of the glutamic acid residue at position B13 with glutamine, resulting in an insulin analog capable of forming stable, zinc-free hexamers.[43] Assembly of the hexamer causes both polar and nonpolar residues to be buried between dimers, although the packing is much looser than in the interface between monomers comprising the dimer. The six monomer subunits of the T_6 insulin hexamer all have B1–B8 residues in an extended conformation, while the B9–B19 regions are α-helical.

Crystallization of insulin conducted in the presence of high concentrations of lyotropic anions such as chloride ion or thiocyanate results in the T_3R_3 hexamer.[37,44] Note that lyotropic

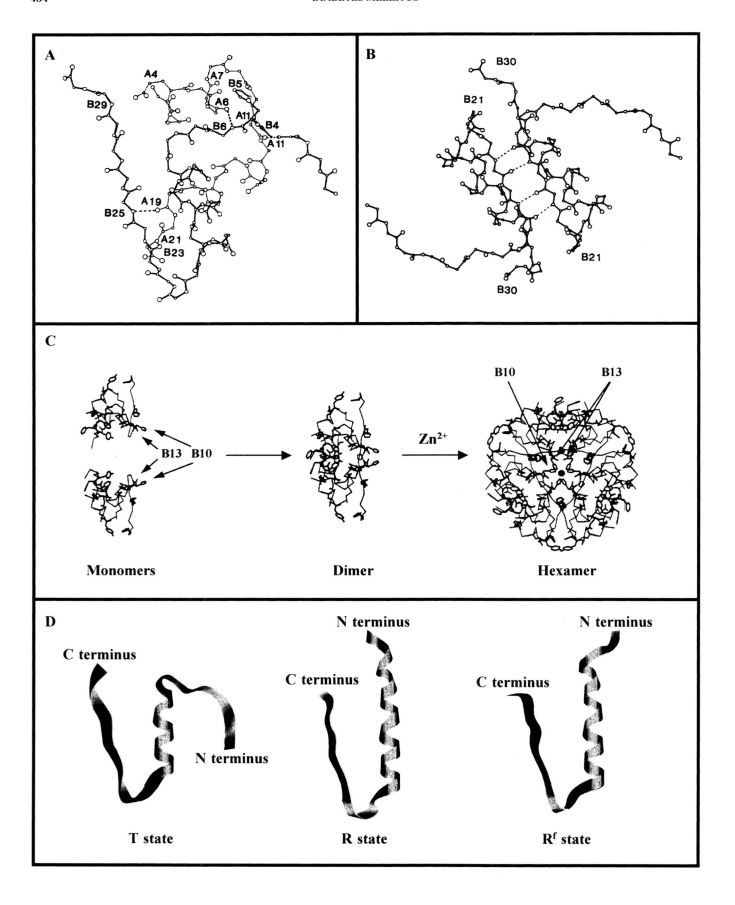

anions cannot drive the T → R transition to completion. In three of the monomer subunits, the N-terminal B1–B8 residues adopt an α-helical conformation producing a continuous α helix from B1–B19, while the monomers in the other half of the hexamer all have an extended chain in this region (Fig. 28-2D). This conformational transition displaces the N terminus of the B chain by more than 30 Å, producing three symmetry-equivalent cavities in the vicinity of the B5 histidine residues. X-ray crystallographic studies indicate that these cavities are either fully or partially occupied by zinc ions coordinated in a tetrahedral geometry involving the side chain of histidine B5, the side chain of histidine B10 positioned in an orientation off the 3-fold axis, and two water molecules.[37] A zinc ion can also be coordinated on the 3-fold axis by another orientation of the three symmetry-related histidine B10 side chains and a chloride ion in a tetrahedral geometry.[37] The other zinc ion in the T-state trimer is octahedrally coordinated by three symmetry-related B10 histidine residues and three water molecules, similar to the geometry observed in the T_6 insulin hexamer.[37]

More recent x-ray crystallographic studies on the T_3R_3 human insulin hexamer have shown that the putative off-axial zinc binding sites do not contain zinc ions, but rather are filled with water molecules.[45] In addition, both of the axial zinc ions exhibit a dual coordination pattern with no evidence for a second orientation of the B10 histidine residue. Most notably, the T → R transition in the R-state trimer results in the formation of a 12-Å-deep channel. The zinc ion lies at the bottom of this channel, isolated from the environment.[45] These authors suggest that zinc dissociation from the hexamer requires conversion of the R-state trimer to the T conformation, allowing solvent access to the metal site. They also observed that the first three N-terminal B-chain residues were extended rather than α-helical in the R-state monomer subunits. The term R^f is now used to distinguish the B1–B3 "frayed" conformation from the fully α-helical R form (see Fig. 28-2D), and the hexamer conformation is referred to as $T_3R_3^f$.[44,46,47]

Some phenolic molecules that are used as antimicrobial agents in pharmaceutical preparations have been shown to bind the insulin hexamer.[21,48] In this hexamer structure, referred to as R_6, the N-terminal B1–B8 residues of all six monomer subunits are α helical, producing a continuous helix from B1–B19. There are two off-axis binding sites at each dimer-dimer interface, and each position contains one phenol molecule. Each phenol molecule donates a hydrogen bond to the A6 cysteine carbonyl oxygen and accepts a hydrogen bond from the A11 cysteine amide nitrogen.[21] The phenol molecules are located in a cavity formed by A-chain residues of one dimer and the B1–B8 helix from an adjacent dimer. This arrangement allows the histidine B5 residue to link the dimer through van der Waals contacts with the phenol molecule. There are two zinc ions located on the hexamer 3-fold axis, both of which are coordinated in a tetrahedral arrangement involving the three

B10 histidine side chains and a chloride ion. The α-helices are extended above the zinc binding sites, limiting accessibility of solvent to the metal ions.[38]

INSULIN SECRETION IN NORMAL INDIVIDUALS

Insulin is matured from preproinsulin and proinsulin, stored and secreted by the β cells of the islets of Langerhans in the pancreas (see Chaps. 3 and 4). The biochemical events associated with these processes and corresponding structural transformations of the insulin molecule are now becoming understood in great detail.[4] In the storage vesicles, insulin hexamers form microcrystals that apparently serve to protect the hormone from proteolytic degradation. Upon release into serum, the insulin microcrystals experience a change in pH ($\approx$5.5 to 7.4) destabilizing favorable hexamer interactions. Dilution of the zinc ions also occurs, causing rapid hexamer dissociation and crystal disintegration. Secreted insulin enters the portal vein and is delivered directly to the liver, where about half is removed by first-pass metabolism. The concentration of insulin in the blood is 10^{-8}–10^{-11} M, ensuring that the hormone circulates and interacts with its receptor as a monomer.[19,33]

Studies conducted in normal subjects have defined the physiological secretion profile in response to various test meals over the course of 24 hours (Fig. 28-3).[6,49,50] The insulin secretion profile is pulsatile and displays both stimulated and basal phases. In the stimulated phase, increases in serum insulin may reach levels of 60–80 μU/mL or more within a few minutes before to 15–30 minutes after a meal is ingested, and decline rapidly to basal levels (5–15 μU/mL) within 120–180 minutes. These elevations in insulin result in disposal of glucose and other nutrients into the peripheral tissues, principally muscle tissue and to a lesser extent into the liver and fat. Between meals and through the night, lower levels of insulin are secreted at approximately 1 unit per hour (note that an international unit of insulin is equal to ~35 μg). Basal insulin secretion restrains but does not totally inhibit hepatic glucose production, assuring adequate substrate for cerebral glucose metabolism.[6]

INSULIN PREPARATIONS: PROPERTIES, PHARMACOLOGY, AND DEFICIENCIES

Pharmaceutical Preparations

Throughout the history of insulin, the desire to optimize subcutaneous injection therapy to more closely simulate the secretion patterns of normal persons has influenced the nature of the pharmaceutical preparations used for treatment. The most significant advances have occurred in the area of pharmaceutical formulation, where excipients have been optimized and approaches defined to

---

FIGURE 28-2. Insulin structure and pattern of self-association. Panel **A** shows the porcine insulin monomer structure with the A chain drawn using thin lines and the B chain drawn using thick lines. Panel **B** shows the antiparallel β sheet and hydrogen bonding structure within the insulin dimer. The pattern of insulin self-association from monomers to dimers and zinc-induced hexamers is depicted in panel **C**. Only backbone and selected side chains important to assembly are shown. The histidine residues at position B10 coordinate the two central zinc ions. The six B13 glutamic acid residues are buried in the hexamer. At neutral pH, the side chains of these residues are negatively charged, and these unfavorable interactions may play a role in hexamer dissociation upon removal of zinc ions. Insulin hexamers adopt various quaternary structures in the presence of certain anions or phenolic molecules. Conformational changes are localized to residues B1–B8 of monomer subunits. For ease of viewing, panel **D** only shows the conformation of insulin B chains in the T state, R state, and R^f state. (*Panels A and B reproduced with permission from Baker* et al[2]; *panel C reprinted with permission from Dodson and Steiner*[4]; *panel D reprinted with permission from Ciszak* et al.[46])

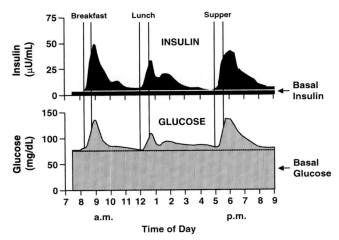

FIGURE 28-3. Mean peripheral plasma insulin and glucose profiles in five normal subjects ingesting 630-kcal meals composed of 40% carbohydrate, 40% fat, and 20% protein. The meals took 15 minutes to ingest. All subjects were ambulatory but did not exercise. The plasma glucose concentration increased only 50% during the meals, whereas the plasma insulin concentration increased approximately 600%. The pattern of the rise in plasma insulin concentration closely matches that of the rise in plasma glucose concentration. *(Reproduced with permission from Schade et al.[49])*

alter pharmacokinetics. Several comprehensive reviews describe the various insulin preparations that have been available over the years.[27,51,52] The specific developments leading to present day insulin preparations are briefly discussed here to provide the necessary background information relating to physical and pharmacologic properties.

Commercial insulin preparations are generally classified depending upon duration of activity as rapid-acting (reaching peak insulin concentrations from approximately 1–3 hours following subcutaneous injection, with a maximum duration of action of 4–6 hours), intermediate-acting (reaching peak insulin concentration at approximately 4–12 hours following subcutaneous injection, with a maximum duration of action of 14–20 hours), or long-acting (minimal peak with a maximum duration of action of 20–30 hours). Rapid-acting preparations are solutions of insulin, while intermediate- and long-acting preparations are composed of amorphous and/or crystalline insulin particles.

Formulation Properties

The earliest insulin preparations were slightly irritating, acidic solutions containing impure insulin isolated from animal pancreata. Because of the low purity of these preparations, patients typically required 4–6 daily injections. A neutral pH, solution preparation of insulin containing NaCl as a tonicity modifier and the preservative methylparaben was not developed until the 1960s.[53] Current, commercially available rapid-acting human insulin preparations are most commonly unbuffered, neutral pH solutions manufactured in 100 U/mL (approximately 3.5 mg/mL insulin) with some 40 U/mL (approximately 1.4 mg/L insulin) strengths. Alternatively, a phosphate buffer (neutral pH) is included specifically for insulin solutions formulated for use with pump devices. Other excipients included in these preparations include Zn^{2+} ions and glycerin as a tonicity modifier. A phenolic preservative, such as m-cresol at a concentration of about 3 mg/mL, is also included to satisfy stringent antimicrobial effectiveness regulatory requirements for multi-

dose parenteral products. The significance of formulation ingredients was not fully appreciated prior to the attainment of a detailed understanding of insulin structure, self-assembly, and phenolic ligand binding propensity. Due to the concentrations of insulin, zinc ions, and phenolic preservative in these preparations, the R_6 hexameric form of insulin likely predominates in solution.

The limited duration of action of the early insulin preparations required inconvenient multiple dosing regimens and carried the risk of overnight hyperglycemia. These deficiencies led to the development of modified formulations with prolonged action, so injection frequency could be reduced and insulin activity maintained through the night. The first successful extended-acting preparation utilized protamine to precipitate insulin as a noncovalent complex.[54,55] Protamine is a highly charged (pI ~13.5), basic peptide consisting of about 30 amino acid residues[56] generally isolated from salmon sperm. Krayenbühl and Rosenberg[57] optimized the insulin-protamine formulation by devising the isophane method for producing a microcrystalline suspension buffered at a neutral pH known as NPH (Neutral Protamine Hagedorn). The term isophane refers to the proper stoichiometric proportions of insulin and protamine (approximately 12:1 on a weight basis) that are used in the process, such that formation of the crystalline complex results in essentially no free amounts of either species in solution. Phenolics, such as m-cresol and phenol, and Zn^{2+} ions are also required to produce the elongated, tetragonal crystals comprising the suspension. The phenolics also serve a dual role as antimicrobial agents. NPH insulin has an intermediate time action and presently remains the most widely used insulin preparation.

After the introduction of NPH, another method for producing extended-acting insulin without the use of protamine was discovered by Hallas-Møller, Petersen, and Schlichtkrull,[58] who determined that the addition of excess zinc ions to formulations having neutral pH and no phosphate buffer produced suspensions displaying protracted effects. The prolonged effect is a result of the molar excess of Zn^{2+} ions that substantially reduces insulin solubility at neutral pH conditions. This finding led to the development of Lente insulins, a series of three suspension preparations having a gradation of extended activity. Semilente, a suspension composed entirely of amorphous particles formed by adjustment of an acidic insulin solution containing excess zinc ions to neutral pH, displays only a moderately retarded effect. Controlled crystallization of insulin at pH 5.5 in the presence of excess zinc ions, high NaCl concentration, and insulin seed crystals results in the formation of rhombohedral insulin crystals of uniform particle size distribution. The entirely crystalline Ultralente suspension is then prepared by diluting these crystals with an aqueous vehicle containing methylparaben and a controlled Zn^{2+} ion concentration followed by adjustment to neutral pH. Ultralente insulin was the longest-acting insulin suspension formulation currently available commercially until the recent development of glargine. Lente insulin is a 3:7 mixture of amorphous and crystalline insulin particles having an intermediate time-action profile. The crystalline component is the Ultralente crystal form while the amorphous part is analogous to Semilente.

Because of the small size and poor crystal quality of Ultralente particles, structural characterization by x-ray crystallography has not been possible. Recent powder diffraction studies on Ultralente crystals have identified the T_6 hexamer conformation.[59] In contrast to these findings, previous x-ray crystallography results on 4-Zn insulin crystals presumed to be representative of the Ultralente suspension identified the T_3R_3 hexamer conformation.[37] As a possible explanation for the extended activity of Ultralente preparations, these authors proposed that conversion of the R-state trimer to the T conformation was required to allow solvent access to the metal site prior to dissociation of the hexamers. However, the recent powder diffraction results indicate T_6 hexamers are more consistent with the actual concentration of sodium chloride used in the Ultralente preparation. Therefore, the time action is unlikely to be influenced by a mechanism involving the R→T conversion. Ultralente crystals contain T_3R_3 hexamers when they are initially grown under high sodium chloride conditions, but the conformation converts to the T_6 form when the salt concentration is diluted for the commercial product.[59]

One of the more recent advances in insulin formulation involves the development of stable mixtures containing rapid- and intermediate-acting insulins. These preparations combine insulin solutions with NPH suspension in various mixture ratios including 10:90, 20:80, 30:70, 40:60, and 50:50 (the 30:70 and 50:50 preparations are available in the U.S.). The basis for such premixed insulins is the convenience of having both meal-related and basal insulin requirements available in a single injection. In addition, the preparations offer better accuracy over extemporaneous mixtures made by the patient. Indeed, one of the most common subcutaneous injection regimens involves twice-daily injections of rapid- and long-acting insulins, making these preparations very popular.[60] A certain portion of the soluble component in these mixtures is known to adsorb to the surface of the NPH crystals.[27,61] However, this predominantly electrostatic interaction is reversible and does not alter the time action of the soluble component.[61] In contrast to the regular/NPH mixtures, combinations of rapid-acting insulin with Ultralente do not have sufficient long-term stability to allow a premixed preparation. The excess zinc present in Ultralente will precipitate the rapid-acting insulin, retarding its onset of action.[62] However, the combination of rapid-acting insulin and Ultralente can be utilized immediately after mixing.

Insulin Purity

Improvements in the overall purity of insulin preparations were first achieved by application of crystallization procedures, most notably those conducted in the presence of Zn^{2+} ions in addition to recrystallization methods. For many years, multiply-recrystallized insulin was thought to be very pure because preparations manufactured in this manner were found to be better tolerated by patients prone to allergic reactions.[27] As advances in analytical methodology progressed and techniques such as polyacrylamide gel electrophoresis and size exclusion chromatography were applied to examine insulin,[63,64] recrystallized insulin was found to contain numerous proinsulin- and insulin-like substances in addition to several noninsulin peptides (e.g., glucagon and pancreatic polypeptide).[27,65] This observation led to the incorporation of chromatographic separation technologies into the purification processes to produce so called single- or mono-component insulin.[65,66] Insulin preparations manufactured with chromatographically-purified insulin helped to reduce the frequency of immunologic complications associated with the therapy, such as allergy, lipoatrophy, and resistance. The subsequent introduction of recombinant human insulin, which is considered to be less immunogenic than either the porcine or bovine forms, further improved the immunologic consequences of diabetes treatment, since insulin antibodies may influence insulin pharmacokinetics.[67] The immunogenic and allergenic aspects associated with insulin therapy have been reviewed elsewhere.[68]

Insulin Sources

Prior to the early 1980s, all commercially available insulin preparations were formulated with either bovine or porcine insulin or a mixture of the two. The complete chemical synthesis of insulin was demonstrated in the 1960s,[69–71] but the inefficiency and poor yields of such a process make it impractical for commercial manufacture of human insulin. A human insulin for use in commercial pharmaceutical preparations was later developed using a semisynthetic process whereby the alanine at position B30 of porcine insulin was exchanged for threonine using a combination of enzymatic and chemical processes.[72,73]

Advances in recombinant DNA technology, demonstrating the ability to express synthetic genes for the A and B chains of human insulin eventually provided a method for producing human insulin biosynthetically.[15] The first biosynthetically manufactured human insulin to receive regulatory approval was prepared by expressing the chemically synthesized genes for the two chains of insulin in *Escherichia coli*.[74,75] This biosynthetic process later was modified to include the initial production of proinsulin that was subsequently converted to human insulin by enzymatic and chemical methods.[76,77] An alternative biosynthetic manufacturing process currently used for commercial human insulin production involves the expression in *Saccharomyces cerevisiae* of a single-chain insulin precursor containing a short amino acid sequence linking the A and B chains.[78] Additional enzymatic and chemical processing complete the conversion to human insulin.

There is some evidence from clinical studies that human insulin preparations are absorbed more rapidly than porcine insulin preparations, although the basis for this difference is not clearly understood. X-ray crystallography studies comparing human and porcine insulin have identified significant shifts in the main chain atoms of B30 at the carboxyl groups and some additional changes in the solvent structure in the region of B28–B30.[79] This difference may account for the greater hydrophilicity of human insulin crystals, suggesting that slightly increased solubility is a possible explanation for the faster absorption of the microcrystalline suspension preparations. Brange and associates[80] have proposed that the small differences in absorption of regular human insulin relative to soluble porcine insulin preparations can be explained by a greater tendency towards dissociation observed in their studies. Based on the x-ray crystallography results, Chawdhury and coworkers[79] suggest that the threonine residue at position B30 in human insulin and the associated structural alterations it causes affect the strength by which dimers are held together within the hexamer. However, the clinical significance of the differences in absorption between human and porcine insulin is debatable.[81] As discussed below, a faster absorption rate for soluble preparations is not necessarily a disadvantage for meal-related insulin requirements, although regular human insulin is not nearly rapid enough to mimic the physiological secretion profile (e.g., see Fig. 28-4). On the other hand, too rapid absorption is generally considered undesirable in terms of basal insulin needs.[82]

Pharmacology of Insulin Preparations

The pharmacologic profiles of the various insulin preparations administered subcutaneously have been reported by numerous investigators.[80,82–92] These studies provide a means for evaluating how well the various insulin preparations simulate physiologic secretion patterns and glucodynamics of insulin. Heinemann and Richter[82] have emphasized that many investigations on insulin

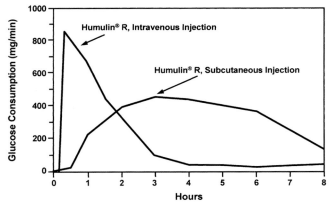

FIGURE 28-4. A comparison of the glucodynamic response of 10 normal volunteers to subcutaneous or intravenous administration of Humulin® R (0.2 U/kg). Glucose consumption was assessed using the glucose clamp technique. Note that the peak effect following subcutaneous administration occurs between 3 and 4 hours and continues for at least 8 hours. *(Reprinted with permission from Galloway et al.[93])*

absorption (pharmacokinetics) and/or insulin action (pharmacodynamics) have involved inappropriate methods and different doses and sites of administration, making it difficult to compare results. Therefore our intent is to provide a general description of the pharmacologic profiles of each insulin preparation rather than a comprehensive examination of all the data on this topic. Of the various methods used to study the pharmacologic properties of insulin preparations, the euglycemic glucose clamp is considered the most ideal for determining pharmacodynamics and pharmacokinetics.[82] The euglycemic glucose clamp procedure involves intravenous glucose infusion to maintain blood glucose concentrations at normal values following administration of insulin. The glucose requirement, therefore, is proportional to the activity of insulin.

Pharmacokinetics and Pharmacodynamics

Prandial (Meal-Related) Insulin

An example of the time course of plasma glucose response in normal subjects following subcutaneous administration of a commercially available solution preparation of regular human insulin (Humulin® R) is illustrated in Fig. 28-4. There is an obvious difference between this profile and the profile for intravenous administration, which better simulates physiologic insulin secretion. First, the rate of glucose consumption is slow, indicating that the plasma insulin concentration does not peak rapidly. Second, there is no real peak in the profile, and the maximal response does not occur until almost 3 hours after injection. Finally, glucose infusion is still required to maintain euglycemia even 8 hours after administration, indicating that plasma insulin concentrations are not rapidly reduced. This glucodynamic profile indicates a situation of relative hypoinsulinemia during the early phase (0.5–3 hours) following injection and relative hyperinsulinemia at later stages (3–8 hours). As a consequence of these abnormal conditions, the early-stage postprandial insulin deficiency causes delayed suppression of endogenous glucose production by the liver and a below-normal increase in the rate of glucose uptake by peripheral tissues, resulting in hyperglycemia soon after meal ingestion. Additionally, the elevated plasma insulin concentration that extends beyond 3 hours after the

meal may lead to conditions of hypoglycemia. Therefore, the pharmacologic properties of regular soluble insulin are more consistent with an intermediate-acting preparation.[6,14,93] In contrast to the profile obtained following subcutaneous injection of regular insulin, intravenous administration better simulates a meal-stimulated secretion pattern.[6,93] As mentioned below, two new soluble insulin analogs have been developed (insulin lispro and insulin aspart) that are quicker-acting with a shorter duration of action than regular human insulins.

Basal Insulins

Another requirement for achieving glycemic control is effective suppression of hepatic glucose production. Normalization of hepatic glucose production can be achieved by simulating the postabsorptive, low levels (5–12 μU/mL) of insulin secretion that occur in healthy nondiabetic individuals. There presently are two approaches in use for satisfying basal insulin requirements, either continuous subcutaneous insulin infusion (CSII) or subcutaneous injection of NPH, Lente, Ultralente, or preferably insulin glargine preparations. For the purposes of this discussion, only the pharmacologic properties of the subcutaneous microcrystalline suspensions are considered. The topic of CSII has been addressed in other reviews (see Chap. 29).[94]

A euglycemic clamp study in normal persons compared the time-action profiles of four widely used NPH insulin preparations.[89] This study showed that the onset of action (defined as half-maximal action) of all the NPH preparations was within 2.5–3 hours (Fig. 28-5). Peak activity was attained after 5–7 hours, and the duration of action (defined as >25% of maximal action) was between 13 and 16 hours. Certain clinical studies have shown differences in the time-action profiles of NPH insulins prepared with human or porcine insulin.[82] In these cases, human insulin NPH displays a more rapid onset and shorter duration of activity. In another euglycemic clamp study in normal subjects, human insulin NPH was found to be absorbed faster than a Lente preparation of human insulin over the course of 8 hours.[88] The peak effect and relatively short duration of activity associated with these intermediate-acting preparations make them ineffective as true basal insulins. Although the premixed NPH/regular insulin preparations are very popular in diabetes treatment, the limitations of their individual pharmacologic properties still exist.

The Ultralente insulin preparation is commonly used as a basal insulin. A euglycemic clamp study evaluating Ultralente preparations manufactured with insulin from either human, porcine, or bovine species have defined the time-action profile and uncovered some interesting differences.[90] Examples of the time-action profiles over the time course of 40 hours following administration of a 0.4 U/kg dose of each preparation are shown in Fig. 28-6. While all of the preparations displayed a duration of activity in excess of 30 hours, human Ultralente displayed plasma insulin levels in excess of 60 μU/mL within 5 hours after injection that persisted for at least 30 hours. The time-action profile of human insulin Ultralente, therefore, is not consistent with a truly basal insulin. In contrast, bovine Ultralente displayed a flat, essentially peakless profile with serum insulin concentrations below 60 μU/mL, although it was noted that a consistent peak was not evident in this case due to the wide variability between subjects. Based on the results of this study, it can be concluded that bovine Ultralente provides a more suitable basal insulin time-action profile. However, the undesirable immunogenicity of bovine insulin[68] limits its usefulness in this

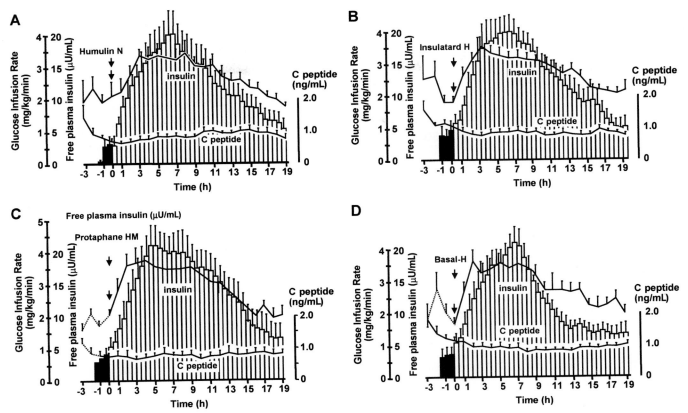

FIGURE 28-5. Glucose infusion rates (**bars**), free plasma insulin, and C peptide concentrations after subcutaneous injection of 12 U of four different NPH insulin preparations (biosynthetic origin: Humulin N [**A**], Eli Lilly; semisynthetic origin: Insulatard® H [**B**] and Protaphane® HM [**C**], Novo/Nordisk; Basal-H® Insulin [**D**], Hoechst AG; all U40) at time 0 during 19-hour euglycemic glucose clamps in six normal subjects. Solid bars show basal glucose infusion rate. (*Reproduced with permission from Starke* et al.[89])

regard. Despite the differences in time-action between the various Ultralente insulins, the authors of this study ultimately concluded that any one of the preparations is suitable to provide basal insulinemia in clinical practice. Conflicting pharmacologic results from a variety of other studies provide no definitive answer to the question of whether the time-action profile of human insulin Ultralente is more consistent with an intermediate-acting rather than a long-acting preparation.[82] Nevertheless, a twice-daily human insulin Ultralente injection regimen has been shown to result in lower fasting blood glucose concentrations.[95,96]

The differences in the time-action profiles of bovine and human Ultralente may be related to solubility[27] or immunogenic potential.[68] In the latter case, insulin released from the crystals may bind to elevated levels of circulating antibodies, further delaying the absorption process. Recent atomic force microscopy studies have provided evidence suggesting that differences in time action between bovine Ultralente compared to either human or porcine Ultralente may be related to packing and orientation of insulin hexamers at the crystal-solution interface.[97] In bovine Ultralente crystals, the hexamers on the predominant faces [(010) and (110)] are oriented "edge-on" to the aqueous medium, limiting solvent penetration into the crystals and consequently further retarding dissolution. Conversely, the predominant exposed crystal surface of human and porcine Ultralente crystals is the (001) crystal plane.

Hexamer orientation on this face allows for easier penetration of solvent through the crystal surface, contributing to more rapid dissolution.

The development of an insulin formulation with the duration of action of bovine Ultralente insulin but without immunogenicity has been a goal of insulin researchers for many years. As described below, a new peakless soluble insulin (insulin glargine) with a long duration of action has recently been introduced that appears to fulfill the desired characteristics of such a basal insulin.

Injection Timing and Clinical Implications

Since it takes between 60 and 90 minutes for subcutaneously injected regular soluble insulin (e.g., Humulin R) to reach peak plasma levels, timing of the injection is critical. Prandial insulin should be administered at least 30 minutes before the meal, to account for the time lag before maximal activity. A number of clinical studies have demonstrated the importance of injection timing for regular insulins.[98,99] The results of one study are presented in Fig. 28-7, which shows that the longer the interval between injection and meal ingestion, the better the simulation of nondiabetic prandial insulin secretion. There are also clinical implications for the long-acting insulin preparations. In clinical practice, injection timing with NPH and Lente insulin preparations is critical to ensuring that metabolic control is effectively maintained through the night.[82]

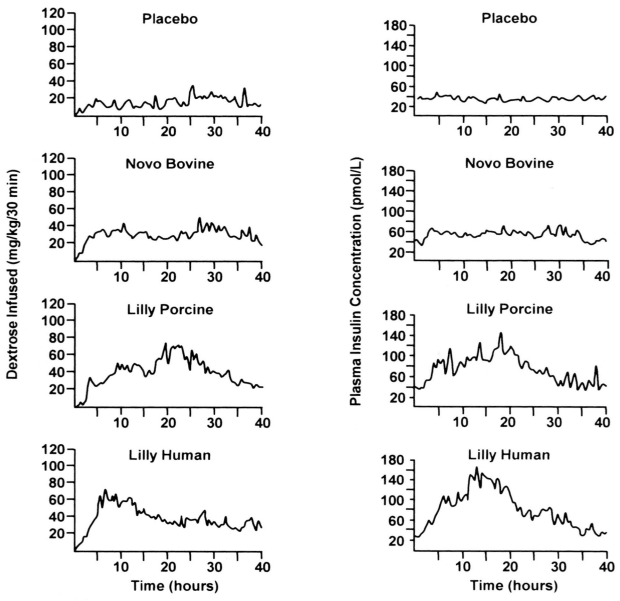

FIGURE 28-6. The plasma insulin and glucodynamic response of 6 or 9 normal volunteers following the subcutaneous administration of placebo and Ultralente bovine, porcine, and human insulin, 0.4 U/kg. *(Reproduced with permission from Seigler et al.[90])*

Thus an evening dose of human insulin NPH is generally injected closer to bedtime. The duration of action of human insulin Ultralente is also not considered substantially longer than NPH, necessitating twice-daily injections of the preparation to achieve basal insulin requirements.[82]

Factors Affecting the Absorption of Insulin

The factors influencing absorption of insulin from the subcutaneous site have been clinically examined, and the topic has been the subject of many reviews.[62,80,85,100,101] These investigations have shown that the region of injection, blood flow, and technique of injection can all influence the absorption process. For example, absorption is faster from the abdominal as opposed to the deltoid, femoral, and gluteal regions. Absorption is also faster with deeper

injections, or if insulin is injected more slowly. As temperature will affect blood flow, increases due to exercise, fever, and massage will also cause faster absorption. Other miscellaneous factors resulting in faster absorption include a lower injection volume or concentration of insulin. The use of NPH instead of Lente insulin in a bolus/basal mixture will also impact absorption because the excess zinc in the Lente preparation will precipitate soluble insulin, causing a blunting of its effect.[83,102]

While some of the factors influencing absorption described above can also impact insulin suspension preparations,[103–105] it is reasonable to suggest that their protracted effects are a result of slow crystal dissolution at the injection site. In these cases, absorption of insulin into the bloodstream presumably can only occur once the hormone is freed from the crystals. This presumption is

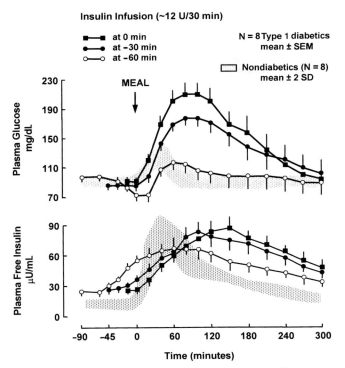

Insulin Infusion (~12 U/30 min)

■——■ at 0 min
●——● at –30 min
○——○ at –60 min

N = 8 Type 1 diabetics
mean ± SEM

▢ Nondiabetics (N = 8)
mean ± 2 SD

FIGURE 28-7. Pre- and postprandial plasma glucose and insulin levels in 8 insulin-dependent diabetic subjects given 30-minute subcutaneous infusions of insulin beginning 60 minutes (open circles), 30 minutes (solid circles), and immediately before (solid squares) ingestion of a standard meal. The shaded area represents one standard deviation above and below the mean of observations in 8 normal individuals. *(Reproduced with permission from Dimitriadis et al.[98])*

substantiated by recent studies, in which monomeric analogs were formulated as either NPH or Ultralente suspensions without significantly altering the pharmacologic properties relative to corresponding human insulin preparations.[59,106] What remains even more elusive is a detailed understanding of the molecular events following subcutaneous injection of regular insulin. In particular, what intrinsic properties of the hormone, if any, influence the absorption process? Greater insight into the subcutaneous absorption mechanism has recently been obtained by considering the potential relationship of insulin self-association to pharmacokinetics and pharmacodynamics[80,107,108] as discussed in the following section.

A Model for Insulin Absorption: Implications of Self-Association

At the β-cell level, the propensity of insulin to self-associate into hexamers is crucial for the hormone's processing and storage.[4,36] This property of insulin has been exploited in pharmaceutical formulation to produce stable, solution preparations and microcrystalline suspensions used for diabetes treatment. Regular insulin preparations contain zinc ions in sufficient concentrations to promote self-association into hexamers, increasing chemical stability.[109] Phenolic compounds, additionally added as antimicrobial agents, have also been shown to have a profound stabilizing effect on deamidation as well as on intermolecular crosslinking reactions.[109] In addition to stabilizing insulin against undesirable chemical degradation, promotion of the hexamer conformation is also beneficial by preventing physical denaturation. Insulin fibrillation,

or nonnative aggregation, is thought to occur by interactions between partially denatured monomers.[110] The addition of excess zinc ions has also been shown to physically stabilize neutral solutions of insulin without affecting the rate of absorption following subcutaneous injection.[111] Thus solution preparations of insulin are formulated to promote hexamer formation, thereby providing the most stable form of the hormone. The implications of this associated state on insulin pharmacology were not fully appreciated until recently.

A scheme describing the putative events in the subcutis following the subcutaneous injection of a soluble insulin preparation is shown in Fig. 28-8A.[7,80,112] As previously described, the predominant associated state of insulin in the formulation is the hexamer with zinc ions and phenolic molecules bound. Diffusion in the interstitial space causes dilution of the insulin concentration, resulting in the progressive dissociation of the hexamer into smaller units.[113] Hexamer dissociation is facilitated by diffusion of the liganded phenolic molecules and zinc ions. The phenolic molecules likely diffuse initially in the process to the surrounding tissues, resulting in the conversion of R_6 hexamers to the T_6 type. Whether or not the R→T conversion plays any significant role in further delaying the dissociation process is not clearly understood. A 50- to 100-fold dilution is required to produce mainly dimers of insulin, whereas the concentration must be reduced at least 1000-fold to achieve a predominant population of monomers. One main feature of this model is that insulin can only be absorbed effectively in its monomeric or dimeric form. It is not known if the insulin hexamer can cross the capillary membrane or whether its size restricts passage relative to the monomer or dimer forms.

NEW HUMAN INSULIN ANALOGS WITH IMPROVED PHARMACOKINETIC AND PHARMACODYNAMIC PROPERTIES

The need for new insulins with improved pharmacokinetic and pharmacodynamic profiles has been well documented.[6,14,28,80,114] In particular, regular soluble insulins act too slowly and last too long, whereas the basal depot insulins do not act long enough and are associated with peak effects rather than providing flat, peakless profiles. With the advent of recombinant DNA technology (human insulin was the first pharmaceutical product derived from recombinant DNA technology in the early 1980s[75]) came the ability to prepare virtually any insulin analog desired. Not only did this new technology provide an important medical product, it gave insulin researchers the wherewithal to design, prepare, and test human insulin analogs for desirable pharmacokinetic and pharmacodynamic properties. Guided by the sophisticated x-ray structural data for insulin crystals and the many physicochemical studies on insulin discussed in the preceding sections, insulin researchers have designed insulin molecules with definite targets. The initial target was the design of insulins capable of giving more rapid serum insulin concentrations with a shorter duration of action compared to the regular soluble insulins.[80] This type of rapid-acting insulin should have the capability of decreasing the magnitude of mealtime glucose excursions while reducing the potential for late hypoglycemia, coupled with improved convenience for the patient with diabetes.[115]

As previously discussed, there is a delay in absorption of insulin upon subcutaneous injection of regular preparations. The absorption of insulin is influenced by a number of factors, many of

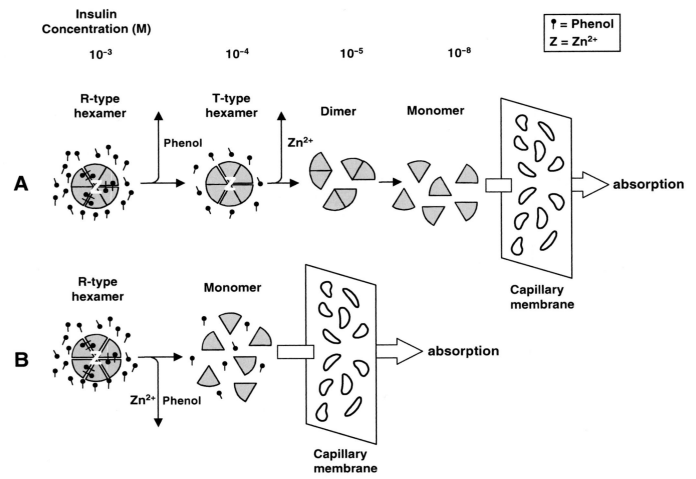

FIGURE 28-8. Schematic representation of the putative events following subcutaneous injection of regular human insulin (**A**) and a formulated monomeric analog [e.g., Humalog, $Lys^{B28}Pro^{B29}$] (**B**). The initial event involves diffusion of phenolic preservative into the surrounding tissue and dissociation of phenolic molecules from the hexamer complexes. Human insulin zinc complexes are relatively stable and require diffusion and dilution for dissociation into smaller absorbable units. A 50- to 100-fold dilution is needed for dissociation to mainly dimers, whereas a further 1000-fold dilution is required to produce predominantly monomeric insulin that can be absorbed. In contrast, both zinc ions and phenolic molecules are required to stabilize the hexameric complex of $Lys^{B28}Pro^{B29}$. Because of the greatly reduced dimerization constant of the analog, hexamer dissociation occurs at much lower dilutions. Thus free $Lys^{B28}Pro^{B29}$ monomers are produced faster than human insulin, resulting in more rapid absorption. The diagrams are based on models proposed in Ciszak and colleagues,[46] Bakaysa and associates,[112] and Brange and coworkers.[80] (*Figure adapted with permission from Brange et al.[7]*)

which also affect the self-association state by facilitating dissociation. For example, dilute insulin concentrations and increased blood flow would be expected to promote faster dissociation of the hexamer. Based on the premise that small molecules diffuse faster and would be unrestricted in passing through the capillary membrane, the absorption process could be accelerated by reducing the self-association state of insulin. This hypothesis forms the basis for designing insulin analogs with reduced propensity towards self-association that would display a more rapid onset of action and shorter duration of action after subcutaneous injection. Two such human insulin analogs were introduced in recent years as very rapid-acting mealtime insulins, namely $Lys^{B28}Pro^{B29}$–human insulin (insulin lispro; Humalog®) and Asp^{B28}–human insulin (insulin aspart; NovoRapid®). Although both of these new insulins exist as stable zinc hexamers in their respective formulations, the

rapid action derives from their quicker dissociation from the hexameric state compared to regular human insulin after subcutaneous injection (see Fig. 28-8).

Another goal was the design of insulins that would produce a more physiologic basal insulin profile, preferably soluble, long-acting insulins capable of duplicating the nearly peakless profile of bovine Ultralente insulin shown in Fig. 28-6.[90] The recently-introduced $Gly^{A21}Arg^{B31}Arg^{B32}$–human insulin (insulin glargine; Lantus®) fits into this category. In this molecule, the two additional positive charges at the C terminus of the B chain increase the isoelectric point from ~5.4 to ~6.7; this allows a soluble formulation at a slightly acidic pH, a formulation that becomes less soluble when injected into the subcutaneous tissue at physiologic pH.[14] These three new insulins are discussed in more detail in the following sections and are illustrated structurally in Fig. 28-9. See also

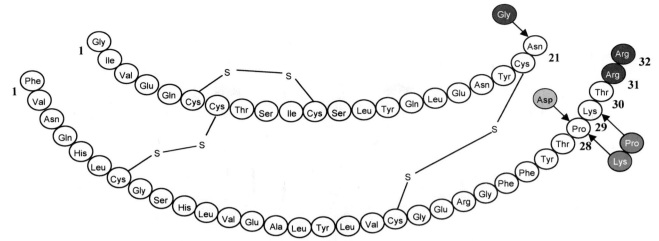

FIGURE 28-9. Primary structure of human insulin in white circles (21-residue A chain connected to 30-residue B chain via disulfide bonds) showing positions of modification for the three human insulin analogs. Modification of human insulin to give the basal human insulin analog Gly^{A21} Arg^{B31} Arg^{B32}-human insulin (insulin glargine or Lantus) is illustrated by **black circles,** whereby glycine replaces A21 asparagine and two arginine residues are attached to the C terminus of the B chain. Aspartic acid replaces proline at position B28 (**stippled circle**) to give the rapid-acting human insulin analog Asp^{B28}-human insulin (insulin aspart or NovoRapid). The modification that creates the rapid-acting human insulin analog Lys^{B28}Pro^{B29}-human insulin (insulin lispro or Humalog) is shown by the **gray circles,** indicating the changes whereby the native sequence Pro^{B28}Lys^{B29} is transposed to Lys^{B28}Pro^{B29}.

recent reviews on the clinical aspects of new insulin analogs and their potential in the management of diabetes mellitus.[14,114]

Lys^{B28}Pro^{B29}–Human Insulin (Insulin Lispro [Humalog])

As shown in Figs. 28-1 and 28-9, the native amino acid sequence of human insulin at positions 28 and 29 in the B chain is Pro-Lys. Researchers found that inverting this sequence to Lys-Pro resulted in an insulin analog with a weakened tendency to self-associate into dimers,[108,116] a characteristic that explains its more rapid onset of action and shorter duration in comparison to regular human insulin.[115,117–121] The physicochemical basis for this rapid activity has been reviewed recently by DeFelippis and colleagues.[28] The Lys^{B28}Pro^{B29} inversion analog has been crystallized in the presence of both zinc ions and phenol at pH 5.9, and its three-dimensional structure as determined by x-ray crystallography to 2.3 Å resolution revealed the T$_3$R$_3$^{f} hexamer conformation.[46] The structure is isomorphous with the uncomplexed native human insulin structure; however, localized structural differences in the C-terminal region of the B chain caused by the sequence inversion result in the elimination of two critical hydrophobic interactions involving Pro^{B28} and weakening (lengthening) of two β-pleated sheet hydrogen bonds that stabilize the dimer.

The x-ray crystallographic results demonstrate that despite modifications to the insulin sequence intended to disrupt self-association, hexamer formation can occur as observed in the solid state. The finding that excipients prone to induce hexamer formation in native insulin also do so for monomeric analogs has important implications for pharmaceutical formulation since the entire design premise is based on eliminating self-association. However, for monomeric analogs to be viable as commercial solution preparations, excipients such as antimicrobial agents are required in the

formulation, and zinc ions might also be included to achieve stability.[109,110] On the other hand, if the addition of such excipients causes comparable self-association of the analog in solution, the potential for delayed dissociation could negatively impact its rapid time action. This situation creates a predicament for the effective formulation of a stable, solution preparation of a monomeric insulin analog, while simultaneously maintaining its desirable pharmacologic attributes. Nevertheless, these practical formulation issues were considered during formulation development of the commercially available monomeric insulin analog Lys^{B28}Pro^{B29}–human insulin (insulin lispro, Humalog) preparation, which contains both zinc ions and m-cresol as excipients. Despite this fact, Lys^{B28}Pro^{B29} maintains its rapid time action properties as shown by the data presented in Fig. 28-10.

The x-ray crystallographic studies on crystals of Lys^{B28}Pro^{B29} grown in the presence of zinc ions and phenol revealed a hexamer conformation.[46] Although the commercial preparation of Lys^{B28} Pro^{B29} (Humalog) is a solution formulation, the structural data obtained in the solid state was used to propose a possible explanation for unaltered time action observed *in vivo*. The authors suggest that the localized structural perturbations of the analog hexamer complex relative to human insulin (see earlier discussion) coupled with the requirement for zinc ions and phenol for stabilization of the hexamer explains why formulated Lys^{B28}Pro^{B29} readily dissociates in subcutaneous tissue. Ciszak and associates[46] hypothesize that initial diffusion of bound phenolic preservative into surrounding tissue destabilizes the analog hexamer, resulting in dissociation into monomer subunits at millimolar concentrations. This hypothesis is supported by a study of the solution-state properties of Lys^{B28}Pro^{B29} in the presence and absence of zinc ions and phenolic compounds monitored by static light scattering.[112] These static light scattering results, monitoring the *in vitro* dissociation of the Lys^{B28}Pro^{B29} complex upon dilution in buffer, showed that the

A

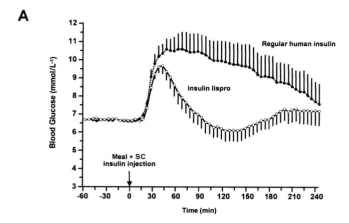

B

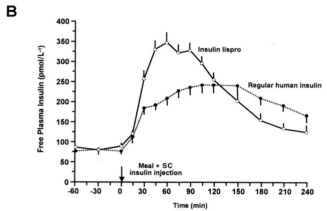

FIGURE 28-10. Blood glucose excursions (**A**) of ten T1DM patients after consumption of a meal rich in rapidly-absorbable carbohydrates [pizza, sugar-sweetened cola, and tiramisu (total caloric content was 1016 kcal)]. After a subcutaneous injection of 15.4 ± 3.5 U at time zero, the meal was eaten within 20 minutes. On one of two study days, insulin lispro (**open circles**) was injected; on the other day regular human insulin (**solid circles**) was injected. Blood glucose was kept constant at 6.7 mmol/L^{-1} in the 3 hours prior to the meal by means of a glucose clamp. Free plasma insulin concentrations (**B**) of ten T1DM patients induced by an intravenous insulin infusion of 0.2 mU•kg^{-1}min^{-1} (maintained throughout the study) and subcutaneous injection immediately prior to the meal at time zero. Injections of insulin lispro (**open circles**) or regular human insulin (**solid circles**) were administered as in A. *(Reproduced with permission from Heinemann et al.[122])*

analog becomes less associated as protein concentration is reduced, whereas human insulin formulated under similar conditions was essentially hexameric regardless of the dilution. Thus these results illustrate the weaker hexamer association of the analog. See Fig. 28-8 for a schematic representation of the putative events following subcutaneous injection of regular human insulin compared to a formulated monomeric insulin analog such as Humalog.

The pharmacokinetics and glucodynamics of insulin lispro have been studied extensively as reviewed recently by Heinemann and Woodworth.[121] The studies showed that subcutaneous administration of clinically relevant doses of insulin lispro gave a more rapid absorption and elimination profile than regular human insulin. After intravenous administration, insulin lispro and regular human insulin gave nearly identical clearance and volumes of distribution, and produced identical metabolic responses, indicating a 1:1 potency ratio.[121] Differences in absorption between insulin lispro and regular human insulin, but equivalence in distribution

and clearance, were observed in healthy volunteers and in patients with type 1 or type 2 diabetes.[121] The authors concluded that the more rapid absorption of insulin lispro allows a better mealtime insulin substitution than regular human insulin.[121] This conclusion was validated by a randomized, double-blind, glucose clamp–controlled study, the results of which are shown in Fig. 28-10. In this study, 10 patients with well-controlled T1DM received subcutaneous injections of either insulin lispro or regular human insulin (15.4 ± 3.5 U; the exact dose selected by the patients based on their own experience), followed immediately by ingestion of a meal rich in rapidly-absorbable carbohydrates.[122] Maximum blood glucose excursions were significantly lower and returned to baseline earlier with insulin lispro than with regular human insulin. The free plasma levels of the analog increased more rapidly and decreased faster than human insulin.

Many of the clinical studies on insulin lispro have been summarized by Anderson and Koivisto[115] and by Bolli and colleagues.[14] Insulin lispro's rapid absorption rate and short duration of action provide several advantages for patients on insulin lispro therapy as compared to regular human insulin. Insulin lispro was developed particularly for mealtime therapy through injection immediately before the meal and when appropriately used in this manner consistently reduces the postprandial rise in blood glucose as compared to regular human insulin in patients with type 1 or type 2 diabetes.[115]

If insulin lispro is administered shortly after a meal, the postprandial rise in blood glucose is no greater than if regular insulin is injected immediately or shortly before a meal as shown by Schernthaner and associates.[123] These clinical investigators studied 18 patients with type 1 diabetes who injected regular human insulin at 40, 20, or 0 minutes before the start of a standardized meal or insulin lispro at 20 or 0 minutes before or 15 minutes after the start of the meal. In this study, the optimal time for bolus injection was immediately before the meal for insulin lispro and 20 minutes before the meal for regular human insulin, based on blood glucose excursions. Insulin lispro injected 15 minutes after the start of the meal was comparable to regular human insulin injected from 40 to 0 minutes before the meal. In their review, Anderson and Koivisto reported that a meta-analysis of over 12,000 patients with T1DM demonstrated a 30% reduction in severe hypoglycemia during insulin lispro therapy.[115] Additionally, insulin lispro appears to be no more immunogenic than regular human insulin as determined in four 1-year international trials including 317 patients with T1DM and 291 patients with T2DM previously treated with regular human insulin.[124] Coupled with a basal insulin therapy adjusted to cover premeal and nocturnal periods, insulin lispro may provide a more physiologic insulin therapy, as emphasized by Bolli and colleagues.[14] Also, insulin lispro administered by a continuous subcutaneous insulin infusion (CSII) regimen is a viable alternative to a multiple daily insulin injection regimen for patients on intensive insulin therapy.[125]

The introduction of Lys^{B28}Pro^{B29} to the commercial market has created interest in exploring other formulations of this analog. Cocrystallization of the analog with protamine produced a suspension called neutral protamine lispro (NPL) with similar physicochemical properties to NPH insulin.[106] The motivation for making this suspension was to allow the preparation of stable mixtures with soluble Lys^{B28}Pro^{B29}. Such preparations could be useful for basal/bolus therapy in type 1 patients. Pharmacologic evaluation of NPL in dogs has shown that the preparation has an intermediate time action.[106] A clinical trial conducted in type 1 diabetic subjects determined that NPL was equally effective as human insulin NPH in controlling overnight glycemia.[126] In a euglycemic glucose clamp study conducted in normal subjects, three mixtures of soluble $Lys^{B28}Pro^{B29}$ combined with NPL in ratios of 75:25, 50:50, and 25:75 were evaluated.[127] The results of this study confirmed that the pharmacokinetic and pharmacodynamic properties of $Lys^{B28}Pro^{B29}$ were maintained in the mixtures. Data from other clinical trials conducted in type 2 patients have reported that the 25:75 analog mixture provides improved postprandial glycemic control relative to a human insulin mixture containing 30% regular insulin and 70% NPH insulin.[128,129]

Asp^B28–Human Insulin (Insulin Aspart [NovoRapid])

Asp^{B28}–human insulin (herein referred to as Asp^{B28} and insulin aspart) was first described in 1988 by Brange and colleagues.[107] As with $Lys^{B28}Pro^{B29}$ insulin, Asp^{B28} was designed as a rapid-acting mealtime insulin with a lesser propensity to self-associate compared to regular insulin. Asp^{B28} refers to an analog prepared by substituting aspartic acid for proline at position 28 in the B chain of human insulin as illustrated in Fig. 28-9. Brange and associates reported on various approaches for producing monomeric insulins.[80,107] In the case of Asp^{B28}, the primary hypothesis was to selectively introduce an amino acid with a negatively-charged side-chain carboxyl group to create charge repulsion and weaken the monomer-monomer interaction. Although charge repulsion may play some role in hindering self-association, a more likely explanation for the more rapid action of this human insulin analog concerns the removal of proline from position B28, which eliminates a key hydrophobic interaction between monomers.[7] The Asp^{B28} analog has recently been crystallized in the presence of zinc and phenol or m-cresol;[130] the analog crystallized as R_6 hexamers with a number of phenolic molecules (m-cresol or phenol) bound at specific sites. This contrasts to $Lys^{B28}Pro^{B29}$ insulin crystal studies, which showed a $T_3R_3^f$ hexamer conformation. The replacement of proline with aspartic acid at position B28 causes increased conformational flexibility in the C terminus of the B chain, resulting in loss of critical intermolecular van der Waals contacts between positions B28 and GlyB23′ at the monomer-monomer interface, explaining the monomeric nature of the analog.[130] As mentioned previously, this explanation is contrary to the original design hypothesis of introducing charge repulsion in the interface.[80,107] However, it has been speculated that charge repulsion may contribute to hexamer destabilization, causing rapid dissociation to monomers.[7]

The pharmacokinetics and pharmacodynamics of Asp^{B28} have been investigated in normal subjects,[131–139] and, as reviewed by Lindholm and Jacobsen,[140] subcutaneously-administered Asp^{B28} showed an absorption profile with a time to reach peak concentration about half that of human insulin, a peak plasma drug concentration approximately twice as high, and a shorter residence time (Fig. 28-11). These observations are similar to those obtained in the insulin lispro studies and are consistent with the notion that more rapid action can be achieved using insulin analogs with impaired self-association characteristics. Similarly, clinical trials in patients with type 1 or type 2 diabetes have demonstrated that insulin aspart, like insulin lispro, is efficacious as a very rapid-acting mealtime insulin, resulting in improved postprandial glucose excursions when compared to the traditional regimen of regular human insulin given approximately 30 minutes before the meal.[140–149] Both insulin aspart and insulin lispro, in conjunction with appropriate basal insulin therapy, appear to more closely mimic the endogenous insulin profile in blood compared with

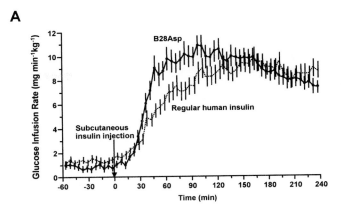

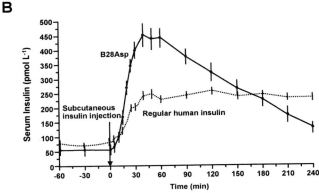

FIGURE 28-11. Glucose infusion rates (**A**) and serum insulin concentrations (**B**) after subcutaneous injection of 0.15 U/kg⁻¹ body weight of Asp^{B28} (———) or regular human insulin (····) into the abdominal region of 14 normal subjects. Baseline insulin concentrations were established by an intravenous insulin infusion of 0.15 mU·kg⁻¹min⁻¹. *(Reproduced with permission from Heinemann et al.[133])*

human insulin.[140,150] Insulin aspart is also an alternative for intensive insulin therapy by CSII,[151] and the analog can be formulated with protamine in a 30:70 mixture.[152–153] Although insulin aspart and insulin lispro are generally assumed to be quite similar in their respective pharmacokinetic and pharmocodynamic properties, there is a paucity of data showing direct comparisons. Hedman and associates[154] designed such a comparison, in which 14 patients with T1DM were administered 10 U of each analog on alternate days immediately before consuming a standardized breakfast in a single blind randomized crossover study. As expected, both insulins were absorbed much faster than human insulin after subcutaneous injection, with higher insulin peaks and shorter duration of action (based on historic data). The main finding in this direct comparison of insulin aspart and insulin lispro is that the free plasma insulin levels resemble each other, with insulin lispro showing a slightly more rapid uptake, reaching the maximum peak concentration earlier, followed by a more rapid decline.

Gly^A21Arg^B31Arg^32–Human Insulin (Insulin Glargine [Lantus]) (also 21^A-Gly-30^Ba-L-Arg-30^Bb-L-Arg-Human Insulin)

This human insulin analog (formerly known as HOE 901) was designed as a soluble, basal insulin. The design concept involved introducing two arginines into the primary structure of human insulin (see Fig. 28-9), thereby shifting the isoelectric point from about 5.5 to a more neutral pH, a maneuver that greatly reduces the solubility of the insulin analog upon injection into the neutral milieu of the subcutaneous tissue. An insulin-like molecule with this characteristic occurs naturally in that diarginyl insulin (insulin–$Arg^{B31}Arg^{B32}$) is one of the intermediate products formed during the proteolytic conversion of proinsulin to insulin in the pancreatic β cell.[155] The same diarginyl insulin is also formed under some manufacturing conditions for recombinant human insulin.[76] The replacement of asparagine with glycine at position 21 in the A chain is necessary to ensure acceptable chemical stability for the slightly acidic, soluble glargine formulation. This is a crucial modification as acidic insulin solutions are known to degrade by mechanisms that involve the COOH-terminal asparagine at position A21.[156]

X-ray crystallographic analysis of $Gly^{A21}Arg;^{B31}Arg^{B32}$–human insulin indicates that the hexamer structure is more stable than the native hormone and that the analog crystallizes as R_6 hexamers in the presence of phenol.[157] Crystal stability is mainly attributed to interactions between neighboring hexamers, and a seventh molecule of phenol was also detected in the structure, located in a surface depression of trimer I.[157] The phenolic hydroxyl group donates a hydrogen bond to the side chain of a glutamic acid residue of a neighboring hexamer in the crystal lattice. This interaction was proposed to increase the attractive interhexamer forces contributing to the stabilization of the analog crystals formed after subcutaneous injection.[157]

The clinical efficacy and safety of insulin glargine have been reported recently in studies with healthy volunteers,[158–159] in patients with T1DM,[160–166] and in patients with T2DM.[167–168] Comparisons were generally made using once-a-day injection for glargine versus once- or twice-a-day injections for NPH. The general consensus is that this new soluble, long-acting insulin provides more stable blood glucose control with a nearly peakless pharmacodynamic profile, in contrast to the peaks seen with NPH insulin (see Fig. 28-12). Also, there appears to be a safety benefit in terms of less nocturnal hypoglycemia. Lepore and coworkers[166] compared insulin glargine against NPH insulin, Ultralente human insulin, and against a CSII regimen. The authors concluded that

glargine is a peakless insulin, that it lasts nearly 24 hours, that it shows lower intersubject variability than NPH and Ultralente, and that it closely mimics CSII. Thus insulin glargine represents a new soluble basal insulin that may be an important part of the basal-bolus equation along with the new mealtime insulins (insulin lispro and insulin aspart).[169] However, because of formulation incompatibility, the acidic insulin glargine formulation should not be mixed with either insulin lispro or insulin aspart formulations.

CONCLUSIONS AND FUTURE OUTLOOK

Physiological insulin secretion in normal individuals is characterized by stimulated and basal phases. The goal of effective diabetes treatment is to simulate this profile with appropriate injections of insulin. While there have been improvements in the area of pharmaceutical formulation, the time-action profiles of the various commercially available insulin preparations do not adequately approximate endogenous secretion. Clinical data indicating that effective blood glucose control reduces the progression of complications associated with diabetes has further driven efforts to optimize subcutaneous injection therapy. Since little more could be done in terms of improving formulation, recent attention has focused on manipulating the properties of the insulin molecule itself. Recombinant DNA technology and continued advancement in insulin structural determinations have provided the tools to explore this new area of research.

Clinical studies have demonstrated that the absorption of subcutaneously injected insulin is influenced by a variety of factors, none of which can be sufficiently controlled by the patient to achieve more physiologic time-action profiles. Until recently, the relationship between the structural properties of insulin and the absorption process were not fully appreciated. The excipients included in soluble regular insulin preparations to impart stability and satisfy other regulatory requirements promote hexamer assembly. Based on the hypothesis that diffusion and dilution of the insulin hexamer at the injection depot may influence pharmacokinetics and pharmacodynamics, insulin analogs with reduced propensity towards self-association were designed and tested. The physico-chemical properties of a number of these analogs confirmed that self-association can be manipulated by selected amino acid modification of the native sequence, and so called "monomeric" insulins could indeed be synthesized. Subsequent *in vivo* testing has demonstrated that the pharmacokinetic and pharmacodynamic properties of these analogs following subcutaneous administration better simulate meal-stimulated secretion compared to human insulin. Two of these analogs (insulin lispro and insulin aspart) have received regulatory approval and are commercially available under the trade names of Humalog and NovoRapid, or Novolog, respectively. Interestingly, a prerequisite for the commercial viability of $Lys^{B28}Pro^{B29}$ was a suitable formulation with the inclusion of excipients found to induce self-association. These formulation conditions appear to undermine the original concept of eliminating hexamer association. However, $Lys^{B28}Pro^{B29}$ hexamers were determined to be destabilized relative to human insulin such that the analog's desirable pharmacokinetic and pharmacodynamic properties are not impacted by formulation. The same is true for insulin aspart.

The strategy of producing monomeric analogs to improve prandial insulin requirements has been very successful. However, basal insulin needs must also be satisfied for effective therapy. NPH and Ultralente suspensions currently used for basal therapy

FIGURE 28-12. Time-action profile of insulin glargine (Lantus) and NPH human insulin, showing the glucose infusion required to maintain plasma glucose concentration at the target of about 130 mg/dL (7.2 mmol/L) in 20 patients with T1DM after injection of either 0.3 U/kg insulin glargine or NPH insulin. The NPH study was terminated at 20 hours because of excessive hyperglycemia. *(Modified with permission from commentary by Bolli et al.[164])*

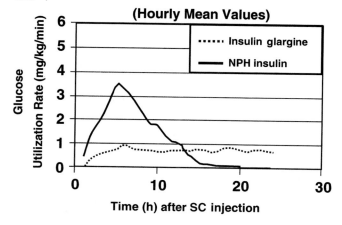

(Hourly Mean Values)

······ Insulin glargine
—— NPH insulin

Glucose Utilization Rate (mg/kg/min)

Time (h) after SC injection

were developed long before physiologic insulin secretion was understood. Pharmacologic studies of these suspensions have demonstrated that the pharmacokinetic and pharmacodynamic properties do not simulate the prolonged, low-level release profile of endogenous insulin secretion. Since these suspensions also require agitation to homogeneously disperse the solid particles prior to injection, they are somewhat more complicated for patients to use. Therefore, the newly-approved, soluble, long-acting insulin preparation insulin glargine (Lantus) is an additional product for patients and diabetes caregivers in the continual quest to obtain the best blood glucose control possible.[169,170] Additional insulin candidates are still in the research stage. One in particular is in clinical development. Insulin detemir [Lys^{B29}(N-tetradecanoyl) des(B30) human insulin] is a soluble insulin derivative being developed as a soluble, basal insulin. Like native insulins, it exists in the formulation primarily in the hexameric state.[171] The fatty acid side chain apparently assists in hexamer aggregation as well as to delay hexamer dissociation and absorption.[172] Also, the fatty acid side chain of the monomeric insulin derivative binds to albumin and subsequently slowly dissociates from the albumin, prolonging time action.[173] While results from an earlier study in normal volunteers gave inconclusive results on the potential use of insulin detemir as a basal insulin,[174] results of clinical studies in patients with T1DM suggest insulin detemir was as effective as NPH in maintaining glycemic control, but only when administered at a higher molar dose.[171]

There appears to be little that can be done to further improve upon the pharmacologic properties of the monomeric analogs for subcutaneous injection therapy. The properties of these analogs are now being exploited in other formulations. For example, in an effort to optimize basal-bolus therapy, intermediate-acting protamine suspensions of insulin lispro and insulin aspart have been developed for use in premixed preparations. The rapid time-action profile of the soluble fraction of the analog is maintained in these preparations. In terms of the promising basal analog formulation, Lantus, the prolongation mechanism involves an *in situ* precipitation at the injection depot rather than injection of a preformed NPH or Ultralente suspension. What potential improvements can be devised to improve upon this approach, or whether a totally different insulin analog concept for improving basal therapy can be created remain to be seen.

Acknowledgement. This chapter was condensed in part from reference 28 with permission.

REFERENCES

1. Banting FG, Best CH: The internal secretion of the pancreas. *J Lab Clin Med* 1922;7:256.
2. Baker EN, Blundell TL, Cutfield JF, *et al*: The structure of 2Zn pig insulin crystals at 1.5Å resolution. *Philes Trans Soc Lond* 1988;B319:369.
3. Steiner DF, Oyer PE: The biosynthesis of insulin and a probable precursor of insulin by a human islet cell adenoma. *Proc Natl Acad Sci USA* 1967;57:473.
4. Dodson G, Steiner D: The role of assembly in insulin's biosynthesis. *Curr Opin Struct Biol* 1998;8:189.
5. Kahn CR, Folli F: Molecular determinants of insulin action. *Horm Res* 1993;39(Suppl 3):93.
6. Galloway JA, Chance RE: Improving insulin therapy: Achievements and challenges. *Horm Metab Res* 1994;26:591.
7. Brange J, Vølund A: Insulin analogs with improved pharmacokinetic profiles. *Adv Drug Delivery Rev* 1999;35:307.
8. Binder C, Brange J: Insulin chemistry and pharmacokinetics. In: Porte D Jr., Sherwin RS, eds. *Ellenberg & Rifkin's Diabetes Mellitus*, 5th ed. Appleton & Lange:1997;689.
9. Zinman B: The physiological replacement of insulin: An elusive goal. *Med Intelligence* 1989;321:363.
10. Lauritzen T, Pramming S, Deckert T, *et al*: Pharmacokinetics of continuous subcutaneous insulin infusion. *Diabetologia* 1983;24:326.
11. Polonsky KS, Byrne MM, Sturis J: Alternative insulin delivery systems: How demanding should the patient be? *Diabetologia* 1997;40(Suppl 2):S97.
12. Chetty DJ, Chien YW: Novel methods of insulin delivery: An update. *Crit Rev Ther Drug Carrier Syst* 1998;15:629.
13. The Diabetes Control and Complications Trial (DCCT) Research Group: The effect of intensive treatment of diabetes on the development and progression of long-term complications in insulin-dependent diabetes mellitus. *N Engl J Med* 1993;329:977.
14. Bolli GB, DiMarchi RD, Park GD, *et al*: Insulin analogues and their potential in the management of diabetes mellitus. *Diabetologia* 1999;42:1151.
15. Goeddel DV, Kleid DG, Bolivar F, *et al*: Expression in *Escherichia coli* of chemically synthesized genes for human insulin. *Proc Natl Acad Sci USA* 1979;76:106.
16. Brandenburg D: Insulin chemistry. In: Cuatrecasas P, Jacobs S, eds. *Insulin*. Springer-Verlag:1990;3.
17. Sanger F: Chemistry of insulin. *Science* 1959;129:1340.
18. Pullen RA, Lindsay DG, Wood SP, *et al*: Receptor-binding region of insulin. *Nature* 1976;259:369.
19. Helmerhorst E, Stokes GB: Self-association of insulin. Its pH dependence and effect of plasma. *Diabetes* 1987;36:261.
20. Bi RC, Dauter Z, Dodson E, *et al*: Insulin's structure as a modified and monomeric molecule. *Biopolymers* 1984;23:391.
21. Derewenda U, Derewenda Z, Dodson EJ, *et al*: Phenol stabilizes more helix in a new symmetrical zinc insulin hexamer. *Nature* 1989;338:594.
22. Roy M, Lee RWK, Brange J, *et al*: ^{1}H NMR spectrum of the native human insulin monomer. *J Biol Chem* 1990;265:5448.
23. Melberg SG, Johnson WC Jr: Changes in secondary structure follow the dissociation of human insulin hexamers: a circular dichroism study. *Proteins: Struct Funct Genet* 1990;8:280.
24. Hefford MA, Oda G, Kaplan H: Structure-function relationships in the free insulin monomer. *Biochem J* 1986;237:663.
25. Mark AE, Berendsen HJC, van Gunsteren WF: Conformational flexibility of aqueous monomeric and dimeric insulin: a molecular dynamics study. *Biochemistry* 1991;30:10866.
26. Derewenda U, Derewenda Z, Dodson EJ, *et al*: X-ray analysis of the single chain B29-A1 peptide-linked insulin molecule. A completely inactive analogue. *J Mol Biol* 1991;220:425.
27. Brange J, Skelbaek-Pedersen B, Langkjaer L, *et al*: *Galenics of Insulin. The Physico-Chemical and Pharmaceutical Aspects of Insulin and Insulin Preparations.* Springer-Verlag:1987.
28. DeFelippis MR, Chance RE, Frank BH: Insulin self-association and the relationship to pharmacokinetics and pharmacodynamics. *Crit Rev Ther Drug Carrier Syst* 2001;18:201.
29. Goldman J, Carpenter FH: Zinc binding, circular dichroism, and equilibrium sedimentation studies on insulin (bovine) and several of its derivatives. *Biochemistry* 1974;13:4566.
30. Grant PT, Coombs TL, Frank BH: Differences in the nature of the interaction of insulin and proinsulin with zinc. *Biochem J* 1972;126:433.
31. Jeffrey PD: Self-association of des-(B26-B30)-insulin. *Biol Chem Hoppe-Seyler* 1986;367:363.
32. Scott DA: Crystalline insulin. *Biochem J* 1934;28:1592.
33. Pekar AH, Frank BH: Conformation of proinsulin. A comparison of insulin and proinsulin self-association at neutral pH. *Biochemistry* 1972;11:4013.
34. Hvidt S: Insulin association in neutral solutions studied by light scattering. *Biophys Chem* 1991;39:205.
35. Schlichtkrull J: *Insulin Crystals* (reprinted). Preben Hoy:1961.
36. Emdin SO, Dodson GG, Cutfield JM, *et al*: Role of zinc in insulin biosynthesis. *Diabetologia* 1980;19:174.
37. Smith GD, Swenson DC, Dodson EJ, *et al*: Structural stability in the 4-zinc human insulin hexamer. *Proc Natl Acad Sci USA* 1984;81:7093.

38. Kaarsholm NC, Ko H-C, Dunn MF: Comparison of solution structural flexibility and zinc binding domains for insulin, proinsulin, and miniproinsulin. *Biochemistry* 1989;28:4427.

39. Krüger P, Gilge G, Çabuk, *et al*: Cooperativity and intermediate states in the T → R-structural transformation of insulin. *Biol Chem Hoppe-Seyler* 1990;371:669.

40. Gross L, Dunn MF: Spectroscopic evidence for an intermediate in the T_6 to R_6 allosteric transition of the Co(II)-substituted insulin hexamer. *Biochemistry* 1992;31:1295.

41. Brader ML: Zinc coordination, asymmetry, and allostery of the human insulin hexamer. *J Am Chem Soc* 1997;119:7603.

42. Jacoby E, Hua QX, Stern AS, *et al*: Structure and dynamics of a protein assembly. ^{1}H-NMR studies of the 36 kDa R_6 insulin hexamer. *J Mol Biol* 1996;258:136.

43. Bentley GA, Brange J, Derewenda Z, *et al*: Role of B13 Glu in insulin assembly. The hexamer structure of recombinant mutant (B13 Glu → Gln) insulin. *J Mol Biol* 1992;228:1163.

44. Wittingham JL, Chaudhuri S, Dodson EJ, *et al*: X-ray crystallographic studies on hexameric insulins in the presence of helix-stabilizing agents, thiocyanate, methylparaben, and phenol. *Biochemistry* 1995;34;15553.

45. Ciszak E, Smith, GD: Crystallographic evidence for dual coordination around zinc in the T3R3 human insulin hexamer. *Biochemistry* 1994;33:1512.

46. Ciszak E, Beals JM, Frank BH, *et al*: Role of C-terminal B-chain residues in insulin assembly: the structure of hexameric Lys^{B28}Pro^{B29}-human insulin. *Structure* 1995;3:615.

47. Smith GD: The phenolic binding site in $T_3R_3{}^f$ insulin. *J Mol Struct* 1998;469:71.

48. Smith GD, Dodson GG: Structure of a rhombohedral R_6 insulin/phenol complex. *Proteins: Struct Funct Genet* 1992;14:401.

49. Schade DS, Santiago JV, Skyler JS, *et al*: *Intensive Insulin Therapy.* Medical Examination Publishing:1983;23.

50. Polonsky KS, Given BD, Van Cauter E: Twenty-four-hour profiles and pulsatile patterns of insulin secretion in normal and obese subjects. *J Clin Invest* 1988;81:442.

51. Schlichtkrull J, Pingel M, Heding LG, *et al*: Insulin preparations with prolonged effect. In: Hasselblatt A, von Bruchhausen F, eds. *Handbook of Experimental Pharmacology*, Vol. 32/2. Springer-Verlag: 1975;729.

52. Costantino HR, Liauw S, Mitragotri S, *et al*: The pharmaceutical development of insulin: historical perspectives and future directions. *ACS Symp S* 1997;675:29.

53. Schlichtkrull J, Munck O, Jersild M: Insulin rapitard and insulin actrapid. *Acta Med Scand* 1965;177:103.

54. Hagedorn HC, Jensen BN, Krarup NB, *et al*: Protamine insulinate. *J Am Med Assoc* 1936;106:177.

55. Scott DA, Fisher AM: Studies on insulin with protamine. *J Pharmacol Exp Ther* 1936;58:78.

56. Hoffmann JA, Chance RE, Johnson MG: Purification and analysis of the major components of chum salmon protamine contained in insulin formulations using high-performance liquid chromatography. *Protein Express Purific* 1990;1:127.

57. Krayenbühl C, Rosenberg T: Crystalline protamine insulin. *Steno Memorial Hospital Rep (Copenhagen)* 1946;1:60.

58. Hallas-Møller K, Petersen K, Schlichtkrull J: Crystalline and amorphous insulin-zinc compounds with prolonged action. *Science* 1952; 116:394.

59. Richards JP, Stickelmeyer MP, Frank BH, *et al*: Preparation of a microcrystalline suspension formulation of Lys^{B28}Pro^{B29}-human insulin with ultralente properties. *J Pharm Sci* 1999;88:861.

60. Davis SN, Thompson CJ, Brown MD, *et al*: A comparison of the pharmacokinetics and metabolic effects of human regular insulin and NPH insulin mixtures. *Diabetes Res Clin Prac* 1991;13:107.

61. Dodd SW, Havel HA, Kovach PM, *et al*: Reversible adsorption of soluble hexameric insulin onto the surface of insulin crystals cocrystallized with protamine: an electrostatic interaction. *Pharm Res* 1995; 12:60.

62. Galloway JA, Spradlin CT, Nelson RL, *et al*: Factors influencing the absorption, serum insulin concentration, and blood glucose responses after injections of regular insulin and various insulin mixtures. *Diabetes Care* 1981;4:366.

63. Mirsky A, Kawamura K: Heterogeneity of crystalline insulin. *Endocrinology* 1966;78:1115.

64. Steiner DF, Hallund O, Rubenstein A, *et al*: Isolation and properties of proinsulin, intermediate forms, and other minor components from crystalline bovine insulin. *Diabetes* 1968;17:725.

65. Chance RE, Root MA, Galloway JA: The immunogenicity of insulin preparations. *Acta Endocrinol* 1976;205:185.

66. Schlichtkrull J, Brange J, Christiansen AA H, *et al*: Clinical aspects of insulin—antigenicity. *Diabetes* 1972;21(Suppl 2):649.

67. Francis AJ, Hanning I, Alberti KGMM: The influence of insulin antibody levels on the plasma profiles and action of subcutaneously injected human and bovine short acting insulins. *Diabetologia* 1985;28:330.

68. Schernthaner G: Immunogenicity and allergenic potential of animal and human insulins. *Diabetes Care* 1993;16(Suppl 3):155.

69. Meienhofer J, Schnabel E, Bremer H, *et al*: Synthese der insulinketten und ihre kombination zu insulinaktiven präparaten. *Z Naturforschg* 1963;18b:1120.

70. Katsoyannis PG: The synthesis of the insulin chains and their combination to biologically active material. *Diabetes* 1964;13:339.

71. Kung Y-T, Du Y-C, Huang W-T, *et al*: Total synthesis of crystalline insulin. *Scientia Sinica* 1966;15:544.

72. Morihara K, Oka T, Tsuzuki H: Semi-synthesis of human insulin by trypsin-catalysed replacement of Ala-B30 by Thr in porcine insulin. *Nature* 1979;280:412.

73. Markussen J, Damgaard U, Pingel M, *et al*: Human insulin (Novo): chemistry and characteristics. *Diabetes Care* 1983;6:4.

74. Chance RE, Kroeff EP, Hoffmann JA, *et al*: Chemical, physical, and biological properties of biosynthetic human insulin. *Diabetes Care* 1981;4:147.

75. Johnson IS: Human insulin from recombinant DNA technology. *Science* 1983;219:632.

76. Frank BH, Pettee JM, Zimmerman RE, *et al*: The production of human proinsulin and its transformation to human insulin and C-peptide. In: Rich DH, Gross E, eds. *Peptides: Synthesis—Structure—Function.* Proceedings of the Seventh American Peptide Symposium. Pierce Chemical Company:1981;729.

77. Chance RE, Frank BH: Research, development, production, and safety of biosynthetic human insulin. *Diabetes Care* 1993;16(Suppl 3):133.

78. Markussen J, Damgaard U, Diers I, *et al*: Biosynthesis of human insulin in yeast via single-chain precursors. In: Theodoropoulos D, ed. *Peptides 1986.* de Gruyter:1987;189.

79. Chawdhury SA, Dodson EJ, Dodson GG, *et al*: The crystal structures of three non-pancreatic human insulins. *Diabetologia* 1983;25:460.

80. Brange J, Owens DR, Kang S, *et al*: Monomeric insulins and their experimental and clinical implications. *Diabetes Care* 1990;13:923.

81. Home PD, Massi-Benedetti M, Shepherd GAA, *et al*: A comparison of the activity and disposal of semi-synthetic human insulin and porcine insulin in normal man by the glucose clamp technique. *Diabetologia* 1982;22:41.

82. Heinemann L, Richter B: Clinical pharmacology of human insulin. *Diabetes Care* 1993;16(Suppl 3):90.

83. Heine RJ, Bilo HJG, Fonk T, *et al*: Absorption kinetics and action profiles of mixtures of short- and intermediate-acting insulins. *Diabetologia* 1984;27:558.

84. Galloway JA, Root MA, Bergstrom R, *et al*: Clinical pharmacologic studies with human insulin (recombinant DNA). *Diabetes Care* 1982; 5:13.

85. Berger M, Cüppers HJ, Hegner H, *et al*: Absorption kinetics and biological effects of subcutaneously injected insulin preparations. *Diabetes Care* 1982;5:77.

86. Gardner DF, Arakaki RF, Podet EJ, *et al*: The pharmacokinetics of subcutaneous regular insulin in type I diabetic patients: assessment using a glucose clamp technique. *J Clin Endocrinol Metab* 1986;64: 689.

87. Olsson PO, Arnqvist H, von Schenck H: Free insulin profiles in insulin-dependent diabetics treated with one or two insulin injections per day. *Acta Med Scand* 1986;220:133.

88. Bilo HJG, Heine RJ, Sikkenk AC, *et al*: Absorption kinetics and action profiles of intermediate acting human insulins. *Diabetes Res* 1987;4:39.

89. Starke AAR, Heinemann L, Hohmann A, *et al*: The action profiles of human NPH insulin preparations. *Diabetic Med* 1989;6:239.

90. Seigler DE, Olsson GM, Agramonte RF, *et al*: Pharmacokinetics of long-acting (ultralente) insulin preparations. *Diabetes Nutr Metab* 1991;4:267.

91. Woodworth JR, Howey DC, Bowsher RR: Establishment of time-action profiles for regular and NPH insulin using pharmacodynamic modeling. *Diabetes Care* 1994;17:64.

92. Roy B, Chou MCY, Field JB: Time-action characteristics of regular and NPH insulin in insulin treated diabetics. *J Clin Endocrinol Metab* 1980;50:475.

93. Galloway JA, Chance RE: Approaches to insulin analogues. In: Marshall SM, Home PD, eds. *The Diabetes Annual/8*. Elsevier Science BV:1994;277.

94. Selam J-L, Charles MA: Devices for insulin administration. *Diabetes Care* 1990;13:955.

95. Tunbridge FKE, Newens A, Home PD, *et al*: A comparison of human ultralente- and lente-based twice-daily injection regimens. *Diabet Med* 1989;6;496.

96. Johnson NB, Kronz KK, Fineberg NS, *et al*: Twice-daily humulin ultralente insulin decreases morning fasting hyperglycemia. *Diabetes Care* 1992;15;1031.

97. Yip CM, DeFelippis MR, Frank BH, *et al*: Structural and morphological characterization of ultralente insulin crystals by atomic force microscopy: Evidence of hydrophobically driven assembly. *Biophys J* 1998;75:1172.

98. Dimitriadis GD, Gerich JE: Importance of timing of preprandial subcutaneous insulin administration in the management of diabetes mellitus. *Diabetes Care* 1983;6:374.

99. Lean MEJ, Ng LL, Tennison BR: Interval between insulin injection and eating in relation to blood glucose control in adult diabetics. *Br Med J* 1985;290:105.

100. Hildebrandt P, Sestoft L, Nielsen SL, *et al*: The absorption of subcutaneously injected short-acting soluble insulin: Influence of injection technique and concentration. *Diabetes Care* 1983;6:459.

101. Binder C, Lauritzen T, Faber O, *et al*: Insulin pharmacokinetics. *Diabetes Care* 1984;7:188.

102. Galloway JA, Spradlin CT, Jackson RL, *et al*: Mixtures of intermediate-acting insulin (NPH and Lente) with regular insulin: An update. In: Skyler JS, ed. *Insulin Update*. Excerpta Medica:1982;111.

103. Thow JC, Johnson AB, Antsiferov M, *et al*: Effect of raising injection-site skin temperature on isophane (NPH) insulin crystal dissociation. *Diabetes Care* 1989;12:432.

104. Thow JC, Johnson AB, Fulcher G, *et al*: Different absorption of isophane (NPH) insulin from subcutaneous and intramuscular sites suggests a need to reassess recommended insulin injection technique. *Diabetic Med* 1990;7:600.

105. Henriksen JE, Vaag A, Hansen IR, *et al*: Absorption of NPH (isophane) insulin in resting diabetic patients: Evidence for subcutaneous injection in the thigh as the preferred site. *Diabetic Med* 1991;8:453.

106. DeFelippis MR, Bakaysa DL, Bell MA, *et al*: Preparation and characterization of a cocrystalline suspension of $[Lys^{B28}, Pro^{B29}]$-human insulin analogue. *J Pharm Sci* 1998;87:170.

107. Brange J, Ribel U, Hansen JF, *et al*: Monomeric insulins obtained by protein engineering and their medical implications. *Nature* 1988;333:679.

108. Brems DN, Alter LA, Beckage MJ, *et al*: Altering the association properties of insulin by amino acid replacement. *Protein Eng* 1992;5:527.

109. Brange J, Langkjaer L: Chemical stability of insulin. 3. Influence of excipients, formulation, and pH. *Acta Pharm Nord* 1992;4:149.

110. Brange J, Andersen L, Laursen ED, *et al*: Toward understanding insulin fibrillation. *J Pharm Sci* 1997;86:517.

111. Brange J, Havelund S, Hommel E, *et al*: Neutral insulin solutions physically stabilized by addition of Zn^{2+}. *Diabetic Med* 1986;3:532.

112. Bakaysa DL, Radziuk J, Havel HA, *et al*: Physicochemical basis for the rapid time-action of $Lys^{B28}Pro^{B29}$-insulin: Dissociation of a protein-ligand complex. *Protein Sci* 1996;5:2521.

113. Hildebrandt P, Sejrsen P, Nielsen SL, *et al*: Diffusion and polymerization determines the insulin absorption from subcutaneous tissue in diabetic patients. *Scand J Clin Lab Invest* 1985;45:685.

114. Owens DR, Zinman B, Bolli GB: Insulins today and beyond. *Lancet* 2001;358:739.

115. Anderson JH Jr., Koivisto VA: Clinical studies on insulin lispro. *Drugs Today* 1998;34(Suppl C):37.

116. Long HB, Baker JC, Belagaje RM, *et al*: Human insulin analogs with rapid onset and short duration of action. In: Smith JA, Rivier JE, eds. *Peptides. Chemistry and Biology*. Proceedings of the Twelfth American Peptide Symposium, June 16–21, 1991, Cambridge, MA. ESCOM:1992;88.

117. DiMarchi RD, Mayer JP, Fan L, *et al*: Synthesis of a fast-acting insulin based on structural homology with insulin-like growth factor I. In: Smith JA, Rivier JE, eds. *Peptides. Chemistry and Biology*. Proceedings of the Twelfth American Peptide Symposium, June 16–21, 1991, Cambridge, MA. ESCOM:1992;26.

118. Howey DC, Bowsher RR, Brunelle RL, *et al*: [Lys(B28), Pro(B29)]-human insulin. A rapidly absorbed analogue of human insulin, *Diabetes* 1994;43:396.

119. Chance RE, Frank BH, Radziuk JM, *et al*: Discovery and development of insulin lispro. *Drugs Today* 1998;34(Suppl C):1.

120. Llewelyn J, Slieker LJ, Zimmermann JL: Preclinical studies on insulin lispro. *Drugs Today* 1998;34(Suppl. C):11.

121. Heinemann, Woodworth J: Pharmacokinetics and glucodynamics of insulin lispro. *Drugs Today* 1998;34(Suppl C):23.

122. Heinemann L, Heise T, Wahl L Ch, *et al*: Prandial glycemia after a carbohydrate-rich meal in type I diabetic patients: using the rapid acting insulin analogue [Lys(B28), Pro(B29)] human insulin. *Diabetic Med* 1996;13:625.

123. Schernthaner G, Wein W, Sandholzer K, *et al*: Postprandial insulin lispro. A new therapeutic option for type 1 diabetic patients. *Diabetes Care* 1998;21:570.

124. Fineberg NS, Fineberg SE, Anderson JH, *et al*: Immunologic effects of insulin lispro [Lys(B28), Pro(B29) human insulin] in IDDM and NIDDM patients previously treated with insulin. *Diabetes* 1996;45:1750.

125. Tsui E, Barnie A, Ross S, *et al*: Intensive insulin therapy with insulin lispro. *Diabetes Care* 2001;24:1722.

126. Janssen MMJ, Casteleijn S, Devillé W, *et al*: Nighttime insulin kinetics and glycemic control in type 1 diabetic patients following administration of an intermediate-acting lispro preparation. *Diabetes Care* 1997;20:1870.

127. Heise T, Weyer C, Serwas A, *et al*: Time-action profiles of novel premixed preparations of insulin lispro and NPL insulin. *Diabetes Care* 1998;21:800.

128. Koivisto VA, Tuominen JA, Ebeling P: Lispro Mix25 insulin as premeal therapy in type 2 diabetic patients. *Diabetes Care* 1999;22:459.

129. Roach P, Yue L, Arora V, *et al*: Improved postprandial glycemic control during treatment with Humalog Mix25, a novel protamine-based insulin lispro formulation. *Diabetes Care* 1999;22:1258.

130. Whittingham JL, Edwards DJ, Antson AA, *et al*: Interactions of phenol and m-cresol in the insulin hexamer, and their effect on the association properties of B28 Pro → Asp insulin analogues. *Biochemistry* 1998;37:11516.

131. Kang S, Brange J, Burch A, *et al*: Subcutaneous insulin absorption explained by insulin's physicochemical properties. Evidence from absorption studies of soluble human insulin and insulin analogues in humans. *Diabetes Care* 1991;14:942.

132. Kang S, Brange J, Burch A, *et al*: Absorption kinetics and action profiles of subcutaneously administered insulin analogues (AspB9GluB27, AspB10, AspB28) in healthy subjects. *Diabetes Care* 1991;14:1057.

133. Heinemann L, Heise T, Jørgensen LN, *et al*: Action profile of the rapid acting insulin analogue B28Asp. *Diabetic Med* 1993;10:535.

134. Heinemann L, Heise T, Ampudia J, *et al*: Action profile of rapid-acting human insulin analogues. In: Berger M, Gries FA, eds. *Frontiers in Insulin Pharmacology*. Thieme Medical Publishers:1993;87.

135. Heinemann L, Kapitza C, Starke AAR, *et al*: Time-action profile of the insulin analogue B28Asp. *Diabetic Med* 1996;13:683.

136. Heinemann L, Weyer C, Rave K, *et al*: Comparison of the time-action profiles of U40- and U100-regular human insulin and the rapid-acting insulin analogue B28 Asp. *Exp Clin Endocrinol Diabetes* 1997;105:140.

137. Heinemann L, Weyer C, Rauhaus M, *et al*: Variability of the metabolic effect of soluble insulin and the rapid-acting insulin analog insulin aspart. *Diabetes Care* 1998;21:1910.

138. Home PD, Barriocanal L, Lindholm A: Comparative pharmacokinetics and pharmacodynamics of the novel rapid-acting insulin analogue, insulin aspart, in healthy volunteers. *Eur J Clin Pharmacol* 1999;55: 199.

139. Mudaliar SR, Lindberg FA, Joyce M, *et al*: Insulin aspart (B28 Asp-Insulin): a fast-acting analog of human insulin. *Diabetes Care* 1999;22:1501.

140. Lindholm A, Jacobsen LV: Clinical pharmacokinetics and pharmaco-dynamics of insulin aspart. *Clin Pharmacokinet* 2001;40:641.

141. Kang S, Creagh FM, Peters JR, *et al*: Comparison of subcutaneous soluble human insulin and insulin analogues (AspB9, GluB27; AspB10; AspB28) on meal-related plasma glucose excursions in type I diabetic subjects. *Diabetes Care* 1991;14:571.

142. Owens DR, Kang S, Luzio S, *et al*: Clinical results of phase I studies with insulin analogues. In: Berger M, Gries FA, eds. *Frontiers in Insulin Pharmacology*. Thieme Medical Publishers:1993;79.

143. Wiefels K, Kuglin B, Hübinger A, *et al*: Insulin kinetics and dynamics in insulin-dependent diabetic patients after injections of human insulin or insulin analogues X14 and X14 + Zn. In: Berger M, Gries FA, eds. *Frontiers in Insulin Pharmacology*. Thieme Medical Publishers:1993;97.

144. Wiefels K, Hübinger A, Dannehl K, *et al*: Insulinkinetic and -dynamic in diabetic patients under insulin pump therapy after injections of human insulin or the insulin analogue (B28Asp). *Horm Metab Res* 1995;27:421.

145. Home PD, Lindholm A, Hylleberg B, *et al*: Improved glycemic control with insulin aspart. A multicenter randomized double-blind crossover trial in type 1 diabetic patients. UK Insulin Aspart Study Group. *Diabetes Care* 1998;21:1904.

146. Lindholm A, McEwen J, Riis AP: Improved postprandial glycemic control with insulin aspart. A randomized double-blind cross-over trial in type 1 diabetes. *Diabetes Care* 1999;22:801.

147. Rosenfalck AM, Thorsby P, Kjems L, *et al*: Improved postprandial glycaemic control with insulin aspart in diabetic patients treated with insulin. *Acta Diabetol* 2000;37:41.

148. Home PD, Lindholm A, Riis A, *et al*: Insulin aspart vs. human insulin in the management of long-term glucose control in type 1 diabetes mellitus: a randomized controlled trial. *Diabetic Med* 2000;17:762.

149. Raskin P, Guthrie RA, Leiter L, *et al*: Use of insulin aspart, a fast-acting insulin analog, as the mealtime insulin in the management of patients with type 1 diabetes. *Diabetes Care* 2000;23:583.

150. Bolli GB: Physiological insulin replacement in type 1 diabetes mellitus. *Exp Clin Endocrinol Diabetes* 2001;109(Suppl 2):S317.

151. Bode BW, Strange P: Efficacy, safety, and pump compatibility of insulin aspart used in subcutaneous insulin infusion therapy in patients with type 1 diabetes. *Diabetes Care* 2001;24:69.

152. Weyer C, Heise T, Heinemann L: Insulin aspart in a 30/70 premixed formulation. Pharmacodynamic properties of a rapid-acting insulin analog in stable mixture. *Diabetes Care* 1997;20:1612.

153. Jacobsen LV, Sogaard B, Riis A: Pharmacokinetics and pharmacody-namics of a premixed formulation of soluble and protamine-retarded insulin aspart. *Eur J Clin Pharmacol* 2000;56:399.

154. Hedman CA, Lindstrom T, Arnqvist HJ: Direct comparison of insulin lispro and aspart shows different plasma insulin profiles after subcuta-neous injection in type 1 diabetes. *Diabetes Care* 2001;24:1120.

155. Hutton JC: Insulin secretory granule biogenesis and the proinsulin-processing endopeptidases. *Diabetologia* 1994;37(Suppl 2):S48.

156. Brange J: Chemical stability of insulin. 4. Mechanisms and kinetics of chemical transformations in pharmaceutical formulation. *Acta Pharmaceutica Nordica* 1992;4:209.

157. Berchtold H, Hilgenfeld R: Binding of phenol to R_6 insulin hexamers. *Biopolymers* 1999;51:165.

158. Heinemann L, Linkeschova R, Rave K, *et al*: Time-action profile of the long-acting insulin analog insulin glargine (HOE901) in compari-son with those of NPH insulin and placebo. *Diabetes Care* 2000;23:644.

159. Owens DR, Coates PA, Luzio SD, *et al*: Pharmacokinetics of ^{125}I-labeled insulin glargine (HOE 901) in healthy men. Comparison with NPH insulin and the influence of different subcutaneous injection sites. *Diabetes Care* 2000;23:813.

160. Pieber TR, Eugène-Jolchine I, Derobert E: Efficacy and safety of HOE 901 versus NPH insulin in patients with type 1 diabetes. The Eu-ropean Study Group of HOE 901 in type 1 diabetes. *Diabetes Care* 2000;23:157.

161. Mohn A, Strang S, Wernicke-Panten K, *et al*: Nocturnal glucose con-trol and free insulin levels in children with type 1 diabetes by use of the long-acting insulin HOE 901 as part of a three-injection regimen. *Diabetes Care* 2000;23:557.

162. Ratner RE, Hirsch IB, Neifing JL, *et al*: Less hypoglycemia with in-sulin glargine in intensive insulin therapy for type 1 diabetes. *Diabetes Care* 2000;23:639.

163. Rosenstock J, Park G, Zimmerman J, *et al*: Basal insulin glargine (HOE 901) versus NPH insulin in patients with type 1 diabetes on multiple daily insulin regimens. *Diabetes Care* 2000;23:1666.

164. Bolli GB, Owens DR: Insulin glargine. *Lancet* 2000;356:443.

165. Raskin P, Klaff L, Bergenstal R, *et al*: A 16-week comparison of the novel insulin analog insulin glargine (HOE 901) and NPH human insulin used with insulin lispro in patients with type 1 diabetes. *Diabetes Care* 2000;23:1666.

166. Lepore M, Pampanelli S, Fanelli C, *et al*: Pharmacokinetics and pharmacodynamics of subcutaneous injection of long-acting human insulin analog glargine, NPH insulin, and Ultralente human insulin and continuous subcutaneous infusion of insulin lispro. *Diabetes* 2000;49:2142.

167. Yki-Jarvinen H, Dressler A, Zieman M: Less nocturnal hypoglycemia and better post-dinner glucose control with bedtime insulin glargine compared with bedtime NPH insulin during insulin combination ther-apy in type 2 diabetes. *Diabetes Care* 2000;23:1130.

168. Rosenstock J, Schwartz SL, Clark CM Jr., *et al*: Basal insulin therapy in type 2 diabetes. *Diabetes Care* 200124:631.

169. Bolli GB: Physiological insulin replacement in type 1 diabetes melli-tus. *Exp Clin Endocrinol Diabetes* 2001;109(Suppl 2):S317.

170. Guthrie R: Is there a need for a better basal insulin? *Clinical Diabetes* 2001;19:66.

171. Hermansen K, Madsbad S, Perrild H, *et al*: Comparison of the soluble basal insulin analog insulin detemir with NPH insulin. *Diabetes Care* 2001;24:296.

172. Whittingham JL, Havelund S, Jonassen I: Crystal structure of a prolonged-acting insulin with albumin-binding properties. *Biochem-istry* 1997;36:2826.

173. Markussen J, Havelund S, Kurtzhals P, *et al*: Soluble, fatty acid acylated insulins bind to albumin and show protracted action in pigs. *Diabetologia* 1996;39:281.

174. Heinemann L, Sinha K, Weyer C, *et al*: Time-action profile of the sol-uble, fatty acid acylated, long-acting insulin analogue NN304. *Dia-betic Med* 1999;16:332.

CHAPTER 29

Intensive Management of Type 1 Diabetes Mellitus

Suzanne M. Strowig

Philip Raskin

INTRODUCTION

The results of the Diabetes Control and Complications Trial (DCCT) resolved any ambiguity regarding the relationship between glycemic control and diabetic microvascular and neuropathic complications.[1] The DCCT showed that an intensive diabetes treatment program that resulted in near-normal glycosylated hemoglobin levels significantly delayed the development and progression of the microvascular complications of diabetes by about 50%. The lowering of the glycosylated hemoglobin level was associated with a curvilinear decrease in the progression of retinopathy (i.e., the lower the level of glycosylated hemoglobin, the less the risk of the development and progression of diabetic complications[2,3]). Based on these data, the DCCT Research Group recommended that intensive diabetes treatment be instituted in most individuals with type 1 diabetes mellitus (T1DM) with the goal of achieving glycemic levels as close to those of nondiabetic individuals as possible.

The value of intensive diabetes treatment was underscored by the recent publication of the findings in DCCT subjects 4 years after the trial ended.[4] At the conclusion of the DCCT, subjects who had received conventional therapy were advised to initiate an intensive insulin treatment program. All subjects received subsequent care from their own physicians, and most were enrolled in the Epidemiology of Diabetes Interventions and Complications (EDIC) trial, a long-term observational study.[5] Although the glycosylated hemoglobin levels were significantly different between the intensively and conventionally treated subjects at the end of the DCCT (7.2% versus 9.1%, respectively), the HbA$_{1c}$ levels in both groups converged during the 4 years following the trial (intensive treatment group, 7.9%; conventional treatment group, 8.2%). Despite this, the subjects who received intensive therapy during the DCCT continued to have a lower risk of retinopathy and nephropathy at the end of year 4 of EDIC compared with those who received conventional therapy during the DCCT. This suggests that the beneficial effect of maintaining near-normal glycemic control persists long after the end of such therapy. Since the DCCT had previously shown that intensive therapy was most effective in preventing complications when introduced during the first 5 years of diabetes, it seems that intensive therapy should be implemented as early as is safely possible, and that such therapy be maintained for as long as possible.

INSULIN REGIMENS

The majority of this chapter describes intensive diabetes treatment techniques. However, since some individuals with T1DM may not be candidates for intensive diabetes treatment or may not be willing to accept the personal commitment inherent in such treatment, other insulin regimens, along with their indications, advantages, and disadvantages, are discussed. In general, insulin injection regimens consist of a combination of basal insulin (intermediate-acting insulin such as NPH or Lente™, or long-acting insulin such as Ultralente™) and short-acting (regular) or rapid-acting insulin (insulin lispro or insulin aspart). Short- or rapid-acting insulin is used before meals to control postprandial blood glucose levels.

Short- and Rapid-Acting Insulin

The optimal time to inject regular insulin to achieve ideal postprandial blood glucose levels is 30–60 minutes before meals. The peak effect of regular insulin is usually achieved 2–6 hours after injection, and its effects may last from 6 hours to as long as 16 hours.[6] However, since the peak glycemic response to a mixed meal has been found to be between 26 and 70 minutes after ingestion, regular insulin may peak too late to control postprandial blood glucose levels.[7] There is also the potential for hypoglycemia to occur several hours after the meal.

The rapid-acting insulin analogues insulin lispro and insulin aspart were developed by modifying the amino acid sequence or composition of the B chain of the insulin molecule. These alterations reduce the stability of the insulin monomer-monomer interaction, leading to a more rapid dissociation and subcutaneous absorption of the insulin.[8] With insulin lispro, lysine and proline at positions 28 and 29 of the B chain of the human insulin molecule have been reversed. In insulin aspart, the proline at position B28 has been replaced by aspartic acid. The pharmacokinetic effects of these modifications in the insulin molecule are: (1) The insulin is absorbed and eliminated faster than regular insulin, producing a shorter duration of action (3 hours versus 6 hours), and (2) the serum concentration peaks more than two times higher and in less than half the time (42 minutes versus 101 minutes) of regular insulin (Fig. 29-1).[9–12] Studies have shown that postprandial blood glucose levels are improved with the use of these insulin analogues,[13–18] although preprandial and fasting blood glucose levels

501

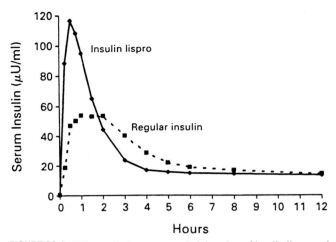

FIGURE 29-1. Effects of subcutaneous administration of insulin lispro and regular insulin on serum insulin concentrations. *(Reproduced with permission from Holleman et al.[9])*

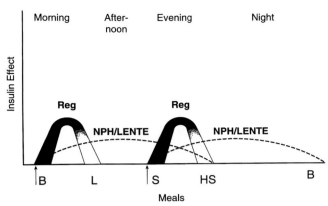

FIGURE 29-2. Representation of idealized periods of insulin effect for a split-and-mixed insulin regimen, consisting of two daily doses of short-acting (regular) and intermediate-acting insulin. Symbols: **B**, breakfast; **L**, lunch; **S**, supper; **HS**, bedtime; **arrows**, time of insulin injection 30 minutes before meal; **Reg**, regular or short-acting insulin effect; **NPH/LENTE**, intermediate-acting insulin effect. *(Reproduced with permission from Hirsch et al.[28])*

may be elevated because of the short duration of action. A reduction in the frequency of hypoglycemia[13,19–21] and an improvement in patient satisfaction[19,22] have been reported with the use of rapid-acting insulin.

There are several clinical considerations associated with the use of rapid-acting insulin. Since the onset of action is fairly rapid, insulin lispro and insulin aspart can be taken within 15 minutes before the meal.[23] Because of its short duration of action, more basal insulin is usually required to control preprandial and fasting blood glucose levels.[24,25] A morning and evening injection of intermediate- or long-acting insulin is usually necessary. Patients may not require between-meal snacks, and in fact may need additional injections of rapid-acting insulin if snacks are desired.[26]

Some practitioners compensate for the shorter duration of action associated with rapid-acting insulin by combining it with regular insulin before meals. At present, there is no evidence to suggest that this combination of insulin provides improved blood glucose control.[27]

Twice-Daily Insulin Injections

Single daily doses of insulin rarely result in 24-hour glycemic control, and are not recommended. A twice-daily insulin injection regimen is usually given as a combination of short- (regular) or rapid-acting (lispro or aspart) insulin and intermediate-acting (NPH or Lente) insulin before breakfast and supper. This regimen provides insulin availability for each meal plus sustained insulin action overnight (Fig. 29-2). The total daily dose of insulin is often determined by body weight, usually between 0.5 and 1.0 U/kg per day.[28] Generally, two-thirds of the total daily dose is given in the morning before breakfast, and one-third is given in the evening before supper, with each injection consisting of two-thirds intermediate-acting insulin and one-third short- or rapid-acting insulin. An insulin algorithm can be employed to adjust the regular insulin or rapid-acting insulin analogues based on prebreakfast and presupper blood glucose levels.

Insulin with a premixed ratio of intermediate- (i.e., NPH) and short- or rapid-acting insulin is available for patients who have physical and cognitive limitations. A patient can draw up a single

dose of insulin from one vial of 70/30 insulin that consists of 70% NPH and 30% regular insulin, or of 75/25 insulin that consists of 75% NPL (neutral protamine lispro) and 25% insulin lispro. Although these mixtures are easy to use, they decrease the flexibility of dose adjustments. For example, 30 units of 70/30 insulin taken before breakfast may contain a sufficient amount of intermediate-acting insulin (21 units) to control presupper blood glucose concentrations, but may provide too much short-acting insulin (9 units) to control prelunch blood glucose levels, resulting in hypoglycemia before lunch. Lowering the dose of 70/30 insulin would correct the hypoglycemia before lunch, but would result in hyperglycemia before supper. In this situation, the patient, if capable, would need to individually draw up the intermediate- and short- or rapid-acting insulin and mix in one syringe.

Adjustments in the short- or rapid-acting insulin component of the prebreakfast dose are made based on the subsequent examination of postbreakfast and prelunch blood glucose concentrations. Changes in the intermediate-acting insulin component of the prebreakfast dose are based on the examination of presupper blood glucose concentrations. Similarly, the subsequent examinations of postsupper and bedtime blood glucose levels determine changes in the short- or rapid-acting insulin component of the presupper insulin dose, whereas the fasting and 3 AM blood glucose levels are used to make changes in the intermediate-acting component of the presupper insulin dose. Insulin dosages should be changed by 10–20% whenever an adjustment is indicated. Once done, it is best to wait several days before making further changes.

Although twice-daily mixed insulin provides adequate insulin availability throughout the day, there are several pitfalls to this regimen. Hypoglycemia late in the afternoon and in the middle of the night related to intermediate acting insulin frequently occurs, especially with the new formulations of biosynthetic human insulin, which have a shorter duration of action than the animal insulins used in the past. Prebreakfast hyperglycemia can also occur because insulin action wanes. Attempts to decrease morning hyperglycemia by increasing the presupper dose of intermediate-acting insulin may only aggravate the frequency and severity of nocturnal hypoglycemia. Correcting prebreakfast hyperglycemia can be resolved by taking the evening dose of intermediate-acting insulin at bedtime. Of course, the patient must now take three insulin injections daily (Fig. 29-3).

A twice-daily insulin injection plan is the least flexible regimen. Insulin must be taken at approximately the same time every day (± 1 hour). Failure to do this creates periods of insulin deficiency and periods of overinsulinization when insulin action overlaps. Meal times must also be consistent since food must be eaten when insulin action peaks. Problems in blood glucose control may result when the patient sleeps late, travels, changes work hours, or eats out. When diabetic patients have a lifestyle that demands flexibility, this regimen is often difficult to manage, and a more intensive regimen involving three or more injections per day or an insulin pump has distinct advantages.

Multiple Daily Insulin Injections

Multiple daily injection (MDI) regimens can be done in a variety of ways. Three injections per day using a mixture of intermediate- and short- or rapid-acting insulin before breakfast, short- or rapid-acting insulin before supper, and intermediate-acting insulin at bedtime can be effective for diabetic patients who experience frequent nocturnal hypoglycemia and prebreakfast hyperglycemia using only two injections per day (Fig. 29-3). This regimen also provides additional control and flexibility for those who do not wish to use the more intensive injection schedules. It may be most suited to individuals who desire better glycemic control and/or flexibility but do not wish to take or frequently forget the prelunch injection. This is often the case in children and adolescents who may find it difficult to take a prelunch injection while at school.

Four daily insulin injections using short- or rapid-acting insulin before each meal and intermediate- or long-acting insulin once or twice a day allows patients more flexibility. A regimen of four daily injections using intermediate-acting insulin at bedtime (Fig. 29-4) avoids problems associated with peak afternoon insulin activity from an injection of intermediate-acting insulin taken before breakfast. Short-acting insulin can be adjusted to adequately

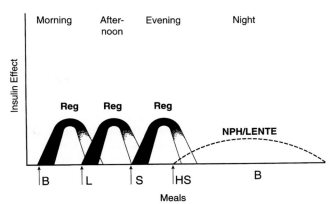

FIGURE 29-4. *Representation of idealized periods of insulin effect for a multiple dosage regimen providing short-acting (regular) insulin before each meal and intermediate-acting insulin at bedtime. Symbols:* **B**, *breakfast;* **L**, *lunch;* **S**, *supper;* **HS**, *bedtime;* **arrows**, *time of insulin injection 30 minutes before meal;* **Reg**, *regular or short-acting insulin effect;* **NPH/LENTE**, *intermediate-acting insulin effect. (Reproduced with permission from Hirsch et al.[28])*

cover each meal, thus controlling postprandial hyperglycemia and facilitating better overall glycemic control throughout the day. However, if rapid-acting insulin (insulin lispro or insulin aspart) is used before meals instead of short-acting insulin, a morning injection of intermediate-acting insulin in addition to the bedtime injection of intermediate-acting insulin will likely be needed. More basal insulin is required when rapid-acting insulin is used because of the short duration of action.[24,25]

Ultralente insulin can be used in MDI regimens in place of intermediate-acting insulin to meet basal insulin needs (Fig. 29-5). Ultralente insulin can be given as one injection in the morning, but is usually divided so that half the dose is taken before breakfast and the other half before supper (preferable when rapid-acting insulin is given before meals). Short- or rapid-acting insulin is given before each meal to provide meal-related insulinemia. Ultralente insulin is considered a sustained, long-acting "peakless" insulin that can provide effective basal insulinemia. There is evidence to

FIGURE 29-3. *Representation of idealized periods of insulin effect for a three-injection-a-day regimen in which split-and-mixed dose is given in the morning, short-acting (regular) insulin before supper, and intermediate-acting insulin is delayed until bedtime. Symbols:* **B**, *breakfast;* **L**, *lunch;* **S**, *supper;* **HS**, *bedtime;* **arrows**, *time of insulin injection 30 minutes before meal;* **Reg**, *regular or short-acting insulin effect;* **NPH/LENTE**, *intermediate-acting insulin effect. (Reproduced with permission from Hirsch et al.[28])*

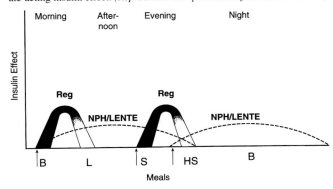

FIGURE 29-5. *Representation of idealized periods of insulin effect for a multiple dosage regimen using premeal short-acting (regular) insulin and basal insulin as Ultralente. Symbols:* **B**, *breakfast;* **L**, *lunch;* **S**, *supper;* **HS**, *bedtime;* **arrows**, *time of insulin injection 30 minutes before meal;* **Reg**, *regular or short-acting insulin effect. (Reproduced with permission from Hirsch et al.[28])*

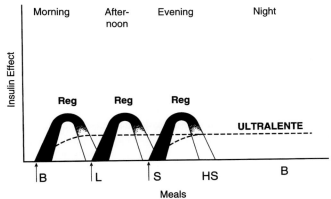

suggest, however, that small peaks in its action occur 15–24 hours after injection, particularly with newer human preparations.[29,30] Since small peaks in the activity of Ultralente insulin are difficult to predict, regimens using Ultralente insulin may be less preferable to those using intermediate-acting insulin.

Insulin analogues that provide more effective basal insulin delivery may make MDI regimens even more successful at achieving glycemic goals. Insulin glargine, recently approved by the FDA, results from two modifications of human insulin. Two arginine molecules which are positively charged are added at the C terminus of the B chain. The aspargine molecule at position 21 in the A chain is replaced by glycine. This leads to a shift of the isoelectric point that results in precipitation at the neutral pH of subcutaneous tissue and thus delayed absorption.[31] Insulin glargine is peakless, lasts nearly 24 hours, and has lower intersubject variability than NPH and Ultralente insulin.[30,32] Studies have shown that insulin glargine given once daily results in lower fasting blood glucose levels and a comparable or lower incidence of hypoglycemia compared with intermediate-acting insulin given one or more times daily.[33,34] Insulin glargine is a clear solution at a pH of 4.0 and cannot be diluted or mixed in a syringe with any other insulin. Patients who are switching from once-daily doses of NPH or Ultralente insulin to a once-daily bedtime dose of insulin glargine should start on the same dose of insulin glargine as was previously used while on intermediate or Ultralente insulin. Patients being switched from twice-daily doses of NPH or Ultralente insulin to a once-daily bedtime dose of insulin glargine should have their insulin glargine dose reduced by 20% from the previous total daily dose of NPH or Ultralente insulin.

Other insulin analogues for basal insulin delivery are under development. One such analogue is insulin detemir, which is created by acylation of LysB29 with a saturated fatty acid, and by removing the amino acid residue at position B30. This analogue has a high affinity for albumin, which results in a delay in the absorption of insulin and a prolonged duration of action.

When four-injection regimens are used, insulin adjustments are made based on blood glucose levels obtained before and after meals, before bed, and periodically at 3 AM. Changes in the bedtime intermediate or long-acting (Glargine)* insulin are based on 3 AM and fasting blood glucose levels. The morning intermediate-acting insulin is adjusted based on the mid- to late-afternoon and presupper blood glucose reading. The premeal short- or rapid-acting insulin doses are adjusted based on the postprandial and premeal blood glucose levels that follow that injection (i.e., the prelunch insulin dose is adjusted based on the blood glucose level after lunch and before supper).

Despite the increased flexibility that multiple insulin injection regimens offer, injections of short-acting insulin should be given within 4–6 hours of one another. Skipping meals and/or injections of short-acting insulin usually results in loss of blood glucose control, although this may be less of a problem with new long-acting insulin analogues. Maintaining this degree of consistency may be a limiting factor for some individuals. In addition, some patients may object to frequent needle injections or having to carry syringes and bottles of insulin with them. Pen-like devices are available (self-contained pens of insulin with a needle attached) that enable a patient to simply dial the desired dose and inject the insulin with relative ease. These devices are simple to use and handy to carry, and may help patients more successfully implement a multiple daily insulin injection regimen.

Inhaled insulin, currently under investigation, may be an option in the future to facilitate implementation of multiple daily doses of insulin. Aerosolized dry powder insulin is inhaled via a device that enhances inhalation and absorption of the insulin through the alveoli of the lungs. The inhaled insulin is a short-acting insulin that can be administered before meals; intermediate- or long-acting insulin must be given via subcutaneous needle injection one or two times daily in addition to the inhaled insulin. Onset of action and maximal action of inhaled insulin appear to occur sooner than subcutaneously administered regular insulin.[35] Preliminary reports suggest that inhaled insulin results in at least comparable levels of glycemic control as subcutaneous insulin.[36] The effect of inhaled insulin on pulmonary function continues to be investigated.

Method for Determining Initial Insulin Dosages for MDI Regimens

The total amount of intermediate-(NPH/Lente) or long-acting (Glargine) insulin at bedtime should be 35–50% of the patient's total daily dose. The total dose of NPH/Lente or ultralente insulin can be divided so that 30–40% is given before breakfast, and the remainder is given at bedtime. This is recommended if rapid-acting insulin instead of short-acting insulin is given before meals. The amount of short-acting insulin before each meal can be calculated as a percentage of the total daily dose as follows: breakfast, 20–25%; lunch, 10–15%; dinner, 15–20%; and bedtime, 3–5%.

For example, an insulin regimen consisting of NPH 20 units and regular 10 units before breakfast and NPH 10 units and regular 5 units before dinner could be converted to a four-injection-per-day regimen as follows:

Bedtime NPH insulin:	40% of 45 units (.40 × 45) = 18 units
Regular insulin:	Breakfast, 9 units (45 × .20)
	Lunch, 7 units (45 × .15)
	Dinner, 9 units (45 × .20)
	Bedtime snack, 2 units (45 × .05)

Premeal dosages of short- or rapid-acting insulin can also be calculated based on the patient's dietary intake using the guidelines described below for insulin pump therapy (i.e., 1–2 units per 10–15 grams of carbohydrate). When a patient switches from short-acting insulin (regular) to rapid-acting insulin (lispro), the dose of rapid-acting insulin may need to be reduced, and the dose of basal insulin (intermediate- or long-acting insulin) may need to be increased.

Continuous Subcutaneous Insulin Infusion

Continuous subcutaneous insulin infusion (CSII) is an alternative to MDI when the patient desires improved blood glucose control or greater flexibility in his or her regimen. Of all options, the insulin infusion device permits the greatest degree of lifestyle flexibility and can therefore facilitate achieving glycemic goals. The reasons for this are (1) the insulin pump uses only short- or rapid-acting insulin, making insulin absorption from subcutaneous tissues more predictable, and (2) insulin delivery is similar to that found in nondiabetic individuals since there is continuous basal insulin delivery supplemented by preprandial increases in plasma insulin levels (Fig. 29-6, Table 29-1).[37]

The pump contains a syringe or reservoir of insulin that connects to a catheter with a 27-gauge needle or teflon cannula at the end. The needle is inserted by the patient into subcutaneous tissue, usually in the abdomen. The user programs the insulin pump to deliver insulin in a basal mode, which is a continuous infusion of insulin usually ranging from 0.5–2.0 U/h. The basal rate is deliv-

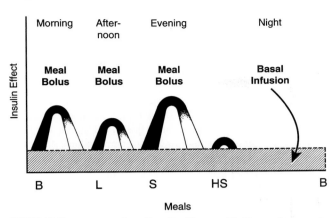

FIGURE 29-6. Representation of insulin effect provided by continuous subcutaneous insulin infusion. A continuous infusion (basal rate) is delivered, with premeal boluses administered before meals. Only short- or rapid-acting insulin is used. Symbols: **B**, breakfast; **L**, lunch; **S**, supper; **HS**, bedtime. *(Reproduced with permission from Hirsch et al.[28])*

ered automatically once programmed. Modern pumps provide the option of automatically delivering multiple different basal rates in a 24-hour period. The majority of patients require one to three basal rates per day, the alternate basal rates being adjusted for lower insulin needs at night or higher insulin needs in the predawn hours. The user programs each premeal bolus before eating.

Although CSII has many advantages, there are several potential problems unique to insulin pump therapy. Interruption of insulin delivery can result in hyperglycemia or ketoacidosis in a matter of hours since there is no depot insulin. Pump malfunction, a dead battery, leakage from the catheter or catheter connections, an empty insulin reservoir, needle displacement, and insulin aggregation in the catheter or in the needle inserted into the abdomen can result in cessation of insulin delivery. Patients must be taught to manage all of the technical components of CSII and be aware of how to deal with problems when they occur. With proper education and follow-up these problems can be avoided. Insulin pumps have alarm systems that warn of pump malfunction, a dead battery, an empty syringe, high pressure, and programming errors.

Another potential problem with CSII is infusion site infections where the needle is inserted. This can be avoided by maintaining good infusion site care and changing the needle every 1–2 days. Infusion site infections are usually resolved with oral antibiotics. Severe infections may have to be surgically incised and drained.

TABLE 29-1. Example of Variable Insulin Dosage Schedule for Insulin Infusion Pump Therapy (Short- or Rapid-Acting Insulin Only)

Blood Glucose (mg/dL)	Units of Insulin			
	Breakfast	Lunch	Supper	Bedtime Snack
<70	4	3	5	0
71–100	6	4	6	0
101–150	7	5	7	1
151–200	8	6	8	2
201–250	9	7	9	2
251–300	10	8	10	3
>300	12	10	12	4

Basal rate = 1.0 U/h.

Other considerations include personal issues related to pump use, such as how to wear the pump with different clothing, how to deal with special occasions, swimming, showering, personal intimacy, and involvement in sports activities. Pump wearers have the option of using a multiple daily insulin injection regimen for occasions when pump use is not desired.

There are three insulin pump manufacturers at present. Since pump technology is constantly changing, there are general characteristics to consider when selecting a pump. These include (1) pump size, (2) type of reservoir used, (3) power source (type of batteries needed), (4) ease of wear, (5) ease of programmability, (6) safety features and alarm systems, (7) special features such as number of programmable basal rates, bolus recall, temporary basal rate options, square wave bolus options, display, and resistance to moisture, (8) warranty, (9) availability of supplies for use with the pump, (10) cost, (11) level of support from the manufacturer for education and dealing with problems as they arise, and (12) record of durability over time. Implantable insulin pumps are under investigation.

Methods for Determining Initial Insulin Dosages for CSII

The insulin pump delivers insulin via a continuous basal rate, and via a bolus, which is a larger amount of insulin taken before a meal. The total 24-hour basal rate is usually 40–50% of the patient's total daily dose. The meal boluses can be estimated as a percentage of the total daily dose as follows: breakfast, 20%; lunch, 10%; dinner, 15%; and snack, 5%.[37] The basal rate should generally be no more than 60% of the patient's total daily dose. If the patient has reasonably good glycemic control, it is advised to take the prepump total daily dose and reduce it by 10% prior to calculating pump dosages since insulin requirements are often lower with insulin pump therapy.

For example, a starting insulin pump dose for a patient who is taking NPH 22 units and regular 8 units before breakfast, and NPH 10 units and regular 6 units before supper, for a total daily dose of 46 units, is as follows:

Basal rate: 46 × 50% (0.50 × 46) ÷ 24 hours = 1.0 U/h
Boluses: Breakfast, 9.0 units (46 × .20)
              Lunch, 4.5 units (46 × .10)
              Dinner, 7.0 units (46 × .15)
              Bedtime snack, 2.0 units (46 × 0.5)

An alternative way to calculate the total daily basal rate is to multiply the patient's weight in kilograms by 0.3. If the patient's weight was 80 kg (176 lb), the basal rate would be (80 × 0.3) ÷ 24 = 1.0 U/h. Assuming the basal rate was 50% of the total daily dose, the boluses would be calculated as above using 48 units as the total daily dose.

Patients using insulin pump therapy have the advantage of programming different basal rates for varying diurnal insulin needs. Patients often need lower basal rates between bedtime and 3:00–5:00 AM and higher basal rates between 3:00–9:00 AM to deal with the so-called "dawn phenomenon." An intermediate basal rate may be needed during the rest of the day. An adjustment of the basal rate by 10–20% is usually recommended. Using the example above, the basal rate profile might be as follows:

* 11:00 PM to 4:00 AM = 0.9 U/h
* 4:00 AM to 8:00 AM = 1.2 U/h
* 8:00 AM to 11:00 PM = 1.0 U/h

After calculating insulin boluses using the above formula, evaluate these starting dosages relative to the patient's meal plan. An average of 1 unit of short- or rapid-acting insulin will dispose of 10–15g of carbohydrate, with a range of 0.5–2.0 units. For a meal containing 60g of carbohydrate, a bolus dose of 4–6 units would be a reasonable place to start. Using the above example, if the breakfast meal plan consisted of 60g of carbohydrate, 9 units of short- or rapid-acting insulin might be too much and a lower starting bolus at breakfast may be indicated. Once initiated, careful blood glucose monitoring must be performed to determine the effectiveness of insulin dosages relative to the meal plan and the patient's usual activity level. Frequent adjustments in the starting insulin dose are usually required during the first 1–3 months of a new regimen.

INTENSIVE DIABETES MANAGEMENT

Intensive diabetes treatment is not simply multiple daily injections of insulin or insulin pump therapy. It is a goal-oriented, comprehensive approach to therapy that consists of frequent blood glucose self-monitoring and a systematic approach to quantifying food and matching insulin to food intake.[38] This treatment approach is designed to achieve near normoglycemia by enabling the patient to change aspects of the regimen as different situations are encountered through day-to-day life. Collaboration among team members including physicians, nurses, dietitians, and mental health professionals is essential.[39,40] Intensive diabetes self-management education is not a single event, but should be integrated into the ongoing care of the patient (see Tables 29-2, 29-4).

Patient Selection

Most patients with T1DM should be given the opportunity to intensify their diabetes treatment. The manner in which this is accomplished and the intensity of the treatment plan and the treatment goals will vary depending on a careful assessment of patient capabilities, resources, personal preferences, and the presence of known risk factors. Based on the results of the DCCT, any improvement in glycemic control will result in a reduction in risk for the development and progression of microvascular complications. However, since the greatest reduction in risk for long-term diabetic complications is accrued with glycosylated hemoglobin levels near the normal range, patients and health care providers need to strive for glycemic control as close to normal as is safely possible.[1,2]

There are patients in whom the risk:benefit ratio of intensive therapy may be less favorable.[1] The major adverse event associated with intensive diabetes treatment in the DCCT was a threefold increase in the risk for severe hypoglycemia.[41] Patients who have repeated severe hypoglycemia or hypoglycemia unawareness should pursue intensive therapy slowly and cautiously. Glycemic goals may need to be modified for these patients to avoid serious sequelae related to hypoglycemia.

The DCCT did not include subjects under 13 years of age. Thus intensive therapy should be implemented with greater caution in children after carefully assessing the child's capabilities and resources. Glycemic goals for children may also need to be modified to increase the safety of the treatment. Patients with advanced complications were not included in the DCCT cohort. Patients with coronary artery disease may be at a higher risk for severe sequelae

TABLE 29-2. Intensive Diabetes Treatment

Treatment plan:	Multiple daily insulin injections or insulin pump therapy
	Blood glucose monitoring 4–7 times daily
	Meal planning based on a systematic approach to quantifying food and matching insulin to food intake
Treatment goals:	Individualized based on capabilities and risk factors
	Ideal glycemic goals:
	Before meals 70–120 mg/dL
	After meals <180 mg/dL
	Bedtime 100–130 mg/dL
	3:00 AM > 70 mg/dL
	Glycated hemoglobin level: nondiabetic range for the assay performed
Characteristics:	Integrates insulin and food preferences into lifestyle practices
	Basic prescription that can be adjusted by the patient
	Liberal, flexible, adapts to changing circumstances, and allows for patient choice
Patient education:	Basic education initially—only what is necessary to implement the treatment plan
	Ongoing education is integrated into each office visit
	Focuses on self-care behaviors and relevant issues within the context of lifestyle practices and experiences
	Emphasizes patient problem solving and decision making
	Emphasizes a systematic approach to matching insulin, food, and exercise rather than a fixed regimen
Interventions:	Nursing, nutrition, behavioral, and medical interventions care provided at each office visit
	Once the treatment plan is prescribed, taught, and implemented, interventions become more behavioral, directed at enabling patients to follow treatment recommendations
Team collaboration:	Team consists of patient, nurse, dietitian, physician, and mental health professional
	Each member contributes equally and is part of the ongoing care of the patient; communication is open and ongoing
	Decisions are made jointly; a unified message is delivered to the patient

from hypoglycemia. In addition, patients with proliferative or severe nonproliferative retinopathy may be at higher risk for transiently accelerated progression of their retinopathy after the start of intensive therapy and should be followed closely by their ophthalmologists. It is unlikely that advanced complications such as renal failure will reverse with intensive therapy. In such patients, the adverse effects of intensive therapy often outweigh any potential benefit.

Once risk factors have been taken into account, the intensity of the treatment plan will depend on the patient's capabilities, motivation, and resources. Blood glucose monitoring at least four times daily is essential for intensive diabetes treatment to be implemented successfully and safely.[38,42] The choice of multiple daily insulin injections or insulin pump will depend on the patient's personal preferences and financial resources. Patients who are reluctant to pursue intensive therapy can implement aspects of an intensive treatment plan in an incremental fashion.[43,44] By making mutually negotiated small changes in the diabetes treatment plan, the patient can demonstrate capabilities and accept aspects of intensive therapy over time.

Methods for Adjusting Insulin Dosage

Insulin Dosage Adjustments Based on Blood Glucose Levels

Intensive treatment regimens commonly utilize insulin algorithms that adjust for premeal blood glucose levels. The algorithm in Table 29-1 assumes that a patient requires about 1.0 units of short- or rapid-acting insulin for every 50 mg/dL of blood glucose. Typically, patients require about 1 unit for every 40–50 mg/dL of blood glucose, but this varies depending on the patient's insulin sensitivity and daily insulin requirements. For example, a patient taking 20 units of insulin per day may require 0.5 units of short- or rapid-acting insulin per 50 mg/dL of blood glucose, whereas a patient taking 80 units of insulin per day may require 2 or 3 units per 50 mg/dL of blood glucose. Patients can also take a supplemental dose of rapid- or short-acting insulin to lower a high blood glucose level in the absence of food intake using the same guideline.[45] When short-acting (regular) insulin is used, taking it 45–60 minutes before a meal instead of 30 minutes may be required if the premeal blood glucose level is elevated.

If the premeal blood glucose level is below normal, patients will often wait less than 15 minutes to eat after administration of short-acting insulin to avoid further hypoglycemia. However, this approach increases the likelihood that postprandial hyperglycemia will occur. The ideal approach in this situation is for the patient to correct the hypoglycemia with a rapidly-absorbed source of carbohydrate and take the bolus or short-acting insulin injection 20–30 minutes before ingesting the meal, based on the corrected blood glucose reading. This situation does not pose a problem when rapid-acting insulin is used, since the patient can eat immediately after taking the insulin injection.

Insulin Dosage Adjustments Based on Food Intake

The American Diabetes Association prioritizes maintenance of near-normal blood glucose levels as the first goal of nutrition therapy,[46] and not necessarily meeting some ideal nutrient content. To achieve this goal, nutrition therapy must be tailored to the patient's lifestyle preferences, and patients should be taught to quantify food intake and adjust insulin for variations in food and exercise.[47–49] No food is prohibited; sucrose and starches have similar effects on glycemia. In addition, reasonable body weight is the level of weight individuals and health care providers acknowledge as achievable and maintainable, not an ideal body weight based on height and frame size.[46,48]

Several dietary approaches can be used to assist patients in quantifying food intake and plan meals. The exchange system is commonly used and involves planning meals based on food groups. Healthy Food Choices is a simplified version of the exchange system. This system can be made even simpler by converting the exchanges to what we refer to as starch equivalents.[37] One starch equivalent is equal to one starch, or one fruit, or one milk, or two meat, or three vegetable exchanges. Carbohydrate counting requires the patient to count grams of carbohydrate and estimate insulin dosage based on carbohydrate intake only. This system assumes a relatively consistent intake of protein and fat. Total available glucose (TAG) defines foods in terms of the amount of glucose derived from foods consumed. This approach assumes that 100% of calories from carbohydrate, 50% of calories from protein, and 10% of calories from fat will contribute to blood glucose.[49] TAG is the most complicated method for estimating food intake and may not be appropriate for most patients.

On average, patients need 1 unit of short- or rapid-acting insulin for every 15 g of carbohydrate (one starch exchange) consumed. However, this can range from 0.5–2.0 units per 15 g of carbohydrate. A more precise estimate of the patient's insulin needs per quantity of food can be determined when the patient achieves normal blood glucose levels while following a specific meal plan and insulin schedule. Prior to initiating a new intensive insulin regimen, the dietitian can create a meal plan based on a patient's 3- to 4-day food record. The meal plan should accurately reflect the patient's personal preferences and should not be based on some "ideal" nutrient content. The patient should follow the meal plan for at least 1 month, until desired blood glucose levels are achieved. During this time, the patient should keep detailed food and insulin records. The food records are useful to determine if the patient understands the meal plan and is quantifying food correctly. When the patient deviates from the meal plan, the food records can be used to teach the patient how to incorporate different foods into the meal plan or how to adjust the insulin for those foods. Food records also help patients identify relationships between food intake and blood glucose levels.

When desired blood glucose levels are achieved, the information from the food and insulin records can be used to determine the insulin dose required per quantity of food. For example, if a patient's meal plan at lunch consists of one fruit exchange, one milk exchange, three bread exchanges, two meat exchanges, and two fat exchanges (72 g of carbohydrate or 6 starch equivalents), and a prelunch insulin dose of 9 units of short- or rapid-acting insulin results in normal postprandial blood glucose levels, the patient requires 1 unit of insulin for every 8 g of carbohydrate or approximately 1.5 units per starch equivalent at lunch. The dosage per quantity of food can be separately calculated for breakfast and dinner, recognizing that insulin requirements may vary at different times of the day. Using this information, the patient can simply estimate the number of grams of carbohydrate or starch equivalents to be consumed at the meal and multiply by the number of units required per quantity of food. The investment of time during the first 2 months to match insulin to the meal plan and determine insulin needs per quantity of food is well worth the effort, as patients tire of the meal plan or encounter situations in which dietary intake will vary. Having a systematic approach to matching insulin to changes in dietary intake enables patients to have flexibility and still maintain near-normal blood glucose control.

Insulin Dosage Adjustments Based on Changes in Activity

Patients must learn to make adjustments in insulin or food intake for changes in activity to keep blood glucose levels near normal and to prevent hypoglycemia. If exercise is planned, insulin dosages can be adjusted. If exercise is unplanned, ingestion of additional carbohydrate will be necessary. Blood glucose testing before, during, and after the activity is recommended to monitor the patient's response to the exercise.[50,51] Special precautions may also be needed depending on the time of the activity. Exercise-induced hypoglycemia can occur many hours after the activity. Nocturnal hypoglycemia can actually occur in response to intense morning or afternoon exercise.[52,53]

Premeal short- or rapid-acting insulin can be decreased 25–50% for moderate levels of planned postprandial activity. If the activity is strenuous, the patient may need additional carbohydrate along with the reduction in premeal short- or rapid-acting insulin.[54] Patients using insulin pumps can temporarily lower the basal rate approximately 20–40% for sustained periods of exercise lasting over 60 minutes. A reduction in the basal rate by 25% during postexercise hours may be necessary to avoid postexercise hypoglycemia.[55] Suspending the basal rate for more than an hour is not recommended. For patients receiving morning NPH insulin, the morning dose of NPH may need to be reduced 15–25% for planned afternoon or evening exercise.[56] Activities such as yard work, shopping, and housework are common events in patients' lives that frequently result in episodes of hypoglycemia. Patients may need to reduce insulin and/or eat an additional snack for these kinds of activities.

If the patient engages in unplanned exercise, additional carbohydrate must be consumed. A useful guideline is to ingest 15–30 g of carbohydrate for every 30–45 minutes of moderate exercise. For sustained periods of moderate to strenuous exercise, one protein exchange prior to the exercise may also be necessary.[54] Patients also need to be reminded to replace fluids during exercise, especially for outdoor activities in warm temperatures. This is particularly true if autonomic dysfunction is present.

Blood Glucose Monitoring

Blood glucose self-monitoring is an essential component of the safe and effective implementation of intensive diabetes treatment. Blood glucose testing is most effective when the technical aspects are mastered and the results are used in a problem-solving fashion to achieve glycemic goals (see Table 29-3). Patients make decisions about elements of the treatment plan in a variety of situations based on blood glucose test results. Evaluating the effectiveness of health care recommendations or of a specific intervention depends upon self-monitored blood glucose levels. Regular and frequent blood glucose testing also provides a means to set glycemic goals and evaluate goal achievement. The patient's blood glucose records enable the patient and health care provider to identify problems and solutions. Feedback from the health care provider regarding blood glucose test results assists the patient to understand the meaning of blood glucose levels and their relationship to specific self-care behaviors.

When intensive treatment is initiated, frequent blood glucose testing before each meal, 1.5–2 hours after each meal, and at bed-

---

TABLE 29-3. Blood Glucose Self-Monitoring

1. Select a blood glucose meter suited to the patient's needs, abilities, resources, and personal preferences. Consider the meter's:
   - Size
   - Display
   - Ease of use
   - Dependence on user technique
   - Type of batteries
   - Calibration procedure
   - Cost
   - Manufacturer support and warranty
   - Accuracy
   - Storage capability for blood glucose results
   - Ability to interface with computer software
2. Provide technical instruction.
3. Monitor the patient's technical competence; i.e., observe technical performance and check patient-obtained results against laboratory results performed simultaneously.
4. Specify the frequency and circumstances under which blood glucose monitoring is to be performed.
5. Specify desired blood glucose targets.
6. Educate the patient on the meaning of blood glucose results; identify the relationship between blood glucose levels and self-care behaviors.
7. Specify guidelines for dealing with blood glucose levels within and outside the desired range.
8. Provide feedback regularly.

---

time provides a profile of fasting and pre- and postprandial glycemia that assists in making insulin dosage adjustments. Blood glucose tests at 3:00 AM several times a week assist in determining the appropriateness of basal insulin delivery or bedtime intermediate-acting insulin. Once glycemic goals have been achieved, blood glucose testing before each meal, at bedtime, and weekly at 3:00 AM is the minimum required for safe and effective intensive diabetes treatment.[1,37,38]

Investigators have shown that a patient's blood glucose records frequently misrepresent the number of blood glucose tests performed as well as the blood glucose levels obtained.[57,58] Meters that have the capacity to store over 100 blood glucose readings as well as the date and time the readings were obtained can be useful to facilitate reliable recordkeeping.[59] Memory meters can also interface with computers so that the data stored in the meter can be retrieved and analyzed. There are several software packages that will analyze parameters such as average blood glucose levels by time of day and day of the week, average number of blood glucose tests per day, and percentage of readings above, below, and within target ranges. Graphic representations of blood glucose readings can also be obtained. These glucose data management systems summarize blood glucose results in a way that is meaningful for patients, and help patients identify patterns and any progress they made. The statistical summaries also give heath care providers tangible ways to share positive feedback with the patient, and can assist in making changes in the treatment plan and setting and evaluating glycemic goals.[60] The use of memory meters and computer-assisted glucose management can also improve glycemic control.[61]

New technologies may facilitate blood glucose monitoring. Several meters allow for alternate-site (e.g., the forearm) capillary blood glucose testing, and require as little as 0.3–1.0 μL of blood. Glucose sensors are at various stages of development. A device manufactured by Minimed is currently available only to physicians, and can monitor a patient's blood glucose readings for up to 3 consecutive days. The device is worn much like a cardiac Holter monitor. It is anticipated that the sensor used in that device will become available for patient use in the future. The sensor is composed of a microelectrode with a thin coating of glucose oxidase beneath several layers of a biocompatible membrane. An introducer needle allows for subcutaneous insertion of the sensor. Glucose is converted into an electronic signal which is transmitted via a wire that is connected to the introducer needle. The wire is attached to a monitor about the size of a beeper which records blood glucose readings every 5 minutes, providing 288 glucose readings per day. The physician can download the stored blood glucose readings to the computer for analysis.

The GlucoWatch® (Cygnus) is another sensor recently made available for patient use. Worn on the wrist like a watch, the sensor provides blood glucose readings every 20 minutes for up to 12 hours. Alarms that warn the user when blood glucose readings go below preset low or high levels can be individually set. To use the GlucoWatch, the patient slides a thin plastic sensor onto the back of the watch. An extremely low-voltage electric current pulls glucose molecules through the skin into gel pads in the sensor. The glucose reacts with glucose oxidase present in the gel pads to form hydrogen peroxide. The biosensor detects the hydrogen peroxide, generating an electronic signal which is converted into the glucose reading.

Both of these devices require at least one conventional blood glucose test per day for calibration.

Prevention and Management of Hypoglycemia

Intensive diabetes treatment designed to achieve near-normal glycemic control carries an increased risk for severe hypoglycemia,[1] as well as a decrease in the signs and symptoms of hypoglycemia, causing so-called hypoglycemic unawareness.[62] This is related to an impaired counterregulatory hormone response to hypoglycemia[63] and/or brain adaptation to glucose uptake at below-normal blood glucose levels.[64,65] Recent antecedent hypoglycemia reportedly reduces autonomic and symptomatic responses to hypoglycemia.[66,67] There is evidence that suggests that avoiding hypoglycemia restores hypoglycemic awareness in patients with T1DM.[68,69] Education and surveillance are important in reducing the incidence and severity of hypoglycemia. Having a systematic approach to matching insulin to food intake and performing frequent blood glucose monitoring provide the foundation for implementing a treatment plan with precision, thus reducing the incidence of hypoglycemia.

Education regarding the prevention and treatment of hypoglycemia should include a discussion of the causes and symptoms of hypoglycemia. Family and friends need to be involved in learning how to recognize hypoglycemia and how to treat it, especially if the patient experiences confusion, coma, or seizure. Family members and/or friends should know how to administer a glucagon injection when patients cannot ingest oral carbohydrates without risk of aspiration. The usual adult dose of glucagon is 0.5–1.0 mg injected intramuscularly.

Treatment for mild hypoglycemia consists of 15–30 g of a rapidly absorbed source of carbohydrate such as juice, sugar-sweetened soft drinks, or commercially prepared tablets or gels. Patients should be instructed to have such sources of carbohydrate with them at all times including at the bedside, in the car, purse or briefcase, desk or locker, and gym bag, and during exercise and travel. The ingestion of carbohydrate should be repeated every 15–20 minutes until the blood glucose level has returned to normal (>70 mg/dL).

Patients need to identify changing symptoms of hypoglycemia. Instruct patients to pay close attention to how they feel when blood glucose levels drop below 70 mg/dL. Often patients describe vague sensations of weakness, emptiness, or just feeling different. If patients become aware of these vague symptoms, they can detect and treat hypoglycemia before becoming confused or lapsing into a coma or seizure.

When patients exercise or deviate from their usual routine, patients should check their blood glucose levels more often to make sure that any adjustment they made in insulin or diet was appropriate. Because the frequency of nocturnal hypoglycemia is often undetected, weekly blood glucose testing at 3:00 AM should be performed to guard against hypoglycemia while the patient is sleeping. Bedtime snacks consisting of some protein and carbohydrate may be necessary to avoid nocturnal hypoglycemia.

All intensively treated type 1 diabetic patients should be advised to check their blood glucose level before operating a motor vehicle. If the patient senses hypoglycemia while driving, the patient should be instructed to pull over to the side of the road, stop the vehicle, treat the hypoglycemia, and resume driving only when the blood glucose level has returned to normal. Patients should not take insulin before driving without eating. When planning to eat out, insulin should be taken after arriving at the restaurant.

Encourage patients to identify situations they are likely to encounter that have a high probability of resulting in hypoglycemia or have resulted in hypoglycemia in the past. Typical activities such as shopping, housework, yard work, or travel can increase the potential for hypoglycemia. Develop a plan to deal with that situation so hypoglycemia is avoided. If an episode of hypoglycemia occurs, assist the patient in identifying the cause of the episode and tell the patient what can be done differently to avoid future episodes. If severe hypoglycemia recurs, glycemic goals may need to be modified.

Educating Patients to Implement Intensive Diabetes Treatment

Diabetes education is not only needed to provide information and training to perform skills such as insulin injections and blood glucose monitoring, but also to assist patients to integrate their regimen into their lifestyle and achieve measurable treatment goals. Health education should motivate and enable patients to change their diabetes self-management behaviors in ways that will lead to measurable improvements in glycemic control.[70] Although diabetes education is an important component of treatment,[71,72] increased knowledge alone does not necessarily result in improved self-management behavior or glycemic control.[73,74] Educational programs that include behavioral strategies are more likely to succeed in achieving treatment goals.

The initial education required for an intensive diabetes treatment plan should include blood glucose monitoring, insulin administration, meal planning, and management of hypo- and hyperglycemia (see Table 29-4).[75] It is neither necessary nor desirable to overwhelm patients with too much information at one time. Focusing on key information until mastery of those concepts is achieved provides patients with a firm foundation upon which to build more advanced problem-solving and decision-making skills.

This initial education can be provided in a number of ways. If a slower, more incremental approach is desired, teaching patients one concept at each outpatient visit spaced at monthly or bimonthly intervals enables the patient to master the skill and demonstrate capabilities.[43] Matching the intervention to the patient's readiness for

TABLE 29-4. Education for Intensive Diabetes Treatment

Initial Education
(3–4 outpatient visits and a 3-day inpatient hospital stay or 3–4 outpatient
visits and a 3- to 7- day intensive outpatient course)
- Blood glucose monitoring
- Insulin administration
- Meal planning and system for quantifying food
- Management of hypoglycemia and hyperglycemia

Education and Management Post initiation
(Biweekly visits and weekly phone calls for 1–2 months)
- Keep food and blood glucose records
- Identify relationship between dietary intake and blood glucose
  readings
- Identify problem areas and revise meal plan as needed
- Educate on how to deal with specific situations
- Adjust insulin dosages as needed to achieve glycemic goals

Ongoing Education and Follow-up
(Monthly for 2–6 months, then every 2–3 months)
- Teach patient to interpret blood glucose readings
- Teach patient to adjust insulin for deviations in dietary intake and
  activity
- Identify problems with implementation of the treatment plan
- Identify strategies for dealing with obstacles that interfere with
  implementing the treatment plan
- Adapt treatment recommendations to lifestyle situations
- Anticipate problems and develop strategies to prevent potential
  problems from interfering with achieving treatment goals

change increases the likelihood that a desired modification in be-havior will occur.[76] Patients can also be taught all of the basic intensive diabetes management skills through a 3- to 7-day course that may be conducted on either an inpatient or outpatient basis.

After the initial education is provided, frequent contact with the patient is required so the newly acquired knowledge can be reinforced as patients integrate the treatment plan into their day-to-day lives. Phone contact is recommended at least weekly during the first 1–2 months of intensive diabetes treatment. Patients can fax or send blood glucose and dietary records to assist in identifying problems and solutions.[77] Visits biweekly for 1–2 months and then monthly may be necessary until the patient has mastered treatment techniques, integrated them into activities of daily life, and achieved glycemic goals. Frequent follow-up and close supervision have been associated with improved outcomes.[44,78,79]

Once competence in the basic skills of intensive diabetes treatment is demonstrated, patients can be taught more advanced problem-solving and decision-making skills. These skills include interpreting blood glucose levels, adjusting insulin for deviations in food intake and activity level, and dealing with a variety of situations the patient may encounter. As the patient's lifestyle changes, treatment recommendations need to be modified. The emphasis is on anticipating insulin needs for different circumstances so blood glucose levels remain within the desired range.

These skills are best taught within the context of the patient's actual experiences. Adults have a problem-centered orientation to learning, and their readiness to learn relates to immediate application of information for a specific problem they are experiencing. Ideally, education should be integrated into every office visit so that problems and solutions can be identified as the problems are encountered. Feedback should be provided soon after a solution is implemented, to determine the effectiveness of the strategy and to reinforce positive changes. New interventions should be based

on an evaluation of the relative success or failure of the previous intervention.[80]

Strategies That Enhance Achieving Diabetes Treatment Goals

Diabetes treatment is complex, and is affected by most daily activities. Adherence to prescribed regimens has been reportedly as low as 12%, with diet being the most difficult component of the treatment plan to master.[81–83] All too often health care providers blame the patient for not achieving treatment goals rather than examining the health care provider's communication style or approach to treatment recommendations that may interfere with a patient's implementation of self-management strategies.[84–86]

Characteristics of a successful approach to intensive diabetes treatment are listed in Tables 29-2 and 29-5. The treatment regimen should be as simple as possible and match the patient's ability and lifestyle. The treatment plan should allow for flexibility and adaptability to the patient's preferences; patients should have as much choice and as many options as possible. For example, patients can fit sweets such as candy bars and doughnuts into their meal plans and/or adjust insulin for these foods to maintain desired blood glucose levels.[87,88] The patient should be encouraged to identify and solve self-management problems, rather than told what to do in a paternalistic fashion.[89,90]

TABLE 29-5. Strategies That Enhance Adherence to Treatment

1. Match the diet and other aspects of the regimen to the patient's current lifestyle, habits, and personal preferences.
2. Design the insulin regimen to match the patient's dietary intake.
3. Keep the treatment plan as simple as possible.
4. Do not overwhelm the patient with too much information at one time; focus on the information the patient needs to implement the treatment plan.
5. Integrate education into every office visit; teach concepts as issues arise and provide information when relevant to a specific situation or experience.
6. Create an environment in which the patient feels comfortable to be honest:
   - Allow the patient to disagree with you.
   - Respect the patients' feelings.
   - Encourage the patient to express his or her own views.
   - Incorporate the patients' views into treatment recommendations.
   - Avoid interrupting the patient.
   - Avoid being critical or judgmental.
   - Avoid an authoritative tone.
7. Allow the patient as much choice and as many options as possible; allow for flexibility.
8. Encourage the patient to be the problem solver and decision maker; ask questions so the patient will identify the solution.
9. Negotiate specific and realistic goals. Establish goals that will lead to success.
10. Assist the patient to change health care behaviors when the patient is ready; make changes one small step at a time.
11. Provide frequent opportunities for positive feedback and encouragement.
12. Help the patient to identify obstacles that can interfere with achieving treatment goals.
13. Help the patient develop a plan to minimize obstacles to implementation of treatment recommendations.
14. Use contracts to define measurable and realistic goals, as well as reward contingencies.

Health care providers also need to create an environment in which the patient feels comfortable enough to be honest. Blood glucose and food records should be viewed as information to help identify and solve diabetes management problems, and should not be used to be critical or judgmental. It is not constructive for patients to make emotional attachments to "bad" or "good" blood glucose readings. Correcting the high or low blood glucose readings is a positive way for the patient to approach blood glucose readings outside the desired range.

Removing Obstacles to Adherence

Most patients can achieve some degree of adherence if the treatment is acceptable, understandable, and manageable. If the patient is not following the treatment plan, there may be a discrepancy between the health care provider's expectations and those of the patient. If the patient's goals are different, they need to be clearly stated and/or renegotiated. If the patient is unhappy with the treatment plan, it should be changed based on an accurate assessment of the patient's needs and abilities. If the patient does not understand the treatment plan or how to carry it out, the patient needs to be reeducated. If the patient understands the treatment plan and wants to implement it, identify obstacles to following the treatment plan.[91]

Obstacles to adherence to a treatment plan may be intrapersonal or interpersonal, or may be related to the patient's social system or the treatment itself.[80] Intrapersonal variables that can influence adherence include the patient's emotions, level of motivation, lack of structure, financial resources, fears, values, thoughts, and beliefs. Interpersonal variables are those that influence the relationship between the patient and the health care provider. The patient may not trust or understand the health care provider or may even be angry about something the health care provider said or did. Social system variables include family pressures, beliefs, and lifestyle practices, such as grocery shopping or timing and content of meals, that are controlled by other family members. Obstacles to adherence can be related to the treatment itself, such as potential for hypoglycemia or weight gain, pain caused by obtaining capillary blood glucose readings, perceived restrictions in food intake or timing of aspects of the regimen, or lack of flexibility to suit lifestyle practices.

Once obstacles are identified, a plan to reduce those obstacles can be developed. The patient may need to verbalize beliefs and evaluate them to determine if they are logical and have importance. Misconceptions should be clarified. Misunderstandings between the patient and health care provider should be reconciled. Interpersonal problems can be prevented by establishing good rapport with patients, listening to them and validating their ideas, engaging in collaborative problem solving and decision making, allowing patients to disagree, and not blaming or criticizing patients. Involve family members in the educational process and clarify their misconceptions. Teaching patients how to talk to family members about their disease and treatment plan can also be helpful.

Treatment obstacles can be dealt with in a number of ways, and health care providers may need to be creative in assisting patients to find ways to overcome barriers to following treatment recommendations. Patients who forget to check blood glucose levels could enter blood glucose testing times into their day planner, link testing to routine daily events, or set the alarm on their watch or PDA. Patients who are making too many visits to the vending machines could leave their loose change at home. Treatment contracts are a tangible way to outline specific and achievable goals and then plan to overcome obstacles. Reinforcement contingencies specified in the contract provide a way to give positive feedback, reinforce implementation of self-management strategies, and enhance the patient's sense of success.

Collaboration Among Members of the Health Care Team

The behavioral and educational nature of the interventions necessary for intensive diabetes treatment requires ongoing collaboration among all of the members of the intensive diabetes treatment team.[92,93] A collaborative team is one in which each member of the team contributes, including the patient. Communication is open and ongoing, opinions are freely discussed, and mutual consensus is reached. Joint decision making is the hallmark of a collaborative team. Patient satisfaction is enhanced when the patient's views are solicited, accepted, and incorporated into health care recommendations.[84]

An example of a collaborative team model is shown in Fig. 29-7. At the center of the team is the patient. The patient is the primary problem solver and decision maker regarding day-to-day diabetes management and relies on the health care team to advise, teach, generate options, and provide support. An experienced diabetes nurse clinician, particularly one who can function as an advanced nurse practitioner, is an ideal primary health care provider for the day-to-day management of the diabetes regimen.[94] Once the plan is prescribed by the physician, the nurse and the dietitian assist the patient to learn the components of the treatment plan and integrate them into existing lifestyle behaviors. The dietitian works closely with the nurse to assess the patient's dietary practices and how they relate to blood glucose levels and insulin requirements. The nurse makes adjustments in the insulin dosage in consultation

FIGURE 29-7. The model represents collaboration among the patient and health care providers in the implementation of chronic diabetes management. The medical condition of the patient, including acute medical problems, is managed by the physician. The physician is a consultant to the chronic diabetes management team and supports the team's interventions. Once the team identifies the treatment plan, the nurse clinician becomes the primary health care provider for chronic diabetes management. The nurse and patient contribute equally in this therapeutic relationship. The patient is the primary problem solver and decision maker, and the nurse educates, advises, provides support, and helps identify problems and generate options for solving self-management problems. The dietitian and mental health professional are consulted as needed and are integrated into the ongoing follow-up of the patient. Communication is equal and ongoing among all team members, and decisions are made jointly.

COLLABORATIVE TEAM MODEL FOR CHRONIC DIABETES MANAGEMENT

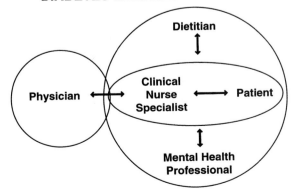

with the physician or independently under physician protocol. Acute medical problems are referred to the physician, who also monitors any physical abnormalities, medications, and abnormal laboratory findings. Referrals to the mental health professional are made for psychosocial problems that interfere with diabetes self-management. Every team member contributes to the ongoing care of the patient, and education is integrated into each office visit.

SUMMARY

Intensive diabetes treatment strategies are necessary to achieve near normoglycemia and prevent or delay the long-term complications of diabetes. Intensive diabetes treatment strategies include multiple daily insulin injections or an insulin pump, frequent blood glucose monitoring, a systematic approach to quantifying food intake, matching insulin to food intake, and education that enables patients to change aspects of the regimen for varying circumstances. Intensive diabetes treatment is flexible and adaptable, and encourages the patient to be the problem solver and decision maker. Frequent feedback, ongoing education with an emphasis on behavioral interventions, and opportunities for self-monitoring and evaluation of goal achievement are important components of an intensive diabetes treatment approach. A team approach that incorporates ongoing input from nursing, nutrition, and counseling, as well as medicine, is essential to achieve measurable improvements in glycemic control. Health care providers need to inform their patients about the influence of glycemic control on the development and progression of diabetes complications, and to encourage and support every patient's efforts at implementing an intensive diabetes treatment plan.

REFERENCES

1. The Diabetes Control and Complications Trial (DCCT) Research Group: The effect of intensive treatment of diabetes on the development and progression of long-term complications in insulin-dependent diabetes mellitus. *N Engl J Med* 1993;329:977.
2. The Diabetes Control and Complications Trial (DCCT) Research Group: The relationship between glycemic exposure (HbA$_{1c}$) and the risk of development and progression of retinopathy in the Diabetes Control and Complications Trial. *Diabetes* 1995;44:968.
3. The Diabetes Control and Complications Trial (DCCT) Research Group: Absence of a glycemic threshold for the development of long-term complications: The perspective in the Diabetes Control and Complications Trial. *Diabetes* 1996;45:1289.
4. The Diabetes Control and Complications Trial and Epidemiology of Diabetes Interventions and Complications Research Group (DCCT/EDIC): Retinopathy and nephropathy in patients with type 1 diabetes four years after a trial of intensive therapy. *N Engl J Med* 2000;342:381.
5. The Epidemiology of Diabetes Interventions and Complications (EDIC) Research Group: Epidemiology of diabetes and intervention: Design, implementation, and preliminary results of a long-term follow-up of the Diabetes Control and Complications Trial cohort. *Diabetes Care* 1999;22:99.
6. Gardner DF, Arakaki RF, Podet EJ, et al: The pharmacokinetics of subcutaneous regular insulin in type 1 diabetic patients: Assessment using a glucose clamp technique. *J Clin Endocrinol Metab* 1986;63:689.
7. Simon C, Follenius M, Brandenberger G: Postprandial oscillations of plasma glucose, insulin and C-peptide in man. *Diabetologia* 1987;30:769.
8. Kang S, Creagh FM, Peters JR, et al: Comparison of subcutaneous soluble human insulin and insulin analogs (AspB9, GluB27, AspB10, AspB28) on meal-related plasma glucose excursions in type 1 diabetic subjects. *Diabetes Care* 1991;14:571.
9. Holleman F, Hoekstra JBL: Insulin lispro. *N Engl J Med* 1997;337:176.
10. Howey DC, Bowsher RR, Brunelle RL, et al: [Lys(B28), Pro (B29)]–human insulin. A rapidly absorbed analogue of human insulin. *Diabetes* 1994;43:396.
11. Mudaliar SR, Lindberg FA, Joyce M, et al: Insulin aspart (B28 Asp-Insulin): A fast-acting analog of human insulin: Absorption kinetics and action profile compared with regular human insulin in healthy nondiabetic subjects. *Diabetes Care* 1999;22:1501.
12. Heinemann L, Kapitza C, Starke AA, et al: Time-action profile of the insulin analog B28Asp. *Diabet Med* 1996;13:683.
13. Anderson JH Jr, Brunelle RL, Koivisto VA, et al: Reduction of postprandial hyperglycemia and frequency of hypoglycemia in IDDM patients on insulin-analog treatment. *Diabetes* 1997;46:265.
14. Ciofetta M, Lalli C, Del Sindaco P, et al: Contribution of postprandial versus interprandial blood glucose to HbA$_{1c}$ in type 1 diabetes on physiologic intensive therapy with lispro insulin at mealtime. *Diabetes Care* 1999;22:795.
15. Renner R, Pfuzner A, Trautmann M, et al: Use of insulin lispro in continuous subcutaneous insulin infusion treatment: Results of a multicenter trial. *Diabetes Care* 1999;22:784.
16. Home PD, Lindholm A, Hylleberg B, et al: Improved glycaemic control with insulin aspart: A multicenter randomized double-blind crossover trial in type 1 diabetic patients. *Diabetes Care* 1998;21:1904.
17. Lindholm A, McEwen J, Riis AP: Improved postprandial glycemic control with insulin aspart. *Diabetes Care* 1999;22:801.
18. Raskin P, Guthrie RA, Leiter L, et al: Use of insulin aspart, a fast-acting insulin analog, as the mealtime insulin in the management of patients with type 1 diabetes. *Diabetes Care* 2000;23:583.
19. Pfutzner A, Kustner E, Forst T, et al: Intensive insulin therapy with insulin lispro in patients with type 1 diabetes reduces the frequency of hypoglycemic episodes. *Exp Clin Endocrinol Diabetes* 1996;104:25.
20. Holleman F, Schmitt H, Rottiers R, et al: Reduced frequency of severe hypoglycemia and coma in well-controlled IDDM patients treated with insulin lispro. *Diabetes Care* 1997;20:1827.
21. Heller S, Colagiuri S, Vaaler S, et al: Reduced hypoglycemia with insulin aspart: A double-blind, randomised, crossover trial in type 1 diabetic patients. *Diabetes* 2001;50(suppl 2):A137.
22. Kotsanos JG, Vignati L, Huster W, et al: Health-related quality of life results from multinational clinical trials of insulin lispro: Assessing benefits of a new diabetes therapy. *Diabetes Care* 1997;20:948.
23. Rassam AG, Zeise TM, Burge MR, et al: Optimal administration of lispro insulin in hyperglycemic type 1 diabetes. *Diabetes Care* 1999;22:133.
24. Ebeling P, Jansson P-A, Smith U, et al: Strategies toward improved control during insulin lispro therapy in IDDM. *Diabetes Care* 1997;20:1287.
25. Lalli C, Ciofetta M, Del Sindaco P, et al: Long-term intensive treatment of type 1 diabetes with the short-acting insulin analog lispro in variable combination with NPH insulin at mealtime. *Diabetes Care* 1999;22:468.
26. Ronnemaa T, Viikari J: Reducing snacks when switching from conventional soluble to lispro insulin treatment: Effects on glycaemic control and hypoglycemia. *Diabet Med* 1998;15:601.
27. Burge MR, Waters DL, Holcombe JH, et al: Prolonged efficacy of short acting insulin lispro in combination with human ultralente in insulin-dependent diabetes mellitus. *J Clin Endocrinol Metab* 1997;82:920.
28. Hirsch IB, Farkas-Hirsch R, Skyler JS: Intensive insulin therapy for treatment of type I diabetes. *Diabetes Care* 1990;13:1265.
29. Seigler DE, Olsson GM, Agramonte RF, et al: Pharmacokinetics of long-acting (ultralente) insulin preparations. *Diabetes Nutr Metab* 1991;4:267.
30. Lepore M, Pampanelli S, Fanelli C, et al: Pharmacokinetics and pharmacodynamics of subcutaneous injection of long-acting human insulin analog glargine, NPH insulin, and ultralente human insulin and continuous subcutaneous infusion of insulin lispro. *Diabetes* 2000;49:2142.
31. Bolli GB, Di Marchi RD, Park GD, et al: Insulin analogues and their potential in the management of diabetes mellitus. *Diabetologia* 1999;42:1151.

32. Dreyer M, Pein M, Schmidt C, *et al*: Comparison of the pharmacokinetics/dynamics of Gly(A21)-Arg(B31,B32)-human-insulin (HOE71GT) with NPH-insulin following subcutaneous injection by using euglycemic clamp technique. *Diabetologia* 1994;37(suppl 1):A78.

33. Raskin P, Klaff L, Bergenstal R, *et al*: A 16-week comparison of the novel insulin analog insulin glargine (HOE 901) and NPH human insulin used with insulin lispro in patients with type 1 diabetes. *Diabetes Care* 2000;23:1666.

34. Ratner RE, Hirsch IB, Neifing JL, *et al*: Less hypoglycemia with insulin glargine in intensive insulin therapy for type 1 diabetes. *Diabetes Care* 2000;23:639.

35. Heinemann L, Klappoth W, Rave K, *et al*: Intra-individual variability of the metabolic effect of inhaled insulin together with an absorption enhancer. *Diabetes Care* 2000;23:1343.

36. Skyler JS, Cefalu WT, Kourides IA, *et al*: Efficacy of inhaled human insulin in type 1 diabetes mellitus: A randomised proof-of-concept study. *Lancet* 2001;357:331.

37. Strowig SM: Initiation and management of insulin pump therapy. *Diabetes Educator* 1993;19:50.

38. The Diabetes Control and Complications Trial (DCCT) Research Group: Implementation of treatment protocols in the Diabetes Control and Complications Trial. *Diabetes Care* 1995;18:361.

39. Eastman RC, Siebert CW, Harris M, *et al*: Implications of the Diabetes Control and Complications Trial. *J Clin Endocrinol Metab* 1993;77:1105.

40. Santiago JV: Lessons from the Diabetes Control and Complications Trial. *Diabetes* 1993;42:1549.

41. The Diabetes Control and Complications Trial (DCCT) Research Group: Hypoglycemia in the Diabetes Control and Complications Trial. *Diabetes* 1997;46:271.

42. American Diabetes Association: Standards of medical care for patients with diabetes mellitus. *Diabetes Care* 2000;23(suppl 1):S32.

43. Rubin RR, Peyrot M: Implications of the DCCT: Looking beyond tight control. *Diabetes Care* 1994;17:235.

44. McCulloch DK, Glasgow RE, Hampson SE, *et al*: A systematic approach to diabetes management in the post-DCCT era. *Diabetes Care* 1994;17:765.

45. American Diabetes Association: *Intensive Diabetes Management*, 1st ed. Farkas-Hirsch R, ed. ADA:1995.

46. American Diabetes Association: Position Statement: Evidence-based nutrition principles and recommendations for the treatment and prevention of diabetes and related complications. *Diabetes Care* 2002; 25(suppl 1):S50.

47. The Diabetes Control and Complications Trial (DCCT) Research Group: Nutrition interventions for intensive therapy in the Diabetes Control and Complications Trial. *J Am Diet Assoc* 1993;93:768.

48. Franz MJ, Bantle JP, Beebe CH, et al: Evidence-based nutrition principles and recommendations for the treatment and prevention of diabetes and related complications [technical review]. *Diabetes Care* 2002;25:148.

49. Delahanty LM, Halford BN: The role of diet behaviors in achieving improved glycemic control in intensively treated patients in the Diabetes Control and Complications Trial. *Diabetes Care* 1993;16:1453.

50. Horton ES: Role and management of exercise in diabetes mellitus. *Diabetes Care* 1988;11:201.

51. Kemmer FW: Prevention of hypoglycemia during exercise in type I diabetes [review]. *Diabetes Care* 1992;15:1732.

52. MacDonald MJ: Postexercise late-onset hypoglycemia in insulin-dependent diabetic patients. *Diabetes Care* 1987;10:584.

53. Campaigne BN, Wallberg-Henriksson H, Gunnarsson R: Glucose and insulin responses in relation to insulin dose and caloric intake 12 h after acute physical exercise in men with IDDM. *Diabetes Care* 1987; 10:716.

54. Schiffrin A, Parikh S: Accommodating planned exercise in type I diabetic patients on intensive treatment. *Diabetes Care* 1985;8:337.

55. Sonnenberg GE, Kemmer FW, Berger M: Exercise in type I (insulin-dependent) diabetic patients treated with continuous subcutaneous insulin infusion. *Diabetologia* 1990;33:696.

56. Richter EA, Turcotte L, Hespel P, *et al*: Metabolic responses to exercise. Effects of endurance training and implications for diabetes. *Diabetes Care* 1992;15(Suppl. 4):1767.

57. Mazze RS, Shamoon H, Pasmantier R, *et al*: Reliability of blood glucose monitoring by patients with diabetes mellitus. *Am J Med* 1984; 77:211.

58. Gonder-Frederick LA, Julian DM, Cox DJ, *et al*: Self-measurement of blood glucose. Accuracy of self-reported data and adherence to recommended regimen. *Diabetes Care* 1988;11:579.

59. Mazze RS, Pasmantier R, Murphy JA, *et al*: Self-monitoring of capillary blood glucose: changing the performance of individuals with diabetes. *Diabetes Care* 1985;8:207.

60. Marrero DG, Kronz KK, Golden MP, *et al*: Clinical evaluation of computer-assisted self-monitoring of blood glucose system. *Diabetes Care* 1989;12:345.

61. Strowig SM, Raskin P: Improved glycemic control in intensively treated diabetic patients using blood glucose meters with storage capability and computer-assisted analyses. *Diabetes Care* 1998;21:1694.

62. Cryer PE, Fisher JN, Shamoon H: Hypoglycemia [technical review]. *Diabetes Care* 1994;17:734.

63. Amiel SA, Tamborlane WV, Simonson DC, *et al*: Defective glucose counterregulation after strict glycemic control of insulin-dependent diabetes mellitus. *N Engl J Med* 1987;316:1376.

64. Nagy RJ, O'Connor A, Robinson B, *et al*: Hypoglycemia unawareness results from adaptation of brain glucose metabolism [abstract]. *Diabetes* 1993;42(suppl 1):133A.

65. McCall AL, Fixman LB, Fleming N, *et al*: Chronic hypoglycemia increases brain glucose transport. *Am J Physiol* 1986;251:E442.

66. Davis MR, Mellman M, Shamoon H: Further defects in counterregulatory responses induced by recurrent hypoglycemia in IDDM. *Diabetes* 1992;41:1335.

67. Lingenfelser T, Renn W, Sommerwerck U, *et al*: Compromised hormonal counterregulation, symptom awareness, and neurophysiological function after recurrent short-term episodes of insulin-induced hypoglycemia in IDDM patients. *Diabetes* 1993;42:610.

68. Fanelli CG, Epifano L, Rambotti AM, *et al*: Meticulous prevention of hypoglycemia normalizes the glycemic thresholds and magnitude of most neuroendocrine responses to, symptoms of, and cognitive function during hypoglycemia in intensively treated patients with short-term IDDM. *Diabetes* 1993;42:1683.

69. Cranston I, Lomas J, Maran A, *et al*: Restoration of hypoglycaemia unawareness in patients with long-duration insulin-dependent diabetes. *Lancet* 1994;344:283.

70. National Institute of Diabetes and Digestive and Kidney Diseases: *Metabolic Control Matters. Nationwide Translation of the Diabetes Control and Complications Trial: Analysis and Recommendations.* NIH Publ. No. 94-3773, May 1994.

71. Brown SA: Studies of educational interventions and outcomes in diabetic adults: A meta-analysis revisited. *Patient Educ Counsel* 1990; 16:189.

72. Padgett D, Mumford E, Hynes M, *et al*: Meta-analysis of the effects of educational and psychosocial interventions on management of diabetes mellitus. *J Clin Epidemiol* 1988;41:1007.

73. Beeney LJ, Dunn SM: Knowledge improvement and metabolic control in diabetes education: Approaching the limits? *Patient Educ Counsel* 1990;16:217.

74. Goodall TA, Halford WK: Self-management of diabetes mellitus: A critical review. *Health Psych* 1991;10:1.

75. American Diabetes Association: Standards and review criteria: National standards for diabetes self-management education programs and American Diabetes Association Review Criteria. *Diabetes Care* 1997;20(suppl 1):S67.

76. Ruggiero L, Prochaska JO: Readiness for change: Introduction. *Diabetes Spectrum* 1993;6:22.

77. Ahring KK, Ahring JPK, Joyce C, *et al*: Telephone modem access improves diabetes control in those with insulin-requiring diabetes. *Diabetes Care* 1992;15:971.

78. Clement S: Diabetes self-management education. *Diabetes Care* 1995;18:1204.

79. Wagner EH: Population based management of diabetes care. *Patient Educ Counsel* 1995;26:225.

80. Becker MH: Patient adherence to prescribed therapies. *Med Care* 1985;23:539.

81. Glasgow RE, McCaul KD, Schafer LC: Self-care behaviors and glycemic control in type I diabetes. *J Chron Dis* 1987;40:399.

82. Glasgow RE, McCaul KD, Schafer LC: Barriers to regimen adherence among persons with insulin-dependent diabetes. *J Behav Med* 1986;9:65.

83. Daschner BK: Problems perceived by adults in adhering to a prescribed diet. *Diabetes Educator* 1986;12:113.

84. Street RL, Piziak VK, Capentier WS, *et al*: Provider-patient communication and metabolic control. *Diabetes Care* 1993;16:714.

85. Anderson LA, Zimmerman MA: Patient and physician perceptions of their relationship and patient satisfaction: A study of chronic disease management. *Patient Educ Counsel* 1993;20:27.

86. Lo R: Correlates of expected success at adherence to health regimen of people with IDDM. *J Adv Nurs* 1999;30:418.

87. Peters AL, Davidson MB, Eisenberg K: Effect of isocaloric substitution of chocolate cake for potato in type I diabetic patients. *Diabetes Care* 1990;13:888.

88. Wise JE, Keim KS, Huisinga JL, *et al*: Effect of sucrose-containing snacks on blood glucose control. *Diabetes Care* 1989;12:423.

89. Anderson RM, Funnell MM, Butler PM, *et al*: Patient empowerment: Results of a randomized controlled trial. *Diabetes Care* 1995;18:943.

90. Williams GC, Freedman ZR, Deci EL: Supporting autonomy to motivate patients with diabetes for glucose control. *Diabetes Care* 1998;21:1644.

91. Basco MR: The cognitive behavior therapist's role in diabetes management. *Behav Therapist* 1993;16:180.

92. The Diabetes Control and Complications Trial (DCCT) Research Group: The impact of the trial coordinator in the Diabetes Control and Complications Trial (DCCT). *Diabetes Educator* 1993;19:509.

93. The Diabetes Control and Complications Trial (DCCT) Research Group: Expanded role of the dietitian in the Diabetes Control and Complications Trial: Implications for clinical practice. *J Am Diet Assoc* 1993;93:758.

94. Funnell MM: Role of nurses in the implementation of intensified management. *Diabetes Rev* 1994;2:322.

CHAPTER 30

Insulin Treatment of Type 2 Diabetes Mellitus

David M. Nathan

INTRODUCTION

The classification of diabetes mellitus into insulin-dependent or type I and non-insulin-dependent or type II diabetes mellitus, and other types, by the National Diabetes Data Group and the World Health Organization more than two decades ago provided a working model of different phenotypes of diabetes.[1,2] The division of the diabetic population into IDDM and NIDDM was based on differences in their clinical characteristics, natural history, and presumed pathogenesis. The absolute dependence of IDDM patients on insulin therapy for survival was connoted by the "insulin-dependent" classification. Unfortunately, many clinicians continued to confuse insulin-treatment with insulin-dependence, and patients who clearly had phenotypic NIDDM, but who were treated with insulin, were often inaccurately described in medical records as having IDDM.

The most recent iteration of the nosologic classification of diabetes by the Expert Committee convened by the American Diabetes Association (ADA) added genotypic information to the classification of diabetes and refined the diagnostic plasma glucose criteria for diabetes, lowering the fasting plasma glucose threshold from 140 to 126 mg/dL.[3] In addition, and in part decrease the misclassification of patients using the old nomenclature, non-insulin-dependent diabetes mellitus was to be called type 2 diabetes (T2DM).

This chapter focuses on the insulin treatment of patients with T2DM. The population of insulin-treated T2DM patients in the U.S. is currently two to three times larger in number than the type 1 diabetic population and is growing at a rapid rate.[4] The worldwide population of T2DM, already pandemic in nature, is projected to reach 300 million in the next 20 years.[5] Although there have been numerous reviews of insulin therapy of type 1 diabetes,[6–10] relatively few major reviews of insulin therapy of T2DM have appeared.[11,12] In this chapter, I review the magnitude of the problem, the pathophysiology of T2DM as it relates to insulin treatment, the goals of therapy including the role of intensive therapy, the relative attributes of insulin therapy compared with other available treatments, the spectrum of insulin regimens and new insulins that have been tested and their relative advantages and disadvantages, the use of combination therapy, and criteria for selecting T2DM patients for insulin therapy. The treatment of T2DM patients who require insulin transiently, such as during perioperative or other stress, is not discussed in this chapter.

BACKGROUND: THE SCOPE OF THE PROBLEM

The identification of T2DM as a specific nosologic entity by the National Diabetes Data Group (NDDG) and WHO was long overdue. Despite the remarkable increase in prevalence of T2DM in the twentieth century, it remained an underrecognized and underdiagnosed disease. The failure of patients to recognize and of clinicians to diagnose T2DM was and continues to be predicated on its subtle clinical presentation compared with type 1 diabetes. [Based on the relatively frequent appearance of long-term complications in "newly diagnosed" T2DM patients, it has been estimated that diabetes has been present for 4–7 years, on average, before it is diagnosed.[13]] T2DM was probably relatively uncommon prior to the extension of life span and the increased obesity and sedentary lifestyle that have accompanied widespread industrialization in the latter part of the twentieth century.[14] The vast majority of descriptions of diabetes mellitus in the older medical literature are of type 1 diabetes, not T2DM. The historic slight against type 2 diabetes persists; even though T2DM represents as much as 90% of all diabetes mellitus, it remains "type 2" diabetes.

The spread of T2DM is reaching pandemic proportions. It currently affects 7% of the adult population in the United States, including 12% of the adult population older than 45 and almost 20% of those older than 65.[3,15] The prevalence of T2DM is similar in Europe as in the United States. In developing countries in Asia and Africa, where T2DM has historically been relatively rare, the shift to more industrial economies with sedentary lifestyles and westernized diets has resulted in a startling increase in T2DM.[5,14]

Currently, at least 2 million T2DM patients in the United States are treated with insulin, compared with an estimated 600,000 to 1.2 million patients with T1DM[4] (Fig. 30-1). This represents approximately 30% of patients with diagnosed T2DM. The increasing size of the T2DM population, the disappointing long-term results with diet therapy[16–18] (the first choice in treating the majority of T2DM patients who are obese), and the relatively high primary and secondary failure rates of sulfonylurea and metformin therapy, which are the mainstay oral hypoglycemic agents,[18–20] strongly suggest that the fraction of the T2DM population and the total number of T2DM patients treated with insulin will increase.

PATHOPHYSIOLOGY OF T2DM: IMPLICATIONS FOR THERAPY

The pathogenesis of T2DM is multifactorial and includes decreased sensitivity to insulin action (insulin resistance) secondary to obesity and genetic factors, and decreased insulin secretion.[21–23] While insulin resistance may be the inherited defect that accompanies most cases of impaired glucose tolerance, progressive worsening of glucose tolerance with the development of fasting hyperglycemia and T2DM is usually preceded by decreased insulin secretion.[22,24] Fasting hyperglycemia is primarily a consequence of increased hepatic

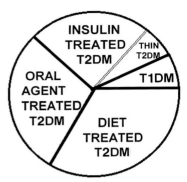

FIGURE 30-1. Prevalence of different types of diabetes mellitus.

glucose output in the setting of relatively low insulin levels. Several studies have suggested that the impaired ability to increase insulin secretion in the face of increasing insulin resistance is also a heritable feature of T2DM.[25,26] In addition to the decrease in insulin secretion that accompanies T2DM, the early stages of glucose intolerance are accompanied by a relatively increased secretion of proinsulin, which has less bioactivity than insulin.[27] Finally, the development of hyperglycemia further compromises insulin secretion and increases resistance Fig. 30-2). This effect of hyperglycemia, termed glucotoxicity, is at least partially reversible if basal glycemia is restored to normal. The beneficial effect of achieving normoglycemia in T2DM (lower glycemia begets further improvement in glycemia with restored endogenous insulin secretion) has been demonstrated with diet, sulfonylurea, and insulin therapy.[28–30]

The implications of these studies with regard to therapy are the following:

1. By the time that T2DM is established, insulin secretion is relatively decreased. In some T2DM patients, the absolute level of insulin secretion may be very low. Insulin secretion as measured by basal and stimulated C-peptide levels often overlaps the levels seen early in the course of type 1 diabetes.[31,32]
2. With longer duration, metabolic control worsens with higher glycemic levels. This is largely attributable to progressive deterioration in insulin secretion.[33]
3. Residual insulin secretion in T2DM, at least early in its course, provides a degree of stability to glucose levels not present in

type 1 diabetes. Insulin regimens need not be as complex in the treatment of T2DM as in the treatment of type 1 diabetes.

4. Although T2DM patients may have severely impaired insulin secretion, they rarely become ketotic. There have been several populations identified, including an African-American population in Flatbush, Brooklyn,[34] and a subset of T2DM patients in Scandinavia,[35] that appear to be more vulnerable to the development of ketoacidosis. Whether some of these "T2DM" patients, especially in Scandinavia where the prevalence of type 1 diabetes is relatively high, are actually misdiagnosed is unclear. In any case, T2DM patients who are thin and/or ketonuric should probably be treated as if they have type 1 diabetes.
5. Correction of fasting hyperglycemia by any means has been demonstrated to result in improved insulin secretion and a modest improvement in resistance. Therapy with insulin early in the course of T2DM may result in remission for as long as several years with no need for hypoglycemic drugs and normal glycemia.[36]
6. Ideally, suppression of increased overnight hepatic glucose output should normalize fasting blood glucose and improve endogenous insulin secretion in response to meals during the day. This effect is presumably mediated by ameliorating the toxic effects of hyperglycemia on the islets.
7. Insulin given in the morning will cover postprandial glucose excursions but may further suppress endogenous insulin secretion during the day.

METABOLIC GOALS OF THERAPY

The Diabetes Control and Complications Trial (DCCT) conclusively established blood glucose goals for type 1 diabetes.[37] Whether similar goals are appropriate for T2DM and the means to achieve those goals have been vigorously debated.[38–40] The similar clinical characteristics of the microvascular and neurologic complications in type 1 and type 2 diabetes, and the similar relationship between the occurrence of long-term complications and level of glycemia demonstrated in epidemiologic studies of type 1 and type 2 diabetes, support a similar benefit in T2DM as demonstrated in the DCCT.[41,42] Two recent clinical trials that have examined the effectiveness of glycemic control in preventing or ameliorating long-term complications in T2DM have provided definitive support for therapies aimed at normalizing glycemia in T2DM.[18,43] The Kumamoto study[43] examined intensive therapy only with insulin, while the United Kingdom Prospective Diabetes Study (UKPDS) tried to establish whether any specific hypoglycemic therapy was advantageous by randomly assigning T2DM patients with relatively recent-onset disease to either sulfonylurea, metformin, or insulin therapy. The UKPDS tried to resolve the uncertainty left by the earlier University Group Diabetes Program (UGDP), which had similar goals.[44] The UGDP, conducted between 1960 and 1969, did not demonstrate a benefit of intensive therapy; moreover, treatment with sulfonylurea or phenformin was associated with excess cardiovascular mortality compared with the insulin-treated and diet-treated groups.

The UKPDS, completed almost 40 years after the UGDP, compared an "active" treatment policy with either sulfonylurea or insulin (or metformin in the obese subjects) with a dietary policy. Over 10–12 years of average follow-up, the active policy, which decreased HbA$_{1c}$ by approximately 1% compared with the dietary policy, was associated with a 12% decreased risk for aggregate diabetes compli-

FIGURE 30-2. Pathophysiology of type 2 diabetes mellitus.

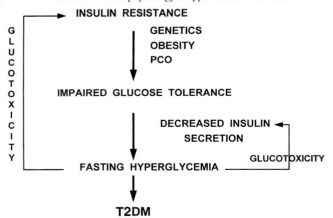

cations. The major effect was mediated through a 25% decrease in microvascular complications. In the Kumamoto study, relatively thin Japanese T2DM patients were treated either intensively or conventionally with insulin. The separation in HbA$_{1c}$ was similar to that achieved in the DCCT, and the magnitude of the reduction in retinopathy and nephropathy also paralleled that seen in the DCCT.[43]

In the aggregate, these studies support the use of intensive therapy, with the goal of achieving near-normal glucose levels, in T2DM. The UKPDS did not definitively establish whether any specific treatment modality was superior, owing to the use of a stepped intervention strategy, which resulted in substantial therapy crossovers.[45] Of note, the UKPDS demonstrated a seemingly inexorable worsening of metabolic control over time, which required the progressive addition of more hypoglycemic agents. Although patients should theoretically always respond to increasing doses of insulin, UKPDS physicians and patients were apparently reluctant to increase insulin to the doses necessary to maintain normal glucose levels.

COMPARISON OF INSULIN WITH OTHER AVAILABLE THERAPIES FOR T2DM

Efficacy

Short-term randomized studies of glycemic response to insulin versus sulfonylurea,[46–50] including one that was double-blind,[50] have demonstrated only modest differences in glycemic control in the first weeks to months of therapy. The vast majority of studies that have examined and compared the metabolic benefits of diet, sulfonylurea, and insulin therapy have been short-term studies; longer-term controlled trials are few in number. Although the longest-term observational studies[17] and controlled clinical trials, including the UGDP,[44] the Kumamoto study,[43] and the UKPDS,[18] are 6–12 years in duration, they are relatively brief for a chronic disease such as T2DM. In concert, these studies demonstrate very limited long-term efficacy of diet therapy. The majority of the benefit with regard to weight loss and lowering of glycemia commonly noted in the first year is lost within 2–3 years with weight regain. In the UKPDS more than 50% of the patients with recent-onset T2DM assigned to diet therapy required subsequent reassignment to pharmacologic therapy in order to maintain even a modicum of glycemic control.[18]

Similarly, the lowering of glycemic levels with sulfonylureas or biguanides is transient, with as many as 50% of sulfonylurea-treated patients failing therapy, either in the first 3 months of therapy (primary failure) or after a salutary initial response (secondary failure).[19,20] Results with either sulfonylurea or biguanides are remarkably similar. In the UGDP and UKPDS, glycemic levels were lowered from baseline for the first several years of therapy, but drifted back to baseline by years 3–5 of therapy.[18,44] In the UKPDS, worsening metabolic control in patients originally assigned to sulfonylurea or metformin occurred despite the addition or substitution of alternative therapies in as much as 30% of the patients originally assigned to the oral hypoglycemics as glycemic levels rose over time.[18] There are no comparable long-term data available with thiazolidinediones or the glitinides.

In contrast to sulfonylureas, biguanides, and thiazolidinediones, insulin has no upper dose limit and can be adjusted over time to achieve normal or near-normal glycemic levels. This attribute of insulin therapy has been demonstrated to provide lower levels of glycemia in oral agent failures[51] or when intensive insulin therapy was compared with a conventional insulin regimen in the

UGDP,[44] Kumamoto,[43] or Veterans Administration Cooperative Study of Diabetes Mellitus (VACSDM).[52] The dose of insulin required to achieve this benefit depends to a great extent on the degree of insulin resistance (or level of obesity as a surrogate) present. In most studies of typically obese patients with T2DM, relatively large doses ranging from 50–200 units per day (usually >0.65 U/kg) are required to achieve near-normal glycemia.(Table 30-1) Insulin doses had to be raised progressively from approximately 25 U/d at baseline to 90 U/d by 2 years in order to maintain stable glycemia in the VACSDM.[52]

Interestingly, the UKPDS, the longest-term study of diabetes therapy, failed to demonstrate substantially lower glycemia with insulin therapy compared with the oral agents. Moreover, HbA$_{1c}$ levels rose over time in the group assigned to doses therapy despite the investigators' intent to raise insulin doses to control glycemia.[18] Of note, the progressive addition of alternative therapies, including insulin, for the patients originally assigned to oral agents, and the apparent reluctance of the UKPDS clinicians and/or patients to raise insulin doses, may explain these findings. In the UKPDS, the median insulin doses rose only modestly, from 22 U at 3 years to 28 U at 6 years, 34 U at 9 years, and 36 U at 12 years. The very obese patients (BMI >35 kg/m^2) were also treated with modest doses of insulin, with median doses of 36 U at 3 years and 60 U at 12 years. These doses are substantially lower than the doses usually required to achieve near-normal glycemia in most studies (Table 30-1).

Other Effects and Adverse Events

A comparison of diet, sulfonylureas, biguanides, and insulin with regard to effects other than glucose control is shown in Table 30-2. Diet therapy has the best benefit risk ratio, with weight loss resulting in improved lipid levels, blood pressure, and other cardiovascular risk factors. Sulfonylureas and insulin share several metabolic benefits other than glycemic control, such as a reduction in free fatty acid levels. Insulin raises HDL cholesterol more than sulfonylurea therapy.[50,53] The frequency of severe hypoglycemia, defined in the DCCT as any episode requiring assistance, is generally low; however, modest weight gain (2–5 kg) is relatively common with insulin or sulfonylurea therapy (Table 30-1). Hypoglycemia associated with sulfonylurea use can be more prolonged and dangerous than the usually self-limited hypoglycemia seen with insulin. Finally, drug-specific complications occur.

Metformin, a relatively old drug that was developed in 1959 but did not become available in the U.S. until 1995, provides several interesting benefits. When used as sole therapy, it has potency similar to that of sulfonylureas, but does not appear to promote weight gain or cause hypoglycemia. The gastrointestinal side effects of bloating and diarrhea that are seen with higher doses and rapid escalation of the dose are usually transient and can be largely eliminated if doses are titrated slowly. The risk of lactic acidosis with metformin is almost nil if patients with decreased renal function, liver disease, severe congestive heart failure, and binge alcohol drinking are excluded from treatment.

The thiazolidinediones are relatively new oral hypoglycemic agents that appear to act by binding to peroxisome proliferator activated receptor α (PPARα) receptors and reducing insulin resistance.[54] They are relatively weak hypoglycemic agents when used alone, but are more efficacious when used in combination with other hypoglycemic medications, including insulin.[55,56] Owing to rare but severe idiosyncratic liver toxicity, the first approved thiazolidinedione, troglitazone, had to be withdrawn from the U.S.

TABLE 30-1. Insulin Treatment Regimens to Achieve Normoglycemia in Patients with Type 2 Diabetes

Duration (Mo)	Subjects (#)	Regimen*	Dose (U/kg)	Glycemia Achieved (HbA$_{1c}$ or HbA$_1$/ upper limit of normal)	Adverse Events[†] (Wt. gain in kg/ severe hypoglycemia)	Reference
9	15	AM NPH	0.66	7.1/6.4	3.8/0	50
4	12	Bedtime NPH	0.86	7.2/6.7	2.4/0	63
120	911	AM UL or NPH[‡]	0.42	7.1/6.2	6/2.3[‡]	18
6	21	BID NPH	0.63	9.5/7.4	4.7/0	73
4	10	BID NPH/REG	0.65	10.6/7.8	4.2/0	70
2	10	BID NPH/REG	NA	5.7/5.0	NA/0	69
6	14	BID NPH/REG	0.98	5.1/NA	8.7/0	68
3	29	BID NPH/REG	0.53	7.9/6.0	1.8/NA	62
6	34	BID 70:30	0.58	8.2/6.2	4.0/0	80
3	30	NPH + TID REG	0.55	8.0/6.0	2.9/NA	62
2	10	NPH + TID REG	NA	5.6/5.0	NA/0	69
27	75	1–3 Injections[§]	NA	7.2/6.1	NA/3.0	52
6	21	TID REG	0.55	9.7/7.0	3.3/0	73
4	10	CSII	0.58	9.2/7.8	4.5/0	70
1	12	CSII	0.81	NA	NA	71
1	12	CSII	0.61	NA	NA	36
12	51	IP Insulin by implantable pump	NA	7.1/6.1	NA/1.0	74
24	3	IV Insulin by implantable pump	0.75	6.2/6.3	9/0	73

* UL, Ultralente insulin; REG, CZI insulin; NPH, neutral protamine Hagedorn insulin; CSII, continuous subcutaneous insulin infusion; NA, information not available.

[†] Defined as hypoglycemia requiring assistance for treatment and including coma, seizures, and/or treatment with glucagon or IV dextrose (episodes/100 pt-yr).

[‡] Daily UL or NPH (+ regular if premeal BG >126 mg/dL). "Major" hypoglycemia in 2.3% of patients.

[§] Stepwise therapy with evening intermediate- or long-acting insulin proceeding to insulin plus to sulfonylurea, to twice per day intermediate-acting insulin, and finally to multiple (≥3) daily injections.

TABLE 30-2. Comparison of Therapies for Type 2 Diabetes Currently Available in the United States When Used as Monotherapy

	Diet	Sulfonylurea	Biguanides	Glycosidase Inhibitors	Thiazolidinediones	Insulin
Metabolic Effects						
Improves resistance	+	+	+ +	+	+ + +	+ +
Secretion	+	+ +	+	+	+	+
Overnight HGO	+	+	+ +	+	+	+
Postprandial excursions	+	+ +	+	+ +	+	+ +
Glycosylated hemoglobin	+	+ +	+ +	+	+	+ + +
Lowers FFA	+	+	+	+	+	+ +
Weight gain	−	+	−	+	+	+ +
Hypoglycemia	−	+	−	−	−	+ +
Allergic phenonema	−	+	+	−	+	+
Other Side Effects						
Antabuse effect	−	+ *	−	−	−	−
Hyponatremia	−	+ *	−	−	−	−
Lactic acidosis[†]	−	−	+	−	−	−
Gastrointestinal	−	−	+	+ +	−	−
Hepatic dysfunction	−	−	−	−	+ [‡]	−

* Very uncommon with second-generation sulfonylureas such as glyburide and glipizide. Most common with chlorpropamide.

[†] Very rare with metformin (<3/100,000 treated patients).

[‡] Severe idiosyncratic liver failure in approximately 1/35,000–50,000 patients treated with troglitazone (discontinued in March, 2000). Rosiglitazone and pioglitazone thought to be less likely to cause hepatic dysfunction.

market. Pioglitazone and rosiglitazone do not appear to suffer from the same problem, although fluid retention can be problematic.

The glitinides are nonsulfonylurea insulin secretagogues that have been introduced recently.[57] With a shorter half-life than the sulfonylureas, they are probably less likely to cause hypoglycemia than sulfonylureas, but need to be administered before each meal.

INSULIN THERAPY

Doses

As noted above, the dose of insulin required to normalize glycemia in T2DM is often more than 60 U/d. More obese, insulin-resistant patients invariably need more insulin. When calculated on the basis of body mass, most studies have required 0.6–1.0 U/kg. In general, insulin treatment is started with conservative doses with empiric adjustment based on glucose levels. Formulaic approaches to selecting an initial dose of insulin have been suggested, with some based on overnight insulin infusions.[18,58] Since most T2DM patients are insulin-resistant, they can usually tolerate fairly high initial doses of insulin without hypoglycemia. On the other hand, hyperglycemia is very diet-responsive in T2DM, and if patients initiate their dietary efforts concurrently with beginning insulin use, they can develop hypoglycemia with relatively small doses. For the reasons above, suggest beginning with 10–15 U of intermediate-acting insulin, at bed or before breakfast. Alternatively, a very long-acting insulin, such as Ultralente or glorcine, can be initiated in the evening. Adjustments can be made relatively quickly, guided by self-monitoring of blood glucose results.

As noted in Table 30-1, many studies attempting to normalize glycemia in T2DM have required large doses of insulin. However, when calculated on the basis of units per kilogram, these doses are only modestly higher than the range of doses used in the DCCT to treat adult T1DM intensively (0.66–0.73 U/kg).[59] The largest doses are generally required in the most obese, most resistant T2DM patients. Insulin requirements in the Pima Indians, whose body mass index—a measure of weight divided by height squared—exceeds 40, are often more than 150 units per day. Similarly high insulin requirements may be seen in very overweight patients of other racial groups. Many physicians remain uncomfortable using the high doses necessary to control glycemia in the near-normal range.

Various rules of thumb have been proposed to guide clinicians in deciding the rate at which to advance insulin doses. With the widespread availability of self-monitoring, which should be implemented in all insulin-treated patients, such rules have been made relatively obsolete. The results of insulin adjustments can be monitored by the patient and the rate and magnitude of further adjustments determined on the basis of self-monitoring. The decision when to split insulin from a single daily dose to two or more doses can also be guided by the results of self-monitoring. For those patients who cannot master self-monitoring, the relative stability of glycemia in T2DM makes possible monitoring of glycemia by visiting nurses or in the office setting to guide adjustment of doses. Timed glucose levels, fasting and/or before dinner, are most useful.

Regimens

Although many insulin treatment regimens have been tried (Table 30-3), most studies achieving glycemic control in the near-normal range, albeit for relatively brief periods of time, have done so with one or two daily insulin injections (Table 30-1). The UKPDS,

TABLE 30-3. Insulin Regimens for Type 2 Diabetes

Morning intermediate*
Bedtime intermediate or very long-acting
Morning intermediate + rapid[†]
Morning intermediate + rapid[‡] with bedtime intermediate
Morning and predinner intermediate and rapid[‡]
Dinner and or morning long-acting (Ultralente) with rapid
Morning and bedtime intermediate and prebreakfast and predinner rapid (multiple daily injection—MDI)
Evening Ultralente with premeal rapid (MDI)
Continuous subcutaneous insulin infusion with an external pump (CSII)
Premeal inhaled insulin with bedtime intermediate
Bedtime intermediate with morning sulfonylurea, or daily metformin, thiazolidinedione, or α-glycosidase inhibitor (combination therapy)

* Intermediate-acting: NPH or Lente.
[†] Rapid-acting: CZI (regular) or lispro (very-rapid acting).
[‡] May be administered as premixed (e.g., 70:30 NPH/regular insulin).

which failed to maintain stable glycemia with its intensive regimen, perhaps owing to inadequate dosing, used a regimen based on a once-per-day Ultralente™ or NPH insulin supplemented with regular insulin as needed.[18] The VACSDM employed increasingly complex regimens based on glycemia.[52] In order to maintain stable glycemia over a 30-month follow-up, 64% of the subjects were advanced to two or three daily injections of insulin by study's end. Whether single injections of intermediate- or long-acting insulin in larger doses will perform as well as split doses has not been adequately studied, but is unlikely.

There are surprisingly few data available on the best timing of the injection. Conventionally, insulin therapy is initiated with morning intermediate-acting insulin, with or without rapid-acting insulin. Predinner intermediate-acting insulin, again with or without rapid-acting insulin, or prebedtime intermediate-acting insulin can be added as needed. As with intensive therapy in type 1 diabetes, the choice of doses of rapid-acting (CZI), or very-rapid-acting (lispro or aspart), insulin before meals is dictated by the results of self-monitoring of blood glucose. However, since blood glucose levels in T2DM are much less labile than in type 1 diabetes, probably mediated by endogenous insulin secretion, frequent adjustment of insulin is less necessary.

The use of nocturnal insulin has been championed[60–62] on the basis of its ability to suppress overnight glucose output and not inhibit endogenous secretion in response to meals; however, there are few studies to recommend it over the more conventional morning regimens.[62] Nevertheless, it is reasonable to initiate insulin therapy with intermediate-acting insulin at bedtime, adjusting the dose until fasting blood glucose levels are in the therapeutic range. This strategy can normalize fasting glucose levels and HbA$_{1c}$ levels.[63] If blood glucose levels during the day remain elevated, morning intermediate-acting insulin, with or without rapid- or very-rapid-acting insulin, can be added. Premixed insulins such as 70:30 or 50:50 mixtures of NPH and rapid-acting or 75:25 mixtures of NPH and very-rapid-acting insulins are available. These mixtures are relatively stable, preserving the individual time action profiles of the components, and can be used in T2DM where day-to-day insulin doses remain relatively stable.

The use of long-acting insulin has also been espoused as a means of supplementing basal indogenous insulin without exogenous peaks which might suppress endogenous secretion.[64] Unfortunately, "peakless" beef-pork Ultralente insulin is no longer available, and human Ultralente insulin has different absorption characteristics that may be problematic.[65] In addition, the relatively long half-life of Ultralente insulin is undesirable when dietary intake is suddenly decreased, for example with hospitalization, when rapid changes in insulin treatment may be required. The UKPDS used human Ultralente insulin.[18] A new insulin analog, glargine, has similar performance characteristics as the old beef-pork Ultralente insulin, with a long half-life and no apparent peak.[66] In clinical trials, it has had little benefit compared with once- or twice-per-day NPH.[67]

Other more complicated regimens including continuous subcutaneous insulin infusion (CSII) with an external pump have been used.[28,29,68–71] Whether they are ever necessary or advantageous compared with less complex regimens is unknown. A crossover study between premeal rapid-acting insulin and twice-per-day (before breakfast and dinner) intermediate-acting insulin revealed no significant benefit of the more frequent injection regimen.[72] Implantable insulin pumps delivering insulin either intravenously at a single rate[73] or by the intraperitoneal route with multiple basal rates and premeal boluses[74] have been used to treat patients with T2DM. The glycemic control was in the near-normal range in these studies, and noteworthy for the relatively low incidence of hypoglycemia. This latter finding has been typical for intensive insulin treatment in T2DM (Table 30-1) regardless of mode of therapy, in contrast to intensive regimens in type 1 diabetes, which are accompanied by a relatively high risk of hypoglycemia (60–100 episodes/100 patient-years).[37,75] Finally, pulmonary delivery of aerosolized insulin before each meal has been used in type 2 diabetes in conjunction with an evening injection of intermediate-acting insulin.[76] The metabolic goals of this "proof of principle" study were modest. Whether long-term therapy with inhaled insulin can achieve and maintain near normoglycemia, and whether such therapy is safe, is unknown.[77]

Intermittent, or short-term, intensive insulin therapy has been tested in clinical studies.[28,29,36] The rationale behind this approach is to lower glycemia to the normal range and, by eliminating glucotoxicity, improve endogenous insulin secretion and decrease insulin resistance. After days to weeks of such therapy, insulin treatment is withdrawn. Glucose levels have been maintained at a near-normal range for as long as 2–3 years. These remissions have been demonstrated most reliably in relatively new onset T2DM.

COMBINATION THERAPY

Insulin has been used in combination with virtually every other therapeutic modality. Conventionally, diet and exercise recommendations accompany insulin therapy. In addition, combination therapy with sulfonylurea (Bedtime Insulin Daytime Sulfonylurea) has also been espoused.[78–80] The rationale behind combination therapy is that nocturnal insulin therapy suppresses overnight glycemia and morning short-acting sulfonylurea stimulates endogenous insulin. The only potential benefit of combining insulin and sulfonylurea, which is more expensive than using insulin alone, is a modest reduction in insulin doses required to achieve a similar level of glycemia.[79] The modest (and lack of additive) effects of combined insulin and sulfonylurea are not surprising since they work by similar mechanisms, i.e. providing increased insulin. I do not favor the use of this two-drug regimen, where compliance may be lower, drug interactions more likely, and expense greater, when insulin alone in adequate doses is effective.

Other combination regimens, using drugs with different primary mechanisms of action than insulin, such as metformin or thiazolidinediones, have been examined. Most studies have not provided for aggressive adjustment of insulin in the insulin-only arm; thus, whether any benefits that occur when oral agents are added are unique to combination therapy, or whether similar results might be obtained merely by adjusting insulin, has not been conclusively established. The glycosidase inhibitor acarbose will lower HbA$_{1c}$ levels achieved with insulin alone by 0.5%.[81] The thiazolidinediones (with most data available using the troglitazone, which is no longer available) can lower HbA$_{1c}$ when added to insulin or maintain HbA$_{1c}$ with lower doses of insulin.[55] Only rarely does thiazolidinedione therapy allow insulin-treated patients to stop their insulin therapy. The use of metformin with insulin has also been investigated. Although HbA$_{1c}$ levels are only modestly lower with additional metformin, weight gain is less with this combination therapy.[82] Whether the added expense, need for additional monitoring of renal and hepatic function (for metformin and thiazolidinediones), the potential for added toxicity and drug interactions, and decreased compliance associated with combination therapy are merited by the modest improvements in HbA$_{1c}$, and limited weight gain (with metformin) is not clear.

HOW TO SELECT T2DM PATIENTS FOR INSULIN THERAPY

As noted above, patients who have evidence of severe insulin deficiency and a catabolic state on the basis of ketonuria, profound weight loss, or dehydration, or who are thin, should be treated as if they have T1DM (Table 30-4). This will protect such patients from more profound metabolic decompensation if, in fact, they have type 1 diabetes, and will rapidly restore all of them to a safe metabolic state. Although criteria based on fasting and stimulated C-peptide levels have been proposed to help identify such patients, the majority of them can be identified on the basis of the clinical criteria listed above. In addition, patients who are symptomatic from hyperglycemia and have not responded initially, or have failed to respond after preliminary success with diet and/or sulfonylurea or metformin, should be treated with insulin. Finally, patients with very elevated triglyceride levels who are at risk for pancreatitis should be treated with insulin and diet, rather than with an oral hypoglycemic agent, as the most effective way to rapidly lower the abnormal lipid levels.

The implications of the UKPDS[18] and Kumamoto[43] studies are that insulin should be started in T2DM patients whose level of glycemia is not in the near-normal range with diet and/or oral agents, regardless of the presence of symptoms. In the past, clini-

TABLE 30-4. Indications for Insulin Therapy in Type 2 Diabetes Mellitus

Presence of ketonuria in unstressed state
Nonobese with persistently elevated glucose levels
Uncontrolled weight loss and hyperglycemia
Dehydration secondary to glycosuria and unresponsive to diet and/or oral agents
Severe hypertriglyceridemia
Diet or oral agent failure with or without symptomatic hyperglycemia
Hyperglycemia with aim of obtaining near-normal glycemia and/or inducing remission

cians have generally implemented stepped intervention of T2DM in a relatively unaggressive fashion, reserving insulin as a last resort, and often after patients had diabetes for many years and had established complications. The now demonstrated beneficial effects of tight control of T2DM and the recognition that dietary and oral agent interventions are, in many cases, temporizing at best, with progressive worsening of metabolic control over time, suggest that insulin treatment should be implemented earlier and aggressively in the course of T2DM. Moreover, reports of "remissions" of T2DM with early and intensive insulin therapy suggest that insulin should be considered as an early, rather than an end-stage, treatment.[36]

CONCLUSIONS

Insulin is the most efficacious pharmacologic treatment for patients with diabetes. The long-awaited approval of metformin in the United States, and the introduction of new agents, such as the glycosidase inhibitors and the thiazolidinediones, are unlikely to decrease the need for insulin in many of the T2DM population, which is rapidly becoming the most common chronic disease in the world. Insulin is ultimately a more powerful drug than any of the other available treatments for T2DM, as well as the only naturally occurring substance used to treat it, and until the high failure rate with diet and oral agents can be abrogated, its frequent use is all but assured.

The anticipated benefits of achieving normoglycemia in T2DM, as in T1DM, should stimulate health care providers and patients alike to use the therapy that provides glycemic control as close to the nondiabetic range as safely possible. When dietary efforts fail, insulin may well be considered the most likely therapy to achieve and maintain those levels of glycemia that are likely to prevent and/or delay long-term complications. Although the best regimen for insulin use in T2DM has yet to be firmly established, a large number of permutations have been investigated. Insulin therapy, with adequate doses and in concert with careful attention to reducing all cardiovascular risk factors, should remain a mainstay of T2DM therapy.

REFERENCES

1. National Diabetes Data Group (NDDG): Classification and diagnosis of diabetes mellitus and other categories of glucose intolerance. *Diabetes* 1979;28:1039.
2. World Health Organization (WHO) Expert Committee: Second report on diabetes mellitus. Technical Report Series No. 646, Geneva, Switzerland, 1980.
3. Expert Committee on the Diagnosis and Classification of Diabetes Mellitus: *Diabetes Care* 1997;20(suppl 1):1183.
4. Personal communication: Vignati L, Eli Lilly and Co., Crossley Study. Roper Starch Co., New York, 1995.
5. King H, Aubert RE, Herman WH: Global burden of diabetes, 1995–2025. *Diabetes Care* 1998;21:1414.
6. Nathan DM: Modern management of insulin-dependent diabetes mellitus. *Med Clin North Am* 1988;72:1365.
7. Zinman B: The physiologic replacement of insulin. *N Engl J Med* 1989;321:363.
8. Hirsch IB, Farkas-Hirsch R, Skyler JS: Intensive insulin therapy for treatment of type I diabetes. *Diabetes Care* 1990;13:1265.
9. Amiel SA: Intensified insulin therapy. *Diabetes Metab Rev* 1993;9:3.
10. Zinman B: Insulin regimens and strategies for IDDM. *Diabetes Care* 1993;16(suppl 3):24.
11. Koivisto V: Insulin therapy in Type II diabetes. *Diabetes Care* 1993; 16(suppl 3):29.
12. Buse JB: The use of insulin alone and in combination with oral agents in type 2 diabetes. *Diabetes* 1999;26:931.
13. Harris MI: Undiagnosed NIDDM. *Diabetes Care* 1993;16:642.
14. Zimmet P: Type 2 (non-insulin-dependent) diabetes—an epidemiological overview. *Diabetologia* 1982;22:399.
15. Harris MI, Hadden WC, Knowler WC: Prevalence of diabetes and impaired glucose tolerance and plasma glucose levels in U.S. population aged 20–74 yr. *Diabetes* 1987;36:523.
16. West K: Diet therapy of diabetes: An analysis of failure. *Ann Intern Med* 1973;79:425.
17. Hadden DR, Blair ALT, Wilson EA, et al: Natural history of diabetes presenting age 40–69 years: A prospective study of the influence of intensive dietary therapy. *J Med* 1986;59:579.
18. UK Prospective Diabetes Study (UKPDS) Group: Intensive blood-glucose control with sulphonylureas or insulin compared with conventional treatment and risk of complications in patients with type 2 diabetes (UKPDS 33). *Lancet* 1998;352:837.
19. Haupt E, Laube F, Loy H: Secondary failures in modern therapy of diabetes mellitus with blood glucose lowering sulfonamides. *Med Klin* 1977;72:1529.
20. Matthews DR, Cull CA, Stratton RR, et al: UKPDS 26: Sulphonylurea failure in non-insulin-dependent diabetic patients over six years. *Diabet Med* 1998;15:297.
21. DeFronzo R: The triumvirate of B-cell, muscle, liver: A collusion responsible for NIDDM. *Diabetes* 1988;37:667.
22. Leahy JL: Natural history of b-cell dysfunction in NIDDM. *Diabetes Care* 1990;13:992.
23. Warram JH, Martin BC, Krolewski AS: Slow glucose removal rate and hyperinsulinemia precede the development of Type II diabetes in the offspring of diabetic parents. *Ann Intern Med* 1990;113:909.
24. Brunzell JD, Robertson RP, Lerner RL, et al: Relationships between fasting plasma glucose levels and insulin secretion during intravenous glucose tolerance tests. *J Clin Endocrinol Metab* 1976;42:222.
25. O'Rahilly S, Turner RC, Matthews DR: Impaired pulsatile secretion of insulin in relatives of patients with non-insulin-dependent diabetes. *N Engl J Med* 1988;318:1225.
26. Eriksson J, Fransilla-Kalunki A, Ekstrand A, et al: Early metabolic defects in persons at increased risk for non-insulin-dependent diabetes mellitus. *N Engl J Med* 1989;321:337.
27. Ward WK, LaCava EC, Pacquette TL, et al: Disproportionate elevation of immunoreactive proinsulin in Type 2 diabetes mellitus and in experimental insulin resistance. *Diabetologia* 1987;30:698.
28. Andrews WJ, Vasquez B, Nagulesparan M, et al: Insulin therapy in obese, non-insulin-dependent diabetes induces improvements in insulin action and secretion that are maintained for two weeks after insulin withdrawal. *Diabetes* 1984;33:634.
29. Garvey WT, Olefsky JM, Griffin J, et al: The effect of insulin treatment on insulin secretion and insulin action in Type II diabetes mellitus. *Diabetes* 1985;34:222.
30. Kosaka K, Kuzuya T, Akanuma Y, et al: Increase in insulin response after treatment of overt maturity onset diabetes is independent of mode of treatment. *Diabetologia* 1980;18:23.
31. Groop L, Schalin C, Fransisila-Kalunki A, et al: Characteristics of non-insulin-dependent diabetic patients with secondary failure to oral antidiabetic therapy. *Am J Med* 1989;87:183.
32. Madsbad S, Krarup T, McNair P, et al: Practical clinical value of the C-peptide response to glucagon stimulation in the choice of treatment in diabetes mellitus. *Acta Med Scand* 1981;21:153.
33. UKPDS Group: UK Prospective Diabetes Study 16: Overview of six years' therapy of type 2 diabetes—a progressive disease. *Diabetes* 1995;44:1249.
34. Banerji MA, Chaiken RL, Huey H, et al: GAD antibody negative NIDDM in adult black subjects with diabetic ketoacidosis and increased frequency of human leukocyte antigen DR3 and DR4. *Diabetes* 1994;43:741.
35. Niskanen L, Karjalainen J, Sarlund H, et al: Five-year followup of islet cell antibodies in type II (non-insulin-dependent) diabetes mellitus. *Diabetologia* 1991;34:402.
36. Ilkova H, Glaser B, Tunckale A, et al: Induction of long-term glycemic control in newly diagnosed type 2 diabetic patients by transient intensive insulin treatment. *Diabetes Care* 1997;20:1353.
37. The Diabetes Control and Complications Trial (DCCT) Research Group: The effect of intensive treatment of diabetes on the development and progression of long-term complications of insulin dependent diabetes mellitus. *N Engl J Med* 1993;329:977.

38. Nathan DM: Inferences and implications: Do the DCCT results apply in NIDDM? *Diabetes Care* 1995;18:251.
39. Lasker RD: The Diabetes Control and Complications Trial—implications for policy and practice. *N Engl J Med* 1993;329:1035.
40. Eastman RC, Siebert CW, Harris M, *et al*: Implications of the Diabetes Control and Complications Trial. *J Clin Endocrinol Metab* 1993; 77:1105.
41. Nathan DM: Long-term complications of diabetes mellitus. *N Engl J Med* 1993;328:1676.
42. Klein R, Klein BEK, Moss SE, *et al*: Wisconsin Epidemiologic Study of Diabetic Retinopathy III. Prevalence and risk of diabetic retinopathy when age at diagnosis is 30 or more years. *Arch Ophthalmol* 1984;102: 527.
43. Ohkubo Y, Kishikawa H, Araki E, *et al*: Intensive insulin therapy prevents the progression of diabetic microvascular complications in Japanese patients with non-insulin-dependent diabetes mellitus: A randomized prospective 6-year study. *Diabetes Res Clin Pract* 1995;28: 103.
44. University Group Diabetes Program: A study of the effects of hypoglycemic agents on vascular complications in patients with adult onset diabetes. *Diabetes* 1970;19(suppl 2):747.
45. Nathan DM: UKPDS. Some answers, more controversy. *Lancet* 1998; 352:832.
46. Peacock I, Tattersall RB: The difficult choice of treatment for poorly controlled maturity onset diabetes. *Br Med J* 1984;596:288.
47. Samanta A, Burden AC, Kinghorn HA: A comparative study of sulfonylurea and insulin treatment in noninsulin dependent diabetics who had failed on diet therapy alone. *Diabetes Res* 1987;4:183.
48. Groop L, Widen E, Fransilla-Kalunki A, *et al*: Differential effects of insulin and oral antidiabetic agents on glucose and energy metabolism in Type II diabetes mellitus. *Diabetologia* 1989;32:599.
49. Firth RG, Bell PM, Rizza RA: Effects of tolazamide and exogenous insulin on insulin action in patients with non-insulin dependent diabetes mellitus. *N Engl J Med* 1986;314:1280.
50. Nathan DM, Roussell A, Godine JE: Glyburide or insulin for metabolic control in non-insulin-dependent diabetes mellitus. *Ann Intern Med* 1988;108:334.
51. Lindstrom T, Eriksson P, Olsson AG, *et al*: Long-term improvement of glycemic control by insulin treatment in NIDDM patients with secondary failure. *Diabetes Care* 1994;17:719.
52. Abraira C, Colwell JA, Nuttall FQ, *et al*: Veterans affairs cooperative study on glycemic control and complications in type II diabetes (VACSDM). *Diabetes Care* 1995;18:1113.
53. Schmidt JK, Harriman K, Poole JR: Modification of therapy from insulin to chlorpropamide decreases HDL cholesterol in patients with non-insulin-dependent diabetes mellitus. *Diabetes Care* 1987;10:692.
54. Saltiel AR, Olefsky JM: Thiazolidinediones in the treatment of insulin resistance and Type 2 diabetes. *Diabetes* 1996;45:1661.
55. Schwartz S, Raskin P, Fonseca V, *et al*: Effect of troglitazone in insulin-treated patients with type II diabetes mellitus. *N Engl J Med* 1998;338:861.
56. Fonseca V, Rosenstock J, Patwardhan R, *et al*: Effect of metformin and rosiglitazone combination therapy in patients with Type 2 diabetes mellitus. *JAMA* 2000;283:1795.
57. Horton ES, Clinnkingbeard C, Gatlin M, *et al*: Nateglinide alone and in combination with metformin improves glycemic control by reducing mealtime glucose levels. *Diabetes Care* 2000;23:1660.
58. Mao CS, Riegelhuth ME, Van Gundy D, *et al*: An overnight insulin infusion algorithm provides morning normoglycemia and can be used to predict insulin requirements in noninsulin-dependent diabetes mellitus. *J Clin Endocrinol Metab* 1977;82:2466.
59. The Diabetes Control and Complications Trial: Implementation of treatment protocols in the Diabetes Control and Complications Trial. *Diabetes Care* 1995;18:361.
60. Riddle MC: Evening insulin strategy. *Diabetes Care* 1990;13:676.
61. Taskinen M-R, Sane T, Helve E, *et al*: Bedtime insulin for suppression of overnight free-fatty acid, blood glucose, and glucose production, in NIDDM. *Diabetes* 1989;38:580.
62. Yki-Jarvinen H, Kauppila M, Kujansuu E, *et al*: Comparison of insulin regimens in patients with non-insulin-dependent diabetes mellitus. *N Engl J Med* 1992;327:1426.
63. Cusi K, Cunningham GR, Comstock JP: Safety and efficacy of normalizing fasting glucose with bedtime NH insulin alone in NIDDM. *Diabetes Care* 1995;18:843.
64. Turner RC, Phillips MA, Ward EA: Ultralente based insulin regimens—clinical applications, advantages, and disadvantages. *Acta Med Scand* 1983;(suppl)671:75.
65. Siegler DE, Olsson GM, Agramonte RF, *et al*: Pharmacokinetics of long-acting (ultralente) insulin preparations. *Diabetes Nutr Metab* 1991;4:267.
66. Lee WL, Zinman B: From insulin to insulin analogs: Progress in the treatment of type 1 diabetes. *Diabetes Rev* 1998;6:73.
67. Raskin P, Klaff L, Bergenstal R, *et al*: A 16 week comparison of the novel insulin analog insulin glargine (HOE 901) and NPH human insulin used with insulin lispro in patients with Type 1 diabetes. *Diabetes Care* 2000;23:1666.
68. Henry RR, Gumbiner B, Ditzler T, *et al*: Intensive conventional insulin therapy for Type II diabetes. *Diabetes Care* 1993;16:21.
69. Lindstrom TH, Arnqvist HJ, von Schenck HH: Effect of conventional and intensified insulin therapy on free-insulin profiles and glycemic control in NIDDM. *Diabetes Care* 1992;15:27.
70. Jennings AM, Lewis KS, Murdoch S, *et al*: Randomized trial comparing continuous insulin infusion and conventional insulin therapy in type II diabetic patients poorly controlled with sulfonylureas. *Diabetes Care* 1991;14:738.
71. Glaser B, Leibovich G, Nesher R, *et al*: Improved beta-cell function after intensive insulin treatment in severe non-insulin-dependent diabetes. *Acta Endocrinologia* 1988;118:365.
72. Taylor R, Foster B, Kryne-Grzebalski D, *et al*: Insulin regimens for the noninsulin dependent: Impact on diurnal metabolic state and quality of life. *Diabet Med* 1994;11:551.
73. Blackshear PJ, Shulman GI, Roussell AM, *et al*: Metabolic response to three years of continuous basal rate intravenous insulin infusion in Type II diabetic patients. *J Clin Endocrinol Metab* 1985;61:753.
74. VA Study Group: Veterans Affairs Implantable Insulin Pump Study: Mean glycemia and hypoglycemia. *Diabetes* 1994;43(suppl 1):61A.
75. Reichard P, Nilsson B-Y, Rosenqvist U, *et al*: The effect of long-term intensified insulin treatment on the development of microvascular complications of diabetes mellitus. *N Engl J Med* 1993;329:304.
76. Cefalu WT, Skyler JS, Kourides IA, *et al*: Inhaled human insulin treatment in patients with Type 2 diabetes mellitus. *Ann Intern Med* 2001; 134:203.
77. Nathan DM: Inhaled insulin for Type 2 diabetes: Solution or distraction? *Ann Intern Med* 2001;134:242.
78. Genuth SM: Treating diabetes with both insulin and sulfonylurea drugs: What is the value? *Clin Diabetes* 1987;5:74.
79. Casner PR: Insulin-glyburide combination therapy for non-insulin dependent diabetes mellitus: A long-term double blind placebo controlled trial. *Clin Pharmacol Ther* 1988;44:594.
80. Wolffenbuttel BHR, Sels J-PJE, Rondas-Colbers GJWM, *et al*: Comparison of different insulin regimens in elderly patients with NIDDM. *Diabetes Care* 1996;19:1326.
81. Chiasson J-L, Josse RG, Hunt JA, *et al*: The effectiveness of acarbose in the treatment of patients with NIDDM. *Ann Intern Med* 1994; 121:928.
82. Yki-Jarvinen H, Ryysy L, Nikkila K, *et al*: Comparison of bedtime insulin regimens in patients with type 2 diabetes mellitus. *Ann Intern Med* 1999;130:389.

Hypoglycemia in Type 1 Diabetes Mellitus: The Interplay of Insulin Excess and Compromised Glucose Counterregulation

Philip E. Cryer

John E. Gerich

SUMMARY

Iatrogenic hypoglycemia is the limiting factor in the glycemic management of diabetes. It is the result of the interplay of therapeutic insulin excess and compromised glucose counterregulation—the clinical syndromes of defective glucose counterregulation and hypoglycemia unawareness—at least in type 1 diabetes mellitus (T1DM). Aggressive attempts to achieve glycemic control increase the risk of severe hypoglycemia about threefold in T1DM, but it is possible to minimize that risk by (1) application of the principles of modern therapy (patient education and empowerment, frequent self-monitoring of blood glucose, flexible insulin regimens, individualized glycemic goals, and ongoing professional guidance and support) and (2) the practice of hypoglycemia risk reduction. Conventional risk factors for hypoglycemia, based on the premise that absolute or relative therapeutic insulin excess is the sole determinant of risk, include insulin excess (dose, timing, and type), decreased food ingestion, increased exercise, other drugs including alcohol, and increased sensitivity to or decreased clearance of insulin. But these explain only a minority of episodes of severe hypoglycemia. More potent risk factors that are clinical surrogates of compromised glucose counterregulation include (1) absolute insulin deficiency (indicating that the first physiological defense against falling glucose levels, a decrease in insulin levels, is lost and implying that the second defense, an increase in glucagon secretion, is also lost) and (2) a history of severe hypoglycemia or aggressive therapy *per se* as evidenced by lower glycemic goals or lower hemoglobin A_{1c} levels, the former indicating and the latter implying recurrent iatrogenic hypoglycemia. Recent antecedent hypoglycemia reduces autonomic responses (including epinephrine, the third defense against falling glucose levels) and symptomatic responses (which normally prompt the behavioral defense) to subsequent hypoglycemia. This is the basis of the concept of *hypoglycemia-associated autonomic failure* in T1DM, which posits that episodes of iatrogenic hypoglycemia cause hypoglycemia unawareness and, in the setting of absent glucagon responses and a defective glucose counterregulation, lead to a vicious cycle of recurrent hypoglycemia. Indeed, as little as 2–3 weeks of scrupulous avoidance of iatrogenic hypoglycemia reverses hypoglycemia unawareness and, at least in part, the reduced epinephrine component of defective glucose counterregulation in most af-

fected patients. Thus while hypoglycemia is a problem for people with diabetes that has not been solved and needs to be addressed vigorously both clinically and investigatively, the goals of improving glycemic control and minimizing hypoglycemia are not incompatible.

THE CLINICAL PROBLEM

Hypoglycemia is the limiting factor in the glycemic management of diabetes mellitus both conceptually and in practice.[1,2] Were it not for the potentially devastating effects of hypoglycemia, diabetes would be rather easy to treat. Administration of enough insulin (or any effective drug) to lower plasma glucose concentrations to or below the normal range would eliminate the symptoms of hyperglycemia and prevent diabetic ketoacidosis or hyperosmolar coma, almost assuredly prevent the long-term specific complications of diabetes (retinopathy, nephropathy, and neuropathy), and likely reduce atherosclerotic risk. But the effects of hypoglycemia on the brain are real, and the management of diabetes is therefore complex.

It is now well established that glycemic control makes a difference for people with diabetes. It prevents or delays the specific long-term complications.[3,4] Nonetheless, over a mean of only 6.5 years diabetic retinopathy developed or progressed in 14% (100 of 711) of patients with T1DM treated intensively (compared with 32% of those treated conventionally) in the Diabetes Control and Complications Trial (DCCT).[3] Similarly, nephropathy and neuropathy developed or progressed in many patients treated intensively (albeit again at lower rates than in those treated conventionally). The occurrence of these complications of diabetes in a substantial portion of people with diabetes over a rather short period of time, despite aggressive attempts to lower circulating glucose levels was largely, perhaps exclusively, the result of the inability to achieve euglycemia in the vast majority of patients. Fewer than 5% of those treated intensively maintained normal hemoglobin A_{1c} levels (<6.05%). The median hemoglobin A_{1c} was 7.2% and mean (±SD) capillary blood glucose levels were 155 ± 30 mg/dL, approximately twice those of nondiabetic individuals. Euglycemia could not be achieved safely in the vast majority of the patients because of the barrier of iatrogenic hypoglycemia. The incidence of severe hypoglycemia (that requiring the assistance of another individual) was more than threefold higher in the patients treated intensively. Clearly, even under the optimized conditions of the DCCT, hypoglycemia was the limiting factor in the management of T1DM. As shown in the United Kingdom Prospective Diabetes Study, that is also the case late in the course of type 2 diabetes mellitus (T2DM).[4,5] Over time, during intensive therapy of T2DM, hypoglycemia became limiting,[5] median hemoglobin A_{1c} levels rose to approximately 8.1%, and complications occurred (e.g., any microvascular endpoint in 8% compared with 11% in the conventional therapy group).[4]

THE CLINICAL CONTEXT

Glycemic control is a fundamentally important component of the management of diabetes.[3,4] The detection and treatment of hypertension, elevated LDL-cholesterol levels, and incipient nephropathy, retinopathy, and neuropathy, and the provision of comprehensive preventive and therapeutic care are also fundamentally important.[6] But the challenge of achieving and maintaining improved glycemic control safely is the focus of this chapter.

Because of the barrier of hypoglycemia, sustained euglycemia is an unrealistic goal for the vast majority of people with T1DM[1,3,7] (and for many with T2DM[1,5]). Aggressive attempts at glycemic control increase the risk of severe, at least temporarily disabling, iatrogenic hypoglycemia (i.e., that requiring the assistance of another individual) more than threefold in T1DM. That was documented in both of the controlled clinical trials with sample sizes large enough to demonstrate beneficial effects of intensive therapy with respect to the long-term complication of diabetes, namely the DCCT[3,7] and the Stockholm Diabetes Intervention Study.[8,9] It was confirmed in a meta-analysis that also included 12 smaller controlled trials of intensive therapy.[10] The key word here is *controlled*. The fact that aggressive attempts to achieve near euglycemia in T1DM increase the risk of iatrogenic hypoglycemia, documented in controlled clinical trials,[3,7,8–10] cannot be negated by reports of uncontrolled series with seemingly low rates of severe hypoglycemia.

Nonetheless, it is possible to reduce the risk of hypoglycemia during aggressive therapy of T1DM. That too was demonstrated in the DCCT. During the feasibility phase of the DCCT the rate of severe hypoglycemia was about sixfold higher in the intensive therapy group compared with the conventional therapy group.[7,11] During the subsequent full scale trial, that was reduced to about threefold.[3,7] As discussed later, minimizing the risk of hypoglycemia in people with T1DM involves both application of the principles of modern aggressive therapy and consideration of the roles of both therapeutic insulin excess and compromised physiological and behavioral defenses against developing hypoglycemia.

THE PHYSIOLOGY OF GLUCOSE COUNTERREGULATION

Systemic Glucose Balance

Glucose is an obligate metabolic fuel for the brain under physiological conditions.[1] This is in contrast to other organs that can oxidize fatty acids as well as glucose. Because of its unique dependence on glucose, and because it cannot synthesize glucose or store more than a few minutes' supply as glycogen, the brain requires a continuous supply of glucose from the circulation. Facilitated diffusion of glucose from the blood to the brain is a direct function of the arterial plasma glucose concentration. At normal plasma glucose concentrations, the rate of blood-to-brain glucose transport exceeds the rate of brain glucose metabolism. However, as the arterial plasma glucose concentration falls below the physiological range (approximately 70–110 mg/dL [3.9–6.1 mmol/L] in the postabsorptive state) blood-to-brain glucose transport becomes limiting to brain energy metabolism, and thus to survival. Given the immediate survival value of maintenance of the plasma glucose concentration, it is not surprising that physiological mechanisms that prevent or rapidly correct hypoglycemia have evolved. Indeed, these are so effective that hypoglycemia is a distinctly uncommon clinical event except in people who use drugs that lower plasma glucose levels (e.g., insulin, sulfonylureas, or alcohol).[1]

Normally, rates of endogenous glucose influx into the circulation and those of glucose efflux out of the circulation into tissues other than the brain are coordinately regulated, largely by the plasma glucose–lowering (regulatory) hormone insulin and the plasma glucose–raising (counterregulatory) hormones glucagon and epinephrine, such that systemic glucose balance is maintained, hypoglycemia (as well as hyperglycemia) is prevented, and a continuous supply of glucose to the brain is assured.[1] This is accomplished despite wide variations in exogenous glucose influx (e.g., after feeding compared with during fasting) and in glucose efflux (e.g., during exercise compared with during rest). Hypoglycemia occurs when rates of glucose appearance in the circulation (the sum of endogenous glucose production, from the liver via both glycogenolysis and gluconeogenesis, and to a lesser extent from the kidneys via gluconeogenesis,[12] and of exogenous glucose delivery from ingested carbohydrates) fail to keep pace with rates of glucose disappearance from the circulation (the sum of ongoing brain glucose metabolism and of variable glucose utilization by tissues such as muscle and fat, as well as the liver and kidneys, among others).

Falling plasma glucose concentrations normally elicit a typical sequence of responses. Arterialized venous glycemic thresholds for several of these[13–15] are listed in Table 31-1. Insulin secretion decreases (favoring increased glucose production as well as decreased glucose utilization by tissues other than the brain) as plasma glucose levels decline within the physiological range. Secretion of counterregulatory hormones including glucagon (which stimulates hepatic glycogenolysis and gluconeogenesis) and epinephrine (which stimulates hepatic glycogenolysis and gluconeogenesis and renal gluconeogenesis[16] and limits glucose utilization by insulin-sensitive tissues) as well as both cortisol and growth hormone (both of which limit glucose utilization and support glucose production) increases as plasma glucose levels fall just below the physiological range. Lower plasma glucose levels cause symptoms and signs of hypoglycemia, and ultimately brain dysfunction.

When the same quantitative method (i.e., the hyperinsulinemic stepped hypoglycemic clamp technique coupled with hyperinsulinemic euglycemic clamps in the same individuals on a separate occasion) is used, the glycemic thresholds for the various responses to falling plasma glucose concentrations in healthy subjects are quite reproducible from laboratory-to-laboratory.[13–15] Nonetheless, these thresholds are dynamic rather than static. They shift to higher plasma glucose concentrations in people with poorly controlled diabetes (who often have symptoms of hypoglycemia at higher-than-normal glucose levels) and to lower plasma glucose concentrations in people who suffer recurrent hypoglycemia, such as those with well-controlled diabetes or with an insulinoma (who often tolerate subnormal glucose levels without symptoms), as discussed later.

Clinical Manifestations of Hypoglycemia

Symptoms of hypoglycemia can be divided into two categories: neuroglycopenic and neurogenic (or autonomic) symptoms.[17] Neuroglycopenic symptoms are the direct result of CNS neuronal glucose deprivation. They include behavioral changes, confusion, fatigue, seizure, loss of consciousness, and if hypoglycemia is severe and prolonged, death. Neurogenic symptoms are the result of the perception of the physiological changes caused by the autonomic nervous system discharge triggered by hypoglycemia. They include adrenergic symptoms such as palpitations, tremor, and anxiety, and cholinergic symptoms such as sweating, hunger, and paresthesias. Adrenergic symptoms are mediated by epinephrine released from the adrenal medullae and norepinephrine released from sympathetic postganglionic neurons, the adrenal medullae, or both. Cholinergic symptoms (at least sweating) are thought to be mediated by acetylcholine released from sympathetic postganglionic neurons.

Common signs of hypoglycemia include pallor and diaphoresis. Heart rate and the systolic blood pressure are typically raised, but these findings may not be prominent. To the extent they are observable, the neuroglycopenic manifestations are often valuable, albeit nonspecific, signs. Transient focal neurological deficits occur occasionally. Permanent neurological damage is uncommon.

Normal Glucose Counterregulation

The principles of glucose counterregulation are as follows. First, the prevention and the correction of hypoglycemia involve both waning of insulin and activation of glucose counterregulatory factors. These are not due solely to dissipation of insulin. Second, whereas insulin is the dominant plasma glucose–lowering factor, there are redundant glucose counterregulatory factors. There is a fail-safe system that prevents failure of the counterregulatory process even when one, or perhaps more of the components of the system fails. Third, there is a hierarchy among the counterregulatory factors. Some are more important than others. The fact that there is a hierarchy of redundant glucose counterregulatory factors

that normally prevent or rapidly correct hypoglycemia is almost assuredly a reflection of the survival value of the prevention of sustained hypoglycemia throughout evolution.

The physiology of glucose counterregulation[1] is also summarized in Table 31-1. The first defense against falling plasma glucose concentrations is decreased insulin secretion. Among the counterregulatory factors, glucagon plays a primary role. Glucose recovery from hypoglycemia is impaired and postabsorptive plasma glucose concentrations decline, but then plateau when glucagon is deficient. Although demonstrably involved, epinephrine is not normally critical, but it becomes critical when glucagon is deficient. Hypoglycemia develops or progresses when both glucagon and epinephrine are deficient and insulin is present, regardless of the actions of the other glucose counterregulatory factors. Thus insulin, glucagon, and epinephrine stand high in the hierarchy of the redundant glucose counterregulatory factors. Growth hormone and cortisol, both of which tend to raise plasma glucose concentrations over several hours, are involved in defense against prolonged hypoglycemia. However, neither is critical to recovery from even prolonged hypoglycemia or to prevention of hypoglycemia after an overnight fast.[1,18] There is some evidence that glucose autoregulation—endogenous glucose production as an inverse function of ambient glucose levels independent of hormonal and neural regulation—is involved, albeit only during very severe hypoglycemia.[1,19] Other hormones, neurotransmitters, or substrates other than glucose may also be involved, but if so they play minor roles.

THE PATHOPHYSIOLOGY OF GLUCOSE COUNTERREGULATION IN DIABETES

Frequency and Impact

Because of the imperfections of all current insulin replacement regimens, coupled with compromised physiological and behavioral defenses against falling plasma glucose concentrations as discussed later, people with T1DM are at ongoing risk for episodes of hypoglycemia.[1] Those attempting to achieve glycemic control suffer untold numbers of episodes of asymptomatic hypoglycemia (plasma glucose levels may be lower than 50 mg/dL [2.8 mmol/L] as much as 10% of the time) and an average of two episodes of symptomatic hypoglycemia per week. They suffer an episode of severe, at least

TABLE 31-1. Physiological Responses to Decreasing Plasma Glucose Concentrations

Response	Glycemic Threshold* (mg/dL)	Physiological Effects	Role in the Prevention or Correction of Hypoglycemia (Glucose Counterregulation)
↓ Insulin	80–85	↑ R$_a$ (↓ R$_d$)†	Primary glucose regulatory factor; first defense against hypoglycemia
↑ Glucagon	65–70	↑ R$_a$	Primary glucose counterregulatory factor; second defense against hypoglycemia
↑ Epinephrine	65–70	↑ R$_a$, ↓ R$_d$	Involved, critical when glucagon is deficient; third defense against hypoglycemia
↑ Cortisol and growth hormone	65–70	↑ R$_a$; ↓ R$_d$	Involve, not critical
Symptoms	50–55	↑ Exogenous glucose	Prompt behavioral defense (food ingestion)
↓ Cognition	<50	—	Compromises behavioral defense

*Arterialized venous, not venous, plasma glycemic thresholds in healthy individuals, 13–15.

†R$_a$, rate of glucose appearance, glucose production by the liver and kidneys.

R$_d$, rate of glucose disappearance, glucose utilization by insulin-sensitive tissues such as skeletal muscle (the glucoregulatory hormones have no direct effect on CNS glucose utilization).

temporarily disabling hypoglycemia, often with seizure or coma, in a given year. Although seemingly complete recovery from the latter is the rule, the possibility of persistent cognitive deficits has been raised and permanent neurological defects can occur. It has been estimated that about 2–4% of deaths of people with T1DM are the result of hypoglycemia.[1,20] In addition, hypoglycemia can cause recurrent or even persistent psychosocial morbidity. The reality of hypoglycemia, the rational fear of hypoglycemia, or both can preclude true glycemic control in T1DM.

Overall, hypoglycemia is a substantially less frequent problem in T2DM.[1] However, it occurs during treatment with sulfonylureas and other insulin secretagogues (and has been reported in patients treated with metformin) or insulin, and its frequency approaches that in T1DM in those who reach the insulin-deficient end of the spectrum of T2DM.[5] In one series the frequency of severe hypoglycemia was similar in patients with T2DM and T1DM matched for duration of insulin therapy.[21] The United Kingdom Prospective Diabetes Study investigators concluded that over time, hypoglycemia becomes limiting in the treatment of T2DM just as it is in the treatment of T1DM.[5]

Altered Glucose Counterregulation in Diabetes

Glucose counterregulation is altered fundamentally in all people with established (i.e., C-peptide negative) T1DM.[1] It is defective in most, and is often associated with unawareness of hypoglycemia.[1]

As the person with T1DM becomes absolutely insulin deficient over the first few months or years of clinical T1DM, circulating insulin levels become totally unregulated; they are a passive function of administered insulin. Thus insulin levels no longer fall as glucose levels fall. The first defense against hypoglycemia is lost. Furthermore, within the same time frame the glucagon response to falling glucose levels, the second defense, is also lost.[22,23] The mechanism of this selective and therefore functional rather than anatomic defect in glucagon secretion is unknown, although it is closely linked to, and potentially attributable to, absolute insulin deficiency.[24] In most patients the third defense against hypoglycemia is compromised when the epinephrine response to hypoglycemia is reduced.[23,25–27] In contrast to the absent glucagon response, the reduced epinephrine response is mainly a threshold abnormality; an epinephrine response can be elicited, but lower plasma glucose concentrations are required.[27] This functional threshold shift is largely the result of recent antecedent hypoglycemia, as discussed shortly, although there may well be an additional anatomic component in patients affected by classic diabetic autonomic neuropathy.[28,29] Thus established T1DM is not just an insulin-deficiency state. From the perspective of defense against hypoglycemia, it is an insulin, glucagon, and epinephrine deficiency state.

The development of an attenuated epinephrine response to falling glucose levels is a critical pathophysiological event. Patients with T1DM who have combined deficiencies of their glucagon and epinephrine responses have the clinical syndrome of *defective glucose counterregulation*,[1] and have been shown in prospective studies to suffer severe hypoglycemia at rates 25-fold or greater higher than those with absent glucagon but intact epinephrine responses during aggressive therapy.[30,31]

Hypoglycemia unawareness is loss of the largely (if not exclusively) neurogenic warning symptoms of developing hypoglycemia that previously prompted the patient to act (e.g., to eat) to abort the episode. Thus the first manifestation of a hypoglycemic episode is neuroglycopenia, and it is often too late for the patient to recognize and self-treat the episode. Hypoglycemia unawareness is

also largely the result of recent antecedent hypoglycemia, as discussed shortly. Reduced β-adrenergic sensitivity has also been reported.[32] It too has been shown in prospective studies to be associated with a high frequency of severe iatrogenic hypoglycemia.[33]

Recent antecedent hypoglycemia reduces autonomic (including adrenomedullary epinephrine) and symptomatic responses (among others) to subsequent hypoglycemia—it actually shifts the glycemic thresholds for these responses to lower plasma glucose concentrations—in nondiabetic individuals[34–38] and in patients with T1DM.[27,39,40] It also impairs physiologic defense against hypoglycemia during hyperinsulinemia in patients with T1DM.[27] Such findings led to the formulation[41] and experimental verification[27,42–45] of the concept of hypoglycemia-associated autonomic failure in T1DM.

The concept of *hypoglycemia-associated autonomic failure* in T1DM (Fig. 31-1) posits that (1) periods of relative or absolute therapeutic insulin excess in the setting of absent glucagon responses lead to episodes of iatrogenic hypoglycemia; (2) these episodes, in turn, cause reduced autonomic (including adrenomedullary) responses to falling glucose concentrations on subsequent occasions; and (3) these reduced autonomic responses result in both reduced symptoms of developing hypoglycemia (i.e., hypoglycemia unawareness) and—because epinephrine responses are reduced in the setting of absent glucagon responses—impaired physiological defense against developing hypoglycemia (i.e., defective glucose counterregulation). Thus a vicious cycle of recurrent hypoglycemia is created and perpetuated.

Perhaps the most compelling support for the concept of hypoglycemia-associated autonomic failure in T1DM is the finding in three independent laboratories[42,46,47] that the syndrome of hypoglycemia unawareness, and at least in part the reduced epinephrine component of the syndrome of defective glucose counterregulation, is reversible after as little as 2 weeks of scrupulous avoidance of iatrogenic hypoglycemia in affected patients with T1DM. While this involves a shift of glycemic thresholds for symptoms, and for the epinephrine response back toward higher plasma glucose concentrations, the basic mechanisms of hypoglycemia-associated autonomic failure remain to be established. Evidence that it is mediated by the cortisol response to previous hypoglycemia[48,49] and involves increased brain glucose uptake[50,51] has been presented although the latter has been challenged.[52]

Consistent with the concept of hypoglycemia-associated autonomic failure, recent antecedent hypoglycemia also shifts glycemic thresholds for cognitive dysfunction during hypoglycemia to lower plasma glucose concentrations,[43–45] and impairs detection of hypoglycemia in the clinical setting in patients with T1DM.[44] In addition to shifting the thresholds for adrenomedullary (plasma epinephrine) and parasympathetic (plasma pancreatic polypeptide) responses, it has been reported to reduce the sympathetic neural response to subsequent hypoglycemia.[38,48,49]

CLINICAL RISK FACTORS FOR HYPOGLYCEMIA IN THE CONTEXT OF THE PATHOPHYSIOLOGY OF GLUCOSE COUNTERREGULATION

The conventional risk factors for iatrogenic hypoglycemia in T1DM, those with which people with diabetes and their caregivers deal regularly, are based on the premise that absolute or relative therapeutic insulin excess—which must occur from time to time because of the pharmacokinetic imperfections of all current insulin

Hypoglycemia-Associated Autonomic Failure

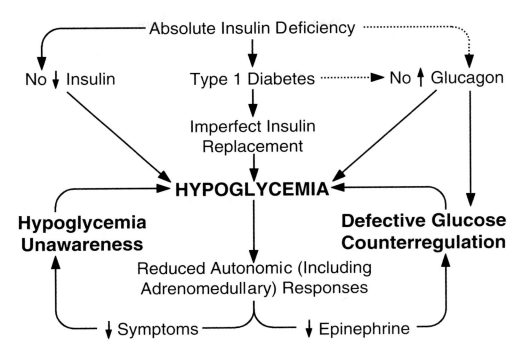

FIGURE 31-1. Schematic diagram of the concept of hypoglycemia-associated autonomic failure in type 1 diabetes.

replacement regimens—is the sole determinant of risk. These risk factors include insulin doses that are excessive, ill-timed, or of the wrong type; decreased food intake; exercise; drugs including alcohol; and increased sensitivity to or decreased clearance of insulin, and are detailed in Table 31-2. However, it became clear early in the DCCT that these conventional risk factors explain only a minority of episodes of severe iatrogenic hypoglycemia.[11] Indeed, in a multivariate model none was a statistically-significant risk factor. Clearly we must look beyond these to understand the majority of episodes.

Iatrogenic hypoglycemia is more appropriately viewed as a result of the interplay of absolute or relative therapeutic insulin excess and compromised glucose counterregulation—compromised physiological and behavioral defenses against developing hypoglycemia—at least in T1DM[1] (Table 31-2). Three clinically well-documented risk factors for iatrogenic hypoglycemia that are statistically more potent than the conventional risk factors are (1) absolute insulin deficiency (i.e., C-peptide negativity);[7,24,53] (2) a history of severe hypoglycemia;[7,53] and (3) aggressive therapy *per se* as evidenced by lower glycemic goals or lower hemoglobin A_{1c} levels.[7,53] These are clinical surrogates of compromised glucose counterregulation, the clinical syndromes of defective glucose counterregulation and hypoglycemia unawareness, and the pathophysiologic construct of hypoglycemia-associated autonomic failure.

Absolute endogenous insulin deficiency indicates that plasma insulin concentrations—which are then simply the result of passive absorption of exogenous insulin—cannot decrease as plasma glucose concentrations fall. Furthermore, absolute insulin deficiency accurately predicts that plasma glucagon levels will not increase as plasma glucose concentrations fall.[24] Thus C-peptide negativity, a potent clinical marker of increased risk of severe hypoglycemia in T1DM, indicates that the first two physiological defenses against developing hypoglycemia—decrease in insulin and increase in glucagon—are lost. Therefore, the patient is dependent upon the third physiological defense, increases in epinephrine.

TABLE 31-2. Conventional Risk Factors for Hypoglycemia in Diabetes

1. Insulin doses excessive, ill-timed, or of the wrong type
2. Decreased influx of exogenous glucose (during the overnight fast or following missed meals or snacks)
3. Increased insulin-independent glucose utilization (during exercise)
4. Decreased endogenous glucose production (alcohol, other drugs, renal failure)
5. Increased sensitivity to insulin (following exercise; middle of the night, with glycemic control; with increased fitness, weight loss, or both; drugs)
6. Decreased insulin clearance (renal failure)

But this third physiological defense (along with the behavioral defense prompted by symptoms) is compromised in patients with the other clinical markers of increased risk: severe hypoglycemia, a history of severe hypoglycemia or aggressive therapy *per se* as evidenced by lower glycemic goals, and lower hemoglobin A_{1c} levels (a history of hypoglycemia indicating an aggressive theraphy implying recurrent episodes of antecedent hypoglycemia). As discussed earlier, hypoglycemia begets hypoglycemia by reducing the autonomic (including epinephrine) and symptomatic responses to subsequent hypoglycemia, thus causing the syndromes of defective glucose counterregulation (reduced epinephrine responses in the setting of absent glucagon responses), and hypoglycemia unawareness (reduced neurogenic symptom responses). This is hypoglycemia-associated autonomic failure in T1DM.

These concepts were developed in people with T1DM. The extent to which they apply to those with T2DM remains to be established critically. It appears that they also apply to patients with relatively long-standing, insulin-requiring T2DM, and in keeping with this, hypoglycemia becomes limiting to glycemic control in such patients.[5]

Hypoglycemia Risk Reduction

Hypoglycemia is a fact of life for people with T1DM (and some with T2DM) who attempt to achieve glycemic control.[3–5,7–11,53] Given the shortcomings of all current insulin replacement regimens, including the most sophisticated regimens available, it is not practical to both maintain euglycemia and eliminate episodes of asymptomatic and even symptomatic hypoglycemia in T1DM. That awaits the ultimate goal of the prevention and cure of diabetes or, probably in the shorter term, development of clinical strategies for perfect or near perfect insulin replacement coupled with measures that prevent, correct, or compensate for compromised glucose counterregulation.[2] Nonetheless, every effort must be made to minimize the risk of hypoglycemia, and eliminate the risk of severe hypoglycemia, while pursuing the greatest degree of glycemic control that can be achieved safely in an individual person with diabetes.

To practice hypoglycemia risk reduction, an approach conceptually analogous to cardiovascular risk reduction, we must first address the issue of hypoglycemia in every patient contact. In addition to asking about episodes of hypoglycemia—and assessing the patient's awareness of developing hypoglycemia—and looking for low values in the patient's self-monitoring of blood glucose (SMBG) log, it is important to determine the extent to which the patient is concerned about the reality or the possibility of hypoglycemia. Fear of hypoglycemia can be a barrier to glycemic control.

The second step in hypoglycemia risk reduction is application of the principles of modern aggressive therapy: patient education

and empowerment, frequent SMBG, flexible insulin replacement regimens, rational individualized glycemic goals, and ongoing professional guidance and support. Successful management of diabetes, particularly glycemic management, is accomplished by a well-informed and empowered patient who receives comprehensive preventive and therapeutic medical care.

The third step in hypoglycemia risk reduction is consideration of both the conventional risk factors for iatrogenic hypoglycemia (Table 31-2) that lead to episodes of absolute or relative therapeutic insulin excess (insulin doses, timing and type, patterns of food ingestion and of exercise, interactions with alcohol or other drugs, and altered insulin sensitivity to or clearance of insulin) and the risk factors for compromised glucose counterregulation that impair physiological and behavioral defenses against developing hypoglycemia (Table 31-3). The principle is that iatrogenic hypoglycemia is the result of the interplay of insulin excess and compromised glucose counterregulation rather than insulin excess alone.

The clinical surrogates of risk attributable to compromised glucose counterregulation include absolute insulin deficiency (which may be apparent from a history of ketosis-prone diabetes requiring insulin therapy from the time of diagnosis, although it is now recognized that insulin deficiency can sometimes develop more gradually) and a history of recurrent hypoglycemia or, absent that, lower glycemic goals, lower hemoglobin A_{1c} levels, or both. It is possible to test for defective glucose counterregulation (with a low-dose insulin infusion test[30,31]), but that is generally not practical. On the other hand, a diagnosis of hypoglycemia unawareness can be made from the history. Clinical hypoglycemia unawareness (which also implies defective glucose counterregulation) is a strong clue to recurrent antecedent hypoglycemia whether or not that has been documented. In the future, documentation will become increasingly possible as continuous glucose monitoring systems become available.

Obviously, with a history of recurrent hypoglycemia, one should identify when it occurs and adjust the treatment regimen accordingly. With a basal-bolus insulin regimen, morning fasting hypoglycemia implicates the long- or intermediate-acting insulin, daytime hypoglycemia implicates the rapid- or short-acting insulin, and nocturnal hypoglycemia may implicate either, all in the context of the other risk factors for insulin excess (Table 31-2). Notably, substitution of preprandial rapid-acting (e.g., lispro or aspart) for short-acting (regular) insulin reduces the frequency of nocturnal hypoglycemia.[54] Similarly, substitution of longer-acting basal insulins (e.g., glargine) for NPH or ultralente insulin may reduce nocturnal hypoglycemia.

A history of severe iatrogenic hypoglycemia—that requiring assistance from another individual—is a clinical red flag. Unless it was the result of an obviously remediable factor, such as a missed meal after insulin administration or vigorous exercise without the appropriate regimen adjustment, a substantive change in the regi-

---

TABLE 31-3. Risk Factors for Hypoglycemia in Diabetes

1. Absolute or relative therapeutic insulin excess (the conventional risk factors)
2. Compromised glucose counterregulation
   - Absolute insulin deficiency (C-peptide negativity)
     β-Cell destruction: No ↓ in insulin response to ↓ glucose
     Unknown: No ↑ in glucagon in response to ↓ glucose
   - History of severe hypoglycemia or aggressive therapy *per se* (lower glucose goals, lower HbA$_{1c}$)
     Episodes of hypoglycemia: Attenuated autonomic (including ↑ epinephrine) activations and symptoms in response to ↓ glucose (defective glucose counterregulation and hypoglycemia unawareness)
   - Hypoglycemia-associated autonomic failure

men must be made. If it is not, the risk of recurrent severe hypoglycemia is unacceptably high.[7,53]

A history of hypoglycemia unawareness implies recurrent hypoglycemia. If that is not apparent to the patient or to his or her family or from the SMBG log, it is probably occurring during the night. Indeed, hypoglycemia, including severe hypoglycemia, occurs most commonly during the night in people with T1DM.[7,11] That is typically the longest interdigestive interval and time between SMBG and the time of maximal sensitivity to insulin.[55] Furthermore, sleep often precludes recognition of warning symptoms of developing hypoglycemia and thus the appropriate behavioral response, and has been reported to further reduce the epinephrine response to hypoglycemia and thus further compromise physiological defense against developing hypoglycemia.[56] Current approaches to the problem of nocturnal hypoglycemia include regimen adjustments, including use of rapid-acting insulin during the day, and administration of bedtime snacks, although the efficacy of the latter is largely limited to the first half of the night.[57] Experimental approaches include bedtime administration of uncooked cornstarch,[58,59] the glucagon-releasing amino acid alanine, or the β_2-adrenergic agonist terbutaline.[57]

The value of uncooked cornstarch is controversial. While Ververs and colleagues[58] using hourly blood sampling found that bedtime administration of a snack that included 0.2–0.8 g/kg body weight of uncooked cornstarch (the equivalent of 14.0–56.0 grams in a 70-kg individual) did not prevent nocturnal hypoglycemia (symptoms, blood glucose <54 mg/dL [3.0 mmol/L], or both) in young T1DM subjects, Kaufman and Devgan[59] reported reduced (as compared to controls) episodes of self-monitored low (<60 mg [3.3 mmol/L]) blood glucose (SMBG) levels at 0200h in young T1DM subjects given a snack that included 5.0–15.0 grams of uncooked cornstarch for 14 days. Thus it remains to be established that bedtime administration of only 5.0 grams of cornstarch (the dose, apparently limited by palatability, in preparations available commercially) would consistently reduce the frequency of hypoglycemia throughout the entire night. Bedtime administration of alanine (with glucose) or terbutaline has been shown to prevent nocturnal hypoglycemia more effectively than a conventional bedtime snack.[57] The limited solubility of alanine in the dose used (40 g) limits its practicability. While bedtime terbutaline can cause metabolic effects (slightly higher lactate, nonesterified fatty acid and perhaps β-hydroxybutyrate levels) and hemodynamic effects (higher heart rates) during the night that are undesirable at least in theory, and can cause hyperglycemia the following morning,[57] the convenience and flexibility of tablet dosing make it an attractive option when other approaches to the problem of nocturnal hypoglycemia are unsuccessful.

Given clinical hypoglycemia unawareness, a 2–3 week period of scrupulous avoidance of hypoglycemia is advisable, and can be assessed by return of awareness.[42,46,47] While this can be accomplished without[46,47] or with minimal[42] compromise of glycemic control, this outcome required substantial involvement of health professionals. In practice it might involve acceptance of somewhat higher glucose levels over the short term. Nonetheless, with the return of symptoms of developing hypoglycemia, empirical approaches to better glycemic control can then be tried.

CONCLUDING COMMENTS

Clearly, hypoglycemia is a problem for most people with T1DM (and some with T2DM) that has not been solved. It is now established that comprehensive treatment reduces morbidity and mortality in people with diabetes. Comprehensive treatment includes glycemic control that at a minimum prevents or delays the specific long-term complications of diabetes[3,4] to the extent that can be accomplished with relative safety. Aggressive attempts at glycemic control increase the risk of iatrogenic hypoglycemia, but it is possible to minimize that risk by applying the principles of modern aggressive therapy and practicing hypoglycemia risk reduction. Thus the goals of improving glycemic control and minimizing hypoglycemia are not incompatible.

Acknowledgments The authors gratefully acknowledge the contributions of their several colleagues who shaped the work that led to the views expressed in this chapter, the assistance of the staffs of our General Clinical Research Centers in the performance of our studies, and the assistance of Ms. Karen Muehlhauser in the preparation of this manuscript. Dr. Cryer's work cited was supported in part by U.S.P.H.S. grants R01 DK27085, M01 RR00036, P60 DK20579, and T32 DK01720, and by a grant and a fellowship award from the American Diabetes Association. Dr. Gerich's work cited was supported in part by U.S.P.H.S. grants R01 DK20411 and M01 RR00044.

REFERENCES

1. Cryer PE: *Hypoglycemia. Pathophysiology, Diagnosis and Treatment.* Oxford University Press:1997.
2. Cryer PE: Hypoglycemia-associated autonomic failure in diabetes. *Am J Physiol* 2001;281:E1115.
3. The Diabetes Control and Complications Trial Research Group (DCCT): The effect of intensive treatment of diabetes on the development and progression of long-term complications in insulin-dependent diabetes mellitus. *N Engl J Med* 1993;329:977.
4. The United Kingdom Prospective Diabetes Study Group (UKPDS): Intensive blood-glucose control with sulfonylureas or insulin compared with conventional treatment and risk of complications in patients with type 2 diabetes. *Lancet* 1998;352:837.
5. The United Kingdom Prospective Diabetes Study Group (UKPDS): A 6-year, randomized, controlled trial comparing sulfonylurea, insulin and metformin therapy in patients with newly diagnosed type 2 diabetes that could not be controlled with diet therapy. *Ann Intern Med* 1998;128:165.
6. American Diabetes Association: Standards of medical care for patients with diabetes mellitus. *Diabetes Care* 1999;22(Suppl 1):S32.
7. The Diabetes Control and Complications Trial Research Group (DCCT): Hypoglycemia in the Diabetes Control and Complications Trial. *Diabetes* 1997;46:271.
8. Reichard P, Berglund B, Britz A, et al: Intensified conventional insulin treatment retards the microvascular complications of insulin-dependent diabetes mellitus: The Stockholm Diabetes Intervention Study after 5 years. *J Intern Med* 1990;230:101.
9. Reichard P, Nilsson B-Y, Rosenqvist U: The effect of long-term intensified insulin treatment on the development of microvascular complications of diabetes mellitus. *N Engl J Med* 1993;329:304.
10. Egger M, Davey Smith G, Stettler C, et al: Risk of adverse effects of intensified treatment in insulin-dependent diabetes mellitus: A meta-analysis. *Diabetic Med* 1997;14:919.
11. The Diabetes Control and Complications Trial Research Group (DCCT): Epidemiology of severe hypoglycemia in the Diabetes Control and Complications Trial. *Am J Med* 1991;90:450.
12. Gerich J E, Meyer C, Woerle H J, Stumvoll M: Renal gluconeogenesis. *Diabetes Care* 2001;24:382.
13. Schwartz NS, Clutter WE, Shah SD, et al: Glycemic thresholds for activation of glucose counterregulatory systems are higher than the threshold for symptoms. *J Clin Invest* 1987;79:777.
14. Mitrakou A, Ryan C, Veneman T, et al: Hierarchy of glycemic thresholds for counterregulatory hormone secretion symptoms and cerebral dysfunction. *Am J Physiol* 1991;260:E67.

15. Fanelli C, Pampanelli S, Epifano L, *et al*: Relative roles of insulin and hypoglycemia on induction of neuroendocrine responses to, symptoms of, and deterioration of cognitive function in hypoglycaemia in male and female humans. *Diabetologia* 1994;37:797.

16. Meyer C, Dostou JM, Gerich JE: Role of the human kidney in glucose counterregulation. *Diabetes* 1999;48:943.

17. Towler DA, Havlin CE, Craft S, *et al*: Mechanisms of awareness of hypoglycemia: Perception of neurogenic (predominantly cholinergic) rather than neuroglycopenic symptoms. *Diabetes* 1993; 42:1791.

18. Boyle PJ, Cryer PE: Growth hormone, cortisol, or both are involved in defense against, but are not critical to recovery from, hypoglycemia. *Am J Physiol* 1991;260:E395.

19. Bolli G, De Feo P, Perriello G, *et al*: Role of hepatic autoregulation in defense against hypoglycemia in humans. *J Clin Invest* 1985; 75:1623.

20. Laing SP, Swerdlow AJ, Slater SD, *et al*: The British Diabetic Association Cohort Study. II. Cause-specific mortality in patients with insulin-treated diabetes mellitus. *Diabet Med* 1999;16:466.

21. Hepburn DA, MacLeod KM, Pell ACH, *et al*: Frequency and symptoms of hypoglycaemia experienced by patients with type 2 diabetes treated with insulin. *Diabet Med* 1993;10:231.

22. Gerich JE, Langlois M, Noacco C, *et al*: Lack of glucagon response to hypoglycemia in diabetes: Evidence for an intrinsic pancreatic alpha cell defect. *Science* 1973;182:171.

23. Bolli G, De Feo P, Compagnucci P, *et al*: Abnormal glucose counterregulation in insulin dependent diabetes mellitus. Interaction of anti-insulin antibodies and impaired glucagon and epinephrine secretion. *Diabetes* 1983;32:134.

24. Fukuda M, Tanaka A, Tahara Y, *et al*: Correlation between minimal secretory capacity of pancreatic β-cells and stability of diabetic control. *Diabetes* 1988;37:81.

25. Boden G, Reichard GA Jr., Hoeldtke RD, *et al*: Severe insulin-induced hypoglycemia associated with deficiencies in the release of counterregulatory hormones. *N Engl J Med* 1981;305:1200.

26. Hirsch BR, Shamoon H: Defective epinephrine and growth hormone responses in type 1 diabetes are stimulus specific. *Diabetes* 1987;36:20.

27. Dagogo-Jack SE, Craft S, Cryer PE: Hypoglycemia-associated autonomic failure in insulin dependent diabetes mellitus. *J Clin Invest* 1993;91:819.

28. Bottini P, Boschetti E, Pampanelli S, *et al*: Contribution of autonomic neuropathy to reduced plasma adrenaline responses to hypoglycemia in IDDM. *Diabetes* 1997;46:814.

29. Meyer C, Grobmann R, Mitrakou A, *et al*: Effects of autonomic neuropathy on counterregulation and awareness of hypoglycaemia in type 1 diabetic patients. *Diabetes Care* 1998;21:1960.

30. White NH, Skor DA, Cryer PE, *et al*: Identification of type 1 diabetic patients at increased risk for hypoglycemia during intensive therapy. *N Engl J Med* 1983;308:485.

31. Bolli GB, De Feo P, De Cosmo S, *et al*: A reliable and reproducible test for adequate glucose counterregulation in type 1 diabetes. *Diabetes* 1984;33:732.

32. Korytkowski MT, Mokan M, Veneman T, *et al*: Reduced β-adrenergic sensitivity in IDDM patients with hypoglycemia unawareness. *Diabetes Care* 1998;21:1939.

33. Gold AE, MacLeod KM, Frier BM: Frequency of severe hypoglycemia in patients with type 1 diabetes with impaired awareness of hypoglycemia. *Diabetes Care* 1994;17:697.

34. Heller SR, Cryer PE: Reduced neuroendocrine and symptomatic responses to subsequent hypoglycemia after one episode of hypoglycemia in nondiabetic humans. *Diabetes* 1991;40:223.

35. Davis M, Shamoon H: Counterregulatory adaptation to recurrent hypoglycemia in normal humans. *J Clin Endocrinol Metab* 1991;73:995.

36. Widom B, Simonson DC: Intermittent hypoglycemia impairs glucose counterregulation. *Diabetes* 1992;41:1597.

37. Veneman T, Mitrakou A, Mokan M, *et al*: Induction of hypoglycemia unawareness by asymptomatic nocturnal hypoglycemia. *Diabetes* 1993;42:1233.

38. Davis SN, Shavers C, Mosqueda-Garcia R, *et al*: Effects of differing antecedent hypoglycemia on subsequent counterregulation in normal man. *Diabetes* 1997;46:1328.

39. Davis MR, Mellman M, Shamoon H: Further defects in counterregulatory responses induced by recurrent hypoglycemia in type I diabetes. *Diabetes* 1992;41:1335.

40. Lingenfelser T, Renn W, Sommerwerck U, *et al*: Compromised hormonal counterregulation, symptom awareness, and neurophysiological function after recurrent short-term episodes of insulin-induced hypoglycemia in IDDM patients. *Diabetes* 1993;42:610.

41. Cryer PE: Iatrogenic hypoglycemia as a cause of hypoglycemia-associated autonomic failure in IDDM: A vicious cycle. *Diabetes* 1992;41:255.

42. Dagogo-Jack SE, Rattarasarn C, Cryer PE: Reversal of hypoglycemia unawareness, but not defective glucose counterregulation, in IDDM. *Diabetes* 1994;42:1426.

43. Hvidberg A, Fanelli CG, Hershey T, *et al*: Impact of recent antecedent hypoglycemia on hypoglycemic cognitive dysfunction in nondiabetic humans. *Diabetes* 1996;45:1030.

44. Ovalle F, Fanelli CG, Paramore DS, *et al*: Brief twice weekly episodes of hypoglycemia reduce detection of clinical hypoglycemia in type 1 diabetes mellitus. *Diabetes* 1998;47:1472.

45. Fanelli CG, Parmore DS, Hershey T, *et al*: Impact of nocturnal hypoglycemia on hypoglycemic cognitive dysfunction in type 1 diabetes mellitus. *Diabetes* 1998;47:1920.

46. Fanelli CG, Pampanelli S, Epifano L, *et al*: Long-term recovery from unawareness, deficient counterregulation and lack of cognitive dysfunction during hypoglycemia following institution of rational intensive therapy in IDDM. *Diabetologia* 1994;37:1265.

47. Cranston I, Lomas J, Maran A, *et al*: Restoration of hypoglycemia unawareness in patients with long duration insulin-dependent diabetes mellitus. *Lancet* 1994;344:283.

48. Davis SN, Shavers C, Costa F, *et al*: Role of cortisol in the pathogenesis of deficient counterregulation after antecedent hypoglycemia in normal humans. *J Clin Invest* 1996;98:680.

49. Davis SN, Shavers C, Davis B, *et al*: Prevention of an increase in plasma cortisol during hypoglycemia preserves subsequent counterregulatory responses. *J Clin Invest* 1997;100:429.

50. Boyle PJ, Nagy R, O'Connor AM, *et al*: Adaptation in brain glucose uptake following recurrent hypoglycemia. *Proc Natl Acad Sci USA* 1994;91:9352.

51. Boyle PJ, Kempers SF, O'Connor AM, *et al*: Brain glucose uptake and unawareness of hypoglycemia in patients with insulin dependent diabetes mellitus. *N Engl J Med* 1995;333:1726.

52. Segel SA, Fanelli CG, Dence CS, *et al*: Blood-to-brain glucose transport, cerebral glucose transport, cerebral glucose metabolism and cerebral blood flow are not increased following hypoglycemia. *Diabetes* 2001;50:1911.

53. Mühlhauser I, Overmann H, Bender R, *et al*: Risk factors for severe hypoglycaemia in adult patients with type 1 diabetes—a prospective population based study. *Diabetologia* 1998;41:1274.

54. Ahmed ABE, Home PD: The effect of the insulin analogue lispro on nighttime blood glucose control in type 1 diabetic patients. *Diabetes Care* 1998;21:32.

55. Perriello G, De Feo P, Torlone E, *et al*: The dawn phenomenon in type 1 (insulin dependent) diabetes mellitus: Magnitude, frequency, variability, and dependence on glucose counterregulation and insulin sensitivity. *Diabetes* 1991;34:21.

56. Jones TW, Porter P, Sherwin RS, *et al*: Decreased epinephrine responses to hypoglycemia during sleep. *N Engl J Med* 1998;338:1657.

57. Saleh TY, Cryer PE: Alanine and terbutaline in the prevention of nocturnal hypoglycemia in IDDM. *Diabetes Care* 1997;20:1231.

58. Ververs MTC, Rouwé C, Smit GPA: Complex carbohydrates in the prevention of nocturnal hypoglycaemia in diabetic children. *Eur J Clin Nutr* 1993;47:268.

59. Kaufman FR, Devgan S: Use of uncooked cornstarch to avert nocturnal hypoglycemia in children and adolescents with type 1 diabetes. *J Diabetes Complications* 1996;10:84.

CHAPTER 32

The Oral Antidiabetic Agents

Sunder Mudaliar

Robert R. Henry

Type 2 diabetes (T2DM) is a chronic disease characterized by hyperglycemia and numerous other metabolic abnormalities. This disabling metabolic disorder affects more than 16 million people in the United States[1] and more than 150 million people worldwide.[2] Three major pathophysiologic abnormalities are associated with T2DM: impaired insulin secretion, excessive hepatic glucose output, and insulin resistance in skeletal muscle, liver, and adipose tissue.[3] The treatment goals are the alleviation of symptoms through normalization of blood glucose levels and the prevention of acute and long-term complications.[4] These goals can be achieved through pharmacologic and nonpharmacologic means. Nonpharmacologic measures include diabetes education and lifelong diet management, exercise, and weight loss. Although diet and exercise remain the cornerstones of treatment, in the vast majority of patients with T2DM, pharmacologic agents are invariably needed to achieve optimal glycemic control and reduce the incidence of microvascular and possibly macrovascular complications, as shown in the United Kingdom Prospective Diabetes Study (UKPDS).[5]

Four major classes of oral pharmacologic agents are available for treatment. They act as follows at the major sites of defects in T2DM: (1) by increasing insulin availability (the secretagogues, i.e., sulfonylureas and meglitinides); (2) by suppressing excessive hepatic glucose output (the biguanides, i.e., metformin); (3) by improving insulin sensitivity (thiazolidinediones or glitazones, i.e., rosiglitazone and pioglitazone); and finally (4) by delaying gastrointestinal glucose absorption (the α-glucosidase inhibitors acarbose and miglitol) (Fig. 32-1). The therapeutic objectives recommended by the American Diabetes Association (ADA) include fasting plasma glucose (FPG) 80–120 mg/dL, bedtime plasma glucose 100–140 mg/dL, and glycosylated hemoglobin (HbA$_{1c}$) < 7%[4] (Table 32-1). All of the above agents are effective as monotherapy in suitable patients and help to maintain optimal glycemic control in the initial stages. However, since T2DM is a progressive disease, over a period of time glycemic control inevitably deteriorates, and eventually combination oral therapy or (in many patients) insulin therapy will be needed to achieve optimal glycemic levels. This was clearly demonstrated in the UKPDS.[5] Here we review the pharmacology, mode of action, and clinical applications of the various antidiabetic agents alone and in combination.

INSULIN SECRETAGOGUES

The insulin secretagogues have potent hypoglycemic effects through stimulation of insulin secretion from the pancreatic β cell. This class of agents includes the sulfonylureas and the meglitinides.

Sulfonylureas

Sulfonylureas have been available for the treatment of T2DM since the 1950s. They continue to be used as initial pharmacologic therapy, particularly when hyperglycemia is pronounced and evidence of impaired insulin secretion is present. Furthermore, sulfonylureas are often the foundation of combination therapy because of their ability to increase or maintain insulin secretion. They have a long history of use and few serious side effects (including hypoglycemia) and are relatively inexpensive. The major disadvantage is secondary failure, which may occur with all oral agents due to the progressive nature of T2DM. Placebo-controlled studies have shown that sulfonylureas reduce FPG levels by about 54–72 mg/dL and HbA$_{1c}$ levels by 1.5–2% in patients with long-standing T2DM.[6–8]

Although all sulfonylurea antidiabetic agents exhibit similar hypoglycemic mechanisms, there are quantitative differences in their individual pharmacokinetic properties that distinguish them. Chlorpropamide, acetohexamide, tolazimide, and tolbutamide are classified as first-generation agents, and glyburide, glipizide, and glimepiride as second-generation agents. In Europe and other parts of the world, glibenclamide and gliclazide are marketed as the equivalent of glyburide and glipizide. Second-generation agents like glyburide and glipizide are thought to bind nonionically to plasma proteins; the first-generation sulfonylureas are thought to bind by both ionic and nonionic mechanisms.[9,10] *In vitro*, acidic drugs such as warfarin and aspirin displace sulfonylureas with ionic binding to a much greater extent than sulfonylureas with nonionic binding. It was once thought that these differences in binding might cause certain agents such as glyburide to have a better drug interaction profile than some of the other sulfonylureas. This has not been proved clinically. A list of the sulfonylureas is given in Table 32-2.

TABLE 32-1. Goals for Glycemic Control

Biochemical Index	Normal	Goal	Action Suggested
Fasting/preprandial plasma glucose (mg/dL)	<110	80–120	<80 or >140
Bedtime plasma glucose (mg/dL)	<120	100–140	<100 or >160)
Glycosylated hemoglobin (%) (normal range 4–6)	<6	<7	>8

Source: American Diabetes Association.[4]

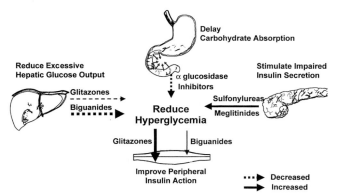

FIGURE 32-1. The major sites of action of the various classes of oral antidiabetic agents.

Mechanism of Action

The hypoglycemic action of the sulfonylureas is due to stimulation of ATP-dependent K^+ channels (K_{ATP} channels) in the pancreatic islet cells (Fig. 32-2). When sulfonylureas bind to the receptors, they close these K_{ATP} channels. This results in a decrease in K^+ permeability of the β-cell membrane, depolarizes the membrane, and opens voltage-dependent Ca^{2+} channels, leading to an increase in intracellular calcium.[11] The calcium ions bind to calmodulin, resulting in the exocytosis of insulin-containing secretory granules. Recently, it has been demonstrated that the K_{ATP} channel is a complex of a 140-kd sulfonylurea receptor (SUR) and an inward rectifier channel protein (KIR6.2).[12] The K_{ATP} channels

are also inhibited by glucose and other islet ATP-generating fuels.[13] Sulfonylureas can increase insulin secretion at substimulatory concentrations of glucose, suggesting an enhancement of β-cell response, and when β cells are exposed to maximally effective glucose concentrations, demonstrating an additive effect independent of glucose concentrations.[13] Incidentally, ATP-dependent K^+ channels binding sulfonylureas are also present in the myocardium, vascular smooth muscle, adipose tissue, and brain, in addition to the β cell. The role of these receptors in vascular and cardiac tissue is discussed below; the significance of sulfonylurea binding in the brain remains to be defined.

Prolonged administration of the sulfonylureas may also produce extrapancreatic effects that contribute to its hypoglycemic activity. These effects include reduction of basal hepatic glucose production and an enhanced peripheral sensitivity to insulin secondary to intracellular signaling events that follow insulin receptor binding. The relative importance of each of these actions to the overall therapeutic effect of the drugs varies among sulfonylureas and from patient to patient. Although a main effect of sulfonylureas appears to be stimulation of basal insulin secretion, these antidiabetic agents also stimulate the secretion of insulin throughout the duration of a meal.[13]

All the sulfonylureas bind to the same receptor site, and differences in potency may relate, in part, to differences in binding affinity. Sulfonylureas also vary widely in their rates of absorption, biotransformation, and elimination, all of which account for the differing potencies and dosages of the various agents in this class. These drugs are not effective in the absence of functioning β cells, as occurs in T1DM, or when the number of viable β cells is low, as occurs in those with long-standing T2DM.

TABLE 32-2. First- and Second-Generation Sulfonylurea Compounds

Name	Initial Dose (mg/day)	Daily Dose Range (mg/day)	Recommended Maximum Daily Dose (mg/day)	Doses/Day
First generation				
Tolbutamide	500–1500	500–3000	3000	2–3
Chlorpropamide	100–250	100–500	500	1
Tolazamide	100–250	100–1000	1000	1–2
Acetohexamide	250–500	250–1500	1500	1–2
Second generation				
Glyburide	1.25–2.50	1.25–20	20	1–2
Micronized formulation	0.75–1.50	0.75–12	12	1
Glibenclamide	1.25–2.50	1.25–2.50	20	1–2
Glipizide	2.5–5	2.5–40	40	1–2
Glipizide XL	5	5–20	20	1
Gliclazide	40	40–320	320	1–2
Glimepiride	1–2	4–8	8	1

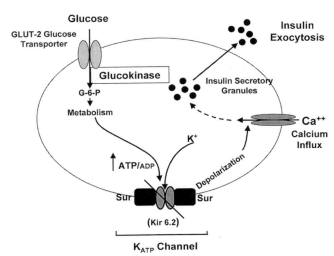

FIGURE 32-2. Sulfonylureas bind to receptors (Sur) on the β-cell membrane, cause decreased permeability of K$^+$ channels, and depolarize the membrane. This causes the voltage-dependent Ca$^+$ channels to open, leading to an increase in intracellular calcium and the exocytosis of insulin-containing secretory granules. The K$_{ATP}$ channel is a complex of a 140-kd sulfonylurea receptor (Sur) and an inward rectifier channel protein (Kir 6.2). The Sur subunit contains unique binding sites for glyburide and repaglinide.

Pharmacokinetics

All the sulfonylureas are rapidly absorbed from the GI tract after oral administration. The pharmacokinetics and metabolism of the sulfonylureas are shown in Table 32-3. It is noteworthy that the half-life of chlorpropamide is very long, ranging from 25–60 hours, with a duration of action of 24–72 hours.

Clinical Use and Efficacy

Sulfonylureas have been used as oral hypoglycemic agents for approximately 50 years,[14] and despite the availability of multiple classes of oral agents, these drugs continue to be used frequently as initial pharmacologic therapy, particularly when hyperglycemia is pronounced and evidence of impaired insulin secretion is present. Furthermore, because of their ability to increase or maintain insulin secretion, these agents are often the foundation of combination therapy. Placebo-controlled studies have shown that sulfonylureas reduce FPG levels by about 54–72 mg/dL in patients with long-

standing T2DM.[6–8] The plasma glucose–lowering effect is slightly better in patients who have been recently diagnosed.[6] Glycosylated hemoglobin levels are reduced on the average of 1.5–2% with use of these agents.[6–8]

Although similar in efficacy to first-generation agents (tolbutamide, chlorpropamide, tolazamide, and acetohexamide), second-generation sulfonylureas (glyburide, glipizide, and glimepiride) are more potent and lack some of the side effects seen with older agents. As a result, they have largely replaced first-generation agents in the clinical setting. Of the second-generation sulfonylureas available, two formulations (glipizide extended release and glimepiride) have the convenience of maximum effectiveness with once-a-day dosing and the potential for greater long-term compliance. Glipizide extended release (Glucotrol XL®) provides controlled release of the short-acting sulfonylurea. Once-daily administration provides effective control of plasma glucose concentrations throughout the 24-hour dosing interval, with less peak-to-trough fluctuation than conventional glipizide.[8] A multicenter, open-label, randomized, two-way crossover study[8] demonstrated that extended-release glipizide is as effective as conventional glipizide in lowering postprandial plasma glucose levels but is significantly more effective in reducing FPG levels than conventional glipizide at week 8 of treatment. In addition, extended-release glipizide exerts its glycemic effect at lower insulin and C-peptide levels, which suggests enhanced insulin sensitivity. Extended-release glipizide lowers HbA$_{1c}$ levels and both fasting and postprandial glucose over a dose range of 5–60 mg/day, with maximal efficacy achieved at a dose of 5 mg for HbA$_{1c}$ and 20 mg for FPG.[15]

The second-generation agent glyburide is also available in a micronized (smaller particle size) formulation (Glynase® PresTab® tablets) that offers improved bioavailability over conventional glyburide and can be administered once or twice daily. A 12-week double-blind, randomized trial demonstrated no significant differences in glycemic or glycosylated hemoglobin levels between patients receiving 5-mg tablets of original glyburide versus 3-mg tablets of micronized glyburide.[16] However, because of the difference in bioavailability, patients should be retitrated when they are switched from original to micronized glyburide. The incidence of side effects is similar for the two agents.

Glimepiride (Amaryl®) is the most potent sulfonylurea on a per-milligram basis and appears to be as effective as other sulfonylureas in reducing glucose levels when administered at 1–8 mg daily.[7,17,18] Glimepiride, like other sulfonylureas, can be used alone

TABLE 32-3. Metabolism of Sulfonylureas

Compound and Date of Introduction	Biologic Plasma Half-Life (h)	Duration of Hypoglycemic Action (h)	Mode of Metabolism	Activity of Metabolites	Excreted in Urine (%)
Tolbutamide	4–6.5	6–10	Hepatic carboxylation	Inactive	100
Chlorpropamide	36	60	Hepatic hydroxylation or side chain cleavage	Active	80–90
Tolazamide	7	12–14	Hepatic metabolism	Three inactive	85
Acetohexamide	4–6	12–18	Hepatic reduction to 1-hydroxyhexamide	Three week 2.5 × original	60
Glyburide (glibenclamide)	4–11*	24	Hepatic metabolites	Mostly inactive	50
Glipizide	2.5–4.7	Up to 24	Hepatic metabolites	Inactive	50
Gliclazide	8–11	Up to 24	Hepatic metabolites	Probably inactive	60–70

*Micronized in 4 hours.

Source: Data from Gerich,[9] Groop,[10] and Zimmerman.[14]

or in combination with other anti-hyperglycemic agents. It is also the only sulfonylurea approved for use as an adjunct to insulin therapy. Maximal efficacy is achieved at 4–8 mg daily.[7] In clinical studies, once-daily doses of 1–8 mg significantly reduced FPG by 43–74 mg/dL and HbA$_{1c}$ values by 1.2–1.9% compared with placebo.[18] In 1-year clinical studies, although glimepiride was similar in efficacy to glibenclamide and glipizide, it appeared to reduce blood glucose more rapidly than glipizide over the first few weeks of treatment. There is now preliminary evidence that although all sulfonylureas bind to the same ATP-dependent K$^+$ channels, glimepiride exhibits different binding behavior to these channels, particularly in the heart (discussed later). Thus, in one study, compared with glibenclamide, glimepiride was able to maintain ischemic myocardial preconditioning during balloon angioplasty.[19]

Since they have potent insulin secretory effects, primary failure of sulfonylurea therapy is uncommon if patients are carefully selected. It is possible that some patients failing sulfonylurea therapy have unrecognized T1DM.[20] When recognized, these patients should always be treated with insulin. Secondary failure of sulfonylurea therapy is also a major long-term therapeutic problem and seems to relate mainly to the natural history of T2DM and decreasing β-cell function. The incidence of secondary failure is also difficult to ascertain since its definition varies from study to study, but it is generally reported to range from 5 to 10% per year.[21] There have been suggestions that the secondary failure of sulfonylureas may be due to exhaustion of the pancreatic β cells. This hypothesis, however, has no evidence to support it. In the UKPDS, β-cell deterioration occurred at the same rate in diet-treated, metformin-treated, and sulfonylurea-treated patients.[22] It appears difficult to identify clinical features predicting secondary failure to sulfonylureas.[23] The primary predictive factor appears to be the duration of diabetes. Studies conducted to see whether a temporary reduction in hyperglycemia with insulin therapy restores the effectiveness of sulfonylurea therapy have not been successful.[24,25] Patients who fail to achieve ADA target goals should be started on combination therapy with any of the other oral agents or on insulin.

Extrapancreatic Effects

Over time, patients with T2DM who are treated with sulfonylureas have an improvement in β-cell function and a reduction of insulin resistance. However, it is known that improvement of hyperglycemia by other treatment methods also results in similar improvements in β-cell function and insulin resistance. Thus it is possible that the improvement is nonspecific and the result of a reduction of glucose or metabolic toxicity rather than a direct effect of sulfonylureas.[26] Even so, interest persists in possible extrapancreatic effects of sulfonylureas because, during chronic sulfonylurea therapy, acute insulinotrophic actions appear to be reduced.[27]

The sulfonylureas possess extrapancreatic effects that have been studied both *in vitro* and *in vivo*, in animal and human studies.[28] In rat L6 cultured skeletal muscle cells, tolazamide enhances glucose uptake by increasing the number of functioning cellular glucose transport molecules by 70%.[29] Glyburide has also been shown to stimulate glucose transport in cultured L6 muscle cells by a protein kinase C–mediated pathway that requires new protein synthesis. In this study, the authors speculated that although intracellular Ca^{2+} metabolism may be involved in this process, the initial step in the mechanism of action is probably different between pancreatic β cells and muscle cells.[30] In isolated insulin-resistant rat adipocytes, glimepiride activates glucose transport by stimulation of GLUT-1 and GLUT-4 translocation via interference at a site downstream of the putative molecular defect in the signaling cascade between the insulin receptor and the glucose transport system induced by high concentrations of glucose and insulin. This molecular site of glimepiride action is related to GLUT-4 phosphorylation/dephosphorylation.[31] Gimepiride also increases cardiac glucose uptake in isolated rat cardiomyocytes, by an insulin-independent pathway most probably involving an increased protein expression of GLUT-1 and GLUT-4.[32]

In human studies, Prigeon and colleagues[33] in their study in 15 patients with T2DM found that glyburide treatment did not have any effect on peripheral glucose uptake, as measured by the insulin sensitivity index. On the other hand, Beck-Nielsen and colleagues[34] demonstrated that sulfonylurea treatment of obese patients with T2DM enhances insulin-stimulated peripheral glucose utilization in both adipose tissue and skeletal muscle, in part through a potentiation of insulin action on adipose tissue glucose transport and lipogenesis and skeletal muscle glycogen synthase. Recently, Shi and coworkers[35] have demonstrated that human adipocytes express a sulfonylurea receptor (SUR1) that regulates intracellular calcium and controls lipogenesis and lipolysis.

Cardiac Effects

Ever since the results of the University Group Diabetes Program (UGDP) study were published, there has been controversy regarding the potentially harmful cardiac effects of sulfonylureas.[36] In the UGDP, approximately 1000 patients with T2DM were randomized to diet and either placebo, tolbutamide, phenformin, standard-dose insulin, or a variable-dose insulin regimen. Unexpectedly, in 1969, after 7 years of follow-up, the tolbutamide arm was discontinued because of an observed and unexpected increase in cardiovascular and all-cause mortality.[37] There was widespread criticism of this study, which included insufficient patient characterization for baseline cardiovascular risk factors (e.g., cigarette smoking), as well as methodologic and interpretive problems in the study protocol.[38] Even so, the UGDP results fueled the long-standing controversy related to the potentially harmful cardiac effects of sulfonylurea drugs.[39] This is because the myocardium K$_{ATP}$ channels mediate ischemic preconditioning, which is critical to myocardial protection and limitation of infarct size.[40–42] These channels are normally closed; they open during ischemia in an adaptive response that protects the myocardium and induces vasodilation. Sulfonylurea binding to the channels has been shown to inhibit the response to ischemia, potentially delay the recovery of contractile function, and increase infarct size during a myocardial infarction.[41,42] In a recent study, sulfonylurea therapy was associated with an increase in in-hospital mortality among patients undergoing direct angioplasty for myocardial infarction.[43]

On the other hand, several studies have reported no link between long-term sulfonylurea use and increased mortality.[44–48] The UKPDS clearly documented that long-term sulfonylurea therapy is not associated with increased cardiovascular morbidity or mortality.[5] A recent study from the Mayo Clinic[47] did not find increased long-term mortality over 8.4 years in a group of 102 T2DM patients treated with either insulin or sulfonylureas at the time of admission to hospital with an acute myocardial infarction.

To add to the controversy further, it is known that the prevention of K$_{ATP}$ channel opening during ischemia reduces potassium efflux from myocardial cells and also reduces the occurrence of ventricular fibrillation during ischemia.[49–52] Indeed, in a recent study from Europe, sulfonylurea therapy was actually associated with reduced postinfarct morbidity and mortality in patients with diabetes.[48] It is also possible that the increased cardiovascular risk may not be a class effect with sulfonylureas. There is a variable efficacy with which sulfonylurea drugs inhibit cardioprotective K_{ATP} channels. In experimental animals, inhibition of the cardiac K_{ATP} channel with glibenclamide has been shown to increase ischemia-reperfusion damage,[53] whereas gliclazide, a sulfonylurea with pronounced *in vivo* antioxidative properties, prevented such damage.[54] In blood flow studies in the human forearm, significant interaction with the vascular K_{ATP} channel was found for glibenclamide, whereas the effect was much less pronounced for tolbutamide[55] and even absent for the new drug glimepiride.[56] In a recent survey from Australia, glibenclamide-treated patients had significantly less ventricular fibrillation than those receiving gliclazide or insulin.[57]

Thus, the interaction between sulfonylurea drugs and K_{ATP} channels during metabolic stress is complex, with various factors governing sulfonylurea-inhibitory gating of the channel.[58,59] The net clinical effects of the seemingly opposing myocardial actions of sulfonylureas may not be deleterious.[60] Further, the UKPDS has clearly documented that long-term sulfonylurea treatment is not associated with increased cardiovascular morbidity or mortality.[5] Whether some sulfonylureas (glipizide or glimepiride) or the other antidiabetic agents (especially the insulin sensitizers) are more beneficial for the cardiovascular consequences of T2DM remains to be determined.

Effects on Lipids

Unlike the insulin sensitizers, sulfonylurea treatment probably does not possess lipid-lowering effects other than that due to improved glycemic control. In one study, Panahloo and coworkers[61] examined the effects of sulfonylurea and insulin treatment on glycemia, insulin sensitivity, and lipid concentrations in 20 poorly controlled, diet-treated T2DM subjects who were given sulfonylurea or insulin each for a period of 16 weeks in a randomized crossover study, with a 4-week washout period between each treatment. Subjects were studied at the baselines (B1 and B2) and after each treatment. Expectedly, although treatment with both sulfonylureas or insulin resulted in equal improvement in insulin sensitivity (measured by the metabolic clearance of glucose) and glycemia (HbA$_{1c}$ declined from $11.7 \pm 2.1\%$ to $8.5 \pm 0.9\%$ with sulfonylurea treatment and to $8.6 \pm 1.2\%$ on insulin), surprisingly, there were no differences in lipid concentrations either with improved glycemia or between therapies. However, the potentially atherogenesis-promoting intact proinsulin levels and plasminogen activator inhibitor-1 (PAI-1) antigen activity were higher on sulfonylurea treatment.[61]

Prevention of Type 2 Diabetes

A limited number of studies have attempted to determine whether the use of sulfonylurea agents in high-risk subjects can prevent or delay the onset of T2DM. Most of these were of short duration and were generally statistically underpowered. The English Bedford Study did not demonstrate a benefit of tolbutamide 500 mg bid to prevent progression to diabetes.[62] However, the study by Sartor and colleagues[63] did show that tolbutamide 500 mg tid decreased the development of diabetes over 10 years compared with placebo. This study was undermined by a failure to follow an intention-to-treat analysis. In a recent English study, Holman and colleagues[64] randomized 227 self-referred subjects at increased risk of developing diabetes (FPG between 99 and 139 mg/dL on

two consecutive occasions 2 weeks apart) to either sulfonylurea therapy (gliclazide $\leq$ 160 mg daily) or a control group allocated either to double-blind placebo or to no tablets. Subjects were also randomly allocated to reinforced or basic healthy-living advice in a factorial design. A total of 201 subjects were evaluated after 1 year in three English and two French centers. Sulfonylurea treatment resulted in a significant reduction in median FPG (by 7 mg/dL) and HbA$_{1c}$ (by 0.2%) compared with the control group. There was no change in insulin sensitivity and β-cell function between groups. Side effects in the sulfonylurea group included weight gain and hypoglycemia. The study is being extended to determine whether sulfonylurea therapy prevents progression to T2DM. It should be mentioned here that the National Institutes of Health (NIH) is presently conducting the 6-year Diabetes Prevention Program in which subjects with impaired glucose tolerance who are at increased risk of developing T2DM are being studied to determine whether intensive lifestyle measures or metformin can prevent or delay the onset of T2DM. There is no sulfonylurea arm in this study. The study completed randomization of 3000 subjects,[65a] and results were published in 2002.[65] They demonstrated a 58% reduction in diabetes incidence with lifestyle intervention and 31% reduction with metformin treatment after 3 years followup.

Dosing

The initial starting dose of the sulfonylurea agent depends on the prevailing level of hyperglycemia (Table 32-2). If the initial FPG is <200 mg/dL, sulfonylureas should be started at the lowest dose and titrated upward at weekly intervals so as to achieve an FPG of $\leq$120 mg/dL. If the initial FPG >200 mg/dL, higher initial doses of sulfonylureas may be used. If a patient presents with marked symptoms and hyperglycemia, the sulfonylurea agent may be started at the highest dose and the patient closely followed up.[66] Studies have shown that the sulfonylureas are better absorbed and are more effective if given about 30 minutes before a meal.[14] This may, however, create a compliance problem for the patients, since it is difficult to remember to take a pill 30 minutes before eating. The goal should be an FPG of $\leq$120 mg/dL and an HbA$_{1c}$ of <7%. All patients should monitor their blood glucose on a regular basis (self-monitored blood glucose [SMBG]), and dosage adjustments in small increments should be made every week depending on SMBG. For once-daily agents, the dose should be given with breakfast or the main meal of the day. Glipizide is best administered 30 minutes before a meal to ensure maximum reduction in postprandial hyperglycemia. However, the sustained-release dosage form should be given with breakfast. In elderly adults over 65 years, patients with hepatic disease, or other patients who may be more sensitive to hypoglycemic drugs, the lowest initial dose should be used and dose adjustments should be made more conservatively.

Special care needs to be taken when transferring a patient from chlorpropamide to any other sulfonylurea therapy. Since chlorpropamide's effects can persist for 1–2 weeks following the discontinuation of therapy, hypoglycemia can result from additive effects of the two agents. The normal starting dose of a sulfonylurea may be used when transferring patients from sulfonylureas (other than chlorpropamide). Patients should be retitrated on micronized glyburide when transferring from conventional glyburide or other oral hypoglycemic agents.

Some patients with T2DM being treated with insulin can be switched successfully to oral sulfonylurea therapy. For patients being treated with <20 U of insulin per day, a lower starting dose of the sulfonylurea once daily may be tried. For patients being treated with 20–40 U of insulin per day, a higher starting dose (half-maximal) may be tried. For patients being treated with >40 U of insulin per day, it is recommended that the daily insulin dose be decreased 50% and the sulfonylurea be initiated at half-maximal dose.

Side Effects

Sulfonylurea antidiabetic agents are generally well tolerated and have a low incidence of side effects. Hypoglycemia is the most common side effect during sulfonylurea therapy and manifests as hunger, pallor, nausea/vomiting, fatigue, diaphoresis, headache, palpitations, numbness of the mouth, tingling in the fingers, tremors, muscle weakness, blurred vision, hypothermia, uncontrolled yawning, irritability, mental confusion, sinus tachycardia, shallow breathing, or loss of consciousness. Hypoglycemia can be a result of excessive dosage, but it also could be due to other factors such as improper diet or excessive physical activity. Sulfonylurea-induced hypoglycemia can be severe and requires immediate re-evaluation and adjustment of both dosage and the patient's diet. The risk of hypoglycemia is also increased in the elderly and when there is poor nutrition, alcohol intake, gastrointestinal disease, or impaired renal function.

Other adverse sulfonylurea effects occur infrequently, typically during the first 6 weeks of therapy. Mild GI effects are common, whereas skin reactions and hematologic complications are rare.[10,67] Patients often experience some weight gain with use of sulfonylureas. Withdrawal of sulfonylurea therapy due to adverse reactions occurs in <2% of patients. Minor adverse reactions include nausea/vomiting, heartburn, dyspepsia, diarrhea, headache, abdominal pain or cramps, constipation, and paresthesias. These symptoms may subside following a reduction in dosage. Administering the total daily dose in two equally divided doses may also alleviate some of the adverse GI effects. However, severe adverse GI effects may necessitate discontinuance of the drug.

Allergic skin reactions to sulfonylurea include maculopapular rash, urticaria, erythema, and pruritus. These reactions are usually mild, but if they persist or become severe, the drug should be discontinued. Rarely, skin eruptions have progressed to erythema multiforme and exfoliative dermatitis; porphyria cutanea tarda and photosensitivity reactions have been reported. Cholestatic jaundice has also been reported with sulfonylurea therapy, and (rarely) hepatic porphyria has been precipitated by sulfonylureas. The drug should be discontinued if this occurs. Sulfonylureas can cause leukopenia, thrombocytopenia, pancytopenia, agranulocytosis, aplastic anemia, and/or hemolysis, which can lead to hemolytic anemia. These effects are usually mild and typically subside following discontinuance of the drug.

The syndrome of inappropriate secretion of antidiuretic hormone (SIADH) has occurred in patients receiving chlorpropamide. Chlorpropamide occasionally can also cause hyponatremia and water intoxication, which is indistinguishable from SIADH. Although rare, hyponatremia and SIADH have also occurred in patients receiving other sulfonylureas. Most of these affected patients had other variables, which may have been responsible or contributory.

Contraindications

Sulfonylurea use is contraindicated in pregnancy since there are no adequate human studies of effects on the fetus, although animal reproduction studies have shown some adverse fetal effects. If they are used at all, the decision to administer sulfonylurea drugs must weigh the potential risks to the fetus against the potential benefits to the mother. Because abnormal glucose concentrations are themselves a risk factor for congenital abnormalities, insulin is recommended to maintain blood glucose as close to normal as possible. However, in a recent study, Langer and coworkers[68] randomized 404 women with gestational diabetes (between 11 and 33 weeks of pregnancy) who were unable to achieve adequate metabolic control with diet and exercise alone to either glyburide or insulin therapy. Adequate control was obtained with significantly less hypoglycemia in the glyburide group than in the insulin group. (Only 4% of glyburide women had to go on insulin.) More importantly, there was no evidence of any of the complications feared to result from fetal or neonatal hyperinsulinemia due to transplacental passage of the sulfonylurea drug. There were no differences between the groups in cord serum insulin concentrations or in the incidence of macrosomia, cesarean delivery, or neonatal hypoglycemia. Glyburide was not detected in the cord serum of any infant, despite measurable serum concentrations in some of their mothers. However, this study does not permit us to draw firm conclusions about the teratogenicity of oral hypoglycemic drugs in early pregnancy (when organogenesis occurs) and thus whether women with T2DM who become pregnant can safely continue oral sulfonylurea agents. Also, since it is not known whether sulfonylureas are excreted in breast milk, it is recommended that sulfonylureas not be used in women who are breastfeeding, to avoid hypoglycemia in nursing infants.

All sulfonylureas are contraindicated in patients with a known sulfonylurea hypersensitivity. Allergic reactions such as angioedema, arthralgia, myalgia, and vasculitis have been reported. Sulfonylureas are also contraindicated in all patients with T1DM and those in acute stress conditions like major surgery, acute myocardial infarction, or trauma.

Renal impairment or *hepatic disease* can cause elevations in sulfonylurea blood concentrations, and hepatic disease can also reduce gluconeogenic capacity[69]; both problems increase the risk of hypoglycemia, and sulfonylureas should be administered carefully in these patients. Some sulfonylureas like chlorpropamide and acetohexamide can exacerbate hepatic porphyria and should be used cautiously in patients with a history of this condition.

Elderly patients may be more susceptible to the hypoglycemic effects of sulfonylureas. Chlorpropamide can cause prolonged and serious hypoglycemia in the elderly, as well as SIADH. Therefore, this medication is not recommended for use in the geriatric population. The use of sulfonylureas has not been studied systematically in children with T2DM.

Drug Interactions

Although drug interactions for the second-generation sulfonylureas (glyburide and glipizide) are theoretically less of a concern than for the first-generation agents, interactions due to displacement have been reported, and caution should be used if any of the following drugs are prescribed to patients receiving oral sulfonylureas due to the potential for protein-binding interactions and hypoglycemia: clofibrate, salicylates, NSAIDs, and sulfonamides. Also, the interaction between oral anticoagulants and oral sulfonylureas is complex, and it is wise for clinicians to monitor coagulation parameters closely when sulfonylureas and warfarin are used together.[70]

Beta blockers promote hyperglycemia by inhibiting insulin secretion and decreasing tissue sensitivity to insulin. Selective beta blockers may cause fewer problems with blood glucose regulation, although all beta blockers can still mask the tachycardic response to hypoglycemia. Monoamine oxidase inhibitors (MAOIs) interfere with the compensatory adrenergic response to hypoglycemia and cause clinically significant hypoglycemia in patients receiving oral antidiabetic agents such as glyburide.

Patients on weight loss medication (sibutramine or orlistat) or weight loss diets should be followed closely and often require a reduction in dose or discontinuation of antidiabetic drug therapy coincident with weight loss.[71]

Chlorpropamide has been associated with a disulfiram-like reaction after ingestion of ethanol.[9] Patients who take other oral hypoglycemics and consume ethanol should be counseled on this reaction. In addition, ethanol is known to inhibit gluconeogenesis, and it is possible that hypoglycemia may occur more readily after ethanol ingestion in patients receiving oral hypoglycemics. Miconazole has been reported to inhibit the metabolism of oral antidiabetic agents. Patients should be monitored for hypoglycemia if miconazole is added. It is not clear whether other azole antifungals interact in the same manner.

Repaglinide

Repaglinide is a carbamoylmethyl benzoic acid (CMBA) derivative that belongs to a new class of antidiabetic agents, structurally related to meglitinides (previously known as the nonsulphonylurea moiety of glibenclamide) (Fig. 32-3). Like the sulfonylureas, repaglinide is an insulin secretagogue, and its mechanism of action involves ATP-sensitive K$^+$ channels.[72] Repaglinide is unique in that it has a rapid onset and short duration of action; when taken just prior to meals, it replicates physiologic insulin profiles. It has been shown to lower HbA$_{1c}$ levels by 1.6–1.9%. Repaglinide is available as Prandin™ in the United States, Actulin® in Canada, and NovoNorm® in Europe. Prandin was approved by the FDA in December 1997.

Mechanism of Action

Repaglinide binds a characterizable site on the β-cells in the pancreas and closes ATP-dependent potassium channels. The intracellular uptake of repaglinide is very limited; however, intracellular uptake is not required to stimulate insulin secretion.[73] Repaglinide's activity is both dose-dependent and glucose-dependent. From *in vitro* studies utilizing mouse islet cells, it has been observed that

FIGURE 32-3. Structure of repaglinide.

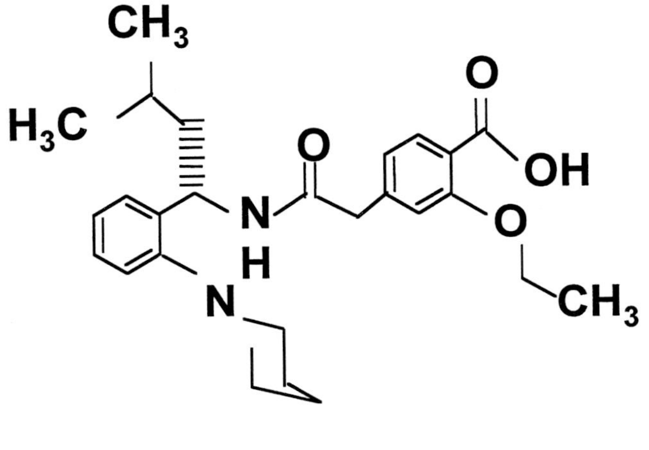

repaglinide was more potent at stimulating insulin secretion than the oral sulfonylurea glyburide in the presence of moderate concentrations of glucose; however, in the absence of glucose, glyburide, but not repaglinide, stimulated insulin secretion. Although repaglinide and glyburide are equally potent as potassium channel blockers, the activity of repaglinide on the potassium channel diminishes as glucose concentrations rise from moderate to high.[73] In addition, repaglinide does not mimic a second action of glyburide on calcium-dependent insulin exocytosis. This secondary action of glyburide may explain why glyburide is more potent than repaglinide at high glucose concentrations. Repaglinide is not effective in the absence of functioning β cells, as occurs in TIDM.

Pharmacokinetics

Repaglinide is administered orally and is rapidly and completely absorbed from the GI tract. The mean absolute bioavailability is 56%, and peak plasma levels are achieved within 1 hour of administration. More than 98% of the drug is protein bound and is metabolized in the liver by the cytochrome P-450 enzyme system 3A4. There are three major metabolites of the parent compound, but none of them have glucose-lowering activity. Elimination of repaglinide is also rapid, with a half-life of 1 hour. Approximately 92% of repaglinide and its metabolites is excreted in the feces, and the remaining 8% is eliminated in the urine. Caution should be used in patients with impaired hepatic function, and longer dosing intervals should be used to assess the extent of glucose control accurately.

Clinical Use and Efficacy

In a 24-week U.S. trial, 361 patients with T2DM were randomized to premeal treatment with placebo or repaglinide 1 or 4 mg. At 6 months, repaglinide 1 or 4 mg decreased mean FPG values by 47 and 49 mg/dL and HbA$_{1c}$ by 1.8–1.9%. In the placebo group, FPG increased by 19 mg/dL. There were no events of severe hypoglycemia, and nearly all those with hypoglycemic symptom episodes had blood glucose levels above 45 mg/dL.[74]

In another U.S. study,[75] repaglinide was shown to provide glycemic control that was at least as effective and potentially safer than that provided by glyburide. In this prospective, 1-year, multicenter, double-blind, randomized, parallel-group study, 576 patients with T2DM of at least 6 months' duration were randomized to receive monotherapy with repaglinide or glyburide. Repaglinide patients received a starting dose of 0.5 mg three times a day preprandially, adjusted as necessary to 1, 2, or 4 mg before breakfast, lunch, and dinner. Glyburide patients received a starting dose of 2.5 mg before breakfast and increased as necessary to 10 mg bid. The glucose-lowering effect of repaglinide was most pronounced in pharmacotherapy-naive patients, who showed rapid and marked decreases in mean HbA$_{1c}$ levels from baseline (9.4%) to month 3 (7.6%) and month 12 (7.9%). Mean FPG levels also decreased overall in this group, from 222 mg/dL at baseline to 175 mg/dL at month 3 and to 188 mg/dL at month 12. At endpoint, morning C-peptide levels had increased significantly in glyburide-treated patients compared with those treated with repaglinide, but morning fasting insulin levels did not differ significantly between the two groups. Repaglinide efficacy was sustained over 1 year and was not influenced by age or gender. Overall safety and changes in lipid profile and body weight were similar with both agents. However, weight gain data for the subset of pharmacotherapy-naive patients suggested that patients on repaglinide gained less weight than those given glyburide. Thus, patients in this study using repaglinide received the same therapeutic benefits as those using glyburide and may have received additional benefits.

In addition to its efficacy when used as monotherapy, repaglinide is also useful as combination therapy. Several studies have documented that combination treatment with repaglinide and metformin provides superior glycemic control compared with monotherapy with either agent alone.[76,77] In combination with metformin, HbA$_{1c}$ levels are further reduced by ~1.4% and FPG levels by ~40 mg/dL.

Since repaglinide is quickly absorbed and has a short half-life, it may be advantageous in subjects who are prone to delayed or missed meals. Indeed, results from one study[78] suggest that treatment with repaglinide in well-controlled T2DM patients who miss or delay a meal is superior to treatment with longer-acting sulfonylurea drugs (such as glyburide) with respect to the risk of hypoglycemic episodes (Fig. 32-4). This double-blind randomized study was designed to compare diurnal blood glucose excursions and the effects of accidental dietary noncompliance in T2DM patients who were well controlled on either repaglinide or glyburide treatment. Repaglinide was administered preprandially with each meal, and glyburide was administered in two daily doses before breakfast and dinner, regardless of whether lunch had been omitted. The diurnal blood glucose levels on a day in which three meals were eaten were compared between the two groups, and the minimum blood glucose concentration (BG$_{min}$) measurements were compared between lunch and dinner on days with three and two meals. Although the results showed no significant differences between the repaglinide and glyburide groups in average blood glucose levels from fasting blood glucose, the influence on the mean BG$_{min}$ of omitting a meal differed significantly between the repaglinide and glyburide groups. In the latter group, BG$_{min}$ decreased from 77 to 61 mg/dL as a result of omitting lunch, whereas in the repaglinide group, BG$_{min}$ was unchanged for the two-meal day (78 mg/dL) and the three-meal day (76 mg/dL). All hypoglycemic events occurred in the glyburide group on the two-meal day, in connection with omitting lunch. No hypoglycemic events were recorded in the repaglinide group.

Extrapancreatic Effects

So far, there have been no studies on the extrapancreatic effects of repaglinide on insulin sensitivity or other parameters.

Dosage

Since repaglinide has a rapid and short-acting pharmacodynamic profile, it is most effective when given before meals. For

treatment-naive patients or patients whose HbA$_{1c}$ is less than 8%, therapy may be initiated with a dose of 0.5 mg (immediately before a meal or 15 or 30 minutes prior to eating) and, depending on the response (aiming at postprandial glucose < 160 mg/dL), increased to 2 mg before meals up to four times a day. For patients who have taken oral hypoglycemic agents and whose HbA$_{1c}$ is >8%, a higher initial dose of 1 or 2 mg may be used prior to each meal. After each dose adjustment, at least 1 week should elapse to assess effectiveness. The maximum dose of repaglinide is 4 mg taken with every meal up to four times a day (total 16 mg in a 24-hour period). If a sulfonylurea agent is to be replaced by repaglinide, repaglinide should be started the day after the final dose of the other agent is given. Since overlapping effects are possible, close monitoring for hypoglycemia should be maintained for up to 1 week. If monotherapy alone fails to achieve glycemic goals, combination therapy with metformin (approved by the FDA) or with glitazones (not yet approved by the FDA) may be initiated.

Patients with Hepatic Impairment

Repaglinide is metabolized mainly in the liver, and its clearance is significantly reduced in patients with hepatic impairment. Also, hepatic disease can reduce gluconeogenic capacity, and hence repaglinide should be carefully administered in these patients to avoid the risk of hypoglycemia.

Patients with Renal Impairment

Repaglinide is safe and well tolerated in subjects with varying degrees of renal impairment.[79] Although adjustment of starting doses of repaglinide is not necessary for renal impairment or renal failure, severe impairment may require more care when upward adjustments of dosage are made. Hemodialysis does not significantly affect repaglinide clearance.

Contraindications/Caution

Repaglinide is contraindicated in patients with a known hypersensitivity to the drug and also in patients with T1DM, as it is not effective in the absence of functioning pancreatic β cells.

There are no adequate human studies regarding the effects of this drug on the fetus, and repaglinide is contraindicated in pregnancy, as are all other oral antidiabetic agents. It is not known whether repaglinide is excreted in breast milk. Because of the possibility of hypoglycemia in nursing infants, it is recommended that repaglinide not be used in women who are breastfeeding. Repaglinide has also not been studied in children and should not be used in them. In the elderly, debilitated, or malnourished, who are more susceptible to the hypoglycemic effects of repaglinide, the drug should be administered with caution and at lower initial doses.

Side Effects

Since repaglinide is an insulin secretagogue like the sulfonylureas, hypoglycemia is the most common side effect. During clinical trials, hypoglycemic occurrences due to repaglinide tended to be lower (16%) than those caused by sulfonylureas (20%). Proper patient selection, dosage, and instructions are important to avoid hypoglycemic episodes. Hypoglycemia may manifest as hunger, pallor, nausea/vomiting, fatigue, perspiration, headache, palpitations, numbness of the mouth, tingling in the fingers, tremors, muscle weakness, blurred vision, hypothermia, uncontrolled yawning, irritability, mental confusion, sinus tachycardia, shallow breathing, and loss of consciousness.

FIGURE 32-4. The minimum blood glucose concentrations (BG) measured between lunch and dinner on days with 3 and 2 meals/day among patients in the repaglinide group and the glyburide group. *, $p < 0.05$ compared with glyburide. (*Data from* Damsbo et al.[78])

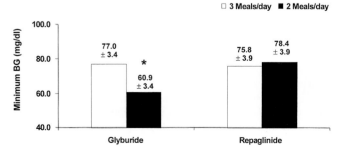

After hypoglycemia, upper respiratory tract infections (16%) and headache (11%) are the two most common adverse reactions for repaglinide in clinical studies. Sinusitis and arthralgia were reported by 6% of the people, whereas GI disturbances such as nausea/vomiting, diarrhea, constipation, and dyspepsia were less common. Back pain and chest pain were experienced by 5% and 3%, respectively.

Drug Interactions

Repaglinide is metabolized in the liver by the cytochrome P-450 enzyme CYP3A4. Drugs that are involved in the induction or suppression of this enzyme system may alter the expected hypoglycemic action of this agent. The metabolism of repaglinide may be inhibited by antifungal agents such as ketoconazole or miconazole, as well as antibacterial agents such as erythromycin. The result of this enzyme inhibition is a greater hypoglycemic effect from repaglinide. On the other hand, hyperglycemia may occur in patients taking repaglinide concomitantly with CYP3A4 inducers like barbiturates, carbamazepine, and rifampin.

Highly protein bound agents may also potentiate the hypoglycemic effects of repaglinide. These include beta blockers, chloramphenicol, MAOIs, NSAIDs, probenecid, salicylates, sulfonamides, and warfarin, which may lower serum glucose levels when used concomitantly with repaglinide. However, drug interaction studies in healthy volunteers demonstrate that repaglinide has no clinically relevant effect on the pharmacokinetic properties of digoxin, theophylline, or warfarin. The coadministration of cimetidine with repaglinide also did not significantly alter the absorption or disposition of repaglinide.

Nateglinide (Starlix®)

Nateglinide (a D-phenylalanine derivative) is a newly approved nonsulfonylurea insulin secretagogue; like repaglinide, it exerts its glucose-lowering effect through binding to the SUR receptor in the pancreatic β cells and closure of the K_{ATP} channels (Fig. 32-5). Like repaglinide, nateglinide's pharmacokinetic features include rapid absorption and elimination. However, its unique faster kinetics may be explained by the relatively low binding affinity of the drug for the SUR receptor.

Effects on Glycemia

In a recent randomized, double-blind study, Horton and colleagues[79a] evaluated the efficacy and tolerability of nateglinide and metformin (alone and in combination) in patients with T2DM inadequately controlled by diet (HbA_{1c} level between 6.8% and 11.0%). After a 4-week placebo run-in period, subjects received 24

weeks' treatment with 120 mg nateglinide before meals ($n = 179$), 500 mg metformin three times a day ($n = 178$), combination therapy ($n = 172$), or placebo ($n = 172$). At the end of the study, HbA_{1c} was significantly reduced from baseline with nateglinide and metformin but was increased with placebo (-0.5, -0.8, and $+0.5\%$, respectively). Combination therapy with nateglinide and metformin was additive with decreases in HbA_{1c} of 1.4% and FPG of 43 mg/dL. In this study, after a Sustacal® challenge, there was a greater reduction in mealtime glucose with nateglinide monotherapy compared with metformin monotherapy or placebo. The authors of this study concluded that nateglinide and metformin monotherapy each improved overall glycemic control, but by different mechanisms. Nateglinide decreased mealtime glucose levels, whereas metformin primarily affected FPG. In combination, nateglinide and metformin had complementary effects, improving HbA_{1c}, FPG, and postprandial hyperglycemia.

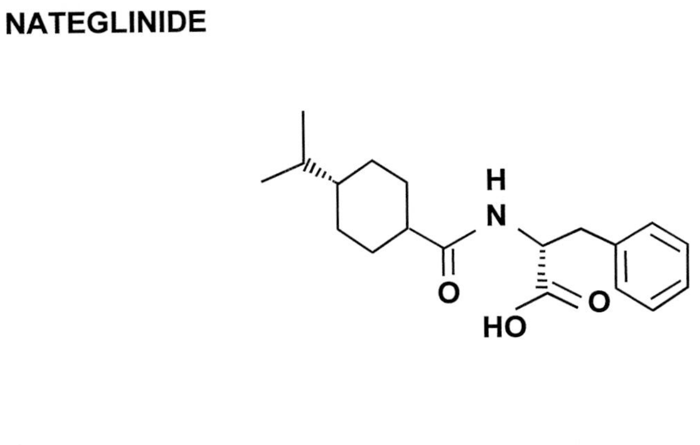

Extrapancreatic Effects

In a recent study, Hu and coworkers[79b] assessed the tissue specificity of nateglinide by examining its effect on K_{ATP} channels in rat tissue. Data from this study indicated that nateglinide has a 300-fold greater selectivity for pancreatic K_{ATP} channels compared with cardiovascular K_{ATP} channels. This property may be of potential benefit, since at concentrations effective in stimulating insulin secretion, nateglinide among the insulin secretagogues is least likely to cause detrimental cardiovascular effects via blockade of cardiovascular K_{ATP} channels.

BIGUANIDES

Phenformin and metformin are oral biguanide agents (Fig. 32-6) that were introduced for the treatment of T2DM in the late 1950s.[80] Phenformin was withdrawn from clinical use in the late 1970s because of an association with lactic acidosis. The risk for lactic acidosis is considerably lower with metformin. Its use was continued in many other countries until it was approved for use in the United States in 1995 for the treatment of T2DM either as monotherapy or in combination with sulfonylureas, α-glucosidase inhibitors, or insulin. Subsequently, it has also been approved for use in combination with rosiglitazone, pioglitazone, and repaglinide.

FIGURE 32-6. Structure of metformin.

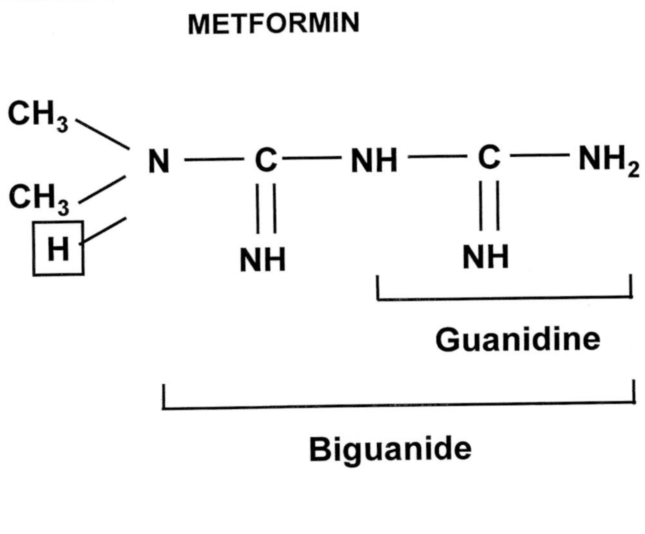

FIGURE 32-5. Structure of nateglinide.

NATEGLINIDE

Mechanism of Action

Although its mechanism of action has not been clearly determined, decreased hepatic gluconeogenesis is thought to be the primary therapeutic effect of metformin in T2DM.[80] In addition, metformin appears to improve utilization of glucose in skeletal muscle and adipose tissue by increasing cell membrane glucose transport. This effect may be due to improved binding of insulin to insulin receptors since metformin is not effective in diabetics without some residual functioning pancreatic islet cells.[80] Another effect of metformin that may contribute to its glucose-lowering properties is its ability to decrease fatty acid oxidation.[80] Other mechanisms may include decreased intestinal glucose absorption; however, this has only been observed in animals.[80] Thus, in insulin-resistant patients with T2DM, metformin increases insulin sensitivity by both decreasing hepatic glucose output and enhancing peripheral glucose uptake. It has no direct effects on insulin secretion[80,81] and hence, in contrast to sulfonylureas, which have a hypoglycemic effect, metformin does not generally cause hypoglycemia when given alone. In clinical practice, metformin demonstrates more of an anti-hyperglycemic action than a hypoglycemic action. Unlike phenformin, metformin does not inhibit the mitochondrial oxidation of lactate unless plasma concentrations of metformin become excessive (i.e., in patients with renal failure) and/or hypoxia is present.[82]

In a recent study, 3 months of metformin treatment reversed the increased activity of lymphocyte plasma cell differentiation antigen (PC-1) found in T2DM.[83] PC-1 is an inhibitor of insulin receptor tyrosine kinase activity and has been implicated in the pathogenesis of insulin resistance in T2DM. Data from this study were consistent with a role of PC-1 in insulin resistance and suggest a new mechanism of action for metformin via PC-1 inhibition.[83]

Pharmacokinetics

The bioavailability of metformin is 50–60%. Food decreases the extent and slightly delays the absorption of metformin; however, it should be taken with meals.[80] Metformin is distributed rapidly into peripheral body tissues and fluids and appears to distribute slowly into erythrocytes and to a deep tissue compartment (most likely GI tissues). The highest concentrations of metformin are found in the GI tract (10 times the concentrations in the plasma) and lower concentrations in the kidney, liver, and salivary gland tissue. Metformin does not bind to liver or plasma proteins. It is not metabolized by the liver, which may explain why the risk of lactic acidosis is much less for metformin than for phenformin.[81] Metformin is excreted by the kidneys, largely unchanged, through an active tubular process. Approximately 30% of an oral dose is excreted in the feces, presumably as unabsorbed metformin, and about 90% of a dose is excreted by the kidneys within 24 hours. The plasma half-life is approximately 6.2 hours, and the blood half-life is approximately 17.6 hours in patients with normal renal function. Half-life is increased in patients with renal impairment. Metformin is removed with hemodialysis.

Clinical Use and Efficacy

Metformin is approved for use as monotherapy and also in combination with sulfonylureas, repaglinide, α-glucosidase inhibitors, and glitazones. Several controlled clinical studies of metformin monotherapy have demonstrated significant reductions in both fasting blood glucose levels (60–70 mg/dL) and HbA$_{1c}$ levels (1–2%) compared with placebo in patients poorly controlled by diet alone.[84–91] The efficacy of metformin in reducing plasma glucose levels in a predominantly overweight population is comparable to that seen with sulfonylureas.[85,88,89] Because of its potential to ameliorate insulin resistance, prevent weight gain, and improve lipid levels, metformin may be best suited for initial monotherapy in obese patients with more severe insulin resistance and dyslipidemia. In these patients, metformin does not cause weight gain and, in fact, may cause a modest weight loss due to drug-induced anorexia. Metformin also decreases plasma VLDL triglycerides, resulting in modest decreases in plasma triglycerides and total cholesterol. Patients receiving metformin show significant improvement in FPG and HbA$_{1c}$ levels and a tendency toward improvement in the lipid profile, especially when baseline values are abnormally elevated.

When monotherapy alone does not result in acceptable glycemic control, metformin should be combined with a sulfonylurea and/or other oral antidiabetic oral agents. In 423 patients failing sulfonylurea treatment (FPG 249 mg/dL), the addition of metformin decreased the FPG by 63 mg/dL and the HbA$_{1c}$ value by 1.7%.[86] Nearly 25% of these patients whose disease was poorly controlled achieved an HbA$_{1c}$ value of <7% with the addition of metformin therapy. These results indicate that the hypoglycemic action of metformin is additive to that of the sulfonylureas. In sulfonylurea-treated patients with T2DM who do not achieve optimal control or who experience secondary failure, it is important not to discontinue sulfonylurea therapy, but to add metformin. Discontinuation of sulfonylurea therapy and substitution of metformin will not decrease the FPG below that observed with sulfonylurea monotherapy alone. The sulfonylurea is continued with metformin to maintain its effect on pancreatic insulin secretion.

Although primarily thought of as a drug for the overweight, it should be noted that, as with sulfonylureas, glycemic improvement is also demonstrated in patients who are not obese.[80,91]

Effects on Insulin Sensitivity

In addition to improving glycemia, metformin has been shown to have insulin-sensitizing effects in humans using the hyperinsulinemic glucose clamp technique. Most studies have documented an increase of ~20–30% in insulin-mediated glucose uptake. This increase in glucose uptake is mainly due to stimulation of nonoxidative glucose disposal (primarily glycogen synthesis).[91] However, as an insulin sensitizer, metformin is less potent than the glitazones in stimulating insulin-mediated glucose uptake into muscle tissue. In a head-to-head comparison, after 3 months of therapy, despite equivalent glucose lowering, the mean rate of glucose disposal increased by 54% during troglitazone therapy and 13% during metformin therapy. Endogenous glucose production, however, decreased during metformin therapy by a mean of 19%, whereas it was unchanged by troglitazone therapy[90] (Fig. 32-7).

Effects on Insulin Secretion

In clinical studies, metformin does not appear to have a direct effect on β-cell function. In metformin-treated patients with diabetes, both fasting and postprandial insulin levels decrease,[80,91] secondary to the normal compensatory response of the pancreas to lower prevailing glucose levels and enhanced insulin sensitivity.

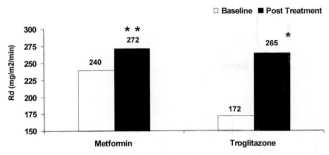

FIGURE 32-7. Maximum glucose disposal rate (Rd) obtained during the hyperinsulinemic clamp technique, before and after 3 months of therapy with metformin and troglitazone. *, $p = 0.006$; **, $p = 0.03$. (*Data from Inzucchi et al.[90]*)

Also, studies to date with the hyperglycemic clamp technique have failed to demonstrate any effect of metformin on either total insulin secretion or first- or second-phase insulin secretion in patients with T2DM. Some studies during an oral glucose tolerance test (OGTT) have demonstrated an increase in insulin secretion after metformin treatment.[91] However, these increases in insulin secretion have been small and probably secondary to amelioration of glucose toxicity.

A recent report notes a direct effect of metformin on pancreatic β cells. Patane and colleagues[92] demonstrated that in rat pancreatic islets whose secretory function has been impaired by chronic exposure to elevated free fatty acids (FFAs) or glucose levels, metformin was able to restore the intracellular abnormalities of glucose and FFA metabolism and to restore a normal secretory pattern. These data raise the possibility that, in diabetic patients, metformin (in addition to its peripheral effects) may have a direct beneficial effect on β-cell secretory function.[92] Interestingly, metformin treatment has also been shown to lower concentrations of intact and des 31,32 proinsulin in T2DM.[93] These molecules have been postulated to play a role in the development of atherosclerosis, and the long-term effect of metformin treatment on proinsulin-like molecules and atherogenesis needs to be assessed further.

Effects on Weight

Unlike the insulin secretagogues and the thiazolidinediones, metformin therapy does not result in weight gain in patients with T2DM who receive metformin alone or in combination with other oral agents or insulin.[81,89,90,94,95] Most studies show modest weight loss (2–3 kg) during the first 6 months of treatment.[81] Metformin therapy is also associated with weight loss in nondiabetic subjects.[96] The exact mechanisms by which metformin prevents weight gain or induces weight loss have not been determined. Several mechanisms have been postulated by which metformin might prevent weight gain or induce weight loss. These include a decrease in food consumption, increase in energy expenditure, and reduction of hyperinsulinemia.[91] Some animal studies suggest an anorectic effect, but in human studies, it has not been possible to differentiate between a central effect of metformin in decreasing calorie intake versus an increase in energy expenditure.[91] Incidentally, in nondiabetic and polycystic ovary syndrome (PCOS) subjects, metformin therapy is associated with a reduction in leptin levels and restoration of menses.[97–99]

Effects on Lipids

In addition to its glycemic effects, metformin is known to have favorable effects on plasma lipids, in both diabetic and nondiabetic subjects.[91] As monotherapy, metformin decreases plasma triglyceride and LDL cholesterol levels by 10–15%[100,101] and also reduces postprandial hyperlipemia, plasma FFA levels, and FFA oxidation. The decrease in plasma triglyceride concentration is independent of changes in the plasma glucose level since metformin reduces triglyceride levels in nondiabetic patients with hypertriglyceridemia.[100,101] Metformin therapy does not appear to affect HDL cholesterol levels consistently, which either do not change or increase slightly after metformin therapy.[91]

Effects on Blood Pressure

In some clinical studies, metformin treatment has been associated with a modest drop in blood pressure in patients with T2DM.[91] However, most studies have failed to demonstrate any decrease in systemic blood pressure with metformin treatment.[91]

Effects on Other Cardiovascular Risk Factors

Insulin resistance is known to be associated with a hypercoagulable state[102] and an increase in many cardiovascular risk factors, including PAI-1. Metformin has many beneficial effects on cardiovascular risk factors.[84,103,104] Elevated PAI-1 levels are decreased with metformin therapy in patients with and without diabetes.[91] In the French Biguanides and the Prevention of the Risk of Obesity (BIGPRO) 1 trial, metformin therapy also reduced tissue-type plasminogen activator (tPA) antigen and von Willebrand factor (vWF) levels. These two factors are mainly secreted by endothelial cells, and metformin therapy appeared to have suppressive effects on the production or metabolism of these two hemostatic proteins.[105] In another 18-month study, metformin treatment in elderly T2DM patients was associated with significant reductions in markers of platelet function, thrombin generation, and fibrinolysis inhibition (PAI-1 activity, PAI-1 antigen).[106] However, in this study, increases in some fibrinolytic activation markers (tPA and antithrombin (AT)-III; $p < 0.01$) were also observed.

Effects on Cardiovascular Disease

The long-term effects of metformin on serum lipids and other metabolic risk factors appear to have cardiovascular benefits. In the UKPDS, metformin therapy in obese, newly diagnosed patients with T2DM was associated with a significant decrease in cardiovascular and all-cause mortality.[107] Whether this benefit with metformin treatment was due to the absence of weight gain or other beneficial effects on the metabolic syndrome of diabetes remains to be determined. It must also be remembered that in the UKPDS, when metformin treatment was added in patients who had failed sulfonylurea therapy, there was a significant and paradoxic increase in cardiovascular and all-cause mortality (Fig. 32-8). This question was addressed in a subsequent analysis by Turner and colleagues, [107a] who found that all the relative increase in mortality observed in the patients who received sulfonylurea plus metformin compared with those who received sulfonylurea alone resulted from a significant reduction in the expected number of deaths in the latter group; there was no increase in mortality in the sulfonylurea plus metformin group. In absolute terms, the number of fatal heart

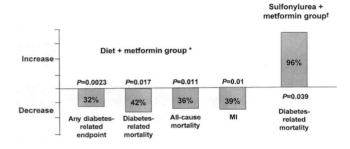

FIGURE 32-8. Risk reduction with metformin monotherapy and in combination with sulfonylureas in the UKPDS. MI, myocardial infarction. (*Data from Turner et al.[107a]*)

attacks actually decreased in the sulfonylurea plus metformin group compared with the expected number of deaths.[107a] The investigators also performed a meta-analysis of all patients receiving sulfonylurea plus metformin in the UKPDS and reported significant reductions in all diabetes-related endpoints and for myocardial infarction.

Effects on PCOS

Women with PCOS are characterized by chronic anovulation and infertility due to excessive androgen production. There is evidence to suggest that this hyperandrogenism may be secondary to insulin resistance and chronic hyperinsulinemia.[108] Several, but not all, studies have shown that in patients with PCOS, metformin improves glucose tolerance and insulin sensitivity and also normalizes plasma sex hormone binding and free testosterone levels.[109,110] In a recent study in 43 amenorrheic women with PCOS, metformin treatment for 6 months was found to reduce the endocrinopathy of PCOS and allow resumption of normal menses in most (91%) previously amenorrheic women with PCOS.[99]

Effects on Prevention of Type 2 Diabetes

Most patients with T2DM have impaired glucose tolerance (IGT) for several years before progressing to diabetes. Persons with IGT tend to have both insulin resistance and β-cell dysfunction; their FPG values during a 75-g OGTT are ≤140 mg/dL, and their 2-hour postglucose values are between 140 and 199 mg/dL.[111] Metformin is known to improve insulin sensitivity, lower plasma insulin levels and blood pressure, and improve lipid profiles in nondiabetic insulin-resistant individuals.[91,112] Hence, metformin therapy is one of the arms of the Diabetes Prevention Program, which is a large randomized placebo-clinical trial being conducted by the NIH to determine whether it is possible to prevent or delay the development of T2DM in high-risk individuals with IGT using intensive lifestyle measures or pharmacologic treatment. The study recruitment of 3000 subjects[65] was completed in 2002[65a] with a 31% reduction in the incidence of T2DM after 3 years of treatment with metformin.

Dosing

Metformin should be taken with meals, and the starting dose (500 or 850 mg with breakfast or 500 mg with breakfast and dinner) and

be increased slowly at weekly or biweekly intervals to minimize GI side effects.[80] Metformin lowers fasting plasma glucose and HbA_{1c} in a dose-related manner, and although benefits are observed at lower doses, significant glycemic responses to metformin are usually seen at doses of approximately 1500 mg/day or greater. Data from one study suggest that most patients will achieve maximal efficacy at a daily dosage of 2000 mg (1000 mg bid), although some patients may achieve additional benefit if the dosage is increased to 2500 mg.[87] The maximum daily dose of metformin is 2550 mg. Doses above 2000 mg daily may be better tolerated when given 3 times a day with meals. The glycemic goal should be an FPG ≤ 120 mg/dL and HbA_{1c} < 7%. If adequate glycemic control is not achieved with maximum doses of metformin (HbA_{1c} > 8%), combination therapy should be considered.

Side Effects

Adverse GI effects are seen in approximately 30% of patients taking metformin. These include anorexia, nausea/vomiting, abdominal discomfort, dyspepsia, flatulence, diarrhea, and metallic taste. These side effects tend to decline with continued use and can be minimized by initiating therapy with low doses of metformin. The risk of hypoglycemia is much less common with metformin than with the sulfonylureas.[80] However, hypoglycemia has been reported with metformin.[80] Since metformin reverses insulin resistance, and subsequently causes a decrease in insulin concentrations, metformin-induced hypoglycemia is usually mild and does not necessitate the discontinuation of therapy. Hypoglycemia is more common when metformin is coadministered with other oral hypoglycemic agents or when there is deficient caloric intake or strenuous exercise not compensated by caloric supplementation. Asymptomatic vitamin B_{12} deficiency was reported with metformin monotherapy in 9% of patients during clinical trials. Serum folic acid concentrations did not decrease significantly. Five cases of megaloblastic anemia have been reported with metformin (none in the United States). Annual screening for hematologic changes is recommended during therapy with metformin. Weight loss may occur during therapy with metformin, perhaps as a result of its ability to cause anorexia. In contrast, sulfonylureas and insulin tend to cause weight gain. Up to 5% of patients cannot tolerate metformin and require discontinuation of this medication.

Contraindications/Caution

Since metformin is largely eliminated unchanged in the urine via glomerular filtration and tubular secretion, it is contraindicated in patients with renal disease or renal impairment (serum creatinine > 1.5 mg/dL in men and > 1.4 mg/dL in women). In patients with reduced muscle mass, such as elderly patients (especially those older than 80 years of age), the serum creatinine concentration may underestimate the glomerular filtration rate, and creatinine clearance should be determined. If the creatinine clearance is <70 mL/min, metformin should not be given.[93] Renal dysfunction also increases the risk of adverse reactions such as lactic acidosis from metformin. Lactic acidosis can also occur in patients predisposed to lactic acidosis such as those with hepatic disease, cardiac disease (e.g., heart failure or acute myocardial infarction), severe infection, severe trauma, dehydration, severe burns, hyperosmolar nonketotic coma, major surgery, or alcoholism. Metformin is contraindicated in these patients.[80]

Metformin should also not be used in diabetic patients with congestive heart failure requiring pharmacologic therapy because in this situation, decreased renal perfusion and glomerular filtration rate can impair metformin excretion. Metformin should also be withheld at the time of or prior to the performance of x-ray procedures involving intravenous radiographic contrast agents because of an increased risk of renal impairment and possible lactic acidosis. Metformin should be reinstituted only after renal function has been reevaluated after 48 hours and found to be normal. In addition, caution should be used in patients with blood glucose levels persistently >300 mg/dL, since this level of hyperglycemia can impair kidney function.[113]

The safety of metformin in pregnant and lactating women has not been established. In one report of metformin use in pregnancy from South Africa, the neonatal mortality rate was lower in patients receiving metformin than in mildly diabetic controls.[114] In another report, slightly higher incidences of polycythemia and necrotizing enterocolitis were noted in the metformin group, and the most frequently encountered problems in the neonate were jaundice, polycythemia, and hypoglycemia.[115]

Recently, metformin has received approval from the FDA for use in adolescents with T2DM.

Drug Interactions

Cimetidine decreases the renal clearance of metformin secondary to a decrease in metformin renal tubular secretion. However, metformin has little effect on the pharmacokinetics of cimetidine. Other cationic drugs that are excreted via renal tubular transport may also interfere with the clearance of metformin. These drugs include amiloride, digoxin, morphine, procainamide, quinidine, quinine, ranitidine, triamterene, trimethoprim, and vancomycin. Concomitant administration of furosemide increases plasma metformin concentrations without any significant change in metformin renal clearance. On the other hand, metformin decreases furosemide plasma and blood maximum concentrations by 31% and 12%, respectively. Furosemide's terminal half-life was also decreased by 32% without any significant change in renal clearance. Nifedipine, and possibly other calcium channel blockers, increases the absorption of metformin. Although the clinical implications of these interactions are minimal, patients on the above drugs and metformin should be closely monitored.

Metformin can also inhibit the absorption of cyanocobalamin (vitamin B_{12}) by competitively blocking the calcium-dependent binding of the intrinsic factor–vitamin B_{12} complex to its receptor. Patients should be monitored for possible development of anemia.

α-GLUCOSIDASE INHIBITORS

There are two α-glucosidase inhibitors currently marketed in the United States, acarbose (Precose®) and miglitol (Glyset®) (Fig. 32-9) The first, acarbose, was approved in the United States in 1995 for use as monotherapy or in combination with insulin, metformin, or sulfonylureas. Miglitol was approved by the FDA in December 1996 but was not marketed until mid-1999. Miglitol is only approved for use as monotherapy and in combination with sulfonylureas. At recommended doses, both agents have only modest effects on HbA_{1c} levels (mean 0.5–1.0% reductions). α-Glucosidase inhibitors are suitable alternatives in patients with mild to moderate hyperglycemia (especially postprandial hyperglycemia) and, be-

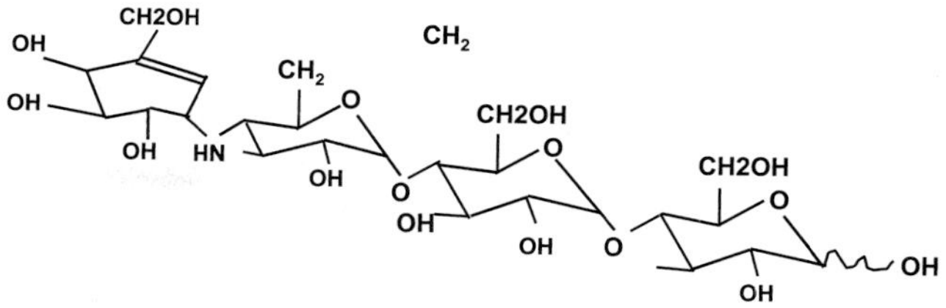

FIGURE 32-9. Structure of miglitol.

cause of their relative safety, are often useful as monotherapy in the elderly T2DM patient. In addition, although not FDA-approved for T1DM, acarbose has been utilized as an adjunct to insulin therapy to reduce postprandial plasma glucose levels in these patients.

Mechanism of Action

Acarbose and miglitol are potent inhibitors of the α-glucosidase enzymes present in the brush border of the enterocytes located in the proximal portion of the small intestine.[116,117] Although the mechanisms of action for the α-glucosidase inhibitors are similar, they are not identical. Both agents significantly inhibit glycoamylase, followed by sucrase, maltase, and dextranase. However, miglitol is a more potent inhibitor of sucrase and maltase than is acarbose. Both drugs also inhibit isomaltase but, in contrast to acarbose, miglitol does not inhibit pancreatic α-amylase. The inhibition of sucrase (which prevents the conversion of sucrose to fructose and glucose), glycoamylase, maltase, and isomaltase results in delayed carbohydrate digestion and absorption throughout the small intestine. Clinically, this leads to delayed intraluminal production of monosaccharides (i.e., glucose), delayed and prolonged postprandial rises in plasma glucose, and a blunted plasma insulin response. In addition to the above actions, miglitol (but not acarbose) interacts weakly with the intestinal sodium-dependent glucose transporter, but this does not appear to affect the physiologic absorption of glucose clinically. Miglitol (unlike acarbose) also minimally inhibits the lactase enzyme, but this does not produce clinical lactose intolerance. When used as monotherapy, both agents do not enhance insulin secretion and in overdose will not result in hypoglycemia.

Pharmacokinetics

The two agents differ significantly in their rate of systemic absorption. Systemic absorption of active acarbose is only about 2%, whereas after oral administration of a 25-mg dose of miglitol, there is rapid and nearly complete systemic absorption of the drug. Low systemic absorption of acarbose is therapeutically desirable, since the drug acts locally in the GI tract. Acarbose is metabolized within the GI tract, and metabolism occurs principally by intestinal microbial flora, intestinal hydrolysis, and the activity of digestive enzymes. At least 13 metabolites have been identified, with approximately 34% of the major metabolite fractions being absorbed systemically and appearing in the urine as sulfate, methyl, and glucuronide conjugates. One metabolite has α-glucosidase–inhibitory effects. This active metabolite, along with the parent compound, is recovered in the urine and accounts for about 2% of the total administered dose. Plasma elimination half-life of acarbose is about 2 hours in healthy adults, and most of an oral dose (~51%) is excreted through the feces.

Unlike acarbose, miglitol is systemically absorbed via a jejunal transport mechanism similar to that of glucose absorption. Oral absorption of miglitol is saturable at high doses; only 50–70% of a 100-mg dose is systemically absorbed. There is no evidence at this time that systemic absorption is required for miglitol activity, but it appears that miglitol concentrates in intestinal enterocytes to exhibit its action locally in the GI tract.[117] The drug distributes primarily into extracellular fluid and is minimally protein-bound. Unlike acarbose, miglitol is not metabolized in any way and is excreted unchanged by the kidneys. More than 95% of a 25-mg dose is recovered in the urine within 24 hours; at higher doses, the cumulative percentage recovered is somewhat less due to lower bioavailability of the higher doses. The plasma elimination half-life of miglitol is about 2 hours in healthy adults. In patients with severe renal impairment (i.e., CrCl < 25mL/min), both acarbose and miglitol attain systemic peak and AUC concentrations that are roughly 5–6 times and 2 times higher, respectively, than in patients with normal renal function. Thus patients with renal failure are expected to accumulate both drugs to some degree. The pharmacokinetics of acarbose have not been studied in patients with cirrhosis. Because miglitol is not metabolized by the liver, the pharmacokinetics in patients with cirrhosis are not altered. For both drugs, no significant differences in pharmacokinetics have been observed based on age, race, or gender.

Clinical Use and Efficacy

Acarbose is approved for use as monotherapy or in combination with insulin, metformin, or sulfonylureas.[116,117] Miglitol is only approved for use as monotherapy and in combination with sulfonylureas. To be maximally effective, both drugs must be administered at the start of a main meal. This is because they are competitive inhibitors and must be present at the site of enzymatic action at the same time the carbohydrates are present in the small intestine. The affinity of the α-glucosidase inhibitors for the α-glucosidase receptors is much greater than that of the oligo- or disaccharides in foods. Taking the medication before or more than 15 minutes after the start of the meal reduces the impact of the medication on postprandial blood glucose. Also, to be clinically effective, the patient must be consuming a diet high in complex carbohydrates (roughly ≥ 50% of calories)[117] since the glycemic response to acarbose and miglitol is dependent on the carbohydrate content of the diet. Several randomized, double-blind, placebo-controlled trials have demonstrated that the addition of acarbose or miglitol to diet therapy significantly reduces postprandial glucose and HbA$_{1c}$ levels compared with placebo.[116–122] Monotherapy with these agents lowers mean postprandial glucose levels by ~40–60 mg/dL and mean fasting glucose levels by 10–20 mg/dL; overall, mean HbA$_{1c}$ levels are reduced 0.5–1.0%[116–122] Fig. 32–10.

In combination therapy with sulfonylureas, metformin, and insulin, acarbose further reduces mean HbA$_{1c}$ between 0.3 and 0.5% and mean postprandial glucose between 25 and 30 mg/dL from baseline.[123–125] Miglitol in combination therapy with sulfonylureas reduces mean HbA$_{1c}$ by 0.7% and mean 1-hour postprandial glucose by ~60–70 mg/dL. Compared with sulfonylureas or metformin, acarbose and miglitol possess less potent effects on fasting glucose and are typically reserved for use as monotherapy in patients with mild-to-moderate hyperglycemia, particularly postpran-

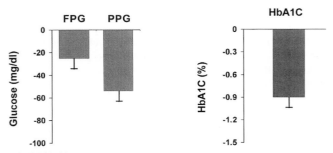

FIGURE 32-10. Mean changes in fasting glucose (FPG), post-prandial glucose (PPG) and HbA, C in acarbose- and miglitol-treated patients. (*Data from refs. 116–122.*)

dial hyperglycemia. In addition, the absence of hypoglycemia with these agents when used as monotherapy makes them particularly useful and relatively safe in elderly T2DM patients.[126]

Effects in Type 1 Diabetes

Although α-glucosidase inhibitors are not FDA-approved for use in T1DM, acarbose has been utilized in these patients as an adjunct to insulin therapy to reduce postprandial plasma glucose levels.[127,128] Riccardi and colleagues[127] evaluated the efficacy and safety of acarbose in the treatment of T1DM in a placebo-controlled, double-blind, multicenter Italian study. After a 6-week run-in, 121 patients with T1DM were randomized to acarbose or placebo and to a high- or low-fiber diet for 24 weeks. The acarbose dose was 50 mg tid for the first 2 weeks and 100 mg tid for the subsequent weeks. At the end of 24 weeks of treatment, an intention-to-treat analysis showed that acarbose decreased 2-hour postprandial plasma glucose levels (220 ± 15 mg/dL versus 268 ± 15 mg/dL; $F = 6.1, p < 0.02$) compared with placebo. There was no significant effect of acarbose on HbA$_{1c}$ or the number of hypoglycemic episodes. Interestingly, in this study, the effect of acarbose on blood glucose control was not influenced by the amount of carbohydrate and/or fiber intake. As expected, the incidences of adverse GI events were 75% and 39% in acarbose and placebo groups, respectively. The authors concluded that acarbose in combination with insulin reduces postprandial plasma glucose levels in T2DM patients who are not satisfactorily controlled with insulin alone.

In another double-blind, placebo-controlled, crossover study, Koch and associates[128] investigated in a German study whether acarbose therapy enables patients with T1DM to administer insulin injections at the same time as meals without adverse glycemic consequences, thus negating the need for an injection-meal interval (IMI). Results from this study provided strong evidence that acarbose prevents the marked increase in postprandial glucose level normally observed when regular insulin is administered with, rather than before, a meal. Acarbose may thus be useful for patients with T1DM who find IMIs inconvenient.

Effects on Insulin Sensitivity

Although studies in animal models suggest that long-term treatment with an α-glucosidase inhibitor (miglitol) improves insulin sensitivity and may have vascular protective effects in obese insulin-resistant rats,[129] studies in human insulin-resistant T2DM subjects using the insulin/glucose clamp method have yielded conflicting results. One study showed that miglitol-induced improvement in postprandial hyperglycemia was not associated with improved insulin sensitivity,[130] whereas in a recent study, acarbose at up to 300 mg daily for 12 months was associated with significant improvements in insulin sensitivity as measured by the hyperglycemic clamp technique and by homeostasis model assessment (HOMA) along with reduced glycemia.[130a]

Effects in Reactive Hypoglycemia and the Dumping Syndrome

α-Glucosidase inhibitors appear to have beneficial effects in people with reactive hypoglycemia and those with the dumping syndrome. In one study[131] of 21 nonobese patients (6 males, 15 females) with reactive hypoglycemia, acarbose treatment for 3 months blunted post-OGTT increases in insulin and C-peptide levels and reduced the frequency of hypoglycemic attacks from four times a week to one. Similar beneficial effects were reported in another study.[132]

Cardiac Effects

In rabbits,[133] miglitol appears to have a dose-dependent effect on reducing myocardial infarct size. Inhibition of glycogenolysis and lactate formation has been suggested to be the responsible mechanism. As yet, there are no human studies in this field.

Effects on Weight

Due to polysaccharide metabolism by colonic microflora and the capacity of the large bowel to conserve calories, there is minimal calorie loss associated with acarbose and miglitol therapy. Hence, in clinical practice, dramatic weight loss is not commonly associated with acarbose or miglitol therapy (in contrast to animal studies).[117] Weight loss, if it occurs, is typically mild (i.e., 0.8–1.4 kg over 1 year in clinical studies). In humans, acarbose and miglitol also appear to offset the insulinotropic effects and weight gain associated with sulfonylurea treatment when they are added to combination therapy.[117] The exact metabolic or pharmacologic mechanism(s) responsible for α-glucosidase–induced weight loss remains unknown.

Effects on Lipids

In some studies, α-glucosidase inhibitors are associated with decreases in triglyceride levels.[117, 134,135] In a study from Japan[134] of 20 patients with T2DM, acarbose not only inhibited the postprandial increase of both plasma glucose and insulin but also significantly suppressed the postprandial increase of serum triglycerides and serum remnant-like cholesterol particles. In addition, acarbose inhibited the postprandial decline of apolipoprotein C-II, and decreased postprandial serum apolipoprotein C-III levels. There is also evidence that acarbose may reduce triglyceride levels in nondiabetics, and the drug may be a useful adjunct to dietary therapy in nondiabetic patients affected by severe hypertriglyceridemia.[135]

Prevention of Type 2 Diabetes

Currently, an international study (the STOP-NIDDM Trial) is evaluating the efficacy of an α-glucosidase inhibitor to prevent or delay the development of T2DM in a population with impaired glucose tolerance (IGT) who are at increased risk of developing T2DM.[136] A total of 1418 subjects diagnosed with IGT according to the

World Health Organization's criteria with an FPG of ≥100 mg/dL will be randomized in a double-blind fashion to receive either acarbose (100 mg tid) or placebo for a median follow-up period of 3.9 years. The primary endpoint is the development of T2DM diagnosed using a 75-g OGTT according to the current diagnostic criteria. The secondary endpoints are changes in blood pressure, lipid profile, insulin sensitivity, cardiovascular events, and morphometric profile. The study is ongoing and hopefully may answer the question of whether acarbose can prevent or delay the progression of IGT to T2DM.

Dosage

Acarbose and miglitol are administered with the first bite of each main meal. If patients do not have oral dietary intake, they should not take these agents. To minimize GI side effects, both acarbose and miglitol should be started at 25 mg po 3 times per day, taken with the first bite of each main meal. To reduce GI side effects further, some patients may benefit from an initial dose of 25 mg po once daily for 1 week, titrated up as tolerated to 25 mg po three times per day. After 4–8 weeks of the 25-mg po three times daily dose, the dosage may be increased if needed to 50 mg po three times daily. One-hour postprandial glucose levels throughout treatment and an HbA$_{1c}$ level at 3 months should be used to determine response to therapy. If at 3 months the HbA$_{1c}$ level is not satisfactory, the dose may be titrated to the maximum recommended dose of 100 mg po three times per day. The usual maintenance dose range is 50–100 mg po three times per day. One-hour postprandial glucose levels should be used to determine response to therapy and to titrate dose. In adults weighing <60 kg, the maximum recommended dose of acarbose is 50 mg tid. Patients who do not respond to monotherapy should be changed to another form of therapy or considered for oral combination therapy in order to achieve optimal glycemic goals.

Patients with Renal Impairment

There is no experience with either acarbose or miglitol in patients with serum creatinine >2 mg/dL, and treatment of these patients with acarbose or miglitol is not recommended.

Contraindications

Acarbose and miglitol are contraindicated in patients with inflammatory bowel disease, colonic ulceration, ileus, partial or predisposition to GI obstruction, or GI disease involving disorders of absorption or digestion. Both drugs should be used cautiously in patients with hiatal hernia or other conditions that might be exacerbated by increased formation of gas. If a patient has poor oral intake, continual vomiting, or diarrhea, acarbose and miglitol therapy should be withheld until adequate oral dietary intake resumes. Since miglitol elimination is dependent on glomerular filtration, the drug may accumulate in patients with renal impairment. Hence the drug should not be used in patients with CrCl < 25 mL/min or serum creatinine ≥ 2.0 mg/dL. Acarbose is contraindicated for use in patients with cirrhosis. If hepatic enzyme elevations occur during acarbose therapy, dose reduction or discontinuation of acarbose may be necessary, particularly if such elevations persist. However, there are two studies whose results document the good tolerability and efficacy of acarbose therapy in patients with chronic liver disease.[137,138]

Acarbose and miglitol have not been studied in pregnancy and should not be used in pregnant or lactating women. The safety and effectiveness of acarbose and miglitol in children have not been established.

Side Effects

Hypoglycemia

When used as monotherapy, acarbose and miglitol do not enhance insulin secretion and hence in overdose do not cause hypoglycemia. However, when these agents are used in combination with insulin or other insulin secretagogues (sulfonylureas or repaglinide), hypoglycemia may occur. It is important to remember that this hypoglycemia associated with the use of acarbose or miglitol plus insulin or a insulin secretagogue should be treated with oral glucose (dextrose) and not sucrose or other complex carbohydrates, which may be ineffective. The hydrolysis of sucrose (cane sugar) to fructose and glucose is inhibited by acarbose, and thus products containing sucrose are unsuitable for the rapid correction of hypoglycemia. Patients should be aware of the need to have a readily available source of glucose (dextrose, d-glucose) to treat hypoglycemic episodes. In severe hypoglycemia, intravenous dextrose or glucagon injections may be required.

Gastrointestinal

The most common adverse reactions to acarbose and miglitol are gastrointestinal in nature, including abdominal discomfort, increased flatulence, and diarrhea.[116,117] These symptoms occur with the highest incidence during initiation of therapy and abate or decrease in intensity with continued use. Roughly 50–60% of patients receiving acarbose and miglitol experience the above adverse GI reactions, which are caused primarily by an increase in gas formation secondary to fermentation of unabsorbed carbohydrate in the large intestine. In clinical studies, increased flatulence has been reported to occur in up to 74% of patients on acarbose versus 29% receiving placebo and in up to 41.5% of patients on miglitol versus 12% receiving placebo. Abdominal pain reported as discomfort occurred in 12–19% of patients on acarbose/miglitol versus 5–9% receiving placebo. Diarrhea occurred in 29–31% of patients on acarbose/miglitol versus 10–12% receiving placebo. Borborygmi may also occur along with flatulence. In clinical trials, the use of antacids or fibrous substances to modify the adverse GI side effects of acarbose has not been successful. Proper dosage titration, however, may help improve patient tolerance of GI-related adverse events (see Dosage above).

Systemic adverse events with acarbose are relatively rare. In one U.S. study, asymptomatic elevations of hepatic enzymes occurred in 3.8% of patients receiving acarbose versus 0.9% of those receiving placebo.[126] In long-term studies (up to 12 months), elevations of serum transaminases (AST and/or ALT) above the upper limit of normal that required emergency treatment were asymptomatic, reversible, more common in females, and, in general, not associated with other evidence of liver dysfunction. Serum transaminase elevations also appeared to be dose-related, with an increased frequency in those on >300 mg/day. Two patients in Japan died of fulminant hepatitis; however, the relationship to acarbose is unclear.

Miglitol and acarbose are known to decrease iron absorption slightly, but in most cases the reduction in iron indices appears to be clinically insignificant.[117,139] In clinical trials, low serum iron levels were more commonly noted in patients treated with miglitol (9.2%) versus placebo (4.2%). In most cases, miglitol was not associated with reductions in hemoglobin or other hematologic indices, and in many cases the effect on iron concentrations was transient. Long-term use of acarbose has also been associated with anemia in roughly 1% of patients. Rare dermatologic findings include an unusual report of serum eosinophilia associated with generalized erythema multiforme and histologic tissue eosinophilia with acarbose therapy.[140] Skin rash (generally transient in nature) also occurred in 4.3% of patients on miglitol versus 2.4% of placebo-treated patients in clinical trials.

Drug Interactions

Digestive enzyme preparations containing carbohydrate-splitting enzymes (e.g., amylase, pancreatin, and pancrelipase) may reduce the pharmacologic effect of α-glucosidase inhibitors (e.g., acarbose or miglitol) and should not be administered concurrently. Since sucrase hydrolyzes sucrose into glucose and fructose, it would antagonize the effects of acarbose or miglitol in the intestine. Charcoal is an intestinal adsorbent that may reduce the effects of the α-glucosidase inhibitors (e.g., acarbose or miglitol) and hence should not be taken concomitantly. It is also possible that concomitant administration of acarbose or miglitol with bile acid sequestrants, such as cholestyramine or colestipol, may decrease the effects of these antidiabetic agents. Also, oral neomycin may eliminate gut bacteria responsible for metabolism of carbohydrates and therefore enhance the reduction in postprandial glucose as well as exacerbate GI adverse effects. Clinical documentation of such interactions, however, is lacking. Antacids are not known to affect acarbose action.

α-Glucosidase inhibitors may also impair the oral absorption of digoxin and lead to subtherapeutic serum digoxin concentrations in some patients. Clinical reports of this interaction have been published, but the mechanism of the interaction is not well understood. It is recommended that these agents be administered 6 hours after an oral digoxin dose to ensure time for adequate digoxin absorption.[141] In addition, patients should be closely observed for the loss of clinical effect of digoxin therapy if either acarbose or miglitol is added to the medication regimen. In some cases, digoxin serum concentration monitoring may be helpful. Caution should also be exercised in patients on concomitant warfarin therapy, and prothrombin times should be closely observed during the first month of acarbose and miglitol therapy. Any dosage adjustments should be made according to individual patient response.

The combination of acarbose with acetaminophen and ethanol should be avoided since both alcohol and acarbose augment the activity of the hepatic isoenzyme CYP2E1, which is responsible for metabolism of acetaminophen to a toxic reactive metabolite.[142]

THIAZOLIDINEDIONES

The thiazolidinediones or glitazones are oral antidiabetic agents that are also termed *insulin sensitizers*; they act primarily by reducing insulin resistance, which is thought to be central to the development of T2DM and its cardiovascular complications. These agents are chemically and functionally unrelated to the other oral antidiabetic agents. Two compounds in this class are presently approved for use in the United States (Fig. 32–11). Rosiglitazone (Avandia®) was approved on May 25, 1999, and pioglitazone (Actos®) was granted approval on July 16, 1999. The first agent in

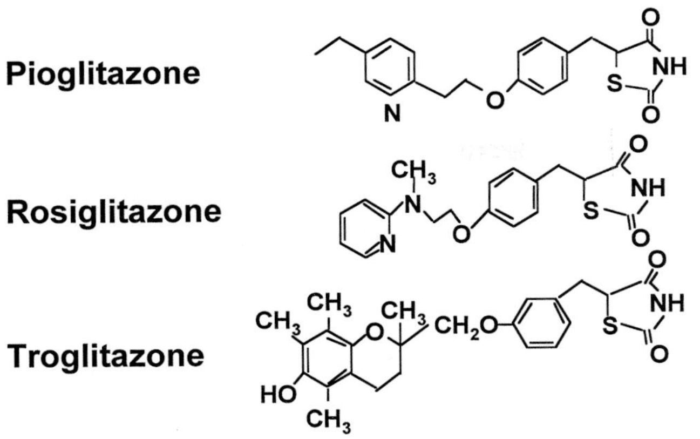

FIGURE 32-11. Structure of the thiazolidinediones.

this class, troglitazone (Rezulin®), was marketed in the United States from March 1997 until it was withdrawn in March 2000, when the FDA determined that the risk of idiosyncratic hepatotoxicity associated with troglitazone therapy outweighed its potential benefits. In clinical use so far, rosiglitazone and pioglitazone appear to be devoid of fulminant hepatotoxicity. Monotherapy with the glitazones results in significant improvements in FPG by 59–80 mg/dL and in HbA$_{1c}$ by 1.4–2.6% compared with placebo. Rosiglitazone is approved for use as monotherapy and in combination with metformin and sulfonylurea. Pioglitazone is approved for use as monotherapy and also in combination with insulin, metformin, or a sulfonylurea.

Mechanism of Action

The thiazolidinediones are highly selective and potent agonists for the peroxisome proliferator-activated receptor γ (PPARγ).[143] PPARs are a family of nuclear receptors comprised of three subtypes designated PPARα, PPARγ, and PPARδ (previously termed PPARβ, FAAR, or NUC-1).[144] PPARγ receptors are found in key target tissues for insulin action such as adipose tissue, skeletal muscle, and liver, and evidence to date indicates that these receptors may be important regulators of lipid homeostasis, adipocyte differentiation, and insulin action.[143,144] A close relationship has been shown to exist between the ability of various thiazolidinediones to stimulate PPARγ and its antidiabetic action.[145] Most of the studies on the mechanism of action of the glitazones have been done with troglitazone.

Thiazolidinediones have been shown to stimulate GLUT-1 and GLUT-4 gene expression[146] and to reduce ob gene, tumor necrosis factor-α (TNF-α), and hepatic glucokinase expression through activation of PPARγ.[147] In obese Zucker rats, treatment with the thiazolidinedione troglitazone resulted in a reduction in leptin levels and lower ob gene and TNF-α expression. Associated with this effect was apoptosis of large adipocytes and an increase in the number of small adipocytes (with no net change in adipose tissue weight).[148] Both TNF-α and leptin (an ob gene product) have been associated with insulin resistance, and it is plausible that with the reduction in large adipocytes and lower TNF-α and leptin levels, there is amelioration of insulin resistance. Moreover, the increase in the number of small adipocytes may also contribute to the reduction of insulin resistance. Small adipocytes take up more glucose than large adipocytes at submaximal insulin levels and are also more sensitive to the antilipolytic action of insulin.[149,150] This

could potentially result in lower FFA and triglyceride levels and improved insulin sensitivity. Although the results from this study suggest that troglitazone exerts potent effects in adipose tissue, another study[151] has demonstrated beneficial effects of troglitazone on glucose and lipid metabolism independent of adipose tissue in aP2/DTA mice whose white and brown fat was virtually eliminated by fat-specific expression of diphtheria toxin. In this study, despite the absence of adipose tissue, beneficial metabolic changes were seen in muscle and liver.

In freshly isolated human adipocytes, rosiglitazone increased p85 α-phosphatidylinositol 3-kinase (p85αPI-3K) and uncoupling protein-2 (UCP) mRNA levels and decreased leptin expression. p85αPI-3K is a major component of insulin action, and the induction of its expression might explain, at least in part, the insulin-sensitizing effect of the thiazolidinediones.[152] In vitro, pioglitazone has been shown to reverse insulin resistance induced by TNF-α in liver cells.[153]

Some studies indicate that the glitazones also have direct effects in skeletal muscle. In human skeletal muscle culture systems, troglitazone treatment markedly increases PPARγ protein expression along with other genes involved in glucose and lipid metabolism.[154] This increase of PPARγ and associated changes in other genes may account, in part, for the insulin-sensitizing effect of troglitazone in skeletal muscle. In the same skeletal muscle culture system, troglitazone has been demonstrated to have acute effects on glucose uptake and chronic effects on glucose uptake and glycogen synthase activity.[155] Concomitant increases in GLUT-1 mRNA and protein were noted, with no change in GLUT-4 or glycogen synthase mRNA or protein.

The hypotensive and antiatherosclerotic effects of the glitazones may also occur through PPARγ agonism.[156–158] Human and rat vascular smooth muscle cells express mRNA and nuclear receptors for PPARγ 1.[156,158] These receptors are upregulated during vascular injury and are present in early human atheroma and precursor lesions. Pharmacologic activation of PPARγ with troglitazone and rosiglitazone inhibits vascular smooth muscle cell proliferation and migration, with the potential to limit restenosis and atherosclerosis. Also, both troglitazone and pioglitazone inhibit vasopressin and PDGF-induced Ca^{2+} entry and proliferation in rat vascular smooth muscle cells.[156]

Thus, the thiazolidinediones act, at least in part, by binding with PPARγ in various tissues to influence the expression of a number of genes encoding proteins involved in glucose and lipid metabolism, endothelial function, and atherogenesis.[156–159] In the near future, it is likely that the expression of numerous other genes will be identified that are affected by thiazolidinediones and contribute to the insulin-sensitizing, lipid-lowering, hypotensive, and antiatherosclerotic effects of these compounds.

Pharmacokinetics

After oral administration, both rosiglitazone and pioglitazone are rapidly absorbed, and peak serum concentrations occur within 1 hour for rosiglitazone and within 2 hours for pioglitazone. Food does not alter the pharmacokinetics of rosiglitazone, but it slightly delays the time to peak serum concentration of pioglitazone to 3–4 hours, although total absorption is unchanged. Steady-state serum concentrations of both drugs are achieved within 7 days and are highly protein-bound (>99%), primarily to serum albumin. Rosiglitazone is extensively metabolized, with no unchanged drug detected in urine. The major routes of metabolism include

N-demethylation and hydroxylation, followed by conjugation with sulfate and glucuronic acid. *In vitro* data show that rosiglitazone is predominantly metabolized by the cytochrome P-450 (CYP) isoenzyme 2C8, with CYP2C9 serving as a minor pathway. Metabolites are active but have significantly less activity than the parent compound. On the other hand, pioglitazone is extensively metabolized by hydroxylation and oxidation. The major hepatic cytochrome P-450 enzymes involved are CYP2C8 and CYP3A4. In animal studies, the metabolites M-II and M-IV (hydroxy derivatives of pioglitazone) and M-III (keto derivative of pioglitazone) are pharmacologically active. The metabolites M-III and M-IV are the principal drug-related species found in human serum following multiple dosing. At steady state, serum concentrations of the metabolites M-III and M-IV are equal to or greater than serum concentrations of pioglitazone. The plasma half-life ranges from 3 to 4 hours for rosiglitazone and from 3 to 7 hours for pioglitazone and 16 to 24 hours for pioglitazone metabolites.

Clinical Use and Efficacy

Rosiglitazone is at present approved for use as monotherapy and in combination with metformin and sulfonylureas.[160] In two U.S. placebo-controlled clinical trials in patients with T2DM, rosiglitazone at doses of 4 and 8 mg/day (as a single daily dose or two divided daily doses) for 26 weeks improved FPG by 25–35 and 42–55 mg/dL and HbA$_{1c}$ by 0.3 and 0.7%, respectively, compared with baseline. In these studies, when administered at the same daily dose, rosiglitazone was generally more effective in reducing FPG and HbA$_{1c}$ when administered in divided doses twice daily compared with once-daily doses. However, for HbA$_{1c}$, the difference between the 4-mg once-daily and the 2 mg twice-daily doses was not statistically significant. In another U.S. study, when compared directly with maximum stable doses of glyburide, rosiglitazone reduced FPG by 25 mg/dL (4 mg/day) and 41 mg/dL (8 mg/day) compared with a reduction of 30 mg/dL for glyburide (15 mg/day). Although the initial fall in FPG was greater with glyburide in this study, the improvement in glycemic control with rosiglitazone was maintained through week 52 of the study. Importantly, in patients treated with rosiglitazone, C-peptide, insulin, and proinsulin levels were significantly reduced compared with an increase of these hormones in the glyburide-treated patients.

The addition of rosiglitazone 2–8 mg/day to existing sulfonylurea, metformin, or insulin therapy also achieves further reductions in FPG and HbA$_{1c}$. In a double-blind, placebo-controlled trial, 348 patients with T2DM were randomized to receive 2500 mg g/day of metformin plus either placebo or 4 or 8 mg/day of rosiglitazone. After 26 weeks, compared with the metformin-placebo group, FPG levels decreased by 40 and 53 mg/dL, and mean HbA$_{1c}$ levels decreased by 1.0 and 1.2% in the 4-mg/day metformin-rosiglitazone group and the 8-mg/day metformin-rosiglitazone groups, respectively. Of patients receiving 8 mg/day of metformin-rosiglitazone, 28.1% achieved an HbA$_{1c}$ level of <7%. In addition, β-cell function, measured by the HOMA model, improved significantly with metformin-rosiglitazone therapy in a dose-dependent manner.[161] Compared with baseline, the combination of rosiglitazone (2 mg bid) and a sulfonylurea decreases FPG by 38 mg/dL and HbA$_{1c}$ by 0.9% (Fig. 32–12A); in combination with insulin, rosiglitazone at 4 mg bid reduces FPG by 55 mg/dL and HbA$_{1c}$ by 1.3%.[162]

The other currently marketed thiazolidinedione, pioglitazone, is the only glitazone approved by the FDA for use as monotherapy and in combination with sulfonylureas, metformin, and insulin. In

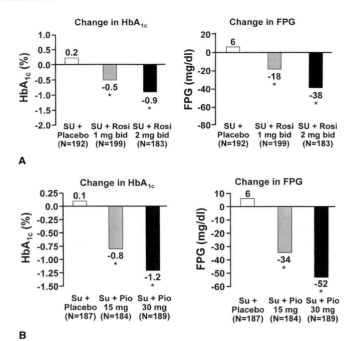

FIGURE 32-12 A. Mean changes in glycemic control at 6 months produced by the addition of rosiglitazone to a sulfonylurea (SU). FPG, fasting plasma glucose; Rosi, rosiglitazone. *, $p < 0.001$ vs. sulfonylurea. (*Data from Wolffenbuttel* et al.[162].) **B.** Mean changes in glycemic control at 6 months produced by the addition of pioglitazone (Pio) to a sulfonylurea. *, $p \leq 0.05$ vs. sulfonylurea. (*Data from Schneider* et al.[164])

the absence of head-to-head studies, it is not possible to evaluate which glitazone is more potent in clinical use. Pioglitazone has been demonstrated to improve glycemia when used as monotherapy. In U.S. studies, after 26 weeks, mean FPG levels were reduced by 30 mg/dL (on pioglitazone 15 mg/day), 32 mg/dL (on pioglitazone 30 mg/day), and, 56 mg/dL (on pioglitazone 45 mg/day) compared with an increase of 9 mg/dL in the placebo group. Concurrent with FPG, the HbA$_{1c}$ levels also decreased by 0.3% with pioglitazone 15 and 30 mg daily and 0.9% with pioglitazone 45 mg daily. HbA$_{1c}$ levels increased 0.7% in the placebo group.[163] In another double-blind study, compared with baseline, pioglitazone 15 and 30 mg daily (when added to a sulfonylurea regimen) reduced FPG by 34 and 52 mg/dL and HbA$_{1c}$ by 0.8 and 1.2%, respectively, after 16 weeks of therapy. In the placebo group, there was an increase of 6 mg/dL in FPG and 0.1% in HbA$_{1c}$[164] (Fig. 32–12B). Pioglitazone is also an useful option when used in combination with metformin. In a large 16-week study, compared with placebo, pioglitazone 30 mg daily significantly reduced mean FPG levels by 38 mg/dL and HbA$_{1c}$ levels by 0.8%.[165] Another significant use for pioglitazone is in the treatment of patients on insulin therapy. In a 16-week study, Rubin and coworkers[166] demonstrated that the addition of pioglitazone 15 and 30 mg daily to patients receiving a median daily dose of 60.5 U of insulin resulted in mean FPG reductions of 36 and 49 mg/dL and HbA$_{1c}$ reductions of 0.7 and 1.0%, respectively, compared with placebo.

Other Beneficial Effects

The glitazones have been shown to have multiple beneficial effects not only on peripheral insulin sensitivity, hepatic glucose metabolism, and lipid metabolism, but also on endothelial function, atherogenesis, fibrinolysis, and ovarian steroidogenesis.[159]

Effects on Insulin Sensitivity

Most of the human studies on the insulin-sensitizing effects of the thiazolidinediones *in vivo* have been done with troglitazone, which is no longer available. These studies have documented troglitazone's *in vivo* effects on peripheral insulin action not only in patients with T2DM but also in other insulin-resistant states like impaired glucose tolerance (IGT), polycystic ovary disease, previous gestational diabetes, and Werner's syndrome.[167–172] Some of these studies used the euglycemic clamp and the frequently sampled intravenous glucose tolerance test (FSIGTT) to quantitate changes of insulin sensitivity, whereas other studies used less direct methods, including the insulin tolerance test and the intravenous or oral glucose tolerance test, to assess troglitazone effects on insulin resistance. In all studies, troglitazone in doses ranging from 200 to 600 mg daily enhanced insulin-mediated peripheral glucose utilization in both obese and lean subjects by approximately 30–100%.

Two Japanese studies have documented the insulin-sensitizing effects of pioglitazone in patients with T2DM. In a double-blind, placebo-controlled clinical trial, Kawamori and colleagues[173] evaluated the effect of pioglitazone on insulin resistance in patients with T2DM. Insulin sensitivity (measured as insulin-stimulated glucose disposal [R_d] by the hyperinsulinemic clamp technique) and splanchnic glucose uptake (SGU) both increased significantly after 3 months of pioglitazone treatment. Placebo treatment produced no significant changes in either R_d or splanchnic glucose uptake. The authors concluded that pioglitazone is effective in ameliorating insulin resistance in T2DM by enhancing splanchnic glucose uptake as well as peripheral glucose uptake.[173] In another Japanese study, Yamasaki and colleagues[174] also evaluated the effect of pioglitazone on R_d in 20 patients with T2DM. After oral administration of pioglitazone (30 mg/day) for 3 months, in addition to improvement in glycemic control and fasting insulin, C-peptide, and lipid levels, the R_d significantly improved by >50%. In this study, the change in R_d before and after pioglitazone administration correlated with baseline values of FPG ($\rho = 0.633$), serum insulin ($\rho = 0.653$), and body mass index ($\rho = 0.456$).[174] In a recent study in the United States, Miyazaki and colleagues[174a] demonstrated that pioglitazone therapy for 4 months in obese patients with T2DM significantly improved glycemic parameters and also enhanced hepatic and peripheral (muscle) sensitivity, despite a significant increase in body fat content and body weight of 3.6 ± 1.4 kg (Fig. 32–13).

Effects on Lipids

In T2DM, the major quantitative change in lipid levels is an elevation in triglyceride-rich lipoproteins and a decrease in HDL cholesterol concentrations and LDL cholesterol levels that are often quantitatively similar to that in the general population.[175] However, qualitative changes in the composition of the LDL molecule (including an increase in the proportion of small, dense LDL, which is prone to glycation and oxidation) tend to make it more atherogenic.[175] This diabetic dyslipidemic profile is closely related to underlying insulin resistance and may be partly responsible for the increased cardiovascular morbidity and mortality in T2DM patients.[176] By improving glucose tolerance and reducing insulin resistance, the glitazones have the potential to influence diabetic dyslipidemia favorably. However, from the data presently available,

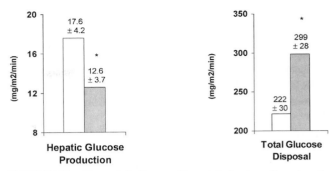

FIGURE 32-13. Effects of pioglitazone 45 mg daily for 4 months on hepatic glucose production and glucose disposal rate in patients with type 2 diabetes. Open bars, baseline; gray bars, after treatment; *, $p < 0.01$. (*Data from Miyazaki* et al.[174a])

there appear to be differences in the lipid-modifying abilities of the various glitazones. Pioglitazone has been shown to lower triglycerides by ~9% and increase HDL levels by ~12–19%.[177,178] Troglitazone also was shown to lower triglyceride levels by ~15–20%[159] and increase HDL cholesterol levels by ~5–8%.[159]

Reduction in triglyceride levels appears to result from several mechanisms, including reduced FFA substrate availability, decreased hepatic triglyceride synthesis, and enhanced peripheral clearance.[159] In the case of rosiglitazone, however, despite a significant decrease in FFA levels by up to 22%, initial studies demonstrated no significant lowering of triglycerides, although HDL levels do increase by up to 19%. The reasons for these differences are not clear at present. In addition, with all the glitazones studied so far, there is an increase in LDL cholesterol levels, which is of concern. In the case of troglitazone, it has been shown that this increase in LDL cholesterol of ~10%[159] occurs without change in atherogenic apolipoprotein B levels.[159] Moreover, following troglitazone treatment, the LDL particles became larger, more buoyant, and less prone to oxidative modification.[179,180] Data on LDL particle size and apolipoprotein B levels are still not available for rosiglitazone and pioglitazone. Long-term follow-up will be needed to see whether the rise in LDL has a negative impact on atherosclerosis and cardiovascular mortality.

In addition to the above data, one report by Japanese investigators[181] found a significant increase in lipoprotein (a) [Lp(a)] levels after 4 weeks of troglitazone treatment at 400 mg daily in a small group of 10 T2DM subjects (despite significant improvements in glucose and insulin sensitivity parameters). No change was found in a control group of sulfonylurea-treated patients. This increase in Lp(a) levels persisted for 12 weeks after discontinuation of troglitazone treatment and then returned to baseline values. Since Lp(a) may be associated with the development of coronary artery disease, further larger, long-term studies are needed to confirm and evaluate the significance of elevated Lp(a) levels in thiazolidinedione-treated diabetic patients.

Effects on Adipose Tissue

At the tissue level, troglitazone has been demonstrated to specifically promote the differentiation of preadipocytes into adipocytes in subcutaneous, but not omental fat.[182] In clinical use, troglitazone at 400 mg/day for 6 months in 30 mildly obese Japanese patients with T2DM not only improved glycemia and increased body mass index but also resulted in fat accumulation in the subcutaneous rather than the visceral adipose tissue depot. The authors speculated that this shift of energy accumulation from the visceral to the subcutaneous adipose tissue might contribute to troglitazone-mediated amelioration of insulin resistance.[183] In another double-blind, randomized trial Kelley and colleagues[184] demonstrated that troglitazone therapy for 12 weeks significantly decreased intra-abdominal fat mass as measured by MRI. In this study, there were no significant changes in total body fat and body weight compared with placebo. In a recent study using MRI analysis, Miyazaki and coworkers[184a] demonstrated that although pioglitazone treatment at 45 mg daily for 4 months was associated with a significant increase in subcutaneous fat area, this was accompanied by a significant decrease in visceral fat area and a concomitant decrease in the ratio of visceral to subcutaneous fat (Fig. 32–14).

Hypertension and Cardiac Function

The prevalence of hypertension in diabetic patients is 1.5–2-fold higher than in nondiabetic individuals,[185] and hypertension is one of the components of the insulin resistance syndrome. In T2DM and other insulin-resistant states, there is impaired insulin-induced vasodilation,[186] and it is possible that by enhancing insulin action, the thiazolidinediones may enhance the tonic vasodilator response to insulin and thereby reduce peripheral vascular resistance and blood pressure. Additionally, by reducing hyperinsulinemia and plasma insulin levels, these agents may reduce the potential blood pressure–raising actions of insulin, such as renal sodium retention and increased sympathetic activity.[185–188] Limited data show that the glitazones may have beneficial effects on blood pressure. Rosiglitazone 4 mg bid over 52 weeks was associated with a significant decrease in systolic BP of 3.5 mmHg and diastolic BP of 2.7 mm Hg.[189] No data are yet available for pioglitazone.

Effects on Atherogenesis

Increased concentrations and activity of PAI-1 are known to be associated with a prothrombotic state. Levels of PAI-1 are increased in patients with T2DM and are strongly correlated with body mass index, insulin resistance, and fasting levels of insulin, triglycerides, and HDLs.[190] Only troglitazone so far has been shown to decrease PAI-1 levels to near-normal levels in diabetic

patients.[190] Pioglitazone has been shown to decrease PAI-1 levels in cultured human umbilical vein endothelial cells.[191] No data are available for rosiglitazone. Platelet aggregation is also increased in diabetic subjects,[192] and only troglitazone so far has been shown to have potent inhibitory effects on human platelet aggregation via suppression of thrombin-induced activation of phosphoinositide signaling in platelets.[193] This effect was not reproducible with pioglitazone and hence may be due to troglitazone's unique structure, which included an α-tocopherol moiety.

Another factor that is correlated with the pathogenesis and progression of atherosclerosis and restenosis is the proliferation and migration of vascular smooth muscle cells from the media to the intima. Troglitazone and pioglitazone both inhibited vascular smooth muscle cell growth and migration in preclinical studies.[156,194–196] Also, improvements in vascular reactivity have been shown for troglitazone in human and animal studies and for pioglitazone in animal studies (in vitro only).[197,198]

Intimal-medial thickness (IMT), a measure of atherosclerotic progression, is correlated with insulin levels in patients with and without T2DM.[199,200] In clinical trials, troglitazone reduced intimal hyperplasia in T2DM patients with and without coronary stent implants.[199,201] Effects were seen in as little as 3 months and were more profound than previously reported data for pravastatin, an HMG-CoA reductase inhibitor[202,203] (Fig. 32–15). Pioglitazone has shown similar results in animal studies.[204] There is evidence to suggest that IMT is negatively related to insulin sensitivity,[205] and it is possible that the reduction in insulin resistance after troglitazone treatment translates to regression of both carotid and coronary IMT. This effect of troglitazone, if confirmed with the other available glitazones and shown to persist in the long term, could be highly beneficial, delaying or preventing development of the accelerated atherosclerosis of diabetes.

Effects on β-Cell Function

An elevated ratio of proinsulin (PI) to immunoreactive insulin (IRI) is often present in T2DM and may reflect dysfunctional β-cell processing of the prohormone and associated reduced β-cell secretory capacity.[206] Troglitazone therapy has been shown to be associated with a decrease in the PI:IRI ratio suggestive of direct effects on the β cell.[206] In a recent study, rosiglitazone therapy for 52 weeks was shown to decrease significantly the PI:IRI ratio.[207] (Fig. 32–16).

FIGURE 32-14. Effects of pioglitazone 45 mg daily for 4 months on abdominal fat distribution in patients with type 2 diabetes. Open bars, baseline; gray bars, after treatment. *, $p < 0.01$; †, $p < 0.05$. (Data from Miyazaki et al.[184a])

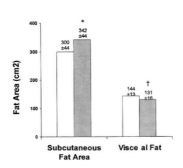

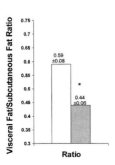

FIGURE 32-15. Effects of troglitazone 400 mg daily on carotid intimal medial thickening (IMT) in patients with type 2 diabetes. (Data from Minamikawa et al.[199])

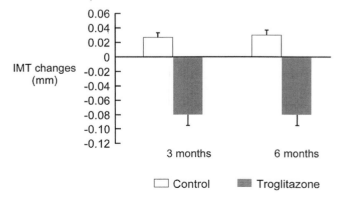

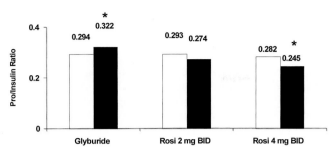

FIGURE 32-16. Effects of rosiglitazone (Rosi) administration for 52 weeks on the proinsulin (Pro):insulin ratio in patients with type 2 diabetes. Open bars, baseline; black bars, after treatment. *, $p < 0.05$ compared with baseline. (*Data from Porter et al.*[207])

Effects on Diabetes Prevention

Consistent with their ability to increase insulin sensitivity and improve insulin secretion, the glitazones have the potential to be used as agents to prevent T2DM. In a recent study, Buchanan and colleagues[207a] observed that troglitazone at 400 mg daily for up to 5 years reduced the incidence of T2DM by 50% in high-risk Hispanic women with a recent history of gestational diabetes mellitus. Indeed, in the NIH-sponsored Diabetes Prevention Study (DPP), troglitazone along with metformin and intensive lifestyle intervention was one of the intervention arms.[65] The troglitazone arm was discontinued after reports of idiosyncratic hepatoxicity associated with its use.

Effects on Cancer Cells

There is preliminary evidence that the thiazolidinediones (through their action on PPARγ) may have adverse effects on cancer cells. Estrogen biosynthesis is catalyzed by aromatase cytochrome P-450, and adipose tissue is the major site of estrogen biosynthesis in postmenopausal women. Rubin and colleagues[208] have demonstrated in tissue culture that the PPARγ ligands troglitazone and rosiglitazone inhibit aromatase expression in cultured breast adipose stromal cells stimulated with oncostatin M or TNF-α plus dexamethasone in a concentration-dependent manner. This action of PPARγ agonism may have potential therapeutic benefit in the treatment and management of breast cancer. Takahashi and colleagues[209] from Japan have also shown that human gastric cancer cells express PPARγ and that activation of PPARγ with troglitazone inhibits cell growth and induces apoptosis in gastric cancer cells. Similar results were obtained by Tsubouchi and colleagues using human lung cancer cells.[210]

On the other hand, there is evidence of tumor-inducing effects of the glitazones in a murine model for familial adenomatous polyposis and sporadic colon cancer. Hence it is recommended that these drugs not be prescribed for people from families with adenomatous polyposis coli.[211] Long-term studies are needed to monitor effects on the development of sporadic colon tumors.

Dosage

The usual starting dose of rosiglitazone is 4 mg po given as either a single dose once daily or in divided doses twice daily. For patients who respond inadequately after 12 weeks of initial treatment with rosiglitazone, the dose may be increased to 8 mg po given as a single dose once daily or in divided doses twice daily. For pioglitazone, therapy may be initiated at 15 or 30 mg po once daily. For patients who respond inadequately to the initial dose, the dose can be increased in increments up to 45 mg po once daily. Patients not responding adequately to monotherapy with either rosiglitazone and pioglitazone should be considered for combination therapy with other antidiabetic agents. The safety and efficacy of both drugs in adolescents and children have not yet been established.

Patients with Hepatic Impairment

If a patient exhibits clinical or laboratory evidence of active liver disease or increased serum transaminase levels (ALT > 2.5 times the upper limit of normal) at start of therapy, rosiglitazone or pioglitazone therapy should not be initiated (see Contraindications below).

Patients with Renal Impairment

There are no clinically relevant differences in the pharmacokinetics of rosiglitazone or pioglitazone in patients with mild-to-severe renal impairment or in hemodialysis-dependent patients compared with patients who have normal renal function. Hence dosage adjustments are not required in patients receiving these agents alone. However, since metformin is contraindicated in patients with renal impairment, concomitant administration of rosiglitazone or pioglitazone with metformin is also contraindicated in patients with renal impairment.

Side Effects

During double-blind clinical trials, the most frequently reported adverse reactions in nearly 2600 patients receiving rosiglitazone monotherapy included back pain, diarrhea, fatigue, headache, hyperglycemia, hypoglycemia, injury, sinusitis, and upper respiratory tract infection. In pioglitazone-treated patients, the most frequently reported adverse reactions during placebo-controlled clinical trials were headache, hyperglycemia, myalgia, pharyngitis, sinusitis, tooth disorder, and upper respiratory tract infection. Overall, the types of adverse experiences reported when rosiglitazone was used in combination with metformin were similar to those during monotherapy with rosiglitazone. Similarly, when pioglitazone was used in combination with metformin, sulfonylureas, or insulin, the types of adverse experiences reported were similar to those during pioglitazone monotherapy (except for an increase in edema in the pioglitazone-insulin combination study). Overall, the incidence of withdrawals from clinical trials due to an adverse event other than hyperglycemia was similar for patients receiving placebo or a glitazone.

The glitazones increase plasma volume by 6–7%, and edema is often associated with their use. In U.S. clinical trials, edema has been reported more frequently in pioglitazone-treated patients than placebo-treated patients. In monotherapy studies, edema was reported at 4.8% in pioglitazone-treated patients vs. 1.2% of placebo-treated patients; in the pioglitazone-insulin combination study, nearly 15.3% of pioglitazone-treated patients developed edema compared with 7.0% of placebo-treated patients. Edema was also reported in 4.8% of patients receiving rosiglitazone compared with 1.3% on placebo, 1% on sulfonylureas, and 2.2% on metformin. Since an increase in plasma volume can worsen or precipitate congestive heart failure (CHF), patients with Class III and IV CHF should not receive glitazone therapy. Also, all patients on glitazone treatment should be regularly monitored for signs and symptoms of CHF.

Weight gain has also been reported more frequently with glitazone therapy. In the 26-week rosiglitazone clinical trials, the mean weight gain in patients treated with rosiglitazone monotherapy was 1.2 kg (on 4 mg daily) and 3.5 kg (on 8 mg daily). When rosiglitazone was administered in combination with metformin, weight gain was 0.7 kg (on 4 mg daily) and 2.3 kg (on 8 mg daily). There was a mean weight loss of about 1 kg in both placebo and metformin-alone groups in these studies. In the 52-week glyburide controlled study, there was a mean weight gain of 1.75 and 2.95 kg for patients treated with 4 and 8 mg of rosiglitazone daily, respectively, versus 1.9 kg in glyburide-treated patients. Similarly, in clinical studies, pioglitazone treatment is accompanied by weight gain in a dose-related manner. The change in average weight in U.S. placebo-controlled monotherapy trials ranged from 0.5 to 2.8 kg for pioglitazone-treated patients, compared with a weight loss of 1.3–1.9 kg in placebo-treated patients. In combination with a sulfonylurea, the change in average weight was 1.9 and 2.9 kg for 15 and 30 mg of pioglitazone, respectively, and −0.8 kg for placebo. The change in average weight in combination with insulin was 2.3 and 3.7 kg for 15 and 30 mg of pioglitazone, respectively, and no weight change for placebo. Even in combination with metformin, the increase in average weight was 1.0 kg for 30 mg of pioglitazone versus −1.4 kg for placebo.

Due to increases in plasma volume and a dilutional effect, decreases in hemoglobin and hematocrit also occur in a dose-related fashion in patients treated with rosiglitazone and pioglitazone alone or in combination. These changes occur primarily during the first 4–12 weeks of therapy and remain relatively constant thereafter. These changes have not been associated with any significant hematologic clinical effects. Reports of anemia (7.1%) were greater in patients treated with a combination of rosiglitazone and metformin; however, lower pretreatment hemoglobin/hematocrit levels in patients taking metformin concurrently may have contributed to the higher reporting rate of anemia in these studies. For pioglitazone, in U.S. double-blind studies, anemia was reported in 0.3–1.6% of pioglitazone-treated patients and 0–1.6% of placebo-treated patients in monotherapy and combination studies. Rosiglitazone-treated patients also experience slight decreases in white blood cell counts, which may be related to the increased plasma volume.

In controlled trials, 0.2% of patients treated with rosiglitazone had reversible elevations in ALT >3 times the upper limit of normal compared with 0.2% on placebo and 0.5% on active comparator agents. Hyperbilirubinemia was reported in 0.3% of patients treated with rosiglitazone compared with 0.9% treated with placebo and 1% in patients treated with other agents. During placebo-controlled clinical trials in the United States, 4 of 1526 (0.26%) pioglitazone-treated patients and 2 of 793 (0.25%) placebo-treated patients had ALT values >3 times the upper limit of normal. After pioglitazone discontinuation, all patients with follow-up lab values had reversible elevations in ALT. In the population of patients treated with pioglitazone, mean values for bilirubin, AST, ALT, alkaline phosphatase, and GGT were decreased at the final visit compared with baseline. Fewer than 0.12% of pioglitazone-treated patients were withdrawn from clinical trials in the United States due to abnormal liver function tests. In preapproval clinical trials, there were no cases of idiosyncratic drug reactions leading to hepatic failure reported for either rosiglitazone or pioglitazone.

The thiazolidinediones do not stimulate insulin secretion and hence when used as monotherapy are not expected to cause hypo-glycemia. However, mild-to-moderate hypoglycemia can occur and has been reported during combination therapy with sulfonylureas or insulin. Hypoglycemia was reported for 1% of placebo-treated patients and 2% of patients receiving pioglitazone in combination with a sulfonylurea. In combination with insulin, hypoglycemia was reported for 5% of placebo-treated patients, 8% of patients treated with pioglitazone 15 mg, and 15% of patients treated with pioglitazone 30 mg.

During required laboratory testing in the pioglitazone clinical trials, sporadic, transient elevations in creatine phosphokinase levels without symptoms were observed. A single, isolated elevation to >10 times the upper limit of normal (values of 2150–8610) was noted in seven patients. Five of these patients continued to receive pioglitazone, and the other two patients had completed study medication at the time of the elevated value. These elevations resolved without any apparent clinical sequelae, and the relationship of these events to pioglitazone therapy is unknown.

Drug Interactions

There are significant differences in drug interactions among the glitazones. Both pioglitazone and troglitazone induce the cytochrome P-450 isoform CYP3A4, which is partly responsible for their metabolism. Thus, safety and efficacy could possibly be affected when pioglitazone is coadministered with other drugs metabolized by this enzyme. In contrast, at clinically relevant concentrations, rosiglitazone has no drug interactions with any drugs metabolized by any of the major cytochrome P-450 enzymes. *In vitro* data demonstrate that rosiglitazone is predominantly metabolized by CYP2C8, and to a lesser extent by 2C9. Drugs metabolized by the cytochrome P-450 isoform CYP3A4 include alfentanil, alprazolam, astemizole, carbamazepine, cisapride, some corticosteroids, cyclosporine, diazepam, diltiazem, donepezil, erythromycin, felodipine, fexofenadine, indinavir, lidocaine, lovastatin, midazolam, nifedipine, quinidine, saquinavir, simvastatin, sirolimus, tacrolimus, terfenadine, triazolam, trimetrexate, and verapamil. Blood glucose should be monitored more carefully in patients receiving pioglitazone in combination with the above drugs and also when administered with inhibitors of CYP3A4 such as ketoconazole or itraconazole. *In vitro*, ketoconazole appears to inhibit the metabolism of pioglitazone significantly. It is recommended that patients receiving both pioglitazone and ketoconazole be evaluated more frequently with respect to glycemic control. Studies with itraconazole, which also inhibits CYP enzymes, have not been performed.

Pioglitazone may also reduce the bioavailability of oral contraceptives containing ethinyl estradiol and norethindrone by induction of CYP3A4, and coadministration of pioglitazone with oral contraceptives may reduce the effectiveness of these agents. Oral contraceptive concentrations were reduced by up to 30% with the coadministration of troglitazone. Higher-dosage oral contraceptive formulations may be needed to increase contraceptive efficacy during pioglitazone use. Alternatively, the use of an alternative or additional method of contraception is recommended. On the other hand, multiple dose studies have shown that rosiglitazone has no clinically relevant effect on the pharmacokinetics of oral contraceptives (ethinyl estradiol and norethindrone).

Repeat dosing with rosiglitazone had no clinically relevant effect on the steady-state pharmacokinetics of either warfarin, nifedipine, digoxin, or ranitidine in healthy volunteers, nor did the administration of these medications alter the pharmacokinetics of rosiglitazone. Also in healthy volunteers, coadministration of pioglitazone with either digoxin, glipizide, metformin, or warfarin for 7 days did not alter the steady-state pharmacokinetics of these medications. Coadministration of acarbose (100 mg three times daily) for 7 days in healthy volunteers had no clinically relevant effect on the pharmacokinetics of a single oral dose of rosiglitazone. A single administration of a moderate amount of alcohol did not increase the risk of acute hypoglycemia in T2DM patients treated with rosiglitazone.

Large doses of aspirin should be used cautiously in patients receiving glitazones. Salicylates inhibit prostaglandin E_2 synthesis, indirectly increase insulin secretion, and in toxic doses may cause hypoglycemia. Also in toxic doses, salicylates may uncouple oxidative phosphorylation, deplete hepatic and muscle glycogen, and cause hyperglycemia and glycosuria acutely. Bexarotene (used in the treatment of cutaneous manifestations of T-cell lymphoma [mycosis fungoides]) may enhance the action of pioglitazone. Patients should be closely monitored while receiving bexarotene in combination with pioglitazone.

Contraindications/Precautions

Troglitazone, the first glitazone marketed in the United States, was associated with idiosyncratic hepatotoxicity and rare cases of liver failure, liver transplants, and death, which led to its recall from clinical use in March 2000. In clinical trials with rosiglitazone and pioglitazone, the incidence of hepatotoxicity and ALT elevations has been similar to that of placebo. In clinical use to date, there have been two reports of hepatotoxicity associated with rosiglitazone use.[212,213] Thus, although the risk of hepatotoxicity is much lower, it is prudent that rosiglitazone and pioglitazone be used cautiously in patients with hepatic disease, since both rosiglitazone and pioglitazone are structurally very similar to troglitazone.

Liver enzymes should be checked prior to the initiation of therapy with rosiglitazone or pioglitazone in all patients. Therapy with glitazones should not be initiated in patients with increased baseline liver enzyme levels (ALT > 2.5 times the upper limit of normal). In patients with normal baseline liver enzymes, following initiation of therapy with rosiglitazone or pioglitazone, it is recommended that liver enzymes be monitored every 2 months for the first 12 months and periodically thereafter. Patients with mildly elevated liver enzymes (ALT levels 1–2.5 times the upper limit of normal) at baseline or during therapy with rosiglitazone or pioglitazone should be evaluated to determine the cause of the liver enzyme elevation. Initiation of, or continuation of, therapy with a glitazone in patients with mild liver enzyme elevations should proceed with caution and should include appropriate close clinical follow-up, including more frequent liver enzyme monitoring, to determine whether the liver enzyme elevations resolve or worsen.

If at any time ALT levels increase to >3 times the upper limit of normal in patients on therapy with rosiglitazone or pioglitazone, liver enzyme levels should be rechecked as soon as possible. If ALT levels remain >3 times the upper limit of normal, glitazone therapy should be discontinued. If any patient develops symptoms suggesting hepatic dysfunction, which may include unexplained nausea, vomiting, abdominal pain, fatigue, anorexia, and/or dark urine, liver enzymes should be checked. The decision of whether to continue the patient on therapy with rosiglitazone or pioglitazone should be guided by clinical judgment pending laboratory evaluations. If jaundice is observed, drug therapy should be discontinued. There are no data available to evaluate the safety of rosiglitazone or pioglitazone in patients who experience liver abnormalities, hepatic dysfunction, or jaundice. Neither one should be used in patients who experienced jaundice while taking troglitazone. For patients with normal hepatic enzymes who were switched from troglitazone to rosiglitazone or pioglitazone, a 1-week washout is recommended before starting therapy with either drug.

Caution should also be exercised when using pioglitazone or rosiglitazone in premenopausal anovulatory females with insulin resistance who may resume ovulation as a result of glitazone therapy. These patients may be at risk of becoming pregnant if adequate contraception is not used. In the case of pioglitazone, those who use oral contraceptive therapy may also be at risk due to CYP3A4 enzyme induction (see above).

Due to increases in plasma volume, both glitazones should be used cautiously in patients with peripheral edema or early congestive heart failure. Rosiglitazone has been associated with preload-induced cardiac hypertrophy in animal studies. In two ongoing echocardiographic clinical studies (a 52-week study using rosiglitazone 4 mg po twice daily and a 26-week study using rosiglitazone 8 mg po once daily) in patients with T2DM, no deleterious alterations in cardiac structure or function have been observed. These studies were designed to detect a change in left ventricular mass of 10% or more. Patients with severe congestive heart failure, defined as New York Heart Association (NYHA) functional Class III and IV, were not studied. As a result, patients with NYHA Class III or IV heart failure should not receive glitazones unless the expected benefit is judged to outweigh the potential risk.[160,178]

Rosiglitazone and pioglitazone are contraindicated in pregnancy. Although animal data suggest no teratogenic effects, there are no adequate and well-controlled studies in pregnant women. Also, it is unknown whether these drugs are secreted in human milk, and hence they should not be administered to breastfeeding women.

Thiazolidinediones are only active in the presence of insulin. They should not be used to treat either diabetic ketoacidosis or T1DM.

NEWER ORAL AGENTS

Several new oral agents including insulin secretagogues and insulin sensitizers are being developed for the treatment of T2DM, and many are in the late phases of clinical studies.[211,214,215] Insulin sensitizers undergoing clinical studies for the treatment of T2DM include several thiazolidinedione and nonthiazolidinedione PPARγ and PPARα agonists. These include G1262570 (a Glaxo compound), which is a novel, nonthiazolidinedione, L-tyrosine-based, highly selective PPARγ agonist. G1262570 is prepared from naturally occurring L-tyrosine and does not contain the 2-4 thiazolidinedione structure common to the other glitazones.[211] (See Chapter 57).

TREATMENT STRATEGIES IN TYPE 2 DIABETES

Insulin resistance is a major abnormality in patients with T2DM, and in addition to hyperglycemia, diabetic patients often manifest hyperlipidemia, hypertension, and a hypercoagulable state. These abnormalities have collectively been referred to as the deadly quartet and comprise the *insulin resistance syndrome* or the *cardiovascular dysmetabolic syndrome*.[102] Hence, in addition to treating hyperglycemia in these patients, we must also strive to ameliorate the other abnormalities of the metabolic syndrome. The goal for glycemic control is an HbA_{1c} of $\leq 7\%$; the goal for lipid control is LDL $\leq$ 100 mg/dL, HDL $\geq$ 45 mg/dL, triglycerides $\leq$ 200 mg/dL (statins are possible first-line agents); the goal for blood pressure control is <130/85 mmHg or 120/75 mmHg (if there is proteinuria; ACE inhibitors are probable first-line agents); and for the hypercoagulable state, all T2DM patients >21 years old should be on aspirin (if not contraindicated).[4]

The first line of therapy for T2DM includes the use of diet management to provide both optimal composition and caloric content so as to assist in achieving desirable body weight. Diet therapy with weight loss is the most effective form of therapy in the obese T2DM patient, but long-term compliance remains poor. Exercise therapy has additional and independent benefits on the metabolic syndrome of diabetes and facilitates the success of diet. When diet, exercise, and weight loss are unable to achieve the glycemic goals outlined above, the usual next step is to proceed to oral antidiabetic medications, alone or in combination. When adequate glycemic control cannot be achieved with oral agents, insulin is then added or substituted as sole therapy.

Monotherapy

The choice of initial oral agents in patients with diabetes is dictated by many factors including patient profile, initial level of hyperglycemia, and economic and formulary considerations (Fig. 32-17 and Table 32-4). A summary of the reported glucose-lowering effects of monotherapy is given in Table 32-5. Since these were not simultaneous trials, the comparative data are only a rough approximation of the relative effectiveness: Stage, severity of hyperglycemia, and type of patient studied varied.

In general, patients with marked hyperglycemia (>300 mg/dL), ketonuria, or ketonemia, pregnant patients, and patients with acute myocardial infarction and all acute situations should all be treated with insulin. In most other patients, a sulfonylurea (in lean patients) or metformin (in obese patients) may be initiated and titrated upward every 1–2 weeks depending on the response. It is extremely important that patients regularly monitor their fingerstick blood glucose. The goal for fasting capillary blood glucose is between 80–120 mg/dL and that of postprandial capillary blood glucose 100–140 mg/dL. In elderly patients and those with irregular meal profiles, a short-acting secretagogue like repaglinide may be preferable to a sulfonylurea, which may cause hypoglycemia with missed meals. In those with predominant postprandial hyperglycemia, acarbose or miglitol may be good choices. Obese patients with renal insufficiency may be started with a glitazone instead of metformin, which is contraindicated in these patients. Some of the other metabolic effects of the oral antidiabetic agents used as monotherapy are shown in (Table 32-6).

Unfortunately, due to the progressive nature of T2DM and the continued decline in β-cell function, monotherapy eventually fails to provide adequate glucose control in most patients with T2DM and combination therapy is frequently a necessity,[5] especially if one is to achieve optimal glycemic control ($HbA_{1c} < 7\%$). In the UKPDS, the progressive deterioration of glucose control was such that after 3 years, only about 50% of subjects attained a goal of $HbA_{1c} < 7\%$ with monotherapy, and after 9 years this declined to <25% (Fig. 32-18). It is important to rule out first the possibility that secondary treatment failure is due to noncompliance; doing so will avoid the need for additional agents.

There is also an emerging concept that it may be advantageous to begin combination therapy earlier in the course of the disease rather than escalate the dose of a single current agent in order to achieve greater glucose-lowering effect. Such a practice is based on the belief that therapy directed at more than one mechanism of action may provide more rapid, sustained, and cost-effective glycemic control. Further studies will be necessary to confirm the clinical utility of this practice.

Combination Therapy

The goal of combination therapy is to take advantage of the differing mechanisms of action of the various pharmacologic agents and create an individualized treatment plan for achieving effective glycemic control. The combination of two agents often results in a synergistic rather than a mere additive glucose-lowering effect. In some cases, lower doses of both agents can be used, which can further minimize side effects. Oral combination therapy is advantageous because it can often delay the need for insulin. Ideally, combination therapy should be instituted prior to manifestation of hyperglycemic symptoms. A comparison of some of the trials is shown in Table 32-7. It must be emphasized that heterogeneity of patients and severity and stage of disease make comparisons only approximate.

Combination of an Insulin Secretagogue and an Insulin Sensitizer

The combination of a secretagogue and an insulin sensitizer is synergistic and addresses two of the major pathophysiologic abnormalities in T2DM. If monotherapy with a sulfonylurea or metformin fails to achieve the desired level of glycemic control, the other second oral agent (if not contraindicated) should be added, with dose escalation over 4–8 weeks to the maximum. Indeed, the use of a sulfonylurea plus metformin is the most widely and extensively studied combination of oral agents and lowers HbA_{1c} by an additional 1.7%.[91] The combination of a sulfonylurea and a glitazone is also useful. The addition of rosiglitazone 4 mg bid to a sulfonylurea resulted in a reduction of FPG by 38 mg/dL and the HbA_{1c} by 0.9% over 6 months.[216] Similarly, pioglitazone 30 mg daily, when added to a sulfonylurea, decreased FPG by 52 mg/dL and HbA_{1c} by 1.2% after 26 weeks.[217]

When a glitazone is used in combination with a sulfonylurea, the current dose of the sulfonylurea should be continued, and the glitazone should be initiated at the lowest dose. If the response is not adequate, the dose can be increased after approximately 2–4 weeks to the maximum. If patients experience hypoglycemia in combination with a sulfonylurea, the sulfonylurea dose may be lowered as necessary to optimize therapy. The addition of the nonsulfonylurea secretagogue repaglinide to metformin has also been shown to confer significantly better glycemic control than monotherapy with either agent. With combination treatment, mean FPG decreased 39 mg/dL and mean HbA_{1c} levels decreased 1.4% from baseline, compared with decreases of 5–9 mg/dL and 0.3–0.4% on therapy with either agent alone.[218] There are no studies evaluating the efficacy of repaglinide in combination with pioglitazone or rosiglitazone.

Combination of Two Insulin Sensitizers

Since both metformin and the glitazones act through different mechanisms, their combination may be expected to be more efficacious. Moreover, since metformin predominantly restrains hepatic glucose production and the glitazones act primarily on insulin resistance in muscle and adipose tissue, their combination also ame-

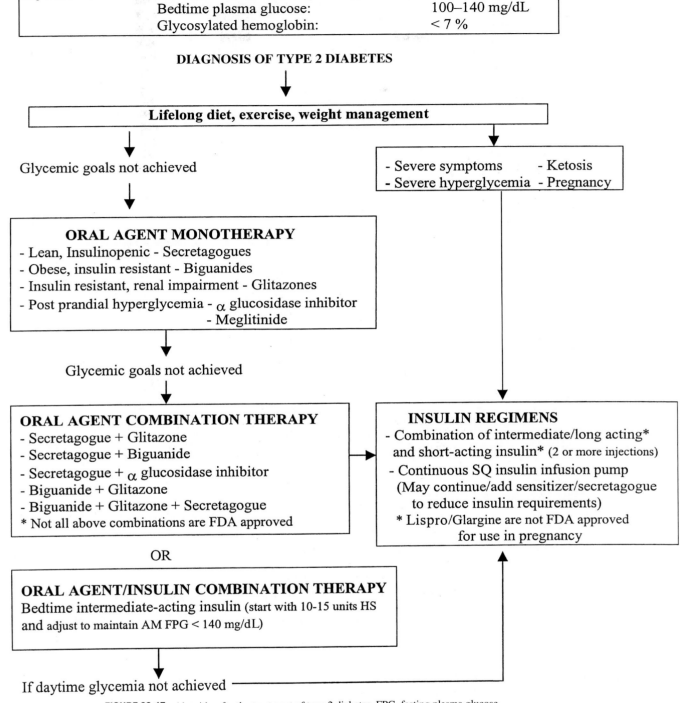

Glycemic Goals:	Fasting and preprandial plasma glucose:	80–120 mg/dL
	Bedtime plasma glucose:	100–140 mg/dL
	Glycosylated hemoglobin:	< 7 %

FIGURE 32-17. Algorithm for the treatment of type 2 diabetes. FPG, fasting plasma glucose.

liorates two major pathophysiologic abnormalities in T2DM. The combination of metformin and rosiglitazone 8 mg daily for 26 weeks reduced FPG by 54 mg/dL and HbA$_{1c}$ by 1.3% compared with placebo.[160] The combination of metformin and pioglitazone 30 mg daily decreased FPG by 38 mg/dL and HbA$_{1c}$ by 0.8% compared with placebo, after 26 weeks.[178]

Other Oral Combinations

The addition of acarbose to sulfonylurea or metformin therapy represents another option for improving glycemic control in patients with T2DM, particularly those with significant postprandial hyperglycemia; it also lowers HbA$_{1c}$ a further 0.5–1%.[219] It should be reiterated that although acarbose monotherapy does not cause

TABLE 32-4. Oral Antidiabetic Agents as Initial Monotherapy

Agent	Major Mechanism(s) of Action	Most Suitable Patient Profile	Glycemic Benefit
Insulin secretagogues			
Sulfonylureas	↑↑ Day-long pancreatic insulin secretion	Lean/insulinopenic	Fasting and postprandial glycemia
Meglitinides	↑↑ Postprandial pancreatic insulin secretion	Lean/insulinopenic	Postprandial glycemia
Biguanide (metformin)	↓↓ Hepatic glucose production ↓ Peripheral glucose utilization	Obese/insulin resistant	Fasting and postprandial glycemia
α-glucosidase inhibitors (acarbose/miglitol)	↓ Postprandial carbohydrate absorption	Lean/insulinopenic or obese/insulin resistant	Postprandial glycemia
Thiazolidinediones/glitazones (rosiglitazone/pioglitazone)	↑↑ Peripheral glucose utilization ↓ Hepatic glucose production	Obese/insulin resistant	Fasting and postprandial glycemia

Source: Data from refs. 9, 10, 14, 80, 91, 117, and 159.

TABLE 32-5. Relative Efficacy of Oral Antidiabetic Agents as Monotherapy (Change from Placebo)*

Agent	Reduction in Fasting Plasma Glucose (mg/dL)	Reduction in HbA$_{1c}$ (%)	Reduction in Postprandial Plasma Glucose (mg/dL)
Insulin secretagogues			
Sulfonylureas (various agents/doses)	54–70	1.5–2.0	92
Repaglinide	61	1.7	104
Metformin (2550 mg/day)	59–78	1.5–2.0	83
Rosiglitazone (8 mg/day)	62–76	1.5	—
Pioglitazone (45 mg/day)	59–80	1.4–2.6	—
Acarbose (300 mg/day)	20–30	0.5–1.0	40–50
Miglitol (300 mg/day)	—	0.5–0.8	40–60

*Since the data were not obtained from simultaneous trials, the comparative data are only a rough approximation of the relative effectiveness; stage, severity of hyperglycemia, and type of patients studied varied in the different studies.

Source: Data from refs. 6–8, 80, 91, 94, 116, 117, 159, 160, and 178.

TABLE 32-6. Metabolic Effects of Oral Antidiabetic Agents as Monotherapy

Parameter	Sulfonylureas/Meglitinides	Acarbose	Metformin	Rosiglitazone/Pioglitazone
Weight	↑	↔	↓ or ↔	↑
LDL cholesterol	↔	↔	↓	↔ or ↑
HDL cholesterol	↔	↔	↑ or ↔	↑↑
Triglycerides	↔	↔	↓	↔ or ↓

Source: Data from refs. 10, 67, 75, 80, 91, 160, 177, and 178.

FIGURE 32-18. Percent of obese subjects achieving a target HbA$_{1c}$ < 7% on diet/monotherapy in the UKPDS. (*Data from UKPDS 49.*[224a])

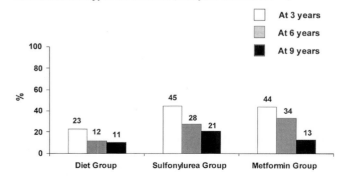

hypoglycemia, combination with sulfonylureas may increase the hypoglycemic potential of the sulfonylurea. This hypoglycemia should be treated with dextrose, and not sucrose, which, as mentioned earlier, may not be effective.

Some physicians may choose to add bedtime insulin to oral agent monotherapy rather than add a second oral agent. However, it has been shown that the addition of metformin to ongoing sulfonylurea therapy in patients experiencing secondary failure achieves reductions in FPG and HbA$_{1c}$ that are not statistically different from those achieved with the addition of insulin to the current therapy or complete switchover to insulin.[220] Thus, use of this combination may delay the need to use insulin.

If combination therapy with two oral agents does not achieve the desired goal, available options include (1) adding a third oral

TABLE 32-7. Relative Efficacy of Oral Agents in Combination

Agents	Reduction in Fasting Plasma Glucose (mg/dL)	Reduction in HbA$_{1c}$ (%)	Reduction in Postprandial Plasma Glucose (mg/dL)
Sulfonylurea + metformin	64	1.7	87
Sulfonylurea + acarbose	—	0.5–1.0	85
Sulfonylurea + rosiglitazone (8 mg)	38	0.9	—
Sulfonylurea + pioglitazone (30 mg)	52	1.2	
Metformin + acarbose	—	0.8	38
Metformin + repaglinide	39	1.4	
Metformin + rosiglitazone (8 mg)	54	1.3	—
Metformin + pioglitazone (30 mg)	38	0.8	—

Source: Data from refs. 77, 91, 117, 160, and 178.

agent; (2) adding bedtime insulin while maintaining therapy with one or both oral agents; or (3) switching the patient to a mixed-split (short-acting plus long-acting insulin given in two to four daily injections) insulin regimen.[221] Although the use of combination therapy may require greater patient adaptability and compliance, most patients would prefer combination therapy to the alternative of exclusive insulin use. Thus, it is important to individualize therapy on the basis of patient preferences.

Triple Oral Combination Therapy

The combination of a sulfonylurea, metformin, and a glitazone, or a sulfonylurea, metformin, and acarbose, is often used in clinical practice. The unique mechanisms of action of these agents can potentially complement each other to improve glycemic control in patients with T2DM. This combination may obviate the need for insulin therapy, but issues of effectiveness, cost, benefit, and compliance have yet to be determined. Future studies will be required to test the efficacy of these various combinations.

Adding Insulin to Oral Therapy

In the not-so-distant past, patients who were not adequately controlled with sulfonylureas were switched over to insulin exclusively. Numerous studies in the late 1980s and in the early part of this decade demonstrated a modest yet significant improvement in glycemic control with combined sylfonylurea-insulin therapy over that seen with insulin alone.[222,223] Continuation of the sulfonylurea in this instance resulted in better glycemic control, primarily owing to the effect of evening insulin in restraining hepatic glucose output during the night and early morning periods (a characteristic feature of T2DM). Once fasting hyperglycemia is controlled, it appears that the daytime sulfonylureas are better able to maintain daytime postprandial glycemia. The use of these two agents simultaneously allows one to start with a low dose of insulin and results in better glycemic control during the transition. Combination sulfonylurea-insulin therapy also reduces the day-to-day variability in fasting glucose levels compared with a single insulin injection.

The addition of intermediate insulin at bedtime to ongoing sulfonylurea therapy has been shown to offer glycemic control comparable to that of various insulin regimens and insulin-sulfonylurea combinations.[224] Moreover, administration of insulin at bedtime resulted in less weight gain and reduced hyperinsulinemia. This regimen, known as bedtime-insulin/daytime-sulfonylurea (BIDS) therapy, may be better than daytime insulin therapy because hepatic glucose overproduction is typically most abnormal during the night.

Patient selection is an important determinant in the success of a BIDS regimen and is more likely to be successful in obese patients who have been diagnosed with diabetes after the age of 35, have had diabetes for less than 10–15 years, and have glucose values consistently <250–300 mg/dL. To implement BIDS therapy, the patient's current sulfonylurea therapy is continued, and intermediate-acting insulin (0.1–0.2 U/kg) is administered at bedtime (usually 9–11 PM). The insulin dose is adjusted until the morning FPG level is <120 mg/dL. The sulfonylurea dose should be reduced if daytime hypoglycemia is a problem. Patients who continue to experience hyperglycemia before supper despite acceptable fasting glucose levels may require a switch to multiple insulin injections and discontinuation of the sulfonylurea. There are few, if any, apparent benefits to maintaining sulfonylureas when patients are on multiple doses of insulin. The above regimen is also suitable for use in those patients who have failed a combination of a sulfonylurea and metformin. Metformin is retained in this regimen since its insulin-sparing effect, along with its favorable effect on the lipid profile, may be beneficial in ameliorating cardiovascular risk.

Adding Oral Agents to Insulin Therapy

If the oral agent–insulin combination therapies described above fail, the patient is typically switched over to insulin exclusively; intermediate-acting insulin (NPH or Lente™) may be administered twice daily (morning and bedtime). However, a combination of intermediate-acting and regular insulin (morning and supper) is more commonly used for optimal control. In some cases, multiple (three or more) injections may be necessary to achieve acceptable glycemic control. Several specific insulin regimens to treat T2DM are available.[221]

Until recently, the only option for patients not adequately controlled with insulin was to increase their insulin dose. However, this practice further increases the likelihood of hyperinsulinemia and weight gain. There has been ongoing research in this area, and it appears that adding oral agents such as acarbose, metformin, or a glitazone to insulin therapy—alone or in combination—is a feasible way of improving or normalizing glycemic control in a significant number of patients[224a] (Fig. 32-19). It may even be possible to discontinue insulin therapy in selected patients and reinitiate combination oral hypoglycemic treatment.

Insulin and Metformin

Metformin may be a useful adjunct in patients poorly controlled with insulin after sulfonylurea agents have achieved

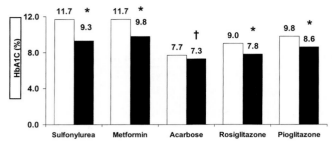

FIGURE 32-19. Improvement in glycemic control (change in HbA_{1c}) with the addition of various oral agents to insulin therapy in patients with type 2 diabetes. *, $p < 0.05$; †, $p < .07$, compared with insulin only. (*Data from Mudaliar* et al.[221])

maximal effect. In these patients, metformin offers an advantage in that it does not stimulate insulin secretion and thereby exacerbate hyperinsulinemia. Metformin also does not contribute to weight gain, which can exacerbate insulin resistance. In a recent study in 96 patients with T2DM poorly controlled with oral sulfonylurea therapy, Yki-Jarvinen and colleagues[225] demonstrated that combination therapy with bedtime insulin plus metformin not only prevents weight gain but also seems superior to other bedtime insulin regimens with sulfonylureas with respect to improvement in glycemic control and frequency of hypoglycemia.

In a patient on a full insulin regimen achieving suboptimal glycemic control, one can attempt to initiate and titrate metformin up to 500 mg three times a day. If the FPG remains <120 mg/dL consistently, the dose of metformin can be further increased gradually to a maximum of 850 mg three times a day (or 1000 mg twice a day). If glycemic control is adequate (FPG remains <120 mg/dL on 2 consecutive days), one can attempt to reduce the dose of insulin by 25% and closely monitor blood glucose values for decompensation. If this occurs or if glycemic control is not adequate on the maximum dose of metformin and lower doses of insulin, there is the option of adding a once-daily sulfonylurea (glipizide extended release or glimepiride) and titrating the dose as required. The addition of a glitazone and acarbose to the above regimen also remains an option to the alternative of exclusive insulin treatment. The issues of cost effectiveness and compliance remain to be determined.

Insulin and Acarbose

The addition of acarbose to insulin therapy may be an option when postprandial hyperglycemia continues to be a problem. Chiasson and colleagues[219] demonstrated a decrease in HbA_{1c} of 0.4% by acarbose in patients poorly controlled on insulin therapy. Acarbose may be initiated in patients on insulin treatment by starting with a low dose of 25 mg with breakfast and titrating up by 25 mg weekly to 50–100 mg three times daily with meals (100 mg tid dose for patients >60 kg in weight), depending on GI tolerance and efficacy.

Insulin and a Glitazone

Glitazones primarily improve insulin sensitivity and thus are well suited for use in insulin-resistant patients with T2DM. In a 26-week, placebo-controlled study,[226] the addition of 4 mg bid of rosiglitazone to insulin therapy in patients poorly controlled on insulin alone (HbA_{1c} ~9%) resulted in a significant reduction of FPG by 44 mg/dL (42 mg/dL on 2 mg bid) and HbA_{1c} by 1.2% (0.6% on

2 mg bid) compared with baseline. In addition, there was a reduction in insulin dose by 9 U on 4 mg bid (5 U on 2 mg bid). The addition of pioglitazone also results in similar reductions.[227] After 16 weeks, the combination of 30 mg of pioglitazone and insulin decreased FPG by 48 mg/dL (35 mg/dL on 15 mg/day) and HbA_{1c} by 1.26% (1% on 15 mg/day). All patients remained on a median of 60.5 U of insulin daily.

When initiating glitazone treatment in T2DM subjects on insulin and suboptimal glucose control, the current insulin dose should be continued, and the lowest dose of a glitazone (4 mg of rosiglitazone or 15 mg of pioglitazone) should be added once daily. If FPG levels remain consistently above 120 mg/dL, the dose of the glitazone should be increased every 2–4 weeks, up to a maximum of 8 mg daily for rosiglitazone and 45 mg daily for pioglitazone until FPG levels are consistently within the target range. At that time, one may attempt to lower the total daily dose of insulin by 10–25%. It must be mentioned here that at the present time, rosiglitazone is not approved by the FDA for use in combination with insulin. Increased weight gain has been observed with this combination.

Reinitiation of Oral Therapy in Insulin-Treated Patients

The recent availability of newer oral antidiabetic agents has allowed the possibility of discontinuing insulin treatment and reinitiating oral agents in selected patients with T2DM. This therapeutic strategy, however, is still under investigation. In a recent pilot study, out of 55 patients with T2DM who were on twice-daily insulin treatment for <10 years and had a random C-peptide level >0.8 ng/mL, 42 patients were successfully able to switch over to a combination of glyburide and metformin and discontinue insulin treatment.[228] This change to a combination of oral agents was accomplished with significantly better glycemic control (a decrease in HbA_{1c} of 1.3%) and decrease in body weight (5 lbs) over 6 weeks. In this study,[228] significant factors predicting a successful switch to oral agents in the responders included a lower body mass index ratio (30 versus 34.8), lesser duration of insulin treatment (5.0 versus 8.6 years), and lesser total daily dose of insulin (0.8 versus 1.2 U/kg body weight).

CONCLUSIONS

Until 1994, the pharmacologic management of T2DM (non-insulin-dependent diabetes mellitus [NIDDM], as it was then called) was quite straightforward. Only two classes of agents were available. Upon initial diagnosis, a sulfonylurea was prescribed, and when patients became too symptomatic or were markedly hyperglycemic, insulin treatment was added or substituted. In the last 6 years, however, two major developments have occurred. First, we now have unequivocal evidence from major long-term studies like the UKPDS that tight control of hyperglycemia in T2DM has significant benefits on the prevention and progression of microvascular and possibly macrovascular disease. Second, to achieve this optimal control, several new classes of oral antidiabetic agents have become available for use as monotherapy: insulin secretagogues (sulfonylureas, repaglinide, nateglinide), biguanides (metformin), α-glucosidase inhibitors (acarbose and miglitol), and thiazolidinediones (rosiglitazone and pioglitazone). However, T2DM is a progressive disease, and over the years tight control of blood glucose often involves combination therapy as a means of optimizing glycemic control. Combinations of oral agents can often delay the need for insulin. Oral agents can also be used in combination with insulin to aid in achieving glycemic goals and reducing hyper-insulinemia.

Which combination of oral agents or insulin is more beneficial is at present not clear, and studies to answer this question are in progress. Several new insulin sensitizer agents are also in development, and the feasibility of inhaled or even buccal insulin may soon become a reality. The ultimate objective, of course, is the prevention of diabetes. The Diabetes Prevention Program is looking into this very question and has randomized more than 3000 subjects into either an intensive lifestyle arm, a placebo arm, or a metformin treatment arm.[65] The finding of a significant preventive effect of lifestyle and metformin have indicated that delay and perhaps prevention is possible.[65a,66] This outcome is exciting indeed for those who take care of patients with T2DM and even more hopeful for those at high risk for the disease.

Acknowledgements. This work was supported by the Department of Veterans Affairs and the VA San Diego Healthcare System, California.

REFERENCES

1. Harris MI, Flegal KM, Cowie CC, *et al*: Prevalence of diabetes, impaired fasting glucose and impaired glucose tolerance in US adults. *Diabetes Care* 1998;21:518.
2. King H, Aubert, Herman W: Global burden of diabetes, 1995–2025: prevalence, numerical estimates, and projections. *Diabetes Care* 1998;21:1414.
3. DeFronzo RA, Bonadonna RC, Ferrannini E: Pathogenesis of NIDDM: a balanced overview. *Diabetologia* 1992;35:389.
4. American Diabetes Association: Clinical practice recomendations. *Diabetes Care* 2002;25(suppl 1):S33.
5. UK Prospective Diabetes Study (UKPDS) Group: Intensive blood-glucose control with sulphonylureas or insulin compared with conventional treatment and risk of complications in patients with type 2 diabetes (UKPDS 33). *Lancet* 1998;352:837.
6. Harrower AD: Comparison of efficacy, secondary failure rate, and complications of sulfonylureas. *J Diabetic Complications* 1994; 8:201.
7. Draeger E. Clinical profile of glimepiride. *Diabetes Res Clin Pract* 1995;28(suppl):S139.
8. Berelowitz M, Fischette C, Cefalu W, *et al*: Comparative efficacy of a once-daily controlled-release formulation of glipizide and immediate-release glipizide in patients with NIDDM. *Diabetes Care* 1994;17:1500.
9. Gerich JE: Oral hypoglycemic agents. *N Engl J Med* 1989; 321:1231.
10. Groop LC: Sulfonylureas in NIDDM. *Diabetes Care* 1992;15:737.
11. Seino S, Inagaki N, Namba N *et al*: Molecular biology of the beta-cell ATP-sensitive K(+) channel. *Diabetes Rev* 1996;4:177.
12. Inagaki N, Gonoi T, Clement JP, *et al*: Reconstitution of IATP: an inward rectifier subunit plus the sulphonylurea receptor. *Science* 1995;270:1166.
13. Panten M, Schwanstecher M, Schwanstecher C: Sulfonylurea receptors and the mechanism of sulfonylurea action. *Exp Clin Endocrinol Diabetes* 1996;104:1.
14. Zimmerman BR: Sulfonylureas. *Endocrinol Metab Clini North Am* 1997;26:511.
15. Simonson DC, Kourides IA, Feinglos M, *et al*: Efficacy, safety, and dose-response characteristics of glipizide gastrointestinal therapeutic system on glycemic control and insulin secretion in NIDDM. *Diabetes Care* 1997;20:597.
16. Carlson RF, Isley WL, Ogrinc FG, *et al*: Efficacy and safety of reformulated, micronized glyburide tablets in patients with non-insulin-dependent diabetes mellitus: A multicenter, double-blind, randomized trial. *Clin Ther* 1993;15:788.
17. Rosenstock J, Samols E, Muchmore DB, *et al*: Glimepiride, a new once-daily sulfonylurea. A double-blind placebo-controlled study of NIDDM patients. Glimepiride Study Group. *Diabetes Care* 1996; 19:1194.
18. Campbell RK: Glimepiride: Role of a new sulfonylurea in the treatment of type 2 diabetes mellitus. *Ann Pharmacother* 1998;32: 1044.
19. Klepzig H, Kober G, Matter C, *et al*: Sulfonylureas and ischaemic preconditioning: A double-blind, placebo-controlled evaluation of glimepiride and glibenclamide. *Eur Heart J* 1999;20:439.
20. Borissova AM, Koev DG, Minev MG, *et al*: Factors for development of secondary failure to sulfonylurea drugs in non-insulin-dependent diabetes mellitus. *Acta Diabetol Latina* 1991;28:91.
21. Stryjek-Kaminska D, Pacula P, Janeczko E *et al*: Analysis of secondary failure to sulfonylureas in type 2 diabetics: A retrospective study for 1976–1987. *Diabetes Res Clin Pract* 1989;7:149.
22. UK Prospective Diabetes Study Group: UK prospective diabetes study 16. Overview of 6 years' therapy of type II diabetes: A progressive disease. *Diabetes* 1995;44:1249.
23. Groop L, Schalin C, Franssila-Kallunki A, *et al*: Characteristics of non-insulin dependent diabetes patients with secondary failure to oral anti-diabetic therapy. *Am J Med* 1989;87:183.
24. Fery F, Desir D, Mockel J: Residual effects of a short-term intensified insulin therapy in type 2 diabetic patients with oral drug failure. *Diabete Metab* 1991;17:525.
25. Groop L, Widen E: Treatment strategies for secondary sulfonylurea failure. Should we start insulin or add metformin? Is there a place for intermittent insulin therapy? *Diabete Metab* 1991;17:218.
26. Robertson RP, Olson LK, Zhang HJ: Differentiating glucose toxicity from glucose desensitization: A new message from the insulin gene. *Diabetes* 1994;43:1085.
27. Farber OK, Beck-Nielsen H, Binder C, *et al*: Acute actions of sulfonylurea drugs during long-term treatment of NIDDM. *Diabetes Care* 1990;13(suppl3):26.
28. Muller G, Satoh Y, Geisen K: Extrapancreatic effects of sulfonylureas—a comparison between glimepiride and conventional sulfonylureas. *Diabetes Res Clin Pract* 1995;28(suppl):S115.
29. Wang PH, Moller D, Flier JS, *et al*: Coordinate regulation of glucose transporter function, number, and gene expression by insulin and sulfonylureas in L6 rat skeletal muscle cells. *J Clin Invest* 1989; 84:62.
30. Davidson MB, Molnar IG, Furman A, *et al*: Glyburide-stimulated glucose transport in cultured muscle cells via protein kinase C-mediated pathway requiring new protein synthesis. *Diabetes* 1991; 40:1531.
31. Muller G, Wied S: The sulfonylurea drug, glimepiride, stimulates glucose transport, glucose transporter translocation, and dephosphorylation in insulin-resistant rat adipocytes in vitro. *Diabetes* 1993; 42:1852.
32. Eckel J: Direct effects of glimepiride on protein expression of cardiac glucose transporters. *Horm Metab Res* 1996;28:508.
33. Prigeon RL, Jacobson RK, Porte D Jr, *et al*: Effect of sulfonylurea withdrawal on proinsulin levels, B cell function, and glucose disposal in subjects with non insulin-dependent diabetes mellitus. *J Clin Endocrinol Metab* 1996;81:3295.
34. Pedersen O, Hother-Nielsen O, Bak J, *et al*: Effects of sulfonylureas on adipocyte and skeletal muscle insulin action in patients with non-insulin-dependent diabetes mellitus. *Am J Med* 1991;90:22S.
35. Shi H, Moustaid-Moussa N, Wilkison WO, *et al*: Role of the sulfonylurea receptor in regulating human adipocyte metabolism. *FASEB J* 1999;13:1833.
36. Engler RL, Yellon DM: Sulfonylurea K-ATP blockade in type 11 diabetes and preconditioning in cardiovascular disease: Time for reconsideration. *Circulation* 1996;94:2297.
37. Klimt CR, Knatterud GL, Meinert CL, *et al*: A study of the effects of hypoglycemic agents on vascular complications in patients with adult-onset diabetes. *Diabetes* 1970;19:747.
38. Kilo C, Miller JP, Williamson JR: The Achilles heel of the University Group Diabetes Program. *JAMA* 1980;243:450.
39. Terzic A, Jahangir A, Kurachi Y: Cardiac ATP-sensitive K(+) channels: Regulation by intracellular nucleotides and potassium opening drugs. *Am J Physiol* 1995;38:C525.
40. Gross G: ATP-sensitive potassium channels and myocardial preconditioning. *Basic Res Cardiol* 1995;90:85.

41. Grover GJ: Protective effects of ATP-sensitive potassium-channel openers in experimental myocardial ischemia. *J Cardiovasc Pharmacol* 1994;24:S18.

42. Cleveland JC, Meldrum DR, Cain BS, *et al*: Oral sulfonylurea hypoglycemic agents prevent ischemic preconditioning in human myocardium: Two paradoxes revisited. *Circulation* 1997;96:29.

43. Garratt KN, Hassinger N, Grill DE, *et al*: Sulfonylurea drug use is associated with increased early mortality during direct coronary angioplasty for acute myocardial infarction among diabetic patients. *J Am Coll Cardiol* 1997;29:493A.

44. Paasikivi J, Wahlberg F: Preventive tolbutamide treatment and arterial disease in mild hyperglycemia. *Diabetologia* 1971;7:323.

45. Sator G, Schersten B, Carlstrom S, *et al*: Ten-year follow-up of subjects with impaired glucose tolerance: Prevention of diabetes by tolbutamide and diet regulation. *Diabetes* 1980;29:41.

46. Smits P, Thien T: Cardiovascular effects of sulphonylurea derivatives: Implications for the treatment of NIDDM? *Diabetologia* 1995;38:116.

47. Brady PA, Al-Suwaidi J, Kopecky SL, *et al*: Sulfonylureas and mortality in diabetic patients after myocardial infarction. *Circulation* 1998;97:709.

48. Klaman A, Sarfert P, Launhardt V, *et al*: Myocardial infarction in diabetic vs non-diabetic subjects. Survival and infarct size following therapy with sulfonylureas (glibenclamide). *Eur Heart J* 2000; 21:220.

49. Wolleben CD, Sanguinetti MC, Siegl PK: Influence of ATP-sensitive potassium channel modulators on ischemia-induced fibrillation in isolated rat hearts. *J Mol Cell Cardiol* 1989;21:783.

50. Billman GE, Avendano CE, Halliwill JR, *et al*: The effects of the ATP-dependent potassium channel antagonist, glyburide, on coronary blood flow and susceptibility to ventricular fibrillation in unanesthesized dogs. *J Cardiovasc Pharmacol* 1993;21:197.

51. Schaffer SW, Warner BA, Wilson GL: Effects of chronic glipizide treatment on the NIDDM heart. *Horm Metab Res* 1993;25:348.

52. Lomuscio A, Vergani D, Marano L, *et al*: Effects of glibenclamide on ventricular fibrillation in non-insulin-dependent diabetics with acute myocardial infarction. *Coron Artery Dis* 1994;5:767.

53. Cole W, McPherson C, Sontag D: ATP-regulated K+ channels protect the myocardium against ischemic/reperfusion damage. *Circ Res* 1991;69:571.

54. Shimabukuro M, Nagamine F, Murakami K, *et al*: Chronic gliclazide treatment affects basal and post-ischemic cardiac function in diabetic rats. *Gen Pharmacol* 1993;25:697.

55. Bijlstra PJ, Russel FGM, Thien T, *et al*: Effects of tolbutamide on vascular ATP-sensitive potassium channels in humans. *Horm Metab Res* 1996;28:512.

56. Bijlstra PJ, Lutterman JA, Russel FG, *et al*: Interaction of sulphonylurea derivatives with vascular K_{ATP} channels in man. *Diabetologia* 1996;39:1083.

57. Davis TME, Parsons RW, Broadhurst R, *et al*: Arrhythmias and mortality after myocardial infarction in diabetic patients: Relationship to diabetes treatment. *Diabetologia* 1996;39(suppl 1):A51.

58. Findlay I: Sulphonylurea drugs no longer inhibit ATP-sensitive K+ channels during metabolic stress in cardiac muscle. *J Pharmacol Exp Ther* 1993;266:456.

59. Brady PA, Zhang S, Lopez JR, *et al*: Dual effect of glyburide, an antagonist of K_{ATP} channels, on metabolic inhibition-induced Ca^{2+} loading in cardiomyocytes. *Eur J Pharmacol* 1996;308:343.

60. Leibowitz G, Cerasi E: Sulphonylurea treatment of NIDDM patients with cardiovascular disease: A mixed blessing? *Diabetologia* 1996;39:503.

61. Panahloo A, Mohamed-Ali V, Andres C, *et al*: Effect of insulin versus sulfonylurea therapy on cardiovascular risk factors and fibrinolysis in type II diabetes. *Metab Clin Exp* 1998;47:637.

62. Keen H, Jarrett RJ, McCartney P: The ten-year follow-up of the Bedford survey (1962–1972): Glucose tolerance and diabetes. *Diabetologia* 1982;22:73.

63. Sartor G, Schersten B, Carlstrom S, *et al*: Ten-year follow-up of subjects with impaired glucose tolerance: Prevention of diabetes by tolbutamide and diet regulation. *Diabetes* 1980;29:41.

64. Karunakaran S, Hammersley MS, Morris RJ, *et al*: The Fasting Hyperglycaemia Study III. Randomized controlled trial of sulfonylurea therapy in subjects with increased but not diabetic fasting plasma glucose. *Metab Clin Exp* 1997;46(12 suppl 1):56.

65. The Diabetes Prevention Program: Design and methods for a clinical trial in the prevention of type 2 diabetes. *Diabetes Care* 1999; 22:623.

65a. Knowles WC, Barrett-Connor E, Fowler SE, *et al*. Reduction in the incidence of type 2 diabetes with lifestyle intervention or metformin. *N Engl J Med* 2002;346:393.

66. Peters AL, Davidson MB: Maximal dose glyburide therapy in markedly symptomatic patients with type 2 diabetes. A new use for an old friend. *J Clin Endocrinol Metab* 1996;81:2423.

67. American Diabetes Association: The pharmacological treatment of hyperglycemia in NIDDM (consensus statement). *Diabetes Care* 1996;19(suppl 1):S54.

68. Langer O, Conway D, Berkus MD, *et al*: A comparison of glyburide and insulin in women with gestational diabetes mellitus. *N Engl J Med* 2000;343:1134.

69. Krepinsky J, Ingram AJ, Clase CM: Prolonged sulfonylurea-induced hypoglycemia in diabetic patients with end-stage renal disease. *Am J Kidney Dis* 2000;35:500.

70. Wells PS, Holbrook AM, Crowther NR, *et al*: Interaction of warfarin with drugs and food. *Ann Intern Med* 1994;121:676.

71. Hollander PA, Elbein SC, Hirsch IB, *et al*: Role of orlistat in the treatment of obese patients with type 2 diabetes. A 1-year randomized double-blind study. *Diabetes Care* 1998;21:1288.

72. Malaisse WJ: Mechanism of action of a new class of insulin secretagogues. *Exp Clin Endocrinol Diabetes* 1999;107(suppl 4):S140.

73. Fuhlendorff J, Rorsman P, Kofod H, *et al*: Stimulation of insulin-release by repaglinide and glibenclamide involves both common and distinct processes. *Diabetes* 1998;47:345.

74. Jovanovic L, Dailey G, Huang WC, *et al*: Repaglinide in type 2 diabetes: A 24-week, fixed-dose efficacy and safety study. *J Clin Pharmacol* 2000;40:49.

75. Marbury T, Huang WC, Strange P, *et al*: Repaglinide versus glyburide: A one-year comparison trial. *Diabetes Res Clin Pract* 1999; 43:155.

76. Moses R: Repaglinide in combination therapy with metformin in Type 2 diabetes. *Diabetes* 1999;107(suppl 4):S136.

77. Moses R, Slobodniuk R, Boyages S, *et al*: Effect of repaglinide addition to metformin monotherapy on glycemic control in patients with type 2 diabetes. *Diabetes Care* 1999;22:119.

78. Damsbo P, Clauson P, Marbury TC, *et al*: A double-blind randomized comparison of meal-related glycemic control by repaglinide and glyburide in well-controlled type 2 diabetic patients. *Diabetes Care* 1999;22:789.

79. Marbury TC, Ruckle JL, Hatorp V, *et al*: Pharmacokinetics of repaglinide in subjects with renal impairment. *Clin Pharmacol Ther* 2000;67:7.

79a. Horton ES, Clinkinbeard C, Gatlin M, *et al*: Nateglinide alone and in combination with metformin improves glycemic control by reducing mealtime glucose levels in 2 diabetes. *Diabetes Care* 2000;23:1660.

79b. Hu S, Wang S, Dunning BE: Tissue selectivity of antidiabetic agent nateglinide: Study on cardiovascular and beta-cell K(ATP) channels. *J Pharmacol Exp Ther* 1999;291:1372.

80. Bailey CJ, Turner RC: Metformin. *N Engl J Med* 1996;334:574.

81. Stumvoll M, Nurjahan N, Perriello G, *et al*. Metabolic effects of metformin in non-insulin-dependent diabetes mellitus. *N Engl J Med* 1995;333:550.

82. Lalau JD, Lacroix C, Compagnon P, *et al*: Role of metformin accumulation in metformin-associated lactic acidosis. *Diabetes Care* 1995;18:779.

83. Stefanovic V, Antic S, Mitic-Zlatkovic M, *et al*: Reversal of increased lymphocyte PC-1 activity in patients with type 2 diabetes treated with metformin. *Diabetes Metab Res Rev* 1999;15:400.

84. Nagi DK, Yudkin JS: Effects of metformin on insulin resistance, risk factors for cardiovascular disease, and plasminogen activator inhibitor in NIDDM subjects. *Diabetes Care* 1993;16:621.

85. Hermann LS, Schersten B, Bitzén P-O, *et al*: Therapeutic comparison of metformin and sulfonylurea, alone and in various combinations. *Diabetes Care* 1994;17:1100.

86. DeFronzo RA, Goodman AM, Multicenter Metformin Study Group: Efficacy of metformin in patients with non-insulin-dependent diabetes mellitus. *N Engl J Med* 1995;333:541.

87. Garber AJ, Duncan TG, Goodman AM, *et al*: Efficacy of metformin in type II diabetes: Results of a double-blind, placebo-controlled, dose-response trial. *Am J Med* 1997;103:491.

88. Campbell IW, Menzies DG, Chalmers J, et al: One year comparative trial of metformin and glipizide in type 2 diabetes mellitus. Diabetes Metab 1994;21:394.

89. UK Prospective Diabetes Study (UKPDS) Group: Effect of intensive blood-glucose control with metformin on complications in overweight patients with type 2 diabetes (UKPDS 34). Lancet 1998; 352:854.

90. Inzucchi SE, Maggs DG, Spollett GR, et al: Efficacy and metabolic effects of metformin and troglitazone in type II diabetes mellitus. N Engl J Med 1998;338:867.

91. Cusi K, De Fronzo RA: Metformin: A review of its metabolic effects. Diabetes Rev 1998;6:89.

92. Patane G, Piro S, Agata M, et al: Metformin restores insulin secretion altered by chronic exposure to free fatty acids or high glucose: A direct metformin effect on pancreatic beta-cells. Diabetes 2000; 49:735.

93. Nagi DK, Ali VM, Yudkin JS: Effect of metformin on intact proinsulin and des 31,32 proinsulin concentrations in subjects with non-insulin-dependent (type 2) diabetes mellitus. Diabet Med 1996; 13:753.

94. Campbell IW, Howlett HC: Worldwide experience of metformin as an effective glucose-lowering agent: A meta-analysis. Diabetes Metab Rev 1995;11(suppl 1):S57.

95. Lee A, Morley JE: Metformin decreases food consumption and induces weight loss in subjects with obesity and type II non-insulin dependent diabetes mellitus. Obes Res 1998;6:47.

96. Fontbonne A, Charles MA, Juhan-Vague I, et al: The BIGPRO Study Group: The effect of metformin on the metabolic abnormalities associated with upper-body fat distribution. Diabetes Care 1996;19:920.

97. Paolisso G, Amato L, Eccellente R, et al: Effect of metformin on food intake in obese subjects. Eur J Clin Invest 1998;28:441.

98. Morin-Papunen LC, Koivunen RM, Tomas C, et al: Decreased serum leptin concentrations during metformin therapy in obese women with polycystic ovary syndrome. J Clin Endocrinol Metabol 1998;83:2566.

99. Glueck CJ, Wang P, Fontaine R, et al: Metformin-induced resumption of normal menses in 39 of 43 (91%) previously amenorrheic women with the polycystic ovary syndrome. Metab Clin Exp 1999; 48:511.

100. Jeppesen J, Zhou MY, Chen YD, et al: Effect of metformin on postprandial lipemia in patients with fairly to poorly controlled NIDDM. Diabetes Care 1994;17:1093.

101. Reaven GM, Johnston P, Hollenbeck CB, et al.: Combined metformin-sulfonylurea treatment of patients with noninsulin-dependent diabetes in fair to poor glycemic control. J Clin Endocrinol Metab 1992;74:1020.

102. Fagan TC, Deedwania PC: The cardiovascular dysmetabolic syndrome. Am J Med 1998;105:77S.

103. Palumbo PJ: Metformin: Effects on cardiovascular risk factors in patients with non-insulin-dependent diabetes mellitus. J Diabetes Complications 1998;12:110.

104. Charles MA, Eschwege E, Grandmottet P, et al: Treatment with metformin of non-diabetic men with hypertension, hypertriglyceridaemia and central fat distribution: The BIGPRO 1.2 trial. Diabetes Metab Res Rev 2000;16:2.

105. Charles MA, Morange P, Eschwege E, et al: Effect of weight change and metformin on fibrinolysis and the von Willebrand factor in obese nondiabetic subjects: The BIGPRO1 Study. Biguanides and the Prevention of the Risk of Obesity. Diabetes Care 1998;21:1967.

106. Gregorio F, Ambrosi F, Manfrini S, et al: Poorly controlled, elderly Type 2 diabetic patients: The effects of increasing sulphonylurea dosages or adding metformin. Diabet Med 1999;16:1016.

107. UK Prospective Diabetes Study (UKPDS) Group: Effect of intensive blood-glucose control with metformin on complications in overweight patients with type 2 diabetes (UKPDS 34). Lancet 1998; 352:854.

107a. Turner RC, Holman R, Stratton I: Correspondence. The UK Prospective Diabetes Study. Lancet 1999;352:1934.

108. Franks S: Polycystic ovary syndrome. N Engl J Med 1995;333:853.

109. Ehrmann D, Cavaghan M, Imperial J, et al: Effects of metformin on insulin secretion, insulin action and ovarian steroidogenesis in women with PCOS. J Clin Endocrinol Metab 1997;82:524.

110. Unluhizarci K, Kelestimur F, Bayram F, et al: The effects of metformin on insulin resistance and ovarian steroidogenesis in women with polycystic ovary syndrome. Clin Endocrinol 1999;51:231.

111. WHO Expert Committee on Diabetes Mellitus. Second Report. WHO Technical Report Series No. 646. WHO:1980.

112. Widen EIM, Eriksson JG, Groop LC: Metformin normalized nonoxidative metabolism in insulin-resistant normoglycemic relatives of patients with NIDDM. Diabetes 1992;41:354.

113. Guerguian J, Green L, Misbin RI, et al: Efficacy of metformin in non-insulin-dependent diabetes mellitus [letter]. N Engl J Med 1996;334:269.

114. Coetzee EJ, Jackson WP. Oral hypoglycaemics in the first trimester and fetal outcome. South Afr Med J 1984;65:635.

115. Pregnancy in established non-insulin-dependent diabetics. A five-and-a-half year study at Groote Schuur Hospital. South Afr Med J 1980;58:795.

116. Campbell LK, White JR, Campbell RK: Acarbose: Its role in the treatment of diabetes mellitus. Ann Pharmacother 1996;30:1255.

117. Lebovitz HE: Alpha-glucosidase inhibitors as agents in the treatment of diabetes. Diabetes Rev 1998;6:132.

118. Segal P, Feig PU, Schernthaner G, et al: The efficacy and safety of miglitol therapy compared with glibenclamide in patients with NIDDM inadequately controlled by diet alone. Diabetes Care 1997; 20:687.

119. Johnston PS, Lebovitz HE, Coniff RF, et al: Advantages of alpha glucosidase inhibition as monotherapy in elderly type 2 diabetics. J Clin Endocrinol Metab 1998;83:1515.

120. Coniff RF, Shapiro JA, Seaton TB: Long term efficacy and safety of acarbose in the treatment of obese subjects with non-insulin-dependent diabetes mellitus. Arch Intern Med 1994;154:2502.

121. Coniff RF, Shapiro JA, Robbins D, et al: Reduction of glycosylated hemoglobin and postprandial hyperglycemia by acarbose in patients with NIDDM. Diabetes Care 1995;18:817.

122. Hanefeld M, Fischer S, Schulze J, et al: Therapeutic potentials of acarbose as first-line drug in NIDDM insufficiently treated with diet alone. Diabetes Care 1991;14:732.

123. Holman RR, Cull CA, Turner RC: A randomized double-blind trial of acarbose in type 2 diabetes shows improved glycemic control over 3 years. Diabetes Care 1999;22:960.

124. Kelly DE, Bidot P, Freedman Z, et al: Efficacy and safety of acarbose in insulin-treated patients with type 2 diabetes. Diabetes Care 1998;21:2056.

125. Rosenstock J, Brown A, Fischer J, et al: Efficacy and safety of acarbose in metformin-treated patients with type 2 diabetes. Diabetes Care 1998;21:2050.

126. Hollander P: Safety profile of acarbose, an alpha-glucosidase inhibitor. Drugs 1992;44(suppl):47.

127. Riccardi G, Giacco R, Parillo M, et al: Efficacy and safety of acarbose in the treatment of Type 1 diabetes mellitus: A placebo-controlled, double-blind, multicentre study. Diabet Med 1999; 16:228.

128. Koch HH, Wudy A, Eberlein G, et al: Use of acarbose for eliminating the interval between meal consumption and insulin injection in patients with Type 1 diabetes. Diabetes Nutr Metab 1999;12: 195.

129. Russell JC, Graham SE, Dolphin PJ: Glucose tolerance and insulin resistance in the JCR:LA-corpulent rat: Effect of miglitol (Bay m1099). Metabolism 1999;48:701.

130. Johnson AB, Taylor R: Does suppression of postprandial blood glucose excursions by the alpha-glucosidase inhibitor miglitol improve insulin sensitivity in diet-treated type II diabetic patients? Diabetes Care 1996;19:559.

130a. Meneilly G, Ryan EA, Radziuk J, et al: Effect of acarbose on insulin sensitivity in elderly patients with diabetes. Diabetes Care 2000; 23:1162.

131. Ozgen AG, Hamulu F, Bayraktar F, et al: Long-term treatment with acarbose for the treatment of reactive hypoglycemia. Eat Weight Disord 1998;3:136.

132. Hasegawa T, Yoneda M, Nakamura K, et al: Long-term effect of alpha-glucosidase inhibitor on late dumping syndrome. J Gastroenterol Hepatol 1998;13:1201.

133. Minatoguchi S, Arai M, Uno Y, et al: A novel anti-diabetic drug, miglitol, markedly reduces myocardial infarct size in rabbits. Br J Pharmacol 1999;128:1667.

134. Kado S, Murakami T, Aoki A, *et al*: Effect of acarbose on postprandial lipid metabolism in type 2 diabetes mellitus. *Diabetes Res Clin Pract* 1998;41:49.

135. Malaguarnera M, Giugno I, Ruello P, *et al*: Acarbose is an effective adjunct to dietary therapy of hypertriglyceridemias. *Br J Clin Pharmacol* 1999;48:605.

136. Chiasson JL, Gomis R, Hanefeld M, *et al*: The STOP-NIDDM Trial: An international study on the efficacy of an alpha-glucosidase inhibitor to prevent type 2 diabetes in a population with impaired glucose tolerance: Rationale, design, and preliminary screening data. Study to Prevent Non-Insulin-Dependent Diabetes Mellitus. *Diabetes Care* 1998;21:1720.

137. Gentile S, Turco S, Guarino G, *et al*: Non-insulin-dependent diabetes mellitus associated with nonalcoholic liver cirrhosis: An evaluation of treatment with the intestinal alpha-glucosidase inhibitor acarbose. *Ann Ital Med Int* 1999;14:7.

138. Kihara Y, Ogami Y, Tabaru A, *et al*: Safe and effective treatment of diabetes mellitus associated with chronic liver diseases with an alpha-glucosidase inhibitor, acarbose. *J Gastroenterol* 1997;32:777.

139. Yoo WH, Park TS, Baek HS: Marked weight loss in a type 2 diabetic patient treated with acarbose. *Diabetes Care* 1999;22:645.

140. Kono T, Hayami M, Kobayashi H, *et al*: Acarbose-induced generalized erythema multiforme. *Lancet* 1999;354:396.

141. Ben-Ami H, Krivoy N, Nagachandran P, *et al*: An interaction between digoxin and acarbose. *Diabetes Care* 1999;22:860.

142. Wang PY, Kaneko T, Wang Y, *et al*: Acarbose alone or in combination with ethanol potentiates the hepatotoxicity of carbon tetrachloride and acetaminophen in rats. *Hepatology* 1999;29:161.

143. Saltiel AR, Olefsky JM: Thiazolidinediones in the treatment of insulin resistance in type 2 diabetes. *Diabetes* 1996;45:1661.

144. Lemberger T, Desvergne B, Wahli W: Peroxisome proliferator-active receptors: A nuclear receptor signaling pathway in lipid physiology. *Annu Rev Cell Dev Biol* 1996;12:335.

145. Willson TM, Cobb JE, Cowan DJ, *et al*: The structure-activity relationship between peroxisome-proliferator-activated receptor agonism and the antihyperglycemic activity of thiazolidinediones. *J Med Chem* 1996;39:665.

146. Bahr M, Spelleken M, Bock M, *et al*: Acute and chronic effects of troglitazone (CS-045) on isolated rat ventricular cardiomyocytes. *Diabetologia* 1996;39:766.

147. De Vos P, Lefebvre AM, Miller SG, *et al*: Thiazolidinediones repress ob gene expression in rodents via activation of peroxisome proliferator activated receptor *J Clin Invest* 1996;98:1004.

148. Szalkowski D, White-Carrington S, Berger J, *et al*: Antidiabetic thiazolidinediones block the inhibitory effect of tumor necrosis factor alpha on differentiation, insulin stimulated glucose uptake, and gene expression in 3T3-L1 cells. *Endocrinology* 1995;136:1474.

149. Okuno A, Tamemoto H, Tobe K, *et al*: Troglitazone increases the number of small adipocytes without the change of white adipose tissue mass in obese Zucker rats. *J Clin Invest* 1998;101:1354.

150. Olefsky JM: The effects of spontaneous obesity on insulin binding, glucose transport and glucose oxidation of isolated rat adipocytes. *J Clin Invest* 1976;57:842.

151. Burant CF, Sreenan S, Hirano K, *et al*: Troglitazone action is independent of adipose tissue. *J Clin Invest* 1998;100:2900.

152. Rieusset J, Auwerx J, Vidal H: Regulation of gene expression by activation of the peroxisome proliferator-activated receptor gamma with rosiglitazone (BRL 49653) in human adipocytes. *Biochem Biophys Res Commun* 1999;265:265.

153. Solomon SS, Mishra SK, Cwik C, *et al*: Pioglitazone and metformin reverse insulin resistance induced by tumor necrosis factor-alpha in liver cells. *Horm Metab Res* 1997;29:379.

154. Park KS, Ciaraldi TP, Lindgren K, *et al*: Troglitazone effects on gene expression in human skeletal muscle of type 2 diabetic subjects involve upregulation of PPAR gamma. *J Clin Endocrinol Metab* 1998;83:2830.

155. Park KS, Ciaraldi TP, Carter LA, *et al*: Troglitazone regulation of glucose metabolism in human skeletal muscle cultures from obese type 2 diabetic subjects. *J Clin Endocrinol Metab* 1998;83:1636.

156. Law RE, Goetze S, Xi XP, *et al*: Expression and function of PPARgamma in rat and human vascular smooth muscle cells. *Circulation* 2000;101:1311.

157. Asano M, Nakajima T, Iwasawa K, *et al*: Troglitazone and pioglitazone attenuate agonist-dependent Ca^{2+} mobilization and cell proliferation in vascular smooth muscle cells. *Br J Pharmacol* 1999;128:673.

158. Benson S, Wu J, Padmanabhan S, *et al*: Peroxisome proliferator-activated receptor (PPAR)-gamma expression in human vascular smooth muscle cells: Inhibition of growth, migration, and c-fos expression by the peroxisome proliferator-activated receptor (PPAR)-gamma activator troglitazone. *Am J Hypertens* 2000;13:74.

159. Saleh YM, Mudaliar SR, Henry RR: Metabolic and vascular effects of the thiazolidinedione, troglitazone. *Diabetes Rev* 2000;7:55.

160. Avandia (prescribing information). Smith Kline Beecham Pharmaceuticals, April 2000.

161. Fonseca V, Rosenstock J, Patwardhan R, *et al*: Effect of metformin and rosiglitazone combination therapy in patients with type 2 diabetes mellitus: A randomized controlled trial. *JAMA* 2000;283:1695.

162. Wolffenbuttel BH, Gomis R Squatrito S, *et al*: Addition of low-dose rosiglitazone to sulphonylurea therapy improves glycemic control in Type 2 diabetic patients. *Diabet Med* 2000;17:40.

163. Aronoff S, Rosenblatt S, Braithwaite S, *et al*: The Pioglitazone 001 Study Group. Pioglitazone hydrochloride monotherapy improves glycemic control in the treatment of patients with type 2 diabetes: A 6-month randomized placebo-controlled dose-response study. *Diabetes Care* 2000;23:1605.

164. Schneider R, Egan J, Houser V, *et al*: Combination therapy with pioglitazone and sulfonylurea in patients with type 2 diabetes. *Diabetes* 1999;47(suppl 1):A106.

165. Egan J, Rubin C, Mathiesen, A, *et al*: Combination therapy with pioglitazone and metformin in patients with type 2 diabetes. *Diabetes* 1999;47(suppl 1):A117.

166. Rubin C, Egan J, Schneider R, *et al*: Combination therapy with pioglitazone and insulin in patients with type 2 diabetes. *Diabetes* 1999;47(suppl 1):A110.

167. Suter SL, Nolan JJ, Wallace P, *et al*: Metabolic effects of new oral hypoglycemic agent CS-045 in NIDDM subjects. *Diabetes Care* 1992;15:193.

168. Nolan JJ, Ludvik B, Beerdsen P, *et al*: Improvement in glucose tolerance and insulin resistance in obese subjects treated with troglitazone. *N Engl J Med* 1994;331:1188.

169. Berkowitz K, Peters R, Kjos SL, *et al*: Effect of troglitazone on insulin sensitivity and pancreatic beta-cell function in women at high risk for NIDDM. *Diabetes* 1996;45:1572.

170. Dunaif A, Scott D, Finegood D, *et al*: The insulin-sensitizing agent troglitazone improves metabolic and reproductive abnormalities in the polycystic ovary syndrome. *J Clin Endocrinol Metab* 1996;81:3299.

171. Yano M, Okuno S, Uotani S, *et al*: The effect of a new oral antihyperglycemic drug (CS-045) on insulin resistance in Werner's syndrome. *Int Congr Series Excerpta Med* 1992;997:357.

172. Takino H, Oghuni S, Uotani S, *et al*: Increased insulin responsiveness after C-045 treatment in diabetes associated with Werner's syndrome. *Diabetes Res Clin Pract* 1994;24(3)167.

173. Kawamori R, Matsuhisa M, Kinoshita J, *et al*: Pioglitazone enhances splanchnic glucose uptake as well as peripheral glucose uptake in non-insulin-dependent diabetes mellitus. AD-4833 Clamp-OGL Study Group. *Diabetes Res Clin Pract* 1998;41:35.

174. Yamasaki Y, Kawamori R, Wasada T, *et al*: Pioglitazone (AD-4833) ameliorates insulin resistance in patients with NIDDM. AD-4833 Glucose Clamp Study Group, Japan. *Tohoku J Exp Med* 1997;183:173.

174a. Miyazaki Y, Mahankali A, Matsuda M, *et al*: Effect of pioglitazone on glucose metabolism in sulfonylurea-treated patients with type 2 diabetes. *Diabetes* 2000;48(suppl 1):A 117:476P.

175. Garg A: Dyslipoproteinemia and diabetes. *Endocr Metab Clin North Am* 1998;27:613.

176. Haffner SM, Miettinen H: Insulin resistance implications for type II diabetes and coronary artery disease. *Am J Med* 1997;103:152.

177. Shaffer S, Rubin CJ, Zhu E. Study Group—Pioglitazone 001. The effects of pioglitazone on the lipid profile in patients with type 2 diabetes. *Diabetes* 2000;48(suppl 1):508P.

178. Actos (prescribing information). Elli Lilly, July 1999.

179. Tack CJJ, Smits P, Demacker PNM: Troglitazone decreases the proportion of small dense LDL and increases the resistance of LDL to oxidation in obese subjects. *Diabetes Care* 1998;21:796.

180. Hirano T, Yoshino G, Kazumi T: Troglitazone and small low-density lipoprotein in type 2 diabetes. *Ann Intern Med* 1998;129:162.

181. Matsumoto K, Miyake S, Yano M, *et al*: Increase of lipoprotein (a) with troglitazone. *Lancet* 1997;350:1748.

182. Adams M, Montague CT, Prins JB, *et al*: Activators of peroxisome proliferator-activated receptor-gamma have depot-specific effects on human preadipocyte differentiation. *J Clin Invest* 1997; 100:3149.

183. Mori Y, Murakawa Y, Okada K, *et al*: Effect of troglitazone on body fat distribution in type 2 diabetic patients. *Diabetes Care* 1999; 22:908.

184. Kelly IE, Han TS, Walsh K, *et al*: Effects of a thiazolidinedione compound on body fat and fat distribution of patients with type 2 diabetes [published erratum appears in *Diabetes Care* 1999;22:536]. *Diabetes Care* 1999;22:288.

184a. Miyazaki Y, Mahankali A, Matsuda M, *et al*: Effect of pioglitazone on abdominal fat distribution and insulin sensitivity in patients with type 2 diabetes mellitus. *Diabetes* 2000;48(suppl 1):A299.

185. Simonson DC: Etiology and prevalence of hypertension in diabetic patients. *Am J Hypertens* 1995;8:316.

186. Baron AD: Hemodynamic actions of insulin. *Am J Physiol* 1994; 267:E187.

187. Laakso M, Edelman SV, Brechtel G, *et al*: Impaired insulin-mediated skeletal muscle blood flow in patients with NIDDM. *Diabetes* 1992;41:1076.

188. Anderson EA, Balon TW, Hoffman RP, *et al*: Insulin increases sympathetic activity but not blood pressure in borderline hypertensive humans. *Hypertension* 1992;19:621.

189. Bakris GL, Dole JF, Porter LE, *et al*: Rosiglitazone improves blood pressure in patients with type 2 diabetes. *Diabetes* 2000;48(suppl 1)388P.

190. Fonseca VA, Reynolds T, Hemphill D, *et al*: Effect of troglitazone on fibrinolysis and activated coagulation in patients with non-insulin-dependent diabetes mellitus. *J Diabetes Complications* 1998;12:181.

191. Kato K, Satoh H, Endo Y, *et al*: Thiazolidinediones down-regulate plasminogen activator inhibitor type 1 expression in human vascular endothelial cells: A possible role for PPARgamma in endothelial function. *Biochem Biophys Res Commun* 1999;258:431.

192. Colwell JA, Winocour PD, Lopes-Virella M, *et al*: New concepts about the pathogenesis of atherosclerosis in diabetes mellitus. *Am J Med* 1983;75:67.

193. Ishizuka T, Itazya S, Wada H, *et al*: Differential effect of the antidiabetic thiazolidinediones troglitazone and pioglitazone on human platelet aggregation mechanism. *Diabetes* 1998;47:1494.

194. Igarashi M, Takeda Y, Ishibashi N, *et al*: Pioglitazone reduces smooth muscle cell density of rat carotid arterial intima induced by balloon catheterization. *Horm Metab Res* 1997;29:444.

195. Marx N, Schonbeck U, Lazar MA, *et al*: Peroxisome proliferator-activated receptor gamma activators inhibit gene expression and migration in human vascular smooth muscle cells. *Circ Res* 1998; 83:1097.

196. Morikang E, Benson SC, Kurtz TW, *et al*: Effects of thiazolidinediones on growth and differentiation of human aorta and coronary myocytes. *Am J Hypertens* 1997;10:440.

197. Buchanan TA, Meehan WP, Jeng YY, *et al*: Blood pressure lowering by pioglitazone. Evidence for a direct vascular effect. *J Clin Invest* 1995;96:354.

198. Ogihara T, Rakugi H, Ikegami H, *et al*: Enhancement of insulin sensitivity by troglitazone lowers blood pressure in diabetic hypertensives. *Am J Hypertens* 1995;8:316.

199. Minamikawa J, Tanaka S, Yamaguchi M, *et al*: Potent inhibitory effect of troglitazone on carotid arterial wall thickness in type 2 diabetes. *J Clin Endocrinol Metab* 1998;83:1818.

200. Folsom AR, Eckfeldt JH, Weitzman S, *et al*: Relation of carotid artery wall thickness to diabetes mellitus, fasting glucose and insulin, body size, and physical activity. *Stroke* 1994;25:66.

201. Takagi T, Yoshida K, Akasaka T, *et al*: Troglitazone reduces intimal hyperplasia after coronary stent implantation in patients with type 2 diabetes mellitus: A serial intravascular ultrasound study [abstract]. *J Am Coll Cardiol* 1999;33(suppl A):100A.

202. Mercuri M, Bond MG, Sirtori CR, *et al*: Pravastatin reduces carotid intima-media thickness progression in an asymptomatic hypercholesterolemic meditgerranean population: The Carotid Atherosclerosis Italian Ultrasound Study. *Am J Med* 1996;101: 627.

203. Salonen R, Nyyssönen K, Porkkala E, *et al*: Kupio atherosclerosis prevention study (KAPS): A population-based primary preventive trial of the effect of LDL lowering on atherosclerotic progression in carotid and femoral arteries. *Circulation* 1995;92:1758.

204. Yoshimoto T: Vasculo-protective effects of insulin-sensitizing agent pioglitazone in neointimal thickening and chronic hypertension. *J Hypertens* 1998;165(suppl 2):S153.

205. Howard G, O'Leary DH, Zaccaro D, *et al*: Insulin sensitivity and atherosclerosis. *Circulation* 1996;93:1809.

206. Prigeon RL, Kahn SE, Porte D: Effect of troglitazone on B cell function, insulin sensitivity and glycemic control in subjects with type 2 diabetes mellitus. *J Clin Endocrinol Metab* 1998;83:819.

207. Porter LE, Freed MI, Jones NP, *et al*: Rosiglitazone improves beta-cell function as measured by proinsulin/insulin ratio in patients with type 2 diabetes. *Diabetes* 2000;48(suppl 1):A122.

207a. Buchanan, TA, Xiang AH, Peters RK, *et al*. Protection from type 2 diabetes persists in the TRIPOD cohort eight months after stopping troglitazone. *Diabetes* 2001:50(suppl 1):A81.

208. Rubin GL, Zhao Y, Kalus AM, *et al*: Peroxisome proliferator-activated receptor gamma ligands inhibit estrogen biosynthesis in human breast adipose tissue: Possible implications for breast cancer therapy. *Cancer Res* 2000;60:1604.

209. Takahashi N, Okumura T, Motomura W, *et al*: Activation of PPARgamma inhibits cell growth and induces apoptosis in human gastric cancer cells. *FEBS Lett* 1999;455:135.

210. Tsubouchi Y, Sano H, Kawahito Y, *et al*: Inhibition of human lung cancer cell growth by the peroxisome proliferator-activated receptor-gamma agonists through induction of apoptosis. *Biochem Biophys Res Commun* 2000;270:400.

211. Schoonjans K, Auwerx J: Thiazolidinediones: An update. *Lancet* 2000;355:1008.

212. Al-Salman J, Arjomand H, Kemp DG, *et al*: Hepatocellular injury in a patient receiving rosiglitazone. A case report. *Ann Intern Med* 2000;132:121.

213. Forman LM, Simmons DA, Diamond RH: Hepatic failure in a patient taking rosiglitazone. *Ann Intern Med* 2000;132:118.

214. Hu S, Wang S, Dunning BE: Tissue selectivity of antidiabetic agent nateglinide: Study on cardiovascular and beta-cell K(ATP) channels. *J Pharmacol Exp Ther* 1999;291:1372.

215. Shibata T, Matsui K, Yonemori F, *et al*: Triglyceride-lowering effect of a novel insulin-sensitizing agent, JTT-501. *Eur J Pharmacol* 1999;373:85.

216. Gomis R, Jones NP, Vallance SE, *et al*: Low dose rosiglitazone provides additional control when combined with sulfonylureas in type 2 diabetes. *Diabetes* 1999;47(suppl 1):abstract A63-0266.

217. Schneider R, Egan J, Houser V, *et al*: Combination therapy with pioglitazone and sulfonylurea in patients with type 2 diabetes. *Diabetes* 1999;47(suppl 1):abstract A106-0458.

218. Moses R, Slobodniuk R, Donnelley T, *et al*: Additional treatment with repaglinide provides significant improvement in glycemic control in NIDDM patients poorly controlled on metformin. *Diabetes* 1997;46(suppl):93A.

219. Chiasson J-L, Josse RG, Hunt JA, *et al*: The efficacy of acarbose in the treatment of patients with non-insulin-dependent diabetes mellitus: A multicenter controlled clinical trial. *Ann Intern Med* 1994;121:928.

220. Haupt E, Knick B, Koschinsky T, *et al*: Oral antidiabetic combination therapy with sulfonylureas and metformin. *Diabete Metab* 1991;17(suppl 1):224.

221. Mudaliar S, Edelman SV: Intensive insulin therapy for type 2 diabetes mellitus. In: LeRoith D, Taylor SI, Olefsky JM, eds. *Diabetes Mellitus: A Fundamental and Clinical Text*, 2nd ed. Lippincott Williams & Wilkins:2000;811.

222. Peters AL, Davidson MB: Insulin plus a sulfonylurea agent for treating type 2 diabetes. *Ann Intern Med* 1991;115:50.

223. Pugh JA, Wagner ML, Sawyer J, *et al*: Is combination sulfonylurea and insulin therapy useful in NIDDM patients? A meta-analysis. *Diabetes Care* 1992;15:953.

224. Yki-Järvinen H, Kauppila M, Kujansuu E, *et al*: Comparison of insulin regimens in patients with non-insulin-dependent diabetes mellitus. *N Engl J Med* 1992;327:1426.

224a. UKPDS Study Group: Glycemic control with diet, sufonylurea, metformin or insulin in patients with type 2 diabetes mellitus: Progressive requirement for multiple therapies (UKPDS 49). *JAMA* 1999;281:2005.

225. Yki-Jarvinen H, Ryysy L, Nikkila K, *et al*: Comparison of bedtime insulin regimens in patients with type 2 diabetes mellitus. A randomized, controlled trial *Ann Intern Med* 1999;130:389.

226. Raskin P, Dole JF, Rappaport EB, *et al*: Rosiglitazone improves glycemic control in poorly controlled insulin-treated type 2 diabetics. *Diabetes* 1999;47(suppl 1):A94-0404.

227. Rubin C, Egan J, Schneider R, *et al*: Combination therapy with pioglitazone and insulin in patients with type 2 diabetes. *Diabetes* 1999;47(suppl 1):A110-0474.

228. Bell DSH, Mayo MS: Outcome of metformin-facilitated reinitiation of oral diabetic therapy in insulin-treated patients with non-insulin-dependent diabetes mellitus. *Endocr Pract* 1997;3:73.

Behavioral and Family Aspects of the Treatment of Children and Adolescents with Type 1 Diabetes

Margaret Grey

William V. Tamborlane

Type 1 diabetes mellitus (T1DM) is a complex metabolic disease that requires constant attention from the patient, the family, and the provider to achieve treatment goals. Even before the results of the Diabetes Control and Complications Trial[1,2] were available, treatment of diabetes was thought to be difficult and onerous for families. Since release of the DCCT findings, the standards of care as published by the American Diabetes Association[3] recommend that all children be treated with intensive therapy, with the goal of achieving levels of metabolic control as close to normal as possible, so as to delay and/or prevent the development of the long-term complications of diabetes. Intensive therapy, which involves frequent blood glucose monitoring, three or more injections of insulin per day or use of continuous subcutaneous insulin infusion (CSII), carbohydrate counting, and more frequent visits to health care providers, thus requires a significant effort on the part of the patient and family to achieve treatment goals. Furthermore, those who are most successful in achieving treatment goals may be most at risk for the acute complications of intensive treatment—severe hypoglycemia and clinically significant weight gain. Finally, the occurrence of a chronic illness such as type 1 diabetes in a developing child may put the child and family at significant risk for the development of behavioral and social problems.[4,5] Thus, T1DM in childhood has the potential to have a significant negative impact on the developing child and the family. Conversely, the challenges provided by diabetes may strengthen and enhance adaptive behaviors in the child and the family.

DEVELOPMENTAL AND FAMILY ISSUES IN T1DM

Two developmental progressions are important in children with diabetes. Type 1 diabetes progresses through four distinct stages: diagnosis, partial remission or the honeymoon period, intensification, and total diabetes care. Furthermore, children and adolescents themselves are developing through several phases: infancy and young childhood (up to 5 years of age), school-age and preadolescent (6–11 years), adolescent (12–18 years), and young adults (19–24 years). According to Erikson's[6] psychosocial theory, the developing person experiences a crisis at each life stage that may result in a positive outcome and transition to the next phase of psychosocial development, or a negative outcome. These developmental phases interact with the phase of the disease and both must be con-

sidered in managing children with diabetes and their families, as shown in Table 33-1. In addition, developmental status might impact on the effectiveness as well as the appropriateness of various interventions.

Infancy and Young Childhood

Diabetes in infants is relatively rare; nonetheless it does occur, with less than 1.5 cases per 100,000 reported.[7] According to Erikson, the major psychosocial task of infancy is "Trust versus Mistrust."[6] During this phase, the infant must develop a foundation of trust of the world, and this trust is established primarily through the establishment of a relationship with a dependable caregiver. The infant needs to learn to trust the environment that surrounds him or her through learning to trust the mother or primary caregiver. This task becomes extremely difficult when painful injections and fingersticks are a consistent part of the infant's day. The mother may also report anxiety at the thought of causing pain to her own infant. Cognitively, the infant learns to separate self from others and learns basic trust in the world.[8] The infant lacks the cognitive ability to understand that painful procedures are necessary and in the best interest of the child. For the infant, both the hospitalization and the ongoing treatment disrupt home routines that are so important in establishing trust. These events interfere with the infant's efforts to master the developmental tasks of behavioral organization and regulation and basic trust. Thus it is extremely important for caregivers to establish ritualistic routines for infants with diabetes that enhance the development of regulation and trust.

These developmental issues are often compounded since the diagnosis of diabetes may be delayed in infants, and when the diagnosis is made, the infant may be quite ill. In addition to the crisis engendered by the serious illness and hospitalization of their infant, parents must now adapt to the diagnosis and learn the myriad skills of daily management. The tremendous responsibility of care and fear of hypoglycemia is extremely stressful for young families.[9] Banion and colleagues[9] found that the younger the child with diabetes, the greater the concern about hypoglycemia. Since infants do not exhibit the classic catecholamine response to hypoglycemia and are unable to communicate sensations associated with hypoglycemia, the risk of severe hypoglycemia, with seizures or coma, is highest in this age group. Moreover, since the brain is

TABLE 33-1. Major Developmental Issues and Their Effect on Diabetes in Children and Adolescents

Developmental Stage	Developmental Issue	Diabetes Management Issues	Psychosocial Complications
Infancy	Trust vs. Mistrust	Hypoglycemia	Failure to gain trust
Toddler	Autonomy vs. Shame and Doubt	Toilet training	Discipline
		Fear of hypoglycemia	Temper tantrums
		Irregular food intake	Burden on families
Preschooler	Initiative vs. Guilt	Child care	Magical thinking
		Unpredictable activity	Regression
School-age	Industry vs. Inferiority	Beginning participation in self-care	Depression, withdrawal
		Cognitive effects of hypoglycemia	Peer acceptance
Adolescence	Identify vs. Role Confusion	Rapid physical growth	Rebellion, family conflict
		Insulin resistance	Depression
		Lack of self-care	Eating disorders

still developing in infants, the adverse consequences of severe hypoglycemia are also greater than in older children. Parents struggle with the balance between the risk of long-term complications versus their fear of severe hypoglycemia and the risk of neuropsychological complications.

During the toddler years, ages 1–3, the diagnosis of type 1 diabetes is more common, although the incidence is still fairly low compared to older age groups. The toddler's major psychosocial task is to develop a sense of autonomy.[6] As toddlers develop more control of their bodies, they begin to explore and experience various aspects of the world. Erikson suggested that if the toddler is not allowed to develop this sense of autonomy and power over the environment, a sense of shame and doubt can develop. This achievement of autonomy relates primarily to the accomplishment of toilet training and mobility, and if diabetes control is not optimal, toilet training may be delayed. Toddlers love to explore and need to be given the freedom, within limits, to explore their world. In terms of cognitive skills, toddlers are able to participate in diabetes care minimally, choosing a finger for a fingerstick, for example. Because they don't understand the need for painful procedures, toddlers are extremely frightened of them. To begin to understand their autonomy, toddlers must begin to incorporate the knowledge of their illness into their emerging sense of self. The toddler begins to experience a sense of power that he or she can effect change in the environment. This sense of power may be reflected in temper tantrums and other behaviors that are indicative of a refusal to cooperate. Especially problematic at this age are the finicky eating habits and food jags associated with this age group.

As with infants, parents carry the burden of management of toddlers totally. Parents also report that hypoglycemia is a constant fear, especially when the child refuses to eat. An important issue at this age is discipline and temper tantrums. It is difficult for a parent to tell the difference between normal developmental opposition and hypoglycemia, and therefore the parent must be taught to check blood sugar before ignoring a temper tantrum. Parents may be overly cautious and interfere with the child's ability to try out new things.

Preschoolers (age 3–5) need to accomplish what Erikson called "Initiative versus Guilt."[6] In other words, they need to gain confidence in their ability to accomplish certain tasks. Cognitively, their style is preoperational and characterized by magical thinking.[8] This developmental stage involves a child's explanations, perceptions, and imaginations of the world. Because of their limited understanding, children may associate the illness or its painful treatment with punishment; in other words, they have diabetes because they were bad. Further, the child believes that the illness can be cured at any time magically by an adult. These factors may contribute to a child developing guilt rather than initiative. Energetic learning helps to promote the child's sense of purpose and direction, giving him or her a sense of accomplishment and satisfaction with activities. If diabetes is diagnosed during the preschool years, the child may regress to clinging, bedwetting, or nightmares. Assisting them to maintain their self-esteem by continuing usual activities and rewarding positive behaviors can be helpful. Preschoolers want to please others. They have boundless energy, but still lack the fine motor control necessary to be an active participant in most diabetes care.

For the most part, parents provide the care for preschoolers, but others, such as child care providers, may be involved in the care. Sharing care of young children with diabetes is often difficult for parents, who may fear that others will not know what to do.[9] Parents of preschoolers have similar anxieties and frustrations as those of younger children. Undetected hypoglycemia remains a concern because of the variations in activity associated with this age group, as well as the unpredictable appetite and food choices, and because of continuing concerns regarding the adverse effects of hypoglycemia on brain development and function.

School Age

Diabetes is the most common endocrine disorder of middle childhood.[10] Thus the incidence of diabetes in school-age children is substantially higher than in earlier age groups. In this stage, which Erickson calls "Industry versus Inferiority," school-aged children strive to develop a sense of industry at school and at home.[6] The child is involved in new ideas and tasks or takes on a sense of inferiority in which he or she feels incapable of accomplishing anything. Between the ages of 7 and 11, the child is better able to think, learn, remember, listen, and communicate.[8] Cognitive processes are becoming more logical and less egocentric. They are learning concrete cognitive operations; they now understand rules and follow them closely. They are able to deal with symbols and begin to master classifications. As children deal with the challenges of school, they begin to turn their attention away from the home environment, and the peer group becomes more important. Each of these skills may affect the adaptation to diabetes.

Several authors have examined the influence of the new diagnosis of diabetes on children in this age group. Kovacs and colleagues[11] studied a cohort of school-aged children with newly diagnosed diabetes for 6 years and found that during the 6 months after diagnosis, children reported mild depression and anxiety, but these usually resolved by 6 months after diagnosis. They also found that after the first year, there was an increase in depressive symptoms, and anxiety decreased for boys but increased for girls over the first 6 years after diagnosis.[11] Similarly, Grey and colleagues[4] found that after an initial period of adjustment characterized by depression and mild anxiety, children with newly diagnosed diabetes were psychosocially similar to age- and gender-matched peers until the period between 1 and 2 years post-diagnosis, when depression markedly increased in the diabetes group. This increase in depression may be associated with the end of the physiologic honeymoon period as well as with the stage of psychosocial adjustment to the disease, when children come to realize that the disease will not go away and that it is more difficult to manage.

Both longitudinal and cross-sectional studies have suggested that school-age children with diabetes may have difficulties in psychosocial adjustment. In general, the majority of children will do well, but diabetes may become a risk factor for the development of psychosocial difficulties in a relatively small percentage of children, often estimated at approximately 10–20%.[5] In most studies of overall adjustment, however, children with diabetes were found to score within the normal range or similarly to age- and gender-matched controls in such areas as behavior,[12] temperament,[13] and self-competence and self-esteem.[4,11] In those who do demonstrate psychosocial difficulties in the school-age years, children tend to be more depressed, withdrawn, and quiet, and their metabolic control may also be compromised.[4]

Although the majority of children do well, some children have difficulty, and researchers have examined several areas that may help to predict those children. How children cope with having diabetes as well as other stressors in their lives has been investigated in a number of studies. Kovacs and her colleagues[11] reported that during the first year after diagnosis, children used instrumental and problem-focused coping strategies, including seeking diabetes-related information. Early in the course of the illness, these authors did not find a correlation between coping behaviors and psychologic adjustment. On the other hand, Grey and associates[14] found that behaviors and lack of self-care of the diabetes were associated with poorer psychosocial adjustment 1 year after diagnosis.

The complexity of the diabetes regimen requires adherence to a multitude of tasks. There have been several studies that examined adherence to the diabetes regimen in school-age children with diabetes. In a study of an onset cohort of children with diabetes, initial assessment of patient coping was found to be associated with the level of patient adherence over 4 years of study.[12] Coping strategies, such as problem-focused coping, contributed significantly to treatment responsibility among children with diabetes, and higher levels of avoidance coping were associated with poorer metabolic control.[15]

Another factor associated with regimen adherence is the involvement of the family. Earlier approaches to diabetes management advocated early transition of care responsibilities to children with diabetes. Fonagy and coworkers[16] studied factors associated with poorer metabolic control and found that a child's early and independent participation in the diabetes regimen was significantly associated with poorer control. This finding was replicated in a later study,[17] so that current recommendations for care emphasize shared care responsibilities between parents and children.

It is clear that the diagnosis of diabetes in a child has a significant impact on parents and families. As part of their prospective study of school-aged children with newly diagnosed diabetes, Kovacs and associates[18] interviewed parents as well as children and found that the initial strain of living with diabetes elicited mild and subclinical depression, anxiety, and overall distress, especially in mothers. By the end of the first year, most mothers came to terms with the diabetes, and other areas of parental functioning such as the quality of the marriage were not affected. Nonetheless, parents remain concerned with their ability to manage the diabetes regimen and cope with restraints imposed by the illness, and this coping had psychological effects, such as anxiety and depression, on the parents.

Such parental distress may be associated with child adjustment, demonstrating the transactional nature of relationships in these families.[19] Parental conflict, cohesion, and organization in the first year after diagnosis have been found to be associated with adherence to the diabetes regimen in children.[20] Furthermore, as children age, the influence of family and parental environment on metabolic control may decrease.

Both children and parents fear hypoglycemia and the potential for hypoglycemia to interfere with learning. Even mild hypoglycemia causes acute alterations in cognitive function, especially associative learning, attention, and mental flexibility.[21] A single episode of hypoglycemia causes both lower plasma glucose thresholds for autonomic activation and symptoms and lower nadir plasma glucose concentrations during moderate hyperglycemia.[22] Thus the potential for further acute events increases. Cognitive deficits associated with the acute phase of hypoglycemia include transient reduction in mental efficiency, altered electroencephalogram, and increased regional cerebral blood flow.[23] There is some evidence that some cognitive deficits persist beyond the acute phase. Several investigations have found that while diabetes itself is not associated with cognitive deficits, cognitive dysfunction may be increased in children and adolescents who have experienced severe hypoglycemia.[24,25] Recent data suggest that some of the learning difficulties in children who have experienced severe hypoglycemia earlier in life may be due to difficulties in delayed spatial memory.[26] In addition, the occurrence of hypoglycemia leads to fear of the next episode of hypoglycemia. Researchers have suggested that fear of hypoglycemia is a legitimate consequence of hypoglycemia in children and that the aversive nature of severe hypoglycemia may lead patients and parents to institute behavioral changes to maintain higher blood glucose, overtreatment of initial symptoms, and poorer metabolic control. Further, fear of hypoglycemia may be associated with poorer psychological status and adaptation as well.[27] For some children, the ability to use avoidance behaviors, such as raising the blood glucose target levels, may not be under their control. Parents also report substantial anxiety and fear of hypoglycemia, and they too may engage in behaviors that serve to avoid hypoglycemic events.[28]

School-age children with diabetes can begin to assume some of the daily diabetes management tasks, such as insulin injections and blood glucose testing. However, they will still need significant assistance from their families for management decisions. It is important to encourage school-age children to attend school regularly and to participate in school activities and sports to facilitate the development of normal peer relationships. Children with diabetes often feel that they are different from their peers because of the diabetes and may be at risk for difficulties with social competence.[29]

Adolescent

Adolescence is a period of rapid biological change accompanied by increasing physical, cognitive, and emotional maturity. Adolescents are struggling to find their own identity separate from their families. If they have difficulty with identity formation, Erikson[30] describes it as role confusion. Many of the diabetes care–related tasks can interfere with the adolescent's drive for independence and peer acceptance. Peer pressure may generate strong conflicts. In this age group, there is a mighty struggle for independence from parents and other adults that is often manifested as poorer adherence to the diabetes regimen. Cognitively, adolescents are beginning to attain the skill of formal operations.[8] Formal operations allow adolescents to "think about their own thinking," transfer information from one situation to another, deal efficiently with complex problems, plan realistically for the future, and conceptualize more abstract ideas. Perhaps because adolescents often manifest more difficulties in diabetes management and more overt psychosocial problems than younger children, the great majority of psychosocial and behavioral literature deals with adolescents.

Hormonal changes trigger the onset of puberty and the development of secondary sexual characteristics, ultimately resulting in the attainment of adult stature and proportion. During this period, adolescents are narcissistic, being preoccupied with their bodies and the changes occurring to them. Second, teens evolve from concrete thinkers into abstract thinkers, making understanding of the relationship of self-care to outcomes difficult. The period is also marked by feelings of ambivalence, impulsiveness, and mood swings, associated with the struggle with separation from parents and the need to be accepted by peers. Finally, adolescents engage in experimentation and risk-taking behaviors which may adversely affect self-care and clinical outcomes as well.

Metabolic control tends to deteriorate in adolescence as a result of several factors: the natural decrease to zero of the production of insulin by the pancreas; the hormonal changes of adolescence, which are associated with insulin resistance and the corresponding need for very large doses of insulin;[31] and adolescent rebellion, which is associated with poorer adherence to the treatment regimen.[32] To further complicate matters, adolescents who are most successful in lowering plasma glucose levels are at the greatest risk for severe hypoglycemic events.[2]

For the most part, it is accepted that diabetes is a risk factor for adolescent psychiatric disorder.[33] Approximately three times more adolescents with diabetes have psychiatric disorders than their age-mates, with rates as high as 33%. This increased morbidity is primarily associated with the incidence of major depression (approximately 27.5%)[34] and generalized anxiety disorder (18.4%), rather than psychiatric behavioral disorders.[33] Furthermore, a substantial number of adolescents with diabetes consider suicide after the onset of the disease.[35] The rate of suicidal ideation has been found to be higher than would be expected (26.4%), but in contrast, the number of suicide attempts was only 4.4%, which is a rate comparable to the general population of adolescents.[36] In addition, adolescents who have recurrent diabetic ketoacidosis may be more likely to have psychiatric disorders, especially anxiety and depression, than those without recurrent hospitalization.[37] These studies are important because not only is psychiatric illness a serious complication of diabetes, it may be associated with poorer metabolic control.

Eating disorders have also been associated with diabetes in adolescents. This topic has been studied for nearly 20 years with mixed findings. Several studies have suggested that adolescents with diabetes are at no higher risk for eating disorders than their peers without diabetes,[38,39] whereas other studies have found rates of both anorexia and bulimia to be higher in youths with T1DM, and have described a specific type of eating disorder seen in these patients, insulin omission to control weight.[40] Youths, especially girls, with such eating disorders are more likely to have other psychiatric morbidity, as well as poorer metabolic control of diabetes[41] and recurrent hospitalizations.[42]

How individuals cope with the burdens of a chronic condition has an important impact on the effectiveness of therapy. Coping with the demands of self-management can be a formidable task. These demands include both the physical demands of management as well as the emotional and social demands of adaptation. A variety of studies have demonstrated that the period of adolescence is often associated with neglect of self-monitoring, dietary recommendations, and pharmacologic treatments. Such neglect in self-management is usually not associated with a deficit in knowledge; rather the cognitive and developmental characteristics of adolescence make appropriate decision making more complex. Thus adolescents are at high risk for poorer clinical outcomes, hospitalization, and eventually, the development of long-term complications.[14,43]

While a smaller percentage of adolescents with diabetes manifest significant psychiatric problems, many have difficulty in psychosocial adjustment. The presence of diabetes in adolescence may hinder normal adolescent development by limiting the development of independence. One recent study[44] examined the personal meaning and perceived impact of diabetes on 54 adolescents and found that youths felt that diabetes controlled or limited their freedom and independence. Girls have been found to report more symptoms of anxiety and depression related to these restrictions and to be in worse metabolic control than boys.[45]

Because difficulties in regimen adherence are so common in adolescents,[32] and poorer regimen adherence is associated with poorer metabolic control,[46] there have been a number of studies that have examined factors associated with adherence. Such factors may be internal, such as coping behaviors or styles,[47] gender,[45,48] age,[32,49] and motivations,[50] or external, such as the supportiveness of the family[51] and the health care system.[52] Adolescents who frequently neglect self-management have less motivation and less support and believe that nonadherence is an issue of personal freedom.[53]

Adolescence is also a period of intense experimentation with risky behaviors. Interestingly, although youths with diabetes frequently experiment with diabetes mismanagement through nonadherence, the rates at which they report other risky behaviors, such as alcohol use, smoking cigarettes, drug use, and unprotected intercourse, are lower than the general population of adolescents.[54] These rates are still substantial, however, and many of these behaviors can interfere with diabetes self-management as well. Furthermore, while girls are more likely to participate in diabetes mismanagement, boys are more likely to engage in risky behaviors.[48]

Although adolescents are struggling to define their own identity apart from the family, the family has continued and profound effects on the adolescent with diabetes. A number of studies provide support for the association between family cohesion and better metabolic control in adolescents,[55] but there is some evidence that this relationship may be attenuated by disease duration.[55]

Other researchers have also shown that adolescents whose parents maintain some guidance and control in the management of diabetes have better metabolic control.[17,56] Thus, continuing to involve parents appropriately, with shared management, is associated with improved control. The challenge is to find the degree of parental involvement that is comfortable for all involved, without risking poorer control from overinvolvement or underinvolvement.[57] Such involvement in diabetes management in this developmental stage can affect parent-adolescent relationships. Parent-child conflict has been associated with poorer diabetes outcomes in several studies.[58,59]

Transition to Young Adulthood

It is only recently that the issues related to the long-term outcomes of youths who have chronic conditions have received attention in the literature, much of it concerned with the differences in approaches between pediatric care and adult care.[60] Bussing and Aro surveyed adolescents in a school at age 16 and again at age 22 and compared individuals with chronic conditions to those without chronic conditions, to determine the effect of the chronic condition on a variety of functional outcomes.[61] They found that adolescents with chronic health conditions attained levels of well-being, education, and marriage or dating as young adults similar to their peers without chronic conditions. Their findings also suggest, however, that males with a chronic condition may be at higher risk for depression than females or those without chronic conditions. Wysocki and colleagues studied 81 young adults with diabetes and found higher rates of psychopathology compared to others, and that poorer metabolic control and poorer adjustment to diabetes in adolescence are associated with poorer status in early adulthood.[62] On the other hand, Pless and colleagues retrospectively surveyed 431 young adults (aged 18–34 years) and found that efforts to achieve better metabolic control during childhood, whether successful or not, were not associated with psychosocial problems later in life.[63] In one of the few longitudinal studies of youths with chronic conditions, Jacobson and colleagues[64] found that DM patients had lower perceived competence, self-worth, and sociability than young adults without chronic illness. All of these studies, however, were conducted prior to the release of the findings of the Diabetes Control and Complications Trial (DCCT) and the recommendations for intensive treatment for all youths. Since improved metabolic control is achieved earlier as a result of intensive therapy, it may be that such regimens will be associated with improved status over time, but this assumption has not been evaluated.

INTERVENTIONS AND IMPLICATIONS FOR TREATMENT

Team Management

Given the complexity of diabetes management, children and adolescents with T1DM should be routinely cared for at a diabetes center that employs a multidisciplinary team of practitioners who are knowledgeable about and experienced in the management of young patients.[65] Such teams should ideally consist of pediatric endocrinologists, diabetes nurse specialists or practitioners, dietitians, social workers or psychologists, and referral resources for eye, renal, neurologic, and other problems. Such teams need to project a positive, upbeat approach to treatment, communicate well among themselves, and be self-critical of their own performance.

Databases that track overall clinic performance with respect to important outcomes can be very useful.

Psychosocial Interventions

There have been a number of studies on the effects of psychosocial interventions for children and adolescents with diabetes. Reports on psychosocial interventions include those that focused on coping skills training, stress management and relaxation, and social support in groups or camps.

A series of studies have been conducted using coping skills training for children and adolescents with diabetes. Coping skills training is designed to increase competence and mastery by retraining inappropriate or nonconstructive coping styles and patterns of behavior into more constructive behaviors. Coping skills training for youths with diabetes is based on the hypothesis that improving coping skills will improve the ability of youths to cope with the problems faced on a day-to-day basis in managing diabetes.

In an experimental study that combined both instruction in blood glucose management and coping skills training called Stress Management Training in Adolescents, Boardway and associates[66] found that while diabetes-specific stress was decreased in the experimental group, there were no differences in metabolic control as measured by HbA$_{1c}$, coping styles, self-efficacy, life events, or adherence over 9 months. In contrast, Grey and colleagues[67] reported on the results of a larger randomized clinical trial, with a sufficient sample to achieve statistical power, to determine both metabolic and psychosocial effects of coping skills training. These studies focused on adolescents initiating intensive insulin therapy after the results of the DCCT were released.[2] In their study of 77 youths, they found significant improvements in metabolic control, general self-efficacy, and quality of life as compared to the control group over 12 months of follow-up.[67]

Two studies were found that used meditation and other forms of stress reduction as a method to improve diabetes care and outcomes. Since stress has been found to be associated with alterations in metabolic control, it is hypothesized that such interventions will assist those with diabetes to have better metabolic control. Mendez and Belendez[68] conducted a quasi-experiment of stress management in 37 adolescents and compared this program to routine medical care. The program consisted of 12 sessions that included review, information, and practicalities of diabetes management, with a focus on stress and coping with stress, including problem solving. Results showed posttest improvements in diabetes information, adherence, daily hassles, social responses, skills, frequency of testing, and errors in blood glucose testing, as measured by observation, and negative family support. There were no effects on self-reported dietary and physical exercise behavior or metabolic control. When retested at 13 months after the intervention, knowledge, barriers to adherence, hassles, and social interactions remained better in the stress management group.

Over the years, a number of studies have suggested that social support is associated with improved adherence and metabolic control in adolescents with diabetes, but despite the understanding that social support is important, there have been relatively few investigations of socially supportive interventions.[52] These interventions differ from group approaches used to teach coping skills and other approaches in that the goal is to improve the supportiveness of the environment rather than to attain specific skills. Interventions that focus on the family as the unit of social support are discussed below under family interventions.

Dr. Barbara Anderson and colleagues[69] examined the effectiveness of a peer group intervention for young adolescents to attempt to prevent the usual decline in metabolic control associated with adolescence. They hypothesized that providing peer support and education in making adjustments in the diabetes regimen according to self-monitored blood glucose results would prevent this decline. In this intervention, small groups of adolescents met at each of their clinic visits. Emphasis was placed on the use of blood glucose data and peer support to improve control. Results indicated that metabolic control was significantly better in the experimental group, who reported more adjustments for exercise, diet, and insulin dose based on blood glucose testing than did those who received routine follow-up care.

Others are interested in social support provided over the telephone or by adult mentors for younger youths. Daley[70] paired adults with T1DM with adolescents with newly diagnosed diabetes to improve adolescents' adjustment to diabetes. The sample for this study differs from many intervention studies, in that it is approximately 44% minority (Hispanic and African-American). The 54 subjects ranged in age from 12–16 years, and the sponsor intervention was provided for 10 months. Results indicated that for the most part, there were no differences (metabolic control, behavior, adjustment, anxiety) between the sponsorship group and the control group, but subjects in the sponsorship group reported an increase in social acceptance and romantic appeal. Furthermore, in qualitative interviews, subjects in the experimental group reported that the sponsors provided an important source of previously unavailable support.

In summary, there have been a number of psychosocial approaches studied for children and adolescents with diabetes, but the majority have been conducted with adolescents. Little attention has been paid to younger children and to the families and extended families of these children. Many of these reports are not rigorous experimental designs, but case control studies or one-group pretest-posttest preexperimental designs. Nonetheless, where adequate controlled studies have been done, interventions such as coping skills training and peer support have been demonstrated to lead to improved adjustment or quality of life as well as improved metabolic control.

Family interventions are those in which the target of the intervention is the family members of a child or adolescent with diabetes rather than the index child. Reviews of the literature on family aspects of chronic illness reinforce the view that while there have been methodological problems in studying families of individuals with chronic illness, families have an important influence on children and adolescents with diabetes.[71]

Studies of family intervention include those whose intervention was targeted on family members, primarily parents, and did not focus on outcomes in children, adolescents, or parents alone. Satin and associates[72] conducted an experimental study of a multifamily group intervention of support and guidance, and a multifamily group intervention plus parent simulation of diabetes, and compared outcomes with a control group of adolescents and families who received routine care. A total of 32 families participated and were randomly assigned to the three groups. The interventions consisted of six weekly sessions that included adolescents and their parents, in which guidance and support were provided, using principles of group therapy. For the group who received the multifamily intervention plus simulation, the parents simulated having diabetes and doing all of the self-care for 1 week. Controls received routine care. Results indicated that the group who received the

multifamily intervention with simulation had the best improvement in metabolic control. Parents in both intervention groups had more positive perceptions of teens with diabetes, but no differences were found on estimates of self-care or family environment.

Wysocki and colleagues[73,74] conducted experimental studies that compared the effectiveness of Behavioral Family Systems Therapy with that of education and support groups for families of adolescents in reducing parent-adolescent conflict in diabetes management. This intervention focused on families with pretest scores demonstrating at least moderate general or diabetes-specific family conflict. Behavioral Family Systems Therapy targets parent-adolescent conflict by focusing on family problem solving and communication skills, the degree to which family members hold extreme beliefs about one another's behavior, and the extent of family structural or systemic anomalies. The experimental treatment consisted of 10 sessions with parents and adolescents that emphasized problem solving for conflict resolution, communication skills training for parent-adolescent communications, cognitive restructuring for family members' beliefs and attributions, and functional or structural family therapy to target maladaptive characteristics of family functioning. A total of 119 families with adolescents with diabetes participated in these studies. Using scales developed and validated for this study, results demonstrated that the Behavioral Family Systems Therapy showed more improvement in parent-adolescent relationships, diabetes-specific family conflicts, treatment adherence, metabolic control (in boys and younger girls only), and treatment evaluation as compared to education and support groups. By 6 months, the improvements in parent-adolescent relationships were maintained, but those related to adherence or metabolic control were not.

As parents and children negotiate responsibilities in diabetes management, and as these responsibilities change over time, it is likely that parent-adolescent conflict will develop. Anderson and colleagues[75] developed an office-based intervention aimed at maintaining parent-adolescent teamwork in diabetes management tasks without increasing diabetes-related family conflict. In a study of 85 adolescent patients and their parents, they found that the brief intervention carried out in quarterly office visits for 12 months led to no decrease in parental involvement in insulin administration and blood glucose testing, with significantly less family conflict as compared to usual care. Over a 24-month follow-up period, average levels of glycosylated hemoglobin did not differ between the groups, but more teens in the teamwork group had improved control than in the comparison group.

SUMMARY

Clearly, type 1 diabetes diagnosed in childhood has a profound effect on children and their families. Diabetes requires constant vigilance to maintain good metabolic control without increasing the risk of severe hypoglycemia. Both parents and children struggle with this awesome responsibility, and they may need special interventions to assist in not only maintaining good metabolic control, but also improving their quality of life.

REFERENCES

1. Diabetes Control and Complications Trial (DCCT) Research Group:
   The effect of intensive treatment of diabetes on the development and

progression of long-term complications in insulin-dependent diabetes mellitus. *N Engl J Med* 1993;329:977.

2. Diabetes Control and Complications Trial (DCCT) Research Group: Effect of intensive insulin treatment on the development and progression of long-term complications in adolescents with insulin-dependent diabetes mellitus: Diabetes Control and Complications Trial. *J Pediatr* 1994;125:177.

3. American Diabetes Association: Clinical practice recommendations. *Diabetes Care* 2000;23:53.

4. Grey M, Cameron ME, Lipman TH, *et al*: Psychosocial status of children with diabetes over the first two years. *Diabetes Care* 1995; 18:1330.

5. Bennett DS: Depression among children with chronic medical problems: A meta-analysis. *J Pediatr Psychol* 1994;19:149.

6. Erikson EH: *Childhood and Society*, 2nd ed. W.W. Norton:1964.

7. Lipman TH: The epidemiology of type 1 diabetes in children 0–14 yrs of age in Philadelphia. *Diabetes Care* 1993;16:922.

8. Piaget J: *The Origins of Intelligence in Children*. International Universities:1952.

9. Banion CR, Miles MS, Carter MC: Problems of mothers in management of children with diabetes. *Diabetes Care* 1983;6:548.

10. National Institutes of Diabetes, Digestive, and Kidney Diseases (NIDDK): *Diabetes in America*. Government Printing Office:1995.

11. Kovacs M, Iyengar S, Goldston D, *et al*: Psychological functioning of children with insulin-dependent diabetes mellitus: A longitudinal study. *J Pediatr Psychol* 1990;15:619.

12. Jacobson AM, Hauser ST, Lavori P, *et al*: Adherence among children and adolescents with insulin-dependent diabetes mellitus over a four-year longitudinal follow-up: 1. The influence of patient coping and adjustment. *J Pediatr Psychol* 1990;15:511.

13. Weissberg-Benchell J, Glasgow A: The role of temperament in children with insulin-dependent diabetes mellitus. *J Pediatr Psychol* 1997;22:795.

14. Grey M, Cameron ME, Lipman TH, *et al*: The relationship of initial coping behaviors to adjustment one year later in children with IDDM. *Nurs Res* 1997;46:312.

15. Reid G, Dubow EF, Carey TC, *et al*: Contribution of coping to the medical adjustment and treatment responsibility among children and adolescents with diabetes. *Dev Behav Pediatr* 1994;15:327.

16. Fonagy P, Moran GS, Lindsay MKM, *et al*: Psychological adjustment and diabetic control. *Arch Dis Child* 1987;62:1009.

17. Follansbee DS: Assuming responsibility for diabetes management. What age? What price? *Diabetes Educator* 1989;15:347.

18. Kovacs M, Finkelstein R, Feinberg TL, *et al*: Initial psychologic responses of parents to the diagnosis of insulin-dependent diabetes mellitus in their children. *Diabetes Care* 1985;8:568.

19. Chaney JM, Mullins LL, Frank RG, *et al*: Transactional patterns of child, mother, and father adjustment in insulin-dependent diabetes mellitus. *J Pediatr Psychol* 1997;22:229.

20. Hauser ST, Jacobson AM, Lavori P, *et al*: Adherence among children and adolescents with insulin-dependent diabetes mellitus over a four year longitudinal follow-up: II. Immediate and long-term linkages with the family milieu. *J Pediatr Psychol* 1990;15:527.

21. Draelos MT, Jacobson AM, Weinger K, *et al*: Cognitive function in patients with insulin dependent diabetes mellitus during hyperglycemia and hypoglycemia. *Am J Med* 1995;98:135.

22. Cryer PE: Iatrogenic hypoglycemia in IDDM: Consequences, risk factors, and prevention. In: Home PD, Marshall S, Alberti KGMM, *et al*, eds. *Diabetes Annual*. Elsevier:1993.

23. Ryan CM, Becker DJ: Hypoglycemia in children with type 1 diabetes—Risk factors, cognitive function, and management. *Endocrinol Metab Clin North Am* 1999;28:883.

24. Northam EA, Anderson PJ, Werther GA, *et al*: Neuropsychological complications of IDDM in children 2 years after disease onset. *Diabetes Care* 1998;21:379.

25. Rovet J, Alvarez M: Attentional functioning in children and adolescents with IDDM. *Diabetes Care* 1997;20:803.

26. Hershey T, Bhargava N, Sadler N, *et al*: Conventional versus intensive diabetes therapy in children with type 1 diabetes: Effects on memory and motor speed. *Diabetes Care* 1999;22:1318.

27. Hepburn DA, Deary IJ, MacLeod KM, *et al*: Structural equation modeling of symptoms, awareness and fear of hypoglycemia, and personality in patients with insulin-treated diabetes. *Diabetes Care* 1994; 17:1273.

28. Marrero DG, Guare JC, Vandagriff JL, *et al*: Fear of hypoglycemia in the parents of children and adolescents with diabetes: Maladaptive or healthy response? *Diabetes Educator* 1997;23:281.

29. Nassau JH, Drotar D: Social competence in children with IDDM and asthma: Child, teacher, and parent reports of children's social adjustment, social performance, and social skills. *J Pediatr Psychol* 1995; 20:187.

30. Erikson EH: *Identity: Youth and Crisis*. W.W. Norton:1968.

31. Amiel SA, Sherwin RS, Simonson DC, *et al*: Impaired insulin action in puberty: A contributing factor to poor glycemic control in adolescents. *N Engl J Med* 1986;315:215.

32. Weissberg-Benchell J, Glasgow AM, Tynan WD, *et al*: Adolescent diabetes management and mismanagement. *Diabetes Care* 1995;18:77.

33. Kovacs M, Goldston D, Obrosky DS, *et al*: Psychiatric disorders in youth with IDDM: Rates and risk factors. *Diabetes Care* 1997;20:36.

34. Kovacs M, Obrosky DS, Goldston D, *et al*: Major depressive disorder in youths with IDDM: A controlled prospective study of course and outcome. *Diabetes Care* 1997;20:45.

35. Goldston D, Kovacs M, Ho V, *et al*: Suicidal ideation and suicide attempts among youth with insulin-dependent diabetes mellitus. *J Am Acad Child Adolesc Psychiatry* 1994;33:240.

36. Goldston DB, Kelley AE, Reboussin DM, *et al*: Suicidal ideation and behavior and noncompliance with the medical regimen among diabetic adolescents. *J Am Acad Child Adolesc Psychiatry* 1997;36:1528.

37. Liss DS, Waller DA, Kennard BD, *et al*: Psychiatric illness and family support in children and adolescents with diabetic ketoacidosis: A controlled study. *J Am Assoc Child Adolesc Psychiatry* 1998;37:536.

38. Peveler RC, Fairburn CG, Boller I, *et al*: Eating disorders in adolescents with IDDM. *Diabetes Care* 1992;15:1356.

39. Striegel-Moore RH, Nicholson TJ, Tamborlane WV: Prevalence of eating disorder symptoms in preadolescent and adolescent girls with IDDM. *Diabetes Care* 1992;15:1361.

40. Polonsky WH, Anderson BJ, Lohrer PA, *et al*: Insulin omission in women with IDDM. *Diabetes Care* 1994;17:1178.

41. Pollock M, Kovacs M, Charron-Prochownik D: Eating disorders and maladaptive dietary/insulin management among youths with childhood-onset insulin-dependent diabetes mellitus. *J Am Acad Child Adolesc Psychiatry* 1995;34:291.

42. Cohn BA, Cirillo PM, Wingard DL, *et al*: Gender differences in hospitalizations for IDDM among adolescents in California, 1991: Implications for prevention. *Diabetes Care* 1997;20:1677.

43. Austin JK, Huster GA, Dunn DW, *et al*: Adolescents with active or inactive epilepsy or asthma: A comparison of quality of life. *Epilepsia* 1996;37:1228.

44. Kyngas H, Barlow J: Diabetes: An adolescent's perspective. *J Adv Nurs* 1995;22:941.

45. LaGreca AM, Swales T, Klemp S, *et al*: Adolescents with diabetes: Gender differences in psychosocial functioning and glycemic control. *Children's Health Care* 1995;24:61.

46. Rosilio M, Cotton JB, Wieliczko MC, *et al*: Factors associated with glycemic control. *Diabetes Care* 1998;21:1146.

47. Murphy LMB, Thompson RJ, Morris MA: Adherence behavior among adolescents with type I insulin-dependent diabetes mellitus: The role of cognitive appraisal processes. *J Pediatry Psychol* 1997;22:811.

48. Hanna KM, Guthrie DW: Involvement in health behaviors among youth with diabetes. *Diabetes Educator* 1999;25:211.

49. Bond GG, Aiken LS, Somerville SC: The Health Belief Model and adolescents with insulin-dependent diabetes mellitus. *Health Psychol* 1992;11:190.

50. Hentinen M, Kyngas H: Diabetic adolescents' compliance with health regimens and associated factors. *Int J Nurs Stud* 1996;33:325.

51. LaGreca AM, Auslander WF, Greco P, *et al*: I get by with a little help from my family and friends: Adolescents' support for diabetes care. *J Pediatr Psychol* 1995;20:449.

52. Burroughs TE, Harris MA, Pontious SL, *et al*: Research in social support in adolescents with IDDM: A critical review. *Diabetes Educator* 1997;23:438.

53. Kyngas H, Hentinen M: Meaning attached to compliance with self-care, and conditions for compliance among young people. *J Adv Nurs* 1995;21:729.

54. Frey MA, Guthrie B, Loveland-Cherry C, *et al*: Risky behavior and risk in adolescents with IDDM. *J Adolesc Health* 1997;20:38.

55. Hanson CL, DeGuire MJ, Schinkel AM, *et al*: Empirical validation for a family-centered model of care. *Diabetes Care* 1995;18:1347.

56. Grey M, Boland EA, Yu C, et al: Personal and social factors associated with quality of life in adolescents with IDDM. *Diabetes Care* 1998;21:909.

57. Seiffge-Krenke I: The highly structured climate in families of adolescents with diabetes: Functional or dysfunctional for metabolic control. *J Pediatr Psychol* 1998;23:313.

58. Miller-Johnson S, Emery RE, Marvin RS, et al: Parent-child relationships and the management of insulin-dependent diabetes mellitus. *J Consult Clin Psychol* 1994;62:603.

59. Wysocki T: Associations among teen-parent relationships, metabolic control, and adjustment to diabetes in adolescents. *J Pediatr Psychol* 1993;18:441.

60. Rosen D: Between two worlds: Bridging the cultures of child health and adult medicine. *J Adolesc Health* 1995;17:10.

61. Bussing R, Aro H: Youth with chronic conditions and their transition to adulthood. *Arch Pediatr Adolesc Med* 1996;150:181.

62. Wysocki T, Hough BS, Ward KM, et al: Diabetes mellitus in the transition to adulthood: Adjustment, self-care, and health status. *Dev Behav Pediatr* 1992;13:194.

63. Pless IB, Heller A, Belmonte M, et al: Expected diabetic control in childhood and psychosocial functioning in early adult life. *Diabetes Care* 1988;11:387.

64. Jacobson AM, Hauser ST, Willett JB, et al: Psychological adjustment to IDDM: 10-year follow-up of an onset cohort of child and adolescent patients. *Diabetes Care* 1997;20:811.

65. Tamborlane WV, Gatcomb P, Held N, et al: Implications of the DCCT results in treating children and adolescents with diabetes. *Clin Diabetes* 1994;12:115.

66. Boardway RH, Delameter AM, Tomakowsky J, et al: Stress management training for adolescents with diabetes. *J Pediatr Psychol* 1993;18:29.

67. Grey M, Boland EA, Davidson M, et al: Coping skills training has long-lasting effects on metabolic control and quality of life in adolescents on intensive therapy. *J Pediatr*; 12:179.(in press).

68. Mendez FJ, Belendez M: Effects of a behavioral intervention on treatment adherence and stress management in adolescents with IDDM. *Diabetes Care* 1997;20:1370.

69. Anderson BJ, Wolf FM, Burkhart MT, et al: Effects of peer-group intervention on metabolic control of adolescents with IDDM: Randomized outpatient study. *Diabetes Care* 1989;12:179.

70. Daley BJ: Sponsorship for adolescents with diabetes. *Health Soc Work* 1992;17:173.

71. Glascow R, Anderson BJ: Future directions for research on pediatric chronic disease management: Lessons from diabetes. *J Pediatr Psychol* 1995;20:389.

72. Satin W, LaGreca AM, Zigo MA, et al: Diabetes in adolescence: Effects of a multifamily group intervention and parent simulation of diabetes. *J Pediatr Psychol* 1989;14:259.

73. Wysocki T, Harris MA, Greco P, et al: Social validity of support group and behavior therapy interventions for families of adolescents with insulin dependent diabetes mellitus. *J Pediatr Psychol* 1997;22:635.

74. Wysocki T, Greco P, Harris M, et al: Behavior therapy for families of adolescents with IDDM: Maintenance of treatment effects. *Diabetes Care* 2001;24:441.

75. Anderson BJ, Brackett J, Ho J, et al: An office-based intervention to maintain parent-adolescent teamwork in diabetes management. *Diabetes Care* 2001;24:441.

Diabetic Ketoacidosis

Elizabeth Delionback Ennis

Robert A. Kreisberg

Diabetic ketoacidosis (DKA) is an important and serious complication of decompensated diabetes mellitus. Each year there are approximately 798,000 individuals with newly diagnosed diabetes mellitus (DM).[1] By 1998, there were an estimated 15.7 million persons in the U.S. (5.9% of the total population) with diabetes mellitus.[1]

In 1994, the most recent year for which data are available, there were 113,000 hospital discharges in which DKA was listed and 89,000 in which it was the primary diagnosis.[1] Although impressive, these data underestimate the true incidence of DKA since mild diabetic ketoacidosis is often treated in a physician's office or an emergency department. In 1997, $1.324 billion out of a total of $44.138 billion spent on diabetes was expended for treatment of acute metabolic conditions (~3% of the total).[1] Based on the reported 1994 prevalence of DKA, this leads to a calculated cost of $12,000–$15,000 per episode.[1]

DKA is the presenting manifestation of type 1 diabetes mellitus in only 20–25% of cases, and most cases of DKA do not occur in individuals with new-onset diabetes mellitus.[2,3] Eighty percent of DKA episodes occur in patients who are known to have diabetes mellitus. Since the majority of the episodes of DKA occur in patients with known diabetes mellitus and 20% of patients with DKA have multiple annual episodes, better patient education is needed.

DKA occurs with equal frequency in men and women; however, it does not occur with equal frequency in all races.[1] African-Americans have an excess DKA burden and data from 1980–1994 show that African-Americans had 2.3 times more hospital discharges for DKA than whites (15.7 episodes versus 6.8 episodes per 1000 diabetic population).[1] Additionally, the rate of DKA increased in African-Americans from 1980-1994, while during the same time it decreased in whites.[1]

Overall, the DKA death rate did not change from 1980–1994.[1] Each year there are approximately 1800 deaths in which DKA is the primary diagnosis.[1] There are an additional ~2800 deaths yearly in which DKA is a contributing cause of death.[1] From 1980–1994 the age-adjusted DKA death rate decreased 34%.[1] The highest DKA death rates are in persons >75 years of age, likely due to their comorbid medical conditions, and in persons <45 years of age.[1] African-American men have the highest DKA death rates, followed by African-American women and whites.[1] DKA mortality data are not available for many other ethnic groups such as Native Americans and Hispanics in whom diabetes is a prevalent condition.

Ketoacidosis is generally thought to be a problem of young diabetics; however, the average age of patients with ketoacidosis is 43 years and 50–85% of the episodes of DKA occur in adults.[3,4] Since these data were collected when the terms juvenile-onset and adult-onset diabetes were still being used, the results cannot be directly extended to type 1 diabetes mellitus (T1DM) and type 2 diabetes mellitus (T2DM). Some older patients have T1DM and are predisposed to the development of DKA just as are younger patients. Many patients with DKA probably have T2DM since 19% of the patients in one series were obese.[3]

Although the entities of DKA and hyperglycemic hyperosmolar syndrome (HHS) are often discussed as separate problems, many authors believe they represent states of decompensated diabetes that differ only by the magnitude of dehydration and the severity of acidosis. Careful review of large numbers of patients with decompensated diabetes mellitus suggests a continuum of decompensation with DKA at one extreme and HHS at the other.[5] Among patients with decompensated diabetes, 22% have DKA, 45% have HHS, and 33% have features of both.[6]

DKA may not be obvious at admission; in one series 20% of patients were not initially recognized to have ketoacidosis and were admitted to the hospital for a primary diagnosis other than diabetes mellitus.[3]

PATHOGENESIS OF DIABETIC KETOACIDOSIS

Although DKA is a complex metabolic disturbance of glucose, fat, and protein metabolism, the signs and symptoms are primarily due to abnormalities in the metabolism of carbohydrate and fat. The biochemistry of ketogenesis, which is critical in DKA, is discussed in detail in Chap. 2.

Hyperglycemia and consequently hyperosmolality occur as a result of overproduction of glucose by the liver and underutilization of glucose by peripheral tissues. When the blood glucose concentration exceeds the threshold for renal tubular reabsorption of glucose, glucosuria occurs and, as a result of the osmotic diuresis, water is lost in excess of electrolyte. Glomerular filtration is initially increased as water moves from the intracellular to the extracellular compartment due to the increase in extracellular osmolality. With the development of marked hypovolemia, glomerular filtration and renal glucose losses diminish, resulting in more severe hyperglycemia.

Because of the tight metabolic coupling of hepatic gluconeogenesis to ketogenesis, ketone body production is activated in DKA; its magnitude usually parallels that of glucose production. Ketoacidosis is primarily due to the overproduction of ketoacids by the liver, although underutilization of ketones makes a minor contribution to the ketonemia. The increase in ketoacid production causes the loss of bicarbonate and other body buffers, resulting in the development of metabolic acidosis.

DKA develops as a consequence of a deficiency of insulin and an excess of the glucose counterregulatory hormones catecholamines, cortisol, glucagon, and growth hormone.[7–9] The insulin deficiency may be relative rather than absolute. Insulin concentrations in patients with DKA are $\sim$10 μU/mL,[9] values that are clearly normal under basal conditions in a euglycemic individual, but are inappropriately low for the hyperglycemia that exists in patients with ketoacidosis. Glucose counterregulatory hormone concentrations are increased in DKA, as a result of coexistent physical and emotional stress or illness,[9] or simply as a consequence of insulin deficiency.[8] The concentrations of some of these hormones increase when insulin therapy is withdrawn under controlled experimental conditions that minimize stress and hypovolemia.[8,10] The administration of specific counterregulatory hormones to patients with T1DM who continue to receive intravenous insulin at rates that maintain basal insulin concentrations increases glucose and ketone body concentrations.[9] The development of DKA in patients who continue to take their insulin further emphasizes that the balance between insulin and the counterregulatory hormones is very important in the pathogenesis of ketoacidosis. The predisposition of the patient with diabetes to ketoacidosis is further amplified by the accentuated release of the glucose counterregulatory hormones that occurs in poorly controlled diabetes. The poorly controlled diabetic develops higher concentrations of certain counterregulatory hormones for any given level of stress than does the nondiabetic.[11,12] In addition, the biologic response to a given concentration or dose of a glucose counterregulatory hormone is exaggerated in DKA.[13] Studies conducted in animals and humans for the purpose of understanding stress hyperglycemia demonstrate that the glucose counterregulatory hormones interact in a synergistic, rather than additive, manner (see Chap. 9).[14,15]

Glucagon is of particular importance in the development of DKA, because it influences both gluconeogenesis and ketogenesis (see Chap. 7). At physiologic concentrations, glucagon does not inhibit glucose utilization by peripheral tissues nor does it increase fat mobilization. When there is an absolute or relative deficiency of insulin, glucagon directly stimulates gluconeogenesis and ketogenesis. Glucagon secretion is increased in DKA and the magnitude of ketone body production directly correlates with the plasma glucagon concentration.[8] A deficiency of insulin and/or an excess of catecholamines, cortisol, and growth hormone augments hepatic

glucose production, inhibits peripheral glucose utilization, increases fat mobilization, and stimulates ketogenesis.[16–22] Free fatty acids (FFAs) provide the substrate necessary to support glucagon-stimulated hepatic ketogenesis. Glucagon can directly increase ketone body production in the absence of increased FFA release from adipose tissue by activating lipolysis of hepatic triglyceride. However, sustained production of ketone bodies requires an adequate supply of substrate FFAs.[23] The central role of glucagon in the development of ketoacidosis is emphasized by the attenuation that occurs in the rates of gluconeogenesis and ketogenesis when glucagon secretion is inhibited with somatostatin.[24,25] When insulin is withdrawn from diabetic patients, the major hormonal factors leading to DKA are probably insulin deficiency and glucagon excess.

The presence of increased concentrations of cortisol, epinephrine, growth hormone, and norepinephrine accentuates the impairment in peripheral glucose utilization and enhances lipolysis produced by insulin deficiency. In this way, the glucose counterregulatory hormones directly or indirectly increase ketone body production. In addition, epinephrine and cortisol are capable of increasing hepatic glucose production, through both glycogenolysis and gluconeogenesis.

The withdrawal of insulin from well-controlled patients with T1DM results in a prompt increase in hepatic glucose and ketone production.[8] Glucose utilization increases transiently, probably due to enhanced glucose utilization by non-insulin-dependent tissues, but glucose clearance is markedly reduced.[8] When insulin is readministered to these patients, glucose and ketone production decrease promptly, as do the plasma glucose and ketone body concentrations. However, these are controlled conditions in which hypovolemia and other stress factors are not present. Consequently, the roles of cortisol, epinephrine, and growth hormone in the development of DKA are minimized.

The withdrawal of insulin from previously well-controlled diabetics leads to progressive increases in the concentrations of epinephrine and glucagon.[8] These hormones are considerably more important in the development of ketoacidosis under everyday circumstances when illness, physical and emotional stress, and hypovolemia are coexistent factors. Although it is likely that the elevated concentrations of glucose counterregulatory hormones may themselves play an important role in the metabolic decompensation of DKA, their elevation may be due solely to insulin withdrawal. Whatever the role of the glucose counterregulatory hormones, they are clearly capable of further intensifying the metabolic defects that exist in DKA. Stress leading to the release of the glucose counterregulatory hormones can precipitate DKA in the presence of the usual insulin dose, whereas omission of insulin and its ensuing deficiency can result in the release of glucose counterregulatory hormones that further aggravate the metabolic effects of insulin deficiency.

TABLE 34-1. Effects of Insulin and Insulin Counterregulatory Hormones

	Gluconeogenesis Liver	Ketogenesis Liver	Glucose Utilization Muscle	Lipolysis Adipose Tissue
Insulin	↓	↓	↑	↓
Glucagon	↑	↑	→	→
Epinephrine	↑	↑	↓	↑
Cortisol	↑	↑	↓	↑
Growth hormone	→	↑	↓	↑

Glucose counterregulatory hormones decrease tissue responsiveness to insulin beyond the binding of insulin to its receptor (i.e., postreceptor or postbinding defect). Thus normal basal concentrations of insulin are less effective when there are increased concentrations of the glucose counterregulatory hormones. The biologic effects of these hormones are summarized in Table 34-1.

Recently, the possibility that prostaglandins (PGI$_2$ and PGE$_2$) may play a role in DKA was considered because their production is increased in experimental models of insulin deficiency.[26–28] In particular, it has been suggested that PGI$_2$ may contribute to the nausea, vomiting, abdominal pain, and "warm shock" commonly seen in patients with DKA.[26]

PRECIPITATING FACTORS

Intercurrent illness and discontinuation of insulin represent the two most readily identifiable factors that lead to the development of DKA.[4,29,30] Coexistent medical illness is the most common factor, accounting for 50–60% of the causes of DKA.[4,29,30] Infection is a common precipitating factor in patients with DKA. The inadvertent or unsuspected interruption of insulin administration due to pump malfunction in patients on continuous subcutaneous insulin infusion (CSII) is relatively common in some centers.[31,32] For example, in one study approximately 30% of patients treated with CSII developed ketoacidosis; half of the episodes were due to unnoticed interruption of insulin delivery, whereas the other half were associated with infection.[32] Fasting of moderate duration may potentiate the ketosis that occurs with insulin deficiency in T1DM patients while reducing the degree of hyperglycemia.[33]

In approximately 20–30% of patients with DKA, no precipitating factor can be found. This suggests that emotional stress may contribute to the development of DKA in certain patients.[34] Although recent studies have not supported the importance of psychological stress as a precipitating factor,[35] the stress models used in these studies do not duplicate the type of personal stress that individual patients may encounter in daily living.[36] A criticism of these studies is that the attempt to evaluate whether stress significantly alters diabetic control was conducted in well-controlled diabetics. It would be far more useful to study the effects of stress in patients whose diabetes is poorly controlled.

Recently, insulin omission as a feature of eating disorders was highlighted in a study of 341 women with T1DM who were 13–60 years of age.[37] Thirty-one percent of the women reported intentionally omitting insulin. This practice was most common among women aged 15–30 years (40.2%). Thirty percent of women aged 31–45 years and 19.7% of women aged 46–60 years reported insulin omission.[37] Sixteen percent of women aged 15–30 years, 4.3% of women aged 31–45 years, and 6.1% of women aged 46–60 years reported routine insulin omission.[37] The women who omitted insulin had significantly more eating attitude and eating behavior problems (fear that good glycemic control would lead to weight gain or feeling bloated), higher hemoglobin A$_{1c}$ values, more diabetes-related hospitalizations, increased emergency room visits, and a higher rate of neuropathy and retinopathy.[37] Omission of insulin is used by these girls and women to control their weight. A significant number of women reported omitting insulin to the point that they developed ketonuria. Although contrary to many studies, eating disorders have been shown to be twice as common in adolescent girls with T1DM than in those without diabetes.[38]

In urban African-Americans, poor compliance with medical regimens and substance abuse have been identified as important precipitating causes of diabetic decompensation.[39] In a recent prospective study of 144 consecutive DKA patients and 23 HHS patients in a large inner-city hospital, poor compliance with insulin therapy was found to be the major precipitating factor for DKA, found in 49% of patients.[39] Thirty-five percent of the DKA patients had confounding alcohol abuse and 13% had cocaine abuse, both of which may lead to poor compliance with medical regimens and compound economic stresses.[39] In another study of DKA in cocaine users, cocaine was associated with frequent omission of insulin and absence of a precipitating cause of DKA other than drug use.[40] Cocaine is associated with recidivism and recurrent episodes of DKA.[40] The mechanisms by which cocaine, in particular, may precipitate DKA are numerous and include effects on glucose counterregulatory hormones in addition to the direct central nervous system effects of the drug.[40]

An atypical form of ketoacidosis has been described in young, obese African-Americans, but has recently also been seen in other races and ethnic groups.[41–43] There is no history of preexistent diabetes mellitus and no obvious precipitating event. Their C peptide levels are normal and anti–islet cell antibodies are negative.[44] Because of the absence of autoimmune markers and its lack of association with specific HLA alleles and increased insulin secretion, it appears to be a form of T2DM. This is supported by the high prevalence of coexistent hypertension. Following control of DKA, these patients can often be initially managed with diet and low doses of sulfonylurea agents.[45]

In menstruating women, menstruation is associated with an increased incidence of DKA. Of 200 women studied, 76 reported changes in diabetic control related to menstruation.[46] Fifty-three women reported deterioration of glycemic control during menstruation and 23 reported improved control and increased hypoglycemia.[46] DKA has also been associated with sauna use, the ingestion of "ecstasy" followed by prolonged exercise, gestational diabetes, the use of glucocorticoids in a patient with gestational diabetes, and in glucagonoma.[47–50]

DIAGNOSIS

Traditionally, DKA is defined by a glucose level $\geq$300 mg/dL, HCO$_3^-$ $\leq$18 mEq/L, and a pH $\leq$7.30. A pH less than 7.35 in a patient with ketonemia and a glucose concentration greater than 300 mg/dL identify mild DKA. Because acute hyperventilation can lower the serum bicarbonate by as much as 5 mEq/L,[51] the presence of a bicarbonate less than 18–19 mEq/L in a patient with appropriate hyperglycemia should also suggest this diagnosis. The blood glucose concentration used as a criterion for DKA is difficult to define because there are patients with blood glucose concentrations above 300 mg/dL who have no evidence of DKA and a substantial number of patients with established DKA whose blood glucose concentrations are less than 300 mg/dL.[52] This emphasizes the variable expression of diabetic decompensation. Hyperglycemia need not be striking, and approximately 15% of patients with DKA have glucose concentrations of less than 350 mg/dL. Low glucose concentrations may be seen in settings where there may be inhibition of gluconeogenesis, such as with the use of alcohol, and in settings where glucose utilization is not completely insulin dependent, such as in women who are pregnant in whom the fetoplacental unit uses glucose in the absence of insulin. Fasting

TABLE 34-2. Calculations

Anion gap = [Na$^+$ − (Cl$^-$ + HCO$_3^-$)]	Normal = 8–14 mEq/L
	Average = 5–12 mEq/L

ΔGap = [patient gap − 12]
Primary gap acidosis − Δ anion gap/HCO$_3^-$ ≥ 0.8
Primary nongap acidosis = Δ anion gap/HCO$_3^-$ ≤ 0.4
Na$^+_{corr}$ = SNa$^+$ + 1.5 [(glucose − 150)/100]

may also be an important factor in the patient with DKA and mild hyperglycemia. Fasting in the setting of insulin deficiency is associated with less severe hyperglycemia and more severe ketoacidosis.[33] It is important to realize that despite relative "euglycemia," patients may be critically ill as a result of severe metabolic acidosis.

The pH of a patient with DKA depends on the degree of respiratory compensation as well as the presence of coexistent acid-base disturbances. The metabolic acidosis that occurs in DKA is one in which there is an increase in the anion gap. The anion gap is calculated by subtracting the sum of the chloride and bicarbonate concentrations from the "uncorrected" sodium concentration [Na$^+$ − (Cl$^-$ + HCO$_3^-$)][53] (Table 34-2). This difference represents the unmeasured anions that are present in plasma, primarily albumin and phosphate. The normal range is from 8–14 mEq/L; a value of 12 mEq/L is usually used to determine whether the anion gap is increased. In DKA, the increase in the anion gap is usually equal to the reduction in the bicarbonate concentration. However, many patients with DKA may deviate from this pattern and demonstrate varying degrees of anion-gap and hyperchloremic metabolic acidoses.[54] Wide variability in the type of metabolic acidosis will be detected if the increase in the anion gap is compared to the reduction in bicarbonate concentration (assuming that a normal baseline bicarbonate level existed before ketoacidosis developed) in DKA patients. At presentation ~46% of patients with DKA have a predominant anion-gap acidosis, 43% have a mixed anion-gap and hyperchloremic acidosis, and 11% have a predominantly hyperchloremic metabolic acidosis[54] (Table 34-3). Thus, in contrast to traditional thinking, at presentation approximately 55% of the patients have a hyperchloremic metabolic acidosis or a component of hyperchloremia.[54] The variable degree of hyperchloremia in DKA correlates with the magnitude of the hypovolemia that exists in the patient.[54] Patients with severe hypovolemia develop the typical reciprocal change in the anion gap and the bicarbonate concentration, due to retention of both the hydrogen ion and the ketoacid anion. In contrast, those patients who can maintain adequate volume and glomerular filtration while developing DKA excrete the ketoacid

anions in the urine while reabsorbing chloride, which leads to hyperchloremia.

The coexistence of other acid-base disturbances—such as metabolic alkalosis from nausea and vomiting or diuretic use, respiratory alkalosis from fever, infection, sepsis, or pneumonia, and hyperchloremic metabolic acidosis from diarrhea—can confound the diagnosis of DKA.[51]

Thus patients with coexistent medical problems may not have simple acid-base disturbances. For example, a hypochloremic, hypokalemic metabolic alkalosis induced by diuretic use may produce offsetting changes in systemic pH in a patient with DKA, which could erroneously suggest that the acidosis is mild when it is severe. An increase in the anion gap that is greater than the calculated reduction in the bicarbonate concentration should suggest coexistent metabolic alkalosis or respiratory acidosis in a patient with hypochloremia. The magnitude of the coexistent alkalosis may be even greater than that of the acidosis, so that the pH of the patient will be alkalemic ("diabetic ketoalkalosis").[55] If patients become alkalemic during recovery, a coexistent metabolic alkalosis should be considered. The presence of a chronic respiratory acidosis would minimize changes in bicarbonate concentrations while intensifying the acidemia.

In an uncomplicated patient with DKA, the respiratory response may be capable of reducing the P$_{CO_2}$ to 10 mm Hg, and the bicarbonate concentration may be as low as 5 mEq/L. More severe reductions in the bicarbonate concentration or less than optimum reduction in the P$_{CO_2}$ indicates the coexistence of other acid-base disturbances.

The osmolal gap (difference between the measured and calculated serum osmolality) may be increased in DKA. This value is usually <10 mOsm/L. When increased, it suggests the presence of low-molecular-weight alcohols, which also cause a "gap acidosis." The increase appears to be due in part to acetone and amino acids and in part to hemoconcentration.[56]

LABORATORY AND WATER ABNORMALITIES

Substantial deficits of sodium, potassium, magnesium, phosphorus, and water can develop in patients with DKA (Table 34-4). However, despite these deficits most patients have normal or elevated plasma concentrations of potassium, magnesium, and phosphorus at the time of presentation (Tables 34-5 and 34-6).[57,58] The presence of normal or increased electrolyte concentrations should not be interpreted to mean that body stores of these elements are normal or increased. The deficit in potassium is the most important;

TABLE 34-3. Acid-Base Disturbances in DKA at Admission and During Therapy

	Hyperchloremic Acidosis	Mixed Acidosis	Anion-Gap Acidosis
Gap/HCO$_3^-$ *	<0.4%	0.4–0.8%	>0.8%
Admission	11	43	46
4 Hours	46	36	17
8 Hours	72	19	9

* Gap = calculated anion gap (mEq/L) − 12.

ΔHCO$_3^-$ = 24 mEq/L − measured HCO$_3^-$.

Source: Reprinted with permission from Adrogue *et al.*[54]

TABLE 34-4. Average Deficits of Water and Electrolytes in DKA

Parameter	DKA
Water (L)	6
Water (mL/kg)*	100
Na (mEq/kg)	7–10
Cl (mEq/kg)	3–5
K (mEq/kg)	3–5
Mg (mEq/kg)	1–2
PO$_4$ (mmol/kg)	1–1.5
Calcium (mEq/kg)	1–2

* Per kilogram of body weight.

Source: Reprinted with permission from Ennis *et al.*[5]

TABLE 34-5. Serum Electrolyte Levels at Entry and After Therapy in Patients with DKA

	Entry			12 Hours		
	% Low	% Normal	% High	% Low	% Normal	% High
Sodium	67	26	7	26	41	38
Chloride	33	45	22	11	41	48
Bicarbonate	100	0	0	46	50	4
Calcium	28	68	4	73	23	4
Potassium	18	43	39	63	33	4
Magnesium	7	25	68	55	24	21
Phosphate	11	18	71	90	10	0

Source: Reprinted with permission from Martin et al.[58]

recognition and treatment of potassium deficiency is of major therapeutic importance.

The deficit of potassium in patients with DKA is 3–5 mEq/kg. During the course of therapy, the serum potassium concentration rapidly decreases, reaching a nadir at approximately 4–12 hours after beginning insulin therapy.[58] The deficit of potassium will become obvious during the course of therapy, particularly if potassium is not administered in adequate amounts. The hyperkalemia that exists in patients with DKA is usually attributed to a shift of hydrogen ion from the extracellular to the intracellular compartment and of potassium from the intracellular to the extracellular compartment. Other factors have been identified that may be more important determinants of the potassium concentration in DKA.[59] The potassium concentration in patients with DKA correlates best with the severity and magnitude of the existing ketoacidosis and hyperglycemia.[59] The administration of glucose to produce hyperglycemia in normal animals stimulates insulin release and the movement of potassium into the intracellular compartment. When insulin release is blocked in the presence of hyperglycemia, such as with the infusion of somatostatin to normal subjects, the serum potassium increases.[60] Thus, insulin deficiency is a major cause of the hyperkalemia that develops in patients with DKA. In normal animals, ketoacid infusion increases the secretion of insulin, elevates portal vein insulin concentrations, stimulates hepatic uptake of potassium, and lowers serum potassium concentrations.[61] In

contrast, the infusion of mineral acid stimulates the release of glucagon but not of insulin, increases hepatic potassium release, and causes hyperkalemia. Lastly, when volume contraction becomes sufficiently severe so as to reduce the glomerular filtration rate, decreased excretion of both potassium and glucose in the urine accentuates the hyperkalemia. Thus the tendency for the serum potassium concentration to decrease rapidly during therapy may be a reflection of the direct action of insulin on cellular potassium uptake, alterations in systemic pH, a reduction in the serum glucose concentration and associated hyperosmolality, and enhanced renal potassium excretion.

A deficit of phosphorus occurs during the development of DKA and may reach 1.0–1.5 mmol/kg of body weight.[57] However, since total body phosphorus stores are 6000–8000 mmol, this represents a mild degree of phosphorus deficiency. The hyperphosphatemia that exists at diagnosis of DKA is attributed to the effects of metabolic acidosis on cellular function and the release of phosphate.

While hypophosphatemia often develops during the course of therapy, adverse effects are rare.[62–64] Serious complications of hypophosphatemia are encountered only when the serum phosphate concentration falls to less than 1 mg/dL.[65] Nonetheless, studies have shown that diaphragmatic and skeletal muscle function may be adversely affected by more modest reductions in the phosphate concentration,[66,67] and that hypophosphatemia may lead to impaired myocardial contractility.[68] The routine use of phosphate supplementation has not been demonstrated to alter morbidity or mortality and is not recommended.[62–64]

Hyponatremia is seen in approximately two-thirds of patients with advanced DKA despite an osmotic diuresis and loss of water in excess of electrolyte. The presence of hyponatremia is due to the effect of hyperglycemia and hyperosmolality on the distribution of water in the intra- and extracellular compartments. Hypernatremia would be expected because of the osmotic diuresis and excretion of water in excess of solute, but the hyperglycemia holds a relative excess of water in the extracellular compartment and contributes to the persistence of hyponatremia until the water deficit is extreme. Thus a disproportionate amount of body water exists in the extracellular compartment in the face of volume contraction (hypovolemia). The shift of water from the intracellular to the extracellular compartment would be expected to produce a predictable lowering in the serum sodium concentration if the water remained exclusively within the extracellular compartment; however, because it is excreted in the urine, this relationship is less precise. As a rule, a 1.6–1.8-mEq/L reduction in the serum sodium concentration can be expected for every 100 mg/dL increase in the glucose concentration[69] (Table 34-2). Recently, it has been suggested that

TABLE 34-6. Average Laboratory Findings in DKA

Glucose (mg/dL)	475
S_{osm} (mosm/kg)	309
Na (mEq/L)	131
K (mEq/L)	4.8
HCO_3 (mEq/L)	9
BUN (mg/dL)	21
Anion gap (mEq/L)	29
ΔGap (anion gap $-$ 12) (mEq/L)	17
pH	<7.3
Ketonuria	≥3+
Growth hormone (ng/mL)	7.9
Cortisol (μg/dL)	49
FFA (mmol/L)	2.26
Glucagon (pg/mL)	400–500
Lactate (mmol/L)	4.6
β-Hydroxybutyrate (mmol/L)	13.7
Catecholamines (ng/mL)	1.78 ± 4

Source: Reprinted with permission from Ennis et al.[5]

the serum sodium decreases by ~2.4 mEq/L for hyperglycemia ≤400 mg/dL and by 4.0 mEq/L for glucose concentrations >400 mg/dL.[70] These data suggest that the change in the serum sodium due to hyperglycemia is underestimated by using a factor of 1.6–1.8 mEq/L.[70] This approximation is valuable because it allows identification of those patients whose degree of hyponatremia is excessive for the prevailing hyperglycemia. Serum sodium concentrations that are less than 120 mEq/L are uncommon, and when present, suggest the presence of hypertriglyceridemia or other disorders that are associated with hyponatremia. In insulin-deficient states, lipoprotein lipase activity is decreased.[71] This leads to a marked reduction in the clearance of triglyceride from the plasma. Serum sodium, potassium, and chloride levels are spuriously decreased in the presence of extremely elevated triglycerides.[71–73] Similarly, "pseudonormoglycemia" has been reported.[71–73] This occurs because electrolytes and glucose are present in the aqueous portion of plasma or serum, whereas concentrations are measured and reported per total volume of sample. In addition, some spectrophotometric methods and bedside blood glucose testing kits may underestimate the glucose value due to lipemic interference with assay methods.[72] Ultracentrifugation of samples will allow the accurate measurement of electrolytes and glucose; however, this usually is not possible. It is essential that the laboratory report the presence of lipemia so that the spurious nature of unanticipated low concentrations of electrolytes and glucose can be appreciated.

Severe hyponatremia may be encountered in patients with end-stage renal disease in whom neither the glucose nor the water, which has shifted out of the cell, can be excreted. In such individuals, lowering the glucose concentration with insulin may be all that is necessary to correct the hyponatremia.[74] When the serum sodium concentration is normal or increased in a patient with DKA, lowering the serum glucose concentration may be associated with the development of hypernatremia, particularly in those patients who receive large volumes of isotonic saline. This is due to loss of water from the extracellular to the intracellular compartment as the glucose concentration falls and to the increased renal tubular reabsorption of sodium induced by volume contraction.

Although magnesium deficiency develops in patients with DKA,[75] the deficit is not usually significant. It is rarely associated with signs or symptoms, and generally corrects itself when a regular diet is resumed. Because magnesium deficiency impairs both the secretion and action of parathyroid hormone,[76,77] patients may develop symptomatic hypocalcemia if they receive phosphate supplements.[78] The phosphate reduces the plasma ionized-calcium concentration, which cannot be restored to normal because of magnesium deficiency. Such patients require calcium supplementation to acutely correct symptomatic hypocalcemia and magnesium replacement to maintain a normal serum calcium.

Hyperamylasemia may occur in patients with DKA.[79–81] Because DKA is often associated with abdominal pain, the presence of hyperamylasemia is of considerable clinical importance. Isoenzyme studies indicate that the amylase in DKA patients is frequently nonpancreatic in origin.[80] The presence of hyperamylasemia correlates poorly with abdominal complaints or physical findings in patients with DKA.[79,80] In addition, hyperamylasemia may occur in 30% of patients with metabolic acidosis who do not have pancreatitis,[82] indicating that it is specific neither for pancreatitis nor an intra-abdominal medical problem. Previously, if pancreatitis was suspected, a serum lipase measurement was obtained. However, the value of lipase measurements in DKA is uncertain. Marked hyperlipasemia, in the absence of clinical or radiographic evidence of pancreatitis, has been demonstrated in patients with DKA.[83,84] Total amylase levels are negatively correlated with bicarbonate levels and serum pH levels.[84] Pancreatic amylase and lipase correlate with glucose and BUN and are negatively correlated with serum bicarbonate levels.[84] The clinical evaluation of the patient is important with regard to the possibility of an intra-abdominal problem or pancreatitis. At the outset, signs and symptoms suggesting an intra-abdominal problem should be pursued aggressively. If there is hyperamylasemia, or hyperlipasemia, but there are no physical findings to suggest another intra-abdominal process, the patient should be followed carefully. The diagnosis of pancreatitis or an intra-abdominal process should be established based on appropriate clinical features. Abdominal pain commonly disappears in patients with DKA as the metabolic acidosis resolves.[85]

BLOOD KETONES

In DKA, the plasma concentrations of β-hydroxybutyrate (B), acetoacetate (A), and acetone are increased. The ratio of B to A (B:A), representing the mitochondrial redox state, shows considerable interindividual variability; however, the mean value for the ratio is only mildly elevated when all patients with DKA are considered.[86] Infrequently, the B/A ratio may be very high and the acidosis due almost exclusively to β-hydroxybutyrate.[87] This is an important diagnostic problem because quantitative plasma ketone measurements are not routinely available, whereas qualitative tests, which detect acetoacetate, may be negative or weakly positive in this situation. The tendency toward a higher B:A ratio in DKA is attributed to the more reduced redox state of the cell that accompanies increased FFA metabolism. The increased B:A ratio may also reflect impairment of β-hydroxybutyrate conversion to acetoacetate and the reduced utilization of ketones that occurs with insulin deficiency. The B:A ratio is shifted toward β-hydroxybutyrate when a more reduced intracellular redox state exists, such as with lactic acidosis resulting from low flow and tissue hypoxia, or from the use of alcohol.[87] Patients with alcoholic ketosis may have significant ketosis, but a negative or weakly positive plasma ketone test.[88] The presence of a combined keto- and lactic acidosis could be overlooked under these circumstances.[87]

Plasma acetone concentrations are markedly elevated in patients with DKA.[89,90] Acetone, a water-soluble and freely diffusible compound, is distributed throughout total body water so that the acetone pool is markedly expanded. Acetone is of low toxicity, but in large concentrations may produce narcosis. It has been suggested that the drowsiness of some patients with DKA is due to high plasma acetone concentrations. The plasma acetone concentration may remain elevated for up to 48 hours, long after the glucose, β-hydroxybutyrate, and acetoacetate concentrations return to normal.[88] This likely explains the ketonuria that has been observed for several days following successful therapy of DKA.

Plasma and urinary ketones are detected and semiquantitated by the use of the nitroprusside reaction. The nitroprusside reagent does not react with β-hydroxybutyrate, and on a molar basis is only one-twentieth as reactive with acetone as with acetoacetate.[91] Thus despite concentrations that are three- to fourfold greater than those of acetoacetate, acetone contributes only minimally to the color reaction. Acetoacetate, therefore, is the predominant determinant of the nitroprusside reaction. Thus, for a variety of reasons, this test correlates poorly with the degree of ketonemia. Additionally, several drugs have been associated with false-positive tests using the nitroprusside reaction.[92] Drugs that contain a sulfhydryl group such as captopril, dimercaprol, mesna, acetylcysteine, and penicillamine may give a false-positive result.[92] Additionally, very high intake of ascorbic acid may cause urinary acidification and result in a false-negative nitroprusside reaction.[92]

Recently, semiquantitative tests for β-hydroxybutyrate have become available. They are rapid and accurate and may be helpful in selected patient situations. To prevent the interference of acetoacetate with the measurement of β-hydroxybutyrate by the Keto-Site™ assay, the serum sample must be diluted.[93] Use of this test to define resolution of ketoacidosis (β-hydroxybutyrate ≤ 1.1 mmol/L) reveals that about one-half of patients still have positive serum Acetest™ results,[94] probably reflecting the slow elimination of acetone. Routine monitoring of ketones during treatment of DKA has not been shown to provide significant additional data to that provided by measuring the anion gap and glucose.

Following institution of therapy with insulin, the concentration of β-hydroxybutyrate decreases promptly while that of acetoacetate remains unchanged or increases slightly.[86] Later, the concentration of acetoacetate also decreases, reflecting the improved metabolic status. The preferential decrease in β-hydroxybutyrate reflects both decreased production and increased utilization. The shift in B:A ratio, however, particularly when the concentration of acetoacetate increases, accounts for the clinical observation that the plasma or urine Acetest reaction may become positive if initially negative, or more positive during the early phases of therapy.

TREATMENT OF DIABETIC KETOACIDOSIS

Successful treatment of DKA requires vigilant patient care as well as the use of effective doses of insulin, correction of volume deficits, and appropriate electrolyte supplementation. Adherence to these guidelines has resulted in a significant reduction in mortality from DKA (Table 34-7).

Until 1972, large doses of insulin were used in the treatment of DKA. The initial insulin dose and all subsequent doses were determined by the degree of hyperglycemia, the severity of the acidosis and ketonemia, or both. Complicated schemes were developed for the selection of insulin doses. Large doses of insulin were thought to be necessary because of the transient increased insulin resistance that resolved during therapy in most patients. In 1973, articles appeared in the literature demonstrating the effectiveness of small doses of insulin administered either by continuous intravenous infusion or intramuscularly. Most authorities recommend the use of low-dose insulin therapy for the treatment of DKA.

Although patients have been treated successfully with as little as 2 U of regular insulin per hour by continuous intravenous infusion, such doses provide an unacceptable rate of glucose reduction and are not recommended.[95] Despite variable rates of insulin administration, low doses (5–10 U/h, intramuscularly or intravenously) are effective in the treatment of most DKA patients. Although the rate at which the glucose concentration decreases varies considerably from patient to patient, it is fairly constant in any given patient. The average decline in the blood glucose concentration is 75–100 mg/dL/h and occurs at a predictable rate. Insulin can be administered either intramuscularly or intravenously, and at these doses produces plasma concentrations that are well within the maximum physiologic range (100–200 μU/mL).[96,97] Although most patients respond to these doses of insulin, there are some who

will not. Patients who are resistant to low doses of insulin cannot be identified prospectively by any clinical or laboratory parameter; consequently, low-dose insulin regimens require monitoring of patients at hourly intervals so that those who fail to respond can be detected at the earliest possible moment.

In the majority of DKA patients, large doses of insulin (50 U/h) administered intravenously do not reduce the blood glucose concentration more rapidly than doses of 5–10 U/h.[98] In the presence of infection, the rate of decrease in the blood glucose may be reduced by 50% to approximately 50 mg/dL/h. During the course of therapy, the plasma glucose concentration reaches a target of 250–300 mg/dL in approximately 4–6 hours, whereas correction of the acidosis (pH ≥ 7.30 or a bicarbonate concentration of ≤ 18 mEq/L) requires approximately 8–12 hours. During therapy, plasma ketone and bicarbonate concentrations change in a reciprocal fashion. The rate of resolution of hyperglycemia and ketoacidosis is not appreciably faster when high-dose and low-dose intramuscular regimens are compared[98] and is comparable to low-dose intravenous administration. Intramuscular insulin is no more effective than intravenous insulin when correction of hyperglycemia and acidosis is considered, and large doses may put patients at risk for hypoglycemia and hypokalemia.

Hypoglycemia and hypokalemia occurred in 25% of a group of patients receiving high doses of insulin during treatment of DKA.[98] If the glucose and potassium levels are monitored carefully, these problems usually can be avoided. The tendency of patients treated with large doses of insulin to develop hypokalemia may reflect their greater predisposition to hypoglycemia and excessive reentry of potassium into the intracellular compartment as it accompanies glucose, or may be a reflection of the direct effect of insulin on cellular potassium uptake. Since the rates at which the acidosis and hyperglycemia are corrected are similar, with 50 U/h and 5–10 U/h, it seems unlikely that the tendency toward hypokalemia reflects the effect of pH on the distribution of potassium between the intra- and extracellular compartments.

The low-dose intravenous and intramuscular insulin regimens appear to be equally effective for resolving hyperglycemia and acidosis. However, intramuscular low-dose insulin administration is not recommended in the severely hypovolemic patient owing to unpredictable absorption. Subcutaneous insulin administration should not be used.

The early decrease in plasma glucose concentrations will be largely a consequence of fluid administration, and therefore cannot be used as an indication of the adequacy of the insulin dose. The blood glucose concentration may decrease by as little as 9 mg/dL/h or as much as 90 mg/dL/h from rehydration.[99] Adequate rehydration contributes significantly to the decrease in the blood glucose concentration, not only as a consequence of dilution of glucose in a larger volume and improved GFR, but because it may also diminish the stimulus to release glucose counterregulatory hormones. During the initial phases of therapy, rehydration alone and dilution of glucose in the glucose space may account for 30–50%, and perhaps as much as 50–75%, of the reduction that occurs in the glucose concentration.[100–102] Glucosuria accounts for approximately 15–20% of the decrease in the glucose concentration when insulin and rehydration are used together.[103] The actual effects of insulin on glucose metabolism during treatment of DKA are rather small and are due primarily to inhibition of hepatic glucose production (accounts for 75% of insulin's effect) and not to increased glucose utilization (accounts for 25% of insulin's effect).[102]

TABLE 34-7 Therapy of DKA

INSULIN

1. 0.1 U/kg body weight regular insulin as intravenous bolus followed by 0.1 U/kg/h (5–10 U/h) thereafter as a continuous infusion until glucose concentration is 250–300 mg/dL and the pH $\geq$ 7.3 or HCO_3^- $\geq$ 18 mEq/L.

   OR

   10 U of regular insulin intravenously as a loading dose followed by 5–10 U/h intramuscularly.

2. Decrease administration to 2–3 U/h when the plasma glucose is 250–300 mg/dL *and* the HCO_3^- $\geq$ 18 mEq/L.

FLUIDS

0–1 hour

   1000–2000 mL 0.9% saline for prompt correction of hypotension/hypoperfusion.

1–4 hours

   750–1000 mL/h 0.9% saline or 0.45% saline based on intake, urinary output, clinical assessment of volume status, and laboratory measurements.

Glucose

   When the plasma glucose reaches 250–300 mg/dL, administer glucose at a rate of 5–10 g/h, either as a separate infusion or combined with saline.

ELECTROLYTE REPLACEMENT*

Potassium (replace as the chloride or phosphate)[†]

   Assure urinary output prior to potassium supplementation

   Maintain K^+ between 4 and 5 mEq/L

   $K^+ > 5.0$ mEq/L; no supplementation

   $K^+ = 4$–5 mEq/L; 20 mEq/L of replacement fluid

   $K^+ = 3$–4 mEq/L; 30–40 mEq/L of replacement fluid

   $K^+ \leq 3.0$ mEq/L; 40–60 mEq/L of replacement fluid

Phosphate

   Not routinely recommended; if indicated, 30–60 mmol of phosphate as potassium phosphate (K_2PO_4) over 24 hours.

Magnesium

   If $Mg^{++} < 1.8$ mEq/L or tetany present, give magnesium sulfate ($MgSO_4$), 5 g in 500 mL 0.45% saline over 5 hours.

Calcium

   For symptomatic hypocalcemia, give 10–20 mL of 10% calcium gluconate (100–200 mg elemental calcium as indicated).

Bicarbonate

   Not routinely recommended in the treatment of DKA. Consider if other indications present.

LABORATORY

Comprehensive admission profile

Arterial blood gases

Serum/urine ketone measurements

Check glucose every hour[‡]

Check electrolytes every 4 hours[‡]

Check Ca^{++}, Mg^{++}, phosphate every 4 hours

Cultures of blood, urine, sputum as indicated

GENERAL CARE

ECG prior to administration of supplemental potassium

Review urine output, vital signs, neurologic status, and laboratory data hourly

Frequent assessment of clinical status and repeat physical examination

Protection of the airway in the unconscious patient

Nasogastric suction as indicated for ileus, emesis, or obtundation with vulnerable airway

Chest radiograph and other imaging studies as needed

Consider CVP, Swan-Ganz catheterization in selected patients

---

* Drug doses should be modified in the patient with significant renal impairment.

[†] Dosage suggested using KCl.

[‡] Modified as necessary depending on clinical assessment.

Source: Modified with permission from Ennis *et al.*[5]

Changes in systemic pH usually do not occur for at least 1–2 hours after the onset of therapy.[103] Therefore, it is reasonable to continue the same dose of insulin for approximately 3–4 hours. If there has not been a substantial reduction in the glucose concentration and improvement in pH, larger doses of insulin should be used.

The success of low-dose insulin regimens is somewhat difficult to understand in light of previous claims that patients with DKA were severely insulin-resistant. The aggressive use of fluids in the therapy of patients may have contributed to the apparent sensitivity of patients to low doses of insulin. If fluid deficits are inadequately addressed, persistent hypovolemia continues to stimulate the re-

lease of counterregulatory hormones as well as impair glucose excretion in the urine. The sensitivity of patients with DKA to relatively low doses of insulin should not be interpreted to mean that these patients are insulin-sensitive and that no insulin resistance exists.[104] Patients with DKA who receive 5–10 U/h of insulin are obviously insulin-resistant. In a normal subject, the infusion of insulin at a rate of approximately 8 U/h requires the concomitant administration of 40 g of glucose per hour to maintain a constant blood glucose concentration.[104] When a normal subject is made hyperglycemic, but infused with somatostatin to prevent the release of endogenous insulin, the administration of exogenous insulin at a rate of 6 U/h is associated with a glucose disposal rate of about

60 g/h.[104] Thus 6–8 U/h can effectively metabolize 40–60 g of glucose per hour. In patients with DKA who are receiving insulin at 6–10 U/h, the glucose disposal rate is approximately 10 g/h, half of which is excreted in the urine.[104] Thus DKA patients are only one-tenth as insulin sensitive as nondiabetic patients.

The mechanisms of the insulin resistance in DKA patients are poorly understood. Glucose counterregulatory hormone levels are markedly increased in DKA. Hyperosmolality decreases insulin-mediated glucose utilization, but its effects are relatively modest.[105] Acidemia decreases receptor-mediated glucose metabolism, and phosphate deficiency produces a mild postbinding defect in glucose utilization.[106,107] Ketoacids, independent of pH, may also induce a postbinding abnormality in insulin action.[106] Therefore, the resistance may be multifactorial.

A rare cause of extreme insulin resistance in patients with DKA is the presence of anti-insulin antibodies that bind insulin. Since the maximum biologic response to insulin is significantly reduced in the postbinding type of insulin resistance, and because resistance resolves slowly, it is not clear how or why large doses of insulin overcome unusual insulin resistance within the brief period of treatment of DKA. Changes occur slowly (over 96 hours) in insulin sensitivity and in glucose metabolism following the achievement of euglycemia.[108] This leads to the frequent clinical observation that it takes more insulin to get patients under control than to keep them in control.

The discrepancy between the rates of correction of hyperglycemia and acidemia has important clinical implications. Insulin administration must be continued despite relative euglycemia until the pH and bicarbonate targets have been achieved. Consequently, glucose must be administered to "buffer" a further decrease in the glucose concentration during the continued administration of insulin. Because glucose disposal is 5–10 g/h under these circumstances, glucose should be administered initially at these rates. If the glucose concentration increases, then the rate of glucose administration should be reduced; if the glucose concentration continues to decrease, additional glucose is needed. Occasionally, the plasma glucose concentration is less than 300 mg/dL at the initiation of therapy and glucose must be incorporated into the initial fluids used for correction of hypovolemia. Although there has been considerable discussion over whether hypotonic or isotonic fluid should be used in DKA, most would agree that hypovolemia should be corrected with isotonic saline, 2–4 L. Thereafter, the decision to use 0.45% or 0.9% saline solution should be guided by hemodynamic considerations, fluid balance, and the prevailing serum sodium and chloride concentrations. In adult patients without severe volume deficits, a lower rate of saline infusion is associated with more rapid recovery of the plasma bicarbonate.[109]

Alternative intravenous solutions containing magnesium, potassium, and reduced chloride content (i.e., Plasmalyte™, Travenol/Baxter) have been advocated for use in the DKA patient, to provide a solution that closely resembles physiologic fluid replacement.[110,111] Their use is not routinely recommended. Insulin should be administered at a rate that ensures optimum or slightly greater than optimum concentrations of plasma insulin (100–200 mU/mL). This can be attained by administration of intramuscular or intravenous insulin at a rate of 5–10 U/h, particularly if an intravenous loading dose is administered as part of the intramuscular regimen. Formerly, recommendations advised that insulin be diluted with protein-containing solutions (plasma or albumin) to minimize the loss of insulin by adsorption to glassware and plastic tubing. This is unnecessary because the insulin-adsorbing capacity of plastic tubing can be saturated by discarding 50–100 mL of a 5-U/dL insulin solution. If this technique is not used or protein is not added to the solution, a lower rate of insulin administration occurs and may contribute to apparent insulin resistance.

Adjuvant therapies for severe insulin resistance are being explored. Reports have described the use of octreotide to suppress ketogenesis in resistant T1DM patients.[112] Octreotide administration suppresses endogenous glucagon secretion, thereby ameliorating the permissive effects of glucagon on the development of DKA. Recently, octreotide (50 μg every 6 hours subcutaneously) has been shown to improve resolution of ketonuria in DKA patients.[113] Suppression of glucagon release is a principal mechanism by which this occurs.[113] However, there was no improvement in the time to resolution of the DKA-associated hyperglycemia and acidosis.[113] Therefore, the use of octreotide cannot be advocated as an adjunct therapy for DKA. Treatment of severe insulin-resistant DKA with IGF-1 (insulin-like growth factor 1) has been found to reverse the hyperglycemia and ketoacidosis and to improve insulin sensitivity in a single patient.[114]

ACID-BASE CHANGES DURING THERAPY

Systemic pH is unchanged during the first hour after starting therapy with insulin and fluids.[103] Thereafter, the pH begins to increase, and by 6–12 hours it is usually between 7.25 and 7.35.[98] After 24 hours, the systemic pH is normal or near-normal, but arterial Pco_2 and bicarbonate are still reduced, a pattern consistent with compensated mild metabolic acidosis. It is unusual for the respiratory rate and therefore the Pco_2 to normalize during the first 24 hours, because the respiratory center continues to drive ventilation.[103] Alkalosis should be avoided because it reduces cerebral blood flow and increases the affinity of hemoglobin for oxygen, thereby reducing oxygen delivery to tissues. It also predisposes to hypokalemia and hypophosphatemia.[65]

There is some controversy concerning the routine use of bicarbonate in the treatment of DKA. Under normal circumstances, the pH of the intracellular compartment is substantially lower than that of the extracellular space and is relatively well protected against the adverse effects of acidemia in acute metabolic acidosis. Whereas bicarbonate equilibrates slowly across the cell membrane, CO_2 equilibrates rapidly. Thus when extracellular pH falls, respiration is stimulated and the Pco_2 decreases, minimizing intracellular pH changes. In fact, intracellular pH may actually increase acutely. While hepatic intracellular pH is markedly reduced in DKA owing to the production of metabolic acid at that site, other cells within the body are initially protected against the adverse effects of acidemia.

Because hemodynamic abnormalities begin to appear when the pH falls below 7.1–7.2, bicarbonate use may be considered in patients with acidemia of this severity.[115,116] On the other hand, some investigators do not recommend bicarbonate supplements unless the pH is less than 7.0.[117] In retrospective studies, no significant differences could be demonstrated with regard to correction of hyperglycemia, acidosis, and level of consciousness among patients treated with bicarbonate and those not treated with bicarbonate.[118–120] Interestingly, both ketone and lactate concentrations decreased more slowly in the patients who were treated with bicarbonate, but were of no apparent clinical consequence.[119] In a more recent prospective randomized study of 21 patients with severe DKA, bicarbonate had no effect on recovery or other metabolic parameters.[121] In a recent retrospective study of patients with severe DKA (pH values between 6.83 and 7.08), bicarbonate therapy (120 mEq $\pm$ 40 mEq) did not improve the time to DKA resolution.[122] However, the patients treated with bicarbonate required significantly greater potassium supplementation for hypokalemia during therapy.[122] Thus the routine use of bicarbonate in DKA appears to offer no therapeutic advantage. It should be noted, however, that in those patients with a marked reduction of the bicarbonate concentration and maximal respiratory compensation, any further reduction in the bicarbonate concentration is associated with a drastic shift in pH. Consequently, the use of small quantities of bicarbonate in individuals whose plasma bicarbonate is of the order of 5–10 mEq/L might be prudent. In addition to exacerbating hypokalemia, it is reasonable to ask whether there is a theoretical disadvantage to the use of bicarbonate. Bicarbonate has been demonstrated to increase ketoacid production in the setting of starvation.[123,124] Bicarbonate supplementation of subjects fasted for 5–7 days increased the plasma ketone concentrations as well as urinary ketoacid excretion, indicating that bicarbonate increased ketoacid production.[124] The exact mechanism for this effect is not clear, but is associated with a reduction in urinary nitrogen excretion and may be a mechanism by which protein breakdown is minimized in the fasting subject. The lack of effect of bicarbonate treatment on pH as well as the slower rate of decrease of the plasma ketone concentrations is consistent with these observations and suggests that bicarbonate may have increased ketoacid production. Although there may be a theoretical advantage to using bicarbonate in fasting subjects to minimize protein breakdown, there is no therapeutic advantage in the setting of DKA.

Patients recovering from DKA commonly demonstrate hyperchloremia and develop a non-anion-gap metabolic acidosis.[54,125] During the treatment of DKA, the anion-gap metabolic acidosis resolves quickly and is replaced by a mixed metabolic acidosis in which features of both an anion-gap and a hyperchloremic metabolic acidosis are present. The hyperchloremic metabolic acidosis begins to develop with therapy, and evolves progressively until it becomes the dominant acid-base disturbance. During the course of recovery, patients with a hyperchloremic metabolic acidosis at presentation may have a lower final bicarbonate concentration than those who present with the typical anion-gap metabolic acidosis.[54] The development of the hyperchloremic metabolic acidosis during the recovery phase is attributed to several factors: (1) The bicarbonate and buffer deficit in such patients is greater than is apparent from the reduction in the plasma bicarbonate concentration because buffer in bone and other tissues has also been lost; (2) the availability of substrate (ketones) for regeneration of bicarbonate is less than that required to stoichiometrically replace the buffer that has been lost, because considerable quantities of ketones have already been lost in the urine; (3) rapid volume expansion further increases the excretion of ketones in the urine, accentuating the deficit in substrate availability required to regenerate bicarbonate; (4) increased proximal tubular chloride reabsorption occurs, owing to limited bicarbonate availability; and perhaps, (5) if volume replacement is excessive, there is also decreased proximal tubular reabsorption of bicarbonate. Though persistence of acidemia in the early phases of the treatment of DKA is an indication for the continued administration of insulin, it is important to recognize that this recommendation does not hold for the hyperchloremic metabolic acidosis that emerges toward the end of active therapy when the other metabolic abnormalities have been corrected. When the hyperglycemia has been controlled, the pH has reached

7.3, and the patient is feeling well without any signs or symptoms of DKA, the rate of insulin administration can be reduced. The acquired hyperchloremic metabolic acidosis will resolve over several days as the kidneys adjust acid secretion and bicarbonate is regenerated.

ALTERATIONS IN CENTRAL NERVOUS SYSTEM FUNCTION AND STRUCTURE

There has been great interest in the central nervous system of patients with DKA. This is a result of the infrequent but devastating development of cerebral edema in some patients recovering from DKA.[126] Though rare, the syndrome of cerebral edema usually occurs during treatment of the first episode of ketoacidosis, but its mechanisms are poorly understood. Neurologic collapse may occur as early as 3.5 hours after implementation of therapy or as late as 22 hours. Neither hyponatremia nor the rate of fluid administration appears to be a precipitating factor. Most patients have corrected sodium concentrations (130 mEq/L), and cerebral edema has developed in patients who were rehydrated with oral fluids. Excessive lowering of the glucose concentration during therapy is probably not important, since it is less than 200 mg/dL in only ~25% of patients who develop this complication.[126] An etiologic role for the rate at which the hyperglycemia is corrected cannot be demonstrated.

During the course of therapy of DKA, the cerebrospinal fluid pressure increases to high levels without any obvious adverse effect.[127] The increase in pressure occurs during the first 10 hours of therapy, and values as high as 600 mm H_2O may be reached without fatal outcome. Papilledema is not observed. The cerebrospinal fluid pressure returns to normal within 9–10 hours. The complication of cerebral edema, if it develops, will usually do so within 14–16 hours of the initiation of therapy.[126]

In patients with coexistent hyponatremia, the plasma osmolality may be normal or just modestly elevated despite the presence of severe hyperglycemia. Correction of hyperglycemia during therapy without simultaneous elevation of the plasma sodium concentration permits adverse osmolar gradients to be created that favor the shift of fluid into the intracellular compartment of the brain and the development of cerebral edema. Careful intake and output measurements indicate that simple fluid overload is unlikely to be responsible for this problem. Large doses of glucocorticoids or mannitol or both[128] have been recommended as therapy, but there is little experience with the problem and it is difficult to know whether such an approach is beneficial.

Several theories have been proposed to explain this phenomenon. Paradoxical development of cerebrospinal fluid/central nervous system acidosis during treatment and altered central nervous system oxygenation resulting from increased hemoglobin affinity for oxygen and diminished cerebral blood flow during treatment of DKA seem unlikely causes of this complication. Development of an unfavorable osmotic gradient during therapy that favors excessive intracellular movement of water and overhydration of the central nervous system is the most plausible theory, but there are serious limitations with this theory as well.

The hypothesis has been postulated that the cerebral edema that occurs during the treatment of DKA is due to activation of the sodium-hydrogen exchanger in the cell membrane that regulates cytoplasmic pH.[129] Cytoplasmic acidification from high levels of organic acids activates sodium-hydrogen exchange, cellular sodium entry, and the exit of hydrogen from the cell. Cell volume increases and swelling occurs as a consequence of acidification of the cytoplasmic compartment. The hypothesis suggests that the cell swelling is asymptomatic prior to the initiation of therapy. During therapy, extracellular proton concentrations fall, thus decreasing the competition between extracellular sodium and hydrogen for transport, sodium uptake increases, and osmotic swelling occurs. Correction of the hyperglycemia produces a decrease in the extracellular osmolality that further accentuates the osmolar gradient between the extracellular and intracellular compartment and favors the movement of water into the cell. Last, insulin may also directly activate the exchanger on the surface of cells, thereby aggravating central nervous system swelling. Other investigators have disputed this theory.[130] At present the hypothesis remains unproved and little additional information is available.

The theory that unfavorable osmotic gradients develop during DKA therapy is more strongly supported than any other at the present time. In dogs, sudden correction of sustained hyperglycemia leads to increased cerebrospinal fluid pressure and cerebral edema. The theory that sustained hyperglycemia produces increased quantities of central nervous system sorbitol via the polyol pathway, and that the accumulation of this slowly metabolizable sugar within the brain results in cerebral edema when the blood glucose concentration is abruptly reduced, is not entirely correct. Measurement of sorbitol and other osmotically active sugars in brain tissue reveals that there are insufficient quantities of these substances to account for the increased intracellular osmolality that develops in the face of sustained hyperglycemia. Several interesting observations relevant to this theory are derived from studies in rabbits.[131,132] Acute hyperglycemia in rabbits will initially produce a loss of water from the brain and intracellular volume contraction. When the hyperglycemia is sustained, however, central nervous system volume and hydration are restored to normal. Thus mechanisms that protect the brain from water loss in the presence of sustained hyperosmolality appear to be operative.[133] The identity of these osmotically active particles, originally thought to be sorbitol but subsequently disproved, is still unknown, and they have been referred to as "idiogenic" osmoles.[131,134] In a rat model of streptozocin-induced DKA, preservation of brain water content despite severe volume depletion is partly explained by an increase in brain taurine content.[135] Taurine has been previously shown to function as an osmoprotector in several mammalian brain models. Additionally, its role as an inhibitory neurotransmitter, increasing the seizure threshold, may be important in DKA.[135]

When the blood glucose concentration is reduced by insulin from 55 mmol/L to less than 14 mmol/L (~300 mg/dL) over 4–6 hours, cerebral edema ensues. When the osmotic gradient between the brain and plasma is greater than 30 mOsm/kg, cerebral edema develops;[136] this gradient does not occur unless the blood glucose concentration is reduced to less than 14 mmol/L within 4 hours.[131] It is particularly interesting that cerebral edema does not develop when dialysis is used to reduce the blood glucose concentration instead of insulin.[131] With insulin, brain osmolality falls more slowly than plasma osmolality, favoring the formation of a significant gradient. In contrast, the decline in intra- and extracellular osmolality is parallel and proportional with dialysis. When insulin is used to correct the hyperglycemia, brain tissue analysis reveals that 50% of the osmotic gradient is due to electrolytes, including potassium, and 45% is due to unidentified particles. Brain water, sodium, and potassium are significantly increased by insulin. In view of its effects on electrolyte transport in other tissues, insulin may be important in the pathogenesis of this problem.[137] The recommendation that the glucose concentration not be acutely reduced to less than 250–300 mg/dL during the active phase of treatment of DKA is derived from these studies. Nonetheless, cerebral edema has developed in patients whose plasma glucose concentrations remained above 250–300 mg/dL.[126]

Cerebral edema is often unpredictable; however, 50% of patients in one series had prodromal headache, confusion, incontinence, changes in arousal and behavior, pupillary changes, blood pressure changes, bradycardia, disturbed temperature regulation, or seizures.[130] Therapy was successful in 50% of patients who had premonitory symptoms.[130] The development of headache or confusion during the course of therapy, particularly in a young patient or one being treated for the first episode of DKA, suggests incipient cerebral edema and the need for aggressive intervention. These symptoms usually occur at a time when there has been considerable metabolic improvement. In a recent study of six children with DKA, treatment was associated with mild cerebral edema in all patients, but none developed neurologic signs or symptoms.[138] They received combinations of isotonic and hypotonic saline with glucose at rates of administration that varied from 3.1–7.95 L/m²/24 h. Computed tomography demonstrated narrowing of the third and lateral ventricles, with a reduction in the subarachnoid space. Sensory evoked potentials may be prolonged within 2 hours after starting therapy for DKA in patients without obvious clinical manifestations, suggesting transient dysfunction during treatment.[139] Thus cerebral edema may be a common subclinical occurrence during the course of treatment of DKA. If this supposition is true, then the difference between those who do and those do not develop symptomatic cerebral edema is quantitative and not qualitative. All patients may develop cerebral edema, but only those with the greatest degree of cerebral edema are likely to have clinical complications. The issue of cerebral edema has been recently reviewed and its cause remains controversial and unresolved.[140–142]

MISCELLANEOUS COMPLICATIONS

It is well known that the P_{O_2} of patients presenting with DKA is significantly elevated and may decrease dramatically during the course of therapy.[143] Hypoxemia has been noted in 53% of patients during the treatment of DKA. In association with the marked reduction that occurs in plasma colloid oncotic pressure during therapy, the arterial P_{O_2} may decrease by a mean of 33 mm Hg and the P_{AO_2}–P_{aO_2} gradient may indicate pulmonary dysfunction, of which pulmonary edema may be one of several causes. The development of noncardiac pulmonary edema as a complication of DKA treatment has been described.[144] A reduction in plasma oncotic pressure in combination with reduced pleural pressure may predispose the patient to the development of pulmonary edema. Pulmonary edema has also been described in patients with chronic renal failure during therapy of DKA.[145]

Aspiration of gastric contents with subsequent respiratory problems or death is a rare complication of the treatment of DKA.[146] Gastric decompression may prevent this complication in selected patients.

The presence of hypothermia in patients with DKA is associated with a poor outcome. Despite hypothermia or absence of temperature elevation, a search for infection and consideration of concomitant endocrinopathy (i.e., myxedema) as a precipitating event for DKA is warranted. Mortality rates of 30–60% have been encountered in hypothermic patients.[147,148] Fulminant malignant hyperthermia has also been associated with DKA and coma.[149]

MORBIDITY AND MORTALITY

There is a common misconception that the mortality rate in DKA is low. Because a substantial number of patients with DKA are elderly, some mortality is expected.[6,150] Intercurrent illnesses are likely to be more serious in elderly patients with coexistent multisystem disease. In the elderly, the intercurrent illness is often the factor limiting survival, not the ketoacidosis.

Although the mortality rate of DKA has decreased, in 1994 DKA was the primary cause of 20 deaths per 100,000 diabetic patients.[1] There remains an excess DKA burden in the African-American population, which has a 2.3-fold increase in DKA.[1] Educational and economic resources must be allocated to this segment of the population to improve the mortality rate from DKA.[151,1] Fortunately, children under age 15 years rarely have fatal DKA[151] unless cerebral edema develops. Above the age of 15 years, DKA mortality increases progressively, reaching 15–28% in patients over the age of 65 years.[150]

Although coma is now infrequently encountered in patients with DKA, its presence is a bad prognostic sign and high mortality should be expected.[3] Mortality may approach 45% when coma is present.[150]

Prevention of DKA through improved recognition of precipitating factors, early diagnosis and therapy, and education should decrease the incidence of DKA and further improve its associated morbidity and mortality.

REFERENCES

1. Centers for Disease Control and Prevention: *Diabetes Surveillance, 1997.* U.S. Department of Health and Human Services:1997.
2. DeFronzo RA, Matsuda M, Barrett EJ: Diabetic ketoacidosis: A combined metabolic-nephrologic approach to therapy. *Diabetes Rev* 1994; 2:209.
3. Faich GA, Fishbein HA, Ellis SE: The epidemiology of diabetic acidosis: A population-based study. *Am J Epidemiol* 1983;117:551.
4. Johnson DD, Palumbo PJ, Chu CP: Diabetic ketoacidosis in a community-based population. *Mayo Clin Proc* 1980;55:83.
5. Ennis ED, Stahl EJvB, Kreisberg RA: The hyperosmolar hyperglycemic syndrome. *Diabetes Rev* 1994;1:115.
6. Wachtel TJ, Tetu-Mouradjian LM, Goldman DL, *et al*: Hyperosmolarity and acidosis in diabetes mellitus: A three-year experience in Rhode Island. *J Gen Intern Med* 1991;6:495.
7. Foster DW, McGarry JD: The metabolic derangements and treatment of diabetic ketoacidosis. *N Engl J Med* 1983;309:159.
8. Miles JM, Gerich JE: Glucose and ketone body kinetics in diabetic ketoacidosis. *J Clin Endocrinol Metab* 1983;12:303.
9. Schade DS, Eaton RP: Pathogenesis of diabetic ketoacidosis: A reappraisal. *Diabetes Care* 1979;2:296.
10. McRae JR, Day RP, Metz SA, *et al*: Prostaglandin E_2 metabolite levels during diabetic ketoacidosis. *Diabetes* 1985;34:761.
11. Christensen NJ: Plasma norepinephrine and epinephrine in untreated diabetics, during fasting and after insulin administration. *Diabetes* 1974;23:1.
12. Tamborlane WV, Sherwin RS, Koivisto V, *et al*: Normalization of the growth hormone and catecholamine response to exercise in juvenile onset diabetics treated with a portable insulin infusion pump. *Diabetes* 1979;28:785.
13. Weiss M, Keller U, Stauffacher W: Effect of epinephrine and somatostatin-induced insulin deficiency on ketone body kinetics and lipolysis in man. *Diabetes* 1984;33:738.

14. Eigler N, Sacca L, Sherwin RS: Synergistic interactions of physiologic increments of glucagon, epinephrine and cortisol in the dog: A model for stress-induced hyperglycemia. *J Clin Invest* 1979;63:114.
15. Shamoon H, Hendler R, Sherwin RS: Synergistic interactions among anti-insulin hormones in the pathogenesis of stress hyperglycemia in humans. *J Clin Endocrinol Metab* 1981;52:1235.
16. Schade DS, Eaton RP: The regulation of plasma ketone body concentration by counter-regulatory hormones in man. III. Effects of norepinephrine in normal man. *Diabetes* 1979;28:5.
17. Deibert DC, DeFronzo RA: Epinephrine-induced insulin resistance in man—A beta receptor mediated phenomenon. *J Clin Invest* 1980;65: 717.
18. Sacca L, Vigorito C, Cicala M, *et al*: Mechanisms of epinephrine-induced glucose intolerance in normal humans. *J Clin Invest* 1982;69: 284.
19. Schade DS, Eaton RP, Standefer J: Glucocorticoid regulation of plasma ketone body concentration in insulin deficient man. *J Clin Endocrinol Metab* 1977;44:1069.
20. Rizza RA, Mandarino LJ, Gerich JE: Cortisol-induced insulin resistance in man: Impaired suppression of glucose production and stimulation of glucose utilization due to a postreceptor defect of insulin action. *J Clin Endocrinol Metab* 1982;54:131.
21. Bratusch-Marrain PR, Smith D, DeFronzo RA: The effect of growth hormone on glucose metabolism and insulin secretion in man. *J Clin Endocrinol Metab* 1982;55:973.
22. Rizza RA, Mandarino LJ, Gerich JE: Effects of growth hormone on insulin action in man. Mechanisms of insulin resistance, impaired suppression of glucose production and impaired stimulation of glucose utilization. *Diabetes* 1982;31:663.
23. Miles JM, Haymond MW, Nissen SL, Gerich JE: Effects of free fatty acid availability, glucagon excess, and insulin deficiency on ketone body production in postabsorptive man. *J Clin Invest* 1983;71:1554.
24. Gerich JE, Lorenzi M, Schneider V, *et al*: Effects of somatostatin on plasma glucose and glucagon levels in human diabetes mellitus. Pathophysiologic and therapeutic implications. *N Engl J Med* 1974; 291:544.
25. Gerich JE, Lorenzi M, Bier DM, *et al*: Prevention of human diabetic ketoacidosis by somatostatin. Evidence for an essential role of glucagon. *N Engl J Med* 1975;292:985.
26. Axelrod L: Diabetic ketoacidosis. *Endocrinologist* 1992;2:375.
27. Axelrod L, Shulman GI, Blackshear DI, *et al*: Plasma level of 13,14-dihydro-15-keto-PGE_2 in patients with diabetic ketoacidosis and in normal fasting subjects. *Diabetes* 1986;35:1004.
28. Quyyumi AA, Iaffaldano R, Guerrero JL, *et al*: Prostacyclin and pathogenesis of hemodynamic abnormalities of diabetic ketoacidosis in rats. *Diabetes* 1989;38:1585.
29. Hockaday TD, Alberti KG: Diabetic coma. *J Clin Endocrinol Metab* 1972;1:751.
30. Schade DS, Eaton RP, Alberti KGMM, *et al*: *Diabetic Coma: Ketoacidosis and Hyperosmolar*, 1st ed. University of New Mexico Press: 1981;106.
31. Mecklenburg RS, Benson EA, Benson JW Jr, *et al*: Acute complications associated with insulin infusion pump therapy. Report of experience with 161 patients. *JAMA* 1984;252:3265.
32. Peden NR, Braaten JT, McKendry JB: Diabetic ketoacidosis during long-term treatment with continuous subcutaneous insulin infusion. *Diabetes Care* 1984;7:1.
33. Burge MR, Hardy KJ, Schade DS: Short-term fasting is a mechanism for the development of euglycemic ketoacidosis during periods of insulin deficiency. *J Clin Endocrinol Metab* 1993;76:1192.
34. MacGillivray MH, Bruck E, Voorhess ML: Acute diabetic ketoacidosis in children: Role of the stress hormones. *Pediatr Res* 1981;15:99.
35. Kemmer FW, Bisping R, Steingruber HJ, *et al*: Psychological stress and metabolic control in patients with type I diabetes mellitus. *N Engl J Med* 1986;314:1079.
36. Carter WR, Gonder-Frederick LA, Cox DJ, *et al*: Effect of stress on blood glucose in IDDM. *Diabetes Care* 1984;8:411.
37. Polonsky WH, Anderson BJ, Lohrer PA, *et al*: Insulin omission in women with IDDM. *Diabetes Care* 1994;17:1178.
38. Jones JM, Lawson ML, Daneman D, *et al*: Eating disorders in adolescent females with and without type 1 diabetes: Cross sectional study. *Br Med J* 2000;320:1563.
39. Umpierrez GE, Kelly JP, Navarrete JE, *et al*: Hyperglycemic crises in urban blacks. *Arch Intern Med* 1997;157:669.

40. Warner EA, Greene GS, Buchsbaum MS, *et al*: Diabetic ketoacidosis associated with cocaine use. *Arch Intern Med* 1998;158:1799.

41. Umpierrez GE, Casals MMC, Gebhart SSP, *et al*: Diabetic ketoacidosis in obese African-Americans. *Diabetes* 1995;44:790.

42. Pinhas-Hamiel O, Dolan LM, Zeitler PS: Diabetic ketoacidosis among obese African-American adolescents with NIDDM. *Diabetes Care* 1997;20:484.

43. Tan KCB, MacKay IR, Zimmet PZ, *et al*: Metabolic and immunologic features of Chinese patients with atypical diabetes mellitus. *JOURNAL?* 2000;23:335.

44. Umpierrez GE, Woo W, Hagopian WA, *et al*: Immunogenetic analysis suggests different pathogenesis for obese and lean African-Americans with diabetic ketoacidosis. *Diabetes Care* 1999;22:1517.

45. Umpierrez GE, Clark WS, Steen M: Sulfonylurea treatment prevents recurrence of hyperglycemia in obese African-American patients with a history of hyperglycemic crisis. *Diabetes Care* 1997;20:479.

46. Walsh CH, Malins JM: Menstruation and control of diabetes. *Br Med J* 1977;2:177.

47. Bienvenu B, Timsit J: Sauna-induced diabetic ketoacidosis. *Diabetes Care* 1999;22:1584.

48. Seymour HR, Gilman D, Quin JD: Severe ketoacidosis complicated by "ecstasy" ingestion and prolonged exercise. *Diabetic Med* 1996;13:908.

49. Bedalov A, Balasubramanyam A: Glucocorticoid-induced ketoacidosis in gestational diabetes: Sequela of the acute treatment of preterm labor. *Diabetes Care* 1997;20:922.

50. Anthony LB, Sharp SC, May ME: Case report: Diabetic ketoacidosis in a patient with glucagonoma. *Am J Med Sci* 1995;309:326.

51. Narins RG, Jones ER, Stom MC, *et al*: Diagnostic strategies in disorders of fluid, electrolyte and acid-base homeostasis. *Am J Med* 1982;72:496.

52. Munro JF, Campbell IW, McCuish AC, *et al*: Euglycaemic diabetic ketoacidosis. *Br Med J* 1973;2:578.

53. Emmett M, Narins RG: Clinical use of the anion gap. *Medicine* 1977;56:38.

54. Adrogue HJ, Wilson H, Boyd AE 3rd, *et al*: Plasma acid-base patterns in diabetic ketoacidosis. *N Engl J Med* 1982;307:1603.

55. Sanders G, Boyle G, Hunter S, *et al*: Mixed acid-base abnormalities in diabetes. *Diabetes Care* 1978;1:362.

56. Davidson DF: Excess osmolal gap in diabetic ketoacidosis explained. *Clin Chem* 1992;38:755.

57. Atchley DW, Loeb RF, Richards DW, *et al*: On diabetic acidosis: A detailed study of electrolyte balances following the withdrawal and reestablishment of insulin therapy. *J Clin Invest* 1933;12:297.

58. Martin HE, Smith K, Wilson IL: The fluid and electrolyte therapy of severe diabetic acidosis and ketosis. *Am J Med* 1956;20:376.

59. Adrogue HJ, Lederer ED, Suki WN, *et al*: Determinants of plasma potassium levels in diabetic ketoacidosis. *Medicine* 1986;65:163.

60. DeFronzo RA, Sherwin RS, Dillingham M, *et al*: Influence of basal insulin and glucagon secretion on potassium and sodium metabolism. *J Clin Invest* 1978;61:472.

61. Adrogue HJ, Chap Z, Ishida T, *et al*: Role of the endocrine pancreas in the kalemic response to acute metabolic acidosis in conscious dogs. *J Clin Invest* 1985;75:798.

62. Becker DJ, Brown DR, Steranka BH, *et al*: Phosphate replacement during treatment of diabetic ketosis. Effects on calcium and phosphorus homeostasis. *Am J Dis Child* 1983;137:241.

63. Fisher JN, Kitabchi AE: A randomized study of phosphate therapy in the treatment of diabetic ketoacidosis. *J Clin Endocrinol Metab* 1983;57:177.

64. Kebler R, McDonald FD, Cadnapaphornchai P: Dynamic changes in serum phosphorus levels in diabetic ketoacidosis. *Am J Med* 1985;79:571.

65. Knochel JP: The pathophysiology and clinical characteristics of severe hypophosphatemia. *Arch Intern Med* 1977;137:203.

66. Aubier M, Murciano D, Lecocguic Y, *et al*: Effect of hypophosphatemia on diaphragmatic contractility in patients with acute respiratory failure. *N Engl J Med* 1985;313:420.

67. Gravelyn TR, Brophy N, Siegert C, *et al*: Hypophosphatemia-associated respiratory muscle weakness in a general inpatient population. *Am J Med* 1988;84:870.

68. O'Connor LR, Wheeler WS, Bethune JE: Effect of hypophosphatemia on myocardial performance in man. *N Engl J Med* 1977;297:901.

69. Katz MA: Hyperglycemia-induced hyponatremia—calculation of expected serum sodium depression. *N Engl J Med* 1973;289:843.

70. Hillier TA, Abbott RD, Barrett EJ: Hyponatremia: Evaluating the correction factor for hyperglycemia. *Am J Med* 1999;106:399.

71. Rumbak MJ, Hughes TA, Kitabchi AE: Pseudonormoglycemia in diabetic ketoacidosis with elevated triglycerides. *Am J Emerg Med* 1991;9:61.

72. Baldwin L, Price L, Henderson A, *et al*: Spurious euglycaemia in severe diabetic ketoacidosis. *Lancet* 1992;340:1407.

73. Kaminska ES, Pourinotabbed G: Spurious laboratory values in diabetic ketoacidosis and hyperlipidemia. *Am J Emerg Med* 1993;11:77.

74. Ryder REJ, Hayes TM: Normo-osmolar, nonketotic, hyponatremic diabetic syndrome associated with impaired renal function. *Diabetes Care* 1983;6:402.

75. Levin GE, Mather HM, Pilkington TR: Tissue magnesium status in diabetes mellitus. *Diabetologia* 1981;21:131.

76. Anast CS, Winnacker JL, Forte LR, *et al*: Impaired release of parathyroid hormone in magnesium deficiency. *J Clin Endocrinol Metab* 1976;42:707.

77. Freitag JJ, Martin KJ, Conrades MB, *et al*: Evidence for skeletal resistance to parathyroid hormone in magnesium deficiency. Studies in isolated perfused bone. *J Clin Invest* 1979;64:1238.

78. Zipf WB, Bacon GE, Spencer ML, *et al*: Hypocalcemia, hypomagnesemia, and transient hypoparathyroidism during therapy with potassium phosphate in diabetic ketoacidosis. *Diabetes Care* 1979;2:265.

79. Knight AH, Williams DN, Ellis G, *et al*: Significance of hyperamylasaemia and abdominal pain in diabetic ketoacidosis. *Br Med J* 1973;3:128.

80. Warshaw AL, Feller ER, Lee KH: On the cause of raised serum-amylase in diabetic ketoacidosis. *Lancet* 1977;1:929.

81. Vinicor F, Lehrner LM, Karn RC, *et al*: Hyperamylasemia in diabetic ketoacidosis: Sources and significance. *Ann Intern Med* 1979;91:200.

82. Eckfeldt JH, Leatherman JW, Levitt MD: High prevalence of hyperamylasemia in patients with acidemia. *Ann Intern Med* 1986;104:362.

83. Nsien EE, Steinberg WM, Borum M, *et al*: Marked hyperlipasemia in diabetic ketoacidosis. A report of three cases. *J Clin Gastroenterol* 1992;15:117.

84. Vantyghem MC, Haye S, Balduyck M, *et al*: Changes in serum amylase, lipase and leukocyte elastase during diabetic ketoacidosis and poorly controlled diabetes mellitus. *Acta Diabetol* 1999;36:39.

85. Campbell IW, Duncan LJ, Innes JA, *et al*: Abdominal pain in diabetic metabolic decompensation. Clinical significance. *JAMA* 1975;233:166.

86. Stephens JM, Sulway MJ, Watkins PJ: Relationship of blood acetoacetate and 3-hydroxybutyrate in diabetes. *Diabetes* 1971;20:485.

87. Marliss EB, Ohman JL Jr, Aoki TT, *et al*: Altered redox state obscuring ketoacidosis in diabetic patients with lactic acidosis. *N Engl J Med* 1970;283:978.

88. Fulop M, Hoberman HD: Alcoholic ketosis. *Diabetes* 1975;24:785.

89. Sulway MJ, Malins JM: Acetone in diabetic ketoacidosis. *Lancet* 1970;2:736.

90. Reichard GA Jr, Skutches CL, Hoeldtke RD, *et al*: Acetone metabolism in humans during diabetic ketoacidosis. *Diabetes* 1986;35:668.

91. Nash J, Lister J, Vobes DH: Clinical test for ketonuria. *Lancet* 1954;1:801.

92. Laffel L: Ketone bodies: A review of physiology, pathophysiology and application of monitoring to diabetes. *Diabetes Metab Res Rev* 1999;15:412.

93. Foreback CC: β-Hydroxybutyrate and acetoacetate levels. *Am J Clin Pathol* 1997;108:602.

94. Umpierrez GE, Watts NB, Phillips LS: Clinical utility of beta-hydroxybutyrate determined by reflectance meter in the management of diabetic ketoacidosis. *Diabetes Care* 1995;18:137.

95. Kitabchi AE, Math R, Murphy MB: Optimal insulin delivery in diabetic ketoacidosis (DKA) and hyperglycemic, hyperosmolar nonketotic coma (HHNC). *Diabetes Care* 1982;5(suppl 1):78.

96. Schade DS, Eaton RP: Dose response to insulin in man: Differential effects on glucose and ketone body regulation. *J Clin Endocrinol Metab* 1977;44:1038.

97. Guerra SM, Kitabchi AE: Comparison of the effectiveness of various routes of insulin injection: Insulin levels and glucose response in normal subjects. *J Clin Endocrinol Metab* 1976;42:869.

98. Kitabchi AE, Ayyagari V, Guerra SM: The efficacy of low-dose versus conventional therapy of insulin for treatment of diabetic ketoacidosis. *Ann Intern Med* 1976;84:633.

99. Waldhausl W, Kleinberger G, Korn A, *et al*: Severe hyperglycemia: Effects of rehydration on endocrine derangements and blood glucose concentration. *Diabetes* 1979;28:577.

100. Owen OE, Licht JH, Sapir DG: Renal function and effects of partial rehydration during diabetic ketoacidosis. *Diabetes* 1981;30:510.

101. West ML, Marsden PA, Singer GG, *et al*: Quantitative analysis of glucose loss during acute therapy for hyperglycemic hyperosmolar syndrome. *Diabetes Care* 1986;9:465.

102. Luzi L, Barrett EJ, Groop LC, *et al*: Metabolic effect of low dose insulin therapy on glucose metabolism in diabetic ketoacidosis. *Diabetes* 1988;37:1470.

103. King AJ, Cooke NJ, McCuish A, *et al*: Acid-base changes during treatment of diabetic ketoacidosis. *Lancet* 1974;1:478.

104. Barrett EJ, DeFronzo RA, Bevilacqua S, *et al*: Insulin resistance in diabetic ketoacidosis. *Diabetes* 1982;31:923.

105. Bratusch-Marrain PR, DeFronzo RA: Impairment of insulin-mediated glucose metabolism by hyperosmolarity in man. *Diabetes* 1983;32:1028.

106. Van Putten JP, Wieringa T, Krans HM: Low pH and ketoacids induce insulin receptor binding and postbinding alterations in cultured 3T3 adipocytes. *Diabetes* 1985;34:744.

107. DeFronzo RA, Lang R: Hypophosphatemia and glucose intolerance: Evidence for tissue insensitivity to insulin. *N Engl J Med* 1980;303:1259.

108. Foss MC, Vlachokosta FV, Cunningham LN, *et al*: Restoration of glucose homeostasis in insulin-dependent diabetic subjects. An inducible process. *Diabetes* 1982;31:46.

109. Adrogue HJ, Barrero J, Eknoyan G: Salutary effects of modest fluid replacement in the treatment of adults with diabetic ketoacidosis. Use in patients without extreme volume deficit. *JAMA* 1989;262:2108.

110. Matz R: Intracellular magnesium deficiency. *Diabetes Care* 1992;15:1825.

111. Matz R: Refractory potassium repletion due to magnesium deficiency. *Arch Intern Med* 1992;152:2346.

112. Diem P, Robertson RP: Preventive effects of octreotide (SMS 201-995) on diabetic ketogenesis during insulin withdrawal. *Br J Clin Pharmacol* 1991;32:563.

113. Yun YS, Lee HC, Park CS, *et al*: Effects of long-acting somatostatin analogue (Sandostatin) on manifest diabetic ketoacidosis. *J Diabetes Complications* 1999;13:288.

114. Usala AL, Madigan T, Burguera B, *et al*: Brief report: Treatment of insulin-resistant diabetic ketoacidosis with insulin-like growth factor I in an adolescent with insulin-dependent diabetes. *N Engl J Med* 1992;327:853.

115. Narins RG, Bastl CP: Bicarbonate therapy in severe diabetic ketoacidosis. *Ann Intern Med* 1987;106:635.

116. Riley LJ Jr, Ilson BE, Narins RG: Acute metabolic acid-base disorders. *Crit Care Clin* 1987;3:699.

117. Schade DS, Eaton RP, Alberti KGMM, *et al*: *Diabetic Coma: Ketoacidosis and Hyperosmolar*, 1st ed. University of New Mexico Press: 1981;171.

118. Assal JP, Aoki TT, Manzano FM, *et al*: Metabolic effects of sodium bicarbonate in management of diabetic ketoacidosis. *Diabetes* 1974;23:405.

119. Hale PJ, Crase J, Nattrass M: Metabolic effects of bicarbonate in the treatment of diabetic ketoacidosis. *Br Med J* 1984;289:1035.

120. Lever E, Jaspan JB: Sodium bicarbonate therapy in severe diabetic ketoacidosis. *Am J Med* 1983;75:263.

121. Morris LR, Murphy MB, Kitabchi AE: Bicarbonate therapy in severe diabetic ketoacidosis. *Ann Intern Med* 1986;105:836.

122. Viallon A, Zeni F, Lafond P: Does bicarbonate therapy improve the management of severe diabetic ketoacidosis? *Crit Care Med* 1999;27:2690.

123. Hannaford MC, Leiter LA, Josse RG, *et al*: Protein wasting due to acidosis of prolonged fasting. *Am J Physiol* 1982;243:E251.

124. Hood VL, Danforth E Jr, Horton ES, *et al*: Impact of hydrogen ion on fasting ketogenesis: Feedback regulation of acid production. *Am J Physiol* 1982;242:F238.

125. Adrogue HJ, Eknoyan G, Suki WK: Diabetic ketoacidosis: Role of the kidney in the acid-base homeostasis re-evaluated. *Kidney Int* 1994;25:591.

126. Rosenbloom AL, Riley WJ, Weber FT, *et al*: Cerebral edema complicating diabetic ketoacidosis in childhood. *J Pediatr* 1980;96:357.

127. Clements RS Jr, Blumenthal SA, Morrison AD, *et al*: Increased cerebrospinal-fluid pressure during treatment of diabetic ketosis. *Lancet* 1971;2:671.

128. Franklin B, Liu J, Ginsberg-Fellner F: Cerebral edema and ophthalmoplegia reversed by mannitol in a new case of IDDM. Case report. *Pediatrics* 1982;69:87.

129. Van der Meulen JA, Klip A, Grinstein S: Possible mechanism for cerebral oedema in diabetic ketoacidosis. *Lancet* 1987;2:306.

130. Rosenbloom AL: Intracerebral crises during treatment of diabetic ketoacidosis. *Diabetes Care* 1990;13:22.

131. Arieff AI, Kleeman CR: Studies on mechanisms of cerebral edema in diabetic comas. Effects of hyperglycemia and rapid lowering of plasma glucose in normal rabbits. *J Clin Invest* 1973;52:571.

132. Arieff AI, Kleeman CR: Cerebral edema in diabetic comas. II. Effects of hyperosmolality, hyperglycemia and insulin in diabetic rabbits. *J Clin Endocrinol Metab* 1974;38:1057.

133. Prockop LD: Hyperglycemia, polyol accumulation, and increased intracranial pressure. *Arch Neurol* 1971;25:126.

134. Guisado R, Arieff AI: Neurologic manifestations of diabetic comas. Correlation with biochemical alterations in the brain. *Metabolism* 1975;24:665.

135. Harris GD, Lohr IW, Fiordalisi I, *et al*: Brain osmoregulation during extreme and moderate dehydration in a rat model of severe DKA. *Life Sci* 1993;53:185.

136. Fulop M, Tannenbaum H, Dreyer N: Ketotic hyperosmolar coma. *Lancet* 1973;2:635.

137. DeFronzo RA, Cooke CR, Andres R, *et al*: The effect of insulin on renal handling of sodium, potassium, calcium and phosphate in man. *J Clin Invest* 1975;55:845.

138. Krane EJ, Rockoff MA, Wallman JK, *et al*: Subclinical brain swelling in children during treatment of diabetic ketoacidosis. *N Engl J Med* 1985;312:1147.

139. Eisenhuber E, Madl C, Kramer L, *et al*: Subclinical brain dysfunction in patients with diabetic ketoacidosis. *Diabetes Care* 1996;19:1455.

140. Rosenbloom AL: Cerebral edema in diabetic ketoacidosis. *J Clin Endocrinol Metab* 2000;85:507.

141. Finberg L: Appropriate therapy can prevent cerebral swelling in diabetic ketoacidosis. *J Clin Endocrinol Metab* 2000;85:508.

142. Muir A: Cerebral edema in diabetic ketoacidosis: A look beyond rehydration. *J Clin Endocrinol Metab* 2000;85:509.

143. Fein IA, Rachow EC, Sprung CL, *et al*: Relation of colloid osmotic pressure to arterial hypoxemia and cerebral edema during crystalloid volume loading of patients with diabetic ketoacidosis. *Ann Intern Med* 1982;96:570.

144. Brun-Buisson CJL, Bonnet F, Bergeret S, *et al*: Recurrent high permeability pulmonary edema associated with diabetic ketoacidosis. *Crit Care Med* 1985;13:55.

145. Catalano C, Fabbian F, DiLandro D: Acute pulmonary oedema occurring in association with diabetic ketoacidosis in a diabetic patient with chronic renal failure. *Nephrol Dial Transplant* 1998;13:491.

146. Soler NG, FitzGerald MG, Bennett MA, *et al*: Intensive care in the management of diabetic ketoacidosis. *Lancet* 1973;1:951.

147. Gale EA, Tattersall RB: Hypothermia: A complication of diabetic ketoacidosis. *Br Med J* 1978;2:1387.

148. Guerin JM, Meyer P, Segrestaa JM: Hypothermia in diabetic ketoacidosis. *Diabetes Care* 1987;10:801.

149. Wappler F, Roewer N, Köchling A, *et al*: Fulminant malignant hyperthermia associated with ketoacidotic diabetic coma. *Intensive Care Med* 1996;22:809.

150. Center for Disease Control: Diabetes Control Demonstration Projects. 1978 Phase I Assessment Summary, June 1979.

151. Holman RC, Herron CA, Sinnock P: Epidemiologic characteristics of mortality from diabetes with acidosis or coma, United States, 1970–78. *Am J Public Health* 1983;73:1169.

CHAPTER 35

Hyperglycemic Hyperosmolar Syndrome

Robert Matz

In 1886 Dreschfeld[1] described two clinical types of a usually fatal acute or subacute complication of uncontrolled diabetes. The most common syndrome is now recognized as diabetic ketoacidosis. The less frequent form of the disease was typically seen in "older diabetics who are still stout and well nourished at the time of the attack"[1] and was characterized by a more insidious onset of drowsiness, eventuating in frank coma. This entity was sporadically recognized by clinicians[2] under a variety of names, and is now best characterized as the *hyperglycemic hyperosmolar syndrome* (HHS).[3]

DEFINITION

The entity is characterized by severe hyperglycemia (plasma glucose ≥600 mg/dL or ≥34 mmol/L), hyperosmolarity (effective osmolarity ≥320 mOsm/L), and dehydration in the absence of significant ketoacidosis (the presence of some ketonuria or mild ketonemia and an arterial pH as low as 7.3 or a serum bicarbonate as low as 15 mEq/L do not preclude the diagnosis) (Table 35-1). It occurs more frequently in the elderly, often mild, type 2 diabetic; develops more insidiously than diabetic ketoacidosis (DKA); is frequently associated with central nervous system dysfunction; is typically associated with severe fluid depletion and renal functional impairment; and has been claimed to have an extraordinarily high mortality. It is part of a clinical spectrum of severe hyperglycemic disorders[2-4] that ranges from hyperglycemic hyperosmolarity without ketosis to full-blown DKA, with a significant degree of overlap.

The term *diabetic coma* is a carryover from the preinsulin era, when coma was a frequent terminal event in the uncontrolled diabetic and over half of these patients on presentation were already comatose. Currently, only 10% of decompensated diabetics present in coma and more than 20% have no alteration of their state of consciousness. Any definition by laboratory values such as serum bicarbonate or serum ketone levels, plasma glucose, or serum osmolarity is arbitrary, and the term diabetic coma should be dropped.

HYPERGLYCEMIC HYPEROSMOLAR SYNDROME (HHS)

Early reports stressed the rarity and high mortality of HHS; however, pure hyperosmolar hyperglycemic diabetes is responsible for one-third to one-half of episodes of uncontrolled diabetes, and hyperosmolarity is present in an additional one-fifth to one-third of episodes, which we have termed *mixed HHS*.[2,4] Therefore, 50–75% of uncontrolled diabetic patients present with significant hyperosmolarity.

Life-threatening hyperosmolarity is not restricted to patients with diabetes mellitus, and is seen, for example, in association with diabetes insipidus and in the elderly with a variety of illnesses, or as severe hypernatremia with a mortality exceeding 40%. Hyperglycemic hyperosmolarity may follow the administration of many medications or a variety of acute illnesses. The precipitants are similar to those responsible for DKA.[3]

While it has been called nonketotic and nonacidotic, this is incorrect since as many as half of the adults and most children with hyperglycemic hyperosmolarity exhibit some degree of metabolic acidosis, with an increased anion gap reflecting excess lactate, azotemia, or a mild degree of ketonemia.[5,6]

The normal serum osmolarity is 290 ± 5 mOsm/L. A rough approximation of the actual value can be obtained as follows:

$$\text{Serum osmolarity (mOsm/L)} = 2[Na^+\ (mEq/L) + K^+\ (mEq/L)]$$
$$+ \frac{\text{plasma glucose (mg/dL)}}{18} + \frac{\text{BUN (mg/dL)}}{2.8}$$

In some calculations the serum K^+ is omitted.[3] Because urea is freely diffusible across cell membranes, it contributes little to the effective serum osmolarity relative to the intracellular space, and it is the effective osmolarity that is the critical determinant in hyperosmolar states. While HHS is referred to as "hyperosmolar" diabetes, the distinction should be made between osmolarity, which is the concentration of an osmolar solution, and tonicity, which is the osmotic pressure of a solution. Tonicity more appropriately reflects what we refer to as the *effective osmolarity* or Eosm.[5]

The effective serum osmolarity (Eosm) is calculated as follows:

$$Eosm = 2[Na^+\ (mEq/L) + K^+\ (mEq/L)]$$
$$+ \frac{\text{plasma glucose (mg/dL)}}{18}$$

When Eosm exceeds 320 mOsm/L, significant hyperosmolarity exists; when Eosm exceeds 350 mOsm/L, severe hyperosmolarity is present.

TABLE 35-1. Hyperglycemic Hyperosmolar Syndrome

- Blood glucose $\geq$ 600 mg/dL or $\geq$ 34 mmol/L
  - Eosm $\geq$ 320 mosm/L
  - Arterial pH $\geq$ 7.30
  - SERUM BICARBONATE > 15 mEq/L

  Eosm = Effective osmolarity

  $$= 2\,[Na^+ + K^+\,(mEq/L)] + \frac{Blood\ glucose\ (mg/dL)}{18}$$

Some authors omit the serum K^+ when calculating the Eosm.

PATHOGENESIS

Emphasis should be placed on the most common precipitants of uncontrolled diabetes. Infection,[3,5] omission or withdrawal of insulin from known diabetics, lack of adequate free water intake (vomiting, restraints, side rails, extremes of age, excessive seda-tion), a variety of physiologic stresses, and a growing number of medications must be considered, sought, and corrected (Fig. 35-1). Social isolation, especially in the elderly, is a major predisposing factor.[6]

The hyperglycemic hyperosmolar syndrome is restricted primarily to the infirm, neglected, very young, very old, institutionalized (in hospitals and nursing homes), mentally deficient, or impaired patients, and those who cannot recognize thirst or express their need for water. It is also seen in patients with major unreplaced fluid losses, usually secondary to a massive glucosuric osmotic diuresis, and following gastrointestinal fluid losses with a limited intake. These patients typically have type 2 diabetes mellitus (T2DM) or are not known to have diabetes prior to the hyperosmolar episode. Rarely, this syndrome may present in a type 1 diabetic at any age.

The critical initiating event is the development of a persistent glucosuric diuresis. Glucosuria develops when the amount of glucose presented to the proximal tubule is greater than 225 mg/min.

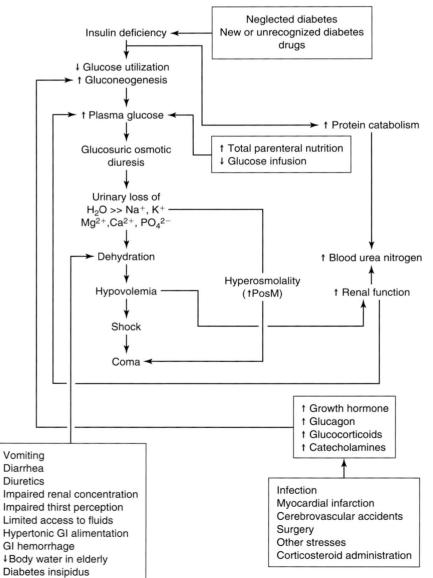

FIGURE 35-1. Pathogenesis of hyperglycemic hyperosmolar syndrome.

To achieve this tubular load, the plasma glucose must exceed 180 mg/dL at a normal glomerular filtration rate (GFR) of 125 mL/min. This level is the plasma renal threshold for glucose (the level beyond which, at normal GFR, glucose first appears in the urine). As the GFR decreases with renal insufficiency or intravascular volume depletion, greater levels of plasma glucose will be necessary to provide a tubular load of 225 mg/min. Thus, at a GFR of 62.5 mL/min, the plasma glucose would have to exceed 360 mg/dL to achieve this tubular load. When the tubular load of glucose exceeds 320 mg/min (the tubular maximum for glucose reabsorption or TmG), almost all of the glucose reaching the tubules above this amount is lost in the urine. As long as fluid intake is adequate and intravascular volume and GFR are maintained, loss of glucose above the threshold and the TmG functions as a renal safety valve, by preventing accumulation in the extracellular fluid (ECF) of nondiffusible glucose and associated life-threatening hyperosmolarity. If the GFR is normal (180 L/d), the filtered load of glucose is 1800 g/d at a plasma concentration of 1000 mg/dL. Since the normal kidney is capable of reabsorbing about 500 g of glucose per day, approximately 1300 g of glucose would be excreted per 24 hours. Thus a normally perfused kidney will not permit marked hyperglycemia to be present even for short periods of time. Since most patients with HHS do not have renal failure after treatment, their GFR must be reduced by a reversible mechanism, namely a marked contraction of the extracellular volume. It is failure to maintain adequate renal function due to primary kidney disease or secondary to intravascular volume depletion and the associated fall in GFR that results in remarkable elevations of the plasma glucose.

These patients may not respond to the stimulus of thirst because of incapacity, confusion, stroke, or age. Often they are unable to take or retain fluids due to restraints, sedation, coma, nausea and vomiting, or diarrhea. They may be receiving hyperosmotic nasogastric tube feedings or total parenteral nutrition with inadequate provision of free water, or have impaired renal function with inability to concentrate their urine or respond to antidiuretic hormone and conserve water. In any event, they do not ingest or retain sufficient quantities of free water to meet the demands of the glucosuric osmotic diuresis. These patients are losing electrolytes plus water, but the losses of water exceed those of electrolytes.[8] If these losses are not replaced, hypovolemia, intra- and extracellular dehydration, and hyperosmolarity develop, setting the stage for the sequence already outlined.

Some of these patients on presentation have an adequate urine output that declines to oliguric levels after plasma glucose levels are lowered to the 250–350-mg/dL range. Patients may suffer from the "latent shock of dehydration"[6] that can be made manifest by rapid correction of hyperglycemic hyperosmolarity without adequate volume replacement. If the plasma glucose concentration falls rapidly, the intracellular space, which is severely depleted of water and in osmotic equilibrium with the extracellular compartment, takes up water freed by the metabolism of glucose along an osmotic gradient favoring the movement of water from the extracellular to the intracellular space. This leaves behind a contracted intravascular space with concomitant hypotension and oliguria. Prevention is achieved by the infusion of larger volumes of crystalloid solutions early in therapy or at the first recognition of the complication. Controlled studies have not demonstrated the superiority of colloid over crystalloid solutions in this situation, and show no evidence that albumin administration reduces mortality in critically ill patients with hypovolemia, while suggesting that it may actually increase mortality.[9]

There is an age-related reduction in renal concentrating ability associated with a low-grade arginine vasopressin (ADH) resistance in the aged kidney.[10] Additional changes that occur with aging include a 30–50% decrease in GFR, renal blood flow (RBF), and kidney mass by age 70. The elderly also have a reduced total body water content. A young individual is approximately 70% water, whereas the elderly are 60% water by weight. This means that a 70-kg (155-lb) 30-year-old has 7–8 L more total body water than a 75-year-old of the same weight. The elderly have less total body water with which to buffer losses in water and changes in osmolarity, and a decreased sense of or response to thirst at serum osmolarities at which younger individuals are driven to drink, so they may not voluntarily drink water to correct significant hyperosmolarity and dehydration. Thus the elderly, for multiple reasons, are more vulnerable to and have limited ability to deal with an osmotic diuresis or any major loss of free water.

CLINICAL MANIFESTATIONS

The liver's ability to produce sugar in the diabetic exceeds 1 kg per day.[6] This gluconeogenic-induced hyperglycemia causes a massive solute diuresis, total body water depletion, and intracellular dehydration resulting in the classic features of uncontrolled diabetes mellitus: polyuria and polydipsia leading to hypovolemia, hypotension, organ hypoperfusion, and tachycardia. The osmotic diuresis results in loss of glucose, water, and multiple electrolytes. In the hyperosmolar nonacidotic patient, the entire syndrome evolves over a longer period of time (usually days to weeks) as compared to classical DKA, and ketosis either does not supervene or is a minor part of the picture.

The typical patient is over 60 years old,[3,4] but HHS may be seen in infants, children, or young adults.[2] Often the patient is not a previously known diabetic or the disease is mild and managed by diet, an oral hypoglycemic agent, or a small amount of insulin. Presentation may include a depressed mental status. In our series[2] 45% of the patients presenting with an Eosm >350 mOsm/L were comatose. The history is one of days to weeks of increasing thirst, polyuria, and frequently, in the background, a disease such as a stroke or renal insufficiency. Patients present with heavy glucosuria and minimal or no ketonuria or ketonemia. A history of weight loss, weakness, visual disturbances, and leg cramps during the preceding days or weeks may be elicited. Patients usually, but not invariably, appear severely ill. Physical examination demonstrates profound dehydration, poor tissue turgor, soft sunken eyeballs, cool extremities, and at times, a rapid thready pulse. In contrast to DKA, respirations are not Kussmaul in nature, and the aroma of acetone cannot be appreciated on the breath.

Nausea, vomiting, and abdominal pain occur less frequently than in DKA, while constipation and anorexia are occasionally seen. Gastric stasis and ileus is less frequent than in classical DKA. Hyperglycemia (levels >250 mg/dL) slows gastric emptying and gastric motility,[11] but cannot alone explain the nausea and vomiting seen in the uncontrolled diabetic. Mild gastrointestinal bleeding from hemorrhagic gastritis occurs in as many as 25% of patients. These findings are typically reversed by hydration and insulin. The occurrence of abdominal pain, tenderness, nausea and vomiting, lack of bowel sounds, and ileus in uncontrolled diabetes must not obscure possible intra-abdominal processes requiring urgent attention (e.g., mesenteric ischemia or cholecystitis). The response to therapy and the history are of critical importance.

Findings secondary to uncontrolled diabetes usually improve dramatically following the rapid infusion of fluids and insulin, and their development follows the onset of the symptoms of uncontrolled diabetes rather than preceding them. Another cause of abdominal pain and tenderness in the uncontrolled diabetic is fatty infiltration of the liver resulting in distension of Glisson's capsule. Liver function tests are abnormal in up to one-third of patients, and both liver functional abnormalities and hepatic size return to normal following treatment.

Hypothermia (rectal temperature $\leq$96.8°F or 36°C, or an oral temperature below 95°F or 35°C) or normothermia is the rule in DKA,[12] and deep hypothermia is a poor prognostic sign in the presence of ketoacidosis.[13] In HHS the average rectal temperature on admission in our series of 130 patients was 99.8°F (37.7°C) and in the fatal episodes 100.7°F (38.2°C).[3]

The dehydration encountered in the hyperosmolar patient has been thought responsible for the absence of physical (rales) or x-ray (infiltrates) evidence of pneumonia until rehydration is achieved, but this is a rarity and more often than not unauthenticated. However, evidence of congestive heart failure may be absent until the patient has been volume repleted. Therefore, patients with HHS should have a periodic repeat physical examination and, when indicated, x-ray examination, during the course of treatment.

The development of acute respiratory distress syndrome (ARDS) in uncontrolled diabetes has been fully described by Carroll and Matz,[13,14] but has been seen in only one patient with pure HHS. Nevertheless, 75% of the patients with this complication have had an Eosm exceeding 320 mOsm/L.

Few patients with HHS or DKA now present in true coma, and many have no clouding of consciousness. Investigators[15] have concluded that the depth of stupor in uncontrolled diabetes does not correlate with acidemia, but rather parallels the hyperglycemia and best correlates with the degree of hyperosmolarity. Acidosis has been claimed to correlate with the level of consciousness, but this relationship has not been confirmed.[16] Hyperosmolarity is not sufficient for the development of stupor in these patients.[15] The additional factor is the rapidity with which hyperosmolarity develops. Others[17] have proposed that the serum sodium concentration corrected for the concomitant serum glucose concentration provides a better index of cerebral hydration and identifies patients at risk for neurological impairment.[18] If the effect of urea is removed and the "effective osmolality" or "tonicity" is calculated, patients with Eosm levels of $\geq$320 mOsm/L may be comatose, whereas those with lower levels are typically not.

In summary, coma in the uncontrolled diabetic is primarily the result of hyperglycemia and hyperosmolarity and not acidosis. Coma rarely occurs unless the measured osmolarity exceeds 340 mOsm/L[5] or the Eosm is >320 mOsm/L,[2,17] and most comatose or stuporous patients have an Eosm >350 mOsm/L. The absence of hyperosmolarity (in the absence of hypoglycemia) in an obtunded diabetic suggests that the alteration in consciousness is not due to metabolic decompensation, and another cause must be sought.

Patients with HHS present with neurologic abnormalities that are rarely observed in DKA not accompanied by hyperosmolarity.[19] Up to 19% manifest grand mal or focal seizures and/or transient hemiparesis, and may have an extensor plantar reflex (Babinski) leading to the erroneous diagnosis of stroke. Additional findings may include aphasia, homonymous hemianopsia, hemisensory deficits, visual hallucinations, muscle fasciculations, opsoclonus-myoclonus, central hyperthermia, nystagmus, delirium, acute quadriplegia, and the exacerbation of a previous organic

mental syndrome.[6] The neurologic signs may be focal, often reflecting sites of prior central nervous system damage. Most of these neurologic abnormalities resolve with correction of the hyperosmolarity. Seizures, when present, should not be treated with anticonvulsants, especially diphenylhydantoin, because anticonvulsants are relatively ineffective in metabolic seizures and diphenylhydantoin has been responsible for precipitating HHS.[20] Seizures usually respond quickly to correction of hyperosmolarity.

Hypotension may be present on admission or develop subsequently if body water and intravascular volume are not adequately repleted.[6] This should be rare with early recognition of the syndrome and the more aggressive use of large volume infusions.

Vascular occlusions have been reported as the most important complication of HHS. These include mesenteric artery occlusion, low-flow syndrome, and disseminated intravascular coagulation. Arterial thromboses are claimed to be responsible for 33% of the deaths in comatose diabetics,[21] and there is speculation about the potential benefits of using anticoagulants and inhibitors of platelet function in these patients.[21,22] Recommendations for low-dose heparin in elderly comatose patients or those with severe hyperosmolarity have been made.[6] We[2] have found the incidence of vascular occlusions to be low (2%), and these events occurred in the presence of severe hypotension, dehydration with associated hemoconcentration, and hyperviscosity associated with low flow in an already compromised circulation. Since platelet aggregation is increased in diabetic subjects,[23] insulin-mediated vasodilation via endothelial release of nitric oxide is impaired in insulin-resistant states, and both type 2 diabetes and insulin resistance are associated with impaired fibrinolysis[23–25] and elevated plasminogen activator inhibitor-1 (PAI-1) levels, the invocation of an additional coagulopathy in HHS is questioned. Heme-positive gastric contents are seen in up to 25% of uncontrolled diabetes.[6] If full anticoagulation becomes routine, an increase in the incidence and severity of gastrointestinal hemorrhage might ensue. Aggressive volume repletion and Mg^{++} replacement[2,26] (which has a platelet antiaggregant effect) may account for the infrequency of thromboembolic complications in our series.[2] No prospective studies have demonstrated the safety or benefit of prophylactic full anticoagulation or of low-dose heparin. As in any acutely ill, bedridden, elderly patient with compromised circulatory status, underlying vascular disease, and a hypercoagulable state, low-dose heparin or low-molecular-weight heparin may be beneficial if there are no contraindications and the peripheral circulation is adequate to permit absorption. If there are specific indications for full anticoagulation, its use should be based on weighing the benefits versus the risks.

Rarely, pleural, pleuropericardial, and pericardial friction rubs and pain may occur in severely dehydrated patients with ketoacidosis, as well as in hyperglycemic hyperosmolar patients. Transient ST and T wave changes compatible with pericarditis maybe seen in patients with HHS with DKA. These evanescent findings are typically seen on presentation and rapidly resolve with hydration.[27,28]

LABORATORY FINDINGS

The laboratory characteristics of HHS are influenced by the criteria chosen for the definition. In two large series, the average plasma glucose was 998 mg/dL, HCO_3 was 21.6 mEq/L, Na^+ was 143 mEq/L, K^+ was 5.0 mEq/L, and the anion gap was 23.4 mEq/L.

A polymorphonuclear leukocytosis with a count in the 12,000–15,000/mm^3 range is the rule, and it may exceed 50,000/mm^3. In most patients the hematocrit will be increased secondary to intravascular volume contraction, with values over 55% commonly seen. A normal hematocrit on presentation should lead the clinician to anticipate anemia when volume has been restored. When the mean corpuscular hemoglobin concentration (MCHC) and hematocrit are determined by the Coulter technique, results may be artificially elevated in patients with hyperosmolarity, since the diluting fluid used during the analysis is isosmotic with normal serum and will cause swelling of hyperosmolar red cells. Abnormal liver function tests and multiple abnormalities of a variety of serum enzymes have been seen in 20–65% of patients with either DKA or HHS. Patients with uncontrolled diabetes develop the "euthyroid sick syndrome," with low levels of T_3, T_4, and TSH, plus elevated levels of reverse T_3.[29] Triglyceride and cholesterol levels are elevated in uncontrolled diabetes. The serum may appear lactescent and lipemia retinalis on funduscopy may be present.

Lipemia may cause methodologic interference with a number of laboratory tests. The problem previously referred to as "pseudo-hyponatremia," or a falsely low serum sodium seen in the presence of severely elevated triglycerides and chylomicrons when serum electrolytes were determined volumetrically, should no longer be an issue in laboratories where ion-specific electrodes are in use. Where older volumetric methods are utilized, pseudohyponatremia may still be seen.

The serum amylase may be elevated in DKA in the absence of acute pancreatitis, but this is uncommon in HHS, and in fact the amylase determination may be falsely low due to interference from serum triglycerides.

TREATMENT

Generally accepted aspects of therapy include searching for correctable precipitants, such as infection, and treating them promptly. In older patients and those with cardiovascular disease, a central venous line capable of monitoring the central venous pressure or a Swan-Ganz catheter is often warranted. If the patient is alert and capable of voiding, an indwelling urinary catheter should be avoided; however, in obtunded patients an indwelling catheter is necessary until they can void on demand, and urine output should be continuously monitored (Table 35-2).

Nasogastric intubation may be required since ileus, gastric distension, and mild gastrointestinal bleeding occur in a number of patients, and the obtunded patient is liable to vomit and aspirate gastric contents, further complicating therapy.

Neither body temperature nor white blood counts are reliable indicators of infection in these patients. Once appropriate cultures are obtained, if an infection is strongly suspected, conventional wisdom dictates antibiotic therapy.

If hypotension is present, large volumes of a crystalloid solution or a volume expander should be administered, and correction of hypoperfusion takes precedence over all other considerations. If necessary, pressors should be added to the regimen when the hypotension is refractory to volume replacement. When the hyperosmolar patient becomes hypotensive, there is no volume reserve to call upon since the hyperosmolar state has already effected maximum removal of water from the intracellular space to maintain the integrity of the intravascular compartment. This "autotransfusion" serves to preserve vascular volume and organ perfusion at the expense of intracellular volume.[5] Therefore, when shock supervenes, water must be rapidly replaced to restore the integrity of the circu-

lation. If hypotension persists after large volume infusions and/or pressors, other causes must be considered (e.g., myocardial infarction, sepsis, pancreatitis, or gastrointestinal hemorrhage).

While insulin resistance is present in virtually every diabetic and although hyperosmolarity results in impairment of insulin-mediated glucose metabolism and reduced pancreatic insulin secretion,[6] the large doses of insulin previously used to treat uncontrolled diabetes are unnecessary. If there is any question about the adequacy of peripheral perfusion, the intravenous route of insulin administration is most reliable. The use of intramuscular or subcutaneous insulin is acceptable as long as perfusion of the injection site is adequate and the clinician remembers that both the onset as well as cessation of action of insulin given in this manner is delayed. Repetitive intravenous insulin bolus treatment of the uncontrolled diabetic is inefficient and unreliable. We recommend an intravenous bolus of approximately 10–15 U of regular insulin to provide a rapid blood level, followed by a continuous infusion of 0.1 U/kg/h (in the average adult, 5–10 U/h). With all reported regimens, the rate of plasma glucose decline is linear and predictable at between 75 and 150 mg/dL/h, provided no other complicating features are present. The amount of insulin required to treat HHS is comparable to that required in DKA.

Once intravenous insulin is discontinued and intermittent subcutaneous insulin begun, management typically defaults to "sliding-scale" insulin coverage. This method of treatment has never undergone objective scrutiny and violates what is known about the physiology of insulin action, which indicates preemptive administration is needed to control hyperglycemia and repair the metabolic chaos of the uncontrolled diabetic state. It is intellectually, intuitively, and practically impossible to regulate blood glucose retroactively, and sliding-scale coverage, while it relieves the tired physician of the necessity to contemporaneously evaluate each glucose level, delays the establishment of a suitable prospective treatment regimen and prolongs hospitalization.

Because of the "safety-valve" function of the normal kidney[7] in the presence of plasma glucose concentrations exceeding the TmG, significant hyperglycemia can occur only if RBF and GFR are reduced (in the absence of an obstructive uropathy). When uncontrolled diabetics are rehydrated and renal blood flow is reestablished, the loss of glucose in the urine should rapidly lower the serum glucose to a level somewhere between the renal threshold and the TmG (i.e., between 180 and 350 mg/dL). Early in treatment the primary mechanism for glucose disposal is urinary excretion rather than insulin-mediated enhancement of glucose utilization.[21] Three mechanisms account for the early fall in plasma glucose in HHS. Dilution by infused fluids accounts for 24–34% of the total reduction, while glucosuria in those with a preserved GFR and the least reduced ECF accounts for most of the reduction (a 29–76% fall in the glucose pool[6]). Raising the GFR in the presence of a high plasma glucose results in excretion of larger amounts of glucose. The remaining early fall in blood glucose concentration is due to non-insulin-dependent glucose metabolism in organs such as the brain and kidney.

The fall in plasma glucose concentration during the early hours of treatment serves as an index of the adequacy of rehydration and the restoration of renal blood flow. Failure of the plasma glucose to fall implies either inadequate volume expansion or renal functional impairment. Therefore, the clinician must be wary of patients with uncontrolled diabetes and renal failure.[21] Patients with either HHS or hyperglycemia in the presence of renal failure may present with high plasma glucose, BUN, and

TABLE 35-2. Treatment of Hyperglycemic Hyperosmolar Syndrome

General
- Perform directed history and physical examination.
- Obtain plasma glucose, P, K^+, Ca^{++}, Mg^{++}, BUN, creatinine, electrolytes, CBC, urinalysis, chest x-ray, electrocardiogram, appropriate cultures, and ABGs.
- Aspirate stomach if patient is nauseated or vomiting, or if distension or bowel sounds are absent. Leave nasogastric tube in place on suction if large volume of gastric contents is obtained or if contents are guaiac-positive.
- Insert urinary catheter if unable to void or obtunded. Monitor urine output hourly.
- Administer thiamine and vitamin B complex IV.
- Administer antibiotics as appropriate for infection or suspected infection.
- Check for hypotension, state of consciousness (coma, stupor, or obtundation), hypothermia, or hyperthermia.
- Other directed studies as indicated (e.g., lumbar puncture if meningitis is suspected).
- Consider airway protection in obtunded or unconscious patients.

Fluids
- Administer 0.5 N electrolyte solution if Eosm >320 mOsm/L, at a rate of 1500 mL/h (15–30 mL/kg/h) for first hour, 1000 mL/h for second and third hours, and 500–750 mL/h for fourth hour.
- When Eosm <320 mOsm/L, crystalloid fluid prescription should be changed to 1 N concentration (isotonic).
- If hypotensive, give 2000 mL/h of electrolyte solution (osmolarity dependent on Eosm as above).
- If hypotension is unresponsive to crystalloids, consider use of colloid and pressors.
- May require central venous pressure and/or pulmonary capillary wedge pressure monitoring to guide treatment. (In complicated cases, monitoring of cardiac output, peripheral resistance, and other parameters may be essential.)
- Add 5% D5W when plasma glucose is 250–300 mg/dL.
- Caution! Reduce fluid administration in presence of renal failure.

Insulin
- Give 15-U regular insulin bolus intravenously followed by intravenous (or intramuscular or subcutaneous) infusion of regular insulin at a rate of 0.1 U/kg/h (5–10 U/h).
- Decrease dose to 2–3 U/h when plasma glucose is 250–300 mg/dL.
- If plasma glucose fails to decrease over 2–4 hours and urine output, fluid administration, and blood pressure are adequate, double insulin dose hourly.

Potassium
- Administer no K^+ if plasma K^+ >5.0 mEq/L.
- Administer 20 mEq/h of K^+ as one-half potassium acetate and one-half potassium phosphate if plasma K^+ is 4–5 mEq/L.
- Administer 40 mEq K^+/h two times if plasma K^+ is 3–4 mEq/L, then administer 20 mEq/h while rechecking K^+.
- Administer 60 mEq/h one time if plasma K^+ <3.0 mEq/L, and then 40 mEq/h one time while plasma K^+ is rechecked.
- Monitor ECG hourly (leads V_4 and V_5) for T waves to assist in guiding therapy between K^+ determinations.

Phosphate
- Administer 0.1 mmol/kg/h (5–10 mmol/h) to maximum of 80–120 mmol/24 h.
- If serum P falls below 1.0 mg/dL, increase infusion to 0.15 mmol/kg/h (10–15 mmol/h).
- If tetany develops, stop phosphate infusion, administer Ca^{++}/Mg^{++}, and check Ca^{++} and Mg^{++} levels.
- Do not use in presence of renal failure.

Magnesium
- Utilize physiologic multielectrolyte solutions containing Mg^{++} (3–5 mEq/L) as standard intravenous fluid vehicle.
- Administer 0.05–0.1 mL/kg of 20% $MgSO_4$ intramuscularly (or IV) (i.e., 4–8 mL of 20% $MgSO_4$ [0.08–0.16 mEq/kg]).
- If Mg^{++} is low or tetany develops, administer 500 mL of 2% $MgSO_4$ solution intravenously over 4 hours plus additional IM doses of 6–12 mEq every 6–8 hours.
- Do not use in presence of renal failure.

Calcium
- If Ca^{++} is low or tetany develops, administer 10 mEq as an intravenous bolus and repeat as indicated.

Comments
- Repeat K^+ hourly or as indicated.
- Repeat Na^+, venous bicarbonate, BUN every 2–4 hours.
- Once plasma glucose is <600 mg/dL, utilize bedside fingerstick blood glucose testing hourly to monitor. Confirm with chemistry lab values every 2–4 hours.
- Monitor blood pressure, pulse rate, temperature, and respiratory rate hourly until stable for 2–4 hours.
- Repeat pertinent physical exam as necessary, with special concentration on neurologic (mental) status; repeat exam of lungs for evidence of pneumonia, CHF, or ARDS; perform abdominal exam if NG tube has been inserted.
- Monitor intake and output hourly for at least 8 hours or until stable.
- Repeat pertinent tests as clinically indicated: ABGs, Hb/Hct, Mg^{++} chest x-ray.
- In the absence of contraindications, consider prophylactic low-dose heparin or low-molecular-weight heparin.

creatinine. If renal failure is unrecognized and rapid fluid replacement is begun, pulmonary edema and/or congestive heart failure is inevitable. For hyperglycemia accompanying renal failure, therapy with insulin alone, often in high doses, is appropriate. Insulin will reduce elevated potassium levels and as plasma glucose falls, the water freed will move out of the ECF into the intracellular space, thus decreasing the manifestations of circulatory congestion. Sudden loss of control of diabetes in the presence of advanced renal failure may cause pulmonary edema and life-threatening hyperkalemia, both reversible by the use of insulin alone.

The fluid losses in HHS range from 4.8 to 12.6 L with a mean of 9.1 L.[6] The fluid lost is hypotonic with respect to electrolytes. Therefore, the losses should be replaced with a hypotonic electrolyte solution (0.45% NaCl or a 0.5 N balanced electrolyte solution). Half-normal balanced electrolyte solutions (e.g., Plasmalyte™, Isolyte S™, Normosol™ or lactated Ringer's) avoid the administration of excess chloride that occurs when saline is used to replace the lost free water. Isotonic solutions, while initially hypotonic to the patient's serum, provide excessive amounts of sodium, and in the case of saline, excess chloride, resulting in hypernatremia or hyperchloremia while aggravating the tendency toward insulin-induced edema. The time has come to replace normal saline and 0.5 N saline with these physiological solutions in the therapy of the uncontrolled diabetic. Until the initial tonicity of the serum (Eosm) can be calculated, especially if the patient is hypotensive, isotonic fluid resuscitation with 1 or 2 L of crystalloid may be used. However, once evidence of significant hyperosmolarity is obtained, hypotonic replacement is safe, effective, and sensible.[3,30]

The arguments against the use of hypotonic solutions in HHS include the concerns that there will be too rapid a fall in ECF osmolarity,[22] that isotonic solutions are already hypotonic with respect to the hyperosmolar fluid compartment of the patient, and that isotonic saline provides a better means of maintaining adequate ECF volume. While isotonic saline initially lowers the osmolarity, it provides more sodium and chloride relative to water than the hypertonic patient needs. As the water freed from the osmotic hold of glucose pours into the hyperosmolar intracellular space, the osmotically active particles of glucose are replaced by equally osmotically active sodium, with resultant prolongation of the hyperosmolar state and development of hypernatremia, which carries a 42% mortality rate,[6] considerably greater than the mortality associated with hyperglycemic hyperosmolarity of comparable severity. While early efforts at treatment and fluid replacement continue, the hyperglycemic hyperosmolar diabetic is still undergoing a massive osmotic diuresis that continually removes water in excess of electrolytes until the glucosuria is curbed. This adds to the body's need for free water without electrolytes or osmoles.[31]

Genuth[30] suggests that the increase in serum Na$^+$ levels, sometimes to 160–170 mEq/L, during therapy of HHS and the occasional persistence of hypernatremia in the 150–155-mEq/L range for days after correction of hyperglycemia in some patients is associated with an elevated serum creatinine, high ADH levels, and unresponsiveness to exogenous AVP, all of which suggest temporary nephrogenic diabetes insipidus. In these patients provision of additional free water in the form of hypotonic solutions may be essential to correct the elevated Na$^+$. Of course, D5W with sufficient insulin to maintain glucose metabolism will provide the necessary free water.

If isotonic replacement solutions are used initially, frequent monitoring of serum concentrations of sodium and chloride are essential to avoid replacing hyperglycemia with hypernatremia and iatrogenic hyperchloremia. If hypotonic solutions are delayed until later in treatment, by the time they are administered the intracellular space may no longer be as hyperosmolar as it was initially, and it will no longer provide a sink for any excess infused fluids, paving the way for circulatory overload. Early in the therapy of the hyperosmolar dehydrated patient, the hypertonic intracellular space, which is huge in comparison to the ECF and intravascular space, acts like a sponge soaking up the fluid administered, thus preventing volume overload. This capacity progressively diminishes with fluid repletion, so that attempts to "catch up" and reduce persistently elevated serum osmolarities late in the course of treatment are hazardous. The first few hours of fluid replacement are key to rapidly replacing water and electrolyte losses in their proper proportion.

The estimated total body water losses in HHS range between 100 and 200 mL/kg with an average of 150 mL/kg (Table 35-2). It must be emphasized that an aggressive volume replacement regimen must not be applied to the oliguric patient with renal failure and hyperglycemia. Several patients who developed pulmonary edema during the treatment of HHS have been successfully managed by infusion of distilled water into their central venous systems.[32]

Electrolyte losses are a major component of the uncontrolled diabetic state.[6] Sodium losses are 5–13 mEq/kg (average, 7.0 mEq/kg); chloride losses are 3–7 mEq/kg (average, 5.0 mEq/kg); and potassium losses are 5–15 mEq/kg, with the average requirement to fully replete potassium stores around 10 mEq/kg. The loss of phosphorus is about 70–140 mg, Ca^{++} 50–100 mEq, and Mg^{++} 50–100 mEq.

Phosphate is lost as a result of vomiting, anorexia, and the glucosuric osmotic diuresis which precedes HHS, while concurrent hypokalemia and hypomagnesemia impair renal phosphate retention. Initial serum phosphate levels may be elevated, but with fluid and insulin therapy the serum levels fall even if phosphate deficiency is not present. Findings associated with hypophosphatemia include weakness, rhabdomyolysis, coma, convulsions, hyporeflexia, and hemolytic anemia. Symptoms of hypophosphatemia are never seen at serum levels above 2 mg/dL, and significant morbidity is rare unless the level is persistently below 0.5 mg/dL. We routinely administer monobasic potassium phosphate unless a specific contraindication exists. While a beneficial effect from the routine use of phosphate in the uncontrolled diabetic has not been demonstrated, this was studied in acute DKA, where the mean nadir of phosphate levels in those patients not given supplemental phosphate was only moderately hypophosphatemic.[6] In HHS, where the development of the full-blown syndrome occurs over a longer period and is associated with a prolonged osmotic diuresis, phosphate stores may be more extensively depleted and warrant routine supplementation.[33] The most frequent cause of hypophosphatemia is internal redistribution commonly seen during glucose administration to nondiabetic hospitalized patients[33] resulting in increased insulin secretion, during recovery from uncontrolled diabetes, and during refeeding of malnourished patients. Intracellular redistribution occurs due to the formation of phosphorylated glycolytic intermediates, and when superimposed on the losses already incurred in chronically poorly controlled diabetics or malnourished patients, significant falls in the serum phosphate routinely occur. Repletion may be important to restore normal metabolic pathways and to prevent the occasional case of symptomatic severe hypophosphatemia. Since potassium and magnesium, the intracellular cations, do not readily enter the cell accompanied by chloride, an alternative anion, phosphate, must be present to allow the timely restoration of the intracellular milieu.[34] Hypocalcemia, clinically manifested as tetany, may complicate the use of phosphate in DKA.[6] We have never seen symptomatic tetany associated with phosphate administration and attribute this to routine use of magnesium replacement.[2]

Calcium losses in the 50–100-mmol range are common, and after 12 hours of treatment serum calcium levels tend to be at the lower end of normal. If phosphate replacement is given without magnesium, one may expect more frequent symptomatic hypocalcemia and the clinician must be alert to this possibility. Magnesium losses are common and tend to parallel those of potassium,[22] but with the exception of an occasional episode of tetany associated with phosphate infusion, no clinical reports of symptomatic magnesium deficiency in diabetic coma are available. Glycosuria is associated with increased urinary losses of magnesium and low serum levels are found in decompensated diabetes after 12 hours of therapy. Symptoms ascribable to magnesium deficiency are primarily neurologic and include lethargy, weakness, mental changes, convulsions, stupor, and coma. Nausea, vomiting, and refractory cardiac arrhythmias may occur.[6] The effects of magnesium and potassium deficiency are similar and may be impossible to differentiate. Indeed, potassium deficiency refractory to replacement therapy may be a result of a hypomagnesemic effect on the renal tubules, and hypocalcemia may also result from magnesium deficiency. We have noted the potential beneficial effects of Mg^{++} in prevention of thromboembolic events in the uncontrolled diabetic state. With recognition that the administration of Mg^{++} is safe, the evidence of its preventive effect on arrhythmias, possible platelet antiaggregation, and enhancement of K^+ retention, we currently routinely administer Mg^{++} to all uncontrolled diabetics unless renal failure or hypermagnesemia is present (Table 35-2).

Potassium losses in HHS occur due to the severe catabolic state and loss of intracellular water rich in potassium as part of the osmotic diuresis. Hypomagnesemia may worsen the potassium losses. The losses in HHS exceed those in DKA and, without replacement therapy, hypokalemia will be seen in most patients after 4–12 hours of treatment. The symptoms of hypokalemia are well known and include neuromuscular weakness, ileus, ECG abnormalities, cardiac conduction system defects, and rhabdomyolysis. Fatal hypokalemia is associated with cardiac arrest and respiratory paralysis. As treatment of uncontrolled diabetes continues, urinary potassium losses and those from nasogastric suction, especially if magnesium deficiency is present, may approach 50% of the amount being administered.

The objective of potassium replacement is to maintain normokalemia. The huge body deficits cannot and should not be replaced acutely. Total body deficits require days to weeks to completely correct. Even in the presence of renal insufficiency, early potassium replacement may be indicated, because with the exception of the urinary losses, all of the other factors that drive the serum potassium down in the treated diabetic are present. Caution must be exercised in patients with diabetic nephropathy, who may have renal tubular acidosis associated with hypoaldosteronism and hyporeninemia. Here serum potassium concentrations may be elevated and rise further when potassium is administered.

Potassium replacement begins in the first hour if urinary output is adequate, the ECG shows no evidence of hyperkalemic changes, and the serum K^+ is less than 5.0 mEq/L (Table 35-2). Potassium is given as the acetate, phosphate, or a combination of these rather than as the chloride salt, to avoid administering excessive chloride.

Sodium is lost due to the osmotic glucosuric diuresis and the absence of insulin essential for distal tubular sodium reabsorption. Since sodium losses are proportionally lower than water losses, the patient may present with hypernatremia. Since in the absence of insulin glucose is largely restricted to the extracellular space, an increase in its concentration causes water to flow out of the cells down an osmotic gradient into the ECF space, diluting the extracellular sodium. For each 100-mg/dL increment in plasma glucose above normal levels, the serum sodium concentration can be expected to decrease by 1.6 mEq/L, based on the analysis by Katz.[35] Recently Hillier and colleagues[36] demonstrated that the serum Na^+ will be decreased by 2.4 mEq/L for every 100-mg/dL increase in plasma glucose concentration. This correction factor brings the corrected Na^+ closer to the calculated Eosm than does the Katz correction, and its adoption is supported. Insulin has a direct antinatriuretic effect on the kidney. Following treatment with crystalloid solutions and insulin, significant edema ("insulin edema") may develop. Occasionally, in patients with preexisting cardiovascular disease, frank congestive heart failure, pulmonary edema, or hypertension may be a consequence.[6]

Because the rapid anabolism of glucose may cause thiamine deficiency (Wernicke's encephalopathy, beriberi) in patients with borderline thiamine stores, thiamine (100 mg) should be routinely administered. The B vitamins are critical cofactors in many intermediate metabolic reactions, and the catabolic state associated with uncontrolled diabetes predisposes to deficiencies; thus intravenous administration of B-vitamin preparations is prudent and advocated. HHS typically develops over days to weeks, during which time the patient is catabolic and may demonstrate many of the features of protein-calorie undernutrition. When malnourished patients are first given nutritional support, they may develop what has been called the "refeeding syndrome."[37] This term describes the sequelae of rapid refeeding, and includes hypophosphatemia (with associated rhabdomyolysis, hemolysis, neurologic dysfunction, and muscle weakness), hypokalemia, hypomagnesemia (which may contribute more to the clinical syndrome than hypophosphatemia or hypokalemia), vitamin deficiency (especially thiamine), congestive heart failure, and benign refeeding edema (which may share pathogenetic features with insulin edema). This syndrome is well described in chronically malnourished patients (e.g., concentration camp victims), chronic alcoholics, and in anorexia nervosa, but also develops after as few as 7–10 days of hypermetabolic stress with inadequate nutritional support[38] (or its equivalent, the inability to anabolize nutrients). Uncontrolled diabetes, especially the hyperosmolar syndrome, and its subsequent treatment may be a common cause of the refeeding syndrome.[39] It may go unrecognized when only parts of the biochemical (e.g., hypokalemia, hypophosphatemia, hypomagnesemia) or clinical (e.g., insulin edema, muscle weakness) picture are present, but prophylaxis is prudent. A sample of potential pitfalls which may occur during treatment of HHS and an approach to their analysis are provided in Table 35-3.

COMPLICATIONS

Cerebral edema occurring in patients dying of otherwise uncomplicated DKA is well described.[40–42] Most of the patients with this syndrome are young and have DKA rather than HHS, which runs counter to expectations. This complication accounts for at least 50% of DKA-associated deaths and over 30% of all deaths in dia-

TABLE 35-3. Potential Pitfalls During Therapy of Hyperglycemic Hyperosmolar Syndrome

Problem	Consider	Approach
1. Hypotension	(a) Myocardial infarct, sepsis, bleeding (b) Internal redistribution of fluid as hyperglycemia is corrected (c) Total body fluid depletion due to osmotic diuresis with inadequate volume replacement (d) Ongoing osmotic diuresis	(a) Std. work-up/specific therapy (b–d) Increase IV fluids
2. Worsening level of consciousness	(a) Meningitis, CVA, drugs, head trauma (b) Hypovolemia/hypoperfusion (c) Increasing Eosm (increasing S_{Na^+}) (d) Cerebral edema (very rare in HHS) (e) Hypoglycemia (f) Wernicke's encephalopathy (refeeding syndrome) (g) $\downarrow Mg^{++}$	(a) Std. work-up/specific therapy (b) Increase IV fluids (c) Give hypotonic fluids (d) Mannitol IV/steroids IV/$\downarrow$insulin (e) Give glucose; reduce insulin (f) Thiamine/B-complex vitamins (g) Give Mg^{++}
3. Seizures	(a) CVA, prior seizure disorder, withdrawal, drugs, etc. (b) Early in HHS (seen in ~19%) (c) Cerebral edema (very rare in HHS) (d) $\downarrow P$, $\downarrow Mg^{++}$	(a) Std. work-up/specific therapy (avoid diphenylhydantoin) (b) Insulin/hypotonic IV fluids (c) Mannitol IV/steroids IV/$\downarrow$insulin (d) Replace P, Mg^{++}
4. Tetany	(a) $\downarrow Ca^{++}$, $\downarrow Mg^{++}$ (b) P infusion (causing $\downarrow Ca^{++}$, Mg^{++}); rare when Mg^{++} is given routinely/proactively	(a) Replace Ca^{++}, Mg^{++} (b) Stop P; replace Ca^{++}/Mg^{++} (c) Proactive Mg^{++} replacement
5. Muscle weakness (may be associated with respiratory failure)	(a) $\downarrow K^+$, $\downarrow Mg^{++}$, $\downarrow P$ (b) Rhabdomyolysis (commonly asymptomatic)	(a) Replace K^+, Mg^{++}, P (b) Obtain creatine kinase (CK); if CK > 1000 watch for ATN/renal failure and maintain high urine output (c) Respiratory failure may require mechanical ventilation
6. Cardiac/ECG abnormalities	(a) Peaked precordial T waves, prolonged PR, Vfib: $\uparrow K^+$ (b) Ectopy, tachyarrhythmias, (+)U waves, flat T waves: $\downarrow K^+$ (c) Wide QRS: $\downarrow K^+$, $\downarrow Ca^{++}$ (d) Short QT: $\uparrow Ca^{++}$ (e) Prolonged QT^c: $\downarrow Ca^{++}$, $\uparrow Mg^{++}$ (f) Vtach: $\uparrow Mg^{++}$ (g) Underlying heart disease (in presence of arrhythmias, CHF, etc.) (h) CVA (especially subarachnoid hemorrhage) with deeply inverted precordial T's. (i) ST segment elevation; friction rubs (underlying pericarditis vs. severe dehydration)	(a)–(f) Monitor ECG hourly, especially T waves. Measure K^+, Mg^{++}, Ca^{++}, correct as necessary; routinely administer K^+, Mg^{++} unless levels are very high (g) Std. work-up/specific therapy (h) Std. work-up/specific therapy (i) If due to severe dehydration, especially with DKA, will rapidly resolve with fluid repletion
7. Persistent hyperglycemia	(a) Inadequate fluid infusion or oliguria (b) Renal failure (chronic or acute rhabdomyolysis) (c) Insulin resistance	(a) Increase fluids—hypotonic (b) May need to reduce fluids and increase insulin (c) Double insulin dose hourly
8. Persistent hyperosmolarity	(a) Persistent hyperglycemia (b) Hypernatremia—unmasked as glucose falls or excess Na^+ in infused isotonic solutions or inadequate free water replacement (c) Nephrogenic diabetes insipidus related to HHS (resistance to ADH)	(a) See 7 above (b) Increase IV fluids; use hypotonic electrolyte solutions (c) Maintain high-volume hypotonic fluid intake

TABLE 35-3. Potential Pitfalls During Therapy of Hyperglycemic Hyperosmolar Syndrome *(Continued)*

Problem	Consider	Approach
9. Oliguria	(a) Renal vascular occlusion or urinary obstruction or papillary necrosis	(a) Std. work-up/specific therapy
	(b) Chronic renal failure (CRF)	(b) History; reduce IV fluids; use caution in volume replacement; $\uparrow$dose of insulin
	(c) Acute renal failure (ARF)	(c) Std. work-up; if trial of increased volume infusion fails, treat as CRF (above)
	(d) Hypovolemia: Internal fluid redistribution as hyperglycemia is corrected, inadequate volume replacement, ongoing osmotic diuresis, or a combination of these	(d) Increase IV fluid replacement
	(e) Rhabdomyolysis ($\uparrow\uparrow$CK)	(e) Check K^+, P, Mg^{++} and correct; adjust IV fluid volume to attempt to sustain high urine output
10. Edema	(a) Underlying cardiac, hepatic, renal, or GI disease	(a) History/std. work-up/specific therapy
	(b) Excess Na^+/H_2O administration (especially in elderly)	(b) Restrict Na^+ and/or H_2O; diuretics
	(c) "Insulin edema"	(c) If asymptomatic, recognize, reassure, and observe; if symptomatic or severe, give diuretics and restrict Na^+
11. Hyperchloremia	(a) Underlying renal disease; RTA	(a) History/std. work-up/specific therapy
	(b) DKA with ketonuria resulting in Cl^- retention	(b) Use physiologic (hypotonic if associated with HHS) electrolyte solutions; avoid use of NaCl and KCl
	(c) Administration of excess Cl^- in treatment (e.g., use of NaCl and KCl^- solutions)	(c) See (b) above. Use Plasmalyte, Isolyte, Normosol, lactated Ringer's, etc.; for K^+ replacement use K acetate/K phosphate
12. Hypokalemia	(a) Typical of catabolic state of uncontrolled diabetes and unmasked as anabolism begins	(a) Begin K^+ repletion at outset of therapy unless hyperkalemia, ECG changes, or renal failure present
	(b) Insulin (and refeeding syndrome)	(b) Proactive and therapeutic K^+ replacement
	(c) Ongoing catabolism, osmotic diuretic losses and, in DKA, as cation accompanying ketoacids in urine	(c) Insulin plus K^+
	(d) Hypomagnesemia (refractory hypokalemia)	(d) Replace K^+ plus Mg^{++}
	(e) Exogenous diuretic therapy	(e) History; stop diuretic; replace K^+
	(f) Bicarbonate administration	(f) Stop HCO_3^-; replace K^+
13. Hypophosphatemia	(a) Catabolic depletion	(a)–(c) Give P; it is the necessary intracellular anion to enable K^+ and Mg^{++} to cross cell membranes and enter cell during anabolism; Cl^- does not cross cell membranes easily or facilitate translocation of K^+ and Mg^{++} to cell interior
	(b) Internal redistribution (insulin/glucose)	
	(c) As part of refeeding syndrome [see (a) & (b) above]	
	(d) If severe, may cause hemolysis	(d) Administer P
14. Hypomagnesemia	(a) Chronic catabolic deficiency state seen in >50% of poorly controlled diabetics	(a)–(c) Replace Mg^{++}; it is a component of over 300 critical enzyme systems and of all energy generating systems in the body
	(b) Osmotic diuretic loss	
	(c) Internal redistribution (refeeding syndrome)	
15. Anemia	(a) Preexistent; may become manifest after rehydration	(a) Std. work-up/specific therapy
	(b) Hemolysis: (1) G-6-PD deficiency, (2) $\downarrow$P	(b) (1) Primarily seen in African-Americans and persons of Mediterranean descent (2) Measure P and replace; usually not seen unless P is <0.5 mg/dL
	(c) Bleeding; may see "coffee grounds" gastric contents in up to 25% of DKA/HHS	(c) Std. work-up/specific treatment; hemorrhagic gastritis resolves with treatment; may require NGT drainage

TABLE 35-3. Potential Pitfalls During Therapy of Hyperglycemic Hyperosmolar Syndrome *(Continued)*

Problem	Consider	Approach
16. Thrombotic events	(a) Hyperviscosity, low flow, hypotension	(a) Rapid large-volume crystalloid infusions; pressors if necessary, Mg^{++}; low-dose heparin prophylaxis
	(b) Hypercoagulable state (seen in diabetes mellitus in general) not necessarily specific to HHS	(b) Consider anticoagulation as necessary, appropriate, and safe
17. Respiratory distress	(a) Pneumonia, CHF	(a) Std. work-up/specific therapy
	(b) Renal failure	(b) History; reduce fluids if CRF and increase insulin; insulin may improve general circulatory and pulmonary fluid overload by redistribution of fluid to intracellular compartments
	(c) Pneumothorax (iatrogenic due to central lines)	(c) CXR; specific therapy
	(d) Pneumomediastinum or pneumothorax in DKA	(d) CXR; specific therapy
	(e) ARDS	(e) Central monitoring to exclude CHF or circulatory overload; supportive therapy and std. ICU monitoring; prognosis poor
	(f) Rhabdomyolysis	(f) Check CK; supportive therapy
	(g) $\downarrow$P, $\downarrow$K$^+$, $\downarrow$Mg^{++}	(g) Monitor serum levels and replace as necessary
	(h) Pulmonary embolism	(h) Std. work-up/specific therapy
18. Hypoxemia	(a) Pneumonia, pulmonary embolus, CHF	(a) Std. work-up/specific therapy
	(b) ARDS, especially with DKA	(b) Poor prognosis; monitor with PCWP to differentiate from CHF; supportive care
	(c) Pneumonthorax, spontaneous in DKA	(c) CXR; specific therapy
19. Hypothermia	(a) Sepsis/infection	(a) Std. work-up/specific therapy
	(b) Hypoglycemia	(b) Monitor plasma glucose, administer glucose
	(c) DKA	(c) Poor prognostic sign in DKA
20. Abdominal pain	(a) Acute surgical abdomen (e.g., appendicitis, pancreatitis, cholecystitis, mesenteric ischemia)	(a) Std. work-up/specific therapy
	(b) Fatty liver	(b) Monitor LFTs; hydration plus insulin usually resolves this problem
	(c) DKA	(c) Especially in children may mimic acute surgical abdominal condition; rapidly responds to hydration and insulin
21. Hyperamylasemia/hyperlipasemia	(a) Pancreatitis, bowel infarction	(a) Std. work-up/specific therapy
	(b) DKA	(b) Responds to hydration/insulin
22. Leukocytosis	(a) Sepsis	(a) Std. work-up/specific therapy
	(b) DKA	(b) Resolves with hydration/insulin

betic patients under 20 years of age.[43] Asymptomatic cerebral edema and arterial hypoxemia have been reported in a number of young adults with DKA during routine therapy,[44] and subclinical brain swelling detected by CT occurs in children during the treatment of DKA.[45] Most adults[44,46] and probably children[45] develop subclinical or "benign" cerebral edema[6] during standard therapy for DKA. The majority of young patients with DKA have brain edema by CT scan on presentation prior to the initiation of any therapy.[18] Most of these patients were not significantly hyperosmolar and none received hypotonic intravenous fluids, thus arguing against the osmotic gradient theory of the pathogenesis of cerebral edema. The overwhelming majority of diabetics who develop overt cerebral edema are young adults or children with DKA. The same is true of the rare patient with HHS who develops fatal cerebral edema. Indeed, only one such adult has been documented.[47] The

cerebral atrophy that accompanies the aging process may allow cerebral edema in the elderly diabetic to remain clinically silent by accommodating excess cerebral water without significant damage.

An increasing number of pediatric patients are being encountered with HHS. Rother and Schwenk[48] identified 22 reported cases in infants and children between the ages of 6 weeks and 12 years. Most pediatricians treating patients with DKA recommend following the "corrected" sodium concentration as a guide to the speed of correction and the tonicity of the fluids used.

As many as 4000 persons die annually in the United States from DKA and HHS, whereas fatal cerebral edema is virtually unseen. It therefore becomes indefensible to base therapeutic recommendations on the prevention of this rarely encountered complication in light of the potential dire consequences of undertreatment, especially since no one has ever demonstrated that slower correction of hyperosmolar hyperglycemia produces the desired benefit. Many more patients die because of undertreatment than from overtreatment of uncontrolled diabetes. Thus any recommendation that would reduce the rate of correction of hyperglycemia risks increasing the mortality rate and should be viewed with alarm.[6]

Other complications seen in HHS include thromboembolic events and possible disseminated intravascular coagulation, pulmonary aspiration of gastric contents in the presence of gastric stasis and obtundation, and the remarkably rare occurrence of renal failure and rhabdomyolysis.

Creatine kinase elevations of greater than 1000 IU/L have been described in over 25% of patients with HHS in the absence of stroke, myocardial infarction, or end-stage renal disease.[49] Thus subclinical rhabdomyolysis is not uncommon in HHS, but clinical manifestations are mild or absent.[50] The reason that acute tubular necrosis (ATN) and acute renal failure are uncommon despite the frequency of rhabdomyolysis, at times with very high CK levels, may be attributable to the high-volume osmotic diuresis that is the pathogenetic hallmark of HHS. Nevertheless, the presence of a CK greater than 1000 IU/L is associated with an increased mortality rate in HHS.[49]

Pancreatitis[5] is said to be a complication as well as an etiology of the hyperosmolar state. It has been suggested that hyperosmolarity may reduce blood flow to the pancreas, resulting in pancreatitis that becomes evident several days after admission. However, abdominal pain, leukocytosis, gastric stasis, vomiting, and an elevated amylase may all be secondary to uncontrolled diabetes, and renal impairment may also elevate the amylase. If such an entity does occur, it may be related to the vascular occlusions seen in some series[21,22] or to the occasional marked hypertriglyceridemia seen in this setting. In this regard, marked hyperlipasemia with hyperamylasemia has uncommonly been reported[51] in several hyperglycemic (>1000 mg/dL) hyperosmolar ketoacidotic patients, both with and without abdominal findings and without ultrasound and CT evidence of any pancreatic abnormality. Further, in these patients hyperamylasemia and hyperlipasemia were prolonged well after clinical recovery from HHS.

PROGNOSIS

The best prognostic indicator in uncontrolled diabetes is the age of the patient. Based on two large series of HHS,[2,52] advanced age, a higher BUN, and a higher Na^+ concentration are predictors of a poor outcome. In these series the mortality for HHS was 10–17%.

The availability of someone who is knowledgeable about the problems presented by the uncontrolled diabetic and facile in directing therapy is an essential element in improving the outcome of this metabolic emergency.

PREVENTION

Improvement in the outcome of this potential metabolic disaster requires an effective preventive strategy. Patients with HHS are elderly, have type 2 diabetes, and often live alone,[6] and social isolation is a precipitant in 25–30% of episodes. The availability of a knowledgeable significant other (friend, neighbor, or family member) who maintains daily contact with the elderly diabetic is essential.[2] They should be educated to recognize alterations in the patient's

mental status and symptoms of loss of diabetic control, and to promptly report these to the physician. Public education about the presenting symptoms of diabetes will help reduce the one-quarter to one-third of patients who have HHS at presentation.

Residence in nursing homes predisposes to HHS,[4] and nursing home residents are prone to develop dehydration and hyperosmolarity, so education of nursing home staff members in prevention and detection of this syndrome is essential. Prompt recognition and treatment of infections and the use of Pneumovax™ and annual influenza immunizations are important preventive measures in the elderly diabetic.

Providers should take into account the potential for medications prescribed for the elderly to cause or worsen glucose intolerance; aggressively apply home blood glucose monitoring in elderly diabetics; intensify efforts to improve blood glucose control; and reinforce education of patients and families regarding compliance with diet and hypoglycemic agents.

REFERENCES

1. Dreschfeld J: The Bradshawe lecture on diabetic coma. *Br Med J* 1886;2:358.
2. Carroll P, Matz R: Uncontrolled diabetes mellitus in adults: Experience in treating diabetic ketoacidosis and hyperosmolar nonketotic coma with low-dose insulin and a uniform treatment regimen. *Diabetes Care* 1983;6:579.
3. Ennis D, Stahl EJvB, Kreisberg RA: The hyperosmolar hyperglycemic syndrome. *Diabetes Rev* 1994;2:115.
4. Wachtel TJ: The diabetic hyperosmolar state. *Clin Geriatric Med* 1990;6:797.
5. Siperstein MD: Diabetic ketoacidosis and hyperosmolar coma. *Endocrinol Metab Clin North Am* 1992;21:415.
6. Matz R: Hyperosmolar nonacidotic diabetes (HNAD). In: Porte D, Sherwin RS, eds. *Ellenberg and Rifkin's Diabetes Mellitus: Theory and Practice*, 5th ed. Appleton & Lange:1987;845.
7. Matz R, Drapkin A: Hyperosmolar coma in diabetes. *Lancet* 1966;1:1101.
8. Brodsky WA, Rapoport S, West CD: The mechanism of glycosuric diuresis in diabetic man. *J Clin Invest* 1950;29:1021.
9. Cochrane Injuries Group Albumin Reviewers: Human albumin administration in critically ill patients: Systematic review of randomized controlled trials. *Br Med J* 1998;317:235.
10. Davis PJ, Davis FB: Water excretion in the elderly. *Endocrinol Metab Clin North Am* 1987;16:867.
11. Barnett JL, Owyand C: Serum glucose concentration as a modulator of interdigestive gastric motility. *Gastroenterology* 1988;94:739.
12. Matz R: Hypothermia in diabetic acidosis. *Hormones* 1972;3:36.
13. Carroll P, Feinstein S, Nierenberg S, et al: The adult respiratory distress syndrome complicating diabetic ketoacidosis. *Cardiovasc Rev Rep* 1986;7:801.
14. Carroll P, Matz R: Adult respiratory distress syndrome complicating severely uncontrolled diabetes mellitus: Report of nine cases and a review of the literature. *Diabetes Care* 1982;5:574.
15. Fulop M, Rosenblatt H, Kreitzer SM, et al: Hyperosmolar nature of diabetic coma. *Diabetes* 1974;24:594.
16. Brandt KR, Miles JM: Relationship between severity of hyperglycemia and metabolic acidosis in diabetic ketoacidosis. *Mayo Clin Proc* 1988;63:1071.
17. Daugirdas JT, Kronfol NO, Tzamaloukas AH, et al: Hyperosmolar coma: Cellular dehydration and the serum sodium concentration. *Ann Intern Med* 1989;110:855.
18. Durr JA, Hoffman WH, Sklar AH, et al: Correlates of brain edema in uncontrolled IDDM. *Diabetes* 1992;41:627.
19. Guisado R, Arieff AI: Neurologic manifestations of diabetic comas: Correlation with biochemical alterations in the brain. *Metabolism* 1975;24:665.
20. Thomas RJ: Seizures and epilepsy in the elderly. *Arch Intern Med* 1997;157:605.

21. Clements RS Jr, Vourgant B: Fatal diabetic ketoacidosis: Major causes and approaches to their prevention. *Diabetes Care* 1978;1:314.

22. Alberti KGMM, Hockaday TDR: Diabetic coma: A reappraisal after five years. *Clin Endocrinol Metab* 1977;6:421.

23. Colwell JA, Winocur PD, Lopes-Virella M, *et al*: New concepts about the pathogenesis of atherosclerosis in diabetes mellitus. *Am J Med* 1993;75:67.

24. Laakso M, Edelman SV, Brechtel G, *et al*: Impaired insulin-mediated skeletal muscle blood flow in patients with NIDDM. *Diabetes* 1992; 41:1076.

25. Scherrer U, Randin D, Vollenweider P, *et al*: Nitric oxide accounts for insulin's vascular effects in humans. *J Clin Invest* 1994;94:2511.

26. Matz R: Magnesium: Deficiencies and therapeutic uses. *Hosp Pract* 1993;28:79.

27. Matz R: Diabetic coma. Guidelines in therapy. *NY State J Med* 1974; 74:642.

28. Campbell IW, Duncan LJP, Clarke BF: Pericarditis in diabetic ketoacidosis. *Br Heart J* 1977;39:110.

29. Reasner CA: Autoimmune thyroid disease and type 1 diabetes. *Diabetes Rev* 1993;1:343.

30. Genuth SM: Diabetic ketoacidosis and hyperglycemic hyperosmolar coma. *Curr Ther Endocrinol Metab* 1997;6:438.

31. Gennari FJ, Kassirer JP: Osmotic diuresis. *N Engl J Med* 1974;291: 714.

32. Worthley LIG: Hyperosmolar coma treated with intravenous sterile water. A study of three cases. *Arch Intern Med* 1986;146:945.

33. Bohannon NJV: Large phosphate shifts with treatment for hyperglycemia. *Arch Intern Med* 1989;149:1423.

34. Weisinger JR, Bellorin-Font E: Magnesium and phosphorus. *Lancet* 1998;352:391.

35. Katz MA: Hyperglycemia-induced hyponatremia—calculation of expected serum sodium depression. *N Engl J Med* 1973;289:843.

36. Hillier TA, Abbott RD, Barrett EJ: Hyponatremia: Evaluating the correction factor for hyperglycemia. *Am J Med* 1999;106:399.

37. Weinsier RL, Krumdieck CL: Death resulting from overzealous total parenteral nutrition: The refeeding syndrome. *Am J Clin Nutr* 1981; 34:393.

38. Mizock BA: Avoiding common errors in nutritional management. Which critical illnesses warrant changes in nutritional support? *J Crit Illness* 1993;8:1116.

39. Matz R: Parallels between treated uncontrolled diabetes and the refeeding syndrome with emphasis on fluid and electrolyte abnormalities. *Diabetes Care* 1994;17:1209.

40. Dillon ES, Riggs HE, Dyer WW: Cerebral lesions in uncomplicated fatal diabetic acidosis. *Am J Med Sci* 1936;192:360.

41. Young E, Bradley RF: Cerebral edema with irreversible coma in severe diabetic ketoacidosis. *N Engl J Med* 1967;276:665.

42. Taubin H, Matz R: Cerebral edema, diabetes insipidus and sudden death during the treatment of diabetic ketoacidosis. *Diabetes* 1968;17: 108.

43. Rosenbloom AL: Intracerebral crises during treatment of diabetic ketoacidosis. *Diabetes Care* 1990;13:22.

44. Fein IA, Rackow EC, Sprung CL, *et al*: Relation of colloid osmotic pressure to arterial hypoxemia and cerebral edema during crystalloid volume loading of patients with diabetic ketoacidosis. *Ann Intern Med* 1982;96:570.

45. Krane EJ, Rockoff MA, Wallman JA, *et al*: Subdural brain swelling in children during treatment of diabetic ketoacidosis. *N Engl J Med* 1985;312:1147.

46. Winegrad AI, Kern EFO, Simmons DA: Cerebral edema in diabetic ketoacidosis. *N Engl J Med* 1985;312:1184.

47. Arieff AI: Cerebral edema complicating nonketotic hyperosmolar coma. *Miner Electrolyte Metab* 1986;12:383.

48. Rother KI, Schwenk WF II: An unusual case of the nonketotic hyperosmolar syndrome during childhood. *Mayo Clin Proc* 1995;70:62.

49. Wang LM, Tsai ST, Holt LT, *et al*: Rhabdomyolysis in diabetic emergencies. *Diabetes Res Clin Prac* 1994;26:209.

50. Pravin CS, Mirel A, Jayanti V: Rhabdomyolysis in the hyperosmolar state. *Am J Med* 1990;88:9.

51. Nsien EE, Steinberg WM, Borum M, *et al*: Marked hyperlipasemia in diabetic ketoacidosis. A report of three cases. *J Clin Gastroenterol* 1992;15:117.

52. Wachtel TJ, Silliman RA, Lamberton P: Prognostic factors in the diabetic hyperosmolar state. *J Am Geriatric Soc* 1987;35:737.

CHAPTER 36

Host Defense and Infections in Diabetes Mellitus

Brian P. Currie

Joan I. Casey

GENERAL PROBLEM OF INFECTION IN DIABETIC PATIENTS

Literature reviews examining the association of infections with diabetes mellitus are often difficult to interpret and fraught with contradictions. A major contributory factor is that diabetes mellitus is a heterogeneous disease and so study populations need to be carefully identified in order to allow comparisons between studies (e.g., type 1 versus type 2 diabetes, well-controlled disease versus poorly controlled disease). In addition, diabetes mellitus is a relatively common disease, and as a consequence, anecdotal reports of various infections in diabetic patients can lead to spurious associations. Nonetheless, it is well established that certain infections occur almost exclusively in diabetic patients and that diabetic patients have a worse prognosis than nondiabetic patients after acquiring certain infections, such as acute pyelonephritis complicated by papillary necrosis or emphysematous pyelonephritis.[1,2]

The morbidity and mortality associated with infectious diseases in diabetic patients are obvious in a study of patients admitted to an intensive care unit with diabetic ketoacidosis. Of the episodes of ketoacidosis, 28% were caused by infections. The mortality for the whole group was 6%, but in 43% of the patients who died, infection was considered the cause of death.[3] Infection was considered the precipitating cause of ketoacidosis in 77% of patients admitted to hospitals in Dallas, Texas.[4] While it is generally believed that diabetic patients with poor metabolic control have an increased susceptibility to infections, the previously mentioned studies indicate that in many cases the poor metabolic control may be the result of the infection, rather than the cause.

While antibiotics may be secondary only to insulin in increasing the life span of the diabetic patient, infection cannot be discounted now or in the foreseeable future as a major cause of morbidity and mortality among patients with diabetes. A knowledge of the normal host defense mechanisms and of those that are abnormal in the diabetic individual may be helpful in understanding the unusual predilection for certain infectious diseases among diabetic patients.

NORMAL HOST DEFENSE MECHANISMS

Skin

Normal skin is impenetrable to most bacteria, and infection rarely occurs unless the skin is damaged. The normal bacterial flora of the skin maintain an environment that is hostile to most pathogenic bacteria. The nerve supply of the skin is important in maintaining the integrity of the mechanical barrier by warning of potential injury from prolonged pressure or penetration by foreign bodies.

Blood Supply

Maintenance of normal nutrition and oxygen tension to tissues, as well as delivery of the humoral and cellular components of the immune system, is dependent on an adequate blood supply.

Humoral Immunity

The two major components of humoral immunity are antibodies and the complement system. Antibodies may neutralize the effect of bacteria, bacterial toxins, or viral capsids by combining with the organisms and preventing their attachment to cell surfaces. Other antibodies act by agglutinating organisms, thereby increasing clearance by the reticuloendothelial system, or by lysing bacteria. Opsonins, antibodies that may be specific or nonspecific, coat bacteria and enhance phagocytosis. Most of these reactions require or are enhanced by the action of complement, through either the classic or the alternate (properdin) pathway.

Phagocytic Function

This component of the immune response is mainly related to polymorphonuclear cells and macrophages. The latter cells are either wandering (alveolar, peritoneal, and skin macrophages and tissue histiocytes) or fixed to vascular endothelium in the liver, spleen, and lymph nodes. Various functions of phagocytes have been recognized, including random migration, chemotaxis and attachment, ingestion, and intracellular killing of bacteria. After ingestion of bacteria by phagocytic cells, a vigorous burst of oxidative metabolism leads to the production of hydrogen peroxide, which combines with myeloperoxidase and halogen (iodide or chloride). This results in rapid killing of most pathogenic bacteria.

Lymphocytes

There is considerable information about the types and functions of lymphocytes and the substances elaborated by these cells when exposed to antigens or mitogens. There are at least three types of lymphocytes now recognized. These are the thymus-derived or T lymphocytes, the bone marrow-derived or B lymphocytes, and the non-B, non-T lymphocytes. The B cells can transform into antibody-secreting or plasma cells, whereas the T cells are regarded as the cells responsible for cell-mediated defense against viruses, fungi, and mycobacteria. T cells may help or suppress the immune functions of other cells such as the B lymphocytes, usually by the production of lymphokines.

ABNORMALITIES OF HOST DEFENSE IN DIABETES MELLITUS

Skin

Although the level of glucose in skin is directly related to that of the blood, there is no evidence that diabetic patients with skin infection have particularly high ratios of skin to blood glucose.[5] Nasal and skin flora of diabetic patients have been studied frequently with varying results. Smith and coworkers[1] found that 53% of type 1 diabetic adults were nasal carriers of *Staphylococcus aureus* compared with 34% of nondiabetic adults and 35% of type 2 diabetic adults. Of diabetic children, 76% were nasal carriers compared with 44% of nondiabetic children. Tuzaon and associates also found a high rate of skin carriage of *S. aureus* in type 1 diabetic patients.[1] In contrast, Somerville and Lancaster-Smith did not find a high carriage rate for *S. aureus* in diabetic patients, but they unfortunately did not include nondiabetic controls.[6] Peripheral neuropathy in diabetic patients can permit undetected disruption of the dermal barrier, which can serve as a portal of entry for pathogens. This decreased sense of touch prevents warning of potential injury from prolonged pressure or penetration injuries. In addition, once dermal barrier disruption occurs and infection is established, this decreased sense of touch contributes to delayed recognition and treatment (Table 36-1).

TABLE 36-1. Relationship of Host Defense Deficit to Disease Syndrome in Diabetic Patients

Host Defense Deficit	Disease Syndrome
Skin integrity	Erythrasma, cellulitis
Neuropathy	Infections secondary to trauma and ulceration; bladder infections
Blood supply	Peripheral vascular disease with ulcers, gangrene, and synergistic infections; invasion of vessels with bacteria and fungi resulting in malignant otitis or mucormycosis; possibility periodontal disease
Humoral immunity	Possibly bacterial infections due to *Pseudomonas* and group B *Streptococcus*

Blood Supply

Vascular problems in diabetic patients, secondary to both the microangiopathy of diabetes and the accelerated course of atherosclerosis in these patients, may predispose them to infection by disrupting normal nutrient and oxygen delivery, as well as disrupting normal immune function.

Recent evidence presented by Williamson and colleagues[7] suggests that the hyperglycemia seen in poorly controlled diabetic subjects may result in an increased tissue cytosolic ratio of free NADH/NAD[1] (in spite of normal O_2 tensions) that mimics the effects of true hypoxia on vascular and neural function. Termed *pseudohypoxia,* the phenomenon is thought to play an important role in the pathogenesis of diabetic complications via a branching cascade of metabolic imbalances that can inflict injury on vascular tissue. Decreased adherence of polymorphonuclear cells and decreased diapedesis have been described in diabetic subjects, and there is evidence that this activity is a function of blood vessel endothelial cells, as well as of the polymorphonuclear cell itself.[8] This oxidative stress contributes to disruption of normal vascular function and its potential impact on immune function.

In addition, poor metabolic control may result in increased vascular permeability, leading to increased diffusion of nutrients and edema formation.[9] This provides an ideal milieu for proliferation of organisms, particularly streptococci.

Finally, a reduction in blood supply can translate into a reduction in delivery of antibiotics when treating established infections in diabetic patients. This could theoretically result in decreased efficacy and treatment failure. Seabrook and associates[10] studied 16 diabetic patients receiving antibiotic and surgical therapy for foot infections and documented that the antibiotics administered in 9 patients provided no effective therapy against infection because of subtherapeutic tissue levels of antibiotic. Furthermore, adequate serum antibiotic levels did not guarantee therapeutic tissue antibiotic levels when tissue was sampled from postoperative viable tissue margins in these patients.

Humoral Immunity

Antibody production after exposure to a variety of bacterial antigens has been studied in diabetic patients. Decreased agglutinating antibodies to *Salmonella typhi,*[11] *Escherichia coli,*[12,13] and *S. aureus*[13] and decreased antitoxin antibodies to *S. aureus*[14] and *Corynebacterium diphtheriae*[13] have been reported in diabetics relative to nondiabetic persons. However, other studies, including those using pneumococcal polysaccharide, have shown that diabetic patients respond well to vaccines. Beam and coworkers[15] studied 40 type 1 diabetic patients and 10 nondiabetic controls. They found that diabetic patients responded as quickly and as well as the controls. There was no correlation between antibody response and age, mean glucose concentration, or duration of diabetes.

Conflicting results have been reported when the bactericidal capacity of diabetic blood has been studied. Richardson[11] found defects in the killing of many bacterial pathogens, but Balch and colleagues[12] found no significant deficiency. The opsonic capacity of diabetic blood was also found to be impaired by Richardson.[11]

Baker and associates[16] studied opsonization of group B streptococci in neonates, type 1 diabetic patients, and healthy adults using type II group B streptococci. They found that inefficient bactericidal activity occurred among neonatal and diabetic sera com-

TABLE 36-2. Summary of Potential Leukocyte Dysfunction Reported Among Diabetic Patients

Neutrophils	↓ Leukocytosis
	↓ Chemotaxis
	↓ Phagocytosis
	↓ Intracellular killing
	↓ Metabolic burst
Lymphocytes	↓ Antibody function/opsonization
	↓ Chemotactic factor
	↓ Lymphokines

pared to normal sera. Only 6 of 15 diabetic patients had sera with efficient bactericidal activity for type II group B streptococci. While bactericidal activity was not dependent on the level of antibody, type-specific antibody did have the capacity to correct certain opsonophagocytic deficiencies.

The majority of studies of serum complement in diabetic patients have found normal or elevated levels so that impaired opsonic capacity of the blood is not necessarily related to deficient complement levels.[11,12]

Phagocytic Function

Although opsonization was considered under humoral immunity, one should keep in mind that phagocytosis of bacteria cannot occur in the absence of opsonization except in unusual circumstances. Indeed, many of the problems in interpreting the inconsistent data relating to phagocytic function in diabetic patients may be due to the fact that there are so many separate steps in this process.

To begin with, random migration of leukocytes, which is probably the first step in the process of phagocytosis, has been reported to be abnormal in type 1 diabetic persons Table 36-2).[17] The ability of polymorphonuclear cells and macrophages to get to an area of infection also depends on their ability to adhere to and migrate through the endothelium of the capillary walls. As noted previously, this diapedesis of phagocytic cells could be dependent in part on the vessel wall. Migration and chemotaxis of cells have been tested by using the Rebuck skin window, and two studies have indicated a significant delay in response to skin abrasion in diabetic patients who were ketoacidotic. In the study of Perillie and coworkers, the defect was corrected in three of four patients by correction of the acidosis.[18] Brayton and colleagues tested both ketoacidotic and nonketotic patients and found impaired responses in both groups.[19] Bagdade and associates tested the adherence of polymorphonuclear cells from ten diabetic patients to nylon fiber columns and found it to be only 53% of normal. By lowering blood glucose levels of the patients, the defect was partly, but not fully corrected.[20] More recently, Anderson and associates[8] examined neutrophil adherence to bovine aortic endothelial cells in 26 diabetic patients compared to age- and sex-matched healthy controls and found that a subset of 16 diabetic patients demonstrated highly significant decreases in basal adhesion. This study also indicated that an adherence-augmenting factor in diabetic plasma increased adherence of both diabetic and control neutrophils in the basal state. The adhesive effects of the factor were mediated through alterations in endothelium rather than neutrophils. Chemotaxis of polymorphonuclear cells from diabetic and nondiabetic subjects was studied by Donovan and coworkers[21] using time-lapse microcinematography and video techniques, which revealed that diabetic cells move at normal rates. These authors collected cells for

these experiments by means of their adherence to glass coverslips. Since diabetic cells have poor adherence properties, this method of collecting cells could have resulted in the loss of those cells with poor chemotactic properties as well. There may be a mixed population of polymorphonuclear cells, some of which have normal adherence and chemotactic properties and others that do not. Other in vitro studies have been reported in which delayed chemotaxis was noted in both type 2[22] and type 1 diabetic patients.[17,22] In these studies, polymorphonuclear cells showed significantly decreased chemotaxis, and sera from diabetic patients were found to be deficient in chemotactic activity. These defects were unrelated to blood glucose levels, and although addition of insulin and glucose resulted in in vitro correction of the defect in two of the studies, chemotaxis was not improved in children given insulin.[22] Molenaar and colleagues also found that chemotactic activity was significantly lower in polymorphonuclear cells of first-degree relatives of patients with type 1 diabetes mellitus when compared with other nondiabetic subjects.[23] McMullen and coworkers[24] found a positive correlation between a family history of diabetes and neutrophil chemotactic defects in 13 of 24 prediabetic subjects. These data suggest that the abnormality in chemotaxis may be intrinsic to the polymorphonuclear cell and possibly to the genetic makeup of the diabetic person.

Defects in phagocyte engulfment and intracellular killing of bacteria have been reported by several authors. In studies in which S aureus was used, ingestion of organisms was found to be normal in the diabetic patients, except for those with ketoacidosis.[25] Tan and associates[26] demonstrated impaired phagocytosis in 11 of 31, an intracellular killing defect in 3 of 31, and a combined defect in 3 of 31 diabetic patients using a S aureus challenge. There was no relationship between blood glucose levels and defects noted. Nolan and coworkers[27] found impaired engulfment and intracellular killing of S aureus among diabetic patients. Data from these latter studies suggest that improved control of blood glucose levels improves resistance to bacterial infections. Repine and colleagues[28] demonstrated that neutrophils from infected nondiabetic patients have an increased capacity to kill S aureus when compared to noninfected nondiabetic persons. Neutrophils from infected diabetic patients, however, failed to show this enhanced bactericidal capacity. This defect was seen in well controlled as well as in poorly controlled diabetic patients. They also noted that neutrophils from poorly controlled uninfected diabetic patients did not kill S aureus as well as those from well-controlled diabetic patients or nondiabetic persons. Impairment of ingestion of Streptococcus pneumoniae has also been reported, and this defect was partially corrected by improved metabolic control of the diabetes.[22] In a later study, Bagdade and associates[29] suggested that the defect was related to serum factors, because it was partially corrected by serum from normal controls, whereas the diabetic serum caused impairment of phagocytic function in cells from nondiabetic controls. Crosby and Allison[30] were unable to demonstrate any impairment of ingestion of S. pneumoniae in diabetic patients who were not ketoacidotic.

Lymphocytes

Cell-mediated immunity, as measured by blast transformation of peripheral blood lymphocytes, has been measured in diabetic patients. When the mitogen phytohemagglutinin was used, the response of diabetic patients in good metabolic control was normal, whereas that of hyperglycemic patients was depressed.[22,31] Impaired metabolism of glucose through the direct oxidative pathway has been noted in lymphocytes from diabetic patients. The lymphocyte response to *Candida* antigen was reported to be normal in diabetic subjects;[32] however, Plouffe and coworkers[33] found positive skin test reactions to *Candida* antigen in only 44% of diabetic patients compared to 88% of nondiabetic subjects. These authors also found the lymphocyte response to streptokinase-streptodornase to be impaired in diabetic subjects with poor glucose control and noted that this defect normalized with institution of metabolic control. When staphylococcal antigen was used in the blast transformation assay, the response of lymphocytes from both type 1 and type 2 diabetic subjects was less than that of nondiabetic subjects. This impaired response to staphylococcal antigen appeared to be unrelated to serum factors or metabolic control.[34,35] Studies in streptozocin-induced and mutant diabetic animals demonstrate impairment of cell-mediated immunity by measurements of granuloma formation, intracellular killing of *Listeria monocytogenes*, and footpad swelling, all of which were less than normal in the diabetic animals.[36,37]

Summary

Although the data are contradictory and inconclusive, there is strong evidence suggesting multiple immune defects in subsets of diabetic patients. As noted, much of the confusion is related to the fact that diabetes mellitus is a heterogeneous disease and that study populations have been poorly defined. The strongest evidence regarding an immune defect in diabetic patients is related to abnormalities of neutrophil function in patients with poor metabolic control (ketoacidosis or hyperglycemia). Studies using *in vitro* systems have documented impaired chemotactic responses and phagocytic activity of neutrophils in these subsets of diabetic patients. However, even among these patients the mechanisms of the defects have not been identified, and the clinical significance of impaired neutrophil function remains to be determined.

In addition, it has become clear that there is a complex interaction between polymorphonuclear cells, endothelial cells, and serum factors that control neutrophil function. Lack of control for these factors can also explain contradictory results.

SERIOUS INFECTIONS CAUSING MORBIDITY AND MORTALITY IN DIABETES MELLITUS

Although the entire immune system is probably alerted to defense against microbial invasion, certain defects may be more directly associated with certain types of infections. Some of the infections to which diabetic patients seem particularly vulnerable may well be related to some or all of the previously described defects, whereas others are still unexplained.

Skin and Soft Tissue Infections

Whether or not staphylococcal infections of the skin are more common in diabetic than nondiabetic persons is a controversy that has never been resolved. The increased skin and nasal carriage that is described in diabetic persons could lead to increased susceptibility to infection. Farrer and MacLeod[38] found staphylococcal infections to be twice as common among diabetic than nondiabetic patients who had other severe debilitating diseases. They also found more diabetic than nondiabetic patients among people admitted to hospitals with severe staphylococcal infections. A paper by Williams[39] is frequently quoted as proof that skin infections caused by *S aureus* are not more common among diabetic than nondiabetic persons. In that paper, he describes 8 of 330 diabetic patients with boils and carbuncles and 166 nondiabetics with similar infections among 26,879 patients without diabetes. These data do not seem to justify the conclusion that staphylococcal skin infections occur no more frequently in diabetic than nondiabetic persons.

Candidal skin infections commonly occur in moist, warm areas around the breasts, thighs, and genitalia. This is especially common in diabetic patients who are overweight or who have been on antibiotics. These infections can cause extreme discomfort to the patient, and the resultant breakdown of skin may allow entry of *Candida* itself or more virulent organisms.

Diabetic foot infections account for at least one-quarter of all diabetic hospital admissions and are the most common cause of partial or complete foot amputations.[40] Most of these infections probably begin with soft tissue injury, which is unrecognized, secondary to peripheral neuropathy. Subsequent tissue edema, inflammation, and necrosis disrupt the dermal barrier and allow a portal of entry for infection. Concomitant peripheral vascular disease contributes to reduced healing and the onset of chronic infections. The resulting infected diabetic foot ulcer frequently involves deeper tissues, and a chronic underlying osteomyelitis can be established. The infections are characteristically polymicrobial and include aerobic gram-positive or gram-negative organisms coupled with microaerophilic and anaerobic organisms. Peptostreptococci can be recovered from 32–80% of diabetic foot ulcers, and *P magnus* is the most commonly isolated species.[41] Krepel and coworkers[41] demonstrated that 94% of *P magnus* isolated from diabetic foot ulcers produced collagenase, as opposed to 18% of isolates from intra-abdominal infections, and suggested that collagenase production from *P magnus* may be a significant pathogenic factor contributing to the establishment of infected diabetic foot ulcers.

Serious and often life-threatening infections of the skin and underlying tissues can occur when aerobic gram-positive (e.g., *S aureus* or streptococci) or gram-negative (e.g., Enterobacteriaceae or *Pseudomonas*) microorganisms act synergistically with microaerophilic or anaerobic gram-positive (e.g., peptococci or peptostreptococci) or gram-negative (eg, *Bacteroides*) microorganisms to produce necrotizing infections of the skin or underlying soft tissues. This syndrome is probably related to the neuropathy and peripheral vascular disease that allows minor infections to become established; the aerobic organisms consume the already compromised oxygen supply and allow anaerobic organisms to thrive. In this situation, the disease is frequently persistent and destructive. The initial presentation may range from that of an indolent ulcer to a fulminant infection, causing marked systemic toxicity and death.

Stone and Martin described 63 patients with necrotizing cellulitis of whom 47 were diabetic.[42] The mortality rate was 85% for diabetic patients and 44% for nondiabetics. These patients presented with high fever, toxicity, and skin ulcers draining thin serosanguineous pus. Variable amounts of skin necrosis were noted, but gangrene was not necessarily extensive. Exquisite local tenderness inconsistent with the amount of skin involvement is characteristic. Subcutaneous gas may or may not be present. Infection of muscle and fascia is common, and necrosis of skin occurs as the underlying vessels become thrombosed.

These infections may begin in the perianal or pelvic regions, where anaerobic organisms are common, or in the extremities, where the vascular supply is compromised. Deep fascial planes of the neck may be infected from infected teeth or tonsils. The study of Bessman and associates of polymicrobial abscesses in diabetic and nondiabetic mice demonstrated that these abscesses persisted for longer periods in diabetic mice.[43] Of added importance was their finding that enterococci were more synergistic for the growth of *B, fragilis* than of *E, coli*. In mixed infections, enterococci are sometimes regarded as nuisances rather than true pathogens, but this study clearly indicated that this is not the case. A variant of this disease, in which the synergistic organisms are usually all aerobes, has been called *necrotizing fasciitis* by some authors. This may lead to confusion because extensive involvement of skin, subcutaneous tissues, and deep fascia can occur in both syndromes and some authors use the terms interchangeably.[42,44]

Bessman and Wagner described 48 diabetic patients with nonclostridial gas gangrene of the lower extremities.[45] Of the 83 organisms cultured from these patients, only three were anaerobic. Nonclostridial gas gangrene is much more common in the diabetic than is clostridial gas infection. It is important to make the distinction because the organisms are very different in their antibiotic sensitivities. *Clostridium perfringens* is sensitive to penicillin, whereas the anaerobes such as *Bacteroides* usually require metronidazole, clindamycin, cefoxitin, or possibly ticarcillin/clarulinic acid or imipenem. The Enterobacteriaceae may be sensitive to a variety of antibiotics such as aminoglycosides, third-generation cephalosporins, extended spectrum penicillins, or imipenem. Extensive surgical debridement is usually necessary and should be done early in the course of these infections.[42–45]

Goodman and coworkers[46] described risk factors for complications in 172 diabetic patients undergoing local operations for diabetic gangrene. Increased severity of infection, as measured by temperature, total white cell count, and subcutaneous gas, was associated with failure. During the 4.5 years of the study, improvement in outcome was achieved mainly with improvement in preoperative management of infection. The authors suggest delay of surgical procedures until medical control of infection has occurred. However, it should be emphasized that medical control must be accomplished as rapidly as possible, because extensive surgical debridement is usually necessary and should be done as early as possible in the course of these infections.[42–45]

Infections of the hands, although not as common as those of the lower extremities, nevertheless require comment because of the serious nature of the problem. Again, possibly because of the neuropathy and poor vision, the diabetic patient may be unaware of the onset of infection in the hand. Of 20 diabetic patients admitted to the hospital with hand infections, 6 required amputation to control infection and 1 because of impaired function of the extremity. Only 6 patients regained normal function. Most of these infections were synergistic.[47] Skin and soft tissue infections of diabetic persons are frequently complicated by osteomyelitis of contiguous bones.

Erythrasma is an unusual disease of the skin caused by *Corynebacterium minutissimum* (a gram-positive rod). In 19 patients with extensive erythrasma, 9 were known to be diabetic and 6 others had clinical evidence of diabetes.[48] As with many other infections to which the diabetic patient is predisposed, there is a predilection for this disease among alcoholic patients as well.

Malignant Otitis Externa

This disease is well named because associated mortality is over 50%. Over 90% of cases have occurred in diabetic patients over 35 years of age. Swimming and use of a hearing aid are additional predisposing factors. *Pseudomonas aeruginosa* is the usual infecting agent and only rarely are other organisms involved. The presenting manifestations are those of chronic ear infection (i.e., pain and purulent drainage). However, the presence of tenderness and swelling of the surrounding tissues, and in particular polyps or granulation tissue in the floor of the external canal strongly suggest this diagnosis. The infection spreads via the clefts between cartilage and bone in the auditory canal to involve the deep soft tissues, parotid gland, the temporomandibular joint, the mastoid bone, and eventually the cranial nerves. Infection can also spread outward to involve the entire pinna. *P aeruginosa* invades small vessels and produces an infectious vasculitis that compounds the microangiopathy of diabetes and makes this infection particularly virulent. The earliest neurologic complication is facial nerve palsy, and in these patients mortality is highest. Diagnosis is often delayed for 6–8 weeks because patients are misdiagnosed with noninvasive otitis externa. A high index of suspicion and early diagnosis are essential for successful treatment. Parenteral antibiotics (usually a beta-lactam with activity against *Pseudomonas* and an aminoglycoside), topical antipseudomonal ear drops, and surgical debridement are the mainstays of therapy.

Mucormycosis

This is another unusual but highly virulent infection that occurs most commonly in patients with diabetes, in particular those with ketoacidosis. The organism is the same ubiquitous gray-black mold as that found on bread and vegetables. The particular susceptibility of the diabetic for this infection may be related to the decreased leukocyte mobilization previously described and also noted by Sheldon and Bauer,[49] who infected diabetic rabbits with *Rhizopus* and *Mucor* species. Artis and colleagues[50] have shown that ketoacidotic sera from diabetic patients have poor iron-binding capacity. They suggest that the free iron enhances growth of *Rhizopus oryzae* and that this may be a mechanism for the increased susceptibility of ketotic diabetic subjects to this fungus. It is also noteworthy that this organism is capable of invading blood vessels, and the combination of factors found in diabetic hosts may explain why these patients are particularly vulnerable to this infection.

The organism probably first colonizes the nose or paranasal sinuses and spreads by direct extension to the orbit and surrounding tissues. Invasion of the cribriform plate and cranial cavity may occur rapidly. The clinical presentation is usually acute with periorbital pain, induration and discoloration of the lid, and bloody nasal discharge. Ischemic infarction of the lid and orbital contents may follow vessel invasion. Blindness and loss of sensation in the distribution of the ophthalmic division of the trigeminal nerve are diagnostic clues because these are unusual with other orbital infections. Black necrotic tissue may be seen in the nose or posterior hard palate. The internal jugular vein or the cavernous sinus may become thrombosed, and chemosis, proptosis, and retinal hemorrhage may occur.

Although this disease resembles malignant otitis externa in that blood vessels are invaded and progressive infection occurs, extension to the meninges and brain is more common in mucormycosis. Rarely the presentation of this disease is chronic. Morbidity and mortality from this infection are very high, and therapy may have to be started on the basis of clinical findings even in the absence of supporting laboratory evidence for mucormycosis. Biopsy of nasal turbinates or pharyngeal tissues must be done early for diagnostic purposes. Extensive surgical debridement is necessary. Amphotericin is currently the only well-tested drug, and even with early and optimal therapy the disease is extensively disfiguring.

Oral Infections

The problem of periodontal disease in diabetic patients has received significant attention in the dental literature. It was found that this disorder was more common and more severe in diabetic than nondiabetic patients. Associated factors were the age of the patient, the duration of diabetes, the occurrence of complications, and the severity of hyperglycemia. In a study of patients with rapidly progressive periodontitis, 48% were found to have impaired leukotaxis. This leukotactic defect was also noted in alloxan-diabetic rats, and Lavine and coworkers suggest that decreased chemotactic factors or the altered basement membrane of the capillaries could account for the diminished accumulation of leukocytes and the increased numbers of anaerobic organisms found in the gingival crevice of these animals.[51] Manouchehr-Pour and associates[52] also demonstrated significantly reduced chemotactic responses of polymorphonuclear cells from diabetic patients with severe periodontal disease relative to cells from diabetic and nondiabetic subjects with mild periodontal disease or nondiabetic patients with severe periodontal disease.

Oral candidiasis is a well-recognized problem in diabetic patients. Carriage rate and density of *Candida albicans* in the mouth were higher in the diabetic than nondiabetic patients in a study with 50 persons in each group. Among the diabetic patients, no differences could be detected that correlated with degree of control, method of treatment, duration of disease, or age of the patients. Smoking and continuous use of dentures were associated with an increased prevalence of *Candida* colonization.[53]

Gastrointestinal Infections

Telzak and coworkers[54] recently investigated the largest nosocomial food-borne outbreak of *Salmonella enteritides* ever described in the United States and sought to determine host factors that increased the risk of infection after exposure to *S enteritides* in a case control study. Cases consisted of 75 patients with stool culture-confirmed salmonellosis randomly selected from 274 patients with culture-confirmed disease, and controls consisted of 80 randomly selected asymptomatic culture-negative patients. Investigation of multiple potential risk factors indicated that diabetes (defined as a patient treated with insulin or an oral hypoglycemic agent) was the only independent risk factor identified for developing infection after exposure to a *Salmonella*-contaminated meal (odds ratio = 3.8, 95% confidence interval = 1.4, 10.5). When the case definition was restricted to culture-positive patients with symptomatic disease, diabetes remained a risk factor. While noting that diabetic patients may have granulocyte and T cell function abnormalities, the authors suggest that diabetes-associated decreased gastric acid production and decreased bowel motility may be contributory factors. Even more recently, an association between *Campylobacter* gastroenteritis and diabetes has also been described.[55]

Additional studies are needed to corroborate these findings to determine if there is an increased risk of gastrointestinal infection for diabetic patients from other bacterial pathogens, and to determine if hyperglycemia is related to the risk and severity of these infections in patients with diabetes.

Urinary Tract Infections

The data relating to urinary tract infections in diabetic patients have been examined in two authoritative reviews which reached contradictory conclusions. Wheat states that the majority of controlled studies noted a two- to fourfold higher incidence of bacteriuria in diabetic women,[56] whereas Gocke and Grieco conclude that in well-controlled diabetes, urinary tract infections are no more likely in diabetics than in nondiabetic patients.[22] Several studies support both views.[57,58] In diabetic children, a prevalence rate similar to that of nondiabetic children is found, and the same appears to be true for diabetic men.[59–61] Among patients with hospital-acquired urinary tract infections, diabetic patients are more susceptible than nondiabetic patients.[62]

Thus it appears that within populations in whom the prevalence of urinary tract infections is known to be high, the diabetic is even more likely than the nondiabetic to develop a urinary tract infection. Some of the reasons for this are that the diabetic patient may have a neurogenic bladder with urinary stasis, may be catheterized frequently, may have underlying renal disease, and may have impaired host defenses, all of which are predisposing factors for urinary tract infection. The diabetic leukocyte may be compromised by the hyperosmolar milieu in the renal medulla, which impairs phagocytosis even in the normal leukocyte.[63]

There is universal agreement that urinary tract infections are more likely to cause serious complications for the diabetic patient than for others. Among bacteriuric pregnant women with diabetic retinopathy, a 50% perinatal death rate was found compared with 15% for women with microangiopathy without bacteriuria.[59] Studies done to localize the anatomic site of bacterial involvement in diabetic patients with asymptomatic bacteriuria document high rates of upper tract involvement. Ooi and colleagues found that 63% of diabetic women with asymptomatic bacteriuria had upper tract involvement, whereas Forland and associates found 80% of such patients had upper tract involvement.[22] However, a prospective study suggested that asymptomatic bacteriuric diabetic women do not have an increased incidence of subsequent symptomatic urinary tract infection, including pyelonephritis.[64]

Data suggest that diabetic patients may experience higher complication rates when they do develop renal infections. In a series of 52 patients with perinephric abscesses, 36 were diabetic. This diagnosis should be suspected in any diabetic patient who does not respond to adequate antibiotic therapy within 3 or 4 days. An abdominal or flank mass is a helpful diagnostic sign, but is present in only about 50% of cases. The organisms are usually those associated with urinary tract infections, although *S. aureus* can cause cortical abscesses by the hematogenous route. Although there are some data that these infections may respond to antibiotics alone, incision and drainage of the abscess are usually required.[65]

A well-known, but now rather uncommon complication of urinary tract infection in diabetic patients is renal papillary necrosis. This disease is probably related to renal ischemia and is usually accompanied by rapidly deteriorating renal function, as well as fever, flank pain, and a poor response to antibiotic therapy. Obstructive uropathy or analgesic use may be concomitant factors in the pathogenesis of this disease. Diagnosis is made by x-ray, and the retrograde pyelogram is preferred over the intravenous pyelogram in the diabetic patient with renal impairment.

Gas-forming infections of the kidney, renal pelvis, ureter, or bladder are uncommon, but not rare, and most occur in diabetic patients. The severity of this disease is related to the site of infection. When gas is confined to the collecting system, survival rates are much better than when the renal parenchyma is involved. Less severe disease can be managed with either antibiotic therapy alone or in conjunction with percutaneous drainage. Greater disease severity may warrant nephrectomy. Overall mortality approaches 18.8%.[66] As with the other renal complications, this disease should be suspected in any diabetic patient not responding quickly to appropriate antibiotics. Nausea, vomiting, and diarrhea in patients with urinary tract infections may give a clue to this disease. Tenderness, a palpable mass, or rarely, crepitus may be felt in the costovertebral angle. Diagnosis is made by abdominal CT scan, since plain radiographs identify gas in only one-third of patients.[65] The pathogenesis of this disease is obscure but is thought to be related to the ability of organisms such as *E coli* or *Klebsiella pneumoniae* to utilize glucose with subsequent formation of carbon dioxide and hydrogen. When infection with these organisms occurs in an area with vascular insufficiency, a severe necrotizing infection can occur. What is not clear is why it happens so infrequently, considering the frequent occurrence of urinary tract infections in diabetic patients with vascular disease and hyperglycemia.

Fungal infections of the urinary tract are not uncommon in diabetic patients. This may be a result of the use of antibiotics for bacterial infections and subsequent overgrowth of *Candida* species, or the fungus may spread from perineal candidal infection. The distinction between colonization and infection is often difficult to assess in these patients. Goldberg and coworkers suggested that patients who have *Candida* colony counts of greater than 10,000/mL in a clean-catch specimen should be catheterized, and if the count is still greater than 10,000/mL, the patient has actual urinary tract infection and not just colonization.[67] If infection is present in a diabetic patient, then treatment should be initiated. Oral fluconazole (200 mg the first day followed by 3–5 days of 100 mg/d) is highly efficacious in the treatment of *Candida albicans* cystitis. However, *C krusei* are routinely resistant to fluconazole. Alternatively, 5 days of continuous bladder irrigation of 50 mg of amphotericin in 1 liter of sterile water per day via a triple-lumen Foley catheter is reported to have resulted in cure rates of 70%. Oral flucytosine can be considered, but about 50% of candidal strains are resistant to this drug and bone marrow toxicity may occur in patients with renal impairment. Ketoconazole is poorly excreted in urine and should not be considered as a therapeutic option. Cases of candidal cystitis resistant to these treatment regimens may respond to low-dose intravenous amphotericin, but upper urinary tract disease or systemic infection should always be suspected in these cases and may require more extensive therapy.

Pneumonia

While hematogenous spread from sites of peripheral infection is one mechanism for development of pneumonia, the more usual route of infection is by inhalation of pathogenic organisms that colonize the oropharynx. The susceptibility of diabetic patients to *S aureus* and *K pneumoniae* pneumonias reported by Khurana and coworkers[68] could be related to the increased nasal carriage of *S aureus* or oropharyngeal carriage of *K pneumoniae*. Patients with chronic illness appear to experience a change from the so-called normal oropharyngeal flora (i.e., from gram-positive organisms to gram-negative rods), and this could predispose patients to gram-negative rod pneumonia. Among alcoholics, 40% were found to be colonized with *K pneumoniae*,[69] and pneumonia with this organism is another disease that appears to be particularly common among alcoholic and diabetic subjects.

Phagocytosis by the pulmonary macrophage is the major defense mechanism against inhaled bacteria, and this may well be defective in the diabetic patient. Acidosis impairs the bactericidal mechanisms of the lung, and this could be an added factor in the uncontrolled diabetic patient.[70]

Infections with either *S aureus* or aerobic gram-negative rods can produce severe, necrotizing pneumonias. Antibiotic therapy for 2–4 weeks is usually necessary and the mortality rate is 40–50%.

There is no documented evidence that pneumococcal pneumonia is more common in diabetic than nondiabetic hosts; nevertheless, the serious nature of this disease in any patient with chronic disease warrants the use of pneumococcal vaccine in these patients, especially those in the older age groups.

Emphysematous Cholecystitis

Although it is difficult to document an increased incidence of cholecystitis among diabetic patients, the more severe and fulminating infection with gas-producing organisms occurs frequently in diabetic patients. In 136 cases of emphysematous cholecystitis, diabetes mellitus was found in 38%. This disease differs from emphysematous pyelonephritis in that *C perfringens* is isolated in about one-half of the cases. In one series of 109 cases in which gall bladder bile was cultured, 95 were culture positive, with *Clostridia* spp isolated from 46% and *E coli* from 33%.

The clinical presentation of this disease resembles that of acute cholecystitis, but the outcome is radically different. Gall bladder perforation and gangrene are frequent, and the mortality rate is 3–10 times higher than in acute cholecystitis. The male to female ratio is about 3:1, the reverse of that seen in acute cholecystitis. Diabetic vascular disease is thought to be a factor in the pathogenesis of this unusual syndrome as it is with the other gas-forming infections. The diagnosis is made by finding radiographic evidence of gas in the gall bladder wall. Since the presence of gas may be seen in the first 48 hours of infection and spread to surrounding tissues in the next 48 hours, Wheat[56] suggests that diabetic patients with evidence of acute cholecystitis have abdominal x-rays each day for at least 4 days. This advice would seem particularly applicable if the patient is a diabetic male. Antibiotic coverage includes the triple combination of ampicillin (or an extended-spectrum penicillin such as piperacillin or mezlocillin), metronidazole, and an aminoglycoside. Imipenem may be useful for alternative antibiotic coverage because it is active against anaerobic bacteria, aerobic gram-negative rods, and *Enterococcus faecalis*. This drug does not have the nephro- or ototoxicity of the aminoglycosides, an important consideration in the diabetic patient. As with the other gas-forming infections, antibiotic coverage is useful only when used in association with early surgical therapy.

Bacteremia

While bloodstream invasion may result from infection with most bacterial pathogens, certain bacteria have been reported to pose a particular threat to diabetic patients. These will be discussed in detail.

Staphylococcal Bacteremia

It has long been suggested that diabetic patients are predisposed to staphylococcal bacteremia, but this has never been established by controlled studies. Diabetes has been recognized as an underlying disease in 8–36% of patients with staphylococcal bacteremia, but studies designed to specifically evaluate the frequency of staphylococcal bacteremia in diabetic and nondiabetic patients have yet to be performed.[1] Although a number of studies have reported higher mortality rates associated with staphylococcal bacteremia in diabetic relative to nondiabetic patients, the most recent information suggests that there is no increased risk of mortality associated with these infections among diabetic patients. Cooper and Platt compared the presentation and course of 27 episodes of *S aureus* bacteremia in diabetic patients with 34 episodes in nondiabetic patients, and although they found no increased mortality in diabetic patients, when a primary focus of infection was present, they found diabetic patients were more likely to develop endocarditis than nondiabetic subjects.[1] It is possible that both granulocyte deficiencies and impaired cell-mediated immunity might be responsible for this increased severity of staphylococcal disease among diabetic patients.

Group B Streptococcal Bacteremia

Beta-hemolytic streptococci of the Lancefield group B have emerged as a leading cause of sepsis of neonates and pregnant women. However, in a population-based assessment of invasive disease due to group B streptococci, Farley and colleagues found that 68% of cases occurred among adult men and nonpregnant women.[71] Of these patients, 31% were diabetic. This striking predilection for diabetic patients confirmed previous reports that noted the association between these two diseases.[72,73] Bayer and associates[73] described 22 patients with bacteremic group B streptococcal infections, of whom 10 were diabetic patients. Pneumonia was the initial infection in five of these patients and cellulitis and pyelonephritis in two each.

The carriage rate of group B streptococci was studied in a group of diabetic compared to nondiabetic subjects.[74] No differences were found between the two groups. The studies by Baker and coworkers[16] described above, showing inefficient opsonization of group B streptococci in diabetic patients, suggest at least one reason for these infections in diabetic patients.

The drug of choice for treatment of group B streptococcal infection is penicillin. The organism is less sensitive to penicillin than group A streptococci and therefore higher doses may be required. In a patient allergic to penicillin, sensitivities must be obtained from the laboratory because several of the strains are resistant to clindamycin, erythromycin, and tetracycline. Cephalosporins could be used, but there is a 10% risk of cross-reaction in cases of penicillin allergy.

Gram-Negative Rod Bacteremia

Bacteremia with aerobic gram-negative rods usually results from urinary tract infections, gastrointestinal disease, gallbladder disease, or in the hospitalized patient, intravenous catheters. In the diabetic patient, synergistic gangrene and gram-negative rod pneumonias are an additional hazard. Several studies document a high prevalence of diabetes among patients with gram-negative rod bacteremias. In their series of patients with *Proteus* bacteremia at the

Boston City Hospital, Adler and associates[75] found that 25% of the patients had diabetes. An investigation by Lewis and Fekety[76] of patients with gram-negative rod bacteremias at Johns Hopkins Hospital found that 20% of these patients had diabetes. The mortality rate among the diabetic patients was almost twice the overall mortality rate. Infection with gram-negative rods frequently requires the use of an aminoglycoside, and these antibiotics may be especially toxic in diabetic patients with compromised renal function. Dosage of these drugs should be carefully monitored, drug levels should be measured, and renal function tests should be done every day or every other day.

Tuberculosis

Whether there is an increased risk of primary tuberculosis after exposure for diabetic patients relative to nondiabetic patients has never been investigated, but diabetes and alcoholism have been suggested as potential risk factors for reactivation of latent tuberculosis.[77] Zack and coworkers[78] noted a 41% abnormal glucose tolerance rate among 256 nondiabetic patients hospitalized with tuberculosis. Unfortunately, long-term follow-up was not conducted, and the significance of this association remains obscure. Interestingly, a recent study comparing 5290 cases of tuberculosis to 37,366 controls diagnosed with deep venous thrombosis, pulmonary embolism, or acute appendicitis, identified diabetes mellitus as a risk factor for tuberculosis, especially among middle-aged Hispanics.[79] This association awaits further confirmation. Previous anecdotal reports describing a tendency for severe lower lobe tuberculosis in diabetic subjects have not been borne out.

Systemic Fungal Infections

Several fungal diseases that are uncommon in the general population seem to be more common in the diabetic population. Cryptococcosis is a disease caused by an encapsulated yeast that is inhaled. In the majority of cases, the host defenses of the lung are sufficient to prevent infection. In immunocompromised patients, pneumonia, meningitis, or disseminated disease may occur. Diabetes has been suggested to be a risk factor for cryptococcal infection, but this is not well established. Coccidioidomycosis, a fungal disease found in certain regions of California and Arizona, seems to be particularly virulent in people of certain genetic backgrounds, such as African-Americans or Asians. Baker and coworkers reported that the disease was particularly severe in patients with type 1 diabetes.[80] Rare cases of septic shock have been seen in patients with candidemia and diabetes.

SUMMARY

Despite advances in the knowledge of host defense in diabetes, there are numerous aspects of the complex host-pathogen interrelationship in diabetic subjects that remain unexplained. Why diabetic patients appear to have increased problems with pyogenic organisms such as *S aureus* and group B streptococci and not with common pathogens such as pneumococci has not been elucidated. Despite numerous unanswered questions, there is clear evidence of increased morbidity and mortality from infectious agents in the diabetic population. A knowledge of these problems coupled with appropriate preventive and therapeutic measures may lessen the impact of these diseases in the diabetic host.

REFERENCES

1. Breen JD, Karchmer AW: *Staphylococcus aureus* infections in diabetic patients. *Inf Dis Clin* 1995;9:11.
2. Patterson JE, Andriole VT: Bacterial urinary tract infections in diabetes. *Inf Dis Clin* 1997;11:735.
3. Soler NG, Bennett MA, Fitzgerald MG, *et al*: Intensive care in the management of diabetic ketoacidosis. *Lancet* 1973;1:951.
4. Muller WA, Faloona GR, Unger RH: Hyperglucagonemia in diabetic ketoacidosis. *Am J Med* 1973;54:52.
5. Peterka ES, Fusaro RM: The skin glucose content of fasting diabetics with and without infection. *J Invest Dermatol* 1966;46:549.
6. Somerville DA, Lancaster-Smith M:. The aerobic and cutaneous microflora of diabetic subjects. *Br J Dermatol* 1973;89:395.
7. Williamson JR, Chang K, Frangos M, *et al*: Hyperglycemic pseudohypoxia and diabetic complications. *Diabetes* 1993;42:801.
8. Anderson B, Goldsmith GH, Spagnulo PJ: Neutrophil adhesive dysfunction in diabetes mellitus: The role of cellular and plasma factors. *J Lab Clin Med* 1988;110:275.
9. Macmillan DE: Pathophysiology of diabetic vascular disease. In: *Diabetes in Review*. Clinical Conference American Diabetes Association, 27th Post Graduate Course, Atlanta:1980.
10. Seabrook GR, Edmiston CE, Schmitt DD, *et al*: Comparison of serum and tissue antibiotic levels in diabetes-related foot infections. *Surgery* 1991;110:671.
11. Richardson R: Immunity in diabetes: Influence of diabetes on the development of antibacterial properties in the blood. *J Clin Invest* 1933; 12:1143.
12. Balch HH, Water M, Kelly D: Blood bactericidal studies and serum complement in diabetic patients. *J Surg Res* 1963;3:199.
13. Eibl LM, Schernthaner G, Erd W, *et al*: Humoral immunodeficiency to bacterial antigens in patients with juvenile diabetes mellitus. *Diabetologia* 1976;12:259.
14. Bates G, Weiss C: Delayed development of antibody to staphylococcal toxin in diabetic children. *Am J Dis Child* 1941;62:346.
15. Beam TR Jr., Crigler ED, Goldman JR, *et al*: Antibody response to polyvalent pneumococcal polysaccharide vaccine in diabetics. *JAMA* 1980;244:2621.
16. Baker CJ, Webb BJ, Kasper DL, *et al*: The role of complement and antibody in opsonophagocytosis of type II group B streptococci. *J Infect Dis* 1986;154:47.
17. Hill HR, Sauls HS, Detloff JL, *et al*: Impaired leucotactic responsiveness in patients with juvenile diabetes mellitus. *Clin Immunol Immunopathol* 1974;2:395.
18. Perillie PE, Nolan JP, Finch SC: Studies of resistance to infection in diabetes mellitus: Local exudative cellular response. *J Lab Clin Med* 1962;59:1008.
19. Brayton RG, Stokes PE, Schwartz MS, *et al*: Effect of alcohol and various diseases on leukocyte mobilization, phagocytosis and intracellular killing. *N Engl J Med* 1970;282:123.
20. Bagdade JD, Stewart M, Walters E: Impaired granulocyte adherence: A reversible defect in host defense in patients with poorly controlled diabetes. *Diabetes* 1978;27:677.
21. Donovan RM, Goldstein E, Kim Y: A computer-assisted image-analysis system for analyzing polymorphonuclear leukocyte chemotaxis in patients with diabetes mellitus. *J Infect Dis* 1978;155:737.
22. Gocke TM: Infections complicating diabetes mellitus. In: Grieco MH, ed. *Infections in the Abnormal Host*. Yorke Medical:1980;585.
23. Molenaar DM, Palumbo PJ, Wilson WR, *et al*: Leucocyte chemotaxis in diabetic patients and their non-diabetic first degree relatives. *Diabetes* 1976;25:880.
24. McMullen JA, Van Dyke TA, Horoszewicz HV, *et al*: Neutrophil chemotaxis in individuals with advanced periodontal disease and a genetic predisposition to diabetes mellitus. *J Periodontol* 1981;52:167.
25. Bybee JD, Rogers DE: The phagocytic activity of polymorphonuclear leukocytes obtained from patients with diabetes mellitus. *J Lab Clin Med* 1964;64:1.
26. Tan JS, Anderson JL, Watanakunakorn C, *et al*: Neutrophil function in diabetes mellitus. *J Lab Clin Med* 1975;85:26.
27. Nolan CM, Beatty HN, Bagdade JD: Further characterization of the impaired bactericidal function of granulocytes in patients with poorly controlled diabetes. *Diabetes* 1978;27:889.
28. Repine JE, Clawson CC, Gaetz FC: Bactericidal function of neutrophils from patients with acute bacterial infections and from diabetics. *J Infect Dis* 1980;142:869.
29. Bagdade JD, Root R, Bulger JR: Impaired leucocyte function in patients with poorly controlled diabetes. *Diabetes* 1974;23:9.
30. Crosby B, Allison F: Phagocytic and bactericidal capacity of polymorphonuclear leukocytes recovered from venous blood of human beings. *Proc Soc Exp Biol Med* 1966;123:660.
31. Ragab AH, Hazlett B, Cowan DH: Response of peripheral blood lymphocytes from patients with diabetes mellitus to phytohemagglutinin and candida antigen. *Diabetes* 1978;27:889.
32. Essman V: Effect of insulin on human leucocytes. *Diabetes* 1963; 12:545.
33. Plouffe JF, Silva J, Fekety FR Jr., *et al*: Cell mediated immunity in diabetes mellitus. *Infect Immunol* 1978;21:425.
34. Casey JI, Heeter BJ, Klyshevich K: Impaired response of lymphocytes of diabetic subjects to *Staphylococcus aureus*. *J Infect Dis* 1977; 136:495.
35. Casey J, Sturm CS Jr.: Impaired response of lymphocytes from non-type 1 diabetics to staphylococcal phage and tetanus antigen. *J Clin Microbiol* 1982;15:105.
36. Fernandes G, Handwerger BS, Yunis EJ, *et al*: Immune response in the mutant diabetic C57 Bl/K$_s$ db 1 mouse. *J Clin Invest* 1978;61:243.
37. Mahoud AA, Rodman HM, Mandel MA, *et al*: Induced and spontaneous diabetes mellitus and suppression of cell mediated immune responses. *J Clin Invest* 1976;57:362.
38. Farrer SM, MacLeod CM: Staphylococcal infections in a general hospital. *Am J Hyg* 1960;72:38.
39. Williams JR: Does diabetes mellitus predispose the patient to pyogenic skin infections? *JAMA* 1942;118:1357.
40. Brodsky JW, Schneidler C: Diabetic foot infections. *Orthop Clin North Am* 1991;22:473.
41. Krepel CJ, Gohr CM, Edmiston CE, *et al*: Anaerobic pathogenesis: Collagenase production by *Peptostreptococcus magnus* and its relationship to site of infection. *J Infect Dis* 1991;163:1148.
42. Stone HH, Martin JD Jr.: Synergistic necrotizing cellulitis. *Ann Surg* 1972;175:702.
43. Bessman AN, Sapico FL, Tabatabai M, *et al*: Persistence of polymicrobial abscesses in the poorly controlled diabetic host. *Diabetes* 1986;35:448.
44. Crosthwait RW Jr, Crosthwait RW, Jordan GL: Necrotizing fasciitis. *J Trauma* 1964;4:149.
45. Bessman AN, Wagner W: Nonclostridial gas gangrene. *JAMA* 1975; 233:958.
46. Goodman J, Bessman AN, Taget B, *et al*: Risk factors in local surgical procedures for diabetic gangrene. *Surg Gynecol Obstet* 1976;143:587.
47. Mann RJ, Peacock JM: Hand infections in diabetes mellitus. *J Trauma* 1977;17:376.
48. Montes LF, Dobson H, Dodge BG, *et al*: Erythrasma and diabetes mellitus. *Arch Dermatol* 1969;99:674.
49. Sheldon WH, Bauer H: The development of the acute inflammatory response to experimental cutaneous mucormycosis in normal and diabetic rabbits. *J Exp Med* 1959;110:845.
50. Artis WM, Fountain JA, Delcher HK, *et al*: A mechanism of susceptibility to mucormycosis in diabetic ketoacidosis: Transferrin and iron availability. *Diabetes* 1982;31:1109.
51. Lavine WS, Maderazo EG, Stolman EG, *et al*: Impaired neutrophil chemotaxis in patients with juvenile and rapidly progressing periodontitis. *J Periodont Res* 1979;14:10.
52. Manouchehr-Pour M, Spagnuolo PJ, Rodman HM, *et al*: Impaired neutrophil chemotaxis in diabetic patients with severe periodontitis. *J Dent Res* 1981;60:729.
53. Tapper-Jones LM, Aldred MJ, Walker DM, *et al*: Candidal infections and populations of *Candida albicans* in mouths of diabetics. *J Clin Pathol* 1981;34:706.
54. Telzak EE, Greenberg MSZ, Budnick LD, *et al*: Diabetes mellitus—a newly described risk factor for infection from *Salmonella enteritidis*. *J Infect Dis* 1991;164:538.
55. Neal KR, Slack RCB: Diabetes mellitus, anti-secretory drugs and other risk factors for campylobacter gastro-enteritis in adults: a case control study. *Epidemiol Infect* 1997;119:307.

56. Wheat LJ: Infections and diabetes mellitus. *Diabetes Care* 1980;3:187.

57. Kass EH: Asymptomatic infections of urinary tract. *Trans Assoc Am Physicians* 1956;69:56.

58. O'Sullivan DJ, Fitzgerald MG, Meynell MJ, *et al*: Urinary tract infection: A comparative study in the diabetic and general populations. *Br Med J* 1961;1(suppl):786.

59. Pometta D, Rees SB, Younger D, *et al*: Asymptomatic bacteriuria in diabetes mellitus. *N Engl J Med* 1967;276:1118.

60. Vyslgaard R: Studies on urinary tract infection in diabetes: I. Bacteriuria in patients with diabetes mellitus and in control subjects. *Acta Med Scand* 1966;179:173.

61. Kunin CM, Southall I, Paguin AJ: Epidemiology of urinary tract infection: Pilot study of 3057 school children. *N Engl J Med* 1960;263:817.

62. Stamm WE, Martin SM, Bennet JV: Epidemiology of nosocomial infections due to gram negative bacilli: Aspects relative to development and use of vaccines. *J Infect Dis* 1977;136:5151.

63. Chernew I, Braude AI: Depression of phagocytosis by solutes in concentration found in the kidney and urine. *J Clin Invest* 1962;41:1945.

64. Batalla MA, Balodimos MC, Bradley RF: Bacteriuria in diabetes mellitus. *Diabetologia* 1971;7:297.

65. Joshi N, Caputo G, Weitekamp MR, *et al*: Infections in patients with diabetes mellitus. *N Engl J Med* 1999;341:1906.

66. Huang J, Tseng C: Emphysematous pyelonephritis: clinicoradiological classification, management, prognosis and pathogenesis. *Arch Intern Med* 2000;160:797.

67. Goldberg PK, Kozinn PJ, Wise GJ, *et al*: Incidence and significance of candiduria. *JAMA* 1979;241:582.

68. Khurana RC, Younger D, Ryan JR: Characteristics of pneumonia in diabetes. *Clin Res* 1973;21:629(abs).

69. Fuxench-Lopez Z, Ramirez-Ronda CH: Pharyngeal flora in ambulatory alcoholic patients. *Arch Intern Med* 1978;138:1815.

70. Goldstein E, Green GM, Seamans C: The effect of acidosis on pulmonary bactericidal function. *J Lab Clin Med* 1970;75:912.

71. Farley MM, Harvey RC, Stull T, *et al*: A population-based assessment of invasive disease due to group B streptococcus in nonpregnant adults. *N Engl J Med* 1993;328:1807.

72. Duma RJ, Weinberg AN, Medrek TF, *et al*: Streptococcal infections: A bacteriologic and clinical study of streptococcal bacteremia. *Medicine* 1969;48:87.

73. Bayer AS, Chow AW, Anthony BF, *et al*: Serious infections in adults due to group B streptococci. *Am J Med* 1976;61:498.

74. Casey JI, Maturlo S, Albin J, *et al*: Comparison of carriage rates of group B streptococcus in diabetic and nondiabetic persons. *Am J Epidemiol* 1982;116:704.

75. Adler JA, Burke JP, Martin DF, *et al*: Proteus infections in a general hospital. *Ann Intern Med* 1971;75:531.

76. Lewis J, Fekety FR Jr.: Gram negative bacteremia. *Johns Hopkins Med J* 1969;124:106.

77. Edsall J, Collins JG, Gran JAC: The reactivation of tuberculosis in New York City in 1967. *Am Rev Resp Dis* 1970;102:725.

78. Zack MB, Fulkeson LL, Stein E: Glucose intolerance in pulmonary tuberculosis. *Am Rev Resp Dis* 1973;108:1164.

79. Pablos-Mendez A, Blustein J, Knirsch CA: The role of diabetes mellitus in the higher prevalence of tuberculosis among hispanics. *Am J Pub Health* 1997;87:574.

80. Baker EJ, Hawkins JA, Washow EA: Surgery for coccidioidomycosis in 52 diabetic patients with special reference to related immunologic factors. *J Thorac Cardiovasc Surg* 1978;75:680.

CHAPTER 37

Diabetes and Surgery

Stephanie A. Amiel

K. George M. M. Alberti

The diabetic patient is not protected from the disorders that require surgical intervention in the nondiabetic population. Indeed the chronic complications of diabetes increase the likelihood of the need for surgery, with particular reference to cardiac and peripheral vascular and renal disease. It has been estimated in the past that a diabetic person has a 50% chance of having a surgical procedure during their lifetime.[1] This chance is steadily increasing with the greater life expectancy of diabetic people and the greater proportion undergoing angioplasty and coronary bypass operations.

Surgery in diabetic patients is complicated by the need for metabolic control during surgery itself and in the postoperative period when feeding is reinstated. The chronic complications are also likely to complicate recovery with particular respect to autonomic neuropathy, nephropathy, and macrovascular disease. A further challenge is offered by the greatly increased volume of (ambulatory) day surgery now performed, although it has been shown that diabetic patients are no more likely than nondiabetic patients to require full admission afterwards.[2] The ability to admit patients for stabilization preoperatively has also decreased.

Surgery and anesthesia have profound metabolic effects. These will be exacerbated in diabetes by insulin deficiency or hyposecretion and by insulin insensitivity (see Chap. 8). The poorly controlled diabetic patient will already be in a catabolic state, which will amplify the effects of surgery. There will be diminished phagocyte function with impaired resistance to infection and delayed wound healing. Together with the chronic complications of diabetes, these factors will add to the morbidity and mortality of the surgical procedures themselves. The aim of treatment of the diabetic patient undergoing surgery must therefore be to control the metabolic scenario in such a way that the risks are no greater and the outcome no worse than for the nondiabetic person.

In the remainder of this chapter, the metabolic effects of surgery and anesthesia will be briefly reviewed together with the impact of diabetes on these events. The pre-operative assessment of the diabetic patient, anesthetic management, and peri- and postoperative treatment will then be discussed, together with the management of diabetes in certain special situations such as emergency surgery and cardiopulmonary bypass. For more details the reader is referred to several recent reviews.[3–9]

METABOLIC EFFECTS OF ANESTHESIA AND SURGERY IN THE NORMAL AND DIABETIC STATES

Under normal conditions, metabolic homeostasis is maintained by a fine balance between the anabolic hormone insulin and the major catabolic hormones, glucagon, the catecholamines, cortisol, and to some extent, growth hormone (see Chap. 1). In the fed state the anabolic actions of insulin predominate, with the stimulation of processes leading to fuel storage: glycogenesis, lipogenesis, glycolysis (to promote new fatty acid synthesis in the liver), and protein synthesis.

In starvation the balance is tilted towards catabolism; insulin concentrations fall while those of the catabolic hormones stay the same or rise slightly. There is enhanced production of the oxidizable substrates, glucose, fatty acids, and ketone bodies through stimulation of glycogenolysis, gluconeogenesis, lipolysis, and ketogenesis, which together with increased proteolysis provide gluconeogenic substrates. Insulin plays a key role in restraining these events through its important anticatabolic actions, as they respond to small amounts of insulin and thereby allow controlled release of substrates. These processes become disturbed in stress states such as surgery, particularly if diabetes is superimposed.

Anesthesia

The impact of modern anesthetic agents on metabolic control is relatively small. Epidural anesthesia blocks catecholamine release and can reduce postoperative protein catabolism (see reference 8). In one study, isoflurane was associated with a greater increase in plasma glucose than fentanyl/midazolam with only the former causing increased hepatic glucose production. Nonetheless the effects are relatively small and disappear rapidly postoperatively.[10] Both locoregional and general anesthesia can be used safely. More important is the presence of autonomic neuropathy or cardiovascular disease in the patient.

Surgery

Surgery induces a trauma-like stress state[9] and provides a classic hyperglycemic challenge. The stress response to both the condition for which the surgery is being performed and any associated anxiety includes adrenergic and sympathetic activation and elevations of circulating catecholamines, cortisol, and growth hormone. These may be sufficient to convert well-controlled diabetes into hyperglycemia—even ketoacidosis—particularly when the surgical condition is an acute one. Furthermore, immobility reduces muscle consumption of glucose and confinement to bed causes insulin resistance, contributing to the tendency toward hyperglycemia. Surgery is associated with a reduction in insulin sensitivity that persists for 3 weeks.[11] Using the short insulin-tolerance test, a 50% fall of insulin sensitivity has been demonstrated 24 hours after laparoscopic cholecystectomy.[12] Thorell and associates showed a one-third decrease in sensitivity even after inguinal hernia repair and a 56% decrease after cholecystectomy.[13]

Food deprivation further worsens the catabolic state. In health the small amounts of circulating insulin still present limit the extent of the catabolic processes. Interestingly, it is possible to normalize postoperative insulin sensitivity by perioperative insulin and glucose infusion[14] and to attenuate it with preoperative glucose loading orally or intravenously.[15] In surgery as opposed to starvation, it is noteworthy that the catabolic processes do not result in elevated circulating levels of plasma free fatty acids or ketones, so the body loses the protein-sparing effect of these metabolic fuels and proteolysis continues unabated. This is probably due in part to the elevated insulin levels which are found due to insulin resistance.

Classical stress hormone responses are unlikely to be the sole or perhaps even major cause of surgery-related insulin resistance. A study of healthy subjects undergoing elective surgery found a significant fall in whole-body insulin sensitivity on the first postoperative day to be strongly correlated with elevated levels of the cytokine interleukin-6.[16] Other cytokines did not show this pattern, perhaps because of the relatively limited tissue damage associated with these procedures. It is noteworthy that in a small number of patients, the insulin resistance persisted to at least the fifth postoperative day. Cholecystectomy had notably more effect on insulin sensitivity, stress hormones and IL-6 levels than herniorrhapy, which was not associated with a significant increase in stress hormones by day one.

The molecular mechanisms of the insulin resistance of surgery remain to be elucidated, but a major effect on peripheral glucose utilization has been observed with reductions in glucose transport, nonoxidative glucose disposal and intracellular glycogen synthase demonstrated in muscle tissue sampled on the first postoperative day.[17] It is likely that impaired translocation of the glucose transporter GLUT-4 in response to insulin in muscle is an important mechanism.

Neural effects are also important in the catabolic response. Epidural anesthesia, spinal blocks, and splanchnic nerve block have all been shown to ameliorate the endocrine and metabolic response.[18]

Diabetes

The uncontrolled diabetic patient will already be in a catabolic state. Superimposition of the metabolic stress of surgery will result in a major worsening of this state. Severe hyperglycemia leads to an osmotic diuresis, with loss of salt and water. In extremes, dehydration and hypovolemia may ensue. Hyperglycemia is associated with decreased levels of antioxidants, disturbances of coagulation, including increments in fibrinogen and plasminogen activator inhibitor (PAI-1), and interferes with neutrophil function. Ketosis with severe acidemia may also ensue.

Not surprisingly, few data are available on the absence of treatment of diabetes during surgery. Blood glucose levels have been shown to rise from about 180 mg/dL (10 mmol/L) to about 270 mg/dL (15 mmol/L) postoperatively with ketone body levels rising to about twice the level of nondiabetic controls.[19] The situation is similar metabolically even in patients with type 2 diabetes mellitus (T2DM) undergoing minor surgery that generates a relatively small stress response. Blood glucose levels were again greater than in the nondiabetic, reaching only 180 mg/dL (10 mmol/L). Ketone body and fatty acid levels were also above normal, although not at a dangerous level.[20]

In order to minimize the adverse effects of these metabolic events on the diabetic patient, meticulous attention to metabolic control is required. The response of surgery relates to the severity of the surgery. Patients with type 1 diabetes mellitus (T1DM) will require insulin replacement regardless, but T2DM patients will probably be able to mount an adequate insulin response to minor surgery and insulin therapy may not be required. By contrast, they should receive insulin for major surgery.

Aims of Therapy

The main aim of therapy must be to avoid any excess morbidity and mortality when compared with the nondiabetic population. To achieve this, hypoglycemia, excessive hyperglycemia, increased protein catabolism, and undue electrolyte disturbances should be prevented. In addition, attention should be paid to cardiovascular status and to problems created by the long-term complications of diabetes. These goals are best achieved by controlling the metabolic status of the patient. There is still argument, however, as to how stringent metabolic control should be. The diabetologist may seek to attain normoglycemia, but this has potential dangers in the unconscious patient. In general, it is probably wiser to aim for blood glucose levels at which resistance to infection and phagocyte function are not impaired and at which normal wound healing can take place. The threshold for these effects is probably around 200 mg/dL (11 mmol/L) so the target for glycemia is in the range of 120–180 mg/dL (6.7–10 mmol/L) during the operative period.

Preoperative Management

All patients require a full preoperative assessment. The diabetic patient presenting for surgery is more likely to have comorbidity than the patient without diabetes. In the young person with a relatively short duration of diabetes, the main focus of attention will be glycemic control, but in the older patient with a longer history of diabetes, careful assessment of the possible chronic complications is necessary if the patient is to be well managed perioperatively.

Assessment of glycemic control and current therapeutic regimen is mandatory. The glycated hemoglobin will indicate the patient's habitual control. The random glucose is not useful until the time of starting the peri-operative management.

Cardiovascular status should be assessed by history and resting ECG. Asymptomatic angina is reported in diabetic patients, but a stress test such as an exercise ECG or thallium scan is not routinely indicated. Symptomatic autonomic neuropathy is fortunately uncommon in diabetes, but lesser degrees of cardiac denervation are not. The anesthetist should be aware of potential defects in the normal cardiovascular responses to hypotension in anesthesia induction. A report of an exaggerated pressor response to intubation has been published[21] in ten consecutive patients presenting for vitreous surgery. All had some degree of autonomic dysfunction preoperatively and all failed to show a heart rate increase when blood pressure fell. This is particularly important, because cardiorespiratory arrest is known to occur in patients with autonomic neuropathy and diabetic patients are more likely to have respiratory arrests postoperatively.[22]

Hypertension coexisting with diabetes is common and its management should be optimized prior to surgery. Peripheral vascular disease should be sought by routine palpation of pedal pulses and peripheral neuropathy by history and the patient's inability to sense pinprick, light touch, and temperature and vibration stimuli. The patient with nonpalpable pedal pulses, especially if the feet are insensitive, is very vulnerable to pressure ulceration and contact with bed frames or adjacent radiators must be prevented, as must prolonged contact of the heels with unyielding mattresses. Heel ulceration resulting from compression of the skin over the heel between bone and bed is common in badly managed surgical patients and preventable by proper care.

Retinal status is unlikely to be adversely affected by surgery, although retinal hemorrhage may be precipitated by sudden hypertension or hypoglycemia and sudden tightening of glycemic control may be associated with worsening of retinal status, which should be documented preoperatively and referred for treatment if preproliferative or proliferative.

Renal impairment is a common problem in long duration diabetes and renal status must be assessed preoperatively.

Careful assessment of metabolic status is essential. In T1DM patients, every effort should be made to achieve good glycemic control before admission. Patients should be on short- and intermediate-acting insulins. In T2DM patients, chlorpropamide should be stopped, as should glyburide in the elderly, because of risk of hypoglycemia, and short-acting agents substituted. Metformin should be stopped on the day of operation except in those with abnormal renal function, in whom it should be stopped without delay.

All these measures (Table 37-1) should be undertaken preadmission. Ideally, patients should be admitted one or two days before surgery to allow final assessment. This often does not occur, however, making preadmission screening even more important. It is worth noting that diabetes may be diagnosed for the first time when a patient is admitted for routine surgery. This is particularly true for elderly patients, and T2DM is usually the diagnosis. Operation should be delayed until glycemic control has been achieved and the patient fully assessed. In general, one should aim for fasting glucose levels of <125 mg/dL (7 mmol/L) and postprandial levels of <180 mg/dL (10 mmol/L). For urgent surgery (e.g., for malignant disease), control can be rapidly established in the hospi-

tal in a few days with insulin therapy. In less urgent situations, time can be taken to establish control conventionally with diet, exercise, and oral hypoglycemic agents.

Ideally pre- and postoperative care should be under the joint management of the diabetes, anesthetic, and surgical teams.

Perioperative Management

In T1DM patients, the need for continued insulin replacement is self-evident. In T2DM patients the indications are also clear. In a patient well controlled on diet alone, management may be possible, especially for minor procedures, as with nondiabetic patients, with the exception that blood glucose should be monitored preoperatively and hourly thereafter, and insulin replacement should be instituted if glucose levels rise above 11 mmol/L. With all other diabetic patients on any form of pharmacologic therapy to lower blood glucose, replacement of that therapy with monitored intravenous insulin therapy is mandatory.

Ambulatory surgery offers special challenges, but is best avoided except in well-controlled T2DM patients. Operations under local anesthetic, such as for cataracts, can then safely be undertaken with omission of therapy on the morning of the operation. It has been shown that cataract operations under local anesthesia cause relatively minor hormonal and metabolic disturbance compared with general anesthesia.[23]

Blood Glucose Control

A glycemic target should be determined for each patient. The ideal is normoglycemia (venous plasma glucose between 70 mg/dL [4 mmol/L] and 125 mg/dL [7 mmol/L]), but the risk of hypoglycemia is a concern. The classic signs of hypoglycemia may be masked by anesthesia and may in any case be absent in patients with longstanding diabetes taking insulin. A modified goal of 120–200 mg/dL (6.7–11 mmol/L) is acceptable during surgery and can then be tightened up postoperatively. This will keep glucose levels below those which cause glycosuria and dehydration and will not inhibit phagocyte function and wound healing.

Blood glucose can now be measured reasonably accurately at the bedside and in the operating suite with test strips and a meter, or electrochemically or using a microcuvette. However, it is vital that such machines are calibrated on a regular basis. Blood glucose should be measured on the morning of surgery, every 2 hours until the patient is anesthetized, hourly during surgery, and then every 1–4 hours during the first 24 hours, depending on the seriousness of the procedure.

T1DM Patients

All T1DM patients should be treated with insulin during surgery involving general anesthesia, regardless of the seriousness of the operation (Table 37-2). Operations should be scheduled early in the day, primarily because of the potential need for laboratory services for postoperative monitoring.

Insulin Therapy

Over the years, a variety of different regimens have been advocated for glycemic management during surgery. These have ranged from giving no insulin at all to using a low-dose SC insulin infusion with no added glucose. The former has obvious unwanted catabolic sequelae (see above), while the latter was only safe because patients were hyperglycemic preoperatively and therefore did not become hypoglycemic.

TABLE 37-1. Preoperative Assessment and Preparation of the Diabetic Patient for Surgery

General Measures
  Cardiovascular assessment
    History of angina, infarction
    History of hypertension
    ECG
    Blood pressure
    Full examination including peripheral pulses
  Neurologic assessment
    Peripheral neuropathy
      Autonomic examination: R-R interval
  Renal assessment
    Proteinuria
    Serum creatinine
  Urine culture
  Electrolytes (sodium, potassium)
Metabolic Assessment
  Glucosylated hemoglobin
  Home glucose control
  T1DM: Stop long-acting insulin, substitute BID split and mixed or TID regimens.*
  T2DM: Stop long-acting sulfonylureas (e.g., chlorpropamide). Substitute short-acting agents. Stop metformin on day of surgery.

*For day surgery, omit or use half the dose of intermediate-acting insulin the evening before surgery.

TABLE 37-2. Outline Guide to Management of Diabetes During Surgery

	Diet	Oral agents	Insulin
Minor surgery	Check BG preop. If <200 mg/dL, continue. If >200 mg/dL, start GIK.	Check BG preop. If <200 mg/dL, continue. If >200 mg/dL, start GIK. Omit on day of surgery until first meal.	Check BG preop. If <270 mg/dL, continue. If >270 mg/dL, stabilize on insulin infusion until BG <200 mg/dL and/or delay operation.
Major surgery	Use GIK as for T1DM. If BG >270 mg/dL, stabilize on insulin infusion until BG <200 mg/dL and/or delay operation.	Use GIK as for T1DM. If BG >270 mg/dL, stabilize on insulin infusion until BG <200 mg/dL and/or delay operation. Omit sulfonylureas.	As above,

For GIK patients, monitor BG preoperatively, intraoperatively (if operation >2 h), immediately postoperatively, then every 2 hours until BG stable. For others, check BG pre- and postoperatively. Use test strips + meter for BG monitoring (see text for precautions). GIK: glucose-insulin -potassium or insulin (pump) + glucose:potassium infusion.

The most widely used recommendations, however, are variants on two themes: (1) SC insulin with IV dextrose; and (2) IV infusion of glucose and insulin either separately or together, generally with added potassium.

Subcutaneous Regimens

Several SC regimens are still recommended for use during surgery.[24] SC regimens allow little flexibility and the rate of absorption, which is always variable, may be further compromised by changes in circulation and peripheral perfusion induced by anesthesia. There seems little rationale for their continued use. In a summary of studies several years ago,[25] we showed that plasma glucose levels 0–1 hour postoperatively with subcutaneous regimens ranged widely, between 193–390 mg/dL (10.2–21.7 mmol/L) and 155–310 mg/dL (8.5–172 mmol/L) at 4 hours, compared with a mean of 189 mg/dL (10.5 mmol/L) and 186 mg/dL (10.3 mmol/L), respectively, when intravenous insulin regimens were used. Better outcomes have been reported in cardiac surgical patients using IV infusion of insulin compared with SC insulin.[26] The only exception may be day surgery under local anesthesia.

Intravenous (IV) Regimens

A variety of different routines have been proposed for the use of IV insulin. Some use a fixed infusion rate of insulin, modifying the glucose infusion according to blood glucose levels, whereas the converse method of keeping glucose infusion constant and varying the insulin infusion rate has also been suggested. Others have varied the initial insulin dose according either to preoperative blood glucose level or to previous insulin dose. Another group has devised a series of complex algorithms to determine the rate of insulin administration. We have summarized these different options previously.[27] There is still some support for the use of hourly IV boluses when pumps are not available.[28] This does not seem logical or necessary and has been tested primarily in T2DM patients.

Two main variants of insulin infusion protocols are now recommended. These are: (1) combined insulin and glucose infusions with added potassium (GIK); and (2) insulin given by infusion pump with glucose (and potassium) given by separate infusion (IP/GK). In both cases potassium is necessary as insulin infusion lowers plasma potassium levels. Both regimens have their advantages, with GIK being safest, but both methods utilizing

separate infusions are the gold standard for well-equipped, well-staffed centers.

Glucose, Insulin, and Potassium (GIK) Regimen This system was originally designed for use in average general hospitals and needed to be simple, safe, and reproducible. Safety is ensured by glucose and insulin being in the same infusion so that their rates of infusion will be synchronously variable. It remains in use today essentially as it was first described in 1979.[29] The infusate comprises 10 units regular insulin plus 10 mmol potassium chloride (KCl) in 500 mL 10% dextrose given at 100 mL/h. Interestingly, this was not markedly different from a suggestion made by Galloway and Shuman in 1963.[29] Based on the original data, we subsequently increased the content of insulin to 16 units, giving 0.32 U/g glucose. Since the advent of U100 insulin, this has been modified to 15 units (0.30 U/g glucose). In one study, plasma glucose levels remained within the target range in 82% of cases and unexplained hypoglycemia and severe hyperglycemia were avoided.[30] Few comparative studies have been made, although unequivocally better metabolic control has been shown than with SC insulin.[31] The amount of insulin required varies to some extent, depending on the state of the patient and preexisting conditions. Table 37-3 shows amounts of insulin required in different states. These can be used as starting doses.

Some have recommended the use of 5% rather than 10% dextrose. We prefer the latter because it gives 240 g carbohydrate (960 kcal) per 24 hours, rather than 120 g (480 kcal). It has been suggested that at least 150 g carbohydrate per day plus insulin is needed to inhibit hepatic glucose production and protein catabolism,[32] although this is somewhat arbitrary. Slower rates of administration of more concentrated solutions of glucose are appropriate

TABLE 37-3. Insulin Requirements During Surgery

Condition	Insulin (U)/Glucose (g)
Normal weight	0.25–0.35
Obesity	0.4
Liver disease	0.4–0.6
Steroid therapy	0.4–0.5
Sepsis	0.5–0.7
Cardiopulmonary bypass	0.9–1.2

when it is necessary to restrict fluid administration or when complex fluid replacement regimens are needed for other reasons. Thus 50 mL/h of 20% dextrose or 20 mL/h of 50% dextrose may be used, given through a central line.

There are some disadvantages to the GIK regimen. These include the need to change the whole infusate bag if a change of insulin dose is needed, although this is surprisingly infrequent for routine operations. More important perhaps is that insulin is absorbed into the material that makes up IV fluid bags and infusion sets. The problem can be diminished by flushing the infusate through the infusion set. It is not a major problem in practice, but is avoided by using a more concentrated insulin solution in a syringe pump.

Separate Insulin and Glucose Regimens Many centers, particularly in the U.S., prefer to give insulin separately using an infusion pump following the groundbreaking study of Taitelman and associates.[33] This method certainly assures more precise delivery of insulin and allows speedy change of dose or infusion rate as required. It has also been used extremely effectively in children and adolescents.[34] It is probably the gold standard because of its flexibility, but if it is not carefully monitored, there is a risk of giving glucose without insulin and vice versa. The same dosages of units of insulin per gram of glucose as those above also apply to this method. Interestingly, in one study, separate infusions were preferred by the nursing staff and attained marginally better glycemic control than the GIK method.[35]

Practical Guidelines

Blood glucose and potassium should be checked on the morning of surgery. Glucose can be measured with a test strip and meter, but it is axiomatic that this should be done only by properly trained staff. A simultaneous sample should be sent to the laboratory as a later check. If blood glucose is greater than 270 mg/dL (15 mmol/L), surgery should be delayed, particularly if major surgery is planned. Either an attempt can be made to achieve control rapidly using the GIK infusion with twice the usual insulin content (60 U/L 10% glucose) or surgery may be delayed. Alternatively, insulin can be given at 4–6 U/h by syringe pump. If blood glucose is greater than 400 mg/dL (22.2 mmol/L), then delay and restabilization are mandatory.

The intravenous insulin and glucose infusion can be started when the surgical patient is due for his or her first insulin dose after being made NPO. The patient scheduled for morning surgery who is normally controlled on intermittent insulin injection therapy does not need to start intravenous insulin (with its requirements for hourly blood glucose monitoring) until just before breakfast the day of the procedure, despite stopping eating after the evening meal the day before. This allows the patient a near-normal night's sleep. It is sensible to check the blood glucose at bedtime and at 3.00 AM, as these are the times when the action of the evening's subcutaneous regular and intermediate-acting insulins, respectively, will be waning. Supplemental subcutaneous regular insulin (25–50% of the patient's usual premeal doses) can be prescribed for these times if the blood glucose is over 11 mmol/L, to avoid starting the intravenous insulin in a very hyperglycemic state. Similarly, the patient scheduled for afternoon surgery can be given a light breakfast with a suitably adjusted dose of regular insulin and intravenous insulinization started midmorning.

The GIK regimen can be based on either 10% (preferably) or 5% dextrose (Table 37-4). Careful monitoring of the plasma glu-

TABLE 37-4. Glucose-Insulin-Potassium (GIK) Infusion Protocols

Plasma Glucose mg/dL	Insulin dose (U/L)	
	Protocol A	**Protocol B**
<80	↓ 10	↓ 5
<120	↓ 5	↓ 3
120–180	Leave unchanged	
>180	↑ 5	↑ 3
>270	↑ 10	↑ 5

A. 30 U regular insulin (human) + 20 mmol KCl in 1000 mL 20% dextrose. Give at 100 mL/h.

B. 15 U regular insulin (human) + 20 mmol KCl in 100 mL 5% dextrose. Give at 100 mL/h.

cose is key. The first check after the fasting sample should be at 2 hours or immediately preoperatively, whichever is first. Plasma glucose and potassium are measured again in the recovery room and intraoperatively if it is a long operation.

For the insulin pump regimen, it is usual to make a solution of regular insulin in saline or Gelofusin of 1 unit per mL, by putting 50 units of the insulin in a 50-mL syringe and making the total volume of solution 50 mL by adding the diluent. This means that the pump setting, in mL/h, is numerically the same as the number of units per hour prescribed. More dilute solutions can be made for very insulin-sensitive subjects or children. The dextrose is given as in the GIK regimen—preferably 10% solutions at 50–100 mL/h, each liter containing 20 mmol potassium. The insulin infusion rate is set at slightly less than the patient's usual hourly requirement (total daily subcutaneous insulin doses divided by 24, or 2 U/h for adults if the daily dose is not known) for the a glucose level of 120–180 mg/dL, and adjusted up or down according to hourly plasma glucose measurements made at the bedside (Table 37-5). The scale should be reviewed regularly and adjusted to maintain plasma glucose in the range of 120–180 mg/dL.

T2DM Patients

All patients left on their usual hypoglycemic drugs risk hyperglycemia in response to the stress of surgery and hypoglycemia in response to the lack of food intake. Patients on metformin, an insulin-sensitizing agent, are unlikely to become hypoglycemic,

TABLE 37-5. An Example of the Separate Intravenous Glucose and Insulin Regimen

Plasma Glucose mg/dL	Insulin U/h	Insulin mL/h
<80	0.5	0.5
80–120	1.0	1.0
121–160*	2.0*	2.0*
161–200	3.0	3.0
201–250	4.0	4.0
251–300	5.0	5.0
>300	6.0	6.0

*The regimen should be personalized to the patient, such that this dose is calculated as the patient's usual total daily insulin dose (all regular and intermediate- or long-acting insulin doses taken in one normal day) divided by 24. The doses for measured plasma glucose outside this range are then increased or reduced by 1 U/h for each range above or below this target. The insulin scale can be rewritten if needed to keep plasma glucose in the 121–160 mg/dL range.

Glucose: 10% dextrose containing 20 mmol KCl per liter, 100 mL/h

Insulin: 50 units regular insulin made up to 50 mL in 0.9% saline = 1 U/mL

but any fall in renal perfusion associated with the anesthesia or the surgery increases their risk of lactic acidosis. Sulfonylureas are insulin secretagogues and carry a high risk of hypoglycemia, especially the longer-acting agents such as glyburide, and with this agent hypoglycemia is likely to be both late in onset and prolonged. There are no data on surgery in patients on thiazolidenediones or meglitinides. In all cases the drugs should not be taken on the day of surgery. Long-acting sulfonylureas should perhaps be withdrawn sooner. Our previous recommendation that metformin be stopped two or three days preoperatively are not justified by its pharmacokinetics, and this too can just be withheld on the operative day.[36]

The main determinants of therapy in the T2DM patient are: (1) the seriousness of the surgical procedure; and (2) the metabolic state of the patient on the day of surgery. The exception is the insulin-treated T2DM patient, who should be treated as a T1DM patient.

There is general agreement that the patient who is well controlled on diet alone or diet plus sulfonylureas does not require any specific therapy for minor surgery. Indeed it has been shown that new metabolic abnormalities may be produced by use of insulin infusions in this group,[37] although blood glucose values did reach a mean of 200 mg/dL (10 mmol/L) postoperatively in the untreated patients. In other studies we have shown pre- and postoperative glucose values of 140–155 mg/dL in such patients, well within the desirable target range.

There is more controversy as to how the poorly-controlled T2DM patient should be treated for minor surgery. Some still advocate no specific therapy, but this seems unwarranted and a glucose/insulin infusion regimen would seem appropriate. A fasting plasma glucose of 200 mg/dL (11.1 mmol/L) is an appropriate cutoff, because metabolic deterioration seems to occur with minor surgery only at higher levels.

Many different regimens have been suggested for metabolic control during major surgery in T2DM patients. One group has even suggested no insulin and no glucose.[28] It is logical and simpler, however, to use the same regimen as for T1DM patients. This does give similar results in terms of glycemic regulation.

Practical Guidelines: Minor Surgery

Preoperatively, control should be improved and long-acting sulfonylureas should be stopped as discussed above. On the day of surgery, drug therapy is withheld and fasting blood glucose checked with a test strip and meter. If blood glucose is <200 mg/dL, surgery is carried out as planned. If blood glucose is >200 mg/dL, a standard GIK or IP/GK protocol is commenced and the patient treated as a T1DM patient. It should be noted that many T2DM patients are obese and may need 40 U insulin/L 10% glucose in a GIK regimen rather than the standard 30 U.

Practical Guidelines: Major Surgery

Preoperatively, control should be optimized and short-acting insulin therapy used for the 24–48 hours before operation, if possible, in patients with unsatisfactory glycemic control. On the morning of surgery sulfonylurea therapy is withheld, an infusion regimen is commenced, and the fasting blood glucose level is checked. Thereafter management is as for the T1DM patient.

Postoperative Management

In all patients who have received GIK, blood glucose should be checked every 1–2 hours following surgery until stable glycemia is achieved, and then every 4 hours. Potassium should be checked 6 hours postoperatively and again on the following day, although it is rare to have to change the potassium content of the infusate. The GIK or separate insulin/glucose infusions are continued until the patient begins to eat again. At that time the usual preoperative SC insulin dose is given. The GIK mixture should be continued for another hour or so to allow absorption of some of the SC dose. If resumption of feeding is delayed, then parenteral nutrition can be instituted with insulin still given by the IV route. In this situation it should be given via a separate line using an infusion pump.

In T1DM patients who have not received GIK, their usual therapy is recommended with the first meal. Blood glucose should be monitored immediately postoperatively and pre- and 2-hour post-meal glucose monitoring done until stable values are obtained.

Good glycemic control postoperatively is paramount. It has been clearly shown that wound infections are fewer in better-controlled patients, although a precise threshold has not been established.[38,39]

SPECIAL SITUATIONS

Day Surgery

In recent years there has been a dramatic increase in day or outpatient surgery. Nowadays nearly half of all surgical procedures are performed on a day surgery or outpatient basis, and the proportion is rising worldwide. It is certainly not necessary for all diabetic patients to be excluded from this group.

In T2DM patients, day surgery is appropriate for all minor procedures. However, preoperative assessment a few days before surgery is a sine qua non.[40] Patients should be treated as outlined above and scheduled for operation early in the day. Cataract surgery under local anesthesia in T2DM patients is entirely safe as an outpatient or day procedure.[41]

Insulin-treated patients may present a greater problem, but with appropriate preoperative assessment, the availability of blood glucose monitoring equipment, and good patient education; they can also be treated as day patients. Particular care will be needed for patients using long-acting analogs, the dose and which may need adjusting. The patients should also be scheduled for early operation and should be given IV insulin as discussed above. Subcutaneous insulin is recommended as soon as possible postoperatively and appropriate carbohydrate given. This applies of course to minor surgery. Blood glucose levels should be checked at the bedside hourly.

Emergency Surgery

Emergency surgery is at least as likely in the diabetic as the nondiabetic subject. Management will depend to a large extent on the metabolic condition of the patient. Surgical emergencies, particularly if there is underlying infection, can cause rapid metabolic decompensation with dehydration, hyperglycemia, and ketoacidosis. Uncontrolled diabetes may also be precipitated in patients not previously known to have diabetes. One trap for the unsuspecting is that patients with diabetic ketoacidosis (DKA) can present with symptoms indistinguishable from those of an acute abdomen. In these patients, the signs and symptoms resolve on metabolic correction. A useful rule of thumb is that if such patients are less than 20 years old, the problem is more likely to be metabolic, whereas if they are older, a genuine surgical emergency should be suspected. The sensible approach in such patients is to manage conservatively in the early stages with the emphasis on correction of the metabolic derangement. If the problem is metabolic rather than surgical, then it will resolve in the next 3–4 hours.

Practical Guidelines

In all cases blood should be sent for immediate analysis of glucose, urea, and electrolytes as well as arterial pH and gases if clinically warranted. Plasma, urine, or both should be checked for ketones. It should be remembered that in the DKA patient, a raised white cell count does not necessarily indicate infection, but correlates with stress and blood ketone body levels.

If the patient is in early or established DKA, the first priority is metabolic management. Surgery should be delayed by 3–4 hours if at all possible. This will allow resolution of the pseudoacute abdomen as well as putting the patient in a better state to withstand the stress of surgery. Treatment comprises rapid saline infusion and insulin delivery via an infusion pump at 6 U/h. Potassium should be given in the saline (20 mmol/h), assuming adequate renal function. Glucose should be monitored hourly and electrolytes checked after 2–4 hours. Once blood glucose concentration has fallen below 270 mg/dL (15 mmol/L), a standard GIK or insulin pump regimen can be commenced, but with 40 U insulin/L 10% glucose for GIK or its equivalent because patients will be insulin-resistant. Blood glucose should be monitored hourly and the insulin content of the infusion increased if necessary.

In patients without severe metabolic disturbance, initial diabetic management is with a GIK or IP/GK protocol. Again, a higher-than-usual insulin concentration is likely to be needed.

Cardiopulmonary Bypass Surgery

Diabetic patients have a high prevalence of coronary artery disease and are therefore likely to undergo coronary artery bypass grafting. Morbidity and mortality are higher in the diabetic than the nondiabetic patient[42] and it is possible that the intraoperative management of the diabetes contributes to this. Cardiopulmonary bypass (CPB) surgery involves the use of large volumes of exogenous fluid, hypothermia, and adrenergic agents, all of which can affect metabolic homeostasis. In the past, pump-priming fluids have often contained glucose and lactate. These should be avoided in the diabetic patient and replaced with plasma-like primers.

CPB is known to be associated with severe insulin resistance. When GIK is used for glycemic control, insulin:glucose ratios of 1–1.6 are needed, in contrast to the 0.3–0.4 used for routine elective surgery. Good results may be achieved by infusing insulin alone, with monitoring of blood glucose every 15–30 minutes by the anesthesiologist in the operating suite. Insulin requirements vary between 5 and 12 U/h. GIK is then introduced postoperatively. Clear indication of the benefits of using GIK therapy in diabetic patients undergoing coronary artery surgery has been reported.[43]

It has also been suggested that hyperglycemia is associated with poor outcomes in diabetic patients undergoing cardiovascular surgery,[26,44] particularly in the elderly.[45] This may well reflect effects on the CNS as well as impaired resistance to infection and impaired wound healing.

MORBIDITY AND MORTALITY

Factors influencing outcome in the diabetic include cardiovascular disease, liability to infection and poor wound healing. The latter can be counteracted by good glycemic regulation. However, cardiovascular disease is a major cause of death in the peri- and postoperative periods.

Conflicting data have been published on whether diabetic patients have poorer outcomes following surgery. In general, poor outcome was related to poor glycemic control. Nowadays with good management of the diabetes, morbidity and mortality should be little increased in the diabetic population except in those with severe cardiovascular disease.

SUMMARY AND CONCLUSIONS

Surgery in the diabetic patient poses special problems—not only the metabolic problems of diabetes, but the susceptibility of the patient to cardiovascular disease, neuropathy, and infection also put the patient at special risk. Surgical stress is accompanied by increased secretion of the counterregulatory hormones and cytokines with resultant insulin resistance, inhibition of insulin secretion, and hyperglycemia. In T1DM patients without the ability to secrete more insulin, this will lead to metabolic deterioration. In T2DM patients with sluggish insulin secretion, there is already insulin resistance, and metabolic deterioration will also occur. The extent of the stress response to surgery depends, however, on the severity of the operation. Minor surgery leads to only minor metabolic derangement.

Therefore, in the well-controlled T2DM patient it is sufficient to withhold regular therapy on the day of surgery. In the poorly-controlled T2DM patient and in all T1DM subjects, insulin therapy is required. Many regimens have been proposed. The simplest is the combined glucose-insulin-potassium (GIK) infusion, which can be used from the morning of surgery until the patient is eating again. In better-staffed and -equipped centers, insulin can be given by separate infusion pump. Meticulous monitoring of plasma glucose is essential and appropriate sliding scales used to regulate dosage.

Certain special situations are also found. With proper attention to preoperative assessment, day surgery is safe for diabetic patients for minor operations. Emergency surgery is more common in the diabetic subject. The sine qua non is to correct any severe metabolic disturbance before embarking on surgery. The GIK or insulin pump regimen is then used. Cardiopulmonary bypass surgery is also a particular problem in diabetes patients because of massive insulin resistance. Here insulin is given intraoperatively without accompanying glucose, standard IV insulin being reinstituted postoperatively.

With appropriate care, the outcome of surgery in the diabetic patient should be little worse than in the nondiabetic patient when matched for clinical status, particularly cardiovascular disease.

REFERENCES

1. Root HF: Pre-operative care of the diabetic patient. *Postgrad Med* 1966;40:439.
2. Gold BS, Kitz DS, Locky JH, et al: Unanticipated admission to the hospital following ambulatory surgery. *JAMA* 1989;262:3008.
3. Hirsch IB, Paauw DS: Diabetes management in special situations. *Endocrinol Metab Clin North Am* 1997;26:631.
4. Gill GV, Alberti KGMM: The care of the diabetic patient during surgery. In: Alberti KGMM, Zimmet P, DeFronzo RA, et al, eds. *International Textbook of Diabetes Mellitus*. Wiley:1997;1243.
5. Racoules-Aimé M, Grimaud D: Prise en charge péri-opératoire des sujets à risque. *Les diabétiques. La Presse Medicale* 1998;27:444.

6. McAnulty GR, Robertshaw HJ, Hall GM: Anaesthetic management of patients with diabetes mellitus. *Br J Anaesth* 2000;85:80.
7. Hoogwerf BJ: Postoperative management of the diabetic patient. *Med Clin North Am* 2001;85:1213.
8. Scherpereel PA, Tavernier B: Perioperative care of diabetic patients. *Eur J Anaesthesiol* 2001;18:277.
9. McCowen KC, Malhotra A, Bistrian BR: Stress-induced hyperglycemia. *Crit Care Clin* 2001;17:107.
10. Latterman R, Schricker T, Wachter U, *et al*: Understanding the mechanisms by which isoflurane modifies the hyperglycemic response to surgery. *Anaesth Analg* 2001;93:121.
11. Thorell A, Ljungqvist O, Efendic S, *et al*: Insulin resistance after abdominal surgery. *Br J Surg* 1994;81:59.
12. Hawthorne GC, Ashworth L, Alberti KGMM: The effect of laparoscopic cholecystectomy on insulin sensitivity. *Horm Metab Res* 1994;26:474.
13. Thorell A, Efendic S, Gutniak M, *et al*: Development of postoperative insulin resistance is associated with the magnitude of operation. *Eur J Surg* 1993;159:593.
14. Nygren JO, Thorell A, Soop O, *et al*: Perioperative insulin and glucose infusion maintains insulin sensitivity after surgery. *Am J Physiol Endocrinol Metab* 1998;38:E140.
15. Soop M, Nygren J, Myrenfors P, *et al*: Preoperative oral carbohydrate treatment attenuates immediate post-operative insulin resistance. *Am J Physiol Endocrinol Metab* 2001;280:E576.
16. Thorell A, Loftenius A, Andersson B, *et al*: Postoperative insulin resistance and circulating concentrations of stress hormones and cytokines. *Clin Nutr* 1966;15:75.
17. Thorell A, Nygren J, Hirshman MF, *et al*: Surgery-induced insulin resistance in human patients: relation to glucose transport and utilization. *Am J Physiol Endocrinol Metab* 1999;39:E754.
18. Kehlet H: The stress response to anaesthesia and surgery: Release mechanisms and modifying factors. *Clin Anaesthesiol* 1984;2:315.
19. Alberti KGMM, Thomas DJB: The management of diabetes during surgery. *Br J Anaesth* 1979;51:693.
20. Thompson J, Husband DJ, Thai AC, *et al*: Metabolic changes in the non-insulin-dependent diabetic undergoing minor surgery: Effect of glucose-insulin-potassium infusion. *Br J Surg* 1986;73:301.
21. Vohra A, Kumar S, Charlton AJ, *et al*: Effect of diabetes mellitus on the cardiovascular responses to induction of anaesthesia and tracheal intubation. *Br J Anaesth* 1993;71:258.
22. Rose DK, Cohen MM, Wigglesworth DF, *et al*: Critical respiratory events in the post anaesthesia care unit. *Anaesthesiology* 1994;81:410.
23. Barker JP, Robinson PN, Vafidis GC, *et al*: Metabolic control of non-insulin-dependent diabetic patients undergoing cataract surgery: comparison of local and general anaesthesia. *Br J Anaesth* 1995;74:500.
24. Jacobes SJ, Sowers JR: An update on perioperative management of diabetes. *Arch Intern Med* 1999;159:2405.
25. Alberti KGMM, Marshall SM: Diabetes and surgery. In: Alberti KGMM, Krall LP, eds. *The Diabetes Annual*, 4th ed. Elsevier: 1988; 248.
26. Furnary AP, Zerr KJ, Grunkemeier GL, *et al*: Continuous intravenous insulin infusion reduces the incidence of deep sternal wound infection in diabetic patients after cardiac surgical procedures. *Ann Thorac Surg* 1999;67:352.
27. Alberti KGMM: Diabetes and surgery. In: Porte D, Sherwin RS, eds. *Ellenberg and Rifkin's Diabetes Mellitus*, 5th ed. Appleton & Lange: 1997;875.
28. Racoules-Aimé M, Labib Y, Levrant J, *et al*: Use of i.v. insulin in well-controlled non-insulin-dependent diabetics undergoing major surgery. *Br J Anaesth* 1996;76:198.
29. Galloway JA, Shuman CR: Diabetes and surgery. *Am J Med* 1963; 34: 177.
30. Husband DJ, Thai AC, Alberti KGMM: Management of diabetes during surgery with glucose-insulin-potassium infusion. *Diabetes Med* 1986;3:69.
31. Pezzarossa A, Taddei F, Cimicchi MC, *et al*: Perioperative management of diabetic subjects: Subcutaneous versus intravenous insulin administration during glucose-potassium infusion. *Diabetes Care* 1988;11:52.
32. Racoules-Aimé M, Ichai C, Roussel LJ, *et al*: Comparison of two methods of IV insulin administration in the diabetic patient during the peri-operative period. *Br J Anaesth* 1994;72:5.
33. Taitelman U, Reece EA, Bessman AN: Insulin in the management of the diabetic surgical patient. *JAMA* 1977;237:658.
34. Kaufman FR, Devgan S, Roe TF, *et al*: Perioperative management with prolonged intravenous insulin infusion versus subcutaneous insulin in children with Type 1 diabetes mellitus. *J Diabetes Complications* 1996;10:6.
35. Simmons D, Morton K, Laughton SJ, *et al*: A comparison of two intravenous insulin regimens among surgical patients with insulin-dependent diabetes mellitus. *Diabetes Education* 1994;20:422.
36. Chan NN, Feher MD: Metformin and perioperative risk. *Br J Anaesth* 1999;83:540.
37. Thompson J, Husband DJ, Thai AC, *et al*: Metabolic changes in the non-insulin-dependent diabetic patient undergoing minor surgery: Effect of glucose-insulin-potassium infusion. *Br J Surg* 1986; 73:301.
38. Risum O, Abdelnoor M, Svennevig JL, *et al*: Diabetes mellitus and morbidity and mortality risks after coronary artery bypass surgery. *Scand J Thorac Cardiovasc Surg* 1996;30:71.
39. Pomposelli JJ, Baxter JK III, Babineau TJ, *et al*: Early postoperative glucose control predicts nosocomial infection rate in diabetic patients. *J Parenter Enteral Nutr* 1998;22:77.
40. Kreines K: Diabetes management during same-day surgery or procedures. *Clin Diabetes* 1992;10:52.
41. Watts S, Aburn NS: Day-case surgery for cataracts in diabetic patients. *Practical Diabetes* 1994;11:181.
42. Thourani VH, Weintraub WS, Stein B, *et al*: Influence of diabetes mellitus on early and late outcome after coronary artery bypass grafting. *Ann Thorac Surg* 1999;67:1045.
43. Lazar HL, Chipkin S, Philippides G, *et al*: Glucose-insulin-potassium solutions improve outcomes in diabetics who have coronary artery operations. *Ann Thorac Surg* 2000;70:145.
44. Murkin JM: Tight intraoperative glucose control improves outcome in cardiovascular surgery. *J Cardiothorac Vasc Anesth* 2000;14:475.
45. Rady MW, Ryan T, Starr NJ: Perioperative determinants of morbidity and mortality in elderly patients undergoing cardiac surgery. *Crit Care Med* 1998;26:225.

The Mother in Pregnancies Complicated by Diabetes Mellitus

Boyd E. Metzger

Richard L. Phelps

Sharon L. Dooley

In 1882, in one of the first published reports of diabetes in pregnancy,[1] J. Mathews Duncan qualified his clinical observations with the following prescient caveat:

> The advance of physiology makes it certain that pregnancy brings about important changes in the quantity or constitution of the blood, the bones, the skin, and its appendages, the heart, and the great glands, and makes it highly probable that every solid and fluid constituent of the frame is profoundly modified for the time.

He therefore suggested that the effects of pregnancy upon any disease should only be evaluated in the context of the changes that occur in the course of normal pregnancy. Insofar as normal pregnancy profoundly affects every aspect of intermediary metabolism,[2,3] the comments of J. Mathews Duncan remain particularly germane to the relationships between diabetes and pregnancy.

METABOLIC ADAPTATIONS IN NORMAL PREGNANCY

Clinical Features of Carbohydrate Metabolism in Pregnancy

Alterations in carbohydrate metabolism are especially prominent in the second half of pregnancy.[2] Historically, it was observed that the disposition of administered glucose is only minimally altered in the normal gravida, whereas the hypoglycemic response to insulin is markedly attenuated.[4,5] This dichotomy has long suggested that an enhanced resistance to insulin action exists as part of normal pregnancy, so that an increased elaboration of insulin is required to maintain normal glucose tolerance.[6] Pregnancy is, therefore, a truly physiologic challenge to insulinogenic reserve. The histologic finding of islet cell hyperplasia during normal gestation and clinical experience in subjects with diminished or absent pancreatic β-cell reserve are in accord with this premise. Thus, pregnancy may be attended by onset or first recognition of carbohydrate intolerance (i.e., gestational diabetes mellitus [GDM][7–9]), and substantial increases in the requirements for insulin may supervene in women with known insulin-requiring diabetes (i.e., pregestational diabetes mellitus). The

changes parallel the growth of the conceptus: they become increasingly manifest as the conceptus rapidly increases in mass from weeks 20–24 of pregnancy onward, and they are promptly reversed following expulsion of the conceptus.[10] Accordingly, in the immediate postpartum period, normal glucose tolerance returns in most women with GDM, and insulin requirements decline precipitously to nongravid levels in patients with insulin-requiring pregestational diabetes. These temporal correlations have implicated the conceptus in the diabetogenic challenges that are part of normal pregnancy.[10]

Metabolic Contributions of the Conceptus

The conceptus (fetus and placenta) arises *de novo*; several of its functional properties exert metabolic effects during its development.[11] Maternal insulin does not cross the placenta, although some may be sequestered and bound there.[12] Insulin can also be degraded in the rat and human placenta, and the degradation coincides with accelerated removal of insulin from the maternal circulation in polytocous species, such as the gravid rat.[13,14] In monotocous species such as humans, blood flow to the placenta represents a relatively smaller proportion of cardiac output than it does in rodents.[15] Nevertheless, Catalano and colleagues[16,17] have recently confirmed a moderate increase in insulin clearance in normal pregnancy and in GDM.

In contrast to the modest effects of human pregnancy on insulin turnover, dramatic changes occur in insulin secretion and insulin action.[10] In early pregnancy, basal insulin concentrations are unchanged, and insulin responses to oral or intravenous glucose are only minimally increased.[16,18–20] On the other hand, basal and stimulated values for plasma-immunoreactive insulin are greatly increased in late human pregnancy.[18,20–22] It has been documented that the increase in circulating levels of immunoreactive material truly represents insulin rather than immunoreactive components with lesser biological potency.[23,24] In normal lean subjects, insulin sensitivity begins to decrease by the end of the first trimester of pregnancy[18] and is greatly reduced in late gestation.[17,18,22,25]

Some quantitative estimations have been made. Pooled data from a number of laboratories indicate that the total output of insulin in response to oral glucose increases two- to threefold throughout pregnancy.[10] More detailed recent analyses of intravenous glucose tolerance have shown that during the third trimester the first and second phases of glucose-stimulated insulin release are increased about threefold in normal gravida. This "extra" insulin compensates for a reduction of approximately 40–60% in the responsiveness of the periphery to insulin action.[17,18,22] The temporal patterns of insulin sensitivity before conception and during early and late gestation in normal pregnancy and gestational diabetes mellitus are shown in Fig. 38-1. When the integrated values for insulin secretion in response to glycemic challenge at various points in gestation are expressed as percentages of the values observed with similar challenges in nonpregnant subjects, the curvilinear pattern of progressive increases simulates the growth pattern of the conceptus (Fig. 38-2).[10]

Two properties of the developing conceptus have been implicated in the diminished sensitivity (i.e., the increased resistance) to insulin in late pregnancy: the endocrine function of the conceptus and the effects of the conceptus on maternal fuels. The precise mechanisms through which either of these properties of the conceptus could alter insulin sensitivity have not been fully elucidated.[26] Insulin resistance appears to be present in liver, adipose tissue, and skeletal muscle. The binding of insulin to receptors on circulating monocytes or erythrocytes, hepatocytes, and skeletal muscle is not diminished in human pregnancy, and it is clear that the insulin resistance of late human pregnancy is mediated by events distal to the binding of ligand to receptor.[27–32]

However, efforts to pinpoint specific pathways that are responsible have yielded variable results. Content of GLUT4 transporters have been reported to be unaffected by pregnancy in muscle tissue of humans[33] and rats.[34] By contrast, GLUT4 transporters have reported to be reduced in adipose tissue of pregnant rats[34] and humans with normal pregnancy or GDM.[35] Insulin-stimulated tyrosine kinase activity of hepatic insulin receptors was reported to be decreased in rats during late pregnancy.[31] In another study,[32] autophosphorylation of skeletal muscle insulin receptors was reported to be unaffected by normal pregnancy or GDM. Recently, Shao and coworkers[36] investigated skeletal muscle insulin receptor tyrosine kinase activity in obese women with GDM or normal pregnancy. They found no changes under basal conditions, but insulin-stimulated insulin receptor function was impaired. They attributed this to tyrosine kinase inhibition by increased levels of a cell membrane glycoprotein-1 (PC-1), which resulted in increased rates of serine/threonine phosphorylation and reduced levels of tyrosine phosphorylation.

The Conceptus as an Endocrine Structure

Increased secretion of progesterone, human placental lactogen (HPL; human chorionic somatomammotropin [HCS]), and estrogen by the placenta during pregnancy tends to parallel the growth of the conceptus.[10] Each hormone has been shown to augment islet secretory responsiveness and to alter the sensitivity to insulin action in the periphery, although the status for estrogen remains somewhat controversial.[37] For example, HCS can exert lipolytic effects *in vitro*,[38] may induce insulin resistance in nongravid subjects when infused overnight in amounts designed to simulate the plasma levels that prevail during late gestation,[39] *and has direct effects on islet structure and function.*[40] Similarly, administration of progesterone to nongravid subjects can increase stimulated as well as basal insulin secretion[41] and can augment such metabolic processes as gluconeogenesis. Estrogen can augment hepatic generation of circulating lipoprotein.[42]

Thus, these hormones, which appear in ever-increasing amounts coincident with increasing placental mass, can create a metabolic setting distal to receptor binding in which the efficacy of a given amount of insulin is blunted and islet secretory performance is augmented. Moreover, their elaboration by the placenta is affected only minimally,[43] if at all, by the normal alimentary excursions of circulating nutrients. Consequently, although the acute hyperinsulinemia can offset their contra-insulin potentialities in the fed state, they are relatively unopposed in the fasted state. The finding that intrinsic rates of lipolysis and re-esterification are increased in adipose tissue isolated from rats[44] or humans[45] in late

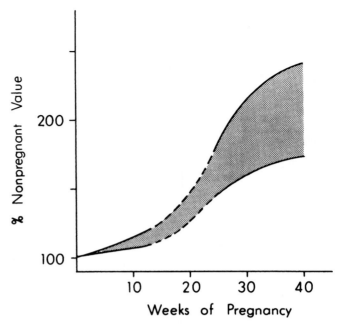

FIGURE 38-2. Effect of pregnancy on stimulated insulin secretion. The increases in plasma insulin above basal values following stimulation with glucose were summated to assess net secretory response. Published values from normal pregnant and nonpregnant women have been employed to derive the comparisons depicted previously. (*Reproduced with permission from Freinkel.*[10])

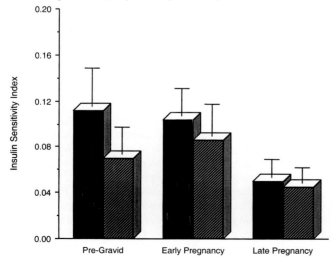

FIGURE 38-1. Longitudinal changes in insulin sensitivity in women with normal pregnancy or gestational diabetes mellitus. Data from before pregnancy (pre-gravid) and early and late pregnancy are expressed as insulin sensitivity index (mean ± SD). **Solid bars,** controls; **hatched bars,** women who developed GDM. (*Adapted with permission from Catalano et al.*[67])

gestation, even when sampling is performed in the fed state,[45] is consistent with this proposition.

Prolactin of pituitary and decidual origin[46] and the human growth hormone variant (hGH-V) of placental origin[47–49] may also play some role in promoting resistance to insulin action.[30,50] However, the precise metabolic contributions of these peptides during pregnancy remain to be defined. Some endocrine influences, not directly of intrauterine origin, may also contribute meaningfully. Glucocorticoids appear to be particularly important in this regard.[30] In human pregnancy, the exposure of maternal tissues to glucocorticoids is increased twofold above nongravid values,[51] and an absolute increase of circulating free cortisol in the mother is well documented.[52] It seems unlikely that these glucocorticoids are of fetal origin, or that autonomously functioning placental corticotrophin or corticotrophin-releasing factor activity[53] are responsible, since normal diurnal rhythms of cortisol secretion are preserved.[52] Instead, maternal hypothalamic-pituitary feedback appears to be operative at a higher setting, perhaps as a result of the increased availability of sex steroids. Currently, potential roles of tissue necrosis factor-α[54] and the recently discovered hormone of adipose tissue origin, leptin, are being investigated intensively.[55]

Effects of the Conceptus on Maternal Fuels

Some abstraction of maternal fuels by the growing conceptus occurs continuously. Many of the nutrients are cleared from the maternal circulation in a concentration-dependent fashion[2] and are deployed for structural growth and development as well as oxidative needs. The fluxes are considerable: glucose utilization by the human fetus at term has been estimated to be 6 mg/kg/min[56] (in contrast to a rate of 2–3 mg/kg/min in normal adults[57]). Growth of the human fetus during the third trimester requires the net transplacental transfer of 54 millimoles of nitrogen per day.[58] Consequently, maternal mechanisms for conserving 3–6-carbon nutrients may be compromised meaningfully as the pregnancy progresses and the fuel needs of placenta and fetus escalate.[11]

Dietary deprivation during the latter half of pregnancy elicits more rapid and profound mobilization of fat[44,59] and exaggerated increases in plasma and urinary ketones.[59] A greater and more rapid fall in maternal blood sugar[59–61] and amino acids[61–64] is also seen coincident with greater activation of intrahepatic gluconeogenesis[59,65,66] and renal ammoniagenesis.[59,61] The reduction in blood sugar may progress to frank hypoglycemia. It has been demonstrated that glucose turnover after overnight fast is increased in late human pregnancy,[67] as previously demonstrated in rodents.[68] This fasting hypoglycemia of pregnancy has been viewed as a *substrate deficiency syndrome*[62] and ascribed to a failure of amino acid mobilization to "keep up" with rates of glucose removal.[62,63] The integrated modifications of the fasted state in late pregnancy have been designated *accelerated starvation*.[10,11]

Such features of "accelerated starvation" as enhanced ketonemia, increased urinary nitrogen, and exaggerated decrements in fasting plasma glucose (FPG) and circulating gluconeogenic amino acids are already manifest during midpregnancy.[61,63,64] Some of the phenomena can be replicated by administering the hormones of pregnancy to nongravid subjects.[69–72] However, in pregnant rats, the difference in the metabolic response to fetectomy vs. hysterectomy suggests that full expression requires the presence of an intact conceptus.[69] Thus, at least part of the "accelerated starvation" must be ascribed to the continued abstraction of essential maternal nutrients by the growing placenta *and* fetus.

There has been some question as to whether "accelerated starvation" occurs under conditions that obtain in standard clinical

practice. However, it has been shown that the increases in plasma free fatty acids (FFAs), glycerol, and ketones and the reductions in plasma glucose and amino acids that are seen just before lunch when breakfast has been withheld are significantly greater in gravid than in nongravid women.[73,74] Thus, the common clinical practice of "skipping breakfast" for laboratory tests or other clinical procedures may not be without meaningful metabolic consequences in late normal pregnancy.

Significant metabolic alterations are also seen in the fed state. The ingestion of glucose after overnight fast in late normal pregnancy elicits a greater and more prolonged increase in blood sugar, a greater increment in plasma very low-density lipoproteins,[10,75] and a greater concurrent fall in plasma glucagon[10,69,75–79] (Fig. 38-3). These changes in circulating glucose concentration are a manifestation of the insulin resistance of late gestation and are attended and perhaps facilitated by a delayed and reduced fall in FFA concentrations.[75,76] This characteristic metabolic response has been designated *facilitated anabolism*.[10,75,76] Since glucose crosses the placenta in concentration-dependent fashion,[80] the exaggerated hyperglycemia after glucose ingestion in late pregnancy results in greater availability of the dietary glucose for transplacental transfer. The increased plasma triglycerides can abet this objective by substituting for some of the circulating glucose as oxidative fuel in the

FIGURE 38-3 Effect of pregnancy on the response to oral glucose after overnight fast. Changes in plasma glucose, triglycerides, immunoreactive insulin, and glucagon are expressed as net increments or decrements from basal values after administration of 100 g oral glucose following a 14-hour overnight fast. The same normal women were used for paired "pregnant" vis-à-vis "postpartum" comparisons. *(Reproduced with permission from Freinkel.[10])*

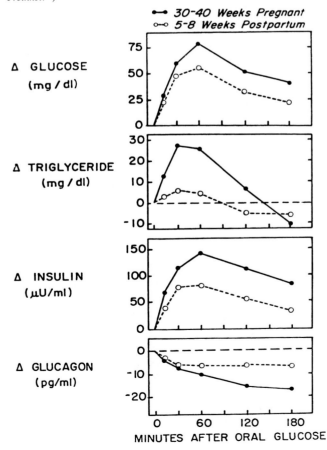

mother and thereby "sparing" glucose for transplacental flux. Moreover, since little if any triglyceride crosses the placenta,[81] the carbohydrate-induced hypertriglyceridemia may also enable some of the ingested glucose to be retained for subsequent recall as triglyceride-glycerol or fatty acid during lipolysis in the fasted state.

Finally, the greater suppression of glucagon[77–79] immediately after glucose ingestion may also "facilitate anabolism" in the fed state: it would blunt the contributions of glucagon to ongoing gluconeogenesis and ketogenesis and so spare ingested amino acids for maternal or fetal access. After disposition of the carbohydrate component of "mixed meals," the well-preserved response of the α cells to amino acid stimulation of glucagon secretion[82,83] could help to to re-establish gluconeogenesis and so prevent exaggerated postprandial hypoglycemia and the full return to accelerated starvation.

PATHOPHYSIOLOGY OF DIABETES AND PREGNANCY

Morbidities associated with diabetes mellitus may affect both the pregnant woman and her offspring. This is illustrated by data from the preinsulin era, when maternal mortality approached 25%.[84] For several years after insulin treatment became widely available, perinatal mortality remained very high.[84] At the present time, maternal deaths have been largely eliminated. Under optimal circumstances, intrauterine fetal deaths are uncommon, and the incidence of neonatal deaths, except for those due to major congenital malformations, approaches that of the general obstetric population. However, other less extreme morbid outcomes continue to be common.

Effects of Diabetes on Pregnancy

Because newborns of pregnancies in which just the father has diabetes appear to develop normally,[85,86] it is believed that morbidities in the offspring are due to abnormalities in the maternal metabolic environment, rather than genetic influences.

The late Jorgen Pedersen was the first to propose a mechanism whereby maternal fuels may exert a direct effect on the fetus. In attempting to explain the "large babies" that were often seen in pregnancies complicated by diabetes, he advanced the *hyperglycemia-hyperinsulinism hypothesis.*[87] He postulated that more maternal glucose gains access to the fetus whenever maternal insulin is inadequate and that this "extra" glucose stimulates insulin release in the fetus and thereby produces an increase of fetal mass. Subsequent work demonstrated that all maternal fuels may be awry in even the mildest forms of gestational diabetes and may increase the nutrients available for fetal growth, β-cell hyperplasia, and the premature activation of insulin secretion that Pedersen postulated. Accordingly, we later proposed that the Pedersen hypothesis be modified to include those maternal fuels besides glucose that are also regulated by maternal insulin (see Chap. 39, Fig. 39-1), and we likened pregnancy to a "tissue culture experience" since most of these fuels cross the placenta in concentration-dependent fashion.[88] Thus, their concentrations in the maternal circulation may determine the quantitative as well as qualitative characteristics of the "incubation medium" in which the conceptus develops.

In his 1980 Banting Lecture,[10] the late Norbert Freinkel formulated the concept of *fuel-mediated teratogenesis* to draw attention to the relationships between maternal metabolism and fetal development throughout gestation. According to this hypothesis, the adverse effects of a metabolic disturbance would be conditioned by

the time in gestation when the event occurred and which cells were undergoing a critical stage of terminal differentiation at the time (Fig. 38-4). Thus, metabolic perturbations during organogenesis might be implicated in congenital malformations; those occurring in the second trimester might initiate pancreatic β-cell hyperplasia or have an impact on CNS development; a surfeit of metabolic fuels in late gestation might augment adipose tissue proliferation, fat synthesis, fetal obesity, and macrosomia. In the intervening two decades, much evidence has been collected in support of this hypothesis.

Congenital Malformations and Early Fetal Loss

Experimental, clinical, and epidemiologic studies indicate that the increased risks of congenital malformations and spontaneous abortions in pregnancies complicated by diabetes are linked to disturbances in maternal metabolism around the time of conception.[10,89–91] The frequency of spontaneous abortions increases in direct proportion to glycohemoglobin concentrations measured in early pregnancy.[92,93] The relationship between metabolic control and the risk of congenital malformations is more difficult to define (Fig. 38-5). The NIH-supported Diabetes in Early Pregnancy (DIEP) study found a 4.9% incidence of birth defects in patients recruited within 21 days of conception, a rate approximately twofold that in the nondiabetic control group (2.1%; $p = 0.027$).[92] Most of the early entry DIEP study subjects were in *fair to good* glycemic control (glycohemoglobin within 7 standard deviations of the mean for controls in 93% of cases) during the first trimester. Green and colleagues[93] reported a prevalence of congenital anomalies of about 5% (almost identical to that of the DIEP Study) until first trimester glycohemoglobin concentrations exceeded the mean control value by 10–12 standard deviations (*poor metabolic control*), beyond which the rate of malformations increased greatly.

Exposure of rodent embryos in culture to marked hyperglycemia or rodent fetuses *in vivo* to severe maternal diabetes is associated with severe alterations of metabolic pathways including disruptions of signaling pathways, oxidative stress, and increased generation of free radicals.[89,90,94–104] Any one or all of these disturbances may contribute importantly to diabetic embryopathy. However, even though the precise time or the duration of exposure to an

FIGURE 38-4. The hypothesis of "fuel-mediated teratogenesis." It has been postulated that phenotypic gene expression in the newly forming cells of the conceptus may be modified by ambient fuels and fuel-related products during intrauterine development. Potential long-range effects will depend on the period in gestation during which maternal fuels and fuel-related products are aberrant and the cells that are undergoing development at that time. (*Adapted with permission from Freinkel.*[10])

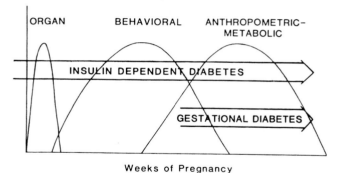

THERAPEUTIC DILEMMA IN EARLY DIABETIC PREGNANCY

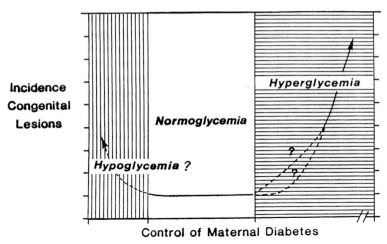

FIGURE 38-5. Therapeutic dilemma in treatment with insulin during early human pregnancy. Hypoglycemia during the period of glycolytic dependence in the rodent embryo has been shown to be teratogenic. Whether the human embryo is similarly vulnerable during the corresponding developmental interval (i.e., about days 16–18 to days 24–25 post conception) has not been established. Moreover, the thresholds for the various factors in maternal serum that account for teratogenesis of diabetes (broadly designated above as "hyperglycemia") have not been ascertained. Thus, the optimal target for metabolic regulation before and during the first 4–6 weeks after conception has not yet been precisely established. *(Adapted with permission from Freinkel.[96]).*

abnormal metabolic environment necessary for adverse events to develop in the human embryo has not been pinpointed, substantial insight has been gained regarding their prevention. Several groups have reported encouraging results from efforts to provide counseling and improved control of diabetes mellitus prior to conception. In such circumstances, rates of major congenital malformations do not appear to be greater than expected in general obstetric populations; however, the studies have not included data on rates of malformation in concurrently examined controls.[105–108] In Denmark, where the majority of pregnancies in women with diabetes are now planned, a nationwide decline in congenital malformations from 7.4 to 2.7% has been reported.[109] These developing trends have stimulated efforts to educate both health care professionals and patients concerning the benefits of preconception care. Unfortunately, the level of compliance in the United States remains substantially below that of the Danish population mentioned above.[110]

Disturbances in Fetal Growth

Neonatal macrosomia (traditionally defined as birthweight in excess of 4000 g or above the 90th percentile for gestational age) is a frequent complication of pregestational as well as GDM. Increased adiposity is the primary component of the macrosomia. Early measurements of fat cell number, size, and lipid content indicated that infants of diabetic mothers may have almost twice as much body fat as infants of normal mothers.[111,112] Skinfold measurements at birth (an index of subcutaneous fat) have been used to document this adiposity and may correlate with the antecedent metabolic regulation.[113,114] Infants of diabetic mothers tend to have significantly increased adiposity at their shoulders,[115] which heightens the likelihood of shoulder dystocia, birth trauma, and cesarean section delivery. Using carefully standardized methods for neonatal anthropometry, Catalano's group[116] has recently demonstrated an increased body fat content in offspring of mothers with GDM, even when total body weight was not increased above that

of the controls. Other insulin-sensitive tissues such as liver and heart are also often enlarged in offspring of diabetic mothers.[112] Although skeletal growth may not be dependent on insulin action, a modest increase in fetal height (length) is commonly found. Head size, although normal, often appears small because of the concurrent truncal obesity.

In lieu of more direct estimates of body fat content, Farquhar[117] first used a simple expression of the relative proportionality between weight and height, which has been termed the symmetry index [SI]) for clinical evaluation of the disparate growth of "insulin-sensitive" tissues. SI is calculated from the relationships between relative weight, Wt_r (i.e., observed weight/50th percentile weight), and relative height, Ht_r (i.e., observed height/50th percentile height), at that time, i.e., $SI = Wt_r/Ht_r$. Thus, whereas in symmetrically grown infants the SI would be expected to approach unity, in macrosomic infants with excessive weight-for-length, the SI is often greater than 1.2.

SI values in offspring of diabetic mothers have correlated with increased levels of several fuels in the maternal circulation in the second as well as the third trimester[118] and with increased insulin or C peptide in amniotic fluid and cord blood, consistent with premature activation of fetal islet function.[119,120] Others have also demonstrated correlation between amniotic fluid insulin or C peptide and neonatal macrosomia and morbidity in diabetic pregnancies.[121,122] Persson and colleagues,[123] like the Northwestern University workers,[118] have found that the premature activation of fetal islets correlates with maternal levels of insulinogenic amino acids as well as glucose.

Most infants who are large for gestational age, based on birthweight as the sole criterion, are born to women with normal carbohydrate tolerance.[124] Thus, gross birthweight is not a specific index of the effects of maternal diabetes on excessive fetal growth in late pregnancy, rather, asymmetric growth (with hypertrophy of insulin-sensitive tissues relative to those tissues whose growth is little influenced by fetal insulin) is the characteristic feature of diabetic fetopathy. This asymmetric growth can be ascertained *in utero* by serial ultrasound measurements of the fetal abdominal circumference, which includes tissues manifesting "insulin-sensitive" growth (e.g., subcutaneous fat, liver), and fetal head circumference or biparietal diameter, which includes tissues whose growth is relatively "insulin-insensitive" (e.g., bony calvarium, brain).[119]

Excessive increase in abdominal circumference in the presence of normal head growth connotes the fetal macrosomia of diabetes mellitus. Fetal humeral soft tissue thickness has been shown to be an even more accurate predictor of asymmetric fetal growth, as confirmed by examination of the neonate.[125] Buchanan and coworkers[126] have used relative increase in abdominal circumference to identify pregnancies in GDM that are at high risk for macrosomic infants and to target this subgroup for more intensive medical therapy with diet and/or insulin. Finally, heavy neonates born to women with diabetes mellitus may not always represent examples of diabetic macrosomia. Keller and colleagues[127] observed a subset of infants of diabetic women in whom birthweights exceeded 4000 g but who had biparietal diameter, length, and birthweight proportionally or symmetrically increased from standard norms, and in whom amniotic fluid insulin concentration was not elevated.

Increase in the rate of insulin secretion in the fetus exposed to the metabolic milieu diabetes mellitus may begin during the second trimester. Histologic and morphometric studies in fetuses of mothers with diabetes delivered at this time have shown islet hypertrophy and hyperplasia.[128] Reiher and colleagues[129] compared stimulated insulin secretion *in vitro* from pancreases of fetuses of varying gestational age from diabetic women in poor metabolic control and nondiabetic women. Fetal insulin secretion was increased as early as 16 weeks of gestation in poorly controlled diabetes. We have found a stronger association between fetal islet function (amniotic fluid insulin [32–38 weeks of gestation] or cord plasma C peptide at delivery) and metabolic control in the second trimester (HbA_{1c} concentration) than in the third trimester.[118] However, visceromegaly and the excessive deposition of fat occur primarily during the third trimester.

Studies in which insulin pumps were implanted in monkey fetuses have shown that hyperinsulinemia *per se* can accelerate the growth of insulin-responsive tissues, even without attendant increases in metabolic fuels.[130] Thus, if increased secretion of insulin from fetal β-cells begins prematurely in midgestation, it is conceivable that hyperinsulinemia and augmented fetal anabolism could continue even in the absence of persistent elevations of maternal nutrients.[118] Although it is clear that insulin has direct effects on fetal tissues, concurrent increases in the levels of the insulin-like growth factors (IGF-I and/or IGF-II) or other growth factors may also be contributory.[131]

In the past, intrauterine growth retardation (IUGR), the converse of macrosomia, was frequently observed in offspring of insulin-dependent diabetic mothers. This was commonly thought to reflect "utero-placental insufficiency" secondary to maternal vascular disease.[132] Current reports indicate that, except for pregnancies complicated by hypertension and/or diabetic nephropathy, IUGR is rarely seen.[133,134] Concurrently, the occurrence of macrosomia in pregestational diabetic pregnancies has markedly increased, reaching rates of 30–40% in some reports. Clinical observations[135] and studies in animal models and in rodent embryo cultures[136] suggest that disturbances in maternal metabolism in early pregnancy may retard growth irreparably, with or without associated birth defects. Better control of diabetes in early pregnancy

and discontinuation of routine delivery before term may account for the rarity of IUGR and the increased prevalence of macrosomia in the newborns of women with pregestational diabetes.

Effects of Pregnancy on Diabetes

Glycemic Control

In normal pregnancy, insulin resistance induced by placental hormone production and the siphoning of maternal fuels by the conceptus (see above) is overcome by major increases in maternal insulin production, such that blood glucose concentrations remain within relatively narrow limits and are close to those seen in nongravid women. With insulin deficiency, substantial increases in blood glucose and other insulin-sensitive fuels will occur unless they are counterbalanced by increased doses of exogenous insulin.

Catalano and coworkers[67] performed measurements of insulin sensitivity by the euglycemic-hyperinsulinemic clamp technique serially before and during pregnancy. Subjects who maintained normal glucose tolerance throughout (controls) showed a small, but significant reduction in insulin sensitivity by late in the first trimester (Fig. 38-1). A group with previous GDM and glucose tolerance in the normal range was somewhat insulin-resistant before pregnancy and showed a small, but significant increase in insulin sensitivity when they were retested late in the first trimester. In women with type 1 diabetes mellitus (T1DM), a mild reduction in insulin dosage is often seen toward the end of the first trimester (approximately 10–14 weeks of gestation).[137] This may be associated with more frequent and severe hypoglycemia. This pattern is most likely to occur in women who have suboptimal metabolic control in early pregnancy. Thus, aggressive efforts to achieve satisfactory glycemic control as quickly as possible may contribute to this tendency. In other cases, morning sickness (nausea and emesis) may result in erratic and unpredictable caloric intake in the first trimester. This may lead to marked swings in glycemic control including episodes of both severe hypo- and hyperglycemia, a problem that is particularly troubling during this period of organogenesis in the fetus. Whatever the factors responsible, it is important for clinicians to be aware of the tendencies toward less stable metabolic control in early pregnancy.

During the second trimester, insulin needs steadily increase, with the major increment occurring between 20 and 30 weeks of gestation, often reaching doses that are two- to threefold greater than in early pregnancy. The last several weeks (32–38 weeks) are characterized by relative stability of glycemic control, often requiring only minor modifications of insulin doses from week to week. In the last 1–2 weeks before delivery, some patients note more frequent hypoglycemia, and insulin doses may need to be reduced, especially those acting overnight. Immediately post partum, normal or supranormal insulin sensitivity is restored. Dramatic reduction of insulin doses (75–90%) may be necessary for several days. After that, insulin requirements usually become similar to what was needed before pregnancy.

Microvascular Disease

Retinopathy

Instances of severe deterioration in diabetic retinopathy during pregnancy have been documented.[138,139] Reports from Northwestern University[139] and elsewhere[140] indicate that severe deterioration of retinopathy during pregnancy rarely, if ever, occurs in subjects with minimal or absent retinopathy prior to conception. Vision-threatening change is primarily confined to patients with severe background retinopathy or untreated proliferative retinopathy already present before pregnancy or discovered in early gestation. By contrast, serious alterations in retinal status rarely occur during gestation in women with proliferative retinopathy who have been treated with photocoagulation and deemed "inactive" prior to conception.[138,141] We, and others, have reported an association between worsening retinopathy during pregnancy and the magnitude of hyperglycemia at enrollment.[139,140] Worsening retinopathy was also related to the magnitude of improvement in diabetic control achieved in the first half of gestation.

This finding suggests that some of the untoward ophthalmologic changes hitherto ascribed to pregnancy may be linked to the *rapid* institution of tight diabetic control in subjects whose diabetes was previously poorly regulated.[139] This phenomenon was noted in nongravid subjects in the Diabetes Control and Complications Trial (DCCT)[142] and elsewhere.[143] Hypertension has also been associated with progression of retinopathy during pregnancy.[144] Recently, analysis of the data from the DCCT[145] indicated that pregnancy does contribute to transient progression of retinopathy. As in previous reports, some subjects developed severe enough retinopathy to require photocoagulation therapy during pregnancy. The analysis of the DCCT experience also indicated that progression of retinopathy can continue after pregnancy or that retinopathy can first appear in the first 6–12 months post partum. However, no permanent adverse affect of pregnancy on retinal status was found.[145] In other words, the tendency for progression that has been observed during gestation is transient.

Although photocoagulation therapy can be used effectively during gestation, it seems prudent to assess retinal status carefully beforehand and to delay conception until stabilization of retinal pathology has been achieved. By this means, the risks of accelerated retinal damage in association with pregnancy may be minimized for most women.

Nephropathy

Normal physiologic adaptations of pregnancy include an increased glomerular filtration rate (GFR), increased renal plasma flow, and afferent arteriolar vasodilation. These changes result in glomerular hyperfiltration, which may be maladaptive in patients with pre-existing renal disease, and an increased systemic pressure transmitted to the glomerulus in the setting of hypertension. In addition, pregnancy is associated with an increase in urinary tract infections and pyelonephritis secondary to ureteral hypomotility with vesicoureteral reflux, physiologic hydronephrosis, and increased urinary nutrient content. This combination of factors may, in certain instances, predispose to accelerated deterioration of renal function in pregnancy. Observations of patients with mild pre-existing diabetic nephropathy (microalbuminuria, proteinuria, or mild renal insufficiency with a creatinine < 1.4 mg/dL [124 mmol/L]) suggest that pregnancy does not permanently accelerate their nephropathy, although there may be a transient worsening of proteinuria and creatinine clearance.[146–148] However, studies of diabetic patients with moderate or severe renal insufficiency raise the concern that pregnancy may accelerate the decline in renal function in such persons,[149,150] as has been seen when patients have moderate renal insufficiency of nondiabetic etiology. In addition, pregnancy in women with more severe degrees of nephropathy may be complicated by exacerbation of hypertension/pre-eclampsia, acceleration of retinopathy, and fetal/neonatal morbidity (prematurity, IUGR).[146,148,150] Prophylactic measures to preserve renal function include maintaining good glycemic and blood pressure control, obtaining frequent urine cultures with antibiotic therapy as needed, and careful monitoring of maternal renal function and fetal well-being.

Neuropathy

Little is known of the effect of pregnancy on diabetic neuropathy, a complication that exists in 7–50% of patients after 1–25 years of diabetes duration, respectively. However, the presence of autonomic neuropathy may have a potentially adverse effect on maternal morbidity[151] and pregnancy outcome.[152] Gastroparesis is of particular concern, as the irregular gastric emptying may result in inadequate nutrition, marked fluctuation in blood glucoses, and maternal aspiration. Genitourinary disturbances in patients who have diabetic nephropathy and bladder dysfunction may result in recurrent urinary tract infection and worsening renal function.

Macrovascular Disease

Patients with macrovascular disease have significant risks of maternal and fetal morbidity. First, pregnancy may exacerbate pre-existing vascular disease. Systolic blood pressure may increase significantly in T1DM women, whereas diastolic blood pressure tends to be higher than in controls at conception and throughout gestation.[153] In a limited number of cases reported, myocardial infarction in pregnancy has been associated with a 50% mortality rate.[141,154,155] Since these reports were published more than 3 decades ago, the outcomes may not reflect risks with current practice. Women with coronary artery disease are also vulnerable to myocardial infarction and congestive heart failure in the immediate postpartum period.

CLASSIFICATION OF DIABETES IN PREGNANCY

Pre-existing insulin-treated diabetes is a complicating event in approximately 0.2–0.5% of all pregnancies in the United States.[156] In some populations, half or more of such pregnancies are in women with type 2 diabetes mellitus (T2DM) rather than T1DM (insulin-dependent). GDM affects an additional 2–6%. These figures are likely to increase in the future, because the incidence of obesity and T2DM seem to be increasing in adolescents and young adults, especially among minority populations. Since there are more than 3,000,000 live births in the United States each year, diabetes during pregnancy constitutes an appreciable and increasing public health problem.

In accord with recommendations of the National Diabetes Data Group,[7] the 1997 Expert Committee on the Diagnosis and Classification of Diabetes Mellitus,[9] and the Fourth International Workshop Conference on GDM,[8] gestational diabetes is defined as "carbohydrate intolerance with onset or first recognition during the present pregnancy." We continue to subdivide GDM on the basis of the severity of the metabolic disturbance[10,120,157,158] and use FPG as the distinguishing characteristic (Table 38-1). To be consistent with changes recently introduced to define an elevated FPG concentration during pregnancy, we designate gravida as GDM Class A_1 when values for FPG are within the normal range for pregnancy, (i.e., <95 mg/dL [5.3 mmol/L]) and as GDM Class A_2 when values equal or exceed this limit.

For epidemiologic purposes, pregnant women with abnormal glucose tolerance who had gestational diabetes with a prior pregnancy are not considered to have gestational diabetes with the current pregnancy. Unless post- or interpartum testing indicated a

TABLE 38-1. Classification of Carbohydrate Intolerance During Pregnancy*

Class	Classification Criteria
Gestational diabetes mellitus (GDM)	Carbohydrate intolerance of varying severity with onset or first recognition during the present pregnancy. Diagnosis as per Tables 38-2 and 38-3. Antepartum subclassification on the basis of values for fasting glucose.
GDM Class A_1	Fasting glucose normal for pregnancy: venous plasma < 95 mg/dL (5.3 mmol/L)
GDM Class A_2	Fasting glucose exceeds normal for pregnancy: venous plasma ≥ 95 mg/dL (5.3 mm/L) on at least two occasions
	Postpartum Reclassification
	Evaluation by fasting plasma glucose or 75 g oral glucose tolerance test to classify according to the criteria of the NDGG and ADA Expert Committee as: "Previous abnormality of glucose tolerance (GDM)" if glucose tolerance normal at this time, or impaired fasting glucose, impaired glucose tolerance (IGT), or diabetes mellitus
Previous GDM	Abnormality of glucose tolerance in a previous pregnancy, without diabetes mellitus having been diagnosed postpartum (postpartum glucose tolerance test normal, impaired fasting glucose, IGT, or not performed)
Previous GDM: Class A_1	(See above for fasting plasma glucose parameters.)
Previous GDM: Class A_2	
Pregestational diabetes mellitus	Diabetes mellitus diagnosed prior to the present pregnancy (according to criteria of the ADA Expert Committee)
Diabetes mellitus type 1	
Uncomplicated	Absence of retinopathy, nephropathy, neuropathy, coronary artery disease, or hypertension
Complicated	Presence of one or more of the above (see footnote for designation and definitions)†
Diabetes mellitus type 2	
Uncomplicated	As for type 1 diabetes
Complicated	As for type 1 diabetes

* Classification is based on prevailing practices in the authors' center and the recommendations of the National Diabetes Data Group (NDDG), the ADA Expert Committee, and the Workshop Conferences on Gestational Diabetes.[7–9]

† BDR, background diabetic retinopathy; PDR, proliferative diabetic retinopathy; NEPH, diabetic nephropathy defined as ≥0.5 g protein in 24-hr urine collection and/or serum creatinine consistently ≥1.2 mg/dL (106 mmol/L); NEUR, neuropathy, defined as known gastroparesis when not pregnant, orthostatic hypotension, or sensory abnormalities in lower extremities detected at bedside examination; CAD, coronary artery disease diagnosed by history, ECG, or stress ECG; HTN, hypertension, defined as BP ≥ 140/90 consistently. (Designations are appended to primary diagnosis as appropriate, e.g., diabetes mellitus-type 2-uncomplicated; diabetes mellitus-type 1-BDR, NEPH, etc.).

Source: From Metzger et al,[137] with permission.

diagnosis of diabetes mellitus, they are classified as Previous GDM and subdivided on the basis of FPG concentration into Class A_1 or Class A_2 (Table 38-1). Patients who had normal or impaired glucose tolerance (IGT) or impaired fasting glucose post partum, as well as patients in whom the interpartum status is unknown, are included in the Previous GDM category.

We, as well as some others, have ceased to use the traditional classification devised several decades ago by White.[159] That scheme is based on the age of onset of diabetes mellitus, its duration, and whether or not micro- or macrovascular complications are present. At the time of its formulation, this was useful in predicting the risk of perinatal loss or serious morbidity. In the present era fetal losses are uncommon, and the degree of metabolic control throughout pregnancy and the presence or absence of vascular complications, independent of maternal age or duration of diabetes mellitus, are more specific predictors of maternal or fetal morbidities. We attempt to distinguish those pregnant patients with T1DM from those with T2DM.[9] Although this distinction cannot be made with certainty in every case, the standard clinical yardsticks are generally reliable. Groups are then subdivided based on whether diabetic complications are known to be present. Abbreviations for the specific complications are added as postscripts (Table 38-1).

MANAGEMENT

Pregestational Diabetes

Preconception Counseling
Under optimal conditions, the management of "pregnancy complicated by diabetes" should begin before pregnancy is even contemplated. Information about the potential complications of pregnancy for mother and offspring should be an essential aspect

of the education of all women with diabetes mellitus. The educational efforts should be initiated as early as possible, ideally by the time of puberty. The precise content and mode of presentation are necessarily tailored to the age and level of maturity of the individual patient. However, it should be repeatedly emphasized that pregnancy may introduce uniquely new problems, if special precautions are not taken in advance. Thus, contraception should be discussed and offered to all women of childbearing age who have diabetes mellitus. Ideally, the woman's satisfaction with her contraceptive practices should be assessed at every contact whether or not that visit is intended as a preconception consultation. An ongoing dialogue with the woman allows reinforcement of the concept that a planned conception after appropriate assessment and improvement of metabolic control will reduce the risk of pregnancy complications such as spontaneous abortion and fetal malformations.

For women seeking preconception advice (ideally offered with the prospective father in attendance), reassessment of maternal health status is undertaken, with particular attention given to possible diabetic vascular complications. In addition to a complete physical examination, including pelvic examination, we recommend ophthalmologic consultation unless diabetes is of short duration and routine funduscopic examination appears to be normal. We also obtain baseline measurements of glycohemoglobin, thyroid-stimulating hormone (TSH), 24-hour creatinine clearance and quantitative urinary protein excretion (micro- or macroalbuminuria as appropriate), complete blood count (CBC), and an automated chemistry screen. Immunity to rubella should also be assessed, with immunization of susceptible individuals. Lifestyle issues should be reviewed for needed adjustments, including assessment of stress, tobacco or alcohol use, and prescription drugs that may need to be discontinued prior to pregnancy. In particular, this often means the discontinuation of angiotensin-converting enzyme (ACE) inhibitors, agents that are increasingly being used early in the treatment of hypertension and microalbuminuria.

Information relating to the potential effects of diabetes on fetal growth and development (see above), including long-range outcomes (see Chap. 39), is reviewed with the prospective parents, emphasizing the benefit of careful diabetic control before and during gestation. The possibility of deleterious effects of pregnancy on maternal vascular complications (see above) is also discussed as the mother's clinical condition warrants. The patient and significant other(s) should also be reminded that prenatal care is intensive and involves a significant time commitment for the greater frequency of prenatal visits and the additional efforts that are needed to maintain optimal metabolic control in the period before conception and during the entire pregnancy. The possibility that fetal and neonatal effects of maternal diabetes (pregestational or gestational) may have a long-range impact on the offspring is an issue with major public health implications. Presently, many studies have focused on the possibilities that obesity, T2DM, and neurobehavioral deficits may be more prevalent in later life in the offspring of diabetic mothers (see Chap. 39).

To minimize the likelihood of birth defects and/or diabetes-related spontaneous abortions, we strive for good, stable metabolic control *before* conception.[90,137] This requires a period of renewed effort for patients already familiar with an intensive management regimen and an introduction to the concept of *tight control* for others. Periconceptional supplementation with folic acid may reduce the risk of neural tube birth defects,[160] and neural tube defects occur at an increased rate when pregnancy is complicated by diabetes. We advise women to start a multivitamin containing 0.8 mg folic acid prior to the intended conception. This should be continued through the first 6 weeks of gestation.

Glucose regulation is assessed by capillary blood sugar measurements performed by the patient and by estimates of HbA_{1c}. We prescribe a diet based on a "exchange system" and set up a multiple-dose insulin injection algorithm for those women who are not currently using an intensive diabetes management program. An experienced caregiver reviews the results of capillary blood glucose tests with the patient at least weekly. Many women, particularly those who use pumps for delivery of insulin, have varying degrees of familiarity with the practice of "carbohydrate counting" wherein the premeal dose (bolus) of short-acting insulin that is given takes into account the grams of carbohydrate that are to be ingested. Many women use this effectively and also maintain a balanced intake of protein, fat, and micronutrients. We do encourage them to maintain more day-to-day consistency in meal time and meal size than they may have done outside of pregnancy. This is particularly helpful during the time of rapidly escalating insulin requirements. Others need more guidance to ensure intake of an adequate number of calories and optimal balance of nutrients. We expect to see corroboration of the improved control by stabilization of glycohemoglobin concentration within or near the normal range before contraception is discontinued. In many cases this entire effort may encompass an interval of 3–4 months.

Management After Conception

T1DM complicates pregnancy infrequently, and expertise in the management of this high-risk population can only be achieved if sufficient numbers of patients are seen on an ongoing basis. Optimally, therefore, such care is provided in specialized referral clinics, employing a team consisting of physician, nurse educator, nutritionist, and social worker (depending on the population served) whose practices and philosophies are consistent and well integrated.

Diet

Diabetes does not alter the basic dietary recommendations for pregnancy, except that complex carbohydrates should be substituted for "free" sugars. Because of the heightened propensity for accelerated starvation,[73,74] inclusion of an evening snack is recommended. Carbohydrate intake is seldom restricted below 200 g/day, and food intake should be distributed throughout the day to avoid periods of fasting in excess of 4–5 hours during the waking hours. The proportion of the daily diet given at specific times can be individualized (within the above constraints) according to patient preference and may also be manipulated to effect stability of metabolic control. However, consistency from day to day is essential for the attainment of excellent diabetic control.

In the interest of simplicity (which we believe enhances adherence to the overall treatment regimen), we usually plan a diet of three major meals and a bedtime snack. Some caregivers recommend multiple small feedings (six to seven) throughout the day in an effort to dampen postmeal hyperglycemia. Whether the mean 24-hour blood glucose is lower with such regimens is unknown. (Dampening postprandial peaks by frequent small meals might be associated with higher premeal glucose concentrations.) Proponents of a multiple-feeding regimen that focuses on control of postprandial hyperglycemia base this approach on the findings in some reports of a stronger correlation between mean values of postprandial glycemia and birthweight than between fasting and premeal glycemia and birthweight.[161,162] However, these were observational findings, not prospectively designed studies. Furthermore, it is not certain what influence day-to-day variability in glycemic control, in contrast to the overall average level of glycemia, may have on perinatal outcome.

Dietary prescriptions are individualized and modified over the course of gestation. The Institute of Medicine of the National Academy of Sciences has published guidelines relating to optimal weight gain during gestation[163]; in the absence of information to the contrary, we consider these recommendations to be appropriate for pregnancy complicated by diabetes. Accordingly, it is recommended that gestational weight gain be inversely proportional to the degree of adiposity in the mother before conception. This may vary from 15 pounds (7 kg), in the very obese, to 40 pounds (18 kg) for underweight women. Adiposity is judged by body mass index (BMI), defined as weight/height^2. A prepregnancy BMI of 19.8–26.0 kg/m^2 is considered normal, in which case a 25–35-pound (11–16 kg) weight gain is judged desirable. For those with BMI < 19.8 kg/m^2, the recommended weight gain is 28–40 pounds, and for those with BMI > 26 kg/m^2, it is 15–25 pounds. Additionally, some experts have estimated that the caloric cost of pregnancy may be only 100–150 kcal/day above requirements outside of pregnancy.[164] This is substantially less than the 250–300-kcal/day figure that was widely accepted in the past as the basis for dietary prescriptions. Thus, we find it very important to monitor weight gain closely during pregnancy and to modify caloric intake to reach the goals that are summarized above.

We base the initial prescription before conception or in early gestation on an estimate of the woman's weight-maintaining caloric intake, or we use an estimate based on 32 kcal/kg ideal body weight (IBW).[165] This is increased to 35–38 kcal/kg IBW after the first trimester, depending on appetite, physical activity, and weight gain. Dietary protein accounts for 1.5–2.0 g/kg IBW, carbohydrates comprise 50–55% of total calories, and fat comprises 30–35%. For women who become pregnant while using carbohydrate counting to guide their dietary intake, care must be taken to achieve an adequate intake of the full spectrum of nutritional needs for pregnancy (see above).

Variations of up to ±25–30% in total calories may be necessary to attain optimal weight gain as described above. In some centers, a relatively large proportion of women with pregestational diabetes have T2DM and are obese. The use of hypocaloric diets to restrict weight gain below the guidelines outlined above has been advocated by some[132] (for review, see ref. 165). Moderate calorie restriction (20–25% below the figure cited above) may reduce hyperglycemia without increasing ketonemia or promoting the development of ketonuria. However, since "around the clock" studies in obese women with GDM whose caloric intake was restricted more than 33% below standard prescriptions have shown significant elevations of FFAs and plasma ketones,[166] we do not advocate this degree of caloric restriction, except in a research setting. High-fiber diets have not been found to be effective in reducing postprandial plasma glucose levels during pregnancy. "Isocaloric diets" containing only 30–40% of calories as carbohydrate (rather than 50–55%) do effect a reduction in hyperglycemia,[167] but the effects of the concomitant increase in dietary protein and fat on maternal amino acids, lipids, and ketones have not been investigated in detail.

Insulin

Optimal therapy necessitates individualization. We have used "intensified" therapy routinely since 1970. We ask our patients to supplement the longer acting insulin (given at breakfast, supper, or bedtime as necessary to maintain *basal* insulinization) with soluble insulin given prior to each meal (to replicate acute postprandial insulin excursions).[10] Lispro insulin (Humalog®), an analog of human insulin, is more rapidly absorbed from subcutaneous tissue than is Regular (soluble) human insulin. Postinjection profiles of circulating Humalog have been shown to mimic the profiles of secreted insulin in normal subjects more closely than the pattern seen after injection of Regular human insulin.[168] Increasing numbers of women are using lispro insulin for their usual treatment and are thus on this therapy when they are seen for evaluation before pregnancy. In nonpregnant subjects, many studies have shown its superiority in controlling postprandial hyperglycemia; it has also resulted in some reduction in the frequency of hypoglycemia. Only limited information is available concerning its efficacy and safety in pregnancy. However, no untoward events have been conclusively ascribed to its use during pregnancy.[169] We do not discourage its use in women who are already using lispro insulin when they are seen for preconception care or when they enroll for prenatal care at our center after they conceive. In many patients, bolus injection of lispro insulin must be supplemented with low doses of intermediate-acting insulin or used in combination with Regular insulin to ensure that hyperglycemia does not ensue before the next meal as a result of complete disappearance of lispro insulin. Other analogs and modified forms of insulin are in development. When they are released for clinical use, there will be uncertainties regarding their use during pregnancy like the circumstances that occurred after the introduction of lispro insulin.

Whatever insulin preparations are used, doses are adjusted in an effort to achieve fasting and premeal blood glucose concentrations of 65–85 mg/dL (3.6–4.7 mmol/L) and 1- or 2-hour postprandial values of <140–150 and 120–130 mg/dL (7.7–8.3 and 6.7–7.2 mmol/L), respectively. Patients are provided with individu-

ally tailored algorithms for adjustments of insulin doses at each injection. These are altered as necessary by telephone or at clinic visits. This variable, multidose regimen provides for greater flexibility in responding to the erratic blood sugar fluctuations that often occur in patients with T1DM. The use of insulin pumps and continuous subcutaneous insulin infusion (CSII) with bolus infusions prior to meals has not been shown to confer any greater benefits in pregnancy than the program of intensified conventional therapy cited above. We continue CSII therapy for patients who have been using it prior to conception; however, we do not initiate its use during pregnancy unless patients are strongly motivated to do so.

Most patients with T2DM retain some endogenous insulin secretion. In such patients, it is often relatively easy to achieve the treatment goals outlined above. This is commonly done using a twice daily "mixed" insulin regimen (combinations of short- and intermediate-acting insulin given before breakfast and supper). If the diet is carefully adhered to, blood glucose levels are quite stable, and insulin dosage modifications are made every 1–2 weeks from a review of fingerstick blood glucose measurements obtained by the patient. Episodes of hyperglycemia are usually caused by temporary lapses in adhering to the prescribed diet.

Patients with near-normal blood sugar values in the first trimester may experience a modest reduction in insulin needs toward the end of this period (10–14 weeks), a time of particular vulnerability to severe hypoglycemic episodes[137] (see above). Subsequently, insulin requirements increase substantially in most patients before seeming to plateau in the third trimester at a level two- to threefold above doses used before pregnancy. A reduction in insulin need is sometimes noted in the week or two before term. The challenge of therapy is to modify the insulin dose in parallel with these alterations in insulin sensitivity.

Monitoring of Diabetes Control

At each outpatient visit, measurements of plasma glucose are obtained from the laboratory simultaneously with patient-determined estimates of capillary blood sugar to check the accuracy of the patient's measurements. Blood sugars are monitored at home before each meal and at bedtime; at least twice weekly, the patient also measures values 1 hour after each meal. As noted above, in women with T1DM, the postprandial values may more closely parallel overall fuel delivery to the fetus and consequently may correlate better with birthweight than fasting values.[161,162] However, we have found premeal blood sugar measurements to be of greater utility in recommending doses of Regular insulin. The limitation on the dose of Regular insulin that can be given before a meal is the nadir blood sugar level that will occur prior to the subsequent meal regardless of the magnitude of the between-meal peak. When postprandial hyperglycemia persists despite normalization of premeal levels, adjustments in meal size and/or frequency of feedings may be beneficial. We rely equally on postprandial and premeal glucose concentrations to assess adequacy of lispro doses. As mentioned above, when using lispro insulin, a premeal concentration that is higher than optimal can reflect either a need for a larger bolus of lispro insulin with the preceding meal or a need for the addition of a longer acting insulin.

Measurements of glycosylated hemoglobin are secured at the first visit during pregnancy and at 4–6-week intervals thereafter, since these supplement but do not replace the information derived from estimates of blood sugar. The initial value for glycosylated hemoglobin can often provide a useful index of the state of maternal fuel metabolism around the time of conception, implantation, and organogenesis (see above), as well as a general indication of the risk of major congenital malformations, helping to guide decisions when elective abortion is a consideration. Measurements of fructosamine or glycosylated albumin may provide information analogous to that of glycosylated hemoglobin and may be desirable when the latter measure is unreliable (e.g., in the presence of hemoglobinopathy or hemolysis).

Patients are asked to test urine for ketones in the first morning urine specimen each day and at any time that premeal estimates of blood glucose exceed 200 mg/dL. These measurements are useful in detecting inadequate dietary intake, particularly of carbohydrate, and providing warning of impending metabolic decompensation. Monitoring urine glucose is unnecessary with the regimen outlined above.

Obstetric Surveillance

Patients are offered serum screening and a comprehensive ultrasound examination as surveillance for fetal anomalies. Serum screening with multiple analytes, performed between 15 and 20 weeks of gestation, typically includes maternal serum α-fetoprotein, estriol, and human chorionic gonadotropin. The α-fetoprotein portion can detect 80–90% of open neural tube defects and may also identify other defects such as gastroschisis and renal agenesis.[170] An abnormal pattern of the three analytes in combination with maternal age can detect approximately 60% of Down's syndrome cases[171] and a similar portion of fetuses with trisomy 18.[172] Regardless of serum screening results, the risk of diverse fetal anomalies in pregnancy complicated by diabetes mellitus warrants a comprehensive fetal anatomic survey by ultrasound. This is best performed after 18 weeks when the size of the fetus is sufficient to facilitate sonographic examination of all fetal structures. The sensitivity of ultrasound in detecting fetal abnormalities varies by anomaly. Gross defects such as hydrocephalus or omphalocele have very high detection rates, whereas others such as cardiac outflow tract anomalies are difficult to ascertain.[173]

Ultrasound examinations during pregnancy permit confirmation of estimated due date as well as an assessment of the pattern of fetal growth. Confirmation of gestational age may be performed in the first trimester as early as convenient after 6 weeks of amenorrhea, at which time both determination of viability and accurate dating can be performed. The presence or absence of evolving fetal macrosomia can be determined by serial measurements of fetal head and abdominal size in conjunction with estimated fetal weight in the late second and third trimesters of pregnancy.[119,125–127]

Intrauterine fetal death in late gestation was a relatively common event prior to the appreciation of the importance of good maternal metabolic control.[84] The etiology of this complication has never been established in human gestation, although data from animal models have suggested that sustained fetal hyperglycemia is associated with increased placental lactate production, increased fetal uptake of glucose and lactate, and stimulated fetal oxygen consumption, ultimately leading to fetal hypoxemia.[174–176] The risk of fetal death may no longer be appreciably increased over background rates in pregnancies attended by excellent metabolic control, particularly in the absence of vascular disease or pregnancy complications.

However, different biophysical methods of fetal assessment may provide objective measures of reassurance.[177] The mainstay of fetal assessment remains the nonstress test. The observation of two or more accelerations of the fetal heart rate in response to spontaneous fetal activity during 20 minutes of continuous fetal heart rate monitoring, designated a reactive test, is highly predictive of fetal well-being. An alternative modality is the biophysical profile by ultrasound, a technique that assesses fetal activity, fetal muscle tone, fetal breathing activity, and amniotic fluid volume, in addition to the nonstress test. A score of 2 is given for each positive finding, with a total possible score of 10; it is sometimes called the intrauterine Apgar score. We have utilized the nonstress test as our primary means of fetal surveillance, reserving use of the biophysical profile for assessment of a nonreactive nonstress test. Although weekly testing is usually initiated by 32 weeks of gestation, earlier and more frequent testing is indicated for pregnancies complicated by significant hypertension or other medical complications that may increase the risk of fetal death.

Meticulous surveillance for pregnancy complications is practiced at frequent prenatal visits, usually on a weekly basis after 30–32 weeks of gestation. It is generally accepted that the risk of preeclampsia is increased in women with diabetes mellitus, particularly for those with pre-existent vasculopathy. The traditional clinical criteria utilized for the diagnosis of pre-eclampsia are abrupt increase in blood pressure and appearance of proteinuria (>300 mg in 24 hours) in association with hyperuricemia. However, women with nephropathy may have a clinical course that can be easily confused with pre-eclampsia, including hypertension, which tends to worsen in the third trimester, increasing proteinuria presumed to be caused by the increased renal plasma flow of pregnancy, as well as hyperuricemia of uncertain origin. Making an accurate diagnosis in such patients requires close surveillance. The diagnosis of pre-eclampsia at or near term warrants consideration of immediate delivery. If pre-eclampsia is suspected in a preterm gestation, hospitalization is prudent for close observation of maternal and fetal status.

Delivery and Postpartum Care

Diabetic Aspects Medical management during either spontaneous or induced labor consists of monitoring blood sugar every 1–4 hours and continuous intravenous infusions of glucose at the rate of 5–10 g/h. Insulin is administered as needed, either as an intravenous infusion via a separate line at the rate of 0.01–0.04 U/h/kg actual body weight (i.e., 0.7–2.8 U/h in a 70-kg woman), or by subcutaneous injection of short-acting (Regular) insulin every 3–6 hours. The need for glucose and/or insulin should be based on the prevailing blood glucose, the time and nature of the last insulin injection, and the time of food ingestion prior to the onset of labor. The "exercise" effect of labor may enhance the rate of glucose utilization.[178] This effect may be partly modulated by the use of a continuous epidural anesthetic during labor. The therapeutic objective is to maintain circulating glucose in the physiologic range (70–120 mg/dL [3.9–6.7 mm/L]) throughout labor. In women who have been in good metabolic "control" throughout their third trimester, we have been unable to demonstrate a relationship between cord blood glucose at delivery and subsequent neonatal hypoglycemia, although such an association has been noted by others.[179]

Elective cesarean sections should be scheduled early in the morning when possible. Neither glucose nor additional insulin is administered if blood sugar is in the range of 70–140 mg/dL (3.9–7.8 mm.L) immediately beforehand. Blood sugar values outside this range necessitate infusion of glucose, insulin, or both. Insulin requirement declines dramatically immediately following delivery (by as much as 75–90%), and the administered dose may have to be reduced temporarily to 25% or less of the total daily antepartum dose. Failure to observe this fall in insulin requirement may be the earliest sign of a postdelivery infection or other obstetric complications. After a variable period, insulin requirements generally return to prepregnancy levels.

Opinions differ about the continuing use of CSII during labor or cesarean delivery. Some physicians feel strongly that the possibility of dislodging the tubing during the exertions of labor, or positioning of patients during delivery and possible alterations in subcutaneous insulin absorption should hypotension or significant hemorrhage occur, for example, speak strongly for use of intravenous insulin in these circumstances. However, patients frequently have a strong desire to continue the use of their insulin pump during delivery, and many physicians are comfortable with using CSII to manage blood glucose concentrations during this time. With either approach, the key to successful management is the frequent measurement of blood sugar concentration throughout the delivery process and post partum.

Women who wish to breastfeed are maintained at, or up to 300 calories above, their caloric intake before pregnancy. Because oral agents may be secreted in breast milk and cause hypoglycemia in the infant, their use is precluded in women with T2DM wishing to breastfeed. Women who do not plan to nurse are returned immediately to a diet appropriate for nongravid women (30–32 kcal/kg IBW [125–135 kjoule/kg]). All patients are encouraged to use the diabetes management skills they acquired during gestation.

Obstetric Aspects   For the woman who has experienced an uncomplicated pregnancy, the goal of obstetric management is vaginal birth of a term infant. Cesarean delivery increases the risk of numerous maternal morbidities, particularly hemorrhage and infection, and should be reserved for standard obstetric indications. Unless spontaneous labor ensures, induction is planned at term (38–40 weeks) when the cervix in considered favorable. Elective preterm delivery is not warranted, as it is well accepted that the sequelae of prematurity are more prevalent in infants of diabetic mothers compared with age-matched infants of nondiabetic mothers. When a term delivery is anticipated, it is not necessary to employ amniocentesis routinely to document fetal pulmonary maturity. This procedure should be utilized if the estimated due date is uncertain or if delivery is performed at <38 weeks of gestation.

Infants are at increased risk of shoulder dystocia when there is an asymmetric increase in upper body size of the fetus relative to head size. This risk is approximately twofold higher for infants of diabetic mothers compared with normal infants at all birthweights.[180] Brachial plexus injury is an uncommon but serious complication of shoulder dystocia, usually presenting as Erb's palsy. Fortunately, >90% of Erb's palsies resolve over a period of time.[181] That the risk of shoulder dystocia rises with increasing absolute fetal weight suggests that this complication may be obviated by planned cesarean delivery for selected patients. Various thresholds have been suggested, most commonly >4500 g in estimated fetal weight. However, formula-based estimates of fetal weight by ultrasound lack precision, with 95% confidence limits generally 15–20% of the estimated weight,[182] and shoulder dystocia may still occur in an infant who is <4000 g actual birthweight. Although protocols may vary in different programs, a combination of ultrasound assessment of the fetus and clinical judgment in assessing the likelihood of an uncomplicated vaginal birth is warranted. Thus, one would not necessarily proscribe vaginal birth in a multipara with anticipated fetal macrosomia if she has had a previous uncomplicated delivery of an infant of similar birthweight.

Gestational Diabetes Mellitus

Definition and Magnitude of the Problem

GDM, defined as "carbohydrate intolerance of variable severity with onset or first recognition during pregnancy,"[7–9] may complicate as many as 2–6% of pregnancies in North American centers, using National Diabetes Data Group (NDDG) criteria.[158,183–186] Even higher figures have been reported when other diagnostic criteria for GDM have been used,[185,187,188] and in some racial and ethnic populations incidences approaching 20% have been found.[189] It is thus >10 times more common than pregestational diabetes during pregnancy.

Studies in the 1970s and early 1980s found the risk of perinatal loss and neonatal morbidity to be increased when GDM was undetected or treated casually.[190–193] However, recent studies have not found an increase in perinatal loss in GDM.[8] This may reflect the concurrent overall improvement in obstetric practice or may be an effect of treatment. Women with GDM are often considered to be at "high risk," even when they are successfully managed with dietary intervention alone. Such a designation may in itself represent a form of intervention because it leads to more intensive obstetric supervision. In addition, home blood sugar monitoring and treatment with insulin if hyperglycemia persists are widely recommended.[8,194] Thus, perinatal loss in GDM[8] and the frequency of some neonatal morbidities (such as hypoglycemia, hypocalcemia, polycythemia, and hyperbilirubinemia) have decreased toward levels found in the general population[195,196] (see Chap. 39). Despite such improvements in outcome, offspring of mothers with GDM remain at risk for fetal hyperinsulinism and attendant excess fetal size (macrosomia), which increases the likelihood of birth trauma and operative delivery,[8,195] and, by implication, persistence of some degree of risk for long-range abnormalities.

Most studies have not found an increased risk of congenital anomalies in GDM. However, some association has been found in a few reports.[197–200] This has been so among populations likely to harbor a substantial proportion of women with unrecognized pregestational T2DM. The above considerations provide incentives for the detection and treatment of GDM using current methods, as well as justification for clinical trials of earlier and more aggressive treatment.

Screening and Diagnosis

GDM is almost always asymptomatic, and selective screening for glucose intolerance on the basis of clinical "risk factors" and/or past obstetric history does not identify one-third to one-half of the affected subjects.[8,184,185,201,202] Random estimates of blood glucose during prenatal visits have been advocated for the detection of asymptomatic glucose intolerance during pregnancy[203]; however, this approach also fails to detect a significant proportion of the cases,[204,205] and measurements of glycosylated hemoglobin[206,207] or fructosamine[208,209] do not provide acceptable diagnostic sensitivity. Screening tests have been studied that assess maternal blood glucose responses to orally administered glucose polymers[210] or mixed meals.[211,212] Measurement of second-trimester amniotic fluid insulin content, although it demonstrates reasonable sensitivity for early diagnosis of GDM,[213,214] is costly and invasive and carries risk.

Participants in the Fourth International Workshop Conference on GDM modified previous recommendations that all women should undergo blood glucose testing for GDM because this approach may not be cost-effective in populations or clinics that

TABLE 38-2. Screening Strategy for Detecting Gestational Diabetes Mellitus (GDM)

Risk	Strategy
	GDM risk assessment should be ascertained at the first prenatal visit
Low	Blood glucose testing not routinely required if *all* of the following characteristics are present:
	Member of an ethnic group with a low prevalence of GDM
	No known diabetes in first-degree relatives
	Age < 25 years
	Weight normal before pregnancy
	No history of abnormal glucose metabolism
	No history of poor obstetric outcome
Average	Perform blood glucose testing at 24–28 weeks using either
	Two-step procedure: 50-g glucose challenge test (GCT) followed by a diagnostic oral
	glucose tolerance test in those meeting the threshold value in the GCT (see text for details)
	One-step procedure: diagnostic oral glucose tolerance test performed on all subjects
High	Perform blood glucose testing as soon as feasible, using the procedures described above.
	If GDM is not diagnosed, blood glucose testing should be repeated at 24–28 weeks, or at
	any time a patient has symptoms or signs suggestive of hyperglycemia

Reproduced from Metzger *et al.*[8]

include a large proportion of subjects at low risk for GDM[8] (Table 38-2). It is recommended that risk assessment be carried out as soon after registration for prenatal care as feasible. To be considered low risk, subjects must have *all* of the following characteristics: member of racial/ethnic group with a low prevalence of GDM; age < 25 years; normal weight; no family history of diabetes; and no personal history of abnormal glucose metabolism or poor obstetric outcome. Those that are designated high risk for GDM should undergo blood glucose testing early in pregnancy. If GDM is not found, testing should be repeated at 24–28 weeks or at any time the patient develops symptoms suggestive of hyperglycemia. All others should be screened at 24–28 weeks of gestational age.[8]

In North America, a two-step screening-diagnostic strategy is most commonly applied. Subjects receive a 50-g oral glucose challenge (GCT) given without regard to time of the last meal or time of day, and venous plasma glucose is measured 1 hour later. A plasma glucose value ≥ 140 mg/dL (7.8 mm/L) is considered positive. Using this threshold, 14–16% of pregnant women at our center screen positive and require further testing.[186] The yield of GDM can be increased by approximately 10% if the screening threshold is reduced to 130 mg/dL (7.2 mmol/L), which might be considered trivial from the epidemiologic cost/benefit perspective in that it increases the proportion who require further testing to 23–25% of women.[185,186,215] Although it is convenient and rapid, measurement of capillary blood sugar with the use of reagent strips and portable meters is not sufficient for this purpose. Intratest variability of

10–15% with such methods lowers both the sensitivity and specificity of the procedure.[216]

A positive screening for GDM is followed by an oral glucose tolerance test (OGTT) for definitive diagnostic evaluation. We use a 100-g load for such diagnostic OGTTs and interpret the venous plasma glucose results according to the criteria of O'Sullivan and Mahan.[183] These criteria for the diagnosis of GDM were originally developed to identify a population of pregnant women who were at high risk for developing diabetes mellitus post partum.[183] In the absence of criteria based on the specific relationships between hyperglycemia and adverse perinatal outcome, the work of O'Sullivan and Mahan has been used as the basis of the criteria recommended by the NDDG,[7] the GDM Workshop Conferences,[8] and the American Diabetes Association[9] because it represents a well-designed, population-based study. The NDDG extrapolated values for Auto-Analyzer-measured plasma glucose from the criteria originally derived from whole blood glucose determination,[7] and Carpenter and Coustan[217] later adjusted the values to approximate more closely the values obtained with the glucose oxidase enzymatic assay of plasma or serum glucose (Table 38-3). Use of the criteria of Carpenter and Coustan labels nearly 50% more subjects as GDM than is the case when the NDDG criteria are applied.[186,188] Data from several populations now indicate that the additional cases diagnosed by Carpenter-Coustan criteria have a risk of perinatal morbidities similar to those of women diagnosed with the NDDG criteria.[188,218–220] Thus, the Fourth International Workshop Conference

TABLE 38-3. Diagnosis of Gestational Diabetes Mellitus (GDM): 100-g Oral Glucose Tolerance Test*

	O'Sullivan-Mahan[183] Whole Blood Somogyi-Nelson (mg/dL [mmol/L])	NDDG[7] Plasma Auto-Analyzer (mg/dL [mmol/L])	Carpenter-Coustan[217] Plasma Glucose Oxidase (mg/dL [mmol/L])
Fasting	90 [5.0]	105 [5.8]	95 [5.3]
1 hour	165 [9.2]	190 [10.6]	180 [10.0]
2 hour	145 [8.1]	165 [9.2]	155 [8.6]
3 hour	125 [6.9]	145 [8.1]	140 [7.8]

The 100-g oral glucose tolerance test is performed in the morning after an overnight fast of at least 8 hours, but not more than 14 hours, and after at least 3 days of unrestricted diet (≥150 g carbohydrate/day) and physical activity. The subject should remain seated and should not smoke throughout the test. Two or more of the venous plasma concentrations must be met or exceeded for a positive diagnosis.

on GDM concluded that the Carpenter-Coustan criteria may be recommended for the interpretation of a 100-g OGTT in pregnancy.[8]

Values for interpretation of 75-g OGTTs have been defined in several study populations in the United States, Europe, Brazil, and Australia.[8] As a general statement, it can be said that the various cutoff values that have been recommended for interpretation of the 75-g OGTT do not differ greatly from the Carpenter and Coustan criteria for the 100-g OGTT. However, studies in which perinatal outcome has been evaluated in large numbers of pregnancies meeting the 75-g OGTT criteria for GDM are lacking. It is anticipated that the currently ongoing study funded by the National Institutes of Health and the American Diabetes Association (Hyperglycemia and Adverse Pregnancy Outcome) will provide data from which criteria can be derived that are based on the relationship between degree of hyperglycemia and risk of adverse perinatal outcome. Therefore, at this time, we suggest that clinics that have established programs for GDM detection and diagnosis continue to use the diagnostic procedure with which they are familiar.

Etiology and Pathogenesis

Although all cases of GDM share the fact that they are first recognized in association with the physiologic insulin resistance of pregnancy, they are also characterized by substantial phenotypic and genotypic heterogeneity.[158,221] The *severity* of the carbohydrate intolerance at the time of diagnosis represents one form of phenotypic heterogeneity, and it has served as the basis for the use of FPG to subclassify GDM (Table 38-1). It is also an important predictor of risk for progression to diabetes outside of pregnancy.[183] There is also appreciable heterogeneity with regard to *age* and *weight*, and it has been long appreciated that women with GDM tend to be older and heavier than unselected "populations" of pregnant women. Finally, GDM is heterogeneous with respect to insulin resistance and β-cell function.

Catalano and coworkers[67] have performed important serial studies of carbohydrate metabolism starting before pregnancy (Fig. 38-5). Women with previous GDM but normal glucose tolerance were insulin-resistant compared with age- and BMI-matched controls. During the first trimester, the GDM group showed a small increase in insulin sensitivity, whereas the controls showed a small decline. In late gestation, the normal subjects had developed marked insulin resistance and the GDM group became more insulin resistant than before gestation. Although both groups were very insulin-resistant in late pregnancy, the women with GDM were on average more insulin-resistant, with considerable overlap. Others have also found somewhat greater insulin resistance in GDM than in normal pregnancy.[26,222] In the Catalano study and in others, women with normal carbohydrate metabolism were found to compensate for the insulin resistance in late gestation with augmentation of β-cell function that was appropriate for the level of insulin resistance. By contrast, those with GDM fail to increase β-cell function adequately and show a large defect in first-phase insulin secretion when challenged with oral or intravenous glucose.[22,26,89,158,221]

On the basis of clinical features, GDM has been classically considered to be a variant of T2DM. However, examinations for certain genetic "markers" suggest that there may be appreciable genotypic heterogeneity in GDM. Some patients exhibit autoimmune phenomenon,[158] with glutamic acid decarboxylase (GAD)[223] or islet cell antibodies[158,224,225] found with variable prevalence depending on the population studied and the methods used. This is more common in Scandinavian countries, where there is greater prevalence of T1DM.[225] These findings suggest that a small proportion of patients with GDM may have evolving T1DM with first appearance in pregnancy. Efforts to identify the specific cases prospectively may be justified in populations with a higher prevalence of T1DM.

Racial/ethnic group differences in prevalence of GDM have been observed that are not fully accounted for by differences in maternal age or obesity.[186,189,226] A small number of women with GDM have been found to have maturity-onset diabetes of the young (MODY) diabetes or defects in mitochondrial DNA. For most women with GDM, however, the specific mechanisms for genetic predisposition remain to be defined.

Management

Diet

Medical nutritional therapy is the cornerstone of management and is implemented as soon as possible after the diagnosis of GDM is established. At Northwestern University, dietary recommendations in the latter half of pregnancy are the same for GDM as in normal pregnancies and in pregnancies complicated by pregestational diabetes (see discussion above).

Insulin

The precise place for insulin in the therapy of GDM is not fully crystallized.[8,194,227] In patients with fasting hyperglycemia diagnostic of diabetes (i.e., FPG ≥ 126 mg/dL [7.0 mm/L]), there is little, if any controversy.[8] At Northwestern University, insulin treatment is started as soon as the diagnosis of GDM is confirmed in these subjects because neonatal risks equal those for patients with pregestational diabetes. Insulin therapy is instituted in all gravidas with GDM and FPG ≥ 105 and < 126 mg/dL (5.8–7.0 mmol/L) persisting on two successive determinations following a brief trial of dietary therapy. At many centers, insulin therapy is initiated if FPG exceeds 94 mg/dL (5.2 mmol/L), the revised upper limit of normal adopted by the Fourth International Workshop Conference on GDM.[8] Many[126] feel that a number of GDM mothers with FPG in the range of 95–104 mg/dL have unaffected offspring. They have suggested that pending the results of the ongoing Hyperglycemia and Adverse Pregnancy Outcome study mentioned above, one should not extend the criteria for initiation of insulin therapy to include this subgroup of subjects.

The use of insulin therapy is more controversial in women with GDM in whom FPG is consistently below the upper limits of "normal," i.e., <95 mg/dL (5.3 mm/L).[228,229] Most patients with GDM fall into this category, and some of their offspring may be at increased risk for macrosomia[88,118,158] and potentially other perinatal difficulties as well as long-range developmental changes.[230–235] Accordingly, some have recommended therapy with insulin in *all* women with GDM who are over 25 years of age, or have offered insulin therapy as a prophylactic option against the possibility of macrosomia in all GDM pregnancies.[236,237] Others have applied strict goals for glycemic control that have resulted in the use of insulin to treat more than half[238] or more than 85%[196] of their subjects with mild GDM. Such aggressive treatment has been shown to reduce average birthweight,[227,228] but the cost/benefits in terms of neonatal morbidity, childhood obesity, and glucose tolerance have not been demonstrated.[8] In the absence of such information, one should restrict the use of insulin treatment in GDM with FPG < 105 mg/dL (5.8 mmol/L), to those with 1-hour post breakfast plasma glucose ≥ 140 mg/dL (7.8 mmol/L) and persisting despite diet therapy.

Defining the optimal criteria for insulin treatment solely by blood glucose values is problematic because other metabolic factors[239] and maternal nutrients in addition to glucose probably impact on fetal growth.[88,118,157] Criteria other than maternal blood sugar levels to determine the need for insulin therapy are being investigated. In uncontrolled trials, Weiss and colleagues[240,241] have reported good fetal outcomes when elevated amniotic fluid insulin levels (which reflect fetal hyperinsulinemia) have been used to determine the need for insulin therapy. Fetal ultrasound to measure shoulder soft tissue[242] or abdominal circumference[126,229,243] have been employed in an effort to select pregnancies with mild hyperglycemia at highest risk for macrosomia, and thus insulin treatment. It is to be hoped that controlled clinical trials designed to assess all these issues and strategies (perhaps on a multicenter basis) will provide the observations necessary for more definitive recommendations.[244]

When insulin is used, doses ranging from 0.5 to 1.4 U/kg of body weight/day are required to maintain fasting and premeal glucose values of 65–85 mg/dL (3.6–4.7 mmol/L) and postprandial values of <140 mg/dL (7.8 mmol/L). A twice-daily "mixed" insulin regimen is usually employed, although multiple injections may be used. Sulfonylurea drugs, as a class, have been avoided during pregnancy because some of them have been shown to cross the placenta, stimulate fetal insulin secretion, and promote neonatal hypoglycemia. Recently, clinical data have been presented by Langer and coworkers[245] indicating that one of these agents, glyburide, is devoid of these properties and is as efficacious as intensive insulin therapy in controlling maternal blood glucose concentration and preventing fetal and neonatal effects of GDM. If these finding are confirmed, glyburide may become an important alternative for the treatment of GDM.

Exercise

Cardiovascular fitness training is known to increase insulin sensitivity and glucose disposal by recruitment of glucose transporter proteins, and it is often used in the treatment of suitable patients. In pregnancy, concerns about increasing uterine contractility, IUGR, prematurity, fetal bradycardia, and ketonuria have overriden the potential beneficial effects of strenuous exercise.[246,247] Two studies employing moderate exercise regimens in GDM, using either arm ergometry[248] or a recumbent bicycle,[249] have found them to be safe and effective in reducing fasting and postprandial glucose to a modest extent. In another trial that explored the effects of moderate exercise on glycemic control, no beneficial response could be demonstrated.[250] Further studies of exercise in GDM are in progress.

Monitoring Carbohydrate Metabolism

Patients with GDM should monitor urinary ketones before breakfast and supper to detect possible deficiencies in dietary carbohydrate. Many women on dietary therapy choose to monitor capillary blood glucose values as well. At each outpatient visit, fasting and 1-hour post-breakfast plasma glucose measurements should be obtained to help determine the need for insulin therapy. All patients who are treated with insulin should monitor capillary blood sugar before meals (4×/day) at home as a guide to making insulin dosage adjustments on a weekly basis in consultation with the physician or nurse practitioner. It is also recommended that patients monitor postprandial blood glucose levels on at least 2 days a week. Monitoring postprandial blood sugar exclusively to guide the selection of insulin doses has been claimed to be superior to a reliance on testing blood glucose concentrations before meals.[251] One approach may not be inherently superior to the other, provided that appropriate target values are set and pursued vigorously. To assess the accuracy on an ongoing basis, patients who perform fingerstick blood glucose testing should have plasma glucose measurements obtained at each prenatal visit to compare with a simultaneously obtained estimate of capillary blood glucose concentration. Some self-monitoring blood glucose systems may consistently over- or underestimate plasma glucose by as much as 10–15%. This must be determined on an individual basis and taken into account when insulin doses are modified.[8]

POSTPARTUM FOLLOW-UP

Carbohydrate Metabolism

The diagnosis of gestational diabetes carries significant implications for long-term maternal health. During pregnancy, one cannot distinguish with certainty between evolving T1- or T2DM and transitory glucose intolerance that will subside post partum. Postpartum reclassification and long-term follow-up are therefore essential (Table 38-1). Within the first year post partum, a significant proportion of our patients with GDM display impaired glucose tolerance or diabetes mellitus by NDDG criteria.[7] For women in whom FPG during pregnancy is elevated to levels that are diagnostic of diabetes, the incidence is 75–90%.[252,253] It is likely that in some of these, abnormalities in glucose tolerance antedate pregnancy.[252,254] Although their testing procedures differed somewhat, workers from Los Angeles,[227,255] East Germany,[256] Australia,[198] and Saudi Arabia[257] have also reported high incidence of impaired glucose tolerance during the first 1 or 2 years of postpartum follow-up. Many others have shown that GDM, based on a variety of diagnostic criteria, identifies women at high risk for the later development of diabetes mellitus and that the incidence increases progressively with time from the index pregnancy.[183,198,199,258–263]

Certain genetic and phenotypic characteristics that are observable during pregnancy convey a higher risk for postpartum glucose intolerance.[227,252,253,255,258,262–264] These include relative insulinopenia; severity of glucose intolerance at diagnosis; obesity; early gestational age at diagnosis; racial/ethnic origin (increased in Hispanics); and family history of maternal diabetes. Using multiple logistic regression, the independent associations between these factors and diabetes mellitus developing early post partum and up to 5 years later were examined.[252,253] Relative deficiency (lower basal insulin levels and blunted acute-phase insulin response to oral glucose) and the severity of antepartum hyperglycemia (fasting and 2-hour values) were independently associated with the presence of diabetes mellitus in the early postpartum period. Obesity (with its associated increased insulin resistance) and blunted integrated insulin responses (area under the curve) were also independent variables in those who developed diabetes mellitus up to 5 years post partum. The other prognostic factors (early gestational age at diagnosis, racial/ethnic origin, and family history of maternal diabetes) are probably mediated through one or more of the independent factors noted above.

Because of the risks outlined above, all women with GDM should receive an assessment of glucose tolerance within 6–12 weeks after delivery. Initial evaluation should be either the measurement of fasting plasma glucose concentration or a 75-g OGTT. Results should be interpreted according to the American Diabetes Association Expert Committee on the Diagnosis and Classification of Diabetes Mellitus.[9] Those who manifest persistent glucose intolerance (impaired fasting glucose, impaired glucose tolerance test, or T2DM) should receive appropriate counseling and/or therapy. At the time of any subsequent pregnancy, their status should be classified as indicated in Table 38-1. Kjos and coworkers[227,255,265–267] have identified postpartum characteristics that predict risks of progression to diabetes at the time of postpartum evaluation. Risk factors include higher level of glycemia at initial postpartum evaluation, further weight gain, use of progestin-only oral contraceptive pills, and subsequent pregnancy.

Individuals with a normal postpartum FPG or OGTT need annual fasting or postload glucose testing and should be aware that glucose intolerance, although not invariable, will probably recur during any future pregnancy, if not before. As yet, only limited data are available from long-term intervention efforts designed to mitigate the development of diabetes under nongravid conditions. Nonetheless, it seems prudent to advise patients to maintain ideal body weight, to exercise regularly, and to avoid the use of progestin-only oral contraceptives, thiazides, niacin, and oral corticosteroids if possible. Clinical trials that include evaluation of pharmacologic agents to "prevent" or delay the development of diabetes in individuals at high risk, including women with previous GDM, are now being carried out. One trial, the Diabetes Prevention Program, includes intensive lifestyle intervention and metformin treatment arms.[268] It will conclude in the year 2002. Another, in which the insulin-sensitizing drug troglitazone was used, has provided encouraging preliminary results.[269] Use of the agent was discontinued when the drug was removed from sale; however, the rate of conversion to diabetes was significantly reduced during the 2 years of exposure to troglitazone. It is not yet known whether this effect persisted after discontinuation of the drug.

Contraception and Other Considerations

The postpartum period is an ideal time to practice preconception counseling, since a recently parous woman, who is of proven fecundity, is likely to conceive again. Behaviors that will promote good health should be discussed, including issues such as weight loss and exercise. These may not have been appropriate interventions to initiate during pregnancy. The benefits of good metabolic control lifelong, especially prior to a planned pregnancy, should be reinforced.[270]

After Pregestational Diabetes

For the woman with T1DM, there are few substantive reasons for selecting one contraceptive method over another, and the woman's desires should be paramount in the decision. Although barrier methods (condom, diaphragm) might be considered ideal choices because of the absence of systemic effects and paucity of side effects, these methods are attended by a failure rate of at least 5% per woman-year.[270] Copper-containing intrauterine devices are equally effective and safe in women with diabetes mellitus but should be reserved for those in a mutually monogamous relationship due to the risk of pelvic infection.

Although the early generations of combination oral contraceptives incurred risks of adverse metabolic effects (e.g., reduced carbohydrate tolerance, lowering of high-density lipoproteins), contemporary formulations have a severalfold reduction in hormonal potency accompanied by an attenuation of metabolic side effects.[270] Preparations containing norethindrone as the progestin appear to have fewer metabolic effects than levonorgestrel. However, the low serum levels manifested with levonorgestrel implants have been shown to effect only minor metabolic changes in nondiabetic women, with excellent protection against pregnancy for up to 5 years. Newer progestins of increased selectivity (e.g., deso-

gestrel) have shown promise of minimal metabolic effects. The use of hormonal contraceptives in women with diabetic vasculopathy remains controversial. However, documented cardiovascular risks of hormonal contraceptives in nondiabetic women, particularly myocardial infarction, have been linked to concurrent smoking and higher dose formulations, and there are no adequately controlled studies in women with diabetes mellitus. Thus, the benefit of excellent contraceptive efficacy must be weighed against theoretical risks.

After GDM

Although contraceptive counseling is similar to that for women with T1DM, there is the concern that oral contraceptives may result in a recrudescence of carbohydrate intolerance.[266,267,270] This concern has not been borne out with use of contemporary low-dose formulations. However, progestin-only oral contraceptive agents have been associated with some increased risk of diabetes after GDM.[266,267] It is prudent to document normal postpartum carbohydrate tolerance before initiating any hormonal contraceptive and to recommend regular surveillance at 6–12-month intervals.

Acknowledgments The authors are grateful to their many collaborators in the Departments of Medicine, Obstetrics, and Pediatrics who have contributed to The Northwestern University Diabetes in Pregnancy Center studies that are cited in this chapter. We thank the nursing staff of the Clinical Research Center at Northwestern Memorial Hospital for help in the testing and clinical management of a number of our patients. This work was supported in part by NIH research grants DK 10699, HD 11021, HD 19070, HD 62903, HD 23141, and RR-48; by Training Grant DK 07169 from the United States Public Health Service; and by a grant from the Ronald McDonald Foundation.

REFERENCES

1. Duncan JM: On puerperal diabetes. *Trans Obstet Soc Lond* 1882;24:256.
2. Freinkel N, Metzger BE: Metabolic changes in pregnancy. In: Foster DW, Wilson JD, eds. *Williams Textbook of Endocrinology*, 8th ed. Saunders:1992;993.
3. Phelps RL, Metzger BE, Freinkel N: Carbohydrate metabolism in pregnancy. XVII. Diurnal profiles of plasma glucose, insulin, free fatty acids, triglycerides, cholesterol, and individual amino acids in late normal pregnancy. *Am J Obstet Gynecol* 1981;140:730.
4. Burt RL: Peripheral utilization of glucose in pregnancy: III. Insulin tolerance. *Obstet Gynecol* 1956;7:658.
5. Knopp RH, Ruder HJ, Herrera E, *et al*: Carbohydrate metabolism in pregnancy. VII. Insulin tolerance during late pregnancy in the fed and fasted rat. *Acta Endocrinol* 1970;65:352.
6. Freinkel N: The effect of pregnancy on insulin homeostasis. *Diabetes* 1964;13:260.
7. National Diabetes Data Group: Classification and diagnosis of diabetes mellitus and other categories of glucose intolerance. *Diabetes* 1979;28:1039.
8. Metzger, BE, Coustan DR, The Organizing Committee: Summary and Recommendations of the Fourth International Workshop-Conference on Gestational Diabetes Mellitus. *Diabetes Care* 1998;21(Suppl 2):161.
9. Kahn R, Expert Committee on the Diagnosis and Classification of Diabetes Mellitus: Report of the Expert Committee on the Diagnosis and Classification of Diabetes Mellitus. *Diabetes Care* 1997;20:1183.
10. Freinkel N: The Banting Lecture 1980: of pregnancy and progeny. *Diabetes* 1980;29:1023.
11. Freinkel N: Effects of the conceptus on maternal metabolism during pregnancy. In: Leibel BS, Wrenshall GA, eds. *On the Nature and Treatment of Diabetes*. Excerpta Medica:1965;679.

12. Posner BI: Insulin metabolizing enzyme activities in human placental tissue. *Diabetes* 1973;22:552.

13. Goodner CJ, Freinkel N: Carbohydrate metabolism in pregnancy: The turnover of I[131] insulin in the pregnant rat. *Endocrinology* 1960;67:862.

14. Katz AI, Lindheimer MD, Mako ME, et al: Peripheral metabolism of insulin, proinsulin, and C-peptide in the pregnant rat. *J Clin Invest* 1975;56:1608.

15. Metzger BE, Rodeck C, Freinkel N, et al: Transplacental extraction ratios for glucose:insulin, glucagon and placental lactogen during normoglycaemia in human pregnancy at term. *Placenta* 1985;6:3474.

16. Catalano PM, Drago NM, Amini SB: Longitudinal changes in pancreatic β-cell function and metabolic clearance rate of insulin in pregnant women with normal and abnormal glucose tolerance. *Diabetes Care* 1998;21:403.

17. Catalano PM, Huston L, Amini SB, et al: Longitudinal changes in glucose metabolism during pregnancy in obese women with normal glucose tolerance and gestational diabetes mellitus. *Am J Obstet Gynecol* 1999;180:903.

18. Catalano PM, Tyzbir ED, Roman NM, et al: Longitudinal changes in insulin release and insulin resistance in nonobese pregnant women. *Am J Obstet Gynecol* 1991;165:1667.

19. Lind T, Billewicz WZ, Brown G: A serial study of changes occurring in the oral glucose tolerance test during pregnancy. *J Obstet Gynaecol Br Commonw* 973;80:1033.

20. Spellacy WN, Goetz FC, Greenberg BZ, et al: Plasma insulin in normal "early" pregnancy. *Obstet Gynecol* 1965;25:862.

21. Bleicher SJ, O'Sullivan JB, Freinkel N: Carbohydrate metabolism in pregnancy. V. The interrelations of glucose, insulin, and free fatty acids in late pregnancy and postpartum. *N Engl J Med* 1964;271:866.

22. Buchanan TA, Metzger BE, Freinkel N, et al: Insulin sensitivity and β-cell responsiveness to glucose during late pregnancy in lean and moderately obese women with normal glucose tolerance or mild gestational diabetes. *Am J Obstet Gynecol* 1990;162:1008.

23. Phelps RL, Bergenstal R, Freinkel N, et al: Carbohydrate metabolism in pregnancy. XIII. Relationships between plasma insulin and proinsulin during late pregnancy in normal and diabetic subjects. *J Clin Endocrinol Metab* 1975;41:1085.

24. Kühl C: Serum proinsulin in normal and gestational diabetic pregnancy. *Diabetologia* 1976;12:295.

25. Cousins L, Rea C, Crawford M: Longitudinal characterization of insulin sensitivity and body fat quantitation in normal and gestational diabetic pregnancies. *Diabetes* 1988;37(Suppl 1):251A.

26. Buchanan TA, Catalano PM: The pathogenesis of GDM: implications for diabetes after pregnancy. *Diabetes Rev* 1995;3:584.

27. Tsibris JCM, Raynor LO, Buhi WC, et al: Insulin receptors in circulating erythrocytes and monocytes from women on oral contraceptives or pregnant women near term. *J Clin Endocrinol Metab* 1980; 51: 711.

28. Moore P, Kolterman O, Weyant J, et al: Insulin binding in human pregnancy: comparisons to the postpartum, luteal and follicular states. *J Clin Endocrinol Metab* 1981;52:937.

29. Puavilai G, Drobny EC, Domont LA, et al: Insulin receptors and insulin resistance in human pregnancy: evidence for a post-receptor defect in insulin action. *J Clin Endocrinol Metab* 1982;54:247.

30. Ryan EA, Enns L: Role of gestational hormones in the induction of insulin resistance. *J Clin Endocrinol Metab* 1988;67:341.

31. Martinez C, Ruiz P, Andres A, et al: Tyrosine kinase activity of liver insulin receptor is inhibited in rats at term gestation. *Biochem J* 1989; 263:267.

32. Damm P, Handberg A, Kühl C, et al: Insulin receptor binding and tyrosine kinase activity in skeletal muscle from normal pregnant women and women with gestational diabetes. *Obstet Gynecol* 1993;82:251.

33. Garvey WT, Maianu L, Hancock JA, et al: Gene expression of GLUT4 in skeletal muscle from insulin-resistant patients with obesity, IGT, GDM and NIDDM. *Diabetes* 1992;41:465.

34. Okuno S, Mawda Y, Yamaguchi Y, et al: Expression of GLUT4 glucose transporter mRNA and protein in skeletal muscle and adipose tissue from rats in late pregnancy. *Biochem Biophys Res Commun* 1993;191:405.

35. Okuno S, Akazawa S, Kawasaki YE, et al: Decreased expression of the GLUT4 glucose transporter protein in adipose tissue during pregnancy. *Horm Metab Res* 1995;27:231.

36. Shao J, Catalano PM, Yamashita H, et al: Decreased insulin receptor tyrosine kinase activity and plasma cell membrane glycoprotein-1 overexpression in skeletal muscle from obese women with gestational diabetes mellitus (GDM): evidence for increased serine/threonine phosphorylation in pregnancy and GDM. *Diabetes* 2000;49:603.

37. Kalkhoff RK, Kissebah AH, Kim H-J: Carbohydrate and lipid metabolism during normal pregnancy: relationship to gestational hormone action. *Semin Perinatol* 1978;2:291.

38. Turtle JR, Kipnis DM: The lipolytic action of human placental lactogen on isolated fat cells. *Biochem Biophys Acta* 1967;144:583.

39. Kalkhoff RK, Richardson BL, Beck P: Relative effects of pregnancy, human placental lactogen and prednisolone on carbohydrate tolerance in normal and sub-clinical diabetic subjects. *Diabetes* 1969;18:153.

40. Sorenson RL, Brelje TC: Adaptations of islets of Langerhans to pregnancy: beta cell growth, enhanced insulin secretion and the role of lactogenic hormones [Review]. *Horm Metab Res* 1997;29:301.

41. Kalkhoff RK, Jacobson M, Lemper D: Progesterone, pregnancy and the augmented plasma insulin response. *J Clin Endocrinol Metab* 1970;31:24.

42. Kekki M, Nikkila EA: Plasma triglyceride turnover during use of oral contraceptives. *Metabolism* 1971;20:878.

43. Surmaczynska B, Nitzan M, Metzger BE, et al: Carbohydrate metabolism in pregnancy. XII. The effect of oral glucose on plasma concentrations of human placental lactogen and chorionic gonadotropin during late pregnancy in normal subjects and gestational diabetics. *Isr J Med Sci* 1974;10:1481.

44. Knopp RH, Herrera E, Freinkel N: Carbohydrate metabolism in pregnancy. VIII. Metabolism of adipose tissue isolated from fed and fasted pregnant rats during late gestation. *J Clin Invest* 1970;49:1438.

45. Elliott JA: The effect of pregnancy on the control of lipolysis in fat cells isolated from human adipose tissue. *Eur J Clin Invest* 1975;5: 159.

46. Riddick DH, Kusmik WF: Decidua: a possible source of amniotic fluid prolactin. *Am J Obstet Gynecol* 1977;127:187.

47. Hill DJ, Hogg J: Growth factors and the regulation of pre-and postnatal growth. *Bailliers Clin Endocrinol Metab* 1989;3:579.

48. Baumann G, Davila N, Shaw MA, et al: Binding of human growth hormone (GH)-variant (placental GH) to GH-binding proteins in human plasma. *J Clin Endocrinol Metab* 1991;73:1175.

49. Goodman HM, Tai L-R, Ray J, et al: Human growth hormone variant produces insulin-like and lipolytic responses in rat adipose tissue. *Endocrinology* 1991; 129:1779.

50. Schernthaner G, Prager R, Punzengruber C, et al: Severe hyperprolactinaemia is associated with decreased insulin binding in vitro and insulin resistance in vivo. *Diabetologia* 1985;28:138.

51. Burke CW, Roulet F: Increased exposure of tissues to cortisol in late pregnancy. *BMJ* 1970;1:657.

52. Nolten WE, Lindheimer MD, Rueckert PA, et al: Diurnal patterns and regulation of cortisol secretion in pregnancy. *J Clin Endocrinol Metab* 1980;51:466.

53. Shibasaki T, Odagiri E, Shizume K, et al: Corticotropin-releasing factor-like activity in human placental extracts. *J Clin Endocrinol Metab* 1982;55:384.

54. Catalano P, Highman T, Huston L, et al: Relationship between reproductive hormones, TNF alpha and longitudinal changes in insulin sensitivity during gestation. *Diabetes* 1996;45(Suppl 2):175A.

55. Highman TJ, Friedman JE, Huston LP, et al: Longitudinal changes in maternal serum leptin concentrations, body composition, and resting metabolic rate in pregnancy. *Am J Obstet Gynecol* 1998;178:1010.

56. Page EW: Human fetal nutrition and growth. *Am J Obstet Gynecol* 1969;104:378.

57. Cahill GF Jr, Owen OE: Some observations on carbohydrate metabolism in man. In: Dickens F, Randle PJ, Whelan WJ, eds. *Carbohydrate Metabolism and Its Disorders*. Academic Press:1968;497.

58. Young M: Placental transfer of glucose and amino acids. In: Camerini-Davalos RA, Cole HS, eds. *Early Diabetes in Early Life*. Academic Press:1975;237.

59. Herrera E, Knopp RH, Freinkel N: Carbohydrate metabolism in pregnancy. VI. Plasma fuels, insulin, liver composition, gluconeogenesis and nitrogen metabolism during late gestation in the fed and fasted rat. *J Clin Invest* 1969;48:2260.

60. Metzger BE, Freinkel N: Regulation of maternal protein metabolism and gluconeogenesis in the fasted state. In: Camerini-Davalos R, Cole H, eds. *Early Diabetes in Early Life*. Academic Press:1975;303.

61. Felig P, Lynch V: Starvation in human pregnancy: hypoglycaemia, hypoinsulinemia, and hyperketonemia. *Science* 1970;170:990.

62. Metzger BE, Hare JW, Freinkel N: Carbohydrate metabolism in pregnancy. IX. Plasma levels of gluconeogenic fuels during fasting in the rat. *J Clin Endocrinol* 1971;33:869.

63. Felig P, Kim YJ, Lynch V, *et al*: Amino acid metabolism during starvation in human pregnancy. *J Clin Invest* 1972;51:1195.

64. Tyson JE, Austin K, Farinholt J, *et al*: Endocrine-metabolic response to acute starvation in human gestation. *Am J Obstet Gynecol* 1976; 125:1073.

65. Metzger BE, Agnoli F, Freinkel N: Effect of sex and pregnancy on formation of urea and ammonia during gluconeogenesis in the perfused rat liver. *Horm Metab Res* 1970;2:367.

66. Metzger BE, Agnoli F, Hare JW, *et al*: Carbohydrate metabolism in pregnancy. X. Metabolic disposition of alanine by the perfused liver of the fasting pregnant rat. *Diabetes* 1973;22:601.

67. Catalano PM, Tyzbir ED, Wolfe RR, *et al*: Carbohydrate metabolism during pregnancy in control subjects and women with gestational diabetes. *Am J Physiol* 1993;264:E60.

68. Ogata ES, Metzger BE, Freinkel N: Carbohydrate metabolism in pregnancy XVI: longitudinal estimates of the effects of pregnancy on D-(6^3H) glucose and D-(6^{14}C) glucose turnover during fasting in the rat. *Metabolism* 1981;30:487.

69. Freinkel N, Phelps RL, Metzger BE: Intermediary metabolism during normal pregnancy. In: Sutherland HW, Stowers JM, eds. *Carbohydrate Metabolism in Pregnancy and the Newborn 1978*. Springer-Verlag:1979;1.

70. Morrow PG, Marshall WP, Kim H-J, *et al*: Metabolic response to starvation. I. Relative effects of pregnancy and sex steroid administration in the rat. *Metabolism* 1981;30:268.

71. Morrow PG, Marshall WP, Kim H-J, *et al*: Metabolic response to starvation. II. Effects of sex steroid administration to pre- and postmenopausal women. *Metabolism* 1981;30:274.

72. Rushakoff RJ, Kalkhoff RK: Effects of pregnancy and sex steroid administration on skeletal muscle metabolism in the rat. *Diabetes* 1981; 30:545.

73. Metzger BE, Ravnikar V, Vileisis RA, *et al*: "Accelerated starvation" and the skipped breakfast in late normal pregnancy. *Lancet* 1982;1:588.

74. Metzger BE, Freinkel N: Accelerated starvation in pregnancy: implications for dietary treatment of obesity and gestational diabetes mellitus. *Biol Neonate* 1987;51:78.

75. Freinkel N, Metzger BE, Nitzan M, *et al*: Facilitated anabolism in late pregnancy: some novel maternal compensations for accelerated starvation. In: Malaise WJ, Pirart J, eds. *Proceedings of the VIIIth Congress of the International Diabetes Federation*. Excerpta Medica International Congress, Series No. 312:1974;474.

76. Freinkel N, Metzger BE: Some considerations of fuel economy in the fed state during late human pregnancy. In: Camerini-Davalos R, Cole H, eds. *Early Diabetes in Early Life*. Academic Press:1975;289.

77. Daniel RR, Metzger BE, Freinkel N, *et al*: Carbohydrate metabolism in pregnancy. XI. Response of plasma glucagon to overnight fast and oral glucose during normal pregnancy. *Diabetes* 1974;23:771.

78. Luyckx AS, Gerard J, Gaspard U, *et al*: Plasma glucagon levels in normal women during pregnancy. *Diabetologia* 1975;11:549.

79. Kühl C, Holst JJ: Plasma glucagon and the insulin:glucagon ratio in gestational diabetes. *Diabetes* 1976;25:16.

80. Simmons MA, Battaglia FC, Meschia G: Placental transfer of glucose. *J Dev Physiol* 1979;1:227.

81. Dawes GS: *Foetal and Neonatal Physiology*. Year Book Medical Publishers:1968;210.

82. Metzger BE, Unger RH, Freinkel N: Carbohydrate metabolism in pregnancy. XIV. Relationships between circulating glucagon, insulin, glucose and amino acids in response to a "mixed meal" in late pregnancy. *Metabolism* 1977;26:151.

83. Kalkhoff RK, Kim H-J: Effects of pregnancy on insulin and glucagon secretion by perifused rat pancreatic islets. *Endocrinology* 1978;102:623.

84. Freinkel N, Dooley SL, Metzger BE: Care of the pregnant woman with insulin-dependent diabetes mellitus. *N Engl J Med* 1985;313:96.

85. Comess LJ, Bennett PH, Man MB, *et al*: Congenital anomalies and diabetes in the Pima Indians of Arizona. *Diabetes* 1969;18:471.

86. Chung CS, Myrianthopoulos NC: Effect of maternal diabetes on congenital malformations. In: Bergsma D, ed. *Factors Affecting Risks of Congenital Malformations*. Stratton:1975;23.

87. Pedersen J: Weight and length at birth of infants of diabetic mothers. *Acta Endocrinol* 1954;16:330.

88. Freinkel N, Metzger BE: Pregnancy as a tissue culture experience: the critical implications of maternal metabolism for fetal development. In: Elliott K, O'Connor M, eds. *Pregnancy Metabolism, Diabetes and the Fetus*. Ciba Foundation #63. Excerpta Medica:1979;3.

89. Freinkel N, Metzger BE: Emerging challenges in diabetes and pregnancy: diabetic embryopathy and gestational diabetes. In: Alberti KGMM, Krall LP, eds. *The Diabetes Annual/4*. Elsevier:1988;179.

90. From research to practice. Diabetes and birth defects: insights from the 1980s, prevention in the 1990s. *Diabetes Spectrum* 1990;3:150.

91. Mills JL, Baker L, Goldman AS: Malformations in infants of diabetic mothers occur before the seventh gestational week: implications for treatment. *Diabetes* 1979;28:292.

92. Mills JL, Simpson JL, Driscoll SG, *et al*: The NICHHD-Diabetes in Early Pregnancy Study: incidence of spontaneous abortion among normal women and insulin-dependent diabetic women whose pregnancies were identified within 21 days of conception. *N Engl J Med* 1988;319:1617.

93. Greene MF, Hare JW, Cloherty JP, *et al*: First trimester hemoglobin A$_1$ and risk for major malformations and spontaneous abortion in diabetic pregnancy. *Teratology* 1989;39:225.

94. Goldman AS, Baker L, Piddington R, *et al*: Hyperglycemia induced teratogenesis is mediated by a functional deficiency in arachidonic acid. *Proc Natl Acad Sci USA* 1985;82:8227.

95. Buchanan T, Schemmer JK, Freinkel N: Embryotoxic effects of brief maternal insulin-hypoglycemia during organogenesis in the rat. *J Clin Invest* 1986;78:643.

96. Freinkel N: Diabetic embryopathy and fuel-mediated organ teratogenesis: lessons from animal models. *Horm Metab Res* 1988;20:463.

97. Sadler TW, Hunter ES III, Wynn RE, *et al*: Evidence for multifactorial origin of diabetes-induced embryopathies. *Diabetes* 1989;38:70.

98. Hod M, Star S, Passonneau JV, *et al*: Glucose-induced dysmorphogenesis in the cultured rat conceptus: prevention by supplementation with myo-inositol. *Isr J Med Sci* 1990;26:541.

99. Weigensberg MJ, Garcia-Palmer F, Freinkel N: Uptake of myo-inositol by early-somite rat conceptus. *Diabetes* 1990;39:575.

100. Strieleman PJ, Connors MA, Metzger BE: Phosphoinositide metabolism in the developing conceptus: effects of hyperglycemia and *scyllo*-inositol in rat embryo culture. *Diabetes* 1992;41:989.

101. Eriksson UJ, Borg LAH: Diabetes and embryonic malformations: role of substrate-induced free-oxygen radical production for dysmorphogenesis in cultured rat embryos. *Diabetes* 1993;42:411.

102. Buchanan TA, Denno KM, Sipes GF, *et al*: Diabetic teratogenesis: in vitro evidence for a multifactorial etiology with little contribution from glucose per se. *Diabetes* 1994;43:656.

103. Lee AT, Reis D, Eriksson UJ: Hyperglycemia-induced embryonic dysmorphogenesis correlates with genomic DNA mutation frequency in vitro and in vivo. *Diabetes* 1999;48:371.

104. Sakamaki H, Akazawa S, Ishibashi M, *et al*: Significance of glutathione-dependent antioxidant system in diabetes-induced embryonic malformations. *Diabetes* 1999;48:1138.

105. Fuhrmann K, Reiher H, Semmler K, *et al*: Prevention of congenital malformations in infants of insulin-dependent diabetic mothers. *Diabetes Care* 1983;6:219.

106. Steel JM, Johnstone FD, Hepburn DA, *et al*: Can prepregnancy care of diabetic women reduce the risk of abnormal babies? *BMJ* 1990; 301:1070.

107. Kitzmiller JL, Gavin LA, Gin GD, *et al*: Preconception care of diabetes. Glycemic control prevents congenital anomalies. *JAMA* 1991;265:731.

108. Kitzmiller JL, Buchanan TA, Kjos S, *et al*: Technical review: preconception care of diabetes, congenital malformations, and spontaneous abortions. *Diabetes Care* 1996;19:514.

109. Damm P, Molsted-Pedersen L: Significant decrease in congenital malformations in newborn infants of an unselected population of diabetic women. *Am J Obstet Gynecol* 1989;161:1163.

110. Herman WH, Janz NK, Becker MP, *et al*: Diabetes and pregnancy: preconception care, pregnancy outcomes, resource utilization and costs. *J Reprod Med* 1999;44:33.

111. Fee BA, Weil WB Jr: Body composition of infants of diabetic mothers by direct analysis. *Ann NY Acad Sci* 1963;110:869.

112. Naeye RL: Infants of diabetic mothers: a quantitative, morphologic study. *Pediatrics* 1965;35:980.

113. Brans YW, Shannon DL, Hunter MA: Maternal diabetes and neonatal macrosomia. II. Neonatal anthropometric measurements. *Early Hum Dev* 1983;8:297.

114. Whitelaw A: Subcutaneous fat in newborn infants of diabetic mothers: an indication of quality of diabetic control. *Lancet* 1977;Jan 1:15.

115. Elliot JP, Garite TJ, Freeman RK: Ultrasonic prediction of fetal macrosomia in diabetic patients. *Obstet Gynecol* 1982;60:159.

116. Catalano PM, Thomas A, Drago NM, *et al*: Body composition and fat distribution in infants of women with normal and abnormal glucose tolerance. *Am J Obstet Gynecol* 1994;170: 386.

117. Farquhar JW: Prognosis for babies born to diabetic mothers in Edinburgh. *Arch Dis Child* 1969;44:36.

118. Metzger BE: Biphasic effects of maternal metabolism on fetal growth: the quintessential expression of "fuel mediated teratogenesis." *Diabetes* 1991;40(Suppl 2):99.

119. Ogata ES, Sabbagha R, Metzger BE, *et al*: Serial ultrasonography to assess evolving fetal macrosomia: studies in 23 pregnant diabetic women. *JAMA* 1980;243:2405.

120. Ogata ES, Freinkel N, Metzger BE, *et al*: Perinatal islet function in gestational diabetes: assessment by cord plasma C-peptide and amniotic fluid insulin. *Diabetes Care* 1980;3:425.

121. Weiss PAM, Hofman H, Winter R, *et al*: Gestational diabetes and screening during pregnancy. *Obstet Gynecol* 1984;63:776.

122. Fallucca F, Gargiulo P, Troili F, *et al*: Amniotic fluid insulin, C peptide concentrations, and fetal morbidity in infants of diabetic mothers. *Am J Obstet Gynecol* 1985;153:534.

123. Persson B, Pschera H, Lunell N-O, *et al*: Amino acid concentrations in maternal plasma and amniotic fluid in relation to trimester of pregnancy in gestational and Type 1 diabetic women and women with small-for-gestational-age infants. *Am J Perinatol* 1986;3:98.

124. Larson G, Spjuth J, Ranstam J, *et al*: Prognostic significance of birth of large infant for subsequent development of maternal non-insulin-dependent diabetes mellitus: a prospective study over 20–27 years. *Diabetes Care* 1986; 9:359.

125. Landon MB, Mintz MC, Gabbe SG: Sonographic evaluation of fetal abdominal growth: predictor of the large-for-gestational-age infant in pregnancies complicated by diabetes mellitus. *Am J Obstet Gynecol* 1989;160:115.

126. Buchanan TA, Kjos SL, Montoro MN, *et al*: Use of fetal ultrasound to select metabolic therapy for pregnancies complicated by mild gestational diabetes. *Diabetes Care* 1994;17:275.

127. Keller JD, Metzger BE, Dooley SL, *et al*: Infants of diabetic mothers with accelerated fetal growth by ultrasonography: are they all alike? *Am J Obstet Gynecol* 1990;163:893.

128. Van Assche FA, Aerts L: The fetal endocrine pancreas. In: Keller PJ, ed. *Contributions to Gynecology and Obstetrics*. Karger:1979;44.

129. Reiher H, Fuhrmann K, Noack S, *et al*: Age-dependent insulin secretion of the endocrine pancreas in vitro from fetuses of diabetic and nondiabetic patients. *Diabetes Care* 1983;6:446.

130. Susa, JB, Neave C, Sehgal P, *et al*: Chronic hyperinsulinemia in the fetal rhesus monkey: effects of physiologic hyperinsulinemia on fetal growth and composition. *Diabetes* 1984;33:656.

131. Verhaeghe J, Van Bree R, Van Herck E, *et al*: C-peptide, insulin-like growth factors I and II and insulin-like growth factor binding protein-1 in umbilical cord serum: correlations with birth weight. *Am J Obstet Gynecol* 1993;169:89.

132. Pedersen J: *The Pregnant Diabetic and Her Newborn. Problems and Management*, 2nd ed. Munksgaard:1977.

133. Rizzo T, Metzger BE, Burns WJ, *et al*: Correlations between antepartum maternal metabolism and intelligence of offspring. *N Engl J Med* 1991;325:911.

134. Neiger R: Fetal macrosomia in the diabetic patient. *Clin Obstet Gynecol* 1992;35:138.

135. Pedersen JL, Molsted-Pedersen L: Early fetal growth delay detected by ultrasound marks increased risk of congenital malformation in diabetic pregnancy. *BMJ* 1981;283:269.

136. Eriksson UJ, Lewis NJ, Freinkel N: Growth retardation during early organogenesis in embryos of experimentally diabetic rats. *Diabetes* 1984;33:281.

137. Metzger BE, Purdy LP, Phelps RL: Diabetes mellitus and pregnancy. In: DeGroot LJ, Jameson JL, Burger H, *et al*, eds. *Endocrinology*, 4th ed. Saunders:2001;2433.

138. Dibble CM, Kochenour NK, Worley RJ, *et al*: Effect of pregnancy on diabetic retinopathy. *Obstet Gynecol* 1982;59:699.

139. Phelps RL, Sakol P, Metzger BE, *et al*: Correlation of changes in diabetic retinopathy during pregnancy with regulation of hyperglycemia. *Arch Ophthalmol* 1986;104:1806.

140. Chew EY, Mills JL, Metzger BE, *et al*: The National Institute of Child Health and Human Development Diabetes in Early Pregnancy Study. Metabolic control and progression of retinopathy: the Diabetes in Early Pregnancy Study. *Diabetes Care* 1995;18:631.

141. Hare JW: Maternal complications. In: Hare JW, ed. *Diabetes Complicating Pregnancy. The Joslin Clinic Method*. Alan R. Liss:1989;81.

142. The Diabetes Control and Complications Trial Research Group: The effect of intensive treatment of diabetes on the development and progression of long-term complications in insulin-dependent diabetes mellitus. *N Engl J Med* 1993;329:977.

143. The Kroc Collaborative Study Group: Blood glucose control and the evolution of diabetic retinopathy and albuminuria. *N Engl J Med* 1984;311:365.

144. Rosenn B, Miodovnik M, Kranias G, *et al*: Progression of diabetic retinopathy in pregnancy: association with hypertension in pregnancy. *Am J Obstet Gynecol* 1992;166:1214.

145. The Diabetes Control and Complications Trial Research Group: Effect of pregnancy on microvascular complications in the Diabetes Control and Complications Trial. *Diabetes Care* 2000;23:1084.

146. Kitzmiller JL, Brown ER, Phillippe M, *et al*: Diabetic nephropathy and perinatal outcome. *Am J Obstet Gynecol* 1981;141:741.

147. Reece EA, Coustan DR, Hayslett JP, *et al*: Diabetic nephropathy: pregnancy performance and fetomaternal outcome. *Am J Obstet Gynecol* 1988;159:56.

148. Miodovnik M, Rosenn BM, Khoury JC, *et al*: Does pregnancy increase the risk for development and progression of nephropathy? *Am J Obstet Gynecol* 1996;174:1180.

149. Biesenbach G, Stoeger H, Zazgornik J: Influence of pregnancy on progression of diabetic nephropathy and subsequent requirement of renal replacement therapy in female type 1 diabetic patients with impaired renal function. *Nephrol Dial Transplant* 1992;7:105.

150. Purdy LP, Hantsch CE, Molitch ME, *et al*: Effect of pregnancy on renal function in patients with moderate-to-severe diabetic renal insufficiency. *Diabetes Care* 1996;19:1067.

151. Macleod AF, Smith SA, Sonksen PH, *et al*: The problem of autonomic neuropathy in diabetic pregnancy. *Diabetic Med* 1990;7:80.

152. Airaksinen KEJ, Anttila LM, Linnaluoto MK, *et al*: Autonomic influence on pregnancy outcome in IDDM. *Diabetes Care* 1990;13:756.

153. Siddiqi T, Rosenn B, Mimouni F, *et al*: Hypertension during pregnancy in insulin-dependent diabetic women. *Obstet Gynecol* 1991;77:514.

154. Reece EA, Egan JFX, Coustan DR, *et al*: Coronary artery disease in diabetic pregnancies. *Am J Obstet Gynecol* 1986;154:150.

155. Hare JW, White P: Pregnancy in diabetes complicated by vascular disease. *Diabetes* 1977;26:953.

156. Connell FA, Vadheim C, Emanuel I: Diabetes in pregnancy: a population based study of incidence, referral for care and perinatal mortality. *Am J Obstet Gynecol* 1985;151:598.

157. Metzger BE, Phelps RL, Freinkel N, *et al*: Effects of gestational diabetes on diurnal profiles of plasma glucose, lipids and individual amino acids. *Diabetes Care* 1980;3:402.

158. Freinkel N, Metzger BE, Phelps RL, *et al*: Gestational diabetes mellitus: heterogeneity of maternal age, weight, insulin secretion, HLA antigens, and islet cell antibodies and the impact of maternal metabolism on pancreatic B-cell and somatic development in the offspring. *Diabetes* 1985;34(Suppl 2):1.

159. White P: Pregnancy complicating diabetes. *Am J Med* 1949;7:609.

160. Centers for Disease Control: Recommendations for the use of folic acid to reduce the number of cases of spina bifida and other neural tube defects. *MMWR* 1992;41:1.

161. Jovanovic-Peterson L, Peterson CM, Reed GF, *et al*: Maternal postprandial glucose levels and infant birth weight: the Diabetes in Early Pregnancy Study. *Am J Obstet Gynecol* 1991;164:103.

162. Combs CA, Gunderson E, Kitzmiller JL, *et al*: Relationship of fetal macrosomia to maternal postprandial glucose control during pregnancy. *Diabetes Care* 1992;15:1251.

163. Committee on Nutritional Status During Pregnancy and Lactation, Food and Nutrition Board, Institute of Medicine, National Academy of Sciences: *Nutrition During Pregnancy, Part I: Weight Gain*. National Academy Press:1990;10.

164. Durnin JVGA: Energy requirements of pregnancy. *Diabetes* 1991; 40(Suppl 2):152.

165. Metzger BE: Pregnancy and diabetes. In: Powers M, ed. *Handbook of Diabetes Nutritional Management*, 2nd ed. Aspen:1996;503.

166. Knopp RH, Magee MS, Raisys V, et al: Metabolic effects of hypocaloric diets in management of gestational diabetes. *Diabetes* 1991; 40(Suppl 2):165.

167. Peterson CM, Jovanovic-Peterson L: Percentage of carbohydrate and glycemic response to breakfast, lunch and dinner in women with gestational diabetes. *Diabetes* 1991;40(Suppl 2):172.

168. Pampanelli S, Torlone E, Lalli C, et al: Improved postprandial metabolic control after subcutaneous injection of a short-acting insulin analog in IDDM of short duration with residual pancreatic β-cell function. *Diabetes Care* 1995;18:1453.

169. Buchbinder A, Miodovnik M, McElvy S, et al: Is insulin lispro associated with the development or progression of diabetic retinopathy during pregnancy? *Am J Obstet Gynecol* 2000;183:1162.

170. Knight GL, Palomaki GE: Maternal serum alpha-fetoprotein and the detection of open neural tube defects. In: Elias S, Simpson JL, eds. *Maternal Serum Screening for Fetal Genetic Disorders.* Churchill Livingstone:1992;41.

171. Haddow JE, Palomaki GE, Knight GJ, et al: Prenatal screening for Down's syndrome with use of maternal serum markers. *N Engl J Med* 1992;327:588.

172. Canick JA, Palomaki GE, Osathanondh R: Prenatal screening for trisomy 18 in the second trimester. *Prenatal Diagn* 1990;12:546.

173. Romero R: Routine obstetric ultrasound. *Ultrasound Obstet Gynecol* 1993;3:303.

174. Philipps A, Dubin JW, Matti PJ, et al: Arterial hypoxemia and hyperinsulinemia in the chronically hyperglycemic fetal lamb. *Pediatr Res* 1982;16:653.

175. Philipps AF, Porte PJ, Stabinsky S, et al: Effects of chronic fetal hyperglycemia upon oxygen consumption in the ovine uterus and conceptus. *J Clin Invest* 1984;74:279.

176. Philipps AF, Rosenkrantz TS, Porte PJ, et al: The effects of chronic fetal hyperglycemia on substrate uptake by the ovine fetus and conceptus. *Pediatr Res* 1985;19:659.

177. Oats JN: Obstetrical management of patients with diabetes in pregnancy. *Baillieres Clin Obstet Gynaecol* 1991;5:395.

178. Jovanovic L, Peterson CM: Insulin and glucose requirements during the first stage of labor in insulin-dependent diabetic women. *Am J Med* 1983;75:607.

179. Light IJ, Kennan WJ, Sutherland JM: Maternal intravenous glucose administration as a cause of hypoglycemia in the infant of the diabetic mother. *Am J Obstet Gynecol* 1972;113:345.

180. Acker DB, Sachs BP, Friedman EA: Risk factors for shoulder dystocia. *Obstet Gynecol* 1985;66:762.

181. Rouse DJ, Owen J: Prophylactic cesarean delivery for fetal macrosomia diagnosed by means of ultrasonography—a Faustian bargain? *Am J Obstet Gynecol* 1999;181:332.

182. McLaren RA, Puckett JL, Chauhan SP: Estimators of birth weight in pregnant women requiring insulin: a comparison of seven sonographic models. *Obstet Gynecol* 1995;85:565.

183. O'Sullivan JB, Mahan CM: Criteria for the oral glucose tolerance test in pregnancy. *Diabetes* 1964;13:278.

184. Amankwah KS, Prentice RL, Fleury FJ: The incidence of gestational diabetes. *Obstet Gynecol* 1977;49:497.

185. Coustan DR, Nelson C, Carpenter MW, et al: Maternal age and screening for gestational diabetes: a population-based survey. *Obstet Gynecol* 1989;73:557.

186. Dooley SL, Metzger BE, Cho NH: Gestational diabetes mellitus: the influence of race on disease prevalence and perinatal outcome in a US population. *Diabetes* 1991;40(Suppl 2):25.

187. Sacks DA, Abu-Fadil S, Greenspoon JS, et al: Do the current standards for glucose tolerance testing in pregnancy represent a valid conversion of O'Sullivan's original criteria? *Am J Obstet Gynecol* 1989; 161:638.

188. Magee MS, Walden CE, Benedetti TJ, et al: Influence of diagnostic criteria on the incidence of gestational diabetes and perinatal morbidity. *JAMA* 1993;269:609.

189. Beischer NA, Oats JN, Henry OA, et al: Incidence and severity of gestational diabetes mellitus according to country of birth in women living in Australia. *Diabetes* 1991;40(Suppl 2):35.

190. O'Sullivan JB, Charles D, Mahan CM, et al: Gestational diabetes and perinatal mortality rate. *Am J Obstet Gynecol* 1973;116:901.

191. Abell DA, Beischer NA: Evaluation of the three-hour oral glucose tolerance test in detection of significant hyperglycemia and hypoglycemia in pregnancy. *Diabetes* 1975;24:874.

192. Roversi GD, Gargiulo M, Nicolini U, et al: Maximal tolerated insulin therapy in gestational diabetes. *Diabetes Care* 1980;3:489.

193. Pettitt DJ, Knowler WC, Baird HR, et al: Gestational diabetes: infant and maternal complications of pregnancy in relation to third-trimester glucose tolerance in Pima Indians. *Diabetes Care* 1980;3:458.

194. American Diabetes Association: Position Statement: Gestational Diabetes Mellitus. *Diabetes Care* 2001;24(Suppl 1):S77.

195. Hod M, Merlob P, Friedman S, et al: Gestational diabetes mellitus: a survey of perinatal complications in the 1980s. *Diabetes* 1991;40 (Suppl 2):74.

196. Drexel H, Bichler A, Sailer S, et al: Prevention of perinatal morbidity by tight control in gestational diabetes mellitus. *Diabetes Care* 1988; 11:761.

197. Schaefer UM, Songster G, Xiang A, et al: Congenital malformations in offspring of women with hyperglycemia first detected during pregnancy. *Am J Obstet Gynecol* 1997;177:1165.

198. Farrell J, Forrest JM, Storey GNB, et al: Gestational diabetes—infant malformations and subsequent maternal glucose tolerance. *Aust NZ J Obstet Gynaecol* 1986;26:11.

199. Jacobson JD, Cousins L: A population based study of maternal and perinatal outcome in patients with gestational diabetes. *Am J Obstet Gynecol* 1989;161:981.

200. Becerra JE, Khoury MJ, Cordero JF, et al: Diabetes mellitus during pregnancy and the risks for specific birth defects: a population based study. *Pediatrics* 1990;85:1.

201. Lavin JP: Screening of high-risk and general populations for gestational diabetes. Clinical application and cost analysis. *Diabetes* 1985; 34(Suppl 2):24.

202. Coustan DR: Screening and diagnosis of gestational diabetes. *Baillieres Clin Obstet Gynaecol* 1991;5:293.

203. Lind T, Anderson J: Does random blood glucose sampling outdate testing for glycosuria in the detection of diabetes during pregnancy. *BMJ* 1984;289:1569.

204. Jowett NI, Samanta AK, Burden AC: Screening for diabetes in pregnancy: is a random blood glucose enough? *Diabetic Med* 1987;4: 160.

205. Nasrat AA, Johnstone FD, Hasan SAM: Is random plasma glucose an efficient screening test for abnormal glucose tolerance in pregnancy? *Br J Obstet Gynaecol* 1988;95:855.

206. Cousins L, Dattel BJ, Hollingsworth DR, et al: Glycosylated hemoglobin as a screening test for carbohydrate intolerance in pregnancy. *Am J Obstet Gynecol* 1984;150:455.

207. Shah BD, Cohen AW, May C, et al: Comparison of glycohemoglobin deterioration and the one-hour oral glucose screen in the identification of gestational diabetes. *Am J Obstet Gynecol* 1982;144:774.

208. Vermes I, Zeyen LJJM, van Roon E, et al: The role of serum fructosamine as a screening test for gestational diabetes mellitus. *Horm Metab Res* 1989;21:73.

209. Roberts AB, Baker JR, Metcalf P, et al: Fructosamine compared with a glucose load as a screening test for gestational diabetes. *Obstet Gynecol* 1990;76:773.

210. Reece EA, Holford T, Tuck S, et al: Screening for gestational diabetes: one-hour carbohydrate tolerance test performed by a virtually tasteless polymer of glucose. *Am J Obstet Gynecol* 1987;156:132

211. Coustan DR, Widness JA, Carpenter MW, et al: The "breakfast tolerance test": screening for gestational diabetes with a standardized mixed nutrient meal. *Am J Obstet Gynecol* 1987;157:1113.

212. Sutherland HW, Pearson DWM, Lean MEJ, et al: Breakfast tolerance test in pregnancy. In: Sutherland HW, Stowers JM, Pearson DWM, eds. *Carbohydrate Metabolism in Pregnancy and the Newborn IV.* Springer-Verlag:1989;267.

213. Weiss PAM, Hofman H, Winter R, Pürstner P, Lichtenegger W: Gestational diabetes and screening during pregnancy. *Obstet Gynecol* 1984;63:776.

214. Carpenter MW, Canick JA, Star J, et al: Fetal hyperinsulinism at 14–20 weeks and subsequent gestational diabetes. *Obstet Gynecol* 1996;87:89.

215. Sacks DA, Abu-Fadil S, Karten GJ, et al: Screening for gestational diabetes with the one-hour 50 g glucose test. *Obstet Gynecol* 1987; 70:89.

216. Carr SR: Screening for gestational diabetes. *Diabetes Care* 1998; 21(Suppl 2):B14.

217. Carpenter MW, Coustan DR: Criteria for screening tests for gestational diabetes. *Am J Obstet Gynecol* 1982;144:768.

218. Berkus MD, Langer O, Piper JM, *et al*: Efficiency of lower threshold criteria for the diagnosis of gestational diabetes. *Obstet Gynecol* 1995;86:892.

219. Rust OA, Bofill JA, Andrew ME, *et al*: Lowering the threshold for the diagnosis of gestational diabetes. *Am J Obstet Gynecol* 1996;175:961.

220. Deerochanawong C, Putiyanun C, Wongsuryrat M, *et al*: Comparison of the National Diabetes Data Group and World Health Organization criteria for detecting gestational diabetes mellitus. *Diabetologia* 1996; 39:1070.

221. Freinkel N, Metzger BE, Phelps RL, *et al*: "Gestational diabetes mellitus": a syndrome with phenotypic and genotypic heterogeneity. *Horm Metab Res* 1986;18:427.

222. Cousins L, Rea C, Crawford M: Longitudinal characterization of insulin sensitivity and body fat quantitation in normal and gestational diabetic pregnancies. *Diabetes* 1988;37(Suppl 1):251A.

223. Beischer NA, Wein P, Sheedy MT, *et al*: Prevalence of antibodies to glutamic acid decarboxylase in women who have had gestational diabetes. *Am J Obstet Gynecol* 1995;173:1563.

224. Catalano PM, Tyzbir ED, Sims EAH: Incidence and significance of islet cell antibodies in women with previous gestational diabetes. *Diabetes Care* 1990;13:478.

225. Buschard K, Buch I, Molsted-Pedersen L, *et al*: Increased incidence of true type I diabetes acquired during pregnancy. *BMJ* 1987;294:275.

226. Green JR, Schumacher LB, Pawson IG, *et al*: Influence of maternal body habitus and glucose intolerance on birth weight. *Obstet Gynecol* 1991;78:235.

227. Kjos SL, Buchanan TA: Current concepts: gestational diabetes mellitus. *N Engl J Med* 1999;341:1749.

228. Langer O: Maternal glycemic criteria for insulin therapy in gestational diabetes mellitus. *Diabetes Care* 1998;21(Suppl 2):B91.

229. Buchanan TA, Kjos SL, Schafer U, *et al*: Utility of fetal measurements in the management of gestational diabetes mellitus. *Diabetes Care* 1998;21(Suppl 2):B99.

230. Pettitt DJ, Baird HR, Aleck KA: Excessive obesity in offspring of Pima Indian women with diabetes during pregnancy. *N Engl J Med* 1983;308:242.

231. Pettitt DJ, Nelson RG, Saad MF, *et al*: Diabetes and obesity in the offspring of Pima Indian women with diabetes during pregnancy. *Diabetes Care* 1993;16:310.

232. Metzger BE, Silverman B, Freinkel N, *et al*: Amniotic fluid insulin concentration as a predictor of obesity. *Arch Dis Child* 1990;65:1050.

233. Pettitt DJ, Aleck KA, Baird HR, *et al*: Congenital susceptibility to NIDDM: role of intrauterine environment. *Diabetes* 1988;37:622.

234. Silverman BL, Cho NH, Metzger BE: Impaired glucose tolerance in adolescent offspring of diabetic mothers: relationship to fetal hyperinsulinism. *Diabetes Care* 1995;18:611.

235. Silverman BL, Purdy LP, Metzger BE: The intrauterine environment: implications for the offspring of diabetic mothers. *Diabetes Rev* 1996; 4:21.

236. Coustan DR, Imarah J: Prophylactic insulin treatment of gestational diabetes reduces the incidence of macrosomia, operative delivery and birth trauma. *Am J Obstet Gynecol* 1984;150:836.

237. Leikin E, Jenkins JH, Graves WL: Prophylactic insulin in gestational diabetes. *Obstet Gynecol* 1987;70:587.

238. Mazze RS, Langer O: Primary, secondary, and tertiary prevention: program for diabetes in pregnancy. *Diabetes Care* 1988;11:263.

239. Catalano PM, Drago NM, Amini SB: Factors affecting fetal growth and body composition. *Am J Obstet Gynecol* 1995;172:1459.

240. Weiss PAM, Hoffmann HMH, Kainer F, *et al*: Fetal outcome in gestational diabetes with elevated amniotic fluid insulin levels. Dietary vs. insulin treatment. *Diabetes Res Clin Pract* 1988;5:1.

241. Weiss PAM, Hofmann HM, Winter RR, *et al*: Diagnosis and treatment of gestational diabetes according to amniotic fluid insulin levels. *Arch Gynecol* 1986;239:81.

242. Landon MB, Sonek J, Foy P, *et al*: Sonographic measurement of fetal humeral soft tissue thickness in pregnancy complicated by GDM. *Diabetes* 1991;40(Suppl 2):66.

243. Bochner CJ, Medearis AL, Williams J, *et al*: Early third trimester ultrasound screening in gestational diabetes to determine the risk of macrosomia and labor dystocia at term. *Am J Obstet Gynecol* 1987; 157:703.

244. Metzger BE: Treatment of mild gestational diabetes mellitus: is it time for a controlled clinical trial? Editorial. *Diabetes Care* 1988;11:813.

245. Langer O, Conway DL, Berkus MD, *et al*: A comparison of glyburide and insulin in women with gestational diabetes mellitus. *N Engl J Med* 2000;343:1134.

246. Sady SP, Carpenter MW: Aerobic exercise during pregnancy-special considerations. *Sports Med* 1989;7:357.

247. Revelli A, Durando A, Massobrio M: Exercise and pregnancy: a review of maternal and fetal effects. *Obstet Gynecol Surv* 1992;47:355.

248. Jovanovic-Peterson L, Durak EP, Peterson CM: Randomized trial of diet versus diet plus cardiovascular conditioning on glucose levels in gestational diabetes. *Am J Obstet Gynecol* 1989;161:415.

249. Bung P, Artal R, Khodiguian N, *et al*: Exercise in gestational diabetes: an optimal therapeutic approach? *Diabetes* 1991;40(Suppl 2):182.

250. Lesser K, Gruppuso P, Terry R, *et al*: Exercise fails to improve postprandial glycemic excursion in women with gestational diabetes. *J Mat Fet Med* 1996;5:211.

251. De Veciana M, Major CA, Morgan MA, *et al*: Postprandial versus preprandial blood glucose monitoring in women with gestational diabetes mellitus requiring insulin therapy. *N Engl J Med* 1995;333: 1237.

252. Metzger BE, Bybee DE, Freinkel N, *et al*: Gestational diabetes mellitus: correlations between the phenotypic and genotypic characteristics of the mother and abnormal glucose tolerance during the first year postpartum. *Diabetes* 1985;34(Suppl 2):111.

253. Metzger BE, Cho NH, Roston SM, *et al*: Pre-pregnancy weight and antepartum insulin secretion predict glucose tolerance five years after gestational diabetes mellitus. *Diabetes Care* 1993;16:1598.

254. Harris MI: Gestational diabetes may represent discovery of preexisting glucose intolerance. *Diabetes Care* 1988;11:402.

255. Kjos SL, Peters RK, Xiang A, *et al*: Predicting future diabetes in Latino women with gestational diabetes: utility of early postpartum glucose tolerance testing. *Diabetes* 1995;44:586.

256. Wollf C, Verlohren H-J, Arlt P, *et al*: Development of metabolic disturbances in patients with gestational diabetes—postgestational classification of carbohydrate tolerance. *Zentralbl Gynakol* 1987;109:88.

257. Al-Shawaf T, Moghraby S, Akiel A: Does impaired glucose tolerance imply a risk in pregnancy? *Br J Obstet Gynaecol* 1988;95:1036.

258. O'Sullivan JB: The interaction between pregnancy, diabetes, and long-term maternal outcome. In: Reece EA, Coustan DR, eds. *Diabetes Mellitus in Pregnancy: Principles and Practice.* Churchill Livingstone:1988;575.

259. Mestman JH, Anderson GV, Guadalupe V: Follow-up study of 360 subjects with abnormal carbohydrate metabolism during pregnancy. *Obstet Gynecol* 1972;39:421.

260. Grant PT, Oats JN, Beischer NA: The long-term follow-up of women with gestational diabetes. *Aust NZ J Obstet Gynaecol* 1986;26:17.

261. Dornhorst A, Bailey PC, Anyaoku V, *et al*: Abnormalities of glucose tolerance following gestational diabetes. *Q J Med* 1990;77:1219.

262. Catalano PM, Vargo KM, Bernstein IM, *et al*: Incidence and risk factors associated with abnormal postpartum glucose tolerance in women with gestational diabetes. *Am J Obstet Gynecol* 1991;165:914.

263. Damm P, Kühl C, Bertelsen A, *et al*: Predictive factors for the development of diabetes in women with previous gestational diabetes mellitus. *Am J Obstet Gynecol* 1992;167:607.

264. Xiang AH, Peters RK, Trigo E, *et al*: Multiple metabolic defects during late pregnancy in women at high risk for Type 2 diabetes. *Diabetes* 1999;48:848.

265. Peters RK, Kjos SL, Xiang A, *et al*: Long-term diabetogenic effect of single pregnancy in women with previous gestational diabetes mellitus. *Lancet* 1996;347:227.

266. Kjos SL, Peters RK, Xiang A, *et al*: Hormonal choices after gestational diabetes. *Diabetes Care* 1998;21(Suppl 2):B50.

267. Kjos SL, Peters RK, Xiang A, *et al*: Contraception and the risk of Type 2 diabetes mellitus in Latino women with prior gestational diabetes mellitus. *JAMA* 1998;280:533.

268. The Diabetes Prevention Program Research Group: The Diabetes Prevention Program. Design and methods for a clinical trial in the prevention of type 2 diabetes. *Diabetes Care* 1999;22:623.

269. Buchanan TA, Xiang AH, Peters RK, *et al*: Response of pancreatic β-cells to improved insulin sensitivity in women at high risk for Type 2 diabetes. *Diabetes* 2000;49:782.

270. Mestman, JH, Schmidt-Sarosi C: Diabetes mellitus and fertility control: contraception management issues. *Am J Obstet Gynecol* 1993; 168:2012.

C H A P T E R   3 9

The Offspring of the Mother with Diabetes

Bernard L. Silverman

Edward S. Ogata

Boyd E. Metzger

PREGNANCY AS A "TISSUE CULTURE EXPERIENCED"

The importance of the intrauterine environment as a determinant of metabolic function throughout the life span is being increasingly recognized.[1] The late Jorgen Pedersen of was the first to propose a mechanism whereby maternal fuels may exert a direct effect on the fetus.[2] In attempting to explain the large babies that are sometimes seen in pregnancies complicated by diabetes, he advanced the hyperglycemia-hyperinsulinism hypothesis. Therein he postulated that more maternal glucose gains access to the fetus whenever maternal insulin is inadequate, and that this extra glucose stimulates insulin release in the fetus and thereby produces an increase of fetal mass.[2,3] Pedersen's hypothesis gained increased credence with the demonstration that the placenta is impermeable to insulin[4] so maternal and fetal insulin (and the metabolic effects of such insulin) are separately compartmentalized.

Subsequent work demonstrated that *all* maternal fuels may be maladjusted in even the mildest forms of gestational diabetes.[5,6] Thus multiple fuels may contribute to the enhanced availability of building blocks for fetal growth and the premature development and functional activation of fetal B-cell secretion that Pedersen postulated.[2,5] Accordingly, the Pedersen hypothesis can be modified to include *maternal fuels besides glucose* that are also regulated by maternal insulin[5,7] (Fig. 39-1). It is then expected[5,8] that the growth enhancing actions of these fuels would affect fetal insulin-sensitive structures[9–13] to a greater degree than structures which are relatively insulin-insensitive.[11–13] Thus the hallmark of diabetic macrosomia should be *asymmetrical* growth in which weight (as an index of adipose stores) would be affected more than biparietal diameter (as an index of cerebral growth) or length (as an index of skeletal growth).[5,14,15] Thus pregnancy can be likened to a "tissue culture experience" since most of these fuels cross the placenta in concentration-dependent fashion (see Chap. 38)[7] so their concentrations in the maternal circulation may determine the quantitative as well as qualitative characteristics of the "incubation medium" in which the conceptus develops.[5,8]

In support of the "tissue culture" formulation and the modified Pedersen hypothesis, it has been shown that even the most minor abnormalities in glucoregulation during pregnancy (i.e., gestational diabetes mellitus class A1; see Chap. 38) are attended by (1) enhanced functional maturation of the β-cells in fetal islets (as judged *in utero* by increased levels of immunoreactive insulin in amniotic fluid during late pregnancy,[15–18] or at birth by elevated C-peptide/glucose ratios in cord blood[15,17,18]); and (2) relatively greater rates of growth in insulin-sensitive than in insulin-insensitive structures (as judged by serial ultrasound patterns *in utero*[15] or weight/length relationships at birth[15,18]). In studies of body composition, Catalano and colleagues have demonstrated increased fat mass in offspring of mothers with gestational diabetes, even at birthweights similar to those of offspring of mothers with normal glucose tolerance.[19] More importantly, these developmental changes can be correlated directly with maternal plasma levels of amino acids and FFA, as well as glucose, during the second or third trimester.[5,20–22] Thus all maternal fuels may be implicated in the altered developmental timetables which appear to affect certain structures more than others, especially in late fetal life.

CLINICAL FEATURES OF SPECIFIC MORBIDITIES

The morbidities in the infants of diabetic mothers (IDMs) are understood most readily in the context of the above alterations in the delivery of multiple building blocks from mother to conceptus and the attendant premature morphological and functional development of the B cells of the fetal pancreas leading to hyperinsulinism. Conversely, extensive clinical experience has documented that both the frequency and the severity of neonatal morbidities are reduced substantially when diabetes mellitus is well controlled throughout gestation.[23,24] However, because of the variability in quality of antepartum metabolic control that is attained, the medical team attending the delivery on an infant of a diabetic mother must remain prepared to deal with a wide spectrum of neonatal morbidities.

Unexplained Fetal Loss During Late Gestation

In the past, difficulties in pinpointing the cause(s) of this major perinatal complication of diabetes in pregnancy or identifying individual pregnancies at highest risk contributed heavily to the practice of arbitrary early delivery. Improvements in metabolic control of diabetes throughout pregnancy and in obstetric assessment of fetal well-being (see Chap. 38) have markedly reduced the frequency of this dreaded complication. Studies with animal mod-

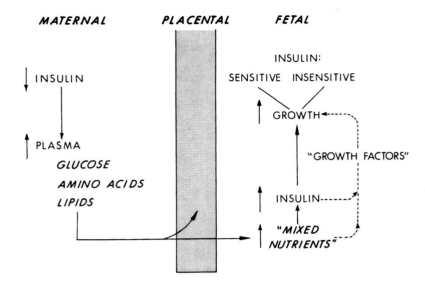

FIGURE 39-1. Effect of maternal fuels on fetus development. The classical "hyperglycemia-hyperinsulinism" hypothesis of Pederson[2,3] has been modified[5,8] to include the contributions of other maternal fuels beside glucose that are also responsive to maternal insulin. All of these can influence the growth of the fetus and the maturation of fetal insulin secretion. Within this formulation, growth will be disparately greater in insulin-sensitive than insulin-insensitive tissues in the fetus.

els have also provided important clues regarding pathophysiology. Philipps and coworkers[25–27] have used the chronically catheterized fetal sheep to demonstrate that sustained fetal hyperglycemia is associated with stimulation of fetal oxygen consumption,[26] increased fetal uptake of substrates (glucose and lactate), and placental lactate production,[27] and can result in fetal hypoxia with consequent metabolic acidosis and fetal demise.[25] While this pathophysiological sequence has not been proven in humans, it could explain some of the increased risk of intrauterine fetal death and poor ability to tolerate labor which remain major concerns when pregnancy complicated by diabetes mellitus has not been optimally controlled.

Birth Defects

Experimental, clinical, and epidemiologic studies indicate that increased risks of congenital malformations and spontaneous abortions in pregnancies complicated by diabetes are linked to disturbances in maternal metabolism around the time of conception. As summarized in Chap. 38, data currently available indicate that predisposition to congenital malformations is unlikely to be explained by a single circulating metabolic agent, but instead may be multifactorial in origin. A number of factors that might mediate "metabolic teratogenesis" have been described (myoinositol depletion, polyol accumulation, arachidonic acid deficiency, free oxygen radical generation). However, alterations in the concentrations of metabolic fuels singly or in combination, do not appear to directly account for the potent dysmorphogenic actions of serum from pregnant diabetic women or diabetic animals.

Although neither the precise time nor duration of exposure to an abnormal metabolic environment necessary for adverse events to develop in the human embryo has been pinpointed, there has been substantial progress towards their prevention. When counseling and improved control of diabetes mellitus are initiated prior to conception, several groups have reported rates of major congenital malformations not higher than expected in the general obstetrical population. Unfortunately, in the United States, the majority of pregnant women with diabetes are not enrolled in regimens of tight metabolic control prior to conception. Consequently major congenital malformations are still commonly encountered.

Neonatal Care of IDMs with Major Malformations

Infants of diabetic mothers (IDMs) with major malformations should be evaluated as if the cause of their malformations might not be maternal diabetes (i.e., fuel-mediated teratogenesis is best considered an etiology of exclusion). For this reason, a genetics consultation might be warranted as chromosomal analysis and other genetic studies may be indicated. In addition, depending on the type of malformation and the findings of a careful physical examination, studies of other organ systems (e.g., ultrasound imaging of the heart, kidneys, etc.) may be important because an anomaly of one organ system may be associated with one in another system. It is appropriate to perform an imaging study of the brain to check for any gross abnormalities. With completion of this evaluation, appropriate plans for care can be implemented.

A multidisciplinary approach to support the family is critically important to address their emotional, social, and financial needs. Every effort must be made to explain the nature of the malformation and treatment options. If necessary, long-term care plans must be devised and all aspects of discharge planning arranged well before the infant leaves the hospital.

Disturbances in Fetal Growth

As noted earlier, alterations in maternal metabolic fuels have a direct influence on the functional state of the fetal pancreatic B cells and the regulation of fetal growth. Normalization of the metabolic milieu throughout pregnancy is the key to prevention of fetal hyperinsulism and diabetic macrosomia. This topic is explored in depth in Chap. 38. Despite the greater insight into the regulation of intrauterine growth, the incidence of large babies has tended to increase in recent years, especially in type 1 diabetes mellitus (T1DM). Better control of diabetes in early pregnancy (thus avoiding early growth retardation) and discontinuation of routine delivery before term may account for the rarity of intrauterine growth restriction and the increased prevalence of macrosomia. Rates of macrosomia as high as 30–40% have been reported in recent years, and the risk of birth trauma (shoulder dystocia) associated with truncal adiposity that is typical of diabetic fetopathy has increased. Thus delivery and neonatal care of IDMs continue to present challenges in perinatal management.

Hypoglycemia

The normal human fetus at term is sufficiently metabolically mature to adapt to extrauterine life. It has adipose tissue, triglyceride stores, hepatic glycogen stores, and gluconeogenic capabilities. These depots interact in homeostatic fashion at birth as catecholamine and glucagon secretions surge while insulin secretion diminishes. The integrated relationships favor the production of endogenous glucose so the neonate can adapt to the sudden cessation of maternally-derived glucose.[28–30] Symptomatic hypoglycemia supervenes whenever this endogenous production of glucose is insufficient to sustain the fuel requirements of the brain.

While cerebral uptake of glucose at a given concentration of circulating glucose can be somewhat variable, determinations of plasma or blood glucose concentrations offer the only clinical means of assessing glucose delivery. From the screening of a large number of infants during the neonatal period, plasma glucose concentrations of 1.4–1.7 mmol/L have often been used as benchmarks of neonatal hypoglycemia. However, it has been suggested that glucose provision to tissues may not always be adequate when plasma glucose concentrations are at these statistically-derived lower limits, and that a value of 2.2 mmol/L is more consistent with safe levels of glucose flux.[31] Within that framework, approximately 20–25% of all IDMs experience neonatal hypoglycemia, usually during the first 4–6 hours. It must be emphasized that the level of plasma glucose concentration corresponding to inadequate provision of glucose to the brain is difficult to assess and that the duration of hypoglycemia necessary to damage the central nervous system has not been determined.[32] Within this framework, transient or persistent hypoglycemia (defined as two or more plasma glucose concentrations <1.7 mmol/L in the first 48 hours of life), when di-

agnosed and treated does not adversely affect cognitive development in IDMs at 2–5 years of age. This emphasizes the importance of optimizing maternal and neonatal care.[33]

The potent role of hyperinsulinism in neonatal hypoglycemia has been verified by isotopic estimates of glucose flux in newborn IDMs.[34,35] Additionally, the hyperplastic[36,37] and hyperfunctioning[15,17,18,38–42] islets of the IDM respond to acute glycemic challenge with brisk insulin secretion rather than the blunted insulin release that constitutes the normal neonatal pattern (Fig. 39-2). The hyperinsulinemia limits hepatic glucose production directly and also enhances tissue uptake of glucose. Hepatic glucose production also may be compromised by an antepartum inhibition of the induction of such key gluconeogenic enzymes as liver phosphoenolpyruvate carboxykinase.[43] Insulin has been shown to block the transcription of mRNA for phosphoenolpyruvate carboxykinase.[44]

The clinical manifestations of neonatal hypoglycemia may vary substantially. Thus hypoglycemic infants may remain asymptomatic or become limp, obtunded, jittery, tremulous, sweaty, or cyanotic. Seizures may develop and profound hypoglycemia may cause brain damage. If hypoglycemia is prolonged, myocardial contractility diminishes and congestive heart failure may develop. Accordingly, all IDMs should be screened for hypoglycemia hourly until the first full feeding and at frequent intervals during the first 24 hours of life. If glucose oxidase-impregnated reagent strips are used to screen for neonatal hypoglycemia, abnormal values must be confirmed with actual plasma or blood determinations in the laboratory. While awaiting laboratory documentation, asymptomatic infants who are capable of oral feeding may receive glucose solution to correct hypoglycemia. Symptomatic infants should be treated with 10–15 mL/kg of 10% glucose solution rather than with more

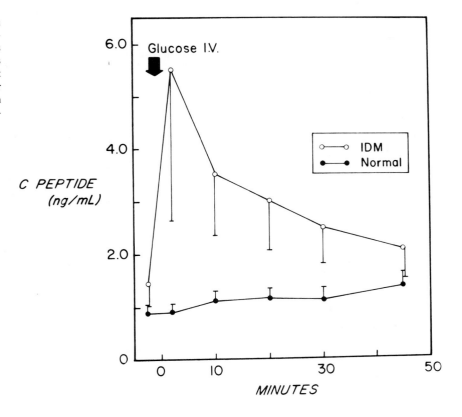

FIGURE 39-2. The effect of intravenous glucose on plasma C peptide in the newborn. The secretory response to glycemic challenge in newborns of mothers with normal carbohydrate metabolism (**solid circles**) is sluggish, characteristic of relatively immature islet function. By contrast, the response is brisk and greater in the IDM (**open circles**), reflecting earlier maturation of stimulus-secretion coupling in fetal islets. (*Reproduced from Phelps et al.[41]*)

concentrated solutions of glucose, that carry the risk of precipitating greater acute insulin release. Follow-up estimates of plasma or blood glucose must always be secured to assure adequacy of therapy and to screen for potential recurrence of hypoglycemia.

Respiratory Distress Syndrome (RDS)

Infants of diabetic mothers have been considered at increased risk for the development of RDS.[45] However, much of this risk may have been eliminated by the recent emphasis on tight control of maternal metabolism (see Chap. 38). The inordinate susceptibility of the offspring of the poorly regulated diabetic mother to RDS has been linked to a delay in the processes leading to fetal lung maturation. Hyperglycemia as well as hyperinsulinism have been implicated[46] due to their inhibitory effects on surfactant synthesis by the pulmonary type II cell. The advent of exogenous surfactant therapy has greatly improved the ability to treat RDS.

Hypocalcemia and Hypomagnesemia

Total plasma or ionized calcium concentrations should be measured after birth in both sick and healthy IDMs since significant hypocalcemia may develop in the neonatal period, even when the effects of prematurity and birth asphyxia are taken into consideration.[47] Parathyroid hormone secretion in IDMs has been reported to be blunted during the first 4 days of life[48,49] compared to infants of normal mothers. Hypomagnesemia which limits parathyroid hormone secretion even in the presence of hypocalcemia may be an important contributing factor.[50] The hypomagnesemia develops in women with diabetes as a result of increased renal losses associated with glucosuria. This in turn causes fetal and neonatal hypomagnesemia.

Clinical signs of hypocalcemia include jitteriness, twitching, or seizures; arrhythmias may also occur. It should be remembered that the neonate may not develop the characteristic prolongation of the QT interval associated with hypocalcemia in the adult. Respiratory distress syndrome and birth stress also increase the risk of hypocalcemia.

Symptomatic hypocalcemia should be treated with an infusion of 10% calcium gluconate (2 mL/kg body weight over 5–10 minutes). During infusion, monitoring with an electrocardiogram is important. IDMs may require from 75–200 mg/kg elemental calcium/day administered either enterally or parenterally. IDMs who are hypocalcemic on the basis of hypomagnesemia will not become normocalcemic until their hypomagnesemia is corrected. A 50% solution of magnesium at a dose of 0.25 mg/kg may be administered intramuscularly to correct hypomagnesemia.

Polycythemia/Hyperviscosity

IDMs are at increased risk for polycythemia and for the development of the neonatal polycythemia/hyperviscosity syndrome. Increased red cell mass is directly correlated with hyperviscosity. Hyperviscosity or red cell sludging can have severe consequences since it can damage any organ. Seizures and gastrointestinal injury are among the major complications of hyperviscosity. Several mechanisms have been proposed but not proven for polycythemia in IDMs. These include increased hematopoiesis, possibly as a consequence of intrauterine hypoxia or enhanced placental transfusion at delivery. The primary therapy for the polycythemia/hyperviscosity syndrome is partial exchange transfusion to reduce red cell mass.

Hyperbilirubinemia

Neonatal hyperbilirubinemia occurs more frequently in IDMs because of increased red cell breakdown.[51] Some of this may be due to increased red cell mass, and diminished red cell distensibility, with a consequent increase in the generation of bilirubin for hepatic conjugation and excretion. The delay in the switch in production from Hgb F to Hgb A may also be a factor. It is also possible that as a consequence of altered maternal metabolic fuel availability, red cell membrane composition in IDMs may differ from normal, resulting in increased susceptibility and hemolysis. In addition, the macrosomia of the IDM can increase the risk of bruising at delivery and thereby also augment bilirubin production.

Hypertrophic Cardiomyopathy

Many IDM neonates have a thickened interventricular septum and left or right ventricular wall.[52] While most such infants are asymptomatic, some develop congestive heart failure as a result of left ventricular outflow obstruction.[53] These abnormalities generally regress over 3–6 months. Since cardiac muscle is responsive to insulin, it has been suggested that the cardiomyopathy represents an acquired defect linked to the increased availability of insulin during fetal life. This possibility is strengthened by the fact that hypertrophic cardiomyopathy has been reported in infants of women with gestational diabetes.[54]

"Lazy Left Colon"

A functional bowel anomaly unique to IDMs may present as neonatal gastrointestinal obstruction. Barium contrast studies are suggestive of aganglionic megacolon. However, unlike Hirschsprung's disease, bowel innervation is normal in this "lazy left colon" or "small left colon" syndrome so that normal bowel function eventually supervenes.[55]

LONG-RANGE IMPLICATIONS OF THE INTRAUTERINE ENVIRONMENT: FUEL-MEDIATED TERATOGENESIS

Some of the above diabetes-related changes affect cells which may be terminally differentiated at birth and thought to undergo relatively limited replication thereafter (e.g., adipocytes, β cells of the pancreas, brain cells, etc.). These relationships prompted Freinkel to suggest that the actions of maternal fuels in developmental biology should be viewed in pharmacological as well as nutritional dimensions.[8,56,57] He proposed that abnormal fuel delivery in utero could exert permanent long-range effects upon the offspring ("fuel-mediated teratogenesis"[8,57]). For example, maternal hyperglycemia, hyperaminoacidemia, or elevated free fatty acids during the second half of pregnancy when fetal adipocytes, muscle cells, pancreatic cells, and neuroendocrine networks are undergoing proliferation and differentiation might confer greater vulnerability for obesity or type 2 diabetes mellitus (T2DM) in later life; abnormal fuel mixtures during the first and second trimester when the brain is established and brain cells are being formed might result in subsequent neurologic, psychologic, or cognitive deficits; and disturbances in the early part of the first trimester during embryogenesis might compromise organogenesis and so produce birth defects (fuel-mediated organ teratogenesis).[8,57]

In recent years, many reports have been published in support of the concept of fuel-mediated teratogenesis. A substantial proportion of the data have come from the long-term follow-up of offspring of diabetic mothers at the Northwestern University Diabetes in Pregnancy Center and the National Institutes of Health Pima Indian studies. These results and others will be summarized in the sections that follow.

Birth Defects

Although the development birth defects in pregnancies complicated by diabetes mellitus provides compelling confirmation of Freinkel's original hypothesis, this topic will not be considered in detail here. As indicated above and in Chap. 38, a metabolic basis for diabetic embryopathy has been established, although neither the precise time nor duration of exposure to an abnormal metabolic environment necessary for adverse events to develop in the human embryo has been pinpointed. It has also been demonstrated that the risk of diabetic embryopathy can be eliminated by good metabolic control around the time of conception. However, because participation in programs that provide such preconception care is far from universal, this form of fuel-mediated teratogenesis continues to be seen with alarming frequency.

Behavioral and Intellectual Functions

The possibility of long-term neurologic deficits in the offspring of diabetic mothers has been recognized for a number of years.[3] Yssing encountered "cerebral handicaps of definite clinical significance" in 18% of neonatally surviving Danish children born between 1946 and 1966 with a birthweight greater than 1000 g.[58] Obvious factors, such as prolonged severe neonatal hypoglycemia, birth trauma, neonatal kernicterus, and others have been implicated in many such cases in the past.[59–61] However, more subtle adverse effects have also been ascribed to fuel metabolism-related pathology. An apparent correlation between acetonuria during pregnancy and diminished IQ in the offspring prompted the suggestion that ketonemia may impair long-term intellectual performance.[62,63] The deleterious effects were attributed to ketones *per se* since they were encountered following all types of acetonuria (i.e., that caused by diabetes as well as malnutrition). These retrospective epidemiologic observations have been challenged,[64] although the demonstration by Shambaugh that ketones can inhibit pyrimidine[65] and purine[66] metabolism in fetal rat brain cells could provide some biochemical basis.

The longitudinal observations of the Northwestern University Diabetes in Pregnancy Center have included detailed analysis of neuropsychological development in offspring of diabetic mothers. On average, these offspring experienced minimally abnormal intrauterine fuel exposures. Significant mental deficiency was no different than national estimates in this group of offspring of mothers with well-controlled gestational and pregestational diabetes. Direct correlations were found between poorer maternal glucoregulation during the second and third trimester and poorer performance at birth in the interactive, motor, and physiologic dimensions of the Brazelton Neonatal Behavioral Assessment Scales.[67,68] Similarly, direct correlations between mild maternal ketonemia in the second and third trimester and poorer performance on both the Mental Development Index of the Bayley Scales of Infant Development at age 2 and the Stanford-Binet Intelligence Scales at ages 3–5 years have been reported.[69] Finally, average scores on the WISC-R Full Scale IQ at ages 7–11 years were inversely correlated with maternal HbA_{1c} in the second trimester and β-OHB in the third trimester. Impaired psychomotor development at 6–9 years of age, as assessed by the Bruininks-Oseretsky Test of Motor Proficiency, is also associated with maternal ketonemia in the second and third trimesters.[70] In these studies, careful perinatal and neonatal care were provided and perinatal morbidities were generally of mild or moderate severity. The perinatal morbidities associated with being an IDM did not appear to be responsible for adverse psychomotor and cognitive outcomes. Analysis of child educational achievement[71] demonstrated lower scores on the arithmetic index that correlated with higher maternal third-trimester free fatty acids, but no other correlations were observed. The above correlations between intrauterine metabolism and development in childhood persist when controlled for socioeconomic status and ethnicity. Moreover, they are not substantially different in gestational than in pregestational diabetes mellitus. Behavioral adjustment scales did not significantly correlate with indices of antepartum maternal metabolism. However, correlations were observed between obesity in the offspring and internalizing behavior problems.[72]

Data reported from Denmark are also consistent with the postulate of congenital fuel-mediated behavioral effects.[73] Denver Developmental Tests in the offspring of diabetic mothers at age 4 were correlated with their prior patterns of early intrauterine growth as measured by ultrasound during weeks 7–14 of pregnancy. Researchers encountered abnormal tests in 32.3% of the 34 4-year-olds who had displayed "early growth delay" (presumably reflective of faulty intrauterine milieu, since such delayed growth occurs in the offspring of mothers with the most elevated values for glycosylated hemoglobin at that time).[74] By contrast, Denver Developmental Tests were abnormal in only 8.0% of the 50 offspring from diabetic mothers whose intrauterine rates of growth had been normal during weeks 7–14 of pregnancy and in 11.6% of 86 4-year-olds from nondiabetic mothers.[73]

Sells and colleagues compared neurodevelopment through 36 months of age in 109 infants of mothers with T1DM and 90 control infants.[75] Mothers who were enrolled in a program of strict glycemic control before or within 21 days of conception had lower glycosylated hemoglobins than mothers enrolled later. Neurodevelopment of the offspring of earlier-enrolled mothers was similar to the control infants, whereas offspring of the later-enrolled mothers scored less well on tests of language development. There were no differences on the Bayley Scales of Infant Development or the Stanford-Binet Intelligence Scale.

Such experiences have not been universal—Several retrospective surveys have failed to disclose an increased incidence of gross neurologic and/or IQ deficits in the offspring of diabetic mothers.[76,77] However, negative reports need not necessarily exclude the possibility of small correlations between perturbations of maternal metabolism at key stages in pregnancy and long-range behavioral and/or intellectual performance.

Obesity

A number of analyses of the offspring of diabetic parents have disclosed disparities in weight relative to height during childhood and adolescence.[60,78–82] Vohr and coworkers observed that this obesity tends to correlate with birthweight.[82,83] However, this association was not found by others.[60] White[80] and more recent workers[84,85] noted that the obesity is far more frequent in the offspring of diabetic mothers than diabetic fathers. However, none of the early reports provided direct correlations with metabolic status during intrauterine development.

In the Northwestern University Diabetes in Pregnancy Center study, neonatal macrosomia in offspring of diabetic mothers disappeared by 1 year of age.[86] This contrasts with data from the general population, where large neonates tend to remain larger than average for at least the first 5 years of life.[87] After 2–3 years of age, offspring of diabetic mothers tend to gain weight faster than other children, and rapid weight gain is observed after 5 years of age.[22] By 8 years of age almost half of the offspring of diabetic mothers in this cohort had a weight greater than the 90th percentile.[88] This trend continues into adolescence, with rather dramatic increases in body mass index for the highest quartile (Fig. 39-3). Significant differences were not observed between offspring of mothers with gestational diabetes mellitus (GDM) when compared to offspring of mothers with pregestational diabetes mellitus (PGDM). Additionally, these studies have provided evidence that fetal islet function may confer predictive insights concerning long-term anthropometrics. Relative obesity in childhood, at ages 6–8 years, is significantly correlated with insulin secretion *in utero* (as judged by amniotic fluid insulin content at week 32–34 of pregnancy),[89] as is relative obesity in adolescence, ages 14–17 years.[86]

In a study of 71 offspring of mothers with T1DM, Weiss and associates found correlations between amniotic fluid insulin measured at 31 ± 2 weeks gestation and body mass index at 5–15 years of age.[90]

Further compelling support for an effect of antepartum maternal glucoregulation on the subsequent anthropometric development of the offspring has come from the Pima Indian Study, an NIH-supported epidemiologic survey initiated in 1965 to secure longitudinal characterizations of diabetes in a relatively pure genetic group having "the highest reported incidence and prevalence of type 2 diabetes."[91] The subjects consist of Pima Indians (and some Papago Indians) who live in the Gila River Indian community of Arizona. As part of that study, each community resident over 5 years of age is asked to have an examination which includes measurements of height and weight and a modified glucose tolerance test approximately every 2 years.

Pettitt and coworkers have correlated the two-hour response of Pima Indian mothers to oral glucose during pregnancy with the occurrence of obesity in their offspring.[85] They have found that obesity (≥140% of standard weight for height) is present at age 15–19 in two-thirds of the offspring who were presumably exposed to an abnormal intrauterine environment by virtue of their mothers being diabetic during gestation. By contrast, they have encountered obesity in only 40% of the 15- to 19-year-olds whose mothers had the genetic propensity for obesity and diabetes, but did not become diabetic until after the pregnancy (i.e., "prediabetic mothers") and in 30% of the offspring whose mothers never became diabetic (i.e., "nondiabetic mothers").[85] Moreover, offspring of diabetic women were heavier than offspring of nondiabetic and prediabetic women regardless of birthweight.[92] Thus although the characterizations of the Pima Indian pregnancies on the basis of a single 2-hour post–glucose load preclude correlations with fuels other than glucose, or with metabolic status throughout pregnancy, the overall experiences are consistent with the theory of fuel-mediated "anthropometric" teratogenesis.[8,57] The report from Italy of greater relative weight-to-height at age 4 in the offspring of diabetic mothers whose control was "poor" rather than "good" during the index pregnancy[93] provides additional support. However, well-controlled, mild gestational diabetes may not increase risk of obesity in offspring before the age of 10 years.[94] Others continue to report an increase in obesity in offspring of women with T1DM.[95] In a study of 200 offspring of diabetic mothers, Plagemann and colleagues found obesity in offspring of mothers with both gestational and T1DM at 1–4 and 5–9 years of age.[96]

Abnormal Glucoregulation and Diabetes Mellitus

Diabetes has been classically viewed as a genetic disorder, and "diabetic genes" have been invoked to explain the increased incidence of diabetes in the offspring of diabetic parents. Attempts to assess whether the "inheritance" may be influenced by congenital factors have been complicated by the failure of early reports to differentiate between parental type 1 and type 2 diabetes (which may differ in patterns of inheritance; see below), and the failure to distinguish between maternal diabetes occurring during the index pregnancy or thereafter (since such temporal factors may have different developmental implications for the conceptus; see above).

Evidence from animal models and epidemiologic studies suggests that disturbance in islet function or development during intrauterine and early postnatal life, produced by a variety of mechanisms, predisposes to metabolic disturbances and impaired glucose tolerance in later life. Thus offspring of rats with streptozocin-induced diabetes during pregnancy develop impaired glucose tolerance and gestational diabetes mellitus.[97] When pregnant rats are made mildly hyperglycemic by glucose infusion in late gestation, the offspring develop impaired glucose tolerance.[98] In crosses between rats with spontaneous T2DM and nondiabetic rats, a greater degree of glucose intolerance was observed in the offspring if the mother was diabetic, rather than the father.[99] Rhesus monkeys made hyperinsulinemic, but euglycemic, *in utero* by infusion of insulin into the fetus develop abnormal glucose tolerance as pregnant adults.[100] In studies of rats, adult offspring of diabetic mothers showed hyperphagia, basal hyperinsulinemia, and impaired glucose tolerance, and were overweight. This was accompa-

FIGURE 39-3. Physical growth of offspring of diabetic mothers expressed as body mass index (BMI). Solid lines indicate percentiles for BMI of normal American children as published by NCHS[130]; dashed lines depict 25th, 50th, and 75th percentiles for ODM. Data were smoothed by fitting to a third order regression.[115]

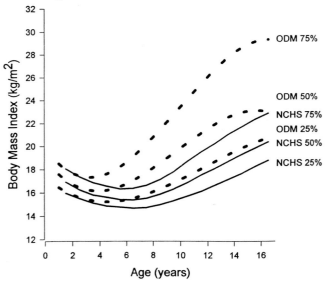

nied by an elevated number of neuropeptide Y neurons and galanin neurons in the arcuate hypothalamic nucleus.[101] Plagemann and colleagues also report disturbed differentiation and organization of distinct hypothalamic nuclei and subnuclei in hyperinsulinemic offspring of diabetic rats, possibly leading to dysfunctions of hypothalamic regulators of body weight and metabolism.[102]

Inferential insights concerning intrauterine fuel exposures and later susceptibilities to diabetogenic challenges can be made by analyzing the family histories of gravida with GDM.[103] T2DM should be present with equal frequency in the mothers and fathers of patients with GDM if sensitivity to the diabetogenic stresses of pregnancy were determined wholly by genetic factors (especially since meaningful sex differences in the incidence of T2DM have not been reported). On the other hand, if some limitations of functional reserve were "acquired"[104] in the course of prior intrauterine experiences,[104–109] a higher incidence of diabetes in the mothers than in the fathers of patients with GDM might be anticipated. A survey disclosed a history of maternal diabetes in 33% of gravidas with GDM, in contrast to a history of maternal diabetes in only 4.8% of normal gravidas.[103] On the other hand, the history of T2DM in the fathers of the two groups of gravidas was not different—8.8% in the women with GDM and 6.0% in the women with normal carbohydrate metabolism.[103] Hence, as first described in animal experiments by Bartelheimer and Kloos,[105] and supported by the pioneering clinical observations of Hoet[106] and Dörner and colleagues,[107,108] some transgenerational vulnerability to diabetogenic challenges may indeed occur as a consequence of prior intrauterine fuel exposures.

Mutations in mitochondrial DNA occur in association with a maternally-inherited form of diabetes and nerve deafness.[110,111] In Japanese subjects with T2DM and a family history of diabetes, a mutation in mitochondrial DNA was found in 60% of those with deafness, but only 2% of individuals with unimpaired hearing.[112] A mutation in mitochondrial DNA was found in only one of 218 unrelated British subjects with T2DM.[113] Since mitochondria are maternally inherited, these mutations may contribute in a rather limited way to the observed excess of maternal diabetes in subjects with T2DM.

Studies in Hattersley's laboratory have determined that up to 6% of gestational diabetes in the United Kingdom is the result of a mutation in the maternal glucokinase gene. In offspring of these mothers, the fetal genotype influences birthweight and glucose at birth. In the presence of a fetal glucokinase mutation, birthweight was reduced by a mean of 640 grams, and glucose was higher by a mean of 1.2 mmol/L.[114]

The offspring of gravidas enrolled in the Northwestern University Diabetes in Pregnancy Center long-term follow-up are demonstrating an increased frequency of impaired glucose tolerance. Plasma glucose and insulin have been measured fasting and 2 hours after oral glucose administration (1.75 g/kg) yearly beginning at 1.5 years of age. At 14–17 years of age, mean fasting glucose concentration in the ODM is no different than in 80 control subjects, and fasting insulin concentrations are identical. However, 2-hour concentrations after a glucose load are 6.5 ± 1.3 mmol/L and 5.7 ± 0.9 mmol/L ($p < 0.001$) respectively, and 2-hour post–glucose load insulin concentrations are 449 (90% CI: 177–1140) pmol/L in the ODM, compared to 331 (90% CI: 140–699) pmol/L in control subjects ($p < 0.01$). Two subjects have developed T2DM that was first detected on yearly glucose tolerance testing. One subject developed T1DM with ketoacidosis. In addition, 28 subjects have had impaired glucose tolerance (2-hour glucose

concentration greater than 7.8 mmol/L) on at least one occasion between 8 and 17 years of age. This is displayed as a cumulative probability (Kaplan-Meir estimator) in Fig. 39-4. On a single test, 2 of 80 control subjects had a 2-hour glucose concentration greater than 7.8 mmol/L. The relative risk of impaired glucose tolerance (2-hour post–glucose load glucose concentration >7.8 mmol/L) is 4.7 (95% CI: 1.7–12.9) for offspring who had an elevated mean amniotic fluid insulin concentration.[115] Plagemann and colleagues also report an increased incidence of impaired glucose tolerance in offspring of mothers with both gestational diabetes and T1DM. Furthermore, they found correlations between insulin:glucose ratios in childhood, and those previously obtained at birth.[116]

In general, populations with a high prevalence of impaired glucose tolerance later become populations with high prevalences of T2DM.[117]

The Pima Indian studies provide additional evidence. Pettitt and associates reported that T2DM is present by age 20–24 in 45.5% of the offspring of "diabetic mothers," but in only 8.6% and 1.4% of the offspring of "prediabetic" or "nondiabetic mothers" respectively (see above for definition of these categories).[118] Moreover, these differences persisted even after taking into account diabetes in the father, age at onset of diabetes in either parent, or obesity in the offspring. In a study of Pima siblings born before or after the mother's development of diabetes, those exposed to maternal diabetes *in utero* had a 3.7-fold greater risk of developing diabetes.[119] Pettitt and coworkers conclude that "the intrauterine environment is an important determinant of the development of diabetes and that its effect is in addition to effects of genetic factors."[118] In another study, Pettitt and colleagues found a lower rate of T2DM in Pima offspring who were exclusively breastfed for the first 2 months of life;[120] however, this report was not specific for offspring of diabetic mothers.

Some of the female offspring of the Pima women in the above studies have been examined during their pregnancies. A significant

FIGURE 39-4. Cumulative probability (Kaplan-Meir estimator) of impaired glucose tolerance (**IGT**) or diabetes in offspring of diabetic mothers.[115]

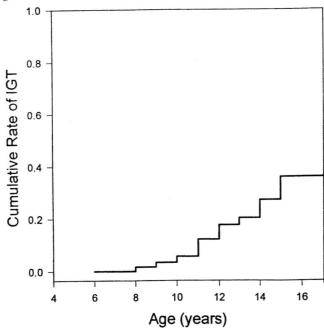

correlation (partial correlation 0.304, $p = 0.011$) was found between 2-hour post–glucose load plasma glucose in 15- to 24-year-old Pima women and their mothers' 2-hour glucose value during pregnancy, after controlling for age.[121] Thus, subsequent generations may be at even greater risk for the development of diabetes than would be predicted on a genetic basis alone.

Converse congenital relationships may also pertain in T1DM. Retrospective studies by Warram and coworkers,[122] in their reanalysis of some of the published reports of others,[123,124] have disclosed a two- to fivefold greater risk for the development of T1DM in the offspring of fathers than mothers with T1DM. These researchers have suggested that the seeming maternal protection against subsequent T1DM may be due to an induction of immunologic tolerance to the autoantigens of the β cells during intrauterine development.[125] Weiss and coworkers examined offspring of diabetic mothers at 5–15 years of age. Upon oral glucose tolerance testing, they find higher glucose, insulin, and C peptide concentrations, especially in those offspring who had higher amniotic fluid insulin concentrations *in utero* at 31 ± 2 weeks.[90] Thus although the directional impacts may be different, current data indicate that nature (as embodied by genetic propensities) may be modified by nurture (as determined by congenital contributions via the intrauterine metabolic environment) in the pathogenesis of T1DM as well as T2DM.

Other Cardiovascular Risk Factors

In the Northwestern Diabetes in Pregnancy Center Study, body mass index, blood pressure, and lipid concentrations were examined in ninety nine offspring of diabetic mothers and 80 controls. ODM were more obese (BMI 22.5 ± 5.6 vs. 20.3 ± 4.0 kg/m^2), and had higher systolic (8 mm Hg) and mean arterial BP (4 mm Hg), but similar diastolic BP compared to controls. ODM had lower fasting concentrations of LDL (2.54 ± 0.67 vs. 2.82 ± 0.70 mmol/L) and total cholesterol (4.01 ± 0.80 vs. 4.40 ± 0.78 mmol/L). In both groups, BMI, triglycerides, and fasting and 2-hour glucose concentrations showed correlations with BP measurements. Fasting insulin correlated with BP readings only in the ODM. Correlations were found between second- and third-trimester maternal free fatty acid concentrations and diastolic and mean arterial BP. Third trimester β-hydroxybutyrate was correlated with mean arterial BP.[126] The increased prevalence of obesity, impaired glucose, and elevated blood pressure may predispose offspring of diabetic mothers to an increased risk of heart disease in adulthood.

As noted above, obesity and impaired glucose tolerance, but not lipid metabolism, are associated with elevated amniotic fluid insulin measured in the third trimester. Thus the cause of physiologic predisposition towards elevated blood pressure may differ from those factors which contribute to elevations in body weight and reduced glucose tolerance.

General Relevance for Development in Later Life

The proposition that maternal fuel metabolism may exert long-range effects on development (i.e., the hypothesis of "fuel-mediated teratogenesis,"[8,57]) is being corroborated by many retrospective and prospective experiences. As such, there are now more reasons than ever to normalize maternal metabolism in all pregnancies complicated by diabetes and for viewing the success of pregnancy outcome in terms of the entire lifetime of the progeny as well as traditional perinatal criteria. Appropriate management of the pregnant diabetic may thereby constitute a meaningful strategy for modifying some of the self-perpetuating, and apparently congenitally-acquired contributions to such public health problems as adult obesity and diabetes mellitus.

Moreover, these fuel-related phenomena need not be limited to pregnancies complicated by diabetes. The same relationships between ambient fuels, fetal insulin secretion, and gene expression *in utero* may well apply to all pregnancies, so the potential for fuel-mediated teratogenesis may be present whenever maternal metabolism is perturbed for any reason.[57,127] Hales and colleagues have found that impaired growth *in utero* and in infancy is associated with impaired glucose tolerance and T2DM in adulthood.[128] McCance and associates, studying the Pima Indian population in Arizona, where most large babies are offspring of diabetic mothers, report a U-shaped relationship between birthweight and the later development of both obesity and diabetes in the offspring, with both extremes of neonatal size inducing abnormalities to a greater degree than those of more normal (average) birthweight.[129] However, in the general population, large babies of normal mothers have a low risk of obesity and diabetes. Thus diabetes in pregnancy has merely served as a paradigm for a more general truism,[127] and the broad ramifications for all of fetomaternal medicine extend far beyond the more parochial preoccupation with diabetes *per se*. To quote Freinkel and Metzger, "No single period in human development provides a greater potential (than pregnancy) for long-range 'payoff' via a relatively short-range period of enlightened metabolic manipulation."[5]

Acknowledgments   The authors are grateful to their many collaborators in the Departments of Medicine, Obstetrics, and Pediatrics who have contributed to The Northwestern University Diabetes in Pregnancy Center studies that are cited in this chapter. This work has been supported in part by NIH research grants DK10699, HD11021, HD19070, HD62903, HD23141 and RR-48; and Training Grant DK07169 from the United States Public Health Service; and a grant from the Ronald McDonald Foundation.

REFERENCES

1. Godfrey KM, Barker DJ: Fetal nutrition and adult disease. *Am J Clin Nutr* 2000;71:1344S.
2. Pedersen J: Weight and length at birth of infants of diabetic mothers. *Acta Endocrinol* 1954;16:330.
3. Pedersen J: *The Pregnant Diabetic and Her Newborn. Problems and Management.* Williams & Wilkins:1977;1.
4. Goodner CJ, Freinkel N: Carbohydrate metabolism in pregnancy. IV. Studies on the permeability of the rat placenta to ^{131}I insulin. *Diabetes* 1961;10:383.
5. Freinkel N, Metzger BE: Pregnancy as a tissue culture experience: The critical implications of maternal metabolism for fetal development. In: Pregnancy Metabolism, Diabetes and the Fetus. CIBA Foundation Symposium No. 63. Excerpta Medica:1979;3.
6. Metzger BE, Phelps RL, Freinkel N, *et al*: Effects of gestational diabetes on diurnal profiles of plasma glucose, lipids and individual amino acids. *Diabetes Care* 1980;3:402.
7. Freinkel N, Metzger B: Metabolic changes in pregnancy. In: Wilson JD, Foster DW, eds. *Williams Textbook of Endocrinology*, 8th ed. Saunders:1992;993.
8. Freinkel N: The Banting Lecture 1980: Of pregnancy and progeny. *Diabetes* 1980;29:1023.
9. Osler M, Pedersen J: The body composition of newborn infants of diabetic mothers. *Pediatrics* 1960;26:985.

10. Fee BA, Weil WB Jr.: Body composition of infants of diabetic mothers by direct analysis. *Ann NY Acad Sci* 1963;110:869.
11. Naeye RL: Infants of diabetic mothers: A quantitative, morphologic study. *Pediatrics* 1965;35:980.
12. Hill DE: Effect of insulin on fetal growth. *Semin Perinatol* 1978; 2:319.
13. Susa JB, McCormick KL, Widness JA, *et al*: Chronic hyperinsulinemia in the fetal rhesus monkey: Effects on fetal growth and composition. *Diabetes* 1979;28:1058.
14. Miller JM Jr, Brown HL, Khawli OF, Pastorek JG 2nd, Gabert HA. Ultra-sonographic identification of the macrosomic fetus. *Am J Obstet Gynecol* 1988;159:1110-4.
15. Ogata ES, Sabbagha R, Metzger BE, *et al*: Serial ultrasonography to assess evolving fetal macrosomia: Studies in 23 pregnant diabetic women. *JAMA* 1980;243:2405.
16. Phelps RL, Metzger BE, Sherman S, *et al*: Amniotic fluid insulin glucose (I/G) and antepartum prediction of neonatal hypoglycemia in infants of diabetic mothers. *Clin Res* 1977;25:397A.
17. Ogata ES, Freinkel N, Metzger BE, *et al*: Perinatal islet function in gestational diabetes: Assessment by cord plasma C-peptide and amniotic fluid insulin. *Diabetes Care* 1980;3:425.
18. Freinkel N, Metzger BE, Phelps RL, *et al*: Gestational diabetes mellitus: Heterogeneity of maternal age, weight, insulin secretion, HLA antigens, and islet cell antibodies and the impact of maternal metabolism on pancreatic B-cell and somatic development in the offspring. *Diabetes* 1985;34(Suppl 2):1.
19. Catalano PM, Thomas A, Drago NM, *et al*: Body composition and fat distribution in infants of women with normal and abnormal glucose tolerance. *Am J Obstet Gynecol* 1994;170(part 2):386.
20. Metzger BE, Freinkel N, Belton A, *et al*: Differential effects of maternal amino acids and glucose on intrauterine development in gestational diabetes mellitus (GDM). *Clin Res* 1986;34:800A.
21. Green OC, Winter RJ, Depp R, *et al*: Fuel-mediated teratogenesis: Prospective correlations between anthropometric development in childhood and antepartum maternal metabolism. *Clin Res* 1987;35:657A.
22. Metzger BE, Silverman BL, Freinkel N, *et al*: Amniotic fluid insulin as a predictor of obesity. *Arch Dis Child* 1990;65:1050.
23. Kitzmiller JL, Gavin LA, Gin GD, *et al*: Preconception care of diabetes. Glycemic control prevents congenital anomalies. *JAMA* 1991; 265:731.
24. Combs CA, Gunderson E, Kitzmiller JL, *et al*: Relationship of fetal macrosomia to maternal postprandial glucose control during pregnancy. *Diabetes Care* 1992;15:1251.
25. Philipps A, Dubin JW, Matti PJ, *et al*: Arterial hypoxemia and hyperinsulinemia in the chronically hyperglycemic fetal lamb. *Pediatr Res* 1982;16:653.
26. Philipps AF, Porte PJ, Stabinsky S, *et al*: Effects of chronic fetal hyperglycemia upon oxygen consumption in the ovine uterus and conceptus. *J Clin Invest* 1984;74:279.
27. Philipps AF, Rosenkrantz TS, Porte PJ, *et al*: The effects of chronic fetal hyperglycemia on substrate uptake by the ovine fetus and conceptus. *Pediatr Res* 1985;19:659.
28. Raiha NC, Lindros KO: Development of some enzymes involved in gluconeogenesis in human liver. *Ann Med Exp Biol Fenn* 1964; 47:146.
29. Shelley HJ: Glycogen reserves and their changes at birth and in anoxia. *Br Med Bull* 1961;17:137.
30. Sperling MA, DeLamater PV, Phelps D, *et al*: Spontaneous and amino acid-stimulated glucagon secretion in the immediate postnatal period: Relation to glucose and insulin. *J Clin Invest* 1974;53:1159.
31. Pagliari AS, Karl IE, Haymond M, *et al*: Hypoglycemia in infancy and childhood. Parts I and II. *J Pediatr* 1973;82:365, 558.
32. Corblath M, Schwartz R, Aynsley-Green A, *et al*: Hypoglycemia in infancy: The need for rational definition. *Pediatrics* 1990;85:834.
33. Rizzo T, Ogata ES, Dooley SL, *et al*: Perinatal complications and cognitive development in 2 to 5 year old children of diabetic mothers. *Am J Obstet Gynecol* 1994;171:706.
34. King K, Tserng KT, Kalhan SC: Regulation of glucose production in newborn infants of diabetic mothers. *Pediatr Res* 1982;16:608.
35. Cowett RM, Susa JB, Giletti B, *et al*: Glucose kinetics in infants of diabetic mothers. *Am J Obstet Gynecol* 1983;146:781.
36. Dubreuil G, Anderodias J: Islets de Langerhans glands chez un nouveau-né issu de mère glycosurique. Comptes rendus des scances de la societe de biologie et de ses filiales. *Coll Roy Soc Biol* 1920;83:1490.
37. Cardell BS: The infants of diabetic mothers: A morphological study. *J Obstet Gynaecol Br Commonw* 1953;60:834.
38. Baird JD, Farquhar JW: Insulin-secretory capacity in newborn infants of normal and diabetic women. *Lancet* 1962;1:71.
39. Isles TE, Dickson M, Farquhar JW: Glucose tolerance and plasma insulin in newborn infants of normal and diabetic mothers. *Pediatr Res* 1968;2:198.
40. Falorni A, Fracassini F, Massi-Benedetti F, *et al*: Glucose metabolism, plasma insulin and growth hormone secretion in newborn infants with erythroblastosis fetalis compared with normal newborns and those born to diabetic mothers. *Pediatrics* 1972;49:682.
41. Phelps RL, Freinkel N, Rubenstein AH, *et al*: Carbohydrate metabolism in pregnancy. XV. Plasma C-peptide during intravenous glucose tolerance in neonates from normal and insulin-treated diabetic mothers. *J Clin Endocrinol Metab* 1978;46:61.
42. Sosenko I, Kitzmiller JC, Loo SW, *et al*: The infant of the diabetic mother. Correlation of increased cord C-peptide levels with macrosomia and hypoglycemia. *N Engl J Med* 1979;30:859.
43. Girard JR, Caquet D, Bal D, *et al*: Control of rat liver phosphorylase, glucose-6-phosphatase and phosphoenolpyruvate carboxykinase activities by insulin and glucagon during the perinatal period. *Enzyme* 1973;15:272.
44. Beale E, Andreone T, Koch S, *et al*: Insulin and glucagon regulate cytosolic phosphoenolpyruvate carboxykinase (GTP) mRNA in rat liver. *Diabetes* 1984;33:328.
45. Robert MF, Neff RK, Hubbell JP, *et al*: Association between maternal diabetes and the respiratory-distress syndrome in the newborn. *N Engl J Med* 1976;294:357.
46. Bourbon JR, Farrell PM: Fetal lung development in the diabetic pregnancy. *Pediatr Res* 1985;19:253.
47. Tsang RC, Kleinman LI, Sutherland JM, *et al*: Hypocalcemia in infants of diabetic mothers. *J Pediatr* 1972;80:384.
48. Tsang RC, Chen I-W, Friedman MA, *et al*: Parathyroid function in infants of diabetic mothers. *J Pediatr* 1975;86:399.
49. Schedewie HK, Odell WD, Fisher DA, *et al*: Parathormone and perinatal calcium homeostasis. *Pediatr Res* 1979;13:1.
50. Noguchi A, Eren M, Tsang R: Parathyroid hormone in hypocalcemia and normocalcemic infants of diabetic mothers. *J Pediatr* 1980;97: 112.
51. Stevenson DK, Bartoletti AL, Ostrander CR, *et al*: Pulmonary excretion of carbon monoxide in the human infant as an index of bilirubin production. II. Infants of diabetic mothers. *J Pediatr* 1979;94:956.
52. Gutgesell HP, Speer ME, Rosenberg HS: Characterization of the cardiomyopathy in infants of diabetic mothers. *Circulation* 1980;61: 441.
53. Walther FJ, Siassi B, King J: Cardiac output in infants of insulin-dependent diabetic mothers. *J Pediatr* 1985;107:109.
54. Mehta S, Nuamah I, Kalhan S: Altered diastolic function in asymptomatic infants of mothers with gestational diabetes. *Diabetes* 1991;40 (Suppl 2):56.
55. Davis W, Allen R, Favara B, *et al*: The neonatal small left colon syndrome. *Am J Roetgenol* 1974;120:322.
56. Freinkel N: The role of nutrition in medicine: Recent developments in fuel metabolism. *JAMA* 1978;239:1868.
57. Freinkel N: Pregnant thoughts about metabolic control and diabetes (editorial). *N Engl J Med* 1981;304:1357.
58. Yssing M: Long-term prognosis of children born to mothers diabetic when pregnant. In: Camerini-Davalos RA, Cole HS, eds. *Early Diabetes in Early Life*. Academic Press:1975;575.
59. Haworth JC, McRae KN, Dilling LA: Prognosis of infants of diabetic mothers in relation to neonatal hypoglycemia. *Dev Med Child Neurol* 1976;18:471.
60. Cummins M, Norrish M: Follow up of children of diabetic mothers. *Arch Dis Child* 1980;55:259.
61. Cowett RM, Schwartz R: The infant of the diabetic mother. *Pediatr Clin North Am* 1982;29:1213.
62. Churchill JA, Berendes HW, Nemore J: Neuropsychological deficits in children of diabetic mothers. *Am J Obstet Gynecol* 1969;105:257.
63. Stehbens JA, Baker GL, Kitchell M: Outcome at ages 1, 3, and 5 years of children born to diabetic women. *Obstet Gynecol* 1977; 127:408.
64. Naeye RL, Chez RA: Effects of maternal acetonuria and low pregnancy weight gain on children's psychomotor development. *Am J Obstet Gynecol* 1981;139:189.

65. Bhasin S, Shambaugh GE III: Fetal fuels. V. Ketone bodies inhibit pyrimidine biosynthesis in fetal rat brain. *Am J Physiol* 1982; 243:E234.

66. Shambaugh GE III, Angulo MC, Koehler RR: Fetal fuels. VII. Ketone bodies inhibit synthesis of purines in fetal rat brain. *Am J Physiol* 1984;247:E111.

67. Rizzo T, Freinkel N, Metzger BE, et al: Fuel-mediated behavioral teratogenesis: Correlations between maternal metabolism in diabetic pregnancies and Brazelton tests in the newborn. *Diabetes* 1988; 37(Suppl 1):86A.

68. Rizzo T, Freikel N, Metzger BE, et al: Correlations between antepartum maternal metabolism and newborn behavior. *Am J Obstet Gynecol* 1990;163:1458.

69. Rizzo T, Metzger BE, Burns WJ, et al: Correlations between antepartum maternal metabolism and child intelligence. *N Engl J Med* 1991; 325:911.

70. Rizzo T, Metzger B, Cho N: Fuel-mediated behavioral teratogenesis: Correlations between antepartum maternal metabolism and child psychomotor development at ages 2 and 6–9 years. *Diabetes* 1994; 43(Suppl 1):425A.

71. Rizzo TA, Metzger BE, Dooley SL, et al: Early malnutrition and child neurobehavioral development: insights from the study of children of diabetic mothers. *Child Dev* 1997;68:26.

72. Rizzo TA, Silverman BL, Metzger BE, et al: Behavioral adjustment in children of diabetic mothers. *Acta Paediatr* 1997;86:973.

73. Petersen MB, Pedersen SA, Greisen G, et al: Early growth delay in diabetic pregnancy: Relation to psychomotor development at age 4. *Br Med J* 1988;296:598.

74. Pedersen JF, Molsted-Pedersen L, Mortensen HB: Fetal growth delay and maternal hemoglobin A$_{1c}$ in early diabetic pregnancy. *Obstet Gynecol* 1984;64:351.

75. Sells CJ, Robinson NM, Brown Z, et al: Long-term developmental follow-up of infants of diabetic mothers. *J Pediatr* 1994;125:S9.

76. Persson B, Gentz J: Follow-up of children of insulin-dependent and gestational diabetic mothers. Neuropsychological outcome. *Acta Paediatr Scand* 1984;73:349.

77. Hadden DR, Byrne E, Trotter I, et al: Physical and psychological health of children of type I (insulin-dependent) diabetic mothers. *Diabetologia* 1984;26:250.

78. Farquhar JW: Prognosis for babies born to diabetic mothers in Edinburgh. *Arch Dis Child* 1969;44:36.

79. Hagbard L, Olow I, Reinand T: A follow-up study of 514 children of diabetic mothers. *Acta Paediatr Scand* 1959;48:184.

80. White P: Childhood diabetes: Its course, and influence on the second and third generations. *Diabetes* 1960;9:345.

81. Breidahl HD: The growth and development of children born to mothers with diabetes. *Med J Aust* 1966;1:268.

82. Vohr BR, Lipsitt LP, Oh W: Somatic growth of children of diabetic mothers with reference to birth size. *J Pediatr* 1980;97:196.

83. Vohr BR, McGarvey ST, Tucker R: Effects of maternal gestational diabetes on offspring adiposity at 4–7 years of age. *Diabetes Care* 1999; 22:1284.

84. Bergmann RL, Bergmann KE, Eisenberg A: Offspring of diabetic mothers have a higher risk for childhood overweight than offspring of diabetic fathers. *Nutr Res* 1984;4:545.

85. Pettitt DJ, Baird HR, Aleck KA, et al: Excessive obesity in offspring of Pima Indian women with diabetes during pregnancy. *N Engl J Med* 1983;308:242.

86. Silverman BL, Rizzo TA, Cho NH, et al: Long-term effects of the intrauterine environment: The Northwestern University Diabetes in Pregnancy Center. *Diabetes Care* 1998;21(Suppl 2):B142.

87. Binkin NJ, Yip R, Fleshood L, et al: Birth weight and childhood growth. *Pediatrics* 1988;82:828.

88. Silverman BL, Rizzo T, Green OC, et al: Long-term prospective evaluation of offspring of diabetic mothers. *Diabetes* 1991;40(Suppl 2): 121.

89. Silverman BL, Landsberg L, Metzger BE: Fetal hyperinsulinism in offspring of diabetic mothers. Association with the subsequent development of childhood obesity. *Ann NY Acad Sci* 1993;699:36.

90. Weiss PA, Scholz HS, Haas J, et al: Long-term follow-up of infants of mothers with type 1 diabetes: evidence for hereditary and nonhereditary transmission of diabetes and precursors. *Diabetes Care* 2000; 23:905.

91. Pettitt DJ, Nelson RG, Saad MF, et al: Diabetes and obesity in the offspring of Pima Indian women with diabetes during pregnancy. *Diabetes Care* 1993;16:310.

92. Pettitt DJ, Knowler WC, Bennett PH, et al: Obesity in offspring of diabetic Pima Indian women despite normal birth weight. *Diabetes Care* 1987;10:76.

93. Gerlini G, Arachi S, Gori MG, et al: Developmental aspects of the offspring of diabetic mothers. *Acta Endocrinol (Copenhagen)* 1986;112 (Suppl 277):150.

94. Whitaker RC, Pepe MS, Seidel KD, et al: Gestational diabetes and the risk of offspring obesity. *Pediatrics* 1998;101:E9.

95. Rodrigues S, Ferris AM, Perez-Escamilla R, et al: Obesity among offspring of women with type 1 diabetes. *Clin Invest Med* 1998;21:258.

96. Plagemann A, Harder T, Kohlhoff R, et al: Overweight and obesity in infants of mothers with long-term insulin-dependent diabetes or gestational diabetes. *Int J Obes Relat Metab Disord* 1997;21:451.

97. Aerts L, Holemans K, Van Assche FA: Maternal diabetes during pregnancy: consequences for the offspring. *Diabetes Metab Rev* 1990; 6:147.

98. Gauguier D, Bihoreau MT, Picon L, et al: Inheritance of diabetes mellitus as consequence of gestational hyperglycemia in rats. *Diabetes* 1990;39:734.

99. Gauguier D, Nelson I, Bernard C, et al: Higher maternal than paternal inheritance of diabetes in GK rats. *Diabetes* 1994;43:220.

100. Susa JB, Sehgal P, Schwartz R: Rhesus monkeys made exogenously hyperinsulinemic *in utero* as fetuses, display abnormal glucose homeostasis as pregnant adults and have macrosomic fetuses (abstract). *Diabetes* 1993;42(Suppl 1):86A.

101. Plagemann A, Harder T, Melchior K, et al: Elevation of hypothalamic neuropeptide Y-neurons in adult offspring of diabetic mother rats. *Neuroreport* 1999;10:3211.

102. Plagemann A, Harder T, Janert U, et al: Malformations of hypothalamic nuclei in hyperinsulinemic offspring of rats with gestational diabetes. *Dev Neurosci* 1999;21:58.

103. Martin OA, Simpson JL, Ober C, et al: Frequency of diabetes mellitus in mothers of probands with gestational diabetes: Possible maternal influence on the predisposition to gestational diabetes. *Am J Obstet Gynecol* 1985;151:471.

104. Aerts L, Van Assche FA: Is gestational diabetes an acquired condition? *J Dev Physiol* 1979;1:219.

105. Bartelheimer H, Kloos K: Die Auswirkung des experimentellen Diabetes auf Gravidität und Nachkommenschaft. *Zeitschrift für die gesamte experimentelle medizin* 1952;119:246.

106. Hoet JP: Carbohydrate metabolism during pregnancy. *Diabetes* 1954; 3:1.

107. Dörner G, Mohnike A, Honigmann G, et al: Zur möglichen Bedeutung eines pränatalen Hyperinsulinismus für die postnatale Entwicklung eines Diabetes mellitus. *Endokrinologie* 1973;61:430.

108. Dörner G, Steindel E, Kohlkoff R, et al: Further evidence for a preventive therapy of insulin-dependent diabetes mellitus in the offspring by avoiding maternal hyperglycaemia during pregnancy. *Exp Clin Endocrinol* 1985;86:129.

109. Dörner G, Plagemann A, Rückert J, et al: Teratogenetic maternofoetal transmission and prevention of diabetes susceptibility. *Endokrinologie* 1988;91:247.

110. Ballinger SW, Shoffner JM, Hedaya EV, et al: Maternally transmitted diabetes and deafness associated with a 10.4 kb mitochondrial DNA deletion. *Nat Genet* 1992;1:11.

111. van der Ouweland JMW, Lemkes HHPJ, Ruitenbeck W, et al: Mutation in mitochondrial tRNALeu(UUR) gene in a large pedigree with maternally transmitted type II diabetes mellitus and deafness. *Nat Genet* 1992;1:368.

112. Kadowaki T, Kadowaki H, Mori Y, et al: A subtype of diabetes mellitus associated with a mutation of mitochondrial DNA. *N Engl J Med* 1994;330:962.

113. Alcolado JC, Majid A, Brockington M, et al: Mitochondrial gene defects in patients with NIDDM. *Diabetologia* 1994;37:372.

114. Spyer G, Allen L, Macleod KM, et al: Fetal genotype is the primary determinant of fetal growth in gestational diabetes due to a mutation in the maternal glucokinase gene. *Diabetes* 2000;49(Suppl 1):A4.

115. Silverman BL, Rizzo TA, Cho NH, et al: Long-term effects of the intrauterine environment: The Northwestern University Diabetes in Pregnancy Center. *Diabetes Care* 1998;21(Suppl 2):B142.

116. Plagemann A, Harder T, Kohlhoff R, *et al*: Glucose tolerance and insulin secretion in children of mothers with pregestational IDDM or gestational diabetes. *Diabetologia* 1997;40:1094.

117. Yudkin JS, Alberti KG, McLarty DG, *et al*: Impaired glucose tolerance. *Br Med J* 1991;301:397.

118. Pettitt DJ, Aleck KA, Baird HR, *et al*: Congenital susceptibility for NIDDM: Role of intrauterine environment. *Diabetes* 1988;37:622.

119. Dabelea D, Hanson RL, Lindsay RS, *et al*: Intrauterine exposure to diabetes conveys risks for type 2 diabetes and obesity: a study of discordant sibships. *Diabetes* 2000;49:2208.

120. Pettitt DJ, Forman MR, Hanson RL, *et al*: Breastfeeding and incidence of non-insulin-dependent diabetes mellitus in Pima Indians. *Lancet* 1997;350:166.

121. Pettitt DJ, Bennett PH, Saad MF, *et al*: Abnormal glucose tolerance during pregnancy in Pima Indian women: long-term effects on the offspring. *Diabetes* 1991;40(Suppl 2):126.

122. Warram JH, Krolewski AS, Gottlieb MS, *et al*: Differences in risk of insulin-dependent diabetes in offspring of diabetic mothers and diabetic fathers. *N Engl J Med* 1984;311:149.

123. Wagener DK, Sacks JM, LaPorte RE, *et al*: The Pittsburgh Study of Insulin-dependent Diabetes Mellitus: Risk for diabetes among relatives of IDDM. *Diabetes* 1982;31:136.

124. Dahlquist G, Gustavsson KH, Holmgren G, *et al*: The incidence of diabetes mellitus in Swedish children 0–14 years of age: A prospective study 1977–1980. *Acta Paediatr Scand* 1982;71:7.

125. Warram JH, Krolewski AS, Kahn CR: Determinants of IDDM and perinatal mortality in children of diabetic mothers. *Diabetes* 1988;37:1328.

126. Cho NC, Silverman BL, Rizzo TA, *et al*: Correlations between the intrauterine environment and blood pressure in adolescent offspring of diabetic mothers. *J Pediatr* 2000;136:587.

127. Freinkel N: Fuel-mediated teratogenesis: Diabetes in pregnancy as a paradigm for evaluating the developmental impact of maternal fuels. In: Serrano-Rios M, Lefebvre PJ, eds. Proceedings of the 12th Congress of the International Diabetes Federation, Madrid, September 23–28, 1985. Elsevier Science:1986;563.

128. Hales CN, Barker DJ, Clark PM, *et al*: Fetal growth and impaired glucose tolerance at age 64. *Br Med J* 1991;303:1019.

129. McCance DR, Pettitt DJ, Hanson RL, *et al*: Birth weight and non-insulin dependent diabetes: thrifty genotype, thrifty phenotype, or surviving small baby genotype? *Br Med J* 1994;308:942.

130. National Center for Health Statistics: Growth Curves for Children: Birth–18 Years. Government Printing Office, 1977 (U.S. Dept. of Health, Education, and Welfare Publ. No. PHS 78-1650, Ser. 11 [165]).

CHAPTER 40

Basic Pathobiology of the Eye and Its Complications

Elia J. Duh

Lloyd P. Aiello

INTRODUCTION

Diabetic retinopathy, a common ocular complication of diabetes mellitus, is the leading cause of blindness in working-age Americans.[1-3] In fact, diabetic retinopathy accounts for 12% of all new cases of blindness in the United States and there are an estimated 148,000 individuals in whom sight-threatening stages of retinopathy occur each year. Indeed, the risk of ocular disease in patients with diabetes is 25 times that of the general population.[4] The prevalence of diabetic eye disease has dramatically increased over the past 40 years, in part due to improvements in managing diabetes that have dramatically extended the life span of these patients.[5]

The mechanisms underlying diabetic retinopathy have been the subject of extensive research for over half a century. Particularly over the last decade, our understanding of the mechanisms of both nonproliferative and proliferative diabetic retinopathy has advanced significantly. These achievements not only improve our knowledge of the basic pathobiology underlying diabetic retinopathy, but also set the stage for the development of novel therapeutic strategies promising significant improvements in clinical care for patients with diabetes.

CLINICOPATHOLOGIC CHANGES IN DIABETIC RETINOPATHY

Diabetic retinopathy is clinically divided into two stages, nonproliferative diabetic retinopathy (NPDR) and proliferative diabetic retinopathy (PDR). However, even before retinopathy becomes clinically apparent, histopathologic changes occur. The earliest known changes are capillary basement membrane thickening (associated with a change in its chemical composition),[6] the loss of the retinal endothelium-supporting pericytes,[7,8] and alterations in retinal blood flow.[9] Pericyte loss potentially contributes to the subsequent formation of microaneurysms (Fig. 40-1) due to weakening of the vessel wall[10] and may also contribute to neovascularization due to the loss of the pericyte's inhibitory effect on endothelial cell growth.[11] Several studies have demonstrated a decrease in retinal blood flow even before retinopathy is clinically apparent[9,12-15] and retinal blood flow increases as diabetic retinopathy progresses.[13,16,17] Autoregulation of retinal blood flow is also significantly impaired before retinopathy becomes clinically apparent.[18-20]

With disease progression, the clinical signs of nonproliferative diabetic retinopathy appear.[5] The classic signs of NPDR include retinal microaneurysms, dot and blot retinal hemorrhages, cotton-wool spots representing infarctions of the nerve fiber layer (Fig. 40-2), venous loops, venous beading, retinal capillary dropout, and intraretinal microvascular abnormalities (IRMAs). Essentially all patients with diabetes will eventually develop NDPR as the incidence approaches 100% after 15 years of disease.[21,22] With the development of NPDR, retinal blood flow begins to increase.[13,16,17]

As NPDR advances, retinal capillary dropout arises, resulting in progressive retinal ischemia. The ischemic retina produces vasoproliferative factors that induce formation of new blood vessels in the retina or iris. This stage of the disease is called proliferative diabetic retinopathy (PDR). The proliferative retinal response is thought to be initiated by decreased oxygen levels as a result of retinal capillary nonperfusion.[23,24] Retinal neovascularization occurs commonly at the borders of perfused and nonperfused retina and is more common and severe in eyes with extensive nonperfusion. Retinal neovascularization also occurs commonly at the optic nerve head (Fig. 40-3) and along the temporal vascular arcades. The new vessels grow along the surface of the retina and along the vitreous scaffold of the posterior vitreous hyaloid. The new vessels are fragile and commonly bleed, resulting in preretinal and vitreous hemorrhage (Fig. 40-4). In addition, glial tissue associated with these new vessels can contract and result in traction on the retina, eventually leading to retinal detachment (Figs. 40-5 and 40-6). Vitreous hemorrhage and traction retinal detachment are responsible for most cases of severe visual loss from diabetic retinopathy.[5]

Macular edema is another important component of diabetic retinopathy. Diabetes causes an increase in retinal vascular permeability. Vessel leakage can occur at any stage of diabetic retinopathy, resulting in edema and thickening of the retina. When present in the macular area of the retina, this thickening is called macular edema. Macular edema is a common cause of moderate visual loss in patients with diabetes[5] and accounts for the majority of all visual loss in patients with DM.

BIOCHEMICAL MECHANISMS UNDERLYING NONPROLIFERATIVE DIABETIC RETINOPATHY

Several biochemical mechanisms have been proposed to explain the adverse systemic effects of hyperglycemia.[25,26] Extracellular glucose has been shown to react nonenzymatically with primary amines of proteins to form intermediate glycation products.[27,28] These intermediate products can further react to form advanced

653

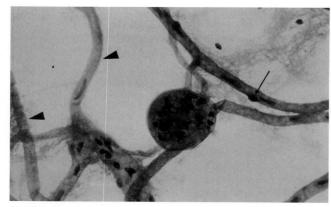

FIGURE 40-1. Trypsin digest preparation of retina from a patient with non-proliferative diabetic retinopathy showing scarcity of pericytes, with small, dark nuclei (**arrow**), relative to endothelial cells; a capillary micro-aneurysm (**center**); and acellular capillaries (**arrowheads**) (original magnification ×160).

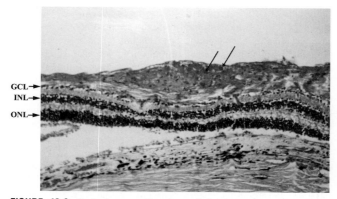

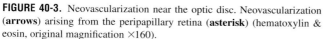

FIGURE 40-2. Retinal nerve fiber layer infarction (cotton-wool spot), showing distended nerve axons (cytoid bodies) (**arrows**). **GCL**, ganglion cell layer; **INL**, inner nuclear layer; **ONL**, outer nuclear layer (hematoxylin & eosin, original magnification ×40).

FIGURE 40-3. Neovascularization near the optic disc. Neovascularization (**arrows**) arising from the peripapillary retina (**asterisk**) (hematoxylin & eosin, original magnification ×160).

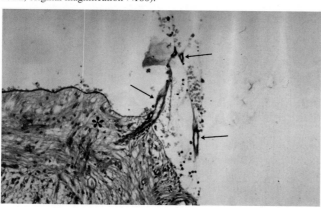

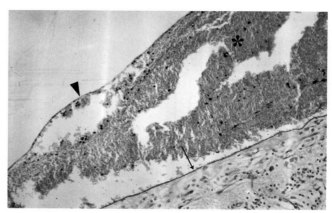

FIGURE 40-4. Preretinal hemorrhage (**asterisk**) located between the vitre-ous (**arrowhead**) and the internal limiting lamina of the retina (**arrow**) (hematoxylin & eosin, original magnification ×100).

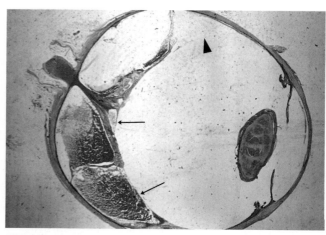

FIGURE 40-5. Proliferative diabetic retinopathy with traction retinal de-tachment with tangential (**arrows**) and anterior-posterior (**arrowhead**) traction bands (hematoxylin & eosin, original magnification ×1.2).

FIGURE 40-6. Retinal detachment. Area where vitreous band (**arrow**) is at-tached to tented-up retina in eye with proliferative diabetic retinopathy with traction retinal detachment (hematoxylin & eosin, original magnification ×100).

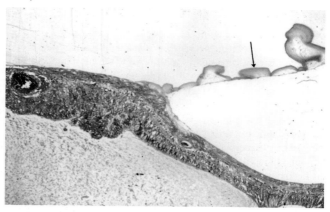

glycation end-products (AGEs). Infusion of AGEs in animals can mimic some of the vascular abnormalities observed in diabetes, particularly basement membrane thickening and changes in vascular contractility.[5] Studies investigating inhibitors of AGE formation, such as aminoguanidine, have demonstrated a reduction in basement membrane thickening and early changes in the retinal vasculature in diabetic rats.[27,29,30]

Excessive extracellular glucose may be transported inside the cell by glucose transporters, where it is metabolized, resulting in a change of redox potential. The resulting increase in oxidative stress has been postulated to be a fundamental factor underlying the biochemical changes associated with complications of diabetes, including diabetic retinopathy. Studies involving antioxidants have demonstrated ameliorative effects on various functions, including normalization of retinal blood flow in human patients with diabetes.[31] Whether antioxidants can be utilized as a therapy to prevent subsequent complications of diabetic retinopathy remains to be determined by prospective clinical trials. Influx of glucose also leads to the production of sorbitol by means of the aldose reductase pathway. Excessive sorbitol production has been postulated to be involved in cataract formation in diabetes.[32] However, a major role for sorbitol in diabetic retinopathy is less likely, since studies to date of aldose reductase inhibitors indicate that they have not prevented retinopathy in diabetic and galactosemic dogs; in addition, such inhibitors have not prevented or delayed the progression of diabetic retinopathy in human clinical trials.[33]

PROTEIN KINASE C AND ITS ROLE IN DIABETIC RETINOPATHY

Hyperglycemia-Induced PKC Activation

The activation of PKC by hyperglycemia and diabetes is related to increases in intracellular diacylglycerol (DAG) levels, the physiologic activator of PKC. In diabetic animal models, DAG levels have been found to be elevated in various tissues, including retina,[34] aorta, heart,[35] renal glomeruli,[36,37] and liver.[38] This elevation in DAG levels appears to be chronic. In diabetic dogs, for instance, DAG levels remain increased even after 5 years of disease.[39] The effect of elevated glucose levels in increasing DAG levels has been confirmed using cultured vascular cells, including retinal endothelial cells.[34]

Although cellular DAG can be increased through several mechanisms, most studies indicate that hyperglycemia-induced DAG results from de novo synthesis.[25,26] In this pathway, glucose-6-phosphate is metabolized through glycolysis to generate glyceraldehyde-3-phosphate, which in turn is further metabolized to generate phosphatidic acid and DAG. This de novo synthesis of DAG production generates DAG containing both saturated and unsaturated fatty acids, which is capable of activating PKC.

Accordingly, the increase in DAG levels is accompanied by PKC activation in diabetes mellitus as demonstrated in retina,[34] aorta, heart,[35] and renal glomeruli.[37] Increased PKC activity has also been observed in cultured cells, including retinal endothelial cells.[34] Diabetes and high glucose levels activate specific PKC isoforms. PKC-β_2 is activated predominantly in the aorta and heart of diabetic rats.[35] PKC-α, -β_1, -β_2, and -ε are activated in the retina of diabetic rats,[34] although PKC-β isoforms show a greater increase than do the others.

Multiple vascular alterations in the retina have been attributed to the activation of DAG and PKC. These include changes in vas-

cular blood flow, capillary basement membrane thickening, vascular permeability, and neovascularization. Retinal blood flow is decreased in animals and patients with short-duration diabetes. Several observations support the role of PKC activation in decreasing retinal blood flow. Intravitreal injection of a PKC agonist, such as phorbol ester, decreases retinal blood flow.[34] Conversely, decreases in retinal blood flow observed in diabetic animals and patients are normalized by PKC inhibitors.[34,36]

Capillary basement membrane thickening is a classical structural change in diabetes, and is present in many tissues including retina, renal glomeruli, heart, and muscle.[6] Aside from providing structural support, the capillary basement membrane is involved in regulating vascular permeability, cell adhesion, proliferation, differentiation, and gene expression. Alterations in basement membrane composition could therefore result in vascular dysfunction.

Most studies of capillary basement membrane changes in diabetes have focused on the renal glomeruli. Histologic studies have demonstrated increases in type IV and VI collagen, fibronectin, and laminin, and decreases in proteoglycans in the mesangium of patients with diabetic nephropathy.[40,41] These changes are also found in cultured mesangial cells incubated in high glucose and were prevented by general PKC inhibitors.[42–47]

Increased vascular permeability is a classic characteristic of diabetic retinopathy. In the retina, vascular leakage can be detected at sites of microaneurysms and retinal exudates (Fig. 40-7). Increased retinal vascular permeability presumably leads to the development of macular edema, which is the leading cause of moderate visual loss from diabetes. In diabetic animals, increased retinal vascular permeability to albumin can occur after only 4–6 weeks of chemically induced diabetes.[48] PKC activation increases the permeability of cultured endothelial cells to albumin and other macromolecules.[49,50]

PKC activation could also increase vascular permeability by its action on growth factors such as vascular endothelial growth factor (VEGF) (see below). VEGF increases in the diabetic retina before extensive retinal ischemia or neovascularization occurs.[51,52] Thus it could play a role in increasing retinal vascular permeability in nonproliferative diabetic retinopathy. In aortic smooth muscle, elevated glucose concentrations increase PKC activation and VEGF expression. This effect is inhibited by PKC inhibitors.[53] Furthermore, intravitreal injection of VEGF activates protein kinase C and increases retinal vascular permeability in rats. Of

FIGURE 40-7. Hard exudates (**asterisks**) in the outer plexiform layer of the macula in a patient with nonproliferative diabetic retinopathy. **GCL**, ganglion cell layer; **INL**, inner nuclear layer; **ONL**, outer nuclear layer (hematoxylin & eosin, original magnification ×100).

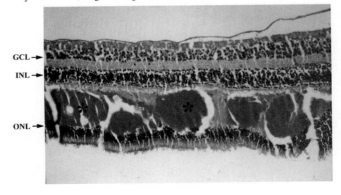

potential therapeutic importance, VEGF-induced permeability is almost completely inhibited by oral administration of a PKC-β selective inhibitor.[54]

Therapeutic Potential for PKC-β Inhibition

From the preceding discussion it is evident that PKC inhibitors may prove therapeutically useful in preventing or delaying ocular complications of DM. Indeed, in diabetic rats, abnormal retinal and renal hemodynamics and increases in albuminuria were normalized by oral administration of a PKC-β isoform selective inhibitor, LY333531. LY333531 inhibited diabetes-induced PKC activation in the retina and renal glomeruli.[36] In addition, LY333531 prevented the overexpression of TGF-β, type IV collagen, and fibronectin in the renal glomeruli of diabetic rats.[55] These studies strongly suggest a role for the PKC-β isoform in mediating diabetic vascular complications in the retina and kidney. As discussed below, inhibition of PKC-β has been shown to prevent growth factor–induced retinal vascular permeability and to normalize diabetes-induced changes in retinal blood flow, further suggesting its potential therapeutic usefulness.

THE ROLE OF GROWTH FACTORS IN PROLIFERATIVE DIABETIC RETINOPATHY

Retinal neovascularization is the principal cause of severe visual loss in patients with diabetes (Fig. 40-8). Neovascularization associated with ischemic retinopathies (such as diabetic retinopathy) is commonly preceded by retinal capillary nonperfusion[56,57] and frequently arises at the border of perfused and nonperfused areas of the retina. Neovascularization is more common and severe in eyes with more extensive retinal capillary nonperfusion.[58] These observations suggest that an angiogenic factor, released by ischemic/hypoxic retina may be responsible for stimulating new blood vessel growth in diabetic retinopathy. This theory was first proposed by Michaelson in 1948[23] and later refined by Ashton and others.

Several growth factors have been evaluated for their potential involvement in stimulating retinal neovascularization.[59] Most notably, these include fibroblast growth factor-2 (FGF-2), growth hor-

mone, and the insulin-like growth factors. More recently, vascular endothelial growth factor (VEGF) has emerged as a principal mediator of neovascularization in diabetic retinopathy.

VASCULAR ENDOTHELIAL GROWTH FACTOR

Vascular endothelial growth factor (VEGF), also known as vasopermeability factor (VPF), is a glycoprotein with both vasopermeability[60,61] and angiogenic activity.[62,63] VEGF is primarily mitogenic for endothelial cells.[64,65] Its expression has been found to be significantly increased in rapidly growing, highly vascularized tumors.[66] Furthermore, hypoxia induces VEGF expression in tumors and glial myogenic tumor cell lines.[67] VEGF binds several high-affinity cell surface tyrosine kinase receptors, the best characterized being fms-like tyrosine kinase (Flt) and fetal liver kinase 1 (Flk-1). VEGF and its receptors are critical for normal embryologic development, since even heterozygous knockout of these genes results in lethal disruption of the macro- and microvasculature.[68,69] These characteristics suggested that VEGF may play a major role in mediating the microvascular complications observed in diabetic retinopathy, which are characterized by tissue ischemia, angiogenesis, and vascular permeability. Indeed, numerous investigations of VEGF in ocular cells, animal models, and patients have implicated VEGF in the etiology of diabetic retinopathy.

Many cell types within the eye produce VEGF, including retinal pigment epithelial cells, pericytes, endothelial cells, glial cells, Müller cells, and ganglion cells.[70,71] Furthermore, hypoxia induces VEGF mRNA expression in various ocular cell cultures.[71] This mRNA induction is reversible following return of the cells to a normoxic environment. Retinal microvascular endothelial cells express high-affinity VEGF receptors on their cell surface at a higher density than many other endothelial cell types.[72] VEGF is capable of stimulating retinal endothelial cell growth in culture.

Investigations of animal models of ischemic retinopathy lend further support to VEGF's underlying role in ocular neovascularization. When neonatal mice,[73] rats,[74] or cats[75] are exposed to elevated concentrations of oxygen at specific times after birth, incomplete vascularization of the retina results. When the animals are returned to room air, the retinas become relatively hypoxic because of the experimentally induced retinal capillary nonperfusion. Neovascularization of the retina and the optic disc subsequently occurs. This neovascularization is clinically and histologically similar to that observed in humans with ischemic retinopathies such as diabetic retinopathy. In the mouse model, VEGF mRNA levels increase over threefold within 12 hours of relative retinal hypoxia and are maintained for many days thereafter, slowly declining as clinically apparent neovascularization regresses.[76] VEGF expression in this model is particularly prominent just anterior to regions of retinal neovascularization. Similar findings have been observed in the rat[74] and cat[75,77] models as well. VEGF mRNA and protein levels also correlate with the development of iris neovascularization in a monkey model of experimentally induced retinal vein occlusion.[78] These models all demonstrate a temporal relationship of increased VEGF expression observed after the onset of retinal hypoxia, but before the development of new vessels.

Clinical Studies

Support for the role of VEGF as a mediator of diabetic retinal neovascularization has been found in clinical studies evaluating the

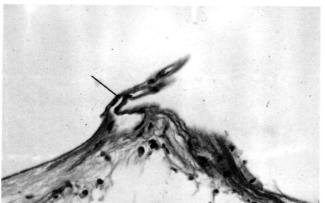

FIGURE 40-8. Early retinal neovascularization, with a new vessel (**arrow**) extending into the vitreous from the retina (hematoxylin & eosin, original magnification ×160).

correlation between proliferative retinopathies (including diabetic retinopathy) and intraocular VEGF concentrations. In one study,[79] ocular fluid specimens were obtained from 164 patients undergoing intraocular surgery, including 31 patients without neovascular disorders and 143 patients with diabetes. Patients in the latter group had different stages of retinopathy, including no retinopathy, nonproliferative retinopathy, quiescent proliferative retinopathy, and active proliferative retinopathy. VEGF concentrations were found to be markedly elevated in both the vitreous and aqueous of patients with active proliferative retinopathy. In contrast, VEGF levels were low in control patients as well as in diabetic patients with no retinopathy, nonproliferative retinopathy, or quiescent proliferative retinopathy. In six patients who underwent successful laser photocoagulation treatment of active proliferative retinopathy, intraocular VEGF levels after treatment were reduced by an average of 75% compared to before treatment. Similar findings were observed in another study[80] measuring vitreous VEGF concentrations in 8 patients with proliferative diabetic retinopathy as compared to 12 patients who underwent vitrectomy for disorders without associated neovascularization. These findings have now been confirmed by numerous studies.[81–86]

Inhibition of VEGF- and Retinopathy-Associated Complications

The establishment of a causal relationship for VEGF in ocular neovascularization has been provided by VEGF inhibition studies in animal models. VEGF inhibitory molecules evaluated in animals include VEGF receptor chimeric proteins, neutralizing antibodies, and antisense phosphorothioate oligodeoxynucleotides.

VEGF receptor chimeric proteins were constructed by joining the extracellular domain of the Flt receptor or the Flk-1 receptor with the heavy chain of IgG.[87] These molecules bind VEGF with the same affinity as native receptors and can therefore act as competitors for VEGF binding. Injection of these chimeric proteins into the mouse model of retinal neovascularization discussed above was performed just when the retinas became hypoxic. Single or dual injections of either chimeric protein significantly reduced retinal neovascularization, with a mean suppression of approximately 50%.[88]

Antisense phosphorothioate oligodeoxynucleotides have been studied in the same model. Two different VEGF antisense molecules were found to reduce VEGF protein levels by 40–66%, while decreasing new blood vessel growth by 25% and 31% as compared to sense or noncomplementary mRNA controls.[89] VEGF neutralizing antibodies have been studied in the primate model of iris neovascularization. Intravitreal injections administered every other day for 2 weeks resulted in inhibition of iris neovascularization as assessed by fluorescein iris angiograms.[90]

These studies suggest that VEGF mediates ocular neovascularization in general and proliferative diabetic retinopathy in particular. For advanced diabetic eye disease, the potential therapeutic implications of modulating these pathways is obvious and the focus of substantial current research efforts.

VEGF and Nonproliferative Diabetic Retinopathy and Macular Edema

Interestingly, recent findings suggest a potential role for VEGF in nonproliferative diabetic retinopathy as well. Increased levels of VEGF were found in a study of postmortem eyes of patients with nonproliferative diabetic retinopathy as compared with nondiabetic controls.[51] In addition, repeated injections of VEGF at high concentrations into primate eyes produced retinal changes resembling nonproliferative diabetic retinopathy, including blood vessel tortuosity, venous beading, capillary abnormalities resembling microaneurysms, intraretinal hemorrhages, capillary closure, and increases in vascular permeability.[91]

VEGF may also play an important role in the pathogenesis of diabetic macular edema, a condition resulting from excessive permeability of retinal vessels in patients with diabetes (Fig. 40-9). In the dermal microvasculature, VEGF is 50,000 times more potent than histamine in producing vasopermeability.[61] VEGF efficiently increases retinal vascular permeability as well.[54,92] The mechanism underlying this response may be related to VEGF downregulation of the interendothelial tight junction protein occludin, and/or to VEGF-induced phosphorylation of the tight junction proteins occludin and zonula occludin 1. Both of these responses have been demonstrated to occur in cultured retinal endothelial cells.[93,94] Since VEGF is increased in the diabetic retina before extensive retinal ischemia or neovascularization occurs,[51,52] it could account for diabetic macular edema that may occur at any stage of diabetic retinopathy.

As discussed above, VEGF-induced increases in vascular permeability in rats can be inhibited by oral administration of a PKC-β selective inhibitor. The mitogenic effects of VEGF on cultured vascular endothelial cells can also be significantly reduced by PKC-β inhibition.[95] Protein kinase C activation therefore appears to also play an important role in diabetic retinal vascular complications through mediating the effect of VEGF.

GROWTH HORMONE AND INSULIN-LIKE GROWTH FACTORS

The role for growth hormone (GH) and its downstream mediators such as insulin-like growth factor-1 (IGF-1) in the pathogenesis of diabetic retinal neovascularization has been extensively evaluated. Based on the observation of regressing proliferative diabetic retinopathy (PDR) after infarction of the pituitary following pregnancy (Sheehans syndrome) and partial responses of PDR following pituitary ablation, the role of GH/IGF-1 has been sought.[96–98] However, conditions in which GH is elevated (e.g., acromegaly) are not necessarily associated with retinal neovascularization.[99,100]

FIGURE 40-9. Diabetic macular edema, with the accumulation of a light-staining proteinaceous material in the outer plexiform (**asterisks**) and inner nuclear (**arrows**) layers of the retina. **GCL**, ganglion cell layer; **INL**, inner nuclear layer; **ONL**, outer nuclear layer (hematoxylin & eosin, original magnification ×100).

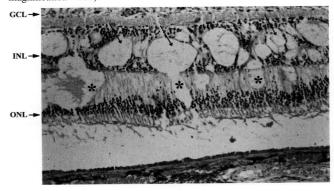

In addition, studies of vitreous and serum levels of IGF-1 have not consistently demonstrated a correlation with retinal neovascularization, in contrast to VEGF.[101–103]

Although the involvement of GH and IGF-1 in initiating diabetic retinal neovascularization may be limited, evidence suggests that they may play a key permissive role in the neovascular process. Studies using the mouse model of retinopathy described above demonstrate this point. Retinal neovascularization was found to be reduced by up to 44% in these mice after systemic administration of an inhibitor of GH secretion, as compared to control animals; similar results were found in transgenic mice expressing a GH antagonist gene. The inhibition was reversed by exogenous IGF-1 administration. Interestingly, a transgenic mouse expressing a GH agonist that results in a giant phenotype did not exhibit an increase in neovascularization.[104]

Another study demonstrated that administration of an IGF-1 receptor antagonist suppressed retinal neovascularization in the mouse model by up to 53%. In addition, this IGF-1 receptor antagonist reduced VEGF activation of the mitogen-activated protein kinase (MAPK) signaling cascade.[105] Taken together, these studies suggest that IGF-1 plays a role in creating a permissive environment for the stimulation of retinal neovascularization by VEGF.

INHIBITORS OF NEOVASCULARIZATION

Recently, attention has been focused on the possible role of endogenous angiogenic inhibitors such as pigment epithelium-derived factor (PEDF) in the eye. PEDF was first isolated from retinal pigment epithelial cells and has been actively studied as a neurotrophic factor.[106,107] It was recently found to potently inhibit corneal neovascularization in a mouse model.[108] PEDF blocks VEGF action in vitro in cultured endothelial cell migration assays. Temporal expression of PEDF in the mouse retina was found to be closely correlated with blood vessel maturation.

PEDF has been found to be present in the cornea and vitreous, two avascular areas of the eye. The ability of corneal extracts and vitreous specimens to inhibit neovascularization was neutralized by antibodies to PEDF. Finally, PEDF was found to be downregulated by hypoxia in a retinoblastoma cell line.[108] This last observation has particularly interesting implications for proliferative diabetic retinopathy. It is possible that ischemia/hypoxia resulting from diabetic microvascular disease may downregulate PEDF, thereby allowing growth factors such as VEGF to stimulate neovascularization.[109]

Transforming growth factor-beta (TGF-β) is another soluble factor that may inhibit blood vessel growth in the eye. The pericyte loss that characterizes early diabetic retinopathy has led to speculation that pericytes may play an inhibitory role in retinal capillary growth.[110] Coculturing capillary endothelial cells and pericytes results in inhibition of endothelial cell proliferation; this inhibition is mediated by TGF-β, which is activated on contact between the cells.[11]

It is probable that other inhibitory factors are also involved in retinal blood vessel regulation. Current views on the pathobiology underlying diabetic retinopathy is that the proliferative complications arise after the relative angiogenic and antiangiogenic balance is tipped in favor of angiogenesis, either by enhancing growth stimuli or reducing antigrowth stimuli. The therapeutic implications of antagonizing angiogenic activity and/or augmenting antiangiogenic activity are currently under investigation.

NEOVASCULAR GLAUCOMA

A particularly destructive complication of proliferative diabetic retinopathy is neovascular glaucoma. In addition to retinal neovascularization, angiogenesis can involve the anterior portion of the eye, including the iris (rubeosis iridis) and the anterior chamber angle (Fig. 40-10). Neovascularization of the angle can obstruct aqueous fluid outflow, resulting in neovascular glaucoma, a severe sight-threatening disorder. As with retinal neovascularization, VEGF is thought to be a major stimulus for neovascularization of the iris and angle. VEGF levels correlate with the development of iris neovascularization in a monkey model of laser-induced retinal vein occlusion.[78] Intravitreal injections of VEGF in primates were sufficient to induce iris neovascularization,[111] while intravitreal injections of antibody against VEGF resulted in inhibition of iris neovascularization. Finally, intraocular concentrations of VEGF are elevated in the eyes of patients with rubeosis iridis.[79]

DIABETIC CATARACT FORMATION

Cataracts are a common cause of visual impairment in patients with diabetes. Two types of cataract are observed in diabetes.[112,113] The true diabetic cataract, or snowflake cataract, occurs in young adults, children, and even infants with severe hyperglycemia. This type of cataract is rarely encountered in the United States today. The senescent cataract is clinically similar to that seen in the normal population, although evidence suggests that patients with diabetes are at increased risk and often develop this type of cataract at a younger age.

The sorbitol-polyol pathway has classically been implicated in cataract formation in diabetes. It has been demonstrated in most cells exposed to high glucose concentrations that glucose can be converted to sorbitol by the enzyme aldose reductase.[114] Although sorbitol can be metabolized into fructose by sorbitol dehydrogenase, this reaction occurs slowly, resulting in cellular accumulation of sorbitol, since sorbitol does not diffuse across cell membranes.[114] Cellular damage could occur as a result of osmotic stress, with influx of water leading to swelling of lens fiber cells. In support of this hypothesis, polyols have been observed to accumu-

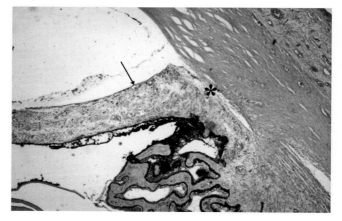

FIGURE 40-10. Eye with proliferative diabetic retinopathy, iris neovascularization (**arrow**), and closure of the anterior chamber angle by peripheral anterior synechiae (**asterisk**) (hematoxylin & eosin, original magnification ×40).

late in the lenses of diabetic animals.[32,115] However, the role of polyols in diabetic cataract formation in humans is less clear. Although sorbitol levels are increased in proportion to the level of hyperglycemia in the lenses of adults with diabetes, these levels may not be high enough to result in significant osmotic effects.[116]

A second mechanism for cataract formation in diabetes is nonenzymatic glycation of lens proteins such as the crystallins. The crystallins represent about 86% of the total lens proteins. Aggregation of these proteins occurs gradually as a normal consequence of aging; the aggregates thus formed lose their ability to transmit light. Diabetes is thought to accelerate nonenzymatic glycation of crystallins, increasing their susceptibility to oxidative damage, which leads to covalent cross-linking of the crystallins via disulfide bonds.[117] An increase in the glycation rate has been observed, particularly in alpha-crystallins.[118] In diabetic rats, glycation of lens proteins increased with time after induction of diabetes and was accompanied by an increase in high-molecular-weight aggregates.[119] Increased glycation of crystallins has also been observed in human diabetic cataracts,[120,121] suggesting that this mechanism may play a role in the pathogenesis of diabetic cataract formation in humans.

CONCLUSIONS

Diabetic retinopathy is a significant cause of morbidity throughout the world, accounting for the majority of severe visual loss among working-age adults in developed countries. Recent discoveries have provided significant insight into the growth factors and signal transduction mechanisms underlying this disease. As a result, we now have a more detailed understanding of the pathobiology of diabetic retinopathy. This knowledge has provided new therapeutic targets currently under investigation. Such studies hold the promise for a possible new age of pharmacologic therapies for the complications of diabetes in the eye.

Acknowledgments.   The authors express their thanks to Dr. W. Richard Green, Ocular Pathologist at the Wilmer Eye Institute, Johns Hopkins Hospital, for providing all of the histopathologic photos in this chapter.

Disclosure

The epidemiology, natural history, and clinical findings of diabetic retinopathy have frequently been presented. In addition, the potential roles of growth factors and underlying mechanisms of diabetic retinopathy have been reviewed extensively in recent years. The reports of fundamental studies and comprehensive reviews of their results are widely quoted and paraphrased. In order to maintain consistent descriptive accuracy of many of these fundamentals, portions of this chapter have been derived from prior publications, including Aiello and colleagues[5] and Aiello.[59]

REFERENCES

1. Klein HA, Moorehead HB: *Statistics on Blindness in the Model Reporting Area, 1969-1970.* U.S. Dept. of Health, Education & Welfare, 1973 (DHEW publ. no. [NIH] 73-427 1970).
2. National Society to Prevent Blindness, Operational Research Department: *Vision Problems in the U.S.: A Statistical Analysis.* National Society to Prevent Blindness:1980. Available from National Society to Prevent Blindness, Schaumburg, Ill.
3. Klein R, Klein BEK: Vision disorders in diabetes. In: Harris MI, Hamman RF, eds. *Diabetes in America.* U.S. Govt. Printing Office: 1985;1 (DHHS publ. no. 85-1468).
4. National Diabetes Data Group: *Diabetes in America.* National Institute of Diabetes and Digestive and Kidney Diseases, National Institutes of Health:1994.
5. Aiello LP, Cavallerano J, Bursell SE: Diabetic eye disease. *Endocrinol Metab Clin North Am* 1996;25:271.
6. Williamson J, Kilo C: Extracellular matrix changes in diabetes mellitus. In: Scarpelli D, Migahi G, eds. *Comparative Pathobiology of Major Age-Related Diseases.* Liss:1984.
7. Engerman RL, Kern TS: Progression of incipient diabetic retinopathy during good glycemic control. *Diabetes* 1987;36:808.
8. Kuwabara T, Cogan D: Studies of retinal vascular patterns. Part 1. Normal architecture. *Arch Ophthalmol* 1960;64:904.
9. Bursell SE, Clermont AC, Kinsley BT, et al: Retinal blood flow changes in patients with insulin-dependent diabetes mellitus and no diabetic retinopathy. *Invest Ophthalmol Vis Sci* 1996;37:886.
10. Cogan D, Toussaint D, Kuwabara T: Retinal vascular patterns. IV. Diabetic retinopathy. *Arch Ophthalmol* 1961;66:366.
11. Antonelli-Orlidge A, Saunders KB, Smith SR, et al: An activated form of transforming growth factor beta is produced by cocultures of endothelial cells and pericytes. *Proc Natl Acad Sci USA* 1989; 86:4544.
12. Wolf S, Arend O, Toonen H, et al: Retinal capillary blood flow measurement with a scanning laser ophthalmoscope. Preliminary results. *Ophthalmology* 1991;98:996.
13. Yoshida A, Feke GT, Morales-Stoppello J, et al: Retinal blood flow alterations during progression of diabetic retinopathy. *Arch Ophthalmol* 1983;101:225.
14. Feke GT, Buzney SM, Ogasawara H, et al: Retinal circulatory abnormalities in type 1 diabetes. *Invest Ophthalmol Vis Sci* 1994;35:2968.
15. Bertram B, Wolf S, Schulte K, et al: Retinal blood flow in diabetic children and adolescents. *Graefes Arch Clin Exp Ophthalmol* 1991; 229:336.
16. Grunwald JE, Riva CE, Baine J, et al: Total retinal volumetric blood flow rate in diabetic patients with poor glycemic control. *Invest Ophthalmol Vis Sci* 1992;33:356.
17. Patel V, Rassam S, Newsom R, et al: Retinal blood flow in diabetic retinopathy. *Br Med J* 1992;305:678.
18. Grunwald JE, Riva CE, Martin DB, et al: Effect of an insulin-induced decrease in blood glucose on the human diabetic retinal circulation. *Ophthalmology* 1987;94:1614.
19. Grunwald JE, Riva CE, Petrig BL, et al: Effect of pure O_2-breathing on retinal blood flow in normals and in patients with background diabetic retinopathy. *Curr Eye Res* 1984;3:239.
20. Riva CE, Grunwald JE, Sinclair SH: Laser Doppler velocimetry study of the effect of pure oxygen breathing on retinal blood flow. *Invest Ophthalmol Vis Sci* 1983;24:47.
21. Rand LI, Krolewski AS, Aiello LM, et al: Multiple factors in the prediction of risk of proliferative diabetic retinopathy. *N Engl J Med* 1985;313:1433.
22. Aiello LM, Rand LI, Briones JC, et al: Diabetic retinopathy in Joslin Clinic patients with adult-onset diabetes. *Ophthalmology* 1981; 88:619.
23. Michaelson IC: The mode of development of the vascular system of the retina, with some observations on its significance for certain retinal disease. *Trans Ophthalmol Soc UK* 1948;68:137.
24. Ashton N, Ward B, Supell G: Effect of oxygen on developing retinal vessels with particular reference to the problem of retrolental fibroplasia. *Br J Ophthalmol* 1954;38:397.
25. Koya D, King GL: Protein kinase C activation and the development of diabetic complications. *Diabetes* 1998;47:859.
26. Ishii H, Koya D, King GL: Protein kinase C activation and its role in the development of vascular complications in diabetes mellitus. *J Mol Med* 1998;76:21.
27. McCance DR, Dyer DG, Dunn JA, et al: Maillard reaction products and their relation to complications in insulin-dependent diabetes mellitus. *J Clin Invest* 1993;91:2470.
28. Brownlee M, Cerami A, Vlassara H: Advanced glycosylation end products in tissue and the biochemical basis of diabetic complications. *N Engl J Med* 1988;318:1315.

29. Hammes HP, Martin S, Federlin K, *et al*: Aminoguanidine treatment inhibits the development of experimental diabetic retinopathy. *Proc Natl Acad Sci USA* 1991;88:11555.

30. Corbett JA, Tilton RG, Chang K, *et al*: Aminoguanidine, a novel inhibitor of nitric oxide formation, prevents diabetic vascular dysfunction. *Diabetes* 1992;41:552.

31. Bursell SE, Clermont AC, Aiello LP, *et al*: High-dose vitamin E supplementation normalizes retinal blood flow and creatinine clearance in patients with type 1 diabetes. *Diabetes Care* 1999;22:1245.

32. Kinoshita JH: Mechanisms initiating cataract formation. Proctor Lecture. *Invest Ophthalmol* 1974;13:713.

33. Sorbinil Retinopathy Trial Research Group: A randomized trial of Sorbinil, an aldose reductase inhibitor, in diabetic retinopathy. *Arch Ophthalmol* 1990;108:1234.

34. Shiba T, Inoguchi T, Sportsman JR, *et al*: Correlation of diacylglycerol level and protein kinase C activity in rat retina to retinal circulation. *Am J Physiol* 1993;265(5 pt 1):E783.

35. Inoguchi T, Battan R, Handler E, *et al*: Preferential elevation of protein kinase C isoform beta II and diacylglycerol levels in the aorta and heart of diabetic rats: Differential reversibility to glycemic control by islet cell transplantation. *Proc Natl Acad Sci USA* 1992;89:11059.

36. Ishii H, Jirousek MR, Koya D, *et al*: Amelioration of vascular dysfunctions in diabetic rats by an oral PKC beta inhibitor. *Science* 1996; 272:728.

37. Craven PA, DeRubertis FR: Protein kinase C is activated in glomeruli from streptozotocin diabetic rats. Possible mediation by glucose. *J Clin Invest* 1989;83:1667.

38. Considine RV, Nyce MR, Allen LE, *et al*: Protein kinase C is increased in the liver of humans and rats with non-insulin-dependent diabetes mellitus: An alteration not due to hyperglycemia. *J Clin Invest* 1995;95:2938.

39. Xia P, Inoguchi T, Kern TS, *et al*: Characterization of the mechanism for the chronic activation of diacylglycerol-protein kinase C pathway in diabetes and hypergalactosemia. *Diabetes* 1994;43:1122.

40. Bruneval P, Foidart JM, Nochy D, *et al*: Glomerular matrix proteins in nodular glomerulosclerosis in association with light chain deposition disease and diabetes mellitus. *Hum Pathol* 1985;16:477.

41. Scheinman JI, Fish AJ, Matas AJ, *et al*: The immunohistopathology of glomerular antigens. II. The glomerular basement membrane, actomyosin, and fibroblast surface antigens in normal, diseased, and transplanted human kidneys. *Am J Pathol* 1978;90:71.

42. Fumo P, Kuncio GS, Ziyadeh FN: PKC and high glucose stimulate collagen alpha 1 (IV) transcriptional activity in a reporter mesangial cell line. *Am J Physiol* 1994;267(4 pt 2):F632.

43. Pugliese G, Pricci F, Pugliese F, *et al*: Mechanisms of glucose-enhanced extracellular matrix accumulation in rat glomerular mesangial cells. *Diabetes* 1994;43:478.

44. Haneda M, Kikkawa R, Horide N, *et al*: Glucose enhances type IV collagen production in cultured rat glomerular mesangial cells. *Diabetologia* 1991;34:198.

45. Ayo SH, Radnik RA, Garoni JA, *et al*: High glucose causes an increase in extracellular matrix proteins in cultured mesangial cells. *Am J Pathol* 1990;136:1339.

46. Ayo SH, Radnik RA, Glass WF II, *et al*: Increased extracellular matrix synthesis and mRNA in mesangial cells grown in high-glucose medium. *Am J Physiol* 1991;260(2 pt 2):F185.

47. Studer RK, Craven PA, DeRubertis FR: Role for protein kinase C in the mediation of increased fibronectin accumulation by mesangial cells grown in high-glucose medium. *Diabetes* 1993;42:118.

48. Williamson JR, Chang K, Tilton RG, *et al*: Increased vascular permeability in spontaneously diabetic BB/W rats and in rats with mild versus severe streptozocin-induced diabetes. Prevention by aldose reductase inhibitors and castration. *Diabetes* 1987;36:813.

49. Lynch JJ, Ferro TJ, Blumenstock FA, *et al*: Increased endothelial albumin permeability mediated by protein kinase C activation. *J Clin Invest* 1990;85:1991.

50. Oliver JA: Adenylate cyclase and protein kinase C mediate opposite actions on endothelial junctions. *J Cell Physiol* 1990;145:536.

51. Amin RH, Frank RN, Kennedy A, *et al*: Vascular endothelial growth factor is present in glial cells of the retina and optic nerve of human subjects with nonproliferative diabetic retinopathy. *Invest Ophthalmol Vis Sci* 1997;38:36.

52. Boulton M, Foreman D, Williams G, *et al*: VEGF localisation in diabetic retinopathy. *Br J Ophthalmol* 1998;82:561.

53. Williams B, Gallacher B, Patel H, *et al*: Glucose-induced protein kinase C activation regulates vascular permeability factor mRNA expression and peptide production by human vascular smooth muscle cells in vitro. *Diabetes* 1997;46:1497.

54. Aiello LP, Bursell SE, Clermont A, *et al*: Vascular endothelial growth factor-induced retinal permeability is mediated by protein kinase C in vivo and suppressed by an orally effective beta-isoform-selective inhibitor. *Diabetes* 1997;46:1473.

55. Koya D, Jirousek MR, Lin YW, *et al*: Characterization of protein kinase C beta isoform activation on the gene expression of transforming growth factor-beta, extracellular matrix components, and prostanoids in the glomeruli of diabetic rats. *J Clin Invest* 1997;100:115.

56. Gartner S, Henkind P: Neovascularization of the iris (rubeosis iridis). *Surv Ophthalmol* 1978;22:291.

57. Henkind P: Ocular neovascularization. The Krill memorial lecture. *Am J Ophthalmol* 1978;85:287.

58. Branch Vein Occlusion Study Group: Argon laser scatter photocoagulation for prevention of neovascularization and vitreous hemorrhage in branch vein occlusion. *Arch Ophthalmol* 1986;104:34.

59. Aiello LP: Clinical implications of vascular growth factors in proliferative retinopathies. *Curr Opin Ophthalmol* 1997;8:19.

60. Senger DR, Galli SJ, Dvorak AM, *et al*: Tumor cells secrete a vascular permeability factor that promotes accumulation of ascites fluid. *Science* 1983;219:983.

61. Senger DR, Connolly DT, Van de Water L, *et al*: Purification and NH2-terminal amino acid sequence of guinea pig tumor-secreted vascular permeability factor. *Cancer Res* 1990;50:1774.

62. Keck PJ, Hauser SD, Krivi G, *et al*: Vascular permeability factor, an endothelial cell mitogen related to PDGF. *Science* 1989;246:1309.

63. Leung DW, Cachianes G, Kuang WJ, *et al*: Vascular endothelial growth factor is a secreted angiogenic mitogen. *Science* 1989; 246:1306.

64. Ferrara N, Houck KA, Jakeman LB, *et al*: The vascular endothelial growth factor family of polypeptides. *J Cell Biochem* 1991;47:211.

65. Plate KH, Breier G, Weich HA, *et al*: Vascular endothelial growth factor is a potential tumour angiogenesis factor in human gliomas in vivo. *Nature* 1992;359:845.

66. Kim KJ, Li B, Winer J, *et al*: Inhibition of vascular endothelial growth factor-induced angiogenesis suppresses tumour growth in vivo. *Nature* 1993;362:841.

67. Shweiki D, Itin A, Soffer D, *et al*: Vascular endothelial growth factor induced by hypoxia may mediate hypoxia-initiated angiogenesis. *Nature* 1992;359:843.

68. Carmeliet P, Ferreira V, Breier G, *et al*: Abnormal blood vessel development and lethality in embryos lacking a single VEGF allele. *Nature* 1996;380:435.

69. Ferrara N, Carver-Moore K, Chen H, *et al*: Heterozygous embryonic lethality induced by targeted inactivation of the VEGF gene. *Nature* 1996;380:439.

70. Adamis AP, Shima DT, Yeo KT, *et al*: Synthesis and secretion of vascular permeability factor/vascular endothelial growth factor by human retinal pigment epithelial cells. *Biochem Biophys Res Commun* 1993; 193:631.

71. Aiello LP, Northrup JM, Keyt BA, *et al*: Hypoxic regulation of vascular endothelial growth factor in retinal cells. *Arch Ophthalmol* 1995; 113:1538.

72. Thieme H, Aiello LP, Takagi H, *et al*: Comparative analysis of vascular endothelial growth factor receptors on retinal and aortic vascular endothelial cells. *Diabetes* 1995;44:98.

73. Smith LE, Wesolowski E, McLellan A, *et al*: Oxygen-induced retinopathy in the mouse. *Invest Ophthalmol Vis Sci* 1994;35:101.

74. Dorey CK, Aouididi S, Reynaud X, *et al*: Correlation of vascular permeability factor/vascular endothelial growth factor with extraretinal neovascularization in the rat. *Arch Ophthalmol* 1996;114:1210.

75. Donahue ML, Phelps DL, Watkins RH, *et al*: Retinal vascular endothelial growth factor (VEGF) mRNA expression is altered in relation to neovascularization in oxygen induced retinopathy. *Curr Eye Res* 1996;15:175.

76. Pierce EA, Avery RL, Foley ED, *et al*: Vascular endothelial growth factor/vascular permeability factor expression in a mouse model of retinal neovascularization. *Proc Natl Acad Sci USA* 1995;92:905.

77. Stone J, Chan-Ling T, Pe'er J, *et al*: Roles of vascular endothelial growth factor and astrocyte degeneration in the genesis of retinopathy of prematurity. *Invest Ophthalmol Vis Sci* 1996;37:290.

78. Miller JW, Adamis AP, Shima DT, *et al*: Vascular endothelial growth factor/vascular permeability factor is temporally and spatially correlated with ocular angiogenesis in a primate model. *Am J Pathol* 1994; 145:574.

79. Aiello LP, Avery RL, Arrigg PG, *et al*: Vascular endothelial growth factor in ocular fluid of patients with diabetic retinopathy and other retinal disorders. *N Engl J Med* 1994;331:1480.

80. Adamis AP, Miller JW, Bernal MT, *et al*: Increased vascular endothelial growth factor levels in the vitreous of eyes with proliferative diabetic retinopathy. *Am J Ophthalmol* 1994;118:445.

81. Malecaze F, Clamens S, Simorre-Pinatel V, *et al*: Detection of vascular endothelial growth factor messenger RNA and vascular endothelial growth factor-like activity in proliferative diabetic retinopathy. *Arch Ophthalmol* 1994;112:1476.

82. Pe'er J, Folberg R, Itin A, *et al*: Upregulated expression of vascular endothelial growth factor in proliferative diabetic retinopathy. *Br J Ophthalmol* 1996;80:241.

83. Ambati J, Chalam KV, Chawla DK, *et al*: Elevated gamma-aminobutyric acid, glutamate, and vascular endothelial growth factor levels in the vitreous of patients with proliferative diabetic retinopathy. *Arch Ophthalmol* 1997;115:1161.

84. Burgos R, Simo R, Audi L, *et al*: Vitreous levels of vascular endothelial growth factor are not influenced by its serum concentrations in diabetic retinopathy. *Diabetologia* 1997;40:1107.

85. Hattenbach LO, Allers A, Gumbel HO, *et al*: Vitreous concentrations of TPA and plasminogen activator inhibitor are associated with VEGF in proliferative diabetic vitreoretinopathy. *Retina* 1999; 19:383.

86. Hernandez C, Burgos R, Canton A, *et al*: Vitreous levels of vascular cell adhesion molecule and vascular endothelial growth factor in patients with proliferative diabetic retinopathy: A case-control study. *Diabetes Care* 2001;24:516.

87. Park JE, Chen HH, Winer J, *et al*: Placenta growth factor. Potentiation of vascular endothelial growth factor bioactivity, in vitro and in vivo, and high affinity binding to Flt-1 but not to Flk-1/KDR. *J Biol Chem* 1994;269:25646.

88. Aiello LP, Pierce EA, Foley ED, *et al*: Suppression of retinal neovascularization in vivo by inhibition of vascular endothelial growth factor (VEGF) using soluble VEGF-receptor chimeric proteins. *Proc Natl Acad Sci USA* 1995;92:10457.

89. Robinson GS, Pierce EA, Rook SL, *et al*: Oligodeoxynucleotides inhibit retinal neovascularization in a murine model of proliferative retinopathy. *Proc Natl Acad Sci USA* 1996;93:4851.

90. Adamis AP, Shima DT, Tolentino MJ, *et al*: Inhibition of vascular endothelial growth factor prevents retinal ischemia-associated iris neovascularization in a nonhuman primate. *Arch Ophthalmol* 1996; 114:66.

91. Tolentino MJ, Miller JW, Gragoudas ES, *et al*: Intravitreous injections of vascular endothelial growth factor produce retinal ischemia and microangiopathy in an adult primate. *Ophthalmology* 1996;103: 1820.

92. Murata T, Ishibashi T, Khalil A, *et al*: Vascular endothelial growth factor plays a role in hyperpermeability of diabetic retinal vessels. *Ophthalmic Res* 1995;27:48.

93. Antonetti DA, Barber AJ, Khin S, *et al*: Vascular permeability in experimental diabetes is associated with reduced endothelial occludin content: Vascular endothelial growth factor decreases occludin in retinal endothelial cells. Penn State Retina Research Group. *Diabetes* 1998;47:1953.

94. Antonetti DA, Barber AJ, Hollinger LA, *et al*: Vascular endothelial growth factor induces rapid phosphorylation of tight junction proteins occludin and zonula occluden 1. A potential mechanism for vascular permeability in diabetic retinopathy and tumors. *J Biol Chem* 1999; 274:23463.

95. Xia P, Aiello LP, Ishii H, *et al*: Characterization of vascular endothelial growth factor's effect on the activation of protein kinase C, its isoforms, and endothelial cell growth. *J Clin Invest* 1996;98:2018.

96. Poulsen JE: Recovery from retinopathy in a case of diabetes with Simmonds' disease. *Diabetes* 1953;2:7.

97. Ray BS, Pazianos AG, Greenberg E, *et al*: Pituitary ablation for diabetic retinopathy. II. Results of yttrium 90 implantation in the pituitary gland. *JAMA* 1968;203:85.

98. Ray BS, Pazianos AG, Greenberg E, *et al*: Pituitary ablation for diabetic retinopathy. I. Results of hypophysectomy (A ten-year evaluation). *JAMA* 1968;203:79.

99. Amemiya T, Toibana M, Hashimoto M, *et al*: Diabetic retinopathy in acromegaly. *Ophthalmologica* 1978;176:74.

100. Ballintine EJ, Foxman S, Gorden P, *et al*: Rarity of diabetic retinopathy in patients with acromegaly. *Arch Intern Med* 1981;141:1625.

101. Grant M, Russell B, Fitzgerald C, *et al*: Insulin-like growth factors in vitreous. Studies in control and diabetic subjects with neovascularization. *Diabetes* 1986;35:416.

102. Dills DG, Moss SE, Klein R, *et al*: Association of elevated IGF-I levels with increased retinopathy in late-onset diabetes. *Diabetes* 1991;40: 1725.

103. Wang Q, Dills DG, Klein R, *et al*: Does insulin-like growth factor I predict incidence and progression of diabetic retinopathy? *Diabetes* 1995;44:161.

104. Smith LE, Kopchick JJ, Chen W, *et al*: Essential role of growth hormone in ischemia-induced retinal neovascularization. *Science* 1997; 276:1706.

105. Smith LE, Shen W, Perruzzi C, *et al*: Regulation of vascular endothelial growth factor-dependent retinal neovascularization by insulin-like growth factor-1 receptor. *Nat Med* 1999;5:1390.

106. Steele FR, Chader GJ, Johnson LV, *et al*: Pigment epithelium-derived factor: Neurotrophic activity and identification as a member of the serine protease inhibitor gene family. *Proc Natl Acad Sci USA* 1993; 90:1526.

107. Tombran-Tink J, Chader GG, Johnson LV: PEDF: A pigment epithelium-derived factor with potent neuronal differentiative activity. *Exp Eye Res* 1991;53:411.

108. Dawson DW, Volpert OV, Gillis P, *et al*: Pigment epithelium-derived factor: A potent inhibitor of angiogenesis. *Science* 1999;285:245.

109. King GL, Suzuma K: Pigment-epithelium-derived factor—a key coordinator of retinal neuronal and vascular functions. *N Engl J Med* 2000;342:349.

110. Kuwabara T, Cogan DG: Retinal vascular patterns. VI. Mural cells of the retinal capillaries. *Arch Ophthalmol* 1963;69:492.

111. Tolentino MJ, Miller JW, Gragoudas ES, *et al*: Vascular endothelial growth factor is sufficient to produce iris neovascularization and neovascular glaucoma in a nonhuman primate. *Arch Ophthalmol* 1996; 114:964.

112. Benson WE, Brown GC, Tasman W: *Diabetes and Its Ocular Complications.* WB Saunders:1988;110.

113. Johns KJ: Diabetes and the lens. In: Feman SS, ed. *Ocular Problems in Diabetes Mellitus.* Blackwell Scientific:1992;221.

114. Greene DA, Lattimer SA, Sima AA: Sorbitol, phosphoinositides, and sodium-potassium-ATPase in the pathogenesis of diabetic complications. *N Engl J Med* 1987;316:599.

115. Kinoshita JH, Kador P, Catiles M: Aldose reductase in diabetic cataracts. *JAMA* 1981;246:257.

116. Varma SD, Schocket SS, Richards RD: Implications of aldose reductase in cataracts in human diabetes. *Invest Ophthalmol Vis Sci* 1979; 18:237.

117. Pennington J, Harding JJ: Identification of the site of glycation of gamma-II-crystallin by (14C)-fructose. *Biochim Biophys Acta* 1994; 1226:163.

118. van Boekel MA, Hoenders HJ: Glycation of crystallins in lenses from aging and diabetic individuals. *FEBS Lett* 1992;314:1.

119. Perry RE, Swamy MS, Abraham EC: Progressive changes in lens crystallin glycation and high-molecular-weight aggregate formation leading to cataract development in streptozotocin-diabetic rats. *Exp Eye Res* 1987;44:269.

120. Liang JN, Hershorin LL, Chylack LT Jr: Non-enzymatic glycosylation in human diabetic lens crystallins. *Diabetologia* 1986;29:225.

121. Lyons TJ, Silvestri G, Dunn JA, *et al*: Role of glycation in modification of lens crystallins in diabetic and nondiabetic senile cataracts. *Diabetes* 1991;40:1010.

CHAPTER 41

Retinopathy and Other Ocular Complications in Diabetes

Ronald Klein

Diabetic retinopathy is an important cause of visual impairment in the United States.[1] While its natural history has been described, its pathogenesis is not known.[2] Available data suggest that good glycemic and blood pressure control reduces the risk of the development and progression of retinopathy.[3–6] Early identification and treatment of proliferative retinopathy or macular edema with photocoagulation may prevent or delay the development of visual loss.[7,8] This chapter describes current concepts about the natural history, pathogenesis, diagnosis, and management of retinopathy as well as other ocular complications of diabetes that may result in visual loss.

DIABETIC RETINOPATHY

Retinal Anatomy

The retina is a thin, transparent neural tissue lining the inner part of the eye.[9] It is in contact with the clear vitreous gel internally and the choroid externally. The retina varies in thickness from 0.1 mm at the fovea and far periphery to 0.55 mm at the macula. There are ten well-defined retinal layers consisting of the nuclei of three sequential neurons, their axons and synaptic connections, and glial supporting cells with little extracellular space. A central retinal artery derived from the ophthalmic artery branches into arterioles at the optic nerve head and supplies blood to the internal two thirds of the retina; the choriocapillaris of the choroid supplies nutrition to the external one third. A blood–retinal barrier comprised of tight junctions of the endothelial cells of the retinal blood vessels and the retinal pigment epithelial cells prevents penetration of all but a few important metabolic products into the retina.

The macular area measures approximately 4 mm in diameter and is centered 4 mm temporal to the optic disk. The fovea, a depression in the inner retinal surface of the macula, is 1.5 mm in diameter (Fig. 41-1). A retinal capillary-free zone of 450–600 μm exists in its center, where the retinal tissue is fed by the choriocapillaris of the choroidal circulation. The central portion of the fovea (or foveola) contains only cone photoreceptors, which are important for the best visual acuity (finest spatial resolution) and highest quality trichromatic color vision.

Natural History

The earliest clinically apparent manifestations of diabetic retinopathy are classified as nonproliferative. During this phase a number of pathophysiologic changes associated with diabetes occur in the microvasculature; these include occlusion, dilation, and increased permeability of the small retinal blood vessels.[10,11] Histologic changes that occur prior to the appearance of retinopathy, early in the course of the disease, are degeneration of retinal capillary pericytes (mural cells) and thickening of the capillary basement membrane.[10,11]

Usually the first changes seen with the ophthalmoscope are retinal microaneurysms, small outpouchings of the retinal capillaries (Fig. 41-1). They appear as small circular red dots, varying in size from about 20–200 μm. Retinal microaneurysms typically arise in areas of capillary closure. These lesions demonstrate abnormal permeability of the endothelial cell wall to fluorescein and possibly to lipoproteins. With time, the walls may thicken with deposition of periodic acid-Schiff (PAS)-positive and lipid material, and stagnant blood may be trapped in the lumen. If there is further thickening of the wall and obliteration of the lumen, the microaneurysm may then appear yellow or white on clinical examination. Occlusion of the feeding capillary or complete hyalinization of the lumen may be responsible for the microaneurysm's ultimate disappearance.[11] Microaneurysms have been reported to have variable survival rates, and their average disappearance rate has been estimated at 3.3%/month.[12]

The number of retinal microaneurysms in an eye is an important predictor of progression of diabetic retinopathy.[13] In the Wisconsin Epidemiologic Study of Diabetic Retinopathy (WESDR), there was an increased risk of progression of diabetic retinopathy over a 4-year period when four or more retinal microaneurysms were present at baseline. Furthermore, the increase in the number of retinal microaneurysms and the ratio of the number of retinal microaneurysms at the 4-year follow-up to the number at baseline were positively associated with the incidence of proliferative retinopathy or clinically significant macular edema at the 10-year WESDR follow-up.[14] Baudoin and coworkers[15] developed a standardized reproducible method for quantitating the number of retinal microaneurysms using fluorescein angiograms. Microaneurysm counts are useful for study of the early natural history of diabetic retinopathy and as an end point in clinical trials to evaluate the effects of treatment or intervention. Retinal microaneurysms generally do not make their appearance until at least 3 years after diagnosis of diabetes.[16,17] They are found in about 69% of people with a history of 10 years of type 1 diabetes mellitus (T1DM).[16] In adults with type 2 diabetes mellitus (T2DM), retinal microaneurysms are present in 55% of the population who have had diabetes for 10 years.[17] Retinal microaneurysms can occur in nondiabetic patients with other conditions associated with retinal ischemia, for example, branch

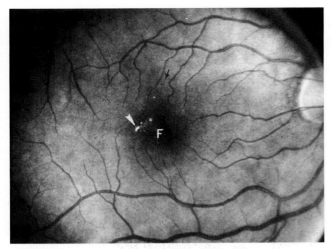

FIGURE 41-1. Fundus photograph of right eye. The foveal area (**F**) corresponds approximately to the dark central portion of the photograph. A retinal microaneurysm (**black arrow**) appears as a small dark spot with sharp margins and retinal hard exudates appear as white deposits with sharp margins just nasal to the foveal area (**white arrowhead**). The visual acuity in this eye is 20/15.

retinal vein occlusion, carotid artery disease, AIDS, and hypertensive retinopathy. Single retinal microaneurysms were found in 3.7% and multiple microaneurysms in 1.2% of eyes in a nondiabetic population.[18] Because hypertension and carotid artery disease are not uncommon in older-onset diabetic people, it may be difficult to determine whether diabetes or the presence of other systemic diseases is the cause of the microaneurysms when they are the only sign of retinopathy in the eyes of older-onset diabetic people.

Retinal microaneurysms by themselves are usually not a threat to vision. However, as the disease progresses, retinal blot hemorrhages and hard exudates appear. Retinal blot hemorrhages are round with blurred edges and result from an extravasation of blood from retinal capillaries or microaneurysms into the inner nuclear layer of the retina (Fig. 41-2). They are not fluorescent on angiography and usually disappear within 3–4 months.

Retinal hard exudates are variable in size, sharply defined, and yellow; they may be scattered, aggregated, or ring-like in their distributions (Figs. 41-1 and 41-2). Hard exudates result from leakage of lipoprotein material from retinal capillaries or microaneurysms into the outer retinal layer; and they may last from months to years.[19] The exudate forms preferentially in the posterior retina, especially temporal to the macula, and may extend into the macula, reducing visual acuity. On ophthalmoscopy, retinal hard exudates are sometimes confused with drusen, which are deposits of PAS-positive material located between the retinal pigment epithelium and Bruch's membrane. Drusen are not characteristic of diabetes, but occur frequently in older individuals. Differentiation between hard exudates and drusen may be difficult in some cases if the examination is done using the direct ophthalmoscope, without stereopsis; drusen are usually rounder, more regular, and less yellow than hard exudates.

In the more advanced stages of nonproliferative retinopathy, closure of the retinal capillaries and arterioles occurs, causing decreased nutrition to the inner layers of the retina. These changes cause whitish or grayish swellings in the nerve fiber layer of the retina, termed "cotton-wool spots" or "soft exudates," which are infarcts of the nerve fiber layer (Figs. 41-2 to 41-4). They remain only a few weeks to months. After their disappearance, the retina may appear normal on ophthalmoscopy, but nonperfusion of retinal arterioles may be seen in fluorescein angiography. In some patients with severe ischemia, occlusion of larger arterioles results in larger areas of irreversible retinal nonperfusion, especially in the retinal midperiphery. Late in the course of the disease, severe ischemia with thin-sheathed sclerotic (white "thread-like") arterioles may appear.

Another manifestation of focal retinal ischemia is the presence of dilated capillaries (intraretinal microvascular abnormalities [IRMAs]) (Fig. 41-3). IRMAs are found in areas of capillary nonperfusion and may be abnormally permeable to plasma proteins;

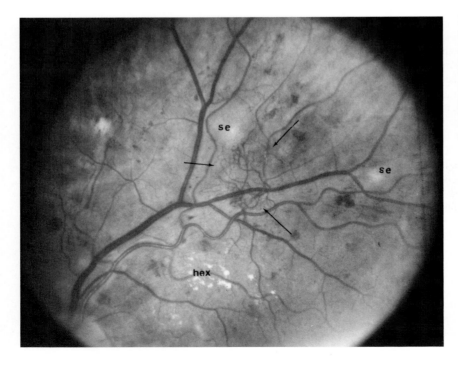

FIGURE 41-2. Fundus photograph of the left eye showing various lesions associated with nonproliferative and proliferative diabetic retinopathy in an area superior and temporal to the macula. Retinal hard exudates (**hex**) appear as white deposits with sharp margins. Soft exudates (**se**) or cotton-wool spots appear as grayish white areas with ill-defined edges. Retinal blot hemorrhages appear as spots of varying size with irregular margins and uneven densities. Retinal new vessels (**long black arrows**) are present.

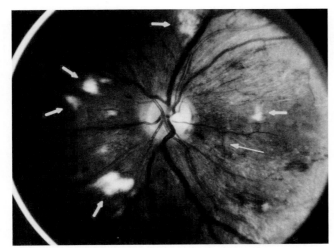

FIGURE 41-3. Fundus photograph of the left eye with preproliferative retinopathy. Soft exudates or cotton-wool spots appear as grayish white areas with ill-defined edges (**small thick white arrows**); intraretinal microvascular abnormalities (**thin white arrow**), venous dilation, and retinal hemorrhages are present. *(Reprinted with permission from Klein R: Retinopathy and other ocular complications in diabetes. In: Olefsky JM, Sherwin R, eds. Diabetes Mellitus: Management and Complications. Churchill Livingstone: 1985;101.)*

they are considered by some to be a compensatory response to hypoxia.[11] Venous beading, duplication, and kinks also occur in response to hypoxia in areas of focal ischemia (Fig. 41-4). These kinks or loops in eyes with diabetic retinopathy are thought to be shunt vessels developed to bypass a nonthrombotic occlusion of larger retinal veins.[20] Many large, dark intraretinal hemorrhages may also appear secondary to retinal ischemia and are thought to represent hemorrhagic infarcts (Fig. 41-4).[10]

FIGURE 41-4. Fundus photograph of the left eye. Retinal venous dilation and beading (**black arrows**) and an area of reduplication are present (**large white arrow**). Slow flow is manifested by "boxcaring" in the small retinal branch vein (**small white arrow**). Intraretinal microvascular abnormalities and a cotton-wool spot (**cw**) are present in this very ischemic retina. *(Reprinted with permission from Klein R: Retinopathy and other ocular complications in diabetes. In: Olefsky JM, Sherwin R, eds. Diabetes Mellitus: Management and Complications. Churchill Livingstone:1985;101.)*

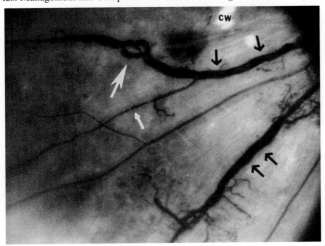

The presence of cotton-wool spots, venous irregularities, IRMAs, and dark intraretinal hemorrhages constitutes what has been called the "preproliferative phase"; eyes with these changes have a significantly increased risk of developing proliferative retinopathy.[10] In the Early Treatment Diabetic Retinopathy Study (ETDRS), eyes with multiple areas of venous beading, severe IRMAs, and large areas of intraretinal hemorrhages (ETDRS Level 55) had a 55% rate of progression to proliferative retinopathy over a 1-year interval.[21] Therefore the appearance of these lesions is considered a warning sign of impending growth of new retinal vessels.

Proliferative diabetic retinopathy is characterized by growth of abnormal blood vessels and fibrous tissue from the optic nerve head (Fig. 41-5) or from the inner retinal surface (usually near or from retinal veins) (Fig. 41-6). The vessels, which appear initially as fine tufts on the surface of the retina, subsequently grow into the outermost layer of the vitreous. Initially they consist of fine "naked"

FIGURE 41-5. Fundus photograph of the right eye. This sequence of photographs demonstrated progression from early proliferative retinopathy manifested initially as fine tufts of retinal new vessels on the optic disk (**A**, dated 2/75) (**black arrows**). There was further growth of retinal new vessels (**B**, dated 4/76) (**black arrows**). *(Reprinted with permission from Klein R: Retinopathy and other ocular complications in diabetes. In: Olefsky JM, Sherwin R, eds. Diabetes Mellitus: Management and Complications. Churchill Livingstone:1985;101.)*

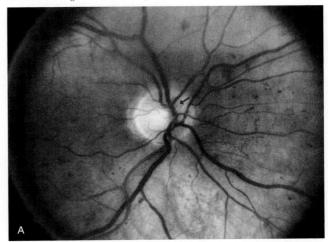

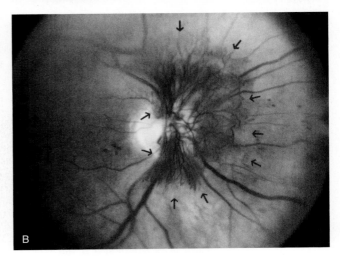

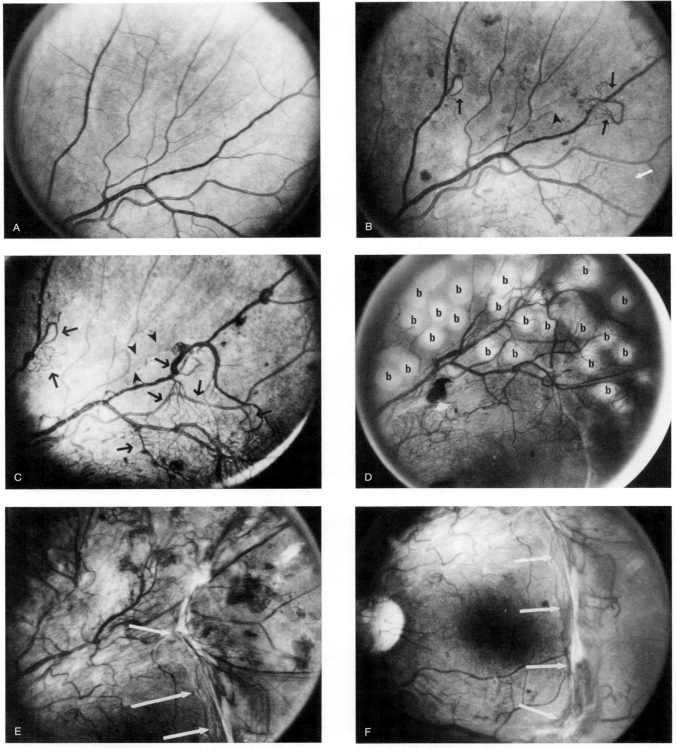

FIGURE 41-6. Fundus photograph of the left eye showing progression from nonproliferative to proliferative diabetic retinopathy in an area superior and temporal to the macula. **A**. When the patient was seen in 11/72 she was 25 years old and had a 14-year history of type 1 diabetic retinopathy. A few dilated capillaries and retinal microaneurysms are present here, and cotton-wool spots and blot hemorrhages were present in the macular area (not in photograph). The visual acuity was 20/15. **B**. In 3/76, flat retinal new vessels (**small black arrows**) are present. An abrupt termination of a branch arteriole (**black arrowhead**), intraretinal microvascular abnormalities (**white arrow**), and venous beading are present. **C**. By 10/76, there is an increase in the size of the retinal new vessels (**black arrows**) and the "feeder" vessel from the vein. The small arterioles above the vein are sheathed and appear white (**small black arrowheads**). **D**. This picture was taken in 2/77, 2 hours after laser treatment; the photocoagulation burns appear white (**b**). A small preretinal hemorrhage, appearing black, is present (**white arrowhead**).

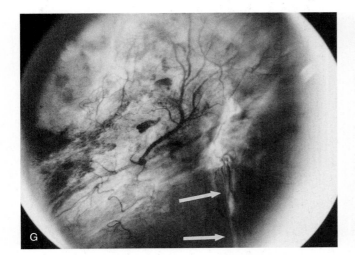

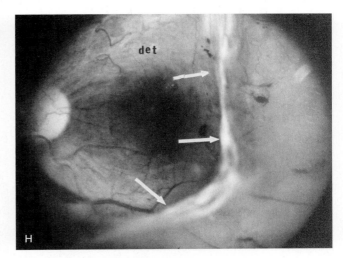

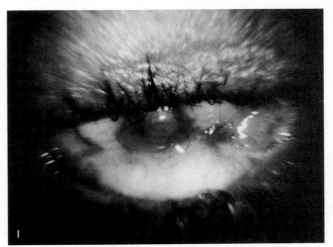

FIGURE 41-6 (continued) E, F. In 6/77 the visual acuity was 20/30. An area of fibrovascular proliferation with traction on the retina superior and temporal to the macula was present (**white arrows**). **G, H**. On 7/15/77 further elevation of fibroproliferative tissue (**white arrows**) led to increased traction with detachment (**det**) of the area above the macula. The visual acuity had dropped to 20/70. **I**. The macular area became detached, and she underwent a vitrectomy and scleral buckle on 7/28/77. Corneal edema and blood in the anterior chamber developed after surgery. Later the eye became phthisical, and she had no light perception when this photograph was taken in 10/78. Her other eye had been enucleated in 4/77 as a result of pain from rubeotic glaucoma, secondary to traction retinal detachment and vitreous hemorrhage. *(Courtesy of Dr. G. Bresnick, University of Wisconsin. Reprinted with permission from Klein R: Retinopathy and other ocular complications in diabetes. In: Olefsky JM, Sherwin R, eds.* Diabetes Mellitus: Management and Complications. *Churchill Livingstone:1985;101.)*

vessels, which are permeable to fluorescein. These vessels may hemorrhage into the vitreous.

The mesenchymal cells responsible for the development of new blood vessels may also form fibrous tissue. Contraction of fibrovascular tissue may result in traction detachment of the retina. Fibrous tissue predominates and may remain as the only evidence of proliferative retinopathy if regression of new vessels occurs later in the course of the disease.

Diabetic Macular Disease

Occlusion or increased permeability of the retinal microvasculature that results in abnormal structure or function of the macular area has been called a primary or intraretinal maculopathy. Traction or dragging of the sensory retina due to shrinkage of fibrovascular vit-

reoretinal membranes causing altered macular function has been called secondary or vitreoretinal maculopathy.[10]

Increased permeability of retinal capillaries and retinal microaneurysms may result in accumulation of extracellular fluid and thickening of the normally compact retinal tissue. Initially, there may be a slight loss of the normal transparency of the retina and the edema may be easily missed by direct ophthalmoscopy. The leakage and resulting edema may be distributed around retinal microaneurysms or be diffuse and in some cases lead to the appearance of cystoid spaces in the outer retina. Focal leakage from retinal microaneurysms or capillaries is usually associated with the deposition of hard exudative material, in either small clumps, rings, or large deposits (Fig. 41-7). The rings of hard exudate usually surround edematous centers of leaking retinal vessels and microaneurysms, and they demarcate the border of nonedematous and

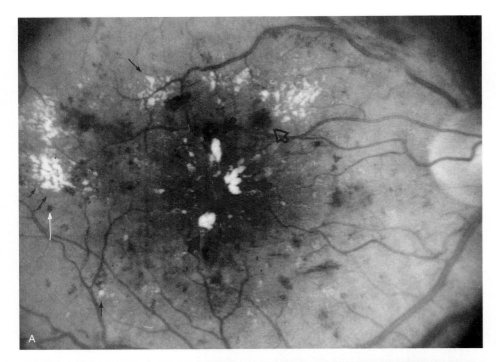

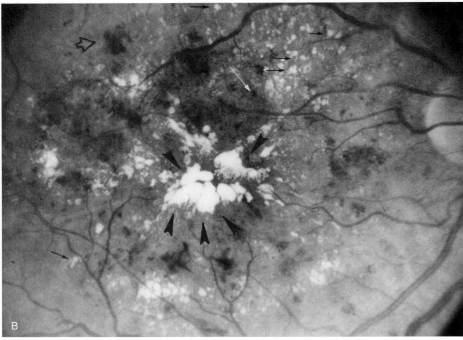

FIGURE 41-7. Fundus photographs of the macular area of the right eye demonstrating retinal hard exudates that appear as white deposits with sharp margins either scattered (**short thin black arrows**), ring-like (**short thick black arrows**), or aggregated in their distributions (**large black arrowheads**). Retinal blot hemorrhages (**white arrows**) and dark intraretinal hemorrhages (**large open black arrows**) are present. At the time photograph **A** was taken, the visual acuity was 20/15; 1 year later, when photograph **B** was taken, the visual acuity had dropped to 20/50. *(Reprinted with permission from Klein R: Retinopathy and other ocular complications in diabetes. In: Olefsky JM, Sherwin R, eds.* Diabetes Mellitus: Management and Complications. *Churchill Livingstone: 1985;101.)*

edematous retina. The accumulation of hard exudate in the macular area is usually gradual and may wax and wane, and spontaneous resolution of the exudate may occur in time.[19]

Macular edema appearing as diffuse thickening of the posterior retina is associated with retinal ischemia, and hard exudate is seldom present. The diffuse leakage of retinal blood vessels is a result of an extensive breakdown of the normally impermeable blood–retinal barrier of the capillary endothelial cells. Patients with diffuse edema have widespread extravasation of fluorescein dye from the capillaries to the retinal tissue during angiography. Based on the results of

the ETDRS,[8] macular edema was defined as either being "clinically or not clinically significant." In that study, clinically significant macular edema was associated with increased risk of loss of vision if left untreated with focal photocoagulation. Clinically significant macular edema was defined as the presence of either of the following: thickening of the retina located 500 μm or less from the center of the macula; or a zone of retinal thickening 1 disk area or larger in size, located within 1 disk diameter of the center of the macula.

Reduced oncotic pressure due to decreased serum albumin levels, increased intravascular fluid load, increased arteriolar perfusion pressure, and tissue hypoxia has been postulated to cause macular edema by exacerbating breakdown of the blood–retinal barrier.[22] Data from some studies suggest that high blood pressure, the presence of cardiovascular disease, and hyperlipidemia contribute to vascular occlusive disease in the retina with retinal ischemia and edema.[23] The presence of untreated diabetic renal failure has been thought to exacerbate the macular edema.[24] However, studies in patients with macular edema often fail to reveal a specific medical abnormality systematically associated with such edema.

Occlusion of small retinal vessels may result in enlargement of the normal 450- to 600-μm diameter foveal avascular zone. This may result in decreased visual acuity in the absence of macular edema.[10]

The vitreoretinal maculopathies all involve traction on the macular area, vary in severity, and result from a number of processes. A grayish or translucent glistening epiretinal glial membrane may be seen on the inner retinal surface, and contraction of this membrane may lead to a wrinkling effect. These membranes are also found in older nondiabetic patients, in diabetic patients with nonproliferative disease, and after panretinal photocoagulation, but they are more common in patients with proliferative retinopathy.

In patients with proliferative retinopathy, shrinkage of fibrovascular tissue and detachment of the posterior vitreous surface may lead to an elevation or displacement of the sensory retina at the macula. A macular detachment may result from traction, leading to a retinal tear with fluid accumulation beneath the retina including the macular area, and a significant decrease in visual acuity.

Classification

Most clinicians, using direct ophthalmoscopy, will classify retinopathy as either absent or present, or as absent, nonproliferative retinopathy present, or proliferative stage present. However, for natural history, epidemiologic studies, and clinical trials, more sensitive and reproducible systems are necessary.

The modified Airlie House classification of diabetic retinopathy[25] and the ETDRS classification for severity of retinopathy,[26] based on the natural history of the disease, have been developed for and used in a number of clinical and epidemiologic studies.[4,7,8,16,17] These systems allow specification of the presence or absence and the severity of major lesions characteristic of diabetic retinopathy, as well as the overall severity. One such severity scale is presented in Table 41-1. Data from the ETDRS demonstrated the validity of the scale. In that study, each stepwise increase in the severity level of retinopathy was associated with an increased risk of progression to proliferative retinopathy 4 years later.[21] In addition, in the WESDR, increasing severity of retinopathy as measured by the ETDRS severity scale at baseline was associated with increased risk of loss of vision over a 10-year follow-up.[27]

The ETDRS severity scale places greater emphasis on the moderate and more severe levels of diabetic retinopathy. Data from the WESDR suggest that microaneurysm counts from gradings of fundus photographs may provide a more sensitive measure of retinopathy severity in the earlier stages of disease.[13] Photographic documentation of retinopathy and use of photographic standards for grading severity of retinal lesions allows detection of early changes, minimizes observer bias by masking the graders with respect to patient characteristics and treatments, provides monitoring of quality control of the documentation, and permits comparisons over time. A number of studies have demonstrated that grading of stereoscopic fundus photographs is more sensitive than ophthalmoscopy in detecting retinopathy.[28] Computer-assisted grading of digitized images has also been used to determine the presence and severity of diabetic retinopathy.[29–32]

Pathogenesis

The exact pathogenesis of diabetic retinopathy is unknown (see Chap. 40). It is assumed that retinopathy is a consequence of hyperglycemia. This is supported by (1) the strong association of

TABLE 41-1.　Modified Early Treatment Diabetic Retinopathy Severity Scale

Retinopathy	Level	Detailed Descriptor
None	Level 10	No retinopathy
Nonproliferative	Level 21	Microaneurysms (Ma) only or retinal hemorrhages (H) or soft exudates (Se) in the absence of microaneurysms
	Level 31	Microaneurysms plus one or more of the following: Venous loops ≥31 μm; questionable Se, intraretinal microvascular abnormalities (IRMA), or venous beading; and retinal hemorrhage
	Level 37	Microaneurysms plus one or more of the following: hard exudate (hex) and Se
	Level 43	Microaneurysms plus one or more of the following: H/Ma ≥ standard photo (SP) #1 in 4–5 fields; H/Ma ≥ SP #2A in 1 field; and IRMA in 1–3 fields
	Level 47	Microaneurysms plus one or more of the following: Both IRMA and H/Ma characteristics from level 43; IRMA in 4–5 fields; H/Ma ≥ SP #2A in 2–3 fields; and venous beading in 1 field
Preproliferative	Level 53	Microaneurysms plus one or more of the following: Any 2–3 of level 47 characteristics; H/Ma ≥ SP #2A in 4–5 fields; IRMA ≥ SP #8A; venous beading in 2 or more fields
Proliferative without DRS high-risk characteristics for severe visual loss (DRS-HRC)	Level 60	Fibrous proliferations only
	Level 61	No evidence of levels 60 or 65 but scars of photocoagulation either in "scatter" or confluent patches, presumably directed at new vessels
	Level 65	Proliferative diabetic retinopathy less than Diabetic Retinopathy Study high-risk characteristics (DRS-HRC). Lesions as follows: New vessels elsewhere (NVE); new vessels on or within 1 disk diameter (NVD) of the disk graded less than SP #10A; and preretinal (PRH) or vitreous hemorrhage (VH) < 1 disk area (DA)
Proliferative with DRS-HRC	Level 71	DRS-HRC, lesions as follows: Vh and/or PRH ≥1 DA; NVE ≥ one-half DA with VH and/or PRH; NVD < SP #10A with VH and/or PRH; and NVD ≥ SP #10A
	Level 75	Advanced PDR, lesions as follows: NVD ≥ SP #10A with VH and/or PRH
Proliferative with DRS-HRC and loss of vision	Level 85	End stage PDR, lesions as follows: Macula obscured by VH and/or PRH; retinal detachment at center of macula; phthisis bulbi; and enucleation secondary to complications of diabetic retinopathy

Source: Klein et al.[78]

retinopathy with increasing duration of disease;[16,17] (2) the finding of retinopathy in secondary diabetes;[33] (3) the production of retinopathy in experimental diabetes in animal models;[34] and (4) the results of the epidemiologic studies and clinical trials that show a strong relationship of glycemia to the incidence and progression of retinopathy.[3,4,35–41] However, the actual mechanism by which high blood glucose levels lead to retinopathy is not known.

There are several hypothesized but unproven pathogenetic explanations.[10,11,42,43] One explanation is that hyperglycemia is an initiator of a number of biochemical changes, including an increase in aldose reductase activity, changes in myoinositol phosphatidylinositol metabolism, increases in 1,2-diacyl-sn-glycerol, nonenzymatic glycosylation, increased protein kinase C activity, decreased heparin sulfate proteoglycan, increased autooxidation, and changes in vasoactive substances such as endothelin, prostanoids, nitrous oxide, and histamine (see Chap. 13).[42]

Aldose reductase–initiated accumulation of sorbitol has been hypothesized to lead to selective degeneration of mural cells in the retinal capillaries.[43] A second role of the polyol pathway in diabetic retinopathy may be its relationship to the development of abnormal basement membrane thickening,[44] which has been hypothesized to cause closure of retinal capillary vessels. This thickening can be prevented by aldose reductase inhibitors in galactosemic rats.[44] Results from clinical trials of aldose reductase inhibitors in galactosemic animals have not been consistent.[45] In a randomized controlled clinical trial in people with T1DM, an aldose reductase inhibitor, sorbinil, was not found to prevent the incidence or progression of early diabetic retinopathy.[46]

The relationship of nonenzymatic or enzymatic glycosylation of proteins to the pathogenesis of retinopathy remains obscure. Clinical trials using aminoguanidine, which blocks glycosylation, have not shown the efficacy of this drug in preventing the progression of moderate to severe nonproliferative retinopathy.

Another proposed mechanism is abnormal release of growth hormone and growth factor changes (increased vascular endothelial and insulin-like growth factors) associated with impaired glucose metabolism.[47] Increased growth hormone has been hypothesized to result in plasma protein abnormalities (increases in alpha-2-globulins, fibrinogen, haptoglobins, and C-reactive proteins), which may be associated with increased plasma viscosity and decreased retinal blood flow. Using cell cultures, D'Amore and associates[48] have demonstrated that growth factors may be important in maintaining the integrity of retinal capillary endothelial and pericyte cells. Randomized controlled clinical trials using inhibitors of growth factors are now underway to determine their effect on the progression to proliferative retinopathy.

Whatever the cause, most proposed pathogenetic mechanisms are based on the assumption that retinal hypoxia is present early in the development of retinopathy.[49] Retinal hypoxia has been hypothesized to result from decreased oxygen release from hemoglobin, as has been reported by Ditzel and Standl in diabetic patients.[50] This has been attributed to decreased red blood cell 2,3-diphosphoglycerate, increased hemoglobin A_1, and increased blood lipids.[49,50] Another explanation for the development of hypoxia is that abnormalities in oxygen delivery result from altered retinal blood flow.[11,49] Abnormalities in retinal blood flow have been found even before the development of ophthalmoscopically-visible diabetic retinopathy.[50] Kohner[51] measured retinal blood flow based on an indicator dilution technique adapted to retinal blood vessels. She reported a decreased transit time of fluorescein dye and an increased volume flow in diabetic patients with no or early retinopathy compared to normal controls. Increased blood flow has also been found in the renal, cerebral, and peripheral circulations in persons with diabetes.[52] Kohner and colleagues have hypothesized that increased retinal blood flow may lead to damage of the retinal capillary pericytes and endothelial cells.[53]

With the appearance of nonproliferative retinopathy, retinal blood flow has been reported to be decreased.[54] Reduction in retinal blood flow in diabetes has been hypothesized to result from abnormalities in plasma viscosity, platelet and red blood cell function, blood vessel wall structure and permeability, and autoregulatory mechanisms.[10,49,50]

The initiation and progression of retinopathy is probably due to a complex relationship among a number of these factors, which vary at different stages in the natural history of retinopathy and from individual to individual. The pathophysiologic findings described above suggest that abnormalities in the diabetic microvasculature may play a primary role in diabetic retinopathy. Metabolic and physiologic alterations in the neuronal retina may also precede or accompany the circulatory changes. This is suggested by retinal functional abnormalities (e.g., color vision defects, electroretinogram changes, and delays in the visually evoked response) in diabetic patients without ophthalmoscopically detectable vascular retinopathy.[55,56]

Why the microvasculature is differentially affected in different organs is still an unanswered question. Although the brain and retina are both neural tissue, it is rare to find microvascular abnormalities in the brains of diabetic patients.

Little is known about the processes responsible for the formation of new retinal blood vessels. Retinal ischemia and resultant hypoxia are hypothesized to liberate retinal angiogenic substances. A number of angiogenic substances have been identified as being present in retinal tissue, but their role in the development of retinal new vessels remains unclear.[57,58] Also unclear is the role of the vitreous gel in inhibiting angiogenesis.

Epidemiology

Knowledge of the prevalence and incidence of diabetic retinopathy and various demographic, genetic, systemic, and ocular factors associated with retinopathy is of great importance in (1) efforts to prevent or modify the course of retinopathy; (2) characterization of the high-risk patient; and (3) estimation of health service needs. A number of epidemiologic studies have provided data about the natural history of diabetic retinopathy and its risk factors.[16,17,35–38,40,41,59–89] Data from one such study, the WESDR, a large geographically defined population of both type 1 and type 2 diabetic persons examined in 1980–1982, in 1984–1986, and again in 1990–1992, and type 1 diabetic persons in 1995–1996 are presented to provide information on the incidence and prevalence of retinopathy.[16,17,76–79] In addition, data from other epidemiologic studies are presented in Table 41-2.

Prevalence of Retinopathy

The prevalence and severity of diabetic retinopathy and macular edema in the baseline WESDR examination in 1980–1982 are presented in Table 41-3.[16,17,90] The highest frequencies of any retinopathy (71%) and of proliferative retinopathy (23%) were found in the younger-onset group, diagnosed prior to age 30 years and taking insulin (n = 996), whereas the lowest frequencies of any retinopathy (39%) and proliferative retinopathy (3%) were

TABLE 41-2. Selected List of Population-Based Studies Describing the Prevalence and/or Incidence of Diabetic Retinopathy

Author/Reference	Site	Type of Diabetes	Number Studied	Duration of Diabetes (y)	Retinopathy Detection*	Crude Prevalence (%)	Crude Incidence
Bennett et al,[59] Nelson et al[35]	Pima Indians, AZ	II	399	0–10+	O	18	—
			279		O		4y = 2.5%
Kahn et al[60]	Framingham, MA	II	229	—	O	18	
West et al,[61] Lee et al[36,37]	Oklahoma Indians	II	973	0–20+	O,P	24	10 − 16 = 72.3% (any)
Houston[62]	Poole, England	I	714	0–30+	O,P	Not reported	—
		II				Severe Ret. 8.3	
King et al[63]	Nauru, Central Pacific	II	343	0–10+	O	24	
Dwyer et al[64]	Rochester, MN	I	75	—	—	—	45.8/1000 person y
Ballard et al[38]	Rochester, MN	II	1060	—	O	—	15.6/1000 person y
Dyck et al[39]	Rochester, MN	I	102	2–64	P	79	—
		II	278	0–62	P	55	—
Danielsen et al[65]	Iceland	I	212	0–20+	P	34	—
Constable et al[66]	Perth, Australia	I	179	0–20+	O,P	33	—
Knuiman et al[67]		II	904	0–20+	O,P	27	—
Sjolie[68]	Country of Fynn, Denmark	I	718	0–30+	O	48	?
Nielsen[69,70]	Falster, Denmark	I	215	0–58	P	66	1 y = 3.7%
		II	333	0–42	P	41	1 y = 3.7%
Teuscher et al[40]	Switzerland	I	105	0–30+	O	51	8 y = 39%
		II	94			9	8 y = 15%
Haffner et al[71]	San Antonio, TX	II	257	0–10+	O,P	45	—
Jerneld[72]	Gotland, Sweden	I	160	0–20+	P	56–65	—
		II	140	0–20+		17	—
Hamman et al[73,74]	San Luis Valley, CO (Hispanics)	II	166	0–5+ 15+	P	19 88	—
McLeod et al[75]	Leicester, England	I	350	0–30+	O,P	41	—
Klein et al[16,17,76,77,78]	South Central, WI	I	996	0–30+	O,P	71	4 y = 59%
		II	1370	0–30+	O,P	39	4 y = 34%
Kostraba et al,[80] Lloyd et al[41]	Allegheny County, PA	I	657	6–38	O,P	86	2 y = 33%
Fujimoto and Fukuda[81]	Seattle, WA (2nd generation Japanese-American men)	I II	78	0–10+	O,P	11.5	
Cohen et al[82]	Oxford, England	II	294	—	O	—	60/1000 person y
Eriksson et al[83]	Narpes, West Finland	I	52	0–10+	O	54	—
		II	268	0–10+	O	12	—
Schachat et al[84]	Barbados, West Indies	II	266	—	O,P	—	—
Sparrow et al[85]	Melton Mowbray	II	145	1–35	O,P	52	—
Wirta et al[86]	Tampere, SW Finland	II	133	<1	O,P	6	—
			125	1–25	O,P	40	—
Falkenberg et al[87]	Kisa, Sweden	II	120	0–20+	O	27	—
Hapnes et al[88]	Eigersund, Norway	I	32	—	P	33	—
		II	178	—	P	10	—
Jones et al[89]	Norway	I	371	6–17	P	33	—
Harris et al[92]	United States	II White	345	0–15+	P	18	—
		Black	261	0–15+	P	27	—
		Hispanic	308	0–15+	P	33	—

* O = ophthalmoscopy; P = photography

Source: Reprinted with permission from Klein R, Klein BEK, Moss S. The Wisconsin Epidemiologic Study of Diabetic Retinopathy: A review. *Diabetes Metab Rev* 1989;5:559.

present in the older-onset group not taking insulin who were diagnosed with diabetes at or after 30 years of age (n = 692). While the proportions of proliferative retinopathy and macular edema were highest in the WESDR younger-onset group, the largest number of people with proliferative retinopathy or macular edema had older-onset diabetes (for proliferative retinopathy, 326 people in the older-onset groups compared with 240 people in the younger-onset group; for clinically significant macular edema, 272 people in the older-onset group compared with 56 people in the younger-onset group). Similar differences in the prevalence of retinopathy in younger- and older-onset diabetes have been reported in other epidemiologic studies (Table 41-2). Based on the WESDR data, it is estimated that in 1980–1982, approximately 700,000 people in the United States with diabetes had proliferative retinopathy, 130,000 of whom had Diabetic Retinopathy Study (DRS) high-risk characteristics for severe visual loss of 5/200 or worse and 325,000 had clinically significant macular edema.

TABLE 41-3. Prevalence and Severity of Retinopathy by Sex at the Baseline Examination in the Wisconsin Epidemiologic Study of Diabetic Retinopathy (1980–1982)

Retinopathy Status	*Younger-Onset Taking Insulin*			*Older-Onset Taking Insulin*			*Older-Onset Not Taking Insulin*		
	Male (%) (n = 512)	Female (%) (n = 484)	Total (%) (n = 996)	Male (%) (n = 321)	Female (%) (n = 352)	Total (%) (n = 673)	Male (%) (n = 313)	Female (%) (n = 379)	Total (%) (n = 692)
None	31.1	27.5	29.3	26.8	32.7	29.9	64.5	58.6	61.3
Early nonproliferative	26.4	34.7	30.4	34.0	27.6	30.6	25.9	28.5	27.3
Moderate to severe nonproliferative	18.2	16.9	17.6	27.7	23.9	25.7	6.4	10.3	8.5
Proliferative without DRS* high-risk characteristics	12.3	14.0	13.2	8.1	9.9	9.1	1.9	1.1	1.4
Proliferative with DRS high-risk characteristics or worse	12.1	6.8	9.5	3.4	6.0	4.8	1.3	1.6	1.4
Clinically significant macular edema	(n = 489) 6.3	(n = 464) 5.4	(n = 953) 5.9	(n = 306) 10.5	(n = 325) 12.6	(n = 631) 11.6	(n = 304) 2.6	(n = 368) 4.6	(n = 672) 3.7

*DRS = Diabetic Retinopathy Study

Source: Klein *et al.*[16]

Incidence and Progression of Diabetic Retinopathy

The highest incidence and progression of retinopathy over the 10 years of the study were found in the younger-onset group, whereas the lowest incidence and progression were found in the older-onset group not taking insulin (Tables 41-4 and 41-5).[76–78] In the younger-onset group, 89.3% without retinopathy and 29.8% without proliferative retinopathy at baseline developed retinopathy and proliferative retinopathy, respectively, by the time of the 10-year follow-up. The 10-year incidence of proliferative retinopathy was 10% in the older-onset group not taking insulin at baseline. The estimates of incident cases of proliferative retinopathy in the 10-year period are higher in the group with older-onset than in the group with younger-onset (387 versus 226). These data emphasize the need for timely referral and appropriate ophthalmologic care for people with older-onset diabetes.

Despite marked changes in the management of insulin-dependent diabetes over the 10-year follow-up period of the WESDR, there were few significant differences in the estimated annual incidence of proliferative diabetic retinopathy over the first 4 years of the study compared to the last 6 years of the study (Fig. 41-8). Based on the WESDR data, it is estimated that over the 10-year period, of the 5,800,000 Americans with known diabetes in 1980, 915,000 will have developed proliferative retinopathy, and 320,000 will have developed proliferative retinopathy with DRS high-risk characteristics.

Risk Factors for Diabetic Retinopathy

Race and Ethnicity

Recent data suggest differences in the prevalence and incidence of diabetic retinopathy among different racial and ethnic groups.[35–37,77] Data from studies in Pima Indians and Oklahoma Indians with

TABLE 41-4. Ten-Year Incidence of any Retinopathy, Improvement or Progression of Retinopathy, or Progression to PDR* by Sex in People with Younger-Onset Diabetes (Type 1). Wisconsin Epidemiologic Study of Diabetic Retinopathy

Ten-Year	Male	Female	Total
No. at risk	142	119	261
Incidence of any retinopathy, %	93.0	84.9	89.3
95% CI	88.6, 97.4	78.2, 91.6	85.4, 93.2
No. at risk	184	200	384
Improvement, %	6.9	12.4	9.8
95% CI	3.1, 10.6	7.8, 17.1	6.7, 12.9
No. at risk	354	358	712
Progression, %	80.2	71.6	75.8
95% CI	75.8, 84.5	66.7, 76.4	72.5, 79.1
Progression to PDR, %	29.0	30.5	29.8
95% CI	24.1, 33.9	25.6, 35.4	26.3, 33.3

* PDR indicates proliferative diabetic retinopathy; CI, confidence interval. Number at risk for incidence of any retinopathy refers to the group that had no retinopathy (level 10/10) at the baseline examination and were at risk of developing retinopathy at the follow-up examination. Number at risk for improvement in retinopathy refers to those with retinopathy levels of 21/21 to 53/53 at the baseline examination who could have a decrease in their retinopathy severity by at least two steps or more at follow-up. Number at risk for no change, progression, or progression to PDR refers to those with retinopathy levels 10/10 to 53/53 who either did not change by two or more steps or progressed by two or more steps.

Source: Klein *et al.*[78]

TABLE 41-5. Ten-Year Incidence of Any Retinopathy, Improvement or Progression of Retinopathy or Progression to PDR* by Sex in People with Older-Onset Diabetes. Wisconsin Epidemiologic Study of Diabetic Retinopathy

Ten-Year	Using Insulin			Not Using Insulin		
	Male	Female	Total	Male	Female	Total
No. at risk	58	88	146	144	157	301
Incidence of any retinopathy, %	76.9	80.4	79.2	69.1	65.3	66.9
95% CI	62.1, 91.7	69.4, 91.3	70.4, 88.0	59.6, 78.5	56.6, 73.9	60.5, 73.3
Improvement, %	18.6	23.7	21.1	17.5	30.0	26.0
95% CI	10.6, 26.6	15.1, 32.4	15.2, 27.0	5.7, 29.3	18.9, 41.0	17.3, 34.6
No. at risk	194	223	417	217	270	487
Progression, %	66.2	70.8	68.7	54.8	51.5	52.9
95% CI	57.6, 74.9	63.2, 78.4	63.0, 74.5	46.3, 63.2	44.1, 58.8	47.4, 58.5
Progression to PDR, %	24.8	22.6	23.6	6.7	11.8	9.7
95% CI	16.8, 32.7	15.8, 29.4	18.4, 28.8	2.5, 10.9	7.0, 16.7	6.4, 13.1

* PDR indicates proliferative diabetic retinopathy; CI, confidence interval. Number at risk for incidence of any retinopathy refers to the group that had no retinopathy (level 10/10) at the baseline examination and were at risk of developing retinopathy at the follow-up examination. Number at risk for improvement in retinopathy refers to those with retinopathy levels of 21/21 to 51/51 at the baseline examination who could have a decrease in their retinopathy severity by at least two steps or more at follow-up. Number at risk for no change, progression, or progression to PDR refers to those with retinopathy levels 10/10 to 51/51 who either did not change by two or more steps or progressed by two or more steps.

T2DM showed a higher risk of developing proliferative retinopathy than found in the non-Hispanic whites with T2DM in the WESDR. In addition, Pima Indians with T2DM are more likely to develop diabetic nephropathy than whites with this disease.[91] The explanation for these differences is not clear. It is possible that Pima and Oklahoma Indians may have been exposed to longer periods of more severe hyperglycemia at a younger age than whites with T2DM.

Few studies have examined racial differences using similar protocols to measure risk factors and to detect diabetic retinopathy. One such study was the Third National Health and Nutrition Examination Survey (NHANES III), in which a representative population-based sample of people age ≥40 years in each of three racial/ethnic groups were examined.[92] Prevalence of diabetic retinopathy in people with diagnosed diabetes was 84% higher in Mexican-Americans compared with non-Hispanic whites. Mexican-Americans also had higher rates of moderate and severe retinopathy and higher levels of many putative risk factors for retinopathy. While controlling for other measures of diabetes severity (duration of diabetes, hemoglo-

bin A_{1c} level, insulin and oral agent use) and systolic blood pressure, the risk of retinopathy in Mexican-Americans was twice that of non-Hispanic whites. Another such study, the San Antonio Study of Diabetic Complications, employed methods similar to those used in the WESDR.[71] After controlling for other known risk factors, Mexican-Americans with T2DM in San Antonio had 1.7 times higher prevalence of any retinopathy than did non-Hispanic whites with T2DM in the WESDR. However, similar frequencies of retinopathy were found in Hispanic whites with T2DM in San Luis Valley, Colorado, and non-Hispanic whites with T2DM in the WESDR, suggesting that geographic and unmeasured factors may result in variations within similar ethnic groups.[73]

Observations from clinical studies suggest a higher frequency of retinopathy in African-Americans attending ophthalmology clinics.[93] However, data from a recent study in St. Louis showed that the prevalence and incidence of retinopathy was lower in blacks than in whites with T1DM.[94] In the NHANES III, the prevalence of retinopathy was 46% higher in non-Hispanic blacks than in non-Hispanic whites.[92] However, while controlling for measures of diabetes severity and blood pressure, non-Hispanic blacks were not at higher risk for retinopathy than non-Hispanic whites. These data suggest that differences in diabetes severity and glycemic control in persons with T2DM may explain black/white differences.

The prevalence of retinopathy in second-generation (Nisei) diabetic Japanese-Americans (12%) in Seattle was significantly lower than that reported in the diabetes clinic at Tokyo University Hospital (49% among patients with an onset of diabetes between 20 and 59 years of age and 47% among those with an onset after 59 years of age) and in diabetic white men not taking insulin reported in the WESDR (36%).[81]

There is a need to compare the distributions of known risk factors to explain the variations of retinopathy incidence and progression in different ethnic and racial groups. This is difficult because of variations from study to study in the detection and definition of diabetes and diabetic retinopathy.

Genetic

The relationships of specific genetic factors to increased susceptibility to diabetic retinopathy are not clear. Support for a

FIGURE 41-8. Estimated annual incidence of proliferative retinopathy in first 4 years and next 6 years in the younger-onset group taking insulin and the older-onset groups taking and not taking insulin in the Wisconsin Epidemiologic Study of Diabetic Retinopathy.

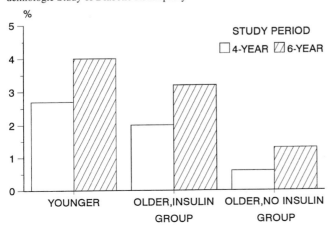

genetic relationship has come from studies that have shown that the severity and onset of retinopathy are similar among concordant identical twins.[95] In the Diabetes Control and Complications Trial (DCCT), familial clustering of diabetic retinopathy was investigated.[96] Familial associations were assessed by comparing the frequency of retinopathy in diabetic relatives of the respective positive versus negative DCCT subjects. There was an increased risk of severe retinopathy (odds ratio 3.1, 95% CI 1.2–7.8) among relatives of retinopathy-positive versus retinopathy-negative DCCT subjects among families of subjects with T1DM in the study. These findings suggest that severity of diabetic retinopathy is influenced by possible genetic factors.

Some studies have found relationships with various HLA antigens while others have not.[97,98] In the WESDR younger-onset group, after adjusting for characteristics associated with proliferative retinopathy such as glycosylated hemoglobin, hypertension, duration of diabetes, and gross proteinuria, the presence of DR4 and the absence of DR3 were associated with a 5.4-fold increase in the odds of having proliferative retinopathy present compared with the absence of both DR4 and DR3.[99] However, in a 6-year follow-up of the same cohort, people with HLA-DR4 were less likely to have progression to proliferative retinopathy during the follow-up than those without this antigen (29.4% versus 43.5%). This relationship remained while controlling for other risk factors. The reasons for this discrepancy with prevalence and incidence data are not known. No other HLA antigens predicted the incidence and progression of retinopathy in the WESDR.

The reasons why specific HLA-DR antigens would increase the risk of developing more severe retinopathy are not apparent. Study of specific genetic factors associated with the pathogenesis of retinopathy, such as glycosylation, aldose reductase activity, collagen formation, and platelet adhesiveness and aggregation may yield a better understanding of the possible causal relationships between genetic factors and diabetic retinopathy.

There is a growing list of candidate genes involved in the pathogenesis of diabetic retinopathy that are being investigated. These include genes involved in inflammation, coagulation, vascular proliferation, glycosylation, metabolism of sugar (such as the polyol pathway), and in regulating vascular tone. Detection of such genes could result in the development of more specific therapeutic approaches for preventing the incidence and progression of retinopathy (see Chaps. 13 and 40).

Sex

Few differences in the prevalence and incidence of retinopathy in men and women with T1DM or T2DM have been reported. In the WESDR, there was a slightly higher prevalence of severe proliferative diabetic retinopathy with high risk for severe visual loss in younger-onset males (12%) compared to females (7%).[16] The prevalence of proliferative retinopathy was similar in men and women with T1DM in Pittsburgh.[80]

Time-Related Variables

Age and Puberty

It is rare to find signs of diabetic retinopathy in children who are less than 10 years of age, regardless of the duration of T1DM.[16,100] After this age, the frequency and severity of retinopathy begins to increase. It has been hypothesized that a protective effect, lost after the start of puberty, is responsible for this.

In the WESDR, menarchal status at the time of the baseline examination was related to the prevalence and severity of retinopathy.[101] After controlling for other risk factors, those who were postmenarchal were 3.2 times as likely to have retinopathy as those who were premenarchal. In a follow-up study of 60 insulin-dependent diabetic children, Frost-Larsen and Starup[102] found the incidence of retinopathy to be higher after puberty than before, independent of duration or metabolic control of diabetes, or type of treatment. These findings have been observed in a number of other studies.[103,104] Increases in growth hormone, insulin-like growth factor I, sex hormones, blood pressure, and poorer glycemic control (due to increased insulin resistance, poorer compliance, and/or inadequate insulin dosage) have been hypothesized to explain the higher risk of developing retinopathy after puberty. Age has less of an effect on the prevalence or incidence of diabetic retinopathy in older-onset diabetics. In the WESDR, few people 75 years of age or older with T2DM developed proliferative retinopathy over the 10 years of follow-up.[78]

Duration of Diabetes

The frequency and severity of diabetic retinopathy, proliferative retinopathy, and macular edema increase with increasing duration of diabetes. The prevalence of retinopathy 3–4 years after diagnosis of diabetes in the WESDR younger-onset group with T1DM was 14.5% in males and 24% in females, and in all cases it was mild (Fig. 41-9).[16] However, in persons with diabetes for

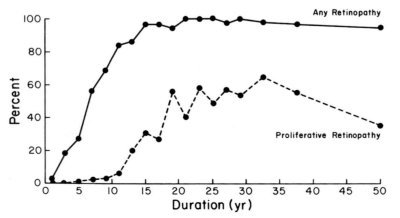

FIGURE 41-9. The frequency of retinopathy or proliferative retinopathy by duration of diabetes in years in 995 insulin-taking persons diagnosed to have diabetes before 30 years of age who participated in the Wisconsin Epidemiologic Study of Diabetic Retinopathy. *(Reprinted with permission from Klein et al.[16])*

19–20 years, 50% of males and 33% of females had proliferative retinopathy. Early after diagnosis of diabetes, retinopathy was more frequent in the older-onset group compared with the younger-onset group (Fig. 41-10).[17] In the first 3 years after diagnosis of diabetes, 23% of the older-onset group not taking insulin had retinopathy, and 2% had proliferative retinopathy. However, after 20 years of diabetes, fewer older-onset persons not taking insulin had retinopathy (60% versus 99%) or proliferative retinopathy (5% versus 53%) than younger-onset people.

Harris and coworkers[105] extrapolated data regarding retinopathy prevalence at different durations of diabetes from older-onset participants in the WESDR and in a study in Australia, to the time when retinopathy prevalence was estimated to be zero. They calculated that the onset of detectable retinopathy occurred about 4–7 years before diagnosis of T2DM in these populations.

In the WESDR, the prevalence of macular edema rose from zero in younger-onset persons with diabetes duration of 5 years to 21% in persons with diabetes duration of more than 20 years.[90] The prevalence of macular edema also varied with increasing duration of diabetes, ranging from 3% at 5 years to 13% at 15 years or more in noninsulin-taking patients. In a referral practice at the Joslin Clinic, macular edema was found to be more common (45%) in type 2 diabetic patients diagnosed after 40 years of age than in type 1 diabetic patients (17%) who were diagnosed before 30 years of age.[106]

In the WESDR, the 4- and 10-year incidence of diabetic retinopathy increased with increasing duration of diabetes at baseline.[76–78] The risk of developing retinopathy in the younger-onset group remained high (74%) even after 10 years of diabetes. The 4-year incidence of proliferative retinopathy varied from zero during the first 3 years after diagnosis of diabetes to 28% in younger-onset people with 13–14 years of diabetes. Thereafter the incidence remained stable.[76] This was also seen in a cohort of type 1 diabetic patients followed at the Joslin Clinic.[107] In the older-onset WESDR groups, 2% of those with less than 5 years' duration and 4.9% of those with 15 or more years of diabetes who were not taking insulin at baseline developed signs of proliferative retinopathy at the 4-year follow-up.[77]

Data from other population-based studies describing the incidence and progression of diabetic retinopathy are presented in Table 41-2. Data from the WESDR and other studies suggest that prior to puberty or within 5 years of diagnosis, younger-onset persons with insulin-dependent diabetes do not need an ophthalmoscopic examination to detect proliferative retinopathy or macular edema.

Age at Diagnosis

Age at diagnosis was not related to incidence or progression of diabetic retinopathy in any of the diabetes groups followed in the WESDR.[76,77] However, after controlling for other risk factors in a cohort with T2DM in Rochester, Minnesota, the development of retinopathy was associated with younger age at diagnosis.[38]

Control of Hyperglycemia

Review of the existing experimental literature using animal models leaves little doubt as to the strong relationship between good glycemic control and less retinopathy.[34,108,109] Epidemiologic studies have consistently demonstrated an association between good glycemic control and the incidence and progression of diabetic retinopathy (Table 41-6).[3,4,35–38,40,41,110,111] The WESDR data demonstrated that lower blood sugar at any stage of retinopathy prior to the proliferative phase and at any duration of diabetes was associated with lower incidence and progression of retinopathy (Figs. 41-11, 41-12, and 41-13).[3] However, the WESDR and other epidemiologic studies could not address the question of underlying severity of the diabetes, independently leading to both poorer control and more severe retinopathy. This could be addressed only by randomized therapeutic trials of metabolic control. The results of these trials suggest that achievement of glycemic control in individuals with previous poor control and nonproliferative retinopathy might be done slowly to potentially minimize the risk of progression to the more severe preproliferative or proliferative phase of the disease.

The DCCT was a large randomized controlled clinical trial of 1441 patients with type 1 diabetes.[4] It showed that intensive

FIGURE 41-10. The frequency of retinopathy or proliferative retinopathy by duration of diabetes in years in 673 insulin-taking and 697 noninsulin-taking persons diagnosed to have diabetes after 29 years of age who participated in the Wisconsin Epidemiologic Study of Diabetic Retinopathy. *(Reprinted with permission from Klein et al.[16])*

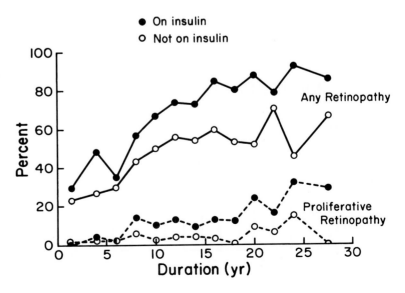

TABLE 41-6 Characteristics Associated with the Prevalence and/or Incidence or Progression of Diabetic Retinopathy from Selected Population-Based Studies

Author/Reference	Type of Diabetes	Hyperglycemia	High Blood Pressure	History of Smoking	History of Renal Disease	High Lipids
Bennett et al,[59] Nelson et al[35]	II	Yes	Yes	—	—	—
West et al,[61] Lee et al[36,37]	II	Yes	No/Yes*	No	Yes/No*	No/Yes*
Houston[62]	I	—	Yes	—	—	—
	II	—	Yes	—	—	—
King et al[63]	II	Yes	Yes	—	—	—
Ballard et al[38]	**II**	**Yes**	**No**	**No**	**No**	**—**
Danielsen et al[65]	I	No	—	—	—	—
Knuiman et al[67]	I	Yes	Yes	—	Yes	No
	II	Yes	Yes	—	Yes	No
Sjolie et al[68]	I	Yes	No	Yes	No	—
Teuscher et al[40]	**I**	**No**	**Yes**	**—**	**—**	**—**
	II	**Yes**	**Yes**	**—**	**—**	**—**
Haffner et al[71]	II	Yes	Yes	No	Yes	—
Jerneld[72]	I	Yes	—	—	Yes	—
	II	Yes	—	—	—	—
Hamman et al[73]	II	Yes	Yes	Yes	—	No
McLeod et al[75]	I	No	Yes	—	—	—
Klein et al[3,16,17,76–78,121,128,132,137]	**I**	**Yes**	**Yes**	**No**	**Yes**	**Yes**
Moss et al[136]	**II**	**Yes**	**Yes/No†**	**No**	**No**	**—**
Kostraba et al,[104] **Lloyd et al[41]**	**I**	**Yes**	**Yes**	**No**	**Yes**	**Yes**
Fujimoto and Fukuda[81]	II	Yes	—	—	—	—

Bold, incidence data

* No relationship of high blood pressure or high cholesterol with prevalence, significant relationship with incidence; relationship of gross proteinuria is significant with prevalence but not incidence or retinopathy.

† Relationship of high blood pressure with prevalence but not 4-year incidence of retinopathy is significant.

Source: Reprinted with permission from Klein R, Klein BEK, Moss SE: The Wisconsin Epidemiological Study of Diabetic Retinopathy: A review. *Diabetes Metab Rev* 1989;5:559.

FIGURE 41-11. Relation of 4-year incidence of diabetic retinopathy by quartiles of glycosylated hemoglobin at baseline in younger-onset persons taking insulin and older-onset persons taking and not taking insulin at baseline in the Wisconsin Epidemiologic Study of Diabetic Retinopathy. The ranges for baseline glycosylated hemoglobin in the younger-onset group (**YO-I**) are first quartile: 6.0–10.8%; second quartile: 10.9–12.2%; third quartile: 12.3–14.1%; and fourth quartile: 14.2–23.3%. The ranges for baseline glycosylated hemoglobin in the older-onset group taking insulin (**OO-I**) are first quartile: 6.9–10.1%; second quartile: 10.2–11.8%; third quartile: 11.9–13.4%; and fourth quartile: 13.5–19.2%. The ranges for baseline glycosylated hemoglobin in the older-onset group not taking insulin (**OO-NI**) are first quartile: 6.2–8.5%; second quartile: 8.6–9.8%; third quartile: 9.9–11.6%; and fourth quartile: 11.7–23.6%.

glycemic control was associated with a reduced risk of incidence and progression of retinopathy, progression to preproliferative and proliferative retinopathy, incidence of macular edema, and the need for panretinal photocoagulation compared to conventional insulin treatment (Table 41-7 and Fig. 41-14). These data indicate a favorable risk:benefit ratio for intensive glycemic control for most people with T1DM with no or early nonproliferative retinopathy. On

FIGURE 41-12. Relation of 4-year progression of diabetic retinopathy by quartiles of glycosylated hemoglobin at baseline in younger-onset persons taking insulin (**YO-I**) and older-onset persons taking (**OO-I**) and not taking (**OO-NI**) insulin at baseline in the Wisconsin Epidemiologic Study of Diabetic Retinopathy.

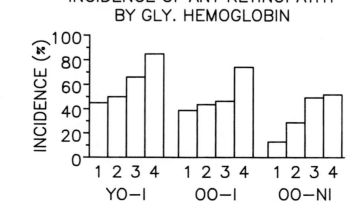

INCIDENCE OF ANY RETINOPATHY BY GLY. HEMOGLOBIN

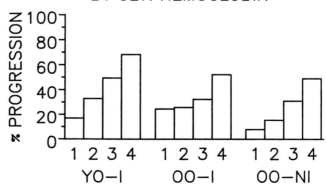

PROGRESSION OF RETINOPATHY BY GLY. HEMOGLOBIN

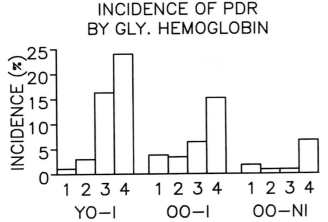

FIGURE 41-13. Relation of 4-year incidence of proliferative diabetic retinopathy by quartiles of glycosylated hemoglobin at baseline in younger-onset persons taking insulin (**YO-I**) and older-onset persons taking (**OO-I**) and not taking (**OO-NI**) insulin at baseline in the Wisconsin Epidemiologic Study of Diabetic Retinopathy.

average, 3 years were required to demonstrate the beneficial effect of intensive treatment. After 3 years, the beneficial effect of intensive insulin treatment increased over time. In addition, the DCCT data did not support the concept of a glycemic threshold regarding progression of retinopathy.

An early worsening of retinopathy in the first year of treatment of the intensive therapy group in the secondary-intervention cohort was observed. This finding was similar to those reported by earlier feasibility clinical trials of intensive treatment in patients with T1DM.[112-114] The results suggest that achievement of glycemic control in individuals with previous poor control and nonproliferative retinopathy might be done slowly to potentially minimize the risk of progression to the more severe preproliferative or proliferative phase of the disease.

The United Kingdom Prospective Diabetes Study (UKPDS) was a randomized controlled clinical trial involving 3867 newly di-

agnosed patients with T2DM.[5,115] After 3 months of diet treatment, patients with a mean of two fasting plasma glucose concentrations of 6.1–15.0 mmol/L were randomly assigned to an intensive glycemic control group with either a sulfonylurea (chlorpropamide, glibenclamide, or glipizide) or with insulin or a conventional glycemic control group with diet. After 10 years of follow-up, hemoglobin A_{1c} was 7.0% in the intensive group and 7.9% in the conventional group. Compared with the conventional group, the risk reduction for progression of diabetic retinopathy (defined as two or more steps on the ETDRS severity scale) over a 12-year period in the intensive group was 21%. In addition, there was a 29% reduction in the need for retinal photocoagulation in the intensive compared to the conventional group. These data conclusively showed that intensive treatment with either sulfonylureas or insulin significantly reduced the risk of progression of retinopathy in persons with T2DM.

C-Peptide Status

Data from studies regarding the relationship between endogenous insulin secretion in those with T2DM, independent of glycemic control, to retinopathy, are not consistent.[116-118] After controlling for characteristics associated with retinopathy in the older-onset group with T2DM in the WESDR, there was no relationship between plasma C peptide and retinopathy.[118] These findings suggest that the level of glycemia and not the level of endogenous C peptide is more important in determining the presence and severity of retinopathy in people with T2DM.

Exogenous Insulin

Exogenous insulin has been postulated to be a possible cause of atherosclerotic vascular disease and retinopathy in people with T2DM.[119] In the WESDR, there was no association between the amount or type of exogenous insulin used and the presence and severity of retinopathy in the older-onset group using insulin whose C peptide was ≥0.3 nmol/L.[118] These data suggest that exogenous insulin itself is probably not causally related to retinopathy in diabetic people with normal C peptide.

TABLE 41-7. Development and Progression of Long-Term Complications of Diabetes in the Study Cohorts and Reduction in Risk with Intensive as Compared with Conventional Therapy*

| Complications | *Primary Prevention* | | | *Secondary Intervention* | | | *Both Cohorts†* |
	Conventional Therapy Rate/100 patient-y	Intensive Therapy Rate/100 patient-y	Risk Reduction % (95% CI)	Conventional Therapy Rate/100 patient-y	Intensive Therapy Rate/100 patient-y	Risk Reduction % (95% CI)	Risk Reduction % (95% CI)
≥3-Step sustained retinopathy	4.7	1.2	76 (62–85)‡	7.8	3.7	54 (39–66)‡	63 (52–71)‡
Macular edema§	—	—	—	3.0	2.0	23 (213–48)	26 (28–50)
Severe nonproliferative or proliferative retinopathy §	—	—	—	2.4	1.1	47 (14–67)¶	47 (15–67)¶
Laser treatment¶ #	—	—	—	2.3	0.9	56 (26–74)‡	51 (21–70)¶

* Rates shown are absolute rates of the development and progression of complications per 100 patient-years. Risk reductions represent the comparison of intensive with conventional treatment, expressed as a percentage and calculated from the proportional-hazards model with adjustment for baseline values as noted, except in the case of neuropathy. CI denotes confidence interval.

† Stratified according to the primary-prevention and secondary-prevention cohorts.

‡ $p \leq 0.002$ by the two-tailed rank-sum test.

§ Too few events occurred in the primary-prevention cohort to allow meaningful analysis of this variable.

¶ $p < 0.04$ by the two-tailed rank-sum test.

# Denotes the first episode of laser therapy for macular edema or proliferative retinopathy.

Source: The DCCT Research Group.[4]

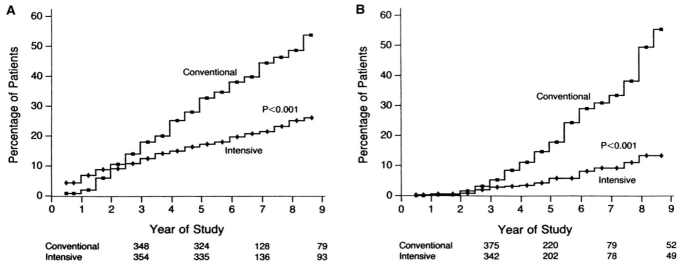

FIGURE 41-14. Cumulative incidence of a sustained change in retinopathy in patients with T1DM receiving intensive or conventional therapy in **A. (left panel)** the primary prevention and **B. (right panel)** the secondary intervention arms of the Diabetes Control and Complications Trial. *(Reprinted with permission from the DCCT Research Group.[4])*

Blood Pressure

Because high blood pressure *per se* can cause many of the lesions associated with diabetic retinopathy (eg, cotton-wool spots, retinal hemorrhages, and microaneurysms), it is not unexpected that a positive association between blood pressure and severity of retinopathy has been reported by a number of investigators.[16,17,59,62,63,67,71,73,75] Increased blood pressure, through an effect on blood flow, has been hypothesized to damage the retinal capillary endothelial cells, resulting in the development and progression of retinopathy.[53] The relative risk (RR) for the presence of retinopathy during the first 10 years of diabetes for the WESDR younger-onset insulin-taking persons with diastolic blood pressure in the highest quartile compared to those in the lowest quartile was about 2; for persons with 10 years or more of diabetes, the RR of proliferative retinopathy in persons whose diastolic blood pressure was in the highest quartile compared to those whose diastolic blood pressure was in the lowest quartile was also about 2.[16] Similarly, the highest risk for retinopathy was reported for persons with highest blood pressure in the older-onset insulin- or noninsulin-taking persons.[17]

Macular edema has also been reported to be associated with increased blood pressure. Deutsch and associates[120] found that patients with macular edema in one clinic in the ETDRS had higher mean blood pressure than patients without edema. Similar findings have been reported in the WESDR for insulin- or noninsulin-taking persons.[90]

In contrast to cross-sectional observation, data regarding the relationship between high blood pressure or hypertension and the development and progression of retinopathy have not yielded consistent findings (Table 41-6).[35–38,40,41,121] In an 8-year follow-up of Swiss patients with T2DM, Teuscher and coworkers[40] found that those with uncontrolled hypertension were more likely to have their retinopathy progress than those whose blood pressure was controlled. In the WESDR, systolic blood pressure was a significant predictor of the 4-year incidence of diabetic retinopathy, diastolic blood pressure was a predictor for the 4-year progression of retinopathy, and both systolic and diastolic blood pressure were

predictors of the incidence of proliferative retinopathy, independent of glycosylated hemoglobin, only in people with younger-onset diabetes (Figs. 41-15 to 41-17).[121] Neither systolic nor diastolic blood pressure was found to be related to the 4- or 10-year incidence or progression of retinopathy in either of the older-onset groups. The failure to find a relationship in the older-onset WESDR groups persisted after controlling for the use of antihypertensive medications.

Whether the relationship between blood pressure and retinopathy is etiologic or both are the result of the effect of diabetes on the microvascular system is difficult to assess from cohort studies. Data from the EURODIAB Controlled Trial of Lisinopril in T1DM (the EUCLID Study Group) study showed a 50% reduction in the

FIGURE 41-15. Relation of 4-year incidence of diabetic retinopathy by quartiles of systolic and diastolic blood pressure at baseline in younger-onset persons in the Wisconsin Epidemiologic Study of Diabetic Retinopathy. The ranges for baseline systolic and diastolic blood pressure, respectively, in the younger-onset group are first quartile: 78–110 and 42–71 mm Hg; second quartile: 111–120 and 72–78 mm Hg; third quartile: 121–134 and 79–85 mm Hg; and fourth quartile: 135–221 and 86–117 mm Hg.

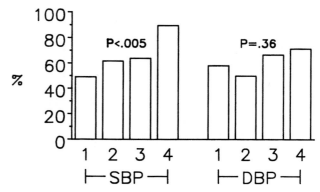

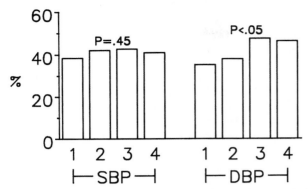

FIGURE 41-16. Relation of 4-year progression of diabetic retinopathy by quartiles of systolic and diastolic blood pressure at baseline in younger-onset persons in the Wisconsin Epidemiologic Study of Diabetic Retinopathy.

progression of retinopathy, after adjustment for glycemic control, in nonhypertensive or mildly hypertensive persons in the Lisinopril treatment group compared to the placebo group.[122]

The UKPDS also sought to determine whether tight control of blood pressure with either a beta blocker or an ACE inhibitor was beneficial in reducing macrovascular and microvascular complications associated with T2DM.[6] They randomized 1148 patients with hypertension (mean blood pressure 160/94 mm Hg) to a regimen of tight control with either captopril or atenolol and another 390 patients to less tight control of their blood pressure. Tight blood pressure control resulted in a 35% reduction in retinal photocoagulation compared to conventional control. After 7.5 years of follow-up, there was a 34% reduction in the rate of progression of retinopathy by two or more steps using the modified ETDRS severity scale, and a 47% reduction in the deterioration of visual acuity by three lines or more using the ETDRS charts (i.e., going from 20/20 to 20/40 or worse on a Snellen chart). The effect was largely due to a reduction in incidence of diabetic macular edema.

FIGURE 41-17. Relation of 4-year incidence of proliferative diabetic retinopathy by quartiles of systolic and diastolic blood pressure at baseline in younger-onset persons in the Wisconsin Epidemiologic Study of Diabetic Retinopathy.

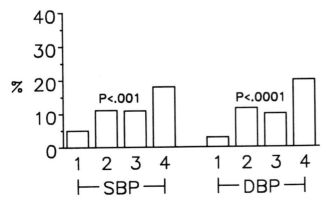

Atenolol and captopril were equally effective in reducing the risk of development of these microvascular complications. The effects of blood pressure control were independent of glycemic control. These findings strongly support tight blood pressure control in people with T2DM as a means of preventing visual loss due to the progression of diabetic retinopathy.

Proteinuria and Diabetic Nephropathy

The prevalence and severity of diabetic retinopathy is associated with the presence of diabetic nephropathy, as manifest by microalbuminuria or gross proteinuria. This is not unexpected, as rheological, platelet, and lipid abnormalities associated with nephropathy may be involved in the pathogenesis of retinopathy.[123]

Diabetic retinopathy is usually seen before clinical detection of nephropathy (measured by proteinuria, increased blood urea nitrogen [BUN], or serum creatinine), although physiologic manifestations of early renal dysfunction (e.g., increased glomerular filtration rate) may be detected early in the course of the disease. Differing underlying pathogenetic or anatomic factors have been postulated to explain such differences.[124] The higher frequency of retinopathy may also be secondary to its easier detection via ophthalmoscopy.

In the WESDR, gross proteinuria was present in 27% of insulin-taking persons diagnosed before 30 years of age who had retinopathy; for persons diagnosed at or after 30 years of age who were not taking insulin, gross proteinuria was present in 19% of those with retinopathy.[16,17] In a study of diabetic Oklahoma Indians, West and colleagues[61] reported that 58% of persons with severe retinopathy had heavy proteinuria.

In WESDR younger-onset persons with 10 years or more of diabetes, proliferative retinopathy was found three times as often in persons with proteinuria as in those without proteinuria; similarly, in noninsulin-taking older-onset persons, proliferative retinopathy was 2.7 times as frequent in the presence of proteinuria as in its absence.[16,17]

In the WESDR, in the younger-onset group taking insulin, the RR of proliferative retinopathy developing over 4 years in those with gross proteinuria at baseline was 2.32 (95% CI 1.40, 3.83) compared with those without gross proteinuria.[125] For the older-onset group taking insulin, it was 2.02 (95% CI 0.91, 4.44), and for those not taking insulin it was 1.13 (95% CI 0.15, 8.50). After controlling for other risk variables, the relationship was of borderline significance ($p = 0.052$) in the younger-onset group with no or early nonproliferative retinopathy at baseline. In Pittsburgh, those with T1DM and microalbuminuria or overt nephropathy at entry had a significantly higher rate of progression to proliferative disease over a 2-year period than people without renal disease.[41] These data suggest that gross proteinuria is a risk indicator for proliferative retinopathy and these patients might benefit from having regular ophthalmologic evaluation.

Most diabetic persons who develop end-stage renal disease that requires dialysis or transplantation have proliferative retinopathy. Ramsey and coworkers[126] reported that 75% of eyes of diabetic patients who were undergoing renal transplantation or dialysis had proliferative retinopathy, and 32% had visual acuity of 20/160 or worse in the better eye.

Patients on dialysis or following renal transplantation usually have a stabilization of visual function.[126] In one study, 54% (165/308) of eyes of diabetic patients had visual acuity of 20/50 or better at the time of their renal transplant for diabetic end-stage renal disease. With a mean follow-up time of 3–5 years, 51% (157/308) of eyes had retained this visual acuity level. Progression of retinopathy was reported (no comparison group) in 38% (30/78) of eyes that had nonproliferative disease before transplantation. However, of eyes that had active proliferative retinopathy at the time of transplantation, 71% (43/61) became inactive and were at lower risk of visual loss after the transplantation. Similar findings were reported for patients on dialysis. However, patients undergoing transplantation are at risk of developing decreased visual acuity due to cataract formation, secondary to systemic corticosteroids, or due to cytomegalovirus retinitis (secondary to immunosuppression).[127]

Patients undergoing hemodialysis have been thought to be at greater risk of vitreous hemorrhage due to heparinization or to rapid metabolic and blood pressure changes.[127] However, Ramsey and associates[126] reported no difference in visual prognosis (if metabolic and blood pressure control is brought about gradually) in diabetic patients managed by peritoneal dialysis compared to chronic hemodialysis. Patients undergoing hemodialysis are also at risk of developing increased intraocular pressure.[127] The mechanism for this is unknown. Monitoring of intraocular pressures of such patients is indicated.

Serum Lipids

Most of the information regarding the relationship of serum lipids to diabetic retinopathy is inconsistent (Table 41-6).[37,41,67,73,128] In the WESDR, higher total serum cholesterol was associated with higher prevalence of retinal hard exudates in both the younger- and older-onset groups using insulin.[128] In the ETDRS, higher levels of serum lipids (triglycerides, LDL cholesterol, and VLDL cholesterol) were associated with an increased risk of developing hard exudates in the macula.[129] Randomized controlled clinical trials to investigate whether statins prevent the incidence and progression of retinopathy and visual loss are underway.

Smoking and Alcohol

Smoking, a known risk factor for cardiovascular disease, has been implicated in some studies as being causally related to retinopathy.[85,130,131] One might anticipate such an association because smoking may cause tissue hypoxia by increasing blood carbon monoxide levels. Additionally, smoking may lead to increased platelet adhesiveness and aggregation. Paetkau and coworkers[130] first reported a positive association between smoking and proliferative diabetic retinopathy in 181 patients referred to a fluorescein angiography unit. Nielsen and Hjollund[131] also found a relationship between severity of retinopathy and cigarette smoking in male, but not in female, T1DM patients. Many subsequent studies have failed to demonstrate an association between the risk of retinopathy and a smoking history.[37,38,41,71,132,133] In the WESDR, cigarette smoking was not associated with the 4-year incidence or progression of diabetic retinopathy.[133]

The few studies that have examined the relationship between alcohol consumption and diabetic retinopathy have not been consistent (Table 41-6).[134–136] A possible protective effect of alcohol, as a result of reduced platelet adhesiveness and aggregation, might be expected. In the WESDR, alcohol consumption was associated with a lower prevalence of proliferative retinopathy.[136] However, there was no relationship between alcohol consumption at the 4-year examination and the incidence and progression of retinopathy 6 years later.

Body Mass (Obesity) and Physical Activity

The severity of retinopathy has been reported to be inversely correlated with body mass index in noninsulin-taking persons.[17,61] This finding is compatible with the concept that obese older-onset noninsulin-taking patients have a milder form of the disease.

In the WESDR, there was no association between physical activity or leisure-time energy expenditure and the prevalence, incidence, and progression of diabetic retinopathy.[137] However, in women diagnosed to have diabetes before 14 years of age, those who participated in team sports were less likely to have proliferative diabetic retinopathy than those who did not.

Socioeconomic Status

There are few data available assessing the relationships between socioeconomic factors and severity of retinopathy. Hanna and colleagues[138] reported a significant association between proliferative retinopathy and occupational status (working class) or a lower income in a case-control study of 49 type 1 diabetic patients. West and coworkers[61] failed to find a relationship of retinopathy with education level in a population of diabetic Oklahoma Indians. Haffner and associates[139] did not find a relationship between lower socioeconomic status (as measured using a combination of the Duncan Index, educational attainment, and income) and more severe retinopathy in 343 Mexican-Americans and 79 non-Hispanic whites with T2DM in San Antonio.

In the WESDR, with the exception of an association of lower incidence of proliferative retinopathy with more education in younger-onset women 25 years of age or older, socioeconomic status (education level and Duncan Socioeconomic Index score) was not related to increased risk of developing proliferative retinopathy.[140] Younger-onset men with proliferative retinopathy at baseline were more likely to become unemployed and younger-onset women were more likely to divorce 4 years later.

Pregnancy

In a review of the literature, Rodman and coworkers[141] found that only 17 (8%) of 201 cases of pregnant diabetic patients with no or early nonproliferative retinopathy at the onset of their pregnancy progressed; only 4 of these 17 developed proliferative diabetic retinopathy. In 127 cases of women known to have proliferative retinopathy at the onset of their pregnancy, 32 (25%) experienced progression during the pregnancy. In a review of the Joslin Clinic data by Beetham[142] in 1950, duration of diabetes before pregnancy was found to be the most important determinant of the progression of retinopathy.

Larinkari and associates[143] in an uncontrolled follow-up series of patients, observed progression of retinopathy in 8 of 42 pregnant diabetic patients. Progression of retinopathy was related to increased duration of diabetes, increased severity of retinopathy at the onset of disease, poor control of blood glucose during the first trimester, and higher serum progesterone concentrations. In a prospective study, Moloney and Drury[144] reported a 40% incidence of retinopathy in patients who were free of retinopathy at the beginning of the pregnancy. There was zero incidence of retinopathy in 120 nonpregnant insulin-dependent control subjects. In patients with background retinopathy at the onset of their pregnancies, progression, manifested by streak or blot hemorrhages, occurred in 53%, and cotton-wool spots occurred in 29%. In comparison, streak or blot hemorrhages occurred in only 8% and soft exudates in none of the diabetic nonpregnant control group. Only one of the pregnant women with nonproliferative retinopathy progressed to proliferative disease. In the pregnant group, ophthalmoscopic manifestations of retinopathy disappeared in 12 (23%) patients after delivery. Development of streak and blot hemorrhages was associated with increased insulin requirement and higher fasting blood glucose and hemoglobin A_1 levels early in pregnancy. Soft exudates were associated with lower fasting blood glucose levels late in pregnancy, but not with hypertension or preeclamptic toxemia.

In a recently completed case-control study of women with T1DM, the frequency of progression to proliferative retinopathy was higher in those who were pregnant compared to those who were not (7% versus 4%).[145] Women in this study were similar in age, duration of diabetes, and retinopathy status at baseline. Pregnancy remained a significant predictor of the progression of diabetic retinopathy after controlling for glycosylated hemoglobin and blood pressure.

With the development of photocoagulation, there has been much change in the management of female diabetic patients since 1950, when Beetham recommended that "in their own best interests, patients presenting a large amount of retinal hemorrhage, or proliferating retinopathy, should not be permitted to undertake pregnancy."[142] Current management recommendations include evaluation by an ophthalmologist of all type 1 diabetic patients considering pregnancy or those who have become pregnant. Those women with no or mild retinopathy, although at low risk of progression, should be followed by an ophthalmologist and seen more frequently than usual during gestation (perhaps every 2–3 months), especially if they develop complications (e.g., toxemia or progression of retinopathy). Because panretinal photocoagulation has been shown to cause significant regression of retinal new blood vessels and prevent serious reduction of vision, women with severe preproliferative or proliferative retinopathy should be referred for possible treatment.[7] There are no data on the benefits of cesarean section as a means of delivery for women with high-risk proliferative retinopathy who do not respond to panretinal photocoagulation treatment.

Severe retinopathy has been shown to be an indicator of higher risk of congenital abnormalities in children born of mothers with T1DM.[146]

Retinopathy, Comorbidity, and Mortality

Severe retinopathy is associated with cardiovascular disease risk factors such as increased fibrinogen, hyperglycemia, hypertension, and increased platelet aggregation.[80] This probably explains in part why people with diabetic retinopathy have been found to have a higher prevalence of coronary disease.[61] Thus it is not surprising that in the WESDR, those with proliferative retinopathy were at increased risk of developing a heart attack, stroke, diabetic nephropathy, and amputation (Table 41-8).

The ETDRS demonstrated that aspirin does not increase the risk of vitreous hemorrhage or loss of vision in persons with proliferative retinopathy.[147] It was also not found to prevent the incidence or progression of retinopathy in the WESDR or the ETDRS.

The probability for survival decreases with increasing severity of retinopathy. In the WESDR, increasing risk of death was found with more severe retinopathy at baseline (Figs. 41-18 and 41-19). These findings are consistent with the association of severe retinopathy with the incidence of cardiovascular disease and diabetic nephropathy. The higher prevalence of systemic conditions (e.g., uremia, coronary heart disease, and hypertension) in patients with severe retinopathy is responsible for the increased risk of death. These data suggest that diabetic patients with retinopathy should be under close medical surveillance for diagnosis and treatment of cardiovascular disease.

Medical Therapy

Aside from oral hypoglycemic agents, insulin, and antihypertensive medications, no drugs have been found to prevent or decrease the progression of diabetic retinopathy.[2,148] Treatment regimens involving androgenic and nonandrogenic anabolic steroids; vitamins B_{12}, C, E, and K; calcium debosilate; calcium phosphate; cyclandelate; anticoagulants; aldose-reductase inhibitors; and aspirin have been proposed, tried, or have not proved to be of therapeutic or preventive value in altering the course of diabetic retinopathy.[2,46,147,148]

Epidemiologic studies, the DCCT, and the UKPDS have clearly demonstrated the significant reduction in the incidence and progression of diabetic retinopathy by reduction of hyperglycemia.[4,5] The findings from the DCCT and UKPDS have strong

TABLE 41-8. The Relative Risk for the Prevalence and Four-Year Incidence of Myocardial Infarction, Stroke, and Amputation of the Lower Extremities Associated with the Presence of Proliferative Retinopathy, Corrected for Age in the Wisconsin Epidemiologic Study of Diabetic Retinopathy

	Myocardial Infarction		*Stroke*		*Amputation of Lower Extremity*	
	RR	**95% CI**	**RR**	**95% CI**	**RR**	**95% CI**
Younger-onset group						
Prevalence	3.5	1.5–7.9	2.6	0.7–9.7	7.1	2.6–19.7
Incidence	4.5	1.3–15.4	1.6	0.4–5.7	6.0	2.1–16.9
Older-onset group taking insulin						
Prevalence	0.8	0.4–1.4	1.2	0.6–2.4	4.2	2.3–7.9
Incidence	1.2	0.5–3.4	2.9	1.2–6.8	3.4	0.9–13.2
Older-onset group not taking insulin						
Prevalence	0.3	0–2.4	2.9	0.9–9.4	5.2	0.6–45.0
Incidence	1.5	0.2–12.5	6.0	1.1–32.6	7.0	0.8–64.4

CI, confidence interval.

RR, relative risk.

Source: Reprinted with permission from Klein R, Klein BEK, Moss SE: The epidemiology of proliferative diabetic retinopathy. *Diabetes Care* 1992;15:1875.

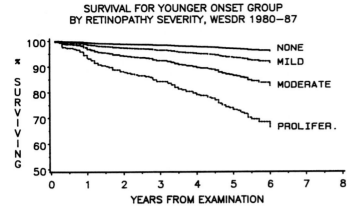

FIGURE 41-18. Age- and sex-adjusted survival curves by diabetic retinopathy status at baseline examination in younger-onset persons participating in the Wisconsin Epidemiologic Study of Diabetic Retinopathy. *(Reprinted with permission from Klein R, Moss SE, Klein BEK, et al: Relation of ocular and systemic factors to survival in diabetes.* Arch Intern Med *1989; 149: 266.)*

public health importance, as only 6.7% of the younger-onset persons, 9.5% of older-onset persons taking insulin, and 34.8% of older-onset persons not taking insulin in the WESDR had glycosylated hemoglobin levels at the baseline examination that fell within two standard deviations from the mean of a nondiabetic comparison group.[3] Ten years after the baseline examination, data from the WESDR continue to show a large number of individuals with poorly controlled diabetes.[149]

The results of the UKPDS and from EUCLID clinical trials suggest that control of blood pressure may also reduce the progression of diabetic retinopathy independent of glycemic control.[6,122] Data from the WESDR also show a significant proportion of people with diabetes whose hypertension is in poor control.

Surgical Therapy

Photocoagulation

The rationale for the use of panretinal photocoagulation resulted from the observation that the eyes of diabetic patients with

FIGURE 41-19. Age- and sex-adjusted survival curves by diabetic retinopathy status at baseline examination in older-onset persons participating in the Wisconsin Epidemiologic Study of Diabetic Retinopathy. *(Reprinted with permission from Klein R, Moss SE, Klein BEK, et al: Relation of ocular and systemic factors to survival in diabetes.* Arch Intern Med *1989;149:266.)*

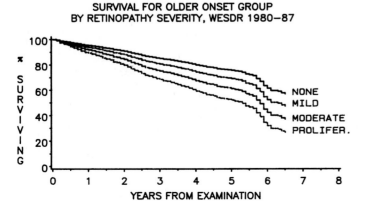

disseminated chorioretinal scars due to trauma or infection had lower rates of retinopathy than the fellow eye without such changes.[2] As a result of these observations, high-energy light sources (xenon arc; ruby, argon, and krypton lasers) have been developed to produce burns leading to scars in the outer layer of the retina.

Despite a number of clinical studies, five of which used concurrent controls, the efficacy of photocoagulation in preventing severe visual loss due to proliferative retinopathy was not widely accepted prior to the onset of the Diabetic Retinopathy Study (DRS) in 1972. That therapeutic trial was sponsored by the National Eye Institute and was conducted between 1972 and 1979.[7] A total of 1758 patients were involved. To be eligible for participation, patients had to have visual acuity of 20/100 or better in each eye, no previous photocoagulation, and proliferative retinopathy in at least one eye or severe nonproliferative or proliferative retinopathy in both eyes. There was random assignment of one eye of each patient to photocoagulation (either xenon arc or argon laser) and the other to follow-up without photocoagulation. The photocoagulation technique involved "scatter" panretinal photocoagulation of retinal new vessels.

The major end point in the DRS was "severe visual loss," defined as a visual acuity of less than 5/200 in two consecutive follow-up visits 4 months apart. The major finding of the DRS was that the risk of severe visual loss in treated eyes was less than one half that in untreated control eyes (Fig. 41-20).[7] The 6-year cumulative event rate for severe visual loss was 38% for untreated and 16% for treated eyes. High-risk retinopathy characteristics for severe visual loss in untreated eyes in the DRS included new vessels at the optic disk equaling or exceeding one-third of the disk area in extent (Fig. 41-21), new vessels at the disk less than one-third of the disk area in extent with preretinal or vitreous hemorrhage, and new vessels more than one disk diameter away from the optic disk greater than one-half the disk area in size associated with preretinal or vitreous hemorrhage. The conclusion reached by the DRS group was that in eyes with such high-risk characteristics, the risk of severe visual loss without treatment was 25% at 2 years and in eyes with treatment it was 12%; this beneficial effect outweighed the risk of harmful treatment effects.[7] The results of the ETDRS suggested that earlier panretinal treatment of eyes with high-risk proliferative retinopathy may result in a 90% decrease in the risk of severe loss of vision.[150]

The ETDRS provided data on panretinal photocoagulation treatment for eyes in which proliferative retinopathy with DRS high-risk characteristics for severe vision loss were not present.[151] The data suggest that in eyes with early or moderate severe nonproliferative retinopathy (Levels 21-47; see Table 41-1) there is little or no reason to treat with panretinal photocoagulation because of the relatively low risk of progression to severe visual loss and the risk of complications associated with such treatment. However, in people in whom both eyes have bilateral severe preproliferative retinopathy or proliferative retinopathy without DRS high-risk complications (Level 53 or 65; see Table 41-1), the data suggest there may be some benefit in prompt initiation of panretinal photocoagulation in at least one eye.

Before undergoing panretinal treatment, the patient is told that photocoagulation may reduce the chances of severe loss of vision (to less than 5/200), but that it does not completely eliminate its possibility. The patient is also told that photocoagulation may cause moderate reduction of visual function as an unavoidable side effect, but that this reduction usually is of minor consequence. Such

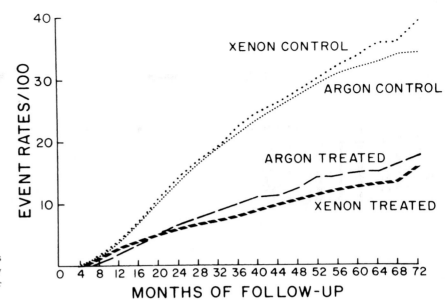

FIGURE 41-20. Cumulative rates of severe visual loss (5/200 or less) in the Diabetic Retinopathy Study Group. *(Reprinted with permission from Diabetic Retinopathy Study Group.[7])*

reduction includes mild loss of central vision (e.g., if the visual acuity was 20/20 before treatment, it might be reduced to 20/25 to 20/30 after panretinal argon laser treatment in 10% of patients), mild constriction of peripheral visual fields (5% of cases with argon laser), impaired night vision, and decreased accommodation.[7,152] The patient is also informed about the rare more severe side effects (e.g., severe constriction of visual fields and severe loss of central vision due to development of vitreous hemorrhage, traction retinal detachment after treatment, or an inadvertent foveal burn).

Panretinal photocoagulation is usually done as an outpatient procedure. To achieve anesthesia, proparacaine drops are applied to the cornea. Rarely, a retrobulbar injection of lidocaine is used. The pupil is dilated, and a contact lens is applied to the cornea. Under

direct visualization of the retina, 800–1800 burns, usually 500-μm diameter in size, are delivered in a grid-like pattern (sparing the central retina) in one or more treatment sessions (Fig. 41-22). A successful treatment usually leads to partial or complete regression of abnormal new preretinal and optic disk blood vessels (Fig. 41-23), in most cases within 4 weeks. If the high-risk characteristics remain, further treatments are usually scheduled. Underlying reasons for failure to respond to laser treatment were not defined in the DRS.

The mechanisms of action of panretinal photocoagulation are not known. A number of theories of how photocoagulation works have been suggested. They include destruction of hypoxic retinal tissue resulting in decreased production of a hypothetical va-

FIGURE 41-21. Fundus photograph of the left eye showing stringy new vessels equaling one-third the disk area in front of the optic disk (**black arrows**). This patient, who is asymptomatic and has normal visual acuity, is at high risk of developing severe visual loss if not treated with panretinal photocoagulation. *(Reprinted with permission from Klein R: Management of eye disease in the insulin-dependent diabetic patient. In: MacDonald M, ed. Managing Diabetes Mellitus in Children and Adolescents. Saunders:1983.)*

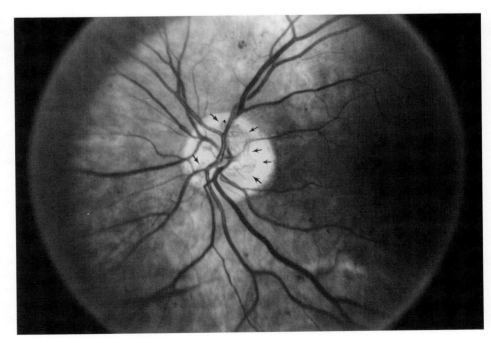

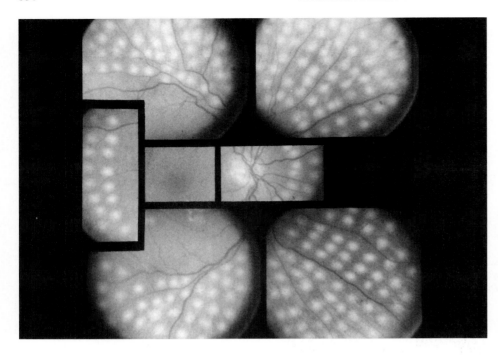

FIGURE 41-22. Fundus photograph of the right eye demonstrating fresh panretinal argon laser photocoagulation burns that have been delivered in a grid-like fashion, sparing the macular area. *(Reprinted with permission from Klein R: Management of eye disease in the insulin-dependent diabetic patient. In: MacDonald M, ed.* Managing Diabetes Mellitus in Children and Adolescents. *Saunders:1983.)*

soproliferative factor, increased oxygenation of untreated retinal tissue leading to vasoconstriction and regression of proliferative tissue, and increased passage of metabolites through the blood–retinal barrier at the level of the retinal pigment epithelium.[10,11]

The ETDRS has demonstrated that treatment of clinically significant macular edema with focal or grid (or both) laser photocoagulation of the macular area reduces doubling of the visual angle (e.g., going from 20/20 to 20/40 or 20/30 to 20/60) to 13% from 30% in untreated eyes (Fig. 41-24).[8]

During treatment for macular edema, a fluorescein angiogram projected on a wall or in a special viewer is used to demonstrate abnormal leakage from retinal blood vessels, which may be responsible for macular edema, as well as for areas of ischemia (closure of retinal capillaries). Topical anesthesia with proparacaine drops is routinely used. Photocoagulation burns of 0.05–0.1 second duration and 100–200 μm in size are directed at leaking retinal microaneurysms as identified on the fluorescein angiograms. Burns of 50 μm may be added to achieve further whitening of the retinal microaneurysms. Nonperfused areas may also be treated in a grid-like pattern to destroy ischemic retina. Follow-up examination is done within 3 months; if the edema persists, the angiogram is repeated and any remaining leaks are treated.

The rationale for photocoagulation for macular edema includes ablation of leaking microaneurysms. Bresnick[22] has suggested that a "debridement" of abnormal retinal pigment epithelial cells with replacement by normal cells may reestablish the blood–retinal barrier, facilitating absorption of retinal edema fluid.

Vitrectomy

Vitrectomy is done to remove vitreous hemorrhage or to cut fibrous bands that cause tractional detachments of the retina due to proliferative disease. Prior to the development of vitrectomy, the only treatment for vitreous hemorrhage was patching of both eyes and elevation of the head. Currently, if a significant vitreous hemorrhage obscures visualization of the retina, bilateral patching and elevation of the head for 24–48 hours is sometimes recommended. The fundus is examined, and if there has been enough settling of the vitreous hemorrhage, panretinal photocoagulation is done if indicated and feasible.

Vitrectomy may be recommended if there has been no clearing of the vitreous hemorrhage after a few months in people with T1DM or after 6–12 months in people with T2DM, or sooner if there is ultrasound or other evidence of a tractional retinal detachment threatening or involving the macular area. The major objectives of vitreous surgery are to clear the optical axis of opacities and to release mechanical traction on the retina.

Vitrectomy is a procedure that may require hospitalization and may be performed under general anesthesia; the average duration of the operation is 2–3 hours. Because the surgery is generally performed on an elective basis, preoperative evaluation includes a thorough examination to diagnose and control numerous medical problems often found in the diabetic patient undergoing vitrectomy. Cardiovascular, renal, and metabolic problems must be managed during and after surgery.

The vitrectomy device and fiberoptic illuminators are introduced into the eye through small openings made in the sclera overlying the pars plana (flat portion) of the ciliary body. Usually the lens is left undisturbed; however, if a cataract is present and prohibits visualization for vitrectomy, the lens may be removed before or during surgery. Under direct observation, the vitrectomy instrument is used to cut and remove fibrous tissues and blood from the vitreous cavity, and vitreous volume is restored with a balanced salt solution. Using special intraocular scissors, the surgeon may cut fibroproliferative tissue and epiretinal membranes, which are responsible for traction on the retina.

In cases in which a prior retinal tear is present or a tear occurs during the procedure, choroidoretinal adhesion is produced around the tear with cryopexy to prevent detachment of the retina. Additionally, air with or without expanding gas mixtures (e.g., sulfur hexafluoride) may be exchanged for the fluid in the vitreous cavity

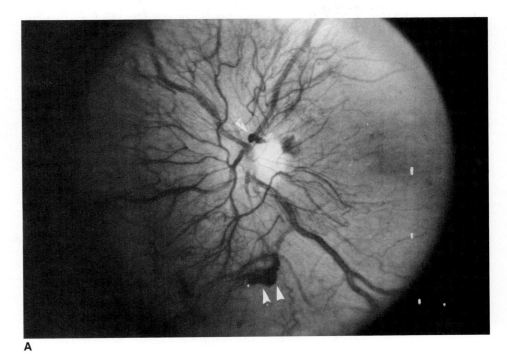

A

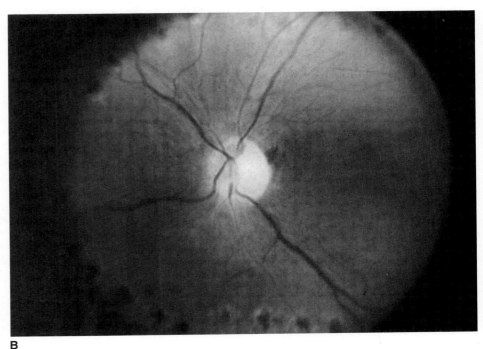

B

FIGURE 41-23. A. Fundus photograph of the left eye demonstrating extensive retinal new vessels in front of the disk and preretinal hemorrhage (**white arrowheads**). **B.** Four weeks after panretinal argon laser photocoagulation there has been a dramatic regression of retinal new vessels. Pigmented photocoagulation scars are present in the periphery of the picture. *(Reprinted with permission from Klein R: Management of eye disease in the insulin-dependent diabetic patient. In: MacDonald M, ed.* Managing Diabetes Mellitus in Children and Adolescents. *Saunders:1983.)*

to tamponade the retinal tear, and the subretinal fluid may be drained during the operation. Scleral buckling (with hard episcleral silicone or sponges) may also be used to indent the sclera, reduce traction further, and thus seal the tear.

In a series of patients undergoing vitrectomy, visual improvement to better than 20/200 was reported in 50% of operated cases.[153] Michaels[154] described a series of 596 consecutive eyes with severe loss of visual acuity and reported a successful result (visual acuity of 5/200 or better and stable anatomic findings) in 384 (66%) of 579 eyes. Successful results after vitrectomy are more likely in

eyes with vitreous hemorrhage alone than in eyes with traction retinal detachment involving the macular area. In the latter, the effects of preexisting anatomic damage to the macular area are more likely to limit visual improvement postoperatively.

Vitrectomy carries with it a number of serious complications, which include iatrogenic retinal tears resulting in retinal detachment, recurrent vitreous hemorrhage, corneal edema, cataract, the development of neovascularization of the iris and rubeotic glaucoma.[155]

Rubeotic glaucoma (secondary to neovascularization of the anterior chamber angle), when it occurs, usually develops within

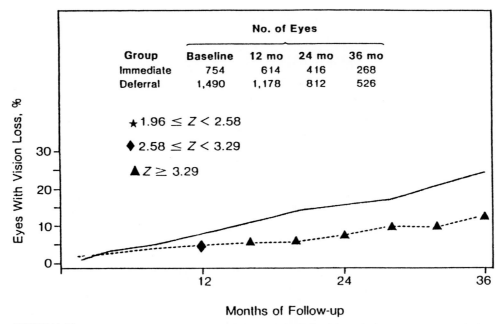

FIGURE 41-24. Comparison of percentage of eyes that experienced visual loss of 15 or more letters (equivalent to at least doubling of initial visual angle or loss of three or more lines) in eyes with macular edema and mild to moderate diabetic retinopathy assigned to either immediate focal photocoagulation (**dashed line**) or deferral of photocoagulation (**solid line**). Z stands for normal deviate. *(Reprinted with permission from ETDRS Research Group.[8])*

6 months of vitrectomy and is more likely to arise in eyes with severe retinal ischemia, retinal detachment, or removal of the lens. Panretinal photocoagulation during (using an endophotocoagulator) or after the procedure may reduce the incidence of this serious complication.

The Diabetic Retinopathy Vitrectomy Study (DRVS) assessed indications, risks, and benefits for early (shortly after the development of vitreous hemorrhage) versus late (a year) vitrectomy.[156] The rationale for early vitrectomy included avoiding prolonged visual disability and possibly avoiding the presumed deleterious effects of long-standing intraocular hemorrhage (possible acceleration of growth of fibroproliferans, exacerbation of retinal vascular occlusive process, and a possible toxic effect of blood on the retina). The rationale for late vitrectomy (at least 1 year after the initial vitreous hemorrhage) included the possibility of spontaneous resolution of hemorrhage and that with time the retinopathy would be stabilized and there would be fewer vision-threatening complications of surgery (e.g., neovascular glaucoma). The DRVS showed that there was a significant benefit in terms of restoring visual acuity by early vitrectomy in those with T1DM.

VISUAL IMPAIRMENT

Diabetes is an important cause of impaired vision.[1,157] It is estimated to account for 5000 new cases of legal blindness (visual acuity of 20/200 or worse in the better eye) in the United States each year. Blindness is 29 times more common in diabetic than in nondiabetic persons (Fig. 41-25). Approximately 8% of people who were legally blind reported diabetes as the etiology of their blindness,[158] and it is estimated that in the United States, more than 12% of new cases of blindness are attributable to diabetes.

Prevalence

The prevalence of blindness in diabetic persons is related to current age.[159] In the WESDR, prevalence of diabetes-related legal blindness increased with increasing age. No cases of legal blindness were found in persons younger than 25 years of age. The prevalence of legal blindness increased in both males and females,

FIGURE 41-25. Percentage of persons with visual acuity of 20/200 or worse in the better eye in the Wisconsin Epidemiologic Study of Diabetic Retinopathy, Health and Nutrition Examination Survey, and the Framingham Eye Study by current age. *(Reprinted with permission from Klein et al.[159])*

VISUAL ACUITY 20/200 OR WORSE IN BETTER EYE IN DIFFERENT POPULATIONS

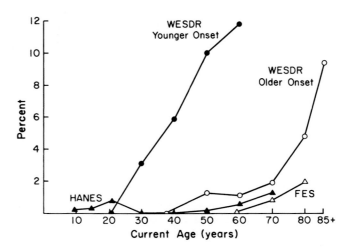

TABLE 41-9. Ten-Year Incidence of Blindness, Visual Impairment, and Doubling of the Visual Angle

Group	Blindness		Visual Impairment		Doubling of the Visual Angle	
	N	%	N	%	N	%
Younger-onset	868	1.8	832	9.4	880	9.2
Older-onset, taking insulin	465	4.0	423	37.2	472	32.8
Older-onset, not taking insulin	490	4.8	454	23.9	494	21.4

Source: Moss et al.[27]

reaching peaks of 14% and 20%, respectively. In the older-onset WESDR group, prevalence of blindness increased with increasing age and accounted for 1.6% in persons taking insulin and 2.2% in those not taking insulin. In a study in Oxford, England, in 1982, 28% of the 188 people 60 years of age or older with known T2DM were visually impaired.[160] The age-specific prevalence of legal blindness in both younger- and older-onset diabetic patients in the WESDR was significantly higher than those estimated for the general United States population in the Health and Nutrition Examination Survey (HANES) or for all participants in the Framingham Eye Study (Fig. 41-25).[158,161,162]

In the WESDR, legal blindness was related to duration of diabetes in both younger- and older-onset groups. In the younger-onset group, legal blindness first occurred in persons having diabetes for about 15 years or more and increased from 3% in those with 15–19 years' duration to 12% in persons with diabetes for 30 or more years. In the older-onset groups, prevalence of legal blindness was lower, only reaching 7% in persons having diabetes for 20–24 years.

In the WESDR, diabetic retinopathy was partially or totally responsible for legal blindness in 86% of eyes of younger-onset persons and in 33% of eyes of older-onset persons with such impairment.

Incidence

In persons 20–79 years of age with T2DM who participated in the University Group Diabetes Program, the 5-year incidence of legal blindness was 4% or less in each treatment group.[111] The incidence of 20/200 or worse visual acuity in either eye was 9% or less in each treatment group at the 5-year follow-up, and rose to about 12% at the 12-year follow-up. Review of earlier data from diabetic patients attending the Radcliffe Infirmary in England provided estimates of incidence of blindness.[2] In diabetic patients diagnosed at 20 years of age, the incidence of blindness was 0.1% after 10 years, 1.6% after 20 years, and 3.5% after 30 years of diabetes. For persons diagnosed at 60 years of age, the incidence of blindness was 1.8% after 10 years and 5.5% after 20 years of diabetes. Sjolie and Green[163] reported an 8-year incidence of 7.6/1000 patient-years in males and 10.2/1000 patient-years in females with T1DM. In Oxford, England, 4.8% of those with T2DM who were 60 years of age or older at baseline became legally blind over a median period of 6 years.[160]

The 10-year incidence of blindness and impaired vision in the WESDR are presented in Table 41-9. The older-onset group taking insulin had the highest 10-year incidence of visual impairment (37.2%). The estimated annual incidence of blindness reported in the WESDR was 3.3 per 100,000 population.[157]

There are few studies that permit determination of trends in the frequency of decreased vision over time. Two studies in England compared rates of registration for blindness benefits attributed to diabetic retinopathy in 1985 with those recorded in England by Sorsby in 1965.[164-166] In Avon the rates remained unchanged over this period while in Leicestershire there was a significant decrease. In the WESDR, the cohort was reexamined 10 years after the baseline examination.[27] There appeared to be a decrease in the estimated annual incidence of blindness in the three WESDR diabetic groups in the last 6 years compared to the first 4 years of the study (Table 41-10). The decrease in the estimated annual incidence of blindness is not explained by changes in the incidence of proliferative retinopathy or an increased frequency of panretinal photocoagulation in the second 6-year period. Higher frequencies of focal photocoagulation for macular edema and lens extraction for cataract in the second 6-year period of the study compared to the first 4 years may explain only part of the decrease in frequency of blindness over time.

TABLE 41-10. Estimated Annual Incidence of Blindness, Doubling of the Visual Angle, and Proliferative Retinopathy in the Periods 1980–1982 to 1984–1986 and 1984–1986 to 1990–1992

End Point	Period	Younger-Onset %	Older-Onset Taking Insulin %	Older-Onset Not Taking Insulin %
Blindness	1980–1982 to 1984–1986	0.38	0.82	0.67
	1984–1986 to 1990–1992	0.05	0.14	0.37
Doubling of the visual angle	1980–1982 to 1984–1986	1.51	3.62	1.87
	1984–1986 to 1990–1992	0.52	3.31	2.50
Proliferative retinopathy	1980–1982 to 1984–1986	2.71	1.98	0.53
	1984–1986 to 1990–1992	3.97	3.17	1.34

Souce: Moss et al.[27]

Risk Factors for Impaired Vision

Diabetic Retinopathy

Eyes with more severe retinopathy have been found to be at higher risk of blindness. The cumulative 5-year rate of blindness (visual acuity of 20/200 or worse) for eyes with good vision (20/60 or better) at the beginning of one study was 2% if retinopathy was not present and 15% if retinal blot hemorrhages, exudates, or both were present.[167] Untreated eyes in the DRS had a cumulative event rate of severe visual loss (less than 5/200) of 14% at 2 years, 27% at 4 years, and 38% at 6 years (Fig. 41-20).[7] In the WESDR, the 4-year incidence of doubling of the visual angle increased with increasing severity of retinopathy at baseline (Fig. 41-26).[157] In the WESDR, the 4-year incidence of doubling of the visual angle was increased in the presence of macular edema at baseline (RR 3.5, 95% CI 1.8, 6.9 in the younger-onset group; RR 2.8, 95% CI 1.8, 4.3 in the older-onset group taking insulin; and RR 5.6, 95% CI 3.2, 9.6 in the older-onset group not taking insulin).

In insulin-dependent younger-onset persons, reduction of vision to 20/200 or worse is more likely to be due to proliferative retinopathy resulting in vitreous hemorrhage or retinal traction detachment involving the macular area.[11] In older-onset persons, similar visual loss in patients with retinopathy is often associated with macular edema.[11,159] In both groups, macular ischemia due to closure of retinal capillaries in the foveal area may also result in a decrease of vision.[10,11]

If proliferative diabetic retinopathy is present, vitreous hemorrhage from fragile abnormal new preretinal blood vessels may result in an acute decrease in vision. In such cases the sudden appearance of a number of small dark floaters, a large spot obscuring vision, or "complete" loss of vision is described. Contraction of fibrous proliferative tissue leading to traction on the macular area may cause distortion in vision. Traction on the retina may also result in retinal detachment; if the macula is involved, severe blurry vision and darkening of vision may result. In some diabetic patients there may be marked fluctuations in vision due to clearing and recurrence of vitreous hemorrhage or macular edema.

In older diabetic patients with macular edema, the visual disturbance may go unnoticed until both eyes are involved. The patient may complain of a blur or distortion in central vision, especially when reading. In the absence of proliferative retinopathy, patients with diabetic maculopathy and loss of central vision are usually left with peripheral vision that is sufficient to navigate, unless glaucoma or severe cataracts are present.

Other Risk Factors for Impaired Vision

In addition to age, duration of diabetes, severity of retinopathy, higher glycosylated hemoglobin, and gross proteinuria were associated with increased 4-year risk of doubling of the visual angle in the WESDR.[157] In the UKPDS, after 9 years of follow-up, tight blood pressure control reduced the risk of doubling of the visual angle by 47%.[6]

Impaired Color Vision

Diabetic patients as a group have poorer color vision than nondiabetic persons. Even before the development of retinopathy, disturbances in yellow-blue hue discrimination may be detected.[56] With progression of maculopathy, manifested by edema or hard exudate, further deterioration in color vision is found. This has therapeutic significance because many patients using home blood glucose

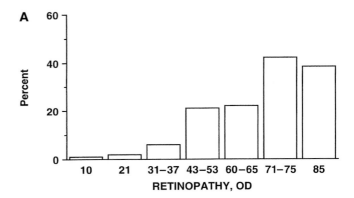

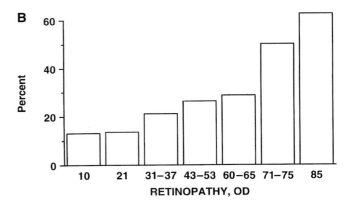

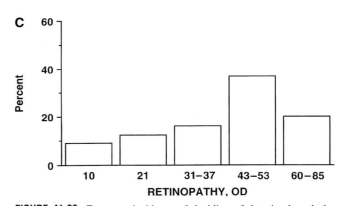

FIGURE 41-26. Four-year incidence of doubling of the visual angle by baseline retinopathy severity (see Table 41-1 for definitions) in the Wisconsin Epidemiologic Study of Diabetic Retinopathy in **A** (**top panel**) the younger-onset group, **B** (**center panel**) the older-onset group taking insulin, and **C** (**bottom panel**) the older-onset group not taking insulin.

monitoring may have difficulty correctly interpreting results of glucose testing. If an impairment in color vision exists, use of alternate devices (e.g., meters with digital display of glucose concentration) when testing glucose should be considered.

Other Causes of Impaired Vision

A frequent cause for sudden change in vision, especially in children and adolescents with diabetes, is related to a change in a refractive medium.[2] In adults this may be one of the presenting symptoms at the time of diagnosis. The patient may complain of blurriness in vision, which can usually be corrected to 20/20 or better with appropriate glasses. Reversible osmotic swelling of the lens due to rapid alterations in blood sugar has been postulated to be responsible for this phenomenon. With better control of the blood sugar, the refraction and acuity return to previous levels.

Cataract

Cataractous lens changes often cause a decrease in vision.[2] This affects a small percentage of young T1DM patients, but occurs more frequently than in age-matched nondiabetic persons. Cataracts in young diabetic patients have been described as vacuolar or snowflake in appearance, involving the cortical or posterior subcapsular area of the lens. In the young, rapidly progressive cataracts have been associated with poor control.[2] It has been suggested that high glucose concentrations in the aqueous humor surrounding the lens enter lens cells and are converted to sorbitol in the polyol pathway.[168] Sorbitol cannot leave the lens cells and so accumulates, leading to osmotic swelling and destruction of cells. The use of aldose-reductase inhibitors has been found to inhibit such cataract formation in poorly controlled diabetic animals.

Prevalence rates of cataracts have been reported to increase with increasing age and are higher for diabetic than nondiabetic persons for each age.[2,169] The association between cataracts and diabetes is stronger at younger ages. In the Beaver Dam Eye Study, after adjusting for age and sex, one type of cataract, cortical opacities, was significantly more common among people with older-onset diabetes compared to the rest of the nondiabetic Beaver Dam population.[170] Posterior subcapsular cataract, another type of lens opacity, was more common in people with diabetes, but the increase was not significant in all age groups. Longer duration of diabetes was associated with increased odds of all kinds of cataracts.

In the WESDR, multivariate analyses indicated that age and duration of diabetes were the most important risk factors for cataract presence. Severity of diabetic retinopathy was associated with a small but significant further increase in risk.[171] In younger-onset persons, diuretic use and glycosylated hemoglobin were also associated with increased risk. In older-onset persons, diuretic use, intraocular pressure, smoking status, and diastolic blood pressure were associated with increased risk of cataract.

Burditt and Caird[172] found a relationship between metabolic control of blood sugar and the frequency of lens opacity for middle-aged men. In the UKPDS, there was a 34% reduction in cataract extraction in those in the intensive glycemic control group compared to the conventional treatment group.[5] These data suggest that glycemic control in persons with T2DM may reduce the progression of cataracts. Potential environmental exposures may also affect rates of cataracts. One such exposure, to aspirin, has not been shown to reduce the prevalence of cataracts in eyes of people with diabetes.[173,174]

If a cataract causes significant visual impairment, the patient may no longer be able to read. Cataract extraction, if successfully performed, usually results in good vision with the use of glasses or contact lenses, assuming that concomitant retinopathy has not affected central vision.

Cataract extraction is a frequent occurrence in people with diabetes. In prevalence data from the WESDR, 3.6% of younger-onset and 8.7% of older-onset persons had such surgery.[171] In the Beaver Dam Eye Study, there were higher frequencies of past cataract surgery in people with diabetes in each age group.[170]

Cataract surgery has been found to be associated with progression of diabetic retinopathy in some studies. Jaffe and Burton[175] reported subsequent progression of the severity of retinopathy in the operated eye of patients with nonproliferative retinopathy prior to cataract extraction. However, others did not find cataract surgery to be associated with progression of retinopathy.[176]

Results of clinical surveys suggest that intraocular lens implants may be used without excess morbidity to the eye in some diabetic patients with no or early nonproliferative retinopathy.[177] Straatsma and coworkers[177] reported no difference in complications or final postoperative visual acuity level between diabetic and nondiabetic patients. They recommended use of an intraocular lens only in diabetic patients 60 years of age or older with a cataract-related decrease in vision that interfered with the patient's activities and if proliferative diabetic retinopathy or rubeosis was not present. These lenses are now commonly used even at younger ages if there are no contraindications present.

Glaucoma

Glaucoma is a disease in which there is loss of vision or visual field from damage to the optic nerve fibers due to absolute or relative elevations in intraocular pressure. Two types of glaucoma, open-angle and rubeotic, are reported to be more common in persons with diabetes.[2,178]

There is conflicting information about the relationship between diabetes and open-angle glaucoma. Most reports describe a higher prevalence of ocular hypertension and open-angle glaucoma in diabetic than in nondiabetic persons. Additionally, patients with open-angle glaucoma or ocular hypertension are reported to have a higher prevalence of diabetes. Data from the 1976–1977 National Health Interview Survey indicate that diabetic persons 20 years of age or older (type unspecified) reported substantially higher rates of glaucoma than did the nondiabetic U.S. population.[158] In the Beaver Dam Eye Study, diabetes was associated with a modest increase in risk of definite and probable glaucoma.[178] Persons in the Framingham Eye Study with intraocular pressure greater than 20 mm Hg were 2–3 times as likely to have diabetes as others,[179] although other investigators have failed to find this relationship.[180]

In the WESDR, the estimated 10-year incidence of glaucoma in the younger-onset group was 4%, in the older-onset group not taking insulin it was 7%, and in those taking insulin it was 12%. In older-onset persons, increasing duration of diabetes was associated with increased risk of glaucoma.[181]

It has been hypothesized that diabetic patients are at increased risk of optic nerve damage owing to vascular factors.[179] Because diabetic patients may be at increased risk of glaucoma, measurement of the intraocular pressure and ophthalmoscopic examination for changes of the cup-to-disk configuration and size is an important part of the ophthalmologic management of these patients. In patients who develop glaucoma, medical intervention is usually successful in preventing or retarding further field and visual loss.

Eyes with severe ischemic retinopathy or detachment of the retina, or eyes that have undergone vitrectomy, are at increased risk of developing rubeotic glaucoma.[10] Abnormal new vessels on the iris and in the anterior chamber angle of the eye may lead to elevations of the intraocular pressure, severe optic nerve damage, and blindness with possible enucleation of the eye if it is painful. In some cases, panretinal photocoagulation may result in regression of the rubeotic vessels and control of the intraocular pressure. Other surgical (cyclocryotherapy and valve implants) or medical interventions (antiglaucoma medications, topical corticosteroids, and mydriatic cycloplegics) for rubeotic glaucoma are rarely successful in preserving vision.

Economic Costs of Blindness

The economic costs associated with blindness due to diabetes have been estimated. Chiang and associates[182] reported that the cost to the federal government was $12,769 for a "person-year" of blindness for a working-age American who becomes blind in adulthood; for those 65 years of age or older, it was $823. These estimates did not include output loss, reduced productivity, societal burdens of rehabilitation, and other nonfederal expenses. Based on the WESDR estimates of prevalence of blindness in 5.8 million people with diagnosed diabetes in the United States in 1980 to 1982, it is estimated that the annual cost of blindness was $500 million per year.

OPHTHALMOLOGIC MANAGEMENT

Health Care Delivery

Because it is possible in many cases to prevent visual loss with photocoagulation, and because proliferative retinopathy and clinically significant macular edema may be present before they affect vision, it is important to identify those diabetic persons in need of ophthalmologic evaluation.[183] The need for careful examination by ophthalmologists has been documented by Sussman and coworkers.[184] They found that internists, diabetologists, and senior medical residents correctly diagnosed the presence of proliferative retinopathy in only 49% of patients they examined (under optimal conditions), whereas ophthalmologists and retinal specialists correctly diagnosed its presence in 96% of cases.

Guidelines have been developed and implemented that suggest that all diabetic patients be informed of the possible ocular complications and of the role of the ophthalmologist in the management (detection and prevention) of these complications (Table 41-11).[185] Because it is rare for young (prepubertal) insulin-dependent patients to develop serious vision-threatening retinopathy during the first 5 years of diabetes,[76,103,104] frequent examinations by an ophthalmologist need not begin until 5 years after diagnosis of diabetes. For older-onset individuals, because the age of onset of diabetes is frequently uncertain and there is a higher frequency of vision-threatening retinopathy at the time of diagnosis,[17,115] regular periodic examinations by an ophthalmologist should begin shortly after diagnosis. Patients who are in poor glycemic control, are pregnant, or who have microalbuminuria or gross proteinuria should be examined by ophthalmologists, as they may be at higher risk for progression of retinopathy.

Recent data suggest that diabetic patients may not be receiving adequate ophthalmologic care.[186–189] In the 1989 National Health Interview Survey, participants 18 years of age or older were asked if they had had a dilated eye examination in the past year.[188] Only 49% reported a dilated eye examination within a year of the interview. People with T2DM were more likely to have had a dilated eye examination if they were older, had a higher socioeconomic status, and had attended a diabetes education class. Receiving a dilated eye examination was not related to race, duration of diabetes, frequency of physician visits for diabetes, or health insurance in that study. Kraft and colleagues[189] identified and surveyed all primary care physicians in Indiana using a questionnaire. Of those surveyed, 1058 (70%) completed the eye care–related questions. The investigators reported that 52% of physicians performed in-office ophthalmoscopy, of which 90% were done through undilated pupils. In addition, nearly 58% of physicians reported that they referred all of their patients with T1DM and 40% reported they referred all of their patients with T2DM to eye care specialists. Physicians who had graduated earlier and those who were either general or family practitioners were less likely to refer their patients to eye care specialists.

In the WESDR in 1980–1982, only 63% of younger-onset and 50% of older-onset diabetic persons had seen an ophthalmologist within the previous 2 years before the examination; 25% of younger- and 36% of older-onset persons had never had an ophthalmologic examination.[186] It was estimated that in 1980–1982 there were 35,000 diabetic Americans with eyes with proliferative retinopathy with high-risk characteristics for severe visual loss and 230,000 with eyes with clinically significant macular edema that were untreated with photocoagulation.

There are a number of possible reasons that explain the high rate of patients with serious retinopathy who are not under the care of an ophthalmologist or who have not received photocoagulation treatment.[186] Physician-related factors include poor ophthalmoscopy skills, ophthalmoscopy through an undilated pupil, lack of knowledge about the benefits of photocoagulation treatment, and no or inadequate referral to ophthalmologists. In addition, there are a number of patient-related factors that explain failure to receive ophthalmologic care. These include the asymptomatic nature of vision-threatening retinopathy, a lack of knowledge about the benefits of timely detection by dilated eye examination and treatment with photocoagulation, lack of motivation or denial, an inability to pay for ophthalmologic care, a lack of time to go for such care, and a lack of availability or accessibility of ophthalmologic care. Findings from the WESDR showed that in persons with 10 or more years of diabetes, in those not having a dilated eye examination in the previous year "79% and 71% of those with Type 1 and Type 2, respectively, reported not having had one because they had no problems with their eyes, and 31% and 35% reported not having been told they needed one. Thirty-two percent and 11% said they were too busy, and 30% and 12% said they could not afford an examination." Persons with T1DM or T2DM were less likely to have had an eye examination if they did not have health insurance that covered such an examination.[190]

TABLE 41-11. Recommendations for Eye Case for Diabetic Patients

PRIMARY-CARE PHYSICIAN INFORMS PATIENT AT TIME OF DIAGNOSIS OF DIABETES THAT:

Ocular complications are associated with diabetes and may threaten sight

Glycemic and blood pressure control reduces risk of developing retinopathy

Timely detection and treatment of retinopathy may reduce the risk of decreased vision

REFERRAL TO AN EYE DOCTOR COMPETENT IN OPHTHALMOSCOPY:

All patients 10–30 years of age who have ≥5 years of diabetes

All diabetic patients diagnosed after 30 years of age at the time of diagnosis or shortly thereafter

REFERRAL TO AN OPHTHALMOLOGIST:

All women with type 1 diabetes mellitus planning pregnancy within 12 months, in the first trimester, and thereafter at the discretion of the ophthalmologist

Patients found to have reduced corrected visual acuity, elevated intraocular pressure, and any other vision-threatening ocular abnormalities

Source: Reprinted with permission from Klein R, Klein BEK, Moss SE: The Wisconsin Epidemiological Study of Diabetic Retinopathy: A review. *Diabetes Metab Rev* 1989;5:559.

A series of studies by Dasbach and colleagues[191] and Javitt and associates[192] in the U.S., and Crijns[193] in the Netherlands, have demonstrated that screening for diabetic retinopathy and obtaining ophthalmologic care results in significant savings in people with younger-onset diabetes. The analyses by Javitt and coworkers[192] predicted an annual savings of an estimated $240.5 million and 138,390 person-years of sight at a 60% screening and treatment rate implementation level. The study by Dasbach and coworkers[191] also found that targeting the younger-onset cohort and the older-onset cohort taking insulin could achieve cost savings.

Screening programs for diabetic eye disease have thus been suggested to reduce blindness due to this disease.[185,192] Other programs involve education. One such program, the National Eye Health Education Program (NEHEP), has been developed by the National Eye Institute. It is directed at patients with diabetes.[194] Its primary aim is to educate diabetic patients and their families regarding the need for dilated eye examinations. It is hoped that the program will lead to a change in behavior regarding pursuing eye care. However, while it has the potential to have an important impact, there is also a need to develop approaches designed to deal with the inability of some patients without health insurance to pay for ophthalmologic care.

Ophthalmologic Care

At each visit,[195] the ophthalmologic examination may include refraction and measurement of the visual acuity, measurement of the intraocular pressure, dilation of the pupil, and examination of the lens by slit-lamp biomicroscopy. Retinal edema is more easily detected using slit-lamp biomicroscopy and a corneal contact lens to provide a magnified stereoscopic view of the retina. Sketches of the retina and color stereoscopic fundus photographs should be obtained to document the presence and severity of the retinopathy. Photographs are used to accurately document the progression of retinal disease. Fluorescein angiography is used when focal photocoagulation treatment is considered and when the extent of retinal ischemia needs to be assessed. The angiograms demonstrate abnormal leakage from retinal blood vessels, which may be responsible for macular edema and may also demonstrate closure of small capillaries or arterioles. More highly specialized procedures, for example, vitreous fluorophotometry, macular recovery time measured with nyctometry, and electrophysiologic testing, are used largely as experimental tools to indicate retinal functional or physiologic abnormalities due to diabetes before the appearance of retinopathy.

REHABILITATION

The visual impairment in diabetes may range from minimal changes in color vision to total blindness and may include periods of rapid or slow progression with fluctuations in vision due to recurrent vitreous hemorrhage or macular edema. The unique problems confronted by visually impaired insulin-taking diabetic patients include identification of the type of insulin, determination of the amount of insulin in the vial, measurement of dose, and location of injection sites. Monitoring glucose levels using blood test strips and foot care become more difficult or impossible for the visually impaired diabetic patient. A number of low-vision aids, devices for insulin administration, and aids in glucose monitoring are available for the visually impaired diabetic patient.[196] Depending on the degree of visual impairment, supportive rehabilitation services, including low-vision clinics, state vocational rehabilitation centers, and schools for the blind, are available. Social workers, psychologists, orientation and mobility instructors, and rehabilitation teachers working as a team are needed to develop successful programs. They must help in handling the anxiety, anger, guilt, depression, loss of self-esteem, and difficulties in social adjustment suffered by the diabetic patients with visual loss.[197,198] Other current or potential systemic problems must be taken into account when planning the program. Helping the patient accept the partial or complete visual loss is an essential step in planning living arrangements and in developing coping strategies.

Acknowledgments. The author acknowledges the support of grant EY03083 from the National Eye Institute. He thanks Dr. Barbara E.K. Klein and Mr. Scot Moss for reviewing the manuscript, Gene Knutson and Michael Neider for preparing the photographs, and Colleen Comeau for secretarial assistance.

REFERENCES

1. Klein R, Klein BEK: Vision disorders in diabetes. In: Hammon R, Harris MWH, eds. *Diabetes in America, Diabetes Data Compiled 1984.* U.S. Public Health Service: NIH Publication No. 85-1468, August 1985;1.
2. Caird FI, Pirie A, Ramsell TG: *Diabetes and the Eye.* Blackwell:1969.
3. Klein R, Klein BEK, Moss SE, et al: Glycosylated hemoglobin predicts the incidence and progression of diabetic retinopathy. *JAMA* 1988;260:2864.
4. The Diabetes Control and Complications Trial (DCCT) Research Group: The effect of intensive treatment of diabetes on the development and progression of long-term complications in insulin-dependent diabetes mellitus. *N Engl J Med* 1993;329:977.
5. UKPDS and blood sugar.
6. UKPDS on blood pressure.
7. Diabetic Retinopathy Study (DRS) Group: Photocoagulation treatment of proliferative diabetic retinopathy: Clinical application of Diabetic Retinopathy Study (DRS) findings. DRS Report No. 8. *Ophthalmology* 1981;88:583.
8. ETDRS Research Group: Photocoagulation for diabetic macular edema. *Arch Ophthalmol* 1985;103:1796.
9. Hogan MJ, Alvarado JA, Weddell JE: *Histology of the Human Eye: An Atlas and Textbook.* Saunders:1971.
10. Bresnick GH: Diabetic retinopathy. In: Peyman GA, Sanders DR, Goldberg MF, eds. *Principles and Practice of Ophthalmology.* Saunders:1977.
11. Kohner EM, McLeod D, Marshall J: Diabetic eye disease. In: Keen H, Jarrett J, eds. *Complications of Diabetes*, 2nd ed. Arnold:1982.
12. Kohner EM, Dollery CT: The rate of formation and disappearance of microaneurysms in diabetic retinopathy. *Eur J Clin Invest* 1970;1:167.
13. Klein R, Meuer SM, Moss SE, et al: The relationship of retinal microaneurysm counts to the 4-year progression of diabetic retinopathy. *Arch Ophthalmol* 1989;107:1780.
14. Klein R, Meuer SM, Moss SE, et al: Retinal microaneurysm counts and 10-year progression of diabetic retinopathy. *Arch Ophthalmol* 1995;113:1386–1391.
15. Baudoin C, Maneschi F, Quentel G, et al: Quantitative evaluation of fluorescein angiograms: Microaneurysm counts. *Diabetes* 1983;32:1.
16. Klein R, Klein BEK, Moss SE, et al: The Wisconsin Epidemiologic Study of Diabetic Retinopathy. II. Prevalence and risk of diabetic retinopathy when age at diagnosis is less than 30 years. *Arch Ophthalmol* 1984;102:520.
17. Klein R, Klein BEK, Moss SE, et al: The Wisconsin Epidemiologic Study of Diabetic Retinopathy. III. Prevalence and risk of diabetic retinopathy when age at diagnosis is 30 or more years. *Arch Ophthalmol* 1984;102:527.
18. Klein R: Retinopathy in a population-based study. *Trans Am Ophthalmol Soc* 1992;90:561.

19. Dobree JH: Simple diabetic retinopathy. Evolution of the lesions and therapeutic considerations. *Br J Ophthalmol* 1970;54:1.

20. Bek T: Venous loops and reduplications in diabetic retinopathy. Prevalence, distribution, and pattern of development. *Acta Ophthalmol Scand* 1999;77:130.

21. Early Treatment Diabetic Retinopathy Study (ETDRS) Research Group: Fundus photographic risk factors for progression of diabetic retinopathy. ETDRS Report No. 12. *Ophthalmology* 1991;98:823.

22. Bresnick GH: Diabetic maculopathy: A critical review highlighting diffuse macular edema. *Ophthalmology* 1983;90:1301.

23. Lopes de Faria JM, Jalkh AE, *et al*: Diabetic macular edema: risk factors and concomitants. *Acta Ophthalmol Scand* 1999;77:170.

24. Aiello LM, Rand LI, Brines JC, *et al*: Nonocular clinical risk factors in the progression of diabetic retinopathy. In: Little HL, Jack RL, Patz A, *et al*, eds. *Diabetic Retinopathy*. Thieme-Stratton:1983.

25. Diabetic Retinopathy Study: Report 7. A modification of the Airlie House classification of diabetic retinopathy. *Invest Ophthalmol* 1981; 7:210.

26. Early Treatment Diabetic Retinopathy Study (ETDRS) Research Group: Grading diabetic retinopathy from stereoscopic color fundus photographs. An extension of the modified Airlie House Classification. ETDRS Report No. 10. *Ophthalmology* 1991;98:786.

27. Moss SE, Klein R, Klein BEK: Ten year incidence of visual loss in a diabetic population. *Ophthalmology* 1994;101:1061.

28. Moss SE, Klein R, Kessler SD, *et al*: Comparison between ophthalmoscopy and fundus photography in determining severity of diabetic retinopathy. *Ophthalmology* 1985;92:62.

29. Cree MJ, Olson JA, McHardy KC, *et al*: A fully automated comparative microaneurysm digital detection system. *Eye* 1997;11:622.

30. Gardner GG, Keating D, Williamson TH, *et al*: Automatic detection of diabetic retinopathy using an artificial neural network: a screening tool. *Br J Ophthalmol* 1996;80:940.

31. Aleynikov S, Micheli-Tzanakou E: Classification of retinal damage by a neural network based system. *J Med Syst* 1998;22:129.

32. Lee SC, Kingsley RM, Lee ET, *et al*: Comparison of diagnosis of nonproliferative diabetic retinopathy between a computer system and human experts. *Arch Ophthalmol* 2001;119:509.

33. Verdonk CA, Palumbo PJ, Gharib H, *et al*: Diabetic microangiopathy in patients with pancreatitic diabetes mellitus. *Diabetologia* 1975;11: 395.

34. Engerman RL: Animal models of diabetic retinopathy. *Trans Am Acad Ophthalmol Otolaryngol* 1976;81:710.

35. Nelson RG, Wolfe JA, Horton MB: Proliferative retinopathy in Type 2. Incidence and risk factors in Pima Indians. *Diabetes* 1989;38:435.

36. Lee ET, Lee VS, Lu M, *et al*: Development of proliferative retinopathy in Type 2, a follow-up study of American Indians in Oklahoma. *Diabetes* 1992;41:359.

37. Lee ET, Lee VS, Kingsley RM, *et al*: Diabetic retinopathy in Oklahoma Indians with Type 2: Incidence and risk factors. *Diabetes Care* 1992;15:1620.

38. Ballard DJ, Melton LJ, Dwyer MS, *et al*: Risk factors for diabetic retinopathy: A population-based study in Rochester, Minnesota. *Diabetes Care* 1986;9:334.

39. Dyck PJ, Kratz KM, Karnes JL, *et al*: The prevalence by staged severity of various types of diabetic neuropathy, retinopathy, and nephropathy in a population-based cohort: The Rochester Diabetic Neuropathy Study. *Neurology* 1993;43:817.

40. Teuscher A, Schnell H, Wilson PWF: Incidence of diabetic retinopathy and relationship to baseline plasma glucose and blood pressure. *Diabetes Care* 1988;11:246.

41. Lloyd CE, Klein R, Maser RE, *et al*: The progression of retinopathy over 2 years: The Pittsburgh Epidemiology of Diabetes Complications (EDC) Study. *J Diabetes Comp* 1995;9:140.

42. Tilton RG, Chang K, Hasan KS, *et al*: Prevention of dysfunction by guanidines: Inhibition of nitric oxide synthase versus advanced glycosylation end-product formation. *Diabetes* 1993;42:221.

43. Frank RN: On the pathogenesis of diabetic retinopathy. A 1990 update. *Ophthalmology* 1991;98:586.

44. Robison WG Jr., Kador PF, Konoshita JH: Retinal capillaries: Basement membrane thickening prevented with aldose reductase inhibitor. *Science* 1983;221:1177.

45. Robison WG Jr., Nagata M, Laver N, *et al*: Diabetic-like retinopathy in rats prevented with an aldose reductase inhibitor. *Invest Ophthalmol Vis Sci* 1989;30:2285.

46. Sorbinil Retinopathy Trial Research Group: A randomized trial of sorbinil, an aldose reductase inhibitor in diabetic retinopathy. *Arch Ophthalmol* 1990;108:1234.

47. Lindback K: Growth hormone's role in diabetic microangiopathy. *Diabetes* 1976;25:845.

48. D'Amore PA, Klagsbrun M: Endothelial cell mitogens derived from retina and hypothalamus, biochemical and biological stimulants. *J Cell Biol* 1984;99:545.

49. Little HL: The role of abnormal hemorrheodynamics in the pathogenesis of diabetic retinopathy. *Trans Am Ophthalmol Soc* 1976;74:574.

50. Ditzel J, Standl E: The problem of tissue oxygenation in diabetes mellitus. 1. Its relation to the early functional changes in the microcirculation of diabetic subjects. *August Krogh Memorial Symposium* 1974:49.

51. Kohner EM: The problems of retinal blood flow in diabetes. *Diabetes* 1976;25:839.

52. Parving HH, Viberti GC, Keen H, *et al*: Hemodynamic factors in the genesis of diabetic microangiopathy. *Metabolism* 1983;32:943.

53. Kohner EM, Porta M, Hyer SL: The pathogenesis of diabetic retinopathy and cataract. In: Pickup J, Williams G, eds. *Textbook of Diabetes*. Blackwell Scientific:1991;564.

54. Blair NP, Feke GT, Morales-Stoppello J, *et al*: Prolongation of the retinal mean circulation time in diabetes. *Arch Ophthalmol* 1983; 100:764.

55. Yonemura D, Kawasaki K: New approaches to ophthalmic electrodiagnosis by retinal oscillatory potentials, drug-induced responses from retinal pigment epithelium and cone potential. *Doc Ophthalmol* 1979; 48:163.

56. Kinnear P, Aspinall P, Lakowski R: The diabetic eye and colour vision. *Trans Ophthalmol Soc UK* 1972;92:69.

57. Glaser BM, D'Amore PA, Michels RG, *et al*: Demonstration of vasoproliferative activity from mammalian retina. *J Cell Biol* 1980;84:298.

58. Glaser BM, Campochiaro PA, Davis JL, *et al*: Retinal pigment epithelial cells release an inhibitor of neovascularization. *Arch Ophthalmol* 1985;103:1870.

59. Bennett PH, Rushforth NB, Miller M, *et al*: Epidemiologic studies of diabetes in the Pima Indians. *Recent Prog Horm Res* 1976;32:333.

60. Kahn HA, Leibowitz HM, Ganley JP, *et al*: The Framingham Eye Study. I. Outline and major prevalence findings. *Am J Epidemiol* 1977;106:17.

61. West KM, Erdreich LJ, Stober JA: A detailed study of risk factors for retinopathy and nephropathy in diabetes. *Diabetes* 1980;19:501.

62. Houston A: Retinopathy in the Poole area: An epidemiological inquiry. In: Eschwege E, ed. *Advances in Diabetes Epidemiology*. Elsevier:1982.

63. King H, Balkau B, Zimmet P, *et al*: Diabetic retinopathy in Nauruans. *Am J Epidemiol* 1983;117:659.

64. Dwyer MS, Melton LJ III, Ballard DJ, *et al*: Incidence of diabetic retinopathy and blindness: A population-based study in Rochester, Minnesota. *Diabetes Care* 1985;8:316.

65. Danielsen R, Jonasson F, Helgason T: Prevalence of retinopathy and proteinuria in type I diabetics in Iceland. *Acta Med Scand* 1982;212: 277.

66. Constable IJ, Knuiman MW, Welborn TA, *et al*: Assessing the risk of diabetic retinopathy. *Am J Ophthalmol* 1984;97:53.

67. Knuiman MW, Welborn TA, McCann VJ, *et al*: Prevalence of diabetic complications in relation to risk factors. *Diabetes* 1986;35:1332.

68. Sjolie AK: Ocular complications in insulin treated diabetes mellitus. An epidemiological study. *Acta Ophthalmol* 1985;172:1.

69. Nielsen NV: Diabetic retinopathy. II. The course of retinopathy in diabetics treated with oral hypoglycemic agents and diet regime alone. A one year epidemiologic cohort study of diabetes mellitus. The Island of Falster, Denmark. *Acta Ophthalmol* 1984;62:266.

70. Nielsen NV: Diabetic retinopathy. I. The course of retinopathy in insulin-treated diabetics. A one-year epidemiological cohort study of diabetes mellitus. The island of Falster, Denmark. *Acta Ophthalmol* 1984;62:256.

71. Haffner SM, Fong D, Stern MP, *et al*: Diabetic retinopathy in Mexican Americans and non-Hispanic whites. *Diabetes* 1988;37:878.

72. Jerneld B: Prevalence of diabetic retinopathy. *Acta Ophthalmol Scand* 1988;188:3.

73. Hamman RF, Mayer EJ, Moo-Young GA, *et al*: Prevalence and risk factors of diabetic retinopathy in non-Hispanic whites and Hispanics with Type 2. San Luis Valley Diabetes Study. *Diabetes* 1989;38:1231.

74. Hamman RF, Franklin GA, Mayer EJ, *et al*: Microvascular complications of Type 2 in Hispanics and non-Hispanic whites. *Diabetes Care* 1991;14:655.

75. McLeod BK, Thompson JR, Rosenthal AR: The prevalence of retinopathy in the insulin-requiring diabetic patients of an English county town. *Eye* 1988;2:424.

76. Klein R, Klein BEK, Moss SE, *et al*: The Wisconsin Epidemiologic Study of Diabetic Retinopathy. IX. Four-year incidence and progression of diabetic retinopathy when age at diagnosis is less than 30 years. *Arch Ophthalmol* 1989;107:237.

77. Klein R, Klein BEK, Moss SE, *et al*: The Wisconsin Epidemiologic Study of Diabetic Retinopathy. X. Four-year incidence and progression of diabetic retinopathy when age at diagnosis is 30 years or more. *Arch Ophthalmol* 1989;107:244.

78. Klein R, Klein BEK, Moss SE, *et al*: The Wisconsin Epidemiologic Study of Diabetic Retinopathy. XIV. Ten-year incidence and progression of diabetic retinopathy. *Arch Ophthalmol* 1994;112:1217.

79. Klein R, Klein BEK, Moss SE, *et al*: The Wisconsin epidemiologic Study of Diabetic Retinopathy. XVII. The 14-year incidence and progression of diabetic retinopathy and associated risk factors in Type 1 diabetes. *Ophthalmology* 1998;105:1801.

80. Kostraba JN, Klein R, Dorman JS, *et al*: The Epidemiology of Diabetes Complications Study. IV. Correlates of diabetic background and proliferative retinopathy. *Am J Epidemiol* 1991;133:381.

81. Fujimoto W, Fukuda M: Natural history of diabetic retinopathy and its treatment in Japan. In: Baba S, Goto Y, Fukui I, eds. *Diabetes Mellitus in Asia*. Excerpta Medica:1976;225.

82. Cohen DL, Neil HAW, Thorogood M, *et al*: A population-based study of the incidence of complications associated with Type 2 diabetes in the elderly. *Diabetic Med* 1991;8:928.

83. Eriksson J, Forsen B, Haggblom M, *et al*: Clinical and metabolic characteristics of type 1 and Type 2 diabetes. An epidemiological study from the Narpes Community in Western Finland. *Diabetic Med* 1992;9:654.

84. Schachat AP, Hyman L, Leske MC, *et al*: Comparison of diabetic retinopathy detection by clinical examinations and photograph gradings. *Arch Ophthalmol* 1993;111:1064.

85. Sparrow JM, McCleod BK, Smith TDW, *et al*: The prevalence of diabetic retinopathy and maculopathy and their risk factors in the non-insulin-treated diabetic patients of an English town. *Eye* 1993;7:158.

86. Wirta OR, Pasternack AI, Oksa HH, *et al*: Occurrence of late specific complications in type II (non-insulin-dependent) diabetes mellitus. *J Diabetes Complications* 1995;9:177.

87. Falkenberg M, Finnstrom K: Associations with retinopathy in Type 2 diabetes: a population-based study in a Swedish rural area. *Diabetes Med* 1994;11:843.

88. Hapnes R, Bergrem H: Diabetic eye complications in a medium sized municipality in Southwest Norway. *Acta Ophthalmol Scand* 1996;74:497.

89. Joner G, Brinchmann-Hansen O, Torres CG, *et al*: A nationwide cross-sectional study of retinopathy and microalbuminuria in young Norwegian type 1 (insulin-dependent) diabetic patients. *Diabetologia* 1992;35:1049.

90. Klein R, Klein BEK, Moss SE, *et al*: The Wisconsin Epidemiologic Study of Diabetic Retinopathy (WESDR). IV. Diabetic macular edema. *Ophthalmology* 1984;91:1464.

91. Nelson RG, Pettit DJ, Carraher MG, *et al*: The effect of proteinuria on mortality in Type 2. *Diabetes* 1988;37:1499.

92. Harris MI, Klein R, Cowie C, *et al*: Is the risk of diabetic retinopathy greater in blacks and Mexican Americans than in non-Hispanic whites with Type 2 diabetes? A U.S. population study. *Diabetes Care* 1998;21:1230.

93. Rabb MF, Gagliano DA, Sweeny NE: Diabetic retinopathy in blacks. *Diabetes Care* 1990;13:1202.

94. Arfken CL, Salicrup AE, Meuer SM, *et al*: Retinopathy in African Americans and Whites with insulin-dependent diabetes. *Arch Intern Med* 1994;154:2597.

95. Pyke DA, Tattersall RB: Diabetic retinopathy in identical twins. *Diabetes* 1973;22:613.

96. The Diabetes Control and Complications Trial (DCCT) Research Group: Clustering of long-term complications in families with diabetes in the Diabetes Control and Complications Trial. *Diabetes* 1997;46:1829.

97. Dornan TL, Ting A, McPherson CK, *et al*: Genetic susceptibility to the development of retinopathy in insulin-dependent diabetics. *Diabetes* 1982;31:226.

98. Bodansky HJ, Cudworth AG, Whitelocke RAF, *et al*: Diabetic retinopathy and its relation to type of diabetes: Review of a retinal clinic population. *Br J Ophthalmol* 1982;66:496.

99. Cruickshanks KJ, Vadheim CM, Moss SE, *et al*: Genetic marker associations with proliferative retinopathy in persons diagnosed with diabetes prior to 30 years of age. *Diabetes* 1992;41:879.

100. Klein R, Klein BEK, Moss SE, *et al*: Retinopathy in young-onset diabetic patients. *Diabetes Care* 1985;8:311.

101. Klein BEK, Moss SE, Klein R: Is menarche associated with diabetic retinopathy? *Diabetes Care* 1990;13:1034.

102. Frost-Larsen K, Starup K: Fluorescein angiography in diabetic children: A follow-up. *Acta Ophthalmol (Copenh)* 1980;58:355.

103. Murphy RP, Nanda M, Plotnick L, *et al*: The relationship of puberty to diabetic retinopathy. *Arch Ophthalmol* 1990;108:215.

104. Kostraba JN, Dorman JS, Orchard TJ, *et al*: Contribution of diabetes duration before puberty to development of microvascular complications in Type 1 subjects. *Diabetes Care* 1989;12:686.

105. Harris MI, Klein R, Welborn TA, *et al*: Onset of Type 2 occurs at least 4–7 years before clinical diagnosis. *Diabetes Care* 1992;15:815.

106. Aiello LM, Rand LI, Briones JC, *et al*: Diabetic retinopathy in Joslin Clinic patients with adult-onset diabetes. *Ophthalmology* 1981;88:619.

107. Krowlewski AS, Warram JH, Rand LI, *et al*: Risk of proliferative retinopathy in juvenile onset type I diabetes: A 40-year follow-up study. *Diabetes Care* 1986;9:443.

108. Engerman RL, Bloodworth JMB, Nelson SL: Relationship of microvascular disease in diabetes to metabolic control. *Diabetes* 1977;26:760.

109. Engerman RL, Kern TS: Progression of incipient diabetic retinopathy during good glycemic control. *Diabetes* 1987;36:808.

110. Chase HP, Jackson WE, Hoops SL, *et al*: Glucose control and the renal and retinal complications of insulin-dependent diabetes. *JAMA* 1989;261:1155.

111. University Group Diabetes Program: A study of the effects of hypoglycemic agents on vascular complications in patients with adult-onset diabetes. *Diabetes* 1982;5:1.

112. Lauritzen T, Frost-Larsen K, Larsen HW, *et al*: Two-year experience with continuous subcutaneous insulin infusion in relation to retinopathy and neuropathy. *Diabetes* 1985;34:74.

113. The Kroc Collaborative Study Group. Diabetic retinopathy after two years of intensified insulin treatment: Follow-up of The Kroc Collaborative Study. *JAMA* 1988;260:37.

114. Dahl-Jorgensen K, Brinchmann-Hansen O, Hanssen KF, *et al*: Effect of near normoglycemia for two years on progression of early diabetic retinopathy, nephropathy, and neuropathy. The Oslo Study. *Br Med J* 1986;293:1995.

115. UKPDS Group: UK Prospective Diabetes Study. Complications in newly diagnosed Type 2 diabetic patients and their association with clinical and biochemical risk factors. *Diabetes Res* 1990;13:1.

116. Sjoberg S, Gunnarsson R, Gjotterberg M, *et al*: Residual insulin production, glycaemic control and prevalence of microvascular lesions and polyneuropathy in long-term type I (insulin dependent) diabetes mellitus. *Diabetologia* 1987;30:208.

117. Madsbad S, Lauritzen E, Faber OK, *et al*: The effect of residual beta cell function on the development of diabetic retinopathy. *Diabetic Med* 1986;3:42.

118. Klein R, Moss SE, Klein BEK, *et al*: Wisconsin Epidemiologic Study of Diabetic Retinopathy. XII. Relationship of C-peptide and diabetic retinopathy. *Diabetes* 1990;39:1445.

119. Serghieri G, Bartolomei G, Pettenello C, *et al*: Raised retinopathy prevalence rate in insulin-treated patients: A feature of obese type II diabetes. *Transplant Proc* 1986;18:1576.

120. Deutsch TA, O'Riodan JF, Ernest JT, *et al*: Systemic blood pressure and diabetic macular edema. *Ophthalmol Vis Sci* 1983;24:80.

121. Klein R, Klein BEK, Moss SE, *et al*: Is blood pressure a predictor of the incidence or progression of diabetic retinopathy? *Arch Intern Med* 1989;149:2427.

122. Chaturvedi N, Sjolie AK, Stephenson JM, *et al*: Effect of lisinopril on progression of retinopathy in normotensive people with type 1 diabetes. The EUCLID Study Group. EURODIAB Controlled Trial of Lisinopril in Insulin-Dependent Diabetes Mellitus. *Lancet* 1998;351:28.

123. Winocour PH, Durrington PN, Ishola M, *et al*: Influence of proteinuria on vascular disease, blood pressure, and lipoproteins in insulin dependent diabetes mellitus. *Br Med J* 1987;294:1648.

124. Feldman JN, Hirsh SR, Beyer MM, *et al*: Prevalence of diabetic nephropathy at time of treatment for diabetic retinopathy. In: Friedman EA, L'Esperance FA, eds. *Diabetic Renal-Retinal Syndrome: Prevention and Management.* Grune & Stratton:1982;2.

125. Klein R, Moss SE, Klein BEK: Is gross proteinuria a risk factor for the incidence of proliferative diabetic retinopathy? *Ophthalmology* 1993;100:1140.

126. Ramsey RC, Knobloch WH, Cantrill HL, *et al*: Visual status in transplanted and dialyzed diabetic patients. In: Friedman EA, L'Esperance FA, eds. *Diabetic Renal-Retinal Syndrome: Prevention and Management.* Grune & Stratton:1982;2.

127. Aiello LM, Rand LI, Brines JC, *et al*: Nonocular clinical risk factors in the progression of diabetic retinopathy. In: Littel HL, Jack RL, Patz A, *et al*, eds. *Diabetic Retinopathy.* Thieme-Stratton:1983.

128. Klein BEK, Moss SE, Klein R, *et al*: The Wisconsin Epidemiologic Study of Diabetic Retinopathy (WESDR). XIII. Relationship of serum cholesterol to retinopathy and hard exudate. *Ophthalmology* 1991;98:1261.

129. Chantry KH, Klein ML, Chew EY, *et al*: Early Treatment Retinopathy Study Research Group: Association of serum lipids and retinal hard exudates in patients enrolled in the Early Treatment Diabetic Retinopathy Study (ETDRS). *Invest Ophthalmol Vis Sci* 1989;30:434.

130. Paetkau ME, Boyd TAS, Winship B, *et al*: Cigarette smoking and diabetic retinopathy. *Diabetes* 1977;26:46.

131. Nielsen MM, Hjollund E: Smoking and diabetic microangiopathy. *Lancet* 1978;2:533.

132. Klein R, Klein BEK, Davis MD: Is cigarette smoking associated with diabetic retinopathy? *Am J Epidemiol* 1983;118:228.

133. Moss SE, Klein R, Klein BEK: Association of cigarette smoking with diabetic retinopathy. *Diabetes Care* 1991;14:119.

134. Kingsley LA, Dorman JS, Doft BH, *et al*: An epidemiologic approach to the study of retinopathy: The Pittsburgh diabetic morbidity and retinopathy studies. *Diabetes Res Clin Pract* 1988;4:99.

135. Young RJ, McCulloch DK, Prescott RJ, *et al*: Alcohol: Another risk factor for diabetic retinopathy? *Br Med J* 1984;288:1035.

136. Moss SE, Klein R, Klein BEK: Alcohol consumption and the prevalence of diabetic retinopathy. *Ophthalmology* 1992;99:926.

137. Cruickshanks KJ, Moss SE, Klein R, *et al*: Physical activity and proliferative retinopathy in persons diagnosed with diabetes before age 30 years. *Diabetes Care* 1992;15:1267.

138. Hanna AK, Roy M, Zinman B, *et al*: An evaluation of factors associated with proliferative diabetic retinopathy. *Clin Invest Med* 1985;8:109.

139. Haffner SM, Hazuda HP, Stern MP, *et al*: Effect of socioeconomic status on hyperglycemia and retinopathy levels in Mexican Americans with Type 2. *Diabetes Care* 1989;12:128.

140. Klein R, Klein BEK, Jensen SC, *et al*: The relation of socioeconomic factors to the incidence of proliferative diabetic retinopathy and loss of vision. *Ophthalmology* 1994;101:68.

141. Rodman HM, Singerman LJ, Arello LM, *et al*: Diabetic retinopathy and its relationship to pregnancy. In: Merkatz ER, Adams PAJ, eds. *The Diabetic Pregnancy: A Perinatal Perspective.* Grune & Stratton:1979.

142. Beetham WP: Diabetic retinopathy in pregnancy. *Trans Am Ophthalmol Soc* 1950;48:205.

143. Larinkari J, Laatikainen L, Mooronen P, *et al*: Metabolic control and serum hormone levels in relation to retinopathy in diabetic retinopathy. *Diabetologia* 1982;22:327.

144. Moloney JBM, Drury MI: The effect of pregnancy on the natural course of diabetic retinopathy. *Am J Ophthalmol* 1982;93:745.

145. Klein BEK, Moss SE, Klein R: Effect of pregnancy on progression of diabetic retinopathy. *Diabetes Care* 1990;13:34.

146. Klein BEK, Klein R, Meuer SM, *et al*: Does the severity of diabetic retinopathy predict pregnancy outcome? *J Diabetes Complications* 1988;2:179.

147. Early Treatment Diabetic Retinopathy Study (ETDRS) Research Group: Effects of aspirin treatment on diabetic retinopathy. ETDRS Report No. 8. *Ophthalmology* 1991;98:757.

148. Rand LJ: Recent advances in diabetic retinopathy. *Am J Med* 1982;70:595.

149. Klein R, Klein BEK, Moss SE, *et al*: The medical management of hyperglycemia over a 10-year period in people with diabetes. *Diabetes Care* 1996;19:744.

150. Ferris FL III: How effective are treatments for diabetic retinopathy? *JAMA* 1993;269:1290.

151. Early Treatment Diabetic Retinopathy Study (ETDRS) Research Group: Early photocoagulation for diabetic retinopathy: ETDRS Report No. 9. *Ophthalmology* 1991;98:766.

152. Little HL: Complications of argon laser photocoagulation in the treatment of diabetic retinopathy. In: Littel HL, Jack RL, Patz A, *et al*, eds. *Diabetic Retinopathy.* Thieme-Stratton:1983.

153. Michaels RG, Rice TA, Rice EF: Vitrectomy for diabetic vitreous hemorrhage. *Am J Ophthalmol* 1983;95:12.

154. Michaels RG: Vitreous surgery for visual loss from proliferative diabetic retinopathy. In: Friedman EA, L'Esperance FA, eds. *Diabetic Renal-Retinal Syndrome: Prevention and Management.* Grune & Stratton:1982;2.

155. Rice TA, Michaels RG: Complications of vitrectomy. In: Littel HL, Jack RL, Patz A, *et al*, eds. *Diabetic Retinopathy.* Thieme-Stratton:1983.

156. Diabetic Retinopathy Vitrectomy Study (DRVS) Research Group: Early vitrectomy for severe vitreous hemorrhage in diabetic retinopathy. Two-year results of randomized trial. DRVS Report No. 2. *Arch Ophthalmol* 1985;92:492.

157. Moss SE, Klein R, Klein BEK: The incidence of vision loss in a diabetic population. *Ophthalmology* 1988;95:1340.

158. Howe LJ, Drury JT: Current estimates from the Health Interview Survey, United States, 1977. National Center for Health Statistics. *Vital and Health Statistics Series 10*, No. 126, 1978.

159. Klein R, Klein BEK, Moss SE: Visual impairment in diabetes. *Ophthalmology* 1984;91:1.

160. Cohen DL, Neil HAW, Thorogood M, *et al*: A population-based study of the incidence of complications associated with Type 2 diabetes in the elderly. *Diabetes Med* 1991;8:928.

161. Roberts J: Monocular visual acuity of persons 4 to 74 years, United States, 1971–72. National Center for Health Statistics. *Vital Health Statistics Series 11*, No. 201, 1977.

162. Leibowitz HM, Krueger DE, Maunder LR: The Framingham Eye Study Monograph. An ophthalmological and epidemiologic study of cataract, glaucoma, diabetic retinopathy, macular degeneration, and visual acuity in a general population of 2,631 adults, 1973–75. *Surv Ophthalmol* 1980;24:335.

163. Sjolie AK, Green A: Blindness in insulin-treated diabetic patients with age at onset <30 years. *Chronic Dis* 1987;40:215.

164. Grey RHB, Burns-Cox CJ, Hughes A: Blind and partial sight registration in Avon. *Br J Ophthalmol* 1989;73:88.

165. Thompson JR, Du L, Rosenthal AR: Recent trends in the registration of blindness and partial sight in Leicestershire. *Br J Ophthalmol* 1989;73:95.

166. Sorsby A: The incidence and causes of blindness in England and Wales 1963–1968. *Reports on Public Health and Medical Subjects.* No. 128. Her Majesty's Stationery Office:1972.

167. Caird FI, Garrett CJ: Prognosis for vision in diabetic retinopathy. *Diabetes* 1963;12:389.

168. Kinoshita JH: Mechanisms initiating cataract formation. *Invest Ophthalmol Vis Sci* 1974;13:713.

169. Ederer F, Hiller R, Taylor HR: Senile lens change and diabetes in two population studies. *Am J Ophthalmol* 1981;91:381.

170. Klein BEK, Klein R, Wang Q, *et al*: Older onset diabetes and lens opacities: The Beaver Dam Eye Study. *Invest Ophthalmol Vis Sci* 1993;34:1065.

171. Klein BEK, Klein R, Moss SE: Prevalence of cataracts in a population-based study of persons with diabetes mellitus. *Ophthalmology* 1985;92:1191.

172. Burditt AF, Caird FI: The natural history of lens opacities in diabetics. *Br J Ophthalmol* 1968;52:433.

173. Seigel D, Sperduto RD, Ferris FL: Aspirin and cataracts. *Ophthalmology* 1982;89:47.

174. Klein BEK, Klein R, Moss SE: Is aspirin use associated with lower rates of cataracts in diabetic individuals? *Diabetes Care* 1987;10:495.

175. Jaffe GJ, Burton TC: Progression of nonproliferative diabetic retinopathy following cataract extraction. *Arch Ophthalmol* 1988;107:745.

176. Pollack A, Leiba H, Bukelman A, *et al*: The course of diabetic retinopathy following cataract surgery in eyes previously treated by laser photocoagulation. *Br J Ophthalmol* 1992;76:228.

177. Straatsma BR, Pettit TH, Wheeler N, *et al*: Diabetes mellitus and intraocular lens implantation. *Ophthalmology* 1983;90:336.

178. Klein BEK, Klein R, Jensen SC: Open angle glaucoma and older onset diabetes. The Beaver Dam Eye Study. *Ophthalmology* 1994;101:1173.

179. Leske MC: The epidemiology of open-angle glaucoma: A review. *Am J Epidemiol* 1983;118:166.

180. Bankes JLK: Ocular tension and diabetes mellitus. *Br J Ophthalmol* 1967;51:557.

181. Klein BEK, Klein R, Moss SE: Incidence of self-reported glaucoma in people with diabetes mellitus. *Brit J Ophthalmology* 1997;81:743.

182. Chiang Y-P, Bassi LJ, Javitt JC: Federal budgetary costs of blindness. *Milbank Mem Fund Q* 1992;70:319.

183. Klein R, Moss SE, Klein BEK: New management concepts for timely diagnosis of diabetic retinopathy treatable by photocoagulation. *Diabetes Care* 1987;10:633.

184. Sussman EJ, Tsiaras WG, Soper KA: Diagnosis of diabetic eye disease. *JAMA* 1982;247:3231.

185. American Diabetes Association: Diabetic retinopathy. *Diabetes Care* 1999;22:S70.

186. Witkin SR, Klein R: Ophthalmologic care for people with diabetes. *JAMA* 1984;251:2534.

187. Sprafka JM, Fritsche TL, Baker R, *et al*: Prevalence of undiagnosed eye disease in high-risk diabetic individuals. *Arch Intern Med* 1990; 150:857.

188. Brechner RJ, Cowie CC, Howie LJ, *et al*: Ophthalmic care for adults with diagnosed diabetes in the U.S. population. *JAMA* 1993;270: 1714.

189. Kraft SK, Marrero DG, Lazaridis EN, *et al*: Primary care physicians—practice patterns and diabetic retinopathy. *Arch Fam Med* 1997;6:29.

190. Moss SE, Klein R, Klein BEK: Factors associated with having eye examinations in persons with diabetes. *Arch Fam Med* 1995;4:529.

191. Dasbach E, Fryback DG, Newcomb PA, *et al*: Cost-effectiveness of strategies for detecting diabetic retinopathy. *Med Care* 1991;29:20.

192. Javitt JC, Canner JK, Frank RG, *et al*: Detecting and treating retinopathy in type I diabetics: A health policy model. *Ophthalmology* 1990; 97:483.

193. Crijns H: *Diabetic Retinopathy. A Cost-Effectiveness Analysis of Ophthalmoscopy and Photocoagulation.* Erasmus University:1993;1 (Doctoral dissertation).

194. National Eye Institute National Eye Health Education Program: From vision research to eye health education. Planning the partnership. Available from NIH, Box 20/20, Bethesda, MD 20892. March 1990.

195. American Academy of Ophthalmology Quality of Care Committee, Retina Panel: *Diabetic Retinopathy: Preferred Practice Patterns.* American Academy of Ophthalmology:1989.

196. The Carroll Center for the Blind: Diabetic control: Equipment for use with vision loss. *Aids Appliances Rev* 1982;6:1.

197. Wulsin LR, Jacobson AM, Rand LI: Psychosocial correlates of mild visual loss. *Psychosomatic Med* 1991;53:109.

198. Wulsin LR, Jacobson AM, Rand LI: Psychosocial adjustment to advanced proliferative diabetic retinopathy. *Diabetes Care* 1993;16: 1061.

Pathophysiology of Renal Complications

Maria Luiza Avancini Caramori

Michael Mauer

Diabetic nephropathy (DN) is the single most common disorder leading to renal failure in adults.[1] The annual cost of caring for these patients in the United States alone exceeds \$6 billion. Forty-four percent of patients entering end-stage renal disease (ESRD) programs in the U.S. are diabetic, most of whom (80% or more) have type 2 diabetes mellitus (T2DM).[1] DN develops in about 25–35% of patients with type 1 diabetic mellitus (T1DM), with a peak in the incidence after about around 15–20 years of disease.[2] Studies in T2DM patients from western Europe[3] and in Pima Indians from Arizona[4] show nephropathy rates similar to or higher than those of T1DM patients. The much higher prevalence of T2DM accounts in part for the greater contribution of these patients to incidence of ESRD. Once overt DN, as manifested as proteinuria, is present, ESRD can be postponed, but in most instances not prevented, by effective antihypertensive treatment[5,6] or careful glycemic control.[7] Moreover, there has been a rapid and continuous increase in the number of diabetic patients entering ESRD programs in the last decade.[1] Thus in the last 10–15 years, there has been intensive research into early predictors of DN risk, pathophysiologic mechanisms of diabetic renal injury, and early intervention strategies. This chapter discusses the current knowledge of the pathology and pathophysiology of DN.

Pathology

T1DM

The changes in kidney structure caused by diabetes are specific, creating a pattern not seen in any other renal disease. The severity of the diabetic lesions is related to diabetes duration, degree of glycemic control, and genetic factors. Ultimately, renal dysfunction results from these progressive structural changes. However, the relationship between duration of T1DM and extent of glomerular pathology is not precise. This is consonant with the marked variability in susceptibility to DN such that some patients may be in renal failure after having diabetes for 15 years or less while others escape complications despite having T1DM for many decades.

Light Microscopy

The earliest renal structural change in T1DM, renal hypertrophy, is not reflected in any specific changes detectable under light microscopy. In many patients, glomerular structure remains normal or near normal despite decades of diabetes.[8–10] Others develop progressive diffuse mesangial expansion seen mainly as increased periodic acid Schiff (PAS)-positive extracellular matrix (ECM) mesangial material (Fig. 42-1). In about 40–50% of patients developing proteinuria, there are areas of extreme mesangial expansion called Kimmelstiel-Wilson nodules or nodular mesangial expansion (Fig. 42-2). Mesangial cell nuclei in these nodules are palisaded around masses of mesangial matrix (MM) material with compression of surrounding capillary lumina. Nodules are thought to result from earlier glomerular capillary microaneurysm formation.[11] Although Kimmelstiel-Wilson nodules are diagnostic of DN, they are not necessary for renal dysfunction to develop. Early changes often include arteriolar hyalinosis lesions involving replacement of the smooth muscle cells of afferent and efferent arterioles with PAS-positive waxy homogenous pink material. The severity of these lesions is directly related to the frequency of global glomerulosclerosis, perhaps as the result of glomerular ischemia. One may also detect, by light microscopy, glomerular basement membrane (GBM) and tubular basement membrane (TBM) thickening, although this is often easier seen by electron microscopy. Finally, usually later in the disease, there is advanced tubular atrophy and interstitial fibrosis, common to most chronic renal disorders.

Immunofluorescence Microscopy

Diabetes is characterized by increased linear GBM, TBM, and Bowman's capsule staining,[12] especially for IgG (mainly IgG$_4$) and albumin.[13] This increased staining is removed only by strong acid conditions, consistent with strong ionic binding of these plasma proteins to GBM ECM constituents. The intensity of staining is not related to the severity of the underlying lesions.[12,13] The immunofluorescence technician should not confuse these findings with antibasement membrane antibody disorders. Diabetic immunohistochemical ECM changes in mesangium, GBM, and TBM through much of the natural history of DN are primarily due to expansion of the intrinsic ECM components normally present at these sites, including type IV and VI collagens, laminin, and fibronectin.[14] However, the exact nature of the accumulated ECM material is not yet known.[15,16] Replacement of these ECM molecules by scar collagens is a very late event.

Electron Microscopy

Glomerular structure is probably normal at onset of diabetes and changes can be detected by morphometric measurements within 1.5–2.5 years after onset.[17] However, since the normal range for glomerular structures, such as GBM width or mesangial

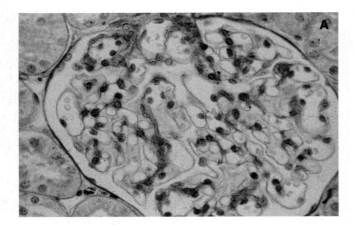

FIGURE 42-1. Light photomicrographs of glomeruli from (**A**) a normal control and from (**B**) a T1DM patient. Note the diffuse mesangial expansion and glomerular basement membrane and Bowman's capsule thickening in the diabetic glomerulus (periodic acid Schiff, ×400).

FIGURE 42-2. Light photomicrographs of glomeruli in sequential kidney biopsies performed at baseline and after 5 and 10 years of follow-up in a longstanding normoalbuminuric T1DM patient with progressive mesangial expansion and renal function deterioration. **A**. Note the diffuse and nodular mesangial expansion and arteriolar hyalinosis in this glomerulus from this patient who was normotensive and normoalbuminuric at the time of this baseline biopsy, 21 years after diabetes onset. The glomerular filtration rate (GFR) was reduced to 74 mL/min/1.73 m^2 (periodic acid Schiff, ×400). **B**. 5-Year follow-up biopsy showing worsening of the diffuse and nodular mesangial expansion and arteriolar hyalinosis in this now microalbuminuric patient with declining GFR (59 mL/min/1.73 m^2) (periodic acid Schiff, ×400). **C**. 10-Year follow-up biopsy showing more advanced diabetic glomerulopathy in this now proteinuric patient with further reduced GFR (29 mL/min/1.73 m^2). Note also the multiple small glomerular probably efferent arterioles in the hilar region of this glomerulus (periodic acid Schiff, ×400), and in the glomerulus in Fig. 42-2A. (*Used with permission from Caramori et al.*[440])

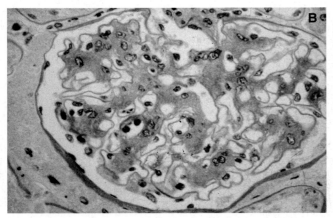

fractional volume [Vv(Mes/glom)] is quite wide, it may take time for some individuals to progress from the normal to the abnormal range. Others develop lesions so rapidly as to result in overt DN in as little as 10 years. However, glomerular changes of longstanding diabetes are always discernible by direct comparison with measures from the patient's nondiabetic identical twin.[18] Using morphometric techniques, the first measurable change is thickening of the GBM (Fig. 42-3).[19] TBM thickening parallels GBM thickening.[18,20] Increase in the relative area of the mesangium may become measurable by 4–5 years (Fig. 42-4). Vv(Mes/glom) increases from about 0.2 in the normal state to about 0.4 when proteinuria begins, and 0.6–0.8 in patients with a glomerular filtration rate (GFR) about 40–50% of normal. In the largest study performed so far,[8] 66 nonproteinuric patients with T1DM duration of at least 10 years (mean of 21 years) were divided on the basis of their albumin excretion rate (AER) into 4 groups: group I, 33 normoalbuminuric patients (AER <15 μg/min); group II, 11 low-level microalbuminuric patients (AER 15–30 μg/min); group III, 13 microalbuminuric patients (AER 31–70 μg/min); and group IV, 9 microalbuminuric patients (AER 71–150 μg/min). Glomerular structural parameters were compared to 52 age- and gender-matched normal controls. All parameters of glomerulopathy were abnormal in the normoalbuminuric group, although approximately one-half of the patients fell into the normal range (Fig. 42-5). Note that in many of group I (normoalbuminuric) patients, Vv(Mes/glom), the structural parameter most closely related to renal functional disturbances in diabetes[9] (see below), overlapped with patients in the microalbuminuric groups (groups III and IV), and in some instances approached levels regularly associated with overt DN. Note also that several of the normoalbuminuric patients (group I) with Vv(Mes/glom) above the normal range had reduced GFR, hypertension, or both (Fig. 42-5A). Evaluating patients with shorter diabetes duration {10.8 (7.5–19.2) years [median (range)]}, Berg and associates[21] found greater GBM width and MM fractional volume [Vv(MM/glom)] in 36 normoalbuminuric adolescents than in normal controls, but did not report an increase in Vv(Mes/glom). Østerby, using pooled data from several studies from her laboratories,[10] also described an increase in GBM width in normoalbuminuric T1DM patients with a mean diabetes duration of 12 years. Vv(Mes/glom) was similar in controls and normoalbuminuric patients in these studies and the different results are best explained by the marked differences in duration of diabetes in the normoalbuminuric patients.

FIGURE 42-3. Electron photomicrographs of GBM from normal control (**A**) and from T1DM patient (**B**) (×11,000). Note the thickening of the glomerular basement membrane in the diabetic patient.

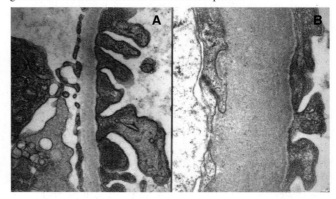

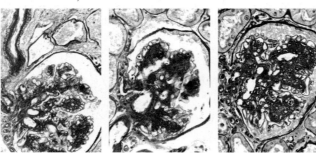

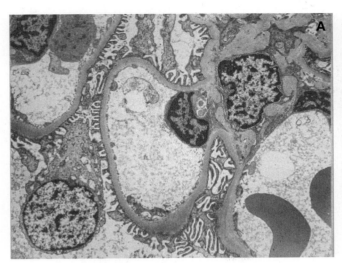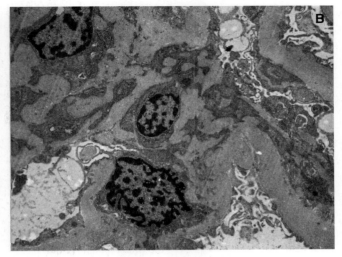

FIGURE 42-4. Electron photomicrographs of mesangial area in normal control (**A**) and in T1DM patient (**B**) (×3900). Note the increase in mesangial matrix and cell content, the GBM thickening, and the decrease in the capillary luminal space in the diabetic patient.

There is, however, general consensus that on average, microalbuminuric patients have increased GBM width and Vv(Mes/glom) compared to normoalbuminuric patients[8,22–24] and controls.[8,23,24] However, all studies have shown wide ranges of glomerular structure among type 1 microalbuminuric patients. Thus GBM width ranges from the upper limits of normal to markedly increased. Moreover, there is no significant increase in GBM width (Fig. 42-5B) in patients with different levels of microalbuminuria.[8] The same is true for Vv(Mes/glom) (Fig. 42-5A), where values in microalbuminuric patients in groups III and IV ranged from the upper limits of normal[8] to levels which overlapped those of patients with proteinuria (unpublished observations). Patients in groups III and IV

had greater Vv(Mes/glom) values (Fig. 42-5A) than patients with lower levels of increased AER (15–30 μg/min; group II) or normoalbuminuric patients (group I), while group I and II overlapped completely.[8] Østerby[10] found some microalbuminuric patients with Vv(Mes/glom) in the normal range. This was also found to be true[8] when patients with AER in the range of 15–30 μg/min were examined (group II; Fig. 42-5A). However, at higher levels of microalbuminuria, Vv(Mes/glom) was increased in virtually all patients. Also, we found that patients with AER above 30 μg/min had a relatively high incidence of hypertension, decreased GFR (<90 mL/min/1.73 m²), or both.[8] Nonetheless, even among these patients, the range of Vv(Mes/glom) was quite wide, and the values in these

FIGURE 42-5. A. Mesangial fractional volume [Vv(Mes/glom)] in the 4 groups of patients. Group I, normoalbuminuric; group II, AER 15–30 μg/min; group III, AER 31–70 μg/min; and group IV, AER 71–150 μg/min. The shaded area represents the mean ± 2 SD in a group of 52 age-matched normal control subjects. Normal BP and GFR (**solid circles**); reduced GFR (<90 mL/min/1.73m²; **open circles**); hypertension (≥140/85; **open squares**); and reduced GFR and hypertension (**circle within square**). *$p < 0.005$ versus groups I and II. **B.** GBM width in the 4 groups of patients. The shaded area represents the mean ± 2 SD in a group of 52 age-matched normal control subjects. Normal BP and GFR (**solid circles**); reduced GFR (<90 mL/min/1.73m²; **open circles**); hypertension (≥140/85; **open squares**); and reduced GFR and hypertension (**circle within square**). *$p < 0.005$ versus groups I and II. (*Both A and B reprinted with permission from Fioretto et al.[8]*)

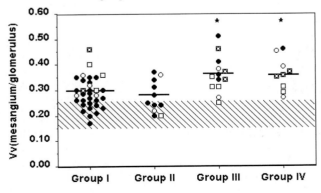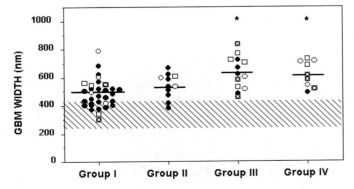

A **B**

microalbuminuric patients overlapped with those of normoalbuminuric patients (Fig. 42-5A). The presence of serious diabetic glomerular lesions in some normoalbuminuric patients suggests that altered glomerular permeability to proteins is not a necessary precondition for the development of these lesions. Moreover, it is unlikely that established diabetic glomerular lesions are of little prognostic value in normoalbuminuric patients. On the contrary, preliminary studies indicate a greater risk of progression in normoalbuminuric patients with more advanced lesions.[25]

Qualitative and quantitative changes in the renal interstitium, the extravascular intertubular compartment with its cellular elements and extracellular substances and spaces, are observed in patients with various renal diseases. Interstitial fibrosis is characterized by an increase in ECM proteins and cellularity.[26] Preliminary studies suggest that the pathogenesis of interstitial changes in DN is different from the MM, GBM, and TBM changes. Initial observations indicate that for all but the later stages of the disease, GBM, TBM, and MM changes represent the accumulation of basement membrane ECM material, while early on, interstitium expansion is largely due to cellular alterations. Only later, when GFR is already compromised, is interstitial expansion associated with increased interstitium fibrillar collagen and peritubular capillary loss.[27] Thus currently available data support the concept that interstitial changes are late contributors to the progressive decline in GFR that follows the initial development of serious glomerular and vascular DN lesions. These conclusions emanate from the following preliminary observations: cortical interstitial composition in patients with T1DM with mild interstitial expansion {cortical interstitial fractional volume [Vv(Int/cortex)] of ≈1.5 times normal} demonstrates a relative increase in the cellular component of interstitium, while a relative increase in collagen fibrils is seen only when Vv(Int/cortex) is about twice normal and patients already have decreased GFR.[27] This is in contrast to early mesangial expansion, where increased mesangial matrix fractional volume [Vv(MM/glom)] dominates.[28] Studies[20] also show that early GBM, TBM, and mesangial changes are correlated to glycemia, while early interstitial changes are not. These differences between glomerular and interstitial changes in T1DM patients may reflect different pathogenetic processes.

T2DM

The rate of development of DN lesions is less clear in patients with type 2 compared with patients with type 1 diabetes, since with the exception of the Pima Indian studies,[29] duration is usually not precisely established in these patients. Nonetheless, GBM width and Vv(Mes/glom) are increased in long-term normoalbuminuric Caucasian,[30] Japanese,[31] and Pima Indian[29] T2DM patients. As in T1DM patients, there is considerable overlap with normal controls, and some normoalbuminuric T2DM patients have relatively advanced glomerular lesions.[30,31] Thus, as is true for T1DM patients, there is a structural basis for explaining the progression to microalbuminuria and proteinuria among some normoalbuminuric T2DM patients. Whether normoalbuminuric T2DM patients with more advanced diabetic renal lesions are at greater risk of progression needs to be determined. In Pima Indians, glomerular structure was no different in microalbuminuric compared with normoalbuminuric patients with long duration, while microalbuminuric patients had more advanced glomerulopathy than normoalbuminuric patients with short duration. These results might explain the observation that some long-term normoalbuminuric patients are at high risk of progression. Further, as discussed below, there are more

varied renal structural patterns and patterns of functional progression among microalbuminuric, and perhaps proteinuric, patients with type 2 as compared with patients with type 1 diabetes, and the ultimate clinical course of these patients remains to be fully described.

A light microscopy study of 34 unselected microalbuminuric T2DM patients found that 10 (29.4%) had normal or near normal renal structure,[32] a finding uncommon in T1DM. Ten patients had renal structural changes typical of those seen in type 1 diabetic patients with more or less balanced severity of glomerular, tubulointerstitial, vascular, and global glomerulosclerosis lesions. However, 14 (41.2%) had atypical patterns of renal injury with absent or only mild diabetic glomerular changes associated with other disproportionately severe renal structural changes, including important tubulointerstitial lesions with or without arteriolar hyalinosis and with or without increased global glomerular sclerosis. Patients with proliferative retinopathy all had typical and well-established DN lesions. None of the patients without retinopathy had typical lesions. However, background retinopathy could be associated with any of the three structural categories defined above. These studies were confirmed by electron microscopy observations,[30] showing that microalbuminuric T2DM patients more frequently had electron microscopy morphometric glomerular structural measures in the normal range and, as a group, had less severe lesions than microalbuminuric T1DM patients. Many of these observations have been confirmed in Japanese type 2 diabetic patients.[31] On the other hand, Pima Indian type 2 diabetic patients, who are known to be at very high risk of ESRD, appear to have lesions more similar to those seen in type 1 diabetic patients.[33] Also, proteinuric type 2 diabetic patients had electron microscopy appearances consistent with typical diabetic glomerulopathy, with an increase in Vv(Mes/glom) and Vv(MM/glom) together with GBM thickening.[34] Interstitial expansion was also observed when these patients were compared to nondiabetic controls.[34] Similar results were seen in an earlier study that included proteinuric type 2 Japanese diabetic patients.[35] Moreover, there are reports that type 2 diabetic patients have an increased incidence of nondiabetic lesions, such as proliferative glomerulonephritis and membranous nephropathy, but this is most likely because biopsies were done in atypical cases. When biopsies are performed for research purposes, the incidence of other definable renal diseases is very low (<5%).[32,36]

It is currently unclear why some studies show more structural heterogeneity in type 2 than in type 1 diabetes[30,31,36] while others do not.[34,35] Whether this is due to differences in patient populations, or to other as yet unknown variables remains to be determined. However, this is an important question since the rate of progression towards ESRD in T2DM appears to be at least in part related to the severity of the classic changes of diabetic glomerulopathy (see below).

STRUCTURAL-FUNCTIONAL RELATIONSHIPS IN DIABETIC NEPHROPATHY

T1DM

Expansion of the mesangium, mainly due to ECM accumulation, is believed to ultimately reduce glomerular capillary luminal space, decreasing glomerular filtration surface and GFR. Vv(Mes/glom) is a good predictor of GFR in type 1 diabetic patients, and it is also related to AER levels and hypertension.[9] The total peripheral capillary filtration surface per glomerulus [Sv(PGBM/glom)] is directly correlated with GFR (Fig. 42-6) and inversely correlated with the

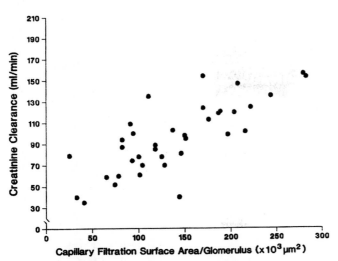

FIGURE 42-6. Relationship between capillary filtration surface area per glomerulus and creatinine clearance (r = 0.78, p < 0.001). *(Reproduced with permission from Ellis et al.[441])*

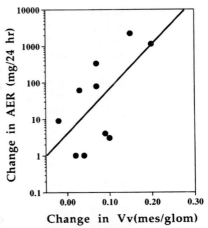

FIGURE 42-8. Correlation between the change in mesangium fractional volume [Vv(Mes/glom)] and the change in albumin excretion rate (AER) over 5 years (r = 0.642, p < 0.05). *(Reproduced with permission from Fioretto et al.[37])*

degree of mesangial expansion (Fig. 42-7). The thickness of the GBM is directly related to AER, but increasing albuminuria appears to be related to increasing mesangial expansion (Fig. 42-8) and not to other structural changes.[37] Percentage of global glomerulosclerosis and interstitial expansion are also correlated with the clinical manifestations of DN (proteinuria, hypertension, and declining GFR). Progressive tubular atrophy, interstitial fibrosis, glomerular arteriolar hyalinosis, arteriosclerosis, and glomerulosclerosis are also important components of DN that probably contribute to the reduction in GFR independently from the glomerular lesions. Finally, larger-vessel atherosclerosis, perhaps especially in T2DM, may lead to ischemic renal tissue damage. In type 1 diabetic patients, these lesions tend to progress more or less in parallel, while in type 2 diabetic patients this is less often the case. As already mentioned, preliminary observations suggest that longstanding normoalbuminuric type 1 diabetic patients who progress to DN have more advanced glomerular lesions than pa-

FIGURE 42-7. Relationship of Vv(Mes/glom) expressed as percentage of total mesangium and S/V of the peripheral capillary surface or Sv(PGBM/glom) (r = −0.86, p < 0.0005). *(Reproduced with permission from Mauer et al.[9])*

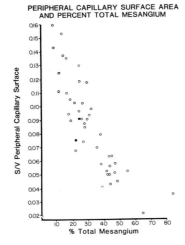

tients that remain normoalbuminuric after long-term follow-up.[25] In this preliminary 5- to 17-year follow-up study of normoalbuminuric patients with longstanding diabetes, patients progressing to microalbuminuria or proteinuria had worse glomerular lesions at baseline than those who remained normoalbuminuric, but these findings are as yet unconfirmed. In longitudinal studies of microalbuminuric type 1 diabetic patients Bangstad and colleagues[38] found that GBM width at baseline biopsy was predictive (r^2 = 0.67; p < 0.0001) of AER after 6 years of follow-up, whereas Vv(Mes/glom) was a significant but less precise predictor.

Changes in interstitium also correlate with functional changes, and interstitial expansion has generally been accepted as the best histologic correlate of renal function in glomerular diseases.[39] Studies have shown that both GFR and serum creatinine at the time of biopsy best correlate with Vv(Int/cortex), while the degree of renal dysfunction may not reflect the severity of glomerular pathology.[40] However, as discussed below, this may depend on how carefully glomerular pathology is measured. Thus, in 96 type 1 diabetic patients with GFR ranging from normal to 45 mL/min/1.73 m² (35 with reduced GFR) and AER from normal to proteinuria (34 with proteinuria), the correlation of Vv(Int/cortex) and Vv(Mes/glom) was only 0.38 (p < 0.01). Both Vv(Int/cortex) (r = 0.49, p < 0.001) and Vv(Mes/glom) (r = 0.41, p < 0.001) correlated inversely with GFR, and were additive in stepwise multiple regression analyses (r = 0.55, p < 0.001).[41] In type 1 and type 2 diabetic patients with overt DN the rate of progression in interstitial fibrosis in the 4-year follow-up biopsy correlated with the rate of GFR decline.[42] However, in type 1 diabetic patients at earlier stages of DN (normoalbuminuria and microalbuminuria), increasing AER correlated with increasing Vv(Mes/glom) in sequential biopsies performed 5 years apart, while Vv(Int/cortex) remained constant.[37] These studies support the view that structural-functional relationships in DN may change as the disease evolves.

T2DM

The structural-functional relationships are less clear in type 2 diabetes. Some studies show weaker structural-functional relationships[30,31] while others reported more typical structural-functional relationships in microalbuminuric and proteinuric type 2 diabetic patients.[34,35] Vv(Mes/glom) and Vv(MM/glom) were correlated with GFR and proteinuria, while GBM width correlated only with proteinuria,[34,35] in a fashion similar to type 1 diabetic patients.[41] Also, as described in type 1 diabetic patients,[41] multiple regression analysis found that GFR was related to both mesangial and interstitial lesions in type 2 diabetic patients.[34] One study argued that the underlying pattern of renal injury does not predict the rate of GFR decline among a Caucasian cohort of proteinuric type 2 diabetic patients.[43] In contrast, a large 4.3-year follow-up study of angiotensin converting enzyme (ACE) inhibitor-treated Caucasian microalbuminuric and proteinuric type 2 diabetic patients found that patients with more rapid GFR decline had greater Vv(Mes/glom) and GBM width at baseline.[44] Also, after 2 years of follow-up of microalbuminuric and proteinuric type 2 diabetic patients, all with typical glomerulopathy, increase in the Vv(Int/cortex) was correlated with changes in proteinuria over the same interval.[45] Thus, as suggested above, it is reasonable to conclude that glomerular lesions are key to the early functional changes of DN, white interstitial and vascular changes may become increasingly important in determining the rate of progression of the disease from established nephropathy to ESRD.

PATHOGENESIS OF DIABETIC NEPHROPATHY

Glycemic Control

Although important modulating factors may exist, DN is secondary to the long-term metabolic aberrations found in diabetes, and exposure to elevated glucose levels appears central to the expression of this disorder. Studies in T1DM and T2DM found that improved glycemic control could reduce the development of DN. The Diabetes Control and Complications Trial (DCCT) demonstrated that the risk of microalbuminuria in type 1 diabetic patients was decreased by strict glycemic control.[46] This study did not show an effect of improved glycemic control in the progression from microalbuminuria to proteinuria, although the study may have had limited power to demonstrate this. The beneficial effects of this 6.3 years of intensive treatment could still be observed 4 years after the end of the study.[47] The United Kingdom Prospective Diabetes Study (UKPDS) also demonstrated a decreased incidence of DN after 10 years of intensive glycemic control in recently diagnosed type 2 diabetic patients.[48] Moreover, a 5-year randomized clinical trial in 48 type 1 diabetic kidney transplant recipients demonstrated that the development of one of the earliest diabetic renal lesions, increased Vv(MM/glom), was prevented by strict glycemic control.[49] Also, intensive insulin treatment for 26–34 months decreased the rate of GBM thickening and increase in Vv(MM/Mes) and matrix star volume in a controlled trial in 18 microalbuminuric type 1 diabetic patients.[50] Finally, regression of established diabetic glomerular lesions has been demonstrated in the native kidneys of 8 type 1 diabetic patients with 10 years of normoglycemia induced by successful pancreas transplantation (Fig. 42-9 and Fig. 42-10).[51] These studies strongly suggest that hyperglycemia is not only necessary for DN lesions to develop, but is also necessary to sustain established lesions. Alleviation of hyperglycemia allows reparative mechanisms to be expressed which ultimately result in healing of the original diabetic glomerular injuries. Studies evaluating the brain-type glucose transporter (GLUT-1) in animals reinforce the pathogenic role of glycemia on the development of DN. High glucose can increase GLUT-1 expression and glucose transport activity in rat mesangial cells.[52] These effects are mediated by transforming growth factor-β (TGF-β).[53] Rat mesangial cells transduced with human GLUT-1 and overexpressing GLUT-1 protein showed increased glucose uptake and ECM synthesis, even in normal glucose concentration.[54] The mechanisms involved in the glomerular injury caused by hyperglycemia will be discussed in detail later.

Hemodynamic Mechanisms

Berkman and Rifkin[55] described a diabetic patient with unilateral renal artery stenosis and marked diabetic lesions in the kidney exposed both to hypertension and diabetes, while the contralateral kidney, protected from hypertension by the narrowed renal artery, had only ischemic changes. A model of unilateral renal artery stenosis in diabetic rats[56] seemed to confirm this human observation, although hypertensive and diabetic changes were not differentiated in this study. Insulin-treated diabetic rats have glomerular hyperfiltration explainable by increased single nephron GFR, which is due to increased single nephron blood flow and, in the Münich-Wistar rat strain, increased glomerular capillary pressure.[57] Thus alterations in intraglomerular hemodynamics could influence the rate at which diabetic lesions develop. Some studies reported that glomerular hyperfiltration was a risk factor for the development of microalbuminuria.[58,59] However, there is still controversy as to whether increased GFR is a predictor of progression.[60,61]

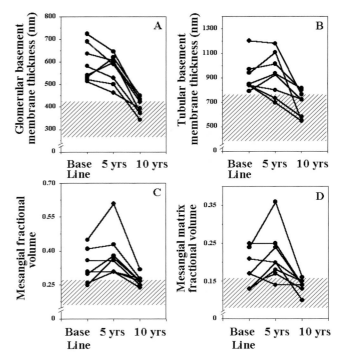

FIGURE 42-9. (**A**) Thickness of the glomerular basement membrane, (**B**) thickness of the tubular basement membrane, (**C**) mesangial fractional volume, and (**D**) mesangial matrix fractional volume at baseline and 5 and 10 years after pancreas transplantation. The shaded areas represent the normal ranges obtained in 66 age- and gender-matched controls (means ± 2 SD). Data for individual patients are connected by lines. (*Reproduced with permission from Fioretto et al.[51]*)

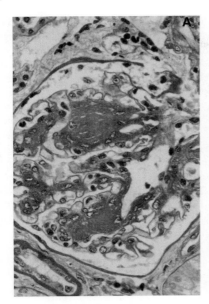
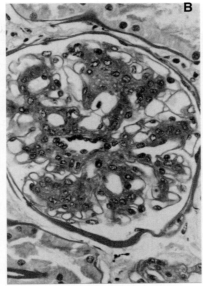
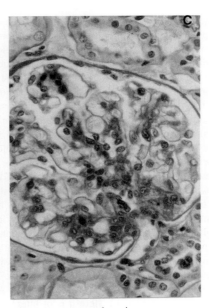

FIGURE 42-10. Photomicrographs of renal biopsy specimens obtained before and after pancreas transplantation in a 33-year-old woman with T1DM of 17 years' duration at the time of transplantation. Panel **A** shows a typical glomerulus from the baseline biopsy specimen, which is characterized by diffuse and nodular (Kimmelstiel-Wilson) diabetic glomerulopathy. Mesangial matrix expansion and the palisading of mesangial nuclei around the nodular lesions are evident. In panel **B**, a typical glomerulus 5 years after transplantation, shows the persistence of the diffuse and nodular lesions. Panel **C** shows a typical glomerulus 10 years after transplantation, with marked resolution of diffuse and nodular mesangial lesions and more open glomerular capillary lumina (periodic acid Schiff, ×120). *(Reproduced with permission from Fioretto et al.[51])*

Several mechanisms have been proposed as mediators of diabetes-induced hyperfiltration. Increased renal tissue and urinary kallikrein levels were associated with increased GFR and renal plasma flow in moderately hyperglycemic diabetic rats,[62] and treatment with a bradykinin B2 receptor antagonist acutely reduced GFR and renal plasma flow in these animals.[63] Urinary kallikrein excretion was also increased in type 1 diabetic patients with glomerular hyperfiltration.[64] The intrarenal renin-angiotensin system within glomeruli and proximal tubules may be activated by hyperglycemia, leading to increased angiotensin II production, which may exert feedback inhibition of systemic renin release.[65,66] Angiotensin II concentration is higher in the glomeruli than systemically.[67] ACE activity is reduced in the renal cortex but enhanced in glomeruli and vessels of diabetic rats[68] and patients,[69] suggesting that renal vessels and glomeruli may be regulated differently from the tubulointerstitial renin-angiotensin system. The genesis of glomerular hyperfiltration has also been associated with increased nitric oxide (NO) generation or action, by a glucose-dependent mechanism.[70,71] The vasodilatation caused by increased NO could enhance the permeability to macromolecules, leading to albuminuria.[72] Furthermore, recent data have shown enhanced NO synthesis by endothelial NO synthase (eNOS) in afferent arterioles and glomerular endothelial cells in diabetic rats, suggesting a pivotal role of NO in preferential afferent arteriolar dilatation, glomerular enlargement, and functional glomerular hyperfiltration in the early stages of DN.[73] Treatment with a nonselective NOS inhibitor normalized GFR and plasma renal flow levels in diabetic rats.[74] NO activity was shown to be increased in microalbuminuric versus normoalbuminuric type 1 diabetic patients or nondiabetic controls, and related to GFR and

AER.[75] Other studies suggest that hyperfiltration may result from an increased proximal tubular fluid reabsorption, and independent of any primary malfunction of the glomerular microvasculature.[76]

However, one cannot explain the *genesis* of DN by hyperfiltration alone. Insulin-treated diabetic rats with hyperfiltration have slower development of diabetic renal lesions than untreated diabetic rats having worse hyperglycemia and relative hypofiltration; in fact, these markedly hyperfiltrating insulin-treated animals do not seem to develop mesangial expansion disproportionate to the size of the glomerulus.[77] Further, reduction in nephron mass in rats by uninephrectomy produces glomerular hemodynamic perturbations[78] that are similar to diabetes,[57] but does not produce the lesions[79] that are classic for DN in animals.[80,81] The central lesion associated with hyperfiltration in rats, focal segmental glomerular sclerosis,[82] is not an important lesion in human or animal diabetes (see the section on pathology). It has been suggested that reduced glomerular number at birth may be a risk factor for progressive renal disease and hypertension.[83] One study in type 2 diabetic patients suggested that reduced glomerular number was associated with increased DN risk.[84] However, studies in type 1 diabetic patients do not confirm these observations. Glomerular number estimated at autopsy was decreased in type 1 diabetic patients only if ESRD was present.[85] No differences in glomerular number were found between type 1 diabetic patients with established DN, but not ESRD, and controls.[85] Another study, evaluating 32 type 1 diabetic patients ranging from normoalbuminuria to proteinuria, and serum creatinine ≤1.5 mg/dL, corroborated these findings.[86] Glomerular number, estimated by morphometric techniques in kidney biopsy tissue, did not correlate with functional or structural parameters.[86] Also, reduced nephron mass, such as in patients with uninephrectomy, has not been documented to produce DN lesions in humans. Moreover, DN lesions may not develop faster in type 1 diabetic kidney transplant recipients (single-kidney diabetic patients) than in type 1 diabetic patients with their native kidneys, matched for diabetes duration.[87] These studies suggest that glomerular number is probably not a crucial variable in the development of DN, although it may be important in progression once clinical findings of DN are present.

Lowering glomerular capillary pressure by long-term ACE inhibitor therapy prevented the development of focal segmental glomerular sclerosis,[88] but did not prevent the GBM widening and increase in Vv(Mes/glom) that occurs in the first 6 months of diabetes in rats.[89] Thus, renin-angiotensin system blockage may not prevent the *development* of specific early DN lesions in diabetic animals[89] and this has not been tested in human diabetes. On the other hand, there are studies which suggest that renin-angiotensin system blockage may slow the rate of progression of established DN lesions and clinical progression in humans. The influences of renin-angiotensin system blockage on clinical progression of DN are discussed in Chap. 43. Here it is of interest to note that ACE inhibitor therapy prevented an increase of GBM width and perhaps changed Mes composition, but had no effect on Vv(Mes/glom), in microalbuminuric type 1 diabetic patients with established diabetic lesions.[90] Cortical interstitial expansion was also prevented in type 1[91] and type 2[45] diabetic patients with already-increased AER. These effects may not be specific to ACE inhibition, as β-blocker therapy in these studies showed similar effects on blood pressure and lesions.[90,91] Taken together these studies could support the hypothesis that hemodynamic abnormalities may be more important in influencing the *progression* of established DN lesions than in serving as the genesis of these structural changes. Thus, occlusion of glomerular capillaries or restriction of filtration surface within nonsclerosed glomeruli, as a consequence of advanced diabetic renal lesions, could cause compensatory enlargement of remaining glomeruli associated with increased intraglomerular pressures and flows and permselectivity alterations.[82] Such abnormal hemodynamic forces could accelerate disruption of the residual glomeruli, thus contributing to a destructive cycle that promotes progressive tissue injury and loss of renal function.[82,92]

Although we are arguing that a case has not been made that currently allows acceptance of the hypothesis that hemodynamic abnormalities are responsible for the *genesis* of the early lesions of DN, it is nonetheless possible that manipulations which can affect glomerular hemodynamics might also affect the development of early diabetic renal lesions through other than hemodynamic influences. For example, the renin-angiotensin system could mediate renal growth responses and renal ECM production and turnover. Angiotensin II stimulates *in vitro* mesangial cell proliferation and fibronectin synthesis.[93] Also, the glucose- stimulated increase in mesangial cell collagen production could be blocked by enalapril.[94] Further, increased glomerular mRNA expression for ECM components including α_1 chains of type I [α_1(I)], III [α_1(III)], and IV [α_1(IV)] collagens, and laminin β_1 were attenuated by ACE inhibitor therapy in streptozocin diabetic rats.[95] Captopril inhibits the 72-kd and 92-kd matrix metalloproteinases (MMP-2 and MMP-9, respectively), two distinct type IV collagenases,[96] thus favoring ECM accumulation. However, lisinopril, a nonsulfydryl ACE inhibitor, inhibited these MMPs only at concentrations 100 times those of captopril.[96] Further, zinc could reverse the inhibitory effect of captopril on metalloproteinases, arguing against a renin-angiotensin system-dependent effect.[96] Thus drugs affecting the renin-angiotensin system might also impact ECM dynamics and thereby renal structure in diabetes. However, the mechanisms of action of these agents appear complex, are incompletely understood, and may in part be independent of the renin-angiotensin system. TGF-β expression may also be regulated in parallel with renin.[97,98] Thus increased juxtaglomerular apparatus prorenin production may be associated with other increased juxtaglomerular apparatus activities such as TGF-β production, and the latter has been linked to glomerular ECM abnormalities in diabetes[99] (see below). Thus glomerular hyperfiltration could promote ECM accumulation by increases in the expression of TGF-β, and this might be modeled *in vitro* by the mechanical stretching of mesangial cells.[100]

Genetics

Genetic predisposition appears to be the most important determinant of DN risk in both T1DM and T2DM. Differences in the prevalence of DN in different patient populations support this view.[1,101,102] Moreover, only about one-half of patients with poor glycemic control develop DN,[103] while some patients do so despite relatively good control, findings consistent with genetically modulated risk.

Familial Clustering of Diabetic Nephropathy

Since the first report about 10 years ago,[104] genetic predisposition to DN has been suggested in multiple cross-sectional studies in type 1[105,106] and type 2[107–110] siblings concordant for diabetes. There is a large difference (300–800%) in the cumulative risk of DN between siblings of probands with or without DN, and some of the data are consonant with a major gene effect, with an autosomal dominant mode of inheritance.[106]

Familial Studies of Blood Pressure, Cardiovascular Disease, and Diabetic Nephropathy

An association between DN and predisposition to hypertension and cardiovascular disease has also been suggested by some,[111–116] but not all[117] studies. Higher blood pressure values were observed in parents of proteinuric patients with T1DM,[111] while a higher prevalence of hypertension has been described in parents of proteinuric and microalbuminuric type 1 diabetic patients.[112,113] Diabetic patients with advanced nephropathy also had higher mean arterial blood pressures during adolescence.[113] Prediabetic blood pressure levels predicted AER after diabetes onset,[114] and presence of hypertension in both parents increased the risk of proteinuria[115] in type 2 diabetic Pima Indians. The prevalence of cardiovascular disease and cardiovascular death was found to be significantly greater in the parents of type 1 diabetic patients with nephropathy,[116] and a positive family history of cardiovascular disease was more frequent in those DN patients who had suffered a cardiovascular event. This study indicates that familial predisposition to cardiovascular disease increases both the risk of nephropathy and the risk of cardiovascular disease in type 1 diabetic patients with nephropathy, linking the pathogenesis of DN to factors also favoring the development of atherosclerosis.[111,112,118] Recent data also suggest that AER and blood pressure are heritable and linked in Caucasian families with T2DM.[119]

Sodium/Lithium Countertransport

Sodium/lithium (Na^+/Li^+) countertransport activity is genetically determined, and has been suggested to be related to hypertension and cardiovascular disease in nondiabetic subjects.[120] Increased Na^+/Li^+ countertransport activity has been reported in diabetic patients with microalbuminuria or overt DN by some[112,121,122] but not all[123] authors, albeit the later study was in type 2 diabetic patients. Increased Na^+/Li^+ countertransport activity has been described in a study of parents of proteinuric type 1 diabetic patients,[124] although not in another.[117] Na^+/Li^+ countertransport activity was similar in 44 identical twin pairs discordant for T1DM,[125] and both values were higher than those of 44 age-matched nondiabetic controls. Interestingly, systolic blood pressure was higher in the diabetic twins, but nondiabetic twins and controls had similar blood pressure values. These findings suggest that raised erythrocyte Na^+/Li^+ countertransport activity seems to be inherited rather than a consequence of diabetes.[125] Raised erythrocyte Na^+/Li^+ countertransport activity was associated with a fourfold increased risk of development of persistent microalbuminuria in type 1 diabetic patients.[126]

Na^+/Li^+ countertransport has parallels with the Na^+/H^+ antiport exchange system that is involved in the regulation of intracellular pH, cell volume and growth, and proximal tubular sodium reabsorption.[127] There is increased Na^+/H^+ antiport activity in leukocytes[128] and cultured skin fibroblasts[129,130] of type 1 and type 2 diabetic patients with microalbuminuria and clinical proteinuria. Also, since cultured skin fibroblast Na^+/H^+ antiport activity is highly correlated among siblings concordant for T1DM and for nephropathy lesions,[131] and independent of environmental factors, it was suggested that these cultured skin fibroblast abnormalities are genetically regulated.

Diabetic Nephropathy Genes

There are ongoing searches for genetic loci related to DN susceptibility through genomic scanning and through candidate gene approaches. Neither approach has yet yielded definitive results, but indications are that multiple genes may be involved.[132,133] Segregation analyses in Pima Indians suggests that a major gene effect with a relatively frequent disease allele is the mode of inheritance of DN in type 2 diabetic patients.[134] Sib-pair linkage analysis in families of type 2 diabetic Pima Indians showed some evidence for linkage with DN in 4 chromosomal regions (chromosomes 3, 7, 9, and 20), the strongest one in chromosome 7.[135] Previous studies in the Caucasian population have shown linkage between DN and chromosome 7q in type 2 diabetic patients[136] and chromosome 3q in type 1 diabetic patients.[137] Recent results of segregation analysis in Caucasian type 2 diabetic families also suggest a major gene effect for AER.[138] Several genes have been proposed as plausible candidates based upon the pathophysiology of DN. Genetic polymorphism affecting background vascular risk in the general population, such as the genes related to the renin-angiotensin system, have been evaluated in many studies in diabetic patients. Polymorphism in the ACE gene, consisting of an insertion or deletion (I/D) of a 287-base pair sequence has also been associated with rate of GFR decline in nondiabetic renal diseases.[139] It is still not clear if ACE polymorphism is important in the *genesis* of DN,[140–144] although a more recent follow-up study supports that this is so.[145]

There is, however, growing evidence that ACE polymorphism can be important in DN progression and response to ACE inhibitor therapy.[146–148] In normo- and microalbuminuric type 1 diabetic patients, AER appears to increase faster in patients with the II genotype,[148] however these patients appear to have the best response to ACE inhibitor therapy.[147,148] On the other hand, D was the risk allele for development of DN in Caucasian type 1 diabetic patients followed for 6 years.[145] Also, the DD genotype was more frequent in normoalbuminuric or microalbuminuric Japanese type 2 diabetic patients who doubled AER or changed AER class (progressors), than in patients who had not progressed after 10 years of follow-up.[146] Despite progression not being associated with ACE genotype in Caucasian normoalbuminuric or microalbuminuric type 2 diabetic patients,[149] patients with II genotype (n = 11) did not decrease GFR after 9 years of follow-up. Moreover, presence of the D allele in Caucasian type 2 diabetic patients was related to the presence of more severe DN lesions.[150] Other studies did not find associations between ACE gene polymorphism and DN[133,151–157] or rate of GFR decline[158] in type 1 or type 2 diabetic patients. One meta-analysis concluded that the D allele was significantly associated with DN in a dominant model (DD + ID versus II) in both type 1 and type 2 diabetic patients.[159] Another one found this association to be significant only in Japanese type 2 diabetic patients, but not in Caucasian type 1 or type 2 diabetic patients.[160] Different definitions of DN patients, different ascertainment strategies, real genetic differences among these populations, or selection bias could have accounted for the different results.

Association with DN risk in type 1 or type 2 diabetic patients and polymorphisms in the angiotensinogen gene was found in some[161,162] but not in all[156,157,163,164] studies. One study observed association between the T-allele angiotensinogen gene and elevated AER only when interaction with the D-allele of the ACE I/D polymorphism was considered.[165] Interaction between ACE and angiotensinogen gene polymorphism has been previously described in cross-sectional[140] but not confirmed in longitudinal[145] studies. A meta-analysis did not find association between angiotensinogen gene polymorphism and DN.[166]

Two large studies did not find a role for angiotensin II type 1 receptor polymorphism in DN,[167,168] while another found this polymorphism to significantly contribute to DN risk in type 1 diabetic patients only when accompanied by poor glycemic control.[169]

Associations with DN risk have also been reported for polymorphisms in the human inducible NOS (iNOS),[170] PC-1,[171] heparan sulfate proteoglycan,[172] paraoxonase 2,[173] MMP-9,[174] TGF-β$_1$,[175] protein kinase C (PKCβ),[176] and haptoglobin[177] genes. Studies of polymorphisms in eNOS,[178–180] aldose reductase,[181–183] plasminogen activator inhibithor-1,[154,184] interleukin-1,[185,186] apolipoprotein E,[187–190] GLUT-1,[191,192] and methylenetetrahydrofolate reductase[193,194] genes showed conflicting results.

Other genes studied include hepatocyte nuclear factor 1α,[195] renin,[196] atrial natriuretic peptide,[197] α$_1$ (IV) collagen,[198] interleukin-1 receptor antagonist,[199] G protein,[200] β$_3$-adrenergic receptor,[201] decorin,[154] Werner syndrome helicase,[154] kallikrein,[202] bradykinin B1-[203] and B2-[204] receptors, paraoxonase 1,[205,206] and insulin.[207]

Thus the genetic determinants of DN risk are still not fully understood. However, it is reasonable to hypothesize that a single gene with a major effect or several genes with moderate or small effects interacting with the metabolic abnormalities of diabetes may be responsible for the genetic susceptibility to DN. Further research in this area is likely to lead to important new information regarding risk factors, pathogenesis, and treatment of DN.

PATHOPHYSIOLOGY OF DIABETIC NEPHROPATHY

The renal lesions of DN are mainly due to accumulation of ECM components, such as collagens, tenascin, and fibronectin,[14] as well as other as yet undescribed molecules. ECM accumulation occurs early in the GBM[19] and TBM,[20] is the principal cause of mesangial expansion, and also contributes to the later stages of interstitial expansion.[27] This ECM accumulation is clearly secondary to an imbalance between synthesis and degradation of ECM components. However, not all renal ECM components change in parallel in DN. Thus, $\alpha_3(IV)$ and $\alpha_4(IV)$ chains persist or increase in density in the GBM of patients developing diabetic renal lesions, while $\alpha_1(IV)$ and $\alpha_2(IV)$ chains are decreasing in density in the peripheral capillary wall and MM in patients with rapid development of DN lesions, but remain unchanged in patients with slow development of DN lesions despite longstanding T1DM.[15,208] Thus the ECM changes in diabetes are highly site-specific, differing in direction in the GBM compared to MM, and suggesting that variables related to cell type (e.g., glomerular epithelial cell for GBM, mesangial cell for MM) are important determinants in the response to the diabetic state. Moreover, these patterns of cell response may be genetically regulated. Type VI collagen, the other major glomerular collagen, is decreased in density of distribution in the endothelial aspect of the GBM and in MM in patients with both slow and fast development of DN lesions, albeit with greater reduction in the latter.[16] Thus the exact ECM component responsible for MM expansion in DN remains to be described.

Mesangial cells cultured in high glucose concentration accumulate various matrix components.[209,210] Matrix metalloproteinases (MMPs) have been implicated in the abnormal *in vitro* degradation of MM by these cells.[211] MMP activity is regulated at several levels, including gene expression, extracellular activation, and inhibition by specific tissue inhibitors of MMPs (TIMPs). MMPs and TIMPs can be modulated by protein kinase C (PKC) agonists, such as cytokines and hormones, and growth factors such as TGF-β.[212–215]

The major hypotheses as to how hyperglycemia causes DN are: (1) increased activity of a variety of growth factors, including TGF-β, growth hormone (GH), insulin-like growth factor (IGF), vascular endothelial growth factor (VEGF), and epidermal growth factor (EGF); (2) activation of PKC isoforms; (3) activation of cytokines, including renin, angiotensin, endothelin, and bradykinin; (4) formation of reactive oxygen species; (5) increased formation of glycation products; (6) increased activity of the aldose reductase pathway, and (7) decreased glycosaminoglycan content in basement membranes ("Steno hypothesis"). The various hypotheses overlap and intersect with one another. Polyol pathway-induced redox changes or hyperglycemia-induced formation of reactive oxygen species could potentially account for most of the other biochemical abnormalities.[216,217] These mechanisms, reviewed below, could be influenced by genetic determinants of susceptibility or resistance to hyperglycemic damage.

Growth Factors

This subject has recently been reviewed in detail by Flyvbjerg[218] and Chiarelli and colleagues[219] and, using a similar organizational scheme, it is summarized here.

TGF-β

TGF-β isoforms (TGF-β_1, TGF-β_2, and TGF-β_3), mRNA, and proteins and TGF-β-receptor mRNA have been demonstrated in all glomerular and proximal tubular cells.[220,221] Glomerular mesangial and epithelial cells exposed *in vitro* to TGF-β demonstrate increased ECM protein synthesis, including type IV collagen, fibronectin, laminin, and proteoglycans, decreased synthesis of MMPs, and increased production of TIMPs.[222–224] TGF-β_1 also stimulates glucose uptake by enhancing the expression of GLUT-1 in mesangial cells,[53] perhaps aggravating the metabolic abnormalities of diabetes. Several pathways can be involved in the elevated TGF-β expression in diabetes, including hyperglycemia, increased intraglomerular pressure, glycated proteins, PKC activation, and mechanical strain.[219] High glucose levels increase TGF-β_1 mRNA levels in mesangial cells[225] and increase synthesis of F2-isoprostane, an arachidonic acid derivative, in glomerular endothelial and mesangial cells *in vitro*. Incubation of glomerular mesangial cells with F2 isoprostane also stimulates TGF-β production.[226] The high glucose-stimulated increase in TGF-β production by mesangial cells is blocked by an inhibitor of isoprostane production. These findings suggest that F2-isoprostane synthesis during diabetes appears to be responsible, at least in part, for the increase in renal TGF-β. TGF-β-neutralizing antibodies reduce the *in vitro* rise in mesangial cell type IV collagen synthesis induced by high glucose levels.[227] Mitogen-activated protein kinases (MAPKs) and PKC may play an important role in the glucose-induced TGF-β-mediated increase in ECM production in these cells.[225,228] Thus, specific PKCβ inhibitors may also have a role as antagonists of the TGF-β system (see below). TGF-β_1 gene overexpression has been described in rat[220,229,230] and human diabetic glomeruli.[99,231,232] Animal models of diabetes show increased TGF-β_1 and TGF-β_2 mRNA levels and TGF-β_2 and TGF-β type II receptor proteins.[221] Glomerular ECM accumulation was observed in a nondiabetic transgenic mouse overexpressing TGF-β_1 in the glomerulus,[233] although the glomerular lesions resembled but did not fully mimic DN lesions. Further, TGF-β antibodies limited the increases in plasma renal TGF-β_1, renal TGF-β_1, TGF-β type II receptor, type IV collagen, and fibronectin mRNA expression, prevented the increase in serum creatinine, and reduced the diabetes-associated renal hypertrophy and MM expansion in diabetic mice.[234,235] ACE inhibitor (enalapril) treatment decreases TGF-β type I, II, and III receptors in the glomerulus, with no changes in TGF-β isoforms, partially prevents renal hypertrophy, and completely prevents AER increase in diabetic rats.[236] Thus ACE inhibitors may regulate the renal TGF-β system through decreases in TGF-β receptors.[236] Interestingly, serum and urinary TGF-β_1 levels were no different between diabetic patients with or without renal impairment, and were similar to levels observed in patients with nondiabetic renal disease.[237]

GH and IGF

Diabetes leads to decreased hepatic production of IGF-1 and the consequent decrease in the serum IGF-I results in excess GH secretion,[238] which in turn can then stimulate local IGF-1 pathways in other tissues, such as the kidney. IGF-1 *in vitro* induces increased mesangial cell proliferation.[239] Mesangial cells from nonobese diabetic (NOD) mice secrete increased amounts of IGF-1,[240] and the consequent reduction in MMP-2 activity[241] could lead to glomerular ECM accumulation. Increased kidney levels of IGF-1 precedes renal growth in diabetic rodents. This IGF-1 renal accumulation is influenced by glycemia,[242] in that strict insulin therapy blocks IGF-1 increase and renal hypertrophy in diabetic rats.[243] Renal accumulation of IGF-1 is more likely to be caused by changes in renal IGF-1 receptors and IGF-1 binding proteins than by an increase in local kidney IGF-1 production.[244,245] Long-acting somatostatin analogues[246] and GH-receptor antagonists[247,248] prevent the rise in renal IGF-1 and IGF binding protein-1 mRNA levels and renal hypertrophy in diabetic animals. An IGF-1-receptor antagonist prevented retinal neovascularization and VEGF increase in a rat model of nondiabetic retinopathy,[249] indicating that VEGF may be a downstream mediator of IGF-1 actions. This hypothesis is further reinforced by the nuclear factor kappa B (NFκB) stimulation by both IGF-1 and VEGF in endothelial cells *in vitro*. NFκB is involved in the upregulation of genes encoding for cytokines, growth factors such as TGF-β, and ECM proteins such as fibronectin.[250]

VEGF

VEGF, a potent mitogen for vascular endothelial cells and a major regulator of angiogenesis, increases microvascular permeability,[251] and has been associated with proliferative retinopathy[252,253] and neoangiogenesis[254,255] in experimental and human diabetes. Hypoxia is a potent VEGF stimulator.[256] In the kidney, VEGF is almost exclusively expressed in glomerular and tubular epithelial cells,[257,258] while the VEGF type 2 receptor (VEGF-R2) is mainly present in glomerular and tubular endothelial cells, but also in interstitial cells.[258] In high-glucose conditions, VEGF and its receptors are also expressed in glomerular endothelial and mesangial cells.[259] Glucose stimulates VEGF expression *in vitro* in vascular smooth[260] and mesangial[261,262] cells, probably through the PKC pathway.[261–263] TGF-β, PKC, and NO enhance VEGF expression in cultured mesangial cells.[218,261,262,264] On the other hand, VEGF stimulates NO production by vascular endothelial cells *in vitro* and *in vivo*, but not by renal mesangial cells *in vitro*.[265] Angiotensin II also stimulates VEGF in human mesangial cells.[266] Mechanical stretching of human mesangial cells *in vitro* induces VEGF production,[266] possibly linking glomerular hemodynamic abnormalities in diabetes to this system. Stretch and angiotensin II have additive effects on increasing VEGF expression. Interestingly, losartan, an angiotensin II receptor antagonist, and anti-TGF-β antibody, have been shown to prevent angiotensin II-induced, but not stretch-induced, VEGF production in human mesangial cells,[266] suggesting that angiotensin II and mechanical stretch can both independently induce VEGF production. Increased proliferation of mesangial cells exposed to VEGF *in vitro* is inhibited by anti-VEGF antibody.[259] VEGF is increased in glomeruli in diabetic animals,[258] and diabetic rats treated with anti-VEGF neutralizing antibody do not hyperfilter and have less AER increase.[267] Plasma and urinary levels of VEGF are increased in microalbuminuric and proteinuric patients with T1DM and T2DM,[255,261,268] but no relationship between VEGF levels and GFR decline was found in proteinuric type 1 diabetic patients followed for 3 years.[255] One study showed that, despite being independently correlated to microalbuminuria and retinopathy, serum VEGF levels were related to glycemic control, and improvement in glycemia resulted in a significant reduction of VEGF levels.[268] No differences in glomerular VEGF mRNA levels were found in microalbuminuric and proteinuric type 2 diabetic patients between patients with typical or atypical diabetic glomerulopathy.[269] Another study found stronger immunostaining of VEGF glomerular epithelial cells in type 2 diabetic patients with mild versus more advanced DN or controls.[261] VEGF staining was markedly decreased or absent in globally sclerotic glomeruli. However, tubular VEGF staining was more intense in advanced than in mild DN. This could be explained by podocyte loss with a consequent decrease in glomerular VEGF expression.[270] Indeed, as is true for neoangiogenesis in diabetic retinopathy,[253] VEGF could also be related to increased vascularization around the glomerular pole in DN. Blood vessel growth has been observed in experimental[271] and human[272] DN. However, the role of VEGF in the pathogenesis of DN is still far from clear, and it is uncertain whether VEGF expression is the cause of pathologic changes, or represents a reparative response to preexisting tissue and functional alterations.

EGF

EGF is synthesized in the kidney, and mesangial, tubular, and interstitial cells all have receptors for this peptide.[273] EGF stimulates *in vitro* tubular cell proliferation[274] and thus may play a role in early diabetic renal hypertrophy.[275] EGF strongly influences the synthesis and turnover of ECM proteins, including collagens, fibronectin, laminin, and glycosaminoglycans.[276] In several cell types, EGF downregulates TGF-β receptor expression,[277,278] suggesting that some EGF activities are indirect. Other growth factors, including platelet-derived, fibroblast, and nerve growth factors can modulate EGF receptor activity.[279] The human EGF receptor-1 is phosphorylated by PKC, reducing the affinity of this receptor for EGF. Interestingly, binding of EGF to its receptor leads to formation of inositol-1,4,5-triphosphate and 1,2 diacylglycerol,[280] stimulating PKC and thus possibly modulating the activity of this system.

PKC

The PKC enzyme regulating Na^+/K^+-ATPase[281] has a role in regulating cell proliferation, vascular contractility and permeability, and basement membrane synthesis. PKC can be activated by diacylglycerol,[282] and thus by high glucose (Fig. 42-11). PKC can increase iNOS expression and regulate NO production in mesangial cells.[283] High glucose-induced PKC activation in glomerular cells *in vitro* is followed by increased TGF-β[284] and MAPK[285] activity. For example, the antioxidant vitamin E inhibits the glucose-induced increase in PKC, TGF-β, and ECM production in mesangial cells *in vitro*, without affecting the exogenous TGF-β-induced increase in ECM production.[284] Increased type IV collagen expression in mesangial cell in high glucose is prevented by nonspecific PKC inhibitors,[286] and treatment of PKC agonists can increase type IV collagen expression.[287] Treatment with a PKCβ inhibitor blocks increases in glomerular TGF-β1 mRNA, MM, GFR, and AER in diabetic rodents.[229,288] In another study, PKCβ inhibition prevented glomerular hypertrophy and albuminuria without affecting the TGF-β axis in diabetic rats,[289] indicating that PKC renal effects in diabetes may at least in part be independent of the TGF-β axis.

Cytokines

As discussed above (see section on hemodynamics), there are *in vitro* and animal model data linking the pathogenesis of DN to the renin-angiotensin system.

Plasma Prorenin Levels and Diabetic Complications

Renin and its inactive precursor, prorenin, are secreted into the circulation from the kidney.[290] Renin is derived almost entirely from the kidney,[290] whereas prorenin, while primarily of renal origin, is also produced in other sites.[290,291] In longstanding diabetes with microvascular complications, plasma prorenin levels tend to be markedly elevated, but renin levels tend to be normal or reduced.[292–294] The pathogenesis of markedly increased plasma prorenin levels in diabetic patients with complications is not completely understood but is likely of renal origin.[295] Followed serially, only 1 of 20 young patients with T1DM with consistently normal prorenin levels developed proteinuria or retinopathy, whereas one or both developed in 8 of 14 patients with increased prorenin levels.[293] Daneman and associates[294] studied 50 adolescents with T1DM for an average of 7 years, 25 of whom had microalbuminuria. Prorenin was highest in the microalbuminuric patients versus the nonmicroalbuminuric patients, and all type 1 diabetic patients combined had higher values than controls. Most interestingly, the nondiabetic siblings of the microalbuminuric patients in this study had higher prorenin values than siblings of the nonmicroalbuminuric type 1 diabetic patients.[294] In another report, type 1 diabetic patients developing microalbuminuria or proteinuria (progressors) had increased total renin content (which is predominantly prorenin) as early as 10 years before onset of microalbuminuria.[296] Increase in plasma prorenin also preceded the development of microalbuminuria in patients with type 1[297] or type 2[298] diabetes. However, this was not confirmed in another study in patients with T2DM.[299] Taken together, these studies suggest that elevated plasma prorenin may be an important predictor of progressive DN.

Angiotensin II

Angiotensin II elevates blood pressure through its direct vasoconstrictor, sympathomimetic, and sodium-retaining (through aldosterone release) activities. Nonhemodynamic effects of angiotensin II on renal cells may contribute to the progression of DN. Glucose may increase mesangial angiotensin II production,[300] and angiotensin II stimulates cellular glucose uptake and transcription of GLUT-1,[301] leading to a high intracellular glucose concentration and its consequences. Angiotensin II also activates PKC in mesangial and tubular cells,[302] and PKC can thus activate TGF-β, promoting mesangial[303] and proximal tubular[304] cell proliferation. Angiotensin II upregulates TGF-β-receptor expression in mesangial cells *in vitro*, which could increase the sensitivity to exogenous TGF-β, enhancing TGF-β fibrogenic actions.[305] Thus angiotensin II can stimulate *in vitro* ECM synthesis through TGF-β activity in mesangial and tubular cells,[304,306] and can inhibit mesangial cell collagenase activity,[307] reducing ECM turnover. These effects are blocked by losartan,[307] an angiotensin II antagonist, and by saralasin,[306] an angiotensin II competitive inhibitor. Angiotensin II-receptor antagonists abolish proliferative growth of murine mesangial cells.[308] Angiotensin II can also stimulate VEGF and endothelin release (see above). Angiotensin II also activates NAD/NADP oxidase and induces superoxide production and hypertrophy by mesangial cells.[309] Many of the angiotensin II actions are indirect, and dependent on TGF-β or VEGF release. Interestingly, diabetic rats deficient in angiotensin type 1 receptors do not show increased renal TGF-β mRNA levels, supporting the hypothesis that the increase in TGF-β in diabetes is mediated by angiotensin II.[310] The relative importance of systemically-derived versus locally-generated angiotensin II in the pathogenesis of tissue injury remains controversial.[311] (see section on hemodynamics).

Bradykinin

Bradykinin, the major effector molecule of the kallikrein-kinin system, could play a role in modulating renal hemodynamics and function. Since this enzyme inhibits angiotensin II formation and also prevents degradation of vasodilatory kinins,[312] increased bradykinin levels could have a protective effect on the progression of renal failure. Bradykinin can also increase NO levels.[313] Alterations in the kallikrein kinin system have been found in experimental[314] and clinical[64] diabetes (see section on hemodynamics). Diabetic rats developing proteinuria and reduced GFR show increased serum and urinary levels of bradykinin compared to control animals.[315] A reduction in renal kallikrein has been found in type 2 diabetic patients, suggesting that an impaired renal kallikrein-kinin system contributes to the development of DN.[316] Under physiologic conditions, most of bradykinin's effects involve bradykinin-B2 receptors.[316] A bradykinin-B2-receptor antagonist had no effect on AER and glomerular ultrastructure [GBM width and Vv(Mes/glom)] when used alone or associated with an ACE inhibitor (ramipril) or an angiotensin II type 1-receptor blocker (valsartan) in diabetic rats.[317] This bradykinin-B2 receptor antagonist had previously been shown to reduce hyperfiltration[63] and AER[318] in diabetic rodents. It has been suggested that changes in the kallikrein-kinin system induced by ACE inhibitors may contribute to the renoprotective effect of these drugs. ACE inhibition reduces angiotensin II formation and induces bradykinin accumulation.[312] However, a randomized, double-blind, crossover clinical trial in 16 patients with T1DM did not find differences in AER, GFR, and 24-hour blood pressure between an ACE inhibitor (enalapril) and an angiotensin II type 1-receptor blocker (losartan) used for 2 months.[319] Both drugs reduced AER and blood pressure when compared to placebo. There was no effect on GFR. These studies suggest that the renoprotective effects of ACE inhibitors are independent of bradykinin, as angiotensin II type 1-receptor blockers do not increase bradykinin levels.

Endothelins

Endothelins, potent vasoconstrictors and positive inotropic and chronotropic myocardial agents, increase the plasma levels of a number of vasoactive hormones, such as atrial natriuretic peptide, aldosterone, and catecholamines. They are produced and secreted by endothelial, epithelial, and mesangial cells.[320] TGF-β, angiotensin, hypoxia, and hemodynamic shear forces increase endothelin synthesis by vascular endothelial cells.[321] On the other hand, endothelins can induce TGF-β synthesis and stimulate mesangial cells, smooth muscle cells, and fibroblast proliferation.[320,321] High glucose levels induce endothelin-1 expression in rat mesangial cells,[322] and endothelin stimulation activates MAPKs [extracellular signal-regulated kinases (ERK1 and ERK2)] in a PKC-dependent mechanism.[323] Thus PKC is necessary, but not sufficient, for mitogenic signaling by endothelin.[324] Reactive oxygen species can also enhance endothelin-1 production by diabetic rat glomeruli, and reactive oxygen species scavengers suppress endothelin-1 production both *in vivo* and *in vitro*.[325] Endothelins can also reduce renal blood flow and GFR.[326] Endothelin-A receptor antagonist,[327] insulin,[328] and enalapril[329] treatment ameliorated the glomerular increase of endothelin-1 mRNA in diabetic rats. Diabetic rats have higher urinary endothelin-1 excretion and AER than controls. Administration of endothelin-A/endothelin-B,[330] but not of endothelin-A,[327] receptor antagonist reduced AER in diabetic rats. Patients with type 1 and type 2 diabetes have higher urinary endothelin-1 excretion than nondiabetic controls, and urinary endothelin-1 is correlated with AER and serum albumin in the diabetic patients.[331,332] However, lower urinary excretion and higher plasma endothelin-1 levels were found in type 2 diabetic patients when compared to controls.[333,334]

To definitively implicate the pathways discussed above (PKC, TGF-β, IGF, VEGF, and others), it is important to demonstrate that they are involved in the genesis of typical DN lesions as defined by well-established electron microscopy morphometric techniques. The lesions studied should include mesangial expansion and GBM thickening. The studies should attempt to demonstrate that these lesions can be caused by activation of these pathways in nondiabetic animals, or prevented by treatment with specific inhibitors of these pathways in animals or humans with diabetes.

Oxidative Stress

Intracellular reactive oxygen species are produced by the mitochondrial electron transport chain in response to hyperglycemia. Indeed, reactive oxygen species may arise from multiple pathways,[335] including (1) glucose autoxidation; (2) hydrogen peroxide (H_2O_2), generated from the oxidation of enediols formed from Amadori products; and (3) superoxide (O_2^-), formed by the mitochondrial oxidation of NADH to NAD^+ or in the formation of prostaglandins, since prostaglandin synthase utilizes NADH (and NADPH) with generation of O_2^-. Both H_2O_2 and hydroxyl radicals (˙OH) may be derived from O_2^-. Mitochondrial superoxide overproduction stimulates aldose reductase activity, thus initiating the *de novo* synthesis of diacylglycerol, activating PKC. Reactive oxygen species can also initiate intracellular formation of advanced glycation end products (AGEs) (Fig. 42-11). Inhibitors of mitochondrial electron transport and manganese superoxide dismutase, an enzyme that leads to reactive oxygen species scavenging in mitochondrial matrix, have been shown to inhibit the production of reactive oxygen species secondary to hyperglycemia. These agents also prevent high glucose-induced PKC and NFκB activation, methylglyoxal-derived AGE formation, and sorbitol accumulation through the polyol-pathway. This strongly suggests that reactive oxygen species are not only necessary for the damage caused by hyperglycemia, but they can also be the link between the several pathophysiologic hypotheses for DN. Methylglyoxal, the most reactive dicarbonyl AGE-intermediate in crosslinking of proteins, can regenerate reactive oxygen species in the course of glycation reactions.[336] *In vitro* studies demonstrated that the antioxidant vitamin E blocks the high glucose-induced increase in PKC, and TGF-β bioactivity, as well as collagen and fibronectin synthesis in mesangial cells.[284] Taurine, another antioxidant, also inhibits the activation of PKC and the increase in TGF-β in response to high glucose levels.[284] In contrast, vitamin E did not alter the mesangial cell increase in matrix protein synthesis induced by TGF-β.[284] However, treatment of diabetic rats with antioxidant agents shows controversial results. Diabetic rats treated with selenium and vitamin E[337] or nitecapone, another antioxidant,[338] showed reduction of AER, hyperfiltration, and glomerular lesions. Intraperitoneal injection of vitamin E also prevented glomerular increase in diacylglycerol content, PKC activity, and filtration rate and fraction, and improved AER in diabetic rats.[339] However, another study found less proteinuria, albuminuria, glomerular hypertrophy, glomerulosclerosis, and tubulointerstitial fibrosis, and preserved glomerular type IV collagen staining in taurine-treated animals, while vita-

min E-treated animals had extremely high mortality and worse renal lesions.[340] Both taurine[341] and vitamin E[284,342] had previously been shown to reduce collagen accumulation in rat mesangial cells exposed to high glucose.

Oxidative stress is increased in diabetes.[343] The debate has been whether oxidative stress has a primary role in the pathogenesis of diabetic complications, occurring at early stages in diabetes, or whether it is merely a consequence of tissue damage, reflecting the presence of complications.[344] Skin fibroblasts from type 1 diabetic patients with DN do not show the expected increase in activity and mRNA expression of the antioxidant enzymes, catalase and glutathione peroxidase, when exposed to a high-glucose condition *in vitro*,[345] while no differences between type 1 diabetic patients with DN and diabetic patients without nephropathy, nondiabetic nephropathic patients, and normal controls were observed when skin fibroblasts were cultured in normal-glucose conditions. Catalase promotes the transformation of hydrogen peroxide to oxygen and water, and glutathione peroxidase reduces peroxide and superoxide levels. Glutathione peroxidase requires a high cellular level of reduced glutathione to be effective. Lipid peroxidation induced by exposure to high glucose was also more pronounced in cells of type 1 diabetic patients with DN. These findings suggest that increased oxidative stress in type 1 diabetic patients with DN is associated with a decreased response of antioxidant enzymes to high glucose. Recent studies have demonstrated increased oxidative stress in families of type 1 diabetic patients,[346] suggesting that an abnormal redox state could even precede diabetes onset. Interestingly, erythrocyte glutathione content is correlated to Na^+/H^+ exchanger (NHE) activity,[347] linking oxidative stress to an ion-transport system associated with DN risk.

There is an association between oxidative stress, altered NO production and action, and endothelial dysfunction.[348,349] Endothelium-derived NO is a potent vasodilator that also has antiatherogenic properties, including decreased platelet and leukocyte adhesion to the endothelium, and inhibition of smooth muscle cell migration.[350] Endothelial NO synthesis can be stimulated by shear stress and pulsatile vessel stretching,[351] hypoxia,[352] and by agonists such as acetylcholine and bradykinin.[353] Exposure to high glucose concentrations increases eNOS gene expression and NO release, with a concomitant increase in superoxide production.[354] Superoxide inactivates and reacts with NO to form peroxynitrite,[354] a potent oxidant, leading to endothelial dysfunction.[355] Normalization of NO-mediated vasorelaxation in high-glucose conditions by superoxide dismutase,[356] a scavenger that transforms superoxide anion into hydrogen peroxide, further adds to this association. NO suppressed TGF-β activity and abolished increases in TGF-β₁ mRNA and collagen synthesis in mesangial cells exposed to high glucose concentration. Endogenous NO produced by glomerular capillary endothelial cells may modulate TGF-β production by these cells and also by mesangial cells.[349] Stimulation of *in vitro* iNOS activity reduces collagen and fibronectin accumulation in rat mesangial cells.[357] NO may also modulate MMP-2 activity in these cells.[358] High glucose *in vitro* enhances EGF- and IGF-1-, but not TGF-β- or VEGF-induced NO production by rat mesangial cells.[265,359] This suggests that growth factors may modulate the inhibitory effects of high glucose on NO production.[359] Decreased basal and stimulated NO release, reduced bioavailability of NO, and decreased vascular smooth cell responsiveness have been shown in diabetes. Hyperglycemia may cause these abnormalities by several mechanisms, including increasing AGE production, polyol pathway, and PKC activities, as well as increasing oxidative stress, as described above. AGEs can quench NO both *in vitro* and *in vivo*,[360] decreasing its bioavailability and impairing NO's antiproliferative effects on mesangial cells.[361] Interestingly, aminoguanidine, an AGE crosslink inhibitor, also inhibits NO[70] and restores endothelium-dependent relaxation in diabetic rats.[360] Increased aldose reductase activity in chronic hyperglycemia causes reduced NADPH, an essential cofactor for NOS, and could thus lead to reduced NO production.[348] Increased PKC could also lead to impaired endothelium-dependent relaxation.[362]

Glycosylation Products

Although the key points are summarized here, the reader is referred to the excellent review by Chen and colleagues[363] and Chap. 13 for greater details on this subject. One of the major metabolic effects of diabetes are the nonenzymatic reactions between reducing sugars, such as glucose, and free amino groups, lipids, or nucleic acids.[364] This interaction, known as the Maillard reaction,[364] is accelerated by hyperglycemia. Many proteins, such as hemoglobin,[365] albumin,[364] low density lipoproteins,[366] erythrocyte membrane proteins,[367] and crystalline lens,[368] undergo nonenzymatic glycosylation in diabetes, leading to altered physiochemical properties of these molecules. This early glycation process proceeds through the labile Schiff base adduct formation and intramolecular Amadori rearrangement, to become a stable glucose-modified protein. Amadori products comprise the majority of plasmatic glucose-modified proteins, and receptors for some of those modified proteins have been defined.[369] Further modifications of Maillard reaction products lead to inter- and intramolecular crosslinks and formation of AGEs. These reactions are complex and the reader is referred to several excellent reviews for greater detail.[370,371] It has been suggested that the accumulation of glycation products may be a major contributor to the development of diabetic complications.[372–374] Increased AGEs can stimulate the synthesis of various growth factors, including IGF-1 and TGF-β. Binding of AGE proteins to AGE receptors on cell surfaces induces an intracellular oxidative response *in vitro*, characterized by increased NFκB.[375] A hallmark of the glomerular changes of diabetes is mesangial expansion, mainly due to increases in ECM. Mesangial cells exposed to high glucose concentration when the matrix is being made, or when the degradation is taking place, have a reduced rate of mesangium degradation.[376] Thus, glycosylated ECM has reduced turnover rates, favoring ECM accumulation.[377] Human and rat mesangial cells exposed to glycated bovine serum albumin showed increased IGF-1 and TGF-β proteins, IGF-1, IGF-2, and TGF-β1 mRNAs, and ECM (laminin, type IV collagen, and fibronectin) proteins and mRNAs. These effects were prevented by aminoguanidine or by an AGE-receptor 1 antagonist.[378] Both high glucose and glycated bovine serum albumin can increase AGE-receptor expression in rat mesangial cells.[379] Diabetes induction also increased glomerular AGE-receptor mRNA expression and increased immunohistochemical staining in diabetic rats.[379] Further, intraperitoneal AGE-modified mouse albumin increases glomerular mRNA for TGF-β1 and ECM components[380] and causes glomerular hypertrophy. These effects are reduced by aminoguanidine.[380] Soulis-Liparota and associates[374] found that aminoguanidine diminished the increased collagen-related fluorescence in diabetic rat aorta, glomeruli, and renal tubules, as well as albuminuria. In this study, GBM width increased in both treated and untreated diabetic rats, while Vv(Mes/glom) increase was prevented by aminoguani-

dine. However, another study found that aminoguanidine ameliorated the GBM thickening but not the Vv(Mes/glom) increase in diabetic rats.[381] In similar studies [M.W. Steffes, M. Mauer, unpublished data], aminoguanidine failed to have any effect on GBM or mesangial expansion in severe longstanding diabetes in rats. More recently, oral treatment with aminoguanidine was also shown to normalize renal mRNA expression of IGF-1 and IGF-binding proteins in diabetic rats,[382] reinforcing a favorable effect of aminoguanidine in DN. Novel inhibitors of advanced glycation have been shown to exhibit renoprotective effects similar to aminoguanidine.[383,384] OPB-9195, a new AGE inhibitor, reduced renal TGF-β1, VEGF, and type IV collagen mRNA expression, glomerular TGF-β1, VEGF, type IV collagen, and AGE immunoreactivity, albuminuria, and progressive glomerulosclerosis without changing glycemia, in an animal model of T2DM.[385,386] Pimagedine, a second-generation AGE inhibitor, reduced urinary protein excretion in proteinuric type 1 diabetic patients, and also decreased the chances of doubling serum creatinine in patients with initial creatinine lower than 1.5 mg/dL.[387] Serum AGE levels were independent predictors of progression of early structural glomerular lesions [Vv(MM/glom)] in microalbuminuric type 1 diabetic patients.[388]

Amadori-Glycated Albumin and Diabetic Nephropathy

Renal cells grown in high glucose have upregulation of the TGF-β[227,389,390] and PKC[287,391] systems, and exhibit ECM overproduction.[286,392] Amadori-glycated proteins, which are earlier products of the glycation process than AGEs, have similar cellular effects even without high-glucose media. For example, glomerular epithelial cells exposed to glycated fetal bovine serum show increased laminin and GBM antigens, unchanged type I collagen and fibronectin, and decreased collagenase activity.[393] Glycated albumin and high-glucose media together cause an even greater *in vitro* increase in TGF-β1 and type II TGF-β-receptor mRNAs than either manipulation alone.[394] Also, mouse mesangial cells incubated in normal glucose media containing glycated serum proteins have increased α_1(IV) collagen and fibronectin mRNA, and these effects are intensified by high-glucose media.[394,395] Moreover, antibody to glycated albumin prevented the increase in fibronectin and type IV collagen expression, and reduced albuminuria in rodent endothelial and mesangial glomerular cells exposed to glycated albumin.[363,395,396] Antiglycated albumin antibody administration lowers plasma glycated albumin concentration, reduces AER, and improves glomerular mesangial pathology in *db/db* diabetic mice.[397,398] Treatment with an inhibitor of glycated albumin formation (EXO-226) reduced AER, prevented GFR decline, and reduced MM accumulation and α_1(IV) collagen cortical mRNA expression in *db/db* mice.[399] Plasma concentrations of glycated albumin were normalized by treatment, despite persistent hyperglycemia.[399] Also, when overall PKC or specifically PKCβ activity are blocked, the glycated albumin-induced increase in type IV collagen production is prevented,[229,288] consistent with the notion that PKC, particularly the β isoform, plays a role in glycated albumin-induced ECM accumulation. Type 1 diabetic patients showed higher plasma levels of glycated albumin than nondiabetic controls, and type 1 diabetic patients with DN showed higher plasma levels of Amadori albumin than normoalbuminuric patients.[400] However, studies examining the role of Amadori-glycated proteins in the progression of diabetic renal disease have reached conflicting conclusions.[401–403] Further studies of glycation's role in pathogenesis and treatment strategies for DN are warranted. However, the fact that glycation is a nonenzymatic process dependent on the duration and magnitude of glycemia, currently leaves unexplained why only about one-half of patients with very poor glycemic control develop clinical DN.[103]

Increased Activity of Aldose Reductase

Aldose reductase, the enzyme that catalyzes the reduction of glucose to sorbitol in the polyol pathway (Fig. 42-11), has been associated with DN and other microvascular complications. Aldose reductase, not present in all mammalian cells, is present in all the target tissues of diabetic complications. These tissues include kidney, lens, retinal capillary wall pericytes, vascular endothelium, and peripheral nerve (Schwann cells). Increased activity of aldose reductase leads to accumulation of sorbitol, which is further converted to fructose by the sorbitol dehydrogenase enzyme, using NAD^+ as substrate. The ratio of NAD^+:NADH decreases and the conversion of glyceraldehyde 3-phosphate to 1,3-bisphosphoglycerate is blocked, leaving more substrate (glyceraldehyde 3-phosphate) for the synthesis of α-glycerol phosphate, a diacylglycerol precursor. Diacylglycerol is a PKC activator that, as discussed, could regulate ECM synthesis and removal. Also, increased activity of aldose reductase consumes NADPH, leading to decreased or depleted glutathione. Glutathione is an antioxidant coenzyme used by glutathione peroxidase to reduce peroxides or superoxide, as described above, yielding oxidized glutathione. Glutathione can also act as a detoxicant for carbonyl compounds.[344] Hypertonicity stimulates aldose reductase gene expression, and kinases (p38-MAPK and ERKs) appear to be involved in the regulation of this response.[404] Both glucose and H_2O_2 activate p38-MAPK *in vitro*, suggesting that increased glucose may contribute to increased aldose reductase expression, independently of hyperosmotic conditions. PKC also has a role in controlling aldose reductase gene transcription.[405] Moreover, reactive oxygen species decrease NO content, which activates aldose reductase. Increased aldose reductase activity may also contribute to impaired renal autoregula-

tion.[406] An aldose reductase inhibitor prevents type IV collagen and fibronectin accumulation in human renal proximal tubular cells exposed to high glucose levels.[407] Treatment of diabetic animals with aldose reductase inhibitors has generated divergent results.[408–410] One study showed prevention of renal and glomerular hypertrophy, but not of GBM thickening,[411] by aldose reductase inhibition, while another reported prevention of mesangial expansion.[412] Tolrestat, an aldose reductase inhibitor, prevented increased GFR, AER, and glomerular hypertrophy, and attenuated the accumulation of basement membrane-like material in diabetic rats, with no effect on mesangium expansion.[413] Peripheral blood mononuclear cell aldose reductase mRNA levels are increased in patients with type 1 diabetes and DN, but not in diabetic patients without nephropathy.[414] Aldose reductase inhibitors have a partial[415,416] or no[417,418] effect in ameliorating renal microvascular complications in human studies.

Steno Hypothesis

According to the Steno hypothesis, albuminuria reflects widespread vascular damage.[419] Heparan sulfate is the main glycosaminoglycan component of glomerular basement membranes.[420] Hyperglycemia can lead to partial depletion of heparan sulfate from both decreased synthesis and reduced sulfation levels.[421] Decreased renal heparan sulfate can diminish the glomerular capillary wall electrostatic charge barrier.[422] Abnormal glomerular charge permselectivity has been observed in diabetic rats[423] and humans,[424] suggesting that loss of glomerular capillary wall proteoglycans may be responsible for the initial increase in the excretion of negatively-charged albumin.[420,425] Changes in heparan sulfate have also been associated with other diabetic complications.[426,427] Administration of a modified heparin glycosaminoglycan preparation to cultured mesangial cells exposed to high glucose caused inhibition of TGF-β_1 overexpression, probably through inhibition of glucose-induced PKC activation.[428] The changes in the balance of α_1(IV) collagen, MMP-2, and TIMP-2 in human and murine cells exposed to high glucose were partially reversed by heparin supplementation.[429] Animal studies have shown that subcutaneous administration of low molecular weight heparin, perhaps by inducing heparan sulfate synthesis, prevented increased AER, GBM, and α_1(IV) collagen expression and deposition in diabetic rats.[430–432] Reduction in AER was also reported after treatment with subcutaneous low molecular weight heparin or similar drugs in microalbuminuric and proteinuric type 1[433–436] and type 2[437] diabetic patients, but the results are still controversial.[438] Danaparoid, a mixture of sulfated glycosaminoglycan consisting mainly of heparan sulfate, not only decreased AER,[435] but also reduced retinal hard exudates in proteinuric type 1 diabetic patients.[439] These studies suggest that decreased glycosaminoglycans can have a pathogenetic role in the development of diabetic complications. However, it is also clear from earlier discussions (see sections on pathology and structural-functional relationships, above) that important DN lesions can develop in patients with normal glomerular permselectivity. Thus, measurably abnormal glomerular permselectivity is not necessary for the genesis of DN lesions.

CONCLUSIONS

Several mechanisms have been proposed to explain the development of renal complications in diabetes. It appears that multiple

FIGURE 42-11. The effects of increased activity of the polyol pathway. The metabolism of glucose to sorbitol and fructose in the polyol pathway decreases the NADPH:$NADP^+$ and NAD^+:NADH ratios. Consumption of the NAD^+ in the conversion of sorbitol to fructose (*) may limit 1,3 bisphosphoglycerate formation (**), resulting in increased diacyglycerol and protein kinase C (**PKC**) activation. The consumption of NADPH in the conversion of glucose to sorbitol (‡) may result in decreased production of glutathione, an antioxidant coenzyme used by gluthathione peroxidase to reduce peroxide and superoxide levels. **PPP**, pentose phosphate pathway.

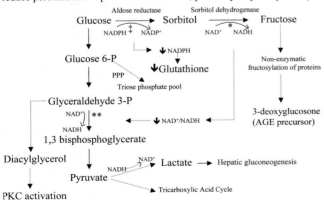

pathways interact and are involved in a process that is probably genetically regulated. Recent advances in molecular biology and genetics should allow us to gain new insight into the molecular mechanisms and genes involved in the development of DN. These advances will allow early identification of patients who are at risk of developing DN, and should lead to the design of specific preventive strategies that are based on this new understanding of the pathophysiologic bases of DN. Moreover, the demonstration that DN lesions are reversible could lead to treatment aimed at stimulating the healing capacities of the kidney, with the goal of restoring lost function or preventing further loss.

REFERENCES

1. The National Institutes of Health, National Institute of Diabetes and Digestive and Kidney Diseases: *USRDS 1999 Annual Data Report*: 1999.
2. Warram JH, Gearin G, Laffel L, *et al*: Effect of duration of type I diabetes on the prevalence of stages of diabetic nephropathy defined by urinary albumin/creatinine ratio. *J Am Soc Nephrol* 1996;7:930.
3. Rychlik I, Miltenberger-Miltenyi G, Ritz E: The drama of the continuous increase in end-stage renal failure in patients with type II diabetes mellitus. *Nephrol Dial Transplant* 1998;13:6.
4. Nelson RG, Meyer TW, Myers BD, *et al*: Course of renal disease in Pima Indians with non-insulin-dependent diabetes mellitus. *Kidney Int* 1997;(Suppl)63:S45.
5. Parving HH, Andersen AR, Smidt UM, *et al*: Early aggressive antihypertensive treatment reduces rate of decline in kidney function in diabetic nephropathy. *Lancet* 1983;1:1175.
6. Lewis EJ, Hunsicker LG, Bain RP, *et al*: The effect of angiotensin-converting-enzyme inhibition on diabetic nephropathy. The Collaborative Study Group. *N Engl J Med* 1993;329:1456.
7. Viberti GC, Bilous RW, Mackintosh D, *et al*: Long term correction of hyperglycaemia and progression of renal failure in insulin dependent diabetes. *Br Med J (Clin Res Ed)* 1983;286:598.
8. Fioretto P, Steffes MW, Mauer M: Glomerular structure in nonproteinuric IDDM patients with various levels of albuminuria. *Diabetes* 1994;43:1358.
9. Mauer SM, Steffes MW, Ellis EN, *et al*: Structural-functional relationships in diabetic nephropathy. *J Clin Invest* 1984;74:1143.
10. Osterby R: Glomerular structural changes in type 1 (insulin-dependent) diabetes mellitus: causes, consequences, and prevention. *Diabetologia* 1992;35:803.
11. Saito Y, Kida H, Takeda S, *et al*: Mesangiolysis in diabetic glomeruli: its role in the formation of nodular lesions. *Kidney Int* 1988;34:389.
12. Miller K, Michael AF: Immunopathology of renal extracellular membranes in diabetes mellitus. Specificity of tubular basement-membrane immunofluorescence. *Diabetes* 1976;25:701.
13. Michael AF, Brown DM: Increased concentration of albumin in kidney basement membranes in diabetes mellitus. *Diabetes* 1981;30:843.
14. Falk RJ, Scheinman JI, Mauer SM, *et al*: Polyantigenic expansion of basement membrane constituents in diabetic nephropathy. *Diabetes* 1983;32(Suppl 2):34.
15. Zhu D, Kim Y, Steffes MW, *et al*: Glomerular distribution of type IV collagen in diabetes by high resolution quantitative immunochemistry. *Kidney Int* 1994;45:425.
16. Moriya T, Groppoli TJ, Kim Y, *et al*: Quantitative immunoelectron microscopy of type VI collagen in glomeruli in type I diabetic patients. *Kidney Int* 2001;59:317.
17. Østerby R: Early phases in the development of diabetic glomerulopathy. *Acta Med Scand* 1974;(Suppl)574:3.
18. Steffes MW, Sutherland DE, Goetz FC, *et al*: Studies of kidney and muscle biopsy specimens from identical twins discordant for type I diabetes mellitus. *N Engl J Med* 1985;312:1282.
19. Osterby R: Morphometric studies of the peripheral glomerular basement membrane in early juvenile diabetes. I. Development of initial basement membrane thickening. *Diabetologia* 1972;8:84.
20. Brito PL, Fioretto P, Drummond K, *et al*: Proximal tubular basement membrane width in insulin-dependent diabetes mellitus. *Kidney Int* 1998;53:754.
21. Berg UB, Torbjornsdotter TB, Jaremko G, *et al*: Kidney morphological changes in relation to long-term renal function and metabolic control in adolescents with IDDM. *Diabetologia* 1998;41:1047.
22. Walker JD, Close CF, Jones SL, *et al*: Glomerular structure in type-1 (insulin-dependent) diabetic patients with normo- and microalbuminuria. *Kidney Int* 1992;41:741.
23. Chavers BM, Bilous RW, Ellis EN, *et al*: Glomerular lesions and urinary albumin excretion in type I diabetes without overt proteinuria. *N Engl J Med* 1989;320:966.
24. Bangstad HJ, Osterby R, Dahl-Jorgensen K, *et al*: Early glomerulopathy is present in young, type 1 (insulin-dependent) diabetic patients with microalbuminuria. *Diabetologia* 1993;36:523.
25. Caramori ML, Fioretto P, Mauer M: Long-term follow-up of normoalbuminuric longstanding type 1 diabetic patients: Progression is associated with worse baseline glomerular lesions and lower glomerular filtration rate [Abstract]. *J Am Soc Nephrol* 1999;10:126A.
26. Eddy AA: Molecular insights into renal interstitial fibrosis. *J Am Soc Nephrol* 1996;7:2495.
27. Katz A, Caramori MLA, Sisson-Ross S, Groppoli T, Basgen J, Mauer M: An increase in the volume fraction of the cortical interstitium occupied by cells antedates interstitial fibrosis in type 1 diabetic patients. *Kidney Int* 2002; in press.
28. Steffes MW, Bilous RW, Sutherland DE, *et al*: Cell and matrix components of the glomerular mesangium in type I diabetes. *Diabetes* 1992;41:679.
29. Pagtalunan ME, Miller PL, Jumping-Eagle S, *et al*: Podocyte loss and progressive glomerular injury in type II diabetes. *J Clin Invest* 1997; 99:342.
30. Dalla Vestra M, Saller A, Bortoloso E, Mauer M, Fioretto P: Structural involvement in type 1 and type 2 diabetic nephropathy. *Diabetes Metab* 2000;26(suppl 4):8.
31. Moriya T, Moriya R, Yajima Y, Steffes M, Mauer M: Urinary albumin as an indicator of diabetic nephropathy lesions in Japanese type 2 diabetic patients. *Nephron* 2002; 77:in press.
32. Fioretto P, Mauer M, Brocco E, *et al*: Patterns of renal injury in NIDDM patients with microalbuminuria. *Diabetologia* 1996;39:1569.
33. Nelson RG, Meyer TW, Myers BD, *et al*: Clinical and pathological course of renal disease in non-insulin-dependent diabetes mellitus: the Pima Indian experience. *Semin Nephrol* 1997;17:124.
34. White KE, Bilous RW: Type 2 diabetic patients with nephropathy show structural-functional relationships that are similar to type 1 disease. *J Am Soc Nephrol* 2000;11:1667.
35. Hayashi H, Karasawa R, Inn H, *et al*: An electron microscopic study of glomeruli in Japanese patients with non-insulin dependent diabetes mellitus. *Kidney Int* 1992;41:749.
36. Parving HH, Gall MA, Skott P, *et al*: Prevalence and causes of albuminuria in non-insulin-dependent diabetic patients. *Kidney Int* 1992; 41:758.
37. Fioretto P, Steffes MW, Sutherland DE, *et al*: Sequential renal biopsies in insulin-dependent diabetic patients: structural factors associated with clinical progression. *Kidney Int* 1995;48:1929.
38. Bangstad HJ, Osterby R, Hartmann A, *et al*: Severity of glomerulopathy predicts long-term urinary albumin excretion rate in patients with type 1 diabetes and microalbuminuria. *Diabetes Care* 1999;22: 314.
39. D'Amico G: Tubulointerstitium as predictor of progression of glomerular diseases. *Nephron* 1999;83:289.
40. Mackensen-Haen S, Bader R, Grund KE, *et al*: Correlations between renal cortical interstitial fibrosis, atrophy of the proximal tubules and impairment of the glomerular filtration rate. *Clin Nephrol* 1981; 15:167.
41. Lane PH, Steffes MW, Fioretto P, *et al*: Renal interstitial expansion in insulin-dependent diabetes mellitus. *Kidney Int* 1993;43:661.
42. Taft JL, Nolan CJ, Yeung SP, *et al*: Clinical and histological correlations of decline in renal function in diabetic patients with proteinuria. *Diabetes* 1994;43:1046.
43. Ruggenenti P, Gambara V, Perna A, *et al*: The nephropathy of non-insulin-dependent diabetes: predictors of outcome relative to diverse patterns of renal injury. *J Am Soc Nephrol* 1998;9:2336.
44. Nosadini R, Velussi M, Brocco E, *et al*: Course of renal function in type 2 diabetic patients with abnormalities of albumin excretion rate. *Diabetes* 2000;49:476.
45. Cordonnier DJ, Pinel N, Barro C, *et al*: Expansion of cortical interstitium is limited by converting enzyme inhibition in type 2 diabetic pa-

tients with glomerulosclerosis. The Diabiopsies Group. *J Am Soc Nephrol* 1999;10:1253.

46. Effect of intensive therapy on the development and progression of diabetic nephropathy in the Diabetes Control and Complications Trial. The Diabetes Control and Complications (DCCT) Research Group. *Kidney Int* 1995;47:1703.

47. The Diabetes Control and Complications Trial/Epidemiology of Diabetes Interventions and Complications Research Group: Retinopathy and nephropathy in patients with type 1 diabetes four years after a trial of intensive therapy. *N Engl J Med* 2000;342:381.

48. UK Prospective Diabetes Study (UKPDS) Group: Intensive blood-glucose control with sulphonylureas or insulin compared with conventional treatment and risk of complications in patients with type 2 diabetes (UKPDS 33). *Lancet* 1998;352:837.

49. Barbosa J, Steffes MW, Sutherland DE, *et al*: Effect of glycemic control on early diabetic renal lesions. A 5-year randomized controlled clinical trial of insulin-dependent diabetic kidney transplant recipients. *JAMA* 1994;272:600.

50. Bangstad HJ, Osterby R, Dahl-Jorgensen K, *et al*: Improvement of blood glucose control in IDDM patients retards the progression of morphological changes in early diabetic nephropathy. *Diabetologia* 1994;37:483.

51. Fioretto P, Steffes MW, Sutherland DE, *et al*: Reversal of lesions of diabetic nephropathy after pancreas transplantation. *N Engl J Med* 1998;339:69.

52. Heilig CW, Liu Y, England RL, *et al*: D-glucose stimulates mesangial cell GLUT1 expression and basal and IGF-I-sensitive glucose uptake in rat mesangial cells: implications for diabetic nephropathy. *Diabetes* 1997;46:1030.

53. Inoki K, Haneda M, Maeda S, *et al*: TGF-beta 1 stimulates glucose uptake by enhancing GLUT1 expression in mesangial cells. *Kidney Int* 1999;55:1704.

54. Heilig CW, Concepcion LA, Riser BL, *et al*: Overexpression of glucose transporters in rat mesangial cells cultured in a normal glucose milieu mimics the diabetic phenotype. *J Clin Invest* 1995;96:1802.

55. Berkman J, Rifkin H: Unilateral nodular diabetic glomerulosclerosis (Kimmelstiel-Wilson): report of a case. *Metabolism* 1973;22:715.

56. Mauer SM, Steffes MW, Azar S, *et al*: The effects of Goldblatt hypertension on development of the glomerular lesions of diabetes mellitus in the rat. *Diabetes* 1978;27:738.

57. Hostetter TH, Troy JL, Brenner BM: Glomerular hemodynamics in experimental diabetes mellitus. *Kidney Int* 1981;19:410.

58. Rudberg S, Persson B, Dahlquist G: Increased glomerular filtration rate as a predictor of diabetic nephropathy—an 8-year prospective study. *Kidney Int* 1992;41:822.

59. Chiarelli F, Verrotti A, Morgese G: Glomerular hyperfiltration increases the risk of developing microalbuminuria in diabetic children. *Pediatr Nephrol* 1995;9:154.

60. Caramori ML, Gross JL, Pecis M, *et al*: Glomerular filtration rate, urinary albumin excretion rate, and blood pressure changes in normoalbuminuric normotensive type 1 diabetic patients: an 8-year follow-up study. *Diabetes Care* 1999;22:1512.

61. Yip JW, Jones SL, Wiseman MJ, *et al*: Glomerular hyperfiltration in the prediction of nephropathy in IDDM: a 10-year follow-up study. *Diabetes* 1996;45:1729.

62. Harvey JN, Jaffa AA, Margolius HS, *et al*: Renal kallikrein and hemodynamic abnormalities of diabetic kidney. *Diabetes* 1990;39:299.

63. Jaffa AA, Rust PF, Mayfield RK: Kinin, a mediator of diabetes-induced glomerular hyperfiltration. *Diabetes* 1995;44:156.

64. Harvey JN, Edmundson AW, Jaffa AA, *et al*: Renal excretion of kallikrein and eicosanoids in patients with type 1 (insulin-dependent) diabetes mellitus. Relationship to glomerular and tubular function. *Diabetologia* 1992;35:857.

65. Burns KD: Angiotensin II and its receptors in the diabetic kidney. *Am J Kidney Dis* 2000;36:449.

66. Correa-Rotter R, Hostetter TH, Rosenberg ME: Renin and angiotensinogen gene expression in experimental diabetes mellitus. *Kidney Int* 1992;41:796.

67. Seikaly MG, Arant BS, Seney FD: Endogenous angiotensin concentrations in specific intrarenal fluid compartments of the rat. *J Clin Invest* 1990;86:1352.

68. Anderson S, Jung FF, Ingelfinger JR: Renal renin-angiotensin system in diabetes: functional, immunohistochemical, and molecular biological correlations. *Am J Physiol* 1993;265:F477.

69. Mizuiri S, Yoshikawa H, Tanegashima M, *et al*: Renal ACE immunohistochemical localization in NIDDM patients with nephropathy. *Am J Kidney Dis* 1998;31:301.

70. Corbett JA, Tilton RG, Chang K, *et al*: Aminoguanidine, a novel inhibitor of nitric oxide formation, prevents diabetic vascular dysfunction. *Diabetes* 1992;41:552.

71. Graier WF, Wascher TC, Lackner L, *et al*: Exposure to elevated D-glucose concentrations modulates vascular endothelial cell vasodilatory response. *Diabetes* 1993;42:1497.

72. Bank N, Aynedjian HS: Role of EDRF (nitric oxide) in diabetic renal hyperfiltration. *Kidney Int* 1993;43:1306.

73. Sugimoto H, Shikata K, Matsuda M, *et al*: Increased expression of endothelial cell nitric oxide synthase (ecNOS) in afferent and glomerular endothelial cells is involved in glomerular hyperfiltration of diabetic nephropathy. *Diabetologia* 1998;41:1426.

74. Veelken R, Hilgers KF, Hartner A, *et al*: Nitric oxide synthase isoforms and glomerular hyperfiltration in early diabetic nephropathy. *J Am Soc Nephrol* 2000;11:71.

75. Chiarelli F, Cipollone F, Romano F, *et al*: Increased circulating nitric oxide in young patients with type 1 diabetes and persistent microalbuminuria: relation to glomerular hyperfiltration. *Diabetes* 2000;49:1258.

76. Thomson SC, Deng A, Bao D, *et al*: Ornithine decarboxylase, kidney size, and the tubular hypothesis of glomerular hyperfiltration in experimental diabetes. *J Clin Invest* 2001;107:217.

77. Rennke HG, Sandstrom D, Zatz R, *et al*: The role of dietary protein in the development of glomerular structural alterations in long term experimental diabetes mellitus [Abstract]. *Kidney Int* 1986;29:289.

78. Azar S, Johnson MA, Hertel B, *et al*: Single-nephron pressures, flows, and resistances in hypertensive kidneys with nephrosclerosis. *Kidney Int* 1977;12:28.

79. Steffes MW, Brown DM, Mauer SM: Diabetic glomerulopathy following unilateral nephrectomy in the rat. *Diabetes* 1978;27:35.

80. Rasch R: Prevention of diabetic glomerulopathy in streptozotocin diabetic rats by insulin treatment. The mesangial regions. *Diabetologia* 1979;17:243.

81. Rasch R: Prevention of diabetic glomerulopathy in streptozotocin diabetic rats by insulin treatment. *Diabetologia* 1979;16:319.

82. Hostetter TH, Olson JL, Rennke HG, *et al*: Hyperfiltration in remnant nephrons: a potentially adverse response to renal ablation. *Am J Physiol* 1981;241:F85.

83. Brenner BM, Chertow GM: Congenital oligonephropathy and the etiology of adult hypertension and progressive renal injury. *Am J Kidney Dis* 1994;23:171.

84. Nielsen FS, Gall MA, Parving HH: Acquired oligonephropathy and diabetic nephropathy. *Am J Kidney Dis* 1995;26:898.

85. Bendtsen TF, Nyengaard JR: The number of glomeruli in type 1 (insulin-dependent) and type 2 (non-insulin-dependent) diabetic patients. *Diabetologia* 1992;35:844.

86. Moriya T, Chow L, Moriya R, *et al*: Does glomerular number influence diabetic nephropathy risk in insulin-dependent diabetes mellitus (IDDM) patients? [Abstract]. *J Am Soc Nephrol* 1997;8:115A.

87. Chang SS, Caramori MLA, Moriya R, Mauer M: Reduced glomerular number as a risk factor for development of diabetic nephropathy in type 1 diabetic patients [Abstract]. *J Am Soc Nephrol* 2001;12:143A.

88. Zatz R, Dunn BR, Meyer TW, *et al*: Prevention of diabetic glomerulopathy by pharmacological amelioration of glomerular capillary hypertension. *J Clin Invest* 1986;77:1925.

89. O'Brien RC, Cooper ME, Jerums G, *et al*: The effects of perindopril and triple therapy in a normotensive model of diabetic nephropathy. *Diabetes* 1993;42:604.

90. Rudberg S, Osterby R, Bangstad HJ, *et al*: Effect of angiotensin converting enzyme inhibitor or beta blocker on glomerular structural changes in young microalbuminuric patients with Type I (insulin-dependent) diabetes mellitus. *Diabetologia* 1999;42:589.

91. Osterby R, Bangstad HJ, Rudberg S: Follow-up study of glomerular dimensions and cortical interstitium in microalbuminuric type 1 diabetic patients with or without antihypertensive treatment. *Nephrol Dial Transplant* 2000;15:1609.

92. Brenner BM: Hemodynamically mediated glomerular injury and the progressive nature of kidney disease. *Kidney Int* 1983;23:647.

93. Ray PE, Bruggeman LA, Horikoshi S, *et al*: Angiotensin II stimulates human fetal mesangial cell proliferation and fibronectin biosynthesis by binding to AT1 receptors. *Kidney Int* 1994;45:177.

94. Ihm CG, Park JK, Ahn JH, *et al*: Effect of angiotensin converting enzyme inhibitor on collagen production by cultured mesangial cells. *Korean J Intern Med* 1994;9:9.

95. Nakamura T, Takahashi T, Fukui M, *et al*: Enalapril attenuates increased gene expression of extracellular matrix components in diabetic rats. *J Am Soc Nephrol* 1995;5:1492.

96. Sorbi D, Fadly M, Hicks R, *et al*: Captopril inhibits the 72 kDa and 92 kDa matrix metalloproteinases. *Kidney Int* 1993;44:1266.

97. Horikoshi S, McCune BK, Ray PE, *et al*: Water deprivation stimulates transforming growth factor-beta 2 accumulation in the juxtaglomerular apparatus of mouse kidney. *J Clin Invest* 1991;88:2117.

98. Ray PE, McCune BK, Gomez RA, *et al*: Renal vascular induction of TGF-beta 2 and renin by potassium depletion. *Kidney Int* 1993;44:1006.

99. Yamamoto T, Nakamura T, Noble NA, *et al*: Expression of transforming growth factor beta is elevated in human and experimental diabetic nephropathy. *Proc Natl Acad Sci USA* 1993;90:1814.

100. Gruden G, Zonca S, Hayward A, *et al*: Mechanical stretch-induced fibronectin and transforming growth factor-beta1 production in human mesangial cells is p38 mitogen-activated protein kinase-dependent. *Diabetes* 2000;49:655.

101. Cowie CC, Port FK, Wolfe RA, *et al*: Disparities in incidence of diabetic end-stage renal disease according to race and type of diabetes. *N Engl J Med* 1989;321:1074.

102. Allawi J, Rao PV, Gilbert R, *et al*: Microalbuminuria in non-insulin-dependent diabetes: its prevalence in Indian compared with Europid patients. *Br Med J (Clin Res Ed)* 1988;296:462.

103. Krolewski M, Eggers PW, Warram JH: Magnitude of end-stage renal disease in IDDM: a 35 year follow-up study. *Kidney Int* 1996;50:2041.

104. Seaquist ER, Goetz FC, Rich S, *et al*: Familial clustering of diabetic kidney disease. Evidence for genetic susceptibility to diabetic nephropathy. *N Engl J Med* 1989;320:1161.

105. Borch-Johnsen K, Norgaard K, Hommel E, *et al*: Is diabetic nephropathy an inherited complication? *Kidney Int* 1992;41:719.

106. Quinn M, Angelico MC, Warram JH, *et al*: Familial factors determine the development of diabetic nephropathy in patients with IDDM. *Diabetologia* 1996;39:940.

107. Freedman BI, Tuttle AB, Spray BJ: Familial predisposition to nephropathy in African-Americans with non-insulin-dependent diabetes mellitus. *Am J Kidney Dis* 1995;25:710.

108. Faronato PP, Maioli M, Tonolo G, *et al*: Clustering of albumin excretion rate abnormalities in Caucasian patients with NIDDM. The Italian NIDDM Nephropathy Study Group. *Diabetologia* 1997;40:816.

109. Canani LH, Gerchman F, Gross JL: Familial clustering of diabetic nephropathy in Brazilian type 2 diabetic patients. *Diabetes* 1999;48:909.

110. Fava S, Azzopardi J, Hattersley AT, *et al*: Increased prevalence of proteinuria in diabetic sibs of proteinuric type 2 diabetic subjects. *Am J Kidney Dis* 2000;35:708.

111. Viberti GC, Keen H, Wiseman MJ: Raised arterial pressure in parents of proteinuric insulin dependent diabetics. *Br Med J (Clin Res Ed)* 1987;295:515.

112. Krolewski AS, Canessa M, Warram JH, *et al*: Predisposition to hypertension and susceptibility to renal disease in insulin-dependent diabetes mellitus. *N Engl J Med* 1988;318:140.

113. Barzilay J, Warram JH, Bak M, *et al*: Predisposition to hypertension: risk factor for nephropathy and hypertension in IDDM. *Kidney Int* 1992;41:723.

114. Nelson RG, Pettitt DJ, Baird HR, *et al*: Pre-diabetic blood pressure predicts urinary albumin excretion after the onset of type 2 (non-insulin-dependent) diabetes mellitus in Pima Indians. *Diabetologia* 1993;36:998.

115. Nelson RG, Pettitt DJ, de Courten MP, *et al*: Parental hypertension and proteinuria in Pima Indians with NIDDM. *Diabetologia* 1996;39:433.

116. Earle K, Walker J, Hill C, *et al*: Familial clustering of cardiovascular disease in patients with insulin-dependent diabetes and nephropathy. *N Engl J Med* 1992;326:673.

117. Jensen JS, Mathiesen ER, Norgaard K, *et al*: Increased blood pressure and erythrocyte sodium/lithium countertransport activity are not inherited in diabetic nephropathy. *Diabetologia* 1990;33:619.

118. Freire MB, Ferreira SR, Vivolo MA, *et al*: Familial hypertension and albuminuria in normotensive type I diabetic patients. *Hypertension* 1994;23:I256.

119. Fogarty DG, Rich SS, Hanna L, *et al*: Urinary albumin excretion in families with type 2 diabetes is heritable and genetically correlated to blood pressure. *Kidney Int* 2000;57:250.

120. Adragna NC, Canessa ML, Solomon H, *et al*: Red cell lithium-sodium countertransport and sodium-potassium cotransport in patients with essential hypertension. *Hypertension* 1982;4:795.

121. Mangili R, Bending JJ, Scott G, *et al*: Increased sodium-lithium countertransport activity in red cells of patients with insulin-dependent diabetes and nephropathy. *N Engl J Med* 1988;318:146.

122. Jones SL, Trevisan R, Tariq T, *et al*: Sodium-lithium countertransport in microalbuminuric insulin-dependent diabetic patients. *Hypertension* 1990;15:570.

123. Gall MA, Rossing P, Jensen JS, *et al*: Red cell Na$^+$/Li$^+$ countertransport in non-insulin-dependent diabetics with diabetic nephropathy. *Kidney Int* 1991;39:135.

124. Walker JD, Tariq T, Viberti G: Sodium-lithium countertransport activity in red cells of patients with insulin dependent diabetes and nephropathy and their parents. *Br Med J* 1990;301:635.

125. Hardman TC, Dubrey SW, Leslie DG, *et al*: Erythrocyte sodium-lithium countertransport and blood pressure in identical twin pairs discordant for insulin dependent diabetes. *Br Med J* 1992;305:215.

126. Monciotti CG, Semplicini A, Morocutti A, *et al*: Elevated sodium-lithium countertransport activity in erythrocytes is predictive of the development of microalbuminuria in IDDM. *Diabetologia* 1997;40:654.

127. Mahnensmith RL, Aronson PS: The plasma membrane sodium-hydrogen exchanger and its role in physiological and pathophysiological processes. *Circ Res* 1985;56:773.

128. Ng LL, Simmons D, Frighi V, *et al*: Leucocyte Na$^+$/H$^+$ antiport activity in type 1 (insulin-dependent) diabetic patients with nephropathy. *Diabetologia* 1990;33:371.

129. Trevisan R, Li LK, Messent J, *et al*: Na$^+$/H$^+$ antiport activity and cell growth in cultured skin fibroblasts of IDDM patients with nephropathy. *Diabetes* 1992;41:1239.

130. Lurbe A, Fioretto P, Mauer M, *et al*: Growth phenotype of cultured skin fibroblasts from IDDM patients with and without nephropathy and overactivity of the Na$^+$/H$^+$ antiporter. *Kidney Int* 1996;50:1684.

131. Trevisan R, Fioretto P, Barbosa J, *et al*: Insulin-dependent diabetic sibling pairs are concordant for sodium-hydrogen antiport activity. *Kidney Int* 1999;55:2383.

132. Adler SG, Pahl M, Seldin MF: Deciphering diabetic nephropathy: progress using genetic strategies. *Curr Opin Nephrol Hypertens* 2000;9:99.

133. Krolewski AS: Genetics of diabetic nephropathy: evidence for major and minor gene effects. *Kidney Int* 1999;55:1582.

134. Imperatore G, Knowler WC, Pettitt DJ, *et al*: Segregation analysis of diabetic nephropathy in Pima Indians. *Diabetes* 2000;49:1049.

135. Imperatore G, Hanson RL, Pettitt DJ, *et al*: Sib-pair linkage analysis for susceptibility genes for microvascular complications among Pima Indians with type 2 diabetes. Pima Diabetes Genes Group. *Diabetes* 1998;47:821.

136. Patel A, Hibberd ML, Millward BA, *et al*: Chromosome 7q35 and susceptibility to diabetic microvascular complications. *J Diabetes Complications* 1996;10:62.

137. Moczulski DK, Rogus JJ, Antonellis A, *et al*: Major susceptibility locus for nephropathy in type 1 diabetes on chromosome 3q: results of novel discordant sib-pair analysis. *Diabetes* 1998;47:1164.

138. Fogarty DG, Hanna LS, Wantman M, *et al*: Segregation analysis of urinary albumin excretion in families with type 2 diabetes. *Diabetes* 2000;49:1057.

139. Harden PN, Geddes C, Rowe PA, *et al*: Polymorphisms in angiotensin-converting-enzyme gene and progression of IgA nephropathy. *Lancet* 1995;345:1540.

140. Marre M, Jeunemaitre X, Gallois Y, *et al*: Contribution of genetic polymorphism in the renin-angiotensin system to the development of renal complications in insulin-dependent diabetes: Genetique de la Nephropathie Diabetique (GENEDIAB) study group. *J Clin Invest* 1997;99:1585.

141. Hsieh MC, Lin SR, Hsieh TJ, *et al*: Increased frequency of angiotensin-converting enzyme DD genotype in patients with type 2 diabetes in Taiwan. *Nephrol Dial Transplant* 2000;15:1008.

142. Doi Y, Yoshizumi H, Yoshinari M, *et al*: Association between a polymorphism in the angiotensin-converting enzyme gene and microvascular complications in Japanese patients with NIDDM. *Diabetologia* 1996;39:97.

143. Jeffers BW, Estacio RO, Raynolds MV, et al: Angiotensin-converting enzyme gene polymorphism in non-insulin dependent diabetes mellitus and its relationship with diabetic nephropathy. *Kidney Int* 1997;52:473.

144. Ohno T, Kawazu S, Tomono S: Association analyses of the polymorphisms of angiotensin-converting enzyme and angiotensinogen genes with diabetic nephropathy in Japanese non-insulin-dependent diabetics. *Metabolism* 1996;45:218.

145. Hadjadj S, Belloum R, Bouhanick B, et al: Prognostic value of angiotensin-I converting enzyme I/D polymorphism for nephropathy in type 1 diabetes mellitus: A prospective study. *J Am Soc Nephrol* 2001;12:541.

146. Oue T, Namba M, Nakajima H, et al: Risk factors for the progression of microalbuminuria in Japanese type 2 diabetic patients—a 10 year follow-up study. *Diabetes Res Clin Pract* 1999;46:47.

147. Parving HH, Jacobsen P, Tarnow L, et al: Effect of deletion polymorphism of angiotensin converting enzyme gene on progression of diabetic nephropathy during inhibition of angiotensin converting enzyme: observational follow up study. *Br Med J* 1996;313:591.

148. Penno G, Chaturvedi N, Talmud PJ, et al: Effect of angiotensin-converting enzyme (ACE) gene polymorphism on progression of renal disease and the influence of ACE inhibition in IDDM patients: findings from the EUCLID Randomized Controlled Trial. EURO-DIAB Controlled Trial of Lisinopril in IDDM. *Diabetes* 1998;47:1507.

149. Huang XH, Rantalaiho V, Wirta O, et al: Angiotensin-converting enzyme insertion/deletion polymorphism and diabetic albuminuria in patients with NIDDM followed up for 9 years. *Nephron* 1998;80:17.

150. Solini A, Vestra MD, Saller A, Nosadini R, Crepaldi G, Fioretto P: The angiotensin-converting enzyme DD genotype is associated with glomerulopathy lesions in type 2 diabetes. *Diabetes* 2002;51:251.

151. Ringel J, Beige J, Kunz R, et al: Genetic variants of the renin-angiotensin system, diabetic nephropathy and hypertension. *Diabetologia* 1997;40:193.

152. Schmidt S, Schone N, Ritz E: Association of ACE gene polymorphism and diabetic nephropathy? The Diabetic Nephropathy Study Group. *Kidney Int* 1995;47:1176.

153. Tarnow L, Cambien F, Rossing P, et al: Lack of relationship between an insertion/deletion polymorphism in the angiotensin I-converting enzyme gene and diabetic nephropathy and proliferative retinopathy in IDDM patients. *Diabetes* 1995;44:489.

154. De Cosmo S, Margaglione M, Tassi V, et al: ACE, PAI-1, decorin and Werner helicase genes are not associated with the development of renal disease in European patients with type 1 diabetes. *Diabetes Metab Res Rev* 1999;15:247.

155. Powrie JK, Watts GF, Ingham JN, et al: Role of glycaemic control in development of microalbuminuria in patients with insulin dependent diabetes. *Br Med J* 1994;309:1608.

156. Chowdhury TA, Dronsfield MJ, Kumar S, et al: Examination of two genetic polymorphisms within the renin-angiotensin system: no evidence for an association with nephropathy in IDDM. *Diabetologia* 1996;39:1108.

157. Dudley CR, Keavney B, Stratton IM, et al: U.K. Prospective Diabetes Study. XV: Relationship of renin-angiotensin system gene polymorphisms with microalbuminuria in NIDDM. *Kidney Int* 1995;48:1907.

158. Bjorck S, Blohme G, Sylven C, et al: Deletion insertion polymorphism of the angiotensin converting enzyme gene and progression of diabetic nephropathy. *Nephrol Dial Transplant* 1997;12:67.

159. Fujisawa T, Ikegami H, Kawaguchi Y, et al: Meta-analysis of association of insertion/deletion polymorphism of angiotensin I-converting enzyme gene with diabetic nephropathy and retinopathy. *Diabetologia* 1998;41:47.

160. Tarnow L, Gluud C, Parving HH: Diabetic nephropathy and the insertion/deletion polymorphism of the angiotensin-converting enzyme gene. *Nephrol Dial Transplant* 1998;13:1125.

161. Rogus JJ, Moczulski D, Freire MB, et al: Diabetic nephropathy is associated with AGT polymorphism T235: results of a family-based study. *Hypertension* 1998;31:627.

162. Freire MB, Ji L, Onuma T, et al: Gender-specific association of M235T polymorphism in angiotensinogen gene and diabetic nephropathy in NIDDM. *Hypertension* 1998;31:896.

163. Tarnow L, Cambien F, Rossing P, et al: Angiotensinogen gene polymorphisms in IDDM patients with diabetic nephropathy. *Diabetes* 1996;45:367.

164. Schmidt S, Giessel R, Bergis KH, et al: Angiotensinogen gene M235T polymorphism is not associated with diabetic nephropathy. The Diabetic Nephropathy Study Group. *Nephrol Dial Transplant* 1996;11:1755.

165. van Ittersum FJ, de Man AM, Thijssen S, et al: Genetic polymorphisms of the renin-angiotensin system and complications of insulin-dependent diabetes mellitus. *Nephrol Dial Transplant* 2000;15:1000.

166. Staessen JA, Kuznetsova T, Wang JG, et al: M235T angiotensinogen gene polymorphism and cardiovascular renal risk. *J Hypertens* 1999;17:9.

167. Tarnow L, Cambien F, Rossing P, et al: Angiotensin-II type 1 receptor gene polymorphism and diabetic microangiopathy. *Nephrol Dial Transplant* 1996;11:1019.

168. Chowdhury TA, Dyer PH, Kumar S, et al: Lack of association of angiotensin II type 1 receptor gene polymorphism with diabetic nephropathy in insulin-dependent diabetes mellitus. *Diabet Med* 1997;14:837.

169. Doria A, Onuma T, Warram JH, et al: Synergistic effect of angiotensin II type 1 receptor genotype and poor glycaemic control on risk of nephropathy in IDDM. *Diabetologia* 1997;40:1293.

170. Johannesen J, Tarnow L, Parving HH, et al: CCTTT-repeat polymorphism in the human NOS2-promoter confers low risk of diabetic nephropathy in type 1 diabetic patients. *Diabetes Care* 2000;23:560.

171. De Cosmo S, Argiolas A, Miscio G, et al: A PC-1 amino acid variant (K121Q) is associated with faster progression of renal disease in patients with type 1 diabetes and albuminuria. *Diabetes* 2000;49:521.

172. Hansen PM, Chowdhury T, Deckert T, et al: Genetic variation of the heparan sulfate proteoglycan gene (perlecan gene). Association with urinary albumin excretion in IDDM patients. *Diabetes* 1997;46:1658.

173. Pinizzotto M, Castillo E, Fiaux M, et al: Paraoxonase2 polymorphisms are associated with nephropathy in type 2 diabetes. *Diabetologia* 2001;44:104.

174. Maeda S, Haneda M, Hayashi K, et al: (A-C)n dinucleotide repeat polymorphism at 5' end of matrix metalloproteinase 9 (MMP9) gene is associated with nephropathy in Japanese subjects with type 2 diabetes [Abstract]. *J Am Soc Nephrol* 1998;118A.

175. Pociot F, Hansen PM, Karlsen AE, et al: TGF-beta1 gene mutations in insulin-dependent diabetes mellitus and diabetic nephropathy. *J Am Soc Nephrol* 1998;9:2302.

176. Araki S, Antonellis A, Canani L, et al: Polymorphism in protein kinase C β (PKCβ) gene and risk of diabetic nephropathy in type 1 diabetes [Abstract]. *Diabetes* 2000;49(Suppl 1):A152.

177. Levy AP, Roguin A, Hochberg I, et al: Haptoglobin phenotype and vascular complications in patients with diabetes. *N Engl J Med* 2000;343:969.

178. Zanchi A, Moczulski DK, Hanna LS, et al: Risk of advanced diabetic nephropathy in type 1 diabetes is associated with endothelial nitric oxide synthase gene polymorphism. *Kidney Int* 2000;57:405.

179. Neugebauer S, Baba T, Watanabe T: Association of the nitric oxide synthase gene polymorphism with an increased risk for progression to diabetic nephropathy in type 2 diabetes. *Diabetes* 2000;49:500.

180. Fujita H, Narita T, Meguro H, et al: Lack of association between an ecNOS gene polymorphism and diabetic nephropathy in type 2 diabetic patients with proliferative diabetic retinopathy. *Horm Metab Res* 2000;32:80.

181. Moczulski DK, Scott L, Antonellis A, et al: Aldose reductase gene polymorphisms and susceptibility to diabetic nephropathy in Type 1 diabetes mellitus. *Diabet Med* 2000;17:111.

182. Maeda S, Haneda M, Yasuda H, et al: Diabetic nephropathy is not associated with the dinucleotide repeat polymorphism upstream of the aldose reductase (ALR2) gene but with erythrocyte aldose reductase content in Japanese subjects with type 2 diabetes. *Diabetes* 1999;48:420.

183. Moczulski DK, Burak W, Doria A, et al: The role of aldose reductase gene in the susceptibility to diabetic nephropathy in Type II (non-insulin-dependent) diabetes mellitus. *Diabetologia* 1999;42:94.

184. Wong TY, Poon P, Szeto CC, et al: Association of plasminogen activator inhibitor-1 4G/4G genotype and type 2 diabetic nephropathy in Chinese patients. *Kidney Int* 2000;57:632.

185. Loughrey BV, Maxwell AP, Fogarty DG, et al: An interleukin 1B allele, which correlates with a high secretor phenotype, is associated with diabetic nephropathy. *Cytokine* 1998;10:984.

186. Tarnow L, Pociot F, Hansen PM, et al: Polymorphisms in the interleukin-1 gene cluster do not contribute to the genetic susceptibility of

diabetic nephropathy in Caucasian patients with IDDM. *Diabetes* 1997;46:1075.

187. Chowdhury TA, Dyer PH, Kumar S, *et al*: Association of apolipoprotein epsilon2 allele with diabetic nephropathy in Caucasian subjects with IDDM. *Diabetes* 1998;47:278.

188. Onuma T, Laffel LM, Angelico MC, *et al*: Apolipoprotein E genotypes and risk of diabetic nephropathy. *J Am Soc Nephrol* 1996; 7:1075.

189. Kimura H, Suzuki Y, Gejyo F, *et al*: Apolipoprotein E4 reduces risk of diabetic nephropathy in patients with NIDDM. *Am J Kidney Dis* 1998;31:666.

190. Araki S, Moczulski DK, Hanna L, *et al*: APOE polymorphisms and the development of diabetic nephropathy in type 1 diabetes: results of case-control and family-based studies. *Diabetes* 2000;49:2190.

191. Liu ZH, Guan TJ, Chen ZH, *et al*: Glucose transporter (GLUT1) allele (XbaI-) associated with nephropathy in non-insulin-dependent diabetes mellitus. *Kidney Int* 1999;55:1843.

192. Gutierrez C, Vendrell J, Pastor R, *et al*: GLUT1 gene polymorphism in non-insulin-dependent diabetes mellitus: genetic susceptibility relationship with cardiovascular risk factors and microangiopathic complications in a Mediterranean population. *Diabetes Res Clin Pract* 1998;41:113.

193. Odawara M, Yamashita K: A common mutation of the methylenetetrahydrofolate reductase gene as a risk factor for diabetic nephropathy. *Diabetologia* 1999;42:631.

194. Neugebauer S, Baba T, Watanabe T: Methylenetetrahydrofolate reductase gene polymorphism as a risk factor for diabetic nephropathy in NIDDM patients. *Lancet* 1998;352:454.

195. Nishigori H, Yamada S, Kohama T, *et al*: Frameshift mutation, A263fsinsGG, in the hepatocyte nuclear factor-1beta gene associated with diabetes and renal dysfunction. *Diabetes* 1998;47:1354.

196. Deinum J, Tarnow L, van Gool JM, *et al*: Plasma renin and prorenin and renin gene variation in patients with insulin-dependent diabetes mellitus and nephropathy. *Nephrol Dial Transplant* 1999;14:1904.

197. Schmidt S, Bluthner M, Giessel R, *et al*: A polymorphism in the gene for the atrial natriuretic peptide and diabetic nephropathy. Diabetic Nephropathy Study Group. *Nephrol Dial Transplant* 1998;13:1807.

198. Chen JW, Hansen PM, Tarnow L, *et al*: Genetic variation of a collagen IV alpha 1-chain gene polymorphism in Danish insulin-dependent diabetes mellitus (IDDM) patients: lack of association to nephropathy and proliferative retinopathy. *Diabet Med* 1997;14:143.

199. Freedman BI, Yu H, Spray BJ, *et al*: Genetic linkage analysis of growth factor loci and end-stage renal disease in African Americans. *Kidney Int* 1997;51:819.

200. Fogarty DG, Zychma MJ, Scott LJ, *et al*: The C825T polymorphism in the human G-protein beta3 subunit gene is not associated with diabetic nephropathy in Type I diabetes mellitus. *Diabetologia* 1998; 41:1304.

201. Tarnow L, Urhammer SA, Mottlau B, *et al*: The Trp64Arg amino acid polymorphism of the beta3-adrenergic receptor does not contribute to the genetic susceptibility of diabetic microvascular complications in Caucasian type 1 diabetic patients. *Nephrol Dial Transplant* 1999;14:895.

202. Yu H, Bowden DW, Spray BJ, *et al*: Identification of human plasma kallikrein gene polymorphisms and evaluation of their role in end-stage renal disease. *Hypertension* 1998;31:906.

203. Knigge H, Bluthner M, Bruntgens A, *et al*: G(-699)/C polymorphism in the bradykinin-1 receptor gene in patients with renal failure. *Nephrol Dial Transplant* 2000;15:586.

204. Schmidt S, Ritz E: Genetic determinants of diabetic renal disease and their impact on therapeutic interventions. *Kidney Int* 1997;63(Suppl): S27.

205. Araki S, Makita Y, Canani L, *et al*: Polymorphisms of human paraoxonase 1 gene (PON1) and susceptibility to diabetic nephropathy in type I diabetes mellitus. *Diabetologia* 2000;43:1540.

206. Ikeda Y, Suehiro T, Inoue M, *et al*: Serum paraoxonase activity and its relationship to diabetic complications in patients with non-insulin-dependent diabetes mellitus. *Metabolism* 1998;47:598.

207. Chowdhury TA, Dyer PH, Mijovic CH, *et al*: Human leucocyte antigen and insulin gene regions and nephropathy in type I diabetes. *Diabetologia* 1999;42:1017.

208. Kim Y, Kleppel MM, Butkowski R, *et al*: Differential expression of basement membrane collagen chains in diabetic nephropathy. *Am J Pathol* 1991;138:413.

209. Ayo SH, Radnik RA, Glass WFD, *et al*: Increased extracellular matrix synthesis and mRNA in mesangial cells grown in high-glucose medium. *Am J Physiol* 1991;260:F185.

210. Pugliese G, Pricci F, Pugliese F, *et al*: Mechanisms of glucose-enhanced extracellular matrix accumulation in rat glomerular mesangial cells. *Diabetes* 1994;43:478.

211. Davies M, Coles GA, Thomas GJ, *et al*: Proteinases and the glomerulus: their role in glomerular diseases. *Klin Wochenschr* 1990;68:1145.

212. Birkedal-Hansen H, Moore WG, Bodden MK, *et al*: Matrix metalloproteinases: a review. *Crit Rev Oral Biol Med* 1993;4:197.

213. Kahari VM, Saarialho-Kere U: Matrix metalloproteinases and their inhibitors in tumour growth and invasion. *Ann Med* 1999;31:34.

214. Matrisian LM: Metalloproteinases and their inhibitors in matrix remodeling. *Trends Genet* 1990;6:121.

215. Bruijn JA, Roos A, de Geus B, *et al*: Transforming growth factor-beta and the glomerular extracellular matrix in renal pathology. *J Lab Clin Med* 1994;123:34.

216. Nishikawa T, Edelstein D, Du XL, *et al*: Normalizing mitochondrial superoxide production blocks three pathways of hyperglycaemic damage. *Nature* 2000;404:787.

217. Du XL, Edelstein D, Rossetti L, *et al*: Hyperglycemia-induced mitochondrial superoxide overproduction activates the hexosamine pathway and induces plasminogen activator inhibitor-1 expression by increasing Sp1 glycosylation. *Proc Natl Acad Sci USA* 2000;97:12222.

218. Flyvbjerg A: Putative pathophysiological role of growth factors and cytokines in experimental diabetic kidney disease. *Diabetologia* 2000;43:1205.

219. Chiarelli F, Santilli F, Mohn A: Role of growth factors in the development of diabetic complications. *Horm Res* 2000;53:53.

220. Nakamura T, Fukui M, Ebihara I, *et al*: mRNA expression of growth factors in glomeruli from diabetic rats. *Diabetes* 1993;42:450.

221. Hill C, Flyvbjerg A, Gronbaek H, *et al*: The renal expression of transforming growth factor-beta isoforms and their receptors in acute and chronic experimental diabetes in rats. *Endocrinology* 2000;141: 1196.

222. Nakamura T, Miller D, Ruoslahti E, *et al*: Production of extracellular matrix by glomerular epithelial cells is regulated by transforming growth factor-beta 1. *Kidney Int* 1992;41:1213.

223. Roberts AB, McCune BK, Sporn MB: TGF-beta: regulation of extracellular matrix. *Kidney Int* 1992;41:557.

224. Marti HP, Lee L, Kashgarian M, *et al*: Transforming growth factor-beta 1 stimulates glomerular mesangial cell synthesis of the 72-kd type IV collagenase. *Am J Pathol* 1994;144:82.

225. Weigert C, Sauer U, Brodbeck K, *et al*: AP-1 proteins mediate hyperglycemia-induced activation of the human TGF-beta1 promoter in mesangial cells. *J Am Soc Nephrol* 2000;11:2007.

226. Montero A, Munger KA, Khan RZ, *et al*: F2-isoprostanes mediate high glucose-induced TGF-beta synthesis and glomerular proteinuria in experimental type I diabetes. *Kidney Int* 2000;58:1963.

227. Ziyadeh FN, Sharma K, Ericksen M, *et al*: Stimulation of collagen gene expression and protein synthesis in murine mesangial cells by high glucose is mediated by autocrine activation of transforming growth factor-beta. *J Clin Invest* 1994;93:536.

228. Inoki K, Haneda M, Ishida T, *et al*: Role of mitogen-activated protein kinases as downstream effectors of transforming growth factor-beta in mesangial cells. *Kidney Int* 2000;58(Suppl 77):S76.

229. Koya D, Haneda M, Nakagawa H, *et al*: Amelioration of accelerated diabetic mesangial expansion by treatment with a PKC beta inhibitor in diabetic db/db mice, a rodent model for type 2 diabetes. *FASEB J* 2000;14:439.

230. Shankland SJ, Scholey JW, Ly H, *et al*: Expression of transforming growth factor-beta 1 during diabetic renal hypertrophy. *Kidney Int* 1994;46:430.

231. Murphy M, Godson C, Cannon S, *et al*: Suppression subtractive hybridization identifies high glucose levels as a stimulus for expression of connective tissue growth factor and other genes in human mesangial cells. *J Biol Chem* 1999;274:5830.

232. Iwano M, Kubo A, Nishino T, *et al*: Quantification of glomerular TGF-beta 1 mRNA in patients with diabetes mellitus. *Kidney Int* 1996;49:1120.

233. Wogensen L, Nielsen CB, Hjorth P, *et al*: Under control of the Ren-1c promoter, locally produced transforming growth factor-beta1 induces accumulation of glomerular extracellular matrix in transgenic mice. *Diabetes* 1999;48:182.

234. Sharma K, Jin Y, Guo J, *et al*: Neutralization of TGF-beta by anti-TGF-beta antibody attenuates kidney hypertrophy and the enhanced extracellular matrix gene expression in STZ-induced diabetic mice. *Diabetes* 1996;45:522.

235. Ziyadeh FN, Hoffman BB, Han DC, *et al*: Long-term prevention of renal insufficiency, excess matrix gene expression, and glomerular mesangial matrix expansion by treatment with monoclonal antitransforming growth factor-beta antibody in db/db diabetic mice. *Proc Natl Acad Sci USA* 2000;97:8015.

236. Flyvbjerg A, Hill C, Grønbæk H, *et al*: Effect of ACE-inhibition on renal TGF-β type II receptor expression in experimental diabetes in rats [Abstract]. *J Am Soc Nephrol* 1999;10:679A.

237. Mogyorosi A, Kapoor A, Isono M, *et al*: Utility of serum and urinary transforming growth factor-beta levels as markers of diabetic nephropathy. *Nephron* 2000;86:234.

238. Janssen JA, Lamberts SW: Circulating IGF-I and its protective role in the pathogenesis of diabetic angiopathy. *Clin Endocrinol (Oxf)* 2000; 52:1.

239. Conti FG, Striker LJ, Lesniak MA, *et al*: Studies on binding and mitogenic effect of insulin and insulin-like growth factor I in glomerular mesangial cells. *Endocrinology* 1988;122:2788.

240. Elliot SJ, Striker LJ, Hattori M, *et al*: Mesangial cells from diabetic NOD mice constitutively secrete increased amounts of insulin-like growth factor-I. *Endocrinology* 1993;133:1783.

241. Lupia E, Elliot SJ, Lenz O, *et al*: IGF-1 decreases collagen degradation in diabetic NOD mesangial cells: implications for diabetic nephropathy. *Diabetes* 1999;48:1638.

242. Flyvbjerg A, Orskov H: Kidney tissue insulin-like growth factor I and initial renal growth in diabetic rats: relation to severity of diabetes. *Acta Endocrinol (Copenh)* 1990;122:374.

243. Flyvbjerg A, Frystyk J, Osterby R, *et al*: Kidney IGF-I and renal hypertrophy in GH-deficient diabetic dwarf rats. *Am J Physiol* 1992; 262:E956.

244. Landau D, Chin E, Bondy C, *et al*: Expression of insulin-like growth factor binding proteins in the rat kidney: effects of long-term diabetes. *Endocrinology* 1995;136:1835.

245. Flyvbjerg A, Kessler U, Kiess W: Increased kidney and liver insulin-like growth factor II/mannose-6-phosphate receptor concentration in experimental diabetes in rats. *Growth Regul* 1994;4:188.

246. Gronbaek H, Nielsen B, Frystyk J, *et al*: Effect of lanreotide on local kidney IGF-I and renal growth in experimental diabetes in the rat. *Exp Nephrol* 1996;4:295.

247. Flyvbjerg A, Bennett WF, Rasch R, *et al*: Inhibitory effect of a growth hormone receptor antagonist (G120K-PEG) on renal enlargement, glomerular hypertrophy, and urinary albumin excretion in experimental diabetes in mice. *Diabetes* 1999;48:377.

248. Segev Y, Landau D, Rasch R, *et al*: Growth hormone receptor antagonism prevents early renal changes in nonobese diabetic mice. *J Am Soc Nephrol* 1999;10:2374.

249. Smith LE, Shen W, Perruzzi C, *et al*: Regulation of vascular endothelial growth factor-dependent retinal neovascularization by insulin-like growth factor-1 receptor. *Nat Med* 1999;5:1390.

250. Ha H, Lee HB: Reactive oxygen species as glucose signaling molecules in mesangial cells cultured under high glucose. *Kidney Int* 2000; 58:19.

251. Connolly DT, Olander JV, Heuvelman D, *et al*: Human vascular permeability factor. Isolation from U937 cells. *J Biol Chem* 1989;264:20017.

252. Lip PL, Belgore F, Blann AD, *et al*: Plasma VEGF and soluble VEGF receptor FLT-1 in proliferative retinopathy: relationship to endothelial dysfunction and laser treatment. *Invest Ophthalmol Vis Sci* 2000; 41:2115.

253. Aiello LP, Avery RL, Arrigg PG, *et al*: Vascular endothelial growth factor in ocular fluid of patients with diabetic retinopathy and other retinal disorders. *N Engl J Med* 1994;331:1480.

254. Miller JW, Adamis AP, Aiello LP: Vascular endothelial growth factor in ocular neovascularization and proliferative diabetic retinopathy. *Diabetes Metab Rev* 1997;13:37.

255. Hovind P, Tarnow L, Oestergaard PB, *et al*: Elevated vascular endothelial growth factor in type 1 diabetic patients with diabetic nephropathy. *Kidney Int* 2000;57(Suppl 75):S56.

256. Shweiki D, Itin A, Soffer D, *et al*: Vascular endothelial growth factor induced by hypoxia may mediate hypoxia-initiated angiogenesis. *Nature* 1992;359:843.

257. Simon M, Rockl W, Hornig C, *et al*: Receptors of vascular endothelial growth factor/vascular permeability factor (VEGF/VPF) in fetal and adult human kidney: localization and [125I]VEGF binding sites. *J Am Soc Nephrol* 1998;9:1032.

258. Cooper ME, Vranes D, Youssef S, *et al*: Increased renal expression of vascular endothelial growth factor (VEGF) and its receptor VEGFR-2 in experimental diabetes. *Diabetes* 1999;48:2229.

259. Thomas S, Vanuystel J, Gruden G, *et al*: Vascular endothelial growth factor receptors in human mesangium *in vitro* and in glomerular disease. *J Am Soc Nephrol* 2000;11:1236.

260. Natarajan R, Bai W, Lanting L, *et al*: Effects of high glucose on vascular endothelial growth factor expression in vascular smooth muscle cells. *Am J Physiol* 1997;273:H2224.

261. Cha DR, Kim NH, Yoon JW, *et al*: Role of vascular endothelial growth factor in diabetic nephropathy. *Kidney Int* 2000;58(Suppl 77): S104.

262. Kim NH, Jung HH, Cha DR, *et al*: Expression of vascular endothelial growth factor in response to high glucose in rat mesangial cells. *J Endocrinol* 2000;165:617.

263. Williams B, Gallacher B, Patel H, *et al*: Glucose-induced protein kinase C activation regulates vascular permeability factor mRNA expression and peptide production by human vascular smooth muscle cells *in vitro*. *Diabetes* 1997;46:1497.

264. Frank S, Stallmeyer B, Kampfer H, *et al*: Differential regulation of vascular endothelial growth factor and its receptor fms-like-tyrosine kinase is mediated by nitric oxide in rat renal mesangial cells. *Biochem J* 1999;338:367.

265. Trachtman H, Futterweit S, Franki N, *et al*: Effect of vascular endothelial growth factor on nitric oxide production by cultured rat mesangial cells. *Biochem Biophys Res Commun* 1998;245:443.

266. Gruden G, Thomas S, Burt D, *et al*: Interaction of angiotensin II and mechanical stretch on vascular endothelial growth factor production by human mesangial cells. *J Am Soc Nephrol* 1999;10:730.

267. De Vriese A, Tilton R, Vanholder R, *et al*: Hyperfiltration and albuminuria in diabetes: Role of vascular endothelial growth factor [Abstract]. *J Am Soc Nephrol* 1999;10:677A.

268. Chiarelli F, Spagnoli A, Basciani F, *et al*: Vascular endothelial growth factor (VEGF) in children, adolescents and young adults with Type 1 diabetes mellitus: relation to glycaemic control and microvascular complications. *Diabet Med* 2000;17:650.

269. Bortoloso E, Del Prete D, Anglani F, *et al*: Vascular endothelial growth factor expression in microdissected glomeruli of type 2 diabetic patients. *Diabetologia* 1999;42(Suppl 1):A273.

270. Shulman K, Rosen S, Tognazzi K, *et al*: Expression of vascular permeability factor (VPF/VEGF) is altered in many glomerular diseases. *J Am Soc Nephrol* 1996;7:661.

271. Nyengaard JR, Rasch R: The impact of experimental diabetes mellitus in rats on glomerular capillary number and sizes. *Diabetologia* 1993; 36:189.

272. Osterby R, Asplund J, Bangstad HJ, *et al*: Neovascularization at the vascular pole region in diabetic glomerulopathy. *Nephrol Dial Transplant* 1999;14:348.

273. Sack E, Talor Z: High affinity binding sites for epidermal growth factor (EGF) in renal membranes. *Biochem Biophys Res Commun* 1988; 154:312.

274. Hamm LL, Hering-Smith KS, Vehaskari VM: Epidermal growth factor and the kidney. *Semin Nephrol* 1993;13:109.

275. Guh JY, Lai YH, Shin SJ, *et al*: Epidermal growth factor in renal hypertrophy in streptozotocin-diabetic rats. *Nephron* 1991;59:641.

276. Cybulsky AV, Bonventre JV, Quigg RJ, *et al*: Extracellular matrix regulates proliferation and phospholipid turnover in glomerular epithelial cells. *Am J Physiol* 1990;259:F326.

277. Jikihara H, Ikegami H, Sakata M, *et al*: Epidermal growth factor attenuates cell proliferation by down-regulating the transforming growth factor-beta receptor in the osteoblastic cell line MC3T3-E1. *Bone Miner* 1991;15:125.

278. Kizaka-Kondoh S, Akiyama N, Okayama H: Role of TGF-beta in EGF-induced transformation of NRK cells is sustaining high-level EGF-signaling. *FEBS Lett* 2000;466:160.

279. Brown AB, Carpenter G: Acute regulation of the epidermal growth factor receptor in response to nerve growth factor. *J Neurochem* 1991; 57:1740.

280. Hepler JR, Nakahata N, Lovenberg TW, *et al*: Epidermal growth factor stimulates the rapid accumulation of inositol (1,4,5)-trisphosphate

and a rise in cytosolic calcium mobilized from intracellular stores in A431 cells. *J Biol Chem* 1987;262:2951.

281. Xia P, Kramer RM, King GL: Identification of the mechanism for the inhibition of Na+,K(+)-adenosine triphosphatase by hyperglycemia involving activation of protein kinase C and cytosolic phospholipase A2. *J Clin Invest* 1995;96:733.

282. Lee TS, Saltsman KA, Ohashi H, *et al*: Activation of protein kinase C by elevation of glucose concentration: proposal for a mechanism in the development of diabetic vascular complications. *Proc Natl Acad Sci USA* 1989;86:5141.

283. Sharma K, Danoff TM, DePiero A, *et al*: Enhanced expression of inducible nitric oxide synthase in murine macrophages and glomerular mesangial cells by elevated glucose levels: possible mediation via protein kinase C. *Biochem Biophys Res Commun* 1995;207:80.

284. Studer RK, Craven PA, DeRubertis FR: Antioxidant inhibition of protein kinase C-signaled increases in transforming growth factor-beta in mesangial cells. *Metabolism* 1997;46:918.

285. Haneda M, Kikkawa R, Sugimoto T, *et al*: Abnormalities in protein kinase C and MAP kinase cascade in mesangial cells cultured under high glucose conditions. *J Diabetes Complications* 1995;9:246.

286. Ziyadeh FN, Fumo P, Rodenberger CH, *et al*: Role of protein kinase C and cyclic AMP/protein kinase A in high glucose-stimulated transcriptional activation of collagen alpha 1 (IV) in glomerular mesangial cells. *J Diabetes Complications* 1995;9:255.

287. Fumo P, Kuncio GS, Ziyadeh FN: PKC and high glucose stimulate collagen alpha 1 (IV) transcriptional activity in a reporter mesangial cell line. *Am J Physiol* 1994;267:F632.

288. Ishii H, Jirousek MR, Koya D, *et al*: Amelioration of vascular dysfunctions in diabetic rats by an oral PKC beta inhibitor. *Science* 1996; 272:728.

289. Flyvbjerg A, Hill C, Nielsen B, *et al*: Effect of protein kinase C β inhibition on renal morphology, urinary albumin excretion and renal transforming growth factor β in experimental diabetes in rats [Abstract]. *J Am Soc Nephrol* 1999;10:679A.

290. Derkx FH, Wenting GJ, Man in 't Veld AJ, *et al*: Control of enzymatically inactive renin in man under various pathological conditions: implications for the interpretation of renin measurements in peripheral and renal venous plasma. *Clin Sci Mol Med* 1978;54:529.

291. Deschepper CF, Mellon SH, Cumin F, *et al*: Analysis by immunocytochemistry and *in situ* hybridization of renin and its mRNA in kidney, testis, adrenal, and pituitary of the rat. *Proc Natl Acad Sci USA* 1986; 83:7552.

292. Luetscher JA, Kraemer FB, Wilson DM, *et al*: Increased plasma inactive renin in diabetes mellitus. A marker of microvascular complications. *N Engl J Med* 1985;312:1412.

293. Wilson DM, Luetscher JA: Plasma prorenin activity and complications in children with insulin-dependent diabetes mellitus. *N Engl J Med* 1990;323:1101.

294. Daneman D, Crompton CH, Balfe JW, *et al*: Plasma prorenin as an early marker of nephropathy in diabetic (IDDM) adolescents. *Kidney Int* 1994;46:1154.

295. Bryer-Ash M, Fraze EB, Luetscher JA: Plasma renin and prorenin (inactive renin) in diabetes mellitus: effects of intravenous furosemide. *J Clin Endocrinol Metab* 1988;66:454.

296. Allen TJ, Cooper ME, Gilbert RE, *et al*: Serum total renin is increased before microalbuminuria in diabetes. *Kidney Int* 1996;50:902.

297. Deinum J, Ronn B, Mathiesen E, *et al*: Increase in serum prorenin precedes onset of microalbuminuria in patients with insulin-dependent diabetes mellitus. *Diabetologia* 1999;42:1006.

298. Anderson PW, Zeidler A, Shaw S, *et al*: Plasma prorenin and diabetic nephropathy in NIDDM. *J Am Soc Nephrol* 1993;4:300.

299. Nielsen S, Schmitz A, Derkx FH, *et al*: Prorenin and renal function in NIDDM patients with normo- and microalbuminuria. *J Intern Med* 1995;238:499.

300. Zhang SL, Filep JG, Hohman TC, *et al*: Molecular mechanisms of glucose action on angiotensinogen gene expression in rat proximal tubular cells. *Kidney Int* 1999;55:454.

301. Tang SS, Diamant D, Rhoads DB, *et al*: Angiotensin II regulates glucose uptake in immortalized rat proximal tubular cells [Abstract]. *J Am Soc Nephrol* 1995;6:748.

302. Liu FY, Cogan MG: Role of protein kinase C in proximal bicarbonate absorption and angiotensin signaling. *Am J Physiol* 1990;258:F927.

303. Wolf G, Thaiss F, Schoeppe W, *et al*: Angiotensin II-induced proliferation of cultured murine mesangial cells: inhibitory role of atrial natriuretic peptide. *J Am Soc Nephrol* 1992;3:1270.

304. Wolf G, Mueller E, Stahl RA, *et al*: Angiotensin II-induced hypertrophy of cultured murine proximal tubular cells is mediated by endogenous transforming growth factor-beta. *J Clin Invest* 1993;92:1366.

305. Kanai H, Centrella M, Noble NA, *et al*: Angiotensin II upregulates the expression of TGF-β type I and type II receptors [Abstract]. *J Am Soc Nephrol* 1997;8:518A.

306. Kagami S, Border WA, Miller DE, *et al*: Angiotensin II stimulates extracellular matrix protein synthesis through induction of transforming growth factor-beta expression in rat glomerular mesangial cells. *J Clin Invest* 1994;93:2431.

307. Singh R, Alavi N, Singh AK, *et al*: Role of angiotensin II in glucose-induced inhibition of mesangial matrix degradation. *Diabetes* 1999; 48:2066.

308. Wolf G, Haberstroh U, Neilson EG: Angiotensin II stimulates the proliferation and biosynthesis of type I collagen in cultured murine mesangial cells. *Am J Pathol* 1992;140:95.

309. Jaimes EA, Galceran JM, Raij L: Angiotensin II induces superoxide anion production by mesangial cells. *Kidney Int* 1998;54:775.

310. Hutchison FN, Cui X, Paul RV, *et al*: Increase in renal transforming growth factor β (TGF-β) in diabetes is angiotensin II (AII) dependent [Abstract]. *J Am Soc Nephrol* 1996;7:1872.

311. Williams B: A potential role for angiotensin II-induced vascular endothelial growth factor expression in the pathogenesis of diabetic nephropathy? *Miner Electrolyte Metab* 1998;24:400.

312. Erdos EG: Conversion of angiotensin I to angiotensin II. *Am J Med* 1976;60:749.

313. Ignarro LJ, Buga GM, Chaudhuri G: EDRF generation and release from perfused bovine pulmonary artery and vein. *Eur J Pharmacol* 1988;149:79.

314. Mayfield RK, Margolius HS, Bailey GS, *et al*: Urinary and renal tissue kallikrein in the streptozocin-diabetic rat. *Diabetes* 1985;34:22.

315. Tschope C, Reinecke A, Seidl U, *et al*: Functional, biochemical, and molecular investigations of renal kallikrein-kinin system in diabetic rats. *Am J Physiol* 1999;277:H2333.

316. Baba T, Murabayashi S, Ishizaki T, *et al*: Renal kallikrein in diabetic patients with hypertension accompanied by nephropathy. *Diabetologia* 1986;29:162.

317. Allen TJ, Cao Z, Youssef S, *et al*: Role of angiotensin II and bradykinin in experimental diabetic nephropathy. Functional and structural studies. *Diabetes* 1997;46:1612.

318. Zuccollo A, Navarro M, Prendes GM, *et al*: Effects of HOE 140 on some renal functions in type I diabetic mice. *Arch Physiol Biochem* 1996;104:252.

319. Andersen S, Tarnow L, Rossing P, *et al*: Renoprotective effects of angiotensin II receptor blockade in type 1 diabetic patients with diabetic nephropathy. *Kidney Int* 2000;57:601.

320. Simonson MS, Dunn MJ: Endothelin peptides and the kidney. *Annu Rev Physiol* 1993;55:249.

321. Sokolovsky M: Endothelins and sarafotoxins: physiological regulation, receptor subtypes and transmembrane signaling. *Trends Biochem Sci* 1991;16:261.

322. Hargrove GM, Dufresne J, Whiteside C, *et al*: Diabetes mellitus increases endothelin-1 gene transcription in rat kidney. *Kidney Int* 2000; 58:1534.

323. Glogowski EA, Tsiani E, Zhou X, *et al*: High glucose alters the response of mesangial cell protein kinase C isoforms to endothelin-1. *Kidney Int* 1999;55:486.

324. Simonson MS, Herman WH: Protein kinase C and protein tyrosine kinase activity contribute to mitogenic signaling by endothelin-1. Cross-talk between G protein-coupled receptors and pp60c-src. *J Biol Chem* 1993;268:9347.

325. Chen HC, Guh JY, Shin SJ, *et al*: Reactive oxygen species enhances endothelin-1 production of diabetic rat glomeruli *in vitro* and *in vivo*. *J Lab Clin Med* 2000;135:309.

326. Simonson MS, Dunn MJ: Renal actions of endothelin peptides. *Curr Opin Nephrol Hypertens* 1993;2:51.

327. Hocher B, Lun A, Priem F, *et al*: Renal endothelin system in diabetes: comparison of angiotensin-converting enzyme inhibition and endothelin-A antagonism. *J Cardiovasc Pharmacol* 1998;31:S492.

328. Fukui M, Nakamura T, Ebihara I, *et al*: Gene expression for endothelins and their receptors in glomeruli of diabetic rats. *J Lab Clin Med* 1993;122:149.

329. Fukui M, Nakamura T, Ebihara I, *et al*: Effects of enalapril on endothelin-1 and growth factor gene expression in diabetic rat glomeruli. *J Lab Clin Med* 1994;123:763.

330. Benigni A, Colosio V, Brena C, *et al*: Unselective inhibition of endothelin receptors reduces renal dysfunction in experimental diabetes. *Diabetes* 1998;47:450.

331. Peppa-Patrikiou M, Dracopoulou M, Dacou-Voutetakis C: Urinary endothelin in adolescents and young adults with insulin-dependent diabetes mellitus: relation to urinary albumin, blood pressure, and other factors. *Metabolism* 1998;47:1408.

332. Shin SJ, Lee YJ, Tsai JH: The correlation of plasma and urine endothelin-1 with the severity of nephropathy in Chinese patients with type 2 diabetes. *Scand J Clin Lab Invest* 1996;56:571.

333. De Mattia G, Cassone-Faldetta M, Bellini C, *et al*: Role of plasma and urinary endothelin-1 in early diabetic and hypertensive nephropathy. *Am J Hypertens* 1998;11:983.

334. Lam HC, Lee JK, Chiang HT, *et al*: Does endothelin play a role in the pathogenesis of early diabetic nephropathy? *J Cardiovasc Pharmacol* 1995;26:S479.

335. Dunlop M: Aldose reductase and the role of the polyol pathway in diabetic nephropathy. *Kidney Int* 2000;58(Suppl 77):S3.

336. Yim HS, Kang SO, Hah YC, *et al*: Free radicals generated during the glycation reaction of amino acids by methylglyoxal. A model study of protein-cross-linked free radicals. *J Biol Chem* 1995;270:28228.

337. Douillet C, Tabib A, Bost M, *et al*: A selenium supplement associated or not with vitamin E delays early renal lesions in experimental diabetes in rats. *Proc Soc Exp Biol Med* 1996;211:323.

338. Lal MA, Korner A, Matsuo Y, *et al*: Combined antioxidant and COMT inhibitor treatment reverses renal abnormalities in diabetic rats. *Diabetes* 2000;49:1381.

339. Koya D, Lee IK, Ishii H, *et al*: Prevention of glomerular dysfunction in diabetic rats by treatment with d-alpha-tocopherol. *J Am Soc Nephrol* 1997;8:426.

340. Trachtman H, Futterweit S, Maesaka J, *et al*: Taurine ameliorates chronic streptozocin-induced diabetic nephropathy in rats. *Am J Physiol* 1995;269:F429.

341. Trachtman H, Futterweit S, Bienkowski RS: Taurine prevents glucose-induced lipid peroxidation and increased collagen production in cultured rat mesangial cells. *Biochem Biophys Res Commun* 1993; 191:759.

342. Trachtman H: Vitamin E prevents glucose-induced lipid peroxidation and increased collagen production in cultured rat mesangial cells. *Microvasc Res* 1994;47:232.

343. Hinokio Y, Suzuki S, Hirai M, *et al*: Oxidative DNA damage in diabetes mellitus: its association with diabetic complications. *Diabetologia* 1999;42:995.

344. Baynes JW, Thorpe SR: Role of oxidative stress in diabetic complications: a new perspective on an old paradigm. *Diabetes* 1999;48:1.

345. Ceriello A, Morocutti A, Mercuri F, *et al*: Defective intracellular antioxidant enzyme production in type 1 diabetic patients with nephropathy. *Diabetes* 2000;49:2170.

346. Matteucci E, Giampietro O: Oxidative stress in families of type 1 diabetic patients. *Diabetes Care* 2000;23:1182.

347. Matteucci E, Giampietro O: Oxidative stress in families of type 1 diabetic patients—Further evidence. *Diabetes Care* 2001;24:167.

348. Chan NN, Vallance P, Colhoun HM: Nitric oxide and vascular responses in Type I diabetes. *Diabetologia* 2000;43:137.

349. Craven PA, Studer RK, Felder J, *et al*: Nitric oxide inhibition of transforming growth factor-beta and collagen synthesis in mesangial cells. *Diabetes* 1997;46:671.

350. Moncada S, Palmer RM, Higgs EA: Nitric oxide: physiology, pathophysiology, and pharmacology. *Pharmacol Rev* 1991;43:109.

351. Lamontagne D, Pohl U, Busse R: Mechanical deformation of vessel wall and shear stress determine the basal release of endothelium-derived relaxing factor in the intact rabbit coronary vascular bed. *Circ Res* 1992;70:123.

352. Pohl U, Busse R: Hypoxia stimulates release of endothelium-derived relaxant factor. *Am J Physiol* 1989;256:H1595.

353. Newby AC, Henderson AH: Stimulus-secretion coupling in vascular endothelial cells. *Annu Rev Physiol* 1990;52:661.

354. Cosentino F, Hishikawa K, Katusic ZS, *et al*: High glucose increases nitric oxide synthase expression and superoxide anion generation in human aortic endothelial cells. *Circulation* 1997;96:25.

355. Tate RM, Morris HG, Schroeder WR, *et al*: Oxygen metabolites stimulate thromboxane production and vasoconstriction in isolated saline-perfused rabbit lungs. *J Clin Invest* 1984;74:608.

356. Tesfamariam B, Cohen RA: Free radicals mediate endothelial cell dysfunction caused by elevated glucose. *Am J Physiol* 1992;263:H321.

357. Trachtman H, Futterweit S, Singhal P: Nitric oxide modulates the synthesis of extracellular matrix proteins in cultured rat mesangial cells. *Biochem Biophys Res Commun* 1995;207:120.

358. Trachtman H, Futterweit S, Garg P, *et al*: Nitric oxide stimulates the activity of a 72-kDa neutral matrix metalloproteinase in cultured rat mesangial cells. *Biochem Biophys Res Commun* 1996;218:704.

359. Trachtman H, Koss I, Bogart M, *et al*: High glucose enhances growth factor-stimulated nitric oxide production by cultured rat mesangial cells. *Res Commun Mol Pathol Pharmacol* 1998;100:213.

360. Bucala R, Tracey KJ, Cerami A: Advanced glycosylation products quench nitric oxide and mediate defective endothelium-dependent vasodilatation in experimental diabetes. *J Clin Invest* 1991;87:432.

361. Hogan M, Cerami A, Bucala R: Advanced glycosylation endproducts block the antiproliferative effect of nitric oxide. Role in the vascular and renal complications of diabetes mellitus. *J Clin Invest* 1992; 90:1110.

362. Tesfamariam B, Brown ML, Cohen RA: Elevated glucose impairs endothelium-dependent relaxation by activating protein kinase C. *J Clin Invest* 1991;87:1643.

363. Chen S, Cohen MP, Ziyadeh FN: Amadori-glycated albumin in diabetic nephropathy: pathophysiologic connections. *Kidney Int* 2000; 58(Suppl 77):S40.

364. Day JF, Thorpe SR, Baynes JW: Nonenzymatically glycosylated albumin. *In vitro* preparation and isolation from normal human serum. *J Biol Chem* 1979;254:595.

365. Bunn HF, Shapiro R, McManus M, *et al*: Structural heterogeneity of human hemoglobin A due to nonenzymatic glycosylation. *J Biol Chem* 1979;254:3892.

366. Gonen B, Baenziger J, Schonfeld G, *et al*: Nonenzymatic glycosylation of low density lipoproteins *in vitro*. Effects on cell-interactive properties. *Diabetes* 1981;30:875.

367. Bailey AJ, Robins SP, Tanner MJ: Reducible components in the proteins of human erythrocyte membrane. *Biochim Biophys Acta* 1976; 434:51.

368. Monnier VM, Stevens VJ, Cerami A: Nonenzymatic glycosylation, sulfhydryl oxidation, and aggregation of lens proteins in experimental sugar cataracts. *J Exp Med* 1979;150:1098.

369. Wu VY, Cohen MP: Evidence for a ligand receptor system mediating the biologic effects of glycated albumin in glomerular mesangial cells. *Biochem Biophys Res Commun* 1995;207:521.

370. Hamada Y, Araki N, Koh N, *et al*: Rapid formation of advanced glycation end products by intermediate metabolites of glycolytic pathway and polyol pathway. *Biochem Biophys Res Commun* 1996;228:539.

371. Raj DS, Choudhury D, Welbourne TC, *et al*: Advanced glycation end products: a nephrologist's perspective. *Am J Kidney Dis* 2000;35:365.

372. Monnier VM, Vishwanath V, Frank KE, *et al*: Relation between complications of type I diabetes mellitus and collagen-linked fluorescence. *N Engl J Med* 1986;314:403.

373. Brownlee M, Cerami A, Vlassara H: Advanced glycosylation end products in tissue and the biochemical basis of diabetic complications. *N Engl J Med* 1988;318:1315.

374. Soulis-Liparota T, Cooper M, Papazoglou D, *et al*: Retardation by aminoguanidine of development of albuminuria, mesangial expansion, and tissue fluorescence in streptozocin-induced diabetic rat. *Diabetes* 1991;40:1328.

375. Yan SD, Schmidt AM, Anderson GM, *et al*: Enhanced cellular oxidant stress by the interaction of advanced glycation end products with their receptors/binding proteins. *J Biol Chem* 1994;269:9889.

376. McLennan SV, Fisher EJ, Yue DK, *et al*: High glucose concentration causes a decrease in mesangium degradation. A factor in the pathogenesis of diabetic nephropathy. *Diabetes* 1994;43:1041.

377. Anderson SS, Kim Y, Tsilibary EC: Effects of matrix glycation on mesangial cell adhesion, spreading and proliferation. *Kidney Int* 1994; 46:1359.

378. Pugliese G, Pricci F, Romeo G, *et al*: Upregulation of mesangial growth factor and extracellular matrix synthesis by advanced glycation end products via a receptor-mediated mechanism. *Diabetes* 1997; 46:1881.

379. Pugliese G, Pricci F, Leto G, *et al*: The diabetic milieu modulates the advanced glycation end product-receptor complex in the mesangium by inducing or upregulating galectin-3 expression. *Diabetes* 2000;49: 1249.

380. Yang CW, Vlassara H, Peten EP, *et al*: Advanced glycation end products up-regulate gene expression found in diabetic glomerular disease. *Proc Natl Acad Sci USA* 1994;91:9436.

381. Ellis EN, Good BH: Prevention of glomerular basement membrane thickening by aminoguanidine in experimental diabetes mellitus. *Metabolism* 1991;40:1016.

382. Bach LA, Dean R, Youssef S, *et al*: Aminoguanidine ameliorates changes in the IGF system in experimental diabetic nephropathy. *Nephrol Dial Transplant* 2000;15:347.

383. Forbes JM, Soulis T, Thallas V, *et al*: Renoprotective effects of a novel inhibitor of advanced glycation. *Diabetologia* 2001;44:108.

384. Degenhardt TP, Alderson NL, Thorpe SR, *et al*: Pyridorin, a post-Amadori inhibitor of advanced glycation reactions, preserves renal function in diabetic rats [Abstract]. *J Am Soc Nephrol* 1998;9:628A.

385. Nakamura S, Makita Z, Ishikawa S, *et al*: Progression of nephropathy in spontaneous diabetic rats is prevented by OPB-9195, a novel inhibitor of advanced glycation. *Diabetes* 1997;46:895.

386. Tsuchida K, Makita Z, Yamagishi S, *et al*: Suppression of transforming growth factor beta and vascular endothelial growth factor in diabetic nephropathy in rats by a novel advanced glycation end product inhibitor, OPB-9195. *Diabetologia* 1999;42:579.

387. Appel G, Bolton K, Freedman B, *et al*: Pimagedine lowers total urinary protein and slows progression of overt diabetic nephropathy in patients with type 1 diabetes mellitus [Abstract]. *J Am Soc Nephrol* 1999;10:A0786.

388. Berg TJ, Bangstad HJ, Torjesen PA, *et al*: Advanced glycation end products in serum predict changes in the kidney morphology of patients with insulin-dependent diabetes mellitus. *Metabolism* 1997; 46:661.

389. Rocco MV, Chen Y, Goldfarb S, *et al*: Elevated glucose stimulates TGF-beta gene expression and bioactivity in proximal tubule. *Kidney Int* 1992;41:107.

390. Han DC, Isono M, Hoffman BB, *et al*: High glucose stimulates proliferation and collagen type I synthesis in renal cortical fibroblasts: mediation by autocrine activation of TGF-beta. *J Am Soc Nephrol* 1999; 10:1891.

391. Ayo SH, Radnik R, Garoni JA, *et al*: High glucose increases diacylglycerol mass and activates protein kinase C in mesangial cell cultures. *Am J Physiol* 1991;261:F571.

392. Ziyadeh FN: The extracellular matrix in diabetic nephropathy. *Am J Kidney Dis* 1993;22:736.

393. Singh AK, Mo W, Dunea G, *et al*: Effect of glycated proteins on the matrix of glomerular epithelial cells. *J Am Soc Nephrol* 1998;9:802.

394. Ziyadeh FN, Han DC, Cohen JA, *et al*: Glycated albumin stimulates fibronectin gene expression in glomerular mesangial cells: involvement of the transforming growth factor-beta system. *Kidney Int* 1998; 53:631.

395. Cohen MP, Ziyadeh FN: Amadori glucose adducts modulate mesangial cell growth and collagen gene expression. *Kidney Int* 1994; 45:475.

396. Cohen MP, Wu VY, Cohen JA: Glycated albumin stimulates fibronectin and collagen IV production by glomerular endothelial cells under normoglycemic conditions. *Biochem Biophys Res Commun* 1997;239:91.

397. Cohen MP, Hud E, Wu VY: Amelioration of diabetic nephropathy by treatment with monoclonal antibodies against glycated albumin. *Kidney Int* 1994;45:1673.

398. Cohen MP, Sharma K, Jin Y, *et al*: Prevention of diabetic nephropathy in db/db mice with glycated albumin antagonists. A novel treatment strategy. *J Clin Invest* 1995;95:2338.

399. Cohen MP, Masson N, Hud E, *et al*: Inhibiting albumin glycation ameliorates diabetic nephropathy in the db/db mouse. *Exp Nephrol* 2000;8:135.

400. Schalkwijk CG, Ligtvoet N, Twaalfhoven H, *et al*: Amadori albumin in type 1 diabetic patients: correlation with markers of endothelial function, association with diabetic nephropathy, and localization in retinal capillaries. *Diabetes* 1999;48:2446.

401. Cavallo-Perin P, Chiambretti A, Calefato V, *et al*: Urinary excretion of glycated albumin in insulin-dependent diabetic patients with micro- and macroalbuminuria. *Clin Nephrol* 1992;38:9.

402. Gragnoli G, Signorini AM, Tanganelli I: Non-enzymatic glycosylation of urinary proteins in type 1 (insulin-dependent) diabetes: correlation with metabolic control and the degree of proteinuria. *Diabetologia* 1984;26:411.

403. Sakai H, Jinde K, Suzuki D, *et al*: Localization of glycated proteins in the glomeruli of patients with diabetic nephropathy. *Nephrol Dial Transplant* 1996;11:66.

404. Nadkarni V, Gabbay KH, Bohren KM, *et al*: Osmotic response element enhancer activity. Regulation through p38 kinase and mitogen-activated extracellular [AQ 2]signal-regulated kinase kinase. *J Biol Chem* 1999;274:20185.

405. Fazzio A, Spycher SE, Azzi A: Signal transduction in rat vascular smooth muscle cells: control of osmotically induced aldose reductase expression by cell kinases and phosphatases. *Biochem Biophys Res Commun* 1999;255:12.

406. Forster HG, ter Wee PM, Hohman TC, *et al*: Impairment of afferent arteriolar myogenic responsiveness in the galactose-fed rat is prevented by tolrestat. *Diabetologia* 1996;39:907.

407. Phillips AO, Steadman R, Morrisey K, *et al*: Exposure of human renal proximal tubular cells to glucose leads to accumulation of type IV collagen and fibronectin by decreased degradation. *Kidney Int* 1997; 52:973.

408. Faiman G, Ganguly P, Mehta A, *et al*: Effect of statil on kidney structure, function and polyol accumulation in diabetes mellitus. *Mol Cell Biochem* 1993;125:27.

409. Isogai S, Inokuchi T, Ohe K: Effect of an aldose reductase inhibitor on glomerular basement membrane anionic sites in streptozotocin-induced diabetic rats. *Diabetes Res Clin Pract* 1995;30:111.

410. Daniels BS, Hostetter TH: Aldose reductase inhibition and glomerular abnormalities in diabetic rats. *Diabetes* 1989;38:981.

411. Osterby R, Gundersen HJ: Glomerular basement membrane thickening in streptozotocin diabetic rats despite treatment with an aldose reductase inhibitor. *J Diabet Complications* 1989;3:149.

412. Itagaki I, Shimizu K, Kamanaka Y, *et al*: The effect of an aldose reductase inhibitor (Epalrestat) on diabetic nephropathy in rats. *Diabetes Res Clin Pract* 1994;25:147.

413. Donnelly SM, Zhou XP, Huang JT, *et al*: Prevention of early glomerulopathy with tolrestat in the streptozotocin-induced diabetic rat. *Biochem Cell Biol* 1996;74:355.

414. Shah VO, Dorin RI, Sun Y, *et al*: Aldose reductase gene expression is increased in diabetic nephropathy. *J Clin Endocrinol Metab* 1997; 82:2294.

415. Passariello N, Sepe J, Marrazzo G, *et al*: Effect of aldose reductase inhibitor (tolrestat) on urinary albumin excretion rate and glomerular filtration rate in IDDM subjects with nephropathy. *Diabetes Care* 1993;16:789.

416. Pedersen MM, Christiansen JS, Mogensen CE: Reduction of glomerular hyperfiltration in normoalbuminuric IDDM patients by 6 mo of aldose reductase inhibition. *Diabetes* 1991;40:527.

417. Ranganathan S, Krempf M, Feraille E, *et al*: Short term effect of an aldose reductase inhibitor on urinary albumin excretion rate (UAER) and glomerular filtration rate (GFR) in type 1 diabetic patients with incipient nephropathy. *Diabetes Metab* 1993;19:257.

418. McAuliffe AV, Brooks BA, Fisher EJ, *et al*: Administration of ascorbic acid and an aldose reductase inhibitor (tolrestat) in diabetes: effect on urinary albumin excretion. *Nephron* 1998;80:277.

419. Deckert T, Feldt-Rasmussen B, Borch-Johnsen K, *et al*: Albuminuria reflects widespread vascular damage. The Steno hypothesis. *Diabetologia* 1989;32:219.

420. Vernier RL, Steffes MW, Sisson-Ross S, *et al*: Heparan sulfate proteoglycan in the glomerular basement membrane in type 1 diabetes mellitus. *Kidney Int* 1992;41:1070.

421. Raats CJ, Van Den Born J, Berden JH: Glomerular heparan sulfate alterations: mechanisms and relevance for proteinuria. *Kidney Int* 2000;57:385.

422. Jensen T: Pathogenesis of diabetic vascular disease: evidence for the role of reduced heparan sulfate proteoglycan. *Diabetes* 1997; 46(Suppl 2):S98.

423. Cohen MP, Klepser H, Wu VY: Undersulfation of glomerular basement membrane heparan sulfate in experimental diabetes and lack of correction with aldose reductase inhibition. *Diabetes* 1988;37:1324.

424. Deckert T, Feldt-Rasmussen B, Djurup R, *et al*: Glomerular size and charge selectivity in insulin-dependent diabetes mellitus. *Kidney Int* 1988;33:100.

425. Yokoyama H, Hoyer PE, Hansen PM, *et al*: Immunohistochemical quantification of heparan sulfate proteoglycan and collagen IV in skeletal muscle capillary basement membranes of patients with diabetic nephropathy. *Diabetes* 1997;46:1875.

426. Jensen T: Albuminuria—a marker of renal and generalized vascular disease in insulin-dependent diabetes mellitus. *Dan Med Bull* 1991; 38:134.

427. Wasty F, Alavi MZ, Moore S: Distribution of glycosaminoglycans in the intima of human aortas: changes in atherosclerosis and diabetes mellitus. *Diabetologia* 1993;36:316.

428. Ceol M, Gambaro G, Sauer U, *et al*: Glycosaminoglycan therapy prevents TGF-ss1 overexpression and pathologic changes in renal tissue of long-term diabetic rats. *J Am Soc Nephrol* 2000;11:2324.

429. Caenazzo C, Garbisa S, Onisto M, *et al*: Effect of glucose and heparin on mesangial alpha 1(IV)COLL and MMP-/2TIMP-2 mRNA expression. *Nephrol Dial Transplant* 1997;12:443.

430. Gambaro G, Cavazzana AO, Luzi P, *et al*: Glycosaminoglycans prevent morphological renal alterations and albuminuria in diabetic rats. *Kidney Int* 1992;42:285.

431. Ceol M, Nerlich A, Baggio B, *et al*: Increased glomerular alpha 1 (IV) collagen expression and deposition in long-term diabetic rats is prevented by chronic glycosaminoglycan treatment. *Lab Invest* 1996; 74:484.

432. Oturai PS, Rasch R, Hasselager E, *et al*: Effects of heparin and aminoguanidine on glomerular basement membrane thickening in diabetic rats. *Apmis* 1996;104:259.

433. Myrup B, Hansen PM, Jensen T, *et al*: Effect of low-dose heparin on urinary albumin excretion in insulin-dependent diabetes mellitus. *Lancet* 1995;345:421.

434. Tamsma JT, van der Woude FJ, Lemkes HH: Effect of sulphated glycosaminoglycans on albuminuria in patients with overt diabetic (type 1) nephropathy. *Nephrol Dial Transplant* 1996;11:182.

435. van der Pijl JW, van der Woude FJ, Geelhoed-Duijvestijn PH, *et al*: Danaparoid sodium lowers proteinuria in diabetic nephropathy. *J Am Soc Nephrol* 1997;8:456.

436. Dedov I, Shestakova M, Vorontzov A, *et al*: A randomized, controlled study of sulodexide therapy for the treatment of diabetic nephropathy. *Nephrol Dial Transplant* 1997;12:2295.

437. Solini A, Vergnani L, Ricci F, *et al*: Glycosaminoglycans delay the progression of nephropathy in NIDDM. *Diabetes Care* 1997;20:819.

438. Myrup B, Jensen T, Gram J, *et al*: No effect of unfractioned or low molecular weight heparin treatment on markers of vascular wall and hemostatic function in incipient diabetic nephropathy. *Diabetes Care* 1997;20:1615.

439. van der Pijl JW, van der Woude FJ, Swart W, *et al*: Effect of danaparoid sodium on hard exudates in diabetic retinopathy. *Lancet* 1997; 350:1743.

440. Caramori ML, Mauer M: Diabetic nephropathy. In: Greenberg, *et al*, eds. *Primer on Kidney Diseases*, 3d ed. Academic Press:2001;212.

441. Ellis EN, Steffes MW, Goetz FC, *et al*: Glomerular filtration surface in type I diabetes mellitus. *Kidney Int* 1986;29:889.

C H A P T E R   4 3

Diabetic Nephropathy

Ralph A. DeFronzo

INTRODUCTION

Renal disease is an all too common occurrence in individuals with diabetes mellitus. Approximately 1 million people in the United States have type 1 (previously called insulin-dependent) diabetes mellitus (T1DM), and of these, 30–40% eventually develop end-stage renal failure.[1] Unfortunately, there is little evidence that the incidence of diabetic nephropathy in type 1 diabetics has changed within the last decade.[2] Type 2 (previously called non-insulin-dependent) diabetes mellitus (T2DM) affects about 16 million people in the United States, but the incidence of renal disease is lower, 5–10%[3–5] However, the incidence of nephropathy in patients with T2DM varies considerably among ethnic groups, being 3–4 times higher in blacks and Hispanics and 7 times higher in Native Americans compared to whites[6–8] (Fig. 43-1). Nevertheless, in absolute terms, more patients with type 2 than type 1 diabetes eventually progress to end-stage renal failure. The magnitude of the problem can be readily appreciated when it is realized that every third patient who is started on dialysis has diabetes mellitus[9] and that the Medicare payment for patients with diabetes is ~$51,000 per year per patient.[10]

DIABETIC NEPHROPATHY

Diabetic nephropathy was first described by Kimmelstiel and Wilson[11] in 1936. Since this original description, numerous studies have documented the renal histologic changes and the clinical course of renal dysfunction, which is characterized by hypertension, edema, severe albuminuria, and a progressive decline in glomerular filtration rate (GFR).[5] Three major histopathologic alterations have been described in the diabetic kidney: glomerulosclerosis, vascular involvement, and tubulointerstitial disease.[12–14]

Glomerulosclerosis

Involvement of the glomeruli is the most characteristic feature of diabetic nephropathy, and proteinuria and/or a reduction in GFR are the most common laboratory abnormalities that signify the presence of glomerular dysfunction. Three distinctive glomerular lesions have been described: diffuse intercapillary glomerulosclerosis, nodular glomerulosclerosis, and glomerular basement membrane (GBM) thickening (Fig. 43-2).

Diffuse and Nodular Lesions

The most common histologic abnormality, diffuse intercapillary glomerulosclerosis, is characterized by increased, periodic acid–Schiff (PAS)-positive, eosinophilic material within the mesangial region (see Fig. 43-2A). The increase in mesangial matrix material is diffuse, involving the entire glomerulus, and generalized, affecting all glomeruli throughout the kidney. With time, there is a progressive expansion of the mesangial material, which encroaches on adjacent capillary lumina. As this process progresses, entire glomeruli become hyalinized. There is no increase in mesangial cell number, but mesangial cell volume is increased.[15] In 40–50% of patients, the increase in mesangial matrix forms large acellular (Kimmelstiel-Wilson) nodules at the center of peripheral glomerular lobules (see Fig. 43-2B). This nodular lesion invariably is associated with the diffuse lesion and is pathognomonic of diabetes mellitus, although it correlates poorly with the severity of clinical renal disease. The best predictor of clinical renal disease is the diffuse increase in mesangial matrix material (see Chap. 42).[13,15]

Immunofluorescent staining of the glomerulus reveals diffuse linear deposition of immunoglobulin G (IgG) along the GBM. Although this linear pattern of immunoglobulin deposition is reminiscent of anti-GBM nephritis, eluted IgG has no affinity for the GBM and most likely represents nonspecific trapping of filtered proteins.

Basement Membrane Thickening

GBM thickening represents an early and characteristic abnormality in patients with diabetic glomerulosclerosis (see Fig. 43-2A). Basement membrane thickening is not limited to the glomerulus and can be observed in capillaries throughout the body, including muscle, skin, and retina.

The GBM is a collagen-like protein that is synthesized by the visceral epithelium of the glomerulus.[12] The integrity of the GBM is maintained by the continuous addition of new material from the epithelial aspect and by the simultaneous removal from the endothelial side by mesangial cells. The half-life of the GBM is about 100 days. Both increased epithelial synthesis and impaired removal by mesangial cells contribute to the basement membrane thickening.

There are significant differences in the collagen and protein content of the normal GBM compared with basement membranes from nonrenal tissues.[16] These differences in chemical composition account for the high glomerular filtration coefficient, which permits a water flux that is 50–100 times greater than in other capillaries, yet totally restricts the passage of serum proteins. The ability to restrict proteins selectively is also related to the strong negative charge provided by heparin sulfate and sialic acid residues within the GBM.

In patients with diabetic nephropathy, a number of biochemical alterations in the composition of the GBM have been described.[16,17]

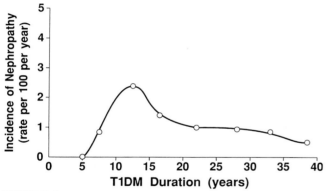

FIGURE 43-1. Incidence of nephropathy according to the duration of type 1 diabetes mellitus. *(Adapted from Krolewski et al.[1])*

In experimental models of diabetes, an increased activity of glucosyltransferase, the enzyme involved in the assembly of hydroxylysine-linked carbohydrate units, has been demonstrated, and restoration of normoglycemia with insulin normalized the activity of this enzyme. These results suggest that the accelerated synthesis of hydroxylysine-glucose-galactose subunits contributes to the GBM thickening. However, other investigators have reported GBM thickening without alteration in amino acid or glucosyl-galactose content in diabetic GBM. This polyantigenic expansion, involving all of the intrinsic components of the GBM and mesangium,[18] suggests an overall increase in the synthetic rate of normal basement membrane, a decrease in its rate of degradation, or some combination thereof. In diabetic patients with advanced nephropathy, the sialic acid and heparin sulfate proteoglycan content of the GBM is uniformly diminished, and this decrease in anionic charge may contribute to the increased clearance of negatively charged macromolecules, such as albumin.[19] *In vitro* studies employing isolated glomeruli have shown that glucose stimulates its own incorporation into capillary basement membrane in a dose-dependent fashion. Excessive glycosylation of the GBM may render collagen more resistant to degradation and contribute to the GBM thickening.

Vascular Involvement

The kidneys of patients with established diabetic nephropathy commonly manifest accelerated renal arteriosclerosis and arteriolosclerosis (see Fig. 43-2B). In the larger arteries, atheromatous changes often are advanced and may contribute to renal failure by causing ischemic parenchymal atrophy. In the smaller renal arterioles, hyaline thickening involves the afferent and efferent vessels, and is believed to play an important role in the development of hypertension. Although arteriosclerosis and arteriolosclerosis may be extensive, neither process correlates with the severity of glomerular change.

Tubulointerstitial Disease

Tubulointerstitial histologic changes (see Fig. 43-2C) are common in the diabetic kidney, and in advanced cases, there is marked tubular atrophy, thickening of the tubular basement membrane, and interstitial fibrosis.[14,20,21] Similar changes also may be observed

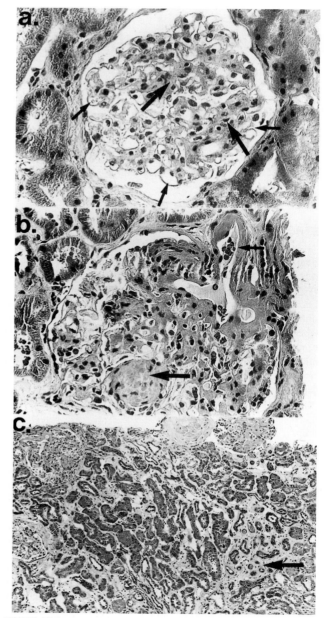

FIGURE 43-2. **a.** Diffuse diabetic glomerulosclerosis with marked mesangial matrix hyperplasia (**thick arrows**) and thickened glomerular basement membranes (**thin arrows**). No hypercellularity is evident. **b.** Nodules (**thick arrows**) usually are observed in the peripheral capillary loops and rarely are seen without the diffuse lesion. Note the prominent arteriolosclerosis in the efferent and afferent arterioles. **c.** Interstitial fibrosis, tubular atrophy (**thick arrows**), and thickening of the tubular basement membranes. *(Reproduced with permission from DeFronzo RA: Diabetes and the kidney: an update. In: Olefsky JM, Sherwin RS, eds. Diabetes Mellitus: Management and Complications. Churchill Livingstone:1985;161.)*

with renal ischemia, but in diabetes, the tubular changes correlate poorly with the degree of vascular involvement and frequently occur in their absence. Immunofluorescent studies have demonstrated deposition of IgG along the tubular basement membrane of the involved tubules. The interstitial area surrounding the tubules is fibrotic and may contain a cellular infiltrate of lymphocytes and plasma cells. These changes progress with increasing duration of the diabetes.[13,14]

Asymptomatic bacteriuria and pyelonephritis are twice as common in patients with diabetes, particularly women, than in patients without diabetes.[22] This increased incidence of urinary tract infection results from a variety of factors, including impaired renal blood flow, bladder dysfunction, interstitial scarring, impaired polymorphonuclear leukocyte function, defective leukocyte chemotaxis, and glucosuria, which enhance bacterial growth. Although patients with diabetes are more likely to develop urinary tract infections, a clear-cut relationship between the frequency or severity of interstitial changes and urinary tract infection has not been demonstrated, and patients whose bacteriuria was not eradicated fared no worse than those in whom the bacteriuria was cured.[23] The tubulointerstitial changes most likely represent a direct manifestation of the altered metabolic milieu that results from insulin lack and/or insulin resistance. The only tubular lesion that is characteristic of the diabetic state is the *Armanni-Ebstein lesion*, a vacuolization of the proximal tubular cells of the pars recta. These vacuoles contain glycogen and are most often observed in poorly controlled patients.

Diabetes mellitus accounts for over half of all reported cases of a special type of interstitial lesion, *papillary necrosis.*[24] Papillary necrosis results from ischemic damage to the inner medulla with eventual infarction and sloughing of part or all of the papilla. Patients with papillary necrosis may present either with an acute fulminant illness, with fever, shock, flank pain, gross hematuria, pyuria, oliguria, and renal failure, or with a more subacute form of the disease that is characterized by microscopic hematuria, pyuria, and indolent renal failure. Urinary tract obstruction and pyelonephritis cause renal papillary necrosis. Because phenacetin has been associated with papillary necrosis, chronic use of this analgesic should be avoided in the diabetic population.

PATHOGENESIS OF DIABETIC GLOMERULOSCLEROSIS

Both genetic and acquired (metabolic/hemodynamic) factors have been invoked to explain the development of diabetic renal disease (Table 43-1). The acquired theory postulates that the renal changes are caused by a combination of metabolic and hemodynamic changes that result from a lack of insulin. The second theory argues that genetic factors are primarily responsible for the alterations in renal structure and function. As discussed below, there is strong evidence to implicate both metabolic/hemodynamic alterations and genetic factors in the pathogenesis of diabetic nephropathy.

Acquired (Metabolic/Hemodynamic) Theory

Many *in vivo* and *in vitro* studies in both humans and animals indicate that diabetic nephropathy is an acquired disorder. First, renal involvement is absent in newly diagnosed diabetic patients (Fig. 43-3). Histologic abnormalities, including basement membrane thickening, expansion of the mesangium, and vascular changes, do not become evident until at least 2–3 years after the onset of diabetes.[12,13,25] Second, all of the characteristic histopathologic changes of diabetic nephropathy occur in patients with pancreatic diabetes (e.g., hemochromatosis, chronic pancreatitis, pancreatectomy),[26] conditions in which genetic factors are not thought to be involved. Third, diabetic nephropathy can be produced in various animal models, including the rat, mouse, dog, and monkey, regardless of the means of induction of diabetes, and treatment of the hyperglycemia with insulin completely reverses or prevents the diabetic renal disease.[27–31] Fourth, transplantation of pancreatic islets into insulinopenic diabetic rats prevents the development of renal lesions.[32,33] Fifth, when rat kidneys with established diabetic nephropathy are transplanted into nondiabetic rats, the renal

TABLE 43-1. Metabolic and Genetic Theories of Diabetic Nephropathy

Metabolic/Hemodynamic (Acquired) Theory	**Genetic Theory**
Renal involvement is absent when diabetes first is diagnosed. Basement membrane thickening and mesangial changes do not become manifest until 2–3 years later.	Marked variation in the incidence of nephropathy among non-insulin-dependent diabetes mellitus patients from different ethnic groups.
Typical changes of diabetic nephropathy have been observed in pancreatic diabetes (hemochromatosis, chronic pancreatitis, pancreatectomy, and cystic fibrosis).	Poor correlation exists between diabetic glomerulosclerosis and the degree of diabetic control as judged by blood glucose levels.
In the dog, monkey, rat, and mouse, lesions similar to those observed in human diabetic nephropathy have been documented after the induction of diabetes.	Excellent glucose control with the insulin pump (artificial pancreas) for 1–2 years has failed to reverse clinically overt proteinuria, and most diabetics have experienced progressive proteinuria and azotemia.
Tight regulation with insulin prevents the development of renal lesions in all diabetic animal models.	Only a minority of pancreatic diabetics develop glomerulosclerosis.
Transplantation of kidneys from diabetic into normal rats cures the renal disease.	Diabetic nephropathy has been reported early in the course of diabetes, in the prediabetic state, and occasionally in patients with normal glucose tolerance.
Tight glycemic control before or during the phase of microalbuminuria can prevent or halt the progression of microalbuminuria.	Diabetic nephropathy clusters within families in individuals with both type 1 and type 2 diabetes mellitus.
Normal human kidneys, transplanted into diabetic patients, develop changes of diabetic nephropathy within 2–5 years.	Sib-pair linkage studies have shown an association between diabetic nephropathy and specific chromosomal regions, although no specific genes have yet been identified.
Transplantation of diabetic kidneys into nondiabetic patients leads to a resolution of the diabetic renal lesion.	
Pancreatic transplantation reverses established lesions of diabetic nephropathy.	

Source: Adapted from DeFronzo RA: Diabetes and the Kidney: An update. In: Olefsky JM, Sherwin RS, eds. *Diabetes Mellitus: Management and Complications*. Churchill Livingstone:

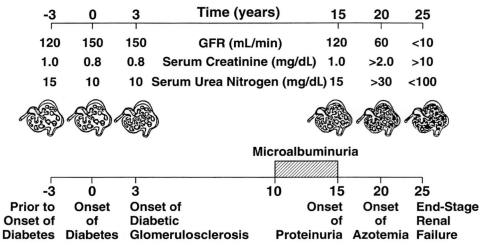

FIGURE 43-3. Natural course of diabetic nephropathy. At the initial diagnosis, renal function and glomerular histology are normal. Within 2–3 years, increased mesangial matrix and basement membrane thickening are observed. Renal function remains normal until 15 years, when proteinuria develops. This is an ominous sign and usually indicates advanced diabetic glomerulosclerosis. Within 5 years after the onset of proteinuria, elevation of the serum urea nitrogen and creatinine levels are observed, and within 3–5 years after the development of azotemia, half of the patients have advanced to end-stage renal insufficiency. **GFR,** glomerular filtration rate. *(Modified from DeFronzo RA: Diabetes and the kidney: an update. In: Olefsky JM, Sherwin RS, eds.* Diabetes Mellitus: Management and Complications. *Churchill Livingstone:1985;169.)*

lesions resolve.[34] Conversely, transplantation of normal kidneys into diabetic rats leads to the development of diabetic nephropathy. Sixth, when kidneys from healthy persons are transplanted into diabetics, all of the typical histologic changes of diabetic nephropathy develop within 2–5 years.[25] The Diabetes Control and Complications Trial (DCCT), in a study carried out in 1441 patients with T1DM, has conclusively demonstrated that intensive insulin therapy can reduce the development of nephropathy.[35] Tight glycemic control reduced the occurrence of microalbuminuria (40–300 mg/d) and of overt albuminuria (>300 mg/d) by 39% and 54%, respectively. Intensified insulin therapy was effective both in primary and secondary prevention of nephropathy (Fig. 43-4).[35]

The importance of the metabolic and hemodynamic environment is underscored by a case report in which kidneys were transplanted from a patient with T1DM with established proteinuria and biopsy-proven diabetic nephropathy into two patients without diabetes.[36] Seven months postrenal transplantation, renal function in both recipients was normal, proteinuria had disappeared, and renal biopsy showed resolution of the diffuse diabetic glomerulosclerosis. Similarly, others have demonstrated the regression of established diabetic nephropathy in patients after pancreatic transplantation. Lastly, pancreatic transplantation has been shown to reverse established lesions of diabetic nephropathy.[37]

Genetic Theory

Several lines of evidence support an important role for genetic predisposition in the development of diabetic nephropathy. Although the level of glycemic control, as documented by the HbA_{1c}, correlates well with the development of proteinuria and diminished GFR,[4,6,35] it is not uncommon to see patients whose glycemic control is quite poor, yet who do not develop diabetic nephropathy. This observation has been cited by proponents of the genetic theory as evidence for the role of genes in the development of diabetic nephropathy. Evidence can be mustered both to support and to refute the role of metabolic control in the pathogenesis of diabetic complications.

In short-term studies with a follow-up of 1–2 years, the achievement of good metabolic control has failed to reverse or ameliorate established nephropathy or to prevent the emergence of new cases of diabetic renal disease.[38–40] This information has been offered in favor of inheritance (genes) as the primary determinant of diabetic nephropathy. However, the follow-up period in these studies was short, less than 2 years, and insulin pump therapy was not initiated until after patients had had their diabetes for many years.[38–40] Major renal hemodynamic and structural changes occur within the initial 2–3 years after the diagnosis of diabetes and, if allowed to persist, may lead to fixed, irreversible alterations that may be responsible for the relentless progression to renal insufficiency.

FIGURE 43-4. Effect of intensive versus conventional glycemic control with insulin on the albumin excretion rate in T1DM patients. Tight glycemic control significantly reduced the risk of developing microalbuminuria (cross hatched area) and macroalbuminuria (stippled area) in normoalbuminuric patients. *(Reproduced with permission from DCCT Research Group.[35])*

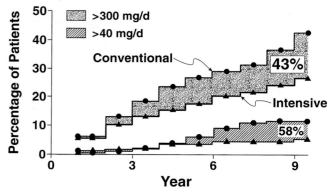

Consistent with this, the Epidemiology of Diabetes Interventions and Complications (EDIC) study (follow-up of the DCCT) failed to demonstrate any decrease in the rate of microvascular complications following 4 years of improved glycemic control in patients with T1DM who had been in poor glycemic control (HbA$_{1c}$ ~9.0%) over the preceding 10 years.[41] On the other hand, after 5–10 years of successful pancreatic transplantation, improvement in renal structure and function has been demonstrated.[37] These results suggest that it takes many years of improved glycemic control to reverse the changes of established diabetic nephropathy. Blood pressure is an important determinant of renal disease in patients with diabetes, and failure to meticulously control both systolic and diastolic hypertension has been shown to offset the benefit of improved glycemic control to slow the progression of established diabetic nephropathy.[42]

Although diabetic glomerulosclerosis has been shown to occur in patients with secondary causes of diabetes (i.e., hemochromatosis, cystic fibrosis, etc.), it occurs in only a minority of such individuals. Moreover, occasional cases of diabetic nephropathy have been shown to occur early in the course of diabetes or in the prediabetic state. Cases of typical diabetic glomerulosclerosis also have been documented in patients without glucose intolerance. Such evidence has been used to argue for a genetic etiology of renal disease in diabetic patients.[26,43] A genetic component to the GBM thickening also has been suggested by the finding of muscle capillary basement membrane thickening in adult T1DM patients at the time of diagnosis.[44] However, this later observations has been refuted by others.[45]

More direct evidence for a genetic etiology of diabetic nephropathy in patients with both type 1 and type 2 diabetes derives from the familial clustering of diabetic nephropathy (Fig. 43-5) and increased albumin excretion rates and hypertension in nondiabetic family members,[46-50] as well as from studies of glomerular structure in sibling pairs of patients with T1DM.[51] Sib-pair linkage analysis has demonstrated several chromosomal regions that are associated with diabetic nephropathy in Pima Indians,[52] who have the highest documented incidence of diabetic renal disease in the world. A number of candidate genes have been proposed and this topic is the subject of a recent review.[53]

In conclusion, it is likely that both metabolic and hemodynamic disturbances play an important role in the development of diabetic nephropathy. The best synthesis of the available data indicates that metabolic derangements operate on a genetic background, which predisposes the kidney to the development of diabetic glomerulosclerosis in patients with poor glycemic control. The marked difference in renal disease among different racial groups[6-8,54] also emphasizes the important role of genetic factors in the etiology of diabetic renal disease.

PATHOGENESIS OF DIABETIC NEPHROPATHY

Two major causative factors have been implicated in the development of diabetic nephropathy: metabolic and hemodynamic[55-60] (Fig. 43-6). In the absence of chronic hyperglycemia, renal disease does not occur and correction of hyperglycemia prevents the subsequent development of diabetic nephropathy.[35,61-67] Hyperglycemia has a direct toxic effect on renal cells and leads to the formation of advanced glycosylation end-products (AGEs), activation of protein kinase C (PKC), increased growth factors, and production of cytokines, which collectively cause an increase in extracellular matrix formation.[55] Of the cytokines, transforming growth factor-β$_1$ (TGF-β$_1$) has been the most extensively studied.[55,57,68,69] It is expressed in all glomerular cells and its production is markedly accelerated in both human and animal models of diabetic nephropathy in response to hyperglycemia, angiotensin II, and AGEs. This has led to the postulate that TGF-β$_1$ may represent a final common element in fibrotic diseases, including diabetic nephropathy. Vascular endothelial growth factor (VEGF) and epidermal growth factor (EGF) also have been implicated in experimental renal disease.[69] Hyperglycemia directly glycosylates proteins in the kidney, and in the presence of reduced GFR, AGEs in the circulation accumulate in the kidney where they are taken up by specific receptors, resulting in the release of growth factors and stimulation of collagen formation.[70,71] PKC, which is activated by hyperglycemia, increases endothelial cell permeability to albumin, stimulates matrix protein synthesis by mesangial cells, and increases the production of vasodilatory prostaglandins, which may contribute to early renal hyperperfusion and hyperfiltration.[55-57] Increased glucose flux through the aldose reductase pathway leads to the accumulation of a variety of polyols and intracellular depletion of myoinositol,

FIGURE 43-5. Prevalence of end-stage renal disease (**ESRD**) and albuminuria in siblings of type 1 diabetic individuals (probands) with and without diabetic nephropathy. (*Reproduced with permission from Seaquist et al.[46]*)

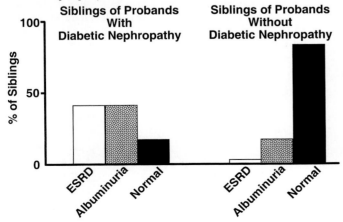

FIGURE 43-6. Pathogenic schema depicting the contribution of metabolic and hemodynamic factors to the development of diabetic nephropathy. **A-II**, angiotensin II; **PKC-βII**, protein kinase C; **VEGF**, vascular endothelial growth factor.

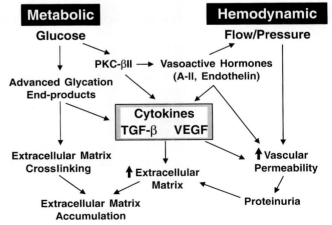

which can lead to the activation of PKC. In various animal models of diabetes, inhibition of the beta II isoform of protein kinase C (PKC-βII) prevents the development of hyperfiltration and albuminuria[72] and PKC inhibitors currently are undergoing clinical testing in humans.

Systemic and local renal hemodynamic factors also play an important role in the development of diabetic nephropathy.[55–57] The important contribution of systemic hypertension was discussed earlier. In diabetic animal models, there is a marked increase in single-nephron glomerular filtration rate, renal plasma flow, and intraglomerular pressure, and this constellation of renal hemodynamic changes is also observed in human diabetes. The increase in intraglomerular pressure results from enhanced sensitivity of the efferent arteriole to angiotensin II. In diabetic rats, these renal hemodynamics changes can be reversed by insulin therapy. Increased single-nephron renal plasma flow and glomerular transcapillary fluid pressure, whether due to non-diabetic renal disease or diabetes mellitus, if sustained over a prolonged period, cause cellular injury, proliferation of mesangial matrix material, and glomerulosclerosis (Fig. 43-6). The elevation in glomerular plasma flow and transcapillary hydraulic pressure leads to increased transcapillary albumin flux, which may further exacerbate the mesangial cell injury and cause the proliferation of mesangial matrix material. At the onset of nephropathy, albuminuria results from changes in either glomerular charge selectivity or altered tubular handling of filtered proteins.[73–75] With progressive renal injury, permselectivity changes in the glomerular barrier occur and further exacerbate the proteinuria.[76] Consistent with this pathogenesis, in diabetic animal models ACE inhibitors decrease intraglomerular pressure, lower GFR and renal plasma flow, reduce proteinuria, and prevent the histologic changes of diabetic nephropathy. Improved renal function also has been observed in both type 1 and type 2 patients who are treated with ACE inhibitors. It should be noted, however, that angiotensin II has a number of nonhemodynamic actions[77] which would be expected to exacerbate diabetic nephropathy. Angiotensin II is a potent growth factor that directly augments mesangial matrix proliferation, stimulates collagen and fibronectin synthesis, causes renal hypertrophy, enhances renal TGF-β expression, and potentiates the effect of a variety of growth factors on the kidney.[78,79] It is likely, therefore, that the renal protective effect of ACE inhibitors is multifactorial in origin.

A parallel view holds that the changes in intrarenal hemodynamics and renal hypertrophy are related to altered sodium transport in the proximal tubule and activation of the tubuloglomerular feedback reflex.[80] In diabetes the increased filtered load of glucose is reabsorbed in concert with sodium in the proximal tubule.[81] The reduction in delivery of salt to the distal tubule activates the tubuloglomerular feedback reflex, leading to vasodilation and increased GFR until distal salt delivery returns to its normal set point. The increased reabsorptive work of the proximal tubule leads to the generation of metabolic growth factors, which cause renal hypertrophy with further augmentation of renal plasma flow and GFR. Most recently, this hypothesis has been challenged by Thomson and associates,[82] who have provided evidence that the initial kidney growth that occurs in response to hyperglycemia is the primary pathogenic disturbance. The resultant renal hypertrophy causes increased proximal tubular reabsorption of sodium, which activates the tubuloglomerular feedback loop, leading to renal vasodilation and hyperfiltration. At present, it remains unresolved whether abnormalities in vascular control (renal vasodilation and early hyperfiltration) represent the primary disturbance and result secondarily in

renal hypertrophy via activation of the tubuloglomerular feedback loop, or whether the renal hypertrophy is primary and leads secondarily to stimulation of tubuloglomerular feedback and elevated renal plasma flow and GFR.[83]

In summary, hyperglycemia sets in motion a number of hemodynamic and metabolic abnormalities that eventuate in the typical histologic and clinical picture that is seen in patients with diabetic nephropathy.

CLINICAL COURSE

Epidemiologic studies have documented that less than half of all patients with T1DM who have had their disease for 20–30 years develop clinically significant renal disease (Fig. 43-7).[1,2,55,84] Unfortunately, at the time of diagnosis, there are no clinical or laboratory findings that predict which patients will progress to end-stage renal failure.[55,85] Although it is often stated that the incidence of glomerulosclerosis is higher in patients with T1DM (30–40%) than in patients with T2DM (5–10%), Pima Indians have the highest incidence of T2DM and diabetic nephropathy in the world.[86,87] Recent studies suggest that the incidence of renal disease may be more similar than previously appreciated in patients with type 1 and type 2 diabetes.[88,89] The dramatic rise in the incidence of renal disease in patients with T2DM may result from enhanced awareness and improved treatment of hypertension and dyslipidemia, which allows patients with T2DM to live longer, thereby exposing them to a greater burden of hyperglycemia.

Early Changes in Renal Function

Early in the course of diabetes (see Fig. 43-3) the GFR is characteristically increased and correlates with increased kidney weight and size, increased glomerular volume, and increased capillary luminal area per glomerulus.[55,86,90] During this same period, renal biopsy has demonstrated the presence of increased mesangial matrix and basement membrane thickening. Institution of intensive short-term (1–2 weeks) blood glucose control normalizes the GFR without any reduction in renal size,[91] suggesting that the augmented GFR is not causally related to the renal hypertrophy. However, within 6 weeks after the start of intensive insulin therapy, a

FIGURE 43-7. The Medicare incidence of end-stage renal failure in Native Americans, African-Americans, Asian-Americans, and white Americans as a function of age. *(Adapted from Teusch S, Newman J, Eggers P: The problem of renal failure in the United States: an overview. Am J Kidney Dis 1989;13:11.)*

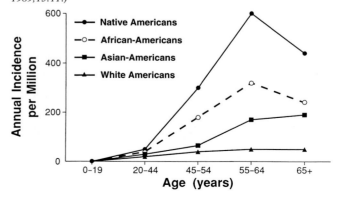

significant reduction in kidney size can be demonstrated in patients with T1DM.[92] Experimental diabetes in animals is also associated with an augmented GFR, which correlates with increased glomerular volume and glomerular capillary length and diameter. All of these changes are reversible with insulin treatment or islet cell transplantation.[29–34]

In early diabetes, no consistent change in renal plasma flow (RPF) has been observed. Although an increase in RPF has been reported by some investigators, most have found blood flow to the kidney to be normal. In all studies, the filtration fraction (GFR/RPF) was elevated.[55]

Late Changes in Renal Function

Patients who are destined to develop renal insufficiency follow a predictable clinical course[55,85,86] (see Fig. 43-3). After the onset of overt diabetes mellitus, there is a long (15–18 years) silent period, during which there is no laboratory evidence of renal dysfunction. However, if one were to perform a renal biopsy, a widespread increase in mesangial matrix material, capillary GBM thickening, interstitial fibrosis, and arteriolosclerosis would be evident. Patients with clinical nephropathy had slightly more mesangial matrix material and fewer open glomerular capillaries than patients with diabetes without clinical nephropathy (see Chap. 42). The increase in mesangial matrix is inversely correlated with the area of open capillary loops. These observations suggest that in the advanced stages of diabetic nephropathy, encroachment of capillary lumina by the expanding mesangial matrix material contributes to the decline in GFR. However, nonstructural factors also must play an important role in the decay of renal function, because the severity of diabetic glomerulosclerosis in patients without clinically evident renal disease can be as marked as in patients with advanced renal insufficiency.[93,94]

STAGING OF DIABETIC NEPHROPATHY

Microalbuminuria is the earliest clinically detectable stage of diabetic nephropathy,[95–97] and patients with microalbuminuria are sometimes said to have *incipient diabetic nephropathy* because of their increased risk of clinical nephropathy.[55,85,86,89] The albumin excretion rate in healthy people ranges from 2.5–25 mg/d, with a mean of approximately 10 mg/d[95] (Table 43-2). The Albustix™ reaction does not become positive until the albumin excretion rate exceeds 300 mg/d. Thus there is a wide subclinical range (30–300 mg/d) in which urinary albumin excretion is increased, but in the past could not be detected by routine laboratory methods. However, sensitive radioimmunoassay techniques have been developed to accurately measure albumin excretion at these lower rates.[98] Patients with an albumin excretion rate of 30–300 mg/d are defined

as having microalbuminuria (Table 43-2). T1DM patients with microalbuminuria have a 20-fold increased likelihood of developing clinical proteinuria (>300 mg/d of albumin) or a diminished GFR within a period of 10 years.[95–97] Patients with high-grade microalbuminuria (>100 mg/d) are at particularly high risk of developing renal impairment.[55,85,86] Microalbuminuria also precedes the development of diabetic nephropathy in patients with T2DM,[55,85,86,89,99–101] although it is not as strong a predictor as in patients with T1DM. Microalbuminuria is a very strong predictor of macrovascular complications (heart attacks, stroke) in all patients with diabetes (Fig. 43-8).[85,99,102–104] A recent review[105] of the relationship between microalbuminuria and the eventual development of clinical proteinuria and reduced GFR underscores the need for the development of other early predictors (i.e., newer imaging techniques, discovery of genes that predict increased risk of diabetic nephropathy, identification of substances in blood and/or urine that signal high-risk patients, measurements of tubular dysfunction, etc.) of diabetic nephropathy.

When interpreting the results of microalbumin excretion, it is important to exercise some clinical judgement. The upper limit of normal should not be considered as absolute, and common sense must be used in judging borderline cases. Many factors (e.g., exercise, high blood pressure, urinary tract infection, and very poor diabetic control) elevate the urinary albumin excretion rate. If such confounding factors are present, the finding of microalbuminuria does not necessarily imply incipient diabetic nephropathy. Although several authors have suggested that exercise-induced microalbuminuria is a harbinger of diabetic renal disease, there are few experimental data to support this claim. Another concern about the clinical interpretation of microalbuminuria centers on its development during the first 5 years in T1DM patients. In these patients, microalbuminuria is unlikely to have the same ominous prognostic significance as microalbuminuria that occurs 10–15 years after the onset of diabetes. This statement is not applicable to T2DM patients, who may have had their disease for many years before the diagnosis of diabetes was established. The interpretation of microalbuminuria in Caucasian type 2 diabetic patients is further complicated, since approximately 25% of such individuals have microalbuminuria, yet the incidence of renal disease in this popula-

FIGURE 43-8. Overall survival in 76 T2DM patients with varying degrees of microalbuminuria based upon the urinary albumin concentration. Patients with microalbuminuria in the moderate to high range (**two right bars**) demonstrated a markedly shortened survival compared to an age-matched control population. (*Reproduced with permission from Mogensen.[99]*)

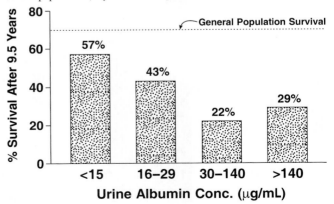

TABLE 43-2. Definition of Microalbuminuria

	Urinary AER (mg/24 h)	Urinary AER (μg/min)	Urine Albumin/Creatinine (mg/mg)
Normoalbuminuria*	<30	<20	<0.02
Microalbuminuria	30–300	20–200	0.02–0.20
Macroalbuminuria	>300	>200	>0.20

*The mean value for urinary albumin excretion rate (AER) in normal individuals is 10 ± 3 mg/d or 7 ± 2 μg/min.

tion is only 5–10%.[85,99–101,104] Therefore, although microalbuminuria is a risk factor for the development of renal disease in type 2 diabetics, it is not as strong a predictor as in type 1 diabetics. Thus, type 2 diabetic patients with microalbuminuria have a fivefold increased risk (as opposed to the 20-fold increase seen in T1DM) of developing proteinuria over a 10-year period. However, in certain ethnic populations with a high incidence of diabetic nephropathy and type 2 diabetes, including Native Americans, Mexican-Americans, and African-Americans, microalbuminuria is a very strong predictor of proteinuria and impaired renal function.[86,103,106]

From the more routine laboratory standpoint, the earliest detectable manifestation of diabetic glomerulosclerosis is Albustix-positive proteinuria (see Fig. 43-3), which begins about 15–18 years after the diagnosis of diabetes.[55,86,89,95–97,99,103] At this time, the GFR may still be normal or even elevated, but within a mean of 5 years after the onset of this level of proteinuria, the GFR begins to decline, and the serum urea nitrogen and creatinine concentrations increase. Within ~3–5 years after an elevation in serum creatinine concentration is documented, about half of the patients will have progressed to end-stage renal insufficiency. Severe proteinuria (>3 g/d) and the nephrotic syndrome are common, occurring in over half of all diabetic patients who progress to end-stage renal failure.

LABORATORY ABNORMALITIES

Proteinuria

The earliest laboratory manifestation of diabetic renal disease is proteinuria. When the urine albumin excretion exceeds 300 mg/d (corresponding to a urine protein excretion of 500 mg/d), the patient is said to have *overt diabetic nephropathy*. Using fractional dextran clearances and urinary albumin/IgG excretion, the increased transglomerular flux of proteins has been shown to result from an augmented transglomerular ultrafiltration pressure gradient and an alteration in the molecular charge of the glomerular barrier, which results from the loss of anionic charges (heparin sulfate and sialic acid residues) from the GBM.[56,57,100,103,107,108] Neither the number of pores in the GBM nor the pore size is altered in the course of diabetic nephropathy. At this stage, loss of barrier charge selectivity, without alteration of pore size diameter, appears to be the primary factor that allows the escape of albumin without change in the clearance of other macromolecules, and improved glycemic control with intensive insulin therapy decreases the albumin excre-

tion rate.[109] More recently, studies by Comper and coworkers[73,74] have demonstrated an important contributory role for impaired tubular handling of albumin in the development of microalbuminuria. With progressive proteinuria and the development of impaired renal function, glomerular charge- and size-selectivity is lost, there is an increase in pore size with the appearance of large-molecular-weight proteins in the urine, due to enhanced transglomerular passage of plasma proteins.

Glomerular Filtration Rate

Prior to the onset of microalbuminuria, the GFR is increased[55–57, 85,86,99–104,110,111] as the result of increased intraglomerular pressure and increased glomerular capillary surface area (Fig. 43-9).[55–57,85] The elevated GFR often persists even though marked renal histologic changes are present. Thus a decline in GFR from elevated to normal values in the absence of an improvement in metabolic control represents an ominous finding (Fig. 43-9). The most commonly used laboratory tests that provide an index of GFR are the serum creatinine and serum urea nitrogen (SUN) concentrations. However, both (especially the SUN) are influenced by prerenal (i.e., extracellular fluid volume depletion) and postrenal (i.e., urinary tract obstruction) factors. The serum creatinine concentration also is dependent on the muscle mass. Consequently, a decrease in muscle mass (as occurs with advancing age) can lead to a reduction in serum creatinine concentration and an underestimation of the severity of renal impairment. More importantly, the GFR may decline by 40–50% before either test increases into the abnormal range. Therefore, many nephrologists and diabetes specialists have advocated serial determinations of the creatinine clearance. In patients with renal failure of diverse etiologies, a plot of the reciprocal of the serum creatinine concentration as a function of time is linear and is useful in following the progression of renal disease. Pragmatically, the author advocates following the creatinine clearance in patients with diabetes with normal serum creatinine levels. Once the serum creatinine concentration becomes elevated, either the reciprocal of the serum creatinine or the creatinine clearance can be followed.

The glomerular filtration rate is determined by two factors: the net transmembrane ultrafiltration pressure and the glomerular ultrafiltration coefficient. The ultrafiltration pressure is governed by the balance of forces between the transmembrane hydraulic pressure, which increases GFR, and the intraglomerular oncotic pressure, which decreases GFR. In animals and man, experimental

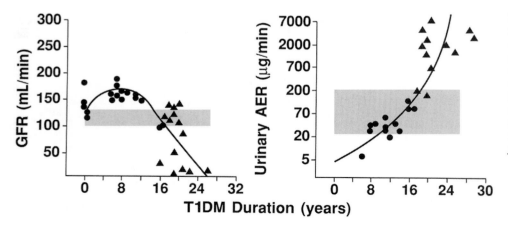

FIGURE 43-9. Natural history of glomerular filtration rate (**GFR**) and urinary albumin excretion rate (**AER**) in 20 type 1 diabetic patients who progressed to overt diabetic nephropathy over a period of 12 ± 3 years. GFR and AER are shown at the time of initial examination (**circles**) and after varying periods of follow-up (**triangles**). Shaded areas show the normal range. *(Reproduced with permission from Mogensen.[131])*

diabetes elevates the transmembrane ultrafiltration pressure.[56,100] Because the glomerular capillary oncotic pressure is normal or reduced in patients with diabetic nephropathy, this factor cannot explain the decrease in GFR. By exclusion, therefore, it has been concluded that the glomerular ultrafiltration coefficient must be reduced. The ultrafiltration coefficient is determined by the surface area available for filtration and the hydraulic permeability. Changes in the latter term have not been evaluated. Early in the course of T1DM, the total glomerular capillary surface area is increased and contributes to the glomerular hyperfiltration. However, in diabetic patients with clinically manifest renal disease, the mesangial matrix is greatly expanded, with obliteration of many capillary lumina.[5] Anatomically, this reduction in surface area for filtration plays a significant role in the decline in GFR in patients with advanced diabetic nephropathy.

Glucosuria

The maximum tubular reabsorptive capacity for glucose (Tm_G) varies inversely with the GFR in healthy individuals, and similar observations have been made in patients with new-onset T2DM.[112] However, in patients with long-term diabetes with reduced GFR and diabetic glomerulosclerosis, the Tm_G is raised. Moreover, even in patients with diabetes without renal disease, glucosuria correlates relatively poorly with the plasma glucose concentration.

Hyperkalemia

The maintenance of normal potassium homeostasis depends on both renal and extrarenal mechanisms (Fig. 43-10).[113] Many factors predispose the patient with diabetes to the development of hyperkalemia. Three hormones play a pivotal role in regulating the distribution of potassium between intracellular and extracellular compartments: insulin, epinephrine, and aldosterone. In patients with longstanding diabetes mellitus, all three of these hormones may be deficient. Therefore, it is not surprising that hyperkalemia

is a commonly encountered clinical problem in the diabetic population.[113] Moreover, in poorly controlled patients the elevated plasma glucose concentration increases tonicity, causing an osmotic shift of fluid and electrolytes, primarily potassium, out of cells. Metabolic acidemia, common in patients with diabetes, also predisposes to hyperkalemia. During the development of metabolic acidemia, about half of a hydrogen ion load is buffered within cells, and this occurs in exchange for potassium ions.[113]

Renal mechanisms also contribute to the development of hyperkalemia. When the GFR declines to less than 15–20 mL/min, the ability of the kidney to excrete potassium may become impaired.[113] Essentially, all of the filtered potassium is reabsorbed by the early- to mid-distal tubule, and the potassium that appears in the final urine represents potassium that is secreted by the late distal tubule and collecting duct. Many patients with diabetes demonstrate a marked interstitial nephritis with prominent tubular atrophy and tubular basement membrane thickening.[14,20,21] Because most urinary potassium is derived from distal and collecting tubular cell secretion, renal potassium excretion becomes impaired.

Hypoaldosteronism is common in patients with diabetes, particularly in those with evidence of impaired renal function (Fig. 43-10).[113,114] Since aldosterone is a key regulator of potassium secretion by the distal tubule and collecting duct, aldosterone deficiency results in impaired potassium excretion. Most patients with hypoaldosteronism are asymptomatic and are diagnosed on routine laboratory screening (by the presence of hyperkalemia) or during evaluation for some other, unassociated illness. The baseline plasma aldosterone concentration is low and fails to increase normally after stimulation with volume contraction. In most patients, the plasma renin level also is reduced and accounts for the hypoaldosteronism. However, in about 20% of patients with hypoaldosteronism, normal basal renin values have been reported.[113-115] Moreover, all patients with the syndrome of hyporeninemic hypoaldosteronism have clinically significant hyperkalemia, which is the most potent stimulus to aldosterone secretion. This suggests that, along with hyporeninemia, there may be a primary adrenal de-

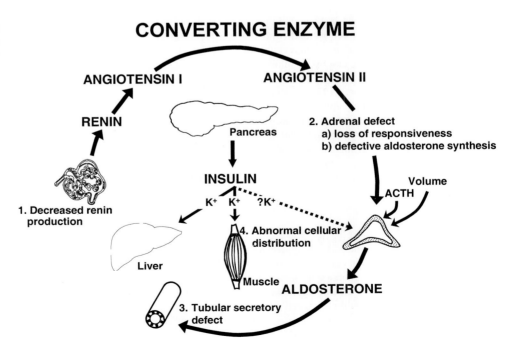

FIGURE 43-10. Hyperkalemia and the renin-angiotensin-aldosterone system. *(Reproduced with permission from DeFronzo et al.[113])*

fect in aldosterone secretion. This hypothesis is supported by the observation that the aldosterone response to angiotensin II and adrenocorticotropic hormone, agents that directly stimulate aldosterone secretion by the zona glomerulosa, is markedly impaired in persons with hypoaldosteronism.[113-115]

The pathogenic factors responsible for the impairment in renin and aldosterone secretion are unknown. Hyporeninemia could result from damage to the juxtaglomerulosal apparatus, impaired conversion of the biologically inactive renin precursor ("big renin") to renin, decreased circulating catecholamine levels or autonomic neuropathy, diminished circulating prostaglandin levels, or chronic extracellular fluid volume expansion secondary to hyperglycemia and sodium retention. However, none of these disturbances can satisfactorily account for the development of hyporeninemia in most diabetics. Impaired aldosterone secretion may be caused by intracellular potassium depletion within the zona glomerulosa of the adrenal gland secondary to insulin deficiency or insulin resistance.[113,114] Several enzymatic steps involved in aldosterone biosynthesis are known to be potassium-dependent.[113] Disruption of the normal tubuloglomerular feedback mechanisms also may lead to suppressed aldosterone secretion.[113] In diabetic patients with fasting plasma glucose levels in excess of 180 mg/dL, there is a large increase in the filtered load of glucose. The resultant osmotic diuresis impairs sodium and chloride reabsorption by all nephron segments, disrupting the normal tubuloglomerular feedback control mechanism and leading to suppression of renin, and secondarily, aldosterone secretion.

The complexity of the alterations in the renin-aldosterone axis in patients with diabetes is underscored by a report in which the aldosterone axis was characterized in 59 normokalemic patients with diabetes with normal GFR.[116] In half of the patients, both the renin and aldosterone responses were normal, 10% of the patients demonstrated diminished aldosterone secretion despite a normal renin response, 20% had impaired renin release with a normal aldosterone response, and 20% manifested impaired secretion of both renin and aldosterone. These results suggest the presence of multiple defects in the renin-aldosterone axis and a multifactorial origin of hyperkalemia.

A number of drugs have been shown to impair aldosterone secretion[113] and, if prescribed for patients with diabetes, require close monitoring of the plasma potassium concentration. Of these medications, the β-blockers and ACE inhibitors are the most widely known. The ACE inhibitors have been advocated for the treatment of diabetic nephropathy. These agents infrequently cause hyperkalemia, and this complication should be monitored closely at the start of therapy.[113] Another widely used class of drugs, the nonsteroidal antiinflammatory prostaglandin inhibitors, causes hyporeninemic hypoaldosteronism and hyperkalemia.[113] The diuretic agents (e.g., spironolactone, triamterene, and amiloride) block potassium secretion by the renal tubular cell[113] and also may result in hyperkalemia.

Metabolic Acidosis

Metabolic acidosis, both anion gap and hyperchloremic (nonanion gap), is commonly observed in patients with diabetes.[113,114,117] The anion gap is calculated by subtracting the concentrations of the major anions (chloride plus bicarbonate) from the major cation (sodium). The difference should not exceed 12 ± 2 mEq/L. If the value is greater than 14 mEq/L, an anion gap acidosis is present.

There are three possible causes of an *anion gap acidosis:* renal insufficiency, ketoacidosis, and lactic acidosis, and all three may occur in diabetic patients. Ketoacidosis and lactic acidosis are discussed in Chap. 34. In diabetic nephropathy, as in other causes of chronic renal disease, when the GFR declines to 20–25 mL/min, the ability of the kidney to excrete titratable acid becomes impaired, and the laboratory manifestation is an anion gap acidosis.

The causes of an anion gap acidosis are well known to the clinician. Less well recognized is the frequent occurrence of a *hyperchloremic* (or *nonanion gap*) *metabolic acidosis.* The syndrome of hypoaldosteronism is commonly observed in patients with diabetes, particularly those with renal impairment.[113–115] Over half of the reported cases of hyporeninemic hypoaldosteronism present with a hyperchloremic metabolic acidosis.[113–115] Aldosterone is an important regulator of ammonia production and hydrogen ion secretion by the distal nephron. Ammomium is an important urinary buffer that prevents the urine pH from dropping to very low levels, which would lead to an inhibition of hydrogen ion secretion by the renal tubule. Because of deficient ammomium secretion, the amount of urinary buffer—and therefore the total amount of hydrogen ion that can be secreted—is reduced in patients with diabetes with hypoaldosteronism. Because aldosterone does not affect urinary acidification, urine pH remains acidic (pH < 5.4). Some patients present with a hyperchloremic metabolic acidosis secondary to a primary renal tubular defect in hydrogen secretion. These individuals have a true distal renal tubular acidosis (i.e., an inability to acidify the urine [pH > 5.4] despite systemic acidemia). This defect may be related to the prominent interstitial nephritis, to the tubular basement membrane thickening, or to an intracellular abnormality in any of the steps involved in hydrogen ion secretion. Other patients with diabetes may present with a hyperchloremic metabolic acidosis due to widespread chronic interstitial nephritis and diffuse tubular injury, resulting in decreased ammonia production. The urine pH in these latter individuals is maximally acidic, indicating that the ability of the distal tubule and collecting duct to generate a steep pH gradient is intact. In these patients, the primary problem is impaired ammonia production, leading to a decrease in the total amount of hydrogen ion that can be excreted. In the absence of ammonia, which is one of the major urinary buffers, the urine pH is maximally acidic. Hyperkalemia may also cause a hyperchloremic metabolic acidosis by inhibiting ammonia synthesis by the renal tubular cell.

CLINICAL CORRELATIONS

Diabetic nephropathy is unusual in the absence of retinopathy, neuropathy, and hypertension. These associations were first popularized by Root and colleagues,[118] who referred to the triopathy of diabetes: nephropathy, retinopathy, and neuropathy. The occurrence of this triad was supported by other studies.[119] However, the validity of this association has also been challenged,[120] and more recent reviews[121–123] suggest a more variable association between the three microvascular complications. Patients with diabetes with nephropathy invariably have retinopathy and the diagnosis of diabetic nephropathy should not be made in the absence of some evidence of retinal involvement. This association has been referred to as the renal-retinal syndrome. However, less than half of the patients with diabetes with retinopathy have clinically evident renal disease. The association between diabetic neuropathy and retinopathy/nephropathy is even more variable, and is clouded by the fact that uremic neuropathy can occur in absence of diabetes.

Diabetic Retinopathy

Diabetic retinopathy (e.g., hemorrhages, exudates, proliferative retinopathy) invariably is present in patients with diabetes with end-stage renal failure who are admitted into dialysis or transplantation programs.[123,124] However, when overt diabetic nephropathy is first diagnosed (i.e., documentation of persistent proteinuria or elevation of the serum creatinine concentration), 30–40% of patients do not have evidence of diabetic retinopathy by routine ophthalmologic examination,[119,120,123,124] even though fluorescein angiography will demonstrate typical diabetic abnormalities in over 80–90% of patients. As the renal disease progresses, however, diabetic retinopathy appears to accelerate.[122–124] In one study, evidence of retinopathy was noted in only 61 of 150 patients when nephropathy was first diagnosed, but retinal involvement developed in another 42 during the follow-up period.[125] In patients placed on hemodialysis, a rapid progression of diabetic retinopathy often ensues. A dissociation between retinopathy and nephropathy is evident if one examines patients with established retinopathy. After 15–20 years, over 80% of patients have evidence of diabetic retinopathy, but as many as 30–50% have no laboratory evidence of renal disease.

Diabetic Neuropathy

The association between diabetic nephropathy and neuropathy is much less striking than that between diabetic nephropathy and retinopathy. In patients who have had diabetes for ≥20 years, only half exhibit clinical evidence of neuropathic involvement.[123,126–128] In patients with end-stage renal failure, the incidence of diabetic neuropathy varies from 50–90%, depending upon how carefully one looks or tests for evidence of diabetic neuropathic involvement. Peripheral neuropathy is more evident clinically than autonomic neuropathy, although in a recent study symptomatic diabetic gastroparesis was observed in ~50% of patients with diabetes treated with dialysis.[129] However, the specificity of these neuropathologic abnormalities, especially those relating to peripheral neuropathy, is questionable because dialysis and transplantation often lead to their reversal,[130] suggesting a uremic etiology. As with retinopathy, uremia appears to exacerbate the progression of diabetic neuropathy. When diabetic nephropathy is first diagnosed, less than half of patients have clinically evident diabetic neuropathy.

Hypertension

The incidence of hypertension, as well as the relationship between hypertension and renal disease, is very different in patients with T1DM and T2DM. In newly diagnosed type 2 patients, approximately 50–60% have hypertension, whereas less than 10% of type 1 patients present with hypertension at the time of initial diagnosis.[55,85,89,131–133] In both T1DM and T2DM patients, the incidence and severity of hypertension progress as the proteinuria becomes more severe. When end-stage renal failure ensues, 70–80% of patients with diabetes are hypertensive.[134] Patients with heavy proteinuria are particularly prone to develop hypertension. In most patients, the hypertension is volume-dependent and becomes easier to control after dialysis is started and dry weight is attained.[135,136]

Edema

The full-blown Kimmelstiel-Wilson syndrome includes edema, hypertension, proteinuria, and azotemia. In patients without renal disease or in those with mild-modest proteinuria (<0.5–1 g/d) and a normal GFR, edema is uncommon. However, when the urinary albumin excretion exceeds 1–2 g/d, and especially when the GFR begins to decline, the incidence of edema increases precipitously. This is caused by decreased oncotic pressure secondary to hypoalbuminemia, sodium retention secondary to renal disease, and altered vascular permeability. When end-stage renal failure ensues, over 50–75% of patients have some evidence of edema.[125,137]

TREATMENT OF DIABETIC NEPHROPATHY

The treatment of patients with *established* diabetic nephropathy is aimed at slowing the progressive decline in GFR. Once overt albuminuria (>300–500 mg/d) is present and the serum creatinine concentration begins to increase, the progression to end-stage renal disease is difficult to halt (Table 43-3). If end-stage renal failure ensues, two options are available: dialysis or transplantation.

Hypertension

Hypertension, even in its mildest form, is associated with decreased survival in patients without diabetes,[138] and this effect is magnified in patients with diabetes (see Chap. 48).[139] Hypertension is the single most important factor that accelerates the progression of diabetic renal disease, and treatment of the hypertension, regardless of the agent employed, markedly slows the progression of renal insufficiency in patients with established renal disease.[55,134,139–141]

Over 25 years ago, it was demonstrated that antihypertensive therapy reduced albuminuria and slowed the rate of decline in GFR in patients with T1DM with established nephropathy.[142] This initial observation has been confirmed by multiple investigators (Fig. 43-11).[55,57,85,134,140,141,143–145] Elevated blood pressure interacts synergistically with poor glycemic control, hypercholesterolemia, and microalbuminuria to accelerate the decline in glomerular filtration rate (Fig. 43-12).[141] In a long-term, randomized, double-blind, prospective study of 409 type 1 diabetic patients with established nephropathy,[146] it was demonstrated that antihypertensive therapy with captopril decreased the doubling time of serum creatinine by 48% and reduced by 50% the combined end points of death, dialysis, and renal transplantation (Table 43-4).

Simple clinical observations have demonstrated the importance of hemodynamic factors in the development of diabetic nephropathy. In type 1 patients with renal artery stenosis, extensive diabetic glomerulosclerosis occurs in the kidney with the patent renal artery, but the kidney with the stenotic renal artery displays only mild diabetic changes.[147] Similar observations have been reported in diabetic rats with Goldblatt kidney hypertension. Conversely, in diabetic rats, dogs, and humans with a single kidney, there is a marked acceleration of diabetic nephropathy, even though systemic hypertension does not develop.[148] This experimental model emphasizes the role of intrarenal hemodynamic factors in the initiation and progression of diabetic glomerulopathy.[55,56] In both T1DM and T2DM patients, genetic factors also have been shown to play an important role in the development of hypertension.[149,150] Hypertension and microalbuminuria also occur as part

TABLE 43-3. Treatment of Diabetic Nephropathy

1. **Hypertension**—the single most important factor shown to accelerate the progression of renal failure.
   a. Angiotensin converting enzyme (ACE) inhibitors, angiotensin receptor blockers, and calcium channel blockers are efficacious and relatively free of side effects. Hyperkalemia and decreased glomerular filtration rate (GFR) may occur with ACE inhibitors.
   b. Because of the development of dyslipidemia and insulin resistance, diuretics should not be considered as first-line agents unless used in very low doses; they are, however, indicated in hypertensive patients with evidence of excessive sodium retention, i.e., edema.
   c. Attempt to avoid propranolol and other β-adrenergic blockers (hyperkalemia, hypoglycemia, hyperglycemia).
2. **Urinary tract infection**—increased incidence, frequent cultures.
3. **Neurogenic bladder**—parasymphatetic/adrenergic drugs, voiding maneuvers.
4. **Intravenous pyelography**—increased incidence of acute renal failure, particularly if heavy proteinuria and renal impairment are present.
5. **Blood glucose control**
   a. Tight blood glucose control, if instituted before or during the phase of microalbuminuria, prevents the development of overt proteinuria and progressive renal failure.
   b. There is little evidence that tight metabolic control prevents or ameliorates the progression of established renal disease (albumin excretion rate >200–300 mg/d or elevated serum creatinine).
   c. Uremia is associated with insulin resistance and increased insulin requirements.
   d. With advanced uremia (GFR <15–20 mL/min), decreased insulin requirements may be observed because kidney removal of secreted insulin is impaired and hepatic degradation of insulin is inhibited.
   e. After the institution of dialysis, the situation is complex. Insulin sensitivity improves (hypoglycemia), but the degradation of insulin is enhanced (hyperglycemia); however, most insulin-treated diabetics who are started on dialysis experience an increase in their daily insulin requirement.
6. **Dialysis**
   a. One in every three patients beginning dialysis in the United States has diabetes.
   b. Diabetic patients do significantly worse on dialysis than do nondiabetic persons.
   c. The increased mortality in diabetic patients treated with dialysis is largely due to cardiovascular deaths resulting from myocardial infarction and stroke. Other complications include peripheral vascular disease, infections, psychiatric problems, and progressive retinopathy and neuropathy.
   d. Diabetic patients treated with peritoneal dialysis appear to do as well as those treated with hemodialysis.
7. **Transplantation**
   a. If a well-matched, living, related donor can be found, renal transplantation is the preferable mode of therapy in most people with diabetes.
   b. Survival statistics with kidneys transplanted from a haplotype-identical relative or unrelated donor are similar to those obtained with hemodialysis.
8. **Protein restriction**
   a. There are good data in animals that show that a low-protein diet slows the progression of diabetic renal disease.
   b. In small uncontrolled studies in humans, a low-protein diet has been shown to slow the progression of established diabetic renal disease.
   c. In a large, well-controlled, prospective study, a low-protein diet did not alter the rate of decline in GFR. In this study, the majority of patients were on an antihypertensive agent (ACE inhibitor or calcium channel blocker). It is likely that a low-protein diet has no added beneficial effect beyond that afforded by the ACE inhibitor or a calcium channel blocker.

Source: Modified from DeFronzo RA: Diabetes and the kidney. In: Olefsky JM, Shewin RS, eds. *Diabetes Mellitus: Management and Complications.* Churchill Livingstone: 1985;189.

of the insulin resistance syndrome,[55,151] which is a common accompaniment in patients with T2DM.

Hypertension markedly accelerates the progression of diabetic nephropathy in both T1DM and T2DM patients.[134,140,141] Therefore, it is essential that all patients with diabetes have their blood pressure normalized. Even mild hypertension (130/90 mm Hg) should not be tolerated in these patients. The Sixth Report of the

Joint National Committee recommends a blood pressure goal of 130/85 mm Hg in patients with diabetes.[152] This is consistent with the recommendation of the American Diabetes Association. The Hypertension Optimal Treatment (HOT) trial, which compared the achievement of a diastolic blood pressure less than 80 versus <85 and <90 mm Hg, concluded that the optimal blood pressure in patients with diabetes in order to prevent macrovascular complica-

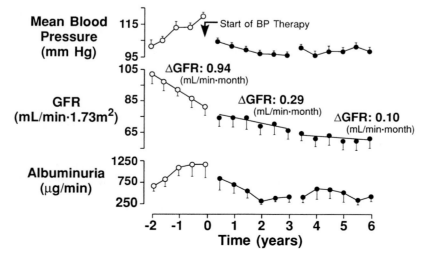

FIGURE 43-11. Effect of antihypertensive treatment (**solid circles**) on blood pressure, glomerular filtration rate, and albuminuria in type 1 diabetic patients. The rate of decline in GFR and the rate of rise in albuminuria before and after the start of antihypertensive therapy (**open circles**) were markedly slowed by effective reduction of the arterial blood pressure. (*Reproduced with permission from Parving et al.[145]*)

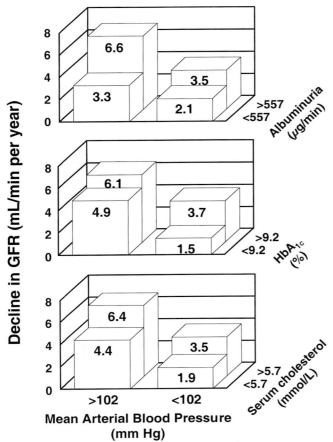

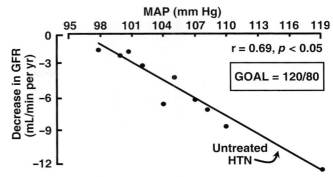

FIGURE 43-13. Relationship between achieved mean arterial blood pressure (**MAP**) control and the decrease in glomerular filtration rate (**GFR**) in nine long-term, antihypertensive clinical trials of diabetic (n = 6) and nondiabetic (n = 3) renal disease. These trials suggest that to maximally preserve renal function, the blood pressure should be reduced to less than 130/85 mm Hg, and ideally to 120/80 mm Hg. (*Adapted from Bakris* et al.[134])

FIGURE 43-12. The decline in glomerular filtration rate (**GFR**) as a function of the mean arterial blood pressure in 301 consecutive type 1 diabetic patients who were followed for 7 years (range = 3–14 years). For any given blood pressure, elevated serum cholesterol and HbA$_{1c}$ levels and an increased rate of urinary albumin excretion accelerated the decline in GFR. (*Reproduced with permission from Hovind* et al.[141])

tions should be less than 120–130/80 mm Hg.[153] The National Kidney Foundation Hypertension and Diabetes Working Group also recommends a diastolic blood pressure of <80–85 mm Hg in patients with diabetes based upon a review of clinical trials relating the achieved blood pressure to decline in GFR (Fig. 43-13).[134] In the author's opinion, the goal of antihypertensive therapy should be to reduce the blood pressure to what the patient's level was before the onset of hypertension or renal disease. In some cases, this may be lower than 120/80 mm Hg. If the patient's blood pressure

before the onset of hypertension or renal impairment is not known, then the goal of 120/80 mm Hg is appropriate. Special care should be taken in normalizing the blood pressure in elderly patients, especially those with underlying cardiovascular disease. Hypertension in patients with diabetes is very volume sensitive. Therefore, a low sodium diet should be used to initiate therapy.[154,155] The characteristics of the ideal antihypertensive drug for the treatment of hypertension in patients with diabetes is shown in Table 43-5. Because hypertension in these patients is very volume sensitive, diuretics would appear to be a logical first-line choice. However, this class of drugs, particularly at higher doses, may aggravate insulin resistance, impair insulin secretion, and cause dyslipidemia.[156,157] Because of these adverse effects on glucose tolerance and plasma lipid levels, if thiazide diuretics are to be used as first-line agents in the treatment of the hypertensive diabetic, they should be used in low doses (i.e., less than 25 mg per day of hydrochlorothiazide), and plasma glucose and lipid levels should be monitored closely after institution of therapy.[149,152,156,157] In patients with edema or renal insufficiency, a diuretic usually is required to normalize the blood pressure. If the serum creatinine concentration is more than 2 mg/dL, a more potent loop diuretic will be required. β-Adrenergic antagonists, especially the nonspecific β-blockers, should be used with caution in diabetic patients. They can impair insulin secretion and worsen glucose tolerance in patients with T2DM. In patients with T1DM, β-blockers may cause hypoglycemia by inhibiting

TABLE 43-4. Effect of Antihypertensive Treatment with Captopril on Renal Function and Outcome in Patients with Renal Insufficiency (Serum Creatinine <2.5 mg/dL) and Proteinuria (>500 mg/d)

	Doubling Time of Serum Creatinine (Months)	Renal Mortality, Dialysis, or Transplantation (No.)
Placebo	25	42
Captopril	43*	23*

*$p < 0.001$ vs. placebo.

Source: Adapted from Lewis *et al.*[146]

TABLE 43-5. The Ideal Antihypertensive Drug in Diabetes Mellitus

Is metabolically "neutral" and does not inhibit:
  Insulin secretion
  Insulin action
  Hepatic glucose production
  Counterregulatory hormone release
Does not:
  Cause or mask symptoms of hypoglycemia
  Aggravate dyslipidemia
  Promote orthostatic hypotension
  Aggravate coronary/peripheral vascular disease
Does:
  Specifically preserve renal function

hepatic glucose production and impairing the counterregulatory hormone response to hypoglycemia. β-Blockers may also mask the clinical symptoms of hypoglycemia, and they can aggravate diabetic dyslipidemia and underlying peripheral vascular disease in both type 1 and type 2 patients. Despite these concerns, the results of the UKPDS[158] demonstrated that after 9 years, treatment with atenolol (a selective β$_1$-antagonist) was as effective as captopril in reducing overall mortality, macrovascular complications (myocardial infarction, stroke, peripheral vascular disease), and microvascular complications (primarily retinopathy). Dyslipidemia and glycemic control were not aggravated by atenolol. The failure to observe any adverse metabolic effects during atenolol treatment most likely is related to its β$_1$ selectivity and the low daily dose that was employed.

Elevated intraglomerular pressure is a characteristic feature of the diabetic kidney, and this alteration in renal hemodynamics is in part related to increased sensitivity of the efferent arteriole to angiotensin II.[56] Consequently, the angiotensin-converting enzyme (ACE) inhibitors have gained widespread acceptance as the drug of choice in the treatment of the hypertensive diabetic, especially if proteinuria or renal insufficiency is present.[55,57,58,85, 90,134,140,144–146,149,154,155] ACE inhibitors also have been shown to retard the progression of albuminuria and decline in GFR in type 1 (Fig. 43-14) and type 2 (Fig. 43-15) patients with microalbuminuria.[55,58,85,90,132,144,146,154,155,159–166] Parving[143,145] has demonstrated a sustained protective effect of captopril in patients with T1DM over a follow-up period of 10 years. In short-term studies the antiproteinuric effect of the angiotensin II receptor blockers and ACE inhibitors has been shown to be similar in patients with and without diabetes with renal disease.[167] An added advantage of the ACE inhibitors is that they may improve insulin sensitivity and may have a beneficial effect on the plasma lipid profile.[156,157,166]

Most recently, two long-term prospective studies have demonstrated the effectiveness of the angiotensin II receptor blockers losartan and irbesartan in slowing the progression of renal failure in patients with T2DM (Fig. 43-16).[168–170] Some authorities have suggested that the angiotensin receptor blockers may be more effective than the ACE inhibitors, since the latter reduce only ACE-dependent angiotensin II production, whereas the receptor blockers inhibit the effect of angiotensin II from any source. However, the renal protective effects of losartan[169] and irbesartan[168,170] appear to

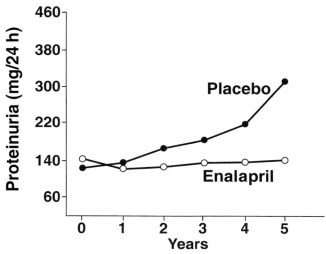

FIGURE 43-15. Effect of enalapril treatment on the progression of microalbuminuria in normotensive type 2 diabetic patients. *(Reproduced with permission from Ravid et al.[160])*

FIGURE 43-16. Effect of irbesartan versus placebo therapy on albumin excretion rate (**AER**), creatinine clearance, and mean arterial blood pressure in 395 hypertensive type 2 diabetic patients with microalbuminuria. Thirty of 201 (15%) placebo-treated and 10 of 194 (5%) irbesartan-treated patients progressed to persistent proteinuria over 2 years (*p* < 0.001). *(From Parving et al.[170])*

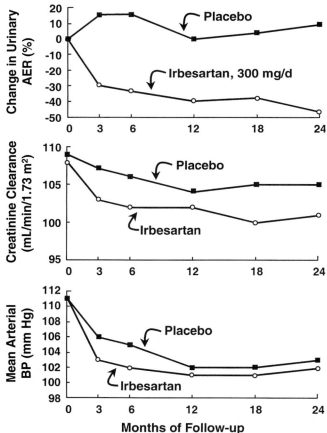

FIGURE 43-14. Effect of captopril versus placebo therapy on albumin excretion rate (**AER**) in 225 type 1 diabetic subjects with microalbuminuria. Twenty-five of 114 (22%) placebo-treated and 8 of 111 (7%) captopril-treated patients progressed to persistent clinical albuminuria over 2 years, (*p* < 0.01). *(Reproduced with permission from The Microalbuminuria Captopril Study Group.[164])*

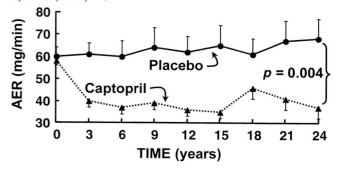

be no greater than those of the ACE inhibitors.[146] Moreover, there is experimental evidence to suggest that elevated kinins (not observed with the angiotensin receptor blockers) may be responsible for some of the renal protective effects of the ACE inhibitors.[171] The evidence from experimental models of diabetic and nondiabetic renal disease indicates that the ACE inhibitors and angiotensin receptor blockers afford equivalent renal protection despite differences in the site of inhibition of the renin-angiotensin system. Although combination therapy with an ACE inhibitor and an angiotensin receptor blocker has been suggested, there are no long-term data in humans to support such an approach.

The calcium channel blockers and postsynaptic α_1-adrenergic blockers also effectively lower blood pressure in patients with diabetes, and have been shown to exert a beneficial effect on renal function in patients with proteinuria.[55,153,154,172–177] Some evidence suggests that an ACE inhibitor plus a calcium channel blocker may provide an additive effect in preventing the progression of renal disease.[178–180] Moreover, when ACE inhibitors are used with calcium channel blockers, this combination has resulted in a reduction in cardiovascular events.[153,181] The calcium channel blockers have no adverse effects on either glucose or lipid metabolism, while the α-blockers improve insulin insensitivity and promote a less atherogenic plasma lipid profile.[172,173]

In summary, the ACE inhibitors or angiotensin receptor blockers, along with the calcium channel antagonists and the α-blockers, should be considered the agents of choice in treating the hypertensive diabetic patient. Since the treatment of hypertension is the single most important factor in preventing the progression of diabetic nephropathy,[55] and since the ACE inhibitors appear to provide a modest additional benefit beyond their antihypertensive action[134,140,159] by their effects on intrarenal hemodynamics[56] and nonhemodynamic mechanisms,[77] it is the author's opinion that the ACE inhibitors are the drugs of choice in treating hypertensive patients with diabetes and evidence of renal disease.

Microalbuminuria

Microalbuminuria (albumin excretion rate of 30–300 mg/d) represents the earliest detectable stage of diabetic nephropathy (Fig. 43-3). Type 1[55,85,86,105] and type 2[55,85,86,99–101,105] patients with microalbuminuria have a 20-fold and a 5-fold increased risk, respectively, of developing clinical proteinuria (>300 mg/d of albumin) or diminished GFR within a period of 10 years. Treatment of microalbuminuria with an ACE inhibitor has been shown to significantly reduce the rate of microalbumin excretion and retard the progression of microalbuminuria to clinical proteinuria (albumin excretion rate >300 mg/d) in both type 1 and type 2 patients.[140,160–162,167,182–192] ACE inhibitors also decrease the incidence of cardiovascular disease in both hypertensive and normotensive individuals with diabetes.[193,194]

At the time that microalbuminuria is first detected, the blood pressure is normal or only modestly elevated. Therefore, in many patients with diabetes, the treatment of microalbuminuria must focus on reducing the level of albumin excretion and not on lowering the blood pressure. All diabetic patients should have an annual test for microalbuminuria. This can be done using a timed urine collection (e.g., over 24 hours) or by checking the microalbumin : creatinine ratio or microalbumin concentration (Micral Dipstix, Roche Diagnostics) on a first-voided morning urine specimen. If microalbuminuria is detected, the author prefers to base future therapeutic interventions on the 24-hour microalbumin excretion rate or on the microalbumin : creatinine ratio (Table 2). After quantitating the rate of microalbumin excretion, the patient is started on the ACE inhibitor of choice (e.g., captopril, 12.5 mg three times a day; enalapril, 5 mg/d; monopril, 10 mg/d) and a repeat urine microalbumin determination is performed in 6–8 weeks. If microalbuminuria is diminished but still present, the dose of the ACE inhibitor should be increased (e.g., captopril by 12.5 mg three times a day; enalapril by 5 mg/d; monopril by 10 mg/d) every 6–8 weeks until the microalbuminuria disappears or the microalbumin excretion rate remains unchanged over three successive dose titrations. The ACE inhibitors produce a maximum or near maximum reduction in microalbumin excretion rate within 6–8 weeks. If a beneficial effect of the ACE inhibitor is observed, therapy should be continued for life, since withdrawal of the ACE inhibitor will lead to a return of the microalbuminuria.

Urinary Tract Infection

The incidence of urinary tract infection is increased in patients with diabetes, especially those with glucosuria. High urine glucose concentrations provide an excellent culture medium for bacteria and inhibit WBC function. Therefore, it is important that a urinalysis be performed on each clinic visit. If white blood cells or bacteriuria are noted, a urine culture should be done. Periodic urine cultures should be obtained, and positive cultures should be treated with an appropriate bactericidal antibiotic.

Neurogenic Bladder

Neurogenic bladder is not uncommon in patients with longstanding diabetes, especially in individuals with other evidence of neuropathy. Since the symptoms may be mistaken for prostatic hypertrophy, the clinician must have a high index of suspicion to establish the diagnosis of neurogenic bladder. In addition to the history, repeated bouts of urinary tract infection should provide a clue to the diagnosis. If the presence of a neurogenic bladder is confirmed by cystometrogram, the patient should receive instruction in the Crede manual voiding maneuver, which should be performed every 6–8 hours. Agents such as bethanechol also may be tried. In some patients with diabetes, adrenergic drugs (i.e., phenoxybenzamine) have proven useful. The success of these various medical interventions can be evaluated by determining the postvoid residual volume. If medical therapy proves unsuccessful, intermittent, straight catheterization should be performed at least 2–3 times daily.

Intravenous Pyelography

Diabetic patients are at increased risk to develop acute renal failure after radiocontrast procedures (e.g., arteriography, cholangiography, intravenous and retrograde pyelography, computed tomographic scanning).[195] This adverse event is observed less frequently with the newer contrast agents, but still remains a concern. Patients with impaired renal function (i.e., serum creatinine >2 mg/dL) or heavy proteinuria are at greatest risk. With the judicious use of ultrasound, radionuclide studies, and computed tomographic scanning without contrast, most of the information necessary to ensure adequate diagnosis and treatment can be obtained. If patients with diabetes must receive radiocontrast dye, hydration with normal saline should be started 12–24 hours prior to the procedure.[196]

Blood Glucose Control

Glycemic Control

Diabetic nephropathy and other microvascular complications (retinopathy and neuropathy) are reduced in individuals who have maintained a lifetime of near normoglycemia. The product of the mean day-long blood glucose concentration (as reflected by the hemoglobin A_{1c}) and the duration of diabetes provides an index of the total hyperglycemic burden and is the best predictor of microvascular complications.[111,197] Poor glycemic control is a major risk factor for diabetic nephropathy in both type 1 and type 2 patients[55,58,85,123,197,198] and diabetic nephropathy is uncommon when the glycosylated hemoglobin is maintained below 7.0%.[61,62] In the Diabetes Control and Complications Trial[35,63] intensive glycemic control with insulin in type 1 patients markedly decreased the risk of microvascular complications (Fig. 43-4). In type 2 patients, improved glycemic control with insulin[64,65] or oral agents[65,66] was equally effective in decreasing the risk of microalbuminuria, as well as other microvascular complications. A similar conclusion was reached from the meta-analysis of several smaller clinical studies.[67] Combined pancreatic and renal transplantation has been shown to prevent the recurrence of diabetic nephropathy in the transplanted kidney as long as the pancreatic transplant functions normally.[199,200] Conversely, the transplantation of kidneys with established diabetic nephropathy into patients without diabetes leads to a reversal of the renal disease.[36] The important role of tight glycemic control in the prevention of diabetic nephropathy has been conclusively established in many animal models of diabetes.[27–32,201]

Despite the encouraging results observed with intensive insulin therapy in diabetic animal models and from pancreatic transplantation in man and animals, the initiation of tight glycemic control after the onset of overt proteinuria (>300 mg/d of albumin) or renal insufficiency generally has been ineffective in halting the relentless progression to end-stage renal failure in T1DM.[55,59,60,125,202,203] These findings suggest that intensive glycemic control in humans is most effective when started early,[25,63–67] i.e., prior to or during the phase of microalbuminuria (30–300 mg/d; see Fig. 43-3) and before the advanced histologic lesions of diabetic nephropathy have become well established. Based upon the available evidence, it is recommended that the hemoglobin A_{1c} in diabetic patients with microalbuminuria and without an elevated creatinine be maintained less than 7% and ideally less than 6% (Table 43-6). In patients with diabetes having normal serum creatinine and albumin excretion rates greater than 300 mg/dL, strict glycemic control (HbA$_{1c}$ <7.0%) is recommended because the level has not been established at which intensified glycemic control of albuminuria is no longer is capable of preventing the progression of renal disease, and because progression of retinopathy and neuropathy still remains a concern. In diabetic patients with renal insufficiency (serum creatinine ≥2.0 mg/dL), a hemoglobin A_{1c} level lower than 7% is desirable, but 7–8% may be acceptable.

Changes in Insulin Degradation and Insulin Sensitivity

In patients without diabetes with renal insufficiency, moderate to severe insulin resistance is a nearly universal finding.[204] The defect in insulin action resides in peripheral tissues, primarily muscle.[204] Therefore it is not uncommon to observe a deterioration in glycemic control with the advent of renal insufficiency in both type 1 and type 2 patients. However, when the GFR decreases to 15–20 mL/min, both the renal (loss of nephron mass) and hepatic (uremia inhibits insulin degradation by the liver) clearance of insulin become markedly reduced. At this stage, it is common to observe an improvement in glucose tolerance because the insulin, which normally would be degraded by the liver and kidneys, is returned to the systemic circulation. If the insulin (or sulfonylurea) dose is not appropriately reduced, hypoglycemia may ensue and some patients may even cease to require insulin (or sulfonylureas). After the institution of hemodialysis therapy, a complex sequence of events ensues. Dialysis enhances the body's sensitivity to insulin, decreasing insulin requirements.[205] However, dialysis also returns hepatic insulin degradation toward normal, increasing the need for insulin.[205] Moreover, the stress of dialysis and a tendency for weight gain may increase insulin requirements. In any given uremic patient with diabetes who is started on dialysis, it is difficult to predict what will happen to the insulin requirements. In general, most patients experience an increase in insulin requirements when dialysis is initiated because of the release of insulin-antagonistic hormones in response to fluid shifts.

From the preceding discussion, it is obvious that the physician must be careful in selecting oral hypoglycemic agents for the treatment of patients with diabetes with impaired renal function.[206] The ideal oral agent should not enhance insulin secretion, and the metabolism of the oral agent should not be influenced by diminished kidney function. Based upon these theoretical considerations, insulin sensitizers, such as thiazolidinediones (rosiglitazone and pioglitazone) appear to be ideal candidates, but there are no published data with this class of drugs in patients with chronic renal failure. Of interest, troglitazone (which is no longer approved for use as monotherapy because of associated liver toxicity) has been shown to correct albuminuria in streptozocin diabetic rats[207] and to halt diabetic glomerulosclerosis by blockade of mesangial expansion.[208] Preliminary studies in human T2DM suggest that the thiazolidinediones also can reduce microalbuminuria. Metformin, an insulin sensitizer, is excreted via the kidneys and should not be used if the serum creatinine is greater than 1.4 mg/dL in females or 1.5 mg/dL in males, corresponding to a GFR of ~70 mL/min.[209] Accumulation of the biguanide in plasma and tissues may lead to lactic acidosis. Until recently, the only truly short-acting insulin secretagogue was glipazide, which is not available in the U.S. Glipizide is almost entirely metabolized by the liver and its metabolites are inactive.[210] Therefore it is well suited for use in patients with diabetes with chronic renal failure (CRF). Glimiperide also can be used in CRF patients.[211] Glyburide should be avoided since it has a long half-life,

TABLE 43-6. Recommend Levels of Glycemic Control in Diabetic Individuals

Control	Normal Control	Type 1 Diabetes: Intensive Control	Type 1 Diabetes: Acceptable Control	Type 2 Diabetes: Intensive	Type 2 Diabetes: Acceptable
Premeal blood glucose (mg/dL)	~90	80–120	<140–160	<110	126
Hemoglobin A_{1c} (%)	4.0–6.0	<6.0	<7.0	<6.0	<7.0

and its metabolites have hypoglycemic activity and are excreted in the urine.[210] Because all sulfonylureas stimulate insulin secretion, titration should be slow (every 2 weeks or more) in patients with CRF. Repaglinide and nateglinide are new nonsulfonylurea insulin secretagogues that belong to the meglitinide class of drugs.[212] These agents are short acting and must be given 3 times per day before meals. The meglitinides undergo hepatic metabolism to inactive products that are excreted in the bile. Because of these characteristics, the meglitinides are well suited for use in diabetic patients with impaired renal function. Acarbose is not approved for use in patients with diabetes with an elevated serum creatinine. Insulin therapy always remains an option for the treatment of patients with chronic renal insufficiency, but the physician must be aware of the alterations in insulin metabolism discussed above. Although HbA$_{1c}$ levels may be slightly reduced in diabetic patients with advanced renal disease because of shortened red blood cell survival, it remains the best tool for assessing glycemic control in diabetic patients.[213]

Hypoglycemia in Chronic Renal Failure and Dialysis Patients

Spontaneous hypoglycemia has been reported in patients with CRF with or without diabetes. However, the pathogenic mechanisms responsible for the hypoglycemia have not been elucidated. In insulin-treated type 1 patients, hypoglycemia most commonly results from excessive insulinemia secondary to impaired insulin degradation by the kidneys and the liver. However, in type 2 patients (who are not on insulin or an oral insulin secretagogue) and in patients without diabetes with chronic renal failure, plasma insulin levels are only modestly elevated, and the hyperinsulinemia cannot explain the profound hypoglycemia that has been reported in some patients with chronic renal insufficiency. It is likely that these patients have a defect in hepatic glucose production. Decreased hepatic glucose production secondary to diminished alanine availability for gluconeogenesis has been documented in a single uremic diabetic patient with spontaneous hypoglycemia.[214] However, the frequency with which decreased alanine availability contributes to spontaneous hypoglycemia is unclear. Severe hypoglycemia also has been reported in patients without diabetes on chronic maintenance hemodialysis[215] in the absence of malnourishment or elevated plasma insulin levels. Of note, all of these patients were on propranolol. Although propranolol can cause hypoglycemia by inhibiting hepatic glucose production, symptomatic hypoglycemia does occur in hemodialysis patients who are not taking β-adrenergic blocking agents.

Peritoneal Dialysis, Glucose Absorption, and Insulin Requirements

Standard hemodialysate solutions contain no glucose. However, there has been considerable interest in continuous ambulatory peritoneal dialysis (CAPD), especially in patients with diabetes. Because dialysis is performed continuously, and the dialysis fluid contains hypertonic glucose, glucose absorption is considerable. During CAPD in patients without diabetes, plasma glucose levels usually do not rise above 160–180 mg/dL. However, in patients with diabetes who are both insulin resistant and insulin deficient, severe hyperglycemia presents a significant problem with this mode of therapy. To prevent the development of excessive hyperglycemia, insulin is added to the dialysis fluid, and intraperitoneal insulin administration has been employed effectively to achieve excellent glucose control. However, insulin requirements usually are increased two- to fourfold with CAPD. In addition to the increased glucose load, the presence of obesity and loss of endogenous insulin secretion (which is related to the duration of diabetes) correlate closely with the increased insulin requirements in CAPD patients.[216] It is best to start patients on CAPD in the hospital setting so that optimal glucose control can be achieved within the shortest time and without hypoglycemic or hyperglycemic complications.

Protein Restriction

Low-protein diets have been advocated to slow the progression of chronic renal failure.[217] The use of protein-restricted diets is based on two assumptions: (1) the "adaptive" increases in intraglomerular pressure and renal blood flow that occur after a reduction in renal mass play a pathogenic role in the progressive injury to remaining nephrons, and (2) the "adaptive" changes in renal hemodynamics can be prevented by protein restriction, leading to the preservation of renal function.

In both diabetic and nondiabetic rats, when renal mass is reduced by a variety of experimental maneuvers, there is an initial stabilization of renal function which results from an increase in single-nephron glomerular plasma flow and intraglomerular pressure. These changes in renal hemodynamics combine to augment the single-nephron GFR.[218] However, on a long-term basis these "adaptive" changes are followed by a progressive decline in GFR secondary to the chronic elevation in intraglomerular pressure, which causes severe glomerular sclerosis and heavy proteinuria. When rats with a single remnant kidney are placed on a low-protein diet, the rises in single-nephron GFR, glomerular plasma flow, and transcapillary hydraulic pressure are prevented, glomerular function is markedly improved, and kidney survival is prolonged. Based on these results in animals, a number of studies have examined whether a low-protein diet in humans also will have a palliative effect on the progression of renal failure.[219–221] Most of these early studies were uncontrolled and involved small numbers of patients, few of whom had diabetes. Nonetheless, the results consistently demonstrated that institution of a low-protein diet slowed the decline in GFR in patients with advanced renal failure. More recently, a well-controlled prospective study involving 840 patients with renal disease of diverse etiology has been completed[222,223] (Fig. 43-17). Insulin-requiring patients with diabetes were not included in the study and diet-treated and sulfonylurea-treated patients were not analyzed separately. After 3 years, no difference in the rate of decline in GFR was observed between the patients receiving

FIGURE 43-17. Effect of low-protein diet on the rate of decline in glomerular filtration rate (**GFR**) in patients with chronic renal disease of diverse etiology, including T2DM. *(Reproduced with permission from Klahr et al.[222])*

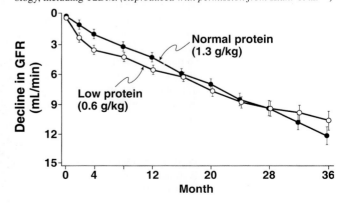

the low-protein diet (0.58 g/kg) and those maintained on a normal protein intake (1.3 g/kg). The failure of this large prospective study[222,223] to demonstrate any beneficial effect of a low-protein diet stands in contrast to many previously published studies with smaller numbers of patients.[219,221] It is likely that any beneficial effect of the low-protein diet in this large prospective study was obscured by the concomitant use of antihypertensive medications, which were taken by 80% of participants. Moreover, 44% of the study population was taking ACE inhibitors, which have a specific renal protective effect in patients with or without diabetes. Based upon these results, it seems prudent to recommend modest protein restriction (~1.0 g/kg/d) in patients with diabetes who are taking an ACE inhibitor or calcium channel blocker, while reserving more severe protein restriction (0.6 g/kg/d) for patients who are not taking any antihypertensive medications. These severely restricted protein diets are associated with poor patient compliance and require close dietary supervision. If a very low protein diet is used, this can lead to negative nitrogen balance and acceleration of muscle protein breakdown, with the development of clinically manifest myopathy.

Dyslipidemia

Type 2 and poorly controlled type 1 patients with normal renal function commonly have dyslipidemia, characterized by hypertriglyceridemia, reduced HDL cholesterol, small dense LDL particles, and postprandial hyperlipidemia.[151] In patients with diabetes and renal insufficiency, the dyslipidemia is aggravated, and in patients with heavy proteinuria, elevated LDL cholesterol and marked hypertriglyceridemia commonly are observed.[224] When patients are started on dialysis, the dyslipidemia usually worsens.[224] Patients with diabetes and impaired renal function are at extremely high risk of developing heart attacks and stroke[99,101,102,225] (Fig. 43-4), and dyslipidemia represents a major risk factor for cardiovascular disease in this population.[226,227] The great majority of patients with diabetes on dialysis have some form of dyslipidemia, and cardiovascular disease is epidemic in this group.[8,228–232] Therefore, it is imperative that all patients with diabetes, whether they have normal renal function, impaired renal function, or are on dialysis, receive aggressive dietary and pharmacologic treatment for their dyslipidemia. The goal of therapy is to reduce the LDL cholesterol and triglycerides to less than 100 mg/dL and 200 mg/dL, respectively. This can be achieved with diet, HMG-CoA reductase inhibitors, and fibric acid derivatives.[224,233] The HDL cholesterol should be increased to at least 45 mg/dL, but this is often difficult to achieve with pharmacologic therapy. Exercise and the thiazolidinediones (although not approved for this indication) are particularly efficacious in increasing the plasma HDL cholesterol concentration.

Hyperlipidemia has also been implicated as a causative factor in the progression of diabetic nephropathy.[233–235] In a number of animal models of progressive renal disease, including diabetic nephropathy, lipogenic diets worsen, while cholesterol-lowering medications ameliorate renal injury.[236–238] Although there has been no large interventional study examining the effect of cholesterol reduction on nephropathy, several small, well-controlled studies have been performed. A meta-analysis of these studies[239] demonstrated that reduction of the plasma cholesterol concentration significantly slowed the rate of decline of GFR, regardless of the lipid-lowering agent that was used or the etiology of the renal disease. Thus patients with diabetes should receive aggressive antilipidemic therapy for the prevention of cardiovascular complications and possible protection against progressive renal deterioration.

Dialysis

Once end-stage renal failure occurs, the patient and physician must choose from one of four options: hemodialysis, peritoneal dialysis, CAPD,[124] or renal transplantation.[231,240]

One of the most important questions that the physician faces is when to initiate dialysis in the patient with diabetes and advanced renal insufficiency. Vascular access and dialysis should be instituted earlier in patients with diabetes than in those without for many reasons. Once the serum creatinine concentration has increased to 3–4 mg/dL, there is a rapid deterioration in renal function, and most patients with diabetes require dialysis within 6–12 months. In general, patients with diabetes tolerate uremia less well than those without diabetes. In particular, there often is a marked acceleration of diabetic retinopathy and neuropathy. Glycemic control becomes more difficult, and negative nitrogen balance, protein wasting, and myopathy may become significant management problems with advancing uremia. Because of sodium retention, hypertension also becomes more difficult to control. All of these complications are easier to manage if dialysis is instituted early.[124] Vascular access should be established when the serum creatinine reaches 4–5 mg/dL, and dialysis initiated at creatinine levels of 6–8 mg/dL. Although hemodialysis is the most frequently employed form of dialysis therapy in all patients with end-stage renal failure, it does not appear to be superior to any other dialysis technique. Morbidity and mortality statistics are similar with intermittent peritoneal and chronic ambulatory peritoneal dialysis.[8,9,229] Regardless of the type of dialysis chosen, survival in patients with diabetes is much worse than in patients without diabetes.[228,229]

Nutritional management of the patient with diabetes on dialysis requires special attention. Many diabetics are malnourished before starting dialysis, and achieving a positive nitrogen balance may be difficult. Patients should receive 37.5–40 kcal/kg of ideal body weight, with about half of the calories given as carbohydrates, primarily complex ones. The achievement of positive nitrogen balance requires at least 1.5 g/kg/d of high-biologic-value protein. With this intake, most insulin-requiring patients on dialysis require a split, mixed insulin regimen to achieve adequate glucose control. A morning and evening injection of long-acting insulin (i.e., NPH) or a single injection of glargine insulin is usually required. The long-acting insulin should be administered with sufficient quantities of regular or very-rapid-acting insulin to cover the postprandial glucose excursions. After dialysis is initiated, the total daily insulin requirement usually increases by 50–100%.[241] Because of frequent, unpredictable fluctuations in glucose control, it is essential that patients with diabetes perform home blood glucose monitoring.

Renal Transplantation

Results from the United States Renal Data System[228,231] indicate that patients with diabetes who are treated by kidney transplantation, especially if the kidney is donated by a living donor, have a much better survival than those who are placed on dialysis. If a human leukocyte antigen (HLA)-identical donor can be found, the chances of long-term patient survival are far superior to those of dialysis. HLA-nonidentical recipients also do better than patients with diabetes treated with dialysis. Long-term survival with cadaveric renal transplantation is slightly better than with dialysis. Therefore, in the absence of an HLA-related donor, the choice between dialysis and transplantation must be individualized for each patient with diabetes. Although combined pancreatic/kidney transplantation is at an early stage, recent results[242,243] suggest that this newer therapeutic option results in lower mortality than dialysis or kidney transplantation alone for patients with T1DM,[242,243] and it may be beneficial in preventing the recurrence of diabetic nephropathy in the transplanted kidney (see Chap. 55).[37] Newer immunosuppressive regimens may bring further improvements in patient survival after cadaveric renal transplantation.

REFERENCES

1. Krolewski AS, Warram JH, Rand LI, et al: Epidemiologic approach to the etiology of type 1 diabetes mellitus and its complications. *N Engl J Med* 1987;317:1390.

2. Krolewski M, Eggers PW, Warram JH: Magnitude of end-stage renal disease in IDDM: A 35 year follow-up study. *Kidney Int* 1997; 50: 2041.

3. Harris MI, Flegal KM, Cowie CC, et al: Prevalence of diabetes, impaired fasting glucose, and impaired glucose tolerance in U.S. adults. The Third National Health and Nutrition Examination Survey, 1988–1994. *Diabetes Care* 1998;21:518.

4. Ballard DJ, Humphrey LL, Nelton LJ, et al: Epidemiology of persistent proteinuria in type II diabetes mellitus: Population-based study in Rochester, Minnesota. *Diabetes* 1988;37:405.

5. Teutsch S, Newman J, Eggers P: The problem of diabetic renal failure in the United States: An overview. *Am J Kidney Dis* 1989;13:11.

6. Pugh JA, Stern MP, Haffner SM, et al: Incidence of end-stage renal disease secondary to diabetes mellitus in Mexican-Americans and non-Hispanic whites. *Am J Epidemiol* 1987;127:135.

7. Hawthorne V, Hamman R, Keen H, et al: Preventing the kidney disease of diabetes mellitus. *Am J Kidney Dis* 1989;13:2.

8. Agodoa LY, Jones CA, Held PJ: End-stage renal disease in the USA: Data from the United States Renal Data System. *Am J Nephrol* 1996; 16:7.

9. United States Renal Data System: USRDS 1998 Annual Data Report. National Institutes of Health, National Institutes of Diabetes and Digestive and Kidney Diseases, Bethesda, MD, 1998. *Am J Kidney Dis* 1998;32(suppl 1):S1.

10. United States Renal Data System: USRDS 1999 Annual Data Report: The economic cost of ESRD and Medicare spending for alternative modalities of treatment. *Am J Kidney Dis* 34(suppl 1):S124.

11. Kimmelstiel P, Wilson C: Intercapillary lesions in glomeruli of kidney. *Am J Pathol* 1936;12:83.

12. Osterby R, Gundersen HJG, Horlyck A, et al: Diabetic glomerulopathy: Structural characteristics of the early and advanced stages. *Diabetes* 1983;32:79.

13. Fioretto P, Steffes MW, Sutherland DER, et al: Sequential renal biopsies in insulin dependent diabetic patients: Structural factors associated with clinical progression. *Kidney Int* 1995;48:1929.

14. Ziyadeh FN: The extracellular matrix in diabetic nephropathy. *Am J Kidney Dis* 1993;22:736.

15. Steffes MW, Bilous RW, Sutherland DER, et al: Cell and matrix components of the glomerular mesangium in type 1 diabetes. *Diabetes* 1992;41:679.

16. Spiro RG: Biochemistry of the renal glomerular basement membrane and its alteration in diabetes mellitus. *N Engl J Med* 1973;288:1337.

17. Wahl P, Depperman D, Hasslacher C: Biochemistry of glomerular basement membrane of the normal and diabetic human. *Kidney Int* 1982;21:744.

18. Falk RJ, Scheinman JI, Mauer SM, et al: Polyantigenic expansion of basement membrane constituents in diabetic nephropathy. *Diabetes* 1983;32:34.

19. Scandling JD, Myers BD: Glomerular size-selectivity and microalbuminuria in early diabetic glomerular disease. *Kidney Int* 1992; 41:840.

20. Lane PH, Steffes MS, Fioretto P, et al: Renal interstitial expansion in insulin-dependent diabetes mellitus. *Kidney Int* 1993;43:661.

21. Brito PL, Fioretto P, Drummond K, et al: Proximal-tubular basement membrane width in insulin-dependent diabetes mellitus. *Kidney Int* 1998;53:754.

22. Vejlsgaard R: Studies on urinary tract infection in diabetics. *Acta Med Scand* 1966;179:173.

23. Batalla MA, Balodimos MC, Bradley RF: Bacteriuria in diabetes mellitus. *Diabetologia* 1971;7:297.

24. Lauler DP, Schreiner GE, David A: Renal medullary necrosis. *Am J Med* 1960;29:132.

25. Mauer SM, Steffes MW, Connett J, et al: The development of lesions in the glomerular basement membrane and mesangium after transplantation of normal kidneys to diabetic patients. *Diabetes* 1983; 32:948.

26. Becker D, Miller M: Presence of diabetic glomerulosclerosis in patients with hemochromatosis. *N Engl J Med* 1960;263:367.

27. Kirose K, Osterby R, Nozawa M, et al: Development of glomerular lesions in experimental long-term diabetes in the rat. *Kidney Int* 1982; 21:689.

28. Bloodworth JMB: Experimental diabetic glomerulosclerosis. II. The dog. *Arch Pathol* 1965;79:113.

29. Rasch R: Prevention of diabetic glomerulopathy in streptozotocin diabetic rats by insulin treatment. Kidney size and glomerular volume. *Diabetologia* 1979;16:125.

30. Hagg E: Influence of insulin treatment on glomerular changes in rats with long-term alloxan diabetes. *Acta Pathol Microbiol Scand* 1974; 82:228.

31. Rasch R: Prevention of diabetic glomerulopathy in streptozotocin diabetic rats by insulin treatment: The mesangial regions. *Diabetologia* 1979;17:243.

32. Mauer SM, Steffes MW, Sutherland DER, et al: Studies of the rate of regression of the glomerular lesions in diabetic rats treated with pancreatic islet transplantation. *Diabetes* 1975;24:280.

33. Federlin K, Bretzel RG, Schmidtchen U: Islet transplantation in experimental diabetes of the rat. V. Regression of glomerular lesions in diabetic rats after intraportal transplantation of isogenic islets. *Horm Metab Res* 1976;8:404.

34. Mauer SM, Steffes MW, Brown DM: Animal models of diabetic nephropathy. In: Hamburger J, Crosnier J, Grunfield JP, et al, eds. *Advances in Nephropathy*, Vol. 8. Year Book Medical Publishers: 1979;23.

35. The Diabetes Control and Complications Trial (DCCT) Research Group: The effect of intensive treatment of diabetes on the development and progression of long-term complications in insulin-dependent diabetes mellitus. *N Engl J Med* 1993;329:977.

36. Abouna GM, Al-Adnani MS, Kremer GD, et al: Reversal of diabetic nephropathy in human cadaveric kidneys after transplantation into non-diabetic recipients. *Lancet* 1983;2:1274.

37. Fioretto P, Steffes MW, Sutherland DER, et al: Reversal of lesions of diabetic nephropathy after pancreas transplantation. *N Engl J Med* 1998;339:69.

38. Kroc Collaborative Study: Blood glucose control and the evaluation of diabetic retinopathy and albuminuria. *N Engl J Med* 1984;311:365.

39. Viberti GC, Bilous RW, Mackintosh D, et al: Long-term correction of hyperglycaemia and progression of renal failure in insulin dependent diabetics. *Br Med J* 1983;286:598.

40. Steno Study Group: Effect of six months of strict metabolic control on eye and kidney function in insulin-dependent diabetics with background retinopathy. *Lancet* 1982;1:121.

41. The Diabetes Control and Complications (DCCT) Trial/Epidemiology of Diabetes Interventions and Complications (EDIC) Research Group: Retinopathy and nephropathy in patients with type 1 diabetes four years after a trial of intensive therapy. *N Engl J Med* 2000; 342:381.

42. Alaveras AE, Thomas SM, Sagriotis A, et al: Promoters of progression of diabetic nephropathy: The relative roles of blood glucose and blood pressure control. *Nephrol Dial Transplant* 1997;2:71.

43. Linner E, Svanborg A, Zelander T: Retinal and renal lesions of diabetic type, without obvious disturbances in glucose metabolism, in a patient with family history of diabetes. *Am J Med* 1971;39:298.

44. Siperstein MD, Unger RH, Madison LL: Studies of muscle capillary basement membranes in normal subjects, diabetic and prediabetic patients. *J Clin Invest* 1968;47:1973.

45. Williamson JR, Kilo C: A common sense approach resolves the basement membrane controversy and the NIH Pima Indian study. *Diabetologia* 1979;17:129.

46. Seaquist ER, Goetz FC, Rich S, et al: Familial clustering of diabetic kidney disease: Evidence for genetic susceptibility to diabetic nephropathy. *N Engl J Med* 1989;320:1161.

47. DCCT Research Group: Clustering of long-term complications in families with diabetes in the Diabetes Control and Complications Trial. *Diabetes* 1997;46:1829.

48. Pettitt DJ, Saad MF, Bennett PH, *et al*: Familial predisposition to renal disease in two generations of Pima Indians with type 2 (non-insulin-dependent) diabetes mellitus. *Diabetologia* 1990;33:438.

49. Faronato PP, Maioli M, Tonolo G, *et al*: Clustering of albumin excretion rate abnormalities in Caucasian patients with NIDDM. The Italian NIDDM nephropathy study group. *Diabetologia* 1997;40:816.

50. Viberti GC, Keen H, Wiseman MJ: Raised arterial pressure in parents of proteinuric insulin-dependent diabetics. *Br Med J* 1987;295:515.

51. Fioretto P, Steffes MW, Barbosa J, *et al*: Is diabetic nephropathy inherited? Studies of glomerular structure in type 1 diabetic sibling pairs. *Diabetes* 1999;48:865.

52. Imperatore G, Hanson RL, Pettitt DJ, *et al*: Sib-pair linkage analysis for susceptibility genes for microvascular complications among Pima Indians with type 2 diabetes mellitus. *Diabetes* 1998;47:821.

53. Krolewski AS: Genetics of diabetic nephropathy: Evidence for major and minor gene effects. *Kidney Int* 1999;55:1582.

54. Cowie CC, Port FK, Wolfe RA, *et al*: Disparities in incidence of diabetic end-stage renal disease according to race and type of diabetes. *N Engl J Med* 1989;321:1074.

55. DeFronzo RA: Diabetic nephropathy: Etiologic and therapeutic considerations. *Diabetes Rev* 1995;3:510.

56. Hostetter TH: Mechanisms of diabetic nephropathy. *Am J Kidney Dis* 1994;23:188.

57. Cooper ME: Pathogenesis, prevention, and treatment of diabetic nephropathy. *Lancet* 1998;352:213.

58. Tuttle KR, DeFronzo RA, Stein JH: Treatment of diabetic nephropathy: A rational approach based on its pathophysiology. *Semin Nephrol* 1991;11:220.

59. Viberti GC, Walker JD: Diabetic nephropathy: Etiology and prevention. *Diabetes Metab Rev* 1988;4:147.

60. Mogensen CE: Prevention and treatment of renal disease in insulin-dependent diabetes mellitus. *Semin Nephrol* 1990;10:260.

61. Norgaard K, Storm B, Graae M, *et al*: Elevated albumin excretion and retinal changes in children with type 1 diabetes are related to long-term poor blood glucose control. *Diabet Med* 1989;6:325.

62. Torffvit O, Agardh E, Agardh CD: Albuminuria and associated medical risk factors: A cross-sectional study in 476 type 1 (insulin-dependent) diabetic patients. Part 1. *J Diabetes Complications* 1991;5:23.

63. The Diabetes Control and Complications Trial (DCCT): The absence of a glycemic threshold for the development of long-term complications: The perspective of the Diabetes Control and Complications Trial. *Diabetes* 1996;45:1289.

64. Ohkubo Y, Kishikawa H, Araki E, *et al*: Intensive insulin therapy prevents the progression of diabetic microvascular complication in Japanese patients with non-insulin-dependent diabetes mellitus: A randomized prospective 6-year study. *Diabetes Res Clin Pract* 1995;28:103.

65. UK Prospective Diabetes Study Group: Intensive blood-glucose control with sulphonylureas or insulin compared with conventional treatment and risk of complications in patients with type 2 diabetes (UKPDS 33). *Lancet* 1998;352:837.

66. UK Prospective Diabetes Study Group: Effect of intensive blood-glucose control with metformin on complications in overweight patients with type 2 diabetes (UKPDS 34). *Lancet* 1998;352:854.

67. Wang PH, Lau J, Chalmers TC: Meta-analysis of effects of intensive blood-glucose control on late complications of type I diabetes. *Lancet* 1993;341:1306.

68. Riser BL, Cortes P, Yee J, *et al*: Mechanical strain- and high glucose-induced alterations in mesangial cell collagen metabolism: Role of TGF-B. *J Am Soc Nephrol* 1998;9:827.

69. Flyvbjerg A: Putative pathophysiological role of growth factors and cytokines in experimental diabetic kidney disease. *Diabetologia* 2000;43;1205.

70. Makita Z, Bucala R, Rayfield EJ, *et al*: Reactive glycosylation end products in diabetic uraemia and treatment of renal failure. *Lancet* 1994;343:1519.

71. Makita Z, Radoff S, Rayfield E, *et al*: Advanced glycosylation end products in patients with diabetic nephropathy. *N Engl J Med* 1991;325:836.

72. Ishi H, Jirousek MR, Koya D, *et al*: Amelioration of vascular dysfunctions in diabetic rats by an oral PKC beta inhibitor. *Science* 1996;272:728.

73. Jerums G, Panagiotopoulos S, Tsalamandris C, *et al*: Why is proteinuria such an important risk factor for progression in clinical trials? *Kidney Int* 1997;52:S87.

74. Osicka TM, Houlihan CA, Chan JG, *et al*: Albuminuria in patients with type 1 diabetes is directly linked to changes in the lysosome-mediated degradation of albumin during renal passage. *Diabetes* 2000;49:1579.

75. Lemley KV, Blouch K, *et al*: Glomerular permselectivity at the onset of nephropathy in type 2 diabetes mellitus. *J Am Soc Nephrol* 2000;11:2095.

76. Deckert T, Feldt-Rasmussen B, Djurp R, *et al*: Glomerular size and change selectivity in insulin-dependent diabetes mellitus. *Kidney Int* 1988;33:100.

77. Wolf G, Ziyadeh FN: The role of angiotensin II in diabetic nephropathy: Emphasis on nonhemodynamic mechanisms. *Am J Kidney Dis* 1997;29:153.

78. Wolf G: Link between angiotensin II and TGF-β in the kidney. *Miner Electrolyte Metab* 1998;24:174.

79. Peters H, Border WA, Noble NA: Targeting TGF-β overexpression in renal disease: Maximizing the antibrotic action of angiotensin II blockade. *Kidney Int* 1998;54:1570.

80. Vallon V, Richter K, Blantz RC, *et al*: Glomerular hyperfiltration in experimental diabetes mellitus: Potential role of tubular reabsorption. *J Am Soc Nephrol* 1999;10:2569.

81. Bank N, Aynedjian HS: Progressive increases in luminal glucose stimulate proximal sodium absorption in normal and diabetic rats. *J Clin Invest* 1990;86:309.

82. Thomson SC, Deng A, Bao D, *et al*: Ornithine decarboxylase, kidney size, and the tubular hypothesis of glomerular hyperfiltration in experimental diabetes. *J Clin Invest* 2001;107:217.

83. Hostetter TH: Hypertrophy and hyperfunction of the diabetic kidney. *J Clin Invest* 2001;107:161.

84. Borch-Johnsen K, Nissen H, Henriksen E, *et al*: The natural history of insulin-dependent diabetes mellitus in Denmark. 1. Long term survival with and without late diabetic complications. *Diabet Med* 1987;4:201.

85. Mogensen CE: Microalbuminuria, blood pressure and diabetic renal disease: Origin and development of ideas. *Diabetologia* 1999;42:263.

86. Nelson RG, Bennett PH, Beck GJ, *et al*: Development and progression of renal disease in Pima Indians with non-insulin-dependent diabetes mellitus. *N Engl J Med* 1996;335:1636.

87. Knowler WC, Bennett PH, Hamman RF, *et al*: Diabetes incidence and prevalence in Pima Indians: A 19-fold greater incidence than in Rochester, Minnesota. *Am J Epidemiol* 1978;108:497.

88. Hasslacher C, Ritz E, Wahl P, *et al*: Similar risk of nephropathy in patients with type I or type II diabetes mellitus. *Nephrol Dial Transplant* 1989;4:859.

89. Ritz E, Orth SR: Nephropathy in patients with type 2 diabetes mellitus. *N Engl J Med* 1999;341:1127.

90. Mogensen CE, Osterby R, Gundersen HJG: Early functional and morphologic vascular renal consequences of the diabetic state. *Diabetologia* 1979;17:71.

91. Wiseman MJ, Saunders AJ, Keen H, *et al*: Effect of blood glucose control on increased glomerular filtration rate and kidney size in insulin-dependent diabetes. *N Engl J Med* 1985;312:617.

92. Tuttle KR, Bruton JL, Perusek MC, *et al*: Effects of strict glycemic control on basal and insulin stimulated renal hemodynamic and kidney size in insulin-dependent diabetes mellitus. *N Engl J Med* 1991;324:1626.

93. Thomsen OF, Andersen AR, Christiansen JS, *et al*: Renal changes in long-term type I (insulin-dependent) diabetic patients with and without clinical nephropathy: A light microscopic, morphometric study of autopsy material. *Diabetologia* 1984;26:361.

94. Kverneland A, Feldt-Rasmussen B, Vidal P, *et al*: Evidence of changes in renal charge selectivity in patients with type I (insulin-dependent) diabetes mellitus. *Diabetologia* 1986;29:634.

95. Viberti GC, Wiseman M, Radmond RS: Microalbuminuria: Its history and potential for prevention of clinical nephropathy in diabetes mellitus. *Diabet Nephropathy* 1984;3:79.

96. Parving HH, Oxenboll B, Svendsen PA, *et al*: Early detection of patients at risk of developing diabetic nephropathy: A longitudinal study of urinary albumin excretion. *Acta Endocrinol (Copenh)* 1982;100:550.

97. Mogensen CE, Christensen CK: Predicting diabetic nephropathy in insulin-dependent patients. *N Engl J Med* 1984;311:89.

98. Mogensen CE, Viberti GC, Preheim E, *et al*: Multicenter evaluation of the micral-test II test strip, an immunologic rapid test for the detection of microalbuminuria. *Diabetes Care* 1997;20:1642.

99. Mogensen CE: Microalbuminuria predicts clinical proteinuria and early mortality in maturity-onset diabetes. *N Engl J Med* 1984; 310:356.

100. Ruggenenti P, Remuzzi G: Nephropathy of type-2 diabetes mellitus. *J Am Soc Nephrol* 1998;9:2157.

101. Gall MA, Rossing P, Skott P, *et al*: Prevalence of micro- and macroalbuminuria, arterial hypertension, retinopathy and large vessel disease in European type 2 (non-insulin-dependent) diabetic patients. *Diabetologia* 1991;34:655.

102. Mattock MB, Morrish NJ, Viberti G, *et al*: Prospective study of microalbuminuria as predictor of mortality in NIDDM. *Diabetes* 1992; 41:736.

103. Nelson RG, Meyer TW, Myers BD, *et al*: Clinical and pathological course of renal disease in non-insulin-dependent diabetes mellitus: The Pima Indians experience. *Semin Nephrol* 1997;17:124.

104. Schmitz A, Vaeth M: Microalbuminuria: A major risk factor in non-insulin dependent diabetes: A 10-year follow-up study of 503 patients. *Diabetic Med* 1988;5:126, 1988.

105. Caramori ML, Fioretto P, Mauer M: The need for early predictors of diabetic nephropathy risk. *Diabetes* 2000;49,1399.

106. Lee JA, Little HL, Myers BD: Consensus statement. *Am J Kidney Dis* 1989;13:2.

107. Friedman S, Jones HW, Golbetz HV, *et al*: Mechanisms of proteinuria in diabetic nephropathy. II. A study of the size selective glomerular filtration barriers. *Diabetes* 1983;32:40.

108. Deckert T, Kofoed-Enevoldsen A, Vidal P: Size and charge selectivity of glomerular filtration in type 1 (insulin-dependent) diabetic patients with and without albuminuria. *Diabetologia* 1993;36:244.

109. Bangstad H-J, Kofoed-Enevoldsen A, Dahl-Jorgensen K, *et al*: Glomerular charge selectivity and the influence of improved blood glucose control in type 1 (insulin-dependent) diabetic patients with microalbuminuria. *Diabetologia* 1992;35:1165.

110. Mogensen CE: Glomerular hyperfiltration in human diabetes. *Diabetes Care* 1994;17:770.

111. Rudberg S, Persson B, Dahlquist G: Increased glomerular filtration rate as a predictor of diabetic nephropathy: Results from an 8-year prospective study. *Kidney Int* 1992;41:822.

112. Mogensen CE: Maximum tubular reabsorption capacity for glucose and renal hemodynamics during rapid hypertonic glucose infusion in normal and diabetic men. *Scand J Clin Lab Invest* 1971;28:101.

113. DeFronzo RA, Smith JD: Disorders of potassium metabolism: Hyperkalemia. In: Arieff A, DeFronzo RA, eds. *Fluid, Electrolyte and Acid-Base Disorders*. Churchill Livingstone:1995;319.

114. DeFronzo RA.: Hyperkalemia and hyporeninemic hypoaldosteronism. *Kidney Int* 1980;17:118.

115. Schambelan M, Sebastian A, Biglieri E: Prevalence, pathogenesis, and functional significance of aldosterone deficiency in hyperkalemic patients with chronic renal insufficiency. *Kidney Int* 1980;17:89.

116. deChatel R, Weidmann P, Flammer J, *et al*: Sodium, renin, aldosterone, catecholamines and blood pressure in diabetes mellitus. *Kidney Int* 1977;12:412.

117. Halperin ML, Bear RA, Hannaford MC, *et al*: Selected aspects of the pathophysiology of metabolic acidosis in diabetes mellitus. *Diabetes* 1981;30:781.

118. Root HF, Porte WH, Frehner H: Triopathy of diabetes: sequence of neuropathy, retinopathy, and nephropathy. *Arch Intern Med* 1984; 94:931.

119. Pirart J: Diabetes mellitus and its degenerative complications: a prospective study of 4400 patients observed between 1944 and 1973. *Diabetes Care* 1978;1:168.

120. Bilous RW, Viberti GC, Christiansen JS, Bilous RW, Viberti GC, Sandahl-Christensen J, Parving H-H, Keen H: Dissociation of diabetic complications in insulin-dependent diabetics: a clinical report. *Diabetic Nephropathy* 1985;4:73.

121. Chahal PS, Kohner EM: The relationship between diabetic retinopathy and diabetic nephropathy. *Diabetic Nephropathy* 1983;2:4.

122. Strowig SM, Raskin P: Glycemic control and the complications of diabetes. *Diabetes Rev* 1995;3:237.

123. Hamman RF: Epidemiology of microvascular complications. In: Alberti KGMM, Zimmet P, DeFronzo RA, eds. *International Textbook of Diabetes Mellitus*. John Wiley 1997;1293.

124. Friedlander MA, Hricik DE: Optimizing end-stage renal disease therapy for the patient with diabetes mellitus. *Semin Nephrol* 1997; 17:331.

125. Goldstein DA, Massry SG: Diabetic nephropathy: clinical course and effect of hemodialysis. *Nephron* 1978;20:286.

126. McCrary RF, Pitts TO, Puschett JB: Diabetic nephropathy: natural course, survivorship, and therapy. *Am J Nephrol* 1981;1:206.

127. Orchard TJ, Dorman JS, Maser RE, *et al*: Prevalence of complications in IDDM by sex and duration. Pittsburgh Epidemiology of Diabetes Complications Study. *Diabetes* 1990;39:1116.

128. Sima AAF, Thomas PF, Ishil D, *et al*: Diabetic neuropathies. *Diabetologia* 1997;40:B74.

129. Eisenberg B, Murata G, Tzamaloukas A, *et al*: Gastroparesis in diabetics on chronic dialysis: Clinical and laboratory associations and predictive features. *Nephrology* 1995;70:296.

130. Najarian JS, Sutherland DER, Simmons RL, *et al*: Kidney transplantation for the uremic diabetic patient. *Surg Gynecol Obstet* 1977; 144:682.

131. Mogensen CE: Prediction of clinical diabetic nephropathy in IDDM patients. Alternatives to microalbuminuria? *Diabetes* 1990;39:761.

132. Mathiesen ER: Prevention of diabetic nephropathy. Microalbuminuria and perspectives for intervention in insulin-dependent diabetes. *Dan Med Bull* 1993;40:273.

133. Nosadini R, Fioretto P, Trevisan R, *et al*: Insulin-dependent diabetes mellitus and hypertension. *Diabetes Care* 1991;14:210.

134. Bakris GL, Williams M, Dworkin L, *et al*: Preserving renal function in adults with hypertension and diabetes: A consensus approach. *Am J Kidney Dis* 2000;36:646.

135. Markell MS, Friedman EA: Care of the diabetic patients with end-stage renal disease. *Semin Nephrol* 1990;10:274.

136. Venkatesan J, Henrich WL: Anemia, hypertension, and myocardial dysfunction in end-stage renal disease. *Semin Nephrol* 1997;17:257.

137. Kjellstrand CM, Whitley K, Comty CM, *et al*: Dialysis in patients with diabetes mellitus. *Diabet Nephropathy* 1983;2:5.

138. Vasan RS, Larson MG, Leip EP, *et al*: Impact of high-normal blood pressure on the risk of cardiovascular disease. *N Engl J Med* 2001; 345,1291.

139. Elving LD, Wetzels JFM, van Lier HJJ, *et al*: Captopril and atenolol are equally effective in retarding progression of diabetic nephropathy. Results of a 2-year prospective, randomized study. *Diabetologia* 1994;37:604.

140. Kshirsagar AV, Joy MS, Hogan SL, *et al*: Effect of ACE inhibitors in diabetic and nondiabetic chronic renal disease: A systematic overview of randomized placebo-controlled trials. *Am J Kidney Dis* 2000;35; 695.

141. Hovind P, Rossing P, Tarnow L, *et al*: Progression of diabetic nephropathy. *Kidney Int* 2001;59:702.

142. Mogensen CE: Progression of nephropathy in long-term diabetics with proteinuria and effect of initial anti-hypertensive treatment. *Scand J Clin Lab Invest* 1976;36:383.

143. Parving H-H: Impact of blood pressure and antihypertensive treatment on incipient and overt nephropathy, retinopathy, and endothelial permeability in diabetes mellitus. *Diabetes Care* 1991;14:260.

144. Mogensen CE: Long-term antihypertensive treatment inhibiting progression of diabetic nephropathy. *Br Med J* 1982;285:685.

145. Parving H-H, Andersen AR, Smidt UM, *et al*: Effect of antihypertensive treatment on kidney function in diabetic nephropathy. *Br Med J* 1987;294:1443.

146. Lewis EJ, Hunsicker LG, Bain RP, *et al*: The effect of angiotensin-converting-enzyme inhibition on diabetic nephropathy. *N Engl J Med* 1993;329:1456.

147. Berkman J, Rifkin H: Unilateral nodular diabetic glomerulosclerosis (Kimmelsteil-Wilson): Report of a case. *Metabolism* 1973;22:175.

148. Steffes MW, Buchwald H, Wigness BD, *et al*: Diabetic nephropathy in the uninephrectomized dog: Microscopic lesions after one year. *Kidney Int* 1982;21:721.

149. Barbosa J, Steffes MW, Sutherland DE, *et al*: Effects of glycemic control on early diabetic renal lesions: A 5-year randomized controlled trial of insulin-dependent diabetic kidney transplant recipients. *JAMA* 1944;272:600.

150. Krolewski AS, Canessa M, Warram JH, *et al*: Predisposition to hypertension and susceptibility to renal disease in insulin-dependent diabetes mellitus. *N Engl J Med* 1988;318:140.

151. DeFronzo RA, Ferrannini E: Insulin resistance: A multifaceted syndrome responsible for NIDDM, obesity, hypertension, dyslipidemia, and ASCVD. *Diabetes Care* 1991;14:173.

152. The Sixth Report of the Joint National Committee on Prevention, Detection, Evaluation, and Treatment of High Blood Pressure. *Arch Intern Med* 1997;157:2413.

153. Hansson L, Zanchetti A, Carruthers SG, *et al*: Effects of intensive blood-pressure lowering and low-dose aspirin in patients with hyper-

tension: Principal results of the Hypertension Optimal Treatment (HOT) randomized trial. *Lancet* 1998;351:1755.

154. Bakris GL: Pathogenesis of hypertension in diabetes. *Diabetes Rev* 1995;3:460.

155. Ismail N, Becker B, Strzelcyzyk P, *et al*: Renal disease and hypertension in non-insulin-dependent diabetes mellitus. *Kidney Int* 1999; 55:1.

156. Elliott WJ, Stein PP, Black HR: Drug treatment of hypertension in patients with diabetes. *Diabetes Rev* 1995;3:477.

157. Bressler P, DeFronzo RA: Drugs and diabetes. *Diabetes Rev* 1994; 2:53.

158. UK Prospective Diabetes Study Group (UKPDS): Tight blood pressure control and risk of macrovascular and microvascular complications in type 2 diabetes: UKPDS 38. *Br Med J* 1998;317:703.

159. Taal MW, Brenner BM: Renoprotective benefits of RAS inhibition: From ACEI to angiotensin II antagonists. *Kidney Int* 2000;57:1803.

160. Ravid M, Savin H, Jutrin I, *et al*: Long-term stabilizing effect of angiotensin-converting enzyme inhibition on plasma proteinuria in normotensive type II diabetic patients. *Ann Intern Med* 1993;188:577.

161. Ravid M, Brosh D, Levi Z, *et al*: Use of enalapril to attenuate decline in renal function in normotensive, normoalbuminuric patients with type 2 diabetes mellitus. A randomized, controlled trial. *Ann Intern Med* 1998;128:982.

162. Mogensen CE: Microalbuminuria, early blood pressure elevation, and diabetic renal disease. *Curr Opin Endocrinol Diabetes* 1994;4:239.

163. Viberti G, Chaturvedi N: Angiotensin converting enzyme inhibitors in diabetic patients with microalbuminuria or normoalbuminuria. *Kidney Int* 1997;52(suppl 63):S-32.

164. The Microalbuminuria Captopril Study Group: Captopril reduces the risk of nephropathy in IDDM patients with microalbuminuria. *Diabetologia* 1996;39:587.

165. Nielsen FS, Rossing P, Gall M-A, *et al*: Long-term effect of lisinopril and atenolol on kidney function in hypertensive NIDDM subjects with diabetic nephropathy. *Diabetes* 1997;46:1182.

166. Lithell HOL: Effect of antihypertensive drugs on insulin, glucose, and lipid metabolism. *Diabetes Care* 1991;14:203.

167. Ganesvoort RT, de Zeeuw D, de Jong PE: Is the antiproteinuric effect of ACE inhibition mediated by interference in the renin-angiotensin system? *Kidney Int* 1994;45:861.

168. Lewis EJ, Hunsicker LG, Clarke WR, *et al*: Renoprotective effect of the angiotensin-receptor antagonist irbesartan in patients with nephropathy due to type 2 diabetes. *N Engl J Med* 2001;345:851.

169. Brenner BM, Cooper ME, De Zeeuw D, *et al*: Effects of losartan on renal and cardiovascular outcomes in patients with type 2 diabetes and nephropathy. *N Engl J Med* 2001;345:861.

170. Parving HH, Lehnert H, Brochner-Mortensen J, *et al*: The effect of irbesartan on the development of diabetic nephropathy in patients with type 2 diabetes. *N Engl J Med* 2001;345:870.

171. Farhy RD, Carretero OA, Ho K-L, *et al*: Role of kinins and nitric oxide in the effects of angiotensin converting enzyme inhibitors on neointima formation. *Circ Res* 1993;72:1202.

172. Giordano M, Matsuda M, Canessa ML, *et al*: The effects of ACE inhibitors, calcium channel antagonists, and alpha adrenergic blockers on glucose and lipid metabolism in type II diabetic patients with hypertension. *Diabetes* 1995;44:665.

173. Giordano M, Sanders LR, Castellino P, *et al*: Effect of alpha-adrenergic blockers, ACE inhibitors, and calcium channel antagonists on renal function in non-insulin dependent diabetic patients. *Nephron* 1996;72:447.

174. Bakris GL, Copley JB, Vicknair N, *et al*: Calcium channel blockers versus other antihypertensive therapies on progression of NIDDM associated nephropathy. *Kidney Int* 1996;50:1641.

175. Zucchelli P, Zuccala A, Borghi M, *et al*: Long-term comparison between captopril and nifedipine in the progression of renal insufficiency. *Kidney Int* 1992;42;452.

176. Kloke HJ, Branten AJ, Huysmans FT, *et al*: Antihypertensive treatment of patients with proteinuric renal diseases: Risks or benefits of calcium channel blockers? *Kidney Int* 1998;53:1559.

177. Velussi M, Brocco E, Frigato F, *et al*: Effects of cilazapril and amlodipine on kidney function in hypertensive NIDDM patients. *Diabetes* 1996;45:216.

178. Munter K, Hergenroder S, Jochims K, *et al*: Individual and combined effects of verapamil or trandolapril on attenuating hypertensive glomerulopathic changes in the stroke-prone rat. *J Am Soc Nephrol* 1996;7:681.

179. Bakris GL, Weir MR, DeQuattro V, *et al*: Effects of an ACE inhibitor/calcium antagonist combination on proteinuria in diabetic nephropathy. *Kidney Int* 1998;54:1283.

180. Stefanski A, Amann K, Ritz E: To prevent progression: ACE inhibitors, calcium antagonists or both? *Nephrol Dial Transplant* 1995; 10:151.

181. Tuomilehto J, Rastenyte D, Birkenhager WH, *et al*: Effects of calcium-channel blockade in older patients with diabetes and systolic hypertension. Systolic Hypertension in Europe Trial Investigators. *N Engl J Med* 1999;340:677.

182. Mathiesen ER, Hommel E, Giese J, *et al*: Efficacy of captopril in postponing nephropathy in normotensive insulin dependent diabetic patients with microalbuminuria. *Br Med J* 1991;303:81.

183. Marre M, Chatellier G, Leblanc H, *et al*: Prevention of diabetic nephropathy with enalapril in normotensive diabetics with microalbuminuria. *Br Med J* 1988;297:1092.

184. Chase HP, Garg SK, Harris S, *et al*: Angiotensin-converting enzyme inhibitor treatment for young normotensive diabetic subjects: A two year trial. *Ann Ophthalmol* 1993;25:284.

185. Viberti G, Mogensen CE, Groop LC, *et al*: Effect of captopril on progression to clinical proteinuria in patients with insulin-dependent diabetes mellitus and microalbuminuria. *JAMA* 1994;271:275.

186. Laffel LMB, McGill JB, Gans DJ: The beneficial effects of angiotensin-converting enzyme inhibition with captopril on diabetic nephropathy in normotensive IDDM patients with microalbuminuria. *Am J Med* 1995;99:497.

187. EUCLID Study Group: Randomized placebo-controlled trial on lisinopril in normotensive patients with insulin-dependent diabetes and normoalbuminuria or microalbuminuria. *Lancet* 1997;349:787.

188. Capek M, Schnack C, Ludvik B, *et al*: Effect of captopril treatment versus placebo on renal function in type 2 diabetic patients with microalbuminuria: A long-term study. *J Clin Invest* 1994;72:961.

189. Bakris GL, Slataper R, Vicknair N, *et al*: ACE inhibitor-mediated reductions in renal size and microalbuminuria in normotensive, diabetic subjects. *J Diabetes Complications* 1994;8:2.

190. Ahmad J, Siddiqui MA, Ahmad H: Effective postponement of diabetic nephropathy with enalapril in normotensive type 2 diabetic patients with microalbuminuria. *Diabetes Care* 1997;20:1576.

191. Crepaldi G, Carta Q, Deferrari G, *et al*: Effects of lisinopril and nifedipine on the progression to overt albuminuria in IDDM patients with incipient nephropathy and normal blood pressure. *Diabetes Care* 1998;21:104.

192. Heart Outcomes Prevention Evaluation (HOPE) Study Investigators: Effects of ramipril on cardiovascular and microvascular outcomes in people with diabetes mellitus: Results of the HOPE study and MICRO-HOPE substudy. *Lancet* 2000;355:253.

193. Heart Outcomes Prevention Evaluation (HOPE) Study Investigators: Effects of an angiotensin-converting-enzyme inhibitor, ramipril, on cardiovascular events in high-risk patients. *N Engl J Med* 2000; 342:145.

194. Hansson L, Lindholm LH, Niskanen L, *et al*: Effect of angiotensin-converting-enzyme inhibition compared with conventional therapy on cardiovascular morbidity and mortality in hypertension: The Captopril Prevention Project (CAPP) randomized trial. *Lancet* 1999;353:611.

195. Bryd L, Sherman RL: Radio-contrast-induced renal failure: A clinical and pathophysiologic review. *Medicine* 1979;58:270.

196. Solomon R, Werner C, Mann D, *et al*: Effects of saline, mannitol, and furosemide to prevent acute decreases in renal function induced by radiocontrast agents. *N Engl J Med* 1994;331:1416.

197. Klein R: Hyperglycemia and microvascular and macrovascular disease in diabetes. *Diabetes Care* 1995;18:258.

198. Microalbuminuria Collaborative Study Group: Microalbuminuria in type I diabetic patients. *Diabetes Care* 1992;15:495.

199. Bilous RW, Mauer SM, Sutherland DER, *et al*: The effects of pancreas transplantation on the glomerular structure of renal allografts in patients with insulin-dependent diabetes. *N Engl J Med* 1989;321:80.

200. Fioretto P, Mauer SM, Bilous RW, *et al*: Effects of pancreas transplantation on glomerular structure in insulin-dependent diabetic patients with their own kidneys. *Lancet* 1993;342:1193.

201. Rasch R: Prevention of diabetic glomerulopathy in streptozotocin diabetic rats by insulin treatment. *Diabetologia* 1979;16:125.

202. Feldt-Rasmussen B: Microalbuminuria and clinical nephropathy in type 1 (insulin-dependent) diabetes mellitus: Pathophysiological mechanisms and intervention studies. *Dan Med Bull* 1989;36:405.

203. The Kroc Collaborative Study Group: Blood glucose control and the evolution of diabetic retinopathy and albuminuria: A preliminary multicenter trial. *N Engl J Med* 1984;311:365.

204. DeFronzo RA, Alvestrand A, Smith D, *et al*: Insulin resistance in uremia. *J Clin Invest* 1981;67:563.

205. DeFronzo RA, Tobin JD, Rowe JW, *et al*: Glucose intolerance in uremia: Quantification of pancreatic beta cell sensitivity to glucose and tissue sensitivity to insulin. *J Clin Invest* 1978;62:425.

206. DeFronzo RA: Pharmacologic therapy for type 2 diabetes mellitus. *Ann Intern Med* 1999;131:281.

207. Fuji M, Takemura R, Yamaguchi M, *et al*: Troglitazone (CS-045) ameliorates albuminuria in streptozocin-induced diabetic rats. *Metabolism* 1997;45:981.

208. McCarthy KJ, Routh RE, Shaw W, *et al*: Troglitazone halts diabetic glomerulosclerosis by blockade of mesangial expansion. *Kidney Int* 2000;58:2341.

209. Sambol NC, Chiang J, Lin ET, *et al*: Kidney function and age are both predictors of pharmacokinetics of metformin. *J Clin Pharmacol* 1995;35:1094.

210. Prendergast BD: Glyburide and glipizide, second-generation oral sulfonylurea hypoglycemic agents. *Clin Pharmacol* 1984;3:473.

211. Rosenkranz B: Pharmacokinetic basis for the safety of glimepiride in risk groups of NIDDM patients. *Horm Metab Res* 1996;28:434.

212. Marbury T, Huang W-C, Strange P, *et al*: Repaglinide versus glyburide: a one-year comparison trial. *Diabetes Res Clin Prac* 1999; 43:155.

213. Tzamaloukas AH: Interpreting glycosylated hemoglobin in diabetic patients on peritoneal dialysis. *Adv Peritoneal Dialysis* 1996;12:171.

214. Garber AJ, Bier D, Cryer PE, *et al*: Hypoglycemia in compensated chronic renal insufficiency: substrate limitation of gluconeogenesis. *Diabetes* 1974;23:982.

215. Grajower M, Walter L, Albin J: Hypoglycemia in chronic hemodialysis patients: association with propranolol use. *Nephron* 1980;26:126.

216. Wong TY-H, Chan JCN, Szeto CC, *et al*: Clinical and biochemical characteristics of type 2 diabetic patients on continuous ambulatory peritoneal dialysis: relationships with insulin requirement. *Am J Kidney Dis* 1999;34:514.

217. Giordano C: Protein restriction in chronic renal failure. *Kidney Int* 1982;22:401.

218. Brenner BM, Meyer TW, Hostetter TH: Dietary protein intake and the progressive nature of kidney disease. *N Engl J Med* 1982;307:652.

219. Zeller KR, Whittaker E, Sullivan L, *et al*: Effect of restricting dietary protein on the progression of renal failure in patients with insulin-dependent diabetes mellitus. *N Engl J Med* 1991;324:78.

220. Pedrini MT, Levey AS, Lau J, Chalmers TC, Wang PH: The effect of dietary protein restriction on the progression of diabetic and non-diabetic renal disease: a meta-analysis. *Ann Intern Med* 1996;124:627.

221. Walker JD, Dodds RA, Murrells TJ, *et al*: Restriction of dietary protein and progression of renal failure in diabetic nephropathy. *Lancet* 1989;ii:1411.

222. Klahr S, Levey AS, Beck GJ, *et al*: The effects of dietary protein restriction and blood-pressure control on the progression of chronic renal disease. *N Engl J Med* 1994;330:877.

223. Modification of Diet in Renal Disease Study Group: Effects of dietary protein restriction on the progression of moderate renal disease in the modification of diet in renal disease study. *J Am Soc Nephrol* 1996; 7:2616.

224. Kasiske BL: Hyperlipidemia in patients with chronic renal disease. *Am J Kidney Dis* 1998;32:S142.

225. Deckert T, Feldt-Rasmussen B, Borch-Johnsen K, Kofoed-Enevoldsen JT: Albuminuria reflects widespread vascular damage. The Steno Hypothesis. *Diabetologia* 1989;32:219.

226. Wilson PWF, Culleton BF: Cardiovascular disease in the general population. Epidemiology of cardiovascular disease in the United States. *Am J Kidney Dis* 1998;32(suppl 3):S89.

227. Wilson PWF: Diabetes mellitus and coronary heart disease. *Am J Kidney Dis* 1998;32(suppl 3)S89.

228. United States Renal Data System: USRDS 1999 Annual Data Report: V. Patient mortality and survival. *Am J Kidney Dis* 1999;34(suppl 1):S74.

229. United States Renal Data System: USRDS 1999 Annual Data Report: VI. Causes of Death. *Am J Kidney Dis* 1999;34(suppl 1):S87.

230. Herzog CA, Ma JZ, Collins AJ: Long-term outcome of dialysis patients in the United States with coronary revascularization procedures. *Kidney Int* 1999;56:324.

231. United States Renal Data System: USRDS 1999 Annual Data Report. VII. Renal transplantation: access and outcomes. *Am J Kidney Dis* 1999;34(suppl 1):S95.

232. Herzog CA: Acute myocardial infarction in patients with end-stage renal disease. *Kidney Int* 1999;56(suppl 71):S130.

233. Oda H, Keane WF: Recent advances in statins and the kidney. *Kidney Int* 1999;56(suppl 71):S-2.

234. Keane WF: Lipids and progressive renal disease: the cardio-renal link. *Am J Kidney Dis* 1999;34:xliii.

235. Krolewski AS, Warram JH, Christlieb AR: Hypercholesterolemia: a determinant of renal function loss and deaths of IDDM patients with nephropathy. *Kidney Int* 1994;45(Suppl 45):S125.

236. Kasiske BL, O'Donnell MP, Schmitz PG, *et al*: Renal injury of diet-induced hypercholesterolemia in rats. *Kidney Int* 1990;37:880.

237. Wellman KF, Volk BW: Renal changes in experimental hypercholesterolemia in normal and subdiabetic rabbits. II. Long-term studies. *Lab Invest* 1971;24:144.

238. Kasiske BL, O'Donnell MP, Cleary MP, *et al*: Treatment of hyperlipidemia reduces glomerular injury in obese Zucker rats. *Kidney Int* 1988;33;667.

239. Fried LF, Orchard TJ, Kasiske BL: Effect of lipid reduction on the progression of renal disease: a meta-analysis. *Kidney Int* 2001;59:260.

240. Ritz E, Rychlik I, Locatelli F, *et al*: End-stage renal failure in type 2 diabetes; a medical catastrophe of worldwide dimensions. *Am J Kidney Dis* 1999;34:795.

241. Comty CM, Leonard A, Shapiro FL: Nutritional and metabolic problems in dialyzed patients with diabetes mellitus. *Kidney Int* 1974; 6:S51.

242. Smets YFC, Westendorp RGJ, van der Pijl JW, *et al*: Effect of simultaneous pancreas-kidney transplantation on mortality of patients with type-1 diabetes mellitus and end-stage renal failure. *Lancet* 1999;353:1915.

243. Lederer E: Pancreas transplants for diabetic nephropathy: a time for reassessment. *Am J Kidney Dis* 2000;35:1238.

CHAPTER 44

Pathogenesis of Diabetic Neuropathy

Martin J. Stevens

Irina Obrosova

Rodica Pop-Busui

Douglas A. Greene

Eva L. Feldman

The classical histologic studies of autopsy and nerve biopsy material from patients with diabetic neuropathy have identified lesions involving peripheral nerve axons. Schwann cells, perineurial cells, and endoneurial vascular elements may contribute to the pathogenesis of the most common form of diabetic neuropathy, distal symmetric peripheral polyneuropathy.[1–10]

PATHOLOGY

Lesions identified include damage to and loss of large and small myelinated nerve fibers with evidence of wallerian degeneration; segmental and paranodal demyelination; and proliferation of endoneurial connective tissue including thickening and reduplication of the basement membranes of nerve fibers, endoneurial blood vessels, and the perineurium. The proximal-to-distal increase in morphologic abnormalities[1,11] and the topographic and temporal distribution of neurologic signs and symptoms in the distal symmetric polyneuropathy of diabetes suggest a primary axonopathy preferentially involving longer myelinated axons.[10,12–15] Nerve biopsies from young diabetic patients characteristically exhibit ultrastructural lesions most consistent with an early primary distal axonal atrophy and degeneration.[8,10,16] However, studies of sural nerve biopsies by Thomas and Lascelles[3,17] and others[7,9] and autopsy studies[6] have emphasized segmental demyelination and remyelination in diabetic distal symmetric polyneuropathy, postulating a primary abnormality of Schwann cells.

Diabetic polyneuropathy may also be characterized by defective axonal regeneration,[18–21] which has been reported to be both positively[18] and negatively[20] correlated with the degree of nerve fiber loss. Progression of diabetic polyneuropathy has been associated with preferential loss of small (<5 μm) myelinated fibers, which may be most sensitive to glucose toxicity.[22] Endoneurial vascular abnormalities such as basement membrane thickening and reduplication, endothelial cell swelling and proliferation, and platelet aggregation resulting in vessel occlusion have been noted in sural nerve biopsies[4,23] and at autopsy[2,5,11,24,25] of diabetic patients. A quantitative increase in these vascular abnormalities in association with focal loss of myelinated fibers in older diabetic subjects has been interpreted to suggest hypoxic or ischemic damage to nerve fibers in diabetic subjects.[1,4,23] Thus, while demonstrating that most tissue elements of peripheral nerve are involved in the disease process at some point, existing studies of human diabetic distal symmetric polyneuropathy provide no consistent evidence as to the location of the initial inciting event.

The neuropathology of diabetic autonomic neuropathy has been less well studied, in part because biopsy material is not readily available. A few reported autopsy studies have demonstrated axonal degenerative changes and fiber loss in the paravertebral sympathetic chain,[13] the vagus nerve, the esophageal and splanchnic nerves,[10,14,15] and the intrinsic nerves of the bladder. Swelling and vacuolization of autonomic ganglionic neurons have been described.[10,14,15]

Relationship of Neuropathy to the Duration and Metabolic Severity of Diabetes in Humans

The relationship of diabetic neuropathy to the severity and duration of hyperglycemia and associated metabolic derangements has important therapeutic as well as pathogenetic implications. A close link between the severity and/or duration of hyperglycemia and the development of diabetic neuropathy would support intensified diabetic control as a potential preventive measure and would implicate glucose- or insulin-related metabolic factors as important pathogenetic elements in the disease process. The Diabetes Control and Complications Trial (DCCT) has provided strong evidence for the importance of insulin deficiency, hyperglycemia, or both in the pathogenesis of diabetic neuropathy.[26] After 5 years, intensive diabetes treatment designed to lower blood glucose to as close to the normal range as possible in nonneuropathic subjects with type 1 diabetes mellitus (T1DM) was able to reduce the prevalence of clinical diabetic neuropathy confirmed by abnormal nerve conduction or autonomic function by 60%.

Pirart's[27] 25-year prospective study of 4400 unselected patients in a diabetic clinic probably provides the most convincing epidemiologic link between the duration and severity of metabolic abnormality and the presence of clinical neuropathy in diabetic patients. Neuropathy, defined as loss of Achilles and/or patellar reflexes combined with diminished vibratory sensation in the presence or absence of "more dramatic polyneuropathy or mono- or multi-neuropathy," was present in 12% of patients when diabetes was diagnosed, with onset of neuropathy tending to cluster in older type 2 diabetic mellitus (T2DM) patients, in whom antecedent undiagnosed hyperglycemia is difficult to exclude. Thereafter, the cumulative prevalence of neuropathy increased linearly with duration of diabetes to nearly 50% after 25 years.[27,28]

The prevalence of neuropathy corrected for duration of diabetes did not differ substantially as a function of age at time of diagnosis,[27] suggesting that the development of neuropathy is similar in T1DM and T2DM despite fundamental differences in the pathogenesis of the underlying metabolic abnormality. On the other hand, the cumulative prevalence of neuropathy increased with duration of diabetes much more rapidly and attained a much higher prevalence in patients whose diabetes was poorly controlled compared with those whose diabetes was moderately or well controlled.[27] Since diabetic neuropathy also occurs in secondary forms of diabetes (pancreatectomy, nonalcoholic pancreatitis, and hemachromatosis),[29] neuropathy would appear to be unrelated to the underlying pathogenetic mechanism(s) of diabetes but would instead constitute a concomitant or consequence of the diabetic state as defined by hyperglycemia. Thus the preventive effect of intensive insulin therapy on neuropathy in T1DM established in the DCCT[26] would be expected to extend to T2DM as well. Indeed, in the United Kingdom Prospective Diabetes Study (UKPDS), intensified diabetes control was associated with less severe deficits of vibration perception threshold after 15 years.[30]

The prevalence of diabetic neuropathy, although initially low, increases progressively with duration and severity of insulin deficiency and hyperglycemia.[27,28,31] However, the relationship between immediately antecedent blood glucose control and the development of diabetic clinical neuropathy is more controversial. The appearance of clinically overt diabetic neuropathy clearly does not uniformly follow a prolonged period of unambiguous severe insulin deficiency and hyperglycemia.[32] Since the development of clinically overt neuropathy merely represents a progression from long-standing underlying subclinical neuropathy, temporal dissociation between the momentary quality of glucose control and the development of clinical signs and symptoms of neuropathy is not entirely unexpected. As mentioned above, neuropathic symptoms and signs in newly diagnosed diabetes are usually confined to T2DM, in which the duration of antecedent occult hyperglycemia may be prolonged.[27] The sometimes reported "paradoxic precipitation of neuropathy following institution of good control"[32] refers primarily to the acute onset of painful neuropathic symptoms that may as likely reflect repair and regeneration of damaged nerve fibers as disease progression.[24,33] Therefore, despite the close epidemiologic association between clinical neuropathy and the duration and severity of hyperglycemia in populations of diabetic patients,[27,31,34] the onset of clinically overt diabetic neuropathy in an individual patient is an unpredictable event, neither necessarily reflecting concurrent metabolic control[35] nor following inexorably from prolonged and severe hyperglycemia.[27]

This somewhat loose clinical association can be understood in terms of the indolent and occult nature of the underlying subclinical nerve damage, but it also may indicate the presence of other independent pathogenetic variables such as genetic, nutritional, toxic (e.g., alcohol[36]), and mechanical (entrapment and compression[31]) factors that may influence the appearance of clinical signs and symptoms in individual patients. Unfortunately, clinical neuro-

pathy was not reassessed in the DCCT until the fifth year after initiation of intensive diabetes therapy, so that the temporal association between the institution of diabetes control and the development of neuropathy could not be determined.[26]

A characteristic neurophysiologic defect in diabetes is slowing of motor and sensory nerve conduction velocity (NCV), which can be attributed to several types of physiologic and anatomic abnormalities. Maximum NCV primarily reflects the integrity of the largest and most rapidly conducting myelinated nerve fibers; it is only modestly decreased with the selective loss of the largest myelinated fibers since smaller fibers conduct only slightly more slowly; on the other hand, conduction is markedly slowed with widespread demyelination.[37] Patients with long-standing, established diabetes exhibit consistent but mild evidence of motor and sensory conduction slowing, whereas patients with clinically overt diabetic neuropathy have slightly more severe electrophysiologic abnormalities than patients with subclinical neuropathy.[38] Motor nerve conduction velocity (MNCV) is slightly reduced at diagnosis of T1DM, but it improves rapidly with and declines rapidly without insulin replacement therapy in a pattern consistent with an initial, direct, and reversible metabolic contribution to motor conduction slowing in newly diagnosed diabetes.[39,40] An initial improvement in motor conduction velocity is accompanied by improved vibratory perception threshold, implying a physiologic significance for this reversible functional defect and evidence that both sensory and motor fibers are involved.[41] Nerve conduction velocity slows progressively but modestly in both T1DM and T2DM as a function of duration of disease.[42,43] In patients with overt diabetic neuropathy, slowing of sensory conduction velocity correlates closely with loss of the largest myelinated fibers, with only a small residual component of conduction slowing attributable to other factors, for example, "metabolic" factors (or possible undetected demyelination).[5] Nerve conduction velocity inversely correlates with the degree of hyperglycemia as measured by the percentage of glycosylated hemoglobin (HbA$_{1c}$).[44]

Because the preponderance of conduction slowing in clinically established (and most likely also chronic subclinical) diabetic neuropathy can be accounted for by poorly reversible loss of large myelinated fibers, improvement of NCV following acute metabolic correction is necessarily confined to that small component of conduction slowing not attributed to nerve fiber loss.[31] Motor conduction velocity improves slightly but proportionately with HbA$_{1c}$ in response to metabolic therapy in chronic stable T2DM.[45] Similarly, intensified insulin treatment that attains near-normoglycemia significantly improves but does not normalize peripheral NCV in T1DM.[46-48] Although consistent with a direct metabolic affect on nerve conduction slowing in established diabetes, these responses, extending over several weeks to months, do not preclude significant structural repair of damaged nerve fibers.

Rapid effects of acute blood glucose normalization on nerve conduction do indeed suggest a small but direct metabolic contribution to nerve conduction slowing in human diabetes. Gallai and associates[49] studied motor and sensory conduction velocities in multiple peripheral nerves in 16 diabetic patients, 8 with and 8 without clinical neuropathy, before and after 3 days of treatment with a microprocessor-controlled "artificial pancreas," the Biostator™. Conduction velocity improved in peroneal and tibial motor and median sensory nerves, but only in those patients with clinical neuropathy. Service and coworkers[50] studied eight hyperglycemic subjects with T1DM before and after 72 hours of Biostator regulation and found improvement in ulnar sensory conduction velocity

($+3.2 \pm 1.4$ m/s) but not in 24 other electrophysiologic parameters measured; they concluded that no consistent improvement in nerve function was demonstrable. Troni and coworkers[51] studied H-reflex conduction velocity (n-HCV; a parameter with less day-to-day variation than standard nerve conduction) in subjects with short-duration T1DM before and during 2 days of Biostator gluco-regulation. Reduced n-HCV was increased from 1 to 3 m/s after 48 hours of Biostator treatment and also increased progressively over 6 months of intensive insulin therapy in other subjects with T1DM in conjunction with improvement in HbA_{1c}.

These observations suggest that a portion of nerve conduction slowing in diabetic patients is rapidly reversible with metabolic therapy and therefore probably reflects a direct biochemical or biophysical contribution related to metabolic abnormalities in peripheral nerve rather than structural abnormalities. Hence, the nerve conduction impairment in diabetes probably reflects the combined effects of rapidly reversible biochemical and somewhat less readily reversible structural abnormalities in peripheral nerve that cannot be easily distinguished by standard electrophysiologic techniques.

Although conduction slowing is usually more pronounced in diabetic patients with clinically overt neuropathy, the predictive value of conduction impairment for either the subsequent development or clinical course of clinical diabetic neuropathy has not been established.[52] Therefore, the promising observation that metabolic intervention rapidly improves nerve conduction in diabetic patients does not constitute evidence that such treatment will prevent or ameliorate the subsequent development of diabetic neuropathy. However, intensive diabetes therapy in the DCCT that prevented the development of neuropathy after 5 years was associated with a demonstrable increase in NCV at 1 year (DCCT Study Group, personal communication).

Clinical improvement in overt diabetic neuropathy following institution of improved metabolic control by intensive insulin therapy[52] would suggest a continuing role for the altered nerve metabolism in established diabetic neuropathy. Although such improvement has been anecdotally reported, appropriately controlled studies that include untreated age- and sex-matched patients with similar type and duration of diabetic neuropathy are not available to confirm the validity of these clinical impressions. Controlled randomized prospective clinical trials comparing treatment strategies that do and do not consistently and predictably lower blood glucose using endpoints that reliably chart the progression of clinically relevant nerve disease are required to establish the efficacy of metabolic therapy in the prevention and treatment of diabetic neuropathy.

Two pilot studies for long-term, randomized controlled prospective intervention trials offered promising results. Holman and colleagues[46] studied 74 T1DM subjects randomly assigned to "usual" or "intensified" insulin and dietary therapy for 24 months. The HbA_{1c} was significantly lowered by intensive insulin therapy. Vibratory sensory threshold over both lateral malleoli and the medial border of the distal phalanx of both great toes was assessed at baseline and yearly thereafter with a biothesiometer. At the completion of the trial, mean vibratory threshold had worsened in the conventionally treated group and improved in the intensively treated group. The authors therefore concluded that intensive insulin therapy prevented deterioration of vibratory sensation that otherwise occurs in subjects with T1DM on conventional insulin therapy. Service and coworkers[47] studied T1DM subjects randomly assigned to either conventional treatment or therapy using continuous subcutaneous insulin infusion (CSII) with an insulin pump. By

8 months, statistically significant differences in nerve conduction and vibratory threshold were found favoring the CSII-treated groups, supporting the observations of Holman and associates.[46] If increasing vibratory perception threshold and/or slowed nerve conduction are true harbingers of clinically overt neuropathy, then long-term intensive insulin therapy should delay or prevent the development of diabetic neuropathy.

More definitive data were provided by the large-scale DCCT. This trial studied the prevalence of clinical diabetic neuropathy confirmed by abnormal nerve conduction or autonomic testing in T1DM subjects randomly assigned to intensive versus conventional diabetes therapy for 5 years. Intensive therapy decreased the risk of development of confirmed clinical neuropathy (diagnosed by neurologic history and physical examination and confirmed by nerve conduction or autonomic function studies) at year 5 by 69% (from 9.8% to 3.1% in the primary prevention cohort) and 57% (from 16.1% to 7.0% in the secondary intervention cohort), with an overall risk reduction of 60%.[53] The DCCT was not designed to test the efficacy of intensive therapy in the treatment of diabetic neuropathy, and patients with clinically significant diabetic neuropathy were excluded from the study. However, 450 patients at baseline had at least one abnormality on clinical examination and were defined as having "possible or definite" clinical neuropathy. The frequency of abnormal nerve conduction was roughly twice as great in patients with possible or definite neuropathy compared with those without neuropathy. The likelihood of having abnormal nerve conduction was significantly reduced in patients with possible or definite neuropathy treated with intensive (37%) versus conventional (56%) therapy at 5 years ($p < 0.001$). Thus, although not designed to examine the question directly, the DCCT is consistent with the belief that intensive diabetes treatment may benefit patients with existing diabetic neuropathy, at least in its very earliest stage.

The results of the DCCT clearly implicate hyperglycemia and related metabolic abnormalities as overriding factors in the development of clinical neuropathy in T1DM. The similar temporal, anatomic, and clinical characteristics of polyneuropathy in T1DM and T2DM would make extrapolation of this conclusion to T2DM not unreasonable. These results unequivocally implicate metabolic abnormalities associated with insulin deficiency and/or hyperglycemia in the pathogenesis of diabetic polyneuropathy in patients with T1DM.

Glucose Control and Diabetic Autonomic Neuropathy

A beneficial effect of metabolic control on the development or progression of cardiovascular diabetic autonomic neuropathy (DAN) should significantly improve the overall prognosis for diabetes. The relationship of metabolic control to progression of abnormalities of autonomic function has been unclear. Improved metabolic control has been reported to slow the progression of heart rate variability (HRV) deficits in T1DM patients in some studies[26,53–55] but not in others.[56,57] As described above, in the DCCT, intensive therapy was able to slow the progression and development of abnormal autonomic tests.[58] The variability of the reported beneficial effects of good glycemic control on the development or progression of DAN could reflect a number of factors including inadequacy of glycemic control, insufficient study duration, too advanced DAN, or insensitivity of the cardiovascular autonomic function tests utilized.

Direct assessment of cardiac sympathetic integrity has become possible with the introduction of radiolabeled analogs of norepinephrine, which are actively taken up by the sympathetic nerve terminals of the heart.[59–64] Quantitative scintigraphic assessment of the pattern of sympathetic innervation of the human heart is possible with either [^{123}I] metaiodobenzylguanidine (MIBG) or [^{11}C] hydroxyephedrine (HED), which may offer greater sensitivity to detect subtle degrees of DAN than is possible by reflex testing. In cross-sectional studies, for example, deficits of left ventricular (LV) [^{123}I] MIBG and [^{11}C] HED retention have been identified in diabetic subjects without abnormalities on cardiovascular reflex testing[61,63] and have been reported even in newly diagnosed diabetes.[62] Widespread abnormalities of myocardial LV MIBG uptake have been reported in metabolically compromised newly diagnosed IDDM subjects; these are partially correctable by intensive insulin therapy[62] and appear to be indicative of a hyperglycemia- or insulin deficiency–induced acute neuronal dysfunction. Recent scintigraphic studies have shown that poor glycemic control has been shown to result in progression of LV sympathetic dysinnervation, which can be prevented[64] or reversed[65] by the institution of near-euglycemia. Thus quantitative scintigraphic imaging techniques such as HED positron emission tomography (PET) and MIBG single-photon emission computed tomography (SPECT) have confirmed the importance of glycemic control in the development, progression, or reversal of myocardial sympathetic dysinnervation.

ANIMAL MODELS OF DIABETIC NEUROPATHY

Studies in a wide range of diabetic animal models also firmly implicate insulin deficiency and/or hyperglycemia in the genesis of biochemical, functional, and structural abnormalities in peripheral nerve that seem to parallel at least the early stages of the development of human diabetic peripheral nerve disease. The first experimental evidence of diabetic neuropathy was the demonstration of acute nerve conduction slowing in alloxan-diabetic rats by Eliasson.[66] Other investigators soon suggested that impaired NCV in rats with experimental diabetes could be improved by insulin treatment.[67] Diabetic animal models have since served as invaluable tools with which to explore relationships among metabolic and microvascular abnormalities, functional deficits, and neuroanatomic changes under strict experimental conditions (Table 44-1). These models can be separated into those in which diabetes is induced by chemical agents cytotoxic to pancreatic β cells (streptozocin and alloxan), and those in which diabetes occurs spontaneously, secondary to genetic mutations (the BB rat, db/db mouse, and Chinese hamster). Both alloxan- and streptozocin-induced diabetes in animals, particularly streptozocin-diabetic (STZ-D) rats, have contributed enormously to our understanding of metabolic events in the diabetic nerve. Alloxan or streptozocin diabetes simulates that seen in insulin-dependent diabetes in humans with respect to the pancreatic β-cell destruction.

Hyperglycemia, the principal clinical finding signifying diabetes mellitus, is thought to be an initiating etiologic event in several complications of diabetes. Because galactose intoxication can produce hyperglycemia (albeit with a different sugar) without a significant hypoinsulinemia, it has been used to assess the role of hyperglycemia *per se* in the pathogenesis of diabetic complications.

Diminished Nerve Conduction Velocity in Diabetic Animal Models

The slowing of NCV in the alloxan-diabetic rat initiated the use of experimentally and spontaneously diabetic rodents in the study of the pathogenesis of diabetic neuropathy. Nerve conduction velocity has subsequently been measured in many animal models of diabetes and is generally found to be decreased.[68–70] The factors influencing the development of impaired sciatic motor NCV in acutely diabetic streptozocin rats were originally investigated by Greene and coworkers.[71] They showed that decreased MNCV in surgically exposed temperature-controlled sciatic nerve developed 2 weeks after streptozocin administration, but only in animals that became hyperglycemic. Insulin treatment prevented impaired MNCV in diabetic animals.[71] These studies were the first to establish conclusively that insulin deficiency, hyperglycemia, or both are primary factors in the development of impaired MNCV in acute experimental diabetes. Subsequent studies in the acutely streptozocin-diabetic rat, the BB rat, and the db/db mouse have confirmed the initial findings by Greene and coworkers.[69,70,72,73]

The evidence that the slowing of nerve conduction in acute experimental diabetes results from metabolic alterations caused by insulin deficiency and hyperglycemia[73] is readily reversible with metabolic (and or nerve perfusion) correction[73] and occurs in the absence of widespread evidence of structural defects such as demyelination, axonal atrophy, or axonal degeneration[74] or contributory vascular abnormalities[75] prompted a search for an underlying biophysical/metabolic mechanism. As discussed below, endoneurial hypoxia, oxidative stress, nerve energy deficits, decreased (Na,K)-ATPase activity, and impaired neurotrophism have emerged as critical mediators of hyperglycemia-induced nerve damage.[73]

TABLE 44-1. Putative Metabolic Initiators and Physiologic Mediators of Glucose Toxicity in Experimental Diabetic Neuropathy

Metabolic Initiator	Tissue Compartment	Physiologic Mediator
Nonenzymatic glycation	Endoneurial microcirculation	Interruption of nerve blood flow
Sorbitol pathway	Perineurial/epineurial vessels	Mitochondrial dysfunction
Glucose auto-oxidation	Dorsal root/anterior horn neurons	Reduced neurotrophic support
Protein kinase C activation	Myelinated/unmyelinated axons	Osmolyte derangements
	Schwann cells	
	Perineurial cells	
	Distal motor/sensory projections	

Source: Reproduced with permission from Greene DA, Obrosova IG, Stevens MJ, *et al:* Pathway of glucose-mediated oxidative stress in diabetic neuropathy. In: Packer L, Rosen P, Tritschler HJ, eds. *Antioxidants in Diabetes Management.* Marcel Dekker: 1999;111.

The Biochemical Pathobiology and Pathophysiology of Diabetic Peripheral Nerve

The observations that the severity of hyperglycemia is a risk factor for the development of neuropathy, that more vigorous metabolic treatment prevents or delays neuropathy[26] and improves nerve function in diabetic subjects, and that hyperglycemia and its metabolic consequences have been linked to abnormal nerve function and biochemistry in laboratory animals have led to a search for possible biochemical mechanisms by which insulin deficiency and/or hyperglycemia might adversely affect peripheral nerve.

Insulin-deficient diabetic subjects exhibit impaired nerve conduction, which is rapidly reversed by insulin replacement.[39,40,51] The rapidity with which metabolic intervention improves nerve conduction in insulin-deficient diabetic subjects[46,47,76] would strongly suggest that a component of nerve conduction slowing in diabetic patients probably reflects a direct biochemical or biophysical contribution related to metabolic factors rather than structural abnormalities. As discussed previously, the analogous rapidly reversible nerve conduction slowing in acutely diabetic animals occurs without fixed alterations of peripheral nerve structure. Therefore, early and reversible slowing of nerve conduction in animal diabetes has been attributed to acute metabolic disturbances that occur in axons, Schwann cells, endoneurial microvessels, and/or their endoneurial environment[77] as a consequence of acute insulin deficiency.[71,78,79] Detailed analysis of the biochemical factors contributing to the acutely reversible slowing of nerve conduction in short-term diabetic animals was viewed as a productive point to initiate studies to identify factors that might contribute to the pathogenesis of diabetic neuropathy. At present, there are six distinct but not mutually exclusive and possibly interrelated hypotheses for the pathogenesis of diabetic neuropathy: the sorbitol, hypoxia-ischemia, nonenzymatic glycation, oxidative stress, apoptosis, and altered neurotrophism hypotheses.

Altered Nerve Metabolism in Acutely Diabetic Rodents

The so-called metabolic hypotheses of diabetic neuropathy argue that metabolic derangements induced by hyperglycemia, insulin deficiency, or both in one or more of the cellular components of peripheral nerve, over time, contribute to progressive functional and structural defects that ultimately culminate in sufficiently severe nerve damage as to produce clinically detectable neurologic deficits. Exploration of the acute effects of diabetes on nerve metabolism and function would constitute a logical venue for the development of specific pathogenetic hypotheses for the disease process. Multiple metabolic and pharmacologic manipulations have recently been shown to modulate the slowing of NCV, reduction of nerve blood flow, resistance of nerve impulse conduction to ischemia, and impaired axonal transport in the acutely diabetic rat (Table 44-2).[73,80,81] Each of these invokes a distinct pathogenetic hypothesis for diabetic neuropathy,[73,81–83] most of which involve alterations in nerve energy metabolism.

Nerve Fuel and Energy Metabolism

Peripheral nerve metabolism shares many characteristics with the central nervous system (CNS).[81–83] Glucose entry into peripheral nerve and brain is neither directly regulated by insulin nor rate-limiting for glucose oxidation (its major metabolic fate),[33,84] so that insulin deficiency should not directly deprive peripheral nerve of adequate metabolic substrate nor should hyperglycemia directly stimulate glycolytic flux by mass action. Glucose uptake

TABLE 44-2. Therapeutic Responses of Neuropathy in Animal Models of Diabetes Mellitus

Treatment	Motor Conduction Velocity	Nerve Blood Flow	Nerve Axoplasmic Transport	Evoked Amplitude
ARIs	+	+	+	—
Insulin	+	−	+	—
Myoinositol	+	+	+	—
Antioxidants	+	+	−	—
Prostaglandin E_1 analog	+	+	−	—
COX-2 inhibitor	+	+	−	—
Protein kinase C B1 inhibitors	+	+	−	—
Essential fatty acids	+	+	—	—
Nitric oxide donors	+	+	−	—
Gangliosides	+	—	+	—
Guanethidine	+	+	—	—
ACE inhibitors	+	+	−	—
Prazosin	+	+	−	—
Potassium channel openers β_2 adrenoreceptor	+	+	−	—
Agonist/α_1 antagonist	+	+	−	—
Islet cell pancreas allotransplantation	+	—	—	+
ACTH (4–9) analog	+	—	—	—
Chronic electrical activation	+	—	—	—
Aminoguanidine	+	+	—	—
Acetylcarnitine	+	+/−	—	+
Acarbose	+	—	—	—
Methylcobalamin-vitamin B mixture	+	—	—	—
Hyperbaric oxygen/oxygen supplementation	+	—	—	—
Piroxicam	—	—	—	+

+, reported effect; − ,not known or no effect. ACE, angiotensin-converting enzyme; ACTH, adrenocorticotropic hormone; ARI, aldose reductase inhibitor; cox, cyclo-oxygenase.

into the sciatic nerve of STZ-D rats has been reported to be decreased,[83] which perhaps reflects posttranslational modification of the principal glucose transporters in sciatic nerve, GLUT-1 and GLUT-3.[85] Nerve adenosine triphosphate (ATP) concentrations have been reported to be unchanged in diabetic rats, and phosphocreatine (PCr) concentrations and PCr:creatine (Cr; a highly sensitive parameter of peripheral nerve energy state)[86,87] ratios reduced in diabetic rats. The decrease in cytoplasmic high-energy phosphate stores parallels the reduction of endoneurial blood flow and endoneurial hypoxia[87] and is sensitive to vasodilator therapy, which corrects these deficits.[88] A report of increased rather than decreased nerve high-energy phosphate compounds in STZ-D rats[89] may be explained by the use of slow-acting systemic anesthesia for such tissue sampling, since increased metabolic substrate for, and adaptation to, anaerobic metabolism may render diabetic nerve more resistant to the bioenergetic effects of anesthetic hypoxia and/or ischemia.[90] β-Hydroxybutyrates, but not long-chain fatty acids, serve as major alternative energy substrates.[33,84] The metabolic role of amino acid oxidation is unclear, although amino acid transport but not content is impaired in diabetic rabbit nerve.[91] On the other hand, carbohydrate metabolism is deranged in diabetic nerve, largely through stimulation of the aldose reductase (AR) or "polyol" pathway, the effect of which has been explored by using specific aldose reductase inhibitors (ARIs) as metabolic probes.

Aldose Reductase and the Sorbitol Pathway

Recent evidence has served to reinforce the link between increased sorbitol pathway flux and the presence of diabetic complications[92,93] including severe neuropathy.[94] The concept that aberrant overexpression of the AR gene may predispose to the development of microvascular complications has received support by the identification of polymorphisms at the 5′ end of the AR gene that are strongly associated with the presence of neuropathy in diabetic subjects.[95]

Two distinct (but not mutually exclusive) biochemical consequences of increased metabolic flux of glucose through the sorbitol pathway have been invoked to explain the short-term and long-term deleterious effects of hyperglycemia on diabetic nerve and other complication-prone tissues. These are the osmoregulatory consequences of sorbitol accumulation (the *osmotic* or *compatible osmolyte hypothesis*)[96] and the effect of the sorbitol pathway on the NADH/NAD and NADPH/NADP redox couples linked, respectively, to sorbitol dehydrogenase (SDH) and AR (the *redox hypothesis*).[97] Studies with specific ARIs strongly implicate this metabolic pathway in the pathogenesis of diabetic peripheral neuropathy (DPN; and perhaps other diabetic complications).[21,22] In experimental diabetic neuropathy in the rat, ARIs prevent, reverse, or moderate various defects in NCV[73,80,81,98–100] and ameliorate nerve fiber damage and loss.[99] In diabetic patients with DPN, potent ARIs improve NCV.[21,22] In multicenter placebo-controlled clinical trials in patients with DPN, doses of potent ARIs that lower sural nerve sorbitol content by 80–85% also reverse the histologic loss of myelinated sensory nerve fibers.[22] The yearly improvements in NCV and myelinated nerve fiber density (MNFD) with effective ARI treatment exceed the magnitude of the yearly loss of MNFD and NCV in untreated diabetic subjects, and they approximate the magnitude of change deemed clinically evident and significant.

The precise mechanisms and the critical loci at which the beneficial effects of ARIs are achieved remain controversial. ARIs correct many fundamental deficits in experimental diabetic neuropathy (EDN), including impaired axonal transport,[101] decreased neurotrophism,[102,103] nerve osmolyte depletion,[73,100] redox disturbances,[104] increased oxidative stress,[73,105] activation of protein kinase c (PKC),[106,107] depressed nerve (Na,K)-ATPase activity,[73,108] depletion of vasoactive agents[109] and nerve blood flow deficits.[109,110] Osmolyte disturbance secondary to sorbitol accumulation and compensatory depletion of taurine and myoinositol (MI) comprise only one limb of AR pathway effects. Redox disturbances resulting from shifts in adenine nucleotide cofactor couples, and nonenzymatic glycation/glycoxidation resulting from fructose production comprise the two other principal pathogenetic pathways that may contribute to the deleterious effects of AR pathway activation.

The Sorbitol-Osmotic Hypothesis

Kinoshita's[111] classical osmotic hypothesis of diabetic complications invoked cell "swelling," particularly in the ocular lens exposed to hyperglycemia, as the direct osmotic consequence of intracellular sorbitol accumulation. A modern revision of the osmotic hypothesis identifies sorbitol as one of a class of nonionic, nonperturbing, "compatible" intracellular osmolytes that include MI, taurine, betaine, and glycerophosphorylcholine.[96] These osmolytes are thought to buffer the cell physiologically against extreme osmotic stress, such as that normally encountered during antidiuresis in the renal medulla. Nonmedullary and even nonrenal cells exposed to hypertonicity exhibit the same compensatory mechanisms even though they rarely if ever encounter such stress *in vivo*. Under hypertonic stress, these compatible osmolytes accumulate intracellularly in a carefully balanced and regulated compensatory fashion through the induction of relevant genes such as AR, the Na-MI and Na-taurine cotransporters, and others.[112]

Osmotic induction of these genes is widespread and may occur in response to much smaller osmotic shifts than previously suspected. Hyperglycemia-induced isotonic sorbitol accumulation is unaccompanied by osmotic induction of other osmoresponsive genes.[113,114] Indeed, the subtle osmotic effects of intracellular sorbitol accumulation (producing a "relative" extracellular hypotonic state) are thought to downregulate the other Na^+-osmolyte cotransporters.[100,115] Osmoregulatory genes are transcriptionally upregulated[116] (but not apparently downregulated)[117] by homologous tonicity elements in their 5' flanking sequence.[116] These respond to a tonicity element binding protein that binds in response to hypertonic stress.[116,117] By raising intracellular osmolality, sorbitol accumulation is presumed to downregulate these compatible osmolyte genes transcriptionally and/or to activate osmolyte efflux posttranslationally through the volume-sensitive osmolyte anion channel (VSOAC).[118] Potentially, sorbitol-induced intracellular osmotic stress may contribute to depletion of reduced glutathione (GSH) and thereby exacerbate oxidative stress. Indeed, GSH depletion is aggravated in complication-prone tissues by therapeutic interventions such as sorbitol dehydrogenase inhibitors, which aggravate sorbitol accumulation,[119] or by overexpression of the AR gene (Fig. 44-1).

AR-mediated oxidative stress may also promote MI and taurine depletion directly via downregulation of sodium-dependent MI transporter (SMIT) and the taurine transporter or indirectly through disruption of the (Na,K)-ATPase–generated Na^+-gradient, which is required for the active uptake of MI and taurine.[117] The ability of the antioxidant α-lipoic acid to correct nerve MI and

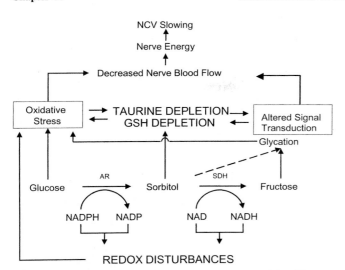

FIGURE 44-1. Potential mechanisms whereby activation of the aldose reductase pathway may exacerbate oxidative stress. Activation of the aldose reductase (AR) pathway consumes NADPH and provokes intracellular sorbitol accumulation, resulting in osmotic stress and the compensatory depletion of the organic osmolytes taurine and myoinositol and perhaps depletion of reduced glutathione (GSH). In turn, this will promote oxidative stress and alterations in signal transduction pathways. Sorbitol oxidation by sorbitol dehydrogenase (SDH) promotes the formation of NADH ("pseudohypoxia") and leads to the formation of fructose, which is a potent glycosylator. Increased oxidative stress results in disruption of vasoactive agents and reduced nerve blood flow, which compromises mitochondrial function, leading to nerve energy deficits and nerve conduction velocity (NCV) slowing.

taurine content[87,120] implicates multiple interconnected pathways by which glucose flux through AR can result in osmolyte depletion. Therefore, in diabetes, AR activation may result in the depletion of intracellular osmolytes, rendering them rate-limiting for normal intracellular metabolism.[80,81] In some cells, MI depletion is profound enough to limit the synthesis of phosphatidylinositol (PI) by cytidine-diphospho-diglyceride-inositol 3-phosphatidyltransferase (PI synthase),[121] secondarily altering phosphoinositide (PPI) turnover and the generation of PI-derived second messengers such as diacylglycerols (DAGs) thought to critically regulate (Na,$^+$K$^+$)-ATPase.[78,122] In concert, depletion of taurine, an important endogenous antioxidant,[123] calcium modulator,[124,125] PKC antagonist,[125] and neurotransmitter,[126] may compound chronic cytotoxicity in diabetes by interaction with a complex matrix of biochemical mechanisms outlined below. However, as described below, ascribing nerve osmolyte depletion entirely to the osmotic stress resulting from exaggerated accumulation of intracellular sorbitol appears to be an oversimplification, as levels of nerve MI and taurine can be changed in diabetic and nondiabetic nerve independently of nerve sorbitol levels.

Depletion of nerve MI has been invoked as an important mediator of the effect of sorbitol pathway activation on NCV slowing in acute experimental diabetes,[69,79,80] although this view has recently been challenged.[109,127,128] Oral 1% MI supplementation, whether given in chow[129] or synthetic diet,[79,80,130] corrects sciatic nerve MI depletion and reproduces the beneficial effects of ARI treatment on slowed NCV,[102,103,131] reduced nerve blood flow,[131] and the development of paranodal axonal swelling[69] in the STZ-D and spontaneously diabetic BB rat models of EDN. The oral dose of MI appears to be critical, since 3% MI supplementation is not efficacious and produces some slowing of MNCV in nondiabetic rats.[109] This may reflect reciprocal depletion of other compatible osmolytes such as taurine.[100] Feeding l-fucose, a competitive inhibitor of SMIT activity, to normal rats reproduces the nerve MI depletion and the impaired nerve electrophysiology and (Na,K)-ATPase activity found in diabetic rats; these are corrected by MI supplementation given simultaneously with l-fucose.[132] SMIT activity in nerve is competitively inhibited by glucose, but it remains diminished in diabetic nerve exposed to normal glucose in vitro,[80,81] suggesting intrinsically impaired SMIT expression or function.

Depletion of intracellular MI has been thought to render it rate-limiting for the membrane PI synthesis and turnover[80] necessary for phospholipase C–mediated, G protein–associated signal transduction. This has been speculated to lead to diminished PI-derived DAG and impaired activation of PKC, which may link altered MI metabolism to defective (Na,K)-ATPase regulation in diabetic nerve. This assertion is based on the observations that (Na,K)-ATPase activity,[80,133] arachidonyl-DAG,[134] and PKC activation[130] are diminished in diabetic nerve and that dietary MI supplementation in vivo[80] or exogenous PKC agonists in vitro[135] correct impaired nerve (Na,K)-ATPase activity. In addition, MI depletion through its effects on signal transduction pathways and fatty acid metabolism may impair nitric oxide synthase (NOS) activity[133,136,137] and/or lipoxygenase/COX pathways,[138] resulting in widespread metabolic and vascular deficits through the disruption of nitric oxide (NO) and prostaglandin metabolism at the level of the sympathetic ganglia, peripheral neuron, or endoneurial vasculature.

Depletion of the β-amino acid taurine (2-aminoethanesulfonic acid)[100,139,140] in complication-prone diabetic tissues including the peripheral nerve[100] has recently emerged as an important mediator of glucotoxicity. Taurine has antioxidant[123,141] properties, and high taurine concentrations are found in tissues subject to oxidative stress, including rat lens,[140,142] kidney,[143] heart,[124,144] and nerve.[100] In the sciatic nerve, taurine levels are depressed in diabetic rats,[100,145] and nerve taurine replacement ameliorates deficits of nerve blood flow, (Na,K)-ATPase activity, and NCV in EDN,[145] suggesting an important modulatory role for taurine on nerve function.

Recently, an important role has emerged for taurine in the regulation of micro- and macrovascular function. Taurine has been demonstrated in the endothelial cells of rat cerebellar cortex capillaries as well as in the perivascular glia and neurons that innervate the vasculature, consistent with a role for taurine in the regulation of microvascular function within the CNS.[146] In human endothelial cells, taurine has also been shown to prevent apoptosis and maintain cell function after exposure to lipopolysaccharide, tumor necrosis factor-α, and calcium ionophore, supporting a role for taurine in antioxidative defense and regulation of intracellular calcium flux[147] in the endothelium. In STZ-D mice, a taurine-supplemented diet has been shown to normalize endothelium-dependent relaxation of aortic rings.[148] Immunohistochemical studies of the distribution of taurine in the peripheral nerve of diabetic rodents have localized taurine to the endothelium of the endoneurial vascular and Schwann cells,[145] consistent with its function in regulating endoneurial blood flow and (Na,K)-ATPase activity.

In addition to its antioxidant effects, taurine modulates intracellular Ca^{2+} flux[124,125,144,149] and PKC activation.[125] Taurine lowers cytosolic Ca^{2+} by stimulating mitochondrial uptake,[125,144] inhibiting PI turnover,[125] and decreasing internal Ca^{2+} flux,[144] thereby inhibiting Ca^{2+}-dependent PKC activation.[125] Thus intracellular taurine depletion in diabetes may contribute to the glucose-induced activation of PKC, which has been invoked in the pathogenesis of diabetic complications[150,151] including DPN.[152,153] In addition, neuronal and glial taurine are thought to function as an osmoregulator, neuromodulator, or inhibitory neurotransmitter,[126,154–156] as well as a neurotrophic agent.[157] Taurine may also modulate neuronal hyperexcitability by producing hyperpolarization or by inhibiting Ca^{2+}/calmodulin-dependent protein kinases, and its depletion may therefore play a role in the pathogenesis of painful neuropathy.[100]

Polyol Pathway and Redox Potential

Glucose flux through AR and SDH oxidizes the NADPH/NADP and reduces the NADH/NAD redox couple, thereby disturbing the adenine nucleotide–linked reaction that functions near the redox equilibrium. Depletion of glutathione secondary to oxidation of the NADPH/NADP couple has been proposed to increase susceptibilty to oxidative stress.[104] Alternatively, the reduction of NADH/NAD coupled to the oxidation of glucose-derived sorbitol to fructose favors lactate production and the diversion of glycolytic intermediates to the synthesis of phospholipid precursors such as α-glycerophosphate, phosphatidic acid, DAG, and cytidine-diphospho-diglyceride (CDP-DG). This flux may also interfere with β-oxidation of long-chain fatty acids, resulting in a metabolic "pseudohypoxia."

Both AR-mediated NADPH oxidation and SDH-mediated NAD reduction have been implicated in diabetes-induced changes in nicotinamide adenine nucleotide homeostasis (increase in free cytosolic $NADP^+$:NADPH and decrease in free cytosolic NAD^+:NADH ratios) as well as the antioxidant and metabolic deficits contributing to diabetic neuropathy, retinopathy, and cataract formation.[97,158–160] In particular, it has been suggested that a deficiency of NADPH, a cofactor shared by AR, glutathione reductase, and NOS, is responsible for diabetes-induced depletion of GSH and total glutathione, and thus enhanced oxidative stress, in the lens and peripheral nerve,[104,133,158] and decreased endoneurial nutritive blood flow.[158] There are a number of findings, however, that are difficult to reconcile with these putative redox cycling mechanisms: (1) the absence of a reciprocal increase of oxidized glutathione (GSSG) levels in concert with the diabetes-induced decrease in GSH levels in the peripheral nerve[161]; (2) a decrease in free cytosolic $NADP^+$:NADPH ratios in the nerve[162] of acutely diabetic rodents; and (3) exacerbated depletion of nonenzymatic antioxidants (GSH and ascorbate) and increased lipid peroxidation in diabetic peripheral nerve by SDH inhibition.[163] None of these three factors are consistent with the possibility that increased redox cycling mechanisms contribute to diabetic complications.

It has been proposed that SDH-mediated NAD-redox imbalances (so-called pseudohypoxia) constitute the principal mechanism responsible for polyol pathway–mediated diabetic complications.[97] This has been explored in rodent models using sorbitol dehydrogenase inhibitors (SDIs),[164,165] as well as SDH-deficient and SDH-knockout mouse models.[160,166] SDH was found to accelerate, rather than retard, the development of autonomic dysfunction.[166] In the peripheral nervous system there have been conflicting results: Some laboratories have found beneficial effects of SDIs on nerve electrophysiologic deficits using a prevention paradigm in diabetic rats,[167] whereas others have failed to find any beneficial effect on neurovascular or functional deficits using an interventional approach.[164] Moreover, the relationship of polyol accumulation

and nerve dysfunction has also been explored in SDH-deficient mutant mice (C57BL/LiA), which have exaggerated sorbitol accumulation but fructose depletion in the peripheral nerve. Diabetic SDH-deficient mice showed MNCV slowing similar to that in normal diabetic mice, thereby suggesting that increased flux through SDH is not responsible for MNCV slowing in experimental diabetes.[165]

Recent reports have reinforced the view that increased flux through SDH cannot account for changes in the dynamic system of nicotinamide nucleotides in complication-prone diabetic tissues. SDI treatment that resulted in >90% inhibition of increased flux through SDH in the nerve failed to ameliorate free cytosolic NAD^+:NADH ratios and actually exacerbated tissue oxidative stress and energy deficiency (manifested by accumulation of lipid aldehydes and further reductions in GSH, PCr, and PCr:Cr ratio in the peripheral nerve of SDI-treated diabetic rats).[163,168] Potentially, diabetes-induced NAD-redox imbalances could promote oxidative stress by resulting in the accumulation of triose phosphates (DHAP and GP), with their subsequent auto-oxidation and formation of methylglyoxal,[169] which generates free radicals and impairs antioxidative defense.[170] Exacerbation of tissue oxidative injury in spite of improvement in NAD^+:NADH ratios coupled with SDI treatment[168] suggests that adverse effects (potentially mediated in part by osmotic disturbances such as taurine depletion) predominate over putative beneficial (NAD-redox) effects of SDH inhibition on oxidative stress.

The ability of other metabolic manipulations to improve nerve conduction or other aspects of the neuropathy associated with diabetes in the rat implies the existence of other contributory factors, some of which may or may not be related to the sorbitol pathway. In particular, various compounds that promote vasodilation improve nerve electrophysiology in experimental diabetes, as do compounds with either neurotransmitter or neurotrophic action. Furthermore, recent observations are consistent with the hypothesis that reductions in cyclic AMP in rat nerve may contribute to impaired (Na,K)-ATPase activity.

Signal Transduction, Nerve Osmolytes, and Nerve Conduction

Glucose-induced alterations in signal transduction pathways are thought to play a critical role in the development of DPN. However, heterogeneous and complex cell-specific relationships between ambient glucose and intracellular signaling have been reported. Hyperglycemia may alter PI signal transduction by two separate mass-action mechanisms with antiparallel effects. In neuronal tissue, glucose-induced, AR-catalyzed sorbitol accumulation and reciprocal MI depletion may diminish PI synthesis and turnover and the subsequent release of PI-derived arachidonyl-DAGs, resulting in decreased PKC activity. Indeed, a reduction in arachidonyl-containing DAGs and PKC activity has been demonstrated in diabetic rat sciatic nerve.[134,135] Inhibition of PKC can also prevent the decrease of sciatic nerve (Na,K)-ATPase but is not able to prevent the decrease in glutathione peroxidase activity that has been reported in diabetic mice.[171]

However, in vascular tissues, including potentially the neurovasculature, the predominant effect of elevated glucose has been reported to be PKC activation.[150,172,173] The importance of glucose-induced activation of PKC in some tissues prone to diabetic complications has received some support by the recent demonstration that a specific PKC β1 inhibitor could correct diabetes-induced retinal and renal dysfunction in the STZ-D rat.[151] Recently, two studies have reported the effects of PKC inhibition on metabolic, neurovascular, and functional deficits in diabetic rats. In STZ-D rats, inhibitors of PKC (WAY151 003 and chelerythrine) dose-dependently corrected deficits of nerve perfusion, (Na,K)-ATPase activity, nerve MI content,[152] and NCV without affecting nerve glutathione content.[153] At high dose, the inhibitors dissociated nerve blood flow (corrected) from nerve conduction (uncorrected) deficits. The beneficial effects were prevented by NOS inhibitor cotreatment.[153]

Since the effects of activation or inhibition of PKC can be expected to have divergent tissue-specific regulatory effects (e.g., on [Na,K]-ATPase activity and NOS activity), tissue nonselective pharmacologic blockade (or activation) of PKC isoforms could be expected to ameliorate the effects of hyperglycemia in some tissues, but they may aggravate glucotoxicity in others.

The concept that depletion of nerve osmolytes in diabetic tissues is simply a result of osmotic compensation for glucose-induced sorbitol accumulation appears to be an oversimplification. This view is supported by the following recently reported data: Nerve acetyl-L-carnitine replacement in STZ-D rats corrects nerve MI levels independently of polyol pathway activity[174]; the chain-breaking antioxidant α-lipoic acid prevents nerve taurine and MI depletion, despite exacerbating nerve sorbitol accumulation; and, in nondiabetic rats,[83,87] nonselective COX inhibition with flurbroben can reproduce diabetes-induced depletion of nerve taurine and MI. These data suggest that nonosmotic metabolic factors may play a critical role in the regulation of nerve organic osmolyte levels. Intracellular levels of taurine and MI are regulated by transmembrane transport mediated by their Na-dependent cotransporters (regulating cellular uptake) and VSOAC (regulating cellular efflux).[104] These transport mechanisms are critically regulated by signal transduction pathways, with PKC activation appearing to have parallel inhibitory effects on transmembrane transport of MI and taurine and stimulation of efflux.[104] Thus the beneficial effects of PKC inhibition on nerve MI content could be explained by direct effects on nerve MI flux.

Recently, a consensus has begun to emerge suggesting that the effects of diabetes on protein kinase signal transduction in the nerve are complex and tissue-specific: PKC activation in the vasculature may contribute to nerve blood flow deficits, whereas a reduction of PKC activity in neuronal tissues may alter nerve metabolism at this site.

(Na,K)-ATPase Activity

The absence of prominent demyelination or nerve fiber degeneration, in association with the nerve conduction slowing in acutely diabetic rats,[74,175] suggested a biochemical or biophysical mechanism, which might also account for the associated paranodal swelling and increased intra-axonal sodium content in diabetic rat nerve.[176] The (Na,K)-ATPase emerged as a possible common denominator for altered energy metabolism, nerve conduction slowing, and paranodal swelling in acute experimental diabetes based on direct measurement of reduced nerve (Na,K)-ATPase activity in diabetic rodents, its correction by multiple metabolic interventions that ameliorate electrophysiologic deficits,[104] and voltage clamp studies documenting a corresponding reduction in the resting axolemmal membrane potential and a four- to fivefold increase in intra-axonal $[Na^1]$.[176] Recent studies have demonstrated that pharmacologic manipulation of nondiabetic rats with agents that decreased nerve (Na,K)-ATPase

activity also reproduces diabetic NCV slowing.[133] Flux through the COX pathway appears to regulate nerve ATPase activity tonically.[177] In EDN, PGE_1 analogs[110] and cilostazol (a phosphodiesterase inhibitor) correct the reduced cAMP levels and prevent the decrease in ATPase activity in STZ-D rats. The potency of nonselective COX-1 and -2 inhibition to disrupt nerve ATPase activity contrasts with its lack of effect on ATPase activity in vascular tissue.[136]

The importance of impaired ATPase activity in mediating the early decrease in motor NCV in EDN is debated, as ouabain-sensitive (Na,K)-ATPase activity is not detectably decreased before 4 weeks of diabetes, and (Na,K)-ATPase activity can be ameliorated without ameliorating MNCV slowing.[174] This discordance may be explained by differences in fiber type and/or differences in an isoform of the ATPase (or phosphorylation of its regulatory domain), which principally contributes to these measurements. For example, MNCV is determined by rapidly conducting large myelinated fibers, in which significant concentrations of ATPase enzyme may be limited to the paranodal Schwann cell processes and the nodal axolemma.[178] In these fibers (and their Schwann cells), the predominant isoform may be the α1, which is highly ouabain-resistant in rodents.[179–181] In contrast, much of the measured composite ouabain-inhibitible (Na,K)-ATPase activity in whole sciatic nerve may reside in the ouabain-sensitive α2 and α3 isoforms[179,180] of the unmyelinated nerve fibers,[181] which contribute little to the measured MNCV. Alternatively, composite ATPase correction may be necessary but not sufficient alone to correct MNCV slowing.

The (Na,K)-ATPase is a heterodimer comprised of an α subunit (112 kd), which contains the catalytic subunit and the ATP- and ouabain-binding site[182] and is the substrate for protein kinases, and a β subunit (35 kd), which may be important for membrane binding. Three different isoforms of the α subunit have been identified (α1, α2, α3), with α1 predominating in peripheral nerve and the Schwann cell.[180] In STZ-D, a marked and rapid insulin-sensitive reduction in the α1 subunit has been demonstrated by Western analysis after 3 weeks of diabetes, the reductions of the other subunits being delayed.[179] More recently, a diabetes-induced decrease in the α2 subunit and an increase in the β2 subunit of the (Na,K)-ATPase has been reported in the Schwann cells (both) and node of Ranvier (α2 only) of diabetic rats.[183] Fish oil selectively corrected the change in the α2 subunit.[183] In general, the effects of experimental diabetes on differential regulation of the (Na,K)-ATPase subunits remain poorly understood.

PKC activation may itself have bidirectional, tissue- and species-specific effects on ATPase activity. Exogenous PKC agonists correct impaired nerve ouabain-sensitive energy metabolism and ATPase activity in vitro.[184] Moreover, PKC activation is without effect on the phosphorylation state of the α subunit in nerves from ND rats,[180] whereas in the STZ-D rat, increased α subunit ^{32}P labeling was observed with PKC activation. However, PKC β1 inhibition has been reported to dose-dependently prevent decreased (Na,K)-ATPase activity in STZ-D rats, and PKC activation has been associated with diminished (Na,K)-ATPase activity in peripheral nerve in the chronically diabetic mouse.[185] Thus, in EDN, the relationships of PKC to (Na,K)-ATPase activity are complex and poorly understood and may be both model- and time-dependent. Potentially chronic stimulation of PKC in EDN could result in compensatory up- or downregulation of its action. Finally, in T1DM subjects, patients with an ATP1 A1 variant of the genes encoding for (Na,K)-ATPase (when detected by Bgl II restriction fragment length polymorphism) were found to have diabetic polyneuropathy more frequently than those without,[186] providing some support in humans for alterations in (Na,K)-ATPase activity in the development of DPN.

The Role of Ischemia and Other Alterations in the Endoneurial Microenvironment in the Pathogenesis of Diabetic Neuropathy

The contributory role of nerve ischemia to diabetic neuropathy has been an area of active investigation, with many modern experts supporting a hypothesis originally generated by Fagerberg[187] over 35 years ago. Originally based on extensive autopsy findings of thickened, para-aminosalicylic acid–positive deposits and luminal occlusion in endoneurial microvessels, the hypothesis in its current form is based on modern morphometric analysis of autopsy or biopsy material,[188,189] sural nerve biopsies,[22,143] and studies in diabetic animals.[80,81] Currently, new efforts have been made to reconcile or merge these two hypotheses, which are not necessarily mutually exclusive.[80,190]

Hemodynamic and oximetric and recent biochemical measurements in diabetic rodents suggest reduced endoneurial blood flow and hypoxia in chronically diabetic rats,[127,191] which may occur as early as 1 week after the induction of diabetes.[127] Decreased nerve blood flow has been reported for both exposed[153,159,164,192–196] and unexposed[197] nerve. In EDN, endoneurial nutritive flow has been reported to be reduced by 45% and nonnutritive flow by 48%.[109] A wide variety of vasoactive agents partially or completely correct NCV slowing in diabetic rats, including those with direct vasodilatory actions such as the α-adrenergic receptor inhibitor prazosin,[128] angiotensin-converting enzyme (ACE) inhibitors,[198] prostaglandin analogs,[110] NO donors,[199] and potassium channel openers,[200] and those with a more indirect vasodilatory action (i.e., ARIs,[80,190] anti-oxidants,[201–203] metal chelators,[204] acetyl L-carnitine,[174,205] PKC inhibitors,[152,153] and evening primrose oil [EPO][206]). Diabetic nerves may be more susceptible to ischemic injury due to imbalance of vasoactive agents.[207] In EDN, 2 weeks of treatment with the β2-AR agonist salbutamol or the α1-AR antagonist doxazosin has recently been shown to partially reverse neurovascular dysfunction and NCV slowing in 8-week STZ-D rats, effects that appeared to be dependent on NO, implicating a role for vasa nervorum α1- and β2-AR in the regulation of nerve blood flow.[208]

ARI treatment prevents or corrects NCV slowing,[80,190] corrects decreased endoneurial blood flow,[109,110] and also impairs endothelium-dependent aortic relaxation (thought to be NO-mediated) in chronically streptozocin-diabetic rats.[209] Indeed, several studies now suggest that microvascular dysregulation in diabetes may primarily involve the endothelial-dependent NO-mediated component.[210,211] Finally, NOS inhibition reproduces the glucose-induced decrease in (Na,K)-ATPase activity in isolated rabbit aortic rings *in vitro*.[136]

These observations together provide the framework for a metabolic-vascular pathogenetic matrix for experimental diabetic neuropathy involving AR, NO, and (Na,K)-ATPase (Fig. 44-2). A role for hyperviscosity as a cause of endoneurial hypoxia has also been proposed and is supported by findings of increased fibrinogen or globulin levels[212] and decreased red cell deformability and/or leukocytosis and leukocyte activation in diabetes, but this area remains extremely controversial.[212]

However, the concept of reduced nerve blood flow and endoneurial hypoxia has not received universal acceptance, since other reports have suggested that blood flow is unchanged[213] or increased[214] and that nerve conduction deficits reflect principally metabolic[215] or other[216] perturbations. A recent report in 12-week

FIGURE 44-2. Interactions of metabolic and vascular defects leading to experimental nerve conduction slowing. Early after the onset of diabetes, aldose reductase (AR) inhibitor–sensitive metabolic defects in the vascular endothelium and/or autonomic ganglia lead to a reduction in nerve blood flow. Acute reduction in nerve blood flow may, in turn, have more distal effects on nerve energy state and nerve metabolism or may lead directly to nerve conduction slowing. Therefore, proximal therapeutic interventions with agents such as ARIs may correct both decreased nerve blood flow and distal defects in nerve metabolism. As indicated, nitric oxide (NO) may mediate and bridge both the metabolic and vascular pathways. PKC, protein kinase C; NCV, nerve conduction velocity.

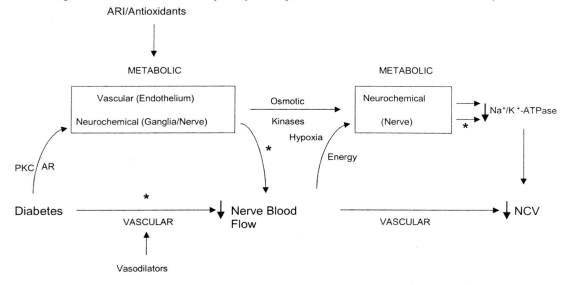

* Potentially NO mediated

STZ-D rats identified an increased number of microvessels supplying the peripheral nerve trunk; it was suggested that these reflected a neovascularity.[207] Recently, evidence in support of endoneurial hypoxia was sought by the determination of biochemical adenine nucleotide–linked redox couples in the nerve. Free NAD^+:NADH ratios in nerve mitochondrial cristae and matrix and cytosol were decreased by 77%, 32%, and 27% after 6 weeks of experimental diabetes in the rat.[217] The diabetes-induced reductions of free NAD^+:NADH ratios in the mitochondrial matrix and cytosol were prevented by treatment with the vasodilator prazosin.[217]

Clinical evidence in support of nerve hypoxia in the development of DPN has been the finding of a reduction of endoneurial oxygen in the sural nerves of diabetic patients with far advanced polyneuropathy[218] and the development of some abnormalities of neural conduction in nondiabetic hypoxic patients with chronic obstructive airway disease.[219] More recently, microlight-guided spectrophotometry has been used to measure intravascular oxygen saturation and blood flow in the sural nerve of diabetic subjects with and without diabetic neuropathy. These studies identified a reduction of nerve oxygenation and impaired nerve blood flow in subjects with diabetic neuropathy.[220] Finally, the ACE inhibitor trandolapril has recently been shown to improve peripheral nerve electrophysiology after 12 months in diabetic subjects with mild neuropathy.[221]

Thus, although hypoxia may play a role in the development of diabetic neuropathy, it probably is not the sole factor. Recently, the importance of the anatomic arrangement of the nerve vasculature has been highlighted in mediating both the diabetes-induced deficits of nerve blood flow and the effects of vasoactive therapeutic interventions. The nerve vascular supply comprises an intrinsic system consisting of microvessels, which are situated longitudinally within the fascicular endoneurium, and an extrinsic system composed of the larger nutritive arteries, arterioles, venules, and epineural vessels. The nerve has only a very limited capacity to autoregulate its vascular supply[222]; perhaps only the epineural and perineural vessels are capable of autoregulation. This means that alterations in system pressure lead to passive fluctuations in perfusion in the nerve,[222] and so assessments of nerve perfusion are best expressed as a "vascular conductance" that corrects for mean blood pressure.[198] Extensive anastomoses (both arteriovenous [AV] and arterioarterial) are formed between the two systems by the epi- and perineural vessels, which, together with the low metabolic requirements of the nerve, confer a resistance to ischemic insults.[223] Extensive perineurial AV anastomoses have recently been demonstrated in neuropathic diabetic subjects and have led to speculation regarding the role of a steal phenomenon, in which the nutritive endoneurial capillary flow is impaired by the high shunt flow.[224] Conversely, whether this putatively increased shunt flow is a result of chronic endoneurial ischemia/sclerosis is unknown. Many successful therapeutic interventions have been shown to regulate endoneurial nutritive and/or AV shunt flow differentially.

Oxidative Stress and EDN

Oxidative stress has recently emerged as a critical factor in the development of chronic diabetic complications[202,225–227] and a leading candidate in the development of nerve blood flow and nerve conduction deficits.[83,87,159,161] Malonyldialdehyde, a degradation product of lipid hydroperoxide, is increased in experimental[228] and human diabetes,[229] and levels of circulating antioxidants including ascorbic acid, platelet vitamin E, and taurine are decreased in human[230,231] and experimental diabetes.[228,232] In recently diagnosed T1DM patients, plasma levels of conjugated lipid dienes have been reported to be elevated, whereas in longer duration diabetes, levels of thiobarbituric acid reactive substances (TBARS) and lipid hydroperoxide were increased additionally.[233] These alterations have been ascribed to increased antioxidant consumption from increased oxidative stress or to transition metal-catalyzed glucose "auto-oxidation."[225,234] Increased oxygen free radical activity in diabetes is reversed by insulin[235] or ARIs[236] and has been ascribed to glucose-protein interactions,[237] to auto-oxidation of glucose,[225,226,234] and to glucose-induced activation of the AR pathway.[236,238]

In the endoneurial vasculature, oxidative stress has been implicated in the development of endoneurial ischemic hypoxia, impaired oxidative metabolism, and nerve energy deficits. Support for this construct has been provided by the recent identification of lipoic acid–sensitive GSH and GSH+GSSG depletion[83,87] and decreased mitochondrial and cytoplasmic NAD^+:NADH ratios,[87,217] together with vasodilator-responsive reductions of PCr:Cr and ATP:ADP ratios[217] in the sciatic nerve of 6-week STZ-D rats. These data are consistent with impaired mitochondrial oxidative phosphorylation, secondary to oxidative stress and ischemic hypoxia.

In EDN, the reduction in nerve blood flow and resultant hypoxia do not appear to be a principal contributer to oxidative stress, since amelioration of nerve blood flow deficits by prazosin does not alter indices of oxidative stress in the sciatic nerve in STZ-D rats.[217] In diabetic rodents, impairment of the blood–nerve barrier,[239] increased nerve conjugated dienes,[240,241] and reduced levels of nerve superoxide dismutase (SOD),[241] glutathione peroxidase,[241] glutathione,[201,242] norepinephrine,[243] and taurine,[100] as well as impaired neurotrophism,[129,244] provide support for the presence of increased oxidative stress. However, the mechanisms leading to paradoxic downregulation of antioxidant defense enzymes in the nerve of diabetic rodents are complex and poorly understood. In STZ-D rats, gene expression of glutathione peroxidase, catalase, cuprozinc superoxide dismutase, and manganese SOD was not decreased in the L4,5 dorsal root ganglion (DRG) and superior cervical ganglion after 3 or 12 months of diabetes.[245] Catalase mRNA was increased, however, after 12 months. Glutathione peroxidase activity is unaffected in the sciatic nerve of STZ-D rats. These observations suggest that glucose-induced posttranslational modifications may play an important role in altered antioxidant defense enzyme activity.

In EDN, increased oxidative stress may decrease nerve blood flow by disruption of signal transduction pathways in the vascular endothelium[150] or in the sympathetic ganglia.[246] Oxidative stress may lead to apoptosis in the vascular endothelium,[247,248] thereby impairing the synthesis or action of local vasodilatory agents. Oxidative stress can perturb prostanoid synthesis (see below)[228] and NO synthesis[249] in diabetes, and impaired endothelium-dependent relaxation in hyperglycemic rabbits can be corrected by probucol.[250] Essential fatty acid metabolism is disrupted by ROS, and therapeutic synergism has been reported between γ-linolenic acid and antioxidants.[159] Attenuation of oxidative stress by the administration of antioxidants can correct nerve blood flow and functional deficits *in vivo*.[86,87,159,161]

The endothelium-derived relaxing factor NO mediates vasodilation, macrophage cytotoxicity, and neurotransmission[251] and is highly susceptible to oxidative stress in diabetes.[251,252] NOS, the enzyme catalyzing the conversion of L-arginine to citrulline and NO at the expense of NADPH, is critically situated in endothelial cells, vascular smooth muscle cells, and sympathetic ganglia. NOS is constitutively expressed in endothelial (eNOS) and neuronal (nNOS) cells, and activity is critically dependent on posttranslational modification by calcium/calmodulin-dependent protein kinases and PKC.[251] Impaired synthesis of NO has been linked to polyol pathway activation through an NADPH-mediated mechanism (via the redox hypothesis), as well as alterations in protein kinase activation and calcium levels (via the osmotic hypothesis). Metabolic competition for NADPH by AR and NOS could precipitate NO depletion[133,209] via both decreasing NO synthesis and increasing levels of superoxide radicals, since NADPH is required for the production of GSH.

Additionally, increased formation of advanced glycosylation end products by glucose and fructose may also quench NO. It has been proposed that heavily glycated proteins in the arterial wall have increased affinity for transition metals, leading to accelerated destruction of NO and persistent vasoconstriction. The beneficial effects of many therapeutic agents on nerve blood flow and MNCV slowing are thought to be mediated by NO, as well as antioxidants, ARIs, EPO, and acetyl L-carnitine.[80,190]

Oxidative stress may also exacerbate nerve metabolic defects in diabetes, by disrupting nerve (Na,K)-ATPase activity,[253] which may lead to disruption of unmyelinated nerve fiber function, and by impairing the function of the Na^+-dependent cotransporters for MI and taurine.[80,190] Support for a role of oxidative stress in EDN is provided by the ability of antioxidants and pro-oxidants to prevent or provoke, respectively, functional nerve deficits. Lipid-soluble antioxidants[201,202,227] (such as probucol, the free radical scavenger and glutathione precursor N-acetylcysteine,[203] glutathione itself,[201] the chain-breaking antioxidant lipoic acid,[86,87,159,161] and the natural antioxidant vitamins C, E, and β-carotene[192]) prevent vascular defects and NCV slowing in diabetic animals. The advanced glycosylation end product (AGE) inhibitor aminoguanidine prevents motor and sensory NCV deficits[196,254,255] in diabetic rats and also prevents the reduction in nerve blood flow.[254] Conversely, aggravation of oxidative stress with primaquine in nondiabetic rats partially reproduces diabetic nerve dysfunction.[227] Impaired peripheral nerve function has been reported to improve in T2DM subjects treated for 6 months with 900 mg/day of vitamin E.[256]

Amelioration of oxidative stress may emerge as the principal mechanism of action of the ARIs.[105] Advanced glycation is exacerbated by high polyol pathway flux, since fructose is a more potent glycating agent than glucose, as are the intermediates and products of the hexose monophosphate shunt that generates NADPH for AR.[257] High flux through the polyol pathway may consume NADPH, required for the reduction of glutathione, which is involved in glutathione peroxidase–catalyzed removal of peroxide formed by the scavenging action of SOD on oxygen free radicals.[227]

A number of observations suggest that the beneficial effects of ARIs in diabetes may involve decreasing oxidative stress by a mechanism that may involve direct antioxidant effects as oxygen free radical scavengers or effects on cellular redox, glutathione, or taurine concentrations.[237] The ARIs sorbinil and rutin[258] inhibited collagen-linked fluorescence and increased vascular permeability in diabetic animals. In diabetic patients, the ARI tolrestat decreases plasma oxygen free radical levels.[238] ARIs may also work partly by binding free copper ions (and thus blocking copper-catalyzed ascorbate oxidation[237]) and by preventing depletion of the endogenous antioxidant taurine.

Therefore, accumulating evidence suggests a central role for increased oxidative stress in the pathogenesis of EDN. The availability of a plethora of naturally occurring and synthetic antioxidants should also accelerate the instigation of clinical trials to evaluate their efficacy in humans.

Nonenzymatic Glycation

Nonenzymatic protein glycation is a widespread biochemical phenomenon by which glucose and its metabolites may alter cellular composition, function, or both in diabetes. Nonenzymatic formation of Schiff base residues between glucose and the amine groups of proteins (with subsequent Amadori rearrangement) yields glycosylated proteins including hemoglobin.[225,226,234,257] More complex heterocyclic carbohydrate-protein adducts (AGEs) in diabetes lead to protein-protein cross-links and liberation of highly reactive free radicals that structurally alter extracellular matrix and promote cytotoxicity, NO quenching, and macrophage activation via the AGE receptor,[259] a cascade central to current thinking regarding the pathogenesis of diabetic complications. Protein glycation could involve the vascular supply, the extracellular matrix, or the cellular constituents of peripheral nerve. Protein glycation could produce vascular damage by generation of free oxygen radicals or through the formation of advanced glycation end products that in turn stimulate cytokine and growth factor release from activated macrophages, resulting in smooth muscle cell proliferation, atherogenesis, and vascular occlusion. Nonenzymatic glycation of extracellular matrix proteins could interfere with their neurotrophic or neurosupportive effects. Involvement in the pathogenesis of DPN is suggested by evidence that glucose-protein adducts on laminin reduce its support of neurite outgrowth in vitro[260] and that aminoguanidine (which among other actions impedes the formation of complex sugar-protein adducts) ameliorates some of the characteristic defects of EDN.[254,255]

Recent studies, however, suggest that glucose has a particularly low glycosylation potential among sugars, especially compared with fructose and its metabolites. In particular, a novel metabolic pathway that enzymatically phosphorylates fructose (and possibly sorbitol) leading to fructose-3-phosphate (and possibly sorbitol-3-phosphate), which subsequently degrades to 3-deoxyglucosone (3DG), a particularly potent glycosylating agent.[261] Thus, AR pathway flux, which converts glucose (with its low glycosylating potential) into fructose and sorbitol, their phosphorylation by a 3-phosphokinase,[261] and subsequent degradation to 3DG would radically accelerate the formation of the complex heterocyclic carbohydrate-protein adducts known as AGE.

Oxidative Stress, Programmed Cell Death, and Diabetic Neuropathy

Generation of ROS has been implicated in the signaling pathway leading to programmed cell death (PCD).[262] PCD leads to the deletion of cells during development or pathogenesis through a gene- and protein-regulated process. The morphologic endpoint of PCD, referred to as apoptosis, results from the degradation of genomic DNA, plasma membrane alterations, and the activation of caspases. PCD has been identified as the mechanism of cell death in a number of human neurodegenerative disorders[263] and has been implicated in the development of chronic diabetic complications. For example, PCD of vascular endothelium has been demonstrated in vivo in the aorta of diabetic rats.[264] In addition, ROS-mediated PCD is induced following glucose exposure in cultured human endothelial cells.[265,266]

Diabetic nephropathy is characterized by DNA fragmentation accompanied by evidence of oxidative stress[267] and also by the downregulation of Bcl-2.[268] The impaired wound healing observed in diabetes is associated with increased DNA fragmentation[269] and dysregulated expression of Bcl-2 and p53[270] in diabetic mice. Retinopathy in human diabetes has been linked to PCD in pericytes of the inner retina through increased expression of Bax and plasma membrane alterations[271] and increased caspase 1 expression.[272] Glucose-induced PCD in pericytes is associated with decreased SOD[272] and GSH,[272] suggesting that pericyte PCD involves oxidative stress. Neurons in the retina also display PCD-associated DNA fragmentation during experimental and human diabetes.[273] In addition to neurons of the retina, sensory neurons also are susceptible to the induction of PCD during hyperglycemia.[82,274,275] Sensory neurons of diabetic, but not normal, rats undergo PCD following axonal injury through an oxidative stress mechanism.[276] Finally, sera from diabetic subjects has been demonstrated to induce apoptosis in cultured neuroblastoma cells.[273,277,278]

Alterations of gene expression, such as increasing p53 or Bax, or decreasing Bcl-2, may be initiating steps in PCD. The relative abundance of the Bcl family of proteins including Bcl-2, Bax and Bcl-x_L,[279] which primarily are located in the inner mitochondrial membrane, appears to critically regulate the threshold for activation of the apoptotic cascade. Bcl-2 is antiapoptotic and inhibits the opening of a large mitochondrial conductance channel.[280] The opening of this channel results in mitochondrial depolarization, expansion of the intermembranous space, outer membrane rupture, and the release into the cytosol[280] of enzymes (such as cytochrome C and/or apoptotic-protease activating factor-1 (Apaf-1)) that activate the caspase cascade. Apoptosis is increased by a shift in the balance toward Bax homodimers, whereas the formation of Bcl-2/Bax or Bcl-x_L/Bax heterodimers inhibit PCD.[281]

Recent reports have suggested that PCD contributes to sensory and autonomic neuron dysfunction in STZ-D rats,[282,283] as well as in acutely hyperglycemic ND rats.[282] In diabetic rats, apoptosis of DRG neurons has been reported to be induced by axonal injury; such injury could be reversed by PGE$_1$ treatment, which promotes axonal regeneration.[276] Increased intracellular calcium has been invoked as a key mediator of apoptosis in DRGs from both diabetic rodents. Indeed, in dorsal horn neurons from diabetic rats, the activity of the N- and L- but not T-type voltage-gated channels has been reported to be increased.[284]

Recently, a pivotal role for the mitochondria has emerged in controlling PCD.[285] In STZ-D, for example, morphologic changes of PCD, such as Schwann cell degeneration, myelin ballooning, reduction of neuronal perikaryal volume, and shrinkage of the axoplasm are associated with markers of mitochondrial dysfunction, such as mitochondrial ballooning and impairment of basal mitochondrial membrane potential.[282,283] Elevated (more positive) mitochondrial membrane potential in diabetic STZ-D rat DRG neurons has been reported as early as 4 weeks after the onset of diabetes.[283] In STZ-D rat DRG neurons, decreased Bcl-2 and translocation of mitochondrial cytochrome C to the cytosol has been pathogenetically associated with activation of the apoptosis cascade, resulting in cleavage of the death effector caspase 3.[282,283] The mechanism underlying the reduction of Bcl-2 abundance is unknown. Unlike Bcl-2, no differences in the abundance of the antiapoptotic protein Bcl-x_L or Bax protein[283] (which promotes hyperglycemia-induced apoptosis in mouse blastocysts[286]) were identified in neurons from diabetic rats.

Many PCD promoters, including toxic agents and radiation, operate through the generation of ROS. The significance of ROS during the induction of PCD has been demonstrated by the ability of antioxidants to inhibit the response. This process, then, becomes significant in diabetes, since hyperglycemia can increase the generation of ROS through several mechanisms, as described above. Since mitochondrial dysfunction in STZ-D rats can be corrected by antioxidant therapy,[87] since ROS-induced PCD may share similar cell death pathways with neurotrophin withdrawal,[287] and since nerve growth factor (NGF) can block mitochondrial oxidative damage,[263,288,289] it is tempting to speculate that diabetes-induced increased oxidative stress is the inciting event that triggers neuronal PCD. The recent discovery that the antiapoptotic Bcl-2 gene product has antioxidant properties lends further support to the importance of oxidative events in PCD.[290,291] Therapeutic strategies such as antioxidants and/or caspase inhibitors may therefore have considerable potential for the prevention or treatment of DPN.

The COX Pathway and Diabetic Neuropathy

Alterations in COX activity and subsequent perturbations in prostanoid metabolism have also been invoked in the pathogenesis of experimental DPN at a neurovascular level. However, in experimental DPN, the effects of COX inhibition on neurovascular and functional deficits have been inconsistent. Initial reports suggested that nonselective COX inhibition could ameliorate certain specific deficits of nerve function in experimental diabetes[292,293]; however, other investigators could not confirm any beneficial effects.[294,295] Nonselective inhibition of the COX pathway with flurbiprofen in nondiabetic (ND) rats has recently been reported to replicate, and in STZ-D rats potentiate, many of the biochemical and physiologic abnormalities of experimental DPN. In contrast, selective COX-2 inhibition did not affect nerve blood flow or nerve conduction in ND rats and prevented MNCV slowing and nerve blood flow deficits in STZ-D rats. A possible explanation for the apparent inconsistency in the effects of different COX inhibitors on both NCV and nerve blood flow deficits in STZ-D rats is unknown, but it may reflect differences in the relative degree of inhibition of the two COX pathways (see below).

Two COX isoforms have been identified.[296] COX-1 is constitutively expressed in a variety of cells and tissues including the vascular endothelium,[297] whereas inducible COX-2 is associated with proinflammatory stimuli, such as cytokines, growth factors, tumor promoters,[298] and oxidative stress.[299] A potential link between oxidative stress and alterations in PG synthesis appears to be the transcription factor NF-κB, which is activated by ROS.[300] Additionally, hypoxia has also been shown to induce COX-2 expression in cultured endothelial cells[301] and rodent brains,[302] suggesting that the effects of oxidative stress on the COX pathway could be mediated by several different pathways.

The interrelationships of COX and ROS are, however, complex, since ROS-induced activation of COX-2 can in itself increase ROS production, during PGG$_2$ to PGH$_2$ conversion, which generates hydrogen peroxide.[297] However, since COX-2 activation can have a protective function on a number of physiologic processes,[303] it is reasonable to conclude that the regulation and consequences of COX-2 expression are highly dependent on both the site of expression and the underlying pathophysiologic condition. Although there is some evidence of COX-2 involvement in brain ischemic and neurodegenerative disorders, to date there have been no published reports regarding altered COX expression in disorders of the peripheral nerve. Preliminary studies in this laboratory suggest that COX-2 protein abundance is significantly elevated in the sciatic nerve of STZ-D rats.[304]

The COX Pathway and Programmed Cell Death

Alterations of the COX-2 pathway have been implicated in the development of PCD. For example, it has been shown that induction of COX-2 mRNA and protein expression precede PCD in *in vivo* and *in vitro* models of neurodegeneration[305] and that enhanced COX-2 protein expression promotes apoptosis in rat neocortex.[306] Nonselective COX inhibitors, including flurbiprofen, which block predominantly the COX-1 pathway, have been shown to upregulate COX-2 gene expression and facilitate flux through this pathway. This has been linked to the induction of apoptosis in cultured rat gastric cells by a mechanism that involves increased oxidative stress.[307] Although the presence of COX-2 induction in neurodegenerative conditions associated with PCD has been documented,[305] its functional significance is still uncertain. It is possible that enhanced COX-2 expression induces neurotoxicity via accumulation of ROS and/or metabolites other than PG.[306] Although most of the published data report a direct causal relationship between COX-2 activation and neuronal PCD, some suggest that COX-2 may be neuroprotective.[308] For instance, COX-2 expression has been demonstrated to inhibit trophic withdrawal apoptosis in NGF-differentiated PC12 cells.[309] It can be concluded, therefore, that the interrelationships of the COX-2 pathway and apoptosis are complex and poorly understood.

We have proposed a model to explain the interrelationships among hyperglycemia, oxidative stress, PCD, and altered COX pathway activity in the development of nerve conduction deficits (Fig. 44-3). Hyperglycemia (through increased glucose autooxidation, advanced glycation end product formation, and activation of the AR pathway) generates increased ROS. Increased ROS, via upregulation of NF-κB, induces COX-2 expression, which facilitates the conversion of arachidonate to vasoconstrictory and proinflammatory PG, thereby favoring endoneurial ischemia and hypoxia. Increased flux through COX-2 may further promote the generation of ROS, resulting in a self-reinforcing cycle. ROS may promote PCD by diminishing neurotrophic support and inducing mitochondrial dysfunction, thereby leading to the release of cytochrome C and activation of the caspase cascade. Increased AR pathway activity and osmolyte depletion contribute to reduced (Na,K)-ATPase activity. Increased oxidative stress, endoneurial ischemia, reduced (Na,K)-ATPase activity, and PCD may result in NCV slowing.

FIGURE 44-3. Proposed interactions of hyperglycemia, oxidative stress, and the cyclo-oxygenase (COX) pathway in experimental diabetic neuropathy. Hyperglycemia through increased auto-oxidation, with subsequent formation of advanced glycation end products, and activation of the aldose reductase (AR) pathway, with secondary NADPH and taurine depletion, generates reactive oxygen species (ROS) and increases oxidative stress. Increased ROS, via modulation of NFκB-induced COX-2 expression, which regulates the conversion of arachidonate to vasoconstrictory and proinflammatory prostaglandin (PG), precipitates the imbalance in thromboxane A_2 (TXA_2)/PGI_2 ratio, therefore favoring vasoconstriction and ischemia. Reciprocally, COX-2 upregulation increases the rate of PGG_2 to PGH_2 conversion and ROS generation, further exacerbating oxidative stress. ROS may promote programmed cell death (PCD) by diminishing the nerve growth factor (NGF) neurotrophic support and by inducing mitochondrial dysfunction, which is thought to lead to caspase activation and cytochrome C release. Increased AR pathway activity and osmolyte depletion contribute to reduced (Na,K)-ATPase activity. Increased oxidative stress, endoneurial ischemia, reduced (Na,K)-ATPase activity, and PCD may result in nerve conduction velocity (NCV) slowing.

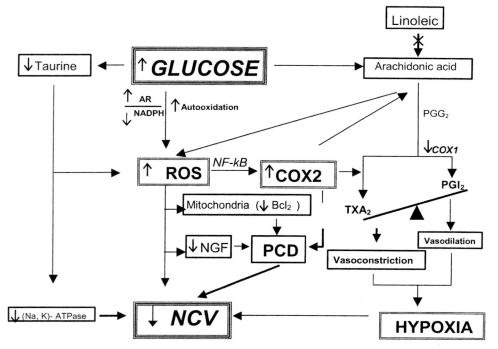

Neurotrophic Growth Factors and Diabetic Neuropathy

Neurotrophic growth factors modulate neuronal outgrowth during development and sustain innervation thereafter. In the mature animal, neurotrophins define the neuronal phenotype and promote local regeneration. An important function of the neurotrophins is to regulate the expression of phenotypic neuropeptides, including substance P and calcitonin gene–related peptide (CGRP), in adult DRG neurons. After nerve injury in the adult, they promote local neurite sprouting and regeneration.[310] Thus, blunting of these neurotrophic responses could mediate diabetic neuropathy if insulin deficiency and/or hyperglycemia (1) decreased growth factor synthesis by target organs or supporting cells, (2) disrupted retrograde transport of growth factors to the neuronal cell body, (3) affected the signal transduction mechanism(s) at the level of the Trk receptors or more downstream signaling cascades, or (4) promoted neuronal cell death.[311]

Mature Schwann cells also synthesize and express growth factors and growth factor receptors during neural development and regeneration,[312] including NGF,[313] ciliary neurotrophic factor (CNTF), a small polypeptide originally purified from chick and rabbit sciatic nerve,[314] and insulin-like growth factor-I (IGF-I).[315] The neurotrophin family[316] has been expanded to include three additional neurotrophic factors, namely, brain-derived neurotrophin factor (BDNF), neurotrophin-3 (NT-3), and neurotrophin-4/5 (NT-4/5).

Recently, the roles of neurotrophins have been explored using knockout mice models. Deletion of the high-affinity NGF receptor Trk A in mice results in extensive loss of sympathetic ganglionic neurons and small neural crest–derived sensory neurons (nociceptive C neurons).[317,318] NT-3 knockout animals are deficient in both type 1a sensory afferents and muscle spindles, whereas BDNF and NT-4/5 null mutants lack neural placode–derived sensory cranial ganglia.[318]

One of the best characterized growth factors is nerve growth factor (NGF), which is relatively specific for sensory and autonomic neurons and their axonal processes. NGF production and gene expression in autonomic and sensory neuronal targets vary reciprocally with the density of innervation by NGF-sensitive neurons.[319] In the rat heart, for example, high levels of NGF mRNA and protein are found in the densely innervated atria, but not in the more sparsely innervated ventricles, although regional ventricular differences have not been reported.[320] Peripherally synthesized NGF is retrogradely transported by the axon from target organs to neuronal cell bodies for normal maintenance and regeneration of the peripheral nervous system. Ganglionic NGF is required for signal transduction, neurotransmitter synthesis, protein phosphorylation, methylation, and gene expression of ras-like proteins in sympathetic and sensory neurons.[321] Retrograde axonal transport is an important modulator of target tissue NGF. For example, total sympathetic denervation in adult rats produces high NGF protein levels in the heart,[322] without affecting tissue mRNA levels.[322,323] NGF has antioxidant properties[324,325] and protects sympathetic neurons from ROS-mediated PCD.[325]

Another family of growth factors thought to be important in the pathogenesis, and potentially the treatment, of diabetic neuropathy[326] is the IGFs. IGF-I and IGF-II are polypeptides essential for normal fetal, neonatal, and pubertal growth. IGFs share many important neurotrophic properties with NGF and have neurotrophic actions in sensory sympathetic[326,327] and motor neurons. These actions can all be affected by diabetes.[328]

IGFs are presently the only known neurotrophic factors that are found in nerve and muscle and are capable of supporting both sensory and motor nerve regeneration in adult animals.[328,329] Glial, but not neuronal, cells express IGF-II mRNAs,[330] unlike IGF-I, which is expressed by both.[330] Both IGF-I and -II increase the numbers of cells with neurites and the lengths of neurites in cultured human neuroblastoma cells[331] and cultured spinal cord motor neurons[332]; they also act as mitogens for the former. IGF receptors are found on the shafts and terminals of axons.[332]

Six IGF binding proteins (BPs) regulate the action of the IGFs[333] and serve as possible targets for disruption by diabetes. IGFBP-II preferentially binds IGF-II and is the predominant IGFBP in the CNS and CSF.[334] IGFBP-III, which binds both IGF-I and -II, is the principal form found in the circulation. Sites of production of IGFBPs include the neurons and glia.[327,333] Local production of IGFs and their binding proteins may stimulate nerve fiber regeneration.[329,335–337] Local production of IGF is probably important in stimulating regeneration, as IGFBPs would tend to block more distant effects.

Neurotrophins bind to a family of tyrosine kinase receptors called Trks (tropomyosin-related kinases).[338] NGF binds to the high-affinity receptor Trk A, whereas Trk B serves as the receptor for both BNDF and NT-4/5, and Trk C binds NT-3. However, neurotrophins can bind and activate more than one receptor. Additionally, an abundant "low"-affinity receptor, termed p75, binds all the neurotrophins.[339] This receptor may serve to modulate neurotrophin sensitivity[339] and determine the survival requirements of mature neurons to the neurotrophins, particularly NGF.[340] p75 may present neurotrophins to high-affinity receptors on the growing axons[339] since it is upregulated by NGF,[341] axonal injury,[342] and collateral sprouting[343] and is expressed in target fields during their innervation.[344]

NGF receptors are expressed by Schwann cells during normal development but decline fivefold with maturation,[345] and NGF production remains suppressed as long as axonal integrity and contact are maintained.[346] Schwann cell NGF receptor expression is increased in human neuropathies associated with active nerve fiber degeneration.[347] IGF-I immunoreactivity is also present in Schwann cell cytoplasm, is increased by sciatic nerve transection,[315] and enhances regeneration in a dose-dependent fashion in lesioned sciatic nerve.[348] The expression of IGF-I and its receptor is markedly suppressed in axotomized diabetic nerve, and this change is associated with significantly impaired nerve fiber regeneration.[349] In STZ-D rats, serum IGF-I levels are diminished,[337,350] as is IGF-I mRNA in liver, kidney, lung, heart, and peripheral nerves.[337,349,351] Thus blunted local neurotrophic effects may contribute to the pathogenesis of diabetic neuropathy, but the magnitude and details of this effect remain to be clarified.

An increasing number of studies have explored the effects of diabetes on neurotrophism in both animal models of DPN and humans. In diabetes, small changes in endogenous NGF levels may be of pathophysiologic significance since endogenous NGF levels are limited,[351] and their NGF receptors are unsaturated.[319] In diabetic rodents, endogenous NGF levels are reduced in some sympathetically innervated target organs,[351] including the sciatic nerve[351] and submandibular glands (the latter displaying decreasing NGF in the superior cervical ganglion).[352] In some target tissues, however, including the atria and ventricles, NGF content increases after the induction of diabetes, which may reflect impaired axonal transport or possibly increased regional synthesis.[351,353]

Retrograde axonal flow of NGF to the cell bodies is altered in STZ-D rats.[353,354] During experimentally induced diabetes, for example, retrograde axonal transport of NGF along the mesenteric nerves (which supply the alimentary tract) to the superior mesenteric ganglion is reduced by approximately half,[354] and these nerves can develop a distal diabetic axonopathy. In a similar fashion, NGF transport is decreased in diabetic somatic sensory neurons.[355] Decreased NGF transport is a component of a generalized transport dysfunction in diabetes that includes proteins, glycoprotein, and neurotransmitters.[354]

Compared with NGF, considerably less is known about the effects of diabetes on other neurotrophins; IGF expression and/or action also appears to be altered in diabetes in both rodents and humans. Schwann cells from genetically diabetic rodents express lowered amounts of IGF-I, IGFI-receptor (IGF-IR), and NGF.[350] In streptozocin-treated rats, there is a decrease in serum IGF-I levels[350,356,357] and a reduction in IGF-I mRNA in sciatic nerve, liver, kidney, lung, and heart.[350,358–361] Recently, a 30–50% decrease in NT-3 and NT-4/5 gene expression was reported in nerves from rodents with experimental diabetes, whereas BDNF was undetectable.[362] Levels of NT-3 are decreased in the leg muscles from diabetic rodents, and its administration is reported to increase the NCV of sensory nerves.[363]

Abnormal neurotrophin receptor expression and/or sensitivity may play an important role in mediated impaired neurotrophic support. In lumbar DRG of diabetic rats, levels of Trk A mRNA, the 110-kd receptor protein,[364,365] and p75 gene expression[366] have been reported to be reduced. Others, however, have reported that DRG-immunoreactive Trk A is not affected by diabetes. NGF gene expression is regulated by glucose-sensitive signal transduction pathways,[367] adrenergic mechanisms,[368] and oxidative stress.[369]

Chronic oxidative stress depletes NGF by inhibiting protein synthesis[369] and may downregulate NGF receptor expression, sensitivity, and transport.[369,370] The chain-breaking antioxidant α-lipoic acid may stimulate NGF synthesis[371] and can prevent NGF protein depletion in sciatic nerve[370] and myocardium of STZ-D rats (Stevens, personal observations). α-Lipoic acid augments NGF-mediated substance P release in STZ-D rats[370] above that of equivalent correction of nerve NGF protein content by exogenous rhNGF alone, perhaps implicating oxidative stress in the downregulation of the NGF sensitivity that complicates diabetes. Some NGF transport defects can be corrected in the diabetic rat by treatment with ARIs, suggesting that increased polyol pathway flux may contribute to these axonal transport defects. In subjects with DAN, serum NGF levels are reduced,[372] and in patients with early diabetic neuropathy, decreased skin axon reflexes, mediated by small sensory fibers, correlate with loss of NGF expression in keratinocytes. In patients with diabetic neuropathy,[373] no change in p75 NGF receptor expression has been reported in sural nerve biopsy specimens.

Limited evidence suggests that neurotrophin treatment may be effective in the management of DPN. In experimental diabetes, NGF treatment protects against the development of diabetic sensory neuropathy[374,375] and ameliorates diabetes-induced decreases in neuropeptide levels *in vivo*[376] and *in vitro*.[377] NGF-treated diabetic rodents retain the ability to respond to noxious thermal stimuli and express normal neuropeptide levels.[375] NGF has been reported to reverse defects in myelinated nerve fiber morphology such as myelin thickness and to increase CGRP and substance P in the DRG and dorsal horn of the spinal cord of diabetic rats. The defects in p75 transport and protein content but not mRNA are reversed by rhNGF.[364] In lumbar DRG, reported deficits of Trk A

mRNA and the 110-kd receptor protein are not sensitive to rhNGF.[364] DRG-immunoreactive Trk A has been reported to be decreased by NGF in healthy control rats.[378] NGF has been reported to restore abnormal sensory C-fiber function in transgenic diabetic mice.[379] Treatment with 4-methylcatechol, which stimulates endogenous NGF synthesis, also ameliorates neuropathy in streptozocin-treated rodents.[380] Treatment of STZ-D rats with IGF-I protects against the development of diabetic neuropathy and restores normal nerve function.[311,328]

Clinical trials in humans, however, have been disappointing to date. For example, a randomized, placebo-controlled trial of s/c NGF did not confirm any beneficial effects on neuropathic symptoms or abnormalities on clinical examination, but small nerve fiber function was inadequately assessed.[381] In humans, studies evaluating the potential of IGF-1 administration as a treatment for diabetic neuropathy have been hampered by the development of toxicity.

SUMMARY AND CONCLUSIONS

Theories of the pathogenesis of diabetic neuropathy continue to evolve; the disease is considered to involve acute functional abnormalities in nerve fibers, followed by more chronic nerve fiber atrophy, injury and loss associated with microvascular dysfunction, and blunted nerve fiber regeneration. These abnormalities can be traced to the metabolic effects of hyperglycemia and/or other effects of insulin deficiency on the various constituents of peripheral nerve, its supporting connective tissue and vascular elements, and possibly the autonomic innervation that controls the endoneurial microvasculature. The polyol pathway, oxidative stress, and/or nonenzymatic glycation affecting one or more cell types in the multicellular constituents of peripheral nerve appears to have an inciting role. The potentially important roles of other factors, such as possible direct neurotrophic effects of insulin and insulin-related growth factors, remain to be explored, as do the more complex and indirect effects of glucose metabolism via the vascular elements of peripheral nerve.

ARIs, which have been proposed as the first mechanistically based treatment for diabetic neuropathy, constitute only the first of many such therapies, each directed against one or more elements in the complex pathogenetic process responsible for diabetic neuropathy. Despite the setbacks of recent clinical trials, the ability of biochemically effective ARIs to improve nerve function in diabetic patients and the evidence that they improve nerve structure and function in patients with early diabetic neuropathy have established the polyol pathway as one likely mediator of nerve dysfunction and damage in human diabetes.

The challenge that lies ahead will be the development of potent therapeutic interventions that can safely be given at high enough doses to prevent the diverse metabolic consequences of hyperglycemia. Animal studies indicate that this may most rapidly be achieved by using combinations of agents to block the diverse metabolic pathways mediating glucose toxicity. However, the evidence that improved metabolic control can prevent the development of clinical neuropathy[83] argues strongly for the hypothesis that hyperglycemia and/or insulin deficiency is at the root of diabetic neuropathy and that improved metabolic control should protect against the development (and probably progression) of the disease.

REFERENCES

1. Porte D, Halter JB: *Textbook of Endocrinology*, 6th ed. Saunders: 1981.
2. Dyck PJ, Lais A, Karnes JL, *et al*: Fiber loss is primary and multifocal in sural nerves in diabetic polyneuropathy. *Ann Neurol* 1986;19:425.
3. Thomas PK: Schwann-cell abnormalities in diabetic neuropathy. *Lancet* 1965;1:1355.
4. Chopra JS, Hurwitz LJ, Montgomery DA: The pathogenesis of sural nerve changes in diabetes mellitus. *Brain* 1969;92:391.
5. Behse F, Buchthal F, Carlsen F: Nerve biopsy and conduction studies in diabetic neuropathy. *J Neurol Neurosurg Psychiatry* 1977;40:1072.
6. Kimura J, Yamada T, Stevland NP: Distal slowing of motor nerve conduction velocity in diabetic polyneuropathy. *J Neurol Sci* 1979;42: 291.
7. Hansen S, Ballantyne JP: Axonal dysfunction in the neuropathy of diabetes mellitus: A quantitative electrophysiological study. *J Neurol Neurosurg Psychiatry* 1977;40:555.
8. Bischoff A: [Diabetic neuropathy. Pathologic anatomy, pathophysiology and pathogenesis on the basis of electron microscopic studies]. *Dtsch Med Wochenschr* 1968;93:237.
9. Yasuda H, Dyck PJ: Abnormalities of endoneurial microvessels and sural nerve pathology in diabetic neuropathy. *Neurology* 1987;37:20.
10. Low PA, Walsh JC, Huang CY, *et al*: The sympathetic nervous system in alcoholic neuropathy. A clinical and pathological study. *Brain* 1975;98:357.
11. Chopra JS, Fannin T: Pathology of diabetic neuropathy. *J Pathol* 1971;104:175.
12. Yagihashi S, Matsunaga M: Ultrastructural pathology of peripheral nerves in patients with diabetic neuropathy. *Tohoku J Exp Med* 1979; 129:357.
13. Appenzeller O, Ogin G: Myelinated fibres in human paravertebral sympathetic chain: White rami communicantes in alcoholic and diabetic patients. *J Neurol Neurosurg Psychiatry* 1974;37:1155.
14. Kristensson K, Nordborg C, Olsson Y, *et al*: Changes in the vagus nerve in diabetes mellitus. *Acta Pathol Microbiol Scand [A]* 1971;79:684.
15. Smith B: Neuropathology of the oesophagus in diabetes mellitus. *J Neurol Neurosurg Psychiatry* 1974;37:1151.
16. Bischoff A: *Report at the Aarhus University 50 Year Jubilee Symposium*. Aarhus (Denmark) University:1978.
17. Thomas PK, Lascelles RG: The pathology of diabetic medicine. *Q J Med* 1966;35:489.
18. Llewelyn JG, Gilbey SG, Thomas PK, *et al*: Sural nerve morphometry in diabetic autonomic and painful sensory neuropathy. A clinico-pathological study. *Brain* 1991;114:867.
19. King RH, Llewelyn JG, Thomas PK, *et al*: Diabetic neuropathy: Abnormalities of Schwann cell and perineurial basal laminae. Implications for diabetic vasculopathy. *Neuropathol Appl Neurobiol* 1989;15: 339.
20. Dyck PJ, Zimmerman BR, Vilen TH, *et al*: Nerve glucose, fructose, sorbitol, myo-inositol, and fiber degeneration and regeneration in diabetic neuropathy. *N Engl J Med* 1988;319:542.
21. Sima AA, Bril V, Nathaniel V, *et al*: Regeneration and repair of myelinated fibers in sural-nerve biopsy specimens from patients with diabetic neuropathy treated with sorbinil. *N Engl J Med* 1988;319:548.
22. Greene DA, Arezzo JC, Brown MB: Effect of aldose reductase inhibition on nerve conduction and morphometry in diabetic neuropathy. Zenarestat Study Group. *Neurology* 1999;53:580.
23. Bischoff A: *Vascular and Neurologic Changes in Early Diabetes*. Academic Press:1973.
24. Williams E, Timperley WR, Ward JD, *et al*: Electron microscopical studies of vessels in diabetic peripheral neuropathy. *J Clin Pathol* 1980;33:462.
25. Faerman I, Glocer L, Celener D, *et al*: Autonomic nervous system and diabetes. Histological and histochemical study of the autonomic nerve fibers of the urinary bladder in diabetic patients. *Diabetes* 1973;22:225.
26. DCCT. The effect of intensive treatment of diabetes on the development and progression of long-term complications in insulin-dependent diabetes mellitus. The Diabetes Control and Complications Trial Research Group [see comments]. *N Engl J Med* 1993;329:977.
27. Pirart J: Diabetes mellitus and its degenerative complications: A prospective study of 4,400 patients observed between 1947 and 1973. *Diabetes Care* 1978;1:168.
28. Pirart J: Diabetic neuropathy: A metabolic or a vascular disease? *Diabetes* 1965;14:1.
29. Thomas PK, Ward JD, Watkins PJ: *Complications of Diabetes*. Arnold:1982.
30. UKPDS: Intensive blood-glucose control with sulphonylureas or insulin compared with conventional treatment and risk of complications in patients with type 2 diabetes (UKPDS 33). UK Prospective Diabetes Study (UKPDS) Group [see comments]. *Lancet* 1998;352:837.
31. Brown MJ, Asbury AK: Diabetic neuropathy. *Ann Neurol* 1984;15:2.
32. Ellenberg M: Diabetic neuropathy: Clinical aspects. *Metabolism* 1976;25:1627.
33. Greene DA, Winegrad AI, Carpentier JL, *et al*: Rabbit sciatic nerve fascicle and 'endoneurial' preparations for in vitro studies of peripheral nerve glucose metabolism. *J Neurochem* 1979;33:1007.
34. Ward JD: *Diabetes Mellitus*. Garland:1981.
35. Winegrad AI, Morrison AD, Greene DA: Late complication of diabetes. In: DeGroot LJ *et al*, eds. *Endocrinology*, Vol. 2. Grune & Stratton:1979;1041.
36. McCulloch DK, Campbell IW, Prescott RJ, *et al*: Effect of alcohol intake on symptomatic peripheral neuropathy in diabetic men. *Diabetes Care* 1980;3:245.
37. Gilliatt RW, Willison RG: Peripheral nerve conduction in diabetic neuropathy. *J Neurol Neurosurg Psychiatry* 1962;25:11.
38. DCCT. Factors in development of diabetic neuropathy. Baseline analysis of neuropathy in feasibility phase of Diabetes Control and Complications Trial (DCCT). The DCCT Research Group. *Diabetes* 1988;37:476.
39. Gregersen G: Variations in motor conduction velocity produced by acute changes of the metabolic state in diabetic patients. *Diabetologia* 1968;4:273.
40. Ward JD, Barnes CG, Fisher DJ, *et al*: Improvement in nerve conduction following treatment in newly diagnosed diabetics. *Lancet* 1971;1:428.
41. Terkildsen AB, Christensen NJ: Reversible nervous abnormalities in juvenile diabetics with recently diagnosed diabetes. *Diabetologia* 1971;7:113.
42. Eng GD, Nellington H, August GP: Nerve conduction velocity determination in juvenile diabetes. *Mod Probl Paediatr* 1975;12:213.
43. Gregersen G: Diabetic neuropathy: Influence of age, sex, metabolic control, and duration of diabetes on motor conduction velocity. *Neurology* 1967;17:972.
44. Graf RJ, Halter JB, Halar E, *et al*: Nerve conduction abnormalities in untreated maturity-onset diabetes: Relation to levels of fasting plasma glucose and glycosylated hemoglobin. *Ann Intern Med* 1979;90:298.
45. Graf RJ, Halter JB, Pfeifer MA, *et al*: Glycemic control and nerve conduction abnormalities in non-insulin-dependent diabetic subjects. *Ann Intern Med* 1981;94:307.
46. Holman RR, Dornan TL, Mayon-White V, *et al*: Prevention of deterioration of renal and sensory-nerve function by more intensive management of insulin-dependent diabetic patients. A two-year randomised prospective study. *Lancet* 1983;1:204.
47. Service FJ, Rizza RA, Daube JR, *et al*: Near normoglycaemia improved nerve conduction and vibration sensation in diabetic neuropathy. *Diabetologia* 1985;28:722.
48. Effect of 6 months of strict metabolic control on eye and kidney function in insulin-dependent diabetics with background retinopathy. Steno Study Group. *Lancet* 1982;1:121.
49. Gallai V, Agostini L, Rossi A, *et al*: Evaluation of the motor and sensory conduction velocity (MCV, SCV) in diabetic patients before and after a three-day treatment with the artificial beta cell (biostator). In: Canal N, Pozza G, eds. *Peripheral Neuropathies*. Elsevier/North-Holland Biomedical:1978;287.
50. Service FJ, Daube JR, O'Brien PC, Dyck PJ: Effect of artificial pancreas treatment on peripheral nerve function in diabetes. *Neurology* 1981;31:1375.
51. Troni W, Carta Q, Cantello R, *et al*: Peripheral nerve function and metabolic control in diabetes mellitus. *Ann Neurol* 1984;16:178.
52. Greene DA, Brown MJ, Braunstein SN, *et al*: Comparison of clinical course and sequential electrophysiological tests in diabetics with symptomatic polyneuropathy and its implications for clinical trials. *Diabetes* 1981;30:139.
53. Group TDR: Effect of intensive diabetes treatment on nerve conduction in the Diabetes Control and Complications Trial. *Ann Neurol* 1995;38:869.

54. Group TDR: The effect of intensive diabetes treatment on the progression of diabetic retinopathy: The Diabetes Control and Complications Trial. *Arch Ophthalmol* 1995;113:36.

55. Jakobsen J, Christiansen JS, Kristoffersen I, *et al*: Autonomic and somatosensory nerve function after 2 years of continuous subcutaneous insulin infusion in type 1 diabetes. *Diabetes* 1988;37:452.

56. Lauritzen T, Frost-Larsen K, Larsen HW, *et al*: Two-year experience with continuous subcutaneous insulin infusion in relation to retinopathy and neuropathy. *Diabetes* 1985;34(suppl 3):74.

57. Ziegler D, Dannehl K, Wiefels K, Gries FA: Differential effects of near-normoglycaemia for 4 years on somatic nerve dysfunction and heart rate variation in type I diabetic patients. *Diabet Med* 1992;9:622.

58. DCCT. The effect of intensive diabetes therapy on measures of autonomic nervous system function in the Diabetes Control and Complications Trial (DCCT). *Diabetologia* 1998;41:416.

59. Stevens MJ, Dayanikli F, Raffel DM, *et al*: Scintigraphic assessment of regionalized defects in myocardial sympathetic innervation and blood flow regulation in diabetic patients with autonomic neuropathy. *J Am Coll Cardiol* 1998;31:1575.

60. Mantysaari M, Kuikka J, Mustonen J, *et al*: Noninvasive detection of cardiac sympathetic nervous dysfunction in diabetic patients using [^{123}I]metaiodobenzylguanidine. *Diabetes* 1992;41:1069.

61. Allman KC, Stevens MJ, Wieland DM, *et al*: Noninvasive assessment of cardiac diabetic neuropathy by C-11 hydroxyephedrine and positron emission tomography. *J Am Coll Cardiol* 1993;22:1425.

62. Schnell O, Muhr D, Weiss M, *et al*: Reduced myocardial ^{123}I-metaiodobenzylguanidine uptake in newly diagnosed IDDM patients. *Diabetes* 1996;45:801.

63. Stevens MJ, Raffel DM, Allman KC, *et al*: Cardiac sympathetic dysinnervation in diabetes: Implications for enhanced cardiovascular risk. *Circulation* 1998;98:961.

64. Ziegler D, Weise F, Langen KJ, *et al*: Effect of glycaemic control on myocardial sympathetic innervation assessed by [^{123}I]metaiodobenzylguanidine scintigraphy: A 4-year prospective study in IDDM patients. *Diabetologia* 1998;41:443.

65. Stevens MJ, Raffel DM, Allman KC, *et al*: Regression and progression of cardiac sympathetic dysinnervation complicating diabetes: An assessment by C-11 hydroxyephedrine and positron emission tomography. *Metabolism* 1999;48:92.

66. Eliasson SG: Nerve conduction changes in experimental diabetes. *J Clin Invest* 1974;43:2353.

67. Preston GM: Peripheral neuropathy in the alloxan-diabetic rat. *J Physiol (Lond)* 1967;189:49P.

68. Sima AA, Brismar T: Reversible diabetic nerve dysfunction: Structural correlates to electrophysiological abnormalities. *Ann Neurol* 1985;18:21.

69. Greene DA, Chakrabarti S, Lattimer SA, *et al*: Role of sorbitol accumulation and myo-inositol depletion in paranodal swelling of large myelinated nerve fibers in the insulin-deficient spontaneously diabetic bio-breeding rat. Reversal by insulin replacement, an aldose reductase inhibitor, and myo-inositol. *J Clin Invest* 1987;79:1479.

70. Jakobsen J: Early and preventable changes of peripheral nerve structure and function in insulin-deficient diabetic rats. *J Neurol Neurosurg Psychiatry* 1979;42:509.

71. Greene DA, De Jesus PV Jr, Winegrad AI: Effects of insulin and dietary myoinositol on impaired peripheral motor nerve conduction velocity in acute streptozocin diabetes. *J Clin Invest* 1975;55:1326.

72. Robertson DM, Sima AA: Diabetic neuropathy in the mutant mouse [C57BL/ks(db/db)]: A morphometric study. *Diabetes* 1980;29:60.

73. Greene DA, Sima AA, Stevens MJ, *et al*: Aldose reductase inhibitors: An approach to the treatment of diabetic nerve damage. *Diabetes Metab Rev* 1993;9:189.

74. Fukuma M, Carpentier JL, Orci L, *et al*: An alteration in internodal myelin membrane structure in large sciatic nerve fibers in rats with acute streptozocin diabetes and impaired nerve conduction velocity. *Diabetologia* 1978;15:65.

75. Zochodne DW, Nguyen C: Increased peripheral nerve microvessels in early experimental diabetic neuropathy: Quantitative studies of nerve and dorsal root ganglia. *J Neurol Sci* 1999;166:40.

76. Pietri A, Ehle AL, Raskin P: Changes in nerve conduction velocity after six weeks of glucoregulation with portable insulin infusion pumps. *Diabetes* 1980;29:668.

77. Clements RS Jr: Diabetic neuropathy—new concepts of its etiology. *Diabetes* 1979;28:604.

78. Winegrad AI: Banting Lecture 1986. Does a common mechanism induce the diverse complications of diabetes? *Diabetes* 1987;36:396.

79. Greene DA, Lattimer SA, Sima AA: Sorbitol, phosphoinositides, and sodium-potassium-ATPase in the pathogenesis of diabetic complications. *N Engl J Med* 1987;316:599.

80. Greene DA, Sima AA, Stevens MJ, *et al*: Complications: Neuropathy, pathogenetic considerations. *Diabetes Care* 1992;15:1902.

81. Stevens MJ, Feldman EL, Thomas T, *et al*: Pathogenesis of diabetic neuropathy. In: Veves A, ed. *Contemporary Endocrinology: Clinical Management of Diabetic Neuropathy*. Humana:1999;13.

82. Greene DA, Stevens MJ, Obrosova I, *et al*: Glucose-induced oxidative stress and programmed cell death in diabetic neuropathy. *Eur J Pharmacol* 1999;375:217.

83. Kishi Y, Schmelzer JD, Yao JK, *et al*: Alpha-lipoic acid: Effect on glucose uptake, sorbitol pathway, and energy metabolism in experimental diabetic neuropathy. *Diabetes* 1999;48:2045.

84. Greene DA, Winegrad AI: In vitro studies of the substrates for energy production and the effects of insulin on glucose utilization in the neural components of peripheral nerve. *Diabetes* 1979;28:878.

85. Magnani P, Cherian PV, Gould GW, *et al*: Glucose transporters in rat peripheral nerve: Paranodal expression of GLUT1 and GLUT3. *Metabolism* 1996;45:1466.

86. Ogawa S, Lee TM, Glynn P: Energy metabolism in rat brain in vivo studied by ^{31}P nuclear magnetic resonance: Changes during postnatal development. *Arch Biochem Biophys* 1986;248:43.

87. Stevens MJ, Obrosova I, Cao X, *et al*: Effects of DL-α-lipoic acid on peripheral nerve conduction, blood flow, energy metabolism, and oxidative stress in experimental diabetic neuropathy. *Diabetes* 2000; 49:1006.

88. Obrosova I, Van Huysen C, Stevens MJ, *et al*: Evaluation of 1-adrenoceptor antagonist on diabetes-induced changes in nerve function, metabolism, and antioxidative defense. *Diabetes* 1999;48 (suppl. 1):A54.

89. Thurston JH, McDouglas DB Jr, Hauhart RE, *et al*: Effects of acute, subacute and chronic diabetes on carbohydrate and energy metabolism in rat sciatic nerve: Relation to mechanisms of peripheral neuropathy. *Diabetes* 1995;44:190.

90. Low PA, Ward K, Schmelzer JD, *et al*: Ischemic conduction failure and energy metabolism in experimental diabetic neuropathy. *Am J Physiol* 1985;248:E457.

91. Greene DA, Lattimer SA, Carroll PB, *et al*: A defect in sodium-dependent amino acid uptake in diabetic rabbit peripheral nerve. Correction by an aldose reductase inhibitor or myo-inositol administration. *J Clin Invest* 1990;85:1657.

92. Dent MT, Tebbs SE, Gonzalez AM, *et al*: Neutrophil aldose reductase activity and its association with established diabetic microvascular complications. *Diabete Med* 1991;8:439.

93. Vinores SA, Campochiaro PA, Williams EH, *et al*: Aldose reductase expression in human diabetic retina and retinal pigment epithelium. *Diabetes* 1988;37:1658.

94. Takahashi Y, Tachikawa T, Ito T, *et al*: Erythrocyte aldose reductase protein: A clue to elucidate risk factors for diabetic neuropathies independent of glycemic control. *Diabetes Res Clin Pract* 1998;42: 101.

95. Heesom AE, Millward A, Demaine AG: Susceptibility to diabetic neuropathy in patients with insulin dependent diabetes mellitus is associated with a polymorphism at the 5' end of the aldose reductase gene. *J Neurol Neurosurg Psychiatry* 1998;64:213.

96. Burg MB, Kador PF: Sorbitol, osmoregulation, and the complications of diabetes. *J Clin Invest* 1988;81:635.

97. Williamson JR, Chang K, Frangos M, *et al*: Hyperglycemic pseudo-hypoxia and diabetic complications. *Diabetes* 1993;42:801.

98. Dvornik D: Hyperglycemia in the pathogenesis of diabetic complications. In: Porte D, ed. *Aldose Reductase Inhibition. An Approach to the Prevention of Diabetic Complications*. Biomedical Information: 1987;69.

99. Sima AA, Prashar A, Zhang WX, *et al*: Preventive effect of long-term aldose reductase inhibition (ponalrestat) on nerve conduction and sural nerve structure in the spontaneously diabetic Bio-Breeding rat. *J Clin Invest* 1990;85:1410.

100. Stevens MJ, Lattimer SA, Kamijo M, *et al*: Osmotically-induced nerve taurine depletion and the compatible osmolyte hypothesis in experimental diabetic neuropathy in the rat. *Diabetologia* 1993;36: 608.

101. Mayer JH, Tomlinson DR: The influence of aldose reductase inhibition and nerve myoinositol on axonal transport and nerve conduction velocity in rats with experimental diabetes. *J Physiol (Lond)* 1983; 340:25P.

102. Mizisin AP, Calcutt NA, DiStefano PS, *et al*: Aldose reductase inhibition increases CNTF-like bioactivity and protein in sciatic nerves from galactose-fed and normal rats. *Diabetes* 1997;46:647.

103. Ohi T, Saita K, Furukawa S, *et al*: Therapeutic effects of aldose reductase inhibitor on experimental diabetic neuropathy through synthesis/secretion of nerve growth factor. *Exp Neurol* 1998;151:215.

104. Greene DA, Stevens MJ: The sorbitol-osmotic and sorbitol-redox hypotheses. In: LeRoith D, Olefsky JM, Taylor S, eds. *Diabetes Mellitus: A Fundamental and Clinical Text*. Lippincott:1997;801.

105. Suarez G, Rajaram R, Bhuyan KC, *et al*: Administration of an aldose reductase inhibitor induces a decrease of collagen fluoresence in diabetic rats. *J Clin Invest* 1988;82:624.

106. Keogh RJ, Dunlop ME, Larkins RG: Effect of inhibition of aldose reductase on glucose flux, diacylglycerol formation, protein kinase C, and phospholipase A2 activation. *Metabolism* 1997;46:41.

107. Ishii H, Tada H, Isogai S: An aldose reductase inhibitor prevents glucose-induced increase in transforming growth factor-beta and protein kinase C activity in cultured mesangial cells. *Diabetologia* 1998;41:36.

108. Greene DA, Lattimer SA: Action of sorbinil in diabetic peripheral nerve. Relationship of polyol (sorbitol) pathway inhibition to a myo-inositol-mediated defect in sodium-potassium ATPase activity. *Diabetes* 1984;33:712.

109. Cameron NE, Cotter MA, Dines KC, *et al*: Aldose reductase inhibition, nerve perfusion, oxygenation and function in streptozocin-diabetic rats: Dose-response considerations and independence from a myo-inositol mechanism. *Diabetologia* 1994;37:651.

110. Yasuda H, Sonobe M, Yamashita M, *et al*: Effect of prostaglandin E1 analogue TFC 612 on diabetic neuropathy in streptozocin-induced diabetic rats. Comparison with aldose reductase inhibitor ONO 2235. *Diabetes* 1989;38:832.

111. Kinoshita JH: Mechanisms initiating cataract formation. Proctor Lecture. *Invest Ophthalmol* 1974;13:713.

112. Kwon HM, Yamauchi A, Uchida S, *et al*: Renal Na-myo-inositol cotransporter mRNA expression in *Xenopus* oocytes: Regulation by hypertonicity. *Am J Physiol* 1991;260:F258.

113. Henry DN, Del Monte M, Greene DA, *et al*: Altered aldose reductase gene regulation in cultured human retinal pigment epithelial cells. *J Clin Invest* 1993;92:617.

114. Stevens MJ, Henry DN, Thomas TP, *et al*: Aldose reductase gene expression and osmotic dysregulation in cultured human retinal pigment epithelial cells. *Am J Physiol* 1993;265:E428.

115. Hosaka Y, Stevens MJ, Porcellati FA, *et al*: Glucose decreases human Na-dependent myo-inositol transporter mRNA levels in cultured human retinal pigment epithelial cells. *Diabetes* 1996;45:A1017.

116. Burg MB: Molecular basis of osmotic regulation. *Am J Physiol* 1995; 268:F983.

117. Rim JS, Atta MG, Dahl SC, *et al*: Transcription of the sodium/myo-inositol cotransporter gene is regulated by multiple tonicity-responsive enhancers spread over 50 kilobase pairs in the 5′-flanking region. *J Biol Chem* 1998;273:20615.

118. Strange K, Morrison R, Shrode L, *et al*: Mechanism and regulation of swelling-activated inositol efflux in brain glial cells. *Am J Physiol* 1993;265:C244.

119. Obrosova IG, Fathallah L, Lang HJ: Interaction between osmotic and oxidative stress in diabetic precataractous lens: Studies with a sorbitol dehydrogenase inhibitor. *Biochem Pharmacol* 1999;58:1945.

120. Low PA, Yao JK, Kishi Y, *et al*: Peripheral nerve energy metabolism in experimental diabetic neuropathy. *Neurosci Res Commun* 1997;21:49.

121. Thomas TP, Feldman EL, Nakamura J, *et al*: Ambient glucose and aldose reductase-induced myo-inositol depletion modulate basal and carbachol-stimulated inositol phospholipid metabolism and diacylglycerol accumulation in human retinal pigment epithelial cells in culture. *Proc Natl Acad Sci USA* 1993;90:9712.

122. Greene DA, Lattimer SA, Sima AA: Are disturbances of sorbitol, phosphoinositide, and (Na,K)-ATPase regulation involved in pathogenesis of diabetic neuropathy? *Diabetes* 1988;37:688.

123. Wright CE, Tallan HH, Lin YY, *et al*: Taurine: Biological update. *Annu Rev Biochem* 1986;55:427.

124. Huxtable RJ: From heart to hypothesis: A mechanism for the calcium modulatory effects actions of taurine. In: Hustable RJ, Franconi F,

Giotti A, eds. *The Biology of Taurine: Methods and Mechanisms*. Plenum:1985;371.

125. Li YP, Lombardini JB: Inhibition by taurine of the phosphorylation of specific synaptosomal proteins in the rat cortex: Effects of taurine on the stimulation of calcium uptake in mitochondria and inhibition of phosphoinositide turnover. *Brain Res* 1991;553:89.

126. Davison AN, Kaczmarek LK: Taurine—a possible neurotransmitter? *Nature* 1971;234:107.

127. Cameron NE, Cotter MA, Low PA: Nerve blood flow in early experimental diabetes in rats: Relation to conduction deficits. *Am J Physiol* 1991;261:E1.

128. Cameron NE, Cotter MA, Ferguson K, *et al*: Effects of chronic alpha-adrenergic receptor blockade on peripheral nerve conduction, hypoxic resistance, polyols, Na(+)-K(+)-ATPase activity, and vascular supply in STZ-D rats. *Diabetes* 1991;40:1652.

129. Tomlinson DR, Mayer JH: Reversal of deficits in axonal transport and nerve conduction velocity by treatment of streptozocin-diabetic rats with myo-inositol. *Exp Neurol* 1985;89:420.

130. Kim J, Rushovich EH, Thomas TP: Diminished specific activity of cytosolic protein kinase C in sciatic nerve of streptozocin-induced diabetic rats and its correction by dietary myo-inositol. *Diabetes* 1991; 40:1545.

131. Stevens MJ, Van Huysen C, Beyer L, *et al*: Amelioration of nerve blood flow deficits by myo-inositol in streptozocin-diabetic rats. *Diabetes* 1996;45:A775.

132. Yorek MA, Wiese TJ, Davidson EP, *et al*: Reduced motor nerve conduction velocity and (Na,K)-ATPase activity in rats maintained on L-fucose diet. Reversal by myo-inositol supplementation. *Diabetes* 1993;42:1401.

133. Stevens MJ, Dananberg J, Feldman EL, *et al*: The linked roles of nitric oxide, aldose reductase and (Na^+,K^+)-ATPase in the slowing of nerve conduction in the streptozocin diabetic rat. *J Clin Invest* 1994; 94:853.

134. Zhu X, Eichberg J: 1,2-diacylglycerol content and its arachidonyl-containing molecular species are reduced in sciatic nerve from streptozocin-induced diabetic rats. *J Neurochem* 1990;55:1087.

135. Kim J, Kyriazi H, Greene DA: Normalization of (Na,K)-ATPase activity in isolated membrane fraction from sciatic nerves of streptozocin-induced diabetic rats by dietary myo-inositol supplementation in vivo or protein kinase C agonists in vitro. *Diabetes* 1991; 40:558.

136. Gupta S, Sussman I, McArthur CS, *et al*: Endothelium-dependent inhibition of (Na,K)-ATPase activity in rabbit aorta by hyperglycemia. Possible role of endothelium-derived nitric oxide. *J Clin Invest* 1992; 90:727.

137. Shindo H, Thomas TP, Larkin DD, et al: Modulation of basal nitric oxide-dependent cyclic-GMP production by ambient glucose, myo-inositol, and protein kinase C in SH-SY5Y human neuroblastoma cells. *J Clin Invest* 1996;97:736.

138. Greene DA, Winegrad AI: Effects of acute experimental diabetes on composite energy metabolism in peripheral nerve axons and Schwann cells. *Diabetes* 1981;30:967.

139. Stevens MJ, Hosaka Y, Masterson JA, *et al*: Downregulation of the human taurine transporter by glucose in cultured retinal pigment epithelial cells. *Am J Physiol* 1999;277:E760.

140. Malone JI, Lowitt S, Cook WR: Nonosmotic diabetic cataracts. *Pediatr Res* 1990;27:293.

141. Halliwell B, Gutteridge JMC: The antioxidants of human extracellular fluids. *Arch Biochem Biophys* 1990;280:1.

142. Obrosova IG, Stevens MJ: Effect of dietary taurine supplementation on GSH and NAD(P)-redox status, lipid peroxidation, and energy metabolism in diabetic precataractous lens. *Invest Ophthalmol Vis Sci* 1999;40:680.

143. Trachtman H, Futterweit S, Prenner J, *et al*: Antioxidants reverse the antiproliferative effect of high glucose and advanced glycosylation end products in cultured rat mesangial cells. *Biochem Biophys Res Commun* 1994;199:346.

144. Lombardini JB: Effects of taurine on protein phosphorylation in mammalian tissues. *Adv Exp Med Biol* 1992;315:309.

145. Pop-Busui R, VanHuysen C, Beyer L, *et al*: Attenuation of nerve vascular and functional defects by nerve taurine replacement in the streptozocin-diabetic rat. *Diabetes* 1998;suppl 1:A537.

146. Gragera RR, Muniz E, Martinez-Rodriguez R: Neuromediators in the cerebellar blood-brain barrier and its microenvironment. Immuno-

cytochemical demonstration of taurine, glycine, serotonin, thiamin and AATase. *J Hirnforsch* 1994;35:31.

147. Wang JH, Redmond HP, Watson RW, *et al*: The beneficial effect of taurine on the prevention of human endothelial cell death. *Shock* 1996;6:331.

148. Kamata K, Sugiura M, Kojima S, *et al*: Restoration of endothelium-dependent relaxation in both hypercholesterolemia and diabetes by chronic taurine. *Eur J Pharmacol* 1996;303:47.

149. Whitton PS, Nicholson RA, Strang RH: Effect of taurine on calcium accumulation in resting and depolarised insect synaptosomes. *J Neurochem* 1988;50:1743.

150. Kunisaki M, Bursell SE, Umeda F, *et al*: Normalization of diacylglycerol-protein kinase C activation by vitamin E in aorta of diabetic rats and cultured rat smooth muscle cells exposed to elevated glucose levels. *Diabetes* 1994;43:1372.

151. Ishii H, Jirousek MR, Koya D, *et al*: Amelioration of vascular dysfunctions in diabetic rats by an oral PKC beta inhibitor [see comments]. *Science* 1996;272:728.

152. Nakamura J, Kato K, Hamada Y, *et al*: A protein kinase C-beta-selective inhibitor ameliorates neural dysfunction in streptozocin-induced diabetic rats. *Diabetes* 1999;48:2090.

153. Cameron NE, Cotter MA, Jack AM, *et al*: Protein kinase C effects on nerve function, perfusion, (Na,K)-ATPase activity and glutathione content in diabetic rats. *Diabetologia* 1999;42:1120.

154. Moriyama T, Garcia-Perez A, Burg MB: Factors affecting the ratio of different organic osmolytes in renal medullary cells. *Am J Physiol* 1990;259:F847.

155. Lerma J, Herranz AS, Herreras O, *et al*: Aminobutyric acid greatly increases the in vivo extracellular taurine in the rat hippocampus. *J Neurochem* 1985;44:983.

156. Uchida S, Nakanishi T, Kwon HM, *et al*: Taurine behaves as an osmolyte in MDCK cells: Protection by polarized, regulated transport of taurine. *J Clin Invest* 1991;88:656.

157. Oja SS, Kontro P: Neuromodulatory and trophic actions of taurine. *Prog Clin Biol Res* 1990;351:69.

158. Cameron NE, Cotter MA: Metabolic and vascular factors in the athogenesis of diabetic neuropathy. *Diabetes* 1997;46(suppl 2):31S.

159. Cameron NE, Cotter MA, Horrobin DH, *et al*: Effects of alpha-lipoic acid on neurovascular function in diabetic rats: interaction with essential fatty acids. *Diabetologia* 1998;41:390.

160. Lee AY, Chung SS: Contributions of polyol pathway to oxidative stress in diabetic cataract. *FASEB J* 1999;13:23.

161. Nagamatsu M, Nickander KK, Schmelzer JD, *et al*: Lipoic acid improves nerve blood flow, reduces oxidative stress, and improves distal nerve conduction in experimental diabetic neuropathy. *Diabetes Care* 1995;18:1160.

162. Obrosova IG, Marvel J, Faller A, *et al*: Reductive stress is a very early metabolic imbalance in sciatic nerve in diabetic and galactose-fed rats. *Diabetologia* 1995;38(suppl 1):A8.

163. Obrosova IG, Lang HJ, Greene D: Antioxidative defense in diabetic peripheral nerve: Effect of DL-α-lipoic acid, aldose reductase inhibitor and sorbitol dehydrogenase inhibitor. In: Dekker M, ed. *Oxidative Stress and Diabetes*. Academic:1999.

164. Cameron NE, Cotter MA, Basso M, *et al*: Comparison of the effects of inhibitors of aldose reductase and sorbitol dehydrogenase on neurovascular function, nerve conduction and tissue polyol pathway metabolites in streptozocin-diabetic rats. *Diabetologia* 1997;40:271.

165. Ng TF, Lee FK, Song ZT, *et al*: Effects of sorbitol dehydrogenase deficiency on nerve conduction in experimental diabetic mice [published erratum appears in *Diabetes* 1998;47:1374]. *Diabetes* 1998;47:96.

166. Lee AYW, Chung SK, Chung SM: Demonstration that polyol accumulation is responsible for diabetic cataracts by the use of transgenic mice expressing the aldose reductase gene in the lens. *Proc Natl Acad Sci USA* 1995;92:2780.

167. Oates P, Schelhorn T, Miller M: Polyol pathway inhibitors dose-dependently preserve nerve function in diabetic rats. *Diabetologia* 1998;41(suppl 1):A271.

168. Obrosova IG, Fathallah L, Lang HJ, *et al*: Evaluation of a sorbitol dehydrogenase inhibitor on diabetic peripheral nerve metabolism: A prevention study. *Diabetologia* 1999;42:1187.

169. Phillips SA, Thornalley PJ: The formation of methylglyoxal from triose phosphates. Investigation using a specific assay for methylglyoxal. *Eur J Biochem* 1993;212:101.

170. Choudhary D, Chandra D, Kale RK: Influence of methylglyoxal on antioxidant enzymes and oxidative damage. *Toxicol Lett* 1997;93:141.

171. Martinez-Blasco A, Bosch-Morell F, Trenor C, *et al*: Experimental diabetic neuropathy: Role of oxidative stress and mechanisms involved. *Biofactors* 1998;8:41.

172. Shiba T, Inoguchi T, Sportsman JR, *et al*: Correlation of diacylglycerol level and protein kinase C activity in rat retina to retinal circulation. *Am J Physiol* 1993;265:E783.

173. King GL, Ishii H, Koya D: Diabetic vascular dysfunctions: A model of excessive activation of protein kinase C. *Kidney Int Suppl* 1997;60:S77.

174. Stevens MJ, Lattimer SA, Feldman EL, *et al*: Acetyl-L-carnitine deficiency as a cause of altered nerve myo-inositol content, (Na,K)-ATPase, and motor conduction velocity in the streptozocin-diabetic rat. *Metabolism* 1996;45:865.

175. Sharma AK, Thomas PK: Peripheral nerve structure and function in experimental diabetes. *J Neurol Sci* 1974;23:1.

176. Brismar T, Sima AA, Greene DA: Reversible and irreversible nodal dysfunction in diabetic neuropathy. *Ann Neurol* 1987;21:504.

177. Pop-Busui R, Van Huysen C, Beyer L, *et al*: Dissociation of nerve blood flow and nerve conduction velocity by acetyl-L-carnitine treatment in streptozocin diabetes. *Diabetes* 1996;45:A12.

178. Powell HC, Garrett RS, Kador PF, *et al*: Fine-structural localization of aldose reductase and ouabain-c sensitive, K(+)-dependent p-nitrophenylphosphatase in rat peripheral nerve. *J Pharmacol Exp Ther* 1991;81:529.

179. Fink DJ, Datta S, Mata M: Isoform specific reductions in (Na,K)-ATPase catalytic (alpha) subunits in the nerve of rats with streptozocin-induced diabetes. *J Neurochem* 1994;63:1782.

180. Borghini I, Geering K, Gjinovci A, *et al*: In vivo phosphorylation of the (Na,K)-ATPase alpha subunit in sciatic nerves of control and diabetic rats: Effects of protein kinase modulators. *Proc Natl Acad Sci USA* 1994;91:6211.

181. Landowne D, Ritchie JM: The binding of tritiated ouabain to mammalian non-myelinated nerve fibres. *J Physiol (Lond)* 1970;207:529.

182. Shull GE, Greeb J, Lingrel JB: Molecular cloning of three distinct forms of the (Na,K)-ATPase alpha-subunit from rat brain. *Biochemistry* 1986;25:8125.

183. Gerbi A, Sennoune S, Pierre S, *et al*: Localization of (Na,K)-ATPase alpha/beta isoforms in rat sciatic nerves: Effect of diabetes and fish oil treatment. *J Neurochem* 1999;73:719.

184. Lattimer SA, Sima AA, Greene DA: In vitro correction of impaired (Na,K)-ATPase in diabetic nerve by protein kinase C agonists. *Am J Physiol* 1989;256:E264.

185. Hermenegildo C, Felipo V, Minana MD, *et al*: Inhibition of protein kinase C restores (Na,K)-ATPase activity in sciatic nerve of diabetic mice. *J Neurochem* 1992;58:1246.

186. Vague P, Dufayet D, Coste T, *et al*: Association of diabetic neuropathy with (Na,K)-ATPase gene polymorphism. *Diabetologia* 1997;40:506.

187. Fagerberg SE: Diabetic neuropathy. *Acta Med Scand* 1959;164:1.

188. Johnson PC, Doll SC, Cromey DW: Pathogenesis of diabetic neuropathy. *Ann Neurol* 1986;19:450.

189. Dyck PJ, Karnes JL, O'Brien P, *et al*: The spatial distribution of fiber loss in diabetic polyneuropathy suggests ischemia. *Ann Neurol* 1986;19:440.

190. Stevens MJ, Feldman EL, Thomas TP, *et al*: The pathogenesis of diabetic neuropathy. In: Veves A, Conn PMC, eds. *Clinical Management of Diabetic Neuropathy*. Humana:1997;13.

191. Tuck RR, Schmelzer JD, Low PA: Endoneurial blood flow and oxygen tension in the sciatic nerves of rats with experimental diabetic neuropathy. *Brain* 1984;107:935.

192. Cotter MA, Love A, Watt MJ, *et al*: Effects of natural free radical scavengers on peripheral nerve and neurovascular function in diabetic rats. *Diabetologia* 1995;38:1285.

193. Low PA, Nickander KK, Tritschler HJ: The roles of oxidative stress and antioxidant treatment in experimental diabetic neuropathy. *Diabetes* 1997;46(suppl 2):38S.

194. Cameron NE, Cotter MA: Neurovascular dysfunction in diabetic rats. Potential contribution of autoxidation and free radicals examined using transition metal chelating agents. *J Clin Invest* 1995;96:1159.

195. Cameron NE, Cotter MA, Dines KC, *et al*: Reversal of defective peripheral nerve conduction velocity, nutritive endoneurial blood flow, and oxygenation by a novel aldose reductase inhibitor, WAY-121,509, in streptozocin-induced diabetic rats. *J Diabetes Complications* 1996;10:43.

196. Dewhurst M, Omawari N, Tomlinson DR: Aminoguanidine—effects of endoneurial vasoactive nitric oxide and on motor nerve conduction velocity in control and streptozocin-diabetic rats. *Br J Pharmacol* 1997;120:593.

197. Stevens EJ, Kalichman MW, Mizisin AP, *et al*: Blood flow in nerve and dorsal root ganglia in experimental diabetes: Effects of insulin. *J. Physiol* 1994;475:86P.

198. Cameron NE, Cotter MA, Robertson S: Rapid reversal of a motor nerve conduction deficit in streptozocin-diabetic rats by the angiotensin converting enzyme inhibitor lisinopril. *Acta Diabetol* 1993;30:46.

199. Cameron NE, Cotter MA: Effects of chronic treatment with a nitric oxide donor on nerve conduction abnormalities and endoneurial blood flow in streptozocin diabetic rats. *Eur J Clin Invest* 1995;25:19.

200. Cameron NE, Hohman TC, Antane M, *et al*: The potassium channel opener, WAY-1 35201, corrects nerve dysfunction in diabetic rats. *Diabetes* 1998;suppl 1:A137.

201. Bravenboer B, Kappelle AC, Hamers FP, *et al*: Potential use of glutathione for the prevention and treatment of diabetic neuropathy in the streptozocin-induced diabetic rat. *Diabetologia* 1992;35:813.

202. Cameron NE, Cotter MA, Maxfield EK: Anti-oxidant treatment prevents the development of peripheral nerve dysfunction in streptozocin-diabetic rats. *Diabetologia* 1993;36:299.

203. Sagara M, Satoh J, Wada R, *et al*: Inhibition of development of peripheral neuropathy in streptozocin-induced diabetic rats with N-acetylcysteine. *Diabetologia* 1996;39:263.

204. Love A, Cotter MA, Cameron NE: Nerve function and regeneration in diabetic and galactosaemic rats: Antioxidant and metal chelator effects. *Eur J Pharmacol* 1996;314:33.

205. Cotter MA, Cameron NE, Keegan A, *et al*: Effects of acetyl- and propionyl-L-carnitine on peripheral nerve function and vascular supply in experimental diabetes. *Metabolism* 1995;44:1209.

206. Stevens EJ, Lockett MJ, Carrington AL, *et al*: Essential fatty acid treatment prevents nerve ischaemia and associated conduction anomalies in rats with experimental diabetes mellitus. *Diabetologia* 1993;36:397.

207. Zochodne DW, Cheng C: Diabetic peripheral nerves are susceptible to multifocal ischemic damage from endothelin. *Brain Res* 1999;838:11.

208. Cotter MA, Cameron NE: Correction of neurovascular deficits in diabetic rats by beta2-adrenoceptor agonist and alpha1-adrenoceptor antagonist treatment: Interactions with the nitric oxide system. *Eur J Pharmacol* 1998;343:217.

209. Cameron NE, Cotter MA: Impaired contraction and relaxation in aorta from streptozocin-diabetic rats: Role of polyol pathway. *Diabetologia* 1992;35:101.

210. Mayhan WG, Simmons LK, Sharpe GM: Mechanism of impaired responses of cerebral arterioles during diabetes mellitus. *Am J Physiol* 1991;260:H319.

211. Kamata K, Miyata N, Kasuya Y: Impairment of endothelium-dependent relaxation and changes in levels of cyclic GMP in aorta from streptozocin-induced diabetic rats. *Br J Pharmacol* 1989;97:614.

212. Lowe GD, Ghafour IM, Belch JJ, *et al*: Increased blood viscosity in diabetic proliferative retinopathy. *Diabetes Res* 1986;3:67.

213. Dines KC, Calcutt NA, Nunag KD, *et al*: Effects of hindlimb temperature on sciatic nerve laser Doppler vascular conductance in control and streptozocin-diabetic rats. *J Neurol Sci* 1999;163:17.

214. Chang K, Ido Y, LeJeune W, *et al*: Increased sciatic nerve blood flow in diabetic rats: Assessment by "molecular" vs. particulate microspheres. *Am J Physiol* 1997;273:E164.

215. Sima AA, Sugimoto K: Experimental diabetic neuropathy: An update. *Diabetologia* 1999;42:773.

216. Mizisin AP, Bache M, DiStefano PS, *et al*: BDNF attenuates functional and structural disorders in nerves of galactose-fed rats. *J Neuropathol Exp Neurol* 1997;56:1290.

217. Obrosova I, Van Huysen C, Fathallah L, *et al*: Evaluation of α 1-adrenoceptor antagonist on diabetes-induced changes in peripheral nerve function, metabolism and antioxidative defense. *FASEB J* 2000; 14:1548.

218. Newrick PG, Wilson AJ, Jakubowski J, *et al*: Sural nerve oxygen tension in diabetes. *BMJ (Clin Res Ed)* 1986;293:1053.

219. Appenzeller O, Parks RD, MacGee J: Peripheral neuropathy in chronic disease of the respiratory tract. *Am J Med* 1968;44:873.

220. Ibrahim S, Harris ND, Radatz M, *et al*: A new minimally invasive technique to show nerve ischaemia in diabetic neuropathy. *Diabetologia* 1999;42:737.

221. Malik RA, Williamson S, Abbott C, *et al*: Effect of angiotensin-converting-enzyme (ACE) inhibitor trandolapril on human diabetic neuropathy: Randomised double-blind controlled trial [see comments]. *Lancet* 1998;352:1978.

222. Takeuchi M, Low PA: Dynamic peripheral nerve metabolic and vascular responses to exsanguination. *Am J Physiol* 1987;253:E349.

223. Adams WE: The blood supply of nerves II. The effects of exclusion of its regional sources of supply on the sciatic nerve of the rabbit. *J Anst* 1943;77:243.

224. Tesfaye S, Harris N, Jakubowski JJ, *et al*: Impaired blood flow and arterio-venous shunting in human diabetic neuropathy: A novel technique of nerve photography and fluorescein angiography [see comments]. *Diabetologia* 1993;36:1266.

225. Baynes JW: Role of oxidative stress in development of complications of diabetes. *Diabetes* 1991;40:405.

226. Wolff SP: Diabetes mellitus and free radicals. Free radicals, transition metals and oxidative stress in the aetiology of diabetes mellitus and complications. *Br Med Bull* 1993;49:642.

227. Cameron NE, Cotter MA, Archibald V, *et al*: Anti-oxidant and pro-oxidant effects on nerve conduction velocity, endoneurial blood flow and oxygen tension in non-diabetic and streptozocin-diabetic rats. *Diabetologia.* 1994;37:449.

228. Karpen CW, Pritchard KA, Arnold JH, *et al*: Restoration of the prostacyclin-thromboxane A2 balance in the diabetic rat: Influence of vitamin E. *Diabetes* 1982;31:947.

229. Sato Y, Hotta N, Sakamoto M, *et al*: Lipid peroxide level in plasma of diabetic patients. *Biochem Med* 1979;21:104.

230. Karpen CW, Cataland S, O'Dorisio TM, *et al*: Interrelation of platelet vitamin E and thromboxane synthesis in type I diabetes mellitus. *Diabetes* 1984;33:239.

231. Franconi F, Bennardini F, Mattana A, *et al*: Plasma and platelet taurine are reduced in subjects with insulin-dependent diabetes mellitus: Effects of taurine supplementation. *Am J Clin Nutr* 1995;61:1115.

232. Luzi L, Castellino P, Simonson DC, *et al*: Leucine metabolism in IDDM. Role of insulin and substrate availability. *Diabetes* 1990;39: 38.

233. Guzel S, Seven A, Satman I, *et al*: Comparison of oxidative stress indicators in plasma of recent-onset and long-term type 1 diabetic patients. *J Toxicol Environ Health* 2000;59:7.

234. Hunt JV, Dean RT, Wolff SP: Hydroxyl radical production and autoxidative glycosylation. Glucose autoxidation as the cause of protein damage in the experimental glycation model of diabetes mellitus and ageing. *Biochem J* 1988;256:205.

235. Morel DW, Chisolm GM: Antioxidant treatment of diabetic rats inhibits lipoprotein oxidation and cytotoxicity. *J Lipid Res* 1989;30:1827.

236. Wohaieb SA, Godin DV: Alterations in free radical tissue-defense mechanisms in streptozocin-induced diabetes in rat. Effects of insulin treatment. *Diabetes* 1987;36:1014.

237. Wolff SP: The potential role of oxidative stress in diabetes and its complications: Novel implications for theory and therapy. In: Crabbe MJC, ed. *Diabetic Complications: Scientific and Clinical Aspects.* Churchill-Livingstone:1987;167.

238. Fondelli C, Signorini AM, Borgogni L, *et al*: Tolrestat and superoxide anion production in type 2 diabetic patients. *Diabetologia* 1993;36: A203.

239. Ohi T, Poduslo JF, Dyck PJ: Increased endoneurial albumin in diabetic polyneuropathy. *Neurology* 1985;35:1790.

240. Low PA, Nickander KK: Oxygen free radical effects in sciatic nerve in experimental diabetes. *Diabetes* 1991;40:873.

241. Godin DV, Wohaieb SA, Garnett ME, *et al*: Antioxidant enzyme alterations in experimental and clinical diabetes. *Mol Cell Biochem* 1988; 84:223.

242. Nickander KK, Schmelzer JD, Rohwer DA, *et al*: Effect of alpha-tocopherol deficiency on indices of oxidative stress in normal and diabetic peripheral nerve. *J Neurol Sci* 1994;126:6.

243. Ward KK, Low PA, Schmelzer JD, *et al*: Prostacyclin and noradrenaline in peripheral nerve of chronic experimental diabetes in rats. *Brain* 1989;112:197.

244. Tomlinson DR, Sidenius P, Larsen JR: Slow component-a of axonal transport, nerve myo-inositol, and aldose reductase inhibition in streptozocin-diabetic rats. *Diabetes* 1986;34:398.

245. Kishi Y, Nickander KK, Schmelzer JD, *et al*: Gene expression of antioxidant enzymes in experimental diabetic neuropathy. *J Peripher Nerv Syst* 2000;5:11.

246. Sasaki H, Schmelzer JD, Zollman PJ, et al: Neuropathology and blood flow of nerve, spinal roots and dorsal root ganglia in longstanding diabetic rats. Acta Neuropathol (Berl) 1997;93:118.

247. Baumgartner-Parzer SM, Wagner L, Pettermann M, et al: High-glucose-triggered apoptosis in cultured endothelial cells. Diabetes 1995;44:1323.

248. Wu QD, Wang JH, Fennessy F, et al: Taurine prevents high-glucose-induced human vascular endothelial cell apoptosis. Am J Physiol 1999;277:C1229.

249. Hattori Y, Kawasaki H, Abe K, et al: Superoxide dismutase recovers altered endothelium-dependent relaxation in diabetic rat aorta. Am J Physiol 1991;261:H1086.

250. Tesfamariam B, Cohen RA: Free radicals mediate endothelial cell dysfunction caused by elevated glucose. Am J Physiol 1992;263:H321.

251. Moncada S, Palmer RM, Higgs EA: Nitric oxide: Physiology, pathophysiology, and pharmacology. Pharmacol Rev 1991;43:109.

252. Gryglewski RJ, Palmer RM, Moncada S: Superoxide anion is involved in the breakdown of endothelium-derived vascular relaxing factor. Nature 1986;320:454.

253. Kowluru RA, Kern TS, Engerman RL, et al: Abnormalities of retinal metabolism in diabetes or experimental galactosemia. III. Effects of antioxidants. Diabetes 1996;45:1233.

254. Cameron NE, Cotter MA, Dines K, et al: Effects of aminoguanidine on peripheral nerve function and polyol pathway metabolites in streptozocin-diabetic rats. Diabetologia 1992;35:946.

255. Kihara M, Schmelzer JD, Poduslo JF, et al: Aminoguanidine effects on nerve blood flow, vascular permeability, electrophysiology, and oxygen free radicals. Proc Natl Acad Sci USA 1991;88:6107.

256. Tutuncu NB, Bayraktar M, Varli K: Reversal of defective nerve conduction with vitamin E supplementation in type 2 diabetes: A preliminary study. Diabetes Care 1998;21:1915.

257. Brownlee M: Glycation products and the pathogenesis of diabetic complications. Diabetes Care 1992;15:1835.

258. Odetti PR, Borgoglio A, De Pascale A, et al: Prevention of diabetes-increased aging effect on rat collagen-linked fluorescence by aminoguanidine and rutin. Diabetes 1990;39:796.

259. Wautier J-L, Zoukourian C, Chappey O, et al: Receptor-mediated endothelial cell dysfunction in diabetic vasculopathy. Soluble receptor for advanced glycation end products blocks hyperpermeability in diabetic rats. J Clin Invest 1996;97:238.

260. Haitoglou CS, Tsilibary EC, Brownlee M, et al: Altered cellular interactions between endothelial cells and nonenzymatically glucosylated laminin/type IV collagen. J Biol Chem 1992;267:12404.

261. Szwergold BS, Kappler F, Brown TR: Identification of fructose-3-phosphate in the lens of diabetic rats. Science 1990;247:451.

262. Verhaegen S, McGowan AJ, Brophy AR, et al: Inhibition of apoptosis by antioxidants in the human HL-60 leukemia cell line. Biochem Pharmacol 1995;50:102.

263. Simonian NA, Coyle JT: Oxidative stress in neurodegenerative diseases. Annu Rev Pharmacol Toxicol 1996;36:83.

264. Lin CP, Lynch MC, Kochevar IE: Reactive oxidizing species produced near the plasma membrane induce apoptosis in bovine aorta endothelial cells. Exp Cell Res 2000;259:351.

265. Du XL, Sui GZ, Stockklauser-Farber K, et al: Introduction of apoptosis by high proinsulin and glucose in cultured human umbilical vein endothelial cells is mediated by reactive oxygen species. Diabetologia 1998;41:249.

266. Ho FM, Liu SH, Liau CS, et al: High glucose-induced apoptosis in human endothelial cells is mediated by sequential activations of c-Jun NH(2)-terminal kinase and caspase-3. Circulation 2000;101:2618.

267. Zhang W, Khanna P, Chan LL, et al: Diabetes-induced apoptosis in rat kidney. Biochem Mol Med 1997;61:58.

268. Ortiz A, Ziyadeh FN, Neilson EG: Expression of apoptosis-regulatory genes in renal proximal tubular epithelial cells exposed to high ambient glucose and in diabetic kidneys. J Invest Med 1997;45:50.

269. Darby IA, Bisucci T, Hewitson TD, MacLellan DG: Apoptosis is increased in a model of diabetes-impaired wound healing in genetically diabetic mice. Int J Biochem Cell Biol 1997;29:191.

270. Kane CD, Greenhalgh DG: Expression and localization of p53 and bcl-2 in healing wounds in diabetic and nondiabetic mice. Wound Repair Regen 2000;8:45.

271. Podesta F, Romeo G, Liu WH, et al: Bax is increased in the retina of diabetic subjects and is associated with pericyte apoptosis in vivo and in vitro. Am J Pathol 2000;156:1025.

272. Li W, Yanoff M, Jian B, et al: Altered mRNA levels of antioxidant enzymes in pre-apoptotic pericytes from human diabetic retinas. Cell Mol Biol (Noisy-le-Grand) 1999;45:59.

273. Barber AJ, Lieth E, Khin SA, et al: Neural apoptosis in the retina during experimental and human diabetes. Early onset and effect of insulin. J Clin Invest 1998;102:78.

274. Russell JW, Feldman EL: Insulin-like growth factor-I prevents apoptosis in sympathetic neurons exposed to high glucose. Horm Metab Res 1999;31:90.

275. Russell JW, Windebank AJ, Schenone A, et al: Insulin-like growth factor-I prevents apoptosis in neurons after nerve growth factor withdrawal. J Neurobiol 1998;36:455.

276. Kogawa S, Yasuda H, Terada M, et al: Apoptosis and impaired axonal regeneration of sensory neurons after nerve crush in diabetic rats. Neuroreport 2000;11:663.

277. Srinivasan S, Stevens MJ, Sheng H, et al: Serum from patients with type 2 diabetes with neuropathy induces complement-independent, calcium-dependent apoptosis in cultured neuronal cells. J Clin Invest 1998;102:1454.

278. Pittenger GL, Liu D, Vinik AI: The apoptotic death of neuroblastoma cells caused by serum from patients with insulin-dependent diabetes and neuropathy may be Fas-mediated. J Neuroimmunol 1997;76:153.

279. Basu A, Haldar S: The relationship between Bcl2, Bax and p53: Consequences for cell cycle progression and cell death. Mol Hum Reprod 1998;4:1099.

280. Kroemer G, Dallaporta B, Resche-Rigon M: The mitochondrial death/life regulator in apoptosis and necrosis. Annu Rev Physiol 1998; 60:619.

281. Kim CN, Wang X, Huang Y, et al: Overexpression of Bcl-X(L) inhibits Ara-C-induced mitochondrial loss of cytochrome c and other perturbations that activate the molecular cascade of apoptosis. Cancer Res 1997;57:3115.

282. Russell JW, Sullivan KA, Windebank AJ, et al: Neurons undergo apoptosis in animal and cell culture models of diabetes. Neurobiol Dis 1999;6:347.

283. Srinivasan S, Stevens M, Wiley JW: Diabetic peripheral neuropathy: evidence for apoptosis and associated mitochondrial dysfunction. Diabetes 2000;49:1932.

284. Voitenko NV, Kruglikov IA, Kostyuk EP, et al: Effect of streptozocin-induced diabetes on the activity of calcium channels in rat dorsal horn neurons. Neuroscience 2000;95:519.

285. Kroemer G: The proto-oncogene Bcl-2 and its role in regulating apoptosis [published erratum appears in Nat Med 1997;3:934]. Nat Med 1997;3:614.

286. Moley KH, Chi MM, Knudson CM, et al: Hyperglycemia induces apoptosis in pre-implantation embryos through cell death effector pathways [see comments]. Nat Med 1998;4:1421.

287. Park DS, Morris EJ, Stefanis L, et al: Multiple pathways of neuronal death induced by DNA-damaging agents, NGF deprivation, and oxidative stress. J Neurosci 1998;18:830.

288. Nistico G, Ciriolo MR, Fiskin K, et al: NGF restores decrease in catalase activity and increases superoxide dismutase and glutathione peroxidase activity in the brain of aged rats. Free Radic Biol Med 1992; 12:177.

289. Delanty N, Dichter MA: Oxidative injury in the nervous system. Acta Neurol Scand 1998;98:145.

290. Hockenbery DM, Oltvai ZN, Yin XM, et al: Bcl-2 functions in an antioxidant pathway to prevent apoptosis. Cell 1993;75:241.

291. Kane DJ, Sarafian TA, Anton R, et al: Bcl-2 inhibition of neural death: decreased generation of reactive oxygen species. Science 1993;262: 1274.

292. Parry GJ, Kozu H: Piroxicam may reduce the rate of progression of experimental diabetic neuropathy. Neurology 1990;40:1446.

293. Zochodne DW, Ho LT: The influence of indomethacin and guanethidine on experimental streptozocin diabetic neuropathy. Can J Neurol Sci 1992;19:433.

294. Pop-Busui R, Van Huysen C, Beyer L, et al: Dissociation of metabolic, vascular and nerve conduction deficits in experimental diabetic neuropathy by cyclooxygenase inhibition and acetyl-L-carnitine administration. Diabetes 2001 (in press).

295. Cameron NE, Cotter MA, Dines KC, et al: The effects of evening primrose oil on nerve function and capillarization in streptozocin-diabetic rats: modulation by the cyclo-oxygenase inhibitor flurbiprofen. Br J Pharmacol 1993;109:972.

296. Williams CS, DuBois RN: Prostaglandin endoperoxide synthase: why two isoforms? *Am J Physiol* 1996;270:G393.

297. O'Neill GP, Ford-Hutchinson AW: Expression of mRNA for cyclo-oxygenase-1 and cyclooxygenase-2 in human tissues. *FEBS Lett* 1993;330:156.

298. Wu KK: Inducible cyclooxygenase and nitric oxide synthase. *Adv Pharmacol* 1995;33:179.

299. Feng L, Xia Y, Garcia GE, *et al*: Involvement of reactive oxygen intermediates in cyclooxygenase-2 expression induced by interleukin-1, tumor necrosis factor-alpha, and lipopolysaccharide. *J Clin Invest* 1995;95:1669.

300. Adderley SR, Fitzgerald DJ: Oxidative damage of cardiomyocytes is limited by extracellular regulated kinases ½-mediated induction of cyclooxygenase-2. *J Biol Chem* 1999;274:5038.

301. Schmedtje JF Jr, Ji YS, Liu WL, *et al*: Hypoxia induces cyclooxyge-nase-2 via the NF-kappaB p65 transcription factor in human vascular endothelial cells. *J Biol Chem* 1997;272:601.

302. Tomimoto H, Akiguchi I, Wakita H, *et al*: Cyclooxygenase-2 is induced in microglia during chronic cerebral ischemia in humans. *Acta Neuropathol (Berl)* 2000;99:26.

303. Lipsky PE, Abramson SB, Breedveld FC, *et al*: Analysis of the effect of COX-2 specific inhibitors and recommendations for their use in clinical practice [editorial] [In Process Citation]. *J Rheumatol* 2000; 27:1338.

304. Pop-Busui R, Marinescu V, Lum M, *et al*: Cox-2 expression is selectively increased in the sciatic nerve of streptozotocin-diabetic rats. *Diabetes* 2001;50:A239.

305. Ho L, Osaka H, Aisen PS, *et al*: Induction of cyclooxygenase (COX)-2 but not COX-1 gene expression in apoptotic cell death. *J Neuroimmunol* 1998;89:142.

306. Bagetta G, Corasaniti MT, Paoletti AM, *et al*: HIV-1 gp120-induced apoptosis in the rat neocortex involves enhanced expression of cyclooxygenase type 2 (COX-2). *Biochem Biophys Res Commun* 1998;244: 819.

307. Kusuhara H, Komatsu H, Sumichika H, *et al*: Reactive oxygen species are involved in the apoptosis induced by nonsteroidal anti-inflammatory drugs in cultured gastric cells. *Eur J Pharmacol* 1999;383:331.

308. Hsu AL, Ching TT, Wang DS, *et al*: The cyclooxygenase-2 inhibitor celecoxib induces apoptosis by blocking Akt activation in human prostate cancer cells independently of Bcl-2. *J Biol Chem* 2000;75: 11397.

309. McGinty A, Chang YW, Sorokin A, *et al*: Cyclooxygenase-2 expression inhibits trophic withdrawal apoptosis in nerve growth factor-differentiated PC12 cells. *J Biol Chem* 2000;275:12095.

310. Thoenen H, Angeletti PU, Levi-Montalcini R, et al: Selective induction by nerve growth factor of tyrosine hydroxylase and dopamine-hydroxylase in the rat superior cervical ganglia. *Proc Natl Acad Sci USA* 1971;68:1598.

311. Brewster WJ, Fernyhough P, Diemel LT, *et al*: Diabetic neuropathy, nerve growth factor and other neurotrophic factors [see comments]. *Trends Neurosci* 1994;17:321.

312. Scarpini E, Ross AH, Rosen JL, *et al*: Expression of nerve growth factor receptor during human peripheral nerve development. *Dev Biol* 1988;125:301.

313. Bandtlow CE, Heumann R, Schwab ME, *et al*: Cellular localization of nerve growth factor synthesis by in situ hybridization. *EMBO J* 1987; 6:891.

314. Lin L-FH, Armes LG, Sommer A, *et al*: Isolation and characterization of ciliary neurotrophic factor from rabbit sciatic nerves. *J Biol Chem* 1990;265:8942.

315. Hansson HA, Dahlin LB, Danielsen N, *et al*: Evidence indicating trophic importance of IGF-I in regenerating peripheral nerves. *Acta Physiol Scand* 1986;126:609.

316. Lindsay R: Role of neurotrophins and trk receptors in the development and maintenance of sensory nerves. *Biol Sci* 1996;351:365.

317. Smeyne RJ, Klein R, Schnapp A, *et al*: Severe sensory and sympathetic neuropathies in mice carrying a disrupted Trk/NGF receptor gene [see comments]. *Nature* 1994;368:246.

318. Barbacid M: The Trk family of neurotrophin receptors. *J Neurobiol* 1994;25:1386.

319. Thoenen H, Bandtlow C, Heumann R: The physiological function of nerve growth factor in the central nervous system: Comparison with the periphery. *Rev Physiol Biochem Pharmacol* 1987;109: 147.

320. Korsching S, Thoenen H: Nerve growth factor in sympathetic ganglia and corresponding target organs of the rat: Correlation with density of sympathetic innervation. *Proc Natl Acad Sci USA* 1983;80:3513.

321. Gorin PD, Johnson EM Jr: Effects of long-term nerve growth factor deprivation on the nervous system of the adult rat: An experimental autoimmune approach. *Brain Res* 1980;198:27.

322. Korsching S, Thoenen H: Treatment with 6-hydroxydopamine and colchicine decreases nerve growth factor levels in sympathetic ganglia and increases them in the corresponding target tissues. *J Neurosci* 1985;5:1058.

323. Clegg DO, Large TH, Bodary SC, *et al*: Regulation of nerve growth factor mRNA levels in developing rat heart ventricle is not altered by sympathectomy. *Dev Biol* 1989;134:30.

324. Jackson GR, Apffel L, Werrbach-Perez K, *et al*: Role of nerve growth factor in oxidant-antioxidant balance and neuronal injury. I. Stimulation of hydrogen peroxide resistance. *J Neurosci Res* 1990;25:360.

325. Jordan J, Ghadge GD, Prehn JHM, *et al*: Expression of human copper/zinc-superoxide dismutase inhibits the death of rat sympathetic neurons caused by withdrawal of nerve growth factor. *Mol Pharmacol* 1995;47:1095.

326. Ishii DN: Implication of insulin-like growth factors in the pathogenesis of diabetic neuropathy. *Brain Res Rev* 1995;20:47.

327. Zackenfels K, Oppenheim RW, Rohrer H: Evidence for an important role of IGF-I and IGF-II for the early development of chick sympathetic neurons. *Neuron* 1995;14:731.

328. Houenou LJ, Li L, Lo AC, *et al*: Naturally occurring and axotomy-induced motoneuron death and its prevention by neurotrophic agents: a comparison between chick and mouse. *Prog Brain Res* 1994;102:217.

329. Glazner GW, Lupien S, Miller JA, *et al*: Insulin-like growth factor II increases the rate of sciatic nerve regeneration in rats. *Neuroscience* 1993;54:791.

330. Rotwein P, Burgess SK, Milbrandt JD, *et al*: Differential expression of insulin-like growth factor genes in rat central nervous system. *Proc Natl Acad Sci USA* 1988;85:265.

331. Caroni P, Grandes P: Nerve sprouting in innervated adult skeletal muscle induced by exposure to elevated levels of insulin-like growth factors. *J Cell Biol* 1990;110:1307.

332. Boyd FT Jr, Clarke DW, Muther TF, *et al*: Insulin receptors and insulin modulation of norepinephrine uptake in neuronal cultures from rat brain. *J Biol Chem* 1985;260:15880.

333. Tseng LY, Brown AL, Yang YW, *et al*: The fetal rat binding protein for insulin-like growth factors is expressed in the choroid plexus and cerebrospinal fluid of adult rats. *Mol Endocrinol* 1989;3:1559.

334. Ishii DN, Glazner GW, Pu SF: Role of insulin-like growth factors in peripheral nerve regeneration. *Pharmacol Ther* 1994;62:125.

335. Kanje M, Skottner A, Sjoberg J, *et al*: Insulin-like growth factor I (IGF-I) stimulates regeneration of the rat sciatic nerve. *Brain Res* 1989;486:396.

336. Near SL, Whalen LR, Miller JA, *et al*: Insulin-like growth factor II stimulates motor nerve regeneration. *Proc Natl Acad Sci USA* 1992; 89:11716.

337. Yang H, Scheff AJ, Schalch DS: Effects of streptozocin-induced diabetes mellitus on growth and hepatic insulin-like growth factor I gene expression in the rat. *Metabolism* 1990;39:295.

338. Bothwell M: Functional interactions of neurotrophins and neurotrophin receptors. *Annu Rev Neurosci* 1995;18:223.

339. Chao MV: The p75 neurotrophin receptor. *J Neurobiol* 1994;25:1373.

340. Lee KF, Davies AM, Jaenisch R: p75-deficient embryonic dorsal root sensory and neonatal sympathetic neurons display a decreased sensitivity to NGF. *Development* 1994;120:1027.

341. Doherty P, Seaton P, Flanigan TP, *et al*: Factors controlling the expression of the NGF receptor in PC12 cells. *Neurosci Lett* 1988;92:222.

342. Taniuchi M, Clark HB, Johnson EM Jr: Induction of nerve growth factor receptor in Schwann cells after axotomy. *Proc Natl Acad Sci USA* 1986;83:4094.

343. Diamond J, Holmes M, Coughlin M: Endogenous NGF and nerve impulses regulate the collateral sprouting of sensory axons in the skin of the adult rat. *J Neurosci* 1992;12:1454.

344. Wyatt S, Shooter EM, Davies AM: Expression of the NGF receptor gene in sensory neurons and their cutaneous targets prior to and during innervation. *Neuron* 1990;4:421.

345. Yan Q, Johnson EM Jr: A quantitative study of the developmental expression of nerve growth factor (NGF) receptor in rats. *Dev Biol* 1987; 121:139.

346. Johnson EM Jr, Taniuchi M, DiStefano PS: Expression and possible function of nerve growth factor receptors on Schwann cells. *Trends Neurosci* 1988;11:299.

347. Sobue G, Yasuda T, Mitsuma T, *et al*: Expression of nerve growth factor receptor in human peripheral neuropathies. *Ann Neurol* 1988;24:64.

348. Sjoberg J, Kanje M: Insulin-like growth factor (IGF-1) as a stimulator of regeneration in the freeze-injured rat sciatic nerve. *Brain Res* 1989;485:102.

349. Levitan I, Henry A, Ristic H, *et al*: Decreased and attenuated gene expression of IGF-I and IGF-IR following sciatic nerve axotomy in BB/W-rat. *Proc Neurodiab IV* 1994;12.

350. Ekstrom AR, Kanje M, Skottner A: Nerve regeneration and serum levels of insulin-like growth factor-I in rats with streptozocin-induced insulin deficiency. *Brain Res* 1989;496:141.

351. Hellweg R, Hartung HD: Endogenous levels of nerve growth factor (NGF) are altered in experimental diabetes mellitus: A possible role for NGF in the pathogenesis of diabetic neuropathy. *J Neurosci Res* 199026:258.

352. Ordonez G, Fernandez A, Perez R, *et al*: Low contents of nerve growth factor in serum and submaxillary gland of diabetic mice. A possible etiological element of diabetic neuropathy. *J Neurol Sci* 1994;121:163.

353. Hellweg R, Raivich G, Hartung HD, *et al*: Axonal transport of endogenous nerve growth factor (NGF) and NGF receptor in experimental diabetic neuropathy. *Exp Neurol* 1994;130:24.

354. Tomlinson DR, Mayer JH: Defects of axonal transport in diabetes mellitus—a possible contribution to the aetiology of diabetic neuropathy. *J Auton Pharmacol* 1984;4:59.

355. Jakobsen J, Brimijoin S, Skau K, *et al*: Retrograde axonal transport of transmitter enzymes, fucose-labeled protein, and nerve growth factor in streptozocin-diabetic rats. *Diabetes* 1981;30:797.

356. Graubert MD, Goldstein S, Phillips LS: Nutrition and somatomedin. XXVII. Total and free IGF-I and IGF binding proteins in rats with streptozocin-induced diabetes. *Diabetes* 1991;40:959.

357. Bornfeldt KE, Arnqvist HJ, Enberg B, *et al*: Regulation of insulin-like growth factor-I and growth hormone receptor gene expression by diabetes and nutritional state in rat tissues. *J Endocrinol* 1989;122:651.

358. Luo JM, Murphy LJ: Differential expression of insulin-like growth factor-I and insulin-like growth factor binding protein-1 in the diabetic rat. *Mol Cell Biochem* 1991;103:41.

359. Ishii DN, Guertin DM, Whalen LR: Reduced insulin-like growth factor-I mRNA content in liver, adrenal glands and spinal cord of diabetic rats. *Diabetologia* 1994;37:1073.

360. Wuarin L, Guertin DM, Ishii DN: Early reduction in insulin-like growth factor gene expression in diabetic nerve. *Exp Neurol* 1994;130:106.

361. Ishii DN, Lupien SB: Insulin-like growth factors protect against diabetic neuropathy: Effects on sensory nerve regeneration in rats. *J Neurosci Res* 1995;40:138.

362. Rodriguez-Pena A, Botana M, Gonzalez M, *et al*: Expression of neurotrophins and their receptors in sciatic nerve of experimentally diabetic rats. *Neurosci Lett* 1995;200:37.

363. Tomlinson DR, Fernyhough P, Diemel LT: Neurotrophins and peripheral neuropathy. *Philos Trans R Soc Lond B Biol Sci* 1996;351:455.

364. Delcroix JD, Michael GJ, Priestley JV, *et al*: Effect of nerve growth factor treatment on p75NTR gene expression in lumbar dorsal root ganglia of streptozocin-induced diabetic rats. *Diabetes* 1998;47:1779.

365. Delcroix JD, Tomlinson DR, Fernyhough P: Diabetes and axotomy-induced deficits in retrograde axonal transport of nerve growth factor correlate with decreased levels of p75LNTR protein in lumbar dorsal root ganglia. *Brain Res Mol Brain Res* 1997;51:82.

366. Maeda K, Fernyhough P, Tomlinson DR: Regenerating sensory neurones of diabetic rats express reduced levels of mRNA for GAP-43, gamma-preprotachykinin and the nerve growth factor receptors, trkA and p75NGFR. *Brain Res Mol Brain Res* 1996;37:166.

367. Neveu I, Jehan F, Houlgatte R, *et al*: Activation of nerve growth factor synthesis in primary glial cells by phorbol 12-myristate 13-acetate: Role of protein kinase C. *Brain Res* 1992;570:316.

368. Kaechi K, Furukawa Y, Ikegami R, *et al*: Pharmacological induction of physiologically active nerve growth factor in rat peripheral nervous system. *J Pharmacol Exp Ther* 1993;264:321.

369. Naveilhan P, Neveu I, Jehan F, *et al*: Reactive oxygen species influence nerve growth factor synthesis in primary rat astrocytes. *J Neurochem* 1994;62:2178.

370. Garrett NE, Malcangio M, Dewhurst M, et al: Alpha-lipoic acid corrects neuropeptide deficits in diabetic rats via induction of trophic support. *Neurosci Lett* 1997;222:191.

371. Murase K, Hattori A, Kohno M, *et al*: Stimulation of nerve growth factor synthesis/secretion in mouse astroglial cells by coenzymes. *Biochem Mol Biol Int* 1993;30:615.

372. Faradji V, Sotelo J: Low serum levels of nerve growth factor in diabetic neuropathy. *Acta Neurol Scand* 1990;81:402.

373. Bradley JL, Thomas PK, King RH, *et al*: Myelinated nerve fiber regeneration in diabetic sensory polyneuropathy: Correlation with type of diabetes. *Acta Neuropathol* 1995;90:403.

374. Fernyhough P, Diemel LT, Hardy J, *et al*: Human recombinant nerve growth factor replaces deficient neurotrophic support in the diabetic rat. *Eur J Neurosci* 1995;7:1107.

375. Apfel SC, Arezzo JC, Brownlee M, *et al*: Nerve growth factor administration protects against experimental diabetic sensory neuropathy. *Brain Res* 1994;634:7.

376. Schmidt Y, Unger JW, Bartke I, *et al*: Effect of nerve growth factor on peptide neurons in dorsal root ganglia after taxol or cisplatin treatment and in diabetic (db/db) mice. *Exp Neurol* 1995;132:16.

377. Sango K, Verdes JM, Hikawa N, *et al*: Nerve growth factor (NGF) restores depletions of calcitonin gene-related peptide and substance P in sensory neurons from diabetic mice in vitro. *J Neurol Sci* 1994;126:1.

378. Unger JW, Klitzsch T, Pera S, *et al*: Nerve growth factor (NGF) and diabetic neuropathy in the rat: Morphological investigations of the sural nerve, dorsal root ganglion, and spinal cord. *Exp Neurol* 1998;153:23.

379. Elias KA, Cronin MJ, Stewart TA, *et al*: Peripheral neuropathy in transgenic diabetic mice: Restoration of C-fiber function with human recombinant nerve growth factor. *Diabetes* 1998;47:1637.

380. Hanaoka Y, Ohi T, Furukawa S, *et al*: The therapeutic effects of 4-methylcatechol, a stimulator of endogenous nerve growth factor synthesis, on experimental diabetic neuropathy in rats. *J Neurol Sci* 1994;122:28.

381. Apfel SC, Kessler JA, Adornato BT, *et al*: Recombinant human nerve growth factor in the treatment of diabetic polyneuropathy. NGF Study Group. *Neurology* 1998;51:695.

Somatosensory Neuropathy

Eva L. Feldman

Martin J. Stevens

James W. Russell

Douglas A. Greene

First identified as a clinical entity more than 200 years ago,[1] diabetic neuropathy is now the most common neuropathy in the Western world.[2–4] Diabetic neuropathy carries a high morbidity and is the leading cause of nontraumatic limb amputations.[5] The Diabetes Control and Complications Trial (DCCT) confirmed the theory that diabetic neuropathy is the result of sustained hyperglycemia.[6] Diabetic neuropathy complicates the secondary forms of diabetes, such as those resulting from pancreatectomy, nonalcoholic pancreatitis, and hemochromatosis, a finding that supports hyperglycemia as the common underlying mechanism for diabetic neuropathy.[7,8]

Diabetic neuropathy is actually composed of several distinct syndromes with differing anatomic distribution, clinical course, and possibly underlying pathogenetic mechanism(s). The overall prevalence of diabetic neuropathy is uncertain, but generally is considered to be approximately 50%, with a clinical course that parallels the duration and severity of hyperglycemia in both type 1 or insulin-dependent diabetes mellitus (T1DM) and type 2 or non-insulin-dependent diabetes mellitus (T2DM).[3,9–16] There are several well-explored metabolic abnormalities in diabetic nerves that result from hyperglycemia and are therefore potential initiating or contributing factors in the pathogenesis of diabetic neuropathy.[8,17–19] The role of specific glucose-linked biochemical processes such as enhanced oxidative stress, polyol-pathway activation, and nonenzymatic glycation in the pathogenesis of neuropathy is the basis of not only intensive investigation, but also the development and testing of new forms of therapy for patients with or at risk of developing diabetic peripheral neuropathy. These abnormalities may occur in several of the cellular constituents of peripheral nerves and their supporting tissues, and may thereby partially account for some of the variability of clinical neuropathy in various subgroups and individual patients with diabetes. Understanding these potential pathogenic mechanisms is essential for the effective management of diabetic neuropathy.[20] These concepts are more fully discussed in Chap. 44 on pathogenesis.

There are three general therapeutic approaches to the treatment of diabetic neuropathy. Preventive management strategies (e.g., education and hygiene) are designed to deal with potential risk factors for the development of neuropathy.[21] Palliative management strategies are designed to alleviate specific symptoms of diabetic neuropathy (e.g., pain, foot deformities, or ulcers).[22,23] Definitive therapeutic strategies are targeted against specific pathogenetic components of diabetic neuropathy.[23–25] Currently, glycemic control is the only effective definitive therapy.[26] The development of future adjunct therapies to prevent and potentially reverse the neurologic damage that underlies the clinical manifestations of diabetic neuropathy awaits clearer understanding of the responsible pathogenetic mechanisms[27] (see Chap. 44).

EPIDEMIOLOGY, IMPACT, AND SCOPE OF DIABETIC NEUROPATHY

Estimates of the impact and frequency of diabetic neuropathy are dependent on the choice of terminology, diagnostic criteria, and study populations. Minor paresthesias may constitute diabetic neuropathy in one study, while others may employ much more rigid criteria, including electrophysiology and quantitative sensory testing. The discrepancies in prevalence estimates reflect the different criteria used to diagnose neuropathy. The sensitivity, specificity, and reliability of simple objective measures to diagnose neuropathy in a person with diabetes are still controversial.[28–31] Nevertheless, certain generalizations are clear from the available data; specifically, neuropathy is a frequent complication of diabetes, and estimated prevalence rates are on average 50% and rise with advancing age.[32]

In a frequently cited prospective study of over 4400 diabetic outpatients, Pirart reported an overall 12% prevalence rate of diabetic neuropathy in patients with newly diagnosed diabetes.[33] The incidence of neuropathy increased with the duration of diabetes, and after 25 years of diabetes, over 50% of patients had diabetic neuropathy.[33] Several cross-sectional multicenter studies of a mixed group of type 1 and 2 diabetic patients have yielded similar results. In the United Kingdom, 6487 diabetic patients were examined for the presence of neuropathy by a simple assessment of ankle reflexes, vibration, pinprick, and temperature sensation, coupled with a 9-point symptoms score. The reported prevalence of neuropathy was 5% in the 20- to 29-year-old group and increased with age, reaching 44.2% in patients between 70 and 79 years of age.[12] A simple screening tool examining ankle reflexes and great toe sensation[34] was administered to 8757 diabetic patients, and

32.3% of patients had abnormalities consistent with diabetic neuropathy.[9] Severity of neuropathy was then graded in the 2033 neuropathic patients using a quantitative assessment of strength, sensation, reflexes, and electrophysiology. Over one-half of all patients had mild to moderate neuropathy, while 20% had borderline and 12% severe neuropathy; in each category, the severity of neuropathy increased with age and duration of diabetes.[9] A similar increase in severity and prevalence of neuropathy with age and duration of diabetes was reported among Spanish patients.[35] In the population-based Rochester Diabetic Neuropathy Study, which commenced in 1986, 54% of type 1 and 45% of type 2 diabetic patients had polyneuropathy,[11] defined as two or more abnormalities from quantitative assessment of symptoms, signs, sensation, autonomic function, and nerve conduction studies.

Several studies evaluated the presence of neuropathy in patients with either T1DM or T2DM. In the Diabetes Control and Complication Trial (DCCT), a cohort of 278 healthy type 1 diabetic patients were examined for the presence of neuropathy, defined as an abnormal neurological examination plus either abnormal nerve conduction studies in two nerves or abnormal autonomic function testing. Using these criteria, 39% of patients had some clinical manifestation of neuropathy.[36] Similarly, in the Pittsburgh Epidemiology of Diabetes Complications Study, the prevalence of neuropathy in T1DM patients was 18% in patients 18–29 years of age, compared to 58% in the >30-year-old group.[37] In the EURO-DIAB complications study, 3250 T1DM patients were examined from 16 European countries, and the overall prevalence of diabetic neuropathy was 28%, with significant correlations with age, duration of diabetes, and quality of metabolic control.[13] Using abnormal nerve conduction studies to define subclinical neuropathy, 87% of type 1 diabetic children were neuropathic, with the majority of abnormalities in the lower limbs.[38] Similar statistics emerge from studying T2DM patients. In a longitudinal study, 8.3% of type 2 patients had neuropathy upon diagnosis of diabetes, with an increased prevalence to 42% after 10 years of diabetes.[10] A separate prospective study of type 2 patients reported that 22% developed diabetic neuropathy after 4 years.[39] In a cohort of type 2 diabetic patients with a mean duration of 12 years of diabetes, 49% had diabetic neuropathy.[40]

This high prevalence of diabetic neuropathy is associated with significant morbidity, including recurrent foot infections, ulcers, and amputations.[41,42] The national annual direct cost of diabetic foot ulcers in the United States is estimated to be $5 billion with an indirect cost of $400 million.[43] Between 1995 and 1996, the average Medicare expenditure for a diabetic patient was $15,309, compared to $5,226 for Medicare patients in general, and 25% of these dollars went to the treatment of foot ulcers.[43] On average, 15% of patients with diabetic neuropathy require an amputation, making diabetic neuropathy the most common cause of nontraumatic amputations in the Western world.[41] Thus diabetic neuropathy is generally conceded to be an extraordinarily common complication of diabetes, causing significant morbidity and carrying a large financial burden.

CLASSIFICATION OF DIABETIC NEUROPATHY

Diabetic neuropathy can be classified into two stages or classes, *subclinical* (class I) and *clinical* (class II) (Table 45-1).[44] *Subclinical diabetic neuropathy* consists of evidence of peripheral nerve dysfunction such as slowed motor and sensory nerve conduction, elevated

TABLE 45-1. Classification and Staging of Diabetic Neuropathy

Class I: Subclinical Neuropathy*

A. Abnormal Electrodiagnostic Tests (EDX)
   1. Decreased nerve conduction velocity
   2. Decreased amplitude of evoked muscle or nerve action potential
B. Abnormal Quantitative Sensory Testing (QST)
   1. Vibratory/tactile
   2. Thermal warming/cooling
   3. Other
C. Abnormal Autonomic Function Test (AFT)
   1. Diminished sinus arrhythmia (beat-to-beat heart rate variation)
   2. Diminished sudomotor function
   3. Increased pupillary latency

Class II: Clinical Neuropathy

A. Diffuse Neuropathy
   1. Distal symmetric sensorimotor polyneuropathy
     a. Primarily small-fiber neuropathy
     b. Primarily large-fiber neuropathy
     c. Mixed
   2. Autonomic neuropathy
     a. Abnormal pupillary function
     b. Sudomotor dysfunction
     c. Genitourinary autonomic neuropathy
       (1) Bladder dysfunction
       (2) Sexual dysfunction
     d. Gastrointestinal autonomic neuropathy
       (1) Gastric atony
       (2) Gallbladder atony
       (3) Diabetic diarrhea
       (4) Hypoglycemia unawareness (adrenal medullary neuropathy)
     e. Cardiovascular autonomic neuropathy
     f. Hypoglycemia unawareness
B. Focal Neuropathy
   1. Mononeuropathy
   2. Mononeuropathy multiplex
   3. Plexopathy
   4. Radiculopathy
   5. Cranial neuropathy

* Neurological function tests are abnormal but no neurological symptoms or clinically detectable neurological deficits indicative of a diffuse or focal neuropathy are present. Class I, Subclinical Neuropathy, is further subdivided into class Ia if an AFT or QST abnormality is present, class Ib if EDX or AFT and QST abnormalities are present, and class Ic if an EDX and either AFT or QST abnormalities or both are present.

Source: Reprinted with permission from American Diabetes Association: Report and recommendations of the San Antonio conference on diabetic neuropathy. Consensus statement. *Diabetes* 1988;37:1000.

sensory perception thresholds that occur in the absence of clinical signs, and/or symptoms of diabetic neuropathy. *Clinical diabetic neuropathy* consists of the superimposition of symptoms and/or clinically detectable neurologic deficits (Table 45-1). Clinically overt diabetic neuropathy manifests itself as the presence of one or more of the individual clinical syndromes, representing either diffuse or focal neuropathy. Although each syndrome has a characteristic presentation and clinical course, they frequently coexist in the same patient, often making classification of individual cases difficult.

Diffuse clinical diabetic neuropathy refers to distal symmetric sensorimotor polyneuropathy and autonomic neuropathy. *Distal symmetric polyneuropathy* is the most commonly recognized form of diabetic neuropathy and features sensory deficits and symptoms that overshadow motor involvement.[31,45] Sensory deficits initially appear in the most distal portions of the extremities and progress proximally in a "stocking-glove" distribution, in the most advanced cases forming vertical bands on the chest as distal portions of truncal nerves become involved.[32,46] The signs, symptoms, and neurologic deficits of distal symmetric polyneuropathy vary depending on the classes of nerve fibers. Loss of large sensory and motor fibers leads to a loss of light touch and proprioception and produces muscle weakness, while loss of small fibers diminishes pain and temperature perception and produces paresthesias, dysesthesias, and/or neuropathic pain.[8,32,47] Diminished or absent deep-tendon reflexes, especially the Achilles tendon reflex, are often an early indication of otherwise mild asymptomatic neuropathy. Undetected but more advanced asymptomatic neuropathy may first present with late complications such as ulceration or neuroarthropathy (Charcot's joints) of the foot.[48] The other diffuse form of clinical diabetic neuropathy is *diabetic autonomic neuropathy* (see Chap. 46). This often but not always accompanies distal symmetric polyneuropathy and can impair virtually any sympathetic or parasympathetic autonomic function.[20,49]

Cardiovascular autonomic neuropathy first compromises cardiac parasympathetic function, diminishing the normal bradycardic responses to sleep and deep inspiration. With progression, sympathetic cardiac and peripheral vascular denervation occurs, interfering with normal cardiovascular response to exercise and sensitizing the heart to circulating catecholamines, which may predispose to tachyarrhythmia and sudden death.[50] Autonomic neuropathy leading to respiratory arrest has also been implicated in sudden death (see Chap. 46). *Gastrointestinal autonomic neuropathy* can involve virtually the entire length of the gastrointestinal tract.[51] It contributes to nonspecific gastrointestinal tract symptoms that afflict the majority of diabetic patients. Esophageal motility impairment and reflux, decreased vagally mediated gastric acid secretion, and delayed gastric emptying produce anorexia, nausea, vomiting, early satiety, and postprandial bloating and fullness.[51] Diabetic enteropathy encompasses the clinical syndromes of diabetic constipation, diabetic diarrhea, and fecal incontinence, which all reflect widespread abnormalities in the intrinsic and extrinsic intestinal autonomic nervous system.[52] *Genitourinary autonomic neuropathy* includes retrograde ejaculation, neuropathic erectile impotence, deficient vaginal lubrication leading to dyspareunia, and diabetic cystopathy.[53] Neuropathic impotence is generally but not always accompanied by other manifestations of diabetic neuropathy (see Chap 46).[53]

Autonomic sudomotor dysfunction produces an asymptomatic distal anhydrosis in a stocking-glove distribution similar to that of distal symmetric polyneuropathy. This diminished thermoregulatory reserve predisposes to heatstroke and hyperthermia, and produces a compensatory central hyperhydrosis that is often bothersome to the patient.[49] All forms of autonomic neuropathy are addressed in detail in Chap. 46.

The *focal forms of diabetic neuropathy* correspond to the distribution of single or multiple peripheral nerves (mononeuropathy and mononeuropathy multiplex), cranial nerves, regions of the brachial or lumbosacral plexuses (plexopathy), or the nerve roots (radiculopathy). With the exception of peripheral nerve mononeuropathies, these focal forms of diabetic neuropathy are relatively uncommon.[11,20] They are frequently of sudden onset, are generally but not always self-limited, and tend to occur in older age groups.[20] Among cranial nerves, the third cranial nerve is often affected, presenting with unilateral pain, diplopia, and ptosis with pupillary

Table 45-2. Diabetes Mellitus: Potential Peripheral Nervous System Complications

A. Mononeuropathy or Mononeuritis Multiplex
   1. Isolated cranial or peripheral nerve involvement (e.g., CN III, ulnar, median, femoral, or peroneal)
   2. If confluent, may resemble polyneuropathy
B. Radiculopathy, Polyradiculopathy, or Plexopathy
   1. Thoracic
   2. Lumbosacral
   3. Diabetic amyotrophy
   4. Lumbosacral plexopathy
C. Autonomic Neuropathy
D. Polyneuropathy
   1. Diffuse sensorimotor
   2. Painful sensory

sparing, in a syndrome termed *diabetic ophthalmoplegia.* Diabetic ophthalmoplegia may occur in the absence of other manifestations of diabetic neuropathy, and may be bilateral, recurrent, or both.[54] Femoral neuropathy, typically seen in older male type 2 diabetic patients, often involves motor and sensory deficits at the level of the lumbar plexus or lumbar roots as well as the femoral nerve, with the relative excess of motor versus sensory involvement differentiating diabetic femoral neuropathy from that seen in other conditions.[55] Thoracic radiculopathies present as band-like thoracic or abdominal pain that is often misdiagnosed as an acute intrathoracic or intra-abdominal emergency.[56] The more common mononeuropathies mimic the compression neuropathies seen in nondiabetic individuals, such as carpal tunnel syndrome or ulnar neuropathy.[57] In summary, distal symmetric polyneuropathy and autonomic neuropathy are common, diffuse, and generally progressive disorders, whereas the focal neuropathies are rare, sudden in onset, often self-limited, and occur primarily in older patients with diabetes. These various forms of diabetic neuropathy are discussed in more detail below and are listed in Table 45-2.

RELATIONSHIP OF NEUROPATHY TO THE DURATION AND METABOLIC SEVERITY OF DIABETES IN MAN

The relationship of diabetic neuropathy to the severity and duration of hyperglycemia has important therapeutic as well as pathogenetic implications. The close link between the severity and/or duration of hyperglycemia with the development of diabetic neuropathy supports intensified glycemic control and implicates glucose or insulin-related metabolic factors as important pathogenetic elements in the disease process. In the Stockholm Diabetes Intervention Study, intensified insulin treatment of T1DM patients prevented the nerve conduction slowing that occurred after 5 years in the regular treatment group,[58] with continued benefit evident at 10 years.[59] The Diabetes Control and Complications Trial (DCCT) provides even stronger evidence for the importance of insulin deficiency, hyperglycemia, or both in the pathogenesis of diabetic neuropathy.[60] Intensive diabetes treatment designed to lower blood glucose to as close to the normal range as possible in nonneuropathic subjects with T1DM was, after 5 years, able to reduce the prevalence of clinical diabetic neuropathy confirmed by abnormal nerve conduction or autonomic function by 60%.[60]

While T2DM is nearly 10 times more common than T1DM, there exists only one prospective trial of type 2 patients and the effects of glycemic control on the development of neuropathy. In the VA cooperative study, 153 men with an average age of 60 and an average known diagnosis of diabetes of 7.8 years were randomly assigned to standard or intensive therapy. After 24 months there was no difference in the overall prevalence of peripheral or autonomic neuropathy.[61] However, these results must be considered in the context of the several large epidemiologic and population-based studies (discussed at the beginning of this chapter) that reveal a strong highly significant association between hyperglycemia and neuropathy.[62] Thus, a large long-duration prospective trial of both men and women with T2DM is required to conclusively address this question. Notwithstanding this fact, the generally held belief is that longer duration and greater extent of hyperglycemia predispose to the development of neuropathy in T2DM patients in a manner similar to that of T1DM patients.[14,16]

The onset of clinically overt diabetic neuropathy in an individual patient is an unpredictable event. This is true despite the close epidemiologic association between clinical neuropathy and the duration and severity of hyperglycemia in populations of diabetic patients. The sometimes-reported "paradoxical precipitation of neuropathy following institution of good control" refers primarily to the acute onset of pain that likely reflects repair and regeneration of damaged nerve fibers. Unfortunately, clinical neuropathy was not reassessed in the DCCT until the fifth year after initiation of intensive diabetes therapy,[60] so the temporal association between the institution of diabetes control and the development of neuropathy could not be determined.

The onset of neuropathy may also be influenced by other independent variables such as genetic, nutritional, and toxic factors.[13,63] Alcohol consumption, even well within the socially accepted norms, appears to be a risk factor for neuropathy.[36,64] In diabetic subjects with absent or very mild clinical neuropathy, nerve conduction parameters are also affected by a variety of features other than the severity and duration of diabetes. These variables include age, height, and gender, as well as pubertal state at the time of diagnosis of diabetes.[36,65]

DIAGNOSIS AND STAGING OF DIABETIC NEUROPATHY

There are three recent areas of active investigation aimed at improving the diagnosis and classification of diabetic neuropathy: (1) the use of quantitative sensory testing and electrodiagnostic studies to quantify neural damage, especially as part of large clinical trials, (2) the use of standardized criteria to diagnose and monitor neuropathy, especially in a research setting, and (3) the development of simple neuropathy screening tools for use in outpatient clinics. This section discusses each area and presents an outpatient program for the diagnosis of neuropathy in the practitioner's office.

Quantitative Sensory Tests

Quantitative tests of nerve function are valuable in evaluating the extent, severity, natural history, and prevalence of diabetic neuropathy.[66] They may also identify patients with unrecognized subclinical or asymptomatic clinical (e.g., signs alone) diabetic neuropathy.[29] Sensory threshold measurements have the advantage over a clinical sensory examination in that reproducible, quantita-

tive, and graded stimuli are administered to the patient. Reproducible algorithms for objectively testing and assessing thresholds are defined and compared to well-established normative values.[67] Abnormal sensory thresholds correlate with the presence of diabetic neuropathy in groups of diabetic patients and in individual patients.[68]

There are several commercial instruments available for the evaluation of quantitative sensory perception thresholds. The sensory stimuli used in these instruments include thermal, touch-pressure, vibratory, tactile, and electrical stimuli.[66] Older methodology and instruments used a ramp technique or a method-of-limits technique, both of which are confounded by response bias. A true alternative forced-choice algorithm minimizes response bias. Stimulus and nonstimulus episodes are presented in pairs, and the patient must identify which episode contained the stimulus. Established algorithms for all commercially available products define threshold as the minimum stimulus correctly detected by the patient 50% of the time.[66] A computer-assisted sensory examination (CASE) is now commercially available and represents the best standardized method for sensory perception threshold testing.[69] It eliminates bias and is the prototype for many of the simpler commercially available products that are less expensive and can be used with a minimal amount of training. Confounding variables that influence sensory perception threshold include age, obesity, ischemia, skin temperature, patient alertness, room ambience, and test anxiety.[66]

Vibratory Perception Threshold

Vibratory perception threshold measures large-nerve fiber integrity and perception and is normally poorer in the lower extremity than the upper extremity. It may be abnormal in the absence of clinical symptoms or deficits and may therefore indicate subclinical neuropathy.[66] More frequently, abnormalities of vibration perception are associated with the loss or reduction of the Achilles tendon reflex. Abnormal vibratory perception threshold is more common than abnormal touch-pressure and temperature threshold in diabetic individuals, and it may therefore be a more sensitive index of subclinical neuropathy.[70] Patients with impaired vibratory sensation are more prone to develop foot ulceration, lending clinical significance to the impairment of vibratory perception.[71–73] Thus vibratory perception threshold is a sensitive and clinically significant index of large-nerve fiber involvement in patients with diabetes.[30,70,71,73]

Thermal Perception Threshold

Thermal perception threshold reflects small-nerve fiber integrity.[66] Because diminished temperature perception predisposes to accidental burns in diabetic individuals, it has important clinical implications. Both warming and cooling can be used to measure thermal perception, although the warming method may have a higher degree of sensitivity than cooling.[74] Both methodologies have been well validated and are easy to perform.[74,75]

Electrodiagnostic Studies

Electrodiagnostic tests have widespread application and are reliable, reproducible measures of peripheral nervous system function relative to disorders of nerve, muscle, and neuromuscular junction.[76] They are objective measures that are relatively independent of patient effort or cooperation.[76] Nerve conduction studies and needle electromyography are well accepted for the evaluation of diabetic neuropathy, including recent use in sequential studies to evaluate disease progression or response to treatment.[46,77] These are sensitive measures, able to detect abnormalities in diabetic patients that may not be clinically apparent.[77]

Test Description

The term *electromyography* technically refers to the needle electrode examination, but it often is used in reference to both nerve conduction measures and the needle examination. Both are important components of the electrodiagnostic examination that have been used since the mid-1950s to evaluate patients with suspected diabetic neuropathy. They are described separately because they evaluate slightly different components of the peripheral nervous system, reflect different abnormalities, and have different applications depending on the question asked.

Nerve Conduction Studies

Nerve conduction studies[76,78] are used to evaluate sensory and motor nerves. In these studies, measures of sensory nerve action potential (SNAP) or compound muscle action potential (CMAP) amplitude, distal latency, and conduction velocity are recorded. Amplitude measures are important in the evaluation of peripheral neuropathy, reflecting in part the size and number of nerve or muscle fibers.

Conduction velocity, as used in conventional electrodiagnostic studies, reflects transmission time in the largest myelinated nerve fibers. It is expressed as a conduction velocity (meters per second; m/s) between two points along the nerve, or as a terminal or distal latency (milliseconds) along a fixed distance at the end of the nerve. For motor conduction studies, the distal latency also includes a neuromuscular transmission latency. The conduction velocity reflects several physiologic components of peripheral nerve function, including nerve size, amount of myelin, nodal and internodal lengths, axonal resistance, and nerve temperature. In addition to the known pathologic findings of primary axonal loss and secondary demyelination and remyelination in diabetic neuropathy, there may be metabolic changes associated with reduced conduction velocity as well. The observation that nerve conduction velocity increased 6 hours after initiating normal glucose levels suggests that nonstructural changes at least partially account for conduction abnormalities in diabetic neuropathy.[79]

Conduction over the entire motor nerve, including its proximal portion, can be approximated by F-wave latency measures. The F wave occurs after antidromic motor nerve stimulation, with resultant activation of a portion of the anterior horn cells from that nerve and transmission of an orthodromic response along those fibers. This response can be recorded directly from a muscle innervated by those fibers and the stimulation-to-response-onset latency determined. Conduction velocity abnormalities in diffuse disorders are accentuated by the long conduction distances, making abnormalities in F-wave latencies very sensitive measures of diabetic neuropathy, as well as in other conditions associated with diabetes, such as diabetic polyradiculopathy.

Needle Electromyography

Needle electromyography[76,78] (EMG) may be the most sensitive indicator of axonal degeneration and may demonstrate abnormality in asymptomatic diabetic patients. Though quantitative measures of motor unit action potential recruitment, amplitude, duration, and configuration are difficult and unreliable compared with nerve conduction measurements, the subjective determination of the presence or absence of fibrillation potentials or positive waves at rest is easily performed and reproducible. The presence of abnormal insertional activity is a very sensitive indicator of axonal degeneration. These may appear prior to development of clinical findings, and prior to development of nerve conduction velocity or SNAP amplitude abnormalities. Most patients feel that the needle examination is more uncomfortable than the conduction studies, and it is rarely used in sequential clinical trials because of poor tolerance. Its most important use in diabetic neuropathy is to document the presence or absence of superimposed diabetic polyradiculopathy, amyotrophy, plexopathy, or other peripheral nerve disorders.[77]

Electrodiagnostic Evaluation of Diabetic Neuropathy

The techniques used in the electrodiagnostic evaluation of diabetic patients must be rigorous. Nerve conduction studies should be performed and reported, together with normal values, using standardized laboratory techniques.[76] Normal values usually are reported as three standard deviations from the mean when the data are normally distributed, or as a normal range or 99th percentile when the distribution is not Gaussian.[76] Different values exist for different age groups and some measures vary according to patient size (height, finger circumference, and limb length).[76] Using appropriately defined normal data, individual diabetic patients or groups of patients may be compared with population normal values.[77] One important source of variability in nerve conduction measurements relates to the influence of limb temperature on amplitude, distal latency, and conduction velocity.[76] Conventional practice is to warm cool limbs into the temperature range used for obtaining normal values, usually 32°–36°C.[77]

Standard Evaluation and Interpretation

The electrodiagnostic examination of diabetic patients must be thorough because a variety of diabetes-related peripheral abnormalities exist, including mononeuropathy, mononeuritis multiplex, plexopathy, polyradiculopathy, and sensorimotor polyneuropathy (Table 45-2). A complete evaluation allows detection and quantification of the peripheral disorder, as well as identifying the predominant pathophysiology. Such an evaluation may allow patient classification into homogeneous groups for treatment trials (e.g., pure sensorimotor polyneuropathy versus polyradiculopathy or polyradiculoneuropathy), while simultaneously identifying patients with superimposed focal or multifocal lesions.

A standard evaluation can be outlined (Table 45-3), although the strategy differs depending on the severity of the disorder. When symptoms or signs are minimal, evaluation is directed toward the most sensitive or susceptible nerves.[77] In diabetic neuropathy, distal lower-extremity studies are more likely to be abnormal than upper-extremity studies, and sensory abnormalities are more common than motor abnormalities.[77] Absent lower-extremity responses cannot be used to document subsequent progression, and because of this, it is important to study less involved nerves.[46,77,78,80]

The needle examination is used in several ways. As a sensitive indicator of axonal degeneration, it may demonstrate the only abnormality in an early diabetic neuropathy.[77] The electromyographer can also use needle electromyography to examine muscles inaccessible or poorly accessible to nerve conduction studies, including paraspinal, abdominal, and proximal extremity muscles. Abnormal findings in such muscles may provide evidence of polyradiculopathy (symptomatic or asymptomatic), amyotrophy,

TABLE 45-3. Polyneuropathy Protocol

I. Conduction Studies*
  A. General
    1. Test most involved site if mild or moderate, least involved if severe.
    2. Warm limb if temperature is <32°C; monitor and maintain temperature throughout study.
    3. Use reproducible recording and stimulation sites (either fixed distances or standard landmarks).
    4. Use supramaximal percutaneous stimulation.
  B. Motor Studies
    1. Peroneal motor (extensor digitorum brevis); stimulate at ankle and knee. Record F-wave latency following distal antidromic stimulation.
    2. Abnormal, tibial motor (abductor hallucis); stimulate at ankle; record F-wave latency.
    3. If no responses: peroneal motor (anterior tibial); stimulate at fibula.
    4. Ulnar motor (hypothenar); stimulate below wrist and elbow. Record F-wave latency.
    5. Median motor (thenar); stimulate wrist and antecubital fossa. Record F-wave latency.
  C. Sensory Studies
    1. Sural sensory (ankle); may occasionally require:
      a. Needle recording
      b. Response averaging
    2. Median sensory (index); stimulate wrist and elbow. If antidromic response absent or focal entrapment suspected, record (wrist) stimulating palm.
    3. Ulnar sensory (5th digit); stimulate wrist. If antidromic response absent or superimposed on motor artifact, perform orthodromic study.
  D. Autonomic Studies
    1. Skin potential responses (palmar and plantar surfaces of hand and foot, respectively); stimulate contralateral median nerve.
  E. Additional
    1. Additional motor or sensory nerves can be evaluated if findings equivocal. Definite abnormalities should result in:
      a. Evaluation of opposite extremity
      b. Proceed to evaluation of specific suspected abnormality.
II. Needle Examination
  A. Representative Muscles
    1. Anterior tibial, medial gastrocnemius, first dorsal interosseous (hand), and lumbar paraspinal muscles.
    2. If normal, intrinsic foot muscles should be examined.
    3. Any abnormalities should be confirmed by examination of at least one contralateral muscle.
  B. Grading
    1. Abnormal spontaneous activity should be graded subjectively [0–4] using conventional criteria.
    2. Motor unit action potential amplitude, duration, configuration, and recruitment graded subjectively.

* Recording sites are in parenthesis.

or other focal disorder.[76] The subjective interpretation of the results of needle electromyography also allows differentiation of acute, subacute, and chronic peripheral disorders. This may be useful in identifying evidence of residual abnormalities, independent from diabetic neuropathy.

    There is a positive relationship between the electrodiagnostic and clinical examinations. Quantitative neurologic measures of sensation, including touch-pressure, vibration, and two-point discrimination, and muscle stretch reflexes and strength correlate with electrodiagnostic measures, including sensory evoked amplitudes and motor conduction velocities.[76] Sural nerve morphology has also been compared with results from nerve conduction studies. Typical findings included loss of large and small myelinated nerve fibers, evidence of segmental remyelination and demyelination, and variable amounts of axonal degeneration. Comparing maximal measured sural conduction velocity with the diameter of the largest axons indicated that conduction velocities were 10–30% slower than expected, based on normal mean values, even in nerves with preserved large fibers.[46] The electrodiagnostic findings in the sural nerve were representative of findings in other nerves. It was concluded that such slowing was due to causes other than fiber loss, whereas more substantial slowing was related to degeneration of large fibers. The reported pathologic findings demonstrate that fiber loss is primary and demyelination with remyelination is secondary.[81–83]

Subclinical Diabetic Neuropathy

Significantly reduced conduction velocity in asymptomatic, neurologically intact patients is not surprising and has been reported in several studies.[46,77] Slowed conduction velocity may reflect segmental demyelination and remyelination without conduction block or substantial axonal degeneration, or it may reflect a metabolic abnormality in diabetic nerve. For example, mean motor conduction velocity differences of 4.6 m/s were found in diabetic patients compared to age-matched controls, averaged for upper- and lower-extremity nerves.[84] Other studies have demonstrated that loss of amplitude of sensory potentials is a sensitive indicator of subclinical involvement, followed by the appearance of fibrillation potentials.[85]

Clinically Evident Diabetic Neuropathy

Conduction velocity slowing has been reported consistently, usually demonstrating a 5–13-m/s difference between diabetic patients with clinically evident neuropathy and age-matched control subjects.[86] The actual difference depends on the nerves studied, the severity of the neuropathy, and other factors, including glycemic control.

    Sensory conduction abnormalities are more pronounced than motor abnormalities (greatest mean deviation from normal), and most pronounced in the distal lower extremities. The overall sensitivity of the electrodiagnostic evaluation has been studied by determining the frequency of abnormality for individual measures for 109 adult diabetic patients under 60 years of age with clinically apparent diabetic neuropathy. The percentage of patients demonstrating abnormality of individual test measures was as follows: abnormal sural amplitude, 91% (absent in 63%; reduced in 16%); abnormal needle examination of intrinsic foot muscles, 88%; reduced tibial and peroneal motor conduction velocities, 75%; reduced median and ulnar motor conduction velocities, 64%; reduced or absent upper-extremity SNAP amplitudes, 57%; and abnormal lumbar paraspinal needle examination, 22%.[86] These findings reflect the experience of most clinical electromyographers, and support the electrodiagnostic protocol outlined in Table 45-3. The most severely impaired patients have the greatest number and greatest magnitude of nerve conduction abnormalities.

Summary

Electrodiagnostic studies are a valuable component of the overall evaluation of patients with known or suspected diabetes. Often abnormal in asymptomatic, clinically intact diabetic patients, these studies are almost invariably abnormal in the presence of clinically evident diabetic neuropathy. A normal electrodiagnostic examination makes the diagnosis of diabetic neuropathy unlikely, even in predominantly small-fiber disease. When properly used, nerve conduction studies and needle electromyography can suggest the underlying pathophysiology, monitor disease progression or improvement, or identify peripheral disorders other than neuropathy that may be causing diagnostic confusion. The use of electrodiagnostic studies in clinical trials is similarly important, although the trials must be sufficiently long to permit physiologic improvement or deterioration.[87]

Standardized Criteria to Diagnose and Monitor Neuropathy for Clinical Trials

A comprehensive set of diagnostic criteria for detection and staging of diabetic neuropathy was first introduced in 1985 by Dyck and colleagues.[88] In response to widespread interest generated by these criteria and by ongoing clinical treatment trials in diabetic neuropathy, the American Diabetes Association and the American Academy of Neurology convened a panel in 1988. Now known as the San Antonio Consensus Conference on Diabetic Neuropathy, this group recommended a set of research guidelines defining subclinical and clinical diabetic neuropathy.[89] The panel suggested that each patient have at least one measure from quantitative tests of (1) clinical symptoms, (2) clinical signs, (3) quantitative sensory testing, (4) autonomic function testing, and (5) electrodiagnostic studies. Results from these tests place patients into definable categories.

The diagnosis of subclinical diabetic neuropathy (Table 45-1, class I) requires the demonstration in a diabetic patient of objective measurement of peripheral neural impairment not attributable to a nondiabetic etiology in the absence of detectable clinical signs or symptoms of neuropathy. The diagnosis of clinical diabetic neuropathy (Table 45-1, class II) requires the demonstration in a diabetic patient of symptoms or signs plus objective measurement of peripheral neural impairment not attributable to a nondiabetic etiology. Since there are no distinguishing features unique to diabetic neuropathy, all other likely causes of peripheral neuropathy or disorders that mimic peripheral neuropathy must be excluded by careful history and physical examination and appropriate diagnostic tests (Table 45-4). Neuropathy must also accompany currently accepted diagnostic criteria for diabetes.[90] Since neuropathic symptoms are often vague and nonspecific, confirmatory clinical signs or objective measurements of peripheral nerve dysfunction (somatic or autonomic) must be present.

OUTPATIENT DIAGNOSIS OF NEUROPATHY

The diagnostic criteria of the San Antonio Conference were developed for research trials and are difficult to employ in routine clinical practice. The Michigan Neuropathy Program is a two-part assessment developed to diagnose and stage diabetic neuropathy in an outpatient setting.[34] In part one, a simple 8-point clinical examination, designated the Michigan Neuropathy Screening Instrument (MNSI), is administered by a health care professional (Fig. 45-1). An MNSI score of >2 indicates the presence of neuropathy with a high specificity (95%) and sensitivity (80%).[86,91] The severity of neuropathy is determined in the second part of the Michigan Neuropathy Program. A focused 146-point neurologic examination is administered by a health care professional (Fig. 45-2), followed by routine nerve conduction studies (sural, peroneal motor, median sensory, and motor and ulnar sensory). The severity of neuropathy

TABLE 45-4. Differential Diagnosis of Diabetic Neuropathy

I. Distal Symmetric Polyneuropathy
  A. Metabolic
    1. Diabetes mellitus
    2. Uremia
    3. Folic acid/cyanocobalamin deficiency
    4. Hypothyroidism
    5. Acute intermittent porphyria
  B. Toxic
    1. Alcohol
    2. Heavy metals (lead, mercury, arsenic)
    3. Industrial hydrocarbons
    4. Various drugs
  C. Infectious or Inflammatory
    1. Sarcoidosis
    2. Leprosy
    3. Periarteritis nodosa
    4. Other connective tissue diseases (e.g., systemic lupus erythematosus)
  D. Other
    1. Dysproteinemias and paraproteinemias
    2. Paraneoplastic syndrome
    3. Leukemias and lymphomas
    4. Amyloidosis
    5. Hereditary neuropathies
II. Pains and Paresthesias without Neurological Deficit
  A. Early small-fiber sensory neuropathy
  B. Psychophysiologic disorder (e.g., severe depression, hysteria)
III. Autonomic Neuropathy without Somatic Component
  A. Shy-Drager syndrome (progressive autonomic failure)
  B. Diabetic neuropathy with mild somatic involvement
  C. Riley-Day syndrome
  D. Idiopathic orthostatic hypotension
IV. Diffuse Motor Neuropathy without Sensory Deficit
  A. Guillain-Barré syndrome
  B. Primary myopathies
  C. Myasthenia gravis
  D. Heavy-metal toxicity
V. Femoral Neuropathy (Sacral Plexopathy)
  A. Degenerative spinal disk disease (e.g., Paget's disease of the spine)
  B. Intrinsic spinal-cord-mass lesion
  C. Cauda equina lesions
  D. Coagulopathies
VI. Cranial Neuropathy
  A. Carotid aneurysm
  B. Intracranial mass
  C. Elevated intracranial pressure
VII. Mononeuropathy Multiplex
  A. Vasculitides
  B. Amyloidosis
  C. Hypothyroidism
  D. Acromegaly
  E. Coagulopathies

is graded in each patient by a composite score consisting of the number of abnormal nerve conductions and total points from the clinical examination (Fig. 45-3). This program has been successfully used in diabetic outpatient clinics for the screening and simple staging of diabetic neuropathy.[9]

The Semmes-Weinstein 5.07 (10-g) monofilament provides a simple screening tool for diabetic neuropathy and is recommended for this use by the International Diabetes Federation and the World Health Organization European St. Vincent Declaration.[92-95] The

			Yes (0)	No (1)
Appearance of feet	Right	Normal	______	______
			If no, check all that apply:	
			______ Deformed	
			______ Dry skin	
			______ Infection	
			______ Ulceration (1)	
			Yes (0)	**No (1)**
	Left	Normal	______	______
			If no, check all that apply:	
			______ Deformed	
			______ Dry skin	
			______ Infection	
			______ Ulceration (1)	

		Present (0)	Present/reinforcement (0.5)	Absent (1)
Ankle reflexes	Right	______	______	______
	Left	______	______	______

		Present (0)	Decreased (0.5)	Absent (1)
Vibration perception at great toe	Right	______	______	______
	Left	______	______	______
			TOTAL	______/8 pts.

FIGURE 45-1. Neuropathy screening instrument. *(Reprinted with permission from Feldman* et al.[34]*)*

monofilament buckles when a 10-g force is applied.[96] In some office settings, patients are tested for the ability to sense the monofilament at 10 sites on the foot.[92,97] Inability to perceive the filament correlates with an insensate foot and diabetic neuropathy.[92,93] A recent study examined the variation and sensitivity of the 10 different sites and found that examining only 2 sites can provide useful information: these are sites 3 and 4, the plantar aspect of the first and fifth metatarsal heads. If a patient can not feel the monofilament in these locations, there is a high sensitivity and specificity (80% and 86%, respectively) that the patient has diabetic neuropathy.[98]

MANAGEMENT APPROACHES TO THE CLINICAL SYNDROMES OF DIABETIC NEUROPATHY

As summarized earlier, clinically evident diabetic neuropathy is subdivided into a series of distinct but not mutually exclusive clinical syndromes that may occur concurrently in individual patients. The diffuse forms of diabetic neuropathy, distal symmetric sensorimotor polyneuropathy, and autonomic neuropathy are by far the most common syndromes, occurring in a large proportion of neuropathic patients. Distal symmetric sensorimotor polyneuropathy usually starts with sensory findings, affecting the distal sensation in a stocking-glove distribution, with later and less prominent motor involvement usually involving the most distal muscle groups. Autonomic neuropathy generally involves multiple organ systems, but clinical presentation and symptoms are often centered within a single organ system. Less common are a variety of focal neuropathic syndromes that either involve single nerves or groups of peripheral nerves, including the cranial nerves, or involve other focal regions of the peripheral nervous system.

The diffuse nature and chronic progressive course of distal symmetric polyneuropathy and autonomic neuropathy suggest metabolic neuropathies, whereas the rapid onset, limited distribution, and self-limited nature of the focal neuropathies suggest a vascular basis. Because the neuropathic syndromes of diabetes are indistinguishable from a variety of other forms of peripheral neuropathy, the diagnosis of diabetic neuropathy is a diagnosis of exclusion, requiring appropriate diagnostic work-up for other causes of neuropathy (Table 45-4).

FOCAL NEUROPATHIES

Focal and multifocal diabetic neuropathies with neurologic deficits confined to the distribution of single or multiple peripheral nerves are termed *diabetic mononeuropathy* and *diabetic mononeuropathy multiplex*, respectively. The appearance of neurologic deficits in the distribution of focal lesions at the level of the brachial or lumbosacral plexuses is termed *diabetic plexopathies*, whereas those conforming to deficits at the level of nerve roots are termed *diabetic radiculopathy.* When diabetic mononeuropathy or mononeu-

Sensory Impairment			
Right	Normal	Decreased	Absent
Vibration at big toe	0	1	2
10 gr filament	0	1	2
Pin prick on dorsum of great toe	Painful 0	Not Painful 2	
Left	Normal	Decreased	Absent
Vibration at big toe	0	1	2
10 gr filament	0	1	2
Pin prick on dorsum of great toe	Painful 0	Not Painful 2	

Muscle Strength Testing				
Right	Normal	Mild to Moderate	Severe	Absent
Finger spread	0	1	2	3
Great toe extension	0	1	2	3
Ankle dorsiflexion	0	1	2	3
Left	Normal	Mild to Moderate	Severe	Absent
Finger spread	0	1	2	3
Great toe extension	0	1	2	3
Ankle dorsiflexion	0	1	2	3

Reflexes			
Right	Present	Present with Reinforcement	Absent
Biceps brachii	0	1	2
Triceps brachii	0	1	2
Quadriceps femoris	0	1	2
Achilles	0	1	2
Left	Present	Present with Reinforcement	Absent
Biceps brachii	0	1	2
Triceps brachii	0	1	2
Quadriceps femoris	0	1	2
Achilles	0	1	2

Total: 146 points

FIGURE 45-2. Diabetic neuropathy score used by the Michigan Neuropathy Program for Neurologic Examination. *(Reprinted with permission from Feldman et al.[34])*

ropathy multiplex involves cranial nerves, it is then termed *diabetic cranial neuropathy.*

Cranial Neuropathies

Isolated cranial neuropathies occur in diabetic patients, especially the aged (but rarely in diabetic children).[54] Signs and symptoms of more generalized diabetic neuropathy may be absent, though the cranial palsies may be recurrent or bilateral. As noted above, the third cranial nerve is most commonly involved, characteristically with pupillary sparing (in contrast to vascular oculomotor compression palsy, where pupillary dilatation is usually an early feature).[54] Patients classically present with unilateral ophthalmoplegia that spares lateral eye movement, and headache. The accompanying pain is typically intense and referred above or behind the eye, but may be mild or absent in 50% of cases.[54] The responsible nociceptors are thought to be either perineurial or in the adjacent first and second divisions of the trigeminal nerve, since the third nerve is essentially

VISIT		Date	Date	Date	Date	Date	
Abnormal Nerves	Clinical Points	Score	Score	Score	Score	Score	CLASS
0–1	0–6 0 1 2 3 4 5 6						0 no neuropathy
	>6						
2	<7						1 mild neuropathy
	7–12 7 8 9 10 11 12						
	>12						
3–4	<13						2 moderate neuropathy
	13–29 13 14 15 16 17 18 19 20 21 22 23 24 25 26 27 28 29						
	>29						
5	<30						3 severe neuropathy
	30–45 30 31 32 33 34 35 36 37 38 39 40 41 42 43 44 45						

FIGURE 45-3. Michigan Diabetic Neuropathy score sheet. *(Reprinted with permission from Feldman et al.[34])*

purely motor.[54] Progressive diminution of pain and return of oculo-motor function is the rule, even in elderly patients.

The intracavernous portion of the third nerve represents a vascular watershed region between the intra- and extracranial circulation, where vascular supply is most tenuous. Focal fusiform central destructive lesions involving the cavernous sinus portion of the third nerve are reported in autopsied cases of isolated diabetic third-nerve palsy. Central nerve fibers were most heavily damaged and demyelinated, while superficial fibers (thought to innervate the pupil) were relatively spared.[99] Differential diagnosis would include lesions of the midbrain or posterior orbit, aneurysm of the internal carotid, cavernous sinus lesions, and tumors of the base of the brain.[54]

Other cranial nerves that are less commonly involved in diabetic neuropathy include the sixth, the fourth (usually in combination with other cranial nerves rather than alone), and the seventh cranial nerves, presumably also on a vascular basis.[54] Other than the third and sixth cranial nerves, there is little evidence to suggest that cranial nerve palsies occur more frequently in diabetic individuals.[54]

Mononeuropathy or Mononeuropathy Multiplex

Isolated peripheral nerve palsies occur more commonly in diabetics, but the causal and coincidental relationships are difficult to differentiate.[57] However, 40% of unselected patients with clinically overt diffuse diabetic neuropathy have either electrophysiologic or clinical evidence of superimposed focal nerve damage at common entrapment or compression sites (e.g., median nerve at wrist and palm, radial nerve in upper arm, ulnar nerve at elbow, lateral cutaneous nerve of the thigh, and peroneal nerve at fibular head), suggesting that diffuse diabetic neuropathy predisposes to focal nerve damage.[57] This contention is further supported by evidence that the risk of developing carpal tunnel syndrome is more than doubled in diabetic subjects.[100] Nerves not commonly exposed to compression or entrapment damage occasionally demonstrate focal impairment in patients with diabetes, but this may simply reflect coincidental occurrence of diabetes and compression neuropathy.[57,100]

Diagnosis of mononeuropathy or mononeuropathy multiplex should be confirmed by electrodiagnostic studies. Other nondiabetic causes of mononeuropathy, mononeuropathy multiplex, or both should be excluded, such as vasculitides, acromegaly, coagulopathies, and hypothyroidism.[57] Compression and entrapment palsies in diabetic patients respond to standard conservative or surgical management (i.e., protection against additional mechanical trauma or surgical release procedures).[57,100] Treatment of other mononeuropathies is the same as for nondiabetic mononeuropathy and is essentially supportive. Improved glucose control has been suggested, but there are no controlled data to suggest that it is specifically helpful.[57,100]

Thoracic Radiculopathy (Intercostal Neuropathy, Truncal Neuropathy)

Diabetic thoracic radiculopathy presents with dermatomal pain and loss of cutaneous sensation. The syndrome may involve multiple dermatomal levels and may be bilateral in some cases.[56] Hypesthesia or paresthesia usually develops during the course of the disorder. Symptoms frequently are attributed to a compressive lesion such as a herniated nucleus pulposus, but radiographic studies and myelography are negative.[56,80] When pain is prominent, truncal radiculopathy is frequently misdiagnosed as an acute intrathoracic or intra-abdominal visceral emergency (e.g., myocardial infarction, cholecystitis, peptic ulcer, or appendicitis), with multiple fruitless diagnostic and/or exploratory surgical procedures performed before the correct diagnosis is recognized.[56,101] Electrodiagnostic studies of the paraspinal muscles are usually diagnostic.[56,77] Although generally ascribed to acute infarction of the nerve root, confirmatory histopathologic evidence is lacking.[56] Signs of diffuse distal symmetric polyneuropathy are often present.[56,80] Spontaneous resolution of both symptoms and signs is the rule, usually within 6–24 months.[56]

Diabetic Polyradiculopathy

In 1953, Garland and Taverner described a syndrome of pain and proximal limb weakness in diabetics, which was later called asymmetric (motor) proximal neuropathy.[55] Among diabetic neuropathies, this syndrome, also known as diabetic amyotrophy, is second only to polyneuropathy in frequency.[55] The pathogenesis of this syndrome is controversial and has been ascribed to lesions of the anterior horn cell, lumbar roots, lumbar plexus, or femoral nerve. Bastron and Thomas[102] attempted to unify the diverse concepts surrounding diabetic amyotrophy by proposing that the syndrome represented a diabetic polyradiculopathy that preferentially involved the high lumbar roots L2, L2, and L4. A recent study by Dyck and associates suggests that ischemic injury secondary to microscopic vasculitis of lumbrosacral roots, plexuses, and nerves underlies the disease process in both diabetic[103] and nondiabetic patients.[104]

In patients with diabetes, the syndrome occurs spontaneously, with pain and sensory impairment and disabling weakness of thigh flexion and knee extension.[55] Pain classically extends from the hip to the anterior and lateral surface of the thigh. The pain may develop insidiously or episodically, and may be worse at night. Muscle weakness most often involves the iliopsoas, quadriceps, and adductor muscles, but usually spares the hip extensors and hamstrings.[55] The anterolateral muscles in the calf may also be involved, mimicking an anterior compartment syndrome. Distal symmetric polyneuropathy is almost always present.[55] Nearly complete recovery is the rule though not universal, and the syndrome may persist for several years or recur.[55]

The syndrome may be distinguished from sciatic neuropathy by a normal straight leg-raising test. Because of the similarities between diabetic polyradiculopathy and that which occurs in association with other conditions, diabetic polyradiculopathy remains a diagnosis of exclusion: space-occupying lesions, trauma, nondiabetic vasculopathies, and skeletal abnormalities must be carefully excluded.[55] Treatment for high lumbar diabetic polyradiculopathy syndrome is supportive pending spontaneous recovery, although several investigators suggest that treatment with intravenous gamma globulin may speed recovery.[105] The beneficial effect of improved diabetic control, though often commented on, remains unsupported.

POLYNEUROPATHY

Distal symmetric polyneuropathy is generally conceded to be the most widely recognized form of diabetic peripheral neuropathy.[3,4,10,12,13] The neurologic deficit is classically distributed over all sensorimotor nerves, but demonstrates a distinct predilection for the most distal innervated sites in a more or less symmetrical fashion.[46,106,107] Similar distributions are shared by other metabolic neuropathies, including uremic and various nutritional neuropathies.[80,108] Neurological impairment begins in the most distal portions of the peripheral nervous system, usually the feet or toes, and extends proximally in both the upper and lower extremities. With continued progression, a coexisting vertical anterior chest band of sensory deficit develops as the tips of the shorter truncal nerves become involved (Fig. 45-4).[106,107,109] As discussed in preceding sections, the diffuseness of peripheral nerve damage in distal symmetric polyneuropathy is evidenced by both electrophysiologic and histologic studies.[110] There is generalized motor and sensory conduction slowing and axonal degeneration and demyelination in patients with distal symmetric polyneuropathy, with slowing of nerve conduction closely paralleling histologic fiber loss.[77,88] Both the histologic and electrophysiologic changes appear earlier and are more pronounced in the most distal components of the peripheral nervous system.[11]

The signs, symptoms, neurologic deficits, and electrophysiologic characteristics of distal symmetric polyneuropathy vary depending on the classes of nerve fibers that are involved. However, the symptoms and signs always initially appear in a distal distribution and spread proximally, with disease progression in a fiber-length-dependent fashion.[8,28] Because the signs and symptoms of diabetic distal symmetric polyneuropathy are identical to those that occur in distal symmetric neuropathies of other etiologies (Table 45-4), the clinical diagnosis is one of exclusion.[20,31,32]

FIGURE 45-4. Sensory deficits in distal symmetric polyneuropathy. *(Reprinted with permission from Low PA, Tuck RR, Takeuchi M: Nerve microenvironment in diabetic neuropathy. In:* Diabetic Neuropathy. Dyck PJ, Thomas PK, Asbury AK, Winegrad AJ, Porte D Jr. Eds. *Saunders:1987; 266.)*

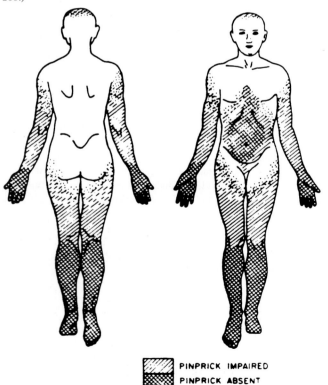

PINPRICK IMPAIRED
PINPRICK ABSENT
HYPERESTHESIA

Clinical Signs and Symptoms of Distal Symmetric Polyneuropathy

As stated earlier, the signs and symptoms of distal symmetric polyneuropathy vary considerably depending on the spectrum of nerve fiber involvement. Large sensory fiber loss produces diminished position and light touch sensation, whereas small-fiber damage produces diminished pain and temperature sensation.[8,20,31,32] Usually both large and small sensory fibers are involved in the neuropathic process to a similar degree, producing a mixed sensorimotor peripheral polyneuropathy. Motor weakness is usually not marked, primarily involving the most distal intrinsic muscles of the hands and feet as a rather late feature. However, diminished deep-tendon reflexes, especially the Achilles tendon reflex, are often an early feature.[11,68,107,109]

Some patients, with more selective fiber damage, present as variations of this general theme. If large-fiber sensory loss predominates, patients present with impaired balance, diminished proprioception and position sense, and absent or reduced vibration sensation. Subjective symptoms of pain, paresthesia, or numbness are usually absent, and the neuropathy may present only via a late neuropathic complication such as a Charcot's joint or a neuropathic ulceration (see below).[106–108,111] With severe large-fiber involvement, loss of position sense may result in a sensory ataxia, which is referred to as a "pseudotabetic" form of diabetic neuropathy. In this variant, nerve conduction slowing is usually clearly demonstrable due to the involvement of the large, rapidly conducting fiber population.[106–108,111] If the neuropathy primarily involves small sensory fibers, then the patient may present with undetected trauma of the extremities (e.g., burns of the fingers from cigarettes, burns of the feet from stepping into hot bath water, or acute abrasions and ulcerations of the feet from small objects retained inside the shoe that go undetected for prolonged periods due to insensitivity to pain). Alternatively, patients with small sensory fiber involvement may present with subjective symptoms of numbness or feelings of "cold feet" or "dead feet."[11,68,107,109]

Several kinds of spontaneous pain may be associated with small-fiber damage in diabetic neuropathy.[68] Most commonly, patients experience typical neuropathic distal paresthesias (spontaneously occurring uncomfortable sensations) or dysesthesias (contact paresthesias).[112] Some patients complain of exquisite cutaneous contact hypersensitivity to light touch. At times the pain is described as superficial and burning, shooting or stabbing, or bone-deep and aching or tearing.[113] Often the pains are more pronounced at night, producing insomnia.[114] At times, pain can become an overriding and disabling feature of diabetic neuropathy. Muscle cramps, which begin distally and slowly ascend, are similar to those reported in other muscle denervation disorders. Because disease involvement in these patients may be primarily confined to the small myelinated nerve fibers, conduction velocity may not be dramatically impaired, vibration sensation may be intact, motor weakness may be absent, and, if the patient's symptoms bring him or her to the physician's attention early in the course of the disease, sensory loss may not be striking.[115] The presence of painful symptoms in the absence of striking neurologic deficit appears somewhat paradoxical; however, painfulness may reflect increased fiber regeneration, which may commence before degeneration is sufficiently severe to present marked sensory deficit.[112,115]

Most patients with diabetic neuropathy experience either no or only slight subjective symptoms and present to the physician with asymptomatic neurologic deficits detected on physical examination, or with complications resulting from the asymptomatic sensory deficits.[11,116] Pure or primarily motor neuropathy is very rare in diabetes, and its presence suggests an alternate etiology such as Guillain-Barré syndrome.[108] A primary motor neuropathy has been associated with insulin-induced hypoglycemia in psychiatric patients and in insulinoma; animal experiments support the concept of a hypoglycemic peripheral neuropathy.[117] Hence recurrent iatrogenic hypoglycemia should be considered in any diabetic presenting with a primarily motor distal neuropathy.[117]

Complications of Distal Symmetric Polyneuropathy

The mechanical and traumatic consequences of distal symmetric polyneuropathy are largely preventable, and as such represent a failure of medical management when they occur.[21] Moreover, they constitute a significant risk to the neuropathic patient.[118] Their prophylaxis is a major target of standard diabetes patient education, especially that dealing with foot care and hygiene.[72,119]

Neuropathic Foot Ulceration

Traumatic damage to the skin and soft tissues of the foot occurs with great frequency in most sensory neuropathies, including diabetic distal symmetric polyneuropathy.[22] Central to all forms of diabetic foot ulceration is insensitivity to pain, although diminished proprioception and muscle strength as well as vascular factors may play contributing roles.[22] In the classic plantar ulcer, neurogenic atrophy of the intrinsic foot muscles, which normally tonically counterbalance the more proximal foot flexors and extensors, results in chronic flexion of the metatarsal-phalangeal joints,

thereby drawing the toes into a curled-up position (claw toe deformity). Weight bearing is then shifted to the now uncovered metatarsal heads, leading to thinning and atrophy of the normal fat pad. In the absence of pain, thick calluses form over the exposed metatarsal bony prominences and protrude from the plantar surface of the foot, further shifting weight bearing to the metatarsal heads (Fig. 45-5).[120,121] The calluses first thicken and then undergo liquefaction. The dry overlying skin breaks down, possibly reflecting in part the diminished lubrication secondary to decreased sudomotor activity of the generally accompanying autonomic neuropathy.[120–122] The resulting central ulcerations may remain unnoticed in the absence of pain sensation, even when secondary infection develops.[22,123] Plantar ulcers, which develop when abnormal foot architecture transfers body weight onto normally non-weight-bearing areas of the foot, are usually located at callused sites of maximal walking pressure. With further architectural deformity due to neuroarthropathy or amputation, plantar ulcers may develop at alternative weight-bearing sites.[124–126]

Neuropathic foot ulcers also develop at other locations through other mechanisms in the absence of callus formation. The deformed neuropathic foot does not conform well to the shape of the standard shoe, leading to pressure lesions and/or abrasions at locations other than weight-bearing sites.[22,121] The generally thin dorsal dermis of the foot may be abraded within hours, so that repeated self-examinations are mandatory when new footwear is worn or with prolonged walking or weight bearing in the absence of pain sensation.[21,22]

Ischemia has been invoked as a factor in diabetic foot ulceration, but its role is controversial. Toe blood pressures have been found to be reduced in patients with neuropathic foot ulceration,

FIGURE 45-5. The pathogenesis of diabetic foot ulcers. *(Reprinted with permission from Kwasnik E:* Surg Clin North Am *1986;66:305.)*

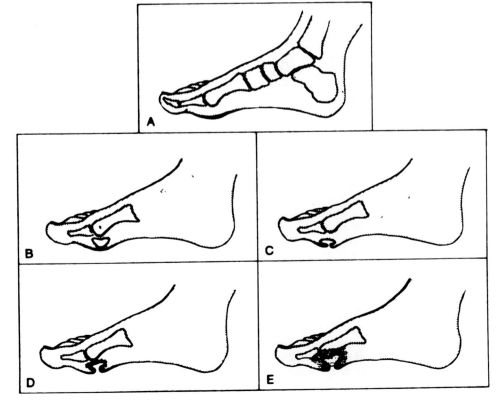

even when the ankle:brachial pressure is normal.[127,128] However, the role of vessel disease of the toes in foot ulceration remains unclear. Frank ischemic gangrene may be hastened in neuropathic feet since ischemic rest pain may go unnoticed.[127,128] Proximal atherosclerotic vascular insufficiency undoubtedly delays healing of neuropathic foot ulcers.[128] However, the neuropathic ulcerated foot is characteristically warm, with easily palpable pulses, mitigating against an important large-vessel ischemic component.[127–129] Doppler flow studies confirm that blood flow to the neuropathic foot is generally increased, and suggest that this increased flow results from abnormal local arteriovenous shunting.[127,128] The role of increased arteriovenous shunting in the pathogenesis of both complications of the diabetic foot, and recently in the development of peripheral neuropathy itself, remains speculative. Increased AV shunting in the foot with diabetic neuropathy is thought to reflect loss of the tonic sympathetic vascular innervation, and there has been debate whether this shunting may precipitate a skin-nutritive capillary steal phenomenon that leads to poor ulcer healing.[127,128] There is little evidence to support such a steal phenomenon, because capillaries are normal in number and patent in diabetic subjects with advanced neuropathy.[127,128] Likewise, an increase in the number of arteriovenous shunts has been directly observed in human sural nerve, but their functional significance in the development of endoneurial ischemia is unclear.[127–129]

Prophylactic treatment of diabetic foot ulcers is accomplished through reinforcement of foot care education in patients with distal symmetric polyneuropathy, identification of abnormal weight bearing and/or callus formation before ulceration occurs, and prescription of appropriate behavioral and mechanical measures to reduce weight bearing.[21,118,130] This would include weight reduction, decreased weight-bearing activity, the use of a cane or cushioned shoes, and specific orthotic devices and inserts to distribute necessary weight bearing in a less threatening fashion.[21,118,130] Once ulcers have occurred, the treatment of diabetic foot ulcers is removal of the traumatic elements that contributed to the ulcer formation.[131] Readjustment of weight bearing with appropriate orthopedic devices is essential. In some cases, partial or complete elimination of weight bearing is required through decreased ambulation, support with a cane or crutches, use of a wheelchair, or enforced bed rest.[130–132] When callus protrusions further disturb weight bearing, then appropriate debridement, trimming, and abrasion are indicated.[131] The application of a walking cast that transfers weight bearing to the upper leg is sometimes helpful; however, the cast must be removed and the leg examined for abrasions or ulcerations at the site to which weight bearing has been shifted.[132] Complicating infection should be treated with antibiotics, including a drug directed against anaerobic bacteria that may be difficult to culture from an open wound.[123] In refractory cases, removal of the offending metatarsal head, sometimes together with amputation of the toe, may be necessary (see Chap. 51).[133]

Neuroarthropathy (Charcot's Joint)

Neuroarthropathy can occur in any nervous system disease that leaves motor function relatively intact but impairs sensation. The primacy of nociceptive impairment in the pathogenesis of neuroarthropathy is supported by its reported occurrence in the "congenital indifference to pain syndrome," where motor and proprioceptive function remain intact. The nociceptive impairment also explains the almost complete absence of pain in many cases of diabetic neuroarthropathy.[134,135] Tabetic neuroarthropathy classically involves the large weight-bearing joints, while diabetic neuroarthropathy primarily involves distal joints of the foot (tarsal-metatarsal or metatarsal-phalangeal) or the ankle.[134] The presentation of recent-onset diabetic neuroarthropathy is usually one of painless swelling and redness of the foot in the absence of fever or leukocytosis, but in the presence of clearly demonstrable distal symmetric sensory deficit and evidence of peripheral autonomic nerve failure.[48] The differential diagnosis is usually cellulitis or osteomyelitis, depending on the extent of radiographic bony destruction.[135]

Unhealed painless fractures are often evident radiographically, and a recent history of painless trauma is frequently but not always elicited. In later stages, the disorder presents as gross architectural distortion of the foot, with shortening and widening of the joint. In its most advanced stage, there are multiple painless fractures accompanied by extensive bone demineralization and reabsorption, so that the foot appears to the examiner as "a bag of bones."[48,134] As with other forms of neuroarthropathy, the pathogenetic mechanism is presumed to be multiple recurrent traumatic insults to the joint and surrounding bony structures that are not noticed by the patient because of insensitivity to pain.[127] Increased bone blood flow due to arteriovenous shunting may also serve to weaken the bone, predisposing the foot to fractures.[127] Prophylactic measures include reinforced education in patients with diminished pain and proprioceptive sensation, especially the avoidance of prolonged weight bearing, the wearing of cushioned shoes, avoidance of strenuous weight-bearing exercise or athletic activities, and ambulating only over well-lighted smooth terrain in well-fitting footwear.[21,130] Therapy is directed at removal of continued trauma by removing the involved extremity from weight bearing, either by decreasing ambulation or by providing other means of weight bearing, for example, a cane, crutches, or a wheelchair.[48,131,132]

Treatment of Neuropathy

Initial treatment strategies in diabetic neuropathy consist of optimal glucose control and foot care. Before the DCCT, the scientific rationale for these therapeutic strategies was based on studies in animal models of diabetes and epidemiologic reports. The DCCT provided direct evidence that optimal glucose control in insulin-dependent diabetic patients can decrease neuropathy frequency, with a reported 60% reduction in the incidence of clinical neuropathy in the combined primary- and secondary-prevention cohorts.[136] Similar results are reported in the Stockholm Diabetes Intervention Study, where intensive insulin treatment of diabetic patients preserved nerve conduction velocities when compared to conventional treatment.[58,59] Optimal glucose control must occur in the setting of rigorous foot care. On a nightly basis, patients are required to carefully inspect their feet for the presence of dry or cracking skin, fissures, plantar callus formation, and signs of early infection in between the toes and the toenails.

A stepwise, systematic treatment plan constitutes the best approach to a patient with painful diabetic neuropathy[131] and has recently been reviewed in detail.[137] Categorization of painful symptoms by duration and potential precipitating causes provides helpful prognostic indicators. Patients with symptoms of less than 6 months' duration associated with alterations in glycemic control have a good prognosis when compared to patients with chronic symptoms lasting longer than 6 months.[26,131] Table 45-5 lists currently available drugs reported to have therapeutic benefits in the treatment of diabetic neuropathy. Nonsteroidal anti-inflammatory drugs can offer pain relief, especially in patients with musculoskeletal or joint abnormalities secondary to long-standing neu-

TABLE 45-5. Drugs Used in the Treatment of Painful Diabetic Neuropathy

1. Nonsteroidal Drugs
   Ibuprofen 600 mg four times a day
   Sulindac 200 mg twice a day
2. Antidepressant Drugs
   Amitriptyline 50–150 mg at night
   Nortriptyline 50–150 mg at night
   Imipramine 100 mg daily
   Paroxetine 40 mg daily
   Trazadone 50–150 mg three times a day
3. Antiepileptic Drugs
   Gabapentin 600–1200 mg three times a day
   Carbamazepine 200 mg four times a day
4. Others
   Tramadol 50–100 mg twice a day
   Mexiletine 150–450 mg daily
   Capsacin 0.075% four times a day
   Transcutaneous electrical nerve stimulation (TENS)

ropathy. In this group of patients, joint deformities may actually be the primary source of pain. A double-blind placebo-controlled fixed-dose study revealed that both ibuprofen (600 mg four times daily) and sulindac (200 mg twice daily) brought substantial pain relief in patients with diabetic neuropathy.[138]

The tricyclic antidepressants are the most commonly used drugs in the treatment of painful neuropathy. They act by blocking the re-uptake of norepinephrine and serotonin, potentiating the inhibitory effect of these neurotransmitters on nociceptive pathways.[139] Double-blind, placebo-controlled trials have reported that both amitriptyline[140,141] and imipramine[142,143] relieve neuropathic pain. After 6 weeks of amitriptyline treatment, patients report significant pain relief, independent of mood but correlating with increasing drug dosage.[144] The side effects of amitriptyline, secondary to its strong anticholinergic properties, include sedation, urinary retention, orthostatic hypotension, and cardiac arrhythmias. If side effects become intolerable, nortriptyline, which is less sedating, can be substituted for amitriptyline.[145] Urinary retention may occur with either amitriptyline or nortriptyline, mandating a change to imipramine therapy. Two double-blind crossover studies have independently reported that imipramine improves neuropathic pain and nocturnal exacerbation of symptoms.[142,143] Additional support for the use of tricyclics for the treatment of neuropathic pain is provided by a recent meta-analysis of 21 trials.[146] In patients with a significant cardiac history, amitriptyline or nortriptyline is contraindicated and therapeutic regimens include either doxepin, the least cardiotoxic tricyclic antidepressant, or desipramine. The topical cream capsaicin can be added to the patient's therapeutic regimen if neuropathic pain persists in spite of treatment with maximally tolerated doses of antidepressant medication.[145] In an outpatient setting, approximately two-thirds of diabetic patients treated with a combination of antidepressant medication and capsaicin cream experience substantial relief of neuropathic pain.

Serotonin reuptake inhibitors may also alleviate neuropathic pain, but the evidence for this is less convincing than that for tricyclic antidepressants. In a randomized, double-blind, crossover study, paroxetine 40 mg per day reduced neuropathic symptoms compared to placebo.[147] Fluoxetine (40 mg per day) was no more effective than placebo except in diabetic patients with depression superimposed on neuropathy in a double-blind, placebo-controlled

study.[148] Open-label sertraline and trazodone are often used empirically, suggesting the possibility that these drugs may have some efficacy in treating painful diabetic neuropathy, but there are no controlled studies.[149,150]

The anticonvulsant gabapentin has recently emerged as the therapy of choice for many clinicians.[151] Gabapentin is more effective than placebo when used in doses ranging from 900–3600 mg per day,[152] although the lower end of this dosage range (900 mg) may be relatively ineffective.[153] Side effects of gabapentin therapy include dizziness, somnolence, headache, diarrhea, confusion, and nausea. A randomized double-blind study comparing the efficacy of gabapentin with amitriptyline found that both drugs provided equal pain relief with no difference between mean pain score and global pain score.[154]

In patients who experience continued pain on combination therapy (i.e., a tricyclic or gabapentin with capsaicin), carbamazepine can be considered and added as a third drug.[155,156] Dizziness, nausea, and a truncal skin rash are the common side effects of this drug, although reports of leukopenia mandate that a patient have a complete blood count with differential weekly for the first month, and monthly for the next 3 months upon beginning carbamazepine therapy.[157] Phenytoin has been used as an alternative to carbamazepine,[158] although a double-blind, crossover study reported that phenytoin provides no significant relief of neuropathic pain in patients with diabetic neuropathy.[159] In patients who experience continued pain on antidepressant medication or gabapentin, capsaicin cream, and carbamazepine, the carbamazepine can be discontinued and a different third drug added to the therapeutic regimen. Choices include oral mexiletine or intravenous lidocaine, both of which are reported to improve neuropathic pain,[160,161] but use of these agents requires clearance from a cardiologist and, in the case of lidocaine, an inpatient hospitalization with cardiac monitoring. Levodopa, gamma-linolenic acid, and dextromethorphan also have reported efficacy.[137] If neuropathic pain persists despite the outlined treatment regimen, addition of a transcutaneous electrical nerve stimulation (TENS) unit, acupuncture, or a series of local nerve blocks may be helpful, although the prognosis for pain relief in these patients is poor.

Acknowledgements. The authors would like to thank Ms. Judith Boldt for excellent secretarial assistance. This work was supported by NIH grants RO1 NS36778 and RO1 NS38849, the Juvenile Diabetes Research Foundation Center for the Study of Complications in Diabetes, and the Program for Understanding Neurological Diseases (PFUND).

REFERENCES

1. Rollo J: *Cases of Diabetes Mellitus.* C. Dilly:1798.
2. Currie CJ, Morgan CL, Peters JR: The epidemiology and cost of inpatient care for peripheral vascular disease, infection, neuropathy, and ulceration in diabetes. *Diabetes Care* 1998;21:42.
3. Morgan CL, Currie CJ, Stott NC, *et al*: The prevalence of multiple diabetes-related complications. *Diabet Med* 2000;17:146.
4. Martyn CN, Hughes RA: Epidemiology of peripheral neuropathy. *J Neurol Neurosurg Psychiatry* 1997;62:310.
5. Thomas PK: Diabetic peripheral neuropathies: Their cost to patient and society and the value of knowledge of risk factors for development of interventions. *Eur Neurol* 1999;41(suppl 1):35.
6. DCCT Research Group. The effect of intensive diabetes therapy on the development and progression of neuropathy. Ann Intern Med, 1995;122:561.

7. Nathan DM: The pathophysiology of diabetic complications: How much does the glucose hypothesis explain? *Ann Intern Med* 1996; 124:86.

8. Zochodne DW: Diabetic neuropathies: Features and mechanisms. *Brain Pathol* 1999;9:369.

9. Fedele D, Comi G, Coscelli C, *et al*: A multicenter study on the prevalence of diabetic neuropathy in Italy. *Diabetes Care* 1997;20:836.

10. Partanen J, Niskanen L, Lehtinen J, *et al*: Natural history of peripheral neuropathy in patients with non-insulin-dependent diabetes mellitus. *N Engl J Med* 1995;333:89.

11. Dyck PJ, Kratz KM, Karnes JL, *et al*: The prevalence by staged severity of various types of diabetic neuropathy, retinopathy, and nephropathy in a population-based cohort: The Rochester Diabetic Neuropathy Study. *Neurology* 1993;43:817.

12. Young MJ, Boulton AJM, Macleod AF, *et al*: A multicentre study of the prevalence of diabetic peripheral neuropathy in the United Kingdom hospital clinic population. *Diabetologia* 1993;36:150.

13. Tesfaye S, Stevens LK, Stephenson JM, *et al*: Prevalence of diabetic peripheral neuropathy and its relation to glycaemic control and potential risk factors: The EURODIAB IDDM Complications Study. *Diabetologia* 1996;39:1377.

14. Molyneaux LM, Constantino MI, McGill M, *et al*: Better glycaemic control and risk reduction of diabetic complications in Type 2 diabetes: Comparison with the DCCT. *Diabetes Res Clin Pract* 1998; 42:77.

15. Payne DM, Rossomando AJ, Martino P, *et al*: Identification of the regulatory phosphorylation sites in pp42/mitogen-activated protein kinase (MAP kinase). *EMBO J* 1991;10:885.

16. Klein R, Klein BE, Moss SE: Relation of glycemic control to diabetic microvascular complications in diabetes mellitus. *Ann Intern Med* 1996;124:90.

17. Stevens MJ, Feldman EL, Thomas T, *et al*: Pathogenesis of diabetic neuropathy. In: Veves A, ed. *Clinical Management of Diabetic Neuropathy*. Humana Press:1998;13.

18. Greene DA, Obrosova I, Stevens MJ, *et al*: Pathways of glucose-mediated oxidative stress in diabetic neuropathy. In: Packer L, Rosen P, Tritschler HJ, *et al*, eds. *Antioxidants in Diabetes Management*. Marcel Dekker:2000;111.

19. Feldman EL, Russell JW, Sullivan KA, *et al*: New insights into the pathogenesis of diabetic neuropathy. *Curr Opin Neurol* 1999;12:553.

20. Windebank AJ, Feldman EL: Diabetes and the nervous system. In: Aminoff MJ, ed. *Neurology and General Medicine*, 3rd ed. Churchill Livingstone:2001;341.

21. Mayfield JA, Reiber GE, Sanders LJ, *et al*: Preventive foot care in people with diabetes. *Diabetes Care* 1998;21:2161.

22. Levin ME: Foot lesions in patients with diabetes mellitus. *Endocrinol Metab Clin North Am* 1996;25:447.

23. Benotmane A, Mohammedi F, Ayad F, *et al*: Diabetic foot lesions: Etiologic and prognostic factors. *Diabetes Metab* 2000;26:113.

24. Litzelman DK, Marriott DJ, Vinicor F: Independent physiological predictors of foot lesions in patients with NIDDM. *Diabetes Care* 1997;20:1273.

25. Dyck PJ, Davies JL, Wilson DM, *et al*: Risk factors for severity of diabetic polyneuropathy: Intensive longitudinal assessment of the Rochester Diabetic Neuropathy Study cohort. *Diabetes Care* 1999;22: 1479.

26. Greene DA, Stevens MJ, Feldman EL: Glycemic control. In: Dyck PJ, Thomas PK, eds. *Diabetic Neuropathy*, 2nd ed. WB Saunders:1998; 297.

27. Greene DA, Stevens MJ, Feldman EL: Diabetic neuropathy: Scope of the syndrome. *Am J Med* 1999;107:2S.

28. Vinik AI, Park TS, Stansberry KB, *et al*: Diabetic neuropathies. *Diabetologia* 2000;43:957.

29. Dyck PJ, O'Brien PC: Quantitative sensation testing in epidemiological and therapeutic studies of peripheral neuropathy. *Muscle Nerve* 1999;22:659.

30. Dyck PJ, Davies JL, Litchy WJ, *et al*: Longitudinal assessment of diabetic polyneuropathy using a composite score in the Rochester diabetic neuropathy study cohort. *Neurology* 1997;49:229.

31. Feldman EL, Stevens MJ, Russell JW, *et al*: Diabetic neuropathy. In: Taylor S, ed. *Current Review of Diabetes*. Current Medicine:1999;71.

32. Feldman EL, Stevens MJ, Greene DA: Diabetic neuropathy. In: Turtle JR, Kaneko T, Osato S, eds. *Diabetes in the New Millennium*. The Endocrinology and Diabetes Research Foundation of the University of Sydney:1999;387.

33. Pirart J: Diabetes mellitus and its degenerative complications; A prospective study of 4,400 patients observed between 1947 and 1973. *Diabetes Care* 1978;1:168.

34. Feldman EL, Stevens MJ, Thomas PK, *et al*: A practical two-step quantitative clinical and electrophysiological assessment for the diagnosis and staging of diabetic neuropathy. *Diabetes Care* 1994;17: 1281.

35. Cabezas-Cerrato J: The prevalence of clinical diabetic polyneuropathy in Spain: A study in primary care and hospital clinic groups. Neuropathy Spanish Study Group of the Spanish Diabetes Society (SDS). *Diabetologia* 1998;41:1263.

36. The Diabetes Control and Complications Trial (DCCT) Research Group: Factors in the development of diabetic neuropathy: Baseline analysis of neuropathy in the feasibility phase of the Diabetes Control and Complications Trial (DCCT). *Diabetes* 1988;37:476.

37. Maser RE, Steenkiste AR, Dorman JS, *et al*: Epidemiological correlates of diabetic neuropathy. Report from Pittsburgh Epidemiology of Diabetes Complications Study. *Diabetes* 1989;38:1456.

38. Meh D, Denislic M: Subclinical neuropathy in type I diabetic children. *Electroencephalogr Clin Neurophysiol* 1998;109:274.

39. Sands ML, Shetterly SM, Franklin GM, *et al*: Incidence of distal symmetric (sensory) neuropathy in NIDDM. The San Luis Valley Diabetes Study. *Diabetes Care* 1997;20:322.

40. de Wytt CN, Jackson RV, Hockings GI, *et al*: Polyneuropathy in Australian outpatients with type II diabetes mellitus. *J Diabetes Complications* 1999;13:74.

41. Frykberg RG: Epidemiology of the diabetic foot: Ulcerations and amputations. *Adv Wound Care* 1999;12:139.

42. Resnick HE, Valsania P, Phillips CL: Diabetes mellitus and nontraumatic lower extremity amputation in black and white Americans: The National Health and Nutrition Examination Survey Epidemiologic Follow-up Study, 1971–1992. *Arch Intern Med* 1999;159:2470.

43. Bloomgarden ZT: American Diabetes Association annual meeting, 1999: Nephropathy and neuropathy. *Diabetes Care* 2000;23:549.

44. Greene DA, Feldman EL, Stevens MJ, *et al*: Diabetic neuropathy. In: Porte D Jr, Sherwin R, eds. *Diabetes Mellitus*, 5th ed. Appleton & Lange:1997;1009.

45. Boulton AJ, Malik RA: Diabetic neuropathy. *Med Clin North Am* 1998;82:909.

46. Dyck PJB, Dyck PJ: Diabetic polyneuropathy. In: Dyck PJ, Thomas PK, eds. *Diabetic Neuropathy*, 2nd ed. WB Saunders:1999;255.

47. Russell J, Karnes J, Dyck P: Sural nerve myelinated fiber density differences associated with meaningful changes in clinical and electrophysiological measurements. *J Neurol Sci* 1996;135:114.

48. Fabrin J, Larsen K, Holstein PE: Long-term follow-up in diabetic Charcot feet with spontaneous onset. *Diabetes Care* 2000;23:796.

49. Freeman R: Diabetic autonomic neuropathy: An overview. In: Veves A, ed. *Clinical Management of Diabetic Neuropathy*. Humana Press: 1998;181.

50. Deliargyris EN, Nesto RW: Autonomic neuropathy and heart disease. In: Veves A, ed. *Clinical Management of Diabetic Neuropathy*. Humana Press:1998;209.

51. Malagelada J-R: Gastrointestinal disorders. In Veves A, ed. *Clinical Management of Diabetic Neuropathy*. Humana Press:1998;243.

52. Meier TJ, Ho DY, Sapolsky RM: Increased expression of calbindin D28k via herpes simplex virus amplicon vector decreases calcium ion mobilization and enhances neuronal survival after hypoglycemic challenge. *J Neurochem* 1997;69:1039.

53. Webster L: Diabetic impotence: Pathogenesis and treatment. In: Veves A, ed. *Clinical Management of Diabetic Neuropathy*. Humana Press: 1998;227.

54. Smith BE: Cranial neuropathy in diabetes mellitus. In: Dyck PJ, Thomas PK, eds. *Diabetic Neuropathy*, 2nd ed. WB Saunders:1999; 457.

55. Said G, Thomas PK: Proximal diabetic neuropathy. In: Dyck PJ, Thomas PK, eds. *Diabetic Neuropathy*, 2nd ed. WB Saunders:1999; 474.

56. Watkins PJ, Thomas PK: Diabetic truncal radiculoneuropathy. In: Dyck PJ, Thomas PK, eds. *Diabetic Neuropathy*, 2nd ed. WB Saunders:1999;468.

57. Wilbourn AJ: Diabetic entrapment and compression neuropathies. In: Dyck PJ, Thomas PK, eds. *Diabetic Neuropathy*, 2nd ed. WB Saunders:1999;481.

58. Reichard P, Berglund B, Britz A, *et al*: Intensified conventional insulin treatment retards the microvascular complications of insulin-dependent

diabetes mellitus (IDDM): The Stockholm Diabetes Intervention Study (SDIS) after 5 years. *J Intern Med* 1991;230:101.

59. Reichard P, Pihl M, Rosenqvist U, *et al*: Complications in IDDM are caused by elevated blood glucose level: The Stockholm Diabetes Intervention Study (SDIS) at 10-year follow up. *Diabetologia* 1996;39: 1483.

60. The Diabetes Control and Complications Trial (DCCT) Research Group: The effect of intensive treatment of diabetes on the development and progression of long-term complications in insulin-dependent diabetes mellitus. *N Engl J Med* 1993;329:977.

61. Azad N, Emanuele NV, Abraira C, *et al*: The effects of intensive glycemic control on neuropathy in the VA cooperative study on type II diabetes mellitus (VA CSDM). *J Diabetes Complications* 1999;13:307.

62. Gaster B, Hirsch IB: The effects of improved glycemic control on complications in type 2 diabetes. *Arch Intern Med* 1998;158:134.

63. Cohen JA, Jeffers BW, Faldut D, *et al*: Risks for sensorimotor peripheral neuropathy and autonomic neuropathy in non-insulin-dependent diabetes mellitus (NIDDM). *Muscle Nerve* 1998;21:72.

64. Adler AI, Boyko EJ, Ahroni JH, *et al*: Risk factors for diabetic peripheral sensory neuropathy. Results of the Seattle Prospective Diabetic Foot Study. *Diabetes Care* 1997;20:1162.

65. Grant IA, O'Brien P, Dyck PJ: Neuropathy tests and normative results. In: Dyck PJ, Thomas PK, eds. *Diabetic Neuropathy*, 2nd ed. WB Saunders:1999;123.

66. Suarez GA, Dyck PJ: Quantitative sensory assessment. In: Dyck PJ, Thomas PK, eds. *Diabetic Neuropathy*, 2nd ed. WB Saunders:1999; 151.

67. Valk GD, Grootenhuis PA, van Eijk JT, *et al*: Methods for assessing diabetic polyneuropathy: Validity and reproducibility of the measurement of sensory symptom severity and nerve function tests. *Diabetes Res Clin Pract* 2000;47:87.

68. Dyck PJ, Larson TS, O'Brien PC, *et al*: Patterns of quantitative sensation testing of hypoesthesia and hyperalgesia are predictive of diabetic polyneuropathy: A study of three cohorts. Nerve growth factor study group. *Diabetes Care* 2000;23:510.

69. Arezzo JC: New developments in the diagnosis of diabetic neuropathy. *Am J Med* 1999;107:9S.

70. Coppini DV, Young PJ, Weng C, *et al*: Outcome on diabetic foot complications in relation to clinical examination and quantitative sensory testing: A case-control study. *Diabet Med* 1998;15:765.

71. Young MJ, Breddy JL, Veves A, *et al*: The prediction of diabetic neuropathic foot ulceration using vibration perception thresholds. A prospective study. *Diabetes Care* 1994;17:557.

72. Pham H, Armstrong DG, Harvey C, *et al*: Screening techniques to identify people at high risk for diabetic foot ulceration: A prospective multicenter trial. *Diabetes Care* 2000;23:606.

73. Abbott CA, Vileikyte L, Williamson S, *et al*: Multicenter study of the incidence of and predictive risk factors for diabetic neuropathic foot ulceration. *Diabetes Care* 1998;21:1071.

74. Dyck PJ, Zimmerman IR, Johnson DM, *et al*: A standard test of heat-pain responses using CASE IV. *J Neurol Sci* 1996;136:54.

75. Lupia E, Elliot SJ, Lenz O, *et al*: IGF-1 decreases collagen degradation in diabetic NOD mesangial cells. *Diabetes* 1999;48:1638.

76. Singleton JR, Russell JW, Feldman EL: Electrodiagnosis of neuromuscular disease. In: Corey-Bloom J, ed. *Adult Neurology*. Mosby-Year Book:1997;37.

77. Daube JR: Electrophysiological testing in diabetic neuropathy. In: Dyck PJ, Thomas PK, eds. *Diabetic Neuropathy*, 2nd ed. WB Saunders:1999;222.

78. Cornblath DR, Chaudhry V: Electrodiagnostic evaluation of the peripheral neuropathy patient. In: Mendell JR, Kissel JT, Cornblath DR, eds. *Diagnosis and Management of Peripheral Nerve Disorders*. Oxford University Press:2001;30.

79. Troni W, Carta Q, Cantello R, *et al*: Peripheral nerve function and metabolic control in diabetes mellitus. *Ann Neurol* 1984;16:178.

80. Mendell JR: Diabetic neuropathies. In: Mendell JR, Kissel JT, Cornblath DR, eds. *Diagnosis and Management of Peripheral Nerve Disorders*. Oxford University Press:2001;373.

81. Dyck PJ, Lais A, Karnes JL, *et al*: Fiber loss is primary and multifocal in sural nerves in diabetic polyneuropathy. *Ann Neurol* 1986;19:425.

82. Dyck PJ, Giannini C: Pathologic alterations in the diabetic neuropathies of humans: A review. *J Neuropathol Exp Neurol* 1996;55:1181.

83. Giannini C, Dyck PJ: Pathologic alterations in human diabetic polyneuropathy. In: Dyck PJ, Thomas PK, eds. *Diabetic Neuropathy*, 2nd ed. WB Saunders:1999;279.

84. Downie AW, Newell DJ: Sensory nerve conduction in patients with diabetes mellitus and controls. *Neurology* 1961;11:876.

85. Lamontagne A, Buchthal F: Electrophysiological studies in diabetic neuropathy. *J Neurol Neurosurg Psychiatry* 1970;33:442.

86. Wilbourn AJ: Diabetic neuropathies. In: Brown WF, Bolton CF, eds. *Clinical Electromyography*, 2nd ed. Butterworth-Heinemann:1993; 477.

87. Pfeifer MA, Schumer MP: Clinical trials of diabetic neuropathy: Past, present, and future. *Diabetes* 1995;44:1355.

88. Dyck PJ, Karnes JL, Daube J: Clinical and neuropathological criteria for the diagnosis and staging of diabetic polyneuropathy. *Brain* 1985; 108:861.

89. American Diabetes Association: Report and recommendations of the San Antonio Conference on Diabetic Neuropathy. *Neurology* 1988; 37:1000.

90. Harris MI: Newly revised classification and diagnostic criteria for diabetes mellitus. In: Taylor S, ed. *Current Review of Diabetes*. Current Medicine:2000;1.

91. Bax G, Fagherazzi C, Piarulli F, *et al*: Reproducibility of Michigan Neuropathy Screening Instrument (MNSI). A comparison with tests using the vibratory and thermal perception thresholds. *Diabetes Care* 1996;19:904.

92. Sosenko JM, Sparling YH, Hu D, *et al*: Use of the Semmes-Weinstein monofilament in the strong heart study. Risk factors for clinical neuropathy. *Diabetes Care* 1999;22:1715.

93. Valk GD, de Sonnaville JJ, van Houtum WH, *et al*: The assessment of diabetic polyneuropathy in daily clinical practice: Reproducibility and validity of Semmes Weinstein monofilaments examination and clinical neurological examination. *Muscle Nerve* 1997;20:116.

94. Kumar S, Fernando DJ, Veves A, *et al*: Semmes-Weinstein monofilaments: A simple, effective and inexpensive screening device for identifying diabetic patients at risk of foot ulceration. *Diabetes Res Clin Pract* 1991;13:63.

95. Mueller MJ: Identifying patients with diabetes mellitus who are at risk for lower-extremity complications: Use of Semmes-Weinstein monofilaments. *Phys Ther* 1996;76:68.

96. McGill M, Molyneaux L, Yue DK: Use of the Semmes-Weinstein 5.07/10 gram monofilament: The long and the short of it. *Diabet Med* 1998;15:615.

97. Duffy JC, Patout CA: Management of the insensitive foot in diabetes: Lessons learned from Hansen's Disease. *Mil Med* 1990;155: 575.

98. McGill M, Molyneaux L, Spencer R, *et al*: Possible sources of discrepancies in the use of the Semmes-Weinstein monofilament. Impact on prevalence of insensate foot and workload requirements. *Diabetes Care* 1999;22:598.

99. Asbury AK, Aldredge H, Hershberg R, *et al*: Oculomotor palsy in diabetes mellitus: A clinico-pathological study. *Brain* 1970;93:555.

100. Freimer M, Brushart TM, Cornblath DR, *et al*: Entrapment neuropathies. In: Mendell JR, Kissel JT, Cornblath DR, eds. *Diagnosis and Management of Peripheral Nerve Disorders*. Oxford University Press:2001;592.

101. Longstreth GF: Diabetic thoracic polyradiculopathy: Ten patients with abdominal pain. *Am J Gastroenterol* 1997;92:502.

102. Bastron JA, Thomas JE: Diabetic polyradiculopathy. *Mayo Clin Proc* 1981;56:725.

103. Dyck PJ, Norell JE: Microvasculitis and ischemia in diabetic lumbosacral radiculoplexus neuropathy. *Neurology* 1999;53:2113.

104. Dyck PJ, Engelstad J, Norell J: Microvasculitis in non-diabetic lumbosacral radiculoplexus neuropathy (LSRPN): Similarity to the diabetic variety (DLSRPN). *J Neuropathol Exp Neurol* 2000;59:525.

105. Jaradeh SS, Prieto TE, Lobeck LJ: Progressive polyradiculoneuropathy in diabetes: Correlation of variables and clinical outcome after immunotherapy. *J Neurol Neurosurg Psychiatry* 1999; 67:607.

106. Martin MM: Diabetic neuropathy. A clinical study of 150 cases. *Brain* 1953;76:594.

107. Mulder DW, Lambert EH, Bastian JA: The neuropathies associated with diabetes mellitus: A clinical and electromyographic study of 103 unselected diabetic patients. *Neurology* 1961;11:275.

108. Thomas PK: Classification, differential diagnosis, and staging of diabetic peripheral neuropathy. *Diabetes* 1997;46(suppl 2):S54.

109. Dyck PJ: Detection, characterization, and staging of polyneuropathy: Assessed in diabetics. *Muscle Nerve* 1988;11:21.

110. Vinik AI: Diagnosis and management of diabetic neuropathy. *Clin Geriatr Med* 1999;15:293.

111. Tesfaye S, Ward JD: Clinical features of diabetic polyneuropathy. In: Veves A, ed. *Clinical Management of Diabetic Neuropathy.* Humana Press:1998;49.

112. Galer BS, Gianas A, Jensen MP: Painful diabetic polyneuropathy: Epidemiology, pain description, and quality of life. *Diabetes Res Clin Pract* 2000;47:123.

113. Belgrade MJ: Following the clues to neuropathic pain. Distribution and other leads reveal the cause and the treatment approach. *Postgrad Med* 1999;106:127.

114. Boulton AJM, Scarpello JHB, Armstrong WD, *et al*: The natural history of painful diabetic neuropathy—a 4-year study. *Postgrad Med J* 1983;59:556.

115. Benbow SJ, Cossins L, MacFarlane IA: Painful diabetic neuropathy. *Diabet Med* 1999;16:632.

116. Franse LV, Valk GD, Dekker JH, *et al*: 'Numbness of the feet' is a poor indicator for polyneuropathy in Type 2 diabetic patients. *Diabet Med* 2000;17:105.

117. Yasaki S, Jakobsen J, Dyck PJ: Hypoglycemic polyneuropathy. In: Dyck PJ, Thomas PK, eds. *Diabetic Neuropathy*, 2nd ed. WB Saunders:1999;445.

118. Litzelman DK, Slemenda CW, Langefeld CD, *et al*: Reduction of lower extremity clinical abnormalities in patients with non-insulin-dependent diabetes mellitus. A randomized, controlled trial. *Ann Intern Med* 1993; 119:36.

119. Smieja M, Hunt DL, Edelman D, *et al*: Clinical examination for the detection of protective sensation in the feet of diabetic patients. International Cooperative Group for Clinical Examination Research. *J Gen Intern Med* 1999;14:418.

120. de Sonnaville JJ, Colly LP, Wijkel D, *et al*: The prevalence and determinants of foot ulceration in type II diabetic patients in a primary health care setting. *Diabetes Res Clin Pract* 1997;35:149.

121. Boyko EJ, Ahroni JH, Stensel V, *et al*: A prospective study of risk factors for diabetic foot ulcer. The Seattle Diabetic Foot Study. *Diabetes Care* 1999;22:1036.

122. Murray HJ, Young MJ, Hollis S, *et al*: The association between callus formation, high pressures and neuropathy in diabetic foot ulceration. *Diabet Med* 1996;13:979.

123. Crane M, Werber B: Critical pathway approach to diabetic pedal infections in a multidisciplinary setting. *J Foot Ankle Surg* 1999;38:30.

124. Sauseng S, Kastenbauer T, Sokol G, *et al*: Estimation of risk for plantar foot ulceration in diabetic patients with neuropathy. *Diabetes Nutr Metab* 1999;12:189.

125. Veves A, Murray HJ, Young MJ, *et al*: The risk of foot ulceration in diabetic patients with high foot pressure: A prospective study. *Diabetologia* 1992;35:660.

126. Frykberg RG, Lavery LA, Pham H, *et al*: Role of neuropathy and high foot pressures in diabetic foot ulceration. *Diabetes Care* 1998;21:1714.

127. Shaw JE, Boulton AJM: The pathogenesis of foot problems. In: Veves A, ed. *Clinical Management of Diabetic Neuropathy.* Humana Press: 1998;291.

128. Akbari CM, LoGerfo FW: The impact of micro- and macrovascular disease on diabetic neuropathy and foot problems. In: Veves A, ed. *Clinical Management of Diabetic Neuropathy.* Humana Press:1998; 319.

129. Frykberg RG, Habershaw GM, Chrzan JS: Epidemiology of the diabetic foot: Ulcerations. In: Veves A, ed. *Clinical Management of Diabetic Neuropathy.* Humana Press:1998;273.

130. Mason J, O'Keeffe C, Hutchinson A, *et al*: A systematic review of foot ulcer in patients with Type 2 diabetes mellitus. II: Treatment. *Diabet Med* 1999;16:889.

131. Feldman EL, Stevens MJ, Greene DA: Clinical management of diabetic neuropathy. In: Veves A, ed. *Clinical Management of Diabetic Neuropathy.* Humana Press:1998;89.

132. Giurini JM, Rosenblum BI, Lyons TE: Management of the diabetic foot. In: Veves A, ed. *Clinical Management of Diabetic Neuropathy.* Humana Press:1998;303.

133. Humphrey LL, Palumbo PJ, Butters MA, *et al*: The contribution of non-insulin-dependent diabetes to lower-extremity amputation in the community. *Arch Intern Med* 1994;154:885.

134. Wilson M: Charcot foot osteoarthropathy in diabetes mellitus. *Mil Med* 1991;156:563.

135. Edmonds ME, Watkins PJ: Plantar neuropathic ulcer and Charcot joints: Risk factors, presentation, and management. In: Dyck PJ, Thomas PK, eds. *Diabetic Neuropathy.* WB Saunders:1998;398.

136. DCCT Research Group. The effect of intensive diabetes therapy on measures of autonomic nervous system function in the Diabetes Control and Complications Trial (DCCT). Diabetologia, 1998;41: 416.

137. Simmons Z, Feldman EL: The treatment of established complications: neuropathy. In: Williams R, Wareham N, Kinmonth AL, *et al*, eds. *The Evidence Base for Diabetes Care.* John Wiley & Sons:2000; in press.

138. Cohen KL, Harris S: Efficacy and safety of nonsteroidal anti-inflammatory drugs in the therapy of diabetic neuropathy. *Arch Intern Med* 1987;147:1442.

139. Joss JD: Tricyclic antidepressant use in diabetic neuropathy. *Ann Pharmacother* 1999;33:996.

140. Max MB, Culnane M, Schafer SC, *et al*: Amitriptyline relieves diabetic neuropathy pain in patients with normal or depressed mood. *Neurology* 1987;37:589.

141. Hoogwerf BJ: Amitriptyline treatment of painful diabetic neuropathy: An inadvertent single-patient clinical trial. *Diabetes Care* 1985;8:526.

142. Kvinesdal B, Molin J, Froland A, *et al*: Imipramine treatment of painful diabetic neuropathy. *JAMA* 1984;251:1727.

143. Kvinesdal B, Molin J, Froland A, *et al*: Antidepressive agents in the treatment of diabetic neuropathy. *Clin Physiol* 1985;5(suppl):97.

144. Morello CM, Leckband CG, Stoner CP, Moorhouse DF, Sahagian GA. Ramdomized double-blind study comparing the efficacy of gabapentin with amitriptyline on diabetic peripheral neuropathy pain. Arch Intern Med, 1999;159:1931.

145. Feldman EL, Stevens MJ, Greene DA: Treatment of diabetic neuropathy. In: Mazzaferri EL, Bar RS, Kreisberg RA, eds. *Advances in Endocrinology and Metabolism.* Mosby Year Book:1994;393.

146. McQuay HJ, Tramer M, Nye BA, *et al*: A systematic review of antidepressants in neuropathic pain. *Pain* 1996;68:217.

147. Sindrup SH, Gram LF, Brosen K, *et al*: The selective serotonin reuptake inhibitor paroxetine is effective in the treatment of diabetic neuropathy symptoms. *Pain* 1990;42:135.

148. Max MB, Lynch SA, Muir J, *et al*: Effects of desipramine, amitriptyline, and fluoxetine on pain in diabetic neuropathy. *N Engl J Med* 1992;326:1250.

149. Khurana RC: Treatment of painful diabetic neuropathy with trazodone. *JAMA* 1983;250:1392.

150. Goodnick PJ, Jimenez I, Kumar A: Sertraline in diabetic neuropathy: Preliminary results. *Ann Clin Psychiatry* 1997;9:255.

151. Backonja MM: Gabapentin monotherapy for the symptomatic treatment of painful neuropathy: A multicenter, double-blind, placebo-controlled trial in patients with diabetes mellitus. *Epilepsia* 1999; 40(suppl 6):S57.

152. Backonja M, Beydoun A, Edwards KR, *et al*: Gabapentin for the symptomatic treatment of painful neuropathy in patients with diabetes mellitus: A randomized controlled trial. *JAMA* 1998;280:1831.

153. Gorson KC, Schott C, Herman R, *et al*: Gabapentin in the treatment of painful diabetic neuropathy: A placebo controlled, double blind crossover trial. *J Neurol Neurosurg Psychiatry* 1999;66:251.

154. Morello CM, Leckband SG, Stoner CP, *et al*: Randomized double-blind study comparing the efficacy of gabapentin with amitriptyline on diabetic peripheral neuropathy pain. *Arch Intern Med* 1999;159: 1931.

155. Rull JA, Quibrera R, Gonzalez-Millan H, *et al*: Symptomatic treatment of peripheral diabetic neuropathy with carbamazepine (Tegretol): Double blind crossover trial. *Diabetologia* 1969;5:215.

156. Chakrabarti AK, Samantaray SK: Diabetic peripheral neuropathy: Nerve conduction studies before, during and after carbamazepine therapy. *Aust N Z J Med* 1976;6:565.

157. Rodin EA: Carbamazepine (Tegretol). In: Browne TR, Feldman RG, eds. *Epilepsy. Diagnosis and Management,* 1st ed. Little, Brown and Company:1983;203.

158. Ellenberg M: Treatment of diabetic neuropathy with diphenylhydantoin. *N Y State J Med* 1968;68:2653.

159. Saudek CD, Werns S, Reidenberg MM: Phenytoin in the treatment of diabetic symmetrical polyneuropathy. *Clin Pharmacol Ther* 1977; 22:196.

160. Oskarsson P, Ljunggren JG, Lins PE: Efficacy and safety of mexiletine in the treatment of painful diabetic neuropathy. The Mexiletine Study Group. *Diabetes Care* 1997;20:1594.

161. Stracke H, Meyer UE, Schumacher HE, *et al*: Mexiletine in the treatment of diabetic neuropathy. *Diabetes Care* 1992;15:1550.

CHAPTER 46

Diabetic Autonomic Neuropathy

Aaron I. Vinik

Tomris Erbas

Michael A. Pfeifer

Eva L. Feldman

Martin J. Stevens

James W. Russell

Diabetic neuropathy is the most common and troublesome complication of diabetes mellitus, leading to great morbidity and mortality and an increase in the economic burden of public health.[1] Diabetic neuropathy is a heterogeneous disorder that encompasses a wide range of abnormalities affecting both proximal and distal, peripheral sensory and motor, and autonomic nervous systems (ANS). The ANS supplies all organs in the body and consists of an afferent and an efferent system, with long efferents in the vagus (cholinergic) and short postganglionic unmyelinated fibers in the sympathetic system (adrenergic). A third component is the neuropeptidergic system, with its neurotransmitters substance P (SP), vasoactive intestinal polypeptide (VIP), calcitonin gene-related peptide (CGRP), and others.

Diabetic autonomic neuropathy (DAN) can cause dysfunction of every part of the body. "Know DAN and you know the whole of medicine." DAN often goes completely unrecognized by patient and physician alike because of its insidious onset and protean multiple organ involvement. Alternatively, the appearance of complex and confusing symptoms in a single organ system due to DAN may cause profound symptoms and receive intense diagnostic and therapeutic attention. Subclinical involvement may be widespread, whereas clinical symptoms and signs may be focused within a single organ. Tests of autonomic function generally stimulate entire reflex pathways. Furthermore, autonomic control for each organ system is usually divided between opposing sympathetic and parasympathetic innervation, so that heart rate acceleration, for example, may reflect either decreased parasympathetic or increased sympathetic nervous system stimulation. The organ systems that most often exhibit prominent clinical autonomic signs and symptoms in diabetes include the ocular pupil, sweat glands, genitourinary system, gastrointestinal tract system, adrenal medullary system, and cardiovascular system (Table 46-1).

ANS disturbances may be functional, e.g., gastroparesis with hyperglycemia and ketoacidosis, or organic, in which nerve fibers are actually lost. This creates inordinate difficulties in diagnosing, treating and prognosticating as well as establishing true prevalence rates.

TABLE 46-1. Clinical manifestations and differential diagnosis of autonomic neuropathy

Clinical Manifestations	Differential Diagnosis
Cardiovascular	**Cardiovascular disorders**
Tachycardia, exercise intolerance	Idiopathic orthostatic hypotension
	Shy-Drager syndrome
Cardiac denervation	Panhypopituitarism
Orthostatic hypotension	Pheochromocytoma
	Hypovolemia
	Congestive heart disease
	Carcinoid syndrome
Gastrointestinal	**Gastrointestinal disorders**
Esophageal dysfunction	Obstruction
Gastroparesis diabeticorum	Bezoars
Diarrhea	Secretory diarrhea (endocrine tumors)
Constipation	Biliary disease
Fecal incontinence	Psychogenic vomiting
	Medications
Genitourinary	**Genitourinary**
Erectile dysfunction	Genital and pelvic surgery
Retrograde ejaculation	Atherosclerotic vascular disease
Cystopathy	Medications
Neurogenic bladder	Alcohol abuse
Neurovascular	**Other causes of neurovascular dysfunction**
Heat intolerance	
Gustatory sweating	Chagas disease
Dry skin	Amyloidosis
Impaired skin blood flow	Arsenic
Metabolic	
Hypoglycemia unawareness	
Hypoglycemia unresponsiveness	
Hypoglycemia associated autonomic failure	
Pupillary	**Pupillary**
Decreased diameter of dark adapted pupil	Syphilis
Argyll-Robertson type pupil	

PREVALENCE

The main subgroups of autonomic disturbances recognized in diabetes mellitus are (1) subclinical DAN, determined by abnormalities in quantative autonomic function tests; and (2) clinical DAN, which presents with symptoms or signs. There are few studies on the prevalence of the two types. The reported prevalence of DAN varies, depending on whether the studies have been carried out in the community, clinic, or a tertiary referral center. This variance also reflects the type and number of tests performed and the presence or absence of signs and symptoms of autonomic neuropathy. Most patients who develop signs of DAN do not become symptomatic. Symptomatic autonomic neuropathy is rare and presents in less than 5% of diabetic patients, except for impotence (5–50%). Clinical symptoms of DAN generally do not occur until long after the onset of diabetes. However, subclinical autonomic dysfunction can occur within a year of diagnosis in type 2 diabetic (T2DM) patients and within 2 years in type 1 diabetic (T1DM) patients.[2]

In the population-based Oxford Community Diabetes Study, 20.9% of T1DM and 15.8% of T2DM individuals had abnormal results in one or more of three autonomic function tests.[3] In a clinic-based study, cardiac autonomic neuropathy was present in 8–22% of T1DM and T2DM patients on screening.[4] The prevalence of autonomic neuropathy was 47% in the EURODIAB IDDM Complications Study.[5]

The major confirmed risk factors are age, duration of diabetes, poor metabolic control, and the presence of retinopathy, nephropathy, and cardiovascular disease. Autonomic neuropathy also involves severe hypoglycemia and severe ketoacidosis.[5,6]

Complications affecting the autonomic nervous system contribute greatly to the morbidity, mortality, reduced quality of life, and activities of daily living of the person with diabetes. They are also major sources of increased cost of caring for the diabetic patient. Among the most troublesome and dangerous of these conditions that are linked to autonomic neuropathy are (1) myocardial ischemia including silent myocardial infarction; (2) cardiac arrhythmias; (3) foot ulceration, gangrene, and amputation; (4) nephropathy; and (5) erectile dysfunction. Parasympathetic nerve dysfunction in T2DM patients is associated with features of the metabolic insulin resistance syndrome, a common risk factor for cardiovascular morbidity and mortality. Patients with parasympathetic neuropathy have elevated fasting C-peptide and triglyceride levels and lowered high-density lipoprotein (HDL) cholesterol levels.[7] Basal hyperinsulinemia is associated with the development of parasympathetic autonomic neuropathy in T2DM. Basal proinsulin and C peptide are also associated with autonomic nerve dysfunction.[8]

The presence of symptomatic autonomic dysfunction is life-threatening, with estimates of mortality ranging from 25 to 50% within 5–10 years of diagnosis; mortality estimates on meta-analysis of nine studies averaged 27% in 2–5 years.[9–13] The 5-year mortality rate of patients with DAN is three times higher than that in diabetic patients without autonomic involvement.[14]

PATHOGENESIS

The pathogenesis of autonomic neuropathy is incompletely understood. There are metabolic, microvascular, and autoimmune theories (see Chap. 44). Persistent hyperglycemia resulting in activation of the polyol pathway and tissue accumulation of sorbitol, fructose, and deficiency of myoinositol, disturbed phosphoinositide metabolism with consequent decreased nerve Na^+/K^+-ATPase activity, increased nonenzymatic glycation, decreased nitric oxide (NO) production leading to impaired endothelium-dependent vasodilation, and finally deficiency in neurotrophic factors have all been proposed as pathogenetic mechanisms for DAN.[15,16]

Although there is increasing evidence that the pathogenesis of DAN involves several mechanisms, the prevailing theory implicates persistent hyperglycemia as the primary factor within the metabolic hypothesis.[17] Persistent hyperglycemia increases polyol pathway activity, with accumulation of sorbitol and fructose in nerves, damaging them by an as yet unknown mechanism. This is accompanied by decreased myoinositol uptake and inhibition of the Na^+/K^+ATPase, resulting in Na^+ retention, edema, axoglial disjunction, and nerve degeneration. Microvascular dysfunction with local ischemia leading to nerve fiber death has been proposed, as well as pseudohypoxia with oxidative stress.[18,19] An immunologic mechanism has also been suggested in the etiology of DAN. Autoantibodies to vagus nerve, sympathetic ganglia, and adrenal medulla are higher in patients with severe symptomatic DAN. Complement-fixing autoantibodies to the vagus nerve, sympathetic ganglion, and adrenal medulla are present in 13.2–30.7% of patients with T1DM.[20] These autoantibodies have been shown to cause apoptosis of adrenergic neurons in culture.[21–23] Antibodies to nerve growth factor (NGF) (important for viability of sympathetic and neuropeptidergic integrity) have been reported in patients with iritis and gastroparesis.[24]

DIFFERENTIAL DIAGNOSIS

The differential diagnosis of DAN depends on the systems involved but generally includes idiopathic orthostatic hypotension, Shy-Drager syndrome, multiple system atrophy, panhypopituitarism, pheochromocytoma, carcinoid syndrome, neuroendocrine tumors, hypovolemia, medications (insulin, vasodilators, and sympathetic blockers), orthostatic hypotension caused by alcoholic neuropathy, congestive heart failure, Chagas' disease in Latin America, the familial forms of amyloidosis in people of Mediterranean origin, and the Argyll-Robertson pupil of syphilis. Specific organ involvement requires consideration of causes within each organ system (Table 46-1).

CARDIOVASCULAR AUTONOMIC NEUROPATHY

Cardiovascular autonomic neuropathy (CAN) is a common form of autonomic neuropathy, embracing abnormalities in heart rate control, and central and peripheral vascular dynamics.[25–28] Parasympathetic activation slows the heart rate, whereas sympathetic activation is both inotrophic and chronotrophic. Sympathetic stimulation of the vasculature tree increases blood pressure, whereas parasympathetic control of the vasculature has only minor effects. Thus, early parasympathetic damage results in resting tachycardia and with the advent of sympathetic damage heart rate slows but not back to normal. Orthostasis may develop and impaired ventricular function occurs.

The prevalence rate of borderline or definite CAN is 8.5 or 16.8% among T1DM patients and 12.2 or 22.1% in T2DM patients attending a general clinic.[4] In the Diabetes Control and Complications Trial (DCCT) cohort of young T1DM patients free of complications, the baseline prevalences of abnormal cardiovascular tests (RR variation and Valsalva ratio) were 1.6% and 6.2%, respectively in the primary prevention cohort, and 6.3% and 5.5%, respectively in the secondary intervention cohort.[29,30] Surveys of clinical endocrine/diabetes practices that include patients with long-standing diabetes have found >40% abnormalities in heart rate variability (HRV).[31] Thus, the prevalence varies with the measurements, the device used and the population being studied.

CAN has been linked to postural hypotension, exercise intolerance, enhanced intraoperative cardiovascular lability, increased incidence of silent ischemia, myocardial infarction, and decreased rate of survival after myocardial infarction.[32-35] CAN cosegregates with impaired vibration perception and higher urinary albumin excretion in T1DM patients. However, in T2DM patients, it is associated with higher body mass index, systolic blood pressure, urinary albumin excretion, and basal insulin levels, i.e., all features of the metabolic syndrome.[3]

Cardiac sympathetic denervation is greater in T2DM than in T1DM patients.[36] In both normal subjects and diabetic patients, reduced autonomic function, measured as loss of HRV, is associated with a high risk of future coronary heart disease predicted either from conventional coronary risk factors or from exercise test parameters.[37] There are links among DAN, higher nocturnal blood pressure levels, increased left ventricular mass, and higher cardiovascular mortality rate. The medical consequences of CAN in diabetes are dramatic: a meta-analysis of 11 studies of CAN among diabetic patients concluded that whereas patients with diabetes without this complication have a mortality of 5% within 5.5 years, mortality among patients with CAN (as determined by abnormal HRV tests) jumps to 27% in that time period.[38] Cardiovascular mortality is increased in diabetic patients with autonomic neuropathy independent of conventional risk factors and glycemia.[39] Autonomic neuropathy is also an independent risk factor for stroke in T2DM patients.[40]

Cardiovascular Symptoms and Signs

In early CAN there is resting tachycardia and loss of beat-to-beat variation in heart rate with deep breathing.[41] A fixed heart rate unresponsive to mild exercise in diabetic patients indicates nearly complete cardiac denervation. Autonomic neuropathy most commonly involves the cardiovascular system, leading to a reduced cardiac ejection fraction and systolic dysfunction, as well as decreased diastolic filling.[26,42] The presence of both asymptomatic and symptomatic coronary artery disease (CAD) is increased in diabetic patients, and subclinical neuropathy is an important cause of silent ischemia in patients with diabetes.[43,44] Indeed, painless ischemia is significantly more frequent in patients with, than in those without, autonomic neuropathy (38% vs. 5%). Diabetic autonomic dysfunction affecting cardiac efferent sympathetic signals is an important determinant of impaired coronary blood flow during increased sympathetic stimulation. Diabetic patients with evidence of cardiac sympathetic nerve dysfunction have impaired sympathetically mediated dilation of coronary resistance vessels. This vasomotor abnormality develops early in the course of DAN, and its severity is related to the degree of cardiac sympathetic nerve dysfunction.[45]

In nondiabetic patients, acute myocardial infarction has a circadian variation, with a significant morning peak. The characteristic diurnal variation in the onset of myocardial infarction is altered in diabetic patients, demonstrating a lower morning peak and a

higher percentage of infarction during evening hours. The blunted morning surge of incidence of myocardial infarction results from altered sympathovagal balance in patients with CAN.[46,47] Chest pain in any location in a patient with diabetes should be considered of myocardial origin until proved otherwise. Moreover, unexplained fatigue, confusion, tiredness, edema, hemoptysis, nausea and vomiting, diaphoresis, arrhythmias, cough, or dyspnea should alert one to a possible silent myocardial infarct.

Prolongation of the QT interval has been suggested as a diagnostic test of DAN and as a prognostic marker of cardiovascular disease.[12] The EURODIAB Type 1 Diabetes Complications Study found that the prevalence of abnormally prolonged corrected QT is 16% in the diabetic population as a whole, 11% in males and 21% in females.[48] Prolonged QTc interval and QT dispersion (the difference between the longest and shortest QT interval) are indicative of an imbalance between right and left sympathetic innervation. Diabetic patients with regional sympathetic imbalance and QTc interval prolongation also may be at greater risk for arrhythmias. Prolonged QT intervals indicate an increased risk of sudden death from autonomic neuropathy, diabetic nephropathy, and coronary heart disease.[49,50]

Regional myocardial autonomic denervation and altered vascular responsiveness in DAN may predispose to malignant arrhythmogenesis and sudden cardiac death. In the resting state, the myocardium is well perfused in subjects with DAN, and thus circulatory deficiencies should not exacerbate arrhythmogenesis under resting conditions. During stress, relative regional ischemia in sympathetically innervated regions with diminished parasympathetic protection may be highly arrhythmogenic.[51,52] In diabetes, excess cardiac death is related to sympathetic hyperactivity or imbalance because these patients experience proportionally greater cardioprotection from beta blockade, with mortality after infarction being decreased by ≤63%.[53,54]

Cardiac Function Testing of the Autonomic Nervous System

The ANS is usually tested by evaluating reflex arcs that involve a stimulus, a receptor, an afferent nerve, central processing, an efferent nerve and an end-organ response.[55] The ideal test must be simple, specific, noninvasive, and easy to perform and undergo, be sensitive, yield reproducible results, suitable for long-term evaluation. The San Antonio Conference concluded that noninvasive tests of ANS function are suitable for routine screening for autonomic dysfunction or for monitoring the progress of autonomic neuropathy.[56] A series of simple noninvasive tests is capable of detecting CAN: resting heart rate, beat-to-beat HRV, Valsalva maneuver, heart rate response to standing, systolic blood pressure response to standing, diastolic blood pressure rise with sustained exercise, and QT interval on ECG (Table 46-2). Reduced 24-hour HRV, a newer measure of cardiac autonomic function, is believed to be a more sensitive measure of cardiac autonomic function that is able to detect dysfunction earlier than standard reflex tests.[57] The abnormal HRV test alone may be useful in diagnosing early-stage autonomic dysfunction. However, with better control of all the variables, an abnormal Valsalva response is more sensitive and reproducible.[31] Combining these with the standing test 30:15 ratio provides greater sensitivity and reveals a higher number of abnormalities.

Absent HRV secondary to DAN is predictive of both left ventricular failure and increased mortality.[58] Thus, due to the large percentage of diabetic patients with CAN complications, HRV

TABLE 46-2. Diagnostic tests of cardiovascular autonomic neuropathy

TEST	METHOD/PARAMETERS
Resting heart rate	>100 beats/min is abnormal.
Beat-to-beat heart rate Variation*	With the patient at rest and supine (no overnight coffee or hypoglycemic episodes), breathing 6 breaths/min, heart rate monitored by EKG or ANSCORE device, a difference in heart rate of >15 beats/min is normal and <10 beats/min is abnormal, R-R inspiration/R-R expiration >1.17. All indices of HRV are age-dependent**.
Heart rate response to Standing*	During continuous EKG monitoring, the R-R interval is measured at beats 15 and 30 after standing. Normally, a tachycardia is followed by reflex bradycardia. The 30:15 ratio is normally >1.03.
Heart rate response to Valsalva maneuver*	The subject forcibly exhales into the mouthpiece of a manometer to 40 mmHg for 15 s during EKG monitoring. Healthy subjects develop tachycardia and peripheral vasoconstriction during strain and an overshoot bradycardia and rise in blood pressure with release. The ratio of longest R-R shortest R-R should be >1.2.
Systolic blood pressure response to standing	Systolic blood pressure is measured in the supine subject. The patient stands and the systolic blood pressure is measured after 2 min. Normal response is a fall of <10 mmHg, borderline is a fall of 10-29 mmHg, and abnormal is a fall of >30 mmHg with symptoms.
Diastolic blood pressure response to isometric exercise	The subject squeezes a handgrip dynamometer to establish a maximum. Grip is then squeezed at 30% maximum for 5 min. The normal response for diastolic blood pressure is a rise of >16 mmHg in the other arm.
EKG QT/QTc intervals	The QTc should be <440 ms.
Spectral analysis	VLF peak ↓ (sympathetic dysfunction) LF peak ↓ (sympathetic dysfunction) HF peak ↓ (parasympathetic dysfunction) LH/HF ratio ↓ (sympathetic imbalance)
Neurovascular flow	Using noninvasive laser Doppler measures of peripheral sympathetic responses to nociception.

* These can now be performed quickly (<15 min) in the practitioners office, with a central reference laboratory providing quality control and normative values. (ANSCORE) Boston Medical Technologies.

testing is a very powerful and useful tool for identifying patients at substantial risk of morbidity and mortality. It is also a sensitive, although not specific, indicator of painless myocardial ischemia. In summary, measuring HRV appears to be an effective means of identifying patients at risk for asymptomatic ischemia and infarction so that treatment may be instituted before a cardiac event occurs.

A 24-hour recording of HRV gives insights into abnormal patterns of circadian rhythms regulated by sympathovagal activity. In frequency domain analysis, very low-frequency (VLF) heart rate fluctuations are thought to be mediated by the sympathetic system; the low-frequency (LF) heart rate fluctuations are under sympathetic control with vagal modulation; and the high-frequency (HF) fluctuations are under parasympathetic control. The balance between the sympathetic and parasympathetic components of autonomic nerve function can be assessed with the LF:HF ratio. The HF component is reduced in diabetic patients with vagal dysfunction. In diabetic patients with sympathetic dysfunction, the VLF and LF components are reduced. The VLF, LF, and HF components, as well as the LF:HF ratio, have been demonstrated to be reduced in diabetic patients with advanced stages of CAN.[38]

Sympathetic innervation of the heart can be visualized and quantified by single-photon emission computed tomography (SPECT) with I^{123} meta-iodobenzylguanidine (MIBG). MIBG is an analog of norepinephrine that shares the same uptake and storage mechanism. MIBG imaging is a valuable tool for the detection of early alterations in myocardial sympathetic innervation in diabetic patients. Diabetic CAN has been directly characterized by reduced or absent myocardial MIBG uptake.[59,60] The regional cardiac sympathetic dysinnervation is mainly in the posterior myocardial region compared with the lateral and apical region, implying a predisposition to arrhythmogenicity.[61] Furthermore, alter-

ations of the sympathetic myocardial innervation are related to subclinical left ventricular dysfunction observed in a large proportion of patients with long-standing T1DM.[62] The sympathetic innervation of the heart can also be visualized with positron emission (PET) imaging using carbon-11 hydroxyephedrine. Defects in carbon-11 hydroxyephedrine uptake have been correlated with CAN and impaired vasodilator response of coronary resistance vessels.[45,63]

Treatment

The DCCT group has shown without question the importance of attention to intensive insulin therapy in preventing the onset and progression of diabetic complications. The DCCT demonstrated that DAN was reduced by 53% in patients with intensive glycemic control. Intensive therapy caused a significant risk reduction in autonomic nerve abnormalities (4 vs. 9%) in the Primary Prevention Group.[29] Furthermore, Burger and colleague[64] showed the effect of strict glycemic control on HRV in T1DM patients with CAN. The response to improved glycemic control is dependent on the degree of autonomic dysfunction at the time when therapy is begun. In patients with early CAN, reversibility is evident by power spectral analysis of HRV as early as 1 year after institution of strict control.[64]

A randomized clinical trial in Japanese patients with T2DM showed that attainment of near-normal glycemia with intensive insulin therapy resulted in improvements in both postural hypotension and the coefficient of variation of R-R.[65] Defects in left ventricular sympathetic innervation can regress in diabetic subjects achieving good glycemic control.[66] The stepwise implementation of intensified multifactorial treatment slowed the progression to autonomic neuropathy in patients with T2DM and microalbumin-

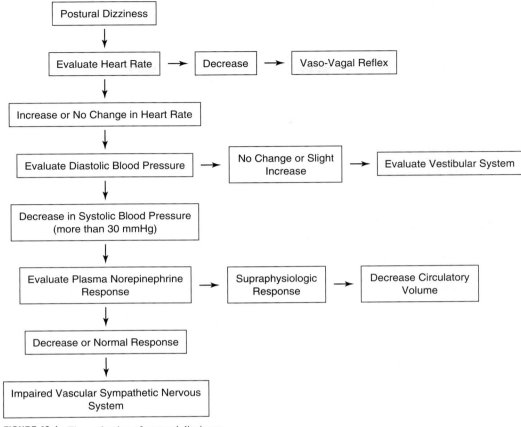

FIGURE 46-1. The evaluation of postural dizziness.

uria.[67] Angiotensin-converting enzyme (ACE) inhibition restores HRV toward normal in those with mild abnormalities. Quinapril increases parasympathetic activity in patients with DAN. Therapies with ACE inhibitors increase vagal tone and decrease sympathetic tone.[68] This may in part explain the salutary effect in the Heart Outcomes Prevention Evaluation (HOPE) and microHOPE trials, in which the decrease in blood pressure was only 3/2 mmHg.[69,70] In addition, a survey of evidence from clinical trials shows that early identification of autonomic neuropathy permits timely initiation of therapy with the powerful antioxidant α-lipoic acid, which slows or reverses progression of CAN.[71]

The progression of DAN may also be reversed by pharmacologic intervention with aldose reductase inhibitors.[72] There is a beneficial effect of low-grade endurance training on HRV in the early stages of diabetic CAN.[73] Combined treatment with C peptide and insulin may improve respiratory HRV in patients with T1DM.[74] The cardioselective and lipophilic beta blockers might modulate the effects of autonomic dysfunction in diabetes (either peripherally by opposing the sympathetic stimulus or by a central acting mechanism) and thereby restore parasympathetic/sympathetic balance.[75]

ORTHOSTATIC HYPOTENSION

Abnormal blood pressure segulation commonly accompanies autonomic neuropathy. The normal nighttime drop in blood pressure is reduced in patients with autonomic neuropathy. Orthostatic hypotension, another sign of autonomic neuropathy, is a fall in systolic blood pressure of (30> mmHg upon standing due to damaged vasoconstrictor fibers, as well as impaired baroreceptor function and poor cardiovascular reactivity. This sign is accompanied by symptoms of dizziness, weakness, faintness, visual impairment, pain in the back of the head, and loss of consciousness (Fig. 46-1).

Two pathophysiologic states cause orthostatic hypotension: autonomic insufficiency and intravascular volume depletion. Physical examination and history should easily rule out volume depletion states. An important point is the exclusion of contributing factors that may be aggravating or unmasking the orthostatic hypotension of DAN. Prominent among these are volume depletion secondary to diuretics, excessive sweating, diarrhea, or polyuria. Other problems occur with antihypertensive medications, beta blockers, tricyclic antidepressants, and phenothiazines. Beta blockers impair heart rate responses, and the last two act through their α-adrenergic blocking properties to impair vasoconstriction.

Diagnosis

There are, however, a group of patients with contracted red cell mass who are not clinically dehydrated and who have orthostatic tachycardia.[76] They may develop modest tachycardia without a fall in pressure and have an exaggerated norepinephrine response.[77] They do respond to erythropoietin.[78] Of particular relevance is the observation that many people with this symptom complex become hypotensive with eating or within 10–15 minutes of taking their insulin injection. The symptoms, which are not unlike those of hypoglycemia, are often incorrectly ascribed to the hypoglycemic action of insulin, but they occur too early and are actually due to a fall in blood pressure. This may be mediated by mild intravascular depletion secondary to increased capillary permeability caused by insulin or by its direct effect on the vasodilation of resistance vessels. Insulin may directly stimulate endothelial release of NO, a potent vasodilator, and may sensitize smooth muscle to the relaxant effects of prostacyclin and NO, thereby causing vasodilation unopposed by the action of norepinephrine.[28] Both an impaired vagal heart rate control and sympathetic nervous dysfunction exaggerate the hemodynamic effects of insulin in patients with diabetes, contributing to insulin-induced hypotension, which therefore tends only to occur with advanced autonomic neuropathy.[79]

Treatment

Orthostatic hypotension in the patient with DAN can present a difficult management problem. Elevating the blood pressure in the standing position must be balanced against preventing hypertension in the supine position. Whenever possible, attempts should be made to increase venous return from the periphery using total body stockings. Patients should be instructed to put them on while lying down and not to remove them until returning to the supine position. Some patients with postural hypotension may benefit from treatment with 9-flurohydrocortisone and supplementary salt 2–6 g daily. Unfortunately, symptoms do not improve until edema occurs, and there is significant risk of developing congestive heart failure and hypertension. If flurohydrocortisone does not work satisfactorily, various adrenergic agonists and antagonists may be used. Patients may be treated with clonidine, which in this setting may paradoxically increase blood pressure. If the preceding measures fail, midodrine, an α adrenergic agonist may help.[27,80] A particularly refractory form of orthostatic hypotension occurs in some patients postprandially and may respond to therapy with octreotide.[81] Care should be taken to avoid higher doses, which could result in hypertension.

GASTROINTESTINAL AUTONOMIC NEUROPATHY

The gastrointestinal tract is innervated by extrinsic parasympathetic and sympathetic neurons and by intrinsic pathways (myenteric or Auerbach's and the submucosal or Meissner's plexus). Movement of food from mouth to the anus involves coordination of sympathetic, parasympathetic, plexus, and dopaminergic pathways. Sympathetic nervous system activity inhibits gastric emptying, parasympathetic nervous system activity stimulates gastric and esophageal peristalsis, and dopaminergic innervation inhibits gastric peristalsis. Neuropeptidergic function, e.g., glucose-dependent, insulin-releasing peptide (GIP) and somatostatin, plays a role in gastric emptying.[82] An aberration in any of these pathways may result in abnormal gastrointestinal function.

Autonomic neuropathy can affect every part of the gastrointestinal tract, i.e., the esophagus, stomach, small intestine, and colon. Thus, the gastrointestinal manifestations are quite variable and include dysphagia, abdominal pain, nausea, vomiting, malabsorption, fecal incontinence, diarrhea, and constipation. Diabetic patients may present with a spectrum of manifestations from mild gastrointestinal symptoms to severe clinical disease.[83] The prevalence of symptoms caused by gastrointestinal dysfunction may reach 76% in a nonselected population of diabetic outpatients. Gastrointestinal tract symptoms and autonomic dysfunction are both common in tertiary referral centers; however, symptoms and objective evidence of neuropathy are not always related.[84] Indeed, many gastrointestinal symptoms relate to depression rather than autonomic disease.[85]

Esophageal Dysfunction

Esophageal motor disorders have been described in 75% of diabetic patients. Despite the frequent motility abnormalities described, symptoms of esophageal disease are rather uncommon in diabetics, and only approximately 30% experience symptoms. Motor abnormalities include impairment of peristaltic activity with double peak and tertiary contractions or impaired peristalsis and diminished lower esophageal sphincteric pressures. These factors may further predispose to gastroesophageal reflux disease, particularly in the setting of impaired gastric emptying. Esophageal dysfunction is detectable through esophageal motility testing and esophageal scintigraphy in diabetic patients.[86]

Gastroparesis Diabeticorum

The prevalence of delayed gastric emptying in patients with long-standing diabetes is not known, due to a lack of population-based studies; it has been shown to occur in up to 50% of selected diabetic patients.[87] It is usually clinical silent, although severe diabetic gastroparesis is one of the most debilitating of all the gastrointestinal complications of diabetes.

Physiology of gastric emptying largely depends on vagus nerve function, which may be grossly disturbed in diabetes. The gastric basal electrical rhythm is initiated by the pacemaker and is conducted circumferentially and longitudinally toward the pylorus. The gastric pacemaker area is located in a region at the junction of the fundus and body on the greater curvature. The interdigestive motor activity of the stomach during fasting is divided into four phases; during the peak activity of the third phase (the migrating motor complex [MMC]), the stomach bursts into contractions with a frequency of three contractions a minute. Liquid emptying is controlled by the fundus and depends on the volume of gastric contents. With impaired vagal function, the proximal stomach is less relaxed, and liquid emptying may actually be faster than normal in diabetic patients. Solid-phase emptying is caused by powerful contractions of the antrum. These contractions grind and mix solid food into particles of <1 mm in size, which then pass through the pylorus into the duodenum. Phase three contractions of the interdigestive MMC are frequently absent in diabetic patients. This results in poor antral grinding and emptying, which may result in gastric retention. Furthermore, there may be disordered integration of gastric and duodenal motor function resulting from disturbances in receptor relaxation of the stomach. Pylorospasm may occur because of disturbed contractility, which causes a functional resistance to gastric outflow. Impaired gastric emptying puts the patient at particular risk for gastric bezoars formation.

The exact pathophysiology of gastric motor disturbances is not certain. It is clear that vagal parasympathetic dysfunction disturbances may occur. The release of the peptide motilin, which regulates gastrointestinal motility, is under vagal control. Motilin stimulates initiation of phase 3 motor activity of the MMC of the stomach and will do so in patients with gastroparesis. Hyperglycemia itself may cause delayed gastric emptying of liquids and solids in both diabetic and healthy individuals.[88] Gastric dysrhythmias, known as functional pathology, are defined as bradygastria and tachygastria. Gastric dysrhythmias have been found in 100% of diabetic patients with meal-related symptoms. Gastric dysrhythmias interfere with the normal gastric peristaltic contractions. Loss of vagal tone and increased sympathetic nervous system activity have been associated with gastric dysrhythmias. Acute hyperglycemia can evoke tachygastria and suppress antral contractions.

The typical symptoms of diabetic gastroparesis are early satiety, nausea, vomiting, abdominal bloating, epigastric pain, and anorexia (Fig. 46-2). Patients with gastroparesis have emesis of undigested food consumed many hours or even days previously. Episodes of nausea and vomiting may last for days to months or occur in cycles.[89] Even with mild symptoms, gastroparesis interferes with nutrient delivery to the small bowel and therefore disrupts the relationship between glucose absorption and exogenous insulin administration. This may result in wide swings of glucose levels and unexpected episodes of postprandial hypoglycemia and "brittle diabetes." Gastroparesis should therefore always be suspected in patients with erratic glucose control. Upper gastrointestinal symptoms should not be attributed to gastroparesis until conditions such as gastric ulcer, duodenal ulcer, gastritis, and gastric cancer have been excluded.

Diagnosis

Scintigraphy is generally regarded as the reference method in the evaluation of disordered gastric emptying in diabetic patients. The measurement of gastric emptying of solids is more sensitive than that of liquids. Hyperglycemia exerts a major influence on gastric motor function in that it slows gastric emptying in diabetic patients. The [^{13}C]octanoic acid breath test represents a suitable measure of delayed gastric emptying in diabetic patients, which is associated with the severity of gastric symptoms but is not affected by the blood glucose level.[90]

Treatment

Initial treatment of diabetic gastroparesis should focus on blood glucose control. Physiologic control of blood glucose levels may improve gastric motor dysfunction. The management of gastroparesis should include multiple small feedings with a reduction in the fat content (<40 g/day), which tends to delay gastric emptying. A low-fiber diet is also advised in diabetic gastroparesis to avoid bezoar formation. Metoclopramide, domperidone and levosulpiride offer potential therapy in the management of gastroparesis. Metoclopramide is a cholinergic and antidopaminergic agent with central antiemetic activity.[91] Central nervous system side effects such as tremor, restlessness, tardive dyskinesia, and drowsiness limit the use of metoclopramide. Other side effects observed with metoclopramide are galactorrhea and hyperprolactinemia. The recommended dosage is 10 mg four times a day, 30–60 minutes before meals and at bedtime. Metoclopramide may be given intravenously or as a liquid or suppository. The drug will not be absorbed when given orally if large gastric residuals secondary to severe gastroparesis are present. In this instance, gastric suctioning and intravenous nutrition, as well as intravenous drug administration, are needed until the stomach begins to empty, at which time oral therapy can be reinstituted. Tachyphylaxis occurs and requires that the drug be stopped temporarily and then restarted.

Domperidone is a peripherally acting dopamine 2-receptor antagonist without cholinergic activity. Domperidone has direct antiemetic activity. Domperidone improves gastrointestinal motility by enhancing antral concentrations. Central nervous side effects are observed less frequently with domperidone than with metoclopramide. The oral dose of domperidone for the treatment of gastroparesis is 20–40 mg, four times a daily, taken 30 minutes before meals and, if necessary, at bedtime.

Levosulpiride is a new prokinetic drug that is a selective antagonist for D_2-dopamine receptors. Recent studies have suggested that patients receiving this medication, given at a dosage of 25 mg

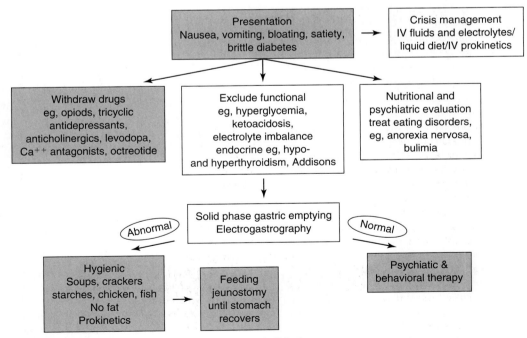

FIGURE 46-2. The evaluation of a patient with gastroparesis diabeticorum.

3 times per day orally, show maintained improvement in gastric emptying and improved glycemic control.

Erythromycin exerts its effect by stimulation of motilin receptors. Erythromycin and its derivatives have improved gastric emptying of solids and liquids and increased antral contraction.[92,93] Erythromycin may cause nausea, abdominal cramps and diarrhea, rash, and allergic manifestations. The oral dose of erythromycin is 250 mg three times daily, taken 30 minutes before meals. Intravenous erythromycin (3 mg/kg/every 8 hours by infusion) is a useful drug for clearance of gastric bezoars. The gastrokinetic efficacy of metoclopramide, domperidone, and erythromycin diminishes during prolonged administration.

If medications fail and severe gastroparesis persists, jejunostomy placement into normally functioning bowel may be needed. Satisfactory relief of intractable vomiting from diabetic gastroparesis is achieved by a percutaneous endoscopic gastrotomy (PEG) or novel radical surgical procedure.[94,95]

Diabetic Diarrhea

Diarrhea may be evident in 20% of diabetic patients, particularly those with known autonomic neuropathy. However, the prevalence of chronic diarrhea in a nonselected heterogeneous diabetic population is 3.7%. Diabetic diarrhea is more common among T1DM than T2DM patients.[96] A number of factors may contribute to the diarrhea, including stasis of bowel contents with bacterial overgrowth, bile acid-induced intestinal hurry, and malabsorption, as well as a diminution in pancreatic exocrine secretions, presumably due to the need for insulin to maintain exocrine pancreatic function and the vagal pancreatic neuropathy. The most frequent cause of chronic nondiabetes-provoked diarrhea has been found to be metformin.[96]

Diagnosis

Autonomic neuropathy-associated diarrhea can be sudden, explosive, nocturnal, and paroxysmal. It is characterized by stool volumes greater than 300 g/day and up to 10–20 bowel movements per day. Fecal incontinence may be associated with severe diabetic diarrhea or may constitute an independent disorder of anorectal dysfunction. Incontinent diabetics have decreased basal sphincteric tone, suggesting abnormal internal and external anal sphincter function.

Treatment

The severe and intermittent nature of diabetic diarrhea makes treatment and assessment difficult. Because afferent denervation may contribute to the problem, a bowel program that includes regular efforts to move the bowels is indicated. Initial therapy of diabetic diarrhea should be directed toward correction of electrolyte/water disturbances and nutrition. Good control of glucose levels is helpful. Treatment should be directed at the identified cause of diabetic diarrhea. A broad-spectrum antibiotic (doxycyline and metronidazole) is usually the treatment of choice for bacterial overgrowth. Retention of bile sometimes occurs, which may be highly irritating to the gut, and chelation of bile salts with 4-g tid cholestyramine mixed with fluid and given orally may be of considerable help. Antidiarrheal agents (loperamide and diphenoxylate) can reduce the number of stools. However, toxic megacolon can occur, and extreme care should be used.

Clonidine may restore adrenergic nerve dysfunction and improve diarrhea. Initial treatment should begin with 0.1 mg twice a day. Clonidine may cause orthostatic hypotension. Topical clonidine may also control diarrhea without causing orthostatic hypotension. Octreotide slows motility and inhibits the release of gastroenteropancreatic endocrine peptides, which may be pathogenetic factors responsible for diarrhea and electrolyte imbalance in diabetic patients. Octreotide has been shown to be effective in improving diarrhea at a dose of 50–75 μ unit = μg sc twice a day.[97]

Constipation

The most common problem associated with diabetic gastrointestinal dysfunction is constipation. Severe constipation may be complicated by ulceration, perforation, and fecal impaction. Precipitous change in bowel habits should prompt colonic evaluation to exclude the possibility of neoplasm and stricture.[98] The most commonly reported drug class associated with constipation in persons with diabetes mellitus is calcium channel blockers. The use of amitryptyline for neuropathic pain is an important cause of constipation in these patients because of its anticholinergic properties. For this reason other agents should be selected.

Treatment

Treatment for constipation should begin with emphasis on good bowel habits, which include regular exercise and maintenance of adequate hydration and fiber consumption. Many constipated patients respond to a high-soluble-fiber diet supplemented with daily hydrophilic colloid. Sorbitol and lactulose may be helpful. Metamucil™ may soften stools, and metoclopramide stimulates colorectal activity. Nonetheless, periodic enemas may be needed, and the anticholinergic drugs used for peripheral neuropathy must be avoided.

Gall Bladder Atony

In diabetic patients with autonomic neuropathy, gallbladder contraction is reduced, because of impaired vagal function. Autonomic neuropathy of the gallbladder results in a stasis of bile salts that may "spill over" into the intestines at inappropriate times. The atony and elevation of cholesterol frequently seen in diabetic patients predispose these patients to cholelithiasis.

Treatment is usually surgical at the time of presentation. However, in patients placed on lithogenic drugs, e.g., somatostatin, ultrasonography is advised prior to starting therapy, with prophylactic stone removal.

GENITOURINARY AUTONOMIC NEUROPATHY

Erectile Dysfunction

The most common form of organic sexual dysfunction in male diabetics is erectile dysfunction (ED). ED is defined as the consistent inability to attain and maintain an erection adequate for sexual intercourse, usually qualified by being present for several months and occurring at least half the time. The incidence of ED in diabetic men has been estimated to be between 35 and 75%.[99]

The etiology of ED in diabetes is multifactorial. Neuropathy, vascular disease, metabolic control, nutrition, endocrine disorders, psychogenic factors, and drugs used in the treatment of diabetes and its complications play a role. ED is a marker for the development of generalized vascular disease and for premature demise from a myocardial infarct, and penile failure may be a portent of upcoming, and possibly preventable, cardiovascular events.[100] Thus, ED in diabetics should alert the physician to perform cardiovascular evaluation.

The relationships among the sympathetic and parasympathetic nervous systems, the endothelium, and smooth muscle function may be disrupted by diseases of blood vessels or nerves, such as occurs in diabetes. In diabetes, the development of autonomic neuropathy is partly responsible for the loss of cholinergic activation of the erectile process. In the penis, acetylcholine acts on the vascular endothelium to release NO and prostacylin, both of which are defective in diabetes. There is also evidence that nonadrenergic/noncholinergic nerve function is hampered, with decreased content of VIP, SP, and other neuropeptide vasodilatator neurotransmitters.

The symptoms of organic ED are gradual in onset and progress with time. The earliest complaints are decreased rigidity with incomplete tumescence before total failure. It occurs with all partners, and there is no loss of libido. Morning erections are lost. Sudden loss of erections with a particular partner, while maintaining morning erections and nocturnal penile tumescence, suggest a psychogenic cause. However, psychogenic factors may be superimposed on organic dysfunction in diabetes.

Diagnosis

Evaluation of diabetic men with erectile dysfunction is complex (Fig. 46-3). Initial assessment of patients with ED should be carried out in the presence of their significant other or sexual partner, if possible. Health care providers should make an attempt to inter-

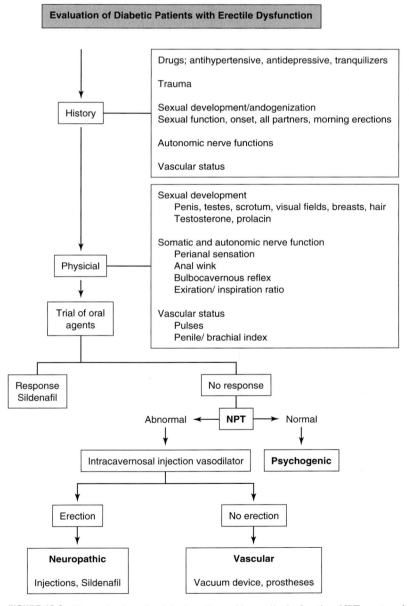

FIGURE 46-3. The evaluation of a diabetic patient with erectile dysfunction. NPT, nocturnal penile tumescence.

view the partner to obtain an impression of the overall relationship and the impact that the return of erections will have on the relationship. Extreme care must be exercised in these situations; in many instances a patient's desire is to be able to have erections but not necessarily to actually have sexual relations.

A thorough work-up for impotence will include medical and sexual history; physical and psychological evaluation; blood tests for diabetes and for testosterone, prolactin, and thyroid hormone levels; test for nocturnal erections (absence of erections during sleep suggests a physical cause of impotence); tests to assess penile, pelvic, and spinal nerve function; and a test to assess penile blood supply and blood pressure. The flow chart provided (Fig. 46-3) is intended as a guide to assist in defining the problem.

The health care provider should initiate questions that will help distinguish the various forms of organic erectile dysfunction from those that are psychogenic in origin. In all instances, a careful history must be taken to determine the rapidity of onset of ED, presence of morning erections, uniformity of sexual dysfunction with all partners, evidence of autonomic nervous dysfunction, vascular insufficiency, hormonal inadequacy, and drugs used in the treatment of satellite disorders.

Physical examination must include an evaluation of the autonomic nervous system, vascular supply, and the hypothalamic-pituitary-gonadal axis.

Autonomic neuropathy causing ED is usually accompanied by loss of ankle jerks and absence or reduction of vibration sense over the large toes. More direct evidence of impairment of penile autonomic function can be obtained by demonstrating normal perianal sensation, assessing the tone of the anal sphincter during a rectal exam, and ascertaining the presence of an anal wink when the area of the skin adjacent to the anus is stroked or contraction of the anus when the glans penis is squeezed, i.e., the bulbo-cavernosus reflex. These measurements are easily and quickly done at the bedside and reflect the integrity of sacral parasympathetic divisions. More sophisticated testing of the autonomic nervous system can be done by measuring the change in postural blood pressure and the change in heart rate with deep breathing.

Vascular disease is usually manifested by buttock claudication but may be due to stenosis of the internal pudendal artery. A penile/brachial index of <0.7 indicates diminished blood supply. A venous leak manifests as unresponsiveness to vasodilators and needs to be evaluated by penile Doppler sonography.

To distinguish psychogenic from organic erectile dysfunction, nocturnal penile tumescence (NPT) testing can be done. Normal NPT defines psychogenic ED, and a negative response to vasodilators implies vascular insufficiency. Application of NPT testing is not so simple. It is much like having a sphygmomanometer cuff inflate over the penis many times during the night while one is trying to have a normal night's sleep including the REM sleep associated with erections. The individual may have to take the device home and become familiar with it over several nights before a conclusion is reached that NPT testing has failed.

Integrity of the penile vasculature is assessed by quantitation of blood flow in response to the potent vasodilator prostaglandin E (alprostadil, 20 μg) given directly into the corpora cavernosa. In patients with psychogenic impotence, erections can be obtained virtually 100% of the time. Similarly, in neurogenic impotence, the response to intracavernosal injection is about 95%. Failure of response implies vascular insufficiency, either arterial or venous in-

competence. It is not surprising that patients with diabetes respond about 65–70% of the time, in keeping with a predominantly neurogenic cause of their ED and compatible with a significant arterial component.

Treatment

A number of treatment modalities are available, each with positive and negative effects; therefore patients must be made aware of both aspects before a therapeutic decision is made. Before considering any form of treatment, every effort should be made to have the patient withdraw from alcohol and eliminate smoking. First and foremost, the patient should be removed, if possible, from drugs that are known to cause erectile dysfunction (Table 46-3). Only three classes of antihypertensives are relatively infrequently associated with erectile dysfunction: α_1-adrenergic blockers, ACE inhibitors, and calcium channel blockers. Metabolic control should be optimized. Direct injection of prostacylin into the corpus cavernosum will induce satisfactory erections in a significant number of men. Also, surgical implantation of a penile prosthesis may be appropriate. The less expensive type of prosthesis is a semirigid, permanently erect type that may be embarrassing and uncomfortable for some patients. The inflatable type is three times more expensive and is subject to mechanical failure, but it avoids the embarrassment caused by other devices.

According to more recent research, relaxation of the corpus cavernosus smooth muscle cells is caused by NO and cGMP, and the ability to have and maintain an erection depends on NO and cGMP. Sildenafil exerts its effect by transiently increasing NO and cGMP levels. Sildenafil is a GMP type-5 phosphodiesterase inhibitor that enhances blood flow to the corpora cavernosae with sexual stimulation. A 50-mg tablet taken orally is the usual starting dose, 60 minutes before sexual activity. Lower doses should be considered in patients with renal failure and hepatic dysfunction. The duration of the drug effect is 4 hours. Before the drug is prescribed, it is important to exclude ischemic heart disease. It is absolutely contraindicated in patients being treated with nitroglycerine or other nitrate-containing drugs. Severe hypotension and fatal cardiac events can occur.[101]

TABLE 46-3. Drugs known to cause erectile dysfunction and commonly used in diabetic patients

Antihypertensive agents
  Beta-blockers
  Thiazide diuretics
  Spironolactone
  Methyldopa
  Reserpine
Agents acting on the central nervous system
  Phenothiazines
  Haloperidol
  Tricyclic antidepressants
Drugs acting on the endocrine system
  Estrogens
  Antiandrogens
  Gonadotropin antagonist
  Spironolactone
  Cimetidine
  Metoclopramide
  Fibric acid derivatives
  Alcohol
  Marijuana

Retrograde Ejaculation

Retrograde ejaculation is caused by damage to efferent sympathetic innervations, which coordinate the simultaneous closure of the internal vesicle sphincter and relaxation of the external vesicle sphincter during ejaculation. Retrograde ejaculation is reported to occur in up to 32% of diabetic men. Lack of spermatozoa in the semen and the presence of motile sperm in a postcoital specimen of urine confirm the diagnosis. Diabetic patients with retrograde ejaculation will require help if pregnancy is to be achieved.

Female Sexual Dysfunction

Despite the severe ravages of autonomic neuropathy on the urogenital system, females with this condition do not suffer from loss of libido and orgasm. Parasympathetic function mediates vaginal lubrication, and, in general, the parasympathetic nervous system is selectively impaired in females with diabetes mellitus. Approximately 30% of diabetic women have some degree of sexual dysfunction. Women with diabetes mellitus have decreased vaginal lubrication, which may lead to vaginal wall atrophy and dyspareunia.[102]

Diagnosis

The diagnosis of female sexual dysfunction requires a conscientious effort to elicit a history of dyspareunia, the use of vaginal lubricants, or both. The value of diagnosis of female sexual dysfunction using vaginal plethysmography to measure lubrication and vaginal flushing has not been well established. Therapy may include use of lubricating agents or estrogen creams.

Treatment

An estrogen cream has the advantage of not only providing the necessary lubrication but also thickening the vaginal walls, thereby possibly decreasing dyspareunia.

Cystopathy

Neural impairment of the bladder includes sympathetic, parasympathetic, and pudendal nerves. Efferent parasympathetic fibers promote bladder contraction during urination. Efferent sympathetic fibers maintain sphincter tone between urinations and decrease their activity during urination. Afferent autonomic fibers transmit sensation of bladder fullness. In DAN, the motor function of the bladder is unimpaired, but afferent fiber damage results in diminished bladder sensation.

The urinary bladder can be enlarged to more than three times its normal size. Patients are seen with bladders filled to their umbilicus, yet they feel no discomfort. Loss of bladder sensation occurs early in DAN, with diminished voiding frequency, and the patient is no longer able to void completely. Consequently, dribbling and overflow incontinence are common complaints. Autonomic neuropathy-associated neurogenic bladder dysfunction may manifest as partial or complete urinary retention, incontinence, or frequent urination including nocturia. Chronic neurogenic bladder can cause vesicoureteric reflux with renal damage. In addition, chronic dysfunction also causes inadequate emptying, with consequent urinary infection. More than two urinary tract infections per year should alert the physician to possible cystopathy and should elicit appropriate diagnostic procedures.

Diagnosis

A postvoiding residual of greater than 150 cc is diagnostic of abnormal bladder function and may be detected by several methods: postvoiding sonography, cystometrogram, postvoiding catheterization, or postvoiding intravenous pyelogram (IVP), which may be injurious to the diabetic kidney. Postvoiding sonography can accurately and noninvasively evaluate the residual urine retained within the bladder. Postvoiding catheterization is invasive and may produce bacteriuria. A cystometrogram is the procedure of choice for evaluating both afferent and efferent bladder function.

Treatment

The principal aims of treatment are improvement of bladder emptying and reduction of risk of urinary tract infection. Patients with cystopathy should be instructed to palpate the bladder and, if they are unable to initiate micturition when the bladder is full, use Crede's maneuver to start the flow of urine every 4 hours. Parasympathomimetics such as bethanechol (10–30 mg three times a day) are sometimes helpful, although frequently they do not help to empty the bladder fully. Extended sphincter relaxation can be achieved with an α_1-blocker such as doxazosin. Self-catheterization can be particularly useful in this setting, with the risk of infection generally being low. If α_1-blockade fails in males, bladder neck surgery may help to relieve spasm of the internal sphincter. Because the somatic supply of the external sphincter remains intact, continence is preserved.

IMPAIRED SKIN BLOOD FLOW

Skin blood flow is important in maintaining nutrition and regional and whole-body temperature and in healing traumatized skin. There are two different types of skin. The first is apical (glabrous) skin, which is present in the palmar surface of the hand, plantar surface of the foot, and the face. Apical skin contains a large number of AV anastomoses or AV shunts and functions in thermoregulation. In contrast, nonapical (hairy) skin is present over most of the body surface. There are relatively few AV shunt vessels, and blood flow is primarily nutritive in function. Microvascular skin flow is under the control of the ANS and is regulated by both the central and peripheral components of the ANS. AV shunts provide a potential low-resistance pathway by which blood flow can be diverted from the arteriolar to the venular circulation, bypassing the capillary bed. The shunts are maintained in a constricted state by sympathetic tone. Loss of this tone due to neuropathy causes the shunts to open, and consequent deviation of blood flow from the skin. Increased venular oxygen levels, apparent ischemic lesions despite the presence of palpable pulses, and raised skin temperatures in the distal extremities are consistent with AV shunting.

In diabetes, the rhythmic contraction of arterioles and small arteries is disordered. Defective blood flow in the small capillary circulation is found, with decreased responsiveness to mental arithmetic, cold pressor, handgrip, and heating (Fig. 46-4). The defect is associated with a reduction in the amplitude of vasomotion and resembles premature aging.[103,104]

There are differences in the glabrous and hairy skin circulations. The vessels in the dorsum of the hand show a moderate endothelial defect and a profound inability to dilate with heat and the added hydrostatic gradient of lowering the limb (Fig. 46-5). In hairy skin, a functional defect is found prior to the development of

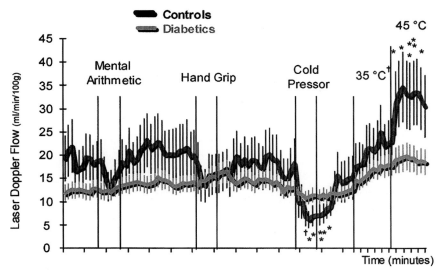

FIGURE 46-4. Impaired skin blood flow in diabetic patients. *(Reproduced with permission from Stansberry et al.[104])*

neuropathy.[105] The factors that contribute to the development of foot ulceration include loss of cutaneous sensitivity to pain and warm thermal stimulation; impairment of sweating with dryness and cracking of the skin; and defective autonomic function with a decrease in blood flow that compromises nerve function and also impairs the supply of essential nutrients and tissue perfusion. It is this constellation that engenders the perfect milieu for the development of foot ulceration and gangrene (see Chap. 51).

Charcot foot may present acutely with severe pain, a warm to hot foot with increased blood flow (despite decreased warm sensory perception and vibration detection), and clear evidence of acute osteopenia.[106–108] An important factor in the development of Charcot joints is equinovarus deformity caused by Achilles tendon shortening.[109] The repetitive trauma in the Charcot foot increases osteoclastic activity and blood flow, with consequent osteopenia.[110]

The osteopenia predisposes the small bones of the foot to small fractures with minimal provocation, especially with the development of equines.

The development of neurovascular dysfunction in diabetic patients involves complex and multifactorial processes. There are three key elements: endothelium, smooth muscle, and nerve supply. Evaluation of each component is essential to understanding the neurovascular dysfunction of diabetes mellitus. The vascular endothelium has a key role in the pathogenesis of microangiopathy and neuropathy by producing important chemicals such as NO, endothelin, and prostacylin.

Diagnosis

The advantage of noninvasive methods for assessing skin blood flow has allowed clinical measurements of the effects of dia-

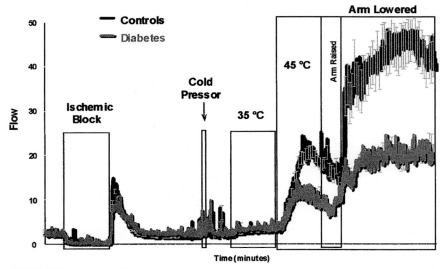

FIGURE 46-5. Abnormal blood flow in hairy skin on dorsum of hand in patients with type 2 diabetes. *(Reproduced with permission from Stansberry et al.[105])*

betes on neurovascular dysfunction. Microvascular blood flow can be accurately measured noninvasively using laser Doppler flowmetry under basal and stimulated conditions. Smooth muscle microvasculature in the periphery reacts to a number of stressor tasks. These may be divided into those dependent on the integrity of the central nervous system—orienting response and mental arithmetic—and those dependent on the distal sympathetic axon—handgrip and cold pressor tests.

Treatment

Drying between the toes after bathing and application of softening creams are critical measures for the prevention of foot ulcers. Daily inspection of the feet is paramount, and patients must be taught proper toenail-cutting techniques. A few studies have examined the ability to alter blood flow in diabetes. In animal models, NGF increases blood flow, but data are not available in humans.[111] A prostaglandin analog, cilastazol, may benefit some people.[112] Altering the rheology of red blood cell viscosity using pentoxifylline has proved disappointing.[113]. Increasing substrate availability for NO generation by ingestion of arginine helps patients with Raynaud's disease, but there are no reports in diabetes mellitus. Changing sensitivity to NO appears to occur with ACE inhibitors and the glitazones, possibly by their action on insulin resistance, but their role needs to be defined.[114,115]

SUDOMOTOR DYSFUNCTION

Hyperhidrosis of the upper body, often related to eating (gustatory sweating) and anhidrosis of the lower body, is a characteristic feature of autonomic neuropathy. Unless careful elicited, a history of abnormal sweating pattern and distal anhidrosis is often unrecognized. Gustatory sweating is thought to be due to axonal regeneration within the autonomic nervous system.[116] Gustatory sweating is much more common among diabetic patients with neuropathy and especially nephropathy. The hyperhidrosis, cracked and dry skin, and increased small blood vessel flow due to autonomic dysfunction create an excellent milieu for infection to take hold and proliferate. Infection develops after skin breaks down and, combined with ischemia, can eventually lead to gangrene.

Treatment

Sudomotor disturbance may respond to treatment with propantheline hydrobromide as scopolamine patches. Anticholinergic drugs have been used successfully for the treatment of gustatory sweating, but anticholinergic agents may be less well tolerated than the condition itself. There is a suggestion that application of glycopyrrolate (an antimuscarinic compound) might benefit diabetic patients with gustatory sweating[117] Intradermal injection of botulinum toxin A is also effective treatment for excessive sweating.[118] Special attention must be paid to foot care. The diabetic patient must pay particular attention to appropriate footwear, padded socks, and hydrating creams.

HYPOGLYCEMIA UNAWARENESS

The counterregulatory hormone responses and awareness of hypoglycemia are reduced in patients with long-standing T1DM (see Chap. 31). The glucagon response is impaired with diabetes duration of 1–5 years, and after 14–31 years of diabetes, the glucagon

response is almost undetectable. The release of catecholamine alerts the patient to take the required measures to prevent coma due to low blood glucose. The absence of warning signs of impending neuroglycopenia is known as **hypoglycemic unawareness**. Hypoglycemic unawareness should not, however, be used as a criterion to make the diagnosis of autonomic neuropathy because it may also occur in diabetes as a result of improved glycemic control in conjunction with recurrent antecedent hypoglycemia. The combined autonomic deficit in heart rate and blood pressure responses to standing is associated with a modest increase in the risk of severe spontaneous hypoglycemia.[119]

Treatment

Patients with hypoglycemia unawareness and unresponsiveness pose a significant management problem for the physician. Although autonomic neuropathy may improve with intensive therapy and normalization of blood glucose, there is a risk to the patient, who may become hypoglycemic without being aware of it and who cannot mount a counterregulatory response. It is our recommendation that if a pump is used, boluses of smaller than calculated amounts should be used; if intensive conventional therapy is used, long-acting insulin with smaller boluses should be given. One should be cautious about attempting to aim for normal glucose and HbA$_{1c}$ levels in these patients and take care to avoid the possibility of hypoglycemia.[120] A remarkable reduction in the frequency of severe hypoglycemia can be achieved with hypoglycemia awareness training.[121]

PUPILLARY ABNORMALITIES

The pupillary iris is dually innervated by parasympathetic and sympathetic fibers. Parasympathetic fibers mediate pupillary constriction, whereas sympathetic fibers mediate pupillary dilation. The sympathetic fibers are most often regulated by changes in arousal, whereas the parasympathetic fibers are activated mainly by change in light intensity. Patients with DAN show delayed or absent reflex response to light and diminished hippus, accounted for by decreased sympathetic activity and a reduced resting pupillary diameter. Autonomic neuropathy of the pupil is often apparent on routine eye examination but can be confirmed by more sophisticated testing using a pupillometer.[122]

Treatment

The pupillary abnormalities do not tend to produce any significant functional defect, except for potential failure of dark adaptation and difficulty with driving at night. Patients should therefore be warned about driving at night.[123]

RESPIRATORY DYSFUNCTION

Respiratory reflexes may be impaired in diabetic patients with autonomic neuropathy. Ventilatory responses to hypoxia and hypercapnia are reduced in DAN.[124] Parasympathetic dysfunction can cause reduced airway tone. Obstructive sleep apnea is more prevalent in diabetic patients with autonomic neuropathy than in those without.[125] Nasal continuous positive airway pressure is an effective therapy for obstructive sleep apnea syndrome.[126] A temporal relationship between sudden cardiac arrest and interference with normal respiration by hypoxia, drugs, or anesthesia has been reported.[124] Sudden cardiopulmonary arrest in diabetic patients with cardiac autonomic neuropathy may be of respiratory origin due to loss of hypoxic respiratory drive.

DEAD IN BED

The undetected autonomic dysfunction, when associated with nocturnal hypoglycemia, may predispose T1DM patients to fatal ventricular dysrhythmia constituting the **dead in bed syndrome**.[127] Possible mechanisms of sudden death are silent ischemia, prolonged QT interval predisposing to ventricular arrhythmias, or abnormal central control of breathing.

SUMMARY

DAN is an extremely important clinical disorder. Although involvement of the ANS is generally diffuse, symptoms may be confined to a single target organ or organ system. Complications affecting these systems contribute greatly to the morbidity, mortality, and reduced quality of life and activities of daily living of the person with diabetes. They are also the major source of increased costs of caring for the diabetic patient. Factors in the pathogenesis are metabolism, vascular insufficiency, loss of growth factor trophism, and autoimmune destruction of nerves in a visceral and cutaneous distribution. We have reviewed the variety of clinical manifestations associated with autonomic neuropathy and have discussed current views related to the symptomatic management of the different abnormalities. Our ability to manage the many different manifestations of DAN successfully depends ultimately on our success in uncovering the pathogenetic processes underlying this disorder and directing therapies at the cause rather than the manifestations. There are also studies in progress suggesting that autonomic nerves can be induced to regenerate, and the future for patients with DAN is less bleak than hithertofore perceived.

REFERENCES

1. Vinik AI, Mitchell BD, Leichter SB, *et al*: Epidemiology of the complications of diabetes. In: Leslie RDG, Robbins DC, eds. *Diabetes: Clinical Science in Practice*. Cambridge University Press;1995:221.
2. Pfeifer MA, Weinberg CR, Cook DL, *et al*: Autonomic neural dysfunction in recently diagnosed diabetic subjects. *Diabetes Care* 1984; 7:447.
3. Neil HAW, Thompson AV, John S, *et al*: Diabetic autonomic neuropathy: the prevalence of impaired heart rate variability in a geographically defined population. *Diabetes Med* 1989;6:20.
4. Ziegler D, Gries FA, Muhlen H, *et al*: Prevalence and clinical correlates of cardiovascular autonomic and peripheral diabetic neuropathy in patients attending diabetes center. The DiaCAN Multicenter Study Group. *Diabete Metab* 1993;19:143.
5. Tesfaye S, Kempler P, Stevens L, *et al*: Prevalence of autonomic neuropathy and potential risk factors in type 1 diabetes in Europe. *Diabetes* 1998;47:A0518.
6. Cohen JA, Jeffers BW, Faldut D, *et al*: Risks for sensorimotor peripheral neuropathy and autonomic neuropathy in non-insulin-dependent diabetes mellitus (NIDDM). *Muscle Nerve* 1998;21:72.
7. Gottsater A, Ahmed M, Fernlund P, *et al*: Autonomic neuropathy in Type 2 diabetic patients is associated with hyperinsulinemia and hypertriglyceridemia. *Diabetic Med* 1999;16:49.
8. Toyry JP, Niskanen LK, Mantysaari MJ, *et al*: Do high proinsulin and C-peptide levels play a role in autonomic nervous dysfunction? Power spectral analysis in patients with non-insulin-dependent diabetes and nondiabetic subjects. *Circulation* 1997;96:1185.
9. Ewing DJ, Boland O, Neilson JM, *et al*: Autonomic neuropathy, QT interval lengthening, and unexpected deaths in male diabetic patients. *Diabetologia* 1991; 34:182.
10. Rathmann W, Ziegler D, Jahnke M, *et al*: Mortality in diabetic patients with cardiovascular autonomic neuropathy. *Diabetic Med* 1993; 10:820.
11. Levitt NS, Stansberry KB, Wynchank S, *et al*: The natural progression of autonomic neuropathy and autonomic function tests in a cohort of people with IDDM. *Diabetes Care* 1996;19:751.
12. Gonin JM, Kadrofske MM, Schmaltz S, *et al*: Corrected Q-T interval prolongation as diagnostic tool for assessment of cardiac autonomic neuropathy in diabetes mellitus. *Diabetes Care* 1990;13:68.
13. Kahn JK, Sisson JC, Vinik AI: Prediction of sudden cardiac death in diabetic autonomic neuropathy. *J Nucl Med* 1988;29:1605.
14. O'Brian IA, McFadden JP, Corrall R: The influence of autonomic neuropathy on mortality in insulin-dependent diabetes. *Q J Med* 1991; 79:495.
15. Vinik AI, Leichter SB, Pittenger GL, *et al*: Phospholipid and glutamic acid decarboxylase autoantibodies in diabetic neuropathy. *Diabetes Care* 1995;18:1225.
16. Vinik AI, Park TS, Stansberry KB, *et al*: Diabetic neuropathies. *Diabetologia* 2000;43:957.
17. Brownlee M: Lilly Lecture 1993. Glycation and diabetic complications. *Diabetes* 1994;43:836.
18. Wolff SP, Jiang ZY, Hunt JV: Protein glycation and oxidative stress in diabetes mellitus and ageing. *Free Radic Biol Med* 199;10:339.
19. Williamson JR, Chang K, Frangos M, *et al*: Hyperglycemic pseudo-hypoxia and diabetic complications. *Diabetes* 1993;42:801.
20. Ejskjaer N, Arift S, Dodds W, *et al*: Prevalence of autoantibodies to autonomic nervous tissue structures in Type 1 diabetes mellitus. *Diabetic Med* 1999;16:544.
21. Pittenger GL, Liu D, Vinik AI: The apoptotic death of neuroblastoma cells caused by serum from patients with insulin-dependent diabetes and neuropathy may be Fas-mediated. *J Neuroimmunol* 1997;76:153.
22. Pittenger GL, Liu D, Vinik AI: The toxic effects of serum from patients with type I diabetes mellitus on mouse neuroblastoma cells: a new mechanism for development of diabetic autonomic neuropathy. *Diabetic Med* 1993;10:925.
23. Pittenger GL, Liu D, Vinik AI: The neuronal toxic factor in serum of type 1 diabetic patients is a complement-fixing autoantibody. *Diabetic Med* 1995;12:380.
24. Zanone MM, Banga JP, Peakman M, *et al*: An investigation of antibodies to nerve growth factor in diabetic autonomic neuropathy. *Diabetic Med* 1994;11:378.
25. Schumer MP, Joyner SA, Pfeifer MA: Cardiovascular autonomic neuropathy testing in patients with diabetes. *Diabetes Spectrum* 1988;11: 227.
26. Zola B, Kahn JK, Juni JE, *et al*: Abnormal cardiac function in diabetic patients with autonomic neuropathy in the absence of ischemic heart disease. *J Clin Endocrinol Metab* 1986;63:208.
27. Vinik AI, Suwanwalaikorn S: Autonomic neuropathy. In: deFronzo R, ed. *Current Therapy of Diabetes Mellitus*. Mosby-Year Book:1997; 165.
28. Vinik AI, Glass LC: Diabetic autonomic Neuropathy. In: Davidson JK, ed. *Clinical Diabetes Mellitus: A Problem-Oriented Approach*, 3rd ed. Thieme:1999;637.
29. The Diabetes Control and Complications Trial Research Group: The effect of intensive diabetes therapy on the development and progression of neuropathy. *Ann Intern Med* 1995;122:561.
30. The Diabetes Control and Complications Trial Research Group: The effect of intensive diabetes therapy on measures of autonomic nervous system function in the Diabetes Control and Complications Trial. *Diabetologia* 1998;41:416.
31. Risk M, Bril V, Broadbridge C, *et al*: Heart rate variability measurement in diabetic neuropathy: review of methods. Diabetes Technol Ther 2001;3:63.
32. Purewal TS, Watkins PJ: Postural hypotension in diabetic neuropathy: a review. *Diabetic Med* 1995;12:192.
33. Storstein L, Jervell J: Response to bicycle exercise testing in long-standing juvenile diabetics. *Acta Med Scand* 1979;205:2227.

34. Burgos LG, Ebert TJ, Asiddao C, *et al*: Increased intraoperative cardiovascular morbidity in diabetics with autonomic neuropathy. *Anaesthesiology* 1989;70:591.

35. Langer A, Freeman MR, Josse RG, *et al*: Detection of silent myocardial ischemia in diabetes mellitus. *Am J Cardiol* 1991;67:1073.

36. Turpeinen AK, Vanninen E, Kuikka JT, *et al*: Demonstration of regional sympathetic denervation of the heart in diabetes. Comparison between patients with NIDDM and IDDM. *Diabetes Care* 1999; 19:1083.

37. May O, Arildsen H, Damsgaard EM: Cardiovascular autonomic neuropathy in insulin-dependent diabetes mellitus: prevalence and estimated risk of coronary heart disease in the general population. *J Intern Med* 2000;248:483.

38. Ziegler D: Cardiovascular autonomic neuropathy: clinical manifestations and measurement. *Diabetes Rev* 1999;7: 342.

39. Toyry JP, Niskanen LK, Mantysaari MT, *et al*: Occurrence, predictors, and clinical significance of autonomic neuropathy in NIDDM. Ten-year follow-up from the diagnosis. *Diabetes* 1996;45:308.

40. Toyry JP, Niskanen LK, Lansimies EA, *et al*: Autonomic neuropathy predicts the development of stroke in patients with non-insulin-dependent diabetes mellitus. *Stroke* 1996;27:1316.

41. Ziegler D, Laux G, Dannehl K, *et al*: Assessment of cardiovascular autonomic function: age-related normal ranges and reproducibility of spectral analysis, vector analysis, and standard tests of heart rate variation and blood pressure responses. *Diabetic Med* 1992;9:166.

42. Kahn JK, Zola B, Juni JE, *et al*: Radionuclide assessment of left ventricular diastolic filling in diabetes mellitus with and without cardiac autonomic neuropathy. *J Am Coll Cardiol* 1986;7:1303.

43. Airaksinen KEJ, Koistinen MJ: Association between silent coronary artery disease, diabetes, and autonomic neuropathy: fact or fallacy? *Diabetes Care* 1992;15:288.

44. Marchant B, Umachandran V, Stevenson R, *et al*: Silent myocardial ischemia: role of subclinical neuropathy in patients with and without diabetes. *J Am Coll Cardiol* 1993;22:1433.

45. Carli MF, Bianco-Batlles D, Landa ME, *et al*: Effects of autonomic neuropathy on coronary blood flow in patients with diabetes mellitus. *Circulation* 1999;100:813.

46. Morning peak in the incidence of myocardial infarction: experience in the ISIS-2 trial. ISIS-2 (Second International Study of Infarct Survival) Collaborative Group. *Eur Heart J* 1992;13:594.

47. Aronson D, Weinrauch LA, D'Elia JA, *et al*: Circadian patterns of heart rate variability, fibrinolytic activity, and hemostatic factors in type I diabetes mellitus with cardiac autonomic neuropathy. *Am J Cardiol* 1999;84:449.

48. Veglio M, Borra M, Stevens LK, *et al*, and the EURODIAB IDDM Complications Study Group: The relation between QTc interval prolongation and diabetic complications. *Diabetologia* 1999;42:68.

49. Sawicki PT, Dahne R, Bender R, *et al*: Prolonged QT interval as a predictor of mortality in diabetic nephropathy. *Diabetologia* 1996;39:77.

50. Sawicki PT, Kiwitt S, Bender R, *et al*: The value of QT interval dispersion for identification of total mortality risk in non-insulin-dependent diabetes mellitus. *J Intern Med* 1998;243:49.

51. Stevens MJ, Dayanikli F, Raffel DM, *et al*: Scintigraphic assessment of regionalized defects in myocardial sympathetic innervation and blood flow regulation in diabetic patients with autonomic neuropathy. *J Am Coll Cardiol* 1998;31:1575.

52. Stevens MJ, Raffel DM, Allman KC, *et al*: Cardiac sympathetic dysinnervation in diabetes: implications for enhanced cardiovascular risk. *Circulation* 1998;98:961.

53. Timolol-induced reduction in mortality and reinfarction in patients surviving acute myocardial infarction. *N Engl J Med* 1981;304: 801.

54. Gundersen T: Secondary prevention after myocardial infarction: subgroup analysis of patients at risk in the Norwegian Timolol Multicenter Study. *Clin Cardiol* 1985;8:253.

55. Kahn R: Proceedings of consensus development conference on standardized measures in diabetic neuropathy. Autonomic nervous system testing. *Diabetes Care* 1992;15:1095.

56. Consensus statement report and recommendation of the San Antonio Conference on diabetic neuropathy. *Diabetes* 1988;37:1000.

57. Bigger JT Jr, Fleiss JL, Steinman RC, *et al*: Frequency domain measures of heart period variability and mortality after myocardial infarction. *Circulation* 1992;85:164.

58. Fava S, Azzopardi J, Muscat HA, *et al*: Factors that influence outcome in diabetic subjects with myocardial infarction. *Diabetes Care* 1993; 16:1615.

59. Ziegler D, Weise F, Langen KJ, *et al*: Effect of glycaemic control on myocardial sympathetic innervations assessed by [^{123}I] metaiodobenzylguanidine scintigraphy: a 4-year prospective study in IDDM patients. *Diabetologia* 1998;41:443.

60. Mantysaari M, Kuikka J, Mustonen J, *et al*: Noninvasive detection of cardiac sympathetic nervous dysfunction in diabetic patients using [^{123}I] metaiodobenzylguanidine. *Diabetes* 1992;41:1069.

61. Schnell O, Muhr D, Weiss M, *et al*: Reduced myocardial ^{123}I-metaiodobenzylguanidine uptake in newly diagnosed IDDM patients. *Diabetes* 1996;45:801.

62. Kreiner G, Wolzt M, Fasching P, *et al*: Myocardial I^{123} meta-iodobenzylguanidine scintigraphy for the assessment of adrenergic cardiac innervation in patients with IDDM. Comparison with cardiovascular reflex tests and relationship to left ventricular function. *Diabetes* 1995; 44:543.

63. Stevens MJ, Raffel DM, Allman KC, *et al*: Cardiac sympathetic dysinnervation in diabetes: implications for enhanced cardiovascular risk. *Circulation* 1998;98:961.

64. Burger AJ, Weinrauch LA, D'Elia JA, *et al*: Effect of glycemic control on heart rate variability in type I diabetic patients with cardiac autonomic neuropathy. *Am J Cardiol* 1999;84:687.

65. Ohkubo Y, Kishikawa H, Araki E, *et al*: Intensive insulin therapy prevents the progression of diabetic microvascular complications in Japanese patients with non-insulin-dependent diabetes mellitus: a randomized prospective 6-year study. *Diabetes Res Clin Pract* 1995;28: 103.

66. Stevens MJ, Raffel DM, Allman KC, *et al*: Regression and progression of cardiac sympathetic dysinnervation complicating diabetes: an assessment by C-11 hydroxyephedrine and positron emission tomography. *Metabolism* 1999;48:92.

67. Gaede P, Vedel P, Parving HH, *et al*: Intensified multifactorial intervention in patients with type 2 diabetes mellitus and microalbuminuria: the Steno type 2 randomised study. *Lancet* 1999;353:617.

68. Kontopoulos AG, Athyros VG, Didangelos TP, *et al*: Effect of chronic quinapril administration on heart rate variability in patients with diabetic autonomic neuropathy. *Diabetes Care* 1997;20:355.

69. Rationale and design of a large study to evaluate the renal and cardiovascular effects of an ACE inhibitor and vitamin E in high-risk patients with diabetes. The MICRO-HOPE Study. Microalbuminuria, cardiovascular, and renal outcomes. Heart Outcomes Prevention Evaluation. *Diabetes Care* 1996;19:1225.

70. Effects of ramipril on cardiovascular and microvascular outcomes in people with diabetes mellitus: results of the HOPE study and MICRO-HOPE substudy. Heart Outcomes Prevention Evaluation Study Investigators. *Lancet* 2000;355:253.

71. Ziegler D, Schatz H, Conrad F, *et al*: Effects of treatment with the antioxidant alpha-lipoic acid on cardiac autonomic neuropathy in NIDDM patients. A 4-month randomized controlled multicenter trial (DEKAN Study). *Diabetes Care* 1997;20:369.

72. Ikeda T, Iwata K, Tanaka Y: Long-term effect of epalrestat on cardiac autonomic neuropathy in subjects with non-insulin dependent diabetes mellitus. *Diabetes Res Clin Pract* 1999;43:193.

73. Howorka K, Pumprla J, Haber P, *et al*: Effects of physical training on heart rate variability in diabetic patients with various degrees of cardiovascular autonomic neuropathy. *Cardiovasc Res* 1997;34:206.

74. Johansson BL, Borg K, Fernqvist-Forbes E, *et al*: Beneficial effects of C-peptide on incipient nephropathy and neuropathy in patients with Type 1 diabetes mellitus. *Diabetic Med* 2000;17:181.

75. Hansen KW: Diurnal blood pressure profile, autonomic neuropathy and nephropathy in diabetes. *Eur J Endocrinol* 1997;136:35.

76. Low PA: Autonomic neuropathies. *Curr Opin Neurol* 1998;11:531.

77. Shannon JR, Flattem NL, Jordan J, *et al*: Orthostatic intolerance and tachycardia associated with norepinephrine-transporter deficiency. *N Engl J Med* 2000;342:541.

78. Hoeldtke RD, Horvath GG, Bryner KD: Treatment of orthostatic tachycardia with erythropoietin. *Am J Med* 1995;99:525.

79. Makimatila S, Mantysaari M, Schlenzka A, *et al*: Mechanism of altered hemodynamic and metabolic responses to insulin in patients with insulin-dependent diabetes mellitus and autonomic dysfunction. *J Clin Endocrinol Metab* 1998;83:468.

80. Hoeldtke RD, Horvath GG, Bryner KD, et al: Treatment of orthostatic hypotension with midodrine and octreotide. *J Clin Endocrinol Metab* 1998;83:339.

81. Hoeldtke RD, Dworkin GE, Gaspar SR, et al: Effect of the somatostatin analogue SMS-201-995 on the adrenergic response to glucose ingestion in patients with postprandial hypotension. *Am J Med* 1989; 86:673.

82. Horowitz M, Edelbroek MA, Wishart JM, et al: Relationship between oral glucose tolerance and gastric emptying in normal healthy subjects. *Diabetologia* 1993;36:857.

83. Feldman M, Schiller LR: Disorders of gastrointestinal motility associated with diabetes mellitus. *Ann Intern Med* 1983;98:378.

84. Maleki D, Loche R, Camilleri M, et al: Gastrointestinal tract symptoms among persons with diabetes mellitus in the community. *Arch Intern Med* 2000;160:2808.

85. Clouse RE, Lustman PJ: Gastrointestinal symptoms in diabetic patients: lack of association with neuropathy. *Am J Gastroenterol* 1989; 84:868.

86. Sundkvist G, Hillcarp B, Lilja B, et al: Esophageal motor function evaluated by scintigraphy, video-radiography, and manometry in diabetic patients. *Acta Radiol* 1989;30:17.

87. Lehmann R, Borovicka J, Kunz P, et al: Evaluation of delayed gastric emptying in diabetic patients with autonomic neuropathy by a new magnetic resonance imaging technique and radio-opaque markers. *Diabetes Care* 1996;19:1075.

88. Rayner CK, Samsom M, Jones KL, et al: Relationships of upper gastrointestinal motor and sensory function with glycemic control. *Diabetes Care* 2001;24;371.

89. Horowitz M, Edelbroek M, Fraser R, et al: Disordered gastric motor function in diabetes mellitus. Recent insights into prevalence, pathophysiology, clinical relevance and treatment. *Scand J Gastroenterol* 1991;26:673.

90. Ziegler D, Schadewaldt P, Pour Mirza A, et al: [^{13}C]octanoic acid breath test for non-invasive assessment of gastric emptying in diabetic patients: validation and relationship to gastric symptoms and cardiovascular autonomic function. *Diabetologia* 1996;39:823.

91. Weber FH, McCallum RW: Gastric motor disorders. In: Snape WJ Jr, ed. *Consultations in Gastroenterology*. Saunders:1996;247.

92. Janssens J, Peeters TL, Vantrappen G, et al: Improvement of gastric emptying in diabetic gastroparesis by erythromycin. Preliminary studies. *N Engl J Med* 1990;322:1028.

93. Erbas T, Varoglu E, Erbas B, et al: Comparison of metoclopramide and erythromycin in the treatment of diabetic gastroparesis. *Diabetes Care* 1993;16:1511.

94. Jacober SJ, Narayan A, Strodel WE, et al: Jejunostomy feeding in the management of gastroparesis diabeticorum. *Diabetes Care* 1986; 9:217.

95. Ejskjaer NT, Bradley JL, Buxton-Thomas MS, et al: Novel surgical treatment and gastric pathology in diabetic gastroparesis. *Diabetic Med* 1999;16:488.

96. Lysy J, Israeli E, Goldin E: The prevalence of chronic diarrhea among diabetic patients. *Am J Gastroenterol* 1999;94:2165.

97. Tsai ST, Vinik AI, Brunner JF: Diabetic diarrhea and somatostatin. *Ann Intern Med* 1986;104:894.

98. Battle WM, Snape WJ Jr, Alavi A, et al: Colonic dysfunction in diabetes mellitus. *Gastroenterology* 1980;79:1217.

99. Mc Culloch DK, Campbell IW, Wu FC, et al: The prevalence of diabetic impotence. *Diabetologia* 1980;18:279.

100. Vinik A, Erbas T, Stansberry K: Gastrointestinal, genitourinary, and neurovascular disturbances in diabetes. *Diabetes Rev* 1999;7; 358.

101. Rendell MS, Rajfer J, Wicker PA, et al: Sildenafil for treatment of erectile dysfunction in men with diabetes: a randomized controlled trial. Sildenafil Diabetes Study Group. *JAMA* 1999;2815:421.

102. Enzlin P, Mathieu C, Vanderschueren, et al: Diabetes mellitus and female sexuality: a review of 25 years' research. *Diabetic Med* 1998; 15:809.

103. Stansberry KB, Shapiro SA, Hill MA, et al: Impaired peripheral vasomotion in diabetes. *Diabetes Care* 1996;19:715.

104. Stansberry KB, Shapiro SA, Hill MA, et al: Impairment of peripheral blood flow responses in diabetes resembles an enhanced aging effect. *Diabetes Care* 1997;20:1711.

105. Stansberry KB, Peppard HR, Babyak LM, et al: Primary nociceptive afferents mediate the blood flow dysfunction in non-glabrous (hairy) skin of type 2 diabetes. A new model for the pathogenesis of microvascular dysfunction. *Diabetes Care* 1999;22:1549.

106. Young MJ, Marshall A, Adams JE, et al: Osteopenia, neurological dysfunction, and the development of Charcot neuroarthropathy. *Diabetes Care* 1995;18:34.

107. Gough A, Abraha H, Li F, et al: Measurement of markers of osteoclast and osteoblast activity in patients with acute and chronic diabetic Charcot neuroarthropathy. *Diabetic Med* 1997;14:527.

108. Childs M, Armstrong DG, Edelson GW: Is Charcot arthropathy a late sequela of osteoporosis in patients with diabetes mellitus? *J Foot Ankle Surg* 1998;37:437.

109. Grant WP, Sullivan R, Sonenshine DE, et al: Electron microscopic investigation of the effects of diabetes mellitus on the Achilles tendon. *J Foot Ankle Surg* 1997;36:272.

110. Shapiro SA, Stansberry KB, Hill MA, et al: Normal blood flow response and vasomotion in the diabetic Charcot foot. *J Diabetes Complications* 1998;12:147.

111. Bennett GS, Garrett NE, Diemel LT, et al: Neurogenic cutaneous vasodilatation and plasma extravasation in diabetic rats: effect of insulin and nerve growth factor. *Br J Pharmacol* 1998;124:1573.

112. Kihara M, Schmelzer JD, Low PA: Effect of cilostazol on experimental diabetic neuropathy in the rat. *Diabetologia* 1995;38:914.

113. Rendell M, Bamisedun O: Skin blood flow and current perception in pentoxifylline-treated diabetic neuropathy. *Angiology* 1992;43:843.

114. Giugliano D, Marfella R, Acampora R, et al: Effects of perindopril and carvedilol on endothelium-dependent vascular functions in patients with diabetes and hypertension. *Diabetes Care* 1998;21:631.

115. Fujishima S, Ohya Y, Nakamura Y, et al: Troglitazone, an insulin sensitizer, increases forearm blood flow in humans. *Am J Hypertens* 1998;11:1134.

116. Shaw JE, Parker R, Hollis S, et al: Gustatory sweating in diabetes mellitus. *Diabetic Med* 1996;13:1033.

117. Shaw JE, Abbott CA, Tindle K, et al: A randomized controlled trial of topical glycopyrrolate, the first specific treatment for diabetic gustatory sweating. *Diabetologia* 1997;40:299.

118. Heckmann M, Ceballos-Baumann AO, Plewig G: Botulinum toxin A for axillary hyperhidrosis (excessive sweating). *N Engl J Med* 2001; 344:488.

119. Stephenson JM, Kempler P, Perin PC, et al: Is autonomic neuropathy a risk factor for severe hypoglycaemia? The EURODIAB IDDM Complications Study. *Diabetologia* 1996;39:1372.

120. Vinik AI: Diagnosis and management of diabetic neuropathy. *Clin Geriatr Med* 1999;15:293.

121. Cox DJ, Gonder-Frederick LA, Kovatchev BP, et al: Biopsychobehavioral model of severe hypoglycemia. II. Understanding the risk of severe hypoglycemia. *Diabetes Care* 1999;22:2018.

122. Karachaliou F, Karavanaki K, Greenwood R, et al.: Consistency of pupillary abnormality in children and adolescents with diabetes. *Diabetic Med* 1997;14:849.

123. Hreidarsson AB, Gundersen HJ: Reduced pupillary unrest. Autonomic nervous system abnormality in diabetes mellitus. *Diabetes* 1988;37:446.

124. Sobotka PA, Liss HP, Vinik AI: Impaired hypoxic ventilatory drive in diabetic patients with autonomic neuropathy. *J Clin Endocrinol Metab* 1986;62:658.

125. Ficker JH, Dertinger SH, Siegfried W, et al: Obstructive sleep apnoea and diabetes mellitus: the role of cardiovascular autonomic neuropathy. *Eur Respir J* 1998;11:14.

126. Veale D, Chailleux E, Hoorelbeke-Ramon A, et al: Mortality of sleep apnoea patients treated by nasal continuous positive airway pressure registered in the ANTADIR observatory. *Eur Respir J* 2000;15:326.

127. Weston PJ, Gill GV: Is undetected autonomic dysfunction responsible for sudden death in Type 1 diabetes mellitus? The 'dead in bed' syndrome revisited. *Diabetic Med* 1999;16:626.

Diabetic Dyslipidemia: Pathophysiology and Treatment

Clay F. Semenkovich

For people with both type 1 and type 2 diabetes mellitus (T1DM and T2DM), the risk of premature death due to atherosclerosis is considerable. Atherosclerosis and its complications account for about 80% of mortality in diabetes. Dyslipidemia is common in diabetic patients and is probably a major contributor to the initiation and propagation of atherosclerotic lesions in these patients. Because of poorly understood interactions between the diabetic state and dyslipidemia, the effects of disturbances in circulating lipid levels are amplified in diabetes. Even modest abnormalities of circulating lipoproteins in diabetics disproportionately increase vascular risk. Since diabetic patients without known coronary artery disease appear to have the same risk for myocardial infarction as nondiabetic patients with previous myocardial infarction,[1] an aggressive approach to lipid management should be considered in every patient with diabetes.

EPIDEMIOLOGY

In poorly controlled T1- and T2DM, patients have elevated levels of triglycerides, low levels of high-density lipoprotein (HDL) cholesterol, and changes in the composition of low-density lipoprotein (LDL) cholesterol that may substantially enhance the atherogenic potential of this particle.

Regardless of the type of diabetes, the hallmark of diabetic dyslipidemia is hypertriglyceridemia. In a compilation of studies comparing mean lipid levels from treated diabetic patients with those from controls matched for age and weight,[2] plasma triglyceride levels were increased in both T1- and T2 DM, and HDL cholesterol was decreased in people with T2DM (Fig. 47-1). In the World Health Organization (WHO) multinational study,[3] serum triglyceride concentrations were related to macrovascular risk using five national sample sets. Triglycerides were more strongly associated with ischemic heart disease than cholesterol. Data from the Multiple Risk Factor Intervention Trial[4] and the Paris Prospective Study[5] also indicate that triglyceride levels better predict vascular risk than total or LDL cholesterol in diabetes. Triglyceride levels increase and HDL cholesterol levels decrease continuously as glucose intolerance increases in nondiabetic cohorts.[6] These data suggest that dyslipidemia predating the development of overt T2DM contributes to the high frequency of coronary heart disease present in these patients at the time of initial diagnosis.

In 1979, the Framingham Study first reported that premenopausal women with diabetes have the same risk for vascular disease as diabetic men,[7] suggesting that the protective effect of being female with respect to heart disease is negated by diabetes.

This observation has been confirmed in economically and racially diverse populations ranging from Evans County, Georgia,[8] to Rancho Bernardo, California.[9] Over the past 30 years, coronary heart disease mortality in the United States has declined for the general population but not for women with diabetes. Recent data from National Health and Nutrition Examination Surveys show that age-adjusted heart disease mortality has declined 27% for nondiabetic women but increased 23% in diabetic women.[10] Smaller declines in mortality were seen for diabetic compared with nondiabetic men.

The poor prognosis for women with diabetes may be explained in part by the effects of diabetes on dyslipidemia in women. The Prospective Cardiovascular Munster study (PROCAM), involving over 50,000 German men and women, reported that diabetic women were more likely than diabetic men to manifest dyslipidemia, especially low HDL cholesterol.[11] The Strong Heart Study is a population-based study of vascular disease that includes over 1400 females and over 800 males with diabetes. In this group, diabetic women compared with their male counterparts had greater decreases in HDL cholesterol and apolipoprotein A1 (apoA1; the major protein component of HDL particles), greater increases in apolipoprotein B (apoB; the major protein component of atherogenic lipoproteins like very-low-density lipoprotein [VLDL], intermediate-density lipoprotein [IDL], and LDL), and greater decreases in the size of LDL particles.[12]

The composition of LDL particles is frequently abnormal in people with diabetes. The most commonly described abnormality is small, dense LDL, a particle that may be particularly atherogenic. In case-control studies of nondiabetics from the Stanford Five-City Project[13] and the Physicians' Health Study,[14] small, dense LDL was shown to be associated with coronary artery disease. The presence of the small LDL phenotype is inversely related to triglyceride levels. Patients with T2DM and insulin resistance have a preponderance of small, dense LDL. T1DM subjects from the Pittsburgh Epidemiology of Diabetes Complications Study[15] and the Diabetes Control and Complications Trial (DCCT)[16] had an increased frequency of the small, dense LDL phenotype, especially in the setting of renal dysfunction.

Although LDL cholesterol levels are usually not classified as elevated in people with diabetes, these "normal" LDL cholesterol levels should be considered elevated given the effects of modest hyperlipidemia in the setting of diabetes. The mean LDL cholesterol level was 109 mg/dL for people with T2DM in the Strong Heart Study. Even at these low levels, LDL cholesterol was a significant independent predictor of vascular disease, with risk increasing linearly from an LDL cholesterol concentration of 70 mg/dL.[17] In the United Kingdom Prospective Diabetes Study (UKPDS),

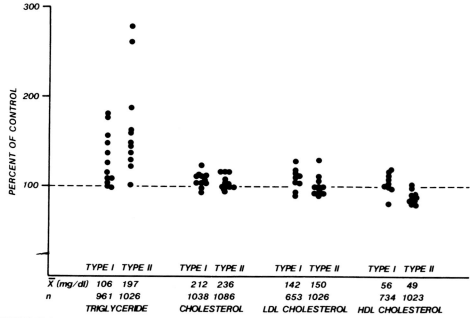

FIGURE 47-1. Plasma lipid levels in treated type 1 and type 2 diabetic patients. Values were obtained from 22 different studies in which age- and weight-matched diabetics were compared with a control group. Each point represents mean values of diabetics divided by mean values of controls. *(Reproduced with permission from Kern.[2])*

the mean LDL cholesterol level was 128 mg/dL for men and 147 mg/dL for women. Even at these relatively "normal" levels, LDL cholesterol was a powerful predictor of coronary artery disease in UKPDS.[18]

GLYCEMIC CONTROL AND DYSLIPIDEMIA

Poor glucose control clearly exacerbates dyslipidemia. Improved glycemic control in both T1- and T2DM improves dyslipidemia. However, most of the improvement in lipid levels occurs after early routine measures to improve diabetic control rather than later after intensive adjustment of hypoglycemic medications.

Glucose promotes hepatic lipogenesis. Since the flux of glucose through the liver is increased in T2DM, glucose alone can increase lipid content and promote dyslipidemia. Glucose can also modify lipoproteins. Like hemoglobin, which becomes glycosylated to form a marker for chronic glycemic control, components of lipoproteins like apoB can become glycosylated. Because the extent of glycosylation is determined by circulating glucose concentrations, it is not surprising that more apoB molecules are glycosylated in LDL from subjects with diabetes compared with nondiabetics. Advanced glycation end products are also found in lipoproteins from people with diabetes.[19] These compositional changes interfere with the clearance of LDL by the LDL receptor and prolong its residence time in the circulation. Glycoxidation of LDL in the vessel wall may contribute to atherogenesis[19] (see Chap. 11).

Type 1 Diabetes Mellitus

In a typical population of 212 people with T1DM treated with conventional therapy, a 1% decrease in glycosylated hemoglobin was associated with an 8% decrease in triglycerides.[20] Ideal therapy of patients with T1DM includes multiple daily injections of insulin or the use of a continuous subcutaneous infusion of in-

sulin. Institution of such therapy lowers triglycerides with near normalization of glucose levels. Changes in LDL and HDL levels are more variable.

In the DCCT, intensive diabetes therapy was associated with a decrease in the incidence of retinopathy, nephropathy, and neuropathy. Intensive therapy was also associated with a decreased incidence of hypercholesterolemia, defined as an LDL cholesterol over 160 mg/dL.[21] Triglyceride levels as well as LDL cholesterol levels were lower with intensive therapy, but HDL cholesterol did not increase.[22] The intensive therapy group manifested other potentially beneficial lipoprotein changes including a decrease in IDL, small, dense LDL, and lipoprotein(a) [Lp(a)].[23] However, weight gain was more common in the intensive therapy group. Patients who experienced the most weight gain with intensive therapy also had more IDL, more dense LDL, and lower concentrations of HDL cholesterol, adverse lipoprotein changes that would be predicted to increase coronary artery risk.[24] These data suggest that intensive insulin therapy alone, at least with current technologies, does not optimally decrease the vascular risk associated with diabetic dyslipidemia in T1DM patients.

Type 2 Diabetes Mellitus

Evaluating the effects of glycemic control on plasma lipoproteins in patients with T2DM is difficult because of the heterogeneous therapeutic approaches to this disease. Substantial effects on dyslipidemia are usually seen when therapy is initiated, regardless of the type of therapy. In previously treated patients for whom new therapies are added, lipoprotein effects are more modest.

Weight loss (as little as 5 kg in some studies) achieved by diet and exercise improves dyslipidemia in patients with T2DM and impaired glucose tolerance.[25,26] T2DM patients gain weight when either sulfonylurea or insulin therapy is initiated. Despite this weight gain, triglycerides decrease and HDL cholesterol increases as glucose levels fall. Acarbose, an α-glucosidase inhibitor that lowers glucose by inhibiting carbohydrate metabolism in the intestine, has been shown to improve triglyceride metabolism.[27]

There are currently two classes of insulin-sensitizing agents, biguanides and the thiazolidinediones. Both have favorable effects on dyslipidemia. These beneficial effects on lipoprotein metabolism may be greater than those seen with sufonylurea therapy because both classes of drugs decrease insulin resistance and insulin concentrations in addition to lowering glucose.

Metformin, a biguanide, has been available for use in the United States since 1995. The molecular mechanism of action for this drug is unknown, but metformin is known to decrease hepatic glucose output, promote insulin-mediated glucose disposal, and decrease fatty acid oxidation, all reflecting improved insulin sensitivity. Metformin decreases triglycerides[28] and may increase HDL cholesterol. Unlike insulin, sulfonylureas, and thiazolidenediones, metformin causes these improvements in dyslipidemia without causing weight gain. Adipose mass may actually decrease in some patients.[29]

Thiazolidenediones include troglitazone, rosiglitazone, and pioglitazone. These drugs are ligands for peroxisome proliferator-activated receptor (PPAR)γ, a nuclear receptor that activates gene transcription, particularly in adipose tissue and macrophages. The most clinical data are available for troglitazone, although this drug was removed from the market in 2000. In insulin-treated patients, the addition of troglitazone has little effect on diabetic dyslipidemia.[30] When used as monotherapy even at low doses, troglitazone causes considerable decreases in triglyceride levels in T2DM but increases LDL levels.[31] Fewer data are available for the other thiazolidenediones, but both compounds lower triglycerides in animals.[32,33] One disadvantage of these compounds is that they can cause striking weight gain (see Chap. 32).

PATHOPHYSIOLOGY

The mechanisms underlying lipoprotein abnormalities in diabetes are complex. However, many of the same mechanisms contribute to metabolic profiles in both T1- and T2DM. In the simplest terms, dyslipidemia in diabetes is caused by the lack of appropriate insulin signaling. In untreated T1DM, the defect is caused by insulin deficiency. In T2DM, the defect is caused by the combination of relative insulin deficiency and the inability of the insulin receptor to transmit its signal appropriately.

Type 1 Diabetes Mellitus

Diabetic ketoacidosis usually causes mild to moderate hypertriglyceridemia. Decreased expression of the enzyme lipoprotein lipase (LPL) appears to be mainly responsible. LPL catalyzes the rate-limiting step in triglyceride metabolism.[34] LPL is made in multiple tissues, but the major sites of expression are cardiac muscle, adipose tissue, and skeletal muscle. The active enzyme is located at the capillary endothelium, where it hydrolyzes triglycerides of circulating lipoproteins. Fatty acids released by this process are available for uptake in muscle, where they are oxidized, and fat, where they are stored. Insulin is required for multiple steps of LPL expression including transcription, translation, and activation of the enzyme, which involves glycosylation of LPL and transport of the protein to heparan sulfate binding sites at the capillary endothelium. In the setting of ketoacidosis, LPL activity is very low, leading to hypertriglyceridemia. Triglyceride levels improve rapidly with institution of appropriate insulin therapy, but mild dyslipidemia can persist for months after a bout of ketoacidosis. In-

sulin rapidly activates available LPL in tissues, but restoration of all the levels of LPL regulation requires chronic insulin treatment.[35]

Although the degree of hypertriglyceridemia in diabetic ketoacidosis (DKA) is usually moderate, severe dyslipidemia can occur rarely with triglycerides exceeding 20,000 mg/dL. In this setting, triglyceride elevations may complicate initial management[36] due to artifactual decreases in glucose and sodium.

Type 2 Diabetes Mellitus

T2DM is usually associated with obesity and insulin resistance. Insulin resistance has multiple effects on lipid metabolism (Fig. 47-2), many of which are also relevant to well-controlled patients with T1DM who may have gained weight due to intensive insulin therapy.

The hydrolysis of triglycerides in adipocytes is mediated by hormone-sensitive lipase (HSL). HSL activity is stimulated by catecholamines producing lipolysis and causing the release of fatty acids from adipocytes. In the absence of insulin resistance, HSL activity is exquisitely sensitive to suppression by insulin, and circulating fatty acid levels are low. In insulin resistance caused by obesity, insulin does not suppress HSL, lipolysis occurs unchecked, and fatty acid levels are elevated (step 1 in Fig. 47-2).

Fatty acids are reesterified into triglycerides in the liver. In the presence of newly synthesized lipid, microsomal transfer protein (MTP) stabilizes apoB and allows the generation of new VLDL particles. In the absence of MTP (as in the rare condition a-beta-lipoproteinemia), no VLDL is secreted from liver. Increased VLDL production driven in part by synthesis of new triglycerides from circulating fatty acids is probably the most important reason for dyslipidema in T2DM (step 2 in Fig. 47-2). Inhibition of MTP activity is an attractive potential therapy for this condition.[37]

Most individuals with T2DM and moderate hypertriglyceridemia have normal LPL activity (step 3 in Fig. 47-2). However, VLDL clearance tends to be decreased in these patients due to the expanded pool size of VLDL triglycerides. LPL at the capillary endothelium becomes saturated at triglyceride levels between 150 and 250 mg/dL. Above these levels, VLDL particles have prolonged circulating times that affect their interaction with HDL, resulting in triglyceride enrichment of HDL particles (see below).

In T2DM patients with marked hypertriglyceridemia, heterozygous LPL deficiency may be responsible for the phenotype. Most humans with heterozygous LPL deficiency have a mild phenotype, but severe hypertriglyceridemia (see below) can be observed when the increased VLDL production rates of T2DM are combined with the impaired VLDL clearance of LPL deficiency.[38] LPL deficiency among people with diabetes does not appear to be common.[39]

IDLs are atherogenic and are increased in diabetes.[40] These particles are metabolized by hepatic lipase (HL; step 4 in Fig. 47-2) to LDL. HL activity is increased in T2DM[41] and probably participates in the conversion of LDL to small, dense LDL.

The atherogenic particles IDL, LDL, and small, dense LDL have access to the subendothelial space of the vascular wall, where their presence contributes to the complicated evolution of atherosclerotic lesions (step 5 in Fig. 47-2). LPL, which hydrolyzes lipoproteins at the capillary endothelium, is also expressed by vessel wall macrophages, where it appears to promote atherosclerosis.[42,43] Lipoproteins in the vessel wall are subject to oxidative modification that promotes their uptake by macrophages, leading to foam cell development. People with diabetes may be more likely to generate oxidized lipoproteins.[44] Oxidized lipoproteins may increase vessel wall matrix components such as proteoglycans.[45]

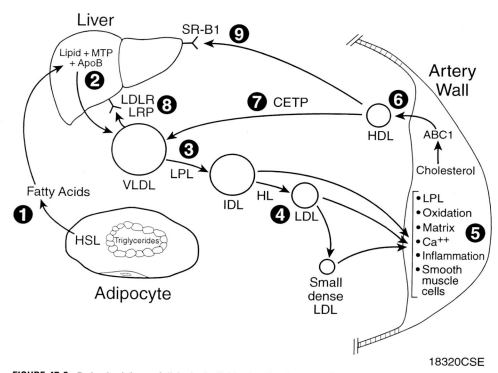

FIGURE 47-2. Pathophysiology of diabetic dyslipidemia. The diagram reflects mechanisms in type 2 diabetes. Many of the same mechanisms are operative in patients with type 1 diabetes. In the setting of insulin resistance, hormone-sensitive lipase (HSL) causes the release of fatty acids from adipocytes (step 1). In normal physiology, HSL is suppressed by low concentrations of insulin. Fatty acids are cleared by the liver, where they are re-esterified to form triglycerides. The synthesis of lipid in liver is associated with the stabilization of apolipoprotein B (apoB), a process mediated by microsomal transfer protein (MTP). ApoB is the major apolipoprotein for very-low-density lipoproteins (VLDLs). The increased production of VLDL is a major cause of diabetic dyslipidemia (step 2). VLDLs are metabolized by lipoprotein lipase (LPL, step 3) to generate intermediate-density lipoproteins (IDLs). These particles are metabolized by hepatic lipase (HL) to generate low-density lipoproteins (LDLs; step 4). HL is also important for the generation of small, dense LDL. IDL, LDL, and small, dense LDL all have access to the subendothelial space of the artery wall, where they initiate a complex series of events (step 5). Reverse cholesterol transport can occur when cholesterol in the vessel wall is transferred to high-density lipoproteins (HDLs), in part through the action of ATP-binding cassette transporter 1 (ABC1; step 6). Cholesterol can be transferred to VLDLs (and other lipoproteins) through the action of cholesteryl ester transfer protein (CETP, step 7). VLDL is then cleared by hepatic receptors such as the LDL receptor (LDLR) and the LDL receptor-related protein (LRP; step 8). Cholesterol can also be transferred to the liver directly through the interaction of HDL with a scavenger receptor (SR-B1; step 9).

Vascular calcification is associated with accelerated mortality in diabetes, and diabetic dyslipidemia activates osteogenic gene expression in diabetic vasculature.[46] Oxidized lipoproteins appear to initiate an inflammatory cascade associated with the released of cytokines and the recruitment of new cells including smooth muscle cells.[47] Inflammatory markers such as high sensitivity C-reactive protein predict vascular risk.[48]

The reverse cholesterol transport system utilizes HDL to move cholesterol from peripheral tissues such as the arterial wall to the liver for excretion. HDL levels are low and the composition of these particles is abnormal in diabetes, suggesting that reverse cholesterol transport is impaired. Recent discoveries of critical proteins involved in reverse cholesterol transport will help to clarify the role of this system in diabetic dyslipidemia.

The removal of cholesterol from tissues requires ATP-binding cassette transporter 1 (ABC1).[49] Mutations in ABC1 are responsible for Tangier disease, characterized by absence of HDL cholesterol. In the presence of ABC1, cholesterol is transferred to HDL

particles (step 6 in Fig. 47-2). HDL delivers cholesterol to the liver by two pathways, an indirect one and a direct one.

The indirect pathway is dependent on the interaction between HDL and triglyceride-rich particles such as VLDL. Cholesteryl ester transfer protein (CETP) moves esterified cholesterol from HDL to VLDL in exchange for triglyceride (step 7 in Fig. 47-2). This process is increased in diabetes.[50] Overexpression of CETP in mice increases experimental atherosclerosis.[51] CETP produces VLDL particles that are enriched in cholesterol, making them more atherogenic. The process also produces triglyceride-enriched HDL particles, making them a better substrate for the elevated levels of hepatic lipase that ultimately metabolize HDL, leading to lower HDL levels.[52] CETP also promotes the formation of small, dense LDL in diabetes. Cholesterol-enriched VLDL can be cleared by the low-density lipoprotein receptor (LDLR) and the LDLR-related protein (LRP) (step 8 in Fig. 47-2).

The direct pathway involves the interaction between HDL and scavenger receptor, class B, type I (SR-BI) (step 9 in Fig. 47-2).

SR-BI is involved in a process that is different from receptor-mediated endocytosis. This receptor binds HDL, the cholesteryl ester in HDL is selectively transferred to the liver, and then the lipid-depleted HDL is released from SR-BI. The receptor can also bind VLDL and LDL. SR-BI knockout mice (genetically modified animals with a mutation in SR-BI) have more experimental atherosclerosis,[53] whereas overexpression of SR-BI suppresses atherosclerosis.[54] The role of SR-BI in diabetic dyslipidemia is unknown.

T2DM may also be characterized by abnormalities of postprandial lipoprotein metabolism.[55] After a fatty meal, chylomicrons are generated by the intestine and rapidly metabolized to chylomicron remnants (similar in composition to IDL) that are cleared by the liver. However, current technologies do not allow the simple clinical evaluation of postprandial lipid metabolism.

TREATMENT

The Chylomicronemia Syndrome

Extreme elevations of triglycerides (usually >2000 mg/dL) can cause a discrete clinical syndrome due to the presence of high concentrations of chylomicrons.[56] The presentation can include pancreatitis, eruptive xanthomas, lipemia retinalis (the appearance of white arterioles and venules at fundoscopy), dyspnea, hepatosplenomegaly, and neurologic defects such as memory loss and carpal tunnel syndrome. Extreme hypertriglyceridemia does not uniformly cause the syndrome. People with uncontrolled diabetes are frequently seen in specialty clinics with documented chronic, extreme hypertriglyceridemia (between 2000 and 10,000 mg/dL) and no symptoms. The mechanisms underlying susceptibility to triglyceride-induced pancreatitis are unknown.

Most patients with the chylomicronemia syndrome have diabetes, but only a small percentage of people with diabetes develop this syndrome. People with diabetes and an underlying genetic hyperlipidemia are most likely to be affected. As noted above, the combination of heterozygous LPL deficiency and diabetes can cause the the syndrome, but familial combined hyperlipidemia (FCH) is a more likely contributor. FCH, an autosomal dominant phenotype that might be influenced by several different genes,[57] is present in about 1-2% of Western populations. It is characterized by the overproduction of hepatic lipoproteins, exacerbating the accelerated VLDL production seen in diabetes. However, chylomicronemia is uncommon even in patients with diabetes and an underlying familial dyslipidemia. Additional factors are usually required. Common antecedents are obesity (which increases VLDL production by poorly defined mechanisms), ethanol, oral estrogens, hypothyroidism (which decreases LPL activity and decreases lipoprotein clearance), thiazide diuretics, β-adrenergic blocking agents (except those with intrinsic sympathomimetic activity), high doses of gluocorticoids, and retinoids.

In patients with no history of the chylomicronemia syndrome, appropriate therapies with potential for elevating triglycerides should not be withheld from diabetics with dyslipidemia. For example, beta blockers (despite their proclivity for raising triglycerides) decrease cardiovascular mortality in people with diabetes. It is prudent to measure serum lipids after instituting such therapy. In women with diabetes and hypertriglyceridemia, transdermal estrogen replacement therapy is preferred over oral estrogens because of the tendency for the latter to increase triglycerides further.

In patients with the chylomicronemia syndrome, conservative therapy for the routine management of pancreatitis is indicated. The cessation of oral intake, the use of intravenous hydration, and treatment of hyperglycemia with insulin usually result in striking decreases in triglycerides within days. Plasmapheresis has been used to treat this disorder.[58] This therapy does not normalize triglycerides, has not been shown to be superior to conservative therapy, alters intravascular volume in the setting of a disorder associated with severe volume shifts, and requires anticoagulation, which might carry additional risk in the patient with pancreatitis.

In those with recurrent triglyceride-induced pancreatitis who anticipate becoming pregnant (which exacerbates hypertriglyceridemia), total parenteral nutrition or low-fat diets supplemented with medium-chain triglycerides may decrease pancreatitis risk. Surgery is not usually recommended for recurrent triglyceride-induced pancreatitis. However, surgically induced fat malabsorption[60] has been used in severe cases with apparently good results.

Clinical Trials Supporting the Use of Lipid-Lowering Medications in Diabetes

Results of clinical trials designed to determine the effects of lipid lowering on cardiac endpoints in people with diabetes are in progress. *Post hoc* analyses of large trials that included subsets of diabetic subjects uniformly support the use of lipid lowering to decrease vascular risk in people with diabetes (Table 47-1).

The Scandinavian Simvastatin Survival Study (4S) randomized men and women with stable angina or a history of myocardial infarction to placebo or simvastatin, an HMG-CoA reductase inhibitor. The trial included 202 people with a clinical history of diabetes.[61] Although data on these individuals are important, they may not be representative of the average person with diabetic dyslipidemia due to the lipid entry criteria of the trial. Participants had total cholesterol values between 212 and 309 mg/dL and triglyceride values <220 mg/dL.

The primary endpoint of the 4S trial was total mortality. There were several secondary endpoints including major coronary events and any atherosclerotic event. The risk of major coronary events was decreased by 55%, the risk of any atherosclerotic event was decreased by 37%, and there was a trend toward less total mortality in simvastatin-treated diabetics. There were an additional 281 patients in 4S with fasting glucose levels consistent with a diagnosis of diabetes, and 678 patients with impaired fasting glucose. An economic analysis of the trial using these larger subsets showed that simvastatin caused the greatest decrease in cardiovascular disease-related hospital days in people with diabetes.[62]

The Cholesterol and Recurrent Events (CARE) Trial also used an HMG-CoA reductase inhibitor, pravastatin, in both men and women with known vascular disease. The trial included 586 diabetics with lower LDL cholesterol levels than those studied in 4S.[63] Lipid lowering in this diabetic subset decreased coronary events by 25%.

Gemfibrozil, a fibrate drug, was used in men with vascular disease and low levels of HDL in the Veterans Affairs HDL Intervention Trial (VA-HIT). There was no effect of drug treatment on LDL cholesterol levels, but HDL levels increased and triglyceride levels decreased. The trial included 630 diabetics, and there was a 24% decrease in death due to coronary heart disease or stroke in the members of this group randomized to gemfibrozil.[64]

Several other trials, including one primary prevention trial,[65] have shown trends toward a reduction in cardiovascular risk with lipid lowering in people with diabetes.

TABLE 47-1. Summary of Important Lipid-Lowering Clinical Trials Including Patients with Diabetes

Trial	Medication	No. of Subjects with Diabetes	Baseline Lipid Values for Diabetics	Lipid Outcomes for Diabetics in the Treatment Group	Clinical Outcome Compared with the Placebo Group
Scandinavian Simvastatin Survival Study (4S)	Simvastatin (HMG-CoA reductase inhibitor)	202 men and women (plus additional 281 with undiagnosed diabetes at entry)	LDL: 176 mg/dL Triglycerides: 153 mg/dL HDL: 42 mg/dL	LDL decreased 36% Triglycerides decreased 11% HDL increased 7%	37% decrease in vascular events in diabetics. Trend favoring less total mortality in treated diabetics
Cholesterol After Recurrent Events (CARE)	Pravastatin (HMG-CoA reductase inhibitor)	586 men and women	LDL: 136 mg/dL Triglycerides: 164 mg/dL HDL: 38 mg/dL	LDL decreased 27% Triglycerides decreased 13% HDL increased 4%	25% decrease in coronary events in diabetics
Veterans Affairs HDL Intervention Trial (VA-HIT)	Gemfibrozil (fibric acid derivative)	630 men	LDL: 111 mg/dL Triglycerides: 161 mg/dL HDL: 32 mg/dL (for the entire study group)	LDL did not change Triglycerides decreased 31% HDL increased 6% (for all subjects treated with gemfibrozil)	24% decrease in death due to coronary heart disease or stroke in diabetics

Dyslipidemia Management

The results of UKPDS indicate that glycemic control has clear beneficial effects on microvascular disease but marginal effects on macrovascular disease.[66] One explanation is that some interventions lower glucose without affecting insulin resistance, a proatherogenic condition. Metformin-treated patients tend not to gain weight and have a reduction in insulin resistance as well as lower levels of triglycerides, making metformin a useful agent for glucose lowering in dyslipidemic T2DM patients with normal serum creatinine. In addition, a small subset in UKPDS had a reduction in cardiovascular endpoints.[67]

Dyslipidemia frequently persists even with excellent glycemic control. Given the risk of coronary events in diabetics, including those with no history of vascular disease, treating dyslipidemia with medications should be considered in every person with diabetes soon after diagnosis, after glucose levels have stabilized.

Optimal lipid levels for adults with diabetes[68] include an LDL cholesterol <100 mg/dL, triglycerides <200 mg/dL, and HDL cholesterol levels >45 mg/dL. Many experts consider a normal triglyceride level to be <150 mg/dL since adverse compositional changes in LDL can be demonstrated above this level. It is useful to base lipid treatment decisions on fasting triglyceride levels.

Triglycerides >1000 mg/dL

The rare patient with triglycerides >1000 mg/dL is at risk for pancreatitis. Marked restriction of dietary fat to <10% of caloric intake is required. Insulin is recommended instead of oral hypoglycemic agents to lower glucose levels in these patients. Fibric acid derivatives such as gemfibrozil (600 mg twice a day taken 30 minutes before meals) or fenofibrate (160 mg once a day with meals) are indicated. Substantial lowering of triglycerides is unlikely without weight loss. For many, the goal is to maintain fasting triglycerides below 1000 mg/dL to decrease the risk of pancreatitis. The use of fish oil capsules (containing n-3 polyunsaturated fatty acids) can also be helpful. Fish oil (supplied as 1 g capsules containing at least 300-500 mg of docosahexanoic acid and eicosapentanoic acid) should be administered as 1 capsule twice a day with food and gradually increased to a total of 6–10 capsules a day. Gastrointestinal side effects are common.

Triglycerides 400–1000 mg/dL

A minority of people with diabetes have fasting triglycerides at this level. Since triglyceride levels are inversely related to HDL cholesterol levels, HDL levels may be very low in these patients.

Diet (see Chap. 26) and exercise counseling are indicated for every person with diabetes. Exercise is generally required for sustained weight loss. It improves dyslipidemia and is known to increase the expression of LPL in human muscle.[69] A graded exercise test is appropriate for sedentary diabetics over the age of 35 before beginning an exercise program. Lower extremity protective sensation should be assessed and non-weight-bearing exercises such as cycling, rowing, or swimming recommended for those with sensory defects. A reasonable goal is 30 minutes of moderate physical activity on most days of the week; on average, 150 minutes a week is recommended. Referral to an exercise physiologist may be helpful, but the physician providing individualized recommendations may enhance compliance. It may be helpful to keep a record of physical activity analogous to recording home blood glucose results.

Fibrates (gemfibrozil or fenofibrate; see above for doses) are appropriate for these patients. These drugs are ligands for the nuclear hormone receptor PPARα.[70] Activation of this receptor increases fatty acid oxidation, leading to decreased hepatic lipogenesis and decreased VLDL secretion. This receptor also increases LPL activity, which clears VLDL particles and promotes the generation of HDL particles. Fibrates lower triglycerides, increase HDL cholesterol, and increase the buoyancy of LDL particles. LDL cholesterol may increase modestly with fibric acid therapy. Fenofibrate may be preferred since it is administered once a day and the drug may be more likely than other fibrates to lower LDL cholesterol. These agents increase the lithogenicity of bile and should be used cautiously in patients with gallstones. Gastrointestinal side effects and erectile dysfunction can occur. The drugs displace warfarin from its binding sites; clotting parameters must be monitored closely, and most patients will require a reduction in warfarin dose. Hepatic dysfunction and myositis can occur, especially when fibrates are used in combination with other lipid-lowering agents.

In the patient already being treated with insulin, extended release niacin is an alternative. Niacin appears to work by decreasing the release of fatty acids from adipocytes (see step 1 in Fig. 47-2), thereby decreasing hepatic lipogenesis and VLDL synthesis. It is the most potent agent for increasing HDL cholesterol. Niacin increases glucose, which can be treated by increasing the insulin dose. In many obese dyslipidemic patients, the effect on glucose metabolism may be small. Flushing is common but not serious for most patients. It can be minimized by taking enteric-coated aspirin before each dose and by avoiding alcohol, spicy foods, and hot beverages. More serious side effects include macular edema (which is rare), hyperuricemia, hepatitis, and myositis. A once-nightly extended-release form of niacin (Niaspan™) appears to be tolerated well. Doses should be gradually increased to 1500–2000 mg a day at bedtime.

Triglycerides 200–400 mg/dL

Many people with T2DM will have levels in this range. Triglycerides at this level are associated with an increase in IDL, more small, dense LDL, and low HDL. Statin drugs (HMG-CoA reductase inhibitors) are the drugs of choice for this group. These drugs inhibit the synthesis of cholesterol, causing the induction of LDL receptors in the liver. Hence, LDL clearance is enhanced. At higher doses, all statins also lower triglycerides. The mechanism may be a combination of enhanced clearance of VLDL particles through the LDL receptor and inhibition of VLDL secretion. Statins also elevate HDL levels.

Diabetics are unlikely to reach therapeutic goals on the standard starting doses of statins. Simvastatin at 40 mg (given with food in the evening), atorvastatin 20 mg (given with food in the evening), and pravastatin 40 mg (taken at bedtime on an empty stomach) may be effective. Patients may complain of sleep disturbances or difficulty concentrating with some statins; pravastatin does not penetrate the central nervous system and may be an option for these individuals.[71] Muscle aches with completely normal muscle enzymes (CPK and aldolase) are common with statin use. The etiology of this effect is unknown. Some patients improve when a different statin drug is used.

Liver dysfunction occurs in <1% of patients who use statins. Myositis is rare. The risk for these side effects increases with concomitant use of erythromycin, cyclosporine, antifungal agents, and protease inhibitors used to treat HIV infection. The risk is also increased in patients treated with statins in addition to other lipid-lowering medications such as fibrates or niacin.

Patients with dyslipidemia and established coronary heart disease are at high risk for subsequent vascular events. Many experts use combinations of lipid-lowering drugs to reach therapeutic goals. Fenofibrate at 160 mg in the morning and simvastatin or pravastatin at 20 mg in the evening can have beneficial effects on multiple lipid parameters in patients with diabetic dyslipidemia. The combination of a statin with niacin may be considered in the patient at very high risk for coronary events who is taking insulin for glucose control. With combination therapy, liver function tests should be followed regularly, and patients should be warned about the symptoms of myositis and hepatitis. Combination therapy should not be used in patients with significant renal dysfunction or in those taking cyclosporine.

Triglycerides <200 mg/dL with LDL cholesterol >100 mg/dL

Statins are the drugs of choice in this group. Bile acid sequestrants are available, but they can increase triglyceride levels, are not as potent as statins for lowering cholesterol, and are not tolerated as well as statins. In addition to statins, it may be appropriate to treat patients in this group, as well as diabetics with higher lipid levels, with fish oils (n-3 polyunsaturated fatty acids). The GISSI-Prevenzione trial showed that low-dose fish oil supplementation (1 g daily) decreased the risk of subsequent cardiovascular events in people with a history of recent myocardial infarction.[72] This trial included 405 diabetics treated with fish oil and 426 diabetics treated with placebo.

Summary of Treatment Recommendations

Diabetics are at high risk for atherosclerotic complications. Treating dyslipidemia may decrease the risk of these complications. Every person with diabetes should receive dietary advice and exercise counseling. Many should also receive a lipid-lowering medication, usually a statin. Lipid management is part of a comprehensive approach to treating vascular risk that should also include counseling for smoking cessation, aspirin therapy, optimal blood pressure control, and consideration of need for an angiotensin-converting enzyme inhibitor.

REFERENCES

1. Haffner SM, Lehto S, Ronnemaa T, et al: Mortality from coronary heart disease in subjects with type 2 diabetes and in nondiabetic subjects with and without prior myocardial infarction. *N Engl J Med* 1998;339:229.
2. Kern PA: Lipid disorders in diabetes mellitus. *Mt Sinai J Med* 1987; 54:245.
3. West KM, Ahuja MMS, Bennett PH, et al: The role of circulating glucose and triglyceride concentrations and their interactions with other "risk factors" as determinants of arterial disease in nine diabetic population samples from the WHO multinational study. *Diabetes Care* 1983;6:361.
4. Shaten BJ, Smith GD, Kuller LH, et al: Risk factors for the development of type II diabetes among men enrolled in the Usual Care group of the Multiple Risk Factor Intervention Trial. *Diabetes Care* 1993; 16:1331.
5. Fontbonne A: A relationship between diabetic dyslipoproteinaemia and coronary heart disease risk in subjects with non-insulin-dependent diabetes mellitus. *Diabetes Metab Rev* 1991;7:179.
6. Meigs JB, Nathan DM, Wilson PWF, et al: Metabolic risk factors worsen continuously across the spectrum of nondiabetic glucose tolerance. *Ann Intern Med* 1998;128:524.
7. Kannel WB, McGee DL: Diabetes and glucose tolerance as risk factors for cardiovascular disease: The Framingham Study. *Diabetes Care* 1979;2:120.
8. Heyden S, Heiss G, Bartel AG, et al: Sex differences in coronary mortality among diabetics in Evans County, Georgia. *J Chron Dis* 1980; 33:265.
9. Barrett-Connor EL, Cohn BA, Wingard DL, et al: Why is diabetes mellitus a stronger risk factor for fatal ischemic heart disease in women than in men? The Rancho Bernardo Study. *JAMA* 1991; 265:627.
10. Ken G, Cowie CC, Harris MI: Diabetes and decline in heart disease mortality in US adults. *JAMA* 1999;281:1291.
11. Assman G, Schulte H: Relation of high-density lipoprotein cholesterol and triglycerides to incidence of atherosclerotic coronary heart disease (the PROCAM experience). *Am J Cardiol* 1992;70: 733.

12. Howard BV, Cowan LD, Go O: Adverse effects of diabetes on multiple cardiovascular disease risk factors in women. *Diabetes Care* 1998; 21:1258.

13. Gardner CD, Fortmann SP, Krauss RM: Association of small low-density lipoprotein particles with the incidence of coronary artery disease in men and women. *JAMA* 1996;276:875.

14. Stempfer MJ, Krauss RM, MA J, *et al:* A prospective study of triglyceride level, low-density lipoprotein particle diameter, and risk of myocardial infarction. *JAMA* 1996;276:882.

15. Erbey JR, Robbins D, Forrest KY, *et al:* Low-density lipoprotein particle size and coronary artery disease in a childhood-onset type 1 diabetes population. *Metabolism* 1999;48:531.

16. Sibley SD, Hokanson JE, Steffes MW, *et al:* Increased small dense LDL and intermediate-density lipoprotein with albuminuria in type 1 diabetes. *Diabetes Care* 1999;22:1165.

17. Howard BV, Robbins DC, Sievers ML, *et al:* LDL cholesterol as a strong predictor of coronary heart disease in diabetic individuals with insulin resistance and low LDL. *Arterioscler Thromb Vasc Biol* 2000; 20:830.

18. Turner RC, Millns H, Neil HAW, *et al:* Risk factors for coronary artery disease in non-insulin dependent diabetes mellitus: United Kingdom Prospective Diabetes Study (UKPDS: 23). *BMJ* 1998;316:823.

19. Semenkovich CF, Heinecke JW: The mystery of diabetes and atherosclerosis: Time for a new plot. *Diabetes* 1997;46:327.

20. Ostlund RE Jr, Semenkovich CF, Schechtman KB: Quantitative relationship between plasma lipid levels and glycohemoglobin in type I diabetes mellitus: A longitudinal study of 212 patients. *Diabetes Care* 1989;12:332.

21. The Diabetes Control and Complications Trial Research Group: The effect of intensive treatment of diabetes on the development and progression of long-term complications in insulin-dependent diabetes mellitus. *N Engl J Med* 1993;329:977.

22. The DCCT Research Group: Effect of intensive diabetes management on macrovascular events and risk factors in the Diabetes Control and Complications Trial. *Am J Cardiol* 1995;75:894.

23. Purnell JQ, Marcovina SM, Hokanson J, *et al:* Effect of intensive diabetes therapy on Lp(a), apo B, and lipoprotein cholesterol distribution in the Diabetes Control and Complications Trial. *Diabetes* 1995; 44:1218.

24. Purnell JQ, Hokanson JE, Marcovina SM, *et al:* Effect of excessive weight gain with intensive therapy of type 1 diabetes on lipid levels and blood pressure: Results from the DCCT. *JAMA* 1998;280:1484.

25. Eriksson J, Lindstrom J, Valle T, *et al:* Prevention of Type II diabetes in subjects with impaired glucose tolerance: The Diabetes Prevention Study (DPS) in Finland. Study design and 1-year interim report on the feasibility of the lifestyle intervention programme. *Diabetologia* 1999;42:793.

26. Halle M, Berg A, Garwers U, *et al:* Concurrent reductions of serum leptin and lipids during weight loss in obese men with type II diabetes. *Am J Physiol* 1999;277:E277.

27. Scott R, Lintott CJ, Zimmet P, *et al:* Will acarbose improve the metabolic abnormalities of insulin-resistant type 2 diabetes mellitus? *Diabetes Res Clin Pract* 1999;43:179.

28. DeFronzo RA, Goodman AM: Efficacy of metformin in patients with non-insulin-dependent diabetes mellitus. *N Engl J Med* 1995; 333:541.

29. Stumvoll M, Nurjhan N, Perriello G, *et al:* Metabolic effects of metformin in non-insulin-dependent diabetes mellitus. *N Engl J Med* 1995;333:550.

30. Schwartz S, Raskin P, Fonseca V, *et al:* Effect of troglitazone in insulin-treated patients with type II diabetes mellitus. *N Engl J Med* 1998;338:861.

31. Maggs DG, Buchanan TA, Burant CF, *et al:* Metabolic effects of troglitazone monotherapy in type 2 diabetes mellitus. *Ann Intern Med* 1998;128:176.

32. Saha AK, Kurowski TG, Colca JR, *et al:* Lipid abnormalities in tissues of the KKAy mouse: Effects of pioglitazone on malonyl-CoA and diacylglycerol. *Am J Physiol* 267:E95, 1994.

33. Edvardsson U, Bergstrom M, Alexandersson M, *et al:* Rosiglitazone (BRL49653), a PPARgamma-selective agonist, causes peroxisome proliferator-like liver effects in obese mice. *J Lipid Res* 1999;40:1177.

34. Coleman T, Seip RL, Gimble JM, *et al:* COOH-terminal disruption of lipoprotein lipase in mice is lethal in homozygotes, but heterozygotes have elevated triglycerides and impaired enzyme activity. *J Biol Chem* 1995;270:12518.

35. Tavangar K, Murata Y, Pedersen M, *et al:* Regulation of lipoprotein lipase in the diabetic rat. *J Clin Invest* 1992;90:1672.

36. Rumbak MJ, Hughes TA, Kitabchi AE: Pseudonormoglycemia in diabetic ketoacidosis with elevated triglycerides. *Am J Emerg Med* 1991; 9:61.

37. Wetterau JR, Gregg RE, Harrity TW: An MTP inhibitor that normalizes atherogenic lipoprotein levels in WHHL rabbits. *Science* 1998; 282:751.

38. Wilson DE, Hata A, Kwong LK, *et al:* Mutations in exon 3 of the lipoprotein lipase gene segregating in a family with hypertriglyceridemia, pancreatitis, and non-insulin-dependent diabetes. *J Clin Invest* 1993;92:203.

39. Elbein SC, Yeager C, Kwong LK, *et al:* Molecular screening of the lipoprotein lipase gene in hypertriglyceridemic members of familial noninsulin-dependent diabetes mellitus families. *J Clin Endocrinol Metab* 1994;79:1450.

40. Watanabe N, Taniguchi T, Taketoh H, *et al:* Elevated remnant-like lipoprotein particles in impaired glucose tolerance and type 2 diabetic patients. *Diabetes Care* 1999;22:152.

41. Tan KC, Shiu SW, Chu BY: Roles of hepatic lipase and cholesteryl ester transfer protein in determining low density lipoprotein subfraction distribution in Chinese patients with non-insulin-dependent diabetes mellitus. *Atherosclerosis* 1999;145:273.

42. Semenkovich CF, Coleman T, Daugherty A: Effects of heterozygous lipoprotein lipase deficiency on diet-induced atherosclerosis in mice. *J Lipid Res* 1998;39:1141.

43. Babaev V, Fazio S, Gleaves LA, *et al.:* Macrophage lipoprotein lipase promotes foam cell formation and atherosclerosis *in vivo. J Clin Invest* 1999;103:1697.

44. Tan KC, Ai VH, Chow WS, et al: Influence of low density lipoprotein (LDL) subfraction profile and LDL oxidation on endothelium-dependent and independent vasodilation in patients with type 2 diabetes. *J Clin Endocrinol Metab* 1999;84:3212.

45. O'Brien KD, Olin KL, Alpers CE, *et al:* Comparison of apolipoprotein and proteoglycan deposits in human coronary atherosclerotic plaques: Colocalization of biglycan with apolipoproteins. *Circulation* 1998;98:519.

46. Towler DA, Bidder M, Latiffe T, *et al:* Diet-induced diabetes activates an osteogenic gene regulatory program in the aortas of low density lipoprotein receptor-deficient mice. *J Biol Chem* 1998;273:30427.

47. Ross R: Atherosclerosis—an inflammatory disease. *N Engl J Med* 1999;340:115.

48. Ridker PM, Hennekens CH, Buring JE, *et al:* C-reactive protein and other markers of inflammation in the prediction of cardiovascular disease in women. *N Engl J Med* 2000;342:836.

49. Orso E, Broccardo C, Kaminski WE, *et al:* Transport of lipids from Golgi to plasma membrane is defective in Tangier disease patients and Abc1-deficient mice. *Nat Genet* 2000;24:192.

50. Riemens S, van Tol A, Sluiter W, *et al:* Elevated plasma cholesteryl ester transfer in NIDDM: Relationships with apolipoprotein B-containing lipoproteins and phospholipid transfer protein. *Atherosclerosis* 1998;140:71.

51. Plump AS, Masucci-Magoulas L, Bruce C, *et al:* Increased atherosclerosis in ApoE and LDL receptor gene knock-out mice as a result of human cholesteryl ester transfer protein transgene expression. *Arterioscler Thromb Vasc Biol* 1999;19:1105.

52. Syvanne M, Ahola M, Lahdenpera S, *et al:* High density lipoprotein subfractions in non-insulin-dependent diabetes mellitus and coronary artery disease. *J Lipid Res* 1995;36:573.

53. Trigatti B, Rayburn H, Vinals M, *et al:* Influence of the high density lipoprotein receptor SR-BI on reproductive and cardiovascular pathophysiology. *Proc Natl Acad Sci USA* 1999;96:9322.

54. Arai T, Wang N, Bezouevski M, *et al:* Decreased atherosclerosis in heterozygous low density lipoprotein receptor-deficient mice expressing the scavenger receptor BI transgene. *J Biol Chem* 1999;274: 2366.

55. Coppack SW: Postprandial lipoproteins in non-insulin-dependent diabetes mellitus. *Diabet Med* 1997;14:S67.

56. Semenkovich CF: Hypertriglyceridemia and combined hyperlipidemia. In: Callow AD, Ernst CB, eds. *Vascular Surgery: Theory and Practice.* Appleton & Lange:1995;105.

57. Pajukanta P, Terwilliger JD, Perola M, *et al:* Genomewide scan for familial combined hyperlipidemia genes in Finnish families, suggesting multiple susceptibility loci influencing triglyceride, cholesterol, and apolipoprotein B levels. *Am J Hum Genet* 1999;64:1453.

58. Lennertz A, Parhofer KG, Samtleben W, *et al*: Therapeutic plasma exchange in patients with chylomicronemia syndrome complicated by acute pancreatitis. *Ther Apheresis* 1999;3:227.

59. Mizushima T, Ochi K, Matsumara N, *et al*: Prevention of hyperlipidemic acute pancreatitis during pregnancy with medium-chain triglyceride nutritional support. *Int J Pancreatol* 1998;23:187.

60. Mingrone G, Henriksen FL, Greco AV, *et al*: Triglyceride-induced diabetes associated with familial lipoprotein lipase deficiency. *Diabetes* 1999;48:1258.

61. Pyorala K, Pedersen TR, Kjekshus J, *et al*: Cholesterol lowering with simvastatin improves prognosis of diabetic patients with coronary heart disease. *Diabetes Care* 1997;20:614.

62. Herman WH, Alexander CM, Cook JR, *et al*: Effect of simvastatin treatment on cardiovascular resource utilization in impaired fasting glucose and diabetes. *Diabetes Care* 1999;22:1771.

63. Goldberg RB, Mellies MJ, Sacks FM, *et al*: Cardiovascular events and their reduction with pravastatin in diabetic and glucose-intolerant myocardial infarction survivors with average cholesterol levels. *Circulation* 1998;98:2513.

64. Rubins HB, Robins SJ, Collins D, *et al*: Gemfibrozil for the secondary prevention of coronary heart disease in men with low levels of high-density lipoprotein cholesterol. *N Engl J Med* 1999;341:410.

65. Downs JR, Clearfield M, Weis S, *et al*: Primary prevention of acute coronary events with lovastatin in men and women with average cholesterol levels: Results of AFCAPS/TexCAPS. *JAMA* 1998; 279:20.

66. UK Prospective Diabetes Study (UKPDS) Group: Intensive blood-glucose control with sulphonylureas or insulin compared with conventional treatment and risk of complications in patients with type 2 diabetes (UKPDS 33). *Lancet* 1998;352:837.

67. UK Prospective Diabetes Study (UKPDS) Group: Effect of intensive blood-glucose control with metformin on complications in over-weight patients with type 2 diabetes (UKPDS 34). *Lancet* 1998; 352:854.

68. American Diabetes Association: Management of dyslipidemia in adults with diabetes. *Diabetes* 2000;23:S57.

69. Seip RL, Mair K, Cole TG, *et al*: Induction of human skeletal muscle lipoprotein lipase gene expression by short term exercise is transient. *Am J Physiol* 1997;272:E255.

70. Staels B, Dallongeville J, Auwerx J, *et al*: Mechanism of action of fibrates on lipid and lipoprotein metabolism. *Circulation* 1998; 98:2088.

71. Knopp RH: Drug treatment of lipid disorders. *N Engl J Med* 1999; 341:498.

72. GISSI-Prevenzione Investigators: Dietary supplementation with n-3 polyunsaturated fatty acids and vitamin E after myocardial infarction: Results of the GISSI-Prevenzione trial. *Lancet* 1999;354:447.

CHAPTER 48

Hypertension and Diabetes

Norman M. Kaplan

Hypertension and diabetes frequently coexist, in large part from underlying obesity. Hypertension is found in over 70% of all diabetic patients,[1] and the risk for developing diabetes is almost doubled by the presence of hypertension even among nonobese people with blood pressure >130/85 mm Hg.[2] When the two coexist, cardiovascular and renal complications occur at a much higher rate, at least twofold more frequently overall, and progressive nephropathy is many times more frequent.

There may be a potential explanation for some of the increased prevalence of hypertension, nephropathy, and diabetes: Hyperglycemia during pregnancy reduces nephrogenesis in the fetus.[3] Just as maternal protein deprivation leads to a reduced number of nephrons, so could hyperglycemia. The infants of women with abnormal glucose tolerance or overt diabetes would then be susceptible to more hypertension, diabetes, and nephropathy.

Beyond the possible contribution to impaired fetal development, there are a number of other reasons for the increasing prevalence of diabetes and hypertension. These include:

* Increasing age of the population
* Rapid growth of more susceptible populations including Hispanic Americans and African-Americans
* Prolonged survival of those with type 1 diabetes
* Expanding reach of medical care
* Increasing prevalence of obesity due to decreased physical activity and increased caloric intake

THE PREDOMINANT ROLE OF OBESITY

The current U.S. population is likely the fattest of all time. Obesity, defined as a body mass index (BMI) >30 kg/m^2, increased from 12% of U.S. adults in 1991 to 17.9% in 1998.[4] The increase occurred in virtually every segment of the population, among both men and women, in teenagers to the elderly, and in all races and socioeconomic strata.

With increasing BMI, the rate of type 2 diabetes mellitus (T2DM) increases markedly. A 5-kg weight gain doubles the risk for diabetes, and the risk further increases with increased duration of being overweight.[5] Not surprisingly, cardiovascular mortality is increased with increasing BMI, with about 300,000 annual deaths attributable to the consequences of obesity in the United States.[6]

The problem often begins in early childhood, when increased weight is associated with hyperinsulinemia, increased blood pressure, and dyslipidemia, particularly in those with greater central (visceral or abdominal) obesity.[7]

Prevention of weight gain in adults is difficult; it may be easier in children if they can be kept physically active, perhaps by turning off the TV and the computer.[8] The clinician should devote greater attention to those who are both diabetic and hypertensive: In a European survey, only about 11% of type 1 diabetics had their hypertension adequately controlled.[9] Moreover, with tighter control of both type 1 diabetes mellitus (T1DM) and T2DM, the associated weight gain may result in an increase in both blood pressure and dyslipidemia.[10]

INCREASING RECOGNITION OF THE PROBLEM

All three recently published guidelines have emphasized the need for both earlier intervention at even lower levels of blood pressure for hypertensives with diabetes, and for more intensive therapy:

* The JNC-6 places all diabetic patients in the highest risk category (group C), wherein immediate drug therapy is indicated if blood pressure is above 130/85 mm Hg.[11]
* The WHO-ISH places all diabetic patients with blood pressure above 140/90 mm Hg into risk group III (high risk), with a 15-20% risk of a major cardiovascular event over the next 10 years; those with blood pressure above 180/110 mm Hg are in risk group IV (very high risk), with a greater than 30% risk over 10 years.[12] Drug therapy is recommended immediately for both groups.
* The British Hypertension Society provides more specific risk assessment and recommends that drug treatment be started at 140/90 mm Hg with a target of below 140/80 mm Hg.[13]

ASSESSMENT OF BLOOD PRESSURE

Before therapy is begun, the presence and degree of blood pressure elevation must be carefully ascertained. Such an assessment should include out-of-the-office readings.

Out-of-Office Measurements

As with all patients, out-of-the-office measurements are needed both to establish the diagnosis and to monitor the management. White-coat hypertension is common, particularly among young type 1 diabetics, and if not recognized, may lead to misdiagnosis.[14]

Ambulatory blood pressure monitoring (ABPM) is best, but it most likely will remain unavailable, because third-party payers often do not reimburse for the procedure. With ABPM, the common lack of a nocturnal drop in pressure in diabetics can be recognized and should lead to more intensive control of the blood pressure.[14]

Recognition of Postural Hypotension

All diabetics, particularly if over age 60, should have their blood pressure measured supine and standing, since postural and postprandial hypotension is common and potentially hazardous. In a study of 204 type 2 diabetic subjects (average age, 58), postural hypotension was found in 28.4% and postural dizziness in 22.5%.[15] If present, postural and postprandial hypotension must be managed before supine and seated hypertension is treated.[16]

NONPHARMACOLOGIC THERAPY

Therapy for all hypertension should begin and continue with lifestyle modifications, even more so in the typically obese type 2 diabetic. Despite the obvious attraction of lifestyle changes, they are hard to accomplish and may not be as protective as drug therapy. The high risk of even diet-controllable T2DM almost mandates early and intensive antihypertensive drug therapy.

Weight Loss

Weight loss lowers blood pressure at least in part by improving insulin sensitivity.[17]

Exercise

Those who are sedentary and unfit may develop more diabetes whether lean or obese. Walking alone, without more vigorous activity, reduces the risk for diabetes and will lower blood pressure.[18]

The manner by which exercise helps both diabetes and hypertension goes beyond a decrease in body weight. Exercise increases glucose uptake into skeletal muscles, making them more insulin sensitive. The effect was seen in mice without muscle insulin receptors, suggesting a phenomenon mediated by nonmuscle cells or by downstream signaling events.[19]

The benefits of exercise in patients with diabetes include improvement in glycemic control, lowering of blood pressure, reduction in levels of triglyceride-rich VLDL, probable improvement in fibrinolytic activity, and reduction in cardiovascular disease.

Moderate Sodium Reduction

Moderate sodium reduction is safe and can be effective,[20] perhaps even more in those diabetics whose hypertension is related to volume expansion from the renal impairment of nephropathy. Moreover, the antiproteinuric effect of ACE inhibitors is markedly enhanced by a lower sodium intake.[21] But even without nephropathy, diabetic subjects need to reduce their sodium intake since insulin-resistant subjects have an impaired natriuretic response to high sodium intake.[22]

The value of moderate sodium reduction is illustrated by a study in 34 type 2 diabetic hypertensive patients. A reduction of sodium intake of 60 mmol/d for 3 months was associated with a 20-mm Hg fall in systolic pressure; when sodium intake was increased, the blood pressure rose 11 mm Hg.[23]

Moderate Alcohol Consumption

Diabetic subjects have been reported to obtain a protective effect against coronary disease by regular, moderate alcohol consumption (no more than 2 drinks a day) similar to that seen in several other groups[24] (Fig. 48-1). In addition to other mechanisms for cardio-

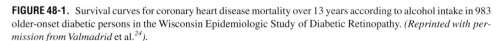

FIGURE 48-1. Survival curves for coronary heart disease mortality over 13 years according to alcohol intake in 983 older-onset diabetic persons in the Wisconsin Epidemiologic Study of Diabetic Retinopathy. *(Reprinted with permission from Valmadrid et al.[24]).*

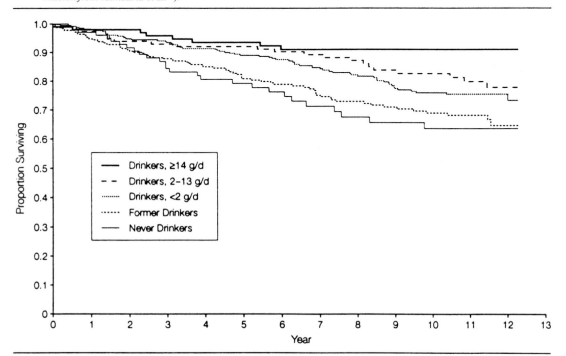

protection provided by alcohol, insulin sensitivity is improved.[25] The risk of T2DM was reduced by 42% among middle-aged Japanese men who drank moderately.[26]

The type of alcoholic beverage is most likely irrelevant. Wine drinkers have the lowest risk for coronary disease, perhaps because of their healthier lifestyle; red wine drinkers have no greater protection than white wine drinkers.[27]

Cessation of Smoking

As the most important lifestyle issue to be addressed, smoking may markedly aggravate insulin resistance in type 2 diabetics.[28]

Others

Dietary Fiber

In a large population of young, healthy subjects, increased dietary fiber intake was associated with lower body weight, lower waist-to-hip ratio, lower fasting insulin, lower blood pressure, and better lipid profiles.[29]

Dietary Magnesium

Low serum magnesium, but not low dietary magnesium intake, was a strong independent predictor of severity in type 2 diabetics in over 12,000 middle-aged people.[30]

ANTIHYPERTENSIVE DRUG THERAPY

The best documentation of the need to lower diastolic blood pressure to 80 mm Hg or below comes from the Hypertension Optimal Treatment (HOT) trial.[31] Among the 19,000 participants in the trial, the only significant benefit to reducing the diastolic blood pressure to near 80 mm Hg was seen among the 1501 diabetic hypertensive subjects. They achieved a greater than 50% reduction in major cardiovascular events (Fig. 48-2). As in the HOT trial, to achieve the necessary goal of blood pressure <130/80 mm Hg usually requires two or more antihypertensive drugs.

In the population of 3642 type 2 diabetics screened for the United Kingdom Prospective Diabetes Study (UKPDS) but not entered into the trial, the progressive reduction in major cardiovascular events seen with progressive reduction of systolic blood pressure from over 160 mm Hg to 110 mm Hg was accomplished by various antihypertensive drugs.[32]

To provide the other essential corrections for concomitant risk factors, multiple nondrug and drug therapies will be needed. The benefits of such intensive therapy are impressive.[33] In this trial, 160 diabetic subjects were randomly assigned to standard or more intensive therapy, the latter requiring a blood pressure below 140/85, HbA$_{1c}$ below 6.5%, total cholesterol below 5 mmol/L, and the use of ACE inhibitors and aspirin plus multiple lifestyle modifications. At the end of 3.8 years of follow-up, those on intensive therapy achieved major benefits (Fig. 48-3). Such intensive therapies, though costly, would not only reduce morbidity and mortality, but also lower lifetime medical costs.[34]

Antihypertensive Drugs

For those diabetic hypertensive patients without proteinuria, a low-dose diuretic may be the appropriate first choice with an angiotensin-converting enzyme (ACE) inhibitor as a second drug and a long-acting calcium channel blocker (CCB) as third. Beta-blockers, and to a lesser extent alpha-blockers, may also be indicated. Rarely, central α_2 agonists may be useful. For those with proteinuria, an ACE inhibitor is mandatory (see Chap. 43). An angiotensin II receptor blocker (ARB) should be substituted if a cough precludes use of an ACE inhibitor.

Diuretics

Low doses of diuretics (e.g., 12.5 mg of hydrochlorothiazide) are effective and safe in diabetic patients, as shown in the Systolic Hypertension in the Elderly Program (SHEP) trial.[35] A thiazide diuretic should be almost always included in the regimen and loop diuretics given only to those with serum creatinine above 1.5 mg/dL.

Beta-Blockers

Despite many warnings about their potential to aggravate diabetes in various ways, beta-blockers may be effective and safe.[36] They are mandatory for those who survive a myocardial infarction.[11] Since they tended to be more protective than ACE inhibitors in the UKPDS trial[37] (Fig. 48-4), their use may increase.

Alpha-Blockers

In addition to their ability to relieve prostatism, alpha-blockers are better than any other class for reducing insulin resistance and improving dyslipidemia.[38]

FIGURE 48-2. The risk for major cardiovascular events in the 1501 diabetic patients in the HOT study according to the target diastolic blood pressure level. *(Adapted with permission from Hansson et al.[31])*

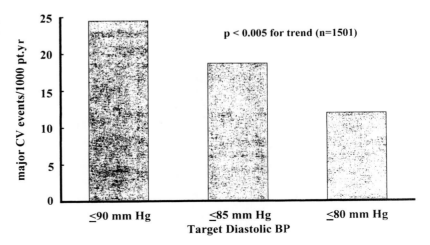

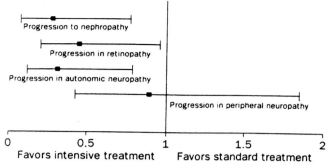

FIGURE 48-3. The development or progression of microvascular complications in the 80 diabetic hypertensives assigned to standard treatment compared to the 80 patients assigned to intensive treatment. *(Reprinted with permission from Gaede et al.[33])*

Calcium Channel Blockers

Concerns persist about the safety of CCBs, particularly the dihydropyridines (DHPs), and particularly in diabetic hypertensive subjects. In their recent review, Abernethy and Schwartz[39] state: "At present, in view of the greater evidence of a benefit of angiotensin-converting-enzyme inhibitors and beta-blockers in patients who have hypertension and diabetes,[37] the relative paucity of data on calcium antagonists in these patients, and the recent finding that the risk of a vascular event may be increased during calcium-antagonist treatment in such patients,[40,41] calcium antagonists cannot be considered as first-line therapy for these patients."

As to their putative effect to increase coronary disease, the problem remains unique to large doses of short-acting agents and does not apply to long-acting agents. The safety of long-acting CCBs in patients with coronary disease was further documented in a 1-year follow-up of over 51,000 patients who were prescribed one of these agents after surviving an acute myocardial infarction.[42]

FIGURE 48-4. Kaplan-Meier plots of proportions of patients who died of diseases related to diabetes (myocardial infarction, sudden cardiac death, stroke, renal failure) in the less tightly controlled group and the more tightly controlled groups based on use of either captopril or atenolol. *(Reprinted with permission from the UKPDS Study Group.[37])*

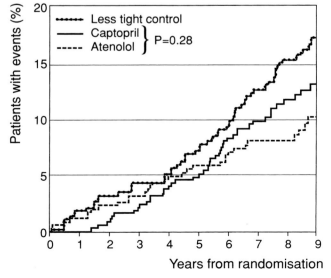

Their relative likelihood of 1-year mortality was no different than those not prescribed a long-acting CCB.

As to their particular effects in diabetes, most of the current evidence of a benefit from antihypertensive therapy in patients with diabetes comes from trials using DHP-CCBs[43] (Table 48-1).

In both the ABCD trial[41] and the FACET study,[44] those diabetic patients given an ACE inhibitor had fewer cardiovascular events than those given a DHP-CCB, although the rates in those on CCBs were not increased beyond the expected numbers in those on no therapy. These results prompted Pahor and associates[45] to state that DHP-CCBs should not be used in diabetic hypertensives.

Birkenhager and Staessen[43] defend the use of DHP-CCBs thusly:

- The excellent protection found in Syst-Eur with nitrendipine was even better than that found in a similar group of hypertensive diabetics given a diuretic in the SHEP trial[46] (Fig. 48-5). The comparability of the two groups of diabetic hypertensive patients is shown by the similar rates of various cardiovascular events in the placebo groups of each study, shown on the right. Of those who were treated, the nitrendipine-based regimen in Syst-Eur provided even better protection than did the chlorthalidone-based regimen in SHEP.
- The major reduction in cardiovascular events in the 1501 diabetic subjects given felodipine-based therapy in the HOT trial[32] (see Fig. 48-2).
- The presumed lack of significant adverse effects in the amlodipine quarter of the ongoing ALLHAT trial, with over 15,000 diabetic patients enrolled, since the Safety Monitoring Committee has not called for a discontinuation of the DHP-CCB limb of the trial, now in its fourth year.
- Multiple defects in both the ABCD and FACET studies, which included protocol breaks, crossovers, and imbalances of other therapies.

Additional evidence in defense of the benefits of CCBs for treatment of hypertensive diabetics comes from the results of the 719 diabetics among the 6614 elderly hypertensives in the Swedish Trial of Old Persons with Hypertension-2 Study (STOP-2), the only completed trial that compared drugs from the three major classes: diuretics/beta-blockers, ACE inhibitors, and CCBs.[46a] A lower rate of CHD and CHF was seen in those taking an ACE inhibitor, but there was a lower rate of stroke and mortality in those on a CCB.

The data now available provide no clear evidence that one class of drug is superior, although CCB-based therapy has been associated with fewer events than either diuretic- or ACE inhibitor–based therapy.

At present, the bottom line seems to be that either DHP-CCBs or non-DHP-CCBs are frequently needed to control hypertension in

TABLE 48-1. Rates of Events per 1000 Patients in the Seven Comparative Trials in Diabetic Hypertensives

	No. Pts.	Total Events per 1000 Patients			
		CHD	**CHF**	**Stroke**	**Mortality**
Diuretic and/or β-Blocker	1903	75	27	62	125
ACE I	1368	87	32	66	121
CCB	1657	71	32	53	83

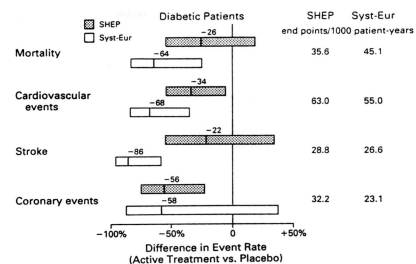

FIGURE 48-5. Outcomes in the diabetic hypertensives enrolled in the Systolic Hypertension in the Elderly Program (SHEP) or the Syst-Eur trial. The two right-hand columns show the number of events per 1000 patient-years in the placebo groups in the two trials. The bars indicate the 95% confidence intervals. The numbers above the bars indicate the benefit of active treatments compared to placebo. *(Reprinted with permission from Tuomilehto et al.[46])*

most diabetics, particularly to prevent the progression of renal damage. They may be renoprotective even if they do not reduce proteinuria. In a 42-month follow-up of 48 proteinuric diabetics, the half given a DHP-CCB, nisoldipine, had no reduction in proteinuria, but a smaller fall in GFR than did the half given an ACE inhibitor.[47]

Angiotensin-Converting Enzyme Inhibitors

An ACE inhibitor should always be used for those patients with proteinuria. This should most likely be expanded to normotensive diabetics with microalbuminuria; over 4 years, 9 of 23 such patients on placebo advanced in diabetic nephropathy, whereas only 2 of 21 given captopril advanced.[48]

Whether an ACE inhibitor should also be the drug of first choice for all diabetic subjects without microalbuminuria is less certain, but this is looking more and more likely. In the Captopril Prevention Project (CAPPP), those diabetic patients given captopril had fewer events than did those given diuretics and beta-blockers, whereas there was no difference in the nondiabetics.[49] On the other hand, the ACE inhibitor was somewhat less protective than the beta-blocker in the UKPDS trial, the largest and longest trial involving type 2 diabetic hypertensives[37] (Fig. 48-4).

The renin-angiotensin system may be set inappropriately high in type 2 diabetics and it also may be less suppressed by high sodium intake,[50] so this could be a theoretical reason to use ACE inhibitors. Certainly ACE inhibitors have been found to be protective in diabetic patients who have survived a myocardial infarction.[51] In the Heart Outcomes Prevention Evaluation (HOPE) trial, the 9297 patients with known cardiovascular disease included 38% with diabetes; over the 4–6 year follow-up, a 17% risk reduction for diabetic complications was reported for those given the ACE inhibitor ramipril compared to those assigned to placebo.[52]

A Markov model simulating the progression of diabetic nephropathy was applied to patients 50 years of age with newly diagnosed T2DM.[53] The analysis found that treating all patients with an ACE inhibitor at a yearly cost of $320 was about $15,000 per patient more expensive than screening for microalbuminuria and then treating with an ACE inhibitor. ACE inhibitor treatment was, however, associated with increased quality-adjusted life expectancy at a cost:effectiveness ratio of $7500 per quality-adjusted life-year gained.

As attractive as they are, ACE inhibitors may cause problems. They interfere with useful actions of angiotensin II such as vasodilator responses in skeletal muscle arterioles,[54] increase the risk of hypoglycemia,[55] and may worsen renal function in patients with diabetic nephropathy.[56] On the other hand, the ACE inhibitor–induced cough, the most common side effect, may protect against aspiration in elderly people with a poor cough reflex, diminishing their incidence of pneumonia.[57]

Angiotensin II Receptor Blockers

For the 10% of patients given an ACE inhibitor who develop cough, an ARB is a logical alternative. Their more widespread usage is not recommended in any of the three recent guidelines,[11–13] but they are being widely promoted for initial therapy.

These agents are in many ways similar to ACE inhibitors, but the renin-angiotensin system has three features that may give rise to differences in the benefits of ARBs versus ACE inhibitors[58] (Fig. 48-6):

1. **Non-ACE alternative pathways** for generation of angiotensin II have been recognized. In particular, the chymotrypsin-like serine protease chymase has been found in heart tissue and shown to have the ability to convert angiotensin I to angiotensin II, even in the presence of natural protease inhibitors.[59]
2. **Beneficial effects of the increased levels of bradykinin** that accompany ACE inhibitors, but not ARBs, have been observed. These include adding to the antihypertensive effect of ACE inhibitors,[60] providing an important source of vasodilation that is NO-mediated. In a rat hypertensive model, enhanced vascular ACE activity was found to induce endothelial dysfunction by impairing the bioavailability of endothelium-derived NO. Both increased angiotensin II formation and decreased brandykinin levels were thought to be at work.[61] ACE inhibitors also inhibit vascular smooth muscle cell growth.[62]
3. **Activation of the angiotensin II receptors.** Most of the adverse effects of the renin-angiotensin system are mediated through the angiotensin I receptors, but increasing evidence supports beneficial effects mediated through the angiotensin II receptor, as shown in Fig. 48-6. Initial concerns that the increased levels of angiotensin II that circulate when the

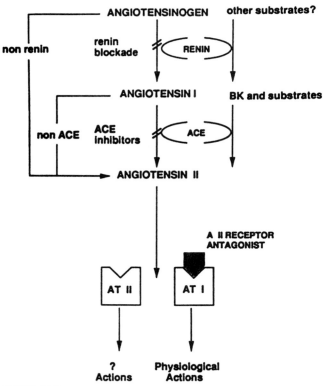

FIGURE 48-6. The renin-angiotensin system with the sites of action of ACE inhibition and angiotensin I receptor blockade.

angiotensin I receptor is blocked could induce deleterious effects have been largely obviated by evidence that angiotensin II receptor stimulation is likely beneficial. For example, over-expression of the angiotensin II receptor activates the vascular kinin system and causes vasodilation.[63]

Clinical Effects of ARBs

The many ARBs now available seem equipotent and equally free of side effects, although angioedema has been noted.[64] Losartan appears to be unique in having a modest uricosuric effect.[65]

ARBs reverse left ventricular hypertrophy[66] and diminish proteinuria.[67] The only published outcome study comparing an ARB against an ACE inhibitor (ELITE I) suggested a better effect of losartan than captopril on heart failure.[68] However, the larger follow-up trial (ELITE II) was reported to show no difference.[69] The apparent failure to confirm the preliminary evidence of a better outcome with losartan than captopril removes the only current evidence for a meaningful difference between ACE inhibitors and ARBs. Another comparative trial in CHF patients, the Randomized Evaluation of Strategies for Left Ventricular Dysfunction (RESOLVD) study found no significant differences between the ARB candesartan and the ACE inhibitor enalapril.[70] The combination of the two was more beneficial in preventing left ventricular remodeling than either alone, whereas there was a trend toward fewer events with enalapril alone (which led to premature termination of the trial).

The Potential for Additive Effects

Since the two classes have different effects on various parts of the renin-angiotensin system, an additive effect may occur. Preliminary evidence has been reported for additive effects of the combination of low doses of lisinopril and losartan on blood pressure.[71]

OTHER DRUGS FOR HYPERTENSIVE DIABETIC SUBJECTS

Antidiabetic Agents

In addition to chronic effects, hyperglycemia will acutely raise blood pressure, probably by activating the renin system.[72] As noted elsewhere, to achieve adequate glycemic control, most patients will require multiple therapies. There may be special vasodilatory effects of glitazones mediated through increased NO synthesis.[73] Any therapy that improves insulin sensitivity or lowers insulinemia should have long-term vascular protective effects.

Statins

The 483 diabetic patients in the Scandinavian Simvastatin Survival Study had as much benefit as the remainder of the subjects.[74] Even though statins may not improve insulin sensitivity, they have vasodilatory effects that may be additive to those provided by ACE inhibitors.[75]

Estrogen Replacement Therapy

At least in Britain, fewer diabetic women were prescribed ERT than nondiabetic women. In a smaller number of obese type 2 diabetics, ERT (with medroxyprogesterone) was associated with reductions in waist circumference, HbA$_{1c}$, and cholesterol levels.[76] However, no data exist to support a cardiovascular protective effect of ERT in postmenopausal women with diabetes.

Aspirin

In the HOT trial[32] aspirin (75 mg/d) reduced major cardiovascular events by 15%, all myocardial events by 36%, and had no effect on stroke. There were more bleeding episodes in the aspirin group, but no more fatal bleeding.

CONCLUSION

Hypertension and diabetes commonly coexist and pose a serious threat. Fortunately, significant protection can be provided, but the benefits may be hard to achieve. Clinicians must be more vigorous in applying more intensive therapy to this rapidly expanding, highly vulnerable population.

REFERENCES

1. Colhoun HM, Dong W, Barakatt MT, *et al*: The scope for cardiovascular disease risk factor intervention among people with diabetes mellitus in England: A population-based analysis from the Health Surveys for England 1991–94. *Diabet Med* 1999;16:35.
2. Hayashi T, Tsumura K, Suematsu C, *et al*: High normal blood pressure, hypertension and the risk of type 2 diabetes in Japanese men. *Diabetes Care* 1999;22:1683.
3. Amri K, Freund N, Vilar J, *et al*: Adverse effects of hyperglycemia on kidney development in rats. *Diabetes* 1999;48:2240.
4. Mokdad AH, Serdula MK, Dietz WH, *et al*: The spread of the obesity epidemic in the United States, 1991–1998. *JAMA* 1999;282:1519.
5. Wannamethee SG, Shaper AG: Weight change and duration of overweight and obesity in the incidence of type 2 diabetes. *Diabetes Care* 1999;22:1266.

6. Allison DB, Fontaine KR, Manson J-AE, *et al*: Annual deaths attributable to obesity in the United States. *JAMA* 1999;282:1530.

7. Morrison JA, Sprecher DL, Barton BA, *et al*: Overweight, fat patterning, and cardiovascular disease risk factors in black and white girls: The National Heart, Lung, and Blood Institute Growth and Health Study. *J Pediatr* 1999;135:458.

8. Robinson TN: Reducing children's television viewing to prevent obesity. *JAMA* 1999;282:1561.

9. Collado-Mesa F, Colhount HM, Stevens L, *et al*: Prevalence and management of hypertension in type 1 diabetes mellitus in Europe: The EURODIAB IDDM complications study. *Diabet Med* 1999;16:41.

10. Purnell JQ, Hokanson JE, Marcovina SM, *et al*: Effect of excessive weight gain with intensive therapy of type 1 diabetes on lipid levels and blood pressure. *JAMA* 1998;280:140.

11. Joint National Committee: The Sixth Report of the Joint National Committee on Prevention, Detection, Evaluation and Treatment of High Blood Pressure. *Arch Intern Med* 1997;157:2413.

12. Guidelines Subcommittee: 1999 World Health Organization-International Society of Hypertension guidelines for the management of hypertension. *Hypertension* 1999;17:151.

13. Ramsay LE, Williams B, Johnston GD, *et al*: British Hypertension Society guidelines for hypertension management 1999: Summary. *Br Med J* 1999;319:630.

14. Holl RW, Pavlovic M, Heinze E, *et al*: Circadian blood pressure during the early course of type 1 diabetes. *Diabetes Care* 1999;22:1151.

15. Wu J-S, Lu F-H, Yang Y-C, *et al*: Postural hypotension and postural dizziness in patients with non-insulin dependent diabetes. *Arch Intern Med* 1999;159:1350.

16. Kaplan NM: Treatment of hypertension: Drug therapy. In: *Clinical Hypertension*, Vol. 8, Lippincott Williams and Wilkins: 2002; 310.

17. Ikeda T, Gomi T, Hirawa N, *et al*: Improvement of insulin sensitivity contributes to blood pressure reduction after weight loss in hypertensive subjects with obesity. *Hypertension* 1996;27:1180.

18. Hu FB, Sigal RJ, Rich-Edwards JW, *et al*: Walking compared with vigorous physical activity and risk of type 2 diabetes in women. *JAMA* 1999;282:1433.

19. Wojtaszewski JFP, Higaki Y, Hirshman MF, *et al*: Exercise modulates post receptor insulin signaling and glucose transport in muscle-specific insulin receptor knockout mice. *J Clin Invest* 1999;104:1257.

20. He J, Ogden LG, Vupputuri S, *et al*: Dietary sodium intake and subsequent risk of cardiovascular disease in overweight adults. *JAMA* 1999;282:2027.

21. Buter H, Hemmelder MH, Navis G, *et al*: The blunting of the antiproteinuric efficacy of ACE inhibition by high sodium intake can be restored by hydrochlorothiazide. *Nephrol Dial Transplant* 1998;13:1682.

22. Facchini FS, DoNascimento C, Reaven GM, *et al*: Blood pressure, sodium intake, insulin resistance and urinary nitrate excretion. *Hypertension* 1999;33:1008.

23. Dodson PM, Beevers M, Hallworth R, *et al*: Sodium restriction and blood pressure in hypertensive type II diabetics: Randomised blind controlled and crossover studies of moderate sodium restriction and sodium supplementation. *Br Med J* 1989;298:227.

24. Valmadrid CT, Klein R, Moss SE, *et al*: Alcohol intake and the risk of coronary heart disease mortality in persons with older-onset diabetes mellitus. *JAMA* 1999;282:239.

25. Kiechl S, Willeit J, Poewe W, *et al*: Insulin sensitivity and regular alcohol consumption: Large, prospective, cross sectional population study (Bruneck study). *Br Med J* 1996;313:1040.

26. Tsumura K, Hayashi T, Suematsu C, et al: Daily alcohol consumption and the risk of type 2 diabetes in Japanese men. *Diabetes Care* 1999; 22:1432.

27. Klatsky AL, Armstrong MA, Friedman GD: Red wine, white wine, liquor, beer, and risk for coronary artery disease hospitalization. *Am J Cardiol* 1997;80:416.

28. Targher G, Alberiche M, Zenere MB, *et al*: Cigarette smoking and insulin resistance in patients with noninsulin-dependent diabetes mellitus. *J Clin Endocrinol Metab* 1997;82:3619.

29. Ludwig DS, Pereira MA, Kroenke CH, *et al*: Dietary fiber, weight gain, and cardiovascular disease risk factors in young adults. *JAMA* 1999; 282:1539.

30. Kao WHL, Folsom AR, Nieto J, *et al*: Serum and dietary magnesium and the risk for type 2 diabetes mellitus. *Arch Intern Med* 1999; 159:2151.

31. Hansson L, Zanchetti A, Carruthers SG, *et al*: Effects of intensive blood-pressure lowering and low-dose aspirin in patients with hypertension: Principal results of the Hypertension Optimal Treatment (HOT) randomised trial. *Lancet* 1998;351:1755.

32. Alder AI, Stratton IM, Neill HAW, *et al*: Association of systolic blood pressure with macrovascular and microvascular complications of type 2 diabetes (UKPDS 36): Prospective observational study. *Br Med J* 2000;321:112.

33. Gaede P, Vedel P, Parving H-H, *et al*: Intensified multifactorial intervention in patients with type 2 diabetes mellitus and microalbuminuria: The Steno type 2 randomised study. *Lancet* 1999;353:617.

34. Elliott WJ, Weir DR, Black HR. Cost-effectiveness of the lower treatment goal (of JNC VI) for diabetic hypertensives. *Arch Intern Med* 2000; 160:1277–1283.

35. Curb JD, Pressel SL, Cutler JA, *et al*: Effect of diuretic-based antihypertensive treatment on cardiovascular risk in older diabetic patients with isolated systolic hypertension. *JAMA* 1996;276:1886.

36. Majumdar SR: Beta-blockers for the treatment of hypertension in patients with diabetes: Exploring the contraindication myth. *Cardiovasc Drugs Ther* 1999;13:435.

37. UK Prospective Diabetes Study Group: Efficacy of atenolol and captopril in reducing risk of macrovascular and microvascular complications in type 2 diabetes: UKPDS 39. *Br Med J* 1998;317:713.

38. Giordano M, Matsuda M, Sanders L, *et al*: Effects of angiotensin-converting enzyme inhibitors, Ca^{2+} channel antagonists and α-adrenergic blockers on glucose and lipid metabolism in NIDDM patients with hypertension. *Diabetes* 1995;44:665.

39. Abernethy DR, Schwartz JB: Calcium-antagonist drugs. *Drug Ther* 1999;341:1447.

40. Byington RP, Craven TE, Furberg CD, *et al*: Isradipine, raised glycosylated haemoglobin and risk of cardiovascular events. *Lancet* 1997;350: 1075.

41. Estacio RO, Jeffers BW, Hiatt WR, *et al*: The effect of nisoldipine as compared with enalapril on cardiovascular outcomes in patients with non-insulin-dependent diabetes and hypertension. *N Engl J Med* 1998; 338:645.

42. Jollis JG, Simpson RJJ, Chowdhury MK, *et al*: Calcium channel blockers and mortality in elderly patients with myocardial infarction. *Arch Intern Med* 1999;159:2341.

43. Birkenhager WH, Staessen JA: Treatment of diabetic patients with hypertension. *Curr Hypertens Rep* 1999;3:225.

44. Tatti P, Pahor M, Byington RB, *et al*: Outcome results of the fosinopril versus amlodipine cardiovascular events randomized trial (FACET) in patients with hypertension and NIDDM. *Diabetes Care* 1998; 21:597.

45. Pahor M, Psaty BM, Furberg CD: Treatment of hypertensive patients with diabetes. *Lancet* 1998;351:689.

46. Tuomilehto J, Rastenyte D, Birkenhager WH, *et al*: Effects of calcium-channel blockade in older patients with diabetes and systolic hypertension. *N Engl J Med* 1999;340:677.

46a.Lindholm LH, Hansson L, Ekbom T, *et al*: Comparison of antihypertensive treatments in preventing cardiovascular events in elderly diabetic patients: Results from the Swedish Trial in Old Patients with Hypertension-2. *J Hypertens* 2000;18:1671.

47. Tarnow L, Rossing P, Jensen C, *et al*: Long-term renoprotective effect of nisoldipine and lisinopril in type 1 diabetic patients with diabetic nephropathy. *J Am Soc Nephrol* 1999;10:134A.

48. Mathiesen ER, Hommel E, Hansen HP, *et al*: Randomised controlled trial of long term efficacy of captopril on preservation of kidney function in normotensive patients with insulin dependent diabetes and microalbuminuria. *Br Med J* 1999;319:24.

49. Hansson L, Lindholm LH, Niskanen L, *et al*: Effect of angiotensin-converting-enzyme inhibition compared with conventional therapy on cardiovascular morbidity and mortality in hypertension: The Captopril Prevention Project (CAPPP) randomised trial. *Lancet* 1999;353:611.

50. Price DA, De-Oliveira JMF, Fisher NDL, *et al*: The state and responsiveness of the renin-angiotensin-aldosterone system in patients with type II diabetes mellitus. *Am J Hypertens* 1999;12:348.

51. Gustafsson I, Torp-Pedersen C, Kober L, *et al*: Effect of the angiotensin-converting enzyme inhibitor trandolapril on mortality and morbidity in diabetic patients with left ventricular dysfunction after acute myocardial infarction. *J Am Coll Cardiol* 1999;34:83.

52. The Heart Outcomes Prevention Evaluation (HOPE) Study Investigators: Effects of an angiotensin-converting-enzyme inhibitor, ramipril,

on death from cardiovascular causes, myocardial infarction, and stroke in high-risk patients. *N Engl J Med* 2000;342:145.

53. Golan L, Birkmeyer JD, Welch HG: The cost-effectiveness of treating all patients with type 2 diabetes with angiotensin-converting enzyme inhibitors. *Ann Intern Med* 1999;131:660.

54. Frisbee JC, Weber DS, Lombard JH: Chronic captopril administration decreases vasodilator responses in skeletal muscle arterioles. *Am J Hypertens* 1999;12:705.

55. Morris AD, Boyle DIR, McMahon AD, et al: ACE inhibitor use is associated with hospitalization for severe hypoglycemia in patients with diabetes. *Diabetes Care* 1997;20:1363.

56. Jaichenko J, Fudin R, Shostak A, *et al*: Use of angiotensin-converting enzyme inhibitors in patients with diabetic and nondiabetic chronic renal diseases: A need for reassessment. *Nephron* 1998;80:367.

57. Kaplan RC, Psaty BM: ACE-inhibitor therapy and nosocomial pneumonia. *Am J Hypertens* 1999;12:1161.

58. Willenheimer R, Dahlof B, Rydberg E, *et al*: AT1-receptor blockers in hypertension and heart failure: Clinical experience and future directions. *European Heart J* 1999;20:997.

59. Takai S, Jin D, Sakaguchi M, *et al*: Chymase-dependent angiotensin II formation in human vascular tissue. *Circulation* 1999;100:654.

60. Gainer JV, Morrow JD, Loveland A, *et al*: Effect of bradykinin-receptor blockade on the response to angiotensin-converting-enzyme inhibitor in normotensive and hypertensive subjects. *N Engl J Med* 1998;339:1285.

61. Goetz RM, Holtz J: Enhanced angiotensin-converting enzyme activity and impaired endothelium-dependent vasodilation in aortae from hypertensive rats: Evidence for a causal link. *Clin Sci* 1999;97:165.

62. Murakami H, Yayama K, Miao RQ, *et al*: Kallikrein gene delivery inhibits vascular smooth muscle cell growth and neointima formation in the rat artery after balloon angioplasty. *Hypertension* 1999;34:164.

63. Tsutsumi Y, Matsubara H, Masaki H, *et al*: Angiotensin II type 2 receptor overexpression activates the vascular kinin system and causes vasodilation. *J Clin Invest* 1999;104:925.

64. van Rijnsoever EW, Kwee-Zuiderwijk WJM, Feenstra J: Angioneurotic edema attributed to the use of losartan. *Arch Intern Med* 1998;158:2063.

65. Puig JG, Mateos F, Ortega R, *et al:* Effect of eprosartan and losartan on uric acid metabolism in patients with essential hypertension. *J Hypertens* 1999;17:1033.

66. Thurmann PA, Kenedi P, Schmidt A, *et al*: Influence of the angiotensin II antagonist valsartan on left ventricular hypertrophy in patients with essential hypertension. *Circulation* 1998;98:2037.

67. Plum J, Bunten B, Nemeth R, *et al*: Effects of the angiotensin II antagonist valsartan on blood pressure, proteinuria and renal hemodynamics in patients with chronic renal failure and hypertension. *J Am Soc Nephrol* 1998;9:2223.

68. Pitt B, Segal R, Martinez FA, *et al*: Randomised trial of losartan versus captopril in patients over 65 with heart failure (Evaluation of Losartan in the Elderly study; ELITE). *Lancet* 1997;349:747.

69. Pitt B, Poole-Wilson PA, Segal R, et al: Losartan heart failure survival study-ELITE II. *Circulation* 1999;100:I-782.

70. McKelvie RS, Yusuf S, Pericak D, *et al*: Comparison of candesartan, enalapril and their combination in congestive heart failure. *Circulation* 1999;100:1056.

71. Fogari R, Zoppi A, Corradi L, *et al*: Adding losartan to lisinopril therapy in patients with hypertension: Assessment by 24-hour ambulatory blood pressure monitoring. *Curr Ther Res* 1999;60:326.

72. Miller JA: Impact of hyperglycemia on the renin angiotensin system in early human type 1 diabetes mellitus. *J Am Soc Nephrol* 1999;10:1778.

73. Hattori Y, Hattori S, Kasai K: Troglitazone upregulates nitric oxide synthesis in vascular smooth muscle cells. *Hypertension* 1999;33:943.

74. Herman WH, Alexander CM, Cook JR, *et al*: Effect of simvastatin treatment on cardiovascular resource utilization in impaired fasting glucose and diabetes. *Diabetes Care* 1999;22:1771.

75. Nazzaro P, Manzari M, Merlo M, *et al*: Distinct and combined vascular effects of ACE blockade and HMG-CoA reductase inhibition in hypertensive subjects. *Hypertension* 1999;33:719.

76. Samaras K, Hayward CS, Sullivan D, *et al*: Effects of postmenopausal hormone replacement therapy on central abdominal fat, glycemic control, lipid metabolism and vascular factors in type 2 diabetes. *Diabetes Care* 1999;22:1401.

CHAPTER 49

Heart Disease in Patients with Diabetes

Lawrence H. Young

Deborah A. Chyun

INTRODUCTION

Cardiovascular disease (CVD) is the leading cause of mortality and a major cause of morbidity in patients with diabetes mellitus. CVD results in large part from macrovascular coronary artery disease (CAD) and hypertension. The most common manifestations of CVD are angina, acute myocardial infarction (MI), heart failure, and sudden death.

Coronary artery atherosclerosis is extremely common in patients with type 2 diabetes mellitus (T2DM) and in patients with long-standing type 1 diabetes mellitus (T1DM). At an early stage, minor atherosclerosis is the nidus for further plaque buildup and the substrate for plaque rupture leading to acute coronary syndromes (unstable angina and acute MI). More advanced atherosclerosis significantly narrows the vessel lumen and restricts blood flow, leading to ischemia during exercise or emotional stress. Ischemia is sometimes associated with angina or dyspnea, but in some diabetic patients may be asymptomatic and therefore may not be detected by either the patient or physician. The first manifestation of CAD in such patients may be acute MI, heart failure, or sudden cardiac death.

CVD in diabetic patients is not restricted simply to the manifestations of CAD. The majority of individuals with T2DM have hypertension, which has an important role in the development of left ventricular dysfunction, heart failure, and atrial fibrillation, as well as being a risk factor for CAD. In addition, patients with diabetes often have impaired endothelial function, a tendency toward thrombosis, and abnormalities in left ventricular function which adversely influence the clinical course of their heart disease once it develops.

CORONARY ARTERY DISEASE

Epidemiology

Patients with both T1DM and T2DM are known to be at risk for the development of CVD. In the Framingham study the age-adjusted risk of CVD was 2–3 times greater in those with diabetes, primarily type 2 patients.[1] The average annual incidence of CVD was 39/1000 in men with diabetes versus 19/1000 in those without diabetes. In women with diabetes, the incidence was 27/1000 as compared to only 10/1000 in women without diabetes. In the recent United Kingdom Prospective Diabetes Study (UKPDS), there was a substantial risk of MI (17/1000 patient-years), stroke (5/1000 pa-

tient-years), angina (7/1000 patient-years) and heart failure (4/1000 patient-years) in conventionally treated T2DM patients.[2]

CVD is also a major cause of death in T1DM, often affecting patients during their fourth and fifth decades of life. In the Wisconsin Epidemiologic Study of Diabetic Retinopathy (WESDR), CVD was responsible for 30% of the deaths in type 1 patients, with the vast majority attributable to CAD.[3] In the Diabetes Control and Complications Trial (DCCT), the risk of cardiac events was 3/1000 patient-years in conventionally treated patients.[4] Diabetes increases the risk of heart disease in all patients, but has a particularly adverse effect in women. In premenopausal women, CAD is extremely unusual except in women with diabetes. In the Nurses' Health Study, women with diabetes diagnosed before the age of 30 had a 12-fold increase in their risk of MI and fatal CAD.[5]

Etiology

The mechanisms responsible for macrovascular CAD in patients with diabetes are complex. Some of the risk for accelerated atherosclerosis in patients with T2DM can be attributed to the presence of multiple known cardiac risk factors, including hypertension, lipid abnormalities, and obesity.[6] These risk factors are also associated with the insulin resistance syndrome and often precede the onset of T2DM. This has led to the "common soil" hypothesis, which postulates that similar genetic and environmental factors predispose both to the development of diabetes and CAD.[7] Strategies to define the genes responsible for insulin resistance are currently underway.[8] In addition to traditional risk factors, microalbuminuria[9,10] and elevation of blood homocysteine levels[11,12] appear to be significant risk factors for CVD in patients with diabetes.

Lipid abnormalities (see Chap. 47) are important contributors to the development of CAD, especially in T2DM. Insulin resistance and T2DM are often associated with reduced high-density lipoprotein (HDL) and increased triglyceride (TG) levels (see Chap. 47).[13] Although elevations in low-density lipoprotein (LDL) cholesterol are not specifically related to diabetes, increased atherogenicity may be related to the presence of oxidized and small dense LDL particles (see Chap. 47).[14] Alterations in lipids are more pronounced in women than in men with T2DM and are associated with more central adiposity, hypertension, and higher fibrinogen levels.[15,16]

Hemostatic abnormalities have a role both in the atherogenic process and in promoting thrombosis once CAD is established. Alterations in factor VIII, von Willebrand factor, plasminogen activator inhibitor, and platelet function are all associated with CAD in patients with diabetes.[17–19] Lipid peroxidation may cause oxidative stress and contribute to increased platelet activation in patients with diabetes.[18] Thus abnormalities in platelet function, thrombosis, and fibrinolysis likely contribute to the increased risk of CAD in patients with diabetes.

Inflammation is also thought to be an important mechanism in the development of atherosclerosis. A number of inflammatory markers are increased in patients with diabetes, including C-reactive protein,[20a] fibrinogen,[19,21] and soluble cell adhesion molecules.[22,23] Hyperglycemia increases the concentration of advanced glycation endproducts (AGEs), which may be responsible in part for inflammation in the vascular wall.[24] Additional cellular mechanisms that have been proposed to contribute to the vascular abnormalities in patients with diabetes include increased flux through the polyol pathway and diacylglycerol-mediated protein kinase C (PKC) activation.[25]

Pathology

Coronary atherosclerosis primarily affects the epicardial or large surface arteries of the heart. Coronary plaques in patients with diabetes have more lipid and macrophages than in control subjects.[26] CAD is generally more widespread in diabetes, with stenoses in a greater number of vessels and more obstructive lesions within each vessel.[27] In addition, diffuse disease involving long segments and/or the distal aspects of the artery may be present (Fig. 49-1). This is a critical finding, since distal disease adversely affects the suitability of the vessels for either percutaneous or surgical revascularization. In many cases, patients with diffusely diseased vessels can only be treated medically. Patients with diabetes also tend to have less collateral blood vessel development to areas supplied by arteries with severe stenoses.[28] This may reflect diminished angiogenesis in the diabetic myocardium. Obstruction of the left main coronary artery is more common in diabetic patients and often requires surgical revascularization.

Small vessel or microvascular disease has also been observed in myocardium from diabetic patients, including perivascular fibrosis, thickening of myocardial capillary basement membranes, and microaneurysms.[29,30] The significance of these abnormalities is uncertain, particularly with regard to whether they limit coronary blood flow. In addition, functional abnormalities in the coronary endothelium are frequently seen in patients with diabetes (see below).[31] Endothelial dysfunction may have an important role in limiting the augmentation of coronary blood flow during stress.

Prevention

The prevention of CVD in patients with diabetes is of paramount importance and requires a multifaceted approach to risk reduction (Table 49-1).[32–39] Lifestyle recommendations should include intensive dietary management, weight control, regular physical activity, moderation in alcohol and sodium consumption, and smoking cessation when indicated. Hypertension (see Chap. 48) and dyslipidemia (see Chap. 47) should be aggressively treated. All patients with diabetes should strive to maintain optimal glycemic control and should be taking daily aspirin.

Exercise is an integral part of the management of both T1DM and T2DM, having beneficial effects on glycemic control, lipids, weight and blood pressure (see Chap. 23). However, individualized exercise recommendations are required in patients with peripheral or cardiovascular autonomic neuropathy, severe retinopathy, or

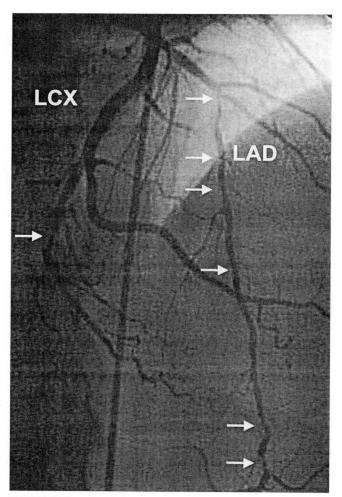

FIGURE 49-1. Diffuse coronary atherosclerosis. Coronary angiogram showing diffuse atherosclerotic narrowing (**arrows**) of the lumen of the mid and distal portions of the left anterior descending (**LAD**) and distal left circumflex (**LCX**) arteries of a 62-year-old patient with T2DM. Note the relatively normal caliber of the proximal portion of the LCX as compared to the diffuse narrowing of the LAD.

known CAD. Because of the possibility of unrecognized CAD, particularly in individuals with T2DM, these patients should generally engage in moderate-intensity exercise regimens. Sedentary individuals should always initiate exercise programs at a low level and gradually increase the intensity of exercise. All patients should be educated about the symptoms of myocardial ischemia and instructed to report them to their physician if they occur. When patients want to engage in high-intensity exercise, those with a long duration of diabetes, multiple CAD risk factors, or known diabetic complications should undergo screening for underlying CAD.[37]

The benefit of hormone replacement therapy in the primary prevention of CVD in postmenopausal diabetic women remains controversial. Although the Heart and Estrogen/Progestin Replacement Study trial raised concern that hormone replacement might increase CVD events in women with known CAD,[40] hormone replacement as primary preventive therapy does not appear to have adverse cardiovascular effects. Case control studies suggest that the incidence of cardiac events may be lower in women who take hormone replacement.[41] The current American Heart Association

TABLE 49-1. Primary Prevention of Cardiovascular Disease in Diabetic Patients

Goal	Strategies
Blood pressure <130/80	Measured at each visit
	Lifestyle modification
	Medication
Lipids	
LDL <100 mg/dL	Tested annually or every 2 years if low-risk
HDL >45 mg/dL in men; >55 mg/dL in women	Medical nutrition therapy
Triglycerides <150 mg/dL	Daily fat intake: <7–10% saturated fat and <200–300 mg cholesterol
	Regular physical activity
	Weight control
	Glycemic control
	Medication
HbA$_{1c}$	
<7%	Tested 2–3 times annually if meeting goal; 4 times annually if above goal or therapy changed
	Medical nutrition therapy
	Weight control
	Regular physical activity
	Self-monitoring of blood glucose
	Education in self-management and problem solving
Physical activity	
Regularly 3–4 times per week for 30 minutes	Routinely assess physical activity and exercise status
	Moderate aerobic regimen
	Increase in daily activities
	With multiple CAD risk factors, complications or long duration of diabetes, consider screening for CAD
	Individualization of prescription
	Caution with peripheral neuropathy or cardiac autonomic neuropathy or proliferative retinopathy
Weight	
BMI 21–25 kg/m^2	Height, weight, BMI, and waist circumference at each visit
Waist circumference <102 cm in men and <88 cm in women	Weight control
	Regular physical activity
Smoking	
Complete cessation	Assess smoking status
	Counseling on prevention and cessation
	Provide counseling, problem-solving or coping skills training, and pharmacotherapy
Aspirin therapy	
Consider	Consider enteric-coated aspiring 75–325 mg/d if age ≥40 years and 1 or more additional CAD risk factors
Estrogen replacement	
Consider	Consider in post-menopausal women with multiple CAD risk factors

BMI, body mass index; CAD, coronary artery disease; HDL, high-density lipoproteins; LDL, low-density lipoproteins.

(AHA) guidelines support the use of estrogen in postmenopausal women,[32] particularly in women with multiple cardiac risk factors. Diabetic women should be taking daily aspirin before initiating hormonal therapy.

Although glucose control is more strongly linked with microvascular complications of diabetes than with macrovascular disease, optimal glucose control is important to the control of lipid levels, and may have an impact on cardiac events (see below).[4,42,43] Both the American Diabetes Association (ADA) and AHA support the intensive treatment of diabetes with patient self-monitoring of blood glucose levels and target HbA$_{1c}$ concentrations <7%.[32]

Asymptomatic Ischemia

Diabetic patients sometimes have unrecognized CAD, causing asymptomatic episodes of myocardial ischemia. Asymptomatic or "silent" ischemia most often occurs in patients who also have symptomatic ischemia with angina, but some patients with diabetes only experience asymptomatic episodes. Ischemia tends to occur more commonly without symptoms in diabetics than in nondiabetics during treadmill testing,[44] ambulatory electrocardiographic monitoring,[45] and coronary angioplasty balloon inflation.[46]

The significance of asymptomatic ischemia depends on the extent of compromised myocardium, with some diabetic patients having only minor regions of ischemia and others having major ischemia. Of particular concern is asymptomatic ischemia which has caused prior MI, decreased left ventricular function, heart failure, or ventricular arrhythmias. These patients are at high risk for subsequent cardiac events and therefore require complete evaluation, usually including coronary angiography.

The mechanisms responsible for asymptomatic CAD in diabetic patients may include cardiac autonomic neuropathy (see Chap. 44).[47] The afferent sympathetic nerves contain fibers responsible for pain awareness during myocardial ischemia. Although this is an appealing explanation for silent ischemia, diabetic patients with painful ischemia also have alterations in cardiac sympathetic innervation.[48] These latter findings suggest that additional factors likely inhibit the diabetic patient's awareness of ischemia.

Diagnosis

Routine electrocardiography sometimes reveals significant Q waves, deep T-wave inversions, or left bundle branch block (LBBB) in asymptomatic patients with diabetes. These findings should raise the possibility of a prior MI. In the Framingham study, 12% of diabetic patients had electrocardiographic evidence of prior MI and no symptoms of CAD.[49] The current ADA recommendations include a yearly electrocardiogram to evaluate older patients for the presence of CAD.[37]

Asymptomatic CAD can also be detected through cardiac testing. Treadmill exercise electrocardiography is perhaps the least expensive and most widely used approach. ST-segment depression occurs in 12–54% of asymptomatic patients.[45,50–52] Abnormal treadmill tests have been associated with retinopathy, male gender, and insulin treatment.[52] However, standard exercise electrocardiography has limitations, including a relatively low sensitivity and a significant incidence of false positive tests (especially in patients with hypertension). In addition, a number of older diabetic patients are unable to exercise adequately, decreasing the utility of the test.

Cardiac assessment with either myocardial perfusion imaging or echocardiography has a greater sensitivity and specificity than exercise testing with electrocardiographic monitoring alone. These techniques can also be used along with pharmacologic stress (adenosine or dobutamine infusions) in patients who are unable to exercise well. The prevalence of asymptomatic myocardial ischemia detected by perfusion imaging ranges from 6–29% in patients with diabetes.[53–55] Predictors of abnormal perfusion studies include increasing age, higher cholesterol level, male gender, proteinuria, and ST-T wave abnormalities on resting electrocardiogram.[55]

Myocardial perfusion imaging not only improves the detection of CAD, but is also a well-recognized predictor of adverse cardiac outcomes in the overall population with either known or suspected CAD.[56] In one study of high-risk patients with T2DM (most of whom were asymptomatic), abnormal thallium perfusion imaging was associated with a 2.9-fold greater risk of nonfatal MI and a 5.7-fold greater likelihood of a major event (MI or death).[57] A greater number of abnormal segments on perfusion imaging pre-dicted a higher incidence of subsequent events. Large, reversible myocardial perfusion defects are sometimes found in asymptomatic diabetic patients and indicate significant areas of potentially jeopardized myocardium (Fig. 49-2).

Screening

The strategy of screening the overall population of patients with diabetes for asymptomatic CAD remains highly controversial. The rationale for screening is that early detection of CAD will lead to interventions that will lower the risk of irreversible cardiac events (MI and death). An effective screening program incorporates tests that not only accurately identify the presence of CAD, but more importantly have predictive value for future cardiac events. Clinical investigations, such as the Detection of Ischemia in Asymptomatic Diabetics (DIAD) study, are under way to address the efficacy of screening for CAD in patients with diabetes.

The identification of asymptomatic CAD has clear implications for the care of the diabetic patient. It strongly reinforces the need to reduce modifiable cardiovascular risk factors, which often requires multiple medications to optimally treat dyslipidemia and hypertension. In some patients it may lead to the initiation of lipid-lowering therapy. Although the ADA recommends that LDL cholesterol levels be less than 100 mg/dL, the current guidelines do not necessarily call for the initiation of pharmacologic therapy for levels between 100 and 130 mg/dL unless macrovascular disease is present.[34] A heightened concern for CAD can motivate efforts at smoking cessation and weight reduction, which otherwise may be difficult to accomplish. Once CAD is identified, physicians are more apt to assure the patient's compliance with daily aspirin treatment and to consider the use of beta-blockers to prevent ischemia. Recommendations for regular exercise are reinforced with limitations placed on very strenuous activity which might place the patient at risk for a cardiac event.

Abnormal noninvasive cardiac testing in patients with diabetes sometimes results in coronary angiography. When critically blocked coronary vessels are detected, patients often undergo coronary revascularization with the rationale that the cardiac event rate will be reduced by such intervention. However, there are risks associated with either percutaneous revascularization or coronary artery bypass grafting which need to be carefully considered (see below). The efficacy of these procedures in improving outcomes in asymptomatic diabetic patients is unproven, although revascular-

FIGURE 49-2. Asymptomatic ischemia. Myocardial perfusion images demonstrating a large defect in the anterolateral region (**arrows**) of the left ventricle on the exercise stress images (**top row**), which has largely resolved in the rest images (**bottom row**). This anterolateral ischemia was due to a 90% stenosis in the middle portion of the left anterior descending artery in an asymptomatic 54-year-old man with T2DM, hypertension, mild obesity, and low HDL cholesterol.

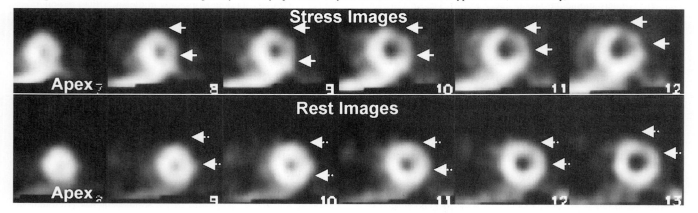

ization does improve outcomes in diabetic patients with mild angina and abnormal cardiac testing.[58,59] The Bypass Angioplasty Revascularization Intervention (BARI) II trial, which is now under way to compare the utility of contemporary medical therapy with or without revascularization in diabetic patients, will help to clarify this important issue. At the current time, revascularization is generally reserved for high-risk patients.

The ADA has published guidelines for CAD screening and risk stratification in high-risk individuals with diabetes.[37] Exercise stress testing with myocardial perfusion imaging or echocardiography is recommended for risk stratification in the patient with cardiac symptoms or evidence of ischemia or MI on electrocardiogram. In the asymptomatic patient with diabetes, screening is considered in patients with peripheral or carotid occlusive disease, cardiovascular autonomic neuropathy, or multiple (2 or more, including microalbuminuria) cardiac risk factors in addition to diabetes.

Medical Treatment

Once the diagnosis of CAD is made in patients with diabetes, an intensive effort is required to modify coronary risk factors, following many of the same principles outlined for the primary prevention of CAD (Table 49-1). A multifaceted approach should include aggressive treatment of dyslipidemia and hypertension, prevention of thrombosis with aspirin, and medications to reduce the occurrence of myocardial ischemia. The goals of this intensive therapy are to decrease the likelihood of subsequent cardiac events and death, to slow the progression of coronary atherosclerosis, and to prevent ischemic symptoms.

Anti-Ischemic Medication

Specific therapy for angina in diabetic patients should include beta-blockers, which prevent ischemia and improve exercise tolerance. Chronic beta-blocker therapy in diabetic patients with CAD reduces the cardiac event rate.[60] The overall benefit of these medications outweighs their potential for worsening glycemic control in patients with T2DM and for masking hypoglycemia in patients requiring insulin. However, they should be used with caution and should be avoided if possible in the presence of bronchospastic lung disease, active heart failure, and significant sinus or atrioventricular node disease.

Angiotensin-converting enzyme (ACE) inhibitors have an important role in the treatment of CAD in diabetic patients, particularly in the presence of heart failure, decreased left ventricular function, or hypertension (see below). However, they may also have a more generalized benefit in preventing cardiac events in diabetic patients with CAD. In the recent Heart Outcomes Prevention Evaluation (HOPE) study, ACE inhibitors decreased cardiac events in a broad group of patients which included diabetics with and without CAD.[61] This benefit may derive from the stabilization of coronary plaques and prevention of unstable coronary syndromes.

Nitrates are useful for the symptomatic relief and prevention of angina, but need to be used with caution in patients with autonomic neuropathy. Calcium channel blockers are also helpful in the treatment of angina and have an important role in controlling blood pressure in hypertensive type 2 diabetics.

Lipids

Treatment of lipid abnormalities is critically important in diabetic patients with CAD. The beneficial effect of lipid lowering is both to stabilize existing plaque and prevent acute coronary syndromes, and to slow the progression of atherosclerosis. Although diabetes does not increase LDL cholesterol, most diabetic patients with CAD benefit from treatment with an HMG-CoA reductase inhibitor (statin). In the Scandinavian Simvastatin Survival Study (4S), treatment with simvastatin decreased the coronary event rate by 40% over 5 years of follow-up in diabetic patients with high LDL cholesterol and known CAD.[62] In the Cholesterol and Recurrent Events (CARE) study, there was a 25% reduction in cardiac event rate in diabetic patients with average LDL cholesterol levels who were treated with pravastatin.[63] Interestingly, in the Atorvastatin versus Revascularization Treatment (AVERT) study, high-dose atorvastatin treatment was as effective as angioplasty in reducing cardiac events and ischemia in mildly symptomatic patients with low-risk stress tests.[64] Although this study included patients with diabetes, whether they had the same benefit as nondiabetic patients was not assessed. In addition, the angioplasty-treated patients did not receive as aggressive lipid-lowering treatment, so it remains uncertain as to whether angioplasty has an additional beneficial effect when combined with intensive lipid-lowering treatment. This issue is currently being evaluated in the ongoing Clinical Outcome Utilizing Revascularization and Aggressive Drug Evaluation (COURAGE) trial.

Many patients with T2DM have pronounced abnormalities in HDL cholesterol and triglycerides with relatively normal concentrations of LDL cholesterol. In these patients, treatment with fibrates may be beneficial in preventing cardiac events. The Helsinki Heart Study suggested that gemfibrozil treatment reduced the incidence of CAD in patients with T2DM.[65] In the Veterans Affairs High-Density Lipoprotein Cholesterol Intervention Trial (VA HIT) study, gemfibrozil decreased cardiac events by 20% in patients with CAD who had low HDL (<40 mg/dL) and average LDL cholesterol (<140 mg/dL) levels.[66] Some diabetic patients have high LDL cholesterol and low HDL/high triglycerides, which remain abnormal after treatment with a statin. In this case, the combined use of a statin and fibrate may be helpful in normalizing the lipid profile. However, there are no outcome data yet showing that this combination of drugs is better than either alone, and there is some potential for the development of myositis with combined therapy.

Antithrombotic Agents

Aspirin inhibits platelet thromboxane synthesis and aggregation, preventing coronary thrombus formation in patients with diabetes. Despite the increased platelet reactivity that occurs in diabetic patients, cardiac events are reduced by relatively low doses of aspirin. In the Physicians Health Study, 325 mg of aspirin every other day reduced the incidence of MI by 60% in diabetic physicians.[67] In the Early Treatment Diabetic Retinopathy Study (ETDRS), 650 mg of aspirin per day reduced the cardiac event rates in diabetic patients.[68] In the Hypertension Optimal Treatment (HOT) trial, 75 mg of aspirin reduced cardiovascular events by 15% and the incidence of MI by 36% in patients with diabetes.[69] Thus it would appear that low-dose aspirin (75–325 mg per day) is effective in reducing cardiac events in diabetic patients with CAD.

A second mechanism involved in thrombosis is ADP-mediated activation of platelets. Agents such as ticlodipine and clopidogrel block this pathway and are effective in inhibiting platelet aggregation. In the Clopidogrel versus Aspirin in Patients at Risk for Ischemic Events (CAPRIE) study, clopidogrel was slightly more effective than 325 mg of daily aspirin in preventing cardiovascular events.[70] Although diabetic patients were included in this study, the analysis did not specifically assess the efficacy of clopidogrel in this subgroup. In addition, these agents are more expensive than aspirin and may rarely cause granulocytopenia and thrombotic thrombocytopenic purpura. These agents are used routinely following coronary stent placement (see below) and in chronic CAD in patients allergic to or unable to take aspirin.

Revascularization

Careful consideration is warranted when deciding whether and by what means a patient with diabetes should undergo coronary artery revascularization. The number, location, morphology, and extent of coronary stenoses are the primary features determining the appropriateness of percutaneous intervention or coronary artery bypass grafting (CABG). The presence of left main stenosis, multivessel disease, or long complex proximal lesions favors the use of CABG. This assumes that the distal vessels are suitable targets with good run-off, and that the patient does not have excessive comorbidity. In the case of a single discrete proximal stenosis, current trends favor the use of percutaneous intervention when technically feasible. In a small number of patients with diabetes, coronary angiography reveals multivessel disease, which is technically suitable for either percutaneous intervention or CABG. Management of these patients remains controversial as discussed below.

Coronary Artery Bypass Grafting

CABG has an important role in the management of CAD patients with diabetes, who generally derive excellent symptomatic improvement from this procedure. In the current era, patients with diabetes have a 95–99% chance of surviving the initial surgery.[71–73] In-hospital mortality is higher in older patients and when surgery is performed on a nonelective basis following presentation with unstable angina or MI.[74] Gender also has an impact on the risk of CABG in patients with diabetes,[74,75] with women having a twofold higher operative mortality than men.[72]

Operative Complications

Diabetic patients are at somewhat increased risk for both cardiac and noncardiac complications associated with CABG. The most serious complications are postoperative MI, stroke, renal failure, and sternal wound infection.[73,76] The development of a new Q-wave MI is a serious complication of CABG that occurs slightly more often in patients with diabetes compared to those without diabetes.[73,77] In the BARI trial, new Q-wave MI was found in 5.8% of the patients with diabetes versus 4.3% of those without diabetes. Potential causes of MI are ischemia prior to cardiopulmonary bypass, an inability to graft diseased vessels, and air or atherosclerotic coronary embolization.

Patients with diabetes are also at increased risk for stroke during CABG. The incidence of stroke is twice as high in diabetics as in nondiabetics and ranges from 2–4% in patients with diabetes.[73] Older patients with diabetes with a history of prior stroke, as well as those with calcification of the ascending aorta or renal failure,[78] are at particular high risk, and these indications sometimes mitigate against proceeding with surgery.

Postoperative renal failure occurs more commonly in patients with diabetes.[79] Those with preoperative renal insufficiency are at particular risk and the use of ACE inhibitors immediately post-CABG may precipitate oliguria in these patients.[80] Preoperative renal insufficiency is also a marker of general risk during CABG, since it often occurs in older patients with diabetes and those with peripheral vascular disease, hypertension, or left ventricular

dysfunction.[81,82] Diabetic patients on dialysis are at particularly high risk, with operative mortalities as high as 10–15%.[83] These patients often require more prolonged mechanical ventilation, and more frequently develop atrial fibrillation and gastrointestinal complications following CABG.

Sternal wound infections occur in 8–10% of diabetic patients undergoing CABG, which is three- to fivefold more often than in nondiabetic subjects.[71,84] The majority of these are successfully treated with antibiotics, but occasionally operative debridement is necessary. The risk of sternal wound infection may be increased when preoperative blood glucose levels are >200 mg/dL.[85,86] Although there is some concern that the use of one or both internal mammary artery (IMA) grafts may devascularize the sternum and predispose to sternal complications in diabetic patients, recent investigations have not found a relationship between the type of graft and infection.[71,87] Antibiotic prophylaxis is given within the 2 hours preceding surgery to minimize the risk of infection.[88]

Long-Term Outcomes

Although most diabetic patients derive significant symptomatic benefit from CABG, they do have somewhat less favorable long-term outcomes than those without diabetes. Compared to nondiabetic subjects, the overall survival of diabetic patients after CABG is reduced from approximately 90% to 80% at 5 years, and from 80% to 65% at 7–10 years.[73,75] This reflects in part their more advanced cardiac disease and comorbidity at the time of surgery. Predictors of worse long-term outcomes following CABG include preoperative stroke, hypertension, heart failure, high glucose levels, proteinuria, multivessel disease, male sex, left ventricular dysfunction, and surgery with less than three grafts.[73,75,89]

A higher incidence of angina and heart failure also occurs following CABG in patients with diabetes.[75] This relates to less complete revascularization due to the presence of diffuse disease, more rapid progression of native disease, increased risk for saphenous vein occlusion, and a tendency to have or develop heart failure (see below). However, the BARI trial reported that over a 7-year period, repeat CABG was performed in only 2% of patients and PTCA in 9% of patients.[90]

The use of an IMA graft during CABG is important in the overall population, but appears to be critical in patients with diabetes.[71,75,77] The long-term patency of the left IMA is superior to that of saphenous vein grafts. In the BARI trial, the 5-year cardiac mortality after CABG was less than 2% in those who received an IMA graft.[77] The 7-year total mortality was 17% when an IMA graft was used, but 45% when only saphenous veins were utilized.[90] This may relate in part to the protection afforded by grafting the left IMA to the left anterior descending artery, which supplies the important anterior wall of the left ventricle. Following revascularization with either CABG or PTCA for multivessel disease, patients with diabetes have an 8% risk of developing a Q-wave MI over the next 5 years. In these patients survival at the time of MI is considerably better if they have had prior CABG.[91]

Percutaneous Transluminal Coronary Angioplasty

Percutaneous coronary intervention most commonly involves PTCA or intracoronary stent placement in patients with diabetes. Coronary atherectomy and laser and rotablator interventions are much less commonly utilized. Percutaneous intervention has an important role in the treatment of single-vessel CAD in diabetic patients. It results in excellent symptomatic improvement in diabetic

TABLE 49-2. Outcomes in Patients with and without Diabetes Following PTCA without Stenting

Series	Follow-Up	Subjects	Survival	MI	CABG	Re-PTCA
Kip et al.[92]	9 years	DM = 281	64%	29%	37%	44%
NHLBI Registry		NonDM = 1833	82%	19%	27%	37%
1985–86						
Marso et al.[97]	2 years	DM = 537	86%			
Registry		NonDM = 2247	93%			
1993–95						
Stein et al.[93]	5 years	DM = 1133	88%	19%	23%	25%
Elective PTCA		NonDM = 9300	93%	11%	14%	21%
Emory						
1980–90						

MI, myocardial infarction; CABG, coronary artery bypass grafting; PTCA, percutaneous transluminal coronary angioplasty; DM, = diabetes mellitus; NHLBI = National Heart, Lung and Blood Institute.

patients with angina. Percutaneous interventions are also attractive in that they avoid the initial complications of CABG in patients at high risk for surgery because of significant comorbidity.

Complications

The primary initial risk of PTCA is coronary occlusion leading to MI. Although the early use of PTCA was associated with increased rates of nonfatal MI and death in diabetic patients,[92] the current results have improved and are comparable to those in nondiabetics. PTCA is now successful in over 99% of diabetic patients, with an overall mortality of 0.4–1%.[77,93,94] The risk of MI (evidenced by an increase in cardiac enzymes) is 3–5%, but significant or Q-wave MI occurs only in 0.5–2% of diabetic patients. The risks are higher in multivessel angioplasty. The use of intensive antiplatelet treatment, including the glycoprotein IIb/IIIa antibody fragment abciximab, has substantially lowered the risk of thrombosis formation, MI, and death during PTCA in diabetics.[94] When PTCA fails, urgent CABG is required in 0.5% of diabetic patients.

In addition to the cardiac risks, percutaneous coronary interventions may cause vascular complications or renal failure, particularly in older diabetic patients with underlying diffuse vascular disease and renal insufficiency. Stroke due to embolization of atheromatous material or thrombus from the aorta is the most serious vascular complication, and occurs in 0.2–0.6% of diabetic patients undergoing PTCA.[77,94] Atheroembolic showering to the kidneys, mesenteric circulation, and periphery rarely occur. Femoral artery catheterization may be complicated by retroperitoneal bleeding, femoral hematoma, femoral or iliac artery occlusion, or pseudoaneurysm formation. Patients with diabetes are also at increased risk for contrast nephropathy, which may be prevented in part by forced diuresis[95] and the administration of the antioxidant acetylcysteine.[96]

Long-Term Outcomes

The long-term outcomes of PTCA in diabetes are less favorable than in nondiabetic patients (Table 49-2).[92,93,97] Following PTCA, mortality was twofold higher in diabetic than in nondiabetic patients over follow-up periods ranging from 2–9 years, with differences evident as soon as 1.5 years after PTCA.[93] Diabetic patients experience more MIs following PTCA than nondiabetic patients. They also have a greater need for CABG and repeat PTCA due to recurrent ischemia.[93] Patients with diabetes, as well as older patients and those with decreased left ventricular function, heart failure, multivessel disease, and proteinuria have decreased survival after PTCA.[92,93,97,98]

A major determinant of the adverse long-term outcomes with PTCA in patients with diabetes has been the high rate of restenosis. Restenosis occurs in 25–40% of diabetics within the first 3–6 months after PTCA and often leads to the recurrence of symptoms.[99–101] In small or diffusely diseased vessels, and in saphenous vein grafts the restenosis rate is in excess of 50%. Restenosis is often symptomatic, requiring repeat PTCA or CABG, but when unrecognized may contribute to long-term mortality in patients with diabetes following angioplasty.

The increased incidence of restenosis following PTCA in diabetics is attributed in part to the smaller intraluminal diameter achieved during the balloon dilatation, and in part to the accelerated neointimal hyperplasia which occurs in these patients.[102,103] The latter reflects greater impairment in endothelial function and increased smooth muscle cell proliferation. Increased thrombus formation at the site of balloon dilatation may trigger the smooth muscle cell response, which may then be enhanced by hyperinsulinemia and insulin-like growth factor-1.

Intracoronary Stents

The use of intracoronary stents has improved the outcome of percutaneous coronary revascularization. With recent progress in the development of stents and device delivery technology, stents are now used in the majority of interventional procedures.[104,105] Coronary stents achieve a greater luminal diameter than PTCA. They also prevent the coronary artery dissection that sometimes complicates PTCA and can lead to complete vessel occlusion and MI. The development of smaller stents has also permitted their more widespread use in patients with diabetes.

The outcomes of intracoronary stents in patients with diabetes have been evaluated in a number of studies over the last 5 years (Table 49-3).[99–101,106,107] Initial reports suggested a 1.5–2 times higher rate of early thrombosis and later restenosis following stent placement in diabetic patients. Increased restenosis in patients with diabetes reflects greater neointimal proliferation through the stent and results in a more frequent need for repeat revascularization. Restenosis is a particular problem in patients treated with insulin, who also have a lower cardiac event–free survival.[100]

Recent studies have demonstrated that diabetic patients benefit from vigorous initial antiplatelet therapy after stent placement. Standard therapy during stent placement includes aspirin, clopidogrel and heparin, followed by aspirin and clopidogrel for 2–4 weeks, and then indefinite aspirin therapy. With the additional use of abciximab prior to device delivery and for 12 hours afterwards, the risks of stent thrombosis and resulting MI have decreased

TABLE 49-3. Restenosis in Patients with and without Diabetes After PTCA with Stenting

Series	Follow-Up	Subjects	Restenosis	
			Angiographic	Clinical
Abizaid et al.[100]	12 months	DM (insulin) = 97		28%*
Consecutive pts.		No insulin = 151		18%
1994–96		Non-DM = 706		16%
Elezi et al.[101]	12 months	DM = 715	38%	23%*
Consecutive pts.		Non-DM = 2839	28%	18%
1992–97				
Gowda et al.[106]	12 months	DM = 77		40%†
Non-Q-wave MI		Non-DM = 299		28%
1992–96				
Silva et al.[107]	6 months	DM = 28		14%*
Acute MI primary stenting		Non-DM = 76		7%
1995–97				
Van Belle et al.[99]	6 months	DM = 56	25%	
Consecutive pts.		Non-DM = 244	27%	
1994–96				

*Target vessel revascularization.

†Any revascularization.

PTCA, percutaneous transluminal coronary angioplasty; DM, diabetes mellitus.

Angiographic restenosis = restenosis determined by routine follow-up angiographic evaluation.

Clinical restenosis = recurrence of symptoms leading to angiography and subsequent revascularization of the initially stented stenosis. Target vessel = vessel initially stented.

TABLE 49-4. Outcomes with the Use of Glycoprotein IIb/IIIa Blockade During Percutaneous Intervention Stenting in Patients with and without Diabetes

Series	Follow-Up	Subjects	Death + MI	Target Vessel Revascularization
Kleiman et al.[94]	6 months	Diabetic		
EPILOG		Placebo = 224	15%	16%
1995		Rx = 414	6%	21%
		Nondiabetic		
		Placebo = 714	10%	19%
		Rx = 1435	6%	15%
Marso et al.[108]	6 months	Diabetic		
EPISTENT		Stent = 173	13%	17%
1996–97		Stent + Rx = 162	6%	8%
		PTCA + Rx = 156	8%	18%
		Nondiabetic		
		Stent = 636	11%	9%
		Stent + Rx = 632	5%	9%
		PTCA + Rx = 640	8%	15%

Rx, abciximab (monoclonal antibody fragment blocking the platelet glycoprotein IIb/IIIa receptor); MI, myocardial infarction; PTCA, percutaneous transluminal coronary angioplasty; target vessel, vessel initially stented or angioplastied.

considerably. In addition, intensive early platelet inhibition may also prevent platelet vessel wall interaction, which is important in initiating the restenosis process. The multicenter Evaluation of Platelet IIb/IIIa Inhibitor for Stenting (EPISTENT) trial also demonstrated that infusion of abciximab reduced by half the need for repeat coronary revascularization during the 6 months following stent placement in diabetic patients (Table 49-4).[94,108] In addition, combined rates of death and MI were also reduced in diabetic patients at 6 months.

The use of stents in diabetic patients is a rapidly evolving field. Although the intermediate-term results are encouraging, long-term outcomes and the use of stents in patients with multivessel CAD remains to be determined. The effect of other glycoprotein IIb/IIIa inhibitors (tirofiban, eptifibatide) on stent outcomes in diabetes needs

to be further evaluated. Finally, biologically-coated stents and brachytherapy (local radiation to prevent neointimal proliferation) are emerging as important approaches to preventing restenosis in diabetic patients.

Multivessel Disease

Patients with diabetes are often found to have multivessel CAD. The majority of these patients are clearly best revascularized by CABG, but a subgroup have localized stenoses that are potentially amenable to either CABG or multivessel percutaneous intervention.

These different strategies have been compared in both randomized clinical trials and observational studies (Table 49-5).[77,91,109–112] A major concern about the use of multivessel

TABLE 49-5. Comparison of Outcomes Following PTCA and CABG for Multivessel Coronary Revascularization in Patients with Diabetes

| | | | | Subsequent | |
Series	Follow-Up	Subjects	Survival	CABG	PTCA
BARI Investigators[77]	5 years	PTCA = 173	66%		
		CABG = 170	81%		
BARI RCT 1988–91					
King et al.[109]	8 years	PTCA = 29	60%		
EAST RCT 1987–90		CABG = 30	76%		
Detre et al.[91]	5 years	PTCA = 182	86%		
BARI Registry 1988–91		CABG = 117	85%		
Barsness et al.[110]	5 years	PTCA = 144	76%	33%	36%
Database 1984–90		CABG = 626	74%	2%	6%
Gum et al.[111]	6 years	PTCA = 279	63%	64%	
Database 1987–90		CABG = 246	70%	8%	
Weintraub et al.[112]	5 years	PTCA = 834	78%	26%	42%
Database		CABG = 1805	76%	2%	6%
1981–94	10 years		45%	49%	53%
			48%	13%	19%

CABG, coronary artery bypass grafting; PTCA, percutaneous transluminal coronary angioplasty; RCT, randomized clinical trail.

PTCA was raised by the BARI trial, which randomized patients to either PTCA or CABG in the late 1980s.[77] In the subgroup of patients with diabetes (on treatment), both the cardiac and overall mortality were higher in those undergoing PTCA than in those treated with CABG after 5 years.[77,113] In contrast, there was no survival difference observed in the nondiabetic patients. In diabetic patients receiving an IMA graft during CABG, the cardiac mortality at 5 years was only 3%, while in those in whom only saphenous vein grafts were used the mortality was 18%, which was similar to that seen with PTCA (21%). The survival advantage associated with CABG in diabetic patients occurred despite a higher risk of Q-wave MI (6% versus 1.4%) and in-hospital mortality (1.2% versus 0.6%) at the time of the initial procedure. Other randomized clinical trials have included patients with diabetes and overall have also shown a survival benefit from CABG.[109,114,115]

The adverse outcomes of PTCA in multivessel CAD in diabetes led to an alert, cautioning about the use of multivessel angioplasty in patients with diabetes,[116] and to the suggestion that multivessel PTCA be abandoned in diabetic patients.[117] However, in nonrandomized studies, the survival with multivessel PTCA and CABG has been equivalent.[110,112] This may be explained in part by the tendency of patients treated with CABG to be at higher risk than those treated with angioplasty in nonrandomized studies. In addition, completeness of revascularization is better in subjects undergoing CABG (79–81%) as compared to those undergoing angioplasty (16–42%).[111,112] Although CABG is often the preferred means of revascularization in diabetics, percutaneous revascularization may be warranted in the future with the use of coronary stents, more effective platelet inhibitors, intensive risk factor management, and careful observation following the initial procedure.

Acute Myocardial Infarction

Acute MI is a common event in patients with diabetes. The incidence of MI in patients with T2DM was approximately 15 per 1000 patient-years in the UKPDS, while the incidence of fatal MI was 7 per 1000 patient-years.[2] MI may occur without the warning of prior angina, and patients may have atypical symptoms which delay their seeking medical attention. In some cases, these patients succumb to ischemic arrhythmias and never reach the hospital.[118,119] In addition, studies have consistently documented a twofold higher mortality and increased morbidity associated with acute MI in patients with diabetes. The poor natural history of MI in diabetic patients is highlighted by studies during the 1960s from the Joslin Clinic, in which early mortality approached 40%.[120] Although early coronary reperfusion, aspirin, beta-blockers, ACE inhibitors, lipid-lowering agents, and coronary revascularization have dramatically improved the survival of diabetic patients with MI, these patients still have a higher risk of complications than nondiabetic patients.

Complications Associated with Acute MI

Patients with diabetes have an increased incidence of complications associated with acute MI. Most problematic of these are heart failure, cardiogenic shock, and postinfarct angina.[121,122] These problems result in part from the more extensive multivessel and left main coronary artery disease found in diabetic patients. Heart block, atrial arrhythmias, and renal insufficiency have also been reported more frequently during the post-MI period in patients with diabetes.[123,124] Recurrent MI is also somewhat more common in individuals with diabetes.[124–127]

Heart failure is a particular problem in diabetic patients during and following acute MI.[125,128] Heart failure develops more commonly, even though the index infarctions are no larger than those in nondiabetic patients.[129] Heart failure may result from more extensive CAD causing ischemia in regions outside the infarct area, or from prior scarring in remote regions. Diabetes-related diastolic dysfunction and impaired systolic reserve (discussed below) may compromise the ability of the heart to cope with the stress of acute infarction. In addition, coexistent hypertension and renal disease may further promote the development of symptomatic heart failure.

Treatment of Acute MI

Overall, patients with diabetes are at high risk during MI and benefit from aggressive therapy, including early reperfusion for ST-segment elevation MI.

Thrombolytic Therapy

Patients with ST-segment elevation MI, in whom there is typically acute thrombotic occlusion of a coronary artery, require prompt treatment to reestablish myocardial reperfusion. In centers without cardiac catheterization facilities, this is achieved with thrombolytic therapy. Support for this approach comes from subgroup analyses of diabetic patients in the large thrombolytic trials carried out in the 1980s and 1990s, including the Thrombolysis and Angioplasty in Myocardial Infarction (TAMI) study,[130] the International Tissue Plasminogen Activator/Streptokinase (TPA/SK) trial,[131] the Second International Study of Infarct Survival (ISIS-2),[132] and the Gruppo Italiano per lo Studio Della Sopravvivenza nell'Infarto Miocardico (GISSI)-2 study.[133] Although thrombolytic therapy improved survival, both in-hospital and late mortality was 1.5- to 2-fold higher in diabetic than in nondiabetic patients. In the patients treated with insulin, and in diabetic women,[125,131] a higher in-hospital and 6-month mortality persists, highlighting the need for improved therapies in these high-risk patients.

Several factors may lead to less-than-optimal responses to thrombolysis in patients with diabetes, including more extensive CAD, diffuse disease with poor run-off in the occluded vessel, and their increased tendency toward thrombosis at the site of plaque rupture. Increased plasminogen activator inhibitor (PAI-1) levels, platelet hyperreactivity, increased concentrations of hemostatic proteins, and endothelial dysfunction promote thrombosis in diabetes. Thus improved strategies of thrombolysis and subsequent antithrombotic treatment to prevent reocclusion are needed in patients with diabetes.

Percutaneous Coronary Reperfusion

In many centers, primary angioplasty or intracoronary stent placement is the preferred treatment for acute MI, in that it provides more effective reperfusion, and definitive information on the extent of CAD, and avoids the use of thrombolytic agents. While the major primary angioplasty and stent trials have included patients with diabetes, in many the outcomes of patients with diabetes have not been specifically evaluated.[134,135] The Global Use of Strategies to Open Occluded Arteries in Acute Coronary Syndromes (GUSTO-IIb) Angioplasty Substudy did report the outcomes of the subgroup of 177 diabetic patients, randomized to thrombolysis (alteplase) or PTCA (8.6% with stent placement) between 1994 and 1996.[136] In the overall cohort of both diabetic and nondiabetic patients, primary PTCA led to better outcomes at 30 days with respect to the primary composite end point of death, reinfarction, and disabling stroke. The diabetic substudy was underpowered, but showed a similar trend in the diabetic patients and a significant reduction in recurrent ischemia and reinfarction with PTCA.[136]

The long-term outcomes after MI treated with primary PTCA are adversely influenced by the presence of multivessel disease, left ventricular dysfunction, and the development of restenosis, all of which are more common in patients with diabetes. In GUSTO-IIb, the 1-year mortality was similar in the diabetic patients treated with thrombolysis or primary PTCA,[136] which may reflect the high incidence of restenosis after PTCA in diabetic patients (see below). At present, myocardial placement of intracoronary stents with adjuvant antithrombotic treatment with glycoprotein IIb/IIIa inhibitors is a common approach to treating ST-segment elevation MI in patients with diabetes. This approach is intended to provide more complete and secure early reperfusion and may diminish the rate of restenosis (see below).

Thus diabetic patients with ST-segment elevation who are within 12 hours of the onset of symptoms should be considered for primary angioplasty with stent placement, particularly when there is evidence of heart failure or hemodynamic stability, where the establishment of secure vessel patency may be critical. Multi-vessel disease is identified more commonly in diabetic than non-diabetic patients at the time of primary angioplasty. While angioplasty or stent placement in the "culprit" lesion is preferable for treatment of the acute MI in most cases, a small number (~5%) of diabetic patients require urgent surgical revascularization.[136] When PTCA or stent placement in the "culprit" lesion leaves significant residual CAD, the presence of recurrent angina or inducible ischemia indicates a need for subsequent revascularization.

Beta-Blockers

Beta-blockers decrease chest pain, limit the amount of myocardial damage, and improve prognosis in the setting of acute MI. In patients with diabetes included in large trials, beta-blockers reduced mortality by 36% during acute MI.[137,138] Contraindications to the use of beta-blockers during MI include bradycardia, hypotension, atrioventricular nodal block, moderate or severe heart failure, or active wheezing. Beta-blockers should be given to patients regardless of administration of thrombolytic therapy or primary PTCA. They are especially useful to treat continuing or recurrent ischemic chest pain or rapid atrial fibrillation. Since diabetic patients often have significant heart failure during MI, patients treated with beta-blockers should be carefully monitored.

ACE Inhibitors

Treatment of patients with ACE inhibitors reduces afterload, prevents adverse myocardial remodeling, and decreases heart failure and mortality following MI. In the GISSI-3 study, in the subgroup of patients with diabetes treated with lisinopril for 6 weeks, the mortality was reduced from 12.4% to 8.7%, and this benefit persisted for 6 months after completion of therapy.[139] ACE inhibitors also appear to have long-term benefit in patients with diabetes following MI, as demonstrated by the subgroup analysis of the Survival and Ventricular Enlargement (SAVE) trial.[140]

Insulin Treatment

The infusion of glucose-insulin-potassium (GIK) during acute MI lowers free fatty acid concentrations, improves myocardial metabolism, and may prevent apoptosis and necrosis.[141] In addition to these early beneficial effects, intensive treatment of diabetes may stabilize the coronary vasculature and prevent recurrent events after acute MI. In the Diabetes Insulin Glucose in Acute MI (DIGAMI) trial, intravenous insulin infusion during the initial 24 hours, followed by intensive insulin treatment for 3 months, reduced mortality at 1 year from 26% to 19%[142] and at 3 years from 44% to 33%.[143] Interestingly, the largest impact was seen in those with a low-risk cardiovascular profile and no previous insulin treatment. The benefit of intensive treatment after discharge may be mediated by favorable effects on platelets, lipoproteins, tissue plasminogen activator-1 activity, vascular reactivity, or ventricular remodeling. However, because DIGAMI was a relatively small study, the current ACC/AHA guidelines caution that routine insulin use is not indicated until confirmatory results have been obtained.[144]

There is some concern that intensive diabetes treatment may cause hypoglycemia and trigger myocardial ischemia in diabetic patients. Hypoglycemia does trigger catecholamine release and increase heart rate and blood pressure. However, these potential negative effects need to be considered within the overall context of the benefits of improved glucose control. Although there was an increased risk of hypoglycemia in intensively treated patients in the DIGAMI study, this risk was outweighed by the benefits of intensive treatment. In addition, diabetic patients presenting with acute MI often are hyperglycemic, and those with poor glucose control are at particularly increased risk.[145,146] Thus improvement in glycemic control is generally considered an important goal in patients during and after acute MI, and further information is needed to determine the optimal means to achieve this goal.

Acute Coronary Syndromes

Unstable angina and non ST-segment MI are now considered part of a spectrum of acute coronary syndromes which have an increased risk for adverse outcomes.[147] These syndromes are characterized by progressive or prolonged anginal symptoms and often result from plaque rupture and intracoronary thrombus formation. The presence of diabetes is an independent risk factor for death, progression to acute ST-segment elevation, myocardial infarction, and subsequent readmission for unstable angina within the next year.[148]

Diabetic patients with unstable angina have coronary vascular instability, as evidenced by a higher incidence of ulcerated plaques and intracoronary thrombi observed during coronary angioscopy.[149] They also have more extensive CAD, involving a greater number and longer segments of vessels and more often involving the left main coronary artery. Particularly difficult to manage are diabetic patients with acute coronary syndromes who have had prior CABG and present with imminent closure of a heavily diseased saphenous vein graft. In these patients, symptoms often persist despite medical therapy and revascularization strategies are less than ideal.

The management and outcomes of patients with acute coronary syndromes in diabetic patients are also complicated by their higher comorbidity. The presence of hypertension, peripheral and cerebral vascular disease, left ventricular hypertrophy (LVH), and heart failure increase their overall risk. Cardiovascular autonomic dysfunction also complicates the management of acute coronary syndromes in patients with diabetes. Autonomic neuropathy may result in an increased heart rate (due to predominant parasympathetic neuropathy) and a decreased awareness of ischemic symptoms.

Treatment

The initial therapy of acute coronary syndromes includes the administration of beta-blockers, aspirin, heparin, and nitrates.

Recent studies suggest that further platelet inhibition by the addition of a glycoprotein IIb/IIIa inhibitor to standard therapy, improves outcomes in patients with unstable angina. In the Platelet Glycoprotein IIb/IIIa in Unstable Angina: Receptor Suppression Using Integrilin Therapy (PURSUIT) trial, eptifibatide reduced the composite end points of death or nonfatal MI at 30 days.[150] In the Platelet Receptor Inhibition in Ischemic Syndrome Management in Patients Limited by Unstable Signs and Symptoms (PRISM-PLUS) study, tirofiban also reduced death or MI at 30 days.[151] Although these trials included patients with diabetes, they were not designed to examine this specific subgroup. However, patients with diabetes have increased platelet reactivity and may derive significant benefit from the addition of these agents, particularly in the presence of significant ischemia or unremitting angina.

Many patients are initially stabilized with anti-ischemic and antithrombotic therapies, but some remain at significant risk for subsequent cardiac events. This has led to the widespread utilization of an invasive strategy with early coronary angiography and revascularization in the management of acute coronary syndromes. However, there has been recent debate as to whether an invasive strategy is preferable to a more conservative strategy with medical therapy and noninvasive testing to detect the subgroup of patients at high risk for subsequent events. In the Veterans Affairs Non-Q-Wave Infarction Strategies in Hospital (VANQWISH) trial, mortality or MI was not significantly different in those randomized to an invasive versus a conservative strategy.[152] In the Fragmin and Fast Revascularization During Instability in Coronary Artery Disease II trial (FRISC II), individuals with unstable angina treated with an invasive strategy had a 30–40% lower risk of death and MI as compared to those treated with a noninvasive strategy.[153] Neither study was powered to evaluate the outcomes specifically in diabetic patients.

In diabetic patients with acute coronary syndromes who respond to initial medical therapy, the decision whether to pursue angiography and revascularization needs to be individualized. The recent American College of Cardiology/American Heart Association (ACC/AHA) guidelines do not make generalized recommendations on the utilization of an initial invasive approach in diabetic patients.[147] An invasive strategy may be preferable in high-risk patients, including those with marked or widespread ST-segment depression, elevated troponin levels prior MI, decreased left ventricular function, or heart failure. A noninvasive approach with further risk stratification based on stress echocardiography or myocardial perfusion imaging may be preferable in lower-risk patients and those with major comorbidity who are at high risk for the invasive approach.

HEART FAILURE

Epidemiology

Heart failure causes substantial morbidity in patients with diabetes, including both exertional limitation and recurrent hospitalizations for shortness of breath. The Framingham Study demonstrated that the age-adjusted risk of developing heart failure was increased 2.4-fold in diabetic men, and 5.1-fold in diabetic women, with an overall incidence of heart failure of 22–27 per 1000 patient years.[154] Although the majority of these patients had T2DM, those treated with insulin had a four- to fivefold increased risk of heart failure compared to nondiabetic patients.

Etiology

The risk of heart failure in patients with diabetes persisted in the Framingham study after adjustment for age, hypertension, hypercholesterolemia, obesity, and clinically evident CAD.[154] However, there were few patients with heart failure who did not have CAD, hypertension, or rheumatic heart disease. Indeed, clinical heart failure is attributed in large part to coexistent CAD and/or hypertension, although abnormalities in left ventricular function related to diabetes may predispose the patient with these conditions to heart failure (see below).

CAD and Heart Failure

Atherosclerotic CAD is the most common cause of heart failure in the U.S. population[155] as well as in patients with diabetes.[154] Although the risk of developing heart failure in patients with diabetes persisted after accounting for clinically-evident CAD in the Framingham study, CAD was excluded only on the basis of absent clinical symptoms and electrocardiographic findings. In addition, the prevalence but not the extent of CAD was evaluated, and it is likely that the diabetic patients had more extensive CAD, which accounted in part for their increased incidence of heart failure. Additional recent cohort studies have also implicated diabetes as a risk factor for heart failure independent of CAD,[156,157] but these studies again excluded CAD only on the basis of clinical history or discharge diagnosis. Unexplained heart failure in a patient with diabetes should prompt evaluation for CAD, often including cardiac catheterization.

Myocardial ischemia resulting from CAD may cause heart failure through impairment in systolic contractile function. In some cases, the diabetic patient presents with a typical dilated ischemic cardiomyopathy where the left ventricle contracts poorly, is enlarged, and has focal regional wall motion abnormalities (Fig. 49-3). Some of these patients have clinically documented or clear electrocardiographic evidence of a prior MI, which has led to fibrosis, progressive left ventricular enlargement, and heart failure.[158] In other cases, more diffuse CAD has caused diffuse patchy fibrosis, without a history or clear electrocardiographic evidence of MI, which nonetheless has caused progressive deterioration in ventricular systolic function.

In some cases there may be a component of the left ventricular dysfunction that may be reversible with revascularization, and therefore is important to identify. Critical CAD may also impair systolic function due to recurrent ischemia in the absence of frank myocardial necrosis, a process referred to as stunned or hibernating myocardium. In addition, diastolic dysfunction is an important mechanism leading to heart failure in patients with CAD.[159] Impaired left ventricular relaxation and compliance may result from myocardial fibrosis or ischemia and increases left ventricular diastolic pressures.

Hypertension and Heart Failure

Hypertension is the most common cause of heart failure in the absence of CAD,[155] and is present in approximately 40–60% of patients with T2DM.[43] In hypertensive patients, diabetes is an independent risk factor for the development of heart failure, increasing the risk 1.8-fold in men and 3.6-fold in women.[160] Thus, the combination of hypertension and diabetes appears to cause heart failure in patients,[30,161–163] as it does in animal models.[164–166]

The combination of diabetes and hypertension is also associated with a greater degree of left ventricular hypertrophy (Fig. 49-4) and diastolic dysfunction. In some populations, diabetes has been associated with an increase in left ventricular mass even in the absence of hypertension.[167,168] Diabetes also increases left ventricular mass in patients with hypertension.[168a] Indeed hyperinsulinemia and insulin resistance, which are common in T2DM, have been correlated with left ventricular mass.[169] This may be related in part to the action of insulin to decrease the rates of protein breakdown in the heart.[170] In addition, patients with diabetes and hypertension may progress to develop a dilated cardiomyopathy with both systolic and diastolic dysfunction.[161] The mechanism responsible for the deterioration in left ventricular systolic function remains uncertain, but once systolic dysfunction becomes established, heart failure can be difficult to treat in these patients.

Diabetic Cardiomyopathy

The diagnosis of diabetic cardiomyopathy is sometimes invoked as the cause of unexplained heart failure or abnormalities in left ventricular function observed in patients with diabetes.

FIGURE 49-3. Ischemic cardiomyopathy. Echocardiogram demonstrating the cross-sectional images of an enlarged and poorly contracting left ventricle. This 65-year-old man with T2DM, dyslipidemia, and CAD had heart failure due to systolic dysfunction.

FIGURE 49-4. Left ventricular hypertrophy. Echocardiogram demonstrating the cross-sectional images of a hypertrophied but normally-contracting left ventricle. This 71-year-old woman with T2DM, hypertension, and obesity had heart failure due to diastolic dysfunction.

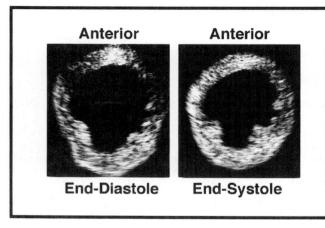

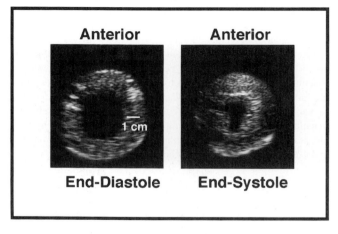

Pathologic Findings

A specific cardiomyopathy related to diabetes was initially proposed 30 years ago.[171] In a small number of patients who died with unexplained heart failure, myofibrillar hypertrophy and diffuse interstitial fibrosis were observed in the absence of significant obstructive CAD. These patients did have diabetic nephropathy, and it is possible that renal insufficiency and undiagnosed hypertension may have contributed to these pathologic findings. Nonetheless, interstitial fibrosis and increased myocardial collagen deposition[30,162,172] may decrease left ventricular compliance and contribute to diastolic dysfunction in patients with diabetes.

In addition, small-vessel changes may play a role in the pathogenesis of diabetic cardiomyopathy, even in the absence of significant large-vessel atherosclerotic CAD. Perivascular fibrosis,[29,173,174] thickening of myocardial capillary basement membranes and microaneurysms[30] have been reported in the diabetic heart. To some extent, these pathologic findings may contribute to the physiologic abnormalities in coronary flow reserve which occur in patients with both type 1[31] and type 2[175] diabetes in the absence of evident CAD. However, abnormal coronary flow reserve also results from endothelial dysfunction, which is related to glycemic control,[176] lipid levels, and a number of other dynamic factors. These functional abnormalities may be more important than the pathologic findings in determining flow reserve. Indeed, abnormalities in flow reserve appear to be associated with diastolic dysfunction in patients with T2DM.[177] Whether this represents a true causal link or simply an association is unclear.

Abnormalities in Cardiac Function

Several series have reported that patients with T1DM and T2DM have asymptomatic abnormalities in cardiac function. These include alterations in left ventricular systolic function (contraction), diastolic function (relaxation), and the ability of the left ventricle to increase its contractility during exercise. Although the preponderance of evidence supports the notion that these abnormalities are primarily related to diabetes or its complications, all of these abnormalities can also occur in the presence of underlying hypertension or CAD. In some series, patients with mild hypertension were included in the analysis, and occult CAD was not rigorously excluded, limiting their conclusiveness. In most studies, patients underwent exercise stress testing, and in some they also had myocardial perfusion imaging, but in very few did patients undergo coronary angiography to exclude occult CAD.

With these caveats in mind, abnormalities in resting systolic function have been reported in patients with diabetes. These include prolongation of the left ventricular pre-ejection interval and shortening of the systolic ejection period,[178] diminished fractional shortening and left ventricular ejection fraction,[179] and increased left ventricular systolic dimension and left ventricular mass.[180,181] However, conflicting information exists, in that other studies have reported increased fractional shortening in diabetic patients,[182] particularly in those with microalbuminuria.[183] Systolic ejection indices are also influenced by preload and afterload, which can vary with glycemic control. Thus in otherwise healthy diabetic patients, resting abnormalities in systolic function are generally not pronounced.

On the other hand, abnormal augmentation of systolic function during exercise has been more commonly observed in diabetic patients. Impaired augmentation of left ventricular ejection fraction (LVEF) during exercise occurs in up to 40% of diabetic patients, including those with T1DM and T2DM.[184–188] Impaired LVEF response has been somewhat variably defined as a decrease, no change, or a subnormal increase (<3–5%) in LVEF with exercise, and is also influenced by changes in afterload and preload. Interestingly, end-systolic indices of contractility and dobutamine-stimulated left ventricular function may be normal in young diabetic patients who have abnormal exercise ejection fractions.[189] These findings suggest that exercise abnormalities may reflect altered loading conditions or autonomic activation during exercise, rather than cardiac muscle dysfunction *per se*, in diabetic patients.

Diastolic function abnormalities have been widely documented in patients with diabetes (Fig. 49-5). These include prolonged isovolumic relaxation time,[190–192] delayed opening of the mitral valve, a

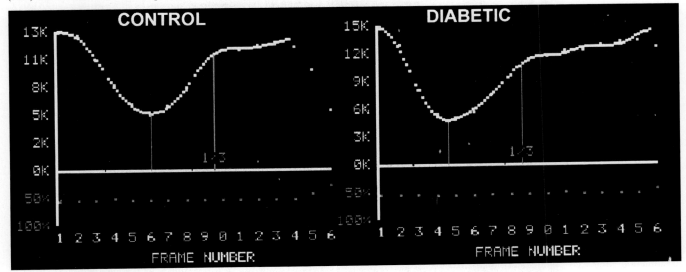

FIGURE 49-5. Diastolic dysfunction. Left ventricular volume measured by radionuclide ventriculography from a healthy control subject and a 37-year-old woman with longstanding T1DM. The curves demonstrate left ventricular emptying during systole (downstroke) and filling during diastole (upstroke). The volume curve from the diabetic patient has a blunted upstroke, which indicates impaired ventricular diastolic filling. The calculated peak diastolic filling rate (PFR) was reduced in the diabetic patient (2.8 volumes/sec) and normal in the control (4.5 volumes/sec).

decreased rate of left ventricular diastolic filling,[193–195] and abnormal transmitral flow velocities.[195–199] In addition, radionuclide ventriculography studies have shown that both left ventricular peak filling rate and the time to peak filling were abnormal in T1DM and T2DM.[187,198,200,201] Diastolic abnormalities may be present earlier than systolic abnormalities in patients with diabetes.[202]

These contractile abnormalities may be related in part to hyperglycemia and insulin deficiency. In some studies, abnormalities in ventricular function resolved with improved glycemic control,[192] indicating that the changes in left ventricular hemodynamics and neurohumoral activation associated with hyperglycemia may contribute to alterations in cardiac function. Abnormal cardiac indices have also been shown to correlate with other diabetes complications such as microangiopathy.[192] Cardiac autonomic neuropathy may contribute to the abnormalities in left ventricular function in diabetics[186,203–205] and will be discussed in more detail below.

Experimental Models

The normal contraction and relaxation of myofibrillar proteins depends on the integrity of the cellular and molecular mechanisms involved in regulating calcium flux, contractile protein function, and substrate and energy metabolism in the heart. Many abnormalities in these essential pathways have been described in experimental animal models of diabetes.[206–208]

Systolic contraction depends on calcium release from the sarcoplasmic reticulum (SR) interacting with calcium binding proteins that modulate the interaction of actin and myosin filaments. Diastolic relaxation of the heart is also an active process, requiring that the SR removes calcium from the cytosol. In experimental animal models of diabetes, alterations in calcium homeostasis include abnormal sarcolemmal calcium binding,[208] decreased calcium pump activity,[209] sodium-calcium exchange,[210] and SR calcium pump activity.[211,212] A diminished peak, but prolonged increase in intracellular calcium concentration occurs in isolated cardiac myocytes from diabetic rats.[213] High extracellular glucose and low insulin concentrations may directly impair relaxation and electromechanical coupling in cultured rat myocytes.[214,215] Of interest, hyperglycemia increases the activity of the important signaling pathway involving protein kinase C, and transgenic models overexpressing this signaling protein develop cardiomyopathy.[216]

Abnormalities in myofibrillar proteins in the diabetic heart may also contribute to impaired contractile function. A shift to the lower activity V3 isoform of the myosin heavy chain leads to diminished cardiac contractility in rodents.[217,218] Altered phosphorylation of troponin I and myosin light chain proteins which regulate contractile protein activity may also interfere with function in the diabetic heart.[219,220] Abnormal collagen crosslinking due to glycosylation products decreases diastolic relaxation.[221]

There are several additional molecular alterations which may lead to contractile dysfunction in diabetes.[206–208] However, animal models of diabetes have limitations with respect to their applicability to human disease. Thus more information is needed to understand the pathophysiology of heart failure in patients with diabetes.

Prognosis and Response to Therapy

The presence of diabetes increases the morbidity and mortality in patients with heart failure. In the Framingham study, diabetes was an independent predictor of death in women with heart failure, increasing their mortality 1.8-fold.[155] The Studies of Left Ventricular Dysfunction (SOLVD) demonstrated that diabetes increased the

risk of heart failure, morbidity, and mortality in patients with low ejection fractions.[222] This risk increased with diabetes duration and was also particularly apparent in women. As discussed above, heart failure is an important cause of the higher morbidity and mortality observed in diabetic patients after MI, as well as following coronary revascularization.[128,223] Thus early detection and management of heart failure are essential for the improvement in clinical outcomes in diabetic patients.

The treatment of heart failure in diabetic patients parallels many of the same strategies utilized in patients without diabetes. The identification and optimal treatment of coexistent hypertension and coronary artery disease is of paramount importance. In the UKPDS, more intensive blood pressure control decreased the incidence of heart failure by 40% in patients with T2DM.[224] Blood pressure should be lowered to below 130/80, and even more aggressive lowering of blood pressure is often indicated to reduce afterload and reverse left ventricular hypertrophy when present.

ACE Inhibitors

ACE inhibitors have a well-established role in the treatment of heart failure. In diabetic patients with reduced systolic function (low LVEF), ACE inhibitors reduce the number of hospitalizations for heart failure and decrease mortality.[222] There are no studies proving the utility of ACE inhibitors in the treatment of heart failure due to diastolic dysfunction (normal LVEF). However, the actions of ACE inhibitors to reduce afterload, decrease neurohumoral responses, and reduce left ventricular mass are all important in the treatment of heart failure due to diastolic dysfunction. In addition, the recent Heart Outcomes Prevention Evaluation (HOPE) study supports the use of ACE inhibitors to decrease cardiac events in diabetic patients, even in the absence of heart failure or known low ejection fractions.[61] Thus in the absence of a clear contraindication (angioedema, severe cough, bilateral renal artery stenosis, or significant hyperkalemia), these drugs should be part of the standard treatment of heart failure in diabetic patients.

Beta-Blockers

Beta-adrenergic receptor blockers are useful in the long-term treatment of patients with heart failure. They are administered after the patient has been stabilized on ACE inhibitors, diuretics, and digoxin, but are contraindicated when overt pulmonary congestion or hypotension are present. Many diabetic patients with heart failure have an underlying ischemic cardiomyopathy, and treatment with beta-blockers clearly improves outcomes in diabetic patients after MI.[137,138] In the overall population with chronic heart failure and systolic dysfunction, beta-blockers also improve left ventricular function, prevent heart failure symptoms, and increase survival.[225,226] A preliminary report on the diabetic patients in the Metoprolol CR/XL Randomized Intervention Trial in Congestive Heart Failure (MERIT-HF), indicates that beta-blockers decrease hospitalization for heart failure and mortality in individuals with class II–III heart failure.[227] Although there are some concerns about potential worsening of glycemic control in T2DM and masking hypoglycemic symptoms in patients receiving insulin, these drugs are generally recommended for diabetic patients with heart failure.

Diuretics

Diuretics are an essential part of the treatment of patients with symptomatic heart failure. In addition to loop diuretics, recent evidence from the Randomized Aldactone Evaluation Study (RALES) indicates that the aldosterone antagonist spironolactone may have an important role in the treatment of advanced symptomatic heart failure.[228] Treatment with spironolactone reduced hospitalizations for heart failure and cardiac mortality. Although this drug is generally used with caution in patients with diabetes or renal insufficiency due to concern for hyperkalemia, there was no increase in the incidence of dangerous hyperkalemia in diabetic patients treated with this medication.[229]

Calcium Channel Blockers

Diastolic dysfunction is an important cause of heart failure in diabetic patients. Calcium channel blockers theoretically may decrease intracellular calcium and improve diastolic relaxation in patients with heart failure due to diastolic dysfunction. However, there is little clinical evidence that these agents are specifically useful in treating diastolic dysfunction. The primary approaches to treat heart failure due to diastolic dysfunction include intensive treatment of hypertension (to reduce afterload and left ventricular mass) and diuretics (to prevent volume overload). In this regard, calcium channel blockers are often useful in treating hypertension in T2DM patients. However, in patients who have heart failure with significant systolic dysfunction, diltiazem and verapamil are contraindicated. In patients who have systolic dysfunction and remain hypertensive despite treatment with an ACE inhibitor, beta-blocker, and diuretic, long-acting dihydropyridine antagonists are often helpful.

Cardiac Transplantation

When conventional heart failure treatment fails in an otherwise healthy diabetic patient with advanced cardiomyopathy, consideration is given for cardiac transplantation. Although insulin-requiring diabetes was once a contraindication to heart transplantation, this is no longer the case at most centers, since the overall survival in the absence of end-organ disease is comparable to those without diabetes. However, end-organ disease, especially nephropathy, increases the risk of unfavorable clinical outcomes after heart transplantation. Diabetic subjects typically require high doses of insulin and other adjuvant hypoglycemic agents during the early phases after transplantation when they are on high doses of corticosteroids.

Diabetes is a risk factor for significant cardiac transplant rejection,[230] although this is a relatively rare occurrence with the use of current immunosuppressive therapies. However, insulin resistance and dyslipidemia increase the risk for transplant vasculopathy, which is the major threat to the transplanted heart.[231] Diabetes also accelerates the development of transplant vasculopathy in animal models.[232] Aggressive lipid-lowering with statins is important to reduce the development of transplant vasculopathy.[233] However, all patients with T2DM require careful surveillance for the development of vasculopathy following heart transplant.

CARDIAC AUTONOMIC NEUROPATHY

Cardiac autonomic neuropathy develops over time in 6–21% of patients with T1DM and in 16–22% of patients with T2DM.[234–240] The reported prevalence rates have varied widely as a result of different methods and criteria used to diagnose autonomic neuropathy. In the DCCT, the prevalence of autonomic neuropathy was 6% in patients with T1DM.[241] In the Oxford Community Diabetes Study, the prevalence of autonomic neuropathy was 16% in T2DM.[240]

Autonomic neuropathy may involve the parasympathetic and sympathetic innervation of the heart and peripheral vasculature, leading to a spectrum of manifestations. In its mildest form, cardiac neuropathy involves the parasympathetic innervation of the heart and may lead to a slightly increased resting heart rate. In advanced cases, autonomic neuropathy causes severe orthostatic hypotension with recurrent lightheadedness, unsteadiness, or syncope.

Diagnosis

The diagnosis of cardiac autonomic neuropathy often requires specific autonomic testing. The standard approach involves analysis of changes in heart rate and blood pressure during provocative measures. These include measuring changes in heart rate during deep breathing, standing, and Valsalva maneuvers, along with blood pressure responses to hand grip and standing. The reliable diagnosis of autonomic neuropathy requires that the procedures are performed in a standardized manner. The test results may be influenced by a number of factors, including recent meals, insulin administration, caffeine, alcohol, smoking, and medications.[242]

Analysis of heart rate variability provides an important approach to the assessment of cardiac autonomic function in the patient with diabetes.[234,243–245] The instantaneous heart rate (R-R interval) varies due to the influence of both parasympathetic and sympathetic modulation. The variability in R-R intervals can be assessed by using either statistical analysis of R-R interval changes (time-domain) or spectral analysis of successive R-R intervals (frequency-domain). The latter approach differentiates to some extent between sympathetic and parasympathetic influences based on the frequency of the heart rate variability. Variations that occur in the high frequency range (0.15–0.40 Hz) are modulated more by parasympathetic activity, while low frequency (0.04–0.15 Hz) variability is modulated more by sympathetic activity. Recently, autonomic analyses have been incorporated into clinical monitoring systems which should facilitate the diagnosis of diabetic autonomic neuropathy.[245a]

Cardiac imaging with radiolabeled ^{123}I-meta-iodobenzylguanidine (MIBG) has also been utilized investigatively to assess the integrity of cardiac sympathetic innervation. Cardiac imaging is performed with single photon emission computed tomography (SPECT), which determines the uptake of the tracer by different regions of the heart. Abnormalities in MIBG uptake in patients with T2DM tend to involve the inferoposterior region of the left ventricle.[246] In type 1 diabetics, MIBG abnormalities are also observed, even in the absence of abnormalities in heart rate variability.[247,248] More recently, heart sympathetic integrity has been assessed by determining the uptake of ^{11}C-ephedrine using positron emission tomography.[249] This approach has demonstrated heterogeneity in myocardial uptake of ^{11}C-ephedrine with diminished activity in the distal inferior and lateral walls.[250]

Significance

Cardiac autonomic neuropathy is a marker of cardiovascular risk in patients with known cardiac disease as well as in diabetics. Early studies demonstrated 5-year mortality rates of 50% in diabetics with symptomatic cardiac autonomic neuropathy.[251] However, more recent evidence indicates a somewhat better prognosis, with mortality rates of ~25%.[252,253] It has been theorized that cardiac neuropathy creates an autonomic imbalance, predisposing to arrhythmic events,[254] or interferes with the perception of angina, predisposing to severe ischemia.[54] However, these concepts remain unproven and cardiac autonomic neuropathy may be associated with other factors predisposing to cardiac events, or to severe CAD or prior MI. Interestingly, cardiac autonomic dysfunction is related to poor glycemic control[241,255] and abnormal lipid levels.[256] The exact mechanism by which autonomic neuropathy contributes to cardiovascular mortality remains uncertain. However, a high level of attention is warranted in diabetic patients with cardiac neuropathy, in whom the presence of significant CAD should be considered.

Cardiac autonomic dysfunction has adverse physiologic consequences, compromising exercise capacity and left ventricular contractile reserve. Peak heart rate and blood pressure responses to exercise are blunted in diabetics with autonomic neuropathy.[257] In addition, peak exercise left ventricular ejection fraction[184–186] and diastolic relaxation are sometimes impaired.[200] These abnormalities occur in the absence of detectable CAD and hypertension. In one study, more than 90% of diabetic patients with exercise-induced systolic dysfunction had cardiac autonomic dysfunction, and more than half of diabetic patients with cardiac autonomic neuropathy had systolic dysfunction.[186] Patients with T1DM who have abnormal contractile reserve also often have abnormal MIBG imaging, indicating abnormal cardiac sympathetic innervation.[258]

Cardiac autonomic neuropathy has been invoked as a potential mechanism of sudden death in patients with diabetes. A number of studies have correlated autonomic neuropathy with prolongation of the QT interval.[259,260] However, few of the patients in these studies have frankly pathologic QT prolongation. QT dispersion reflecting interlead variability in the QT interval may also occur more frequently in individuals with diabetes and autonomic neuropathy.[261,262]

Cardiac autonomic neuropathy may also have a role in the pathogenesis of silent ischemia in patients with diabetes (see above discussion). Early studies showed a high incidence of asymptomatic ischemia in diabetics with cardiac autonomic dysfunction.[54] These patients also have abnormalities in cardiac MIBG uptake.[47] However, silent ischemia during exercise occurs in a substantial number of patients without diabetes or autonomic dysfunction.[44,50,263] Thus the mechanisms responsible for silent ischemia are complex and may involve central as well as autonomic pathways that are currently under investigation.

CONCLUSION

The association between diabetes and heart disease has been recognized for over 100 years. However, in contrast to the overall population, progress in reducing heart disease morbidity and mortality has lagged behind in patients with diabetes.[264] With this recognition, there have been recent efforts to better define the pathophysiology and treatment of heart disease in patients with diabetes. Ongoing research studies promise to answer key clinical questions related to how best to identify and treat CVD in patients with diabetes.

REFERENCES

1. Kannel WB, McGee DL: Diabetes and cardiovascular risk factors: The Framingham Study. *Circulation* 1979;59:8.
2. United Kingdom Prospective Diabetes (UKPDS) Group: Intensive blood-glucose control with sulfonylureas or insulin compared with conventional treatment and risk of complications in patients with type 2 diabetes (UKPDS 33). *Lancet* 1998;352:837.
3. Moss SE, Klein R, Klein BEK: Cause-specific mortality in a population-based study of diabetes. *Am J Public Health* 1991; 81:1158.
4. The Diabetes Control and Complication Trial (DCCT) Research Group: Effect of intensive diabetes management on macrovascular events and risk factors in the DCCT. *Am J Cardiol* 1995;75:894.
5. Manson JE, Colditz GA, Stampfer MJ, *et al*: A prospective study of maturity-onset diabetes mellitus and risk of coronary heart disease and stroke in women. *Arch Intern Med* 1991;151:1141.
6. Stamler J, Vaccaro O, Neaton JD, *et al*: Diabetes, other risk factors, and 12-year cardiovascular mortality for men screened in the Multiple Risk Factor Intervention Trial. *Diabetes Care* 1993;16:434.
7. Stern MP: Diabetes and cardiovascular disease. The "common soil" hypothesis. *Diabetes* 1995;44:369.
8. Stern MP: Strategies and prospects for finding insulin resistance genes. *J Clin Invest* 2000;106:323.
9. Dinneen SF, Gerstein HC: The association of microalbuminuria and mortality in non-insulin-dependent diabetes mellitus: A systematic overview of the literature. *Arch Intern Med* 1997;157:1413.
10. Kuusisto J, Mykkanen L, Pyorala K, *et al*: Hyperinsulinemic microalbuminuria: A new risk indicator for coronary heart disease. *Circulation* 1995;91:831.
11. Stehouwer CD, Gall MA, Hougaard P, *et al*: Plasma homocysteine concentration predicts mortality in non-insulin-dependent diabetic patients with and without albuminuria. *Kidney Int* 1999;55:308.
12. Hoogeveen EK, Kostense PJ, Jakobs C, *et al*: Hyperhomocysteinemia increases risk of death, especially in type 2 diabetes: 5-year follow-up of the Hoorn Study. *Circulation* 2000;101:1506.
13. Stern MP, Haffner SM: Dyslipidemia in type 2 diabetes. *Diabetes Care* 1991;14:1144.
14. Reaven GM, Chen YD, Jeppesen J, *et al*: Insulin resistance and hyperinsulinemia in individuals with small, dense low density lipoprotein particles [see comments]. *J Clin Invest* 1993;92:141.
15. Kannel WB, Wilson PWF: Risk factors that attenuate the female coronary disease advantage. *Arch Intern Med* 1995;155:57.
16. Howard BV, Cowan LD, Go O, *et al*: Adverse effects of diabetes on multiple cardiovascular risk factors in women. *Diabetes Care* 1998; 14:11258.
17. Carmassi F, Morale M, Puccetti R, *et al*: Coagulation and fibrinolytic system impairment in insulin dependent diabetes mellitus. *Thromb Res* 1992;67:643.
18. Davi G, Ciabattoni G, Consoli A, *et al*: *In vivo* formation of 8-iso-prostaglandin F$_2$alpha and platelet activation in diabetes mellitus: effects of improved metabolic control and vitamin E supplementation. *Circulation* 1999;99:224.
19. Saito I, Folsom AR, Brancati FL, *et al*: Nontraditional risk factors for coronary heart disease incidence among persons with diabetes: the Atherosclerosis Risk in Communities (ARIC) Study. *Ann Intern Med* 2000;133:81.
20. Schalkwijk CG, Poland DC, van Dijk W, *et al*: Plasma concentration of C-reactive protein is increased in type I diabetic patients without clinical macroangiopathy and correlates with markers of endothelial dysfunction: evidence for chronic inflammation. *Diabetologia* 1999;42:351.
20a. Tan KC, Chow WS, Tam SC, Ai VH, Lam CH, Lam KS: Atorvastatin lowers C-reactive protein and improves endothelium-dependent vasodilation in type 2 diabetes mellitus. *J Clin Endocrinol Metab* 2002;87:563.
21. Kannel WB, D'Agostino RB, Wilson PW, *et al*: Diabetes, fibrinogen, and the risk of cardiovascular disease: The Framingham experience. *Am Heart J* 1990;120:672.
22. Ribau JC, Hadcock SJ, Teoh K, *et al*: Endothelial adhesion molecule expression is enhanced in the aorta and internal mammary artery of diabetic patients. *J Surg Res* 1999;85:225.
23. Baumgartner-Parzer SM, Tschoepe D: Role of adhesion molecules in diabetes mellitus. *Horm Metab Res* 1997;29:613.
24. Schmidt AM, Yan SD, Wautier JL, *et al*: Activation of receptor for advanced glycation end products: a mechanism for chronic vascular dysfunction in diabetic vasculopathy and atherosclerosis. *Circ Res* 1999;84:489.
25. Caprio S, Wong S, Alberti KG, *et al*: Cardiovascular complications of diabetes. *Diabetologia* 1997;40:B78.
26. Moreno PR, Murcia AM, Palacios IF, Leon MN, Bernardi VH, Fuster V, Fallon JT: Coronary composition and macrophage infil-

tration in atherectomy specimens from patients with diabetes mellitus. *Circulation* 2000;102:2180.

27. Lindvall B, Brorsson B, Herlitz J, *et al*: Comparison of diabetic and non-diabetic patients referred for coronary angiography. *Int J Cardiol* 1999;70:33.

28. Abaci A, Oguzhan A, Kahraman S, *et al*: Effect of diabetes mellitus on formation of coronary collateral vessels. *Circulation* 1999; 99:2239.

29. Zoneraich S, Silverman G, Zoneraich O: Primary myocardial disease, diabetes mellitus, and small vessel disease. *Am Heart J* 1980; 100:754.

30. Factor SM, Minase T, Sonnenblick EH: Clinical and morphological features of human hypertensive-diabetic cardiomyopathy. *Am Heart J* 1980;99:446.

31. Johnstone M, Creager S, Scales K, *et al*: Impaired endothelium-dependent vasodilation in patients with insulin-dependent diabetes mellitus. *Circulation* 1993;88:2510.

32. Grundy SM, Benjamin IJ, Burke GL, *et al*: Diabetes and cardiovascular disease: A statement for healthcare professionals from the American Heart Association. *Circulation* 1999;100:1134.

33. American Diabetes Association: Diabetes mellitus and exercise. *Diabetes Care* 2002;25:S64.

34. American Diabetes Association: Management of dyslipidemia in adults with diabetes. *Diabetes Care* 2002;25:S74.

35. American Diabetes Association: Aspirin therapy in diabetes. *Diabetes Care* 2002;25:S78.

36. American Diabetes Association: Smoking and diabetes. *Diabetes Care* 2002;25:S80.

37. American Diabetes Association: Consensus development conference on the diagnosis of coronary heart disease in people with diabetes. *Diabetes Care* 1998;21:1551.

38. Third Report of the National Cholesterol Education Program (NCEP) Expert Panel on Detection, Evaluation and treatment of high blood cholesterol in adults (Adult Treatment Panel III). NHLBI, NIH Publication No. 01-3670, May 2001

39. American Diabetes Association: Treatment of hypertension in adults with diabetes. *Diabetes Care* 2002;25:1999.

40. Hulley S, Grady D, Bush T, *et al*: Randomized trial of estrogen plus progestin for secondary prevention of coronary heart disease in postmenopausal women. Heart and Estrogen/Progestin Replacement Study (HERS) Research Group. *JAMA* 1998;280:605.

41. Kaplan RC, Heckbert SR, Weiss NS, *et al*: Postmenopausal estrogens and risk of myocardial infarction in diabetic women. *Diabetes Care* 1998;21:1117.

42. Turner RC, Millns H, Neil JAW, *et al*: Risk factors for coronary artery disease in non-insulin dependent diabetes mellitus: United Kingdom Prospective Diabetes Study (UKPDS:23). *Br Med J* 1998; 352:837.

43. The Diabetes Control and Complication Trial (DCCT) Research Group: The effect of intensive treatment of diabetes on the development and progression of long-term complications in IDDM. *N Engl J Med* 1993;329:977.

44. Nesto RW, Phillips RT, Kett KG, *et al*: Angina and exertional myocardial ischemia in diabetic and nondiabetic patients: Assessment by exercise thallium scintigraphy. *Ann Intern Med* 1988; 108:170.

45. Chiarello M, Indolfi C, Cotecchia MR, *et al*: Asymptomatic transient ST changes during ambulatory ECG monitoring in diabetic patients. *Am Heart J* 1985;110:529.

46. Titus BG, Sherman T: Asymptomatic myocardial ischemia during percutaneous coronary angioplasty and importance of prior Q-wave infarction and diabetes mellitus. *Am J Cardiol* 1991;68:735.

47. Langer A, Freeman MR, Josse RG, *et al*: Metaiodobenzylguanidine imaging in diabetes mellitus: Assessment of cardiac sympathetic denervation and its relation to autonomic dysfunction and silent myocardial ischemia. *J Am Coll Cardiol* 1995;25:610.

48. Koistinen MJ, Airaksinen KE, Huikuri HV, *et al*: No difference in cardiac innervation of diabetic patients with painful and asymptomatic coronary artery disease. *Diabetes Care* 1996;19:231.

49. Kannel WB, Abbott RD: Incidence and prognosis of unrecognized myocardial infarction. *N Engl J Med* 1984;311:1144.

50. Chipkin SR, Frid D, Alpert JS, *et al*: Frequency of painless myocardial ischemia during exercise tolerance testing in patients with and without diabetes mellitus. *Am J Cardiol* 1987;59:61.

51. Kurata C, Sakata K, Taguchi T, *et al*: Exercise-induced silent myocardial ischemia: Evaluation by thallium-201 emission computed tomography. *Am Heart J* 1990;119:557.

52. Naka M, Hiramatsu K, Aizawa T, *et al*: Silent myocardial ischemia in patients with non-insulin-dependent diabetes mellitus as judged by treadmill exercise testing and coronary angiography. *Am Heart J* 1992;123:46.

53. Koistinen MJ: Prevalence of asymptomatic myocardial ischaemia in diabetic subjects. *Br Med J* 1990;301:92.

54. Langer A, Freeman MR, Josse RG, *et al*: Detection of silent myocardial ischemia in diabetes mellitus. *Am J Cardiol* 1991;67: 1073.

55. Milan Study on Atherosclerosis and Diabetes Group: Prevalence of unrecognized silent myocardial ischemia and its association with atherosclerotic factors in noninsulin-dependent diabetes mellitus. *Am J Cardiol* 1997;79:134.

56. Hachamovitch R, Berman DS, Shaw LS, *et al*: Incremental prognostic value of myocardial perfusion single-photon emission computed tomography for the prediction of cardiac death. *Circulation* 1998;97:535.

57. Vanzetto G, Halimi S, Hammoud T, *et al*: Prediction of cardiovascular events in clinically selected high-risk NIDDM patients. *Diabetes Care* 1999;22:19.

58. Davies RF, Goldberg D, Forman S, *et al*: Asymptomatic Cardiac Ischemia Pilot (ACIP) Study two-year follow-up. *Circulation* 1997; 95:2037.

59. Weiner DA, Ryan TJ, Parsons L, *et al*: Significance of silent myocardial ischemia during exercise testing in patients with diabetes mellitus: A report from the Coronary Artery Surgery Study (CASS) Registry. *Am J Cardiol* 1991;68:729.

60. Jonas M, Reicher-Reiss H, Boyko V, *et al*: Usefulness of beta-blocker therapy in patients with non-insulin-dependent diabetes mellitus and coronary artery disease. *Am J Cardiol* 1996;77: 1273.

61. Heart Outcomes Prevention Evaluation Study Investigators: Effects of ramipril on cardiovascular and microvascular outcomes in people with diabetes mellitus: Results of the HOPE study and MICRO-HOPE study. *Lancet* 2000;355:253.

62. Scandinavian Simvastatin Survival Study Group: Randomized trial of cholesterol lowering in 4444 patients with coronary heart disease: The Scandinavian Simvastatin Survival Study (4S). *Lancet* 1994;344:1383.

63. Goldberg RB, Mellies MJ, Sacks FM, *et al*: Cardiovascular events and their reduction with pravastatin in diabetic and glucose-intolerant myocardial infarction survivors with average cholesterol levels: subgroup analyses in the cholesterol and recurrent events (CARE) trial. The Care Investigators. *Circulation* 1998;98:2513.

64. Pitt B, Waters D, Brown WB, *et al*: Aggressive lipid-lowering compared with angioplasty in stable coronary artery disease. *N Engl J Med* 1999;341:70.

65. Koskinen P, Manttari M, Manninen J, *et al*: Coronary heart disease incidence in NIDDM patients in the Helsinki Heart Study. *Diabetes Care* 1992;15:820.

66. Rubins HB, Robins SJ, Collins D, *et al*: Gemfibrozil for the secondary prevention of coronary heart disease in men with low levels of high-density lipoprotein cholesterol: Veterans Affairs High-Density Lipoprotein Cholesterol Intervention Trial Study Group. *N Engl J Med* 1999;341:410.

67. Steering Committee of the Physicians' Health Study Research Group: Final report on the aspirin component of the ongoing Physicians' Health Study. *N Engl J Med* 1989;321:129.

68. The Early Treatment Diabetic Retinopathy Study (ETDRS) Investigators: Aspirin effects on mortality and morbidity in patients with diabetes mellitus. *JAMA* 1992;268:1292.

69. Hansson L, Zanchetti A, Carruthers SG, *et al*: Effects of intensive blood-pressure lowering and low dose aspirin on patients with hypertension: principal results of the Hypertension Optimal Treatment (HOT) randomized trial. *Lancet* 1998;351:1755.

70. CAPRIE Steering Committee: A randomised, blinded trial of clopidogrel versus aspirin in patients at risk of ischemic events (CAPRIE). *Lancet* 1996;348:1329.

71. Hirotani T, Kameda T, Kumamoto T, *et al*: Effects of coronary artery bypass grafting using internal mammary arteries for diabetic patients. *J Am Coll Cardiol* 1999;34:532.

72. Cohen Y, Raz I, Merin G, et al: Comparison of factors associated with 30-day mortality after coronary bypass grafting in patients with versus without diabetes mellitus. Am J Cardiol 1998;81:7.

73. Thourani VH, Weintraub WS, Stein B, et al: Influence of diabetes mellitus on early and late outcome after coronary artery bypass grafting. Ann Thorac Surg 1999;67:1045.

74. Abizaid A, Costa MA, Centemero M, Abizaid AS, Legrand VMG, Limet RV, Schuler G, Mohr FW, Lindeboom W, Sousa AGMR, Sousa JE, van Hout B, Hugenholtz PG, Unger F, Serruys PW: Clinical and economic impact of diabetes mellitus on percutaneous and surgical treatment of multivessel coronary disease patients: Insights from the Arterial Revascularization Therapy Study (ARTS) Trial. Circulation 2001;104:533.

75. Morris JJ, Smith LR, Jones RH, et al: Influence of diabetes and mammary artery grafting on survival after coronary bypass. Circulation 1991;84:275.

76. Kuan P, Bernstein SB, Ellestad MH: Coronary artery bypass surgery morbidity. J Am Coll Cardiol 1994;3:1391.

77. BARI Investigators: Influence of diabetes on 5-year mortality and morbidity in a randomized trial comparing CABG and PTCA in patients with multivessel disease: The Bypass Angioplasty Revascularization Investigation (BARI). Circulation 1997;96:1761.

78. John R, Choudhri AF, Weinberg AD, et al: Multicenter review of preoperative risk factors for stroke after coronary artery bypass grafting. Ann Thorac Surg 2000;69:30.

79. Mangano CM, Diamondstone LS, Ramsay JG, et al: Renal dysfunction after myocardial revascularization: Risk factors, adverse outcomes, and hospital resource utilization. Ann Intern Med 1998;128:194.

80. Manche A, Galea J, Busuttil W: Tolerance to ACE inhibitors after cardiac surgery. Eur J Cardio-Thoracic Surg 1999;15:55.

81. Zanardo G, Michielon P, Paccagnella A, et al: Acute renal failure in the patient undergoing cardiac operation: Prevalence, mortality rate and main risk factors. J Thorac Cardiovasc Surg 1994;107:1489.

82. Rao V, Weisel RD, Buth KJ, et al: Coronary artery bypass grafting in patients with non-dialysis-dependent renal insufficiency. Circulation 1997;96:II-38.

83. Khaitan L, Sutter FP, Goldman SM: Coronary artery bypass grafting in patients who require long-term dialysis. Ann Thorac Surg 2000;69:1135.

84. Fietsam RJ, Bassett J, Glover JL: Complications of coronary artery surgery in diabetic patients. Am Surg 1991;57:551.

85. Zerr KJ, Furnary AP, Grunkemeier GL, et al: Glucose control lowers the risk of wound infection in diabetics after open heart surgery. Ann Thorac Surg 1998;63:356.

86. Trick WE, Scheckler WE, Tokars JI, et al: Modifiable risk factors associated with deep sternal site infection after coronary artery bypass grafting. J Thorac Cardiovasc Surg 2000;119:108.

87. Galbut DL, Traad EA, Dorman MJ, et al: Coronary artery bypass grafting in the elderly: Single versus bilateral internal mammary artery grafts. J Thorac Cardiovasc Surg 1993;106:128.

88. Classen DC, Evans RS, Pestotnik SL, et al: The timing of prophylactic administration of antibiotics and the risk of surgical-wound infection. N Engl J Med 1992;326:281.

89. Marso SP, Ellis SG, Gurm HS, et al: Proteinuria is a key determinant of death in patients with diabetes after isolated coronary artery bypass grafting [see comments]. Am Heart J 2000;139:939.

90. BARI Investigators: Seven-year outcome in the Bypass Angioplasty Revascularization Investigation (BARI) by treatment and diabetic status. J Am Coll Cardiol 2000;35:1122.

91. Detre KM, Guo P, Holubkov R, et al: Coronary revascularization in diabetic patients: A comparison of the randomized and observational components of the Bypass Angioplasty Revascularization Investigation (BARI). Circulation 1999;99:633.

92. Kip KE, Faxon DP, Detre KM, et al: Coronary angioplasty in diabetic patients. The National Heart, Lung, and Blood Institute Percutaneous Transluminal Coronary Angioplasty Registry. Circulation 1996;94:1818.

93. Stein B, Weintraub WS, Gebhart SSP, et al: Influence of diabetes mellitus on early and late outcome after percutaneous transluminal coronary angioplasty. Circulation 1995;91:979.

94. Kleiman NS, Lincoff AM, Kereiakes DJ, et al: Diabetes mellitus, glycoprotein IIb/IIIa blockade, and heparin: evidence for a complex interaction in a multicenter trial. EPILOG Investigators. Circulation 1998;97:1912.

95. Stevens MA, McCullough PA, Tobin KJ, et al: A prospective randomized trial of prevention measures in patients at high risk for contrast nephropathy: results of the P.R.I.N.C.E. Study. Prevention of Radiocontrast Induced Nephropathy Clinical Evaluation. J Am Coll Cardiol 1999;33:403.

96. Tepel M, van der Giet M, Schwarzfeld C, et al: Prevention of radiographic-contrast-agent-induced reductions in renal function by acetylcysteine [see comments]. N Engl J Med 2000;343:180.

97. Marso SP, Ellis SG, Tuzcu M, et al: The importance of proteinuria as a determinant of mortality following percutaneous coronary revascularization in diabetics. J Am Coll Cardiol 1999;33:1269.

98. Halon DA, Merdler A, Flugelman MY, et al: Importance of diabetes mellitus and systemic hypertension rather than completeness of revascularization in determining long-term outcome after coronary balloon angioplasty (the LDCMC registry). Lady Davis Carmel Medical Center. Am J Cardiol 1998;82:547.

99. Van Belle E, Bauters C, Hubert E, Bodart J-C, Abolmaali K, Meurice T, McFadden eP, Lablanche J-M, Bertrand ME: Restenosis rates in diabetic patients: A comparison of coronary stenting and balloon angioplasty in native coronary vessels. Circulation 1997;96:1454.

100. Abizaid A, Kornowski R, Mintz GS, et al: The influence of diabetes mellitus on acute and late clinical outcomes following coronary stent implantation. J Am Coll Cardiol 1998;32:584.

101. Elezi S, Kastrati A, Pache J, et al: Diabetes mellitus and clinical and angiographic outcome after coronary stent placement. J Am Coll Cardiol 1998;32:1866.

102. Aronson D, Bloomgarden Z, Rayfield EJ: Potential mechanisms promoting restenosis in diabetic patients. J Am Coll Cardiol 1996;27:528.

103. Kornowski R, Lansky AJ: Current perspectives on interventional treatment strategies in diabetic patients with coronary artery disease. Catheter Cardiovasc Interv 2000;50:245.

104. Al Suwaidi J, Berger PB, Holmes DR Jr.: Coronary artery stents. JAMA 2000;284:1828.

105. Rankin JM, Spinelli JJ, Carere RG, et al: Improved clinical outcome after widespread use of coronary-artery stenting in Canada [see comments]. N Engl J Med 1999;341:1957.

106. Gowda MS, Vacek JL, Hallas D: One-year outcomes of diabetic versus nondiabetic patients with non-Q-wave acute myocardial infarction treated with percutaneous transluminal coronary angioplasty. Am J Cardiol 1998;81:1067.

107. Silva JA, Ramee SR, White CJ, et al: Primary stenting in acute myocardial infarction: Influence of diabetes mellitus in angiographic results and clinical outcome. Am Heart J 1998;138:446.

108. Marso SP, Lincoff AM, Ellis SG, et al: Optimizing the percutaneous interventional outcomes for patients with diabetes mellitus: results of the EPISTENT (Evaluation of platelet IIb/IIIa inhibitor for stenting trial) diabetic substudy [see comments]. Circulation 1999;100:2477.

109. King SBI, Kosinski AS, Guyton RA, et al: Eight year mortality in the Emory Angioplasty vs Surgery Trial (EAST). J Am Coll Cardiol 2000;35;116.

110. Barsness GW, Peterson ED, Ohman EM, et al: Relationship between diabetes mellitus and long-term survival after coronary bypass and angioplasty. Circulation 1997;96:2551.

111. Gum PA, O'Keffe J, James H, et al: Bypass surgery versus coronary angioplasty for revascularization of treated diabetic patients. Circulation 1997;96(suppl II):II-7.

112. Weintraub WS, Stein B, Kosinski A, et al: Outcome of coronary bypass surgery versus coronary angioplasty in diabetic patients with multivessel coronary artery disease. J Am Coll Cardiol 1998;31:10.

113. Chaitman BR, Rosen AD, Williams DO, et al: Myocardial infarction and cardiac mortality in the Bypass Angioplasty Revascularization Investigation (BARI) randomized trial. Circulation 1997;96:2162.

114. CABRI Trial Participants: First year results of CABRI (Coronary Angioplasty versus Bypass Revascularization Investigation). Lancet 1995;46:1184.

115. Ellis SG, Narins CR: Problem of angioplasty in diabetics. Circulation 1997;96:1707.

116. Ferguson JJ: NHLBI BARI clinical alert on diabetics treated with angioplasty. *Circulation* 1995;92:3371.

117. O'Neill WW: Multivessel balloon angioplasty should be abandoned in diabetic patients: [editorial; comment]. *J Am Coll Cardiol* 1998; 31:20.

118. Miettinen H, Lehto S, Salomaa V, *et al*: Impact of diabetes on mortality after the first myocardial infarction. *Diabetes Care* 1998;21: 69.

119. Haffner SM: Coronary heart disease in patients with diabetes [editorial; comment]. *N Engl J Med* 2000;342:1040.

120. Partamian JO, Bradley RF: Acute myocardial infarction in 258 cases of diabetes. *N Engl J Med* 1965;273:455.

121. Jacoby RM, Nesto RW: Acute myocardial infarction in the diabetic patient: Pathophysiology, clinical course and prognosis. *J Am Coll Cardiol* 1992;20:736.

122. Aronson D, Rayfield EJ, Chesebro JH: Mechanisms determining course and outcome of diabetic patients who have had acute myocardial infarction. *Ann Intern Med* 1997;126:296.

123. Chyun DA: The prognostic importance of diabetes mellitus in elderly patients with myocardial infarction. *Dissertation Abstracts International*. Yale University:1998.

124. Malmberg K, Rydén L: Myocardial infarction in patients with diabetes mellitus. *Eur Heart J* 1988;9:256.

125. Abbott RD, Donahue RP, Kannel WB, *et al*: The impact of diabetes on survival following myocardial infarction. *JAMA* 1988;260:3456.

126. Herlitz J, Malmberg K, Karlson BW, *et al*: Mortality and morbidity during a five-year follow-up of diabetics with myocardial infarction. *Acta Med Scand* 1988;224:31.

127. Behar S, Boyko V, Reicher-Reiss H, *et al*: Ten-year survival after acute myocardial infarction: Comparison of patients with and without diabetes. *Am Heart J* 1997;133:290.

128. Stone PH, Muller JE, Hartwell T, *et al*: The effect of diabetes mellitus on prognosis and serial left ventricular function after acute myocardial infarction: Contribution of both coronary disease and diastolic left ventricular dysfunction to adverse prognosis. *J Am Coll Cardiol* 1989;14:49.

129. Jaffe AS, Spadaro JJ, Schechtman K, *et al*: Increased congestive heart failure after myocardial infarction of modest extent in patients with diabetes mellitus. *Am Heart J* 1984;108:31.

130. Granger CB, Califf RM, Young S, *et al*: Outcome of patients with diabetes mellitus and acute myocardial infarction treated with thrombolytic agents. *J Am Coll Cardiol* 1993;21:920.

131. Barbash GI, White HD, Modan M, *et al*: Significance of diabetes mellitus in patients with acute myocardial infarction receiving thrombolytic therapy. *J Am Coll Cardiol* 1993;22:707.

132. ISIS-2 (Second International Study of Infarct Survival) Collaborative G: Randomized trial of intravenous streptokinase, oral aspirin, both, or neither among 17,187 cases of suspected acute myocardial infarction. *Lancet* 1988;2:349.

133. Zuanetti G, Latini R, Maggioni AP, *et al*: Influence of diabetes on mortality in acute myocardial infarction: Data from the GISSI-2 Study. *J Am Coll Cardiol* 1993;22:1788.

134. Grines CL, Browne KF, Marco J, *et al*: A comparison of immediate angioplasty with thrombolytic therapy for acute myocardial infarction. *N Engl J Med* 1993;328:673.

135. Grines CL, Cox DA, Stone GW, *et al*: Coronary angioplasty with or without stent implantation for acute myocardial infarction. Stent Primary Angioplasty in Myocardial Infarction Study Group [see comments]. *N Engl J Med* 1999;341:1949.

136. Hasdai D, Granger CB, Srivatsa SS, *et al*: Diabetes mellitus and outcome after primary coronary angioplasty for acute myocardial infarction: Lessons form the GUSTO-IIb Angioplasty Substudy. Global Use of Strategies to Open Occluded Arteries in Acute Coronary Syndromes. *J Am Coll Cardiol* 2000;35:1502.

137. Gottlieb SS, McCarter RJ, Vogel RA: Effect of beta-blockade on mortality among high-risk and low-risk patients after myocardial infarction. *N Engl J Med* 1998;339:498.

138. Kjekshus J, Gilpin E, Blackey A, *et al*: Diabetic patients and beta-blockers after acute myocardial infarction. *Eur Heart J* 1990;11:43.

139. Zuanetti G, Latini R, Maggioni AP, *et al*: Effect of the ACE inhibitor lisinopril on mortality in diabetic patients with acute myocardial infarction. *Circulation* 1997;96:4239.

140. Moye LA, Pfeffer MA, Wun CC, *et al*: Uniformity of captopril benefit in the SAVE Study: Subgroup analysis. *Eur Heart J* 1994;15:2.

141. Apstein C, Taegtmeyer H: Glucose-insulin-potassium in acute myocardial infarction. *Circulation* 1997;96:1074.

142. Malmberg K, Ryden L, Suad E, *et al*: Randomized trial of insulin-glucose infusion followed by subcutaneous insulin treatment in diabetic patients with acute myocardial infarction (DIGAMI Study): Effects on mortality at 1 year. *J Am Coll Cardiol* 1995;26:57.

143. Malmberg K: Prospective randomised study of intensive insulin treatment on long term survival after acute myocardial infarction in patients with diabetes mellitus. DIGAMI (Diabetes Mellitus, Insulin Glucose Infusion in Acute Myocardial Infarction) Study Group. *Br Med J* 1997;314:1512.

144. Ryan TJ, Antman EM, Brooks NH, *et al*: ACC/AHA guidelines for the management of patients with acute myocardial infarction: Executive summary and recommendations: A report of the American College of Cardiology/American Heart Association Task Force on Practice Guidelines (Committee on Management of Acute Myocardial Infarction). *Circulation* 1999;100:1016.

145. Malmberg K, Norhammar A, Wedel H, *et al*: Glycometabolic state at admission; Important risk marker of mortality in conventionally treated patients with diabetes mellitus and acute myocardial infarction. *Circulation* 1999;138:2626.

146. Capes SE, Hunt D, Malmberg K, *et al*: Stress hyperglycaemia and increased risk of death after myocardial infarction in patients with and without diabetes: a systematic overview [see comments]. *Lancet* 2000;355:773.

147. Braunwald E, Antman EM, Beasley JW, *et al*: ACC/AHA guidelines for the management of patients with unstable angina and non-ST-segment elevation myocardial infarction: executive summary and recommendations. A report of the American College of Cardiology/American Heart Association task force on practice guidelines (committee on the management of patients with unstable angina). *Circulation* 2000;102:1193.

148. Malmberg K, Yusuf S, Gerstein HC, *et al*: Impact of diabetes on long-term prognosis in patients with unstable angina and non-Q-wave myocardial infarction: results of the OASIS (Organization to Assess Strategies for Ischemic Syndromes) Registry. *Circulation* 2000;102:1014.

149. Silva JA, Escobar A, Collins TJ, *et al*: Unstable angina: A comparison of angioscopic findings between diabetic and nondiabetic patients. *Circulation* 1995;92:1731.

150. Pursuit Trial Investigators: Inhibition of platelet glycoprotein IIb/IIIa with eptifibatide in patients with acute coronary syndromes. *N Engl J Med* 1998;339:436.

151. Platelet Receptor Inhibition in Ischemic Syndrome Management in Patients Limited by Unstable Signs and Symptoms (PRISM-PLUS) Study Investigators: Inhibition of the platelet glycoprotein IIb/IIIa receptor with tirofiban in unstable angina and non-Q-wave myocardial infarction. *N Engl J Med* 1998;338:1488.

152. Boden WE, O'Rourke RA, Crawford MH, *et al*: Outcomes in patients with acute non-Q-wave myocardial infarction randomly assigned to an invasive as compared with a conservative management strategy. Veterans Affairs Non-Q-Wave Infarction Strategies in Hospital (VANQWISH) Trial Investigators [see comments] [published erratum appears in *N Engl J Med* 1998;339:1091]. *N Engl J Med* 1998;338:1785.

153. Wallentin L, Lagerquist B, Husted S, *et al*: Outcome at 1 year after an invasive compared with a non-invasive strategy in unstable coronary-artery disease: the FRISC II invasive randomised trial. *Lancet* 2000; 356:9.

154. Kannel WB, Hjortland M, Castelli WP: Role of diabetes in congestive heart failure: The Framingham Study. *Am J Cardiol* 1974;34: 29.

155. Ho KKL, Anderson KM, Kannel WB, *et al*: Survival after the onset of congestive heart failure in Framingham Heart Study subjects. *Circulation* 1993;88:107.

156. Chen YT, Vaccarino V, Williams CS, *et al*: Risk factors for heart failure in the elderly: a prospective community-based study. *Am J Med* 1999;106:605.

157. Chae CU, Pfeffer MA, Glynn RJ, *et al*: Increased pulse pressure and risk of heart failure in the elderly. *JAMA* 1999;281:634.

158. Dash H, Johnson RA, Dinsmore RE, *et al*: Cardiomyopathic syndrome due to coronary artery disease. *Br Heart J* 1977;39:740.

159. Litwin SE, Grossman W: Diastolic dysfunction as a cause of heart failure. *J Am Coll Cardiol* 1993;22:49A.

160. Levy D, Larson MG, Vasan RS, *et al*: The progression from hypertension to congestive heart failure [see comments]. *JAMA* 1996;275:1557.

161. Grossman E, Messerli FH: Diabetic and hypertensive heart disease. *Ann Intern Med* 1996;125:304.

162. van Hoeven KH, Factor SM: A comparison of the pathological spectrum of hypertensive, diabetic, and hypertensive-diabetic heart disease. *Circulation* 1990;82:848.

163. Factor SM, Borczuk A, Charron MJ, *et al*: Myocardial alterations in diabetes and hypertension. *Diabetes Res Clin Pract* 1996;31: S133.

164. Fein FS, Capasso JM, Aronson RS, *et al*: Combined renovascular hypertension and diabetes in rats: a new preparation of congestive cardiomyopathy. *Circulation* 1984;70:318.

165. Fein FS, Sonnenblick EH: Diabetic cardiomyopathy. *Prog Cardiovasc Dis* 1985;27:255.

166. Siri FM, Malhorta A, Factor SM, *et al*: Prolonged ejection duration helps to maintain pump performance of the renal-hypertensive-diabetic rat heart: correlations between isolated papillary muscle dysfunction and ventricular performance in situ. *Cardiovasc Res* 1997; 34:230.

167. Galderisi M, Anderson KM, Wilson PW, *et al*: Echocardiographic evidence for the existence of a distinct diabetic cardiomyopathy (the Framingham Heart Study). *Am J Cardiol* 1991;68:85.

168. Devereux RB, Roman MJ, Paranicas M, *et al*: Impact of diabetes on cardiac structure and function: the strong heart study. *Circulation* 2000;101:2271.

169. Ohya Y, Abe I, Fujii K, *et al*: Hyperinsulinemia and left ventricular geometry in a work-site population in Japan. *Hypertension* 1996; 27:729.

170. McNulty P, Louard R, Deckelbaum L, *et al*: Hyperinsulinemia inhibits myocardial protein degradation in patients with cardiovascular disease and insulin resistance. *Circulation* 1995;92:2151.

171. Rubler S, Dlugash J, Yuceoglu YZ, *et al*: New type of cardiomyopathy associated with diabetic glomerulosclerosis. *Am J Cardiol* 1972;30:595.

172. Regan TJ, Lyons MM, Ahemd SS, *et al*: Evidence for cardiomyopathy in familial diabetes mellitus. *J Clin Invest* 1977;60:885.

173. Blumenthal HT, Alex M, Goldenberg S: A study of lesions of the intramural coronary artery branches in diabetes mellitus. *Arch Pathol* 1960;70:27.

174. Ledet T: Histological and histochemical changes in the coronary arteries of old diabetic patients. *Diabetologia* 1968;4:268.

175. Yokoyama I, Momomura S, Ohtake T, *et al*: Reduced myocardial flow reserve in non-insulin-dependent diabetes mellitus. *J Am Coll Cardiol* 1997;30:1472.

176. Yokoyama I, Ohtake T, Momomura S, *et al*: Hyperglycemia rather than insulin resistance is related to reduced coronary flow reserve in NIDDM. *Diabetes* 1998;47:119.

177. Strauer BE, Motz W, Vogt M, *et al*: Impaired coronary flow reserve in NIDDM: a possible role for diabetic cardiopathy in humans. *Diabetes* 1997;46:S119.

178. Sykes CA, Wright AD, Malins JM, *et al*: Changes in systolic time intervals during treatment of diabetes mellitus. *Br Heart J* 1977;39: 255.

179. Uusitupa M, Siitonen O, Pyorala K, *et al*: Left ventricular function in newly diagnosed non-insulin-dependent (type 2) diabetics evaluated by systolic time intervals and echocardiography. *Acta Med Scand* 1985;217:379.

180. Friedman NE, Levitsky LL, Edidin DV, *et al*: Echocardiographic evidence of impaired performance in children with type I diabetes mellitus. *Am J Med* 1982;73:846.

181. Lababidi ZA, Goldstein DE: High prevalence of echocardiographic abnormalities in diabetic youths. *Diabetes Care* 1983;6:18.

182. Thuesen L, Christiansen JS, Falstie-Jensen N, *et al*: Increased myocardial contractility in short-term type 1 diabetic patients: an echocardiographic study. *Diabetologia* 1985;28:822.

183. Thuesen L, Christiansen JS, Mogensen CE, *et al*: Cardiac hyperfunction in insulin-dependent diabetic patients developing microvascular complications. *Diabetes* 1988;37:851.

184. Mildenberger RR, Bar-Shlomo B, Druck MN: Clinically unrecognized ventricular dysfunction in young diabetic patients. *J Am Coll Cardiol* 1984;4:234.

185. Vered Z, Battler A, Sega P, *et al*: Exercise-induced left ventricular dysfunction in young men with asymptomatic diabetes mellitus (diabetic cardiomyopathy). *Am J Cardiol* 1984;54:633.

186. Zola B, Kahn J, Juni J, *et al*: Abnormal cardiac function in diabetics with autonomic neuropathy in the absence of ischemic heart disease. *J Clin Endocrinol Metab* 1986;63:208.

187. Mustonen JN, Uusitupa MIJ, Tahvanainen K, *et al*: Impaired left ventricular systolic function during exercise in middle-aged insulin-dependent and noninsulin-dependent diabetic subjects without clinically evident cardiovascular disease. *Am J Cardiol* 1988; 62:1273.

188. Arvan S, Singal B, Knapp R, *et al*: Subclinical left ventricular abnormalities in young diabetics. *Chest* 1988;93:1031.

189. Borow KM, Jaspan JP, Williams KA, *et al*: Myocardial mechanics in young adult patients with diabetes mellitus: effects of altered load, inotropic state and dynamic exercise. *J Am Coll Cardiol* 1990; 15:1508.

190. Rynkiewicz A, Semetkowska-Jurkiewicz E, Wyrzykowski B: Systolic and diastolic time intervals in young diabetics. *Br Heart J* 1980;44:280.

191. Shapiro LM, Howat AP, Calter MM: Left ventricular function in diabetes mellitus I: Methodology, and prevalence and spectrum of abnormalities. *Br Heart J* 1981;45:122.

192. Shapiro LM, Leatherdale BA, MacKinnon J, *et al*: Left ventricular function in diabetes mellitus II: Relation between clinical features and ventricular function. *Br Heart J* 1981;45:129.

193. Sanderson JE, Brown DJ, Rivellese A, *et al*: Diabetic cardiomyopathy? An echocardiographic study of young diabetics. *Br Med J* 1978;1:404.

194. Hausdorf G, Rieger U, Koepp P: Cardiomyopathy in childhood diabetes mellitus: incidence, time of onset, and relation to metabolic control. *Int J Cardiol* 1988;19:225.

195. Danielsen R, Nordrehaug JE, Vik-Mo H: Left ventricular function in young long-term type 1 (insulin-dependent) diabetic men during exercise assessed by digitized echocardiography. *Eur Heart J* 1988;9: 395.

196. Zarich SW, Arbuckle BE, Cohen LR, *et al*: Diastolic abnormalities in young asymptomatic diabetic patients assessed by pulsed Doppler echocardiography. *J Am Coll Cardiol* 1988;12:114.

197. Takenaka K, Sakamoto T, Amano K, *et al*: Left ventricular filling determined by doppler echocardiography in diabetes mellitus. *Am J Cardiol* 1988;61:1140.

198. Bouchard A, Sanz N, Botvinick EH, *et al*: Noninvasive assessment of cardiomyopathy in normotensive diabetic patients between 20 and 50 years old. *Am J Med* 1989;87:160.

199. Paillole C, Dahan M, Paycha F, *et al*: Prevalence and significance of left ventricular filling abnormalities determined by doppler echocardiography in type I (insulin-dependent) diabetic patients. *Am J Cardiol* 1989;64:1010.

200. Kahn JK, Zola B, Juni JE, *et al*: Radionuclide assessment of left ventricular diastolic filling in diabetes mellitus with and without cardiac autonomic neuropathy. *J Am Coll Cardiol* 1986;7:1303.

201. Ruddy TD, Shumak SL, Liu PP, *et al*: The relationship of cardiac diastolic dysfunction to concurrent hormonal and metabolic status in type I diabetes mellitus. *J Clin Endocrinol Metab* 1988;66:113.

202. Raev DC: Which left ventricular function is impaired earlier in the evolution of diabetic cardiomyopathy? *Diabetes Care* 1994;17:633.

203. Kahn JK, Zola B, Juni JE, *et al*: Decreased exercise heart rate and blood pressure response in diabetic subjects with cardiac autonomic neuropathy. *Diabetes Care* 1986;9:389.

204. Mustonen J, Uusitupa M, Lansimies E, *et al*: Autonomic nervous function and its relationship to cardiac performance in middle-aged diabetic patients without clinically evident cardiovascular disease. *J Intern Med* 1992;232:65.

205. Scognamiglio R, Avogaro A, Casara D, *et al*: Myocardial dysfunction and adrenergic cardiac innervation in patients with insulin-dependent diabetes mellitus. *J Am Coll Cardiol* 1998;31:404.

206. Taegtmeyer H, McNulty P, Young ME: Adaptation and maladaptation of the heart in diabetes: part I: General concepts. Circulation 2002;105:1727.

207. Young ME, McNulty P, Taegtmeyer H: Adaptation and maladaptation of the heart in diabetes: part II: Potential mechanisms. Circulation 2002;105:1861.

208. Young LH, Russell RR, Chyun DA, Ramahi T: Heart failure in diabetic patients. In Diabetes and Cardiovascular Disease Johnstone M, Veves A, eds. Totowa, NJ, Humana Press, 2001, p. 281–298

209. Heyliger CE, Prakash A, McNeill JH: Alterations in cardiac sarcolemmal Ca^{2+} pump activity during diabetes mellitus. *Am J Physiol* 1987;252:540.

210. Schaffer SW, Ballard-Croft C, Boerth S, *et al*: Mechanisms underlying depressed Na^+/Ca^{2+} exchanger activity in the diabetic heart. *Cardiovasc Res* 1997;34:129.

211. Lopaschuk GD, Tahiliani A, Vadlamudi RVSV, *et al*: Cardiac sarcoplasmic reticulum function in insulin or carnitine-treated diabetic rats. *Am J Physiol* 1983;245:969.

212. Penpargkul S, Fein FS, Sonnenblick EH, *et al*: Depressed cardiac sarcoplasmic reticular function from diabetic rats. *J Mol Cell Cardiol* 1981;13:303.

213. Lagadic-Grossman D, Buckler KJ, Le Prigent K, *et al*: Altered Ca^{2+} handling in ventricular myocytes isolated from diabetic rats. *Am J Physiol* 1996;270:H1529.

214. Davidoff AJ, Ren J: Low insulin and high glucose induce abnormal relaxation in cultured adult rat ventricular myocytes. *Am J Physiol* 1997;272:H159.

215. Ren J, Gintant GA, Miller RE, *et al*: High extracellular glucose impairs cardiac E-C coupling in a glycosylation-dependent manner. *Am J Physiol* 1997;273:H2876.

216. Wakasaki H, Koya D, Schoen FJ, *et al*: Targeted overexpression of protein kinase C beta2 isoform in myocardium causes cardiomyopathy. *Proc Natl Acad Sci USA* 1997;94:9320.

217. Dillmann WH: Diabetes mellitus induces changes in cardiac myosin of the rat. *Diabetes* 1980;29:579.

218. Malhotra A, Penpargkul S, Fein FS, *et al*: The effect of streptozotocin-induced diabetes in rats on cardiac contractile proteins. *Circ Res* 1981;49:1243.

219. Liu X, Takeda N, Dhalla NS: Troponin I phosphorylation in heart homogenate from diabetic rat. *Biochem Biophys Acta* 1996;1316:78.

220. Liu X, Takeda N, Dhalla NS: Myosin light-chain phosphorylation in diabetic cardiomyopathy in rats. *Metabolism* 1997;46:71.

221. Norton GR, Candy G, Woodiwiss AJ: Aminoguanidine prevents the decreased myocardial compliance produced by streptozotocin-induced diabetes mellitus in rats. *Circulation* 1996;93:1905.

222. Shindler DM, Kostis JB, Yusuf S, *et al*: Diabetes mellitus, a predictor of morbidity and mortality in the Studies of Left Ventricular Dysfunction (SOLVD) Trials and Registry. *Am J Cardiol* 1996;77:1017.

223. Halon DA, Merdler A, Flugelman MY, Rennert HS, Weisz G, Shahla J, Lewis BS: Late-onset heart failure as a mechanism for adverse long-term outcome in diabetic patients undergoing revascularization (a 13-year report from the Lady Davis Carmel Medical Center registry). Am J Cardiol 2000;85:1420.

224. United Kingdom Prospective Diabetes Study Group: Tight blood pressure control and risk of macrovascular and microvascular complications in type 2 diabetes: UKPDS 38. *Br Med J* 1998;317:703.

225. Bristow MR, Gilbert EM, Abraham WT, *et al*: Carvedilol produces dose-related improvements in left ventricular function and survival in subjects with chronic heart failure. MOCHA Investigators. *Circulation* 1996;94:2807.

226. Hjalmarson A, Goldstein S, Fagerberg B, *et al*: Effects of controlled-release metoprolol on total mortality, hospitalizations, and well-being in patients with heart failure: Metoprolol CR/XL Randomized Intervention Trial in congestive heart failure (MERIT-HF). MERIT-HF Study Group. *JAMA* 2000;283:1295.

227. Deedwania PC, Giles TD, Ghali JK, *et al*: Safety and efficacy of treatment with metoprolol CR/XL in diabetic patients with heart failure. *Circulation* 2000;102(Suppl II):779.

228. Pitt B, Zannad F, Remme WJ, *et al*: The effect of spironolactone on morbidity and mortality in patients with severe heart failure. Randomized Aldactone Evaluation Study Investigators. *N Engl J Med* 1999;341:709.

229. Pitt B, Perez A: Spironolactone in patients with heart failure. *N Engl J Med* 2000;342:132.

230. Mills RM, Naftel DC, Kirklin JK, *et al*: Heart transplant rejection with hemodynamic compromise: a multi-institutional study of the role of endomyocardial cellular infiltrate. *J Heart Lung Transplant* 1997;16:813.

231. Weis M, von Scheidt W: Cardiac allograft vasculopathy: a review. *Circulation* 1997;96:2069.

232. Hoang K, Chen YD, Reaven G, *et al*: Diabetes and dyslipidemia. A new model for transplant coronary artery disease. *Circulation* 1998;97:2160.

233. Wenke K, Meiser B, Thiery J, *et al*: Simvastatin reduces graft vessel disease and mortality after heart transplantation: a four-year randomized trial [see comments]. *Circulation* 1997;96:1398.

234. Ziegler D: Cardiovascular autonomic neuropathy: clinical manifestations and measurement. *Diabetes Rev* 1999;7:342.

235. Hilsted J, Jeensen SB: A simple test for autonomic neuropathy in juvenile diabetics. *Acta Med Scand* 1979;205:385.

236. Maser RE, Pfeifer MA, Dorman JS, *et al*: Diabetic autonomic neuropathy and cardiovascular risk. Pittsburgh Epidemiology of Diabetes Complications Study III. *Arch Intern Med* 1990;150:1218.

237. Ziegler D, Gries FA, Spuler M, *et al*: The epidemiology of diabetic neuropathy. *J Diabetes Complications* 1992;6:49.

238. Ziegler D, Dannehl K, Volksw D, *et al*: Prevalence of cardiovascular autonomic dysfunction assessed by spectral analysis and standard tests of heart-rate variation in newly diagnosed IDDM patients. *Diabetes Care* 1992;15:908.

239. Barzilay J, Warram JH, Rand LI, *et al*: Risk for cardiovascular autonomic neuropathy is associated with the HLA-DR3/4 phenotype in type I diabetes mellitus. *Ann Intern Med* 1992;116:544.

240. Neil HAW, Thompson AV, John S, *et al*: Diabetic autonomic neuropathy: The prevalence of impaired heart rate variability in a geographically defined population. *Diabet Med* 1989;6:20.

241. DCCT Research Group: The effect of intensive therapy on measures of autonomic nervous system function in the Diabetes Control and Complications Trial (DCCT). *Diabetologia* 1998;41:416.

242. Spallone V, Menzinger G: Autonomic neuropathy: clinical and instrumental findings. *Clin Neurosci* 1997;4:346.

243. Ewing DJ, Borsey DQ, Bellavere F, *et al*: Cardiac autonomic neuropathy in diabetes: comparison of measures of R-R interval variation. *Diabetologia* 1981;21:18.

244. O'Brien IA, O'Hare P, Corrall RJM: Heart rate variability in healthy subjects: effects of age and the derivation of normal ranges for test of autonomic function. *Br Heart J* 1986;55:65.

245. Task Force of the European Society of Cardiology and the North American Society of Pacing and Electrophysiology: Heart rate variability: Standards of measurement, physiological interpretation, and clinical use. *Circulation* 1996;93:1043.

245a. Risk M, Bril V, Broadbridge C, Cohen A: Heart rate variability measurement in diabetic neurophy: review of methods. *Diabetes Technology & Therapeutics* 2001;3:63.

246. Turpeinen AK, Vanninen E, Kuikka JT, *et al*: Demonstration of regional sympathetic denervation of the heart in diabetes. Comparison between patients with NIDDM and IDDM. *Diabetes Care* 1996;19:1083.

247. Schnell O, Kirsch CM, Stemplinger J, *et al*: Scintigraphic evidence for cardiac sympathetic dysinnervation in long-term IDDM patients with and without ECG-based autonomic neuropathy. *Diabetologia* 1995;38:1345.

248. Schnell O, Muhr D, Weiss M, *et al*: Reduced myocardial ^{123}I-metaiodobenzylguanidine uptake in newly diagnosed IDDM patients. *Diabetes* 1996;45:801.

249. Munch G, Nguyen NT, Nekolla S, *et al*: Evaluation of sympathetic nerve terminals with [(11)C]epinephrine and [(11)C]hydroxyephedrine and positron emission tomography. *Circulation* 2000;101:516.

250. Allman KC, Stevens MJ, Wieland DM, *et al*: Noninvasive assessment of cardiac diabetic neuropathy by carbon-11 hydroxyephedrine and positron emission tomography. *J Am Coll Cardiol* 1993;22:1425.

251. Ewing DJ, Campbell IW, Clarke BF: Mortality in diabetic autonomic neuropathy. *Lancet* 1976;5:601.

252. O'Brien IA, McFadden JP, Corrall RJM: The influence of autonomic neuropathy on mortality in insulin-dependent diabetes. *Q J Med* 1991;290:495.

253. Rathman W, Ziegler D, Jahnke M, *et al*: Mortality in diabetic patients with cardiovascular autonomic neuropathy. *Diabet Med* 1993; 10:820.

254. Stevens MJ, Raffel DM, Allman KC, *et al*: Cardiac sympathetic denervation in diabetes: Implications for enhanced cardiovascular risk. *Circulation* 1998;98:961.

255. Porte DJ, Graf RJ, Halter JB, *et al*: Diabetic neuropathy and plasma glucose control. *Am J Med* 1981;70:195.

256. Burger AJ, Hamer AW, Weinrauch LA, *et al*: Relation of heart rate variability and serum lipoproteins in type 2 diabetes mellitus and chronic stable angina pectoris. *Am J Cardiol* 1998;81:945.

257. Hilsted J, Galbo H, Christensen NJ, *et al*: Haemodynamic changes during graded exercise in patients with diabetic autonomic neuropathy. *Diabetologia* 1982;22:318.

258. Scognamiglio R, Fasoli G, Ferri M, *et al*: Myocardial dysfunction and abnormal left ventricle exercise response in autonomic dysfunction in diabetic patients. *Clin Cardiol* 1995;18:276.

259. Bellavere F, Ferri M, Guarini L, *et al*: Prolonged QT period in diabetic autonomic neuropathy: A possible role in sudden cardiac death? *Br Heart J* 1988;59:379.

260. Ewing DJ, Boland O, Neilson JMN, *et al*: Autonomic neuropathy, QT interval lengthening and unexpected deaths in male patients. *Diabetologia* 1991;34:182.

261. Shimabukuro M, Chibana T, Yoshida H, *et al*: Increased QT dispersion and cardiac adrenergic dysinnervation in diabetic patients with autonomic neuropathy. *Am J Cardiol* 1996;78:1057.

262. Naas AA, Davidson NC, Thompson C, *et al*: QT and QTc dispersion are accurate predictors of cardiac death in newly diagnosed non-insulin-dependent diabetes: cohort study. *Br Med J* 1998; 613:745.

263. Abenavoli T, Rubler S, Fisher VJ, *et al*: Exercise testing with myocardial scintigraphy in asymptomatic diabetic males. *Circulation* 1981;63:54.

264. Gu K, Cowie CC, Harris MI: Diabetes and decline in heart disease mortality in US adults. *JAMA* 1999;281:1291.

CHAPTER 50

Peripheral Vascular Disease in the Person with Diabetes

Cameron M. Akbari

Frank W. LoGerfo

Diabetes mellitus is found in over 6% of the U.S. population, and the incidence is rising, with more than half a million new cases diagnosed annually.[1] Many epidemiologic studies spanning several decades have clearly established the link between diabetes and vascular disease. The Framingham Study of over 5000 subjects demonstrated that diabetes is a powerful risk factor for atherosclerotic coronary and peripheral arterial disease, independent of other atherogenic risk factors, with a relative risk averaging twofold in men and threefold for women.[2] The Framingham Study also confirmed that the risk of stroke is at least 2.5-fold higher in patients with diabetes,[3] a finding that has been confirmed in other large epidemiologic studies.[4,5] Moreover, diabetes is strongly associated with atherosclerosis of the extracranial internal carotid artery and thus imparts an additional independent risk of stroke.[6]

PATHOPHYSIOLOGY

The complications of diabetes may best be characterized as alterations in vascular structure and function, with subsequent end-organ damage and death.[7] Specifically, two types of vascular disease are seen in patients with diabetes: a nonocclusive microcirculatory impairment involving the capillaries and arterioles of the kidneys, retina, and peripheral nerves, and a macroangiopathy characterized by atherosclerotic lesions of the coronary and peripheral arterial circulation.[8–11] The former is relatively unique to diabetes, whereas the latter lesions are morphologically and functionally similar in both nondiabetic and diabetic patients.

Retinopathy is the most characteristic microvascular complication of diabetes, and population-based studies have identified a correlation between its development and the duration of diabetes.[12] Similar correlations have been found with nephropathy, neuropathy, and diabetes,[13] with perhaps the strongest evidence coming from the Diabetes Control and Complications Trial (DCCT). The results from the DCCT clearly showed a delay in the development and progression of these microvascular complications with intensive glycemic control, thus supporting the direct causal relationship between hyperglycemia, diabetes, and its microvascular sequelae.[14] These and other clinical trials have provided the rationale for experimental studies investigating the fundamental pathophysiology of micro- and macrovascular disease in diabetes mellitus.

Microvascular dysfunction in diabetes is manifested by an increased vascular permeability and impaired autoregulation of blood flow and vascular tone. These changes culminate in nephropathy, retinopathy, and neuropathy and probably contribute to the cardiovascular complications of diabetes. Although multiple theories have been postulated as to the etiology of accelerated microangiopathy, it is likely that several biochemical derangements exist in the presence of hyperglycemia and diabetes and that these mechanisms work synergistically to cause microvascular dysfunction. These metabolic alterations produce functional and structural changes in many areas at the arteriolar and capillary levels, including the basement membrane,[9] the smooth muscle cell,[15] and, in particular, the endothelial cell.[16]

One of the greatest impediments in understanding and treating vascular disease in patients with diabetes is the misconception that they have an untreatable occlusive lesion in the microcirculation, which has fostered the belief that arterial reconstruction is futile. This idea originated from a retrospective histologic study demonstrating the presence of PAS-positive material occluding the arterioles in amputated limb specimens from diabetic patients.[17] However, subsequent prospective anatomic staining and arterial casting studies[18,19] have demonstrated the *absence* of an arteriolar occlusive lesion. Further evidence comes from physiologic studies of femoro popliteal bypass grafts in diabetic and nondiabetic patients in which direct vasodilator administration into these grafts demonstrates a comparable fall in peripheral resistance between the two groups.[20] Dispelling the notion of "small vessel disease" is fundamental to the principles of limb salvage in patients with diabetes, since arterial reconstruction is almost always possible and successful in these patients.

Although there is no occlusive lesion in the diabetic microcirculation, other structural changes do exist, most notably thickening of the capillary basement membrane. This alteration in the extracellular matrix may represent a response to the metabolic changes related to diabetes and hyperglycemia. However, these changes do not lead to narrowing of the capillary lumen, and arteriolar blood flow may be normal or even increased despite these changes.[21] Capillary basement membrane thickening is the dominant structural change in both diabetic retinopathy and neuropathy. In the kidney, nonenzymatic glycosylation reduces the charge on the basement membrane, which may account for transudation of albumin, an expanded mesangium, and albuminuria.[22] Similar increases in vascular permeability occur in the eye and probably contribute to macular exudate formation and retinopathy.

In the diabetic foot, basement membrane thickening may theoretically impair the migration of leukocytes and the hyperemic response following injury and thus may increase the susceptibility of the diabetic foot to infection.[23,24] Although resting total skin microcirculatory flow is similar in both diabetic and nondiabetic patients, the capillary blood flow is reduced in diabetes, indicating a maldistribution and functional ischemia of the skin.[25] Moreover, studies of skin microvascular flow have demonstrated a reduced maximal hyperemic response in diabetic patients, suggesting that a *functional* microvascular impairment is a major contributing factor for diabetic foot problems. All of these changes result in an inability to vasodilate and achieve maximal blood flow following injury.

Diabetes also affects the axon reflex (Fig. 50-1). Injury directly stimulates nociceptive C fibers, which results in both orthodromic conduction to the spinal cord and antidromic conduction to adjacent C fibers and other axon branches. One function of this axon reflex is the secretion of several active peptides, such as substance P and calcitonin gene–related peptide, which directly and indirectly (through mast cell release of histamine) cause vasodilation and increased permeability. This neurogenic vasodilatory response is impaired in diabetes, further reducing the hyperemic response when it is most needed, that is, under conditions of injury and inflammation.[26]

The above changes contribute to an early functional impairment in vascular reserve in the peripheral, coronary, and cerebral circulation of patients with diabetes. Using positron emission tomography (PET), myocardial blood flow may be measured at rest and after vasodilator administration, and thus coronary flow reserve (as a measure of endothelial function) may be calculated. Reduced coronary flow reserve and impaired coronary reactivity have been observed in diabetic patients with angiographically normal coronary arteries and no other detectable microvascular complications, suggesting an early endothelial dysfunction.[27,28] Similarly, cerebrovascular reactivity and reserve capacity may be assessed using transcranial Doppler and acetazolamide, which causes vasodilation of the brain resistance vessels. Impaired cerebrovascular reserve is

also noted in patients with diabetes, particularly among those patients with other microvascular complications.[29]

There is substantial evidence that endothelial function is abnormal in animal models of diabetes mellitus[30–32] and in patients with both type 1 and type 2 diabetes mellitus (T1- and T2DM),[33,34] thus directly implicating either hyperglycemia or hyperinsulinemia as a possible mediator of abnormal endothelium-dependent responses. A variety of mechanisms responsible for vascular dysfunction have been proposed, principally abnormalities in the nitric oxide pathway, abnormal production of vasoconstrictor prostanoids, intracellular signaling, reduction in Na^+/K^+-ATPase activity, and advanced glycosylated end products.[35–37]

In 1980, Furchgott and Zawadzki[38] discovered that arterial vasodilation was dependent on an intact endothelium and its release of a substance they called endothelium-derived relaxing factor (EDRF), which causes arterial smooth muscle relaxation in response to acetylcholine and other vasodilators. Later identified as endothelial-derived nitric oxide (EDNO), it activates vascular smooth muscle guanylate cyclase, elevates cyclic GMP levels, and may increase Na^+/K^+-ATPase activity.[39]

A variety of substances other than acetylcholine may cause EDNO-mediated vasodilation. Notably, it appears that the vasodilatory effects of insulin are nitric oxide–dependent[40,41] and that insulin mediates vasodilation by modulating the synthesis and release of EDNO. Although hyperglycemia with hyperinsulinemia impairs endothelial-dependent vasodilation, hyperinsulinemia with euglycemia actually potentiates endothelium-dependent vasodilation via enhanced EDNO release, suggesting that hyperglycemia, independent of hyperinsulinemia, contributes to endothelial dysfunction. This has been corroborated by studies performed on healthy individuals, in which ingestion of a glucose load and subsequent acute hyperglycemia impair the endothelial-dependent vasodilation of the macrocirculation and microcirculation.[42]

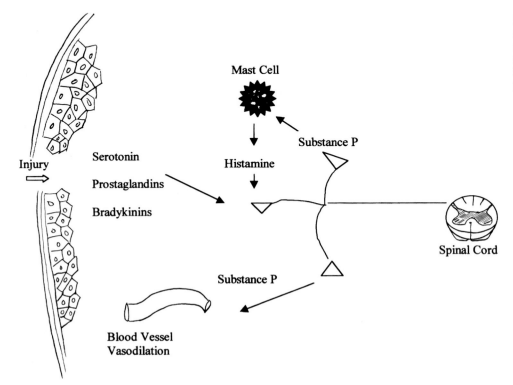

FIGURE 50-1. Illustration of the axon (nociceptive) reflex, in which injury results in vasodilation via secretion of active peptides such as substance P, histamine, and calcitonin gene–related peptide.

Impaired endothelial-dependent vasodilation in certain insulin-resistant states may be instrumental in the pathogenesis of atherosclerosis and hypertension and is postulated to be due to diminished insulin-mediated EDNO production and release.[43] Patients with T1- and T2DM demonstrate impaired endothelium-dependent responses to acetylcholine, but the response to exogenous nitric oxide donors (i.e., sodium nitroprusside) remains intact in T1DM[32,33] (Fig. 50-2).

Although there is considerable controversy regarding the role of free radicals in diabetic vascular disease,[44] an increased production of oxygen-derived free radicals has been described in diabetes and may contribute to endothelial dysfunction.[45] Superoxide anions and other oxygen-derived free radicals directly inactivate EDNO.[46] In animal models, endothelium-derived free radicals impair EDNO-mediated vasodilation, and administration of super-oxide dismutase and other free radical scavengers normalizes EDNO-dependent relaxation in diabetic arteries.[47] Defective endothelium-dependent relaxation in diabetic rat aorta is significantly attenuated by vitamin E, a potent free radical scavenger.[48] In human studies, administration of vitamin C in pharmacologic doses restores and improves endothelium-dependent vasodilation, but not endothelium-independent responses in patients with both T1- and T2DM, thus further suggesting that oxygen-derived free radicals may decrease the bioavailability of EDNO.[49]

A potentially treatable source of oxygen-derived free radicals is hyperlipidemia. Increased levels of low-density lipoprotein (LDL) and very-low-density lipoprotein (VLDL) are common in diabetic patients. Hyperglycemia promotes the oxidation and nonenzymatic glycation of LDL, which has been strongly implicated in atherogenesis by a variety of mechanisms.[50] In animal models of hypercholesterolemia, the vascular endothelium produces several free radicals, presumably through xanthine oxidase activation, and these endothelial-derived free radicals inactivate EDNO.[51] Moreover, flow-mediated vasodilation and reactive hyperemia (endothelium-dependent) are more impaired in patients with T1DM and elevated LDL cholesterol levels, which further supports the relationship of hypercholesterolemia, free radicals, and EDNO.[52]

FIGURE 50-2. In response to acetylcholine, nitric oxide synthetase (NOS) is activated, which leads to nitric oxide (NO) release and vasodilation. The response is endothelium-dependent in that it is dependent on endothelium-derived NOS and NO. In contrast, sodium nitroprusside, an exogenous nitric oxide donor, directly activates cyclic guanosine monophosphate (cGMP) and thus is not dependent on endothelium-derived NOS and NO. TXA_2, thromboxane A_2; PGs, prostaglandins. *(Reproduced from Akbari et al.[7])*

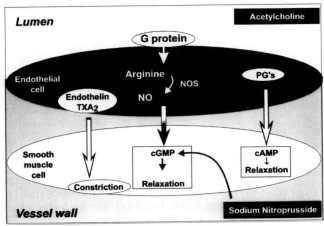

Advanced glycosylation end products (AGEs) have also been implicated in the pathogenesis of diabetic microvascular complications. These are formed from a reversible reaction between glucose and protein to form Schiff bases, which then rearrange to form stable Amadori-type early glycosylation products. Some of these reversible early glycosylation products may undergo complex rearrangements to form irreversible AGEs. In experimental diabetes, AGEs impair the actions of EDNO and cause an impaired endothelium-dependent response, which is ameliorated by administration of an AGE inhibitor.[53]

AGEs also displace disulfide cross-linkages in collagen and scleral proteins, accounting for the diminished charge in the capillary basement membrane. This may contribute to the increased vascular permeability of diabetes, since blockade of a specific receptor for AGE reverses diabetes-mediated vascular hyperpermeability.[54] Moreover, the presence of AGE receptors on both endothelial cells and monocytes, along with AGE deposition in the subendothelium, suggests monocyte deposition into the subendothelial space and secondary complications.[55] In studies using a radioreceptor assay for AGEs in serum and arterial wall, higher AGE levels have been demonstrated in patients with diabetes compared to nondiabetic controls, with the highest levels occurring among diabetic patients with nephropathy.[56] Since at least part of AGE-induced cellular dysfunction is due to an oxidant-sensitive mechanism, which is inhibited by antioxidants, it is likely that both oxygen-derived free radicals and AGEs contribute to cause impaired EDNO-dependent vasodilation in diabetes. Taken together, the effects of AGEs on vascular permeability, subendothelial protein deposition, inactivation of nitric oxide, and modification of LDL provide strong evidence of their important role in diabetic vascular disease.

Experimental studies in diabetic animals have also indicated that abnormal endothelial production of vasoconstrictor prostanoids, notably thromboxane (TX) A_2 and prostaglandin (PG) H_2, may contribute to endothelial cell dysfunction. In humans, however, the role of vasoconstrictor prostanoids is less clear. Flow-dependent vasodilation in healthy subjects, which may be used as an index of endothelial function, is unaffected by aspirin, thus demonstrating that it is entirely mediated by EDNO and independent of vasoactive prostanoids.[57] Moreover, the attenuated endothelium-dependent vasodilation that is observed in diabetic patients following acetylcholine administration is not affected by pretreatment with cyclo-oxygenase inhibitors.

It therefore appears that dysfunction of the microcirculation strongly contributes to the renal, eye, and macrovascular complications of diabetes. Several lines of evidence have indicated that the microcirculation is also implicated in the pathogenesis of diabetic neuropathy, and the etiology of diabetic neuropathy may be a complex interplay among metabolic and microvascular defects involving aldose reductase, Na^+/K^+-ATPase activity, and nitric oxide. Some of these may include EDNO stimulation of Na^+/K^+-ATPase activity, decreased Na^+/K^+-ATPase activity by EDNO inhibitors, and hyperglycemic inhibition of Na^+/K^+-ATPase activity in normal rabbit aorta, which is preventable by administering aldose reductase inhibitors or by raising plasma myoinositol levels.[58,59]

More recent studies using laser Doppler imaging have further defined the relationships among the microcirculation, diabetes, and neuropathy.[60] These findings suggest that the endothelium-dependent vasodilation and the axon reflex are impaired in the presence of diabetes and neuropathy but that the endothelium-independent response is spared, and that this dysfunction may be attributed to an impaired production of nitric oxide. In addition, the nerve axon reflex is reduced in diabetic neuropathic patients with and without vascular disease, while it is intact in diabetic patients without neuropathy. In addition, the expression of endogenous endothelial nitric oxide synthetase (eNOS) activity (taken from the skin of the foot) has been found to be reduced in patients with diabetes and either neuropathy or macrovascular disease, compared with healthy controls.[61] In contrast, the level of von Willebrand factor (an anatomic marker of the endothelium) is comparable among the controls and diabetic patients. Therefore, it appears that in diabetic neuropathic patients, with or without lower extremity ischemia, the eNOS activity is reduced, even though the endothelium is anatomically present and endothelial functional changes may be related to the development of neuropathy.

Current hypotheses regarding the etiology of diabetic neuropathy are centered on a combination of metabolic defects secondary to hyperglycemia and vascular changes that result in nerve hypoxia.[62] Evidence for a hypoxic etiology is considerable and includes reduced endoneurial blood flow, increased vascular resistance, and decreased endothelial production of nitric oxide.[63,64] Although microvascular dysfunction has been mainly implicated, the role of peripheral vascular disease remains considerable, as it appears likely that a decrease in total limb blood flow would potentiate nerve ischemia. This concept has been supported by clinical trials, which have demonstrated a more severe neuropathy in diabetic patients with lower limb ischemia compared with nonischemic diabetic and ischemic nondiabetic patients, and an improvement in nerve function shortly after revascularization.[65,66]

Clinical studies from the authors' laboratory have focused on the effect of arterial reconstruction on the natural history of diabetic neuropathy.[67] Fifty-five patients with diabetes and peripheral vascular disease requiring revascularization were studied. Peroneal nerve conduction velocity was measured prior to arterial bypass and then again at a mean follow-up of 19 months. In the operated leg, the peroneal nerve conduction velocity remained unchanged during the follow-up period (preoperative 35.79 ± 6.02 m/s versus postoperative 35.33 ± 7.51 m/s, p = NS), but deteriorated in the nonoperated leg (36.68 ± 6.22 m/s versus 33.64 ± 7.30 m/s, p < 0.05). The data suggest that reversal of hypoxia in diabetic patients halts the progression of neuropathy, lending further support to the role of localized ischemia in the pathogenesis of nerve dysfunction in diabetes mellitus.[68]

DIABETES AND CEREBROVASCULAR DISEASE

Compelling data from several large clinical studies have demonstrated that diabetes is a major risk factor for stroke, and the incidence of ischemic stroke is at least 2.5-fold higher in diabetic patients.[3–5] Moreover, the mortality and severity of stroke are higher among patients with diabetes.[69,70] The relative risk of stroke increases even further among diabetic patients with established retinopathy, neuropathy, or nephropathy, thus suggesting that the presence of diabetes introduces additional microvascular and cerebrovascular pathophysiology, which may increase the frequency and severity of stroke in these patients.[71,72]

Elevated blood glucose is toxic to infarcted brain tissue, and stroke severity is greater in patients with hyperglycemia.[73,74] Among patients with diabetes, poor glycemic control doubles the risk of ischemic stroke, even after adjustment for other variables.[75]

Morphologic abnormalities in diabetes include arterial endothelial cell necrosis and thickened capillary basement thickening in cerebral vessels; in addition, diabetic patients have shown impaired cerebrovascular reactivity to hypercapnia and blood pressure changes.[76] Abnormal cerebral blood flow may be seen in experimental diabetes, and among patients with diabetes and no history of cerebrovascular disease, single-photon emission computed tomography (SPECT) scanning has demonstrated multiple subclinical alterations in cerebral blood flow.[77] Hyperglycemia alone causes both a decrease in cerebral blood flow and an impaired cerebral vasodilatory response.[78] As noted previously, altered cerebral vascular reactivity occurs among patients with long-standing diabetes and may reflect a generalized cerebrovascular microangiopathy involving the brain resistance arterioles.[28]

Acute hyperglycemia and glucose exposure may also impair the autoregulation of cerebral blood flow. *In vitro* exposure of isolated cerebral arteries to high glucose concentrations causes vasodilation and inhibition of arterial tone, suggesting that both cerebrovascular tone and control of cerebral blood flow may be impaired during acute hyperglycemia.[79] Moreover, since removal of the endothelium abolishes this effect, this appears to be an endothelium-dependent and nitric oxide–mediated mechanism. Impaired cerebral vessel endothelium-dependent relaxation, but not endothelium-independent vasodilation, has also been observed in the presence of diabetes.[80,81] These findings suggest either reduced activity/synthesis of EDNO or increased destruction, the latter possibly mediated by a thromboxane A_2 and prostaglandin H_2 pathway.

Multiple cerebrovascular metabolic abnormalities also contribute to the worse stroke outcome in hyperglycemia and diabetes.[82] Anaerobic metabolism of glucose during ischemia produces lactate, which accumulates inside brain cells and results in lower intracellular pH and may promote cell death. As noted earlier, AGEs accumulate as a consequence of diabetes and may also contribute to the increased stroke severity in diabetic patients, as systemic administration of AGEs into animals with focal brain infarction increases cerebral infarct size and damage.[83]

Because of the worse prognosis of stroke in patients with diabetes, efforts should be directed toward reducing the risk of stroke in these patients, including reduction or elimination of concomitant risk factors. In addition, among selected symptomatic and asymptomatic patients with a high-grade internal carotid artery stenosis, carotid endarterectomy has been shown to reduce the risk of stroke.[84,85] Because diabetes is associated with multiple cerebrovascular abnormalities, the safety of carotid endarterectomy in patients with diabetes may be questioned.[86] A recent report has summarized the experience with carotid endarterectomy in patients with diabetes.[87] Over a 6-year period, 732 carotid endarterectomy procedures were performed, of which 284 (39%) were in patients with diabetes mellitus. The total operative mortality rate was 0.3%. There were 11 perioperative neurologic events (8 strokes, 3 transient ischemic attacks) during the entire period (1.5%), of which 6 (2.1%) were among diabetic patients and 5 (1.1%) among nondiabetic patients, a difference that was not statistically significant. Of the 8 strokes, 3 occurred in diabetic patients (1.0%) and 5 in nondiabetic patients (1.1%), which again was not statistically significant. Moreover, it was demonstrated that diabetes is not an independent risk factor for postoperative cardiac morbidity among patients undergoing carotid endarterectomy. These results show that carotid endarterectomy may be safely performed in diabetic patients, with neurologic morbidity and mortality rates comparable to those of the nondiabetic population.

THE DIABETIC FOOT

Problems of the diabetic foot are the most common cause of hospitalization in diabetic patients, with an annual health care cost of over $1 billion.[88] Diabetes is a contributing factor in half of all lower extremity amputations in the United States, and the relative risk for amputation is 40 times greater in people with diabetes.[89] Diabetic foot ulceration will affect 15% of all diabetic individuals during their lifetime and is clearly a significant risk factor in the pathway to limb loss.[90] The principal pathogenetic mechanisms in diabetic foot disease are neuropathy, infection, and ischemia; acting together, they contribute to the sequence of tissue necrosis, ulceration, and gangrene (Fig. 50-3).

As discussed previously, the etiology of diabetic neuropathy is unknown and most likely multifactorial. Peripheral neuropathy is a common complication of diabetes, afflicting as many as 50–60% of all patients,[91,92] and is present in over 80% of diabetic patients with foot lesions, thus further emphasizing the direct relationship between neuropathy and foot ulceration.[93] Neuropathy is broadly classified as focal or diffuse; the latter is more common and includes the autonomic and chronic sensorimotor polyneuropathies, which both contribute to foot ulceration.

Sensorimotor neuropathy initially involves the distal lower extremities, progresses centrally, and is typically symmetric. Sensory nerve fiber involvement leads to loss of the protective sensation of pain, whereas motor fiber destruction results in small muscle

FIGURE 50-3. The biologically compromised foot. Multiple abnormalities, including sensorimotor neuropathy, altered architecture, microvascular dysfunction, ischemia, and infection contribute to the diabetic foot. *(Reproduced from Akbari et al.[7])*

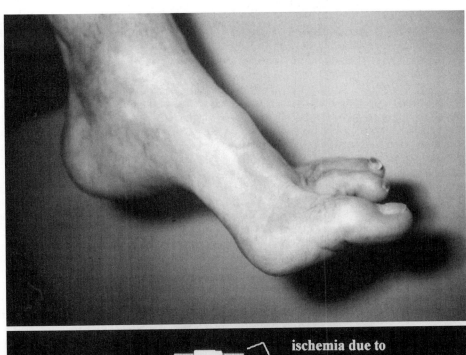
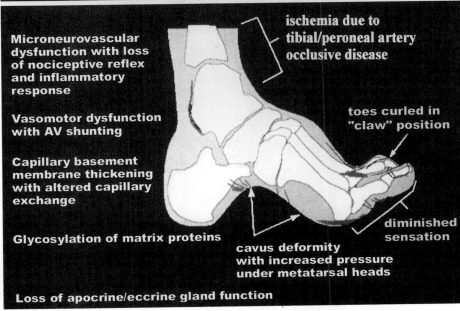

atrophy in the foot. Consequently, the metatarsals are flexed, with metatarsal head prominence and "clawing" of the toes. This causes abnormal pressure points to develop on the bony prominences without sensation, with subsequent callus formation, cracking, erosion, and ulceration. Meanwhile, autonomic neuropathy in the foot causes loss of sympathetic tone, which results in increased arteriovenous shunting and inefficient nutrient flow. Autonomic denervation of oil and sweat glands leads to cracking of dry skin, which further predisposes the diabetic foot to skin breakdown and ulceration.[94]

The spectrum of infection in diabetic foot disease ranges from superficial ulceration to extensive gangrene with fulminant sepsis (Fig. 50-4). Most infections are polymicrobic, with the most common pathogens being staphylococci and streptococci; more complicated ulcers may harbor anaerobes and gram-negative bacilli. Potential sources of diabetic foot infection include a simple puncture wound or ulcer, the nail plate, and the interdigital web space. Untreated infection can lead to bacterial spread along tendon sheaths and fascial planes, destruction of the interosseous fascia, and spread to the foot dorsum. Edema in the foot elevates compartmental pressures, with resultant capillary thrombosis and further impairment of nutrient blood flow.

Classical signs of infection may not always be present in the infected diabetic foot due to the consequences of neuropathy, alterations in the foot microcirculation, and leukocyte abnormalities. Fever, chills, and leukocytosis may be absent in up to two-thirds of diabetic patients with extensive foot infections, and hyperglycemia is often the sole presenting sign.[95] Therefore, a complete examination of the infected areas is mandatory, and the wound should be thoroughly inspected, including unroofing of all encrusted areas, to determine the extent of involvement. Because most infections are polymicrobic, cultures should be obtained from the base or depths of the wound after debridement so that appropriate antibiotic treatment may ensue.

Osteomyelitis is common in diabetic foot ulceration and may be demonstrated by bone biopsies in almost 70% of benign-appearing ulcers.[96] A variety of diagnostic tests may be ordered to assist in the diagnosis, including plain radiographs, a three-phase bone scan, labeled leukocyte scans, CT scans, and magnetic resonance imaging. Criticism may be leveled at the indiscriminate use of these tests and a costly "shotgun" approach to the diagnosis of osteomyelitis. A more cost-effective approach involves the use of a sterile probe to detect bone in an open ulcer.[97] With a positive predictive value of nearly 90%, osteomyelitis should be presumed if bone is palpated on probing, thus rendering other specialized and expensive radiographic tests unnecessary.

A critical step for limb salvage in patients with diabetic foot ulceration is a thorough evaluation for ischemia. The complex milieu of motor and sensory neuropathy, capillary basement thickening, loss of the neurogenic inflammatory response, as well as the wide spectrum of microcirculatory and endothelial abnormalities, results in a biologically compromised foot. Even moderate ischemia may lead to ulceration under these circumstances. Thus the concept of ischemia must be modified in making decisions about arterial reconstruction in the diabetic foot, since the biologically compromised foot requires *maximum* circulation to heal an ulcer. This leads to three significant principles: (1) All diabetic foot ulcers should be evaluated for an ischemic component; (2) correction of a moderate degree of ischemia will improve healing in the biologically compromised diabetic foot; and (3) whenever possible, the arterial reconstruction should be designed to restore normal arterial pressure to the target area. Ultimately, all limb salvage efforts will fail unless ischemia is recognized and corrected.

Treatment of the diabetic foot should be directed toward the pathogenic factors outlined above. The most important treatment guidelines are as follows[98]:

1. Prompt control of infection. This assumes first priority in the management of any diabetic foot problem.
2. Evaluation for ischemia.
3. Prompt arterial reconstruction once active infection has resolved.

FIGURE 50-4. Fulminant sepsis in a 52-year-old with an infected diabetic foot. Corresponding x-rays demonstrated gas within the soft tissues (**white arrow**), consistent with a polymicrobic and opportunistic infection. Note the *absence* of cellulitis, due to, among other factors, the consequences of neuropathy and loss of the nociceptive reflex.

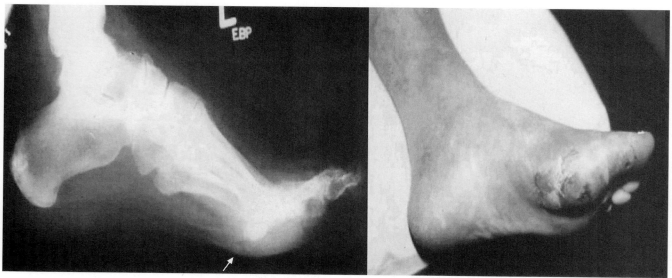

4. Secondary procedures, such as further debridement, toe amputations, local flaps, and even free flaps, may then be carried out separately in the fully vascularized foot.

DIABETES AND LOWER EXTREMITY VASCULAR DISEASE

Lower extremity arterial disease is more common among patients with diabetes. The presence of diabetes is associated with a two- to threefold excess risk of intermittent claudication compared with its absence.[99] Despite significant advances in the prevention and treatment of peripheral vascular disease, diabetes continues to be the single strongest cardiovascular risk factor for the development of critical leg ischemia and limb loss.[100]

Unlike microvascular disease, which is unique to diabetes and its metabolic alterations, the cause of lower extremity ischemia is similar in both diabetic and nondiabetic patients and is due to accelerated atherosclerosis. One notable difference between these populations is the pattern and location of the occlusive atherosclerotic lesion. As noted earlier, there is no evidence for an occlusive lesion at the arteriolar level ("small-vessel disease") in patients with diabetes. However, diabetic patients are more likely to have atherosclerotic disease affecting the infrapopliteal (tibial) arteries, with sparing of the foot arteries,[101] which allows for successful arterial reconstruction to these distal vessels. Conversely, the superficial femoral or popliteal artery is less likely to be affected by the occlusive process, allowing these vessels to serve as a possible inflow source for bypass grafting.

Because the foot vessels are often patent in the diabetic patient, and because of the success of bypass grafting to these vessels, an appropriate evaluation for ischemia is essential in diabetic patients. Unless ischemia is recognized and corrected, limb salvage efforts with the diabetic foot will fail, even if infection and neuropathy have been appropriately treated.

As with any other disease process, evaluation should begin with a detailed history and physical exam. In the patient with a diabetic foot ulcer, it is helpful to consider the duration of the ulcer, the type of treatments utilized, and any past history of foot ulceration and treatment. Although nocturnal rest pain in the foot is strongly suggestive of lower extremity arterial disease in the nondiabetic patient, the variable effects of neuropathy make pain more difficult to evaluate in the diabetic limb. Similarly, claudication symptoms may be entirely absent in the patient with an ischemic diabetic foot ulcer. Long-standing foot ulceration, coexisting cardiac disease (such as angina or heart failure), and sensorimotor neuropathy may all limit the ability to ambulate sufficiently to manifest claudication symptoms.

Physical examination should be directed toward the underlying pathophysiology of foot ulceration. Neuropathy may easily be evaluated: Observation may reveal the morphologic motor abnormalities such as "claw foot" or Charcot's osteoarthropathy; monofilament testing will assess the degree of sensory neuropathy. Noting the location of the ulcer may also be helpful, in that purely ischemic lesions typically occur in the most distal parts of the foot, such as the toes, forefoot, or heel, in contrast to the neuropathic ulcers seen on the weight-bearing areas.

All ulcers, including those with a significant neuropathic component, should be assessed for an ischemic component. The most important observation is the presence or absence of a palpable foot pulse; in simplest terms, if the foot pulses are not palpable, it can be assumed that occlusive disease is present.

A variety of noninvasive arterial tests may be ordered in an effort to quantify the degree of ischemia. However, in the presence of diabetes, *all* of these tests have significant limitations. Although Doppler-derived pressures have proved to be reliable in localizing the degree and level of arterial occlusive disease in nondiabetic patients, their use is limited in the presence of diabetes. Medial arterial calcinosis occurs frequently in diabetic patients and is characterized by a *nonobstructive* calcification of the vessel wall at the media layer; its presence can result in noncompressible arteries with artifactually high segmental systolic pressures and ankle-brachial indices. Medial calcification should be suspected whenever the ankle pressure greatly exceeds arm pressure or when the Doppler signal at the ankle cannot be obliterated with greater than 250 mm Hg pressure. The finding of lower levels of calcification in the toe vessels supports the use of toe systolic pressures as a more reliable indicator of arterial flow to the foot.[102] However, the use of toe pressures is often limited by the proximity of the foot ulcer to the cuff site, the size of the cuff itself, and other extrinsic variables.

Segmental Doppler waveforms and pulsed volume recordings are unaffected by medial calcification. A normal Doppler waveform is triphasic; with proximal obstruction, the waveform becomes monophasic (Fig. 50-5). Pulse volume recordings rely on plethysmographic recordings of the change in volume that occurs with each pulsation. A sharp upstroke, narrow peak, and dicrotic notch characterize a normal recording. With increasing levels of arterial insufficiency, the waveform loses the dicrotic notch, followed by loss of amplitude and blunting of the waveform (Fig. 50-6). Since neither of these tests relies on obliterating flow within

FIGURE 50-5. The normal Doppler tracing on the left illustrates a triphasic flow pattern, with forward flow in systole (**first arrow**), a reversal of flow in early diastole (**second arrow**), and a secondary forward flow in late diastole (**third arrow**). With proximal arterial obstruction, the waveform becomes monophasic (**right**), with loss of the reverse flow component and blunting of the systolic peak.

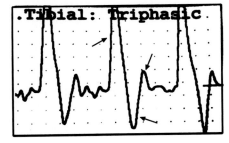

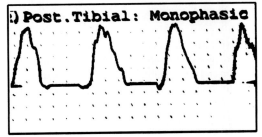

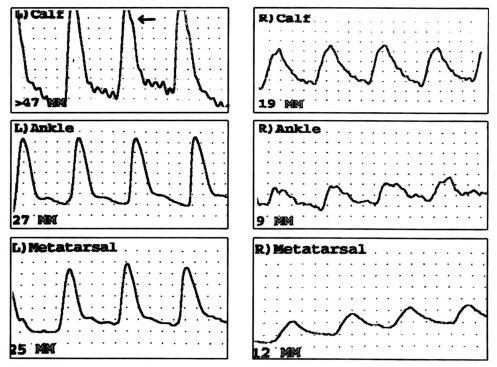

FIGURE 50-6. Normal pulse volume recordings (PVRs) on the left illustrate a brisk, sharp rise to the systolic peak, with a dichrotic notch (indicated by the **arrow on the calf tracing**). With increasing levels of proximal arterial obstruction (**right**), the waveform loses the dichrotic notch, the peak becomes more rounded, and the downslope is prolonged. Severe occlusive disease produces a flattened waveform with a slow upstroke and downstroke.

a vessel (unlike Doppler-derived pressures), they may prove useful in the diabetic patient with suspected arterial insufficiency. However, significant limitations exist in their use, and caution should be exercised when interpreting results. Evaluation of these waveforms is primarily qualitative and not quantitative. A flat forefoot tracing is a convincing demonstration of ischemia, but it is difficult to make clinical decisions based on the magnitude of the waveform. Similarly, severity of arterial insufficiency cannot be accurately interpreted, since no reliable quantitative scoring exists. In addition, the quality of the waveforms is affected by peripheral edema, cuff size, and motion artifact. Finally, the presence of ulceration, especially at the forefoot level, often precludes accurate cuff placement.

Regional transcutaneous oximetry (TcPo$_2$) measurements are also unaffected by medial calcinosis, and recent studies have noted its reliability in predicting healing of ulcers and amputation levels.[103] Limitations, including a lack of equipment standardization, user variability, and a large "gray area" of values, preclude its applicability. Furthermore, TcPo$_2$ measurements are higher in diabetic patients with foot ulcers compared with the nondiabetic population, which further limits the ability of this test to predict ischemia.[104]

The limitations of noninvasive vascular testing in diabetic patients with foot ulceration emphasize the continued importance of a thorough bedside evaluation and clinical judgment. To reiterate, the status of the foot pulse is the most important aspect of the physical exam. In simplest terms, it can be assumed that occlusive disease is present if the foot pulses are not palpable. This finding alone is an indication for contrast arteriography in the clinical setting of tissue loss, poor healing, or gangrene, even if neuropathy may have been the antecedent cause of skin breakdown or ulceration.

Concern for contrast-induced renal failure should not mitigate against a high-quality angiogram of the entire lower extremity circulation. The incidence of contrast nephropathy is not higher in the diabetic patient without preexisting renal disease, even with the use of ionic contrast.[105,106] The more costly nonionic agents should be reserved for the diabetic patient with compromised renal function. Even in this group, the concern for contrast nephropathy should not delay arteriography, as it seldom requires dialysis for treatment. More recently, attention has focused on the roles of magnetic resonance angiography, carbon dioxide angiography, and duplex scanning as replacements for contrast arteriography. However, each has its own limitations, and although we have selectively utilized these modalities, we continue to rely heavily on a high-quality contrast arteriogram for most of our patients requiring distal arterial reconstruction.

Whatever preoperative imaging modality is chosen prior to arterial reconstruction, it is mandatory that consideration be given to the pattern of lower extremity vascular disease in patients with diabetes. Because the foot vessels are often spared by the atherosclerotic occlusive process, even when the tibial arteries are occluded, it is essential that arteriograms not be terminated at the midtibial level. The complete infrapopliteal circulation should be incorporated, including the foot vessels. The advent of digital subtraction angiography, which allows for subtraction of the bones from the final images, has greatly helped in visualizing these distal vessels. Both anteroposterior and lateral foot views should be included to differentiate branch vessels and to visualize all stenoses.

PRINCIPLES OF ARTERIAL RECONSTRUCTION IN THE DIABETIC FOOT

A complete arteriogram will facilitate the choice of an outflow artery that will restore a palpable foot pulse. Proximal bypass to the popliteal or tibioperoneal arteries may restore foot pulses. More often, however, because of the pattern of occlusive disease in the diabetic patient, bypass grafting to the popliteal or even tibial arteries cannot accomplish this goal, due to more distal obstruction. Similarly, although excellent results have been reported with peroneal artery bypass,[107] the peroneal artery is not in continuity with the foot vessels and may not achieve maximal flow, particularly to the forefoot, to achieve healing.

Restoration of the foot pulse is a fundamental goal of revascularization in the diabetic foot. Specifically, autogenous vein grafting to the dorsalis pedis, distal posterior tibial, and plantar arteries incorporates our knowledge of the anatomic pattern of diabetic vascular disease and provides durable and effective limb salvage. The choice of outflow artery should be based on availability of conduit, the location of the foot ulcer, and the quality of the outflow vessel.

The dorsalis pedis bypass represents the single most important advance in our management plan for diabetic limb salvage[108,109] (Fig. 50-7). Fundamental to the success of the dorsalis pedis bypass are meticulous technique and its appropriate use. The principal indication for the pedal graft is when there is no other vessel that has continuity with the foot, particularly in cases with tissue loss. Dorsalis pedis bypass is unnecessary when a more proximal bypass will restore foot pulses and should not be done if there is an inadequate length of autogenous vein. In addition, if the dorsum of the foot is extensively infected and the peroneal artery is of good quality on the preoperative arteriogram, preference should be given to peroneal artery bypass.

Technical feasibility and short-term durability of dorsalis pedis arterial bypass have been demonstrated, with patency and limb salvage rates approaching 90% at 3 years.[110] A more extensive 8-year experience encompassing 384 vein grafts to the dorsalis pedis artery in 367 patients has been reported.[111] Ninety-five percent of the patients had diabetes mellitus, and all procedures were performed for limb-threatening ischemia. Twenty-nine grafts (7.5%) failed within the first 30 days, but 19 were successfully revised when a correctable technical problem was found at reoperation. The perioperative in-hospital mortality rate was 1.8%, and the actuarial primary and secondary patency rates were 68% and 82% at 5-year follow-up. Furthermore, the limb salvage rate was 87% at 5 years, again attesting to the durability of the dorsalis pedis graft.

The distal location of the dorsalis pedis artery theoretically necessitates a long venous conduit, which is often not attainable. However, by using the popliteal or distal superficial femoral artery as an inflow site, a shorter length of vein may be used, with excellent long-term patency.[112] This is particularly true in the diabetic patient, again due to the pattern of atherosclerotic disease. In the authors' institutional experience of 384 pedal bypasses over a 7-year period, 60% of grafts utilized the more distal inflow site, usually the popliteal artery. This avoids dissection in the groin and upper thigh, a common location for wound complications, and also obviates the need for foot extension of the vein harvest incision. The approach is flexible, in that the vein graft to the dorsalis pedis artery can be prepared as an *in situ*, reversed, or nonreversed vein graft, without any significant difference in outcome.[113] With the *in situ* or nonreversed graft, the valves may be lysed blindly or, preferably, cut under direct vision with an angioscope. This also

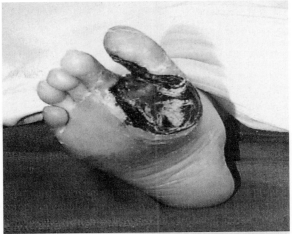

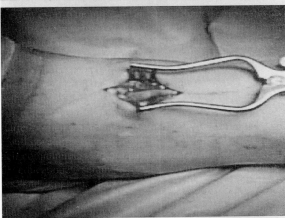

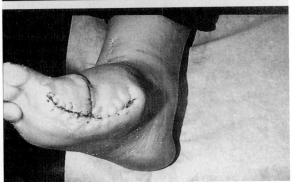

FIGURE 50-7. Temporal photographs illustrating the methodical use of the dorsalis pedis bypass for limb salvage. Evaluation for ischemia in a patient with gangrene (**top photo**) revealed extensive lower extremity arterial occlusive disease and a patent dorsalis pedis artery. A bypass to the dorsalis pedis was performed (**middle photo**). Once the foot was fully revascularized, a local amputation was performed, with resultant adequate healing and limb salvage (**bottom photo**).

allows for concomitant angioscopic assessment of the vein to detect any intraluminal abnormalities.[114]

Active infection in the foot is commonly encountered in the complicated ischemic diabetic foot. However, it is not a contraindication to dorsalis pedis bypass, as long as the infectious process is controlled and located remotely from the proposed incision. Adequate control implies resolution of cellulitis, lymphangitis, and

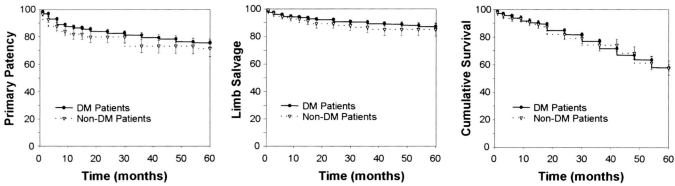

FIGURE 50-8. Vein graft patency, limb salvage, and survival rates for nearly 1000 patients at the authors' institution, all followed for 5 years or more. Note the virtually identical rates for patients with and without diabetes (**DM** and **NON-DM**). *(Reproduced from Akbari et al.[117])*

edema, especially in areas of proposed incisions required to expose the distal artery or saphenous vein. The results of 56 vein bypasses to the dorsal pedal artery in patients with ischemic foot lesions complicated by infection were recently reviewed.[115] This included 15 patients with severe gangrene, osteomyelitis, and/or deep space abscess. The average duration between admission and bypass was 10 days. Although there was a 12% wound infection rate, the primary graft patency was 92% at 36-month follow-up. This aggressive approach to revascularization in the ischemic and infected foot resulted in a limb salvage rate of 98% at the end of 3 years.

In the patient with an ischemic heel ulcer or gangrene, first consideration should be given to the posterior tibial or plantar arteries if they are patent by preoperative imaging. However, the absence of a patent posterior tibial artery is not a contraindication to arterial bypass and limb salvage. The role and efficacy of dorsalis pedis artery bypass in the treatment of ischemic heel lesions was recently examined in 96 patients who had undergone pedal bypass for heel ulceration.[116] Compared with a similar cohort of 336 patients with forefoot lesions undergoing dorsalis pedis bypass, there were no differences at 5 years with respect to primary patency, secondary patency, or limb salvage. More importantly, dorsalis pedis bypass accomplished complete healing in 87% (84/96) of heel lesions, with healing rates being independent of the presence or absence of an intact pedal arch, and it allowed for a limb salvage rate of almost 90% at 5 years.

Despite the technical success of lower extremity bypass in patients with diabetes, concerns continue about long-term patient function and survival. To evaluate the question of *late* graft patency, limb salvage, and survival among diabetic patients, a recent report reviewed the experience with lower extremity revascularization in a largely diabetic population of nearly 1000 patients followed for 5 years or longer.[117] A total of 962 vein grafts were performed on 843 patients, of which 83% (795 grafts) were in patients with diabetes. Minimum follow-up was 5 years and extended up to 9 years. The dorsalis pedis or plantar/tarsal arteries served as the outflow artery in 271 (35%) of the diabetic patients. Cumulative 5-year primary graft patency was 74.7% overall, with no difference among patients with and without diabetes (diabetic 75.6% versus nondiabetic 71.9%). The secondary graft patency rate was 76.2% for the entire cohort and was also similar between the diabetic and nondiabetic group (diabetic 77% versus nondiabetic 73.6%). Most importantly, 5-year limb salvage and survival rates were virtually identical in diabetic and nondiabetic patients. The overall limb salvage rate was 87.1% (diabetic 87.3% versus nondiabetic 85.4%).

Survival at 5 years was 58.1% in the entire cohort (diabetic 58.2% versus nondiabetic 58.0%). These data strongly emphasize that concern for *long-term* mortality, limb loss, and graft patency in diabetic patients is unnecessary and should not prevent the aggressive attempts at distal bypass required for limb salvage (Fig. 50-8).

Following successful revascularization, secondary procedures may be performed for both limb *and* foot salvage. Chronic ulcerations may be treated by ulcer excision, arthroplasty, or hemiphalangectomy. In the patient with extensive tissue loss, both local flaps and free flaps may be used. Due to the architecture of the diabetic foot, underlying bony structural abnormalities are often the cause of ulceration and may be corrected by metatarsal head resection or osteotomy. Heel ulcers may be treated by partial calcanectomy and local (e.g., flexor tendon) or even free flap coverage.

CONCLUSIONS

The patient with diabetes and peripheral vascular disease represents a uniquely complex pathophysiology involving microcirculatory and macrovascular disease. Because much of the disability

FIGURE 50-9. Beginning with the introduction of the pedal bypass in 1984, and concomitant with a rise in all distal lower extremity arterial reconstructions, there has been a significant drop in every category of amputations at the authors' institution. TMA, transmetatarsal amputation; BKA, below-knee amputation; AKA, above-knee amputation. *(Reproduced from LoGerfo et al.[108])*

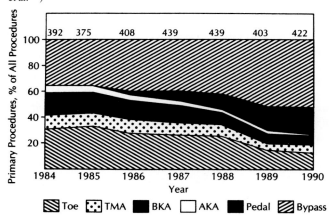

and morbidity of diabetes are directly caused by these vascular changes, an understanding of diabetic vascular disease is critical for reducing the overall morbidity and mortality of diabetes.

Knowledge of diabetic vascular disease should be incorporated into every aspect of the treatment plan. Taking a systematic and aggressive approach to diabetic foot disease has resulted in improved limb and foot salvage. As can be seen in Fig. 50-9, there has been a significant reduction in every category of lower limb amputation since 1984, with a concomitant increase in the number of patients undergoing arterial reconstruction and a greater application of the dorsalis pedis bypass graft. It is very likely, therefore, that further awareness of diabetic peripheral vascular disease can lead to a greater reduction in overall diabetic morbidity and mortality.

REFERENCES

1. American Diabetes Association: *Diabetes: 1993 Vital Statistics.* ADA: 1993.
2. Ruderman NB, Haudenschild C: Diabetes as an atherogenic factor. *Prog Cardiovasc Dis* 1984;26:373.
3. Stokes J, Kannel WB, Wolf PA, *et al*: The relative importance of selected risk factors for various manifestations of cardiovascular disease among men and women from 35 to 64 years old: 30 years of follow-up in the Framingham Study. *Circulation* 1987;75:65.
4. Burchfiel CM, Curb JD, Rodriguez BL, *et al*: Glucose intolerance and 22-year stroke incidence. The Honolulu Heart Program. *Stroke* 1994; 25:951.
5. Jorgensen H, Nakayama H, Raaschou HO, *et al*: Stroke in patients with diabetes. The Copenhagen Stroke Study. *Stroke* 1994;25:1977.
6. Yasaka M, Yamaguchi T, Shichiri M: Distribution of atherosclerosis and risk factors in atherothrombotic occlusion. *Stroke* 1993;24:206.
7. Akbari CM, LoGerfo FW: Diabetes and peripheral vascular disease. *J Vasc Surg* 1999;30:373.
8. Cameron NE, Cotter MA: The relationship of vascular changes to metabolic factors in diabetes mellitus and their role in the development of peripheral nerve complications. *Diabetes Metab Rev* 1994; 10:189.
9. LoGerfo FW, Coffman JD: Vascular and microvascular disease of the foot in diabetes. *N Engl J Med* 1984;311:1615.
10. Williamson JR, Titlon RG, Chang K, *et al*: Basement membrane abnormalities in diabetes mellitus: Relationship to clinical microangiopathy. *Diabetes Metab Rev* 1988;4:339.
11. LoGerfo FW: Vascular disease, matrix abnormalities, and neuropathy: Implications for limb salvage in diabetes mellitus. *J Vasc Surg* 1987; 5:793.
12. Palmberg P, Smith M, Waltman S, *et al*: The natural history of retinopathy in insulin-dependent juvenile-onset diabetes. *Ophthalmology* 1981;88:613.
13. Pirart J: Diabetes mellitus and its degenerative complications: A prospective study of 4400 patients observed between 1947 and 1973. *Diabetes Care* 1978;1:168.
14. DCCT Research Group: The effect of intensive treatment of diabetes on the development and progression of long-term complications in insulin-dependent diabetes mellitus. *N Engl J Med* 1993;329:977.
15. Vanhoutte PM: The endothelium—modulator of vascular smooth-muscle tone. *N Engl J Med* 1988;319:512.
16. Cohen RA: Dysfunction of vascular endothelium in diabetes mellitus. *Circulation* 1993;87:V 67.
17. Goldenberg SG, Alex M. Joshi RA, *et al*: Nonatheromatous peripheral vascular disease of the lower extremity in diabetes mellitus. *Diabetes* 1959;8:261.
18. Strandness DE Jr, Priest RE, Gibbons GE: Combined clinical and pathologic study of diabetic and nondiabetic peripheral arterial disease. *Diabetes* 1964;13:366.
19. Conrad MC: Large and small artery occlusion in diabetics and nondiabetics with severe vascular disease. *Circulation* 1967;36:83.
20. Barner HB, Kaiser GC, Willman VL: Blood flow in the diabetic leg. *Circulation* 1971;43:391.
21. Parving HH, Viberti GC, Keen H, *et al*: Hemodynamic factors in the genesis of diabetic microangiopathy. *Metabolism* 1983;32:943.
22. Morgensen CE, Schmitz A, Christensen CR: Comparative renal pathophysiology relevant to IDDM and NIDDM patients. *Diabetes Metab Rev* 1988;4:453.
23. Flynn MD, Tooke JE: Aetiology of diabetic foot ulceration: A role for the microcirculation? *Diabet Med* 1992;8:320.
24. Rayman G, Williams SA, Spencer PD, *et al*: Impaired microvascular hyperaemic response to minor skin trauma in Type I diabetes. *BMJ* 1986;292:1295.
25. Jorneskog G, Brismar K, Fagrell B: Skin capillary circulation severely impaired in toes of patients with IDDM, with and without late diabetic complications. *Diabetologia* 1995;38:474.
26. Parkhouse N, LeQueen PM: Impaired neurogenic vascular response in patients with diabetes and neuropathic foot lesions. *N Engl J Med* 1988;318:1306.
27. Yokoyama I, Ohtake T, Momomure S, *et al*: Hyperglycemia rather than insulin resistance is related to reduced coronary flow reserve in NIDDM. *Diabetes* 1998;47:119.
28. Pitkanen OP, Nuutila P, Raitakari OT, *et al*: Coronary flow reserve is reduced in young men with IDDM. *Diabetes* 1998;47:248.
29. Fulesdi B, Limburg M, Bereczki D, *et al*: Impairment of cerebrovascular reactivity in long-term type I diabetes. *Diabetes* 1997;46: 1840.
30. Gupta S, Sussman I, McArthur CS, *et al*: Endothelium-dependent inhibition of Na+ − K+ ATPase activity in rabbit aorta by hyperglycemia. Possible role of endothelium-derived nitric oxide. *J Clin Invest* 1992;90:727.
31. Pieper GM, Meier DA, Hager SR: Endothelial dysfunction in a model of hyperglycemia and hyperinsulinemia. *Am J Physiol* 1995;269: H845.
32. Tesfamarian B, Brown ML, Cohen RA: Elevated glucose impairs endothelium-dependent relaxation by activating protein kinase C. *J Clin Invest* 1991;87:1643.
33. Williams SB, Cusco JA, Roddy M, *et al*: Impaired nitric oxide-mediated vasodilation in patients with non-insulin-dependent diabetes mellitus. *J Am Coll Cardiol* 1996;27:567.
34. Johnstone MT, Creager SJ, Scales KM, *et al*: Impaired endothelium-dependent vasodilation in patients with insulin-dependent diabetes mellitus. *Circulation* 1993;88:2510.
35. Tesfamarian B, Brown ML, Deykin D, *et al*: Elevated glucose promotes generation of endothelium-derived vasoconstrictor prostanoids in rabbit aorta. *J Clin Invest* 1990;85:929.
36. Simmons DA, Winegrad AI: Elevated extracellular glucose inhibits adenosine-Na+ − K+ ATPase regulatory system in rabbit aortic wall. *Diabetologia* 1991;34:157.
37. Brownlee M, Cerami A, Vlassare H: Advanced glycosylation end products in tissue and the biochemical basis of diabetic complications. *N Engl J Med* 1988;318:1315.
38. Furchgott RF, Zawadzki JV: The obligatory role of endothelial cells in the relaxation of arterial smooth muscle by acetylcholine. *Nature* 1980; 288:373.
39. Palmer RM, Ferrige AG, Moncada S: Nitric oxide release accounts for the biologic activity of endothelium-derived relaxing factor. *Nature* 1987;327:524.
40. Scherrer U, Randin D, Vollenweider P, *et al*: Nitric oxide release accounts for insulin's vascular effects in humans. *J Clin Invest* 1994; 94:2511.
41. Taddei S, Virdis A, Mattei P, *et al*: Effect of insulin on acetylcholine-induced vasodilation in normotensive subjects and patients with essential hypertension. *Circulation* 1995;92:2911.
42. Akbari CM, Saouaf R, Barnhill DF, *et al*: Endothelium-dependent vasodilatation is impaired in both microcirculation and macrocirculation during acute hyperglycemia. *J Vasc Surg* 1998;28:687.
43. Baron AD: The coupling of glucose metabolism and perfusion in human skeletal muscle. The potential role of endothelium-derived nitric oxide. *Diabetes* 1996;45:S105.
44. Oberly LW: Free radicals in diabetes. *Free Radic Biol Med* 1988; 5:113.
45. Wolff SP, Dean RT: Glucose autoxidation and protein modification: The role of oxidative glycosylation in diabetes. *Biochem J* 1987;245:234.
46. Gryglewski RJ, Palmer RM, Moncada S: Superoxide anion is involved in the breakdown of endothelium-derived vascular relaxing factor. *Nature* 1986;320:454.

47. Diederich D, Skopec J, Diederich A, et al: Endothelial dysfunction in mesenteric resistance arteries of diabetic rats: Role of free radicals. Am J Physiol 1994;266:H1153.
48. Keegan A, Walbank H, Cotter MA, et al: Chronic vitamin E treatment prevents defective endothelium-dependent relaxation in diabetic rat aorta. Diabetologia 1995;38:1475.
49. Timimi FK, Ting HH, Haley EA, et al: Vitamin C improves endothelium-dependent vasodilation in patients with insulin-dependent diabetes mellitus. J Am Coll Cardiol 1998;31:552.
50. Witzum JL: The oxidation hypothesis of atherosclerosis. Lancet 1994;344:793.
51. Ohara Y, Peterson TE, Harrison DG: Hypercholesterolemia increases endothelial superoxide anion production. J Clin Invest 1993;91:2546.
52. Clarkson P, Celermajer DS, Donald AE, et al: Impaired vascular reactivity in insulin-dependent diabetes mellitus is related to disease duration and low density lipoprotein cholesterol levels. J Am Coll Cardiol 1996;28:573.
53. Bucala R, Tracey KJ, Cerami A: Advanced glycosylation end products quench nitric oxide and mediate defective endothelium-dependent vasodilatation in experimental diabetes. J Clin Invest 1991;87:432.
54. Wautier JL, Zoukourian C, Chappey O: Receptor-mediated endothelial cell dysfunction in diabetic vasculopathy. Soluble receptor for advanced glycation end products blocks hyperpermeability in diabetic rats. J Clin Invest 1996;97:238.
55. Schmidt AM, Hori O, Brett J, et al: Cellular receptors for advanced glycation end products. Implications for induction of oxidant stress and cellular dysfunction in the pathogenesis of vascular lesions. Arterioscler Thromb 1994;14:1521.
56. Makita Z, Radoff S, Rayfield EJ: Advanced glycosylation end products in patients with diabetic nephropathy. N Engl J Med 1991;325:836.
57. Joannides R, Haefeli WE, Linder L, et al: Nitric oxide is responsible for flow-dependent dilatation of human peripheral conduit arteries in vivo. Circulation 1995;91:1314.
58. Simmons DA, Winegrad AI: Mechanism of glucose-induced Na+ − K+ ATPase inhibition in aortic wall of rabbits. Diabetologia 1989;32:402.
59. Stevens MJ, Dananberg J, Feldman EL, et al: The linked roles of nitric oxide, aldose reductase and Na+ − K+ ATPase in the slowing of nerve conduction in the streptozotocin diabetic rat. J Clin Invest 1994;94:853.
60. Veves A, Akbari CM, Donaghue VM, et al: The effect of diabetes, neuropathy, Charcot arthropathy, and arterial disease on the foot microcirculation. Diabetologia 1996;39(suppl 1):A3.
61. Veves A, Akbari CM, Primavera J, et al: Endothelial dysfunction and the expression of endothelial nitric oxide synthetase in diabetic neuropathy, vascular disease, and foot ulceration. Diabetes 1997;47:457.
62. Stevens MJ, Feldman EL, Greene DA: The aetiology of diabetic neuropathy: The combined roles of metabolic and vascular defects. Diabet Med 1995;12:566.
63. Tuck RR, Schmelzer JD, Low PA: Endoneurial blood flow and oxygen tension in the sciatic nerves of rats with experimental diabetic neuropathy. Brain 1984;107:935.
64. Tesfaye S, Harris N, Jakubowski JJ, et al: Impaired blood flow and arterio-venous shunting in human diabetic neuropathy: A novel technique of nerve photography and fluorescein angiography. Diabetologia 1993;36:1266.
65. Tesfaye S, Harris N, Jakubowski JJ, et al: Impaired blood flow and arterio-venous shunting in human diabetic neuropathy: A novel technique of nerve photography and fluorescein angiography. Diabetologia 1993;36:1266.
66. Ram Z, Sadeh M, Walden R, et al: Vascular insufficiency quantitatively aggravates diabetic neuropathy. Arch Neurol 1991;48:1239.
67. Akbari CM, Gibbons GW, Habershaw GM, et al: The effect of arterial reconstruction on the natural history of diabetic neuropathy. Arch Surg 1997;132:148.
68. Akbari CM, LoGerfo FW: The micro- and macrocirculation in diabetes mellitus. In: Veves A, ed. A Clinical Approach to Diabetic Neuropathy, 1st ed. Humana:1998;319.
69. Mortel KP, Meyer JS, Sims PA, et al: Diabetes mellitus as a risk factor for stroke. South Med J 1990;83:904.
70. Tuomilehto J, Rastenyte D, Jousilahti P, et al: Diabetes mellitus as a risk factor for death from stroke: Prospective study of the middle-aged Finnish population. Stroke 1996;27:210.
71. Petitti DB, Bhatt H: Retinopathy as a risk factor for nonembolic stroke in diabetic patients. Stroke 1995;26:593.
72. Toyry JP, Niskanen LK, Lansimies EA, et al: Autonomic neuropathy predicts the development of stroke in patients with non-insulin-dependent diabetes mellitus. Stroke 1996;27:1316.
73. Kushner M, Nencini P, Reivich M, et al: Relation of hyperglycemia early in ischemic brain infarction to cerebral anatomy, metabolism, and clinical outcome. Ann Neurol 1990;28:129.
74. Pulsinelli WA, Levy DE, Sigsbee B, et al: Increased damage after ischemic stroke in patients with hyperglycemia with or without established diabetes mellitus. Am J Med 1983;74:540.
75. Lehto S, Ronnemaa T, Pyorala K, et al: Predictors of stroke in middle-aged patients with non-insulin dependent diabetes. Stroke 1996;27: 63.
76. Lee KY, Sohn YH, Baik JS, et al: Arterial pulsatility as an index of cerebral microangiopathy in diabetes. Stroke 2000;31:1111.
77. Quirce R, Carril JM, Jimenez-Bonilla JF, et al: Semi-quantitative assessment of cerebral blood flow with 99m Tc-HMPAO SPET in type I diabetic patients with no clinical history of cerebrovascular disease. Eur J Nucl Med 1997;24:1507.
78. Duckrow RB, Beard DC, Brennan RW: Regional cerebral blood flow decreases during chronic and acute hyperglycemia. Stroke 1987;18:52.
79. Cipolla MJ, Porter JM, Osol G: High glucose concentrations dilate cerebral arteries and diminish myogenic tone through an endothelial mechanism. Stroke 1997;28:405.
80. Mayhan WG, Simmons LK, Sharpe GM: Mechanism of impaired responses of cerebral arterioles during diabetes mellitus. Am J Physiol 1991;260:H319.
81. Fujii K, Heistad DD, Faraci FM: Effect of diabetes mellitus on flow-mediated and endothelium-dependent dilatation of the basilar artery. Stroke 1992;23:1494.
82. Harati Y: Diabetes and the nervous system. Endocrinol Metab Clin North Am 1996;25:325.
83. Zimmerman GA, Meistrell M, III, Bloom O, et al: Neurotoxicity of advanced glycation endproducts during focal stroke and neuroprotective effects of aminoguanidine. Proc Natl Acad Sci USA 1995;92:3744.
84. North American Symptomatic Carotid Endarterectomy Trial Collaborators: Beneficial effect of carotid endarterectomy in symptomatic patients with high-grade carotid stenosis. N Engl J Med 1991;325:445.
85. Executive Committee for the Asymptomatic Carotid Atherosclerosis Study: Endarterectomy for asymptomatic carotid artery stenosis. JAMA 1995;273:1421.
86. Salenius JP, Harju E, Riekkinen H: Early cerebral complications in carotid endarterectomy: Risk factors. J Cardiovasc Surg 1990:31:162.
87. Akbari CM, Pomposelli FB Jr, Gibbons GW, et al: Diabetes mellitus: A risk factor for carotid endarterectomy? J Vasc Surg 1997;25:1070.
88. Grunfeld C: Diabetic foot ulcers: Etiology, treatment, and prevention. Adv Intern Med 1991;37:103.
89. Nathan DM: Long-term complications of diabetes mellitus. N Engl J Med 1993;328:1676.
90. Reiber GE, Boyko EJ, Smith DG: Lower extremity foot ulcers and amputations in diabetes. In: National Diabetes Data Group, ed. Diabetes in America, 2nd ed. National Institutes of Health:1995;409.
91. The DCCT Research Group: Factors in the development of diabetic neuropathy: Baseline analysis of neuropathy in the feasibility phase of the Diabetes Control and Complications Trial (DCCT). Diabetes 1988;37:476.
92. Dyck PJ, Kratz KM, Karnes JL, et al: The prevalence by staged severity of various types of diabetic neuropathy, retinopathy, and nephropathy in a population-based cohort: The Rochester Diabetic Neuropathy Study. Neurology 1993;43:817.
93. Caputo GM, Cavanagh PR, Ulbrecht JS, et al: Assessment and management of foot disease in patients with diabetes. N Engl J Med 1994;331:954.
94. Young MJ, Veves A, Boulton AJM: The diabetic foot: Aetiopathogenesis and management. Diabetes Metab Rev 1993;9:109.
95. Mills JL, Beckett WC, Taylor SM: The diabetic foot: Consequences of delayed treatment and referral. South Med J 1991;84:970.
96. Newman LG, Waller J, Palestro CJ, et al: Unsuspected osteomyelitis in diabetic foot ulcers: Diagnosis and monitoring by leukocyte scanning with indium In 111 oxyquinolone. JAMA 1991;266:1246.
97. Grayson ML, Gibbons GW, Balogh K, et al: Probing to bone in infected pedal ulcers: A clinical sign of underlying osteomyelitis in diabetic patients. JAMA 1995;273:721.

98. Akbari CM, Pomposelli FB Jr: The diabetic foot. In: Perler B, Becker G, eds. *A Clinical Approach To Vascular Intervention*, 1st ed. Thieme: 1998;211.

99. Brand FN, Abbott RD, Kannel WB: Diabetes, intermittent claudication, and risk of cardiovascular events. The Framingham Study. *Diabetes* 1989;38:504.

100. Dormandy J, Heeck L, Vig S: Predicting which patients will develop chronic critical leg ischemia. *Semin Vasc Surg* 1999;12:138.

101. Menzoian JO, LaMorte WW, Paniszyn CC, *et al*: Symptomatology and anatomic patterns of peripheral vascular disease: Differing impact of smoking and diabetes. *Ann Vasc Surg* 1989;3:224.

102. Young MJ, Adams JE, Anderson GF, *et al*: Medial arterial calcification in the feet of diabetic patients and matched non-diabetic control subjects. *Diabetologia* 1993;36:615.

103. Ballard JL, Eke CC, Bunt TJ, *et al*: A prospective evaluation of transcutaneous oxygen measurements in the management of diabetic foot problems. *J Vasc Surg* 1995;22:485.

104. Wyss CR, Matsen FA III, Simmons CW, *et al*: Transcutaneous oxygen tension measurements on limbs of diabetic and nondiabetic patients with peripheral vascular disease. *Surgery* 1984;95:339.

105. Parfrey PS, Griffiths SM, Barrett BJ, *et al*: Contrast material-induced renal failure in patients with diabetes mellitus, renal insufficiency, or both. A prospective controlled study. *N Engl J Med* 1989;321: 395.

106. Schwab SJ, Hlatky MA, Pieper KS, *et al*: Contrast nephrotoxicity: A randomized controlled trial of a nonionic and ionic contrast agent. *N Engl J Med* 1989;320:149.

107. Plecha EJ, Seabrook GR, Bandyk DF, *et al*: Determinants of successful peroneal artery bypass. *J Vasc Surg* 1993;17:97.

108. LoGerfo FW, Gibbons GW, Pomposelli FB Jr, *et al*: Trends in the care of the diabetic foot: Expanded role of arterial reconstruction. *Arch Surg* 1992;127:617.

109. Akbari CM, LoGerfo FW: Distal bypasses in the diabetic patient. In: Yao JST, Pearce WH, eds. *Vascular Surgery—Year 2000*. Appleton & Lange (in press).

110. Pomposelli FB Jr, Jepsen SJ, Gibbons GW, *et al*: Efficacy of the dorsal pedis bypass for limb salvage in diabetic patients: Short-term observation. *J Vasc Surg* 1990;11:745.

111. Pomposelli FB Jr, Marcaccio EJ, Gibbons GW, *et al*: Dorsalis pedis arterial bypass: Durable limb salvage for foot ischemia in patients with diabetes mellitus. *J Vasc Surg* 1995;21:375.

112. Veith FJ, Gupta SK, Samson RH, *et al*: Superficial femoral and popliteal arteries as inflow sites for distal bypasses. *Surgery* 1981;90:980.

113. Pomposelli FB Jr, Jepsen SJ, Gibbons GW, *et al*: A flexible approach to infrapopliteal vein grafts in patients with diabetes mellitus. *Arch Surg* 1991;126:724.

114. Akbari CM, LoGerfo FW: Saphenous vein bypass to pedal arteries in diabetic patients. In: Yao JST, Pearce WH, eds. *Techniques in Vascular and Endovascular Surgery*. Appleton & Lange:1998;227.

115. Tannenbaum GA, Pomposelli FB Jr, Marcaccio EJ, *et al*: Safety of vein bypass grafting to the dorsal pedal artery in diabetic patients with foot infections. *J Vasc Surg* 1992;15:982.

116. Berceli SA, Chan AK, Pomposelli FB Jr, *et al*: Efficacy of dorsal pedal artery bypass in limb salvage for ischemic heel ulcers. *J Vasc Surg* 1999,30:499.

117. Akbari CM, Pomposelli FB Jr, Gibbons GW, *et al*: Lower extremity revascularization in diabetes: Late observations. *Arch Surg* 2000; 135:452.

The Diabetic Foot

William C. Coleman

INTRODUCTION

The history of caring for the feet of persons with diabetes is fraught with frustration for medical professionals, family members, and patients. During the last decade of the twentieth century there has been a continuing refinement of interventional techniques to improve vascular flow to the lower extremities of persons with diabetes. New topical medications and dressings have been introduced to improve the management of foot wounds in diabetic patients. Despite these advances, during this same period of time, there has been a disappointing 22% increase in the total number of amputations performed on this diabetic population.

During the 1980s more than 55,000 diabetic foot amputations were performed annually in the United States.[1] In 1991, the U.S. Department of Health and Human Services set several goals it wanted to achieve by the year 2000. One of these goals was to lower the annual number of amputations of the feet of diabetics by 40%.[2] By the end of the 1990s the annual number of lower extremity amputations in the diabetic population had risen to over 67,000.[3]

In the United States, the majority of these amputations have been done on patients who receive Medicare benefits. Wrobel and colleagues found that diabetes-related amputations were 53% of all amputations within the Medicare population in 1996 and 1997.[4] There were 44,599 major amputations in the Medicare diabetic population, or 3.69 amputations per 1000 patients with diabetes, versus 0.39 amputations per 1000 patients among the nondiabetic patients. The highest rates of amputation among persons with diabetes on Medicare were in California, Texas, New Mexico, and the upper Midwest and mid-Atlantic states.

The answers to reducing the majority of these amputations have been emerging over the past 20 years. Successful amputation prevention practices have been repeatedly confirmed by several studies over the past two decades. At Grady Memorial Hospital from 1972–1974, the amputation rate dropped 50%.[5] The amputation rate declined 44% at Kings College Hospital in London in 2 years.[6] In Memphis, a 68% reduction was achieved in 2 years.[7] Assal applied his principles to the clinical practices of the University Hospital of Geneva, and the rate of below-the-knee amputations dropped 85% in 4 years.[8] The first randomized, blinded, prospective controlled trial was reported by Litzelman and colleagues.[9] Their experimental group was 0.41 as likely to develop serious foot lesions as the control group.

In Spain, 318 diabetic patients with neuropathy were followed by Calle-Pascual and associates for 3–6 years for their compliance with participation in an education and foot monitoring program.[10] The program entailed an extensive educational program, changing from inadequate to more adequate foot care behavior within the first 6 months, regular visits to a routine foot care specialist, at least one foot review every 6 months, and an annual diabetic treatment review. One group (223 patients) complied with all aspects of the continuing program and a second group (95 patients) did not. Seven ulcers developed on six patients in the first group and 30 ulcers appeared on 26 patients of the second group. The second group had 19 lower extremity amputations (LEAs) and the first group had one LEA. The compliant group had a 13 times lower risk of experiencing a first foot ulcer than the less compliant group.

Often, when clinicians hear of the results of these studies, they will develop seminar programs for professionals and patients in their communities. Unfortunately, even with the best intentions, small educational seminars, focus groups of physicians and nurses, and programs that do not target specific professional behavioral changes have failed to improve the morbidity statistics for diabetic foot pathology.[11] As in the case of the goals set by the Department of Health and Human Services in the United States, around the world national programs were developed to decrease amputation rates among diabetic populations throughout the last decade of the twentieth century. All of these large-scale, national initiatives failed to demonstrably decrease national amputation rates.

There are several examples of small-scale, single-institution success. Each of these came as the result of multidisciplinary foot care teams directed by a knowledgeable, influential leader. In all of these studies foot specialists, and/or specialized education techniques on foot care, were incorporated into multidisciplinary programs. In all of them, regular preventive visits were scheduled to help the patients monitor their feet and to reinforce the need for constant protective behavior.

As cited above, the program that has produced the most effective reduction of amputations published to date (85%) was headed by Assal at the University of Geneva. Assal contends that this problem persists because medical education poorly prepares the professional for the management of chronic diseases. The professional education is focused on the diagnosis of the disease followed by the treatment. But the educational process does not prepare the physician for the psychological and sociological problems that emerge when patients have to be constantly active in the management of a lifelong disease. In these chronic diseases a more holistic approach is warranted.[12]

Vasculopathy and Neuropathy

When a medical professional thinks of the spectrum of diabetic foot problems, two major contributing factors come to mind. These are peripheral neuropathy and peripheral vascular disease. In the context of foot management, it is the neuropathy that increases the likelihood that the person will develop a serious foot wound. Peripheral vascular disease rarely increases the chance of injury occurring, but an injury to a limb with severe arterial occlusive disease increases the possibility of limb loss.[13] A moderate vascular impairment may be present without symptoms and may be compatible with the natural life expectancy for the limb. More severe disease may be capable of maintaining the tissues as long as no significant injury occurs. If an ingrown toenail or ulcer then occurs, and remains untreated because of a lack of pain sensation, the infection may spread throughout the foot, creating a gross infection that demands more blood supply than the impaired vessels can provide. The resulting gangrene may demand an amputation. The hospital records may show the cause as diabetic gangrene or vascular insufficiency, and may thus fail to correctly identify the neuropathy that allowed the process to continue undetected by the patient, until it was too late to salvage the limb.

At the center of the success of the programs that are able to achieve significant reductions in their numbers of lower extremity amputations is their ability to manage the ramifications of lower extremity sensory loss.

INJURY PREVENTION

During a meeting of the National Diabetes Advisory Board in 1980, a group of experts was asked to make recommendations that would result in better foot care and prevention of amputation. Those who expected advice on modern medications or vascular surgery were surprised when the first recommendation was for a national campaign to advise doctors to take off the patient's shoes.[14] It was determined that the primary problem was that patients did not complain to their doctors or report the early stages of their foot disability because they had no pain. Therefore, doctors must take the initiative and look for early lesions. Physicians are 3–4 times more likely to examine a patient's feet if the shoes and socks are removed before the doctor enters the examination room.[15]

This aspect is mentioned first because many physicians overlook this simple maneuver. It may seem incredible that a person would walk on a foot and fail to note that it was swollen and infected or that it had an open ulcer on the sole. However, when sensation is lost, individuals commonly lose a sense of identity with their insensitive parts, and thus fail to note obvious problems. An insensitive limb feels like a wooden block fastened to the body and is treated as such. In a sense, such action may be a deep rejection of a "dead" body part.

As the result of following 51 of their regular diabetic foot clinic patients, Mantey and associates found that foot ulcers most frequently recurred in patients with the poorest glycemic control and the most profound distal neuropathy.[16] They also found that those with recurrent ulceration tended to delay reporting early signs and symptoms of the new injury.

Every health professional who wants to help these people needs to know this and to help the person understand the consequences of this neglect. If the patients recognize the danger, they will be able to readjust their mindsets to compensate for this lack of feeling. They can be helped to give very special conscious care to make up for the potential for subconscious neglect. Only with understanding and education will they obey rules of foot care which otherwise might be regarded as unnecessary and unimportant. One session is not enough. Patients need to have their foot consciousness reinforced frequently and in diverse ways, especially if they are thought to have slipped into neglect. Such education and reinforcement must be done with sympathy, understanding, and good humor if it is to succeed. The patient is quick to detect an impatient, angry, or intolerant attitude from the health care professional, and this will only lower the patient's self-image, and may lead to concealment of the problem foot next at the next medical checkup.

Soon after a person has been told that they have diabetes and become aware that it will be with them for the rest of their life, they go through stages of acceptance similar to the psychological adjustment we experience after the death of a close acquaintance.[12] These may include denial, revolt, bargaining, depression, and/or acceptance. The rate at which an individual passes through these stages varies. When the patient is diagnosed with subsequent peripheral neuropathy and learns of the lifestyle changes necessary to successfully protect the feet, in most cases a second period of psychological adjustment is needed. To compound the problem of foot care, very few persons with diabetes lose all of the feeling in their feet. The medical team and family members are faced with the task of effectively achieving compliance with needed lifestyle changes to protect the feet while patients still have some sensation in their feet. Physicians must be aware that these psychological and physical factors can be present and may interfere with successful foot care management.

PROTECTIVE SENSATION

The threshold of sensation that protects a normal foot strikes a very delicate balance. The purpose of pain sensation is not to cause pain, but to allow the body to act to minimize damage. A person who has lost some pain sensation has not lost the ability to feel pain; he or she feels it at a higher level of stress. It takes more pressure, higher temperatures, and more prolonged ischemia before the residual peripheral nerves are activated.

Peripheral, symmetrical, lower extremity sensorimotor polyneuropathy affects approximately 50% of all persons who have had diabetes more than 15 years.[17] It does not take total sensory loss for trophic ulcers to develop in persons with diabetes. Gross testing for pinprick or for touch may reveal remnants of sensation. Therefore, one should not be surprised if breakdown occurs. The problem is that a foot may be vulnerable to damage long before gross sensory loss is noted. The physician or therapist must identify the degree of sensory loss that puts a person at risk. This involves a quantitative test of sensation, which should be repeated at least annually for every person with diabetes. Because sensory mapping is time consuming, we have tried to identify the simplest and fastest test that will discern feet that need protection and that will identify the areas of the foot that are most at risk.

The sensory test used in many specialist clinics is based on the principle of von Frey.[18] He used horse hair of various thicknesses and lengths, and noted that the force needed to bend a given hair was the same every time. This principle could be used to quantify sensibility. Semmes and Weinstein[19] used the same principle with a series of monofilament nylon fibers of varied diameters. These were calibrated to bend when different forces were applied to the ends of the fibers.

In 1986, Birke and Sims published a study of insensitive feet, using selected fibers from the Semmes-Weinstein series.[20] They demonstrated that patients who could feel the filament that bent under a 10-g force (designated 5.07 on the Semmes-Weinstein scale) were unlikely to suffer damage and ulceration to their feet under normal walking conditions. Patients who could not feel that fiber were the ones who had problems. This was a retrospective study, but the 10-g fiber has since been used prospectively to identify patients who need special care and education, as well as special care in choice of shoes. They have found it to be a reliable index of vulnerability. This group now recommends the use of just three fibers for the testing of diabetic feet. These are: (1) the 1-g fiber (Semmes-Weinstein rating of 4.17), which can be felt by normal feet and which identifies the early onset of sensory neuropathy at a stage when special care may not be necessary; (2) the 10-g (5.07 rating) fiber, to identify the areas that need to be protected; and (3) a third fiber (75g), to identify areas that have lost all protective sensation (6.10 rating). Clearly, the 10-g fiber is the important one. Busy diabetic clinics may benefit from frequent tests with one fiber, rather than less frequent full mapping of sensation.

RISK CATEGORIZATION

With the use of a quantifiable test for protective sensation, the clinician can then begin to identify patients most likely to develop neuropathic injury. Several studies have been conducted during the last decade to identify factors that add to the morbidity of the diabetic foot.

In a prospective study of 749 patients, Boyko and coworkers found diabetic foot ulcers develop as the result of multiple factors.[21] These factors included neuropathy, diminished vascular perfusion, foot deformity, higher pressures under the foot, severity of diabetes, and comorbid complications from diabetes. In a study of 225 subjects, Lavery and associates[22] found that persons with diabetes and neuropathy were 1.7 times more likely to develop foot ulceration. If the person also has foot deformity (limited great toe motion, bunion, or toe deformity), the patient is 12.1 times more likely to experience a foot ulcer. If they have an amputation of the lower extremity, their risk of ulceration on the opposite limb increases to 36.4 times normal.

By being aware of these data, the clinician can begin to categorize patients according to their risk of developing foot injury.

Category 0

This category includes all persons diagnosed as having diabetes. These patients need to be monitored periodically for glycemic control and the development of pathology related to their diabetes. These people also need to be made aware of the relationship between glycemic control and the emergence of comorbid consequences. They need to be educated about the signs detailed in previous chapters that indicate that damage to the vasculature or nerves is occurring. This is a good time to begin counseling the person on the need for properly fitting, conservative footwear. These patients should be evaluated each year for signs of lower extremity neuropathy or arterial occlusive disease.

Category 1

A person is placed in this category when they have been identified as having peripheral neuropathy, either by failing to feel the Semmes-Weinstein 10-g monofilament, or because of excessively dry skin. Dryness of the skin is a good indicator of autonomic nerve loss. The authors have found that feet that can sweat normally rarely become ulcerated. This does not mean that it is the loss of the autonomic fibers that makes the foot vulnerable. It suggests that a significant loss of touch sensation occurs at about the same time as the loss of sweating.

These persons are at much higher risk of pedal injury. They need to be educated on the need for daily visual foot inspection. They must be made aware that they can no longer trust the feelings in their feet as an indication of the presence or severity of a wound. They must contact their physician or other medical staff member as soon as possible for assistance with the care of the wound. Their prior experience has not prepared them for managing wounds in the presence of neuropathy.

If at all possible, persons in this category must have a competent professional ensure that all of their shoes fit properly. Tapered-toe shoes, pumps, and other footwear that excessively stress the toes pose a risk to the foot. Toenails and calluses should be maintained by a trained medical professional. These patients should have their feet medically evaluated at least every 6 months.

Category 2

Persons in this category not only have diabetes and neuropathy, but they also have a foot deformity. The deformity may be very subtle, such as a limited subtalar joint range of motion, or very obvious, as in the case of a large bunion deformity. The lesser toes commonly curl into clawed-toe deformity on diabetic patients with neuropathy. Any bony prominence, significant lack of joint motion, or gross malalignment of the foot qualifies as deformity.

The presence of elevated blood glucose results in the glycosylation of many tissues in the body. Zilberberg found a higher density of nonenzymatic, cross-linked pentosidine in the plantar skin of amputated diabetic feet as compared to similar skin from nondiabetic controls.[23] The skin of the feet of persons with diabetes was less flexible. Nonenzymatic glycosylation has been found to affect ligaments, resulting in restricted motion of several joints. This was first noted in the hands, but later was also demonstrated in the subtalar, ankle, and first metatarsal-phalangeal joint. Birke and coworkers found a correlation between first metatarsal-phalangeal motion and a history of ulcers of the first metatarsal head.[24] When a person has limited subtalar range of motion along with neuropathy, significantly higher plantar pressures are found.[25]

Surgical correction of the deformity may be indicated. The presence of neuropathy obviates symptoms as a indication or contraindication for surgery.

Strict adherence to the use of proper footwear at all times is essential for patients in this category. Often, custom footwear or shoe inserts are needed to lower the risk of injury. These patients should see a foot specialist every 3 months for nail and callus care. This professional must examine the foot for changes in shape or mobility, review the patient's footwear, and emphasize the need to report any findings from the patient's self-foot examinations, as well as the need to treat any lesion found as soon as possible.

Category 3

Neuropathic feet most likely to ulcerate have been ulcerated before or have had significant morphologic changes to the foot as the result of Charcot's arthropathy. This places these patients at the highest risk of developing a neuropathic foot wound. Everyone in this category must wear prescription footwear to lower weight-bearing stress at the previous site of ulcer or Charcot's deformity. This footwear must be worn at all times. The clinician must ensure that the patient is aware that barefoot walking, as well as walking in stocking feet, slippers, and nonprescribed footwear, poses a threat to the foot. Every step must be protected. Even the nightly walks for nocturia must be protected by footwear.

These persons should visit the foot clinic every 2 months, and in extreme cases every month. In addition to all of the treatments mentioned in the previous categories, their footwear needs to be examined at every visit for proper fit and function.

IMPACT OF AUTONOMIC NEUROPATHY

Autonomic neuropathy can result in anhidrosis of the pedal skin. In the normal foot, the superficial layer of the skin is kept constantly hydrated by sweat. In the hydrated condition, the keratin of the skin is soft and pliable. If a flake of thickened callus is shaved off a foot and moistened, it can be rolled up like a piece of rubber, or it can be stretched and will spring back to shape. If the same flake of keratinized skin is then allowed to dry in the sun, it becomes hard and brittle and loses all ability to stretch. The same change occurs in the keratin layer *in situ* on the foot in the absence of sweating. When such skin is subject to flexion and extension as occurs at the joint creases of the toes and at the curve of the edge of the sole, the keratin cracks. Early in their development such cracks are limited to the stratum corneum layer of the epidermis, but they do allow a superficial inflammation to develop. This can eventually result in a chronic dermatitis in the lower third of the leg (Fig. 51-1). In the sole, the cracks become inflamed and stimulate build-up of more callus along both margins of the crack. The thickened plates of hard callus allow no flexion or stretch, and thus concentrate and localize all movement to the keratin-free cracks. This makes the condition worsen, until deeper layers of the epidermis become inflamed or even torn open where the crack makes them vulnerable. The final result is often an open ulcer and deep infection.

If keratin cracks have already occurred, they are treated by: (1) paring down the callused edges of keratin buildup, (2) painting the crack with gentian violet to dry the base, and (3) providing some measure of splinting to minimize the movement of the keratin plates. This may be done by splinting an affected toe by making the shoe sole rigid, or by wearing a molded insole that turns up around the edge of the sole or heel. It is also helpful to use an insole that has been molded to the foot. It should offer support up around the edges of the sole and heel where cracks commonly occur (so called "pinch calluses"). These are found wherever the skin is pinched in the unsupported angle between the supported sole and the side-wall of the shoe.

CALLUSES

When subjected to repeated pressure, skin thickens to form callus tissue. Callus strengthens the skin's ability to withstand pressure. Callus is protective if it remains a moderate thickness, as on the

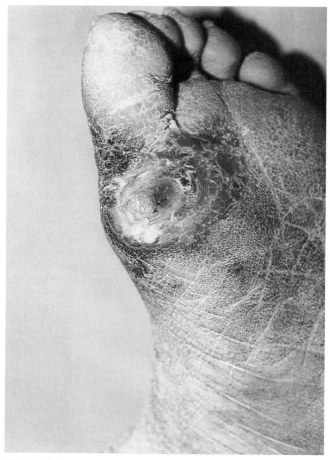

FIGURE 51-1. Dry keratin is not pliable and tends to crack at skin flexion sites. The superficial inflammation that follows can lead to chronic dermatitis or to ulceration.

hands of construction workers. If the callus becomes too thick, it can act as a foreign body. At that point, when pressure is again applied to the area, the callus can contribute to damage in deeper tissues. In a sensate individual, this results in pain, and the person alters their behavior to find ways to relieve the pain, as with the woman who searches for adhesive pads to relieve her toe corns rather than change to more comfortable footwear. In one study of insensate feet on diabetic patients, plantar callus was highly predictive of eventual foot ulceration.[26] These calluses can also add to the increase in stress on the foot. The removal of callus tissue has been shown to reduce these pressures by 29%.[27]

WOUNDS OF THE FOOT

By the time the clinician first examines an ulcerated foot, the initial cause of the problem may be lost from the patient's memory, and it may be hard to diagnose from the appearance of the ulcer. Thus all ulcers are often lumped together under generic terms such as pressure ulcer or diabetic ulcer. Prevention and correction of damage to the insensitive foot requires that the physician and patient understand the actual pathology of the early stages of damage to the foot, and the actual forces that may cause the damage. The focus should be directed toward the external mechanical factors that cause the foot to break down. The insensitive diabetic foot is not really very much weaker than a normal foot; it is just less well protected because of decreased pain sensation.

A foot may be damaged by external forces in one or more of three ways: (1) An unrelenting, low pressure, as from a tight shoe, may cause ischemic necrosis or a pressure sore. Its pathology is similar to that of a decubitus ulcer. (2) A much higher pressure may cause direct mechanical damage, as when a foot lands heavily on a sharp stone, broken glass, or a thumbtack, and the skin is broken or penetrated. (3) Constantly repeated moderate pressure with every step may result in inflammation at high-pressure points, followed by blister or ulcer formation. This is not ischemic necrosis, because the blood supply is not continuously blocked, but is more of an inflammatory enzymatic autolysis. We have termed these three pathogenic factors *ischemia, mechanical disruption, and inflammatory autolysis*.

Ischemic Pressure Ulceration

Decubitus ulcers develop when a section of otherwise healthy skin is subjected to unrelenting pressure. The skin over the sacrum or over the backs of the heels is a common location for this type of wound. A neuropathic foot is also vulnerable to this form of injury. Sustained external pressure that is greater than capillary or local arteriolar blood pressure will occlude these vessels wherever the tissues are compressed between the shoe and an underlying bony structure.

A good deal of experimental work has been done by Branemark,[28] Daly,[29] and Romanus[30] to determine exactly how much external pressure it takes to block the blood flow in peripheral capillaries and produce a state of ischemia. Kosiak and others have studied the relationships between the level of external pressure and the time it takes to produce necrosis or ulceration.[31] Kosiak's diagram (Fig. 51-2) shows that at higher pressures gangrene occurs sooner than at lower pressures.

These studies are not discussed in detail because it has proven impractical to measure these small pressures on the foot in a clinical setting. Also, the structure of the sole of the foot offers mechanical protection to its blood vessels that makes it impossible to standardize thresholds of safety for different parts of the foot. However, some important generalizations about protecting the foot from this type of damage will be discussed.

Localized necrosis of the skin of the foot may occur with pressures as low as 1 pound per square inch (psi). Each member of the diabetic clinical team should demonstrate to himself or herself, and to every patient, how little pressure it takes to produce ischemia. This can be done by pressing a glass slide onto a fingertip or toe until the skin is seen to blanch. This is ischemia. It should be obvious that tight shoes often exceed such a pressure. It is also obvious that such ischemia is painless. Only after an hour or more will pain force normal people to take off their shoes. A person with diabetic neuropathy will keep them on indefinitely.

At pressures of 1–5 psi, such as might be found in a tight shoe (non-weight-bearing), it takes many hours to produce actual necrosis. Although it is not practical to measure pressures inside every shoe, it is very practical to measure time, and it is not difficult to observe the reaction to pressure, such as redness and hyperemia, after removal of a shoe. A new shoe should be worn for only 2–3 hours on the first day. When it is removed, the patient should look carefully for an area of redness and feel for a patch of warmth. If the skin becomes flushed after only 2 hours, it is good evidence that it might become severely damaged if that shoe were worn for 8–10 hours. A leather shoe may be moistened (using a 50% water/50% isopropyl alcohol solution) and stretched on a special last, and may then be worn again for short periods until it is broken in. People with diabetes should be advised to wear only leather shoes, because vinyl and other plastic uppers do not adapt to the shape of the foot to relieve localized pressure.

An excellent habit for a diabetic is the 5-hour shoe change. This involves keeping one pair of shoes at the office or factory. The patient wears one pair of shoes to go to work and at work until lunch time. At lunch, the patient changes shoes and leaves his or her morning shoes in the locker. The second pair is worn until the patient gets home in the evening, when he or she changes into house shoes or slippers, which are worn until bedtime.

Thus each pair of shoes is worn about 5 hours (i.e., 7 AM to noon, noon to 5 PM, and 5 PM to 10 PM). If this habit is developed, the patient will never be in danger of an ischemic pressure ulcer. Even if one pair of shoes is tight, it will not cause necrosis in 5 hours, and the next pair will either not be tight, or may be tight in a different place.

An insensitive foot may develop a pressure ulcer in a previously well-fitting shoe because an insole, pad, or dressing has been added inside the shoe (Fig. 51-3). Bulky dressings of any sort should not be applied to an insensate foot if that person is going to walk. If a foot needs dressing, the patient should probably be in bed or in a cast. If a foot must be in a shoe, it should be a special protective shoe. If a foot needs more than a 1/8 -inch-thick additional insole, an extra-depth shoe should be used (Fig. 51-4).

It is very uncommon for ischemia to cause problems on the sole of the foot. This is because a person with diabetes is generally active; thus pressures from weight bearing are intermittent. The only constant pressure on the foot of an active person is due to circumferential tension from a shoe, strap, or bandage; thus the primary force is tension. Pressure occurs at right angles to the tension (an open shoe may be loose, but when the laces are pulled tight, the foot feels pressure). The simple mechanical rule that links pressure and tension states that tension results in pressure only when the line of tension passes around a curve. The pressure

FIGURE 51-2. Kosiak's classic experiment showing how there is an inverse relationship between the pressure and the time it takes to cause ischemic necrosis. Pressure–time relationship noted in 62 separate experiments on 16 dogs: **X**, ulceration; •, no ulceration. (*Reprinted with permission from Kosiak.[31]*)

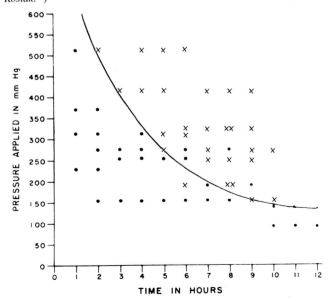

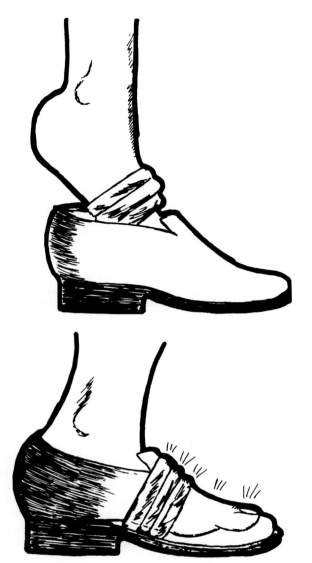

FIGURE 51-3. If a bulky dressing or a thick insole is added and the foot forced back into a previously well-fitting shoe, the increased pressure may result in local gangrene.

that results from tension is inversely proportional to the radius of the curve:

$$Pressure \sim \frac{Tension}{Radius}$$

In the diagram of the transverse section of a forefoot in a shoe (Fig. 51-5), three curves are drawn: (1) the curve of the dorsum of the foot is part of a large circle with a large radius; (2) the curve around the first metatarsal head has a small radius; and (3) the curve of the lateral border of the foot is the smallest and has the smallest radius.

Since the tension in a tight shoe is equal all around the foot, the pressure due to the tension will be least on the dorsum, high on the medial border, and highest on the lateral border (Fig. 51-6). The sole is more or less straight and therefore suffers negligible pressure from tension. The medial border may be curved in two planes

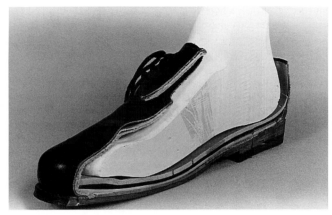

FIGURE 51-4. An extra-deep shoe provides more vertical space for the toes and metatarsal head area. Such shoes are required when insoles exceed 1/8 inch in thickness.

if there is a bunion or hallux valgus, and may thus have a higher pressure than the lateral border. If a patient has a bunion, it is an extra hazard, and surgical correction should be considered if only to prevent future ischemic ulceration.

Although it may seem logical to encourage persons with diabetes to purchase loose shoes, this should be avoided. The danger from friction is as great or greater than that from ischemia. Friction blisters or ulcers may occur behind the heel or around the rim of the shoe because the foot moves up and down due to the loose fit. These blisters and ulcers are prevented by ensuring that the heel is snug and well shaped, and that the lacing or strap over the dorsum reaches far enough up and back over the instep to hold the shoe firmly on the foot.

In summary, to prevent ischemic ulcers, shoes should have leather uppers and be carefully fitted. Feel the medial and lateral borders of the forefoot. New shoes should be worn only 2 hours on the first day, and then the foot should be carefully inspected for areas of redness or heat. Time is an essential element with this form of damage. It takes a long time for low pressure to result in

FIGURE 51-5. Cross section of a forefoot showing that the dorsum is part of a large curve radius (R_1), the medial border is part of a smaller curve radius (R_2), and the lateral border has the smallest curve radius (R_3). The pressures from a single circumferential band of equal tension all around will be slight on the dorsum (P_1), greater on the medial side (P_2), and greatest on the lateral border (P_3). When the tension is equal, $R_1P_1 = R_2P_2 = R_3P_3$.

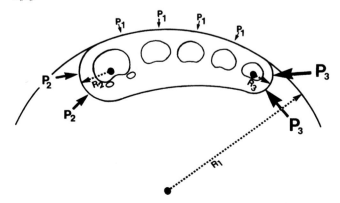

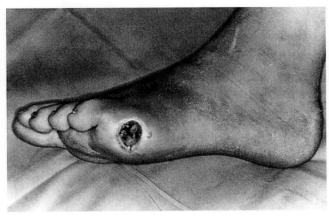

FIGURE 51-6. Pressure necrosis at the lateral border of an insensitive foot due to the wearing of a tight shoe all day.

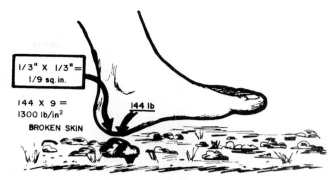

FIGURE 51-8. Barefoot walking is good for the feet, but only if they are sensitive enough to respond to pressure.

ischemic damage. Periodic removal of shoes during the day eliminates this risk. The patient should be advised to change shoes every 5 hours. Routine changing of shoes at noon and 5 PM or other regular intervals can aid the patient to develop an easily remembered routine.

Direct Mechanical Damage

Yamada,[32] in his book on strength of biological materials, quotes Yamaguchi[33] as saying that the skin of the human foot has a tensile breaking load of 2.5 kg/mm and an ultimate tensile strength of 0.95 kg/mm^2. This means that sole skin may be torn by about 100 kg/cm^2 or 1300 psi. Thus it takes about 1000 times more force per unit area to damage skin directly than it does to damage it by ischemia (Fig. 51-7). Direct damage to the sole of the foot might occur if the whole weight of a 144-lb person were to rest on an area of ⅑ of a square inch (Fig. 51-8). A woman wearing stiletto heels could penetrate the skin of a companion's bare foot if she stood on it with just one heel. Actual damage occurs at lower levels of pressure or tension if an element of shear stress is present.

FIGURE 51-7. His weight remains the same, but the area of the stump on which he stands is smaller. Under the foot, damage is caused more readily by narrowing the area of support than by increasing force.

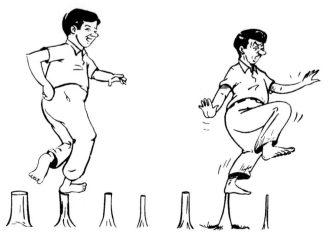

In short, it is unlikely that a person wearing shoes could ever suffer direct damage from any external force unless a small, sharp object were under the foot inside the shoe. However, persons should be extra vigilant when walking around a construction site or a recently roofed building. The risk of stepping on a nail or screw capable of penetrating the shoe sole is much greater in these locations. Insensitive feet are sometimes damaged by walking in stocking feet or barefoot on broken glass, thumbtacks, or sharp stones. Such damage may be avoided completely by a simple rule that all diabetics should follow: "Never walk barefoot, always wear shoes with soles thick enough to prevent a thumbtack from penetrating to the foot, and always shake out your shoes before you put them on." Barefoot walking is very beneficial at all ages, but only when the feet are sensitive to pain.

Along with direct damage from very high forces, direct damage from heat, cold, or corrosive chemicals should be mentioned. All persons with insensitivity need to be alert to such danger and to maintain a margin of safety. They need extra socks when skiing, protective footwear in chemical plants, and special awareness of hot floors in automobiles and trucks. They should be wary of fires or car heaters, and they must never use steam pipes or electric heaters to warm their feet on a cold day.

Moderate Repetitive Stress

Inflammatory autolysis is by far the most common cause of ulceration in the diabetic foot. The pressures that cause it range from 20–70 psi, and are quite similar to the pressures that are ordinarily accepted by normal people who go jogging or walking briskly in firm-soled shoes. Such pressures do not do any harm to normal or diabetic feet unless:

1. They are repeated many thousands of times, day after day, on the same areas of the foot.
2. The tissues are already inflamed as a result of excessive mechanical stress.
3. The tissues are structurally abnormal as a result of previous ulceration and scarring.

The typical diabetic foot ulceration is postulated to begin as a callus on the surface of the skin. Due to repeated impacts to this callus as a result of walking, breakdown occurs between the callus and the deeper tissue.[34] This breakdown comes as the result of the accumulation of inflammatory cells.[35] These cells release lytic enzymes into the tissues. These enzymes lyse the tissues, resulting in a pocket of accumulated fluid. Because the person is insensate, he or she continues to walk on the foot. The inflammation and associated dissolution of tissue becomes exacerbated by hydraulic fluid pressure as the result of stresses on the pocket. This eventually results in the formation of a blister adjacent to the callus or a break in the skin. The hole in the skin will be smaller than the deeper pocket. For the inexperienced clinician, this could result in an underestimation of the extent of damage. When a blister rather than an open wound is found, and the foot is neuropathic, the clinician should appreciate that the real damage is deep to the callus rather than under the blister.

Figure 51-9 shows the histology of rat footpads that were subjected to 10,000 repetitions per day of 20 psi for several days. The rats were lightly anesthetized and had one foot placed in a machine. A piston applied repeated intermittent stress to the footpad to simulate walking or running. The pressure and the number of repetitions per day could be varied. In this experiment the footpads looked normal, though a little swollen, for the first 3 days. They finally broke down and ulcerated about the seventh or eighth day. However, as early as the second or third day, the histology showed invasion of the area by many inflammatory cells. Small foci of necrosis developed in the areas that were crowded with inflammatory cells.

In the inflamed condition, the footpads were swollen and hot, and they had a changed elasticity and viscosity. Thus the same

FIGURE 51-9. **A**. Full thickness of footpad of rat, on second day of program in which 20 psi of pressure was applied 10,000 times per day to the foot of the anesthetized rat. This program simulated the repetitive stress on a human foot jogging 7 miles per day. **B**. Same experiment—third day. Note increased thickness (edema), thickened epithelium, and some inflammation. **C**. Eighth day. Specimen too swollen to fit on slide. Enormous hyperplasia of epithelium. Skin has broken down and ulcerated. This program resulted in ulceration in all of the feet that were involved. **D**. Similar footpad from rat after 6 weeks of a program in which the same pressures were applied, but only 8000 times per day (similar to 5 miles of jogging) and only 5 days per week. Note hyperplasia of epithelium, but footpad is not grossly thickened or inflamed. This program resulted in strong, well-conditioned feet.

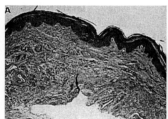
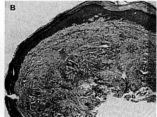
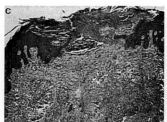
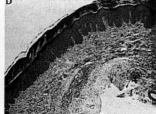

external forces were now more damaging because they were less well absorbed and dissipated by the tissues. Also, the invading inflammatory cells are known to contain lysosomal enzymes. On further mechanical insult, these could have been spilled into the tissues to cause local foci of necrosis. The following conclusions can be derived from these studies:

1. The breakdown of the tissues was the end point of a long process of repeated moderate stress that seemed quite harmless in its early stages.
2. The final breakdown and ulceration could be predicted by the physical signs of local swelling and heat.
3. The breakdown and ulceration could be prevented by discontinuing the repeated stress as soon as the swelling and heat began to persist from one day to the next.
4. The breakdown could be prevented either by decreasing the amount of pressure per repetition (i.e., per step), or by keeping the pressure the same and reducing the number of repetitions.

The early stages of these experiments have been repeated using human fingertips without anesthesia. Repeated pressures of 20 psi were comfortable for several hundred cycles, but then the fingertips gradually became more and more painful until withdrawal became essential. At that stage the fingertip was red, somewhat swollen, and warmer. Within a few minutes it developed a temperature of 4°C higher than the other fingers. The discomfort passed within an hour or so. Upon returning the next day to repeat the experiment on a different finger, the subject could tolerate about the same number of repetitions. However, repeating the stress on the finger that had been exposed the previous day resulted in much more rapid onset of pain. The hyperemia and heat also developed sooner and lasted longer.

By studying the thermographic patterns of the sole of the foot of normal runners (Fig. 51-10), each individual can develop his or her own pattern of "hot spots" that appear on the sole after running a couple of miles. However, after further periods of running, the subject alters his or her gait just enough to spare the now-tender areas of the foot and put more stress on less involved parts of the foot. This constant change of stress patterns on the foot in response to the perception of tenderness and changing thresholds of pain is probably the most important factor that prevents breakdown and ulceration in normal individuals. The fact that persons with diabetes do not appear to limp or change their gait in the early stages of traumatic inflammation may allow them to continue until they develop necrosis, a blister, or ulceration.

Stokes and associates were the first to quantify the correlation between high-pressure points under the insensate foot and ulcer sites.[36] Boulton and coworkers discovered that pressures under insensate feet are usually higher than pressures under normally-sensate feet.[37] It was later found that persons who have limited mobility in major joints of the foot generate the highest pressures and should be considered to be at high risk of ulceration.[25]

WALKING MANAGEMENT

Every person who has insensitive feet needs to be educated about the dangers of repetitive, moderate stress to the feet and the need for extra foot protection to compensate for the reduction in sensation. Preulcerative changes (i.e., blisters, petechiae, erythema, and increased skin temperature) can alert patients and clinicians at a

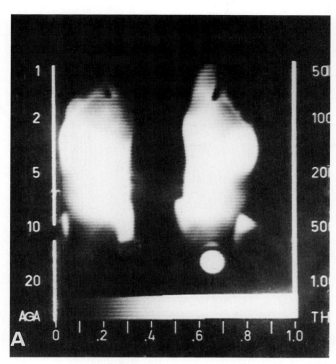
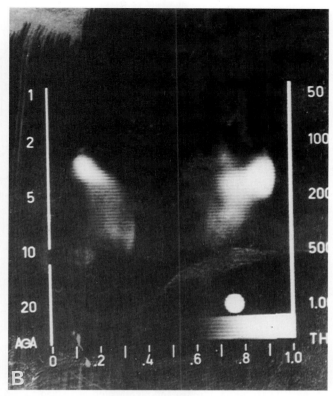

FIGURE 51-10. Thermograph of a normal pair of feet (**A**) immediately after running and (**B**) after a rest. The subject had a button taped to the underside of his foot under the fifth metatarsal head. Note that the area that was over the button remains hot while the rest of the foot cools down.

stage when the foot can be better protected to prevent further damage. Patients need to know that they will be able to walk further if they reduce localized high-pressure areas on the sole. A study by Edmonds and colleagues demonstrated the value of proper footwear in the prevention of recurrent ulceration in a population of diabetics.[6] They found an 83% recurrence of ulceration in patients who reverted to wearing their regular shoes, while only 26% who wore only their prescribed footwear had recurrence. In a controversial study in Italy, Uccioli and associates selected a group of diabetic neuropathic patients and randomly assigned them to either wear their own footwear or footwear with custom-molded inserts in extra-depth shoes for a year.[38] Of those who wore nonprescription footwear, 58.3% developed foot ulcers within a year. Of those who were wearing the custom-molded inserts in extra-depth shoes, 27.7% experienced foot ulcers within the year.

The best way to reduce pressure is to spread the stress over the entire surface of the sole. This may be accomplished in one of three ways: by using a soft sole or insole, a molded insole, and/or a rigid-soled rocker shoe.

$$Pressure = \frac{Force}{Area}$$

In a foot, the force is the weight of the body that is transmitted through the foot to the ground. This force may vary a little in running and jumping, but usually approximates body weight. When a patient is standing still, both feet share the load so that the area under pressure is large, and the pressure itself is thus usually under 20 psi and is harmless. When one foot is off the ground, in the swing phase of the gait, the other foot takes all the force. The pressure is therefore equal to the body weight divided by the total area of foot in contact with the ground (or shoe). This ranges from 10–25 psi, and is usually harmless, even after many repetitions.

While the "swing" foot is moving forward in preparation for the next step, the weight of the body is moving forward over the weight-bearing foot, that now enters the propulsive phase. In this phase, the heel leaves the ground and the entire body weight rests on the forefoot and toes. At this point the pressure is at the peak experienced during the walking cycle. The heel and midfoot bear no weight, and there may be only a few square inches to carry the body weight. This is when pressures under the metatarsal heads or toes may rise to 40, 50, or 60 psi. It is these levels of pressure that will result in inflammation and ulceration if they are repeated too frequently.

SHOE INSERTS

If a soft material is placed under the foot, this results in an increased area of contact over which the force of weight bearing is dispersed. Figure 51-11 shows a tracing taken from five pressure-sensing devices on the sole of a normal foot while the subject was walking freely for four paces. The devices were taped on the great toe, the first, third, and fifth metatarsal heads, and the center of the heel. The pressure from each device was recorded in kg/cm^2 (1 kg/cm^2 = 14.2 psi). The third tracing (from the top in Fig. 51-11) showed the

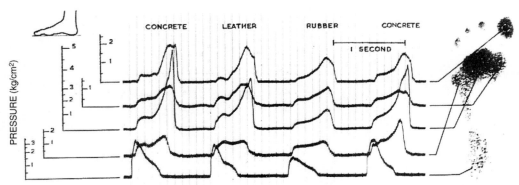

FIGURE 51-11. Pressure tracings of a normal foot on three different surfaces. Note how the use of resilient, compliant materials results in equalization of pressures.

highest pressures. This was derived from the third metatarsal head (i.e., the center of the ball of the foot). At each step, the pressure rises moderately when the foot comes down flat and then rises to a peak when the heel is lifted, prior to the final thrust at toe-off. This subject walked four steps barefoot. His foot came down on a polished concrete floor for the first step, then on a sheet of regular cowhide shoe leather, then on a sheet of $\frac{1}{2}$-inch-thick microcellular rubber, and finally on the concrete floor again. Notice that the peak pressure on concrete was 5 kg/cm^2, on leather was about 3 kg/cm^2, and on microcellular rubber was only about 1.5 kg/cm^2.

In diabetics, a soft insole might offer greater safety than a hard insole because peak pressures would be lower. However, there are limitations to the use of soft insoles in regular shoes. No soft insole can have a great effect on pressure unless it is thick enough for the foot to sink into, so that pressure can spread over a wider area. Regular shoes do not have sufficient room for thick insoles. Also, even if a shoe were deep enough for a $\frac{1}{2}$-inch-thick insole, the foot would move up and down in the shoe as the insole was compressed and decompressed, leading to friction blisters where the foot rubs on the shoe. For this reason, we prescribe thick, soft insoles only for open sandals. Inside a regular shoe, thin, soft insoles may be used, such as a $\frac{1}{8}$-inch-thick Spenco insole, which is made of microcellular rubber covered with stretch nylon. This does reduce local pressure and shear stress, but only to a limited extent. Instead, we usually use a molded insole, so that even when the foot has prominent bones or hollows, the pressure can be spread out.

Thicker soft materials are effective when they are part of the outer shoe sole. Soft-soled athletic footwear has been shown to significantly reduce pressures under the feet 25–30% as compared to leather-soled footwear.[39] The benefit is greatest when the individual has higher-than-normal pressures under the feet when walking.[40]

Molded Insoles

The advantage of molded soles is that the foot does not have to sink down into the material in order to spread the stress. A properly molded sole will meet the foot at every point at which it bears weight. In the past, the danger of using a molded shoe for an insensitive foot was that the shape of the insole might not fit the shape of the sole, and the patient would not know that it was improperly fitted. This was a common cause of secondary problems. For example, an arch support might be too high, or a metatarsal bar might be too far forward, thus increasing the pressure it was intended to relieve.

In the last 30 years there has been a revolution in moldable insole materials. Since the introduction of Plastazote in the 1960s, a whole series of closed-cell polyethylene foams have become available. Many of these materials are heat molded at about 140°C and are poor conductors of heat, so it is possible to mold them directly on the foot without causing burns. This ensures that every insole is a perfect fit, whether made on the foot, or even better, on a plaster model of the foot. The original Plastazote insoles were good, but they were subject to rapid wear and would "bottom out" after a few months. Firmer grades of Plastazote and other materials, such as Aliplast, XPE, and Pelite, now allow a wide choice of texture and lasting quality. It is also possible to make composite insoles with layers of microcellular rubber or polyurethane to support the polyethylene foam and improve durability. In some cases, the innermost layer of the sole may be of leather, wet-molded on a plaster model and backed by cork and latex.

Whatever materials are used, molded insoles should be custom-molded for each individual foot. Prefabricated arch supports or other modular inserts should no longer be prescribed for insensitive feet. Fully-molded insoles take up room in a shoe, and in many cases extra-depth shoes, with an additional $\frac{1}{4}$–$\frac{3}{8}$ inch of vertical room, must be used to accommodate them. These are now available from P.W. Minor, Miller Shoes, Alden Shoe Company, and most recently from SAS (San Antonio Shoes). These shoes look like regular oxford shoes, so patients do not look as though they are wearing orthopedic footwear.

ROCKER-SOLED SHOES

The forefoot suffers maximum vulnerability when (1) the other foot is off the ground, (2) the heel is off the ground, or (3) the weight-bearing part of the foot is bending (causing shear stress). Maximum relief of local pressure and shear stress is obtained by (1) prevention of bending of the foot by making the sole of the shoe rigid, and (2) prevention of localized pressure on the forefoot by keeping ground contact further back, near the center of the shoe.

These criteria are fulfilled by the rocker shoe (Fig. 51-12). Studies by Pollard and associates have shown that a significant reduction of shear stress can be accomplished with a properly constructed rocker-soled shoe.[41] If this shoe is to be custom-made, a plaster model of the foot should be taken with the toes somewhat dorsiflexed, so that the toe of the shoe is turned upward a little. This allows the heel to lift without the toe taking weight while walking.

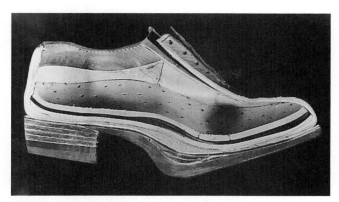

FIGURE 51-12. Construction detail of a custom-made rigid-sole rocker shoe that minimizes pressures in the vulnerable forefoot area.

A regular extra-depth shoe may be made into a rocker by: (1) tilting the toe up a little, (2) adding a steel shank (Fig. 51-13) along the sole to make it more rigid, (3) adding an undersole which is thickened into a rocker behind the metatarsal heads, and (4) adding a molded insole.

PRESSURE FOOTPRINTS

In spite of the great care used in fitting shoes, there will be some patients whose stress is still not relieved, and it may even be worsened by the shoe prescribed. Since the patient cannot feel what is wrong, an objective way to detect pressure problems before the patient leaves the clinic is needed. During the past decade, electronic pressure-sensing tools have become increasingly sophisticated, but their expense and the time needed to conduct these tests still precludes their use as a daily clinical tool. On the other hand, the Harris footprint mat is inexpensive, takes little time to use, and has served well in this regard. It is an inexpensive, practical method that gives a result that the patient and all members of the team can easily understand.

The mat is made of vulcanized rubber and consists of small ridges of three different heights (Fig. 51-14). It is inked with a roller using washable printer's ink and covered with unglazed paper. When a patient stands on it, the part of the sole of the foot that bears the most pressure will flatten the high ridges and will print from the high, medium, and low ridges. Those parts that take less pressure will print only the high and medium ridges, while the

FIGURE 51-13. A regular extra-depth shoe can become a rocker shoe. The sole must be made rigid by adding a steel shank.

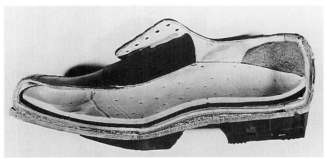

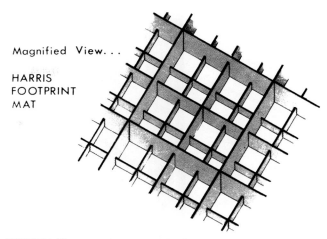

Magnified View...

HARRIS FOOTPRINT MAT

FIGURE 51-14. The multilevel, cross-hatched design of the Harris footprint mat provides differential printing of pressures on the feet.

lowest-pressure points print only from the high ridges. Thus there is an instant record of the pressure pattern that is permanent and can be kept for comparison to subsequent prints (Fig. 51-15). The mat can be used in three ways: the hard footprint, the soft footprint, and the in-the-shoe footprint. All are dynamic and must be taken while the person is walking at a normal pace. An area of floor is set aside for footprints. It may be narrow, but should be long enough for four or five steps.

A line is marked for the start of the walk. The technician demonstrates the technique. The patient takes a practice walk, barefoot or in thin socks. The technician notes exactly where the foot comes down on the second step. He places an inked mat covered with paper on that spot (Fig. 51-16). The patient repeats the walk, lands on the mat, and walks on for two more steps. The footprint is of no value if the patient stops as soon as the footprint is taken. The highest pressure is usually in the propulsive phase of gait, and this is lost if the patient slackens off once the foot is down.

A soft footprint is taken in exactly the same way, except that a sheet of soft insole material, such as Spenco, is placed under the mat. The soft footprint shows just how much pressure reduction in

FIGURE 51-15. The footprint from the Harris mat shows high-pressure areas. The footprint is a valuable patient record.

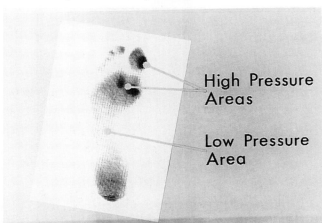

High Pressure Areas

Low Pressure Area

FOOTPRINT TEST...

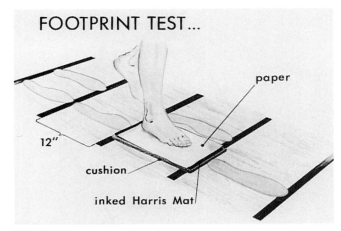

FIGURE 51-16. Premarked footprints may be used to help the patient place feet on the pressure mat. The cushion shown under the Harris mat is used in the soft-footprint test.

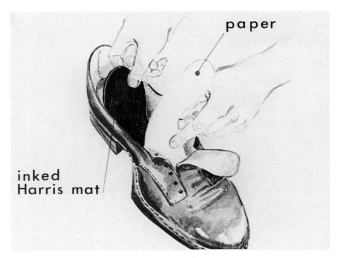

FIGURE 51-18. The thinnest variety of Harris mat is cut into insole-shaped pieces and used to test shoes.

high-pressure areas can be expected from a soft insole, as shown in Fig. 51-17.

A number of precut insoles of the thinnest variety of Harris mat can be used to localize pressure points within the patient's shoe. Two or three different sizes can be cut from a single mat. They are kept and used over and over again indefinitely. An appropriately sized Harris mat insole is inked and covered with paper, which is held in position with small adhesive strips (Figs. 51-18, 51-19, and 51-20). It may be placed in the shoe or on the foot with the sock put on over it. In either case, the shoe is opened widely to allow the foot to step in without smudging the print. The shoes are laced and the patient told to walk briskly and normally for three or four steps. The shoe is opened carefully and the print removed.

This in-the-shoe print is usually creased and smudged; nevertheless, it is extremely valuable. It identifies the real continuing pressures that the patient will experience in the days ahead. Sometimes it is the only device that will convince the patient that their

favorite high-heeled shoe is really dangerous. It may also demonstrate that a simple inexpensive shoe with an insole is really quite appropriate, and expensive special shoes are not needed.

By provision of special shoes, or by minor modification of regular shoes, the patient may spread the pressures of walking as widely as possible (Fig. 51-21). The amount of daily walking must also be limited so that damage can be avoided.

FIGURE 51-19. An example of an unacceptable in-the-shoe footprint when a simple insole was used.

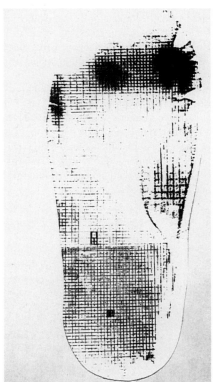

FIGURE 51-17. Comparison of results of hard and soft footprints will demonstrate pressure relief from insole material.

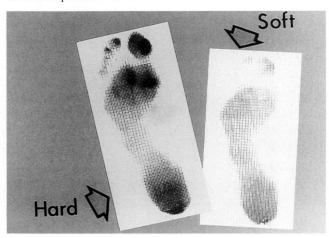

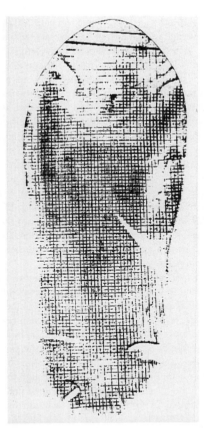

FIGURE 51-20. A second footprint in the same shoe after a molded insole and rocker bar were used.

THE DAILY FOOT EXAMINATION

The person with diabetes is advised to check his or her feet every night before bed. Localized redness, localized heat, and localized callus formation are all good indications of stress. If any of them is progressive, it means that the patient is walking too much or wear-

FIGURE 51-21. Special shoes or modifications to regular shoes can change high-pressure areas (**right**) into a more acceptable pattern of normal pressure distribution (**left**).

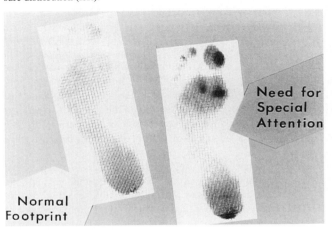

Need for Special Attention

Normal Footprint

ing the wrong kind of shoe. Small areas of increased surface temperature that are still present the next morning represent inflammation. Persons with insensate feet should remove their feet from under the covers 20 minutes before arising for the day. After this time has passed, the temperature of the pedal skin should be evaluated. Localized, elevated skin temperatures greater than 3–4°F can be detected with a little practice. These elevated temperatures on the foot in the morning, before the first steps are taken, are significant. Any finding of significantly increased surface skin temperature should be evaluated by a foot specialist.

The Open Ulcer

If the person with diabetes finds a wound during the daily inspection, he or she must communicate its presence to the foot care team as soon as possible. In addition to the three previously reviewed ways in which the skin may be broken by mechanical force, it may also be damaged by burns, frostbite, ingrown toenails, or during attempts at self-care, such as the cutting of corns. The result of any one of these is an open wound that may lead to infection. At this point, in most cases the condition is correctable. After a few days of rest with pressure eliminated at the site of injury, normal healing will occur. However, in the absence of normal pain thresholds, many people continue to walk on a wounded foot. Infected tissue fluids are squeezed into deeper areas until bones, joints, and tendon sheaths are involved. Now, with spreading cellulitis and deep abscesses, the person seeks medical attention. Unfortunately, serious problems associated with the diabetic foot occur after the skin is broken and a wound or ulcer forms.

In a survey of causal factors that resulted in lower extremity amputation in diabetic patients, Reiber and associates showed that 84% had foot ulceration as the initial pathology.[42] It is important to prevent the wound or ulcer, but it is absolutely essential to concentrate on the care and healing of the foot after it is wounded. Much of the reputation for nonhealing wounds on the feet of persons with diabetes has emerged because such wounds have gone undetected or are allowed to progress with each step for months or even years.

ACUTE CARE

Persons with normal sensation automatically do the right thing whenever they have a wound on the foot. Their intact pain sensation regulates their activity every second the injury is present. These persons will not only avoid stepping on the injured extremity, but they will not move the injured part. The absence of direct pressure and movement allows uninterrupted healing, even though the patient remains otherwise active.

In the absence of pain sensation, it is almost impossible for an active person to avoid at least occasional moments of pressure on, or movement of, the wounded part. One unguarded step may undo the immune system's localization of infection that it has taken hours or days to develop. Successful treatment of a wounded insensitive foot depends on the patient's and physician's ability to provide an environment that protects the foot as well as pain sensation does in a normal foot. The wound must not be subjected to weight bearing, and the joints, tendons, and soft tissues should be immobilized to restrict the extent of inflammation and infection.

The physician must feel the skin around the ulcer. If it is hot and red, the prognosis for healing is good. If it is cool, bluish, or dusky, the limb needs careful evaluation for vascular competence, and it may be a candidate for revascularization, angioplasty, or possible amputation. All necrotic tissue and callus should be debrided from the wound site.

All foot wounds should be probed with a sterile instrument such as a nasal sinus probe to reveal any sinus tracts. The presence of a tract is often masked by granulation or necrotic tissue. Gentle insertion of the sinus probe in several parts of the wound from various angles will reveal the presence of the tract. Grayson and colleagues found in a study of 75 patients that probing for osteomyelitis had a specificity of 85% and a sensitivity of 66%.[43] The predictive value of probing for osteomyelitis was 89% when bone was felt. However, if bone is not felt, osteomyelitis cannot be ruled out. Probing compares very favorably in sensitivity and specificity to radiographic and radionuclide studies. Grayson and coworkers defined bone contact as a gentle probing resulting in the palpation, as felt through the probe, of a solid, often gritty, structure without intervening soft tissue.[43] Early detection of the bone can prevent further destruction by the organism and can often reduce the length of antibiotic therapy. The presence of osteomyelitis requires prolonged antibiotic courses. Probing should not be used as a diagnostic tool when the bone was exposed as the result of surgical debridement. If the opening of the wound on the foot is narrow in proportion to its depth, it should be opened. Dead material may be removed and the wound lightly packed.

A new ulcer or infection may need immediate bed rest and antibiotics. Many publications in the past have contended that all persons with foot infections and diabetes must be hospitalized. However, a prospective study by Lipsky and colleagues has found that diabetic patients with non-limb-threatening infections can be successfully managed on an outpatient basis.[44] If outpatient management is selected, the principles of controlling pressure and motion must be addressed. Patients with foot infections or severe peripheral vascular disease can be managed with posterior splints or other special protective devices such as have been described in detail by Hampton and Birke.[45]

When the acute phase has subsided (with alleviation of fever and swelling), the ulcer may be classified as chronic, and the foot may be treated by providing a plaster cast for ambulation. No topical medication presently available is so beneficial that it obviates the use of devices such as casts to apply it. In the case of insensitive feet, there is an additional reason for treatment in a plaster cast, namely that patients on bed rest will rarely rest their feet completely. In the absence of pain, even in a hospital setting, patients will get out of bed and go to the bathroom and walk on the infected foot. Hospital personnel are often unaware of the risks of allowing a neuropathic patient with a foot wound to ambulate to the bathroom. In a plaster cast, the foot is protected and patients are free to walk a little and be independent.

The Total Contact Cast

The results of several clinical studies of the effectiveness of total contact casting have been published within the past 15 years. It remains the most reliable method for the treatment of these wounds. Several studies now relate that ulcers that have been present for months to years can predictably be healed within 8 weeks with weight-bearing relief provided by these specialized casts.[46] Longer healing times have been attributed to severe compromise to the vasculature or poor patient compliance.[47]

Sinacore and associates were able to heal 82% of plantar foot ulcers in an average of 44 days, and found the technique to be far more reliable than conventional wound management.[48] With casting, Helm and colleagues healed 73% of patients in an average of 38 days.[49] Walker and coworkers healed 80% of patients in 44 days.[50] Most recently, Meyerson and associates were able to heal 90% of patients in an average of 39 days.[51] Location and size of the ulcer correlated with the time it took to close these wounds. Larger ulcers took longer to heal. Forefoot ulcers healed in 30 days, and more posterior plantar ulcers took an average of 63 days to close.

The safe criteria for treatment in a plaster cast are: (1) only feet with adequate blood supply (warm around the wound) should be casted; (2) wait until the infection is localized and systemic symptoms have subsided (e.g., fever, tender glands in the groin); (3) make sure the wound is wide open so there is no danger of skin closing over and leaving a deep pocket of infection; and (4) keep in touch with the patient and remove the cast if any new or recurrent symptoms are noted.[35]

The first cast is usually removed and casting reapplied after 7 days because the limb always shrinks from loss of edema as soon as it is immobilized. If there is obvious swelling at the time the cast was first applied, it should be changed even earlier, because a loose cast is liable to move around and produce friction blisters. The second cast may often be left on for 2 weeks without significant loosening. Never leave a window in a cast. The edges of the window cause shear stress on the tissues that bulge through the window.

The technique for casting does require some practice to lower the risk of secondary complications. The technique is as follows:

1. The patient lies face down with the knee flexed at a right angle and the foot horizontal.
2. The ulcer is covered with a gauze dressing of approximately $\frac{1}{16}$-inch thickness held by paper surgical tape (Fig. 51-22).
3. A tube of stockinette covers the foot and leg. If creases form at the bend in front of the ankle, they are slit and allowed to overlap, and taped to avoid any ridges.
4. Orthopedic felt ($\frac{1}{4}$ inch thick) is used to cover both malleoli and the navicular tuberosity, and a strip of felt is applied anteriorly from top to bottom to facilitate removal of the cast. All felt is beveled at the edges and held with adhesive tape (Fig. 51-23). A layer of foam rubber encloses the toes and metatarsal heads (Fig. 51-24). Thin layers of cast padding are applied under the top edge of the cast and around the heel.
5. A single roll of Gypsona or other very fine plaster bandage is very loosely applied around the foot and leg (Fig. 51-25). It is then rubbed continuously and vigorously into every hollow and around every prominence of the limb until the plaster has set. This inner layer of plaster bandage will be eggshell-thin (consisting of only two or three layers of plaster fabric). The hands of the practitioner who applies it must keep moving constantly. In particular, the plaster on the sole of the foot must be in close contact with every contour of the sole with no padding in between. Padding between the sole of the foot and the sole of the plaster allows movement of the leg in the cast when weight bearing.
6. Once the inner layer of plaster has set, slabs of plaster splint may be applied over it, up and down the posterior calf and sole, and from side to side of the calf under the heel (Fig. 51-26). These may be applied fast and held by encircling plaster or fiberglass bandages; the critical inner layer is already formed. By keeping the leg vertical with the knee flexed, it is easy to

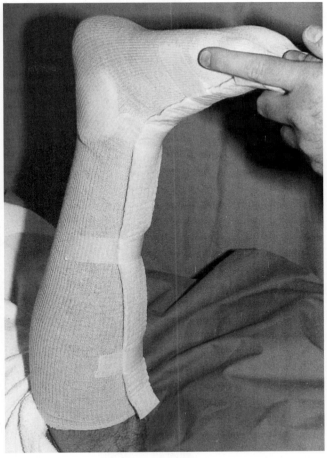

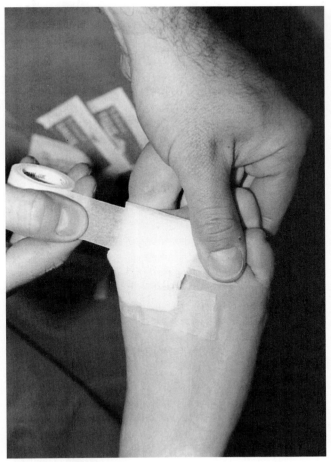

FIGURE 51-22. Gauze dressing over ulcer is secured by paper surgical tape.

FIGURE 51-24. Malleolar pads can be seen through the stockinette. A 1-1/2-inch-wide strip of 1/4-inch felt protects the crest of the tibia and facilitates cast removal.

FIGURE 51-23. Edges of felt pads over malleoli are beveled. Pads are held by paper surgical tape.

FIGURE 51-25. After the eggshell-thin, intimate first layer has set, slabs (five layers of plaster splint) are applied as described in the text to provide support to the cast, but prevent excessive anterior build-up of plaster, thus easing removal.

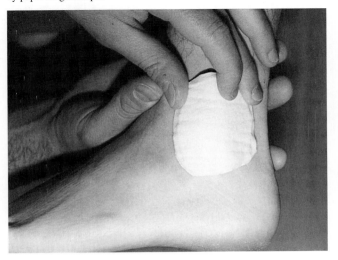

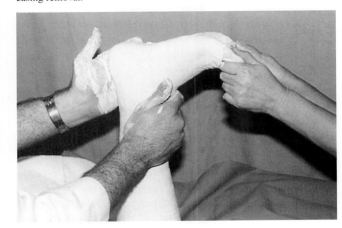

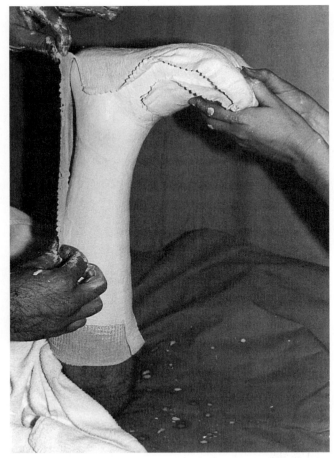

FIGURE 51-26. Assistance is required to maintain ankle at 90 degrees during cast application. Toes are held in extension to prevent toe–ground contact later during walking.

keep the ankle at right angles and air is free to circulate around the cast.

7. A thin ¼-inch plywood sole plate can be laid on the plaster sole, and bunched plaster tucked into the hollows between plaster and wood (Fig. 51-27). Finally, a rocker is applied just behind the center of the sole over the plywood (Fig. 51-28). A rubber heel on a 1¼-inch plywood sole plate is satisfactory (Fig. 51-29).

8. No weight bearing is allowed for 24 hours (Fig. 51-29).

9. The patient is told to report back if the cast begins to feel loose or if pain or fever develops. The cast should then be removed and a new one applied if the only problem is loosening of the original cast. Such an event usually just serves to reassure patient and physician that all is going well.

THE NEWLY HEALED FOOT

When an ulcer has finally epithelialized, the problem is no longer one of infection; it is not necessary to keep the patient in bed or in a cast. However, the foot is not yet completely healed, and walking has to be carefully graded because the scar has not consolidated and the tissues are still friable. When a healed ulcer breaks down

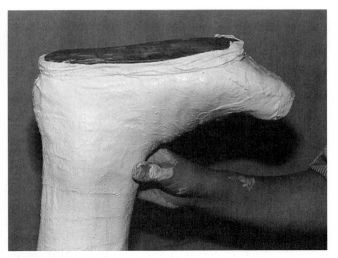

FIGURE 51-27. A 1/4-inch plywood sole plate is placed from the heel to the metatarsal heads to prevent localized pressure under the walking heel. Gaps between plywood and cast should be filled with plaster.

again, it usually occurs in the first month after healing. This has often been attributed to a recurrence of infection, but the real reason is commonly shear stress.

Shear Stress

In mechanical terms, normal stress refers to forces that are at right angles to a surface. Shear stresses are parallel or oblique to the surface. In the sole of the foot, normal stresses tend to compress the tissues between the skin and bone. Deposits of fat are flattened, and forces are redistributed and dispersed to prevent localized high pressure. This process is less efficient when normal tissues are destroyed by ulceration and are replaced by scar tissue. However, the difference is not of great consequence.

Shear stress is a different story. The skin of the sole is attached to the bones of the foot by a complex web of fibrous and elastic bands that allow differential movement of the skin over the bone in a well-defined manner. At rest or under compression, the

FIGURE 51-28. The rubber heel is placed behind the center of the plywood sole plate.

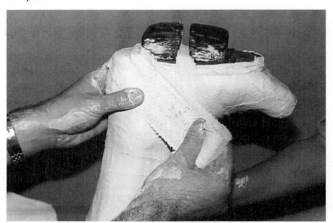

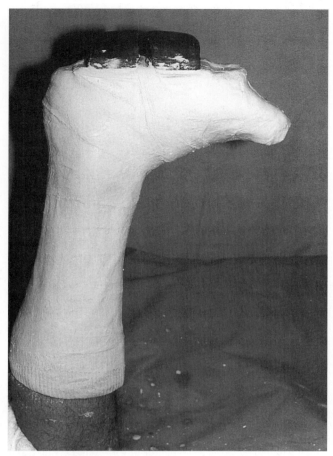

FIGURE 51-29. No weight bearing should be permitted for 24 hours after casting.

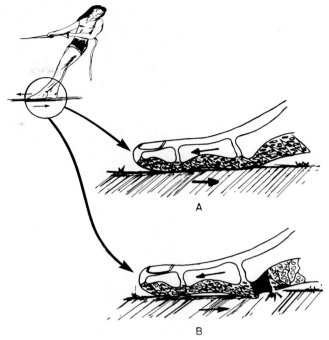

FIGURE 51-30. A. Shear stress in normal intact skin. The continuous network of fibrous and elastic tissue withstands the stress. **B.** Shear stress in presence of scar from a recently healed ulcer. The scar forms a fixed point in the fibrous supportive network. Stresses cause tearing around the junction of mobile and fixed parts of the sole.

THE MANAGEMENT OF NEWLY HEALED PLANTAR ULCERS

Several simple rules should be followed to minimize the recurrence of foot ulcers:

1. The patient must understand the problem; otherwise he or she will make no real attempt to limit activity.
2. Shear stress occurs maximally with fast walking, quick starts and stops, and when making long strides. It also occurs with extension of the toes at the metatarsophalangeal joint when the foot bends at the ball of the foot in the propulsive phase of gait.
3. For the first few weeks after an ulcer heals, the patient should walk as little as possible, slowly and with short steps, preferably with a rigid-soled shoe.
4. Friction between the skin of the sole and the insole of the shoe must be minimized. The inner layer of the insole should be slick and slippery (leather or nylon, rather than rubber or exposed Plastazote). Talcum powder, silicone, or a double layer of socks helps to minimize the extent to which the skin of the foot sticks to the shoe.

SURGICAL INTERVENTION

Elective surgery on the diabetic foot is mainly directed at the prevention of localized pressure and shear. If for any reason it is difficult to avoid high stress to a single aspect of the foot, even with well-fitted shoes, then a foot surgeon should be consulted. Clawed toes or hammer toes may be straightened to avoid stress on the tip

vertical fibers of the sole are slack and loose. When a horizontal thrust is applied to the foot, as when one begins to run or stop suddenly, or when resisting in a tug-of-war (Fig. 51-30), the skin tends to grip the ground and the bones move on the skin until the vertical fibers become oblique, or almost horizontal, and they are then subject to great tension. They have a limited capability to stretch, and after a certain point can yield no more. At that point, either the body moves in relation to the foot or the foot slides along the ground.

The beauty of the normal structure is that during normal activity, all of the restraining fibers of the skin have a similar ability to stretch or to change their obliquity, so that the strain between skin and skeleton is distributed evenly and the tissues can usually handle all the stress they are subjected to. The trouble with a recently healed ulcer is that the flexible elastic sole tissue is replaced at one point by a solid, inflexible scar. The skin at that point cannot move in relation to the bone. What makes this dangerous is the fact that the rest of the skin of the sole retains its normal mobility. Thus when the foot transmits the shear stress of walking, the only restraint is the single small area of adherence, so the shear stress that is ordinarily taken up by some 15 square inches of normal fibers is now taken up by 1 square inch of a new, weak mass of scar tissue. The predictable result is that the newly formed tissues are torn. A hematoma forms under the new skin. The damage is repeated with continued walking until the wound breaks down again.

of the toe or on the dorsal aspect of the interphalangeal joint. Bunions and hallux valgus may need correction. If one metatarsal head is prominent on the sole and is shown to be under undue stress during walking in a well-fitted shoe, it may be useful to do an osteotomy at its neck to allow the head to move into alignment with the other metatarsals. Less often, a metatarsal may be shortened to bring it into line with other already shortened metatarsals. Rarely should a metatarsal be removed. Although it allows the ulcer under it to heal, its removal decreases available weight-bearing surface and increases the stress under other metatarsals and creates new problems.

Sometimes a foot may have an imbalance, such as a foot drop or inversion. If such an imbalance or deformity can be corrected surgically by tendon transfer or by an osteotomy, it may avoid the need for custom-made shoes or braces on a permanent basis.

NEUROPATHIC FRACTURES

The definition of a "Charcot's" fracture has evolved over time. Jean Martin Charcot described arthropathy that developed without known cause in patients with tabes dorsalis or other neuropathies.[52] The term *Charcot's fracture* is now used to describe a fracture in the presence of neuropathy. It should also be extended to include cases in which the tarsus collapses due to ligamentous failure, but no fracture can be identified radiographically.

When confronted with a neuropathic fracture, a physician who rarely sees them can be misled to make an incorrect diagnosis of infection with cellulitis. Frequently, patients with neuropathic fractures in the feet retain this diagnosis of infection for months before the correct diagnosis of fracture is made.

CASE REPORT

A 49-year-old African-American male was referred to the foot clinic by his family physician. The patient had refused to consent to having his left foot amputated. He wanted a second opinion. He had been admitted to his local hospital for foot infection 3 months earlier. No open foot wound had been present prior to his admission at that time.

Three weeks after that admission, radiologic studies were made of the foot. A radiologist interpreted the films as showing signs of osteomyelitis. An exploratory surgery was performed and a bone biopsy was taken. No abscess was found. The bone and soft tissue samples showed no bacterial growth when cultured.

At no time during this hospital stay was the patient advised not to walk on his foot. After surgery the foot became more red and swollen. A second exploratory surgery was performed and again all cultures were negative. Two weeks later the patient was advised to have the foot amputated.

On presentation to the foot clinic he presented with a dorsal foot wound 2 × 10 cm in size. It showed no sign of purulence or necrosis. The foot was red, hot, and swollen. Radiologic studies revealed an anterior-medial pillar Charcot's fracture.[53] He was placed in a rigid posterior splint. He was admitted to the hospital on complete bed rest with bedside commode and orders that he could only be transferred from the bed by wheelchair. He was treated with wet-to-damp normal saline dressings and IV antibiotics. The skin wound healed in 3 weeks. Also by then most of the edema and erythema had subsided. A total contact cast was applied. He was then discharged from

the hospital and antibiotics were discontinued. The cast was changed weekly for 4 weeks. After that casts were changed every 3 weeks. Casting was continued until the surface skin temperature was within 2°C of that of the other foot.

After 3 months of casting, a custom-molded foot-bed was constructed and placed in an off-the-shelf double upright, orthopedic walking boot with Velcro straps. He used this boot for an additional 3 months. He was then gradually rehabilitated from the boot to a custom-molded orthotic device in an extra-depth oxford shoe. He has been maintained in this shoe for the past 10 years. He has occasional small foot injuries. These are quickly addressed in the foot clinic.

The key to success in the treatment of neuropathic joint deformity is early diagnosis. It is frequently at the regular routine checkup of the foot that early cases are detected. This includes the patient's own nightly foot examination. The most constant sign of early joint damage is a patch of localized heat. If the patient feels his or her own feet each morning, he or she will quickly note this hot area, often on the medial aspect of the midfoot. At that stage the x-ray may show early fragmentation of the navicular, the medial cuneiform, or the head of the talus. When any increased heat, redness, or swelling is discovered in an insensitive foot with no open wound present, neuropathic fracture must be considered first.

When confronted with a red, warm, swollen foot on a diabetic patient, and no open wound can be found, the clinician should assume that a Charcot's fracture is present until an alternative diagnosis is conclusively proven. Even if radiologic studies fail to show the presence of a fracture, if the surface skin temperature remains hot, the foot must be immobilized and weight bearing should be supported until the temperature returns to normal.

Harris and Brand described patterns of tarsal disintegration.[53] Any fracture in the presence of neuropathy could be classified as a Charcot's fracture, but they have identified five patterns unique to insensate foot. They are:

1. **Posterior Pillar**—This is a fracture of the posterior portion of the calcaneus. With time, the posterior portion of the fracture is pulled proximally by the Achilles tendon.
2. **Central Body**—This fracture occurs at the inferior part of the talus where it articulates with the calcaneus. Initially, it does not involve the ankle joint. If the person continues to walk on the fracture, the bottom of the leg will get progressively closer to the ground by passing medial to, lateral to, or through the body of the calcaneus.
3. **Anterior Pillar (medial)**—These fractures occur in the head of the talus or at the talar-navicular articulation. They progress to form a rocker-bottom foot or a large exostosis under the medial arch.
4. **Anterior Pillar (lateral)**—These are the rarest pattern and involve the calcaneal-cuboid joint. The foot quickly develops a rocker-bottom shape.
5. **Tarsal/Metatarsal**—These fractures are difficult to diagnose early in their development because they begin as a fracture in the first cuneiform, and radiologically the only evidence is a small increase in the space between the bases of the first and second metatarsals. With continued walking, the fracture extends across the bases of all of the metatarsals. A bony ridge often forms across the top of the foot.

Inflammation results in hyperemia. Prolonged hyperemia can result in local bone absorption. In normally sensate individuals, the pain associated with inflammation will regulate their activity. In the absence of protective sensation, with continued unprotected use, the injury will attain a duration and intensity of inflammation not seen in normal individuals. This degree of inflammation results in the spread of injury, both from the repetitive stress of walking on an open wound and in the case of neuropathic fracture. Successful management of these injuries requires the cessation of the progression of inflammation through relief of weight bearing and immobilization of joints and tendons.

CONCLUSION

The vast majority of lower extremity amputations can be avoided. To accomplish this on a national scale, the medical community must embrace changes in its current approach to this epidemic. The physician must learn to appreciate the unique environment in which neuropathic injuries occur. A multidisciplinary team is needed to successfully manage diabetic foot problems. Injury prevention through education, appropriate footwear, and regularly scheduled clinic visits should be at the heart of such a program. Members of this team should have a knowledge of psychology, social intervention, patient education, footwear and orthoses, biomechanics of the lower extremity, neuropathic wound and fracture care, and diabetes management. The person with diabetes is a patient for life. Professionals who accept the challenges of helping them should be willing and able to provide treatment and rehabilitation for the rest of their patients' lives.

REFERENCES

1. U.S. Department of Health and Human Services, *Diabetes in the United States: A Strategy for Prevention, 1992.* National Center for Chronic Disease Prevention and Health Promotion, Division of Diabetes Translation:1992.
2. Department of Health and Human Services: *Healthy People 2000. National Health Promotion and Disease Prevention Objectives.* Government Printing Office:1991.
3. National Center for Health Statistics: *Healthy People 2000 Review, 1995-1996.* U.S. Public Health Service:1996.
4. Wrobel JS, Mayfield JA, Reiber GE: Geographic variation of lower-extremity major amputation in individuals with and without diabetes in the Medicare population. *Diabetes Care* 2001;24:860.
5. Davidson JK, Alonga M, Goldmith M, *et al*: Assessment of program effectiveness at Grady Memorial Hospital–Atlanta. In: Steiner G, Lawrence PA, eds. *Educating Diabetic Patients.* Springer-Verlag:1981;329.
6. Edmonds ME, Blundell MP, Morris HE, *et al*: Improved survival of the diabetic foot: The role of a specialized foot clinic. *Q J Med* 1986;60:763.
7. Runyan JW: The Memphis chronic disease program. *JAMA* 1975;231:264.
8. Assal J-P, Mulhauser I, Pernat A, *et al*: Patient education as the basis for diabetes care in clinical practice. *Diabetologia* 1985;28:602.
9. Litzelman DK, Slemenda CW, Langefield CD, *et al*: Reduction of lower extremity clinical abnormalities in patients with noninsulin-dependent diabetes mellitus: A randomized, controlled trial. *Ann Intern Med* 1993;119:36.
10. Calle-Pascual AL, Duran A, Benedi A, *et al*: Reduction in foot ulcer incidence. *Diabetes Care* 2001;24:405.
11. Trautner C, Haastert B, Spraul M, *et al*: Unchanged incidence of lower-limb amputations in a German city, 1990-1998. *Diabetes Care* 2001;24:855.
12. Assal J-P: From metabolic crisis to long-term diabetes control: A plea for more efficient therapy. In: Davidson JK, ed. *Clinical Diabetes Mellitus: A Problem Oriented Approach.* Thieme Medical Publishers:2000;799.
13. McNeely MJ, Boyko EJ, Ahroni JE, *et al*: The independent contributions of diabetic neuropathy and vasculopathy in foot ulceration. *Diabetes Care* 1995;18:216.
14. *A Report of the National Diabetes Advisory Board.* NIH Publication No. 81-2284:1980.
15. Cohen S: Potential barriers to diabetes care. *Diabetes Care* 1983;6:499.
16. Mantey I, Foster AVM, Spencer S, *et al*: Why do foot ulcers recur in diabetic patients? *Diabet Med* 1999;16:245.
17. Dyck PJ, Kratz KM, Karnes JL, *et al*: The prevalence by staged severity of various types of diabetic neuropathy, retinopathy, and nephropathy in a population based cohort: the Rochester Diabetic neuropathy study. *Neurology* 1993;43:817.
18. von Frey M: Zur physiologic der judsempfindung, Arch Neurol Physical, 1922;7:142.
19. Semmes S: Tactile sensitivity of the phalanges, In: Perceptical Motor Skills, South University Press:1962;351.
20. Birke JA, Sims DS: Plantar sensory threshold in the ulcerative foot. *Lepr Rev* 1986;57:261.
21. Boyko EJ, Ahroni JH, Stensel V, *et al*: A prospective study of risk factors for diabetic foot ulcer: the Seattle foot study. *Diabetes Care* 1999;22:1036.
22. Lavery LA, Armstrong DG, Vela SA, *et al*: Practical criteria for screening patients at high risk for diabetic foot ulceration. *Arch Intern Med* 1998;158:157.
23. Zilberberg J: *Fluorescence and pentosidine content of diabetic foot skin.* Master's thesis. University Park, Pennsylvania State University:1998.
24. Birke JA, Franks BD, Foto JG: First ray joint limitations, pressure, and ulceration of the first metatarsal head ulceration in diabetes mellitus. *Foot Ankle Int* 1995;16:277.
25. Fernando DJS, Masson EA, Veves A, *et al*: Relationship of limited joint mobility to abnormal foot pressures and diabetic foot ulceration. *Diabetes Care* 1991;14:8.
26. Murray HJ, Young MJ, Boulton AJM: The relationship between callous formation, high pressures and neuropathy in diabetic foot ulceration. *Diabet Med* 1996;13:979.
27. Young MJ, Murray HJ, Boulton AJM: Effect of callous removal on dynamic foot pressure in diabetic patients. *Diabet Med* 1992;9:75.
28. Branemark PI: In: Kenedi RM, Cowden JM, eds. *Bedsore Biomechanics.* Macmillan:1975;69.
29. Daly CH: Chimoskey TE, Holloway, Ga, etal: The effect of pressure loading the blood flow rate of human skin. In: Kenedi RM, Cowden JM, eds. *Bedsore Biomechanics.* Macmillan:1975;69.
30. Romanus EM: Microcirculatory reactions to controlled tissue ischoemic and temperature: A vital microscopic study on the hampsters cheek pouch. In: Kenedi RM, Cowden JM, eds. *Bedsore Biomechanics.* Macmillan:1975;79.
31. Kosiak M: Etiology and pathology of ischemic ulcers. *Arch Phys Med Rehab* 1959;40:62.
32. Yamada H: *Strength of Biological Materials.* Williams & Wilkins:1970;219.
33. Yamaguchi T: Title in Japanese only. *J Kyoto Pref Med Ctr* 1960;67:347.
34. Delbridge L, Ctercteko G, Fowler, *et al*: The aetiology of diabetic neuropathic ulceration of the foot. *Br J Surg* 1985;72:1.
35. *Brand PW: Insensitive Feet: A Practical Handbook on Foot Problems in Leprosy.* The Leprosy Mission:1977.
36. Stokes IAF, Faris IB, Hutton WC: The neuropathic ulcer and loads on the foot in diabetic patients. *Acta Orthop Scand* 1975;46:839.
37. Boulton AJM, Betts RP, Franks CI, *et al*: Abnormal foot pressures in early diabetic neuropathy. *Diabet Med* 1987;4:225.
38. Uccioli L, Faglia E, Monticone G, *et al*: Manufactured shoes in the prevention of diabetic foot ulcers. *Diabetes Care* 1995;18:1376.
39. Kastenbauer T, Sokol G, Stary S, *et al*: Running shoes for relief of plantar pressure in diabetic patients. *Diabet Med* 1998;15:518.
40. Perry JE, Cavanagh PR, Ulbrecht JS: The use of conventional footwear to relieve plantar pressures in the diabetic foot. In: *Proceedings of the May 5–8, 1992 8th Annual East Coast Clinical Gait Laboratories Conference.* Rochester, MN:1993;121.
41. Pollard JP, Le Quesne LP, Tappin JW: Forces under the foot. *J Biomed Eng* 1983;5:37.

42. Reiber GE, Pecararo RE, Koepell TD: Risk factors for amputation in patients with diabetes mellitus: a case control study. *Ann Intern Med* 1992;117:97.

43. Grayson ML, Gibbons GW, Karoly K, *et al*: Probing to bone in infected pedal ulcers: a clinical sign of underlying osteomyelitis in diabetic patients. *JAMA* 1995;273:721.

44. Lipsky BA, Pecararo RE, Wheat LJ: Outpatient management of uncomplicated lower-extremity infections in diabetic patients. *Arch Intern Med* 1990;150:790.

45. Hampton GH, Birke JA: Treatment of wounds caused by pressure and insensitivity. In: McCullough J, ed. *Contemporary Perspectives in Rehabilitation: Wound Healing*. FA Davis:1990.

46. Sinacore DR: Total contact casting for diabetic neuropathic ulcers. *Phys Ther* 1996;76:296.

47. De Block C, van Acker K, de Leeuw I: Chronic diabetic foot ulcers. *Diabetes* 1993;47(suppl 1):A168.

48. Sinacore DR, Mueller MJ, Diamond JE, *et al*: Diabetic ulcers treated by total-contact casting: A clinical report, *Phys Ther* 1987;67:1543.

49. Helm PA, Walker SC, Pullium G: Total contact casting in diabetic patients with neuropathic foot ulcerations. *Arch Phys Med Rehab* 1984;65:691.

50. Walker SC, Helm PA, Pullium G: Total contact casting and chronic diabetic neuropathic foot ulcerations: Healing rates by wound location. *Arch Phys Med Rehab* 1987;68:217.

51. Myerson M, Papa J, Eaton K, *et al*: The total-contact cast for management of neuropathic plantar ulceration of the foot. *J Bone Joint Surg* 1992;74:261.

52. Charcot JM: Lectures on the diseases of the nervous system: Lecture IV. *Proceedings of the New Sydenham Society*. London:1881.

53. Harris JR, Brand PW: Patterns of disintegration of the tarsus in anaesthetic feet. *J Bone Joint Surg* 1966;48B:4.

Diabetes and the GI System

Francisco J. Baigorri

Jamie S. Barkin

Diabetes mellitus affects the entire gastrointestinal system. Therefore as expected, patients with diabetes mellitus are prone to develop a spectrum of clinical symptoms directly related to the effects of diabetes mellitus on their GI tract. This chapter will review these entities, discussing both clinical and pathologic features. In addition, multiple organs may be involved and therefore symptoms may overlap and present a complex picture.

ESOPHAGUS

Esophageal Motor Dysfunction

Esophageal motor dysfunction has been well-documented in patients with diabetes mellitus since Mandelstam and Lieber's cineradiographic study in 1967.[1] They described reduced or absent primary peristaltic waves and occasional tertiary contractions in 12 of 14 diabetic patients with neuropathy. Subsequently, these abnormalities have been characterized using manometry, radiography, and scintigraphy.

Overall, manometric abnormalities occur in over 50% of patients with diabetes. These include increased numbers of spontaneous and repetitive contractions, aperistaltic contractions, reduced lower esophageal sphincter pressure, reduced amplitude of pharyngeal and esophageal contractions, and increased duration of peristaltic contractions. Studies using high-fidelity manometric recordings have demonstrated an aberrant pattern of multipeaked peristaltic pressure complexes in the smooth muscle segment of the esophagus in patients with evidence of diabetic autonomic neuropathy (DAN).[2] This finding was uncommon in patients with diabetic autonomic neuropathy or in other patient groups. However, the multipeaked peristaltic waves moved food boluses through the esophagus effectively, and the diabetic subjects studied lacked clinical symptoms. Other manometric studies have corroborated that despite the demonstration of esophageal manometric abnormalities, clinical symptoms such as dysphagia, chest pain, or heartburn are usually very mild or absent.[3] This may be secondary to an underlying diabetic sensory neuropathy. Therefore, the functional significance of these manometric abnormalities remains unclear.

Video radiography and nuclear scintigraphy are more useful screening tests for evaluating disturbances of esophageal motility. Impaired esophageal transit and emptying was demonstrated in up to 35% of patients with both type 1 (T1DM) and type 2 diabetes mellitus (T2DM).[4-6] Another prospective study demonstrated delayed esophageal emptying in 34 of 50 type 1 diabetic patients. Despite the demonstration of delayed esophageal emptying, most subjects remained asymptomatic. Again, whether this is related to impaired sensory perception or a lack of symptoms of physiologic significance is unclear. However, these patients probably have an increased risk of stasis, including localized pill ulceration of the mucosa and delayed drug absorption.

Gastroesophageal reflux also occurs more often in patients with diabetes. Diminished lower esophageal sphincter pressure has been demonstrated manometrically, and 24-hour pH monitoring has shown that reflux occurs more frequently in diabetic patients than in controls. Using ambulatory pH monitoring, 9 of 20 persons with diabetes had abnormal acid reflux. It was suggested that delayed gastric emptying may have contributed to the reflux. Neural impairment appears to play a significant role in the pathogenesis of esophageal dysmotility. There is a strong correlation between the presence of autonomic and peripheral neuropathy and abnormal esophageal motor function in diabetic patients.[2] Some studies have shown that the duration of disease may correlate with the severity of the neuropathy, yet others have found no significant correlation. An interesting association is the proposed strong relationship between psychiatric illness, especially depression and generalized anxiety, and esophageal motility disturbances, which was independent of the presence of neuropathy.[5]

Physiologic and histologic evidence supports neural dysfunction rather than esophageal smooth muscle impairment as a primary factor in diabetic patients with esophageal motility disturbances. Animal studies have demonstrated intramural neural mechanisms for the control of esophageal peristalsis. The on-contraction (A wave) is controlled by cholinergic excitatory nerves, and the off-contraction (B wave) is elicited by noncholinergic, nonadrenergic inhibiting nerves. Therefore, A waves are atropine sensitive whereas B waves are not. Loo and coworkers demonstrated an aberrant manometric pattern of multipeaked peristaltic pressure complexes in diabetic patients with DAN.[2] These complexes were converted to monophasic waves by administration of a small dose of atropine, whereas administration of edrophonium exaggerated the number and amplitude of these complexes. They concluded that neural dysfunction caused the aberrant motility pattern. Evidence of a neurologic rather than a myopathic disorder includes histologic studies that show abnormalities within prevertebral ganglia, including Schwann cell loss and Wallerian degeneration, whereas myenteric plexus and esophageal musculature remain intact.[4]

Also, monilial esophagitis, reflux esophagitis, and both benign and malignant strictures should be excluded. Obviously, one must exclude a cardiac source of the chest pain and esophageal mucosal disease prior to ascribing it to an esophageal motor disorder.

Monilial Esophagitis

Monilial esophagitis is most commonly found in patients with underlying malignancies, cirrhosis, or reduced immune response. In addition, diabetic patients are predisposed to monilial esophagitis. These patients usually have uncontrolled diabetes or are receiving immunosuppression after undergoing renal transplantation. Symptoms of monilial esophagitis include dysphagia or odynophagia that may be so severe as to prevent swallowing. The dysphagia is usually for solids, but may involve liquids, especially if they are hot. Radiographic findings of candidiasis on barium swallow include a shaggy outline of the esophageal wall or frank ulcerations, intermucosal filling defects, nodular formations, or a combination of these entities. These findings are usually more prominent in the middle or lower third of the esophagus. Esophagoscopy often reveals a yellowish, cheesy exudate on the mucosa, which is erythematous and friable but may be ulcerated. Esophageal brushings reveal yeast forms. Cultures for *Candida* may reveal the organisms, but are unable to distinguish whether there is colonization or invasion of the esophageal mucosa. Biopsies of the esophagus may show buds or hyphae invading the mucosa. Serum agglutinating titers may be valuable when the titer is >160, which usually correlates with severe infection and tissue invasion.

Treatment for monilial esophagitis is dependent on the severity of the infection. Mild cases can be treated with luminally active agents such as nystatin, clotrimazole, or oral amphotericin. In symptomatic or refractory cases, oral medications that reach the systemic circulation such as ketoconazole or fluconazole can be used, and a single dose has been reported to be curative. Fluconazole appears to have fewer side effects than ketoconazole and may be better absorbed in the patient with achlorhydria. Both of these agents may interfere with the metabolism of other drugs, for example, coumadin and cyclosporine. The use of intravenous therapy for monilial esophagitis with amphotericin B and flucytosine is usually reserved for granulocytopenic patients with fungal esophagitis, who have a higher risk of disseminated disease.[7]

STOMACH

Gastroparesis Diabeticorum

Clinical Features

Gastric neuropathy secondary to diabetes was first described by Rundles in 1945[8] and became widely recognized after 1958 when Kassander first used the term **gastroparesis diabeticorum**. Although gastric motor abnormalities can be found in approximately 20–30% of diabetic patients, most studies show very little correlation with clinical complaints. Symptoms predominantly result from (1) gastroesophageal reflux with heartburn and halitosis, (2) gastric stasis with early satiety, pain, nausea, vomiting, and/or anorexia, and (3) distension with hiccups. These are most pronounced postprandially and occur intermittently, punctuated by symptom-free intervals. There may a deterioration and lability of glycemic control due to unpredictable gastric emptying, resulting in hypoglycemic episodes. Moreover, in some diabetic patients

with gastroparesis, the only symptom may be poor glycemic control, without any gastrointestinal symptoms. So gastroparesis can be present without any symptoms, just as myocardial ischemia can occur without symptoms in diabetic patients.[10] Rarely gastric stasis may result in formation of gastic bezoras and bacterial overgrowth.

Pathophysiology

The etiology of delayed gastric emptying due to diabetes mellitus remains unclear. Vagal neuropathy has been proposed because of its role in the reflexes that regulate gastric motility and emptying. In support of this theory, postvagotomy patients demonstrate similar radiographic and clinical findings to patients who have diabetic gastroparesis. Physiologic evidence of vagal dysfunction has been demonstrated by decreased acid output in response to sham feeding and elevated gastrin levels in diabetic patients with gastroparesis.[11] Pharmacologic evidence also exists in that antral contractions are directly stimulated by metoclopramide and bethanechol and are inhibited by atropine in affected patients. Support also rests on histologic abnormalities of the vagus, including lymphocytic infiltration, irregularity or disruption of nerve fibers, and crowding of Schwann cell nuclei, as well as segmental demyelination, that are seen in patients with gastroparesis diabeticorum.[6,12] Evidence against vagal neuropathy is the lack of acceleration of early gastric emptying seen in postvagotomy patients, but not in diabetic patients with gastroparesis. In addition, after surgical vagotomy, there is preservation of the differential rate of emptying of liquids and solids, which is occasionally lost in diabetic patients. Finally, Yoshida and collaborators found no histologic abnormalities of the myenteric plexus or abdominal vagus in diabetic subjects with or without gastroparesis when compared to controls. Coordinated relaxation of the pylorus is essential for chyme to move efficiently from the antrum to the duodenum. Pylorospasm has been reported as a cause of delayed gastric emptying in diabetic patients.[10,13]

Hormonal factors are important in the control of gastric emptying. Motilin, a gut polypeptide, is capable of initiating an interdigestive migrating motor complex (IMMC). Diabetic patients have higher basal levels of motilin,[12] which decrease in response to insulin administration.[14] In normals, metoclopramide-induced IMMC was associated with increased plasma motilin levels that were decreased in diabetic patients.[15] In addition to motilin, diabetic subjects have altered secretion of pancreatic polypeptide, somatostatin, glucagon, and gastrin.[16] Despite these abnormalities, the role of hormonal imbalance in diabetic gastric dysfunction remains unclear.

Several other factors in diabetes may affect gastric motility. These include the level of glycemic control and the occurrence of ketonemia, acidosis, and electrolyte disturbances. Acute hyperglycemia decreases emptying of liquid meals and may contribute to a generalized gastric atony. Acute gastric dilation is frequently seen in patients with diabetic ketoacidosis and may be a result of hyperglycemia, hyperglucagonemia, electrolyte imbalance, ketonemia, acidosis, or an acute reversible autonomic neuropathy. In summary, the etiology of diabetic gastric dysfunction is unclear, but it likely results from an alteration of several interrelated factors.

Diagnosis

Gastroparesis diabeticorum should be suspected clinically if the patient has upper GI tract symptoms or if their diabetes becomes difficult to control without explanation. Roentgenographic and nuclear medicine solid phase gastric emptying studies assist in diagnosis. Contrast studies will likely demonstrate advanced disease, whereas early disease and its quantification are measured by gastric emptying studies. The most common radiologic feature on upper gastrointestinal series is sluggish, ineffectual, and irregular gastric peristalsis. This often may be accompanied by the presence of a significant amount of solid gastric residue despite the preceding 12-hour fasting period. Other features commonly noted on barium study include elongation of the stomach, giving it a sausage-shaped configuration, significant retention of ingested barium (grossly defined as 50% or more of the ingested barium present on the 30-minute follow-up film), and duodenal bulb atonic dilatation without evidence of organic obstruction (Fig. 52-1). The pylorus is widely patent, although it may be necessary for the examiner to externally compress the abdomen in order to force barium into the duodenum to demonstrate pyloric patency.

Radioisotope gastric serial scintiscanning studies allow quantification and accurate measurement of both liquid- and solid-phase emptying. The method for measuring solid-phase emptying uses *in vitro* labeled egg albumin and is usually abnormal in patients with diabetes mellitus and gastroparesis (Fig. 52-2). Conversely, gastric emptying of liquid meals is often normal. The emptying rate of the indigestible solids seems to demonstrate the most profound abnormalities of gastric emptying in patients with gastroparesis diabeticorum.[17] In a healthy control group, most orally ingested markers emptied from the stomach by the fourth postprandial hour, and all ten markers had emptied by 6 hours in 45 of 46 trials. In contrast,

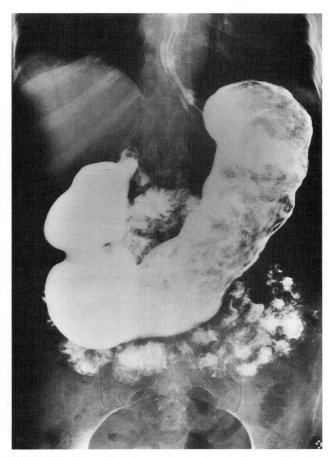

FIGURE 52-1. Upper GI barium study, showing significant solid residue after an overnight fast in an elongated sausage-shaped stomach with retained barium without evidence of mechanical gastric outlet obstruction.

indigestible solid markers were retained in the stomach 6 hours after the meal in 50% of the diabetic patients studied. The gastric emptying rate has been measured by carbon-labeled breath test and compared with scintiscanning studies. [12]C labeled food is absorbed from the intestine as it is emptied from the stomach, and then expired from the lungs where it can be measured. There seems to be a good correlation between the results of the breath test and the scintiscanning test.

Manometric studies of the stomach demonstrate diminished proximal stomach and antral motor activity as well as an absence of gastric interdigestive motor complexes in patients with gastroparesis diabeticorum.[18] Mearin and associates investigated the pyloric activity in diabetic patients who had recurrent nausea or vomiting without evidence of mechanical obstruction.[19] The duration of their total pyloric activity before and after meals was found to be significantly greater than in controls. Further, episodes of unusually prolonged pyloric activity and intense tonic contractions, so-called pylorus spasms, were observed in 14 of 24 diabetic patients versus only one control. They concluded that pyloric dysmotility is part of the widespread disruption of gut motility that affects patients with diabetes. Its pathophysiologic and clinical sequelae are undetermined.

Gastric contractions are normally coordinated by slow waves that migrate distally through the body and antrum of the stomach at a rate of 3 cycles per minute (cpm) in humans.[20] These can be accurately recorded by electrodes placed either on the serosal surface of the stomach or cutaneously.[21] The resulting electrogastrogram (EGG) can detect gastric arrhythmias which are present in disorders such as diabetes mellitus, nausea and vomiting in pregnancy, anorexia nervosa, and motion sickness.[22–25] Interestingly, these arrhythmias can be created in normals by injection of large doses of glucagon.[26] Good correlation has been obtained between symptoms and EGG findings both before treatment and after clinical improvement with directed therapy.[27,28] Although this examination is not widely available, it appears to be promising as a diagnostic test and may be useful for clinical monitoring after treatment.

In summary, the normal emptying of digestible solids from the stomach is dependent on antral motor function, whereas liquid emptying is dependent on the gradient between proximal stomach and duodenum. Diabetic patients with symptomatic gastroparesis do not empty liquids significantly differently from normal patients, whereas digestible and nondigestible solids empty significantly more slowly than normal. The slow emptying of nondigestible solids occurs because of abnormalities of the IMMC. The IMMC is normally associated with a cyclically appearing caudally migrating muscular contraction that acts as a janitorial service to sweep the stomach and upper small bowel of nondigestible products and bacteria. A loss of antral phase three of the IMMC has been found in diabetic patients.[29] Abnormalities of this function may lead to development of gastric bezoars and bacterial overgrowth. The pylorus is especially important in regulating gastric emptying of solids, and pyloric dysmotility may contribute to delayed solid-phase emptying that affects some patients with diabetes mellitus. Finally, abnormal gastric slow-wave activity has been detected by electrogastrography, which in humans originates in the antrum and may be related to nausea symptoms and a delay in gastric emptying.[30]

The diagnosis of gastroparesis diabeticorum requires exclusion of other causes of gastric dysfunction, including functional and mechanical obstruction. Functional disorders that may mimic gastroparesis diabeticorum include parasympathetic loss, such as surgical vagotomy; destruction of the vagus from pulmonary,

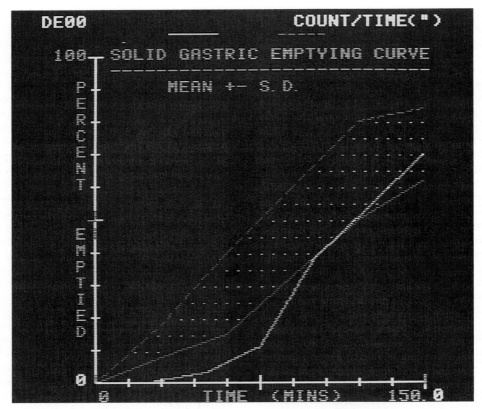

FIGURE 52-2. Delayed emptying on solid-phase nuclear gastric emptying scan in a diabetic patient with gastroparesis.

esophageal, or gastric malignancy; and drug-induced motility dysfunction. The most common drugs include tranquilizers, anticholinergics, ganglionic blocking agents, and tricyclic antidepressants. Symptoms similar to gastroparesis diabeticorum may also be a consequence of gastric mucosal disease, such as peptic ulcer disease, tumor or mechanical obstruction such as pyloric stenosis, or cicatrix.

The diagnostic evaluation of diabetic patients with symptoms suggestive of gastric stasis should begin with upper endoscopy to exclude primary mucosal disease or mechanical obstruction. Parkman and Schwartz found that 55% of their 20 diabetic patients with intractable nausea and vomiting had gastrointestinal disorders other than gastroparesis that could explain their symptoms.[31] Following exclusion of an anatomic cause of obstruction, further evaluation of gastric emptying with a radioisotopic study should be performed. This work-up provides both anatomic and functional evaluation of the stomach and permits exclusion of other causes of gastric dysfunction. Other diagnostic tests that should be performed are a small bowel series and possibly an abdominal CT, the latter to visualize the pancreas. Unfortunately, there is a very poor correlation between gastric emptying and symptoms (Table 52-1).

Treatment

Treatment of gastroparesis diabeticorum is often difficult because hyperglycemia inhibits gastric motility. Conversely, diabetic control may be more difficult because of the delayed gastric emptying. Our approach is to initiate a liquid diet if the patient is an outpatient, or if hospitalized the patient is kept NPO, and intravenous glucose is administered. Once glucose levels have returned

TABLE 52-1. Gastroparesis Diabeticorum: Diagnosis and Management

Diagnosis
  Suspect gastroparesis in patients with nausea, vomiting, reflux, bloating
  Exclude mechanical obstruction and peptic ulcer disease by performing an upper endoscopy
  Exclude drug-induced mechanical obstruction: anticholinergics, tricyclic antidepressants
  Barium studies are sensitive only in patients with advanced disease; also may show
    impaired peristalsis, and retained solid gastric residue despite fasting
  Electrogastrogram: not widely available
  Solid phase radioisotopic study
  Consider CT of the abdomen to evaluate the pancreas
Management
  Optimize glucose control
  Low-fat, low-fiber diet
  Four to six small meals daily
  Metoclopramide
  Domperidone (outside U.S.)
  Cisapride (outside the U.S.)
  Erythromycin
  Erythromycin derivatives (in the future)

to normal, medical therapy is initiated. A low-fat diet (<40 grams per day) and a decreased amount of fiber distributed in 4–6 meals a day may help the symptoms of patients with gastroparesis diabeticorum.[10] Cholinergic agents such as bethanechol and cholinesterase inhibitors such as ambenonium chloride have met with variable success and are often associated with disturbing side effects. The agents most commonly used for the treatment of gastroparesis diabeticorum are promotility drugs such as metoclopramide, domperidone (outside of the United States), cisapride, and erythromycin. Cisapride, which was also used, has been withdrawn from the U.S. market by the Food and Drug Administration because of drug-induced cardiac arrhythmias. These agents stimulate contraction of the smooth muscle of the gastrointestinal tract.

Although metoclopramide's mechanism of action has not been completely elucidated, actions that may be responsible for its effects include: (1) the release of acetylcholine from intrinsic nerve plexus in muscles, (2) antagonism of dopaminergic and tryptaminergic neural transmission, (3) inhibitory effects of dopamine on gastric motility, (4) facilitation of peristaltic reflexes, (5) direct effect on gut smooth muscle, and (6) inhibition of the central nervous system chemoreceptor trigger zone for vomiting. The mechanism of action of domperidone has not been completely elucidated, but it is believed to promote gastric relaxation and enhanced antral contractility through antagonism of peripheral dopamine receptors.[32] Unlike metoclopramide, domperidone does not cross the blood–brain barrier and therefore has no significant effects within the central nervous system (CNS).[33] Erythromycin and other 14-member macrolides are believed to stimulate gastrointestinal motility by mimicking the effects of the gut polypeptide motilin.[34]

Administration of metoclopramide initially increases the rate of gastric emptying in patients with delayed gastric emptying, as evidenced by decreased gastric volumes, decreased recovery of ingested solid foods, and increased rate of gastric emptying of isotopically labeled test meals.[35,36] Several clinical trials of multiple-dose metoclopramide therapy have demonstrated improvement in both symptoms and gastric emptying rate.[37–39] Investigators have noted that a reduction in symptoms was seen in some patients with minimally impaired gastric emptying, suggesting an important role for the antiemetic properties of metoclopramide.[38,39] However, long-term trials have demonstrated a discordance between diminished motility effects and continued symptomatic relief with this agent.[40] Unfortunately, adverse effects occur in approximately 20% of patients after metoclopramide administration and most commonly involve the CNS and GI tract. The CNS effects require monitoring of the patient for development of extrapyramidal symptoms, and rarely, Parkinsonian motor disorders and dystonia,[41] which may not resolve with discontinuance of the drug. Additionally, metoclopramide can produce hyperprolactinemia, resulting in breast tenderness and enlargement, galactorrhea, and menstrual irregularities.[41] The usual adult dosage of metoclopramide for the treatment of diabetic gastroparesis is 10 mg, four times daily given 15–30 minutes before meals and at bedtime. Initially, the patient should be started on liquid metoclopramide to facilitate its absorption. Higher doses are often tolerated, but an increased incidence of adverse effects is likely, particularly in the elderly.[41] Lastly, patients with a creatinine clearance <60 mL/min should have appropriate reductions in dosage.[41]

Domperidone experimentally enhances gastroduodenal contractility and coordination, and clinically increases the rate of gastric emptying.[36,42] Similarly to metoclopramide, domperidone treatment in diabetic patients commonly results in early symptom relief, although quantitative improvement in gastric emptying has been only temporary and statistically insignificant.[27,43] Koch and associates, in an open-label trial, demonstrated normalization of gastric arrhythmias in all six insulin-requiring diabetic patients treated for 6 months with domperidone, 20 mg four times a day.[27] The restoration of the normal gastric myoelectric activity (3 cycles/min) occurred despite the persistence of abnormal solid-phase

gastric emptying, but was associated with symptomatic improvement in these diabetic patients. However, this did not normalize their solid-phase emptying rates, demonstrating another discordance between the clinical and physiologic effects of drug therapy for diabetic gastroparesis. In contrast to metoclopramide, domperidone has poor penetration of the blood–brain barrier and therefore CNS symptoms are exceedingly rare.[33] Cardiac arrhythmias may result from intravenous administration.[44] The usual adult daily dosage ranges from 40–120 mg in three to four divided doses and need not be adjusted for renal dysfunction.[33]

Erythromycin and the other 14-member drugs that are macrolides stimulate increased gastrointestinal motility by acting as competitive agonists for motilin receptors located predominantly above the ligament of Treitz.[45] The initial report of the use of erythromycin in 10 patients with diabetic gastroparesis by Janssens and coworkers revealed that 200 mg administered intravenously 20 minutes postprandially markedly improved the severely impaired gastric emptying of both liquids and solids.[45] In addition, patients receiving erythromycin at a dose of 250 mg orally three times daily before meals for 1 month, showed statistically significant improvement in their emptying of both solids and liquids at 120 minutes after ingestion of a double-isotope test meal. Peeters and associates demonstrated that low-dose IV erythromycin (40 mg) in patients with diabetic gastroparesis induced a premature pattern of contractions that mimicked the naturally occurring gastric phase three of the IMMC.[46] Larger doses (200–350 mg given intravenously) prompted a burst of rhythmic antral contractions at maximal contractile frequency with no propagation to the small bowel and absent phase one IMMC quiescence. Erythromycin and other macrolides with motilinomimetic properties appear to correct both the interdigestive and postprandial motility defects found in patients with diabetic gastroparesis during short-term treatment. It remains unclear whether these physiologic effects will translate into long-term symptomatic improvement. Preliminary studies suggest that erythromycin derivatives may play a role in the therapy of diabetic gastroparesis without the antibacterial effect of erythromycin.[47]

Our treatment approach in a hospitalized patient with intractable symptoms is to initially use an intravenous bolus of erythromycin or metoclopramide. Peristalsis visualized during endoscopy following drug infusion may predict a successful initial therapeutic response. We generally continue intravenous administration of the drug during progressive liberalization of food intake from liquids to semisolids to solids, switching to an oral prokinetic preparation after solids have been tolerated for 24–48 hours. Improved response may be obtained when these drugs are combined because they act physiologically on different areas of the GI tract.

Surgical intervention for refractory diabetic gastroparesis is rare but should arguably provide a means for gastric drainage, decompression, and a route for predictable nutritional support. Drainage procedures alone, such as gastrojejunostomies and pyloroplasties, have only a 50% success rate.[48] Reardon and coworkers reported a patient who underwent a pyloroplasty, decompression gastrostomy, and feeding jejunostomy with significant clinical improvement initially, but then suffered a complication due to the jejunostomy tube, which eventually resulted in death.[48] A feeding jejunostomy, although a valuable tool for nutritional support and glycemic control, is associated with significant complications such as clogging, a "dumping" syndrome related to bolus feedings, and small bowel necrosis due to nonthrombotic occlusion of mesenteric vessels. Alternatively, a percutaneous endoscopically guided jejunostomy (PEJ) can provide a means of both gastric decompression and jejunal feeding without the inherent risks of surgery.

The prognosis for patients with symptomatic gastroparesis diabeticorum is guarded, since these patients usually have advanced complications of diabetes mellitus. The course of patients with asymptomatic gastric motility disturbances is unknown.

Atrophic Gastritis

The gastric mucosa in diabetic individuals becomes atrophic at an earlier age and more frequently than in nondiabetic patients. As many as 85% of diabetic patients have biopsy-proven partial or complete atrophy of the gastric mucosa.[49] The gastritis does not appear to be related to the severity or duration of the diabetes, but instead is age related. With advancing age, the frequency of superficial or atrophic gastritis increases.

Studies of gastric acid secretion of diabetic patients have yielded conflicting results. Several studies have reported a decrease in gastric secretion when compared with nondiabetic individuals, whereas others have found no difference in their maximum acid output.[11,50] One possible explanation is that both hyperglycemia and hyperglucagonemia inhibit gastric acid secretion. Green and associates used sham feeding to evaluate vagal control of gastric acid production compared with pentagastrin stimulation.[51] In contrast to previous findings, a reduced acid secretory response to sham feeding was not consistently found in a diabetic population.[52] In addition, Gramm and coworkers found that acid secretory responses to homogenized food, infused directly into the stomach of diabetics, as well as maximal acid secretion to parenteral pentagastrin, is normal,[52] indicating an intact acid secretory capacity. However, in diabetic subjects, the food-stimulated gastrin response was exaggerated, and this may have been sufficient to permit a normal acid response to food.

Antibodies to gastric components are more frequently found in type 1 diabetic patients than in nondiabetic individuals. Circulating parietal cell antibodies have been found in up to 25% of type 1 diabetic patients compared with 8% of controls. Intrinsic factor antibodies occur in up to 8% of people with diabetes,[53] and these were especially prevalent in young women with type 1 diabetes. As might be expected with time, latent pernicious anemia appears to be more common in this group, affecting 4–5% of middle-aged and elderly type 1 diabetic patients, especially women.[53] Therefore, in type 1 diabetic patients who have peripheral neuropathy, coexisting unsuspected pernicious anemia may be present and should be sought by determining periodic B_{12} levels.

The role, if any, that *Helicobacter pylori* has in diabetic gastritis is unclear and remains to be further elucidated. There appears to be a greater incidence of *H. pylori* infection in diabetics, which correlates better with duration of diabetes than with the chronological age of the patient. Conversely, there is a decreased incidence of *H. pylori* infection in patients with diabetic gastroparesis when compared to patients with normal gastric emptying.

SMALL INTESTINE

Diabetic Diarrhea

Clinical Presentation

Involvement of the small intestine in diabetics is often symptomatic, resulting in diarrhea. The frequency of diarrhea varied from 10–22% in Feldman and Schiller's study. The syndrome of diarrhea in diabetic patients was first described by Bargen and colleagues in 1936. Characteristically, these patients are young adults (20–40 years old), more often men than women (ratio 3:2), with poorly controlled, longstanding type 1 diabetes occurring a mean of 8 years after the onset of diabetes mellitus.[54] There is usually coexistent peripheral or autonomic neuropathy. The diarrhea is usually brown, watery, and voluminous, and may be associated with tenesmus. As many as 75% of diabetic patients with diarrhea have documented steatorrhea. Altered small bowel motor function alone, without any concomitant malabsorption disorder, may produce up to 14 grams per day of fat in the stool.[55] Fecal incontinence may also occur and is distinguished from diabetic diarrhea by frequent stools of low volume, associated with neuropathy of the external and internal[56,57] sphincter. Diabetic diarrhea can occur at any time, but is often nocturnal and may be associated with soiling and fecal incontinence. It is important to distinguish fecal incontinence from true diabetic diarrhea, the latter presenting with an increased stool volume (>200 g daily). In patients with diabetic diarrhea: (1) defecation may be preceded by abdominal distension and borborygmi, (2) the patient may pass up to 20 or more stools daily, and diarrhea is often worse following meals, and (3) the diarrhea is typically episodic, with bouts lasting days to weeks. These episodes are often followed by weeks to months of normal bowel habits, or occasionally constipation. Interestingly, as time passes the diarrhea tends to become less severe. Even with severe diarrhea, body weight is generally maintained. If weight loss is present, it is usually in association with concomitant gastroparesis or steatorrhea.

Pathophysiology

The pathogenesis of diabetic diarrhea is still not completely resolved and is probably multifactorial. Several mechanisms are proposed to explain the structural and functional pathogenic abnormalities involved in diabetic diarrhea. These include (1) visceral autonomic neuropathy,[81] (2) bacterial overgrowth, (3) bile acid malabsorption,[58] (4) pancreatic exocrine insufficiency, and (5) electrolyte imbalance[58] and altered gut hormone production. Overall, it appears that the major contributing factor is the presence of diabetic autonomic neuropathy (DAN).

Several concepts support this postulate. The diarrhea often coexists with other manifestations of DAN, particularly abnormal pupillary responses, impotence, dysfunction of the urinary bladder, anhidrosis, retrograde ejaculation, or orthostatic hypotension. Autonomic dysfunction from causes other than diabetes also result in diarrhea, including vagotomy, sympathectomy, pheochromocytoma, administration of ganglionic blocking agents, and infiltrative processes involving the autonomic ganglia such as amyloidosis.[60] Previously, the only significant autonomic histological finding was a nonspecific dendritic swelling in the sympathetic prevertebral and postvertebral ganglia, which was often present in diabetic patients both with and without diarrhea. Degenerative histologic changes have not been consistently observed in the intestinal plexuses studied by Meissner and Auerbach in diabetic patients, and the intestinal mucosa, muscle, microvasculature, and ganglia are often normal histologically.[61] Occasionally, there is mild lymphocytic infiltration of the lamina propria.

The mechanism by which DAN plays a role in diabetic diarrhea may involve alterations in ion transport as well as impairment of intestinal motility. First, the loss of autonomic regulation of ion transport, which is secondary to the loss of the α_2-adrenergic enterocytic receptors, may lead to diarrhea. These α_2-adrenergic receptors in the small and large intestine enterocytes stimulate sodium chloride absorption and inhibit bicarbonate secretion,[62,63] resulting in a net influx of fluids and ion. Chang and coworkers demonstrated an impaired adrenergic regulation of mucosal ion transport resulting in a net intestinal fluid secretion in streptozocin-induced chronically diabetic rats with diarrhea.[63,64] Clonidine, a specific α_2-adrenergic receptor agonist that enhances mucosal absorption of fluid and electrolytes and inhibits anion secretion, has resulted in decreased diarrhea in uncontrolled trials.[65,66] The prominent side effects of clonidine such as orthostatic hypotension, sedation, and dry mouth have been less frequently found in diabetic patients who receive this drug. In cases where the use of oral clonidine is associated with side effects significant enough to limit treatment, recent case reports have suggested that topical clonidine may be substituted with a similar benefit in the treatment of diabetic diarrhea, with a less pronounced side effect profile.

Gastrointestinal motor abnormalities also affect the small bowel in diabetic patients. Studies have shown considerable variability in small bowel transit time. Thus both delayed and enhanced motility have been observed in studies using radiopaque markers and hydrogen breath tests.[67,68] In view of these conflicting findings, it is likely that the pathophysiology of diabetic diarrhea is diverse. A recent study has shown that even though the transit time is often abnormal in diabetics, patients did not necessarily have diarrhea.[68] It has been suggested that the neuropathic process can induce alterations in the intestinal motility by disturbing the propagation of myoelectric activity.[69] The presence of rapid transit may result in increased fecal propulsion and diarrhea, or conversely, slow transit may lead to stasis and bacterial overgrowth, promoting diarrhea and steatorrhea via a type of blind-loop syndrome.

The three factors that prevent the growth and accumulation of enteric bacteria in the upper small intestinal lumen are intestinal motility, gastric acid, and immunologic or bacteriostatic intestinal secretions. Alteration of one or more of these mechanisms can result in small intestinal bacterial overgrowth. The delayed small bowel transit observed in diabetic patients can therefore lead to bacterial overgrowth. The pathophysiologic basis is that small bowel bacteria deconjugate bile acids, preventing micelle formation, and result in fat malabsorption, steatorrhea, and diarrhea. Indirect support of this proposal comes from a few reports that describe clinical improvement of the diarrheal syndrome with broad-spectrum antibiotics. Bacteriologic evidence has revealed normal bacterial concentrations in most of these patients. However, these studies did not culture for anaerobic bacteria (i.e., bacteroides, enterococcus, and clostridium) which unlike aerobic bacteria, are capable of deconjugating bile salts more effectively.

The gold standard for the diagnosis of bacterial overgrowth is the proper placement of a jejunal tube and culture of the intestinal aspirate. The normal concentration of bacteria in the upper GI tract is $<10^4$ organisms per mL of intestinal contents. Noninvasive breath tests have also been evaluated as a means to detect bacterial overgrowth. Studies have shown that the ^{14}C xylose breath test has a sensitivity and specificity exceeding 90%, and therefore it has become the noninvasive test of choice in the evaluation of patients with suspected bacterial overgrowth. Two recent French studies have demonstrated the efficacy of antibiotics (norfloxacin and amoxicillin-clavulanic acid) in diabetic patients with diarrhea and bacterial overgrowth.[70,71]

Bile acid malabsorption has also been suggested as a contributing factor to diabetic diarrhea on the basis of a decreased bile salt pool. However, measuring fecal $^{14}CO_2$ levels after administering ^{14}C glycocholate revealed that only 15% of diabetic patients with diarrhea had increased fecal bile acid excretion.[72] In addition, the administration of cholestyramine did not show any therapeutic effects in the majority of patients. Therefore the role of bile acid malabsorption is not clearly established and may be related to accelerated small bowel transit or bacterial overgrowth.

Pancreatic exocrine insufficiency, abnormal colonic motility, anorectal dysfunction, and celiac sprue in diabetics are several other mechanisms that may contribute to diarrhea found in a diabetic patient. In addition, consumption of dietetic foods that contain sorbitol, including sugarless chewing gum, dried roasted nuts, meat products, icings, toppings, dairy products, brown sugar, and beverages, may also result in diarrhea. This may be a confounding factor because many diabetics who consume sorbitol are unaware of its presence in the diet.[58]

Management of chronic diarrhea in diabetics should initially be directed toward correction of the imbalance of fluids and electrolytes, control of diabetes, and restoration of nutrition, and subsequently a search for an identifiable cause of the diarrhea is initiated. Small bowel bacterial overgrowth is treated with oral broad-spectrum antibiotics (see above), to include coverage for anaerobic bacteria, such as metronidazole with a quinolone or cephalosporin with tetracycline. Antibiotics are administered for 1 week of every month on a rotating basis to avoid development of bacterial resistance. Other treatable causes of diarrhea in a diabetic patient are a gluten-free diet for celiac disease, pancreatic enzymes for pancreatic insufficiency, and biofeedback mechanisms, which may be effective in controlling diarrhea secondary to fecal incontinence.[73]

Often, however, the pathogenesis of diarrhea in the diabetic patient is not clear, and treatment must be directed at alleviating the patient's symptoms. Antidiarrheal agents such as diphenoxylate, loperamide hydrochloride, or codeine can decrease the number of stools, but usually do not affect stool volume. These agents may be particularly effective in patients with rapid intestinal transit, but may consequently have adverse effects on motility in patients with delayed transit by promoting stasis and bacterial overgrowth. Further investigation with controlled studies is required in establishing their benefit in the management of diabetic diarrhea.

Somatostatin and its long-acting synthetic analogue octreotide acetate have been shown to reduce diarrhea in patients with short bowel syndrome, ileostomy, and tumor-induced secretory diarrhea. It has also been shown to be efficacious in many patients with diabetic diarrhea when conventional therapies failed.[74,75] Physiologically, somatostatin inhibits stimulated water secretion, increases gut absorptive capacity, and suppresses both gastrointestinal hormones that produce diarrhea and counterregulatory hormones that promote hyperglycemia. Octreotide is administered as a subcutaneous injection of 50–75 μg twice daily and may be given with insulin.[74] The role of newer, long-acting somatostatin analogues remains to be determined. The management of chronic diarrhea in diabetic patients is depicted in Table 52-2.

Celiac Disease

The association of type 1 diabetes mellitus with celiac disease has been reported in both children and adults. The incidence of concomitant disease in children and adolescents is estimated at 4.6%,[76] and in adults the incidence has been estimated at 1 in 1700. It is unclear whether this rate applies to all racial groups.[77] Typing of HLA in patients with both celiac disease and diabetes mellitus reveals

TABLE 52-2. Management of Chronic Diarrhea in Diabetic Patients

Concepts
  Distinguish fecal incontinence from true diarrhea
  Exclude bacterial overgrowth, infectious diarrhea, celiac sprue, sorbitol-
    containing food,
    pancreatic insufficiency
Management
  Replace fluid and electrolytes as needed
Steps in Treatment of Diabetic Diarrhea
  Diphenoxylate, loperamide, codeine
  Clonidine (α_2-adrenergic receptor antagonist)
  Somatostatin or octreotide

that the incidence of the histocompatibility antigens HLA-B8, HLA-DR3, and DQW2 are significantly higher in patients with both diseases, and suggests a genetic predisposition to these diseases.[78,79]

Diabetic diarrhea and celiac disease may have similar clinical manifestations. Certain clues, however, may assist in differentiating the two disease entities. Celiac disease occurs more often in women, and the diarrhea often precedes clinical diabetes. Celiac patients often have evidence of malabsorption, weight loss, peripheral edema, and bone pain, and peripheral neuropathy is often absent. An important clue that the diarrhea in a diabetic patient may be due to celiac disease is a history of repeated episodes of hypoglycemia when the diarrhea is troublesome.

The diagnosis of celiac disease is made by demonstrating the characteristic pathology on jejunal biopsy, which typically shows villous atrophy with crypt hyperplasia. In addition, a clinical and histologic response to a gluten-free diet is required to make the diagnosis. Antiendomysial antibodies more than antigliadin antibody determination has been shown to have high levels of sensitivity and specificity in the screening and follow-up of celiac disease. Treatment consists of removal of gluten from the diet and correcting any deficiencies caused by the absorptive defects.

LARGE INTESTINE

Constipation is seen in up to 60% of diabetic patients who have neuropathies.[8] This probably represents an increase in frequency above that seen in the nondiabetic population, even though constipation is a common complaint in the general population. With progressive obstipation and constipation, on occasion a massive amount of fecal material may be found in a large atonic dilated colon and may simulate intestinal obstruction with fecal impaction. This may lead to stercoral ulcerations, the result of subsequent mucosal erosion by feces in the rectum. A study of colonic motility in patients with diabetes mellitus revealed abnormalities related to feeding in the myoelectrical and motor responses of the colon that correlated closely with symptoms of constipation.[80-82] The most consistent abnormality is the absence of the normal rapid increase in colonic spike motor activity within the first 30-minute postprandial period. The colon was found to respond to drugs that stimulate colonic motility, for example, metoclopramide or neostigmine, suggesting that neural control mechanisms were abnormal while colonic muscular activity remained intact.[82]

Like other intestinal motor abnormalities, large bowel motility problems are usually seen in patients with DAN. Treatment is

symptomatic, initially with the use of increased dietary fiber, and regular use of laxatives or stool softeners. Unresponsive patients may benefit from drugs that act at the myoneural junction or directly on the smooth muscle, for example, metoclopramide.[80-82] Impaired anorectal function determined by anorectal manometry occurs in the diabetic population.[83]

Its association with DAN is supported by the finding of an abnormal anorectal reflex in 3 of 11 diabetic patients with DAN and in none of 9 diabetics without DAN. Decreased rectal sensation and impaired function of the external and internal sphincters have been suggested as causes of fecal incontinence in diabetics.[73] Biofeedback is performed by inserting a balloon in the external canal and having the patient squeeze, while allowing the patient to visualize and note the increased balloon pressure on a viewing device. It has been utilized in an effort to lower the threshold of conscious rectal sensation. Good to excellent results, characterized by a 75% or greater reduction in the frequency of soiling episodes, has been reported in 70% of diabetic patients.[73] Incontinence frequently coincides with the onset of diabetic diarrhea and may simply respond to antidiarrheal therapy. According to two recent studies, diabetes mellitus may be associated with an increased risk of colorectal cancer in both men and women after adjusting for other risk factors.[84,85] Thus one cannot assume that a change in bowel habits is related to the diabetes, and therefore such changes require an appropriate evaluation.

BILIARY TRACT

Cholecystopathy

A common feature in diabetic patients is the presence of an enlarged gallbladder, which may increase to three times the normal size. Diabetic neurogenic gallbladder has been characterized using ultrasonography and scintigraphy imaging techniques that evaluate gallbladder motility, and these studies have shown impaired gallbladder contractility and emptying.[86–91]

Eating normally stimulates gallbladder contraction by the mechanisms of (1) cephalic vagal stimulation, (2) mechanical gastrointestinal distension stimulating cholinergic reflexes, and (3) chemical interaction of food and digestive products, causing the release of a complex array of hormones, especially cholecystokinin (CCK), which can modulate gallbladder motor function. DAN, a frequent complication of longstanding diabetes, impairs parasympathetic (vagal) regulation in the gut and other organs. Therefore it is not unexpected that patients with DAN have impaired gallbladder motility that may relate to the severity of the neuropathy.[87,92]

However, other factors may have a pathophysiologic role. Stone and collaborators demonstrated a decreased gallbladder emptying rate in patients with DAN in response to CCK. They postulated that the gallbladder smooth muscle in diabetic patients with autonomic neuropathy may be less sensitive to hormonal stimulation.[91] Mitsukawa and coworkers reported elevated levels of CCK in diabetic patients with DAN compared with controls after ingesting egg yolk,[87] a known stimulant of CCK release. This occurred despite impaired gallbladder emptying in these diabetic patients, and decreased responsiveness of the gallbladder wall to CCK was again proposed. More recently, however, Fiorucci and associates studied gallbladder contractility in response to either a meal or separate cephalic or hormonal stimulation.[93] They found that gallbladder emptying induced by an ordinary meal was comparable in diabetic patients and healthy controls, and were unable to confirm any differences in gallbladder emptying induced by hormonal stimulation with CCK/cerulein. They demonstrated that gallbladder emptying in response to cephalic stimulation is abolished in diabetic patients with DAN, which paralleled reductions of gastric acid secretion and pancreatic polypeptide release induced by vagal stimulation. These functional abnormalities are analogous to vagotomy and atropine infusion, which may impair normal gallbladder contractions in response to a meal. Erythromycin may be effective in reducing gallbladder volume in diabetic patients.[94,95] However, treatment with metoclopramide does not improve gallbladder emptying.[80] Obesity has been associated with an increased incidence of gallstones and may also reduce gallbladder emptying in healthy subjects. However, a recent study contradicted these earlier studies and found no correlation between weight and delayed gallbladder emptying in both healthy and diabetic subjects.[91] This study also demonstrated that the type of treatment of the diabetics, the presence or absence of peripheral neuropathy, and the degree of diabetic control do not appear to be independent risk factors for impaired gallbladder contractility in diabetic patients.[91] Further work is needed to understand these discrepancies.

Cholelithiasis

The presence of diabetes is often mentioned as an independent risk factor for the development of cholelithiasis, along with female gender, obesity, advancing age, and multiparity.[96] Several autopsy studies have reported a higher frequency of cholelithiasis in diabetic individuals than in the general population (30.2% in diabetic patients compared with 11.6% in nondiabetic patients),[97,98] although other reported series were not confirmatory.[99,100] One survey of 641 patients in a health maintenance organization found the incidence of diabetes to be nearly 30% in those with asymptomatic cholelithiasis.[101] However, this observation was not corroborated in several subsequent population-based studies,[102–105] and comorbid conditions including type IV hyperlipidemia and obesity, also risk factors for gallstone formation, may confound the effect of diabetes.[103–108]

The pathogenic mechanism for the proposed increased risk of cholelithiasis in diabetes is believed to involve incomplete gallbladder emptying secondary to the diabetic neurogenic gallbladder as well as supersaturated bile and hyperinsulinemia. One study of type 2 diabetic patients revealed an increase in bile supersaturated with cholesterol and reduced bile acid concentration, which perhaps predisposed these patients to cholesterol precipitation and stone formation.[109] However, patients with type 1 diabetes had normal bile composition. Meinders and colleagues compared bile cholesterol saturation and bile acid composition in 12 nonobese, male type 1 diabetic patients and 28 normal healthy controls, and found that the total bile lipid concentration in the bile-rich duodenal aspirates examined were actually lower in this diabetic population.[110]

Hyperinsulinemia, which is frequently present with type 2 diabetes, may be a factor in gallstone formation.[111] Insulin itself stimulates the enzyme hepatic hydroxymethyl glutamyl co-enzyme A reductase, which is the rate-limiting step in hepatic cholesterol biosynthesis. A case-control study demonstrated significantly higher fasting plasma insulin levels in diabetic patients with gallstones than in diabetic patients without gallstones.[112] Also, insulin therapy may increase bile lithogenicity. Studies in Pima Indians have shown that improved glycemic control with insulin therapy results in a contracted bile acid pool and increased cholesterol saturation index from 114–181%.[113]

The management of asymptomatic gallstones is an evolving issue. Until the 1980s, prophylactic cholecystectomy was recommended in all operable patients in the general population with gallstones because of the perceived risk of potential gallstone complications. However, several recent studies have established that asymptomatic gallstones rarely lead to life-threatening complications, and therefore the risk and expense of surgery outweigh the benefit.[101,114–116] Whether this applies specifically to the diabetic population has been debated. A few questions have been answered and many still remain. The course of treatment for diabetic patients with asymptomatic gallstones requires further examination of these questions.

First we need to know if diabetic patients with silent gallstones are more likely to develop complications. The natural history of cholelithiasis in diabetes is largely unknown because no prospective cohort studies have been undertaken. However, McSherry and associates followed a group of 135 patients, of whom 30% had diabetes with asymptomatic cholelithiasis for 5 years.[101] Outcome data were not broken down; however, the outcome in the diabetic groups appeared to be no different than others in the study. Only 14 patients developed symptoms during their follow-up period and 10 required surgery (mean of 47 months) after diagnosis. Other studies have demonstrated that asymptomatic patients or patients with nonspecific symptoms (e.g., nausea) have a favorable prognosis in their natural history, and were unable to show whether the fate of persons with diabetes is different. Thus it seems that asymptomatic patients with diabetes mellitus are no more likely to develop symptoms than the general population.

Uncertainty remains as to whether diabetic patients with silent gallstones develop complications more frequently; interestingly, the complications that arise are probably more severe than those in nondiabetic patients. As one author states, "it is true that when the silent gallstone speaks in the diabetic, it is usually with a loquacious roar."[116] Rabinowitch first suggested that diabetic patients who develop cholecystitis do worse than nondiabetic patients because of the high risk of infection-related complications of cholelithiasis.[117] Indeed, diabetic patients have a higher susceptibility to infection, secondary to defects in host–defense mechanisms, including abnormal neutrophil chemotaxis, phagocytosis, and bactericidal activity, as well as depressed cell-mediated immunity. Earlier studies reported a 22% incidence of severe gallbladder disease (hydrops, perforation, and empyema),[118] and others concurred, noting a 20–40% rate of advanced inflammation among diabetic patients presenting with acute cholecystitis.[119–121] One review of patients with perforation complicating acute cholecystitis found that 16–25% of the subjects had diabetes.[122] Older age and presence of atherosclerosis were risk factors for perforation. Also, emphysematous cholecystitis is more common in diabetes, and occurs in up to one-third of reported cases. The course of this form of acute cholecystitis is more severe and has been associated with a 30-fold increase of gangrene and a threefold increase of both perforation and death.[122] The gas-forming organisms implicated in its pathogenesis include *Clostridium welchii*, which is cultured most often, as well as anaerobic streptococci, *Escherichia coli, Staphylococcus aureus, Pseudomonas*, and *Klebsiella*.

In the past, diabetic patients with silent gallstones were advised to have cholecystectomy because of the belief that infectious and inflammatory complications were more likely to develop, with subsequent higher morbidity and mortality rates. In the 1960s two reports supported this suspicion. Turill and collaborators, at Los Angeles County Hospital, found the mortality rate to be fivefold higher in diabetic than in nondiabetic patients, with deaths occurring almost exclusively in patients admitted with complicated cholelithiasis undergoing emergent surgery.[123] Advancing age was also a factor because diabetic patients in their fifth and sixth decades of life, undergoing emergency surgery for complicated cholelithiasis, had a 20-fold greater mortality than for nondiabetic patients. In 1962, Mundth compared diabetic and nondiabetic patients operated on for gallstones over a 15-year period[124] and found higher mortality and morbidity in diabetic patients operated on for complicated cholelithiasis, but not in those undergoing elective surgery. Thus oral cholecystography was performed in diabetic patients as a screening measure for gallstones, and early prophylactic cholecystectomy was then performed in all diabetic patients having no surgical contraindications.

The existence of comorbid conditions rather than diabetes as a single risk factor may be a more important predictor of outcome. Haff and coworkers studied 1000 consecutive patients who underwent biliary tract surgery to identify factors that influenced morbidity.[125] Diabetic patients had more complications than nondiabetic patients, but these differences vanished when the data were corrected for the presence of cardiovascular disease and other associated illnesses. Later, Walsh and associates demonstrated that rates of death among diabetic patients and nondiabetic patients undergoing biliary tract surgery were nearly identical.[126] The authors attributed this to advances in antibiotic therapy and postoperative hemodynamic monitoring. The presence of renal and vascular occlusive disease were the two major determinants of postoperative morbidity. In 1988, however, Hickman and colleagues studied the influence of diabetes on morbidity and mortality of patients undergoing surgery for acute cholecystitis, and found that infectious complications occurred threefold more often in diabetic patients than in nondiabetic controls, and all deaths (4.2%) occurred in diabetic patients as a result of sepsis.[127] Concurrent medical disease was more common in diabetic patients than in nondiabetic patients, but did not account for all of the increased morbidity. Ransohoff and associates reviewed the course of acute cholecystitis between 1960 and 1981 in 311 patients.[128] Death occurred in 3 of 46 patients with diabetes and 1 of 263 without diabetes. The difference was not statistically significant. In contrast, patients in this study who had azotemia were found to have a markedly higher mortality rate compared with patients without azotemia (27% compared with 2%).[128] These data support the importance of comorbid diseases and imply that complications of renal or vascular disease are more important in escalating the risk of morbidity and mortality in patients with biliary tract disease than is diabetes alone.

Friedman and coworkers used decision analysis to assess whether diabetic patients with asymptomatic gallstones should have expectant management or prophylactic cholecystectomy.[130] Three variables were studied as to their influence on the optimal choice of therapy: the rate at which diabetic patients develop symptoms, the probability of requiring emergency surgery once symptomatic, and the mortality rate during emergency surgery. Their conclusion favored expectant management over prophylactic cholecystectomy in diabetic patients with asymptomatic gallstones.[129] However, estimates of these variables in some cases were only educated guesses since true data on the natural history of diabetic patients with gallstones are scarce.

Laparoscopic cholecystectomy has now become the procedure of choice as it shortens hospital stay and may reduce the cost of surgery. Less than 5% of patients will require conversion to the standard open cholecystectomy for technical reasons.[130] The mortality associated with laparoscopic cholecystectomy in the 1990s (0–0.1%) was less than the mortality associated with open cholecystectomy (0.17–1.80%) in the 1980s. The incidence of common duct injury associated with laparoscopic cholecystectomy was higher in the 1990s than in the 1980s, when open cholecystectomy was widely used.[131-135] As surgeons become more experienced with laparoscopy, the morbidity associated with the procedure should decrease.

Other therapeutic options are available for patients who are poor operative candidates or who refuse surgery. These include dissolution therapy with oral bile salts or extracorporeal shock-wave lithotripsy. Only a small subset of patients with symptomatic gallstones are appropriate candidates for these therapies. Candidates for treatment with bile salts include those with noncalcified cholesterol gallstones and a patent cystic duct. The composition of stones can be determined indirectly by oral cholecystography or ultrasound. Small stones that appear to float on an oral cholecystograph are mostly cholesterol, and are more likely to dissolve with oral therapy. Success rates for stone dissolution are about 60% for those patients who meet optimal criteria. However, successful dissolution of 30% is more typical, and gallstones frequently recur after bile salt therapy is stopped.[136] In one study of 40 patients who were followed to complete dissolution of their gallstones, 43% had stone recurrence after 4 years, but only 49% had recurrence when observed after 11 years.[137]

Extracorporeal biliary lithotripsy uses high-amplitude sound waves that can fragment gallstones but pass through most soft tissue without harm. A functioning gallbladder is essential to allow emptying of the fragments into the common bile duct and subsequently into the small intestine. Success rates for this therapy depend on (1) stone characteristics of size, number, and composition; (2) energy and number of shock waves administered; (3) use of adjuvant bile acid therapy; and (4) gallbladder emptying.[138]

LIVER

Diabetes Mellitus and Liver Disease

Glycogen-Laden Hepatomegaly

Diabetes mellitus is associated with an increased frequency and variety of hepatic histopathologic lesions. A common lesion is an increase in liver glycogen demonstrated both at autopsy and in biopsy material (Fig. 52-3). This accumulation of glycogen produces a clear appearance in the cytoplasm and vacuolization of the hepatocyte nuclei.[139] It has been reported in up to 80% of both type 1 and type 2 diabetic patients. Increased glycogen infiltration appears to be associated with treatment with large amounts of insulin, particularly in young, brittle diabetic patients. This process resolves with reduction of insulin levels.[140]

Fatty Liver

The accumulation of triglycerides in the liver of diabetic patients may result in steatosis. Fatty liver is especially prevalent in patients with type 2 diabetes, particularly in the presence of obesity. Approximately 50% of obese type 2 diabetics will have biopsy-proven excess fat in their liver.[141] In T1DM, fatty liver is usually found in the setting of inadequate diabetic control[142] and is one-tenth as frequent as in T2DM. The pathophysiologic basis for the development of diabetic fatty liver is poorly understood. Accumulation of fat as intracellular lipid occurs because the rate of

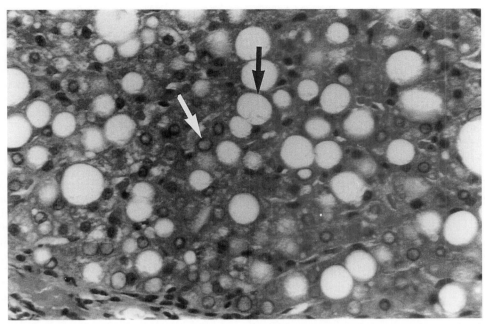

FIGURE 52-3. Liver biopsy in a type 2 diabetic patient demonstrating glycogen deposition (**white arrow**) and fatty metamorphosis (steatosis) (**black arrow**).

triglyceride synthesis exceeds the liver's capacity to secrete newly formed triglyceride as very low density lipoprotein (VLDL).[140]

In T1DM, fat deposition may result from insulin deficiency and hyperglycemia, both of which enhance the release of free fatty acids from adipose tissue. This provides substrate for hepatic triglyceride synthesis. In addition, low insulin levels may lead to reduced triglyceride secretion by the liver.

In T2DM, fatty liver appears to be a manifestation of obesity and insulin resistance rather than hyperglycemia and insulin deficiency. The greater dietary intake of fats and carbohydrates and portal hyperinsulinemia lead to increased synthesis of hepatic triglycerides at a rate that exceeds the liver's capacity to secrete newly formed VLDL. Reducing caloric intake or dietary intake of carbohydrates can reverse the fat deposition.[140,143]

Clinically, steatosis in diabetic patients leads to hepatomegaly, and occasionally tenderness to palpation in T1DM. Liver biochemistries are often normal or minimally elevated. Findings on liver biopsy include large cytoplasmic fat globules that displace the cell nucleus by light microscopy and abnormal mitochondria and displacement of organelles by fat globules on electron microscopy.

A controversial issue has been whether associated obesity rather than diabetes accounts for the fatty infiltration. Observations support the former because (1) similar hepatic histologic changes are seen in nondiabetic obese patients, (2) fatty liver is ten times more frequent in T2DM, where obesity is common, and (3) steatosis in diabetic patients may regress with weight reduction.[144–147]

Cirrhosis

Diabetes mellitus is also associated with cirrhosis of the liver. Recent data suggest that steatosis alone can progress directly to cirrhosis. Diabetic patients with steatosis may have intracytoplasmic hyaline and centrilobular fibrosis by light microscopy, and collagen bundles lining the space of Disse by electron microscopy.[148] These changes may represent the initial fibrotic steps leading to a cir-

rhotic liver. A recent study found that T2DM was significantly more common in cryptogenic cirrhotic patients and nonalcoholic steatohepatitis (NASH) patients than cirrhotic patients with primary biliary cirrhosis (PBC) or hepatitis C. The authors suggest that NASH may be a cause of cryptogenic cirrhosis. A recent study published by the Mayo Clinic found that older age, obesity, diabetes mellitus, and an AST:ALT ratio greater than 1 were good predictors of significant liver fibrosis (bridging/cirrhosis) in patients with NASH.[149]

Conversely, established liver disease from any cause may lead to glucose intolerance. Carbohydrate intolerance is seen in approximately 50% of patients with liver disease and 80% of patients with cirrhosis.[111] This is suggested to be secondary to impaired binding and degradation of insulin by the liver due to a reduced first-pass effect.[110] However, glucose intolerance also occurs in cases of liver disease with low insulin levels. The carbohydrate intolerance is most likely due to a multitude of biochemical and physiologic derangements that accompany liver disease, including portal–systemic shunting of glucose, elevated glucagon[150-153] and growth hormone[154] levels, peripheral and hepatic resistance to insulin, malnutrition, elevated levels of free fatty acids, and hypokalemia.[115]

Hepatitis

A diabetic patient is at increased risk for developing viral hepatitis (B and C) with a rate 2–4 times that of a control population.[155] One study demonstrated an increased HBsAg in diabetics subjects compared with age- and sex-matched controls.[156] Likely factors include frequent hospital exposures[156] and perhaps an increased susceptibility to infection. Previously, the high incidence of hepatitis in diabetes was attributed to frequent needle sticks, but with the advent of sterile disposable syringes, this no longer remains a valid postulate. Furthermore, several retrospective studies have shown a stronger association between hepatitis C infection and diabetes mellitus when compared with other types of hepatitis.[157-160] About 20% of patients with hepatitis C cirrhosis have diabetes mellitus, compared with only about 9% of patients with hepatitis B cirrhosis.[158] Others, however, have not found this association between hepatitis C infection and diabetes [AQ 14]mellitus.[161] Alfa-interferon therapy should be administered with caution in patients with diabetes mellitus. It has been reported that 10% of patients with hepatitis developed insulin autoantibodies after 6 weeks of therapy with INFα.[162] On the other hand, two large studies that examined the adverse effects of INFα in patients with chronic viral hepatitis found that less than 1% develop clinical diabetes mellitus.[163-165] A recent study observed improved glucose tolerance in patients with chronic hepatitis treated with INFα, regardless of whether they had a previous history of diabetes or not.[164]

The treatment of diabetic patients with oral hypoglycemic agents also may increase the risk of hepatic dysfunction. The sulfonylureas (chlorpropamide, tolazide, tolbutamide, and acetohexamide) have each rarely been associated with jaundice. The highest reported incidence occurs with chlorpropamide, at a rate of 0.5–1.0%.[166] The toxic effect is usually cholestasis, but hepatocellular injury or a mixed picture are occasionally seen.[166] Less frequently, hepatocellular necrosis can occur secondary to a hypersensitivity reaction to the central sulfonyl group, which acts as the antigenic stimulus. Rarely, the formation of granulomatous liver disease has been attributed to these agents.[167]

Hemochromatosis

The association between hemochromatosis and diabetes mellitus was first clinically recognized by Trosier in 1871,[168] and later the term "bronze diabetes" was coined by Hanot and Schachmann.[169] This disorder of iron metabolism has a high incidence of concomitant diabetes, with a rate of 75%, according to Saudek[170] (rates in other series range from 14–91%). Different pathogenetic mechanisms have been proposed, and two deserve particular attention.[171]

Theoretically, extensive iron deposits in the pancreas can result in diabetes. Support rests on pathologic changes in the pancreas with extensive hemosiderin deposits in nearly all cases in which hepatic iron deposition is also noted.[171] In addition, other secondary causes of iron overload such as thalassemia and excessive blood transfusions are associated with glucose intolerance or diabetes.[170-172] Third, the glucose intolerance observed with hemochromatosis may improve with phlebotomy.[173] However, it is likely that the development of diabetes is not solely due to pancreatic damage, because other forms of liver disease and cirrhosis are associated with glucose intolerance. Moreover, secondary causes of iron overload have been reported to produce insulin resistance that has been attributed to iron deposition in peripheral tissues. Data suggest that the carbohydrate intolerance results from a combination of iron overload in the liver and pancreas.

It has also been suggested that the association between diabetes mellitus and hemochromatosis is that they are genetically linked or that subclinical diabetes is exaggerated by hemochromatosis. This was first suggested by Balcerzak and coworkers, who studied five separate families with hemochromatosis.[174] Oral glucose tolerance, quantification of iron stores, and measurement of insulin levels was performed in 30 relatives of each of the five cases. They concluded that the association between these diseases was not due to iron overload, based on these observations: (1) diabetes mellitus occurred in 47% of family members with normal iron stores, (2) there was poor correlation between the amount of iron deposition and the presence of diabetes, (3) glucose intolerance appeared in family members despite adequate therapy for the hemochromatosis.[140,174] No correlation with HLA haplotypes between these diseases has been found.[140] However, some studies have shown a higher prevalence of the C282Y mutation of the hemochromatosis gene in patients with T2DM.

PANCREAS

Abnormalities of pancreatic exocrine secretion are seen commonly in diabetic patients. The abnormalities of secretion include decreased volume and amylase content, and at times reduced bicarbonate content. These abnormalities, which are usually not clinically apparent, may be due to vagal neuropathy, deficient stimulation by insulin, or inhibition by glucagon. Although patients with diabetes mellitus frequently have a 50–60% reduction in bicarbonate and enzyme secretion, this deficiency does not result in steatorrhea, nor is it likely to play a role in diabetic diarrhea.[175]

Acute Pancreatitis

Individuals with diabetes are at increased risk for acute pancreatitis. The damage appears to result from hypertriglyceridemia and/or vascular lesions in the diabetic pancreas. Acute pancreatitis may be lethal if it is associated with diabetic ketoacidosis because of a predisposition to hypovolemic shock.[176]

Acute pancreatitis in nondiabetic individuals often results in transient hyperglycemia and may induce glucose intolerance. Only rarely is there a progression to permanent diabetes. However, 21–26% of patients with acute necrotizing pancreatitis subsequently develop diabetes,[177] and 66–100% of those who undergo partial pancreatectomy develop diabetes. Hyperamylasemia occurs in up to 80% of patients with diabetic ketoacidosis. Its origin is purely pancreatic in only half of the cases and there is no correlation between the presence, degree, or type of amylase and gastrointestinal symptoms that occur with diabetic ketoacidosis.[178] Acidosis from any cause may result in nonpancreatic amylase elevation.

Chronic Pancreatitis

Pancreatic exocrine function is diminished in a high percentage of patients with diabetes mellitus, especially in patients with T1DM.[179] In addition, low levels of pancreatic lipase and immunoreactive trypsin have been found in T1DM.[180] Nakanishi and associates compared pancreatic duct morphology via endoscopic retrograde pancreatography in 43 patients with T1DM to that in 334 patients with T2DM.[181] They found that 40% of type 1 and 26% of type 2 diabetic patients had abnormal pancreatograms. A particularly high prevalence of ductal abnormalities was found in those who had slowly progressive T1DM. Pancreatic histopathologic analysis in patients with T1DM showed atrophy of exocrine pancreatic cells and infiltration with CD8 T lymphocytes.[181] In summary, there is increasing evidence of both structural and functional pancreatic exocrine abnormalities in T1DM.

The causes of pancreatic exocrine dysfunction in diabetes remain unknown. It has been postulated that the absence of the local trophic effects of insulin may cause this phenomenon. Diabetic microangiopathy could be a causative factor in diabetic pancreatic exocrine dysfunction, but investigations have found no correlation between pancreatic ductal changes and the extent of vascular abnormalities.[181] Interestingly, patients with diabetes may have autoantibodies to pancreatic cytokeratin, which is found in both the exocrine and endocrine pancreas, suggesting a possible immunologic pathogenesis.[181]

Conversely, chronic pancreatitis frequently results in glucose intolerance or overt diabetes. In Western societies, alcoholic chronic pancreatitis accounts for 0.5% of all diabetes. This results in sclerosis of the pancreatic islets and impaired insulin secretory response.[182] The typical patient with pancreatic diabetes gives a history of alcohol overindulgence for 5–15 years, followed by recurrent episodes of abdominal pain, and then by the appearance of diabetes, steatorrhea, or both, generally 1–20 years later. Patients with diabetes secondary to chronic pancreatitis often are very sensitive to insulin and therefore may be more susceptible to severe hypoglycemia.[183] Higher caloric intake is generally required because of the frequent finding of weight loss, due to malabsorption from associated pancreatic exocrine insufficiency. Therapeutically, these patients generally require pancreatic enzyme replacement as well.

Cystic Fibrosis

Cystic fibrosis is an autosomal recessive disorder that is linked to a gene found on chromosome 7.[184] Moderate to severe glucose intolerance occurs in approximately 40–50% of patients with cystic fibrosis, and virtually all cystic fibrosis patients have a diminished insulin secretory response.[185] The glucose intolerance appears to be a consequence of anatomic disorganization of the islets of Langerhans produced by pancreatic fibrosis. Additionally, studies have shown that patients with diabetes secondary to cystic fibrosis have predominantly pancreatic fibrosis as opposed to the replacement with adipose tissue seen in nondiabetic cystic fibrosis.[186]

Pancreatic Carcinoma

There appears to be an increased association between diabetes mellitus and carcinoma of the pancreas. It is not clear whether there is an increased risk of pancreatic carcinoma in patients with diabetes or whether the early diabetic manifestations are the result of an undiagnosed pancreatic tumor. Ishikawa and coworkers found a significantly higher incidence of hyperplastic and well-differentiated neoplastic changes of the pancreatic duct in patients with diabetes for greater than 2 years, and suggested that diabetes mellitus could be a cofactor for pancreatic carcinogenesis.[186] A recent Italian study found that of 720 patients with pancreatic cancer, 22% had diabetes, compared with only 8% of 720 matched controls.[187] However, when only patients with diabetes of 3 or more years' duration were considered, there was no significant difference between the groups. The study concludes that diabetes is not a risk factor for pancreatic cancer. A clue to the diagnoses of pancreatic carcinoma in a diabetic patient is the onset of weight loss and deterioration of glycemic control. Carbohydrate intolerance may manifest before the emergence of symptoms of pancreatic malignancy. Therefore pancreatic malignancy should be considered when poorly controlled diabetes develops in a thin, middle-aged, or elderly individual, particularly in the absence of a family history of diabetes, regardless of whether unexplained systemic symptoms coexist.

SUMMARY

This chapter has reviewed the relationships between diabetes mellitus and the gastrointestinal system. The protean manifestations of diabetes often eventuate in gastrointestinal problems, principally as a consequence of autonomic visceral neuropathy. The mechanisms, clinical presentations, and treatment strategies for each of these have been explored. In addition, those disorders of the gastrointestinal system that have a special relationship with diabetes were discussed. The physiologic and possible pathophysiologic relationships between gastrointestinal hormones and islet cell function are explored in Chaps. 4 and 6.

REFERENCES

1. Mandelstam P, Lieber A: Esophageal dysfunction in diabetic neuropathy-gastroenteropathy. *JAMA* 1967;201:88.
2. Loo FD, Dodds WJ, Soergel KH, *et al*: Multipeaked esophageal peristaltic pressure waves in patients with diabetic neuropathy. *Gastroenterology* 1985;88:485.
3. Pozzi M, Rivolta M, Gelosa M, *et al*: Upper gastrointestinal involvement in diabetes mellitus: Study of esophagogastric function. *Acta Diabetol Lat* 1988;25:333.
4. Horowitz M, Maddox AF, Wishart JM, *et al*: Relationships between esophageal transit and solid and liquid gastric emptying in diabetes mellitus. *Eur J Nucl Med* 1991;18:229.
5. Clouse RE, Lustman PJ, Reidel WL: Correlation of esophageal motility abnormalities with neuropsychiatric status in diabetics. *Gastroenterology* 1986;90:1146.
6. Smith B: Neuropathy of the oesophagus in diabetes mellitus. *J Neurosurg Psych* 1974;37:1151.
7. Medoff G: Controversial areas in antifungal chemotherapy: Short course and combination therapy with amphotericin B. *Rev Infect Dis* 1987;9:403.
8. Rundles RW: Diabetic neuropathy: General reviews with report of 125 cases. *Medicine* 1945;???:111.
9. Kassander P: Asymptomatic gastric retention in diabetics (gastroparesis diabeticorum). *Ann Intern Med* 1958;48:797.
10. Okanoue T, Sakamoto S, Itoh Y, *et al*: Side effects of high dose interferon therapy for chronic hepatitis C. *J Hepatol* 1996;25:283.
11. Feldman M, Borbett DB, Ramsey EJ, *et al*: Abnormal gastric function in longstanding, insulin-dependent diabetic patients. *Gastroenterology* 1979;77:12.
12. Rothstein RD: Gastrointestinal motility disorders in diabetes mellitus. *Am J Gastroenterol* 1990;85:782.
13. Schiller LR, Santa Ana CA, Schmulen AC, *et al*: Pathogenesis of fecal incontinence in diabetes mellitus: evidence for internal anal sphincter dysfunction. *N Engl J Med* 1982;307:1666.
14. Achem-Karam SR, Funakosh A, Vinik AI, *et al*: Plasma motilin concentration and interdigestive migrating motor complex in diabetic gastroparesis: Effect of metoclopramide. *Gastroenterology* 1985;88:492.
15. Funakosh A, Glowniak J, Owyang C, *et al*: Evidence for cholinergic and vagal noncholinergic mechanisms modulating plasma motilin-like immunoreactivity. *J Clin Endocrinol Metab* 1982;54:1129.
16. Falchuk KR, Conlin D: The intestinal and liver complications of diabetes mellitus. *Adv Intern Med* 1993;38:269.
17. Feldman M, Smith HJ, Simon TR: Gastric emptying of solid radiopaque markers: Studies in healthy subjects and diabetic patients. *Gastroenterology* 1984;87:895.
18. Mazzotta LJ, Go VWL: Gastric motor abnormalities in diabetic and post-vagotomy gastroparesis: Effect of metoclopramide and bethanechol. *Gastroenterology* 1980;78:286.
19. Mearin F, Camilleri M, Malagelada JR: Pyloric dysfunction in diabetics with recurrent nausea and vomiting. *Gastroenterology* 1986;90:1919.
20. Meyer JE: Motility of the stomach and gastroduodenal junction. In: Johnson LR, ed. *Physiology of the Gastrointestinal Tract.* Raven Press:1987;393.

21. Hamilton JW, Bellahsene BE, Reichelderfer M, *et al*: Human electro-gastrograms. Comparison of surface and mucosal recordings. *Dig Dis Sci* 1986;31:33.

22. Abell TL, Camilleri M, Malagelada J-R: High prevalence of gastric electrical dysrhythmias in diabetic gastroparesis. *Gastroenterology* 1985;88(Abstract):1299.

23. Koch KL, Stern RM, Vasey MW, *et al*: Gastric dysrhythmias and nausea of pregnancy. *Dig Dis Sci* 1987;32(Abstract):917.

24. Abell TTL, Malagelada J-R, Lucas AR, *et al*: Gastric electromechanical and neurohormonal function in anorexia nervosa. *Gastroenterology* 1987;93:958.

25. Stern RM, Koch KL, Stewart WR, *et al*: Spectral analysis of tachygastria recorded during motion sickness. *Gastroenterology* 1987; 92:92.

26. Abell TL, Malagelada JR: Glucagon-evoked gastric dysrhythmias in humans shown by improved electrogastrographic technique. *Gastroenterology* 1985;88:1932.

27. Koch KL, Stern RM, Stewart WR, *et al*: Gastric emptying and gastric myoelectric activity in patients with diabetic gastroparesis and effect of long-term domperidone treatment. *Am J Gastroenterol* 1989; 84:1069.

28. Liberski SM, Koch KL, Atnip RG, *et al*: Ischemic gastroparesis: Resolution after revascularization. *Gastroenterology* 1990;99:252.

29. Dooley CP, Newihi HM, Zeidler A, *et al*: Abnormalities of the migrating motor complex in diabetics with autonomic neuropathy and diarrhea. *Scand J Gastroenterol* 1988;23:217.

30. You CH, Lee KY, Chey WY: Gastric electromyography in normal and abnormal states in humans. In: Chey WY, ed. *Functional Disorders of the Digestive Tract*. Raven Press:1983;167.

31. Parkman HP, Schwartz SS: Esophagitis and gastroduodenal disorders associated with diabetic gastroparesis. *Arch Intern Med* 1987; 147:1477.

32. Schuurkes JAJ, Helsen LFM, Van Neuten JM: A comparative study on the effects of domperidone, metoclopramide, clebopride and trimebutine on the gastroduodenal preparation of the guinea pig. *Eur J Pharmacol* 1985;39:123.

33. Brogden RN, Carmine AA, Heel RC, *et al*: Domperidone: A review of its pharmacologic activity, pharmacokinetics and therapeutic efficacy in the treatment of chronic dyspepsia and as an antiemetic. *Drugs* 1982;24:360.

34. Tomomasa T, Kuroume T, Ara H, *et al*: Erythromycin induces migrating motor complex in human gastrointestinal tract. *Dig Dis Sci* 1986; 31:157.

35. Ricci DA, Saltzman MB, Meyer C, *et al*: Effect of metoclopramide in diabetic gastroparesis. *J Clin Gastroenterol* 1985;7:25.

36. Schade RR, Dugas MC, Lhotsky DM, *et al*: Effect of metoclopramide on gastric liquid emptying in patients with diabetic gastroparesis. *Dig Dis Sci* 1985;30:10.

37. McCallum RW, Ricci DA, Rakatansky H, *et al*: A multicenter, placebo controlled clinical trial of oral metoclopramide in diabetic gastroparesis. *Diabetes Care* 1983;6:463.

38. Ricci DA, Saltzman MB, Meyer C, *et al*: Effect of metoclopramide in diabetic gastroparesis. *J Clin Gastroenterol* 1985;7:25.

39. Snape WJ, Battle WM, Schwartz SS, *et al*: Metoclopramide to treat gastroparesis due to diabetes mellitus. *Ann Intern Med* 1982;96:444.

40. Schade RR, Dugas MC, Lhotsky DM, *et al*: Effect of metoclopramide on gastric liquid emptying in patients with diabetic gastroparesis. *Dig Dis Sci* 1985;30:10.

41. Albibi R, McCallum RW: Metoclopramide: Pharmacology and clinical application. *Ann Intern Med* 1983;98:86.

42. Heer M, Moller-Duysing W, Benes I, *et al*: Diabetic gastroparesis: Treatment with domperidone—a double-blind, placebo-controlled trial. *Digestion* 1983;27:214.

43. Davis RH, Clench MH, Mathias JR: Effects of domperidone in patients with chronic, unexplained gastrointestinal symptoms: A double-blind, placebo-controlled study. *Dig Dis Sci* 1988;33:1505.

44. McCallum RW: Review of the current stains of prokinetic agents in gastroenterology. *Am J Gastroenterol* 1985;80:1008.

45. Janssens J, Peeters TL, Vantrappen G, *et al*: Improvement of gastric emptying in diabetic gastroparesis by erythromycin. *N Engl J Med* 1990;22:1028.

46. Peeters TL, Annese V, Depoortere I, *et al*: Effect of erythromycin on gastric motility in controls and in diabetic gastroparesis. *Gastroenterology* 1992;103:72.

47. Ishii M, Nakamura T, Kasai F, et al. Erythromycin derivative improves gastic empting and insulin requirement in diabetic patients with gastroparesis. *Diabetes Care* 1997;1134-1137.

48. Reardon TM, Schnell GA, Smith OJ, *et al*: Surgical therapy of diabetic gastroparesis. *J Clin Gastroenterol* 1989;11:204.

49. Angervall L, Dotevall G, Lehmann KE: The gastric mucosa in diabetes mellitus. A functional and histopathological study. *Acta Med Scand* 1961;169:339.

50. Aylett P: Gastric emptying and secretion in patients with diabetes mellitus. *Gut* 1965;6:262.

51. Green A, Jaspan J, Kavin H, *et al*: Influence of long-term aldose reductase inhibitor therapy on autonomic dysfunction of urinary bladder, stomach and cardiovascular systems in diabetic patients. *Diabetes Res Clin Pract* 1987;4:67.

52. Gramm HF, Reuter K, Costell P: The radiologic manifestations of diabetic gastric neuropathy and its differential diagnosis. *Gastrointest Radiol* 1978;3:151.

53. Ungar B, Stocks AE, Martin FI, *et al*: Intrinsic-factor antibody, parietal-cell antibody, and latent pernicious anaemia in diabetes mellitus. *Lancet* 1968;2:415.

54. Gullo L: Diabetes and the risk of pancreatic cancer. *Ann Oncol* 1999; 10(Suppl 4):S79.

55. Fine KD, Fordtran JS. The effect of diarrhea on fecal fat excretion. *Gastroenterology* 1992;102:1936-1939.

56. Litwin DE: Laparoscopic cholecystectomy. Trans-Canada experience with 2201 cases. *Can J Surg* 1992;35:291.

57. Schiller LR, Santa Ana, CA, Schmulen AC, et al. Pathogenesis of Fecal incontinence in diabetes mellitus: evidence for internal anal sphincter dysfunction. *New Engl J Med* 1982;307:1666-1671.

58. Badiga MS, Jain NK, Casanova C, *et al*: Diarrhea in diabetics: The role of sorbitol. *J Am Coll Nutr* 1990;9:578.

59. Chang EB, Bergenstal RM, Field M: Diabetic diarrhea: Loss of adrenergic regulation of intestinal fluid and electrolyte transport. *Gastroenterology* 1983;84(Abstract):1121.

60. French JM, Hall G, Parish DJ, *et al*: Peripheral and autonomic nerve involvement in primary amyloidosis associated with uncontrollable diarrhea and steatorrhea. *Am J Med* 1965;39:277.

61. Malins JM, Mayne N: Diabetic diarrhea: A study of 13 patients with jejunal biopsy. *Diabetes* 1969;18:858.

62. Ogbonnaya K, Arem R: Diabetic diarrhea: Pathophysiology, diagnosis and management. *Arch Intern Med* 1990;150:262.

63. Chang E, Fedorak R, Field M: Experimental diabetic diarrhea in rats. *Gastroenterology* 1986;91:564.

64. Chang E, Bergenstal R, Field M: Diarrhea in streptozotocin-treated rats. *J Clin Invest* 1985;75:1666.

65. Fedorak RN, Field M, Chang EB: Treatment of diabetic diarrhea with clonidine. *Ann Intern Med* 1985;102:197.

66. Migliore A, Barone C, Manna R, *et al*: Diabetic diarrhea and clonidine. *Ann Intern Med* 1988;109:170(Letter).

67. Yang R, Arem R, Chan L: Gastrointestinal tract complications of diabetes mellitus: Pathophysiology and management. *Arch Intern Med* 1984;144:1251.

68. Keshavarzian A, Iber F: Gastrointestinal involvement in insulin-requiring diabetes mellitus. *J Clin Gastroenterol* 1987;9:685.

69. Ogbonnaya KI, Arem R: Diabetic diarrhea: Pathophysiology, diagnosis and management. *Arch Intern Med* 1990;150:262.

70. Larson GM: Multipractice analysis of laparoscopic cholecystectomy in 1983 patients. *Am J Surg* 1992;163:221.

71. Mulvihill SJ: Laparoscopic management of gallstone disease. *Semin Gastrointest Dis* 1994;5:120.

72. Scarpello JHB, Hague RV, Cullen DR, *et al*: The ^{14}C-glycocholate test in diabetic diarrhea. *Br Med J* 1976;2:673.

73. Wald A, Tunuguntla AK: Anorectal sensorimotor dysfunction in fecal incontinence and diabetes mellitus: Modification with biofeedback therapy. *N Engl J Med* 1984;310:1282.

74. Tsai S-T, Vinik AI, Brunner JF: Diabetic diarrhea and somatostatin. *Ann Intern Med* 1986;104:894(Letter).

75. Dudl RJ, Anderson DS, Forsythe AB, *et al*: Treatment of diabetic diarrhea and orthostatic hypotension with somatostatin analogue SMS 201-995. *Am J Med* 1987;83:584.

76. Walsh CH, Cooper BT, Wright AD, *et al*: Diabetes mellitus and coeliac disease: A clinical study. *Q J Med* 1978;47:89.

77. Maeki M, Hallstoem O, Huuponen T, *et al*: Increased prevalence of coeliac disease in diabetes. *Arch Dis Child* 1984;59:739.

78. Falchuk ZM, Rogentine GN, Strober W: Predominance of histocompatibility antigen HL-A8 in patients with gluten-sensitive enteropathy. *J Clin Invest* 1972;51:1602.

79. Cudworth AG, Woodrow JC: Genetic susceptibility in diabetes mellitus: Analysis of the HLA association. *Br Med J* 1976;2:846.

80. Battle WM, Snape WJ Jr., Alavi A, et al: Colonic dysfunction in diabetes mellitus. *Gastroenterology* 1980;79:1217.

81. Battle WM, Cohen JD, Snape WJ Jr.: Disorders of colonic motility in patients with diabetes mellitus. *Yale J Biol Med* 1983;56:277.

82. Snape WJ Jr.: Myoelectric and motor activity of the colon in normal and abnormal states. *Scand J Gastroenterol* 1984;96(Suppl):55.

83. Caviezel F, Bossi A, Baresi A, et al: Ano-rectal manometry as an evaluating test for impaired ano-rectal function in diabetes mellitus. *Acta Diabetol Lat.* 1986;23:331.

84. Morgenstern L, Wong L, Berci G: Twelve hundred open cholecystectomies before the laparoscopic era. A standard for comparison. *Arch Surg* 1992;127:400.

85. The Southern Surgeons Club: A prospective analysis of 1518 laparoscopic cholecystectomies. *N Engl J Med* 1991;324:1073.

86. Braverman DZ: The lack of effect of metoclopramide on gallbladder volume and contraction in diabetic cholecystoparesis. *Am J Gastroenterol* 1986;81:960.

87. Mitsukawa T, Takemura J, Ohgo S: Gallbladder function and plasma cholecystokinin levels in diabetes mellitus. *Am J Gastroenterol.* 1990; 85:981.

88. Shaw SJ, Hajnal F, Lebovitz Y, et al: Gallbladder dysfunction in diabetes mellitus. *Dig Dis* 1993;38:490.

89. Sarva RP, Schreiner DP, Van Thiel D, et al: Gallbladder function: Methods for measuring filling and emptying. *J Nucl Med* 1985; 26:140.

90. Schreiner DP, Sarva RP, Van Thiel D, et al: Gallbladder function in diabetic patients. *J Nucl Med* 1986;27:357.

91. Stone BG, Gavaler JS, Belk SH, et al: Impairment of gallbladder emptying in diabetes mellitus. *Gastroenterology* 1988;95:170.

92. Ikard R: Gallstones, cholecystitis and diabetes. *Surg Gynecol Obstet* 1990;171:528.

93. Fiorucci S, Bosso R, Sciouti L, et al: Neurohumoral control of gallbladder motility in healthy subjects and diabetic patients with or without autonomic neuropathy. *Dig Dis* 1990;35:1089.

94. Ishii M, Nakamura T, Kasai F, et al: Erythromycin derivative improves gastric emptying and insulin requirement in diabetic patients with gastroparesis. *Diabetes Care* 1997;20:1134.

95. Catnach SM, Ballinger AB, Stevens M, et al. Erythromycin induces supranormal gallbladder contractions in diabetic autonomic neuropathy. *Gut* 1993;34(8):1123-1127

96. Diehl AK: Epidemiology and natural history of gallstone disease. *Gastroenterol Clin North Am* 1991;20:1.

97. Warren S: Recent advances in the pathology of diabetes mellitus. *Rhode Island Med J* 1938;21:117.

98. Lieber MM: The incidence of gallstones and their correlation with other disease. *Ann Surg* 1952;135:394.

99. Zaher Z, Sternley NH, Kagon A, et al: Frequency of cholelithiasis in Prague and Malmo; an autopsy study. *Scand J Gastroenterol* 1974; 9:3.

100. Honore LH: The lack of a positive association between symptomatic cholesterol cholelithiasis and clinical diabetes mellitus: A retrospective study. *J Chron Dis* 1980;33:465.

101. McSherry CK, Ferstenberg H, Calhoun WF, et al: The natural history of diagnosed gallstone disease in symptomatic and asymptomatic patients. *Ann Surg* 1985;202:59.

102. The Rome Group for Epidemiology and Prevention of Cholelithiasis (GREPCO): The epidemiology of gallstone disease in Rome, Italy. II: Factors associated with the disease. *Hepatology* 1988;8:907.

103. Barbara L, Sama C, Labate AM, et al: A population study on the prevalence of gallstone disease: The Sirmione study. *Hepatology* 1987;7:913.

104. Jorgenson T: Gallstones in a Danish population: Relation to weight, physical activity, smoking, coffee consumption and diabetes mellitus. *Gut* 1989;30:528.

105. Kono S, Kochi S, Ohyama S, et al: Gallstones, serum lipids and glucose tolerance among male officials of self-defense forces in Japan. *Dig Dis* 1988;33:839.

106. Maculure KM, Hayes KC, Colditz GA, et al: Weight, diet and the risk of symptomatic gallstones in middle-aged women. *N Engl J Med* 1989;321:563.

107. Thijs C, Knipschild P, Brombacher P: Serum lipids and gallstones: A case control study. *Gastroenterology* 1990;99:843.

108. Ahlberg J, Angelin B, Einarsson K, et al: Prevalence of gallbladder disease in hyperlipoproteinemia. *Dig Dis* 1979;24:459.

109. Ponz de Leon M, Ferenderes R, Carvlli N: Bile lipid composition and bile acid pool size in diabetics. *Am J Dig Dis* 1978;23:710.

110. Meinders AE, Van Berge Henegovwen G, Willekens F, et al: Biliary lipid and bile acid composition in insulin dependent diabetes mellitus. Arguments for increased intestinal bacterial bile acid degradation. *Dig Dis Sci* 1981;26:402.

111. Scragg RG, Calvert GD, Oliver JR: Plasma lipids and insulin in gallstone disease: A case-control study. *Br Med J* 1984;289:521.

112. Laasko M, Schonen M, Julkunen R, et al: Plasma insulin, serum lipids and lipoproteins in gallstone disease in non-insulin diabetic subjects: A case-control study. *Gut* 1990;31:344.

113. Bennion L, Grundy S: Effects of diabetes mellitus on cholesterol metabolism in man. *N Engl J Med* 1977;296:1365.

114. Gracie WA, Ransohoff DR: The natural history of silent gallstones: The innocent gallstone is not a myth. *N Engl J Med* 1982; 307:798.

115. Ransohoff DF, Gracie WA, Wolfenson LB, et al: Prophylactic cholecystectomy of expectant management for silent gallstones: A decision analysis to assess survival. *Ann Intern Med* 1983;99:199.

116. Pattison AC, Turill FL, McCarron MM, et al: Gallstones and diabetes: An ominous association. *Am J Surg* 1961;102:184.

117. Rabinowitch IM: On the mortality resulting from surgical treatment of chronic gallbladder disease in diabetes mellitus. *Ann Surg* 1932; 96:70.

118. Eisele HE: Results of gallbladder surgery in diabetes mellitus. *Ann Surg* 1943;118:107.

119. Turner RJ, Becker WF, Coleman WO, et al: Acute cholecystitis in the diabetic. *South Med J* 1961;102:184.

120. Abramson DJ: Diabetes mellitus and cholecystectomy. *Ann Surg* 1957;145:371.

121. Schein CJ: Acute cholecystitis in the diabetic. *Am J Gastroenterol* 1969;51:511.

122. Roslyn JJ, Thompson JE, Darvin H, et al: Risk factors for gallbladder perforation. *Am J Gastroenterol* 1987;82:636.

123. Turill FL, McCarron MM, Mikkelson WP: Gallstones and diabetes: An ominous association. *Am J Surg* 1961;102:184.

124. Mundth ED: Cholecystitis and diabetes mellitus. *N Engl J Med* 1962; 267:642.

125. Haff RC, Butcher HR, Ballinger WF: Factors influencing morbidity in biliary tract operations. *Surg Gynecol Obstet* 1971;132:195.

126. Walsh DB, Eckhauser FE, Ramsburgh SR, et al: Risk associated with diabetes mellitus in patients undergoing gallbladder surgery. *Surgery* 1982;91:254.

127. Hickman MS, Schwesinger WH, Page CP: Acute cholecystitis in the diabetic. *Arch Surg* 1988;123:409.

128. Ransohoff DF, Miller GL, Forsythe SB, et al: Outcome of acute cholecystitis in patients with diabetes mellitus. *Ann Intern Med* 1987; 106:829.

129. Friedman L, Roberts MS, Brett AS, et al: Management of asymptomatic gallstones in the diabetic patient. *Ann Intern Med* 1988; 109:913.

130. The Southern Surgeon Club: A prospective analysis of 1518 laparoscopic cholecystectomies. *N Engl J Med* 1991;324:1073.

131. Litwin DE, Laparoscopic cholecystectomy. Trans-Canada Experience with 2201 Cases. *Can J Surg* 1992;35:291

132. Larson GM. Multi-practice analysis of laparoscopy cholecystecomy in 1983 patients. *Am J Surg* 1992;163:221.

133. Mulvihill SJ. Laparoscopic management of gallstone. *Semin Gastrontest Dis.* 1994;5:120.

134. Morgenstern L, Wong L, Berci G. Twelve hundred open cholecystectomies before the laparoscopic era. A standard for comparison. *Arch Surg* 1992;127:400.

135. The Southern Surgeons Club. A prospective analysis of 1518 laparoscopic cholecystectomies. *N Engl J Med* 1991;324:1073.

136. Strasberg SM, Clavien PA: Cholecystolithiasis: Lithotherapy for the 1990's. *Hepatology* 1992;16:820.

137. O'Donnell LDJ, Heaton KW: Recurrence and re-recurrence of gallstones after medical dissolution: A long-term follow-up. *Gut* 1988; 20:655.

138. Paumgartner G: Nonoperative management of gallstone disease. In: Sleisenger MH, Fordtran JS, eds. *Gastrointestinal Disease*, 5th ed. Saunders:1993;1844.

139. Glick ME, Hoefs JC, Meshkinpour H: Glucose intolerance and hepatic, biliary tract and pancreatic dysfunction. *Dig Dis* 1987;5:78.

140. Stone BG, van Thiel DH: Diabetes mellitus and the liver. *Semin Liver Dis* 1985;5:8(Review).

141. Goodman JI: Hepatomegaly and diabetes mellitus. *Ann Intern Med* 1953;39:1077.

142. Creutzfeldt W, Frerichs H, Sickinger K: Liver diseases and diabetes mellitus. *Prog Liver Dis* 1970;3:371(Review).

143. Reaven GM, Bernstein RM: Effect of obesity on the relationship between very low density lipoprotein production rate and plasma triglyceride concentration in normal and hypertriglyceridemic subjects. *Metab Clin Exp* 1978;27:1047.

144. Batman P, Schever P: Diabetic hepatitis preceding the onset of glucose intolerance. *Histopathology* 1985;9:237.

145. Adler M, Schaffner F: Fatty liver hepatitis and cirrhosis in obese patients. *Am J Med* 1979;67:811.

146. Keefe E, Adesman P, Stenzel P, *et al*: Steatosis and cirrhosis in an obese diabetic. *Dig Dis Sci* 1987;32:441.

147. Balazs M, Halmos T: Electron microscopic study of liver fibrosis associated with diabetes mellitus. *Exp Pathol* 1985;97:153.

148. Johnson DG, Alberti KG, Faber OK, *et al*: Hyperinsulinism of hepatic cirrhosis: Diminished degradation or hypersecretion? *Lancet* 1977; 1(8001):10.

149 Angulo P, Keach JC, Batts KP, et al. Independent predictors of liver fibrosisi in patients with nonalcoholic steatohepatitis. *Hepatology* 1999;30(6): 1356-62.

150. Samaan NA, Stone DDB, Eckhardt RD: Serum glucose, insulin, and growth hormone in chronic hepatic cirrhosis. *Arch Intern Med* 1969; 124:149.

151. Podolsky S, Zimmerman HJ, Burrows BA, *et al*: Potassium depletion in hepatic cirrhosis. A reversible cause of impaired growth-hormone and insulin response to stimulation. *N Engl J Med* 1973;288:644.

152. Sherwin R, Joshi P, Hendler R, *et al*: Hyperglucagonemia in Laennec's cirrhosis. The role of portal-systemic shunting. *N Engl J Med* 1974;290:239.

153. Shurberg JL, Resnick RH, Koff RS, *et al*: Serum lipids, insulin, and glucagon after portacaval shunt in cirrhosis. *Gastroenterology* 1977; 72:301.

154. Conn HO, Daughaday WH: Cirrhosis and diabetes. V. Serum human growth hormone levels in Laennec's cirrhosis. *J Lab Clin Med* 1970; 76:678.

155. Creutzfeldt W, Frerichs H, Sickinger K: Liver diseases and diabetes mellitus. *Prog Liver Dis* 1970;13:371.

156. Khuri KG, Shamma MH, Abourizk N: Hepatitis B virus markers in diabetes mellitus. *Diabetes Care* 1985;8:250.

157. El-Zayadi AR, Selim OE, Hamdy H, et al. Association of Chronic Hepatitis C infection and diabetes mellitus. *Trop Gastroenterol* 1998; 19(4):141-144

158. Caronia S, Taylor K, Pagliaro L, et al. Futher evidence for an association between non-insulin dependent diabetes mellitus and chronic hepatitis C virus infection. *Hepatology* 1999;30(4):1059-63.

159. Allison ME, Wreghitt T, Palmer CR, Alexander GJ. Evidence for a link between hepatitis C virus infection and diabetes mellitus in a cirrhotic population. *J Hepatology* 1994;21(6):1135-1139.

160. Mason AL, Lau JY, Hoang N, et al. HCV and diabetes mellitus and chronic hepatitis C virus infection. *Hepatology* 1999;29(2):328-333.

161. Mangis A, Schiavone G, Lezzi G, et al. HCV and diabetes mellitus: Evidence for a negative association. *Am J Gastroenterol* 1998;93(12): 2363-2367.

162. Di Cesare E, Previtti M, Russo F, et al. Interferon-alpha therapy may induce insulin autoantibody development in patients with chronic viral hepatitis. *Dig Dis Sci* 1996;41(8):1672-1677,

163. Okanoue T, Sakamoto S, Itoh Y, et al. Side effects of high-dose interferon therapy for chronic hepatitis V. *J Hepatol* 1996;25(3):283-291.

164. Konard T, Vicini P, Zeuzem S, et al. Interferon-alpha improves glucose tolerance in diabetes and non-diabetes patients with HCV-induced liver disease. *Exp Clin Endocrinol* diabetes 1999;107(6):343-349.

165. Fattovich G, Giustina G, Favarato S, et al. A survey of adverse events in 11,241 patients wih chronic viral hepatitis treated with alpha interferon. *J Hepatol* 1996;24(1):38-47.

166. Schneider HL, Hornback KD, Kniaz JL, *et al*: Chlorpropamide hepatotoxicity: Report of a case and review of the literature. *Am J Gastroenterol* 1984;79:721.

167. Bloodworth JMB, Hamwi GJ: Histopathologic lesions associated with sulfonylurea administration. *Diabetes* 1959;10:90.

168. Trosier M: *Bull Soc Anat (Paris)* 1871;44:231.

169. Hanot V, Schachmann M: *Arch Physiol Norm Pathol* 1886;7:50.

170. Saudek CD: Diabetes and the diseases of iron excess. In: Podolsky S, Visnanathan M, eds. *Secondary Diabetes: The Spectrum of the Diabetic Syndromes*. Raven Press:1980.

171. Crosby WH: Hemochromatosis: The unsolved problems. *Semin Hematol* 1977;14:135.

172. Schafer I, Cheron RG, Dluhy R, *et al*: Biological consequences of acquired transfusional iron overload in adults. *N Engl J Med* 1981; 304:319.

173. Williams R, Smith PM, Spicer EJF, *et al*: Venesection therapy in idiopathic hemochromatosis. *Q J Med* 1969;149:1.

174. Balcerzak SP, Mintz DH, Westerman MP: Diabetes mellitus and idiopathic hemochromatosis. *Am J Med Sci.* 1968;255:53.

175. El Newihi H, Dooley CP, Saad C, *et al*: Impaired exocrine pancreatic function in diabetics with diarrhea and peripheral neuropathy. *Dig Dis Sci* 1988;33:705.

176. Trapnell JE, Duncan EH: Patterns of incidence in acute pancreatitis. *Br Med J* 1975;2(5964):179.

177. Eriksson J, Doepel M, Widen E, *et al*: Pancreatic surgery not pancreatitis, is the primary cause of diabetes after fulminant pancreatitis. *Gut* 1992;33:847.

178. Vincor F, Lehrner LM, Karn RC, *et al*: Hyperamylasemia in diabetic ketoacidosis: Sources and significance. *Ann Intern Med* 1979;91: 200.

179. Yokoyama J, Ohno M, Tajima N, *et al*: Evaluation of pancreatic exocrine function with the synthetic peptide BT-PABA in diabetes mellitus. *Mt Sinai J Med* 1982;49:18.

180. Junglee S, De Albarran R, Katarak A, *et al*: Low pancreatic lipase in insulin-dependent diabetics. *J Clin Radiol* 1983;36:200.

181. Nakanishi K, Kobayashi T, Miyashita H, *et al*: Exocrine pancreatic ductograms in insulin-dependent diabetes mellitus. *Am J Gastroenterol* 1994;89:762.

182. Vinik AL, Jackson WPU: Endocrine secretions in chronic pancreatitis. In: Prodolsky S, Viswanathan M, eds. *Secondary Diabetes: The Spectrum of the Diabetic Syndromes*. Raven Press:1980;165.

183. Linde J, Nilsson LH, Barany FR: Diabetes and hypoglycemia in chronic pancreatitis. *Scand J Gastroenterol* 1977;12:369.

184. Rommens JM, Iannuzzi MC, Kerem B, *et al*: Identification of the cystic fibrosis gene: Chromosome walking and jumping. *Science* 1989; 245:1059.

185. Handwerger S, Roth J, Gorden P, *et al*: Glucose intolerance in cystic fibrosis. *N Engl J Med* 1969;281:451.

186. Lohr M, Goertchen P, Nizze H, *et al*: Cystic fibrosis associated islet changes may provide a basis for diabetes. An immunocytochemical and morphometrical study. *Virchows Arch* 1989;414:179.

187. Ishikawa O, Ohhigashi H, Wada A, *et al*: Morphologic characteristics of pancreatic carcinoma with diabetes mellitus. *Cancer* 1989; 64:1107.

188. Gullo L. Diabetes and the risk of pancretic cancer. *Annals of Oncology* 1999;10;Suppl.4:s79-s81.

Diabetes and the Skin

John Olerud

The skin is the largest organ of the body, and it is readily available for inspection and scientific study. Small wonder there have been so many clinical and scientific studies related to the skin in patients with diabetes. The skin is affected in one way or another in essentially 100% of diabetic patients. Dysregulation of glucose, insulin, and lipids leads directly to physical signs in the skin of patients with diabetes.

Chronically elevated blood sugar results in nonenzymatic glycosylation (NEG) of cutaneous proteins, which eventually leads to irreversible advanced glycation end-products (AGEs; see Chap. 13).[1] AGEs have been proposed as the mechanism for clinical phenomena such as thickened skin and scleroderma-like changes seen in patients with diabetes,[2] as well as limited joint mobility (LJM).[3] Structural proteins, such as collagen, that have undergone NEG become insoluble and resistant to degradation.[1] Certain AGEs are clearly related to glycemic control, whereas others change with age as well as with glycemic control.[1,4,5] It is encouraging to note that intensive insulin therapy for patients in the Diabetes Control and Complication Trial (DCCT) resulted in lower levels of skin collagen AGEs in parallel with reduction in HbA$_{1c}$, as well as with reduction in the risk of retinopathy, nephropathy, and neuropathy.[6]

Normal activities of insulin and lipoprotein lipase are necessary for normal production and catabolism of certain plasma lipids, particularly very-low-density lipoproteins (VLDLs). Diabetes is the most common cause of severe hypertriglyceridemia[7] (see Chap. 47). Some individuals with insulin resistance and insufficient levels of insulin have high levels of serum triglycerides with cutaneous xanthomas, particularly the clinical variant known as eruptive xanthomas. On the other hand, individuals with insulin resistance and hyperinsulinemia may have the clinical manifestations of acanthosis nigricans.

In addition to these biochemical and endocrine influences on the skin, there are profound changes in cutaneous structure and function in diabetes based on abnormalities of nerves and blood vessels. Structural studies document that cutaneous sensory innervation is diminished in patients with diabetes compared with controls and even further diminished in diabetic patients with measurable neuropathy.[8] The most striking reduction in sensory innervation occurs in the epidermis.[9] These observations have been documented by functional studies as well.[10] There is a growing body of evidence that nerves and neuropeptides may be important for normal immune function[11] as well as for normal tissue repair.[12–14] Poor tissue repair and infections are contributing factors to skin ulcers. It has been documented that nonhealing ulcers are the most frequent proximal cause of amputation, which, as one would predict, is more common in patients with diabetic neuropathy.[15,16]

The cutaneous microvasculature likewise shows both structural and functional abnormalities and contributes to development of lower extremity ulcers. Structural abnormalities of blood vessels include (1) an increase in the overall thickness of the walls of the microvessels,[17] (2) an increased number of gaps between endothelial cells and pericytes in postcapillary venules,[18] (3) homogeneous basement membrane thickening (BMT) between endothelial cells and pericytes of dermal microvessels,[18,19] and (4) an increase in size and number of the periadventitial fibroblast-like cells (veil cells).[20]

Functional abnormalities of the diabetic microvasculature include (1) increased permeability,[21] increased baseline capillary pressure,[22] and decreased capillary peak blood flow following arterial occlusion[23]; (2) a normal resting blood flow to capillaries in dorsal fingers and toes, but a decreased response to heat-induced hyperemia[24]; and (3) an increased resting cutaneous blood flow in the legs and feet of diabetic patients with neuropathy, but a deficiency in the normal hyperemic response to heating.[25,26] The defective hyperemic response was greater on the legs than arms and correlated with duration of diabetes, retinopathy, and proteinuria.[26] Taken together, the observations regarding functional changes of the microvasculature in diabetes show the vessels to be "leakier," less constricted by the sympathetic nervous system at baseline, and less able to respond maximally to thermal and hypoxemic stress. The lower extremities generally are more affected than upper extremities.

In this chapter, we review the current literature regarding conditions that appear to be directly linked to the endocrine, vascular, neurologic, and immunologic impairment seen in diabetes mellitus (DM). These conditions include ulcers, acanthosis nigricans, diabetic thick skin, cutaneous infections, and cutaneous xanthomas. A number of other clinical conditions associated with diabetes will be reviewed, although the pathobiology of the disorders remains unclear. These include necrobiosis lipoidica, granuloma annulare, diabetic dermopathy, bullosis diabeticorum, and acquired perforating dermatosis. Glucagonoma and complications of insulin injection are reviewed as well because of their special importance in the management of diabetic patients.

DIABETIC ULCERS

Without question, the most important skin lesions in diabetic patients are lower extremity ulcers. Lower extremity ulcers cost the Medicare system $1.5 billion in 1995 (see Chap. 51).[27] Pecoraro and coworkers noted that ulcers were the proximal cause of amputation in 67 of 80 (84%) diabetic patients hospitalized for amputation.[15]

The annual incidence of foot ulcers was nearly 2% in a retrospective cohort study of 8905 patients with diabetes in a health maintenance organization.[28] It has been estimated that 15–24% of diabetic patients with foot ulcers will eventually undergo amputation.[29] A publication by the Centers for Disease Control (CDC) suggests that the vast majority (up to 85%) of lower extremity amputations are preventable.[29] Despite efforts directed at prevention, the rate of amputation in patients with DM continues to rise.[29] This poor result is related in part to the underuse of recommended preventive care practices among patients with DM.[30]

The etiology of diabetic ulcers is multifactorial.[31] In a study by Reiber and colleagues,[31] neuropathy, minor foot trauma, and foot deformity were the commonest causal pathways for lower extremity ulceration, but edema, ischemia, and callus formation were also important contributors. In addition, factors that contribute to lower extremity ulcers in diabetic patients are the same as in patients without diabetes, for example, venous insufficiency, stasis dermatitis, and infection. Occasionally, diabetic patients get ulcerations from conditions associated with diabetes, such as necrobiosis lipoidica and bullosis diabeticorum. When patients with diabetes develop ulcers, healing may be compromised by some of the biochemical, endocrine, neurologic, and microvascular factors discussed above. Nonenzymatic glycosylation (NEG) may affect the function of regulatory or matrix proteins and cells necessary for normal tissue repair.[32–35]

Vasculopathy is a major factor in the pathogenesis of diabetic ulcers. The greatest risk factor for amputation in a study by Reiber and associates[16] was low cutaneous blood flow as measured by transcutaneous oxygen pressure ($TcPo_2$). There was a 16-fold excess risk of amputation if the $TcPo_2$ was below 20 mm Hg. Likewise, when Pecoraro and coworkers assessed risk factors associated with failure of ulcers to heal, they found that the most important predictors of nonhealing were low $TcPo_2$ and high $TcCo_2$ in the skin adjacent to the ulcers. In ulcers that healed directly, the mean time to reepithelialization was 89 days despite aggressive outpatient management, including weekly or biweekly visits for debridement by an experienced ulcer care team.[36]

Sensory neuropathy is also a major factor associated with diabetic ulcers[31] and lower extremity amputation[37] (see Chap. 45). The prevalence of symptomatic sensory neuropathy is 30–40% in diabetic patients compared to about 10% in the nondiabetic population.[38] A case-control study by Reiber and collaborators, to assess risk factors for amputation, showed that diabetic patients lacking vibratory sensation had a 15.5-fold excess risk of amputation compared to diabetic patients with intact vibratory sense.[16] Clinical examination and the use of a 5.07 Semmes-Weinstein filament were the most sensitive tests in identifying patients at risk for foot ulceration in a large prospective multicenter trial.[39] The combination of neuropathy and limited joint mobility was found to be the most important etiologic factor for foot ulcers occurring on high-pressure (friction) areas of patients with diabetes[40,41] (Fig. 53-1). It undoubtedly relates to unperceived trauma such as blisters and ingrown toenails, but it may also relate in part to diminished influences of neuropeptides on skin immunity and tissue repair. Ulcers heal very slowly in diabetic patients with neuropathy. Only approximately 31% of 349 patients with diabetic neuropathic foot ulcers receiving standard treatment healed in 20 weeks.[42]

Management of lower extremity ulcers requires modification of contributing factors. For example, if stasis dermatitis is present, it should be treated with topical steroids on the skin adjacent to the ulcers. Edema control is essential. Peripheral edema was a significant

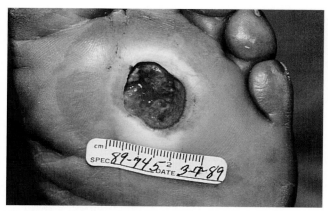

FIGURE 53-1. Diabetic ulcer on an insensate plantar surface. Debridement was done without anaesthesia.

causal factor in the pathway leading to lower extremity ulceration[31] and was associated with amputations in 58% of diabetic patients undergoing amputation in a large series from Sweden.[43] It has also been shown that $TcPo_2$ may improve significantly when leg edema is treated.[44] This may be accomplished by bedrest, leg elevation, sodium restriction, or appropriately used diuretics. Unna boots, ace wraps, compression stockings, and even contact casting may be useful if severe arterial insufficiency does not preclude these interventions. Treatment of underlying local soft tissue infection is important. Approximately 15% of diabetic patients with lower extremity ulcers develop osteomyelitis.[28] Osteomyelitis should be suspected in deep or chronically draining ulcers, particularly if bone is exposed. In a study emphasizing decision and cost-effectiveness analysis, it was suggested that diabetic patients with suspected osteomyelitis from a foot ulcer (without systemic toxicity) might receive a 10-week course of culture-guided antibiotics followed by surgical debridement without obtaining noninvasive imaging studies.[45] Mechanical protection for neuropathic extremities is another key element in therapy of diabetic ulcers. This topic is reviewed in detail in Chap. 51.

Trials of growth-promoting factors and skin equivalents have been under investigation to enhance diabetic ulcer healing.[46–49] Data on treatment for diabetic ulcers were reviewed at an international Consensus Development Conference on Diabetic Foot Wound Care in Boston, Massachusetts.[29] It was concluded that new technologies for the topical treatment of diabetic foot ulcers show "modest benefit" if used with adequate off-loading, debridement, and control of infection. LoGerfo and associates advocate the expanded role of arterial reconstruction for severe diabetic ulceration and gangrene, especially vein bypass grafts to the dorsalis pedis artery (see Chap. 50).[50] Specialized ulcer care teams in outpatient departments have produced impressive results in the prevention and management of lower extremity ulcers as well as the prevention of amputations.[51–53] This team approach to ulcer management will become increasingly important as life expectancy for diabetic patients as well as the general population continues to increase.

Without question, the most important ulcer interventions by physicians and other health care professionals are in the area of prevention. These interventions can be summarized as follows:

1. Implement formal outpatient education that includes teaching daily foot inspection, particularly for neuropathic patients.

2. Advise careful selection of footwear that is not rigid or constricting in design or requiring a break-in period. Ill-fitting shoes or socks were the most common reasons for foot ulcers in a study of 314 diabetic patients with ulcers.[54] Issuing sports shoes to a group of diabetic patients as an experimental variable resulted in a measurable reduction of calluses.[55] Calluses are a sign of excess friction and are often associated with foot ulcers.

3. Advise patients to inspect shoes for foreign bodies before putting them on and to avoid walking barefoot. Figure 53-2 graphically demonstrates problems that can be encountered by patients with insensate feet walking barefoot.

4. Seek early health care attention for calluses, blisters, ingrown toenails, dermatitis, or athlete's foot.

5. Personally inspect the feet of diabetic patients at each visit.

6. Advise patients with a history of ulceration that they are at high risk for reulceration (34% at 1 year, 61% at 3 years, and 70% at 5 years).[56] Redouble education and prevention efforts in this group. Lifelong surveillance is required.

ACANTHOSIS NIGRICANS

Acanthosis nigricans (AN) is a skin disorder that in most cases is a marker for hyperinsulinemia and insulin resistance.[57] The clinical features include a velvety, warty hyperkeratosis, which is black or gray-brown in color, observed on the back and sides of the neck, the axillae, the anogenital region, and other skin folds (Fig. 53-3). The neck is the most consistently affected area[58] and it is also the most reliable area for quantification of AN.[59] AN was previously

FIGURE 53-2. **A.** Nodule on the foot of a diabetic patient with sensory neuropathy. **B.** X-ray showing a needle in the foot that the patient acquired painlessly while walking barefoot.

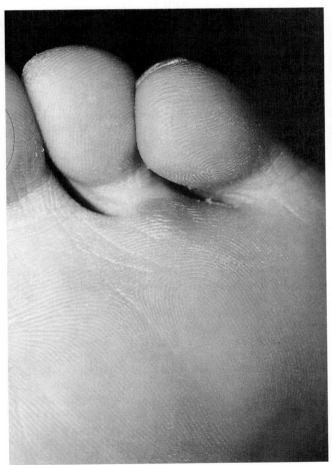

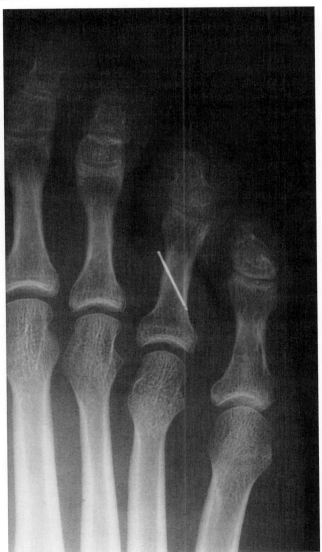

A

B

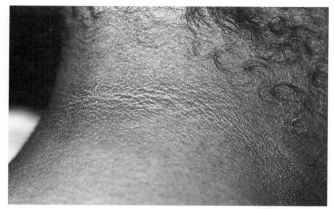

FIGURE 53-3. Acanthosis nigricans on the neck of a black woman with T1DM.

thought to be uncommon or a marker for malignancy, but more recent studies have shown it to be common in certain subpopulations. AN has been observed, for example, with a prevalence of 74% in obese adults,[60] 66% in primary school children weighing 200% of ideal body weight (IBW), and 27% in children weighing 120% of IBW.[61] An overall prevalence of 7.1% was observed for AN in 1412 unselected primary school children, with 0.5% affected in Caucasian children, 5% in Hispanics, and 13% in African-Americans.[61] These differences among ethnic groups have been emphasized.[57] In selected subpopulations of Native Americans the prevalence of AN is 40%.[57] The prevalence of type 2 diabetes mellitus (T2DM) in this subpopulation of Native Americans with AN is 50% in individuals above the age of 40. AN has also been shown to be a risk factor for development of T2DM in a prospective longitudinal study.[62] AN is strongly correlated with hyperinsulinemia,[59] and hyperinsulinemia has been demonstrated to be an independent risk factor for the development of ischemic heart disease.[63] Some investigators have recommended that AN be used as an inexpensive surrogate marker for hyperinsulinemia to identify children and adolescents with a future risk of T2DM and ischemic cardiovascular disease.[58,64]

In conditions of insulin resistance and hyperinsulinemia, excess binding of insulin to insulin-like growth factor (IGF-1) receptors has been proposed as a mechanism for AN as well as for androgen excess.[60,65,66] It is known that high concentrations of insulin stimulate DNA synthesis and cell proliferation *in vitro* through the IGF-1 receptor in fibroblasts,[67] and that keratinocytes have IGF-1 receptors as well.[68] Ovarian cells capable of steroidogenesis have likewise been shown to possess IGF-1 receptors.[66] Molecular biology has been used to identify a number of specific mutations in the insulin receptor gene in patients with AN and type A insulin resistance.[69] These patients have both severe insulin resistance and hyperandrogenemia.

Earlier authors have emphasized the relationship between AN and malignancy.[70] However, the frequency of AN and its lack of specificity for malignancy suggests that when history and physical examination are negative, an extensive cancer work-up is unlikely to be productive. Certain drugs such as nicotinic acid[71] and diethylstilbestrol[72] have been reported to cause AN as well. Treatment for AN is generally ineffective, although disappearance of AN has been observed in obese individuals with weight reduction to IBW[58,60,65] and with discontinuation of offending drugs.[73]

DIABETIC THICK SKIN

In a review of the skin manifestations of diabetes in 1989, Huntley concluded that patients with diabetes generally have thicker skin than their nondiabetic counterparts.[74] He and Walter subsequently presented ultrasound data comparing patients with diabetes (mean age, 44) with control subjects, showing that the skin on the dorsum of the hands and feet was thicker in the diabetic patients.[75] Likewise, Collier and colleagues used ultrasound measurements to show that flexor forearm and medial upper arm skin in patients with diabetes (mean age, 25) was thicker than in controls. Diabetic patients with disease duration greater than 10 years and those with LJM of the hand had the greatest mean skin thickness.[76] Although the contention that patients with diabetes generally have thicker skin has not been shown in an unselected population-based study, two well-characterized syndromes of thick skin in diabetic patients are discussed below.

Scleroderma-Like Syndrome (SLS) and Limited Joint Mobility (LJM)

As reviewed,[77,78] SLS is typically described in children and young adults with type 1 diabetes mellitus (T1DM) in the context of the "diabetic hand syndrome," limited joint mobility (LJM), or "cheiroarthropathy." Skin and joint findings are observed to coexist in a majority of cases, although each may exist independently. Thickening and induration of the skin on the dorsal fingers may be demonstrated by palpation in 8–50% of children with T1DM.[79,80] SLS and LJM typically begin on the fifth finger and progress radially, as well as from distal to proximal. With increasing duration of diabetes, the changes may be seen proximal to the metacarpophalangeal joint. Thickening of the skin has been shown to result from accumulation of connective tissue in the deep dermis.[2]

LJM is thought to result from deposition of connective tissue in the periarticular soft tissues around the joint capsule rather than being the result of a true arthropathy.[81] For study purposes, criteria have been defined for staging the severity of LJM[79] and quantitating restrictions in motion with a goniometer.[82] For clinical purposes, however, LJM may be well demonstrated by the "prayer sign"[79] (Fig. 53-4) or the "table top sign."[82] These signs demonstrate that when the fingers are spread apart, the palmar surface cannot be entirely flattened.

Approximately 50% of adolescent patients with T1DM for more than 5 years are affected.[79] Adults with T2DM may be affected as well.[83] Brik and coworkers[77] summarize the literature on 1845 patients with T1DM and show that for all studies cited, a correlation was found between LJM or SLS and duration of DM. In all of five studies in which microvascular complications were examined, LJM or SLS correlated with retinopathy. Though other signs of microvascular complications have been reported to be associated with LJM or SLS,[77,79,82] retinopathy appears to be the strongest association. In a more recent cross-sectional study, 83 patients with LJM and T2DM were compared with 56 diabetic patients without LJM for evidence of diabetic complications. Patients with LJM were 9.3 times more likely to have proliferative retinopathy, 4 times more likely to have cerebrovascular disease, 3.3 times more likely to have nephropathy, and 3.1 times more likely to have coronary heart disease.[84] Longitudinal control of diabetes as measured by HbA$_{1c}$ was strongly associated with the presence or absence of LJM.[85]

Although the pathogenesis of this condition is controversial,[86,87] evidence for the role of nonenzymatic glycosylation (NEG) of connective tissue is becoming stronger.[88] Advanced gly-

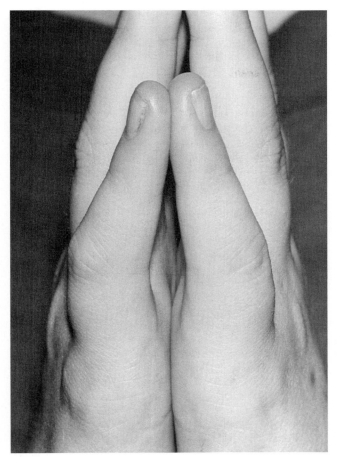

FIGURE 53-4. Prayer sign showing limited joint mobility (LJM) and scleroderma-like (SLS) skin changes. This young woman with T1DM also has severe diabetic retinopathy and nephropathy.

cation end-products (AGEs) extracted from skin correlated significantly with signs of LJM in two studies,[3,88] but not in a third study.[89] The most compelling data come from a longitudinal prospective study showing a two- to threefold excess risk of LJM with HbA$_{1c}$ levels above 8% over a 2-year period. For every 1% increase in HbA$_{1c}$ level, there was a 2.5-fold excess risk of LJM.[85] Evidence is accumulating that intensive insulin therapy may be beneficial in the treatment of LJM and SLS. A study of four patients reported a decrease in skin thickness with tight control of glucose.[90] Monnier and colleagues[6] reported intensive insulin therapy in 122 patients in the DCCT resulted in lower levels of skin collagen AGEs. While evidence was not presented in that study regarding SLS and LJM, the reduction in skin AGEs suggests the effect of intensive insulin therapy may be beneficial. Another study of 2 patients showed improvement in LJM over a 10-year period using aldose reductase inhibition.[91] Physical therapy to preserve range of motion should be considered as well.

Scleredema

Scleredema is usually described as a rare complication of diabetes. However, in two studies the prevalence was reported to be 2.5% of 484 diabetic outpatients in a Veteran Administration Medical Center in the United States[92] and 14% of 100 hospital-based diabetic patients at Kuwait University in Kuwait.[93] Scleredema in diabetic

patients is characterized as firm nonpitting edema of the skin, symmetrically distributed over the posterior neck, upper back, and shoulders. Occasionally, the skin thickness can be so severe as to limit complete range of motion of the neck and shoulders (Fig. 53-5). Usually, however, it is asymptomatic, a fact that could lead to considerable underreporting of the phenomenon by both patients and physicians. A population-based study would provide the best data regarding the true prevalence of scleredema of diabetes.

FIGURE 53-5. **Top**: A man with adult-onset DM with scleredema diabeticorum so severe that it restricts his efforts at neck extension. **Bottom**: A close-up view of the remarkable thickening of skin on his neck.

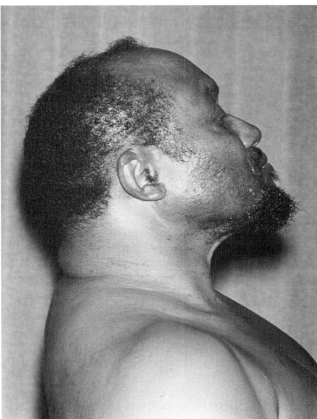

A

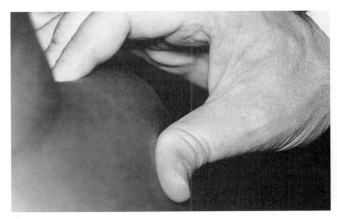

B

Scleredema of diabetes or scleredema diabeticorum[92] is often reported as part of the spectrum of scleredema adultorum.[94] It may be seen in both T1DM and T2DM, but is much more common in type 2 disease.[92,94] The classical Bushke type of scleredema adultorum occurs after a febrile illness, but more commonly scleredema adultorum occurs without a preceding febrile illness. These types of scleredema are similar to the scleredema of diabetes in clinical appearance except they involve the face more often and may resolve spontaneously within 2 years.[94] Monoclonal gammopathy and multiple myeloma have been reported with scleredema.[95] Histopathology shows remarkable thickening of the dermis with acid mucopolysaccharide staining on the majority of biopsies.[96]

The pathogenesis is unclear. Ohta and collaborators[95] showed that serum from patients with scleredema and a paraproteinemia caused enhanced synthesis of extracellular macromolecules in cultured fibroblasts. No consistent pattern of cellular response was observed, however. One patient reported had diabetes. In another diabetic patient with paraproteinemia a sixfold increase in procollagen synthesis was demonstrated in fibroblasts taken from lesional skin.[97] These studies focus on the possibility that circulating serum factors may be responsible for this condition. Similar studies on scleredema of diabetes without paraproteinemia would be of interest. Currently there is no established therapy for the scleredema of diabetes, and it usually persists chronically. Case reports regarding the use of electron beam radiation, penicillin, cyclosporine, bath PUVA, and prostaglandin E_1 have recently been referenced.[98]

CUTANEOUS INFECTIONS

Gilgor extensively reviewed cutaneous infections in diabetic patients and concluded that there is little evidence that well-controlled patients with diabetes are more prone to skin infections.[99] A review of 500 diabetic patients in 1927, before the era of modern metabolic management and antibiotic therapy, contributed to the view that the incidence of furunculosis, carbuncles, erysipelas, and epidermophytosis is increased in diabetic patients.[100] Infection clearly makes diabetes more difficult to manage and, conversely, hyperglycemia and ketoacidosis diminish chemotaxis, phagocytosis, and bactericidal ability of white blood cells. It is difficult, however, to correlate hyperglycemia with skin infections.[99] While population-based studies of prevalence of cutaneous infections are for the most part lacking, we will discuss some of the cutaneous infections that appear to be overrepresented in diabetic patients. A recent review emphasizes these associations.[101]

Bacterial Infections

Both a retrospective and a prospective population-based study have shown diabetes to be a risk factor for invasive group B streptococcal infection in adults.[102,103] Skin and soft tissues were the most common local site of infection. Approximately 30% of the cases occurred in patients with diabetes, and the overall case mortality rate was 21–32%. Diabetes is also associated with a 3.7-fold increased relative risk of invasive group A streptococcal infections.[104]

Malignant external otitis (MEO) is a pyogenic infection of the ear canal, often with *Pseudomonas aeruginosa*, which is characteristically seen in older diabetic patients with purulent discharge, facial swelling, unrelenting pain, hearing loss, and granulation tissue in the ear canal.[101,105] The onset may be indolent, and the diagnosis is often delayed.[101] In a study by Chandler, 68 of 72 patients

had diabetes.[106] In a more recent study, 21 of 30 patients had evidence of diabetes.[107] Aural irrigation with tap water was reported as a preceding event in 8 of 13 patients in a study by Rubin and coworkers.[108] The mortality rate is cited as 20–40% despite appropriate antibiotics.[101,105]

Necrotizing fasciitis is another uncommon but potentially lethal infection seen postoperatively and following minor trauma, as well as at injection sites.[99,101,109] Synergistic infection involving two or more organisms is the rule; however, one organism may cause the condition.[110] Organisms may include facultative streptococci, *Bacteroides*, peptostreptococci, and occasionally staphylococci. The perineum, trunk, abdomen, and upper extremities are the sites most commonly involved. Toxicity is often out of proportion to signs. Redness, induration, cyanosis, and necrosis with overlying bullae may be seen. In a study by Baskin and associates,[110] 12 of 27 patients with necrotizing soft tissue infection had diabetes. Mortality rates of 21–80% have been reported.[99,101,110] The most important aspect of treatment is early aggressive surgical debridement.

The prevalence of staphylococcal infections in diabetic patients has been the source of controversy. Gilgor concluded that no well-controlled studies have proved that furunculosis, boils, or carbuncles are more prevalent in patients with diabetes.[99] In a more recent review, the authors concluded that currently available data do not permit estimation of proportional risk of staphylococcal infection in patients with DM.[111] A large study from a single center demonstrated an increased rate of cutaneous staphylococcal infections in diabetic patients using continuous subcutaneous insulin infusion (CSII).[112] However, an increase in the rate of staphylococcal carriage could not be demonstrated for patients using CSII compared with diabetic patients injecting insulin or normal control subjects.[113] A geographically based study of 551 residents in the San Luis Valley of Colorado also failed to show an increased rate of nasal staphylococcal carriage among patients with diabetes.[114]

Erythrasma is an infection of intertriginous skin with *Corynebacterium minutissimum*. The organism produces a porphyrin pigment that results in characteristic coral red fluorescence when a Wood's lamp is shined on the skin. The infection is of little medical consequence but has been observed in up to 61% of diabetic patients.[99] Each of these bacterial infections may be treated with appropriate systemic antibiotics. Erythrasma may be treated with topical or oral erythromycin.

Fungal and Yeast Infection

Candida albicans causes angular cheilitis, glossitis, vulvovaginitis, balanitis, finger web space infection, and paronychia in diabetic patients.[101] *Candida* infection appears to be more common in poorly controlled patients with diabetes.[99] Clinical evidence of candidal paronychia was observed in 9.6% of 250 diabetic women compared with only 3.4% of 500 nondiabetic women.[115] *Candida* infections may be treated with oral or topical antifungals. In the case of paronychia, it may be even more important to alter the environment of the proximal nail fold by avoiding wetness (e.g., cotton gloves worn under rubber gloves when working in water) and by using drying agents for treatment, such as 15% sulfacetamide in 50% ethanol (3–4 drops four times per day and each time the hands get wet).

The prevalence of toenail onychomycosis appears to be increased in patients with diabetes.[116] The importance of treating dermatophyte infections on the feet of diabetic patients is that they may provide a portal of entry for subsequent bacterial infections. Topical antifungals usually suffice to control fungal infection on skin adjacent to affected nails, but oral agents are needed to clear the onychomycosis.

Mucormycosis is an infection caused by a ubiquitous fungal organism found primarily in soil and decaying vegetation. It has been repeatedly reported in diabetic patients.[99,101] In particular, *Rhizopus* and *Mucor* have been observed complicating skin ulcers on legs and hands in diabetic patients. A destructive nasal mucosa and sinus infection called rhinocerebral mucormycosis (RCM) is particularly devastating. Early manifestations include facial or ocular pain and nasal stuffiness with or without discharge. Later manifestations may include proptosis, necrotic lesions on the palate or nasal turbinate, ophthalmoplegia, and vision loss.[101] Approximately 75–80% of RCM occurs in diabetic patients with uncontrolled disease.[117] Amphotericin B and surgical debridement are the treatments of choice. Mortality rates for RCM have been reported to be 15–34%.[118]

ERUPTIVE XANTHOMAS

Diabetes is the most common cause of acquired hypertriglyceridemia[7] (see Chap. 47). Triglyceride-rich chylomicrons are usually rapidly cleared by the action of lipoprotein lipase; however, lipoprotein lipase activity is decreased in uncontrolled diabetes.[119] Insulin is necessary for normal clearance of plasma lipoproteins.[120] Eruptive xanthomas may develop as the skin manifestations of chylomicrons in hypertriglyceridemic patients.[121,122] Plasma lipoproteins can be shown to enter the skin,[123] where they are phagocytosed by macrophages. These macrophages appear as foam cells in the eruptive xanthomas.[124]

Eruptive xanthomas appear as 1- to 4-mm reddish yellow papules on the extensor surfaces of the arms, legs, and buttocks. They are usually asymptomatic, but are a most important clinical sign because they may be the first indication of diabetes. The hypertriglyceridemia responds rapidly to diet and insulin therapy and the eruptive xanthomas usually resolve completely in 6–8 weeks.[122] Untreated severe hypertriglyceridemia may lead to abdominal pain, pancreatitis, hepatosplenomegaly, lipemia retinalis, hypoxemia, abnormal hemoglobin oxygen affinity, decreased pulmonary diffusing capacities, and psychological changes.[125]

NECROBIOSIS LIPOIDICA (NL)

One of the significant developments in the most recognized skin condition associated with diabetes is its taxonomy. Since Urbach coined the term *necrobiosis lipoidica diabeticorum* in 1932,[126] generations of dermatologists and diabetologists have used the abbreviation "NLD" to refer to this condition. Now in the modern era of computerized literature searches, if one adds the term "diabeticorum" to the search, about 80% of the published papers on the topic for the past 5 years are not retrieved. Many investigators[127] prefer the term *necrobiosis lipoidica*, because many of the patients with this condition do not have diabetes.[128] Perhaps we eventually will get used to this term as well as the abbreviation "NL."

NL was associated with diabetes in approximately two-thirds of 171 cases reported from the Mayo Clinic.[129] Glucose tolerance tests performed on nondiabetic patients revealed another 5–10% with abnormalities in carbohydrate metabolism.[129] A more recent

series of 65 patients with NL revealed that only 11% had been diagnosed with diabetes after 15 years of follow-up.[128] In the converse situation, evaluation of unselected patients with diabetes at the Mayo Clinic revealed that only 3 per 1000 diabetic patients had NL.[129] Similarly, only 3 of 395 patients with diabetes (age 15–55) in a population-based study from Sweden had NL,[130] and the prevalence of NL in children with T1DM was 1 in 1557 patients in the Scottish Study Group for the Care of the Young Diabetic.[131]

The typical clinical presentation is that of multiple (four to eight), asymptomatic, oval, sharply marginated, reddish brown plaques over the anterior legs (bilateral 75% of the time) on young (mean age, 30 years) diabetic women (3:1 female to male ratio).[129] The plaques often slowly enlarge, with the center developing the typical glazed-porcelain sheen with a yellowish hue and prominent telangiectasia (Fig. 53-6). The active margins remain erythematous and slightly elevated. Ulceration occurs in about one-third of diabetic patients with NL, and spontaneous remission is relatively rare (19%).[129] Clinical variants may be solitary and may be seen on the hands, fingers, forearms, face, scalp, and nipple.[127,132] When NL is present, it rarely spares the legs (2% of the time).[129]

The clinical presentation is usually the key to diagnosis, but the histology is also characteristic. At times, however, it is difficult to distinguish NL from other necrobiotic conditions such as granuloma annulare. The histopathologic and immunohistochemical features of NL have been succinctly reviewed[127,133] and contrasted with granuloma annulare (GA).[133] The histologic features of NL include poorly defined histiocytic granulomas with necrobiosis in the middle to deep dermis, periodic acid Schiff (PAS)–positive staining in the areas of necrobiosis, and vascular changes consisting of endothelial swelling, fibrosis, and hyalinization. Nerve staining with S-100 is diminished in lesional skin and in the inflammatory perilesional areas.[134] The latter observation is offered as an explanation for decreased sensation in well-developed plaques of NL.[135]

The pathogenesis of NL remains unknown, but many mechanisms have been proposed and reviewed in detail.[127] Proposed mechanisms include heredity, microangiopathy, increased production of fibronectin by endothelial cells, increased factor VIII–related antigen, abnormal platelet function and prostaglandin synthesis, accelerated collagen aging, and immune-mediated vasculopathy. Most recently, Saarialho-Kere and associates[136] studied the pattern of mRNA expression for tissue inhibitor of metalloproteinase 1 (TIMP-1), interstitial collagenase, and 92-kd gelatinase in

FIGURE 53-6. Plaques of necrobiosis lipoidica. The lesion has a typical glazed-porcelain sheen and yellowish hue with prominent telangiectasia.

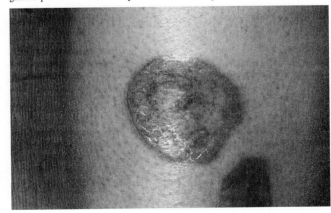

skin biopsies from lesions of NL and GA. Both disorders are characterized by altered extracellular matrix and degenerative changes in collagen and elastic fibers. Expression of metalloproteinases was noted in early lesions, but not later lesions of NL and GA, suggesting that collagenolysis is an early event in these lesions. There is no evidence that poor glycemic control is a factor in NL,[129,137] although this has not been extensively studied using newer techniques for subfractionating AGEs from skin biopsies. TcPo$_2$ values are significantly lower in lesional skin than in adjacent normal skin.[138]

The long list of treatments for NL is evidence that no treatment is the accepted standard of effective care.[127] Studies of NL therapy generally suffer from small numbers of patients, the absence of controls, or both. Our experience with dipyridamol and aspirin has been disappointing, as was that reviewed by Lowitt and Dover.[127] High-potency topical steroids may be useful in the early, inflammatory phase of NL. Likewise, injection of triamcinolone in perilesional skin has been used with success[129]; however, care should be exercised with local steroid use because ulceration may occur. Short-term use of systemic steroids has been advocated,[139] as has pentoxifylline 400 mg three times a day.[140] However, the admonition to "do no harm" may be well advised in this disorder.

The main issues for plaque-type NL are the cosmetic appearance and protection to avoid ulceration. Cover-up products such as Dermablend or Covermark may be useful for special occasions to help cosmetically. Protective padding is well advised for ulcer protection during high-risk activities, and a night-light is useful to prevent inadvertent trauma when using the bathroom at night.[141]

When ulcers occur in NL, the same principles apply as discussed above for diabetic ulcers. Recently, a report of the successful use of cyclosporine for the treatment of persistently ulcerated NL in two patients was published.[142] For very large or recalcitrant ulcers in NL, excision down to fascia with split-thickness skin grafting appears to be effective and the preferred therapy.[143]

GRANULOMA ANNULARE (GA)

Granuloma annulare is a benign self-limited condition characterized by annular plaques usually seen over the dorsal hands, feet, or ankles. The plaques often consist of a ring of papules, red to reddish purple in color, with clearing or flattening in the center. They may be solitary papules, nodules, or plaques, and on rare occasions present as subcutaneous nodules or perforating lesions.[144] About 15% of patients have more than 10 lesions and 7–10% have generalized lesions.[144,145] The localized form tends to come on earlier in life (two-thirds prior to age 30) and usually clears within 2 years,[146] whereas in the generalized form the mean age of onset is 52 years, and it rarely clears spontaneously.[145]

The pathogenesis of GA remains unknown. Its association with diabetes has long been debated.[147] In a large series from the Mayo Clinic in 1989, Dabski and Winkelmann reported diabetes in 9.7% of 1353 patients with localized lesions of GA, and 21% of 100 patients with generalized GA.[145] In two more recent retrospective studies, 11 of 61 patients (18%)[148] and 10 of 84 patients (12%)[149] with GA had diabetes. A large population-based study of patients with DM would be useful to help resolve the relationship between GA and DM, but the more recent data continue to support the arguments in favor of an association.

Treatment with high-potency topical steroids or steroid injection may be effective for localized GA, but it is usually an asymp-

tomatic self-limited process. Generalized GA may be more pruritic and persistent, and it is certainly more cosmetically disabling. Encouraging results for generalized GA have been reported with PUVA.[150] It should be noted, however, that sunburn has been reported as a precipitating factor for some patients with generalized GA.[145] Limited success has been reported with systemic corticosteroids, chloroquine, potassium iodide, sulfones, niacinamide, and chlorpropamide, as reviewed by Dabski and Winkelmann.[145]

A careful history and physical examination should be done with the question of diabetes in mind. It could be argued that a fasting blood sugar should be obtained in older patients with generalized GA. GA lesions have been reported in patients with HIV infection.[151,152] If risk factors for HIV are present, antibody testing should be considered.

DIABETIC DERMOPATHY

Melin is generally credited with describing atrophic circumscribed lesions localized to the lower extremities[153] in diabetic patients. They consist of small (2–10 mm), rounded, brownish, atrophic lesions almost exclusively over the pretibial surface of the legs (Fig. 53-7). They have subsequently been referred to most commonly as

FIGURE 53-7. Atrophic "shin spots" or diabetic dermopathy on the legs of a diabetic man.

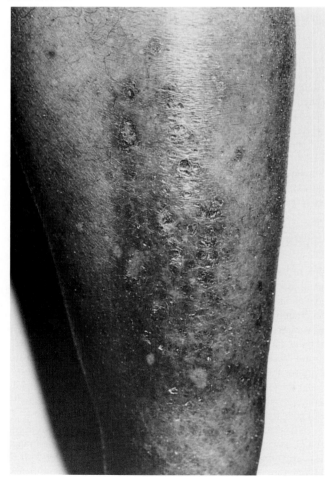

"shin spots"[154] and diabetic dermopathy.[155] Controversy has surrounded this condition regarding the prevalence, the specificity as a cutaneous marker for diabetes, the relationship to other complications of diabetes, and its relationship to trauma.[156]

Prevalence of atrophic shin spots ascertained from diabetic patients in outpatient clinics has ranged from 24–65% for males and 4–39% for females.[153,154,157,158] The prevalence in nondiabetic control groups was 7% of 104 patients in a hypertension clinic,[153] 20% of 183 patients in an endocrine clinic,[154] 3% of 100 patients in a dermatology clinic,[157] and 1.6% of 201 healthy medical students.[154] Perhaps the best prevalence data come from a population-based study in which standard skin examinations were performed on the lower extremities of 96% of 395 patients with known diabetes aged 15–50 years from Umea County, Sweden.[158] It is of interest that the University of Umea is where Melin's report originated in 1964. They observed shin spots in 33% of patients with T1DM and 39% of patients with T2DM, compared with 2% of a control group comprised of 100 healthy people, mainly hospital personnel aged 15–50 years. Most authors agree that though the finding is not specific for diabetes, diabetic dermopathy does occur with greater frequency in patients with diabetes. Additionally, there is agreement that it occurs more frequently in men, and the duration of diabetes is directly related to the prevalence of diabetic dermopathy.

The pathogenesis of the condition is unknown. Trauma has been the leading candidate, even though most patients are unaware of associated trauma and the lesions are asymptomatic. Arguments in favor of trauma are supported by the location on the shins and the increased prevalence in men. Melin was unable to produce lesions on the shins of diabetic patients with a rubber hammer and found no lesions on the shins of normal healthy soccer players.[153] Lithner, however, was able to induce atrophic circumscribed skin lesions at the site of trauma from locally applied heat and cold in patients with diabetes.[159] Perhaps diabetic dermopathy represents a pattern of repair in response to injury or inflammation within the milieu of diabetes.

Melin found an association of atrophic shin spots with other clinical complications of diabetes, including retinopathy, lower extremity vascular disease, and nephropathy.[153] However, in the other large study to look at this question, Danowski and colleagues found no such associations.[154] In the most recent study of 173 patients with DM (69 with atrophic shin spots), a strong statistical relationship with retinopathy, nephropathy, and neuropathy was reported.[160] The histology is not diagnostic. It shows epidermal atrophy and pigment inclusion but no clear-cut evidence for a vasculopathy in lesional skin by either histology or electron microscopy.[161] No treatment is necessary since it is without symptoms or morbidity.

BULLOSIS DIABETICORUM

The abrupt onset of bullae on the extremities has been reported as a rare condition associated with diabetes.[162] The lesions are usually on the toes, feet, and distal lower extremities, but are also observed on the fingers, hands, and forearms. They are unrelated to any apparent trauma or infection and heal without scarring in 2–5 weeks unless they become infected. Although the condition may resolve spontaneously, it may recur over a number of years.[163]

The histopathology is variable, as reviewed by Toonstra.[163] The level of separation resulting in the bulla may be intraepidermal

or subepidermal. The intraepidermal split may occur anywhere from suprabasally to subcorneally, usually without acantholysis, although spongiosis may be present. Direct immunofluorescence is usually negative.[163,164]

Because the pathogenesis is unknown and the treatment is supportive wound care, the main significance of this condition is recognition that it is not one of the other blistering disorders of the skin. The differential diagnosis includes bullous impetigo, bullous pemphigoid, pemphigus vulgaris, epidermolysis bullosa acquisita, porphyria cutanea tarda (PCT), bullous erythema multiforme (e.g., due to drugs), and insect bite reaction. A negative culture for staphylococci, a negative direct immunofluorescence on skin biopsy, and compatible histopathology makes this diagnosis by exclusion relatively certain. A porphyrin screen could be considered if other signs of PCT are present. The diagnosis is important because the treatment of a number of the other blistering diseases involves the use of systemic steroids or immunosuppressive therapy, which confers significant risk of toxicity to diabetic patients.

ACQUIRED PERFORATING DERMATOSIS

Acquired perforating dermatosis (APD) has been reported in association with diabetes and renal failure. Rapini and collaborators[165] reviewed a variety of terms used for this group of conditions. They include Kyrle's disease, reactive perforating collagenosis (RPC), perforating folliculitis, and elastosis perforans serpiginosa. Because histology may vary from location to location on the same patient and the pathogenesis is unclear, it appears more logical to consider these conditions together rather than to emphasize differences.

APD is characterized by transepidermal elimination of what appears to be altered collagen. The clinical appearance consists of pruritic papules and nodules on the upper and lower extremities as well as the trunk and, to a lesser extent, the face. The lesions are often perifollicular, as noted in Fig. 53-8. In review of the literature, Faver and associates[166] were able to describe 22 cases considered to be RPC: 72% (16/22 patients) had diabetes with at least one complication (nephropathy, retinopathy, peripheral vascular disease, or cardiomyopathy), 15 patients had nephropathy, and 10 were on dialysis. In a more recent study in which dialysis patients received prospective skin examinations, 11% (8 of 72 patients) were observed to have APD. Seven of the eight patients had DM.

FIGURE 53-8. Acquired perforating dermatosis in a young woman with T1DM who is on dialysis.

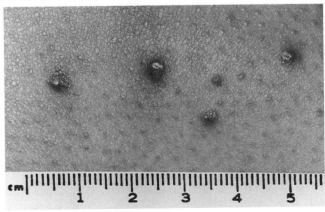

These observations are supportive of the association of APD with DM and chronic renal failure, and it suggests that APD may be more common than previously appreciated.[167] The pathogenesis is unclear, but treatment with glycemic control, ultraviolet light, retinoic acid, or topical steroids is at times effective.

GLUCAGONOMA

Glucagonoma is one cause for diabetes that is potentially curable by surgery; hence it deserves mention even though it occurs rarely. This diagnosis should be considered in diabetic patients with a recalcitrant erosive dermatitis, typically involving the central face, groin, friction areas, and the distal extremities.[168] It is usually seen in the clinical setting of weight loss, diarrhea, glossitis, anemia, hypoalbuminemia, and mild DM. Skin biopsy shows epidermal necrosis, edema, and a split in the upper spinous layer, along with a neutrophilic infiltrate.[169] The clinical and histologic features taken together resulted in the term *necrolytic migratory erythema* (NME).[170]

Glucagonoma is a tumor of the α (alpha) cells of the pancreas, which secrete glucagon. It is malignant in 60–80% of cases and often is metastatic at the time of diagnosis.[171] Early diagnosis is rare because it is not considered by the clinician. Some authors suggest obtaining a glucagon level in any patient with DM and an unexplained rash.[172] The diagnosis is made more difficult by the fact that 15% of patients with glucagonoma do not have DM,[168] and some patients with NME have normal glucagon levels and no evidence of glucagonoma.[173]

In the proper clinical context, the diagnosis can usually be confirmed with a fasting serum glucagon level. The tumors can usually be visualized on CT scan;[174] however, selective celiac axis arteriography is the most useful diagnostic study for localizing the tumor and identifying metastases in the liver.[175,176] Treatment usually includes surgical excision. Even in metastatic disease, cytoreductive surgery often results in long remission.[172] Chemotherapy may be helpful, and long-acting somatostatin analogues result in good symptomatic relief even though they have no effect on tumor size.[177]

INSULIN INJECTION COMPLICATIONS

Strong evidence has been presented that intensive insulin therapy effectively delays the onset and slows the progression of microvascular disease in T1DM[178,179] (see Chap. 54). Multiple daily insulin injections have become the norm, and external insulin pumps are an effective alternative for intensive insulin therapy.[179] Management of the skin complications of insulin therapy may become more problematic with intensive insulin therapy. In older literature, the incidence of skin complications was given as 10% and 56% of all patients with diabetes receiving conventional bovine and pork insulin, respectively.[180] That incidence has decreased substantially with the use of purified pork and bovine insulin as well as with human insulin (HI).[181–183]

Lipoatrophy with less pure, earlier insulin preparations was reported in 16% of patients,[184] whereas with highly purified insulin it occurred in 0–2.5% of cases.[182–184] It is sufficiently uncommon with use of HI that case reports and letters regarding its occurrence continue to appear.[185,186] Lipoatrophy has been attributed to local immune complex formation and complement fixation with release of lysosomal enzymes in response to a presumed antigenic component of the less purified insulins.[187] As noted, however, it does continue to occur with highly purified insulin and HI. Chantelau and coworkers reported a case in which lipoatrophy resulted from injection of intermediate- and long-acting HI. The authors successfully used continuous subcutaneous insulin injection (CSII) with regular HI, and speculated that the shorter-acting insulin may have been responsible for the improvement.[185]

Lipohypertrophy has not decreased with the use of highly purified insulin and HI. In fact, at one center lipohypertrophy was observed in 14% of patients using conventional insulin, whereas 22% of patients injecting highly purified insulin developed lipohypertrophy.[184] At another center lipohypertrophy was observed in 76 of 281 (27%) patients injecting purified insulin.[183] Lipohypertrophy is thought to occur because of a local anabolic effect of insulin that promotes fat and protein synthesis. The problem can usually be alleviated by rotation of injection sites, but the hypertrophic sites are often repeatedly used by the patients because they tend to be less painful. However, patients should be discouraged from using the sites with lipohypertrophy because the insulin absorption can be delayed or inconsistent.[188,189]

Local and systemic allergic reactions have been reported with insulin injections. Fortunately, local reactions are by far the most common. A variety of factors may be involved, including contaminating proteins,[190] zinc,[191] and protamine,[192] as well as insulin itself (including HI).[193] Such allergic reactions are usually IgE-mediated,[194] although patients may have IgE antibodies to insulin without clinical evidence of an adverse reaction,[190,195] and IgE antibodies have been measured in sera from allergic nondiabetic individuals with affinities and concentrations similar to those seen in diabetic patients.[196,197] Local reactions to insulin are often transient and of no major significance. They usually present as a wheal and flare within 30 minutes. Systemic allergic reactions, though rare, are potentially life-threatening. They include urticaria, angioedema, anaphylaxis, and the Arthus reaction.[198] Although highly purified insulin and HI are less immunogenic, allergic reactions are still observed.[193] Intradermal testing may be used to find an insulin preparation to which the patient does not react.[193,199] Desensitization techniques are useful for generalized insulin allergies.[199] Systemic steroids and antihistamines are occasionally required.[181,200]

Nonimmunologic cutaneous reactions have been reported to insulin injection as well. They include infections (e.g., *S. aureus*, *S. epidermidis*, and *M. chelonei*),[112,201] zinc granulomas and sterile abscesses,[202] silicon oil from disposable syringes,[203] and keloid formation, as well as pigmentation that can resemble acanthosis nigricans.[204]

Continuous subcutaneous insulin infusion (CSII) deserves special mention because skin complications are the most common reason the treatment is discontinued.[205] Chantelau and collaborators[206] reported on 116 patients with T1DM followed for a mean period of 4.5 years. They reported 134 cases of skin inflammation or infection during the study period: 51% developed redness at the catheter sites, 19% developed subcutaneous nodules, and 48% had whitish scars secondary to previous infections. In an earlier study, catheters were cultured from 40 patients during 120 separate examinations. *S. epidermidis* was recovered in 42 cases and *S. aureus* in 15 cases.[112] Pyogenic skin inflammation was described by van Faassen and coworkers[113] in 48% of 50 patients treated with CSII, compared with 6% of the insulin-injecting patients and 3% of healthy volunteers. Recommendations regarding skin care with CSII include needle change every 48 hours, no catheter reuse, hand washing before insertion of needles, antiseptic preparation of needle insertion sites, and sterile covering of the needles.[112]

REFERENCES

1. Beisswenger PJ, Moore LL, Curphey TJ: Relationship between glycemic control and collagen-linked advanced glycosylation end products in type I diabetes. *Diabetes Care* 1993;16:689.

2. Buckingham BA, Uitto J, Sandborg C: Sclerederma-like changes in insulin-dependent diabetes mellitus: Clinical and biochemical studies. *Diabetes Care* 1984;7:163.

3. Sell DR, LaPolla A, Odetti P: Pentosidine formation in skin correlates with severity of complications in individuals with long-standing IDDM. *Diabetes* 1992;41:1286.

4. Lyons TJ, Bailie KE, Dyer DG: Decrease in skin collagen glycation with improved glycemic control in patients with insulin-dependent diabetes mellitus. *J Clin Invest* 1991;87:1910.

5. Dyer DG, Dunn JA, Thorpe SR: Accumulation of maillard reaction products in skin collagen in diabetes and aging. *J Clin Invest* 1993;91:2463.

6. Monnier VM, Bautista O, Kenny D, et al: Skin collagen glycation, glycoxidation, and crosslinking are lower in subjects with long-term intensive versus conventional therapy of type 1 diabetes: Relevance of glycated collagen products versus HbA1c as markers of diabetic complications. DCCT Skin Collagen Ancillary Study Group. Diabetes Control and Complications Trial. *Diabetes* 1999;48:870.

7. Chait A, Brunzell JD: Severe hypertriglyceridemia: Role of familial and acquired disorders. *Metabolism* 1983;32:209.

8. Levy DM, Terenghi G, Gu X-H: Immunohistochemical measurements of nerves and neuropeptides in diabetic skin: Relationship to tests of neurological function. *Diabetologia* 1992;35:889.

9. Kennedy WR, Wendelschafer-Crabb G: Utility of skin biopsy in diabetic neuropathy. *Semin Neurol* 1996;16:163.

10. Aronin N, Leeman S, Clements RS: Diminished flare response in neuropathic diabetic patients. Comparison of effects of substance P, histamine, and capsaicin. *Diabetes* 1987;36:1139.

11. McGillis J, Mitsuhashi M, Payan D: Immunologic properties of substance P. In: Ader R, Felten D, Cohen N, eds. *Psychoneuroimmunology*. Academic Press:1991;209.

12. Nilsson J, von Euler AM, Dalsgaard C-J: Stimulation of connective tissue cell growth by substance P and substance K. *Nature* 1985;315:61.

13. Haegerstrand A, Dalsgaard CJ, Jonzon B: Calcitonin gene-related peptide stimulates proliferation of human endothelial cells. *Proc Natl Acad Sci USA* 1990;87:3299.

14. Senapati A, Anand P, McGregor GP: Depletion of neuropeptides during wound healing in rat skin. *Neurosci Lett* 1986;71:101.

15. Pecoraro R, Reiber G, Burgess E: Pathways to diabetic limb amputation: Basis for prevention. *Diabetes Care* 1990;13:513.

16. Reiber G, Pecoraro R, Koepsell T: Risk factors for amputation in patients with diabetes mellitus, a case-control study. *Ann Intern Med* 1992;117:97.

17. Braverman IM, Keh-Yen A: Ultrastructural abnormalities of the microvasculature and elastic fibers in the skin of juvenile diabetes. *J Invest Dermatol* 1984;82:270.

18. Braverman IM, Sibley J, Keh A: Ultrastructural analysis of the endothelial-pericyte relationship in diabetic cutaneous vessels. *J Invest Dermatol* 1990;95:147.

19. Yasuda H, Taniguchi Y, Yamashita M: Morphological characteristics of dermal diabetic microangiopathy. *Diabetes Res Clin Pract* 1990;9:187.

20. Braverman IM, Sibley J, Keh-Yen A: A study of the veil cells around normal, diabetic and aged cutaneous microvessels. *J Invest Dermatol* 1986;86:57.

21. Bollinger A, Frey J, Jäger K: Patterns of diffusion through skin capillaries in patients with long-term diabetes. *N Engl J Med* 1982;307:1305.

22. Sandeman DD, Shore AC, Tooke JE: Relation of skin capillary pressure in patients with insulin-dependent diabetes mellitus to complications and metabolic control. *N Engl J Med* 1992;327:760.

23. Pazos-Moura CC, Moura EG, Bouskela E: Nailfold capillaroscopy in non-insulin dependent diabetes mellitus: Blood flow velocity during rest and post-occlusive reactive hyperaemia. *Clin Physiol* 1990;10:451.

24. Rendell M, Bamisedun O: Diabetic cutaneous microangiopathy. *Am J Med* 1992;93:611.

25. Gaylarde PM, Fonseca VA, Llewellyn G: Transcutaneous oxygen tension in legs and feet of diabetic patients. *Diabetes* 1988;37:714.

26. Rayman G, Hassan A, Tooke JE: Blood flow in the skin of the foot related to posture in diabetes mellitus. *Br Med J* 1986;292:87.

27. Harrington C, Zagari MJ, Corea J, et al: A cost analysis of diabetic lower-extremity ulcers. *Diabetes Care* 2000;23:1333.

28. Ramsey SD, Newton K, Blough D, et al: Incidence, outcomes, and cost of foot ulcers in patients with diabetes. *Diabetes Care* 1999;22:382.

29. American Diabetes Association: Consensus development conference on diabetic foot wound care, April 7–8, 1999, Boston, MA. *Diabetes Care* 1999;22:1354.

30. Beckles GLA, Engelgau MM, Venkat Narayan KM, et al: Population-based assessment of the level of care among adults with diabetes in the U.S. *Diabetes Care* 1998;21:1432.

31. Reiber GE, Vileikyte L, Boyko EJ, et al: Causal pathways for incident lower-extremity ulcers in patients with diabetes from two settings. *Diabetes Care* 1999;22:157.

32. Vlassara H, Brownlee M, Cerami A: Specific macrophage receptor activity for advanced glycosylation end products inversely correlates with insulin levels in vivo. *Diabetes* 1988;37:456.

33. Tarsio J, Wigness B, Rhode TD: Nonenzymatic glycation of fibronectin and alterations in the molecular association of cell matrix and basement membrane components in diabetes mellitus. *Diabetes* 1985;34:477.

34. Brownlee M, Vlassara H, Cerami A: Nonenzymatic glycosylation reduces the susceptibility of fibrin to degradation by plasmin. *Diabetes* 1983;32:680.

35. Kelly SB, Olerud JE, Witztum JL, et al: A method for localizing the early products of nonenzymatic glycosylation in fixed tissue. *J Invest Dermatol* 1989;93:327.

36. Pecoraro RE, Ahroni JH, Boyko EJ: Chronology and determinants of tissue repair in diabetic lower-extremity ulcers. *Diabetes* 1991;40:1305.

37. Adler AI, Boyko EJ, Ahroni JH, et al: Lower-extremity amputation in diabetes. The independent effects of peripheral vascular disease, sensory neuropathy, and foot ulcers. *Diabetes Care* 1999;22:1029.

38. Harris M, Eastman R, Cowie C: Symptoms of sensory neuropathy in adults with NIDDM in the U.S. population. *Diabetes Care* 1993;16:1446.

39. Pham H, Armstrong DG, Harvey C, et al: Screening techniques to identify people at high risk for diabetic foot ulceration: A prospective multicenter trial. *Diabetes Care* 2000;23:606.

40. Masson EA, Hay EM, Stockley I: Abnormal foot pressures alone may not cause ulceration. *Diabet Med* 1989;6:426.

41. Veves A, Murray HJ, Young MJ, et al: The risk of foot ulceration in diabetic patients with high foot pressure: A prospective study. *Diabetologia* 1992;35:660.

42. Margolis DJ, Kantor J, Berlin JA: Healing of diabetic neuropathic foot ulcers receiving standard treatment. A meta-analysis. *Diabetes Care* 1999;22:692.

43. Apelqvist J, Larsson J, Agardh C-D: The importance of peripheral pulses, peripheral oedema and local pain for the outcome of diabetic foot ulcers. *Diabet Med* 1990;7:590.

44. Pecoraro RE: The nonhealing diabetic ulcer—a major cause for limb loss. In: Barbul A, Caldwell MD, Eaglstein WH, et al, eds. *Clinical and Experimental Approaches to Dermal & Epidermal Repair: Normal & Chronic Wounds*. Wiley-Liss:1991;27.

45. Eckman MH, Greenfield S, Mackey WC, et al: Foot infections in diabetic patients: Decision and cost-effectiveness analyses. *JAMA* 1995;273:712.

46. Steed DL, Goslen JB, Holloway GA, et al: Randomized prospective double-blind trial in healing chronic diabetic foot ulcers. CT-102 activated platelet supernatant, topical versus placebo. *Diabetes Care* 1992;15:1598.

47. Apelqvist J, Larsson J, Stenstrom A: Topical treatment of necrotic foot ulcers in diabetic patients: A comparative trial of DuoDerm and MeZinc. *Br J Dermatol* 1990;123:787.

48. Grentzkow GD, Iwasaki SD, Hershon KS, et al: Use of dermagraft, a cultured human dermis, to treat diabetic foot ulcers. *Diabetes Care* 1996;19:350.

49. Knighton DR, Fiegel VD, Austin LL, et al: Classification and treatment of chronic nonhealing wounds: Successful treatment with autologous platelet-derived wound healing factors (PDWHF). *Ann Surg* 1986;204:322.

50. LoGerfo FW, Gibbons GW, Pomposelli FB Jr: Trends in the care of the diabetic foot. Expanded role of arterial reconstruction. *Arch Surg* 1992;127:617.

51. Edmonds ME, Blundell MP, Morris ME, *et al*: Improved survival of the diabetic foot: The role of a specialised foot clinic. *Q J Med* 1986; 60:763.

52. Van Gils CC, Wheeler LA, Mellstrom M, *et al*: Amputation prevention by vascular surgery and podiatry collaboration in high-risk diabetic and nondiabetic patients. *Diabetes Care* 1999;22:678.

53. Dargis V, Pantelejeva O, Jonushaite A, *et al*: Benefits of a multidisciplinary approach in the management of recurrent diabetic foot ulceration in Lithuania: A prospective study. *Diabetes Care* 1999;22:1428.

54. Apelqvist J, Larsson J, Agardh C-D: The influence of external precipitating factors and peripheral neuropathy on the development and outcome of diabetic foot ulcers. *J Diabetes Complications* 1990;4:21.

55. Soulier SM: The use of running shoes in the prevention of plantar diabetic ulcers. *J Am Podiatr Med Assoc* 1986;76:395.

56. Apelqvist J, Larsson J, Agardh C-D: Long-term prognosis for diabetic patients with foot ulcers. *J Intern Med* 1993;233:485.

57. Stuart CA, Driscoll MS, Lundquist KF, *et al*: Acanthosis nigricans. *J Basic Clin Physiol Pharmacol* 1998;9:407.

58. Stuart CA, Gilkison CR, Smith MM, *et al*: Acanthosis nigricans as a risk factor for non-insulin dependent diabetes mellitus. *Clin Pediatr* 1998;37:73.

59. Burke JP, Hale DE, Hazuda HP, *et al*: A quantitative scale of acanthosis nigricans. *Diabetes Care* 1999;22:1655.

60. Hud JA Jr, Cohen JB, Wagner JM: Prevalence and significance of acanthosis nigricans in an adult obese population. *Arch Dermatol* 1992;128:941.

61. Stuart CA, Pate CJ, Peters EJ: Prevalence of acanthosis nigricans in an unselected population. *Am J Med* 1989;87:269.

62. Kekalainen P, Sarlund H, Pyorala K, *et al*: Hyperinsulinemia cluster predicts the development of type 2 diabetes independently of family history of diabetes. *Diabetes Care* 1999;22:86.

63. Despr'es J-P, Lamarche B, Mauriege P, *et al*: Hyperinsulinemia as an independent risk factor for ischemic heart disease. *N Engl J Med* 1996;335:976.

64. Bent KN, Shuster GF, Hurley JS, *et al*: Acanthosis nigricans as an early clinical proxy marker of increased risk of type II diabetes. *Public Health Nurs* 1998;15:415.

65. Cruz PD Jr, Hud JA Jr: Excess insulin binding to insulin-like growth factor receptors: Proposed mechanism for acanthosis nigricans. *J Invest Dermatol* 1992;98:82S.

66. Geffner ME, Golde DW: Selective insulin action on skin, ovary, and heart in insulin-resistant states. *Diabetes Care* 1988;11:500.

67. Flier JS, Usher P, Moses AC: Monoclonal antibody to the type I insulin-like growth factor (IGF-I) receptor blocks IGF-I receptor-mediated DNA synthesis: Clarification of the mitogenic mechanisms of IGF-I and insulin in human skin fibroblasts. *Proc Natl Acad Sci USA* 1986;83:664.

68. Misra P, Nickoloff BJ, Morhenn VB: Characterization of insulin-like growth factor-I/somatomedin-C receptors on human keratinocyte monolayers. *J Invest Dermatol* 1986;87:264.

69. Taylor SI, Cama A, Accli D: Genetic basis of endocrine disease 1. Molecular genetics of insulin resistant diabetes mellitus. *J Clin Endocrinol Metab* 1991;73:1158.

70. Brown J, Winkelmann RK: Acanthosis nigricans: A study of 90 cases. *Medicine (Baltimore)* 1968;47:33.

71. Tromovitch TA, Jacobs PH, Kern S: Acanthosis nigricans-like lesions from nicotinic acid. *Arch Dermatol* 1964;89:222.

72. Banuchi SR, Cohen L, Lorincz AL: Acanthosis nigricans following diethylstilbestrol therapy. *Arch Dermatol* 1974;109:545.

73. Coates P, Shuttleworth D, Rees J: Resolution of nicotinic acid-induced acanthosis nigricans by substitution of an analogue (acipimox) in a patient with type V hyperlipidaemia. *Br J Dermatol* 1992; 126:412.

74. Huntley AC: Cutaneous manifestations of diabetes mellitus. *Dermatol Clin* 1989;7:531.

75. Huntley AC, Walter RM Jr: Quantitative determination of skin thickness in diabetes mellitus: Relationship to disease parameters. *J Med* 1990;21:257.

76. Collier A, Matthews DM, Kellett HA: Change in skin thickness associated with cheiroarthropathy in insulin dependent diabetes mellitus. *Br Med J* 1986;292:936.

77. Brik R, Berant M, Vardi P: The scleroderma-like syndrome of insulin-dependent diabetes mellitus. *Diabetes Metab Rev* 1991;7:121.

78. Rosenbloom AL: Limited joint mobility in insulin dependent childhood diabetes. *Eur J Pediatr* 1990;149:380.

79. Rosenbloom AL, Silverstein JH, Lezotte DC: Limited joint mobility in childhood diabetes indicates increased risk for microvascular disease. *N Engl J Med* 1981;305:191.

80. Buckingham B, Perejda AJ, Sandborg C: Skin, joint and pulmonary changes in type I diabetes mellitus. *Am J Dis Child* 1986;140:420.

81. Seibold J: Digital sclerosis in children with insulin-dependent diabetes mellitus. *Arthritis Rheum* 1982;25:1357.

82. Grgic A, Rosenbloom AL, Weber FT: Joint contracture—common manifestation of childhood diabetes mellitus. *J Pediatr* 1976;88: 584.

83. Jennings AM, Milner PC, Ward JD: Hand abnormalities are associated with the complications of diabetes in type 2 diabetes. *Diabet Med* 1989;6:43.

84. Arkkila PE, Kantola IM, Viikari JS: Limited joint mobility in non-insulin-dependent diabetic (NIDDM) patients: Correlation to control of diabetes, atherosclerotic vascular disease, and other diabetic complications. *J Diabetes Complications* 1997;11:208.

85. Silverstein JH, Gordon G, Pollock BH, *et al*: Long-term glycemic control influences the onset of limited joint mobility in type I diabetes. *J Pediatr* 1998;132:944.

86. Rosenbloom AL: Diabetic thick skin and stiff joints. *Diabetologia* 1989;32:74.

87. Goodfield MJD: The skin in diabetes mellitus. *Diabetologia* 1989; 32:75.

88. Monnier VM, Vishwanath V, Frank KE: Relation between complications of type I diabetes mellitus and collagen-linked fluorescence. *N Engl J Med* 1986;314:403.

89. McCance DR, Dyer DG, Dunn JA: Maillard reaction products and their relation to complications in insulin-dependent diabetes mellitus. *J Clin Invest* 1993;91:2470.

90. Lieberman LS, Rosenbloom AL, Riley WJ: Reduced skin thickness with pump administration of insulin. *N Engl J Med* 1980;303:940.

91. Eaton RP, Sibbitt WL Jr, Shah VO, *et al*: A commentary on 10 years of aldose reductase inhibition for limited joint mobility in diabetes. *J Diabetes Complications* 1998;12:34.

92. Cole GW, Headley J, Skowsky R: Scleredema diabeticorum: A common and distinct cutaneous manifestation of diabetes mellitus. *Diabetes Care* 1983;6:189.

93. Sattar MA, Diab S, Sugathan TN: Scleredema diabeticorum: A minor but often unrecognized complication of diabetes mellitus. *Diabet Med* 1988;5:465.

94. Venencie PY, Powell FC, Su WPD: Scleredema: A review of thirty-three cases. *J Am Acad Dermatol* 1984;11:128.

95. Ohta A, Uitto J, Oikarinen AI: Paraproteinemia in patients with scleredema. *J Am Acad Dermatol* 1987;16:96.

96. Cole HG, Winkelmann RK: Acid mucopolysaccharide staining in scleredema. *J Cutan Pathol* 1990;17:211.

97. Oikarinen A, Ala-Kokko L, Palatsi R: Scleredema and paraproteinemia. *Arch Dermatol* 1987;123:226.

98. Lee MW, Choi JH, Sung KH, *et al*: Electron beam therapy in patients with scleredema. *Acta Derm Venereol* 2000;80:207.

99. Gilgor RS: Cutaneous infections in diabetes mellitus. In: Jelink JE, ed. *The Skin in Diabetes*. Lea & Febiger:1986;111.

100. Greenwood AM: A study of the skin in five hundred cases of diabetes. *JAMA* 1927;89:774.

101. Nirmal J, Caputo GM, Weitekamp MR, *et al*: Infections in patients with diabetes mellitus. *New Engl J Med* 1999;341:1906.

102. Farley MM: A population-based assessment of invasive disease due to group B streptococcus in nonpregnant adults. *N Engl J Med* 1993;328: 1807.

103. Muñoz P, Llancaqueo A, Rodriguez-Créixems M, *et al*: Group B streptococcus bacteremia in nonpregnant adults. *Arch Intern Med* 1997;157:213.

104. Davies HD, McGeer A, Schwartz B, *et al*: Invasive group A streptococcal infections in Ontario, Canada. Ontario Group A Streptococcal Study Group. *N Engl J Med* 1996;335:590.

105. Yu LH, Shu CH, Tu TY, *et al*: Malignant otitis externa. *Chung Hua Hsueh Tsa Chih (Taipei)* 1999;62:362.

106. Chandler JR: Malignant external otitis: Further considerations. *Ann Otolaryngol* 1977;86:417.

107. Shpitzer T, Levy R, Stern Y: Malignant external otitis in nondiabetic patients. *Ann Otol Rhinol Laryngol* 1993;102:870.

108. Rubin J, Kamerer DB, Yu V, *et al*: Aural irrigation with water: A potential pathogenic mechanism for inducing malignant external otitis? *Ann Otol Rhinol Laryngol* 1990;99:117.

109. Eke N: Fournier's gangrene: A review of 1726 cases. *Br J Surg* 2000; 87:718.

110. Baskin LS, Carroll PR, Cattolica EV: Necrotising soft tissue infections of the perineum and genitalia. *Br J Urol* 1990;65:524.

111. Breen JD, Karchmer AW: Staphylococcus aureus infections in diabetic patients. *Infect Dis Clin North Am* 1995;9:11.

112. Chantelau E, Lange G, Sonneberg G: Acute cutaneous complications and catheter needle colonization during insulin-pump treatment. *Diabetes Care* 1987;10:478.

113. van Faasen I, Razenberg PPA, Simoons-Smit AM, *et al*: Carriage of *Staphylococcus aureus* and inflamed infusion sites with insulin-pump therapy. *Diabetes Care* 1989;12:153.

114. Boyko EJ, Lipsky BA, Sandoval R: NIDDM and prevalence of nasal *Staphylococcus aureus* colonization. *Diabetes Care* 1989;12:189.

115. Stone OJ, Mullins JF: Incidence of chronic paronychia. *JAMA* 1963; 186:71.

116. Gupta AK, Konnikov N, MacDonald P, *et al*: Prevalence and epidemiology of toenail onychomycosis in diabetic subjects: A multicentre survey. *Br J Dermatol* 1998;139:665.

117. Batra VK, Gaiha M, Gupta PS: Mucormycosis in a diabetic. *Postgrad Med J* 1982;58:781.

118. Lehrer RI, Howard DH, Sypherd PS: Mucormycosis. *Ann Intern Med* 1980;93:93.

119. Brunzell JD, Porte D Jr, Bierman EL: Abnormal lipoprotein-lipase-mediated plasma triglyceride removal in untreated diabetes mellitus associated with hypertriglyceridemia. *Metabolism* 1979; 28:897.

120. Bagdade JD, Porte D Jr, Bierman EL: Diabetica lipemia. A form of acquired fat-induced lipemia. *N Engl J Med* 1967;276:427.

121. Brunzell JD, Bierman EL: Chylomicronemia syndrome. Interaction of genetic and acquired hypertriglyceridemia. *Med Clin North Am* 1982; 66:455.

122. Parker F: Xanthomas and hyperlipidemias. *J Am Acad Dermatol* 1985;13:1.

123. Scott PJ, Winterbourn CC: Low-density lipoprotein accumulation in actively growing xanthomas. *J Atheroscler Res* 1967;7:207.

124. Parker F, Bagdade JD, Odland GF: Evidence for the chylomicron origin of lipids accumulating in diabetic eruptive xanthomas: A correlative lipid biochemical, histochemical, and electron microscopic study. *J Clin Invest* 1970;49:2172.

125. Chait A, Robertson HT, Brunzell JD: Chylomicronemia syndrome in diabetes mellitus. *Diabetes Care* 1981;4:343.

126. Urbach E: Beitrage zu einer physiologischen und pathologischin chemie der haut. X. Mitteilung. Eine neue diabetische stoffwechsel-dermatose, nekrobiosis lipoidica diabeticorum. *Arch Dermatol Syph* 1932;166:273.

127. Lowitt MH, Dover JS: Necrobiosis lipoidica. *J Am Acad Dermatol* 1991;25:735.

128. O'Toole EA, Kennedy U, Nolan JJ, *et al*: Necrobiosis lipoidica: Only a minority of patients have diabetes mellitus. *Br J Dermatol* 1999; 140:283.

129. Muller SA, Winkelmann RK: Necrobiosis lipoidica diabeticorum. A clinical and pathological investigation of 171 cases. *Arch Dermatol* 1966;93:272.

130. Borssen B, Bergenheim T, Lithner F: The epidemiology of foot lesions in diabetic patients aged 15–50 years. *Diabet Med* 1990;7: 438.

131. De Silva BD, Schofield OM, Walker JD: The prevalence of necrobiosis lipoidica diabeticorum in children with type 1 diabetes. *Br J Dermatol* 1999;141:593.

132. Kavanagh GM, Novelli M, Hartog M: Necrobiosis lipoidica—involvement of atypical sites. *Clin Exp Dermatol* 1993;18:543.

133. Crosby DL, Woodley DT, Leonard DD: Concomitant granuloma annulare and necrobiosis lipoidica. *Dermatologica* 1991;183:225.

134. Boulton AJM, Cutfield RG, Abouganem D: Necrobiosis lipoidica diabeticorum: A clinicopathologic study. *J Am Acad Dermatol* 1988;18: 530.

135. Mann RJ, Harman RRM: Cutaneous anaesthesia in necrobiosis lipoidica. *Br J Dermatol* 1984;110:323.

136. Saarialho-Kere UK, Chang ES, Welgus HG: Expression of interstitial collagenase, 92-kDa gelatinase, and tissue inhibitor of metalloproteinase-1 in granuloma annulare and necrobiosis lipoidica diabeticorum. *J Invest Dermatol* 1993;100:335.

137. Dandona P, Freedman D, Barter S: Glycosylated haemoglobin in patients with necrobiosis lipoidica and granuloma annulare. *Clin Exp Dermatol* 1981;6:299.

138. Brungger A: Transkutane sauerstoff- und kohlendioxiddruckmessung bei necrobiosis lipoidica. *Hautarzt* 1989;40:231.

139. Petzelbauer P, Wolff K, Tappeiner G: Necrobiosis lipoidica: Treatment with systemic corticosteroids. *Br J Dermatol* 1992;126:542.

140. Noz KC, Korstanje MJ, Vermeer BJ: Ulcerating necrobiosis lipoidica effectively treated with pentoxifylline. *Clin Exp Dermatol* 1993; 18:78.

141. Jelinek JE: Skin disorders associated with diabetes mellitus. In: Rifkin H, Porte D, eds. *Diabetes Mellitus*. Elsevier:1990;838.

142. Darvay A, Acland KM, Russell-Jones R: Persistent ulcerated necrobiosis lipoidica responding to treatment with cyclosporin. *Br J Dermatol* 1999;141:725.

143. Dubin BJ, Kaplan EN: The surgical treatment of necrobiosis lipoidica diabeticorum. *Plast Reconstr Surg* 1977;60:421.

144. Dahl MV: Granuloma annulare. In: Fitzpatrick TB, Freedberg IM, Eisen AZ, *et al*, eds. *Dermatology in General Medicine*. McGraw-Hill:1999;1152.

145. Dabski K, Winkelmann RK: Generalized granuloma annulare: Clinical and laboratory findings in 100 patients. *J Am Acad Dermatol* 1989;20:39.

146. Wells RS, Smith MA: The natural history of granuloma annulare. *Br J Dermatol* 1963;75:199.

147. Haim S, Friedman-Birnbaum R, Haim N: Carbohydrate tolerance in patients with granuloma annulare: Study of fifty-two cases. *Br J Dermatol* 1973;88:447.

148. Veraldi S, Bencini PL, Drudi E, *et al*: Laboratory abnormalities in granuloma annulare: A case-control study. *Br J Dermatol* 1997;136: 652.

149. Studer EM, Calza AM, Saurat JH: Precipitating factors and associated diseases in 84 patients with granuloma annulare: A retrospective study. *Dermtaology* 1996;193:364.

150. Kerker BJ, Huang CP, Morison WL: Photochemotherapy of generalized granuloma annulare. *Arch Dermatol* 1990;126:359.

151. Ghadially R, Sibbald RG, Walter JB: Granuloma annulare in patients with human immunodeficiency virus infections. *J Am Acad Dermatol* 1989;20:232.

152. McGregor JM, McGibbon DH: Disseminated granuloma annulare as a presentation of acquired immunodeficiency syndrome (AIDS). *Clin Exp Dermatol* 1992;17:60.

153. Melin H: An atrophic circumscribed skin lesion in the lower extremities of diabetics. *Acta Med Scand* 1964;423(suppl):1.

154. Danowski TS, Sabeh G, Sarver ME: Shin spots and diabetes mellitus. *Am J Med Sci* 1966;251:570.

155. Binkley GW: Dermopathy in diabetes mellitus. *Arch Dermatol* 1965; 92:106.

156. Port M: Diabetic dermopathy. *J Am Podiatr Assoc* 1982;72:418.

157. Bauer ME, Levin NE, Frankel A: Pigmented pretibial patches: A cutaneous manifestation of diabetes mellitus. *Arch Dermatol* 1966; 93:282.

158. Borssen B, Bergenheim T, Lithner F: The epidemiology of foot lesions in diabetic patients aged 15-50 years. *Diabet Med* 1990;7:438.

159. Lithner F: Cutaneous reactions of the extremities of diabetics to local thermal trauma. *Acta Med Scand* 1975;198:319.

160. Shemer A, Bergman R, Linn S, *et al*: Diabetic dermopathy and internal complications in diabetes mellitus. *Int J Dermatol* 1998;37:113.

161. Fisher ER, Danowski TS: Histologic, histochemical, and electron microscopic features of the shin spots of diabetes mellitus. *Am J Clin Pathol* 1968;50:547.

162. Lipsky BA, Baker PD, Ahroni JH: Diabetic bullae: 12 cases of a purportedly rare cutaneous disorder. *Int J Dermatol* 2000;39:196.

163. Toonstra J: Bullosis diabeticorum. Report of a case with a review of the literature. *J Am Acad Dermatol* 1985;13:799.

164. Bernstein JE, Medenica M, Soltani K, *et al*: Bullous eruption of diabetes mellitus. *Arch Dermatol* 1979;115:324.

165. Rapini RP, Hebert AA, Drucker CR: Acquired perforating dermatosis. Evidence for combined transepidermal elimination of both collagen and elastic fibers. *Arch Dermatol* 1989;125:1074.

166. Faver IR, Daoud MS, Su WPD: Acquired reactive perforating collagenosis. Report of six cases and review of the literature. *J Am Acad Dermatol* 1994;30:575.

167. Morton CA, Henderson IS, Jones MC, *et al*: Acquired perforating dermatosis in a British dialysis population. *Br J Dermatol* 1996; 135:671.

168. Higgins GA, Recant L, Fischman AB: The glucagonoma syndrome: Surgically curable diabetes. *Am J Surg* 1979;137:142.

169. Kheir S, Omura EF, Grizzle WE: Histologic variation in the skin lesions of the glucagonoma syndrome. *Am J Surg Pathol* 1986; 10: 445.

170. Wilkinson DS: Necrolytic migratory erythema with carcinoma of the pancreas. *Trans St John's Derm Soc* 1973;59:244.

171. Boden G: Insulinoma and glucagonoma. *Semin Oncol* 1987;14:253.

172. Edney JA, Hofmann S, Thompson JS: Glucagonoma syndrome is an underdiagnosed clinical entity. *Am J Surg* 1990;160:625.

173. Kasper CS, McMurry K: Necrolytic migratory erythema without glucagonoma versus canine superficial necrolytic dermatitis: Is hepatic impairment a clue to pathogenesis? *J Am Acad Dermatol* 1991; 25:534.

174. Breatnach ES, Han SY, Rahatzad MT: CT evaluation of glucagonomas. *J Comput Assist Tomogr* 1985;9:25.

175. Prinz RA, Dorsch TR, Lawrence AM: Clinical aspects of glucagon-producing islet cell tumors. *Am J Gastroenterol* 1981;76:125.

176. Reyes-Govea J, Holm A, Aldrete JS: Response of glucagonomas to surgical excision and chemotherapy. *Am Surg* 1989;55:523.

177. Maton PN, Gardner JD, Jensen RT: Use of long-acting somatostatin analog SMS 201-995 in patients with pancreatic islet cell tumors. *Dig Dis Sci* 1989;34:28S.

178. Reichard P, Nilsson B-Y, Rosenqvist U: The effect of long-term intensified insulin treatment on the development of microvascular complications of diabetes mellitus. *N Engl J Med* 1993;329:304.

179. The Diabetes Control and Complications Trial (DCCT) Research Group: The effect of intensive treatment of diabetes on the development and progression of long-term complications in insulin-dependent diabetes mellitus. *N Engl J Med* 1993;329:977.

180. Goldstein HH: Allergy and diabetes. In: Marble A, White P, Bradley RF, *et al*, eds. *Joslin's Diabetes Mellitus*. Lea & Febiger:1971;701.

181. Anderson JA, Adkinson NF: Allergic reactions to drugs and biologic agents. *JAMA* 1987;258:2891.

182. Wright AD, Walsh CH, Fitzgerald MG: Very pure porcine insulin in clinical practice. *Br Med J* 1979;1:25.

183. McNally PG, Jowett NI, Kurinczuk JJ: Lipohypertrophy and lipoatrophy complicating treatment with highly purified bovine and porcine insulins. *Postgrad Med J* 1988;64:850.

184. Young RJ, Steel JM, Frier BM: Insulin injection sites in diabetes—a neglected area? *Br Med J* 1981;283:349.

185. Chantelau E, Reuter M, Schotes S: Severe lipatrophy with human insulin: Successfully treated by CSII. *Diabet Med* 1993;10:580.

186. Page MD, Bodansky HJ: Human insulin and lipoatrophy[letter]. *Diabet Med* 1992;9:779.

187. Reeves WG, Allen BR, Tattersall RB: Insulin-induced lipoatrophy: Evidence for an immune pathogenesis. *Br Med J* 1980;280:1500.

188. Young RJ, Hannan WJ, Frier BM: Diabetic lipohypertrophy delays insulin absorption. *Diabetes Care* 1984;7:479.

189. Thow JC, Johnson AB, Marsden S: Morphology of palpably abnormal injection sites and effects on absorption of isophane (NPH) insulin. *Diabet Med* 1990;7:795.

190. Kahn CR, Rosenthal AS: Immunologic reactions to insulin: Insulin allergy, insulin resistance, and the autoimmune insulin syndrome. *Diabetes Care* 1979;2:283.

191. Feinglos MN, Jegasothy BV: Insulin allergy due to zinc. *Lancet* 1979; 1:122.

192. Dykewicz MS, Kim HW, Orfan N: Immunologic analysis of anaphylaxis to protamine component in neutral protamine Hagedorn human insulin. *J Allergy Clin Immunol* 1994;93:117.

193. Takatsuki H, Ishii H, Yamauchi T: A case of insulin allergy: The crystalline human insulin may mask its antigenicity. *Diabetes Res Clin Pract* 1991;12:137.

194. Falholt K, Hoskam JAM, Karamanos BG: Insulin-specific IgE in serum of 67 diabetic patients against human insulin (Novo), porcine insulin, and bovine insulin. Four case reports. *Diabetes Care* 1983; 6(suppl 1):61.

195. Small P, Lerman S: Human insulin allergy. *Ann Allergy* 1984;53:39.

196. Fireman P, Fineberg SE, Galloway JA: Development of IgE antibodies to human (recombinant DNA), porcine, and bovine insulins in diabetic subjects. *Diabetes Care* 1982;5(suppl 2):119.

197. Peterson K-G, Khalaf A, Naithani V: IgE antibodies to insulin and related peptides, a result of insulin treatment? *Diabetes Res Clin Pract* 1989;7:41.

198. Jegasothy BV: Cutaneous complications of diabetic treatment. In: Jelinek JE, ed. *The Skin in Diabetes*. Lea & Febiger:1986;217.

199. Thompson DM, Ronco JJ: Prolonged desensitization required for treatment of generalized allergy to human insulin. *Diabetes Care* 1993;16:957.

200. Ganz MA, Unterman T, Roberts M: Resistance and allergy to recombinant human insulin. *J Allergy Clin Immunol* 1990;86:45.

201. Kelly SE: Multiple injection abscesses in a diabetic caused by *Mycobacterium chelonei*. *Clin Exp Dermatol* 1987;12:48.

202. Jordaan HF, Sandler M: Zinc-induced granuloma—a unique complication of insulin therapy. *Clin Exp Dermatol* 1989;14:227.

203. Chantelau E, Berger M, Bohlken B: Silicone oil released from disposable insulin syringes. *Diabetes Care* 1986;9:672.

204. Fleming MG, Simon SI: Cutaneous insulin reaction resembling acanthosis nigricans. *Arch Dermatol* 1986;122:1054.

205. Guinn TS, Bailey GJ, Mecklenburg RS: Factors related to discontinuation of continuous subcutaneous insulin-infusion therapy. *Diabetes Care* 1988;11:46.

206. Chantelau E, Spraul M, Mu;auhlhauser I: Long-term safety, efficacy and side-effects of continuous subcutaneous insulin infusion treatment for type I (insulin-dependent) diabetes mellitus: A one centre experience. *Diabetologia* 1989;32:421.

CHAPTER 54

Relationship of Glycemic Control to Diabetic Complications

Jay S. Skyler

The most important issue facing clinicians who care for patients with diabetes is the extent to which the frequency or severity of chronic complications can be influenced by the degree to which glycemia is controlled. For many years, this was one of the most controversial questions in the field of diabetes. This was in spite of the fact that substantial accumulated evidence demonstrated that the frequency, severity, and progression of retinopathy, nephropathy, and neuropathy are related to the degree of hyperglycemia over time. That evidence came from epidemiologic, clinical, and pathologic studies in human beings; from studies using animal models of diabetes; and from the elucidation of a number of biochemical mechanisms, putatively involved in the pathogenesis of these complications, that are influenced directly by hyperglycemia. Yet controversy on this subject continued, principally because there were no longitudinal prospective randomized intervention studies. That lacuna no longer exists. Now it has been unequivocally established—by randomized controlled clinical trials—that careful control of glycemia indeed can lessen the risk of the microangiopathic and neurologic complications of diabetes. This has been demonstrated for type 1 diabetes mellitus (T1DM) in the landmark Diabetes Control and Complications Trial (DCCT), the Stockholm Diabetes Intervention Study (SDIS), and a number of smaller prospective intervention studies. It also has been demonstrated for type 2 diabetes mellitus (T2DM) by the United Kingdom Prospective Diabetes Study (UKPDS) and the smaller Kumamoto Study from Japan.

A growing number of epidemiologic studies also have shown that there is a relationship between degree of glycemia and the incidence and prevalence of macrovascular complications of diabetes (i.e., cardiovascular disease, cerebrovascular disease, and peripheral vascular disease). Indeed, the relationship between glycemia and macrovascular disease extends throughout the range of glycemia, including nondiabetic individuals. Yet, the large randomized controlled clinical trials have failed to show convincingly that macrovascular disease is impacted by glycemic control. However, some analyses suggest that the DCCT and UKPDS do show such an effect.

In this chapter, the focus will be on intervention studies, specifically, randomized controlled clinical trials. However, because of their historical importance, the WESDR Study and the Brussels study also are discussed.

EPIDEMIOLOGIC AND OBSERVATIONAL STUDIES

Brussels Study

The Brussels Study, reported in 1978, represented a landmark in delimiting the question of the relationship between glycemia and diabetic complications.[1] Between 1947 and 1973, Jean Pirart of Brussels, Belgium, personally followed 4400 patients for up to a quarter century, and meticulously recorded observations on their glycemic control and the appearance of diabetic complications. His striking observations demonstrated that the frequency and severity of diabetic retinopathy, nephropathy, and neuropathy were related to both duration of disease and to cumulative glycemic control. Poor control assessed cumulatively over the years was associated with a higher prevalence and incidence of microangiopathy and neuropathy, especially severe retinopathy. Yet, Pirart did not randomly allocate patients *a priori* to either "good" or "poor" control. Thus it was impossible to exclude the possibility that patients with mild diabetes achieved "good" control and escaped complications, while patients with more severe diabetes achieved "poor" control and suffered more complications. Moreover, the study was conducted in an era prior to the availability of glycated (glycosylated) hemoglobin determinations to assess glycemic control.

Other Epidemiologic and Clinical Studies

Subsequently, many other similar clinical studies, as well as a large number of both cross-sectional and longitudinal epidemiologic studies have reported relationships between glycated hemoglobin and incidence and prevalence of retinopathy, nephropathy, and neuropathy.

Wisconsin Study

One of the longest, largest, and most carefully conducted of these longitudinal epidemiologic studies is the Wisconsin Epidemiologic Study of Diabetic Retinopathy (WESDR).[2–22] The Wisconsin study is a large population-based study which has reported on the evolution of diabetic complications, particularly retinopathy, among diabetic patients receiving community care in 11 counties in southern Wisconsin.[2–6] The sample included all diabetic subjects with onset before 30 years of age (younger-onset cohort; n = 1210) and a probability sample of those with onset after 30 years of age (older-onset cohort; n = 1780 of 5431 patients with a confirmed diagnosis of diabetes). From this sample, 79.1% (n = 2366) underwent baseline evaluation in 1980–1982. Four-year follow-up evaluations were performed in 1984–1986 on 1878 individuals, 95.7% of those evaluated at baseline and still alive. Ten-year follow-up evaluations were performed in 1990–1992 on 1298 individuals, 88.7% of those evaluated at baseline and still alive.[6] Because of the high death rate in the older cohort, only the younger cohort was re-examined at 14 years in 1995–1996, with 634 subjects participating.[11] Some information also was obtained from an additional 309 subjects from the older cohort.[12,19] Evaluations were conducted in a special van, and included collection of historical data, blood pressure, visual acuity, seven-field fundus photography, measurement of glycosylated hemoglobin (HbA_{1c}), and urine protein.

The younger-onset cohort presumably includes mostly individuals with T1DM. For many analyses, the older-onset cohort is divided into those treated with insulin (46.3% of the original probability sample) and those not treated with insulin (53.7% of the original probability sample). Those not treated with insulin presumably have T2DM, while those treated with insulin presumably are a mixed group with most probably having T2DM.

Among the many findings reported by the WESDR investigators, the most notable describe the relationship of hyperglycemia (both baseline HbA_{1c} and change of HbA_{1c} between baseline and 4-year follow-up) and (a) incidence and progression of retinopathy, (b) incidence of nephropathy, (c) nerve function and incidence of lower extremity amputations, (d) hospitalizations, and (e) survival. Most of these analyses evaluated the influence on a given outcome measure of HbA_{1c} divided into quartiles.

In all three cohorts (younger-onset, older-onset treated with insulin, older-onset not treated with insulin), there was at both 4[7] and 10 years' follow-up[8] a statistically significant relationship between baseline HbA_{1c} and (a) incidence of retinopathy, (b) progression of retinopathy by two or more steps on a 15-step scale, and (c) progression to proliferative retinopathy. The 10-year data for progression to proliferative retinopathy are shown in Fig. 54-1, as an example of the relationships observed. At the 10-year follow-up, they also reported a statistically significant relationship between baseline HbA_{1c} and macular edema in the younger-onset cohort and the older-onset cohort considered as a whole,[9] and visual loss in the younger-onset cohort and the older-onset cohort treated with insulin, but not in the older-onset cohort not treated with insulin.[10] In the older-onset cohort, however, nondiabetic causes of visual loss (e.g., cataract, glaucoma, macular degeneration) complicated data interpretation. As noted, at 14 years, only data from the younger-onset cohort have been reported.[11,12] At that time, progression of retinopathy was more likely with elevated HbA_{1c} at baseline, or an increase in HbA_{1c} from the baseline to the 4-year follow-up. Increased risk of proliferative retinopathy or incidence of macular edema was associated with higher HbA_{1c} at baseline, and an increase in HbA_{1c} between the baseline and 4-year follow-up examination. Lower HbA_{1c} at baseline was associated with improvement in retinopathy. Visual loss was associated with higher HbA_{1c} levels.

In both the younger-onset cohort and the older-onset cohort, there was a statistically significant relationship between baseline HbA_{1c} and 4-year incidence of gross proteinuria[13,14] and microalbuminuria,[15,16] and 10-year incidence of gross proteinuria.[2] In the younger-onset cohort, but not in the older-onset cohort, there was a statistically significant relationship between baseline HbA_{1c} and 10-year incidence of decline in creatinine clearance and develop-

FIGURE 54-2. The effect on risk of development of complications of a 1% increase in glycosylated hemoglobin at baseline in (**A**) the younger-onset group, and (**B**) the older-onset group, in the Wisconsin Study. In each case the points are the estimate and the bars represent the 95% confidence interval of the estimate. (*Adapted with permission from Klein.[2]*)

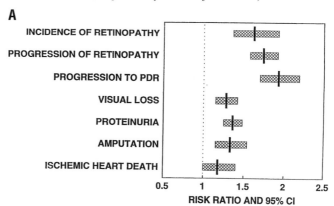

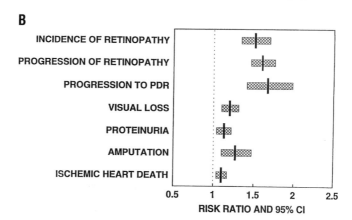

FIGURE 54-1. The relationship of 10-year progression to proliferative diabetic retinopathy (**PDR**) by quartile of glycosylated hemoglobin (1st quartile □, 2nd quartile ▨, 3rd quartile ▦, 4th quartile ■) at baseline in the Wisconsin Study. This is shown in three cohorts: the younger-onset group taking insulin, the older-onset group taking insulin, and the older-onset group not taking insulin. In each cohort the *p* values for the Mantel-Haenszel test of trend are significant. (*Adapted with permission from Klein et al.[8]*)

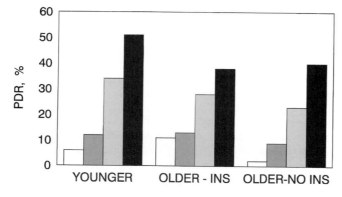

ment of renal insufficiency.[17] The absence of a relationship with glycemia in the older-onset cohort may have been because the overall event rate for renal failure was low (1.8%).

In terms of nerve function, in all three cohorts, there was at 10 years' follow-up a statistically significant relationship between baseline HbA$_{1c}$ and loss of tactile sensation, whereas the relationship between baseline HbA$_{1c}$ and loss of tactile sensation was statistically significant only in the younger-onset cohort and the older-onset cohort on insulin.[3] In both the younger-onset cohort and the older-onset cohort considered as a whole, there was a statistically significant relationship between baseline HbA$_{1c}$ and incidence of lower extremity amputation both at 10 years[18] and 14 years.[19]

Factors from the 4-year examination were studied for their ability to predict hospitalization at the 10-year examination. HbA$_{1c}$ level predicted hospitalization.[20]

In terms of mortality,[3,21] in the younger-onset cohort, after controlling for other risk factors in proportional hazard models and considering underlying cause of death, HbA$_{1c}$ was significantly associated with 10-year mortality from all causes, from diabetes *per se*, and from ischemic heart disease. In the older-onset cohort, HbA$_{1c}$ was significantly associated with 10-year mortality from all causes, from diabetes *per se*, from ischemic heart disease, and from stroke.

The data from the Wisconsin study demonstrate a strong and consistent relationship between glycemia and the incidence and progression of microvascular (diabetic retinopathy, loss of vision, and nephropathy) and macrovascular (amputation and cardiovascular disease mortality) complications in people with both T1DM and T2DM. The relationship was such that the investigators could calculate the effect on risk of development of complications of a 1% increase in baseline glycosylated hemoglobin, as illustrated in Fig. 54-2.[2]

INTERVENTION TRIALS

The Brussels Study mentioned earlier[1] stimulated the initiation of a number of prospective trials designed to examine the influence of improved glycemic control, achieved with intensive insulin therapy (often, but not always, using an insulin infusion pump), in contrast to unchanged conventional therapy. These were generally initiated in the early 1980s, and most (except one from the mid- to late 1970s) have used glycosylated hemoglobin determinations to assess integrated glycemic control. These early trials mostly involved subjects with T1DM.

Three clinical trials have studied subjects with T2DM. One of these, the Veterans Administration Cooperative Study on Glycemic Control and Complications in Type 2 Diabetes Mellitus (VACSDM), was unfortunately aborted after the pilot phase due to lack of funding.[22,23] After a long hiatus, it is finally again under way.[24] The large United Kingdom Prospective Diabetes Study (UKPDS) was completed in 1998. It will be discussed in detail. The smaller Kumamoto Study also will be discussed.

Intervention Trials: Type 1 Diabetes

Meta-Analysis

In 1993, Wang and colleagues[25,26] reported a formal meta-analysis of published randomized controlled trials that evaluated the effects of intensive glycemic control of T1DM on the progression of diabetic retinopathy and nephropathy, and the risks of severe hypoglycemia and diabetic ketoacidosis. These authors performed a search of the English language literature from 1966 through 1991 and identified 32 potential studies. Sixteen reports met their inclusion criteria of being randomized clinical trials with sufficient follow-up data for retinopathy and/or nephropathy to permit analysis. These 16 reports used in the meta-analysis contain data from 12 independent randomized controlled trials. The overall difference in the risk of retinopathy or nephropathy progression was analyzed, and the overall difference in the incidence of hypoglycemia or diabetic ketoacidosis was estimated. Table 54-1 summarizes the results of the meta-analysis. When compared to conventional control, intensive therapy reduced glycosylated hemoglobin (%) by 1.4 with a 95% confidence interval ranging from 1.1–1.8. The analysis showed that compared to conventionally treated patients, after more than 2 years of intensive therapy the risk of retinopathy progression was significantly lower (odds ratio [OR] 0.49; 95% confidence interval, 0.28–0.85). Seeking evidence of early worsening of retinopathy, the analysis found that in the intensive therapy group, the risk of retinopathy progression was insignificantly higher after 6–12 months of intensive control. In studies that assessed albumin excretion rate, the risk of nephropathy progression was decreased significantly in the intensive therapy group (OR 0.34; 95% confidence interval, 0.20–0.58). The authors

TABLE 54-1. Formal Reported Meta-Analysis Results

		Studies	Subjects	OR	95% CI	*p*
Retinopathy	Early: 6–12 mo	5	223	2.11	(0.54, 8.31)	0.29
	Late: >2 yr	6	271	0.49	(0.28, 0.85)	0.011
	PDR or laser	4	186	0.44	(0.22, 0.87)	0.018
Nephropathy	All	8	278	0.32	(0.19, 0.55)	0.000033
	Only AER	7	266	0.34	(0.20, 0.58)	0.000079
				ABS CHG #/100 pt-yr		
Hypoglycemia	Severe	6	347	+9.1	(−1.4, 19.6)	
DKA	In CSII	3	144	+12.6	(8.7, 16.5)	

Comparison of intensive therapy to conventional control (odds ratio [OR]) for retinopathy progression (after 6–12 months of intensive therapy, after more than 2 years of intensive therapy, and for progression to proliferative retinopathy or laser treatment) and for nephropathy progression (including all eligible trials, and limiting analysis to studies that measured changes in albumin excretion rate [AER]). Comparison of intensive therapy to conventional control (absolute change in incidence) for severe hypoglycemia and for diabetic ketoacidosis in those who received continuous subcutaneous insulin infusion (CSII). The 95% confidence interval (CI) and *p* value for significance (where available) are shown.

concluded that long-term intensive glycemic control significantly reduced the risks of diabetic retinopathy and nephropathy progression among T1DM patients when compared with randomly assigned controls.

Review of Studies

The studies discussed in this section are listed in Table 54-2. They include those reviewed in the above meta-analysis (with updated data on some), three trials published since the meta-analysis (Oslo-2A, Oslo-2B, and the DCCT), one apparently missed by the meta-analysis (Italian Multicenter), and one nonrandomized but prospective study (Dallas). Several of these studies have included neurologic endpoints, lipid levels, and other parameters. The bulk of this discussion, however, relates to endpoints in the eyes and kidneys, which are easier to assess.

Steno Studies

Under the leadership of Torsten Deckert, investigators at the Steno Memorial Hospital in Gentofte, Denmark, conducted two independent studies in 70 patients with T1DM.[27-33] In both of these studies, subjects were randomly allocated to either unchanged conventional therapy (CT) or improved metabolic control using continuous subcutaneous insulin infusion (CSII). In the first study, initiated in 1980, 34 subjects were enrolled on the basis of having moderately advanced background diabetic retinopathy. In the second study, initiated in 1983, enrollment (of 36 subjects) was based

on the presence of microalbuminuria. In the retinopathy study, in the CSII group, there was consistent improvement in renal function studies after 6 months, 1 year, and 2 years.[27-29] On the other hand, there was transient deterioration in retinal morphology, characterized by the appearance of soft exudates, indicative of retinal infarction, at the 1-year follow-up in the CSII group. Yet by 2 years, there was a marginally significant trend towards stabilization or improvement in retinal morphology in the CSII group, in contrast to progressive deterioration in the CT group.[29]

In the Steno microalbuminuria study, over 2 years 5 of 18 patients randomized to CT progressed from microalbuminuria to clinical nephropathy, defined as dipstick-positive proteinuria.[30] In contrast, in the CSII group, none of the 18 patients so progressed, a statistically significant difference. Moreover, if one includes in this analysis those subjects in the Steno retinopathy study who also had microalbuminuria at baseline,[31] a total of 10 of 25 subjects treated with CT progressed from microalbuminuria to clinical nephropathy by 2 years, compared to a total of 1 of 26 subjects treated with CSII ($p < 0.001$).[32]

A subsequent report updated these observations after follow-up of 8 years for subjects initially enrolled in the retinopathy study and after 5 years for subjects initially enrolled in the microalbuminuria study.[33] Interestingly, there was sustained difference between the groups in glycemic control. Of the total cohort at long-term follow-up, 12 of 33 assigned to CT had developed proliferative retinopathy, in contrast to 8 of 36 assigned to CSII, but

TABLE 54-2 List of Intervention Studies in Type 1 Diabetes Examining the Effects of Glycemic Control on Diabetic Complication

Study	n* (Start/End)	Age (Start) (years)	Study Duration (months)	Outcomes Assessed†	Glyco-Hb %‡ (Con‡/Int)	Entry Criteria§ Eyes	Entry Criteria§ Kidney	Outcome¶ Eyes	Outcome¶ Kidneys	Outcome¶ Nerves	Refs#
Steno-1	34/29	18–51	24	E	8.5/7.0	NP	N-Cr	Trend	—	Trend	27–30
	30/29		24	K	8.5/7.0			—	Benefit	—	
Steno-2	36/36	18–50	24	K	8.9/7.4	NP	AER >30	—	Benefit	—	31–33
Kroc	68/62	14–60	48	E	—	NP	N-Cr, UPE<1000	No △	—	—	34–37
	68/59		8	K	10.0/8.1			—	Benefit	—	
Oslo-1	45/43	18–42	48	E K N	10.2/8.9	NP	N-Cr, –Dipstick	No △	Benefit	Trend	38–46
Oslo-2A	30/23	14–29	12	K	10.4/9.0	N/NP	AER 22-300	—	Benefit	—	47
Oslo-2B	18/18	18–29	24	K	9.7/8.6	N/NP	AER 22-300	—	Benefit	—	48
SDIS	102/89	31 ± 1	94	E K N	8.5/7.1	NP	N-Cr	Benefit	Benefit	Benefit	49–59
Oxford	74/69	21–60	24	E K N	11.4/10.5	NP	N-Cr	No △	Benefit	Benefit	60
Aarhus-1	24/23	18–41	36	E	8.5/7.2	N/NP	–Dipstick	No △	—	—	61–62
	24/23		12	K	9.1/7.0			—	Benefit	—	
Aarhus-2	24/21	29 ± 1	24	K	8.6/7.2	N/NP	N/↑ AER	—	No △	—	63
Italian MC	38/34	21–55	24	E	8.1/7.3	NP	N-Cr, AER<1000	Trend	—	—	64
Naples	44/38	18–50	60	E	10.7/8.7	NP	UPE<500	No △	—	—	65
Paris	52/42	40 ± 2	50	E	FBG: 195/154	NP	—	Benefit	—	—	66–68
Guy's	12/12	18–43	12	K	11.8/7.1	NP	↑GFR, –Ren Dis	—	Benefit	—	69
Helsinki	65/54	18–57	12	E	10.1/9.9	N/NP/P	UPE<1000	No △	—	—	70
DDPT	57/54	16–42	48	E K N BM	10.4/7.2	N/NP	N-Cr	Benefit	Benefit	Benefit	71–76
DCCT	1441/1422	13–39	108	E K N	9.1/7.2	N/NP	AER<200	Benefit	Benefit	Benefit	77–88
	726					N	AER<40	Benefit	Benefit	Benefit	
	715					NP	AER<200	Benefit	Benefit	Benefit	

*n = number of subjects enrolled at start and available for analysis at end.

†Outcomes assessed: E = eyes, K = kidneys, N = nerves, BM = basement membrane width (muscle capillary).

‡Glyco-Hb% = ending glycated hemoglobin (%) for control (Cont) and intensive (Int) groups (FBG = fasting plasma glucose in mg/dL for study where glyco-Hb not available).

§Entry criteria—for eyes: N = normal, NP = nonproliferative (background) retinopathy, P = proliferative retinopathy; for kidneys: N-Cr = normal serum creatinine, AER = albumin excretion rate (mg/24 h), UPE = urine protein excretion rate (mg/24 h), –Dipstick = dipstick negative for protein, ↑ = increased, GFR = glomerular filtration rate, –Ren Dis = negative history of renal disease.

¶Outcome: for intensive therapy: Benefit = statistically significant benefit; Trend = trend (not statistically significant) of benefit; No △ = no change or no difference.

#Refs = references.

this difference is not significant. On the other hand, the renal data are astounding. It turned out that no subject with low-range microalbuminuria (30–99 mg/24 h) at the outset progressed to proteinuria, regardless of treatment assignment. Among the 19 subjects with high-range microalbuminuria (100–300 mg/24 h) at the outset, all 10 of the subjects on CT had progressed to proteinuria (and had done so by 2 years' follow-up) and 7 of the 10 had developed hypertension, while only 2 of 9 subjects on CSII had similarly progressed to proteinuria and only 1 had hypertension. The differences for proteinuria and hypertension were significant, both with $p < 0.01$.

Kroc Group Study

In 1981 six centers in the United States and United Kingdom, led by Harry Keen of Guy's Hospital in London, combined under the aegis of the Kroc Foundation to conduct a randomized pilot trial comparing CT to CSII in 68 subjects with T1DM and mild to moderate background retinopathy.[34–37] After 8 months, they found deterioration of retinopathy in the CSII group,[34] which again proved to be transient, so that by 2 years' follow-up, the two groups were indistinguishable, with a trend towards lesser deterioration in the CSII group.[36] Moreover, they found that in subjects with microalbuminuria at the outset, there was an improvement in albumin excretion rate in the CSII group with no change in the CT group.[34,37]

Oslo Studies

The original Oslo study was initiated by Kristian Hanssen and his colleagues at the Aker Hospital in Oslo, Norway in 1980. In it, 45 subjects with T1DM were randomized to one of three treatments: conventional (CT) twice-daily insulin, multiple insulin (MI) injections (4–5/d), or CSII.[38–46] The randomization was maintained for 41 months, after which subjects could choose their own treatment. This study also demonstrated a transient deterioration in retinopathy with CSII,[39] with the 2-year data showing less progression of retinopathy in the MI and CSII groups than in the CT group,[40] but no significant difference in retinopathy at 41 months.[41] Follow-up of the original study cohort continued through 8 years, by which time treatment assignment was no longer in effect. That long-term follow-up showed that retinopathy outcome was related to both baseline glycemic control and mean glycemic control over the duration of follow-up.[42]

In the original Oslo study, mean urinary albumin excretion was only slightly elevated at the start of the study, but after 3–4 years showed a statistically significant decline in the CSII group, but not the other two groups.[43] Long-term follow-up of the original cohort after 7 years, by which time treatment assignment was no longer in effect, did show albumin excretion to be related to both baseline glycemic control and mean glycemic control over the 7-year follow-up period.[44,45] Neurologic outcomes were also assessed after 8 years.[46] It was found that there was a significant reduction in peripheral motor and sensory nerve conduction velocity in subjects with poorer glycemic control. Lowering of glycemia retarded the deterioration.

A second Oslo study randomized to CSII or CT 30 subjects with T1DM and early incipient nephropathy manifested by microalbuminuria.[47,48] There have been two reports from these subjects, each assessing novel outcome measures. In one, glomerular charge selectivity was measured in 23 subjects over a 12-month period.[47] The microalbuminuric subjects had reduced (compared to normal) glomerular charge selectivity at baseline, which was cor-rected by improved glycemic control. The second report described the results of serial renal biopsies performed in 18 subjects in this series at baseline and after 24–36 months.[48] With improved glycemic control, there was less increase in basement membrane width. Moreover, in the CT group but not the CSII group there was an increase in matrix/mesangial volume fraction and matrix star volume. There was a close relationship between glycemia and progression of glomerular morphological changes.

Stockholm Study

In this study, the Stockholm Diabetes Intervention Study (SDIS) conducted by Per Reichard and Urban Rosenqvist in Stockholm, Sweden, initially (in 1982) 102 subjects with T1DM, background diabetic retinopathy, normal serum creatinine, and unsatisfactory glycemic control were randomly allocated to either standard insulin treatment or improved metabolic control using intensified insulin treatment. They were evaluated at baseline, at 18 months, at 3 years, at 5 years (n = 96), and at 7.5 years (n = 89).[49–57] Follow-up reports after 10 years also have appeared, although during the last 2.5 years excellent glycemic control was sought in all subjects.[58,59]

In the experimental group with intensive treatment, over the initial 7.5 years of the study, mean glycosylated hemoglobin (HbA$_{1c}$) (upper limit of normal 5.7%) was 7.1% (versus a baseline value of 9.5%), while the control group with standard treatment was 8.5% (versus a baseline value of 9.4%), the difference between groups being highly statistically significant ($p < 0.001$). During the subsequent 2.5 years, the HbA$_{1c}$ values in the two groups converged slightly, with the previous intensive group rising to 7.3% and the previous standard group falling to 8.1%, still a significant difference ($p < 0.001$).

During the active 7.5-year treatment phase, cumulative rates of development of serious retinopathy[51,52,54] (i.e., that requiring laser photocoagulation) were 52% with standard treatment and 27% with intensive treatment, for a risk reduction of 48% with intensive treatment. The risk reduction for decreased visual acuity was 67%. When other variables influencing retinopathy progression were controlled for in logistic regression analysis, the effect of assignment to intensified treatment resulted in a risk reduction of 60%. In multivariate analysis, it was found that for every 1% increase in HbA$_{1c}$ during the period encompassing 6–60 months in the study, there was a 2.4-fold increased risk of developing serious retinopathy.

During the active 7.5-year treatment phase, cumulative rates of development of nephropathy[50,52,54] (i.e., an albumin excretion rate greater than 200 μg/min) were 19.6% with standard treatment and 2.3% with intensive treatment, for a risk reduction of 88% with intensive treatment. When other variables influencing retinopathy progression were controlled for in multivariate analysis, the effect of assignment to intensified treatment resulted in a risk reduction of 90%. Six of the subjects in the standard treatment group and none in the intensive treatment group developed nephropathy with a glomerular filtration rate below the normal range.

There was not a statistically significant difference in the rate of development of clinical neuropathy[54] during the active 7.5-year treatment phase. However, during the course of the study, deterioration in nerve conduction velocities (tibial, peroneal, sural nerves) was greater in the standard treatment group than the intensive treatment group. Cardiovascular autonomic nerve function was associated with lower HbA$_{1c}$, and after a mean of 11.4 years, autonomic function was better in the intensively treated group.[58]

Early indices of atherosclerosis were explored in a subset of SDIS subjects.[57] Carotid arteries were scanned for plaques, intima-media thickness was measured, and arterial wall stiffness was calculated. Patients in the standard treatment group had stiffer arteries ($p = 0.011$) and thicker intimamedia in the common carotid artery ($p = 0.009$) than those in the intensive treatment group. Patients with lower HbA_{1c} generally had better endothelial function ($p = 0.028$) and less stiff arteries ($p = 0.009$).

When the subjects were evaluated after 10 years, cumulative rates of development of serious retinopathy (63% versus 33%, $p = 0.003$), nephropathy (26% versus 7%, $p = 0.012$), and symptoms of neuropathy (32% versus 14%, $p = 0.041$) all were higher in the standard treatment group than the intensive treatment group.[59]

Other than the DCCT, of randomized controlled clinical trials designed to examine the influence of glycemic control on diabetic complications in T1DM, the SDIS is the largest trial and had the longest duration. It demonstrated that intensive insulin treatment retards the development of retinopathy and nephropathy, slows the rate of deterioration of nerve function, and perhaps positively impacts on early changes of atherosclerosis.

Oxford Study

The Oxford/Aylesbury (England) study group report in 1983 involved random assignment of 74 patients with insulin-treated diabetes (type 1 and type 2) and background retinopathy into two groups: usual diabetic care (group U) and more intensive care (group A) using basal Ultralente™ insulin and preprandial regular insulin.[60] Group A achieved lower glycosylated hemoglobin levels than group U. Group A also showed statistically better preservation of renal and sensory nerve function, as manifested by absence of change in creatinine clearance and vibratory perception threshold, parameters which showed some deterioration in group U. There was no significant difference in progression of retinopathy.

Aarhus Studies

The Aarhus (Denmark) group studied 24 subjects with T1DM and minimal or no retinopathy at the outset.[61,62] They were randomly allocated to standard insulin therapy (CIT) or CSII. Both their 1-year and 3-year reports showed minimal progression of retinopathy, with no statistical difference between the groups. The 1-year report found that elevated glomerular filtration rate was significantly improved in the CSII group, which also showed a decrement in albumin excretion rate that failed to reach statistical significance.

A separate study, also conducted in Aarhus, examined the influence of glycemic control on renal function in 24 subjects with T1DM.[63] Prior to intervention, there was hyperfunction manifested by hyperfiltration and nephromegaly. Elevated glomerular filtration rate was significantly reduced in the CSII group, whereas there was no reduction in the elevated renal plasma flow or nephromegaly.

Italian Study

The Italian National Research Council Study Group on Diabetic Retinopathy, comprising investigators at the Universities of Padua, Milan, and Perugia, studied 38 subjects with T1DM and ischemic background retinopathy, who were matched in pairs for gender, age, diabetes duration, and retinal status.[64] The pairs were then randomly assigned to conventional therapy (CT) or CSII, and followed every 6 months for 2 years. Their report in 1989 demonstrated significant difference in glycemic control, and less deterioration of retinopathy in the CSII group.

Naples Study

Another Italian group in Naples randomized 44 subjects with T1DM and mild to moderate background retinopathy to usual conventional therapy (UCT) or intensified conventional therapy (ICT), and admitted them for 24-hour glucose profiles at baseline and after 1, 3, and 5 years.[65] In this study, improved glycemic control did not prevent progression of retinopathy, which was similar in both groups.

Paris Study

An important study from Hotel Dieu in Paris was the first attempt at a prospective randomized study of diabetic retinopathy in T1DM.[66,67] This study evaluated progression of background retinopathy in 52 subjects and reported that attempts at careful control resulted in slower progression over 50 months of follow-up. Unfortunately, the study was marred by both a relatively crude endpoint (number of microaneurysms) and by a high rate of crossover between groups.[68] It also antedated the era of glycosylated hemoglobin measurements.

Guy's Study

A study from Guy's Hospital randomized 12 patients with normal albumin excretion rates, but increased glomerular filtration rates, to CSII or UCIT.[69] They found that after 1 year, improved control in the CSII group resulted in normalization of glomerular filtration rate, but persistence of increased renal size.

Helsinki Study

A study from Helsinki enrolled 65 subjects with T1DM in a crossover study that spanned 1 year.[70] The duration was too short to see a beneficial effect on retinopathy. However, what was evident was an early worsening of retinopathy seen in other studies as a transient deterioration.

Dallas Study

The Dallas Diabetes Prospective Trial (DDPT) was initiated by Philip Raskin and colleagues in the early 1980s.[71–76] Patients with T1DM were offered the opportunity to participate in an intensive treatment program using CSII. Thirty accepted, while 24 declined, remaining on their existing conventional treatment (CT), but agreed to follow-up evaluations over 4 years. Thus the DDPT is a nonrandomized, but prospective study. In it, there was sustained improvement in glycemic control in the CSII group, and no change in the CT group. There have been many reports from this study, and they have demonstrated, among other things, the following statistically significant findings regarding microvascular complications: (1) Measurement of capillary basement membrane (CBM) width, thickening of which is the histologic hallmark of microangiopathy, showed there was thinning of thickened CBMs in the CSII group, in contrast to progressive thickening of CBMs in the CT group;[71,72] (2) there was less progression of retinopathy with CSII (i.e., stabilization or improvement in retinopathy in the CSII group), in contrast to stabilization or deterioration in the CT group;[73,74] (3) among subjects with microalbuminuria at the outset, there was stabilization in the CSII group, and increased albumin excretion in the CT group;[74] and (4) there was improvement in nerve function in the CSII group.[75,76]

The Diabetes Control and Complications Trial (DCCT)

The DCCT examined whether intensive treatment with the goal of maintaining blood glucose concentrations close to the normal range could decrease the frequency and severity of diabetic microvascular and neurologic complications.[77–88] It was conducted under the auspices the U.S. National Institutes of Health—specifically the National Institute of Diabetes, Digestive, and Kidney Diseases (NIDDK)—with the support of the National Heart, Lung, and Blood Institute, the National Eye Institute, the National Center for Research Resources, and various corporate sponsors. The DCCT was designed with sufficient statistical power to draw a relatively firm conclusion. The DCCT was conducted in 29 centers across North America (26 in the United States and 3 in Canada). Enrollment began in the early 1980s. A total of 1441 subjects with T1DM were enrolled. Of these, 726 subjects were recruited within the first 5 years after developing diabetes (mean duration at entry = 2.5 years) and had no evidence of diabetic retinopathy or of microalbuminuria at baseline (the primary prevention cohort). Another 715 subjects were recruited within the first 15 years (mean duration at entry = 8.8 years) after developing diabetes and had mild to moderate background diabetic retinopathy with either normoalbuminuria or microalbuminuria (the secondary intervention cohort). Subjects had to be willing to accept random allocation to treatment group and maintain that treatment assignment for the duration of the study. They were randomly assigned either to intensive therapy or to conventional therapy. Intensive therapy involved insulin administered either by continuous subcutaneous insulin infusion (CSII) with an external insulin pump or by multiple daily insulin injections (MDI) (three or more injections per day), guided by frequent self-monitoring of blood glucose (SMBG) 3–4 times daily, with additional specified samples including a weekly overnight sample; meticulous attention to diet; and monthly visits to the treating clinic. Conventional therapy involved no more than two daily insulin injections, urine glucose monitoring or SMBG no more than twice daily, periodic diet review, and clinic visits every 2–3 months. The subjects were followed for a minimum of 4 years and a maximum of 9 years, with a mean follow-up of 6.5 years (a mean of 6 years in the primary prevention cohort and of 7 years in the secondary intervention cohort), for a total of approximately 9300 patient-years of observation. Of 1430 subjects alive at the end of the study, 1422 came for evaluation of outcomes. Throughout the study, 98–99% of available data were collected.

The experimental group treated with intensive therapy achieved a median glycosylated hemoglobin (HbA$_{1c}$) throughout the study of approximately 7.2% versus a value in the control group treated with conventional therapy of approximately 9.1% ($p < 0.001$) (Fig. 54-3).[77] The upper limit of normal, and treatment target in the intensive group, was 6.05%. Thus even in the intensive group, the goal of normalization of HbA$_{1c}$ was not achieved. Yet the "glycemic separation," or difference between the two groups, was statistically significant throughout the study. The mean blood glucose, obtained on periodic glucose profiles, was 155 mg/dL in the intensive group and 231 mg/dL in the conventional group, whereas the corresponding value for nondiabetic individuals is 110 mg/dL. (During pregnancy, all subjects received intensive therapy. There were a total of 287 pregnancies, among 189 subjects, including 146 pregnancies in the conventional therapy group, during which treatment was temporarily changed, according to the study protocol.)

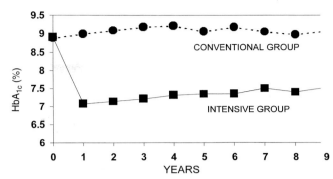

FIGURE 54-3. Measurement of glycosylated hemoglobin (HbA$_{1c}$) in DCCT patients with type 1 diabetes, assigned to intensive or conventional therapy. Median values are shown. Differences are statistically significant at all time points after baseline ($p < 0.001$). *(Adapted with permission from the DCCT Research Group.[77])*

The appearance and progression of retinopathy and other complications were assessed regularly. Retinopathy was assessed by seven-field fundus photography performed every 6 months. Renal function was assessed by annual measurement of creatinine clearance and albumin excretion rate on timed 4-hour urine samples measured in the clinics. Neuropathy was evaluated by clinical examination (neurologic history and physical examination), electrophysiology (peripheral nerve conduction velocities), and autonomic nerve testing. The clinical and electrophysiologic evaluations were performed at baseline, at 5 years, and at study's end. The autonomic testing was done every 2 years.

The primary outcome in the DCCT was progression of diabetic retinopathy. Therefore, the DCCT had been planned to have the statistical power to detect a 33.5% treatment effect for diabetic retinopathy. Many observers had hoped for at best a 40% reduction in event rates in the intensive therapy group versus the conventional therapy group. The results (Table 54-3) dramatically exceeded anyone's wildest expectations.[89] Cumulative 8.5-year rates of clinically important sustained progression of diabetic retinopathy (i.e., three or more steps change on the quantitative grading scale sustained at two consecutive 6-month visits) were 54.1% with conventional treatment and 11.5% with intensive treatment in the primary prevention cohort and 49.2% with conventional treatment and 17.1% with intensive treatment in the secondary intervention cohort (Fig. 54-4). Thus retinopathy progression was significantly reduced by 70.3% in the combined cohorts, by 78.5% for those in the primary prevention cohort with no retinopathy at entry, and by 64.5% for those in the secondary intervention cohort with some retinopathy at entry. The analysis over time suggested that these beneficial effects may actually be underestimated, since event rates increased substantially in the conventional treatment group over time, while changing relatively little in the intensive treatment group.

In the secondary intervention cohort, rates of progression of retinopathy to more severe events were also reduced significantly. Progression to severe nonproliferative retinopathy or worse was reduced by 60.8%. Progression to neovascularization was reduced by 46.3%. The frequency of clinically significant macular edema was reduced by 22.1%, but this did not achieve statistical significance. The need for laser photocoagulation, an index of progression to sight-threatening retinopathy, was significantly reduced by 56% in

TABLE 54-3 DCCT Risk Reduction for Intensive Therapy (versus Conventional Therapy)

Event	Combined Cohorts	Primary Cohort	Secondary Cohort
Diabetic retinopathy			
Clinically important sustained progression	70.3%	78.5%	64.5%
1 yr duration diabetes prior to entry	92%		
5 yr duration diabetes prior to entry	77%		
10 yr duration diabetes prior to entry	64%		
15 yr duration diabetes prior to entry	53%		
Adolescents		53%	70%
Progression to severe nonproliferative retinopathy or worse			60.8%
Progression to neovascularization			46.3%
Clinically significant macular edema			22.1% NS*
Laser photocoagulation	56%		
Initial appearance of *any* retinopathy		27%	
Diabetic nephropathy			
Microalbuminuria AER† >28 μg/min	39%	34%	43%
Adolescents			55%
Sustained microalbuminuria	60%	56%	61%
"Advanced" microalbuminuria	51%	39%	56%
AER ≥70 μg/min			
Sustained "advanced" microalbuminuria	65%	54%	67%
"Clinical grade albuminuria"	54%	44% NS	56%
AER ≥208 μg/min			
Advanced nephropathy	NS		
AER ≥208 μg/min + C$_{cr}$‡ < 70 mL/min / 1.73 m^2 BSA§			
Diabetic neuropathy			
Incidence confirmed clinical neuropathy	64%	71%	61%
Prevalence clinical neuropathy	48%	54%	45%
Prevalence abnormal peripheral NCV¶	44%	59%	38%
Prevalence abnormal ANS#	53%	56%	51%
Microvascular events			
Cardiac and peripheral vascular events combined	41% ($p = 0.06$)		
Elevated LDL**cholesterol > 160 mg/dL	35%		

*NS = not significant.

†AER = albumin excretion rate.

‡C$_{cr}$ = creatinine clearance.

§BSA = body surface area.

¶NCV = nerve conduction velocity.

#ANS = autonomic nervous system testing.

**LDL = low-density lipoprotein.

the combined cohorts. In addition, the initial appearance of any retinopathy (as opposed to clinically significant retinopathy) in the primary prevention cohort was significantly reduced by 27%.

The DCCT investigators noted that the slowing in progression of retinopathy was substantial in magnitude, increased with time, was consistent across all outcome measures assessed, and was present across the spectrum of retinopathy severity enrolled in the DCCT.

At the end of the DCCT, the patients in the conventional therapy group were offered intensive therapy, the care of all patients was transferred to their own physicians, and most were enrolled in the Epidemiology of Diabetes Interventions and Complications (EDIC) study, a long-term observational study.[90–92] Retinopathy was evaluated by fundus photography in 1208 patients during the fourth year after the DCCT ended, and nephropathy was evaluated on the basis of urine specimens obtained from 1302 patients during the third or fourth year, approximately half of whom were from each treatment group. The difference in the median HbA$_{1c}$ values between the conventional therapy and intensive therapy groups during the DCCT (average, 9.1% and 7.2%, respectively) narrowed

during follow-up (median during the first 4 years of follow-up, 8.2% and 7.9%, respectively; $p <0.001$),[91] and by year 6, both groups had HbA$_{1c}$ levels of 8.1%.[92] Nevertheless, during 4.5 years of EDIC follow-up, a smaller proportion of patients in the intensive therapy group than in the conventional therapy group had worsening of retinopathy (76% adjusted odds reduction), progression to proliferative retinopathy (74% adjusted odds reduction), clinically significant macular edema (77% adjusted odds reduction) (all $p <0.001$), and the need for laser therapy (77% adjusted odds reduction) ($p = 0.002$).[91] The EDIC follow-up to DCCT demonstrates that the effects of any level of hyperglycemia increase exponentially over time and continue even after the differences between groups narrow. They suggest that intensive therapy offers a prolonged benefit in terms of reduction in the risk of complications.

Outcome measures related to diabetic nephropathy were also examined, and again dramatic improvements were observed,[77,79] yet these effects were not evident in the first 3–5 years of the study. The incidence of microalbuminuria, a sign of early renal damage, defined as an albumin excretion rate (AER) greater than 28 μg/min (40 mg/24 h), was significantly reduced by 39% in the combined

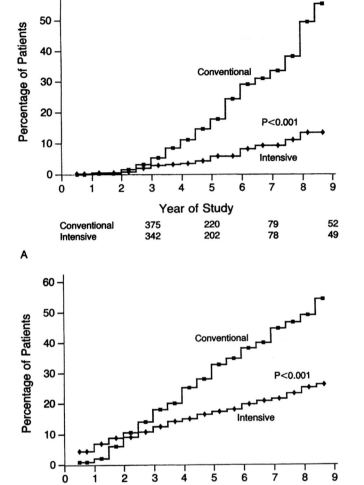

Conventional 375 220 79 52
Intensive 342 202 78 49

A

Conventional 348 324 128 79
Intensive 354 335 136 93

B

FIGURE 54-4. Cumulative incidence in the DCCT of a sustained change in retinopathy (defined as a change in fundus photography of at least three grading scale steps from baseline that was sustained for at least 6 months) in patients with T1DM receiving intensive or conventional therapy in (**A**) the primary prevention cohort, and (**B**) the secondary intervention cohort. *(Adapted with permission from the DCCT Research Group.[77])*

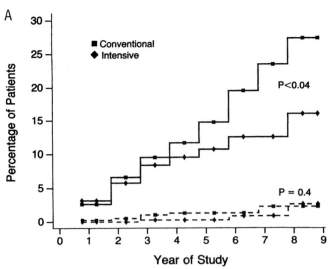

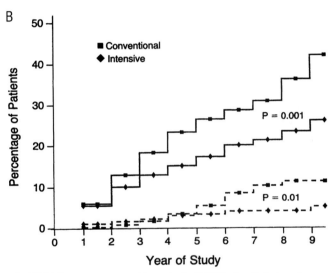

FIGURE 54-5. Cumulative incidence in the DCCT of a clinical nephropathy (urinary albumin excretion ≥300 mg/24 h) (**dashed lines**) and microalbuminuria (urinary albumin excretion ≥40 mg/24 h) (**solid lines**) in patients with T1DM receiving intensive or conventional therapy in (**A**) the primary prevention cohort, and (**B**) the secondary intervention cohort. (Subjects with baseline urinary albumin excretion ≥40 mg/24 h were excluded from the analysis of development of microalbuminuria). *(Adapted with permission from the DCCT Research Group.[77])*

cohorts, by 34% in the primary prevention cohort, and by 43% in the secondary intervention cohort (Fig. 54-5A). The incidence of sustained microalbuminuria (i.e., an AER >28 μg/min on two consecutive annual evaluations) was significantly reduced by 60% in the combined cohorts, by 56% in the primary prevention cohort, and by 61% in the secondary intervention cohort. More severe "advanced" microalbuminuria (i.e., an AER ≥70 μg/min [100 mg/24 h]), which data from the Steno studies suggested is more predictive of evolution into clinical nephropathy,[33] was significantly reduced by 51% in the combined cohorts, by 39% in the primary prevention cohort, and by 56% in the secondary intervention cohort (Fig. 54-5B). The incidence of sustained "advanced" microalbuminuria with an AER ≥70 μg/min on two consecutive annual evaluations,

was significantly reduced by 65% in the combined cohorts, by 54% in the primary prevention cohort, and by 67% in the secondary intervention cohort. Clinically significant renal damage, termed "clinical grade albuminuria" and defined as an AER ≥208 μg/min (300 mg/24 h), was significantly reduced by 54% in the combined cohorts. This event was mostly confined to the secondary intervention cohort, where the reduction was by 56% (both for initial and sustained appearance). In the primary prevention cohort, there was a 44% reduction, but the event rate was so low that this did not achieve statistical significance. Advanced nephropathy, defined as an AER ≥208 μg/min (300 mg/24 h) and a creatinine clearance below 70 mL/min/1.73 m² body surface area, developed very rarely, involving only seven subjects, two in the intensive group and five in the conventional group. In the secondary intervention cohort, after the first year, there was a 6.5%/y increase in AER in the conventional group in contrast to essentially no change (−0.3%/y) in the intensive group. Neither the rate of change of blood pressure nor the appearance of hypertension differed significantly between treatment groups.

During the EDIC follow-up of the DCCT, the proportion of patients with an increase in urinary albumin excretion was significantly lower in the intensive therapy group at both the 4.5- and 6-year time points.[91,92] After 6 years of EDIC, 4.2% of those in the intensive therapy group had newly diagnosed microalbuminuria (during EDIC) versus 12.7% in the conventional therapy group (69% adjusted odds reduction of prevalent microalbuminuria; $p < 0.0001$). Likewise, after 6 years of EDIC, 0.6% were newly diagnosed with clinical albuminuria in the intensive therapy group versus 5.4% in the conventional therapy group (87% adjusted odds reduction; $p = 0.0022$).[92]

Marked improvement in neuropathic outcomes was also seen, despite the fact that most of these were only assessed at baseline, at 5 years, and at study's end.[77,80] (Autonomic nerve testing was done every 2 years.) Confirmed clinical neuropathy was defined as a history and/or physical examination consistent with clinical neuropathy confirmed by either abnormal peripheral nerve conduction or autonomic nerve testing. The incidence of such confirmed clinical neuropathy in the combined cohorts after 5 years of follow-up was 13% with conventional treatment and 5% with intensive treatment. This corresponded to a risk reduction of 64% in the combined cohorts, by 71% for those in the primary prevention cohort, and by 61% for those in the secondary intervention cohort. The prevalence of clinical neuropathy was reduced by 48% in the combined cohorts, by 54% in the primary prevention cohort, and by 45% in the secondary intervention cohort. The prevalence of abnormal peripheral nerve conduction was reduced by 44% in the combined cohorts, by 59% in the primary prevention cohort, and by 38% in the secondary intervention cohort. The prevalence of abnormal autonomic nerve testing was reduced by 53% in the combined cohorts, by 56% in the primary prevention cohort, and by 51% in the secondary intervention cohort. Nerve conduction velocities generally remained stable with intensive therapy, while declining significantly with conventional treatment. On cardiovascular autonomic testing, in the secondary intervention cohort, R-R variation was less abnormal with intensive treatment (7% abnormal at 4–6 years) than conventional treatment (14% abnormal; $p = 0.004$).[81] No statistical difference was seen in the primary prevention cohort ($p = 0.17$), but the difference was significant in the combined cohorts (5% versus 9%; $p = 0.0017$). There were few abnormal Valsalva ratios or postural tests during the trial, and no differences between groups. However, both the R-R variation and the Valsalva ratio had significantly greater slopes of decline over time in the conventional treatment group than the intensive treatment group.

These beneficial effects of intensive therapy were not without associated risks. The chief adverse event associated with intensive therapy was a threefold increase in severe hypoglycemia,[77] defined as those episodes requiring assistance of another person to recover, confirming earlier DCCT reports.[82] This included a threefold increased risk of coma or seizures consequent to hypoglycemia. Emergency room visits or hospitalization for hypoglycemia was increased 2.3-fold in the intensive therapy group. There were no deaths attributable to hypoglycemia among subjects in either treatment group, although a study patient was involved in a motor vehicle accident leading to the death of a nonstudy participant. Impor-

tantly, 53% of severe hypoglycemic episodes occurred during sleep, and 35% occurred without warning symptoms while awake. In the earlier report,[82] it was noted that 23% of severe hypoglycemic episodes were associated with missed meals.

There was also increased weight gain among intensive treatment subjects.[77] This group had a 33% increased risk of becoming overweight, defined as 120% of ideal body weight. Average weight gain was 10.1 lb greater in the intensive group. With intensive treatment, subjects in the fourth quartile of weight gain had the highest body mass index (BMI), blood pressure, and levels of triglyceride, total cholesterol, low-density lipoprotein cholesterol (LDL-C), and apolipoprotein B compared with the other weight gain quartiles, with the greatest difference seen when compared with the first quartile.[83]

Infections at sites of catheters used for continuous subcutaneous insulin infusion (CSII) occurred at a rate of 12 episodes per 100 patient-years of follow-up. Since CSII was only used in the intensive group, all of these infections were in those subjects.

Importantly, there was no difference in frequency of diabetic ketoacidosis between groups, both having an event rate of approximately two episodes per 100 patient-years of follow-up. Moreover, there was no difference between groups in neurobehavioral events, which might be indicative of brain insult consequent to hypoglycemia. Also, there was no difference between groups in psychological symptom scores or quality of life.

The DCCT examined whether the effects of intensive therapy could be demonstrated in the subset of adolescent subjects (13–17 years of age at entry) who participated in the trial.[84] There were 125 adolescent subjects in the primary prevention cohort, and 70 in the secondary intervention cohort. Intensive therapy effectively delayed the onset and slowed the progression of diabetic retinopathy and nephropathy when initiated in adolescent subjects. Among adolescents, intensive therapy decreased the risk of having retinopathy by 53% in the primary prevention cohort, and decreased the risk of retinopathy progression by 70% in the secondary intervention cohort. It also decreased the occurrence of microalbuminuria by 55% in the secondary intervention cohort. Motor and sensory nerve conduction velocities were faster in intensively treated adolescent subjects. As in the entire study sample, the major adverse event with intensive therapy was a nearly threefold increase of severe hypoglycemia.

Macrovascular events, both cardiac and peripheral vascular, were not significantly reduced in the primary analysis.[85] Yet the outcome, when episodes of cardiac and peripheral vascular events are combined, showed a 41% risk reduction, which was just short of being statistically significant ($p = 0.06$). Certainly there was no evidence, as was feared by some critics, of an increased rate of macrovascular events in the intensive treatment group. The risk of developing an elevated LDL cholesterol, defined as a value greater than 160 mg/dL, was significantly reduced by 35% overall. The risk of developing other lipid abnormalities was not significantly affected, yet the original DCCT analysis[77,85] counted first events in any subject. In the context of a meta-analysis that considered the combined risk of all fatal and nonfatal macrovascular events (not just first events), the DCCT results showed risk reductions of 57% in the primary prevention cohort and 71% in the secondary intervention cohort, both of which were statistically significant.[93] Although in this analysis the results were driven by a relatively small number of DCCT patients with multiple events, taken together with the near statistical significance in the primary analysis, it is suggestive of a beneficial effect of intensive therapy on macrovascular complications.

In an analysis primarily focusing on the costs of implementation of intensive therapy, it was calculated that intensive therapy resulted in 15.3 years of living without complications and a gain of 5.1 years in life expectancy.[86]

In subsequent analyses, the DCCT investigators examined the relationship of glycemic exposure to the risk of development and progression of diabetic complications.[87,88] Using multiple regression analyses employing generalized estimating equations, and a number of regression models to assess risks, they found that total glycemic exposure was the dominant factor associated with risk of retinopathy progression (the principal DCCT outcome measure), with comparable results seen with other retinal outcome measures and with renal and neurologic outcome measures. Total glycemic exposure is defined as the baseline HbA_{1c} related to duration of diabetes prior to study entry, the mean study HbA_{1c} related to time in the study, and the interaction between these variables. This is demonstrated in Fig. 54-6, which shows the impact of treatment group and time on absolute risk of sustained retinopathy progression.[88] Within each treatment group, the mean HbA_{1c} during the trial was the dominant predictor of retinopathy progression (and the other outcome measures), with a continuous risk gradient without an apparent glycemic threshold. Figure 54-7[89] shows a stylized model of the kind of continuous risk gradients demonstrated by the DCCT results, in which the event rate for any outcome measure is set to "1" for an HbA_{1c} of 6%.

Risk increased with time in the study in the conventional treatment group but remained relatively constant in the intensive treatment group.[88] In addition, the initial level of HbA_{1c} at eligibility screening and the duration of diabetes at entry were identified as baseline variables that predicted risk of progression. The shorter the duration of disease, the greater the benefit seen. Nevertheless, substantial benefit still accrued regardless of duration of diabetes prior to entry. Whereas retinopathy progression was significantly reduced by 70.3% overall, the risk reduction was 92% for those with only 1 year of diabetes prior to entry, 77% for those with 5 years of diabetes prior to entry, 64% for those with 10 years of diabetes prior to entry, and 53% for those with 15 years of diabetes prior to entry.

Thus intensive therapy effectively delays the onset and slows the progression of diabetic retinopathy, diabetic nephropathy, and diabetic neuropathy in patients with T1DM. It results in increased life expectancy and a prolonged period free of complications.

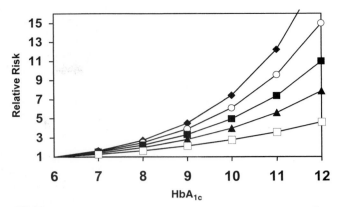

FIGURE 54-7. Stylized relative risks for development of various complications as a function of mean HbA_{1c} during follow-up in the DCCT. For the purposes of illustration, the relative risk of various complications is set to 1 at HbA_{1c} of 6%. The lines depict a stylized relationship for risk of sustained progression of retinopathy (**diamonds**), progression to clinical nephropathy (urinary albumin excretion ≥300 mg/24 h) (**open circles**), progression to severe nonproliferative or proliferative retinopathy (**solid squares**), progression to clinical neuropathy (**solid triangles**), and progression to microalbuminuria (urinary albumin excretion ≥40 mg/24 h) (**open squares**). *(Adapted with permission from Skyler.[89])*

There may be beneficial effects on macrovascular disease, but these have yet to be convincingly demonstrated. The risks of intensive therapy are increased frequency of severe hypoglycemia and greater weight gain. The benefits more than outweigh the risks in most patients with T1DM. Therefore, intensive therapy, with the goal of achieving glucose levels as close to the nondiabetic range as possible, should be employed in most patients with T1DM.

Intervention Trials: Type 2 Diabetes

The Kumamoto Study

The Kumamoto Study was designed to be similar to the DCCT, except the subjects had T2DM.[94–96] Thus the study contrasted intensive insulin therapy (multiple daily injections—preprandial regular and bedtime intermediate-acting insulin) and conventional insulin therapy (once or twice daily intermediate-acting insulin) in two cohorts—a primary prevention cohort and a secondary intervention cohort. A total of 110 thin Japanese patients with T2DM were randomized. Of these, 102 subjects completed the initial 6-year study,[94] with 99 subjects completing 8 years of follow-up,[95] and 97 subjects completing 10 years of follow-up.[96]

Over the initial 6 years of follow-up, the glycemic outcomes and risk reductions were almost identical to those found in the DCCT. In the experimental group with intensive treatment, mean glycosylated hemoglobin (HbA_{1c}; upper limit of normal 6.4%) was reduced from 9.0% to 7.1% versus no change in the control group with standard treatment—9.2% to 9.4% ($p < 0.001$).[94] The 8-year mean HbA_{1c} was similar to that at 6 years—7.2% in the intensive group and 9.4% in the conventional group.[95] The mean blood glucose (over 6 years) was 157 mg/dL in the intensive group and 221 mg/dL in the conventional group, similar to that seen in the DCCT. Likewise, there were significant differences between groups in fasting blood glucose, mean amplitude of glycemic excursions (MAGE), and M value (an index of lability of glycemia).

The 6-year risk reduction[94] for two-step progression of diabetic retinopathy overall was 65% by crude relative risk analysis

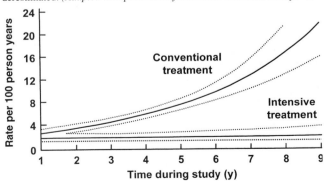

FIGURE 54-6. Absolute risk of sustained retinopathy progression by years of follow-up and treatment group in the DCCT. With time, the curves diverge, suggesting that the beneficial effects of intensive therapy may be underestimated. *(Adapted with permission from DCCT Research Group.[88]).*

and 69% by proportional hazards analysis. The risk reduction was 76% for those in the primary prevention cohort, and 65% for those in the secondary intervention cohort. In addition, in the secondary intervention cohort, progression of retinopathy to proliferative or severe nonproliferative retinopathy was reduced by 40%, and the need for laser photocoagulation also was reduced by 40%. By 10 years, crude relative risk reductions for the combined cohorts were 67% for retinopathy progression, 69% for progression of retinopathy to proliferative or severe nonproliferative retinopathy, and 77% for photocoagulation.[96]

Nephropathy was divided into three stages depending on urinary albumin excretion—normoalbuminuria (<30 mg/24 h), microalbuminuria (30–300 mg/24 h), or clinical grade albuminuria (>300 mg/24 h). Overall risk of nephropathy progression was reduced by 70%—microalbuminuria by 57%, and albuminuria by 100% (a statistical anomaly because no clinical-grade albuminuria appeared in the intensive group).[94] By 10 years, overall crude relative risk reduction for nephropathy progression in the combined cohorts was 66%.[96]

Motor and sensory nerve conduction velocities and vibration thresholds were better in the intensive group than the conventional group at 6 years and 8 years.[94,95] By 10 years, overall crude relative risk reduction for clinical neuropathy in the combined cohorts was 64%.[96]

Macrovascular events—combined cardiac, cerebrovascular, and peripheral vascular events—were said to be reduced by 54% in the original report,[94] but the total number of events was very low. By 10 years, the 95% confidence interval (2–78%) for overall crude relative risk reduction for reduction of macrovascular events in the combined cohorts became significant, with a nominal risk reduction of 54%.[96] Diabetes-related deaths over 10 years were reduced by 81%.[96]

In contrast to the DCCT, hypoglycemia was not a problem. Over the entire study period, six patients in the intensive group and four patients in the conventional group had one or more episodes of mild hypoglycemia, while no patient had seizure, coma, or severe hypoglycemia requiring the assistance of another person. Likewise, weight gain was not a major problem. There was a slight but not significant increase in BMI in both groups from baseline to 6 years.

Thus in this randomized controlled study designed to examine the influence of glycemic control on diabetic complications in T2DM, intensive therapy was found to delay the onset and the progression of early stages of retinopathy, nephropathy, and neuropathy, and to decrease the frequency of macrovascular events.

The United Kingdom Prospective Diabetes Study (UKPDS)

The United Kingdom Prospective Diabetes Study (UKPDS), a randomized, multicenter controlled clinical trial, demonstrated that an intensive treatment policy in T2DM, with the goal of meticulous glycemic control, could decrease clinical diabetic complications.[97–102] The UKPDS was conducted in 23 centers. Enrollment was between 1977 and 1991, and end-of-study evaluations were performed during 1997. UKPDS screened 7616 newly diagnosed patients who had the clinical phenotype of T2DM.[97,98] Of these, 5102 were recruited and completed a 3-month vigorous dietary treatment run-in period. Of these, 744 continued to manifest symptoms and/or had fasting plasma glucose (FPG) greater than 270 mg/dL and were excluded from the main treatment protocol. Another group attained FPG less than or equal to 108 mg/dL and were initially excluded from randomization, but could be randomized

later if their subsequent FPG exceeded 108 mg/dL, with the exception of 149 individuals who were either lost or never reached the 108 mg/dL threshold. Thus a total of 4209 individuals with newly diagnosed T2DM were randomized in the main protocol. At entry, they were 25–63 years of age (median 53 years).

Subjects were randomly assigned either to "intensive treatment policy" (originally called "active treatment policy") or "conventional treatment policy." Intensive policy aimed at achieving fasting plasma glucose of 108 mg/dL using various pharmacologic agents. Conventional policy attempted control with diet alone, adding pharmacologic therapy when symptoms developed or fasting plasma glucose exceeded 270 mg/dL. The randomization was not balanced, as there were several arms in the intervention group. These included insulin, sulfonylureas, and among obese patients, metformin, but it was a bit more complicated than that. In the first 15 (of the 23) centers, the sulfonylureas were either glyburide (glibenclamide) or chlorpropamide, and it was only in these 15 centers that obese patients could receive metformin. In the last eight centers, the sulfonylureas were either glipizide or chlorpropamide. Moreover, in these eight centers the protocol was different and involved early addition of insulin if FPG could not be maintained lower than 108 mg/dL. It is important to note that therapeutic additions (in contrast to dose titrations) could not otherwise be made unless FPG reached 270 mg/dL, with the exception of some subgroups to be discussed later.

The primary outcome measures in the UKPDS were three aggregate end-points—"any diabetes-related endpoint" (sudden death, death from hyperglycemia or hypoglycemia, myocardial infarction, angina, heart failure, stroke, renal failure, amputation, vitreous hemorrhage, retinopathy requiring photocoagulation, blindness in one eye, or cataract extraction), "diabetes-related death" (death from myocardial infarction, stroke, peripheral vascular disease, renal disease, hyperglycemia or hypoglycemia, and sudden death), and all-cause mortality.[97,99] Multiple other individual clinical and surrogate subclinical end-points were also assessed. Additional clinical end-point aggregates were used: myocardial infarction (fatal and nonfatal) and sudden death, stroke (fatal and nonfatal), amputation or death due to peripheral vascular disease, and microvascular complications (retinopathy requiring photocoagulation, vitreous hemorrhage, and renal failure).

The primary analysis was based on the "intention to treat" principle—comparing subjects assigned "intensive policy" or "conventional policy."[99] Inexplicably, those obese subjects randomized to metformin were not included in the primary "intention to treat" analysis. Since these subjects were randomized with the other subjects,[97] there appears to be no reason for them to have been excluded from analysis. Although the investigators claim they never intended to include them in the primary analysis, that might be inappropriate, since a major aspect of the "intention to treat" principle is to include all subjects randomized.

Secondary analyses of the effects of individual treatments also were reported. In one paper, the results of treatment with glyburide, chlorpropamide, or insulin among subjects in the first 15 centers were compared.[99] In a second paper, the results of treatment with metformin among obese subjects in the first 15 centers also were considered.[100]

The intensive policy group achieved a median HbA$_{1c}$ of 7.0% versus 7.9% in the conventional policy group ($p < 0.001$) (Fig. 54-8).[99] Initially, with vigorous dietary therapy during the 3-month run-in period, there was a dramatic reduction of HbA$_{1c}$, from ~9.0% to 7.08%, accompanied by a weight loss of ~5 kg (~11

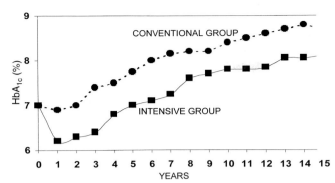

FIGURE 54-8. Measurement of glycosylated hemoglobin (**HbA$_{1c}$**) in UKPDS patients with T2DM assigned to intensive treatment policy or to conventional treatment policy. Median values are shown. Differences over the course of the study are statistically significant ($p < 0.0001$). *(Adapted with permission from UKPDS Group.[99]).*

lb).[98] Over the first few years, the intensive policy group achieved HbA$_{1c}$ levels in the 6% range, while the conventional policy group maintained HbA$_{1c}$ levels in the 7% range. Subsequently, there was a progressive deterioration in glycemia over time. Nevertheless, approximately the same degree of glycemic separation was maintained for 6–20 years, with a median duration of follow-up of 11.1 years.

As noted, the primary outcome measures in the UKPDS were three aggregate end-points—"any diabetes-related endpoint," "diabetes-related death," and all-cause mortality. Of these, only any diabetes-related endpoint was significantly impacted—a 12% risk reduction.[99] In addition, risk reductions were seen for other end-points. Patients assigned intensive policy had a significant 25% risk reduction in microvascular end-points compared with conventional policy ($p < 0.01$), most of which was due to fewer cases of retinal photocoagulation, for which there was a 29% risk reduction ($p < 0.005$).[99] There was also a decreased risk of cataract extraction (24% risk reduction), deterioration in retinopathy (21% risk reduction at 12 years' follow-up), and of microalbuminuria (33% risk reduction at 12 years' follow-up).[99]

The only macrovascular end-point that demonstrated a trend in risk reduction in the main analysis was myocardial infarction (16% risk reduction), which did not quite reach statistical significance ($p = 0.052$).[99] In the metformin subgroup analysis within UKPDS, however, there were significant risk reductions in diabetes-related deaths (42% risk reduction, $p = 0.017$), any diabetes-related endpoint (32% risk reduction, $p = 0.0023$), and myocardial infarction (39% risk reduction, $p = 0.01$).[100] In the metformin subgroup, a combined analysis of all macrovascular end-points (myocardial infarction, sudden death, angina, stroke, peripheral vascular disease) showed a risk reduction of 30% over the conventional therapy group ($p = 0.02$).[100] Had the metformin subjects not been excluded from the primary analysis, the overall risk reduction for myocardial infarction would have been 18%, and likely would have achieved statistical significance.

In analyzing the individual therapies, the major difference was the increased risk reduction for macrovascular disease seen in the relatively small obese subgroup treated with metformin.[100] There was an even smaller subgroup in which metformin was added early to sulfonylurea-treated patients in a randomized design.[100] In this subgroup, there was an inexplicable difference in outcome, particularly diabetes-related deaths, which were higher in the combined

metformin-sulfonylurea group than those who continued on sulfonylureas alone. A subsequent analysis suggested that the expected death rate was higher than that observed in either group, although the sulfonylurea group had a statistically significantly lower rate than either that expected or that seen in the metformin-sulfonylurea combination group.[101] With sulfonylurea therapy, there was no evidence of deleterious effect on myocardial infarction, sudden death, or diabetes-related deaths.[99] With insulin therapy, there was no evidence for more atheroma-related disease.[99] Thus in UKPDS, there was no evidence of an adverse effect of insulin or insulin secretagogues on macrovascular disease, thus negating the erroneous (but widely held) belief that increasing insulin availability may in some way be detrimental to patients with diabetes.

The overall risk reductions found in the UKPDS are shown in Table 54-4.

In a subsequent analysis, performed across all UKPDS subjects, the relationship between exposure to glycemia over time and the risk of macrovascular or microvascular complications was determined.[102] The incidence of clinical complications was significantly associated with glycemia. Each 1% reduction in updated mean HbA$_{1c}$ was associated with reductions in risk of 21% for any end-point related to diabetes ($p < 0.0001$), 21% for deaths related to diabetes ($p < 0.0001$), 14% for myocardial infarction ($p < 0.0001$), 43% for peripheral vascular disease ($p < 0.0001$), and 37% for microvascular complications ($p < 0.0001$). No threshold of risk was observed for any end-point. Figure 54-9 depicts the relationship between updated mean HbA$_{1c}$ (glycemic exposure) and incidence of microvascular disease and myocardial infarction.[102]

Thus the UKPDS provides substantial evidence that glycemic control impacts also on T2DM. The continuous relationship of glycemic exposure to risk of complications, without a threshold,[102] is similar to that seen in T1DM in the DCCT.[87,88] Taken together, these findings suggest that the target for glycemic control should be an HbA$_{1c}$ level as close to normal as feasible.

POST-TRANSPLANTATION STUDIES

Histologic studies on biopsy specimens of transplanted kidneys permit study of the influence on renal structure of the metabolic milieu in which the kidney exists. The University of Minnesota Transplantation Program has provided much of the available data. These human observations, although confined to a few individuals,

TABLE 54-4 UKPDS Risk Reduction for Intensive Therapy (versus Conventional Therapy)

Event	Main Analysis	Metformin Subgroup
Any diabetes-related end-point	12%	32%
Diabetes-related deaths	NS	42%
All-cause mortality	NS	36%
Myocardial infarction	16% ($p = 0.52$)	39%
Microvascular end-points	25%	NS
Fatal myocardial infarction	NS	50%
Laser photocoagulation	29%	NS
Cataract extraction	24%	NS
Retinopathy at 12 years	21%	NS
Microalbuminuria at 12 years	33%	NS

Percentage risk reduction for various UKPDS outcome measures in main analysis and in Metformin Subgroup.

NS = not significant.

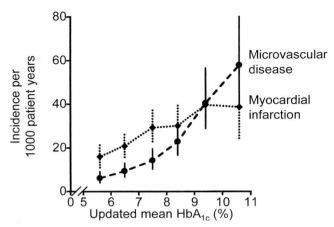

FIGURE 54-9. UKPDS epidemiologic analysis depicting the relationship between updated mean HbA$_{1c}$ (glycemic exposure) and incidence of microvascular disease (**circles**) and of myocardial infarction (**diamonds**). *(Adapted with permission from Stratton et al.[102])*

provide further powerful and persuasive evidence about the relationship between glycemic control and evolution of diabetic complications. Only one randomized intervention study examined renal histology,[48] and it is consistent with a wealth of similar animal data which demonstrate that the metabolic milieu in which the kidney exists influences its histologic structure. In a hyperglycemic milieu, histologic features of diabetic nephropathy unfold. In a normoglycemic metabolic milieu, histologic changes do not appear and existing changes regress. The studies are summarized below.

Kidneys from Nondiabetic Donors in Diabetic Recipients

Michael Mauer, David Sutherland, and their coworkers in Minnesota have demonstrated that typical diabetic histologic changes, both glomerular changes and immunohistologic changes specific for diabetes, invariably develop in normal kidneys transplanted into patients with diabetes, usually within 2 years of transplantation.[103–105] Comparable changes are not seen in kidneys transplanted into nondiabetic individuals.

Kidneys in Pancreas Transplant Recipients

In a series from the University of Minnesota, successful pancreas transplantation which normalized glycemia resulted in significantly less severe diabetic glomerulopathy in the transplanted kidneys of 12 diabetic patients than was seen in 13 matched diabetic patients who received renal allografts but did not have a pancreas transplant.[105] A recent larger confirmatory report from the Stockholm group reports similar findings in 20 diabetic patients after successful combined pancreatic and renal transplantation compared to 30 diabetic recipients after kidney transplantation only.[106] These series were heralded by an early report from Gliedman and colleagues,[107] who in a single patient noted that renal histology remained normal 4 years after combined renal and pancreatic transplantation. In addition, Bohman and associates have described a similar experience in two cases.[108] The Minnesota group also noted that pancreas transplantation results in regression of recurrent early diabetic nephropathy present at the time of pancreas transplantation.[105,109]

Interestingly, in their first report, the Minnesota group noted a failure to see regression of more advanced lesions of diabetic nephropathy in the native kidneys 5 years after having had a pancreas transplant in patients who had not received kidney grafts.[110,111] However, after 10 years, thickness of the glomerular and tubular basement membranes had decreased in comparison to baseline values.[111] Moreover, mesangial fractional volume (the proportion of the glomerulus occupied by the mesangium) had decreased at 10 years, mostly because of a reduction in mesangial matrix.[111]

It should be noted that in contrast to the beneficial effects of pancreas transplantation on renal histology, no effects are seen on retinopathy.[112,113] However, it should be noted that most pancreas transplant recipients have had such advanced retinopathy that they may be beyond the stage of measurable impact.

Kidneys from Diabetic Donors in Nondiabetic Recipients

George Abouna and coworkers from Kuwait have reported dramatic changes in kidneys taken from a diabetic donor and transplanted into two nondiabetic recipients.[114,115] At the time of transplantation, the kidneys showed some histologic features of diabetic nephropathy, although Mauer has cautioned that the histologic changes demonstrated by Abouna and associates are not the lesions most representative of diabetic nephropathy.[116] The renal changes in the donated organs had reversed on biopsies taken 7 months posttransplant, during which both recipients remained euglycemic.[114] Fifteen months after transplant, one of the recipients developed steroid-induced hyperglycemia, and required initiation of insulin therapy. Twelve months later, he developed clinical evidence of renal disease, and on rebiopsy 30 months after transplant, the kidney showed recurrence of diabetic nephropathy.[115]

CONCLUSIONS

There is no doubt that hyperglycemia is essential to the development of diabetic microangiopathy. Multiple randomized controlled intervention studies have convincingly demonstrated that. In particular, the overall results reported by the DCCT dramatically exceeded all expectations. The benefits of intensive therapy include a slowing of the onset and progression of diabetic retinopathy, diabetic nephropathy, and diabetic neuropathy. The risks of intensive therapy are increased frequency of severe hypoglycemia and greater weight gain. These risks clearly must be considered whenever intensive therapy is contemplated. However, although in the DCCT there was a threefold increased risk for hypoglycemia in the intensive therapy group, for coma or seizure this amounts to one episode every 6.25 patient-years of follow-up, versus one episode every 20 patient-years of follow-up in the conventional treatment group. This may very well be tolerable. Thus the benefits of intensive therapy would seem to be worth the risks in most patients with T1DM. Therefore, intensive therapy, with the goal of achieving glucose levels as close to the nondiabetic range as possible, should be the standard management approach in most patients with T1DM.

The analyses from the Wisconsin Epidemiologic Study of Diabetic Retinopathy (WESDR) and similar epidemiologic studies show that the relationship between glycemia and diabetic complications is present in both type 1 and type 2 diabetes. The results of the UKPDS and the Kumamoto Study suggest that meticulous glycemic control also should be the therapeutic goal in T2DM. However, since the major morbidity and mortality in T2DM is a consequence of accelerated atherosclerosis, which is multifactorial in nature and not merely related to prevailing glycemia, attention also needs to be paid to other risk factors, such as high blood pressure, an excess of lipids, and cigarette smoking.

There is also a general relationship between degree of hyperglycemia as manifested by mean level of HbA_{1c} (or glycemia-years, analogous to pack-years of smoking) and the frequency, severity, and progression of microangiopathy. In both the UKPDS and the DCCT, the relationship between glycemic exposure and risk of development of complications was evident across the range of HbA_{1c} and without evidence of a threshold.[87,88,102] In UKPDS, when subjects were examined by HbA_{1c} category, there was a log-linear relationship between HbA_{1c} and risk of complications, without evidence of a threshold.[102] In the DCCT, where the relationship was examined continuously rather than categorically, an exponential relationship was seen between HbA_{1c} and risk of complications,[87,88] again without evidence of a threshold.[88] This supports the view that the lower the glycemic exposure, the lower the risk of complications. However, the quantitation of the relationship between hyperglycemia and microangiopathy in an individual patient may be influenced by other factors, including coexisting hypertension and genetic predisposition. Thus some individuals may be more genetically prone to microangiopathy, and so may develop these complications in the face of little hyperglycemia, while others with less genetic predisposition may escape complications in spite of substantial hyperglycemia. Nevertheless, it would appear that in most cases, regardless of a person's genetic substrate, the degree of hyperglycemia directly influences the risk of microangiopathy.

The evidence that glycemic control makes a difference in diabetic complications should serve to refocus the debate not only on the best means of attaining effective glycemic control, but also on the therapeutic targets that should be sought. Ironically, as noted by Robert Tatersall in his lucid historical review, "The Quest for Normoglycemia," the goal articulated by the DCCT investigators of maintaining glycemic status as close to normal as safely possible is identical to that recommended in 1923, shortly after the discovery of insulin.[117]

It should be noted, however, that no available intervention, save the drastic approach of pancreas transplantation, uniformly permits normalization of glycemia. All of the cited intervention studies achieved statistically significant glycemic separation between groups; none achieved normoglycemia. If normoglycemia is necessary to completely prevent, delay, or slow microangiopathy, then we cannot expect to totally prevent microangiopathy. However, because there is a continuous relationship between prevailing glycemia and risk of progression of complications, any improvement in glycemic control is beneficial. Therefore, a prudent clinical approach is to select treatment goals and treatment strategies that are individualized for each patient and that are designed to achieve the best control reasonably attainable in that patient, without adding unnecessary risk. In striving for meticulous control, we should therefore focus on those patients with longest life expectancy, while being slightly less aggressive in those with increased risk factors for devastating problems consequent to hypoglycemia. Meanwhile, we should expend our best efforts in devising and implementing newer therapeutic strategies that will more closely approximate metabolic normality. When that is accomplished, we have the potential of eliminating the microangiopathic complications of diabetes mellitus.

REFERENCES

1. Pirart J: Diabetes mellitus and its degenerative complications: A prospective study of 4400 patients observed between 1947 and 1973. *Diabetes Care* 1978;1:168,252.
2. Klein R: Hyperglycemia and microvascular and macrovascular disease in diabetes. *Diabetes Care* 1995;18:258.
3. Klein R, Klein BE, Moss SE: Relation of glycemic control to diabetic microvascular complications in diabetes mellitus. *Ann Intern Med* 1996;124(1 pt 2):90.
4. Klein R, Klein BE, Moss SE, et al: The Wisconsin epidemiologic study of diabetic retinopathy. III. Prevalence and risk of diabetic retinopathy when age at diagnosis is 30 or more years. *Arch Ophthalmol* 1984;102:527.
5. Klein R, Klein BEK, Moss SE, et al: The Wisconsin Epidemiologic Study of Diabetic Retinopathy. II. Prevalence and risk of diabetic retinopathy when age at diagnosis is less than 30 years. *Arch Ophthalmol* 1984;102:520.
6. Klein R, Klein BEK, Moss SE, et al: The Wisconsin Epidemiologic Study of Diabetic Retinopathy XIV. Ten-year incidence and progression of diabetic retinopathy. *Arch Ophthalmol* 1994;112:1217.
7. Klein R, Klein BEK, Moss SE, et al: Glycosylated hemoglobin predicts the incidence and progression of diabetic retinopathy. *JAMA* 1988;260:2864.
8. Klein R, Klein BEK, Moss SE, et al: Relationship of hyperglycemia to the long-term incidence and progression of diabetic retinopathy. *Arch Intern Med* 1994;154:2169.
9. Klein R, Klein BE, Moss SE, et al: The Wisconsin Epidemiologic Study of Diabetic Retinopathy. XV. The long-term incidence of macular edema. *Ophthalmology* 1995;102:7.
10. Moss SE, Klein R, Klein BE: Ten-year incidence of visual loss in a diabetic population. *Ophthalmology* 1994;101:1061.
11. Klein R, Klein BE, Moss SE, et al: The Wisconsin Epidemiologic Study of Diabetic Retinopathy: XVII. The 14-year incidence and progression of diabetic retinopathy and associated risk factors in type 1 diabetes. *Ophthalmology* 1998;105:1801.
12. Moss SE, Klein R, Klein BE: The 14-year incidence of visual loss in a diabetic population. *Ophthalmology* 1998;105:998.
13. Klein R, Klein BEK, Moss SE: The incidence of gross proteinuria in people with insulin-dependent diabetes mellitus. *Arch Intern Med* 1991;151:1344.
14. Klein R, Klein BEK, Moss SE: Incidence of gross proteinuria in older-onset diabetes: A population-based perspective. *Diabetes* 1993;42:381.
15. Klein R, Klein BEK, Linton KLP, et al: Microalbuminuria in a population-based study of diabetes. *Arch Intern Med* 1992;152:153.
16. Klein R, Klein BE, Moss SE: Prevalence of microalbuminuria in older-onset diabetes. *Diabetes Care* 1993;16:1325.
17. Klein R, Klein BE, Moss SE, et al: The 10-year incidence of renal insufficiency in people with type 1 diabetes. *Diabetes Care* 1999;22:743.
18. Moss SE, Klein R, Klein BE: The prevalence and incidence of lower extremity amputation in a diabetic population. *Arch Intern Med* 1992;152:610.
19. Moss SE, Klein R, Klein BE: The 14-year incidence of lower-extremity amputations in a diabetic population. The Wisconsin Epidemiologic Study of Diabetic Retinopathy. *Diabetes Care* 1999;22:951.
20. Moss SE, Klein R, Klein BE: Risk factors for hospitalization in people with diabetes. *Arch Intern Med* 1999;159:2053.
21. Klein R, Moss SE, Klein BEK, et al: The association of glycemia and cause-specific mortality in a diabetic population. *Arch Intern Med* 1994;154:2473.
22. Abraira C, Emanuele N, Colwell J, et al: Glycemic control and complications in type II diabetes. *Diabetes Care* 1992;15:1560.
23. Abraira C, Colwell JA, Nuttall FQ, et al: Veterans Affairs Cooperative Study on glycemic control and complications in type II diabetes (VA CSDM). Results of the feasibility trial. Veterans Affairs Cooperative Study in Type II Diabetes. *Diabetes Care* 1995;18:1113.

24. Duckworth WC, McCarren M, Abraira C: Glucose control and cardio-vascular complications: The VA Diabetes Trial. *Diabetes Care* 2001; 24:942.

25. Wang PH, Lau J, Chalmers TC: Meta-analysis of effects of intensive blood glucose control on late complications on Type I diabetes. *Lancet* 1993;341:1306.

26. Wang PH, Lau J, Chalmers TC: Meta-analysis of effects of intensive glycemic control on late complications on Type I diabetes mellitus. *Online J Curr Clin Trials* 1993;Document Number 60:May 21, 1993.

27. Steno Study Group: Effect of 6 months of strict metabolic control on eye and kidney function in insulin-dependent diabetics with back-ground retinopathy. *Lancet* 1982;1:121.

28. Lauritzen T, Frost-Larsen K, Larsen HW, et al: Effect of one year of near-normal blood glucose levels on retinopathy in insulin-dependent diabetes. *Lancet* 1983;1:200.

29. Lauritzen T, Frost-Larsen K, Larsen HW, et al: Two-year experience with continuous subcutaneous insulin infusion in relation to retinopa-thy and neuropathy. *Diabetes* 1985;34(suppl 3):74.

30. Feldt-Rasmussen B, Mathiesen ER, Deckert T: Effect of two years of strict metabolic control on the progression of incipient nephropathy in insulin-dependent diabetes. *Lancet* 1986;2:1300.

31. Deckert T, Lauritzen T, Parving H-H, et al: Effect of two years of strict metabolic control on kidney function in long-term insulin-dependent diabetics. *Diabetic Nephropathy* 1983;2:6.

32. Deckert T, Feldt-Rasmussen B, Borch-Johnsen K, et al: Natural his-tory of diabetic complications: Early detection and progression. *Diabet Med* 1991;8(suppl):S33.

33. Feldt-Rasmussen B, Mathiesen ER, Jensen T, et al: Effect of im-proved metabolic control on loss of kidney function in Type I (insulin-dependent) diabetic patients: An update of the Steno Studies. *Diabetologia* 1991;34:164.

34. Kroc Collaborative Study Group: Blood glucose control and the evo-lution of diabetic retinopathy and albuminuria. *N Engl J Med* 1984; 311:365.

35. Rodger NW, ed.: Proceedings of a conference on insulin pump ther-apy in diabetes: Multicenter study of effect on microvascular disease. *Diabetes* 1985;35(suppl 3):1.

36. Kroc Collaborative Study Group: Diabetic retinopathy after two years of intensified insulin treatment. *JAMA* 1988;260:37.

37. Bending JJ, Viberti GC, Bilous RW, et al: Eight-month correction of hyperglycemia in insulin-dependent diabetes mellitus is associated with a significant and sustained reduction of urinary albumin excre-tion rates in patients with microalbuminuria. *Diabetes* 1985;35(suppl 3):69.

38. Dahl-Jorgensen K, Brinchmann-Hansen O, Hanssen KF, et al: Near-normoglycemia retards the progression of early diabetic retinopathy and neuropathy. *Br Med J* 1985;290:811.

39. Brinchmann-Hansen O, Dahl-Jorgensen K, Hanssen KF, et al: Effects of intensified insulin treatment on various lesions of diabetic retinopa-thy. *Am J Ophthalmol* 1985;100:644.

40. Dahl-Jorgensen K, Brinchmann-Hansen O, Hanssen KF, et al: Effect of near nomoglycaemia for two years on progression of early diabetic retinopathy, nephropathy, and neuropathy: The Oslo Study. *Br Med J* 1986;293:1195.

41. Brinchmann-Hansen O, Dahl-Jorgensen K, Hanssen KF, et al: Dia-betic retinopathy through 41 months with multiple insulin injections, insulin pumps and conventional insulin therapy. *Arch Ophthalmol* 1988;106:1242.

42. Brinchmann-Hansen O, Dahl-Jorgensen K, Sandvik L, et al: Blood glucose concentrations and progression of diabetic retinopathy: The seven year results of the Oslo Study. *Br Med J* 1992;304:19.

43. Dahl-Jorgensen K, Hanssen KF, Kierulf P, et al: Reduction of urinary albumin excretion after 4 years of continuous subcutaneous insulin in-fusion in insulin-dependent diabetes mellitus. The Oslo Study. *Acta Endocrinologica* 1988;117:19.

44. Dahl-Jorgensen K, Bjoro T, Kierulf P, et al: Long-term glycemic con-trol and kidney function in insulin-dependent diabetes mellitus. *Kid-ney Int* 1992;41:920.

45. Hanssen KF, Bangsted HJ, Brinchmann-Hansen O, et al: Blood glu-cose control and microvascular complications: Long-term effects of near-normoglycemia. *Diabet Med* 1992;9:697.

46. Amthor KF, Dahl-Jorgensen K, Berg TJ, et al: The effect of eight years of strict glycemic control on peripheral nerve function in IDDM patients: The Oslo Study. *Diabetologia* 1994;37:579.

47. Bangstad HJ, Kofoed-Enevoldsen A, Dahl-Jorgensen K, et al: Glomerular charge selectivity and the influence of improved blood glucose control. *Diabetologia* 1992;35:1165.

48. Bangstad HJ, Osterby R, Dahl-Jorgensen K, et al: Improvement of blood glucose control retards the progression of morphological changes in early diabetic nephropathy. *Diabetologia* 1994;37:483.

49. Reichard P, Britz A, Cars I, et al: The Stockholm Diabetes Interven-tion Study (SDIS): 18 months' results. *Acta Med Scand* 1988;224: 115.

50. Reichard P, Rosenqvist U: Nephropathy is delayed by intensified in-sulin treatment in patients with insulin dependent diabetes mellitus and retinopathy. *J Intern Med* 1989;226:81.

51. Reichard P, Britz A, Carlsson P, et al: Metabolic control and compli-cations over 3 years in patients with insulin dependent diabetes (IDDM): The Stockholm Diabetes Intervention Study (SDIS). *J In-tern Med* 1990;228:511.

52. Reichard P, Berglund B, Britz A, et al: Intensified conventional insulin treatment retards the microvascular complications in insulin depend-ent diabetes mellitus (IDDM): The Stockholm Diabetes Intervention Study (SDIS). *J Intern Med* 1991;230:101.

53. Reichard P: Risk factors for progression of microvascular complica-tions in the Stockholm Diabetes Intervention Study (SDIS). *Diabetes Res Clin Pract* 1992;16:151.

54. Reichard P, Nilsson BY, Rosenqvist U: The effect of long-term inten-sified insulin treatment on the development of microvascular compli-cations of diabetes mellitus. *N Engl J Med* 1993;329:304.

55. Reichard P, Pihl M: Mortality and treatment side effects during long-term intensified conventional insulin treatment in the Stockholm Dia-betes Intervention Study (SDIS). *Diabetes* 1994;43:313.

56. Reichard P: Glycemic thresholds for diabetes complications. *J Dia-betes Complications* 1995;9:25.

57. Jensen-Urstad KJ, Reichard PG, Rosfors JS, et al: Early atherosclero-sis is retarded by improved long-term blood glucose control in pa-tients with IDDM. *Diabetes* 1996;45:1253.

58. Reichard P, Jensen-Urstad K, Ericsson M, et al: Autonomic neuropa-thy—a complication less pronounced in patients with Type 1 diabetes mellitus who have lower blood glucose levels. *Diabet Med* 2000;17: 860.

59. Reichard P, Pihl M, Rosenqvist U, et al: Complications in IDDM are caused by elevated blood glucose level: The Stockholm Diabetes In-tervention Study (SDIS) at 10-year follow up. *Diabetologia* 1996;39: 1483.

60. Holman RR, Dornan TL, Mayon-White V, et al: Prevention of deteri-oration of renal and sensory-nerve function by more intensive man-agement of insulin-dependent diabetic patients. *Lancet* 1983;1:204.

61. Beck-Nielsen H, Richelsen B, Mogensen CE, et al: Effect of insulin pump treatment for one year on renal function and retinal morphology in patients with IDDM. *Diabetes Care* 1985;8:585.

62. Olsen T, Richelsen B, Ehlers N, et al: Diabetic retinopathy after 3 years' treatment with continuous subcutaneous insulin infusion (CSII). *Acta Ophthalmologica* 1987;65:185.

63. Christensen CK, Christiansen JS, Schmitz A, et al: Effect of continu-ous subcutaneous insulin infusion on kidney function and size in IDDM patients: A 2 year controlled study. *J Diabetes Complications* 1987;1:91.

64. The Italian National Research Council Study Group on Diabetic Retinopathy: The effects of continuous insulin infusion as compared with conventional insulin therapy in the evolution of diabetic retinal ischemia: Two years report. *Diabetes Nutr Metab* 1989;2:209.

65. Verrillo A, De Teresa A, Martino C, et al: Long-term correction of hy-perglycemia and progression of retinopathy in insulin-dependent dia-betes. A five-year randomized prospective study. *Diabetes Res* 1988; 8:71.

66. Job D, Eschwege E, Guyot-Argenton C, et al: Effect of multiple daily insulin injections on the course of diabetic retinopathy. *Diabetes* 1976;25:463.

67. Eschwege E, Job D, Guyot-Argenton C, et al: Delayed progression of diabetic retinopathy by divided insulin administration: A further fol-low-up. *Diabetologia* 1978;16:13.

68. Ashikaga T, Borodic G, Sims EAH: Multiple daily insulin injections in the treatment of diabetic retinopathy—the Job Study revisited. *Dia-betes* 1978;26:592.

69. Wiseman MJ, Saunders AJ, Keen H, et al: Effect of blood glucose control on increased glomerular filtration rate and kidney size in in-

sulin-dependent diabetes. *N Engl J Med* 1985;312:617.

70. Helve E, Laatikainen L, Merenmies L, *et al*: Continuous insulin infusion therapy and retinopathy in patients with Type I diabetes. *Acta Endocrinologica* 1987;115:313.

71. Raskin P, Pietri AO, Unger R, *et al*: The effect of diabetic control on the width of skeletal-muscle capillary basement membrane in patients with Type I diabetes mellitus. *N Engl J Med* 1983;309:1546.

72. Rosenstock J, Challis P, Strowig S, *et al*: Improved diabetes control reduces skeletal muscle capillary basement membrane width in insulin-dependent diabetes mellitus. *Diabetes Res Clin Pract* 1988;4:167.

73. Friberg TR, Rosenstock J, Sanborn G, *et al*: The effect of long-term near normal glycemic control on mild diabetic retinopathy. *Ophthalmology* 1985;92:1051.

74. Rosenstock J, Friberg T, Raskin P: Effect of glycemic control on microvascular complications in patients with Type I diabetes mellitus. *Am J Med* 1986;81:1012.

75. Pietri AO, Ehle AL, Raskin P: Changes in nerve conduction velocity after six weeks of glucoregulation with portable insulin infusion pumps. *Diabetes* 1980;29:668.

76. Ehle AL, Raskin P: Increased nerve conduction in diabetics after a year of improved glucoregulation. *J Neurol Sci* 1986;74:191.

77. The Diabetes Control and Complications Trial (DCCT) Research Group: The effect of intensive treatment of diabetes on the development and progression of long-term complications in insulin-dependent diabetes mellitus. *N Engl J Med* 1993;329:977.

78. The Diabetes Control and Complications Trial (DCCT) Research Group: The effect of intensive treatment of diabetes on the progression of diabetic retinopathy in insulin-dependent diabetes mellitus: Diabetes Control and Complications Trial. *Arch Ophthalmol* 1995;113:36.

79. The Diabetes Control and Complications Trial (DCCT) Research Group: Effect of intensive therapy on the development and progression of diabetic nephropathy in the Diabetes Control and Complications Trial. *Kidney Int* 1995;47:1703.

80. The Diabetes Control and Complications Trial (DCCT) Research Group: The effect of intensive diabetes therapy on the development and progression of neuropathy. *Ann Intern Med* 1995;122:561.

81. The Diabetes Control and Complications Trial (DCCT) Research Group: The effect of intensive diabetes therapy on measures of autonomic nervous system function in the Diabetes Control and Complications Trial (DCCT). *Diabetologia* 1998;41:416.

82. The Diabetes Control and Complications Trial (DCCT) Research Group: Epidemiology of severe hypoglycemia in the Diabetes Control and Complications Trial. *Am J Med* 1991;90:450.

83. Purnell JQ, Hokanson JE, Marcovina SM, *et al*: Effect of excessive weight gain with intensive therapy of type 1 diabetes on lipid levels and blood pressure: Results from the DCCT. Diabetes Control and Complications Trial. *JAMA* 1998;280:140.

84. Diabetes Control and Complications Trial Research Group: Effect of intensive diabetes treatment on the development and progression of long-term complications in adolescents with insulin-dependent diabetes mellitus: Diabetes Control and Complications Trial. *J Pediatr* 1994;125:177.

85. The Diabetes Control and Complications Trial (DCCT) Research Group: Effect of intensive diabetes management on macrovascular events and risk factors in the Diabetes Control and Complications Trial. *Am J Cardiol* 1995;75:894.

86. The Diabetes Control and Complications Trial (DCCT) Research Group: Lifetime benefits and costs of intensive therapy as practiced in the Diabetes Control and Complications Trial. The Diabetes Control and Complications Trial Research Group. *JAMA* 1996;276:1409.

87. The Diabetes Control and Complications Trial (DCCT) Research Group: The relationship of glycemic exposure (HbA$_{1c}$) to the risk of development and progression of retinopathy in the Diabetes Control and Complications Trial. *Diabetes* 1995;44:968.

88. The Diabetes Control and Complications Trial (DCCT) Research Group: The absence of a glycemic threshold for the development of long-term complications: The perspective of the Diabetes Control and Complications Trial. *Diabetes* 1996;45:1285.

89. Skyler JS: Diabetic complications: Glucose control is important. *Endocrinol Metab Clin North Am* 1996;25:243-254.

90. Epidemiology of Diabetes Interventions and Complications (EDIC) Research Group: Epidemiology of Diabetes Interventions and Complications (EDIC): Design, implementation, and preliminary results of a long-term follow-up of the Diabetes Control and Complications Trial cohort. *Diabetes Care* 1999;22:99.

91. The Diabetes Control and Complications Trial/Epidemiology of Diabetes Interventions and Complications Research Group: Retinopathy and nephropathy in patients with Type 1 diabetes four years after a trial of intensive therapy. *N Engl J Med* 2000;342:381.

92. Steffes MW, Molitch ME, Chavers BM, *et al*: Sustained reduction in albuminuria six years after the Diabetes Control and Complications Trial (DCCT). *Diabetes* 2001;50(suppl 2):254.

93. Diem P, Steffes MW, Egger M, *et al*: Macrovascular disease in Type 1 diabetes mellitus: Effects of intensified insulin treatment. *Diabetes* 2001;50(suppl 2):A252.

94. Ohkubo Y, Kishikawa H, Araki E, *et al*: Intensive insulin therapy prevents the progression of diabetic microvascular complications in Japanese patients with non-insulin-dependent diabetes mellitus: A randomized prospective 6-year study. *Diabetes Res Clin Pract* 1995;28:103.

95. Shichiri M, Kishikawa H, Ohkubo Y, *et al*: Long-term results of the Kumamoto Study on optimal diabetes control in type 2 diabetic patients. *Diabetes Care* 2000;23(suppl 2):B21.

96. Wake N, Hisashige A, Katayama T, *et al*: Cost-effectiveness of intensive insulin therapy for type 2 diabetes: A 10-year follow-up of the Kumamoto study. *Diabetes Res Clin Pract* 2000;48:201.

97. UK Prospective Diabetes Study Group: UK Prospective Diabetes Study. VIII. Study design, progress and performance. *Diabetologia* 1991;34:877.

98. Turner R, Cull C, Holman R: United Kingdom Prospective Diabetes Study 17: A 9-year update of a randomized, controlled trial on the effect of improved metabolic control on complications in non-insulin-dependent diabetes mellitus. *Ann Intern Med* 1996;124(1 pt 2):136.

99. UK Prospective Diabetes Study (UKPDS) Group: Intensive blood glucose control with sulphonylureas or insulin compared with conventional treatment and risk of complications in patients with type 2 diabetes (UKPDS 33). *Lancet* 1998;352:837.

100. UK Prospective Diabetes Study (UKPDS) Group: Effect of intensive blood-glucose control with metformin on complications in overweight patients with type 2 diabetes (UKPDS 34). *Lancet* 1998;352:854.

101. Turner RC, Holman R, Stratton I: The UK Prospective Diabetes Study [letter]. *Lancet* 1998;352:1934.

102. Stratton IM, Adler AI, Neil HAW, *et al*: Association of glycaemia with macrovascular and microvascular complications of type 2 diabetes (UKPDS 35): Prospective observational study. *Br Med J* 2000;321:405.

103. Mauer SM, Barbosa J, Vernier J, *et al*: Development of diabetic vascular lesions in normal kidneys transplanted into patients with diabetes mellitus. *N Engl J Med* 1976;295:916.

104. Mauer SM, Steffes MW, Connett J, *et al*: The development of lesions in the glomerular basement membrane and mesangium after transplantation of normal kidneys to diabetic patients. *Diabetes* 1983;32:948.

105. Bilous RW, Mauer SM, Sutherland DER, *et al*: The effects of pancreas transplantation on the glomerular structure of renal allografts in patients with insulin dependent diabetes. *N Engl J Med* 1989;321:80.

106. Wilczek HE, Jaremko G, Tyden G, *et al*: Evolution of diabetic nephropathy in kidney grafts. Evidence that a simultaneously transplanted pancreas exerts a protective effect. *Transplantation* 1995;59:51.

107. Gliedman ML, Tellis VA, Soberman R, *et al*: Long-term effects of pancreatic transplant function in patients with advanced juvenile-onset diabetes. *Diabetes Care* 1978;1:1.

108. Bohman SO, Tyden G, Wilczek H, *et al*: Prevention of kidney graft diabetic nephropathy by pancreas transplantation in man. *Diabetes* 1985;34:306.

109. Sutherland DER, Goetz FC, Moudry KC, *et al*: Pancreatic transplantation: A single institution's experience. *Diabetes Nutr Metab* 1988;1:57.

110. Fioretto P, Mauer SM, Bilou RW, *et al*: Effects of pancreas transplantation on glomerular structure in insulin-dependent diabetic patients with their own kidneys. *Lancet* 1993;342:1193.

111. Fioretto P, Steffes MW, Sutherland DER, *et al*: Reversal of lesions of diabetic nephropathy after pancreas transplantation. *N Engl J Med* 1998;339:69.

112. Ramsay RC, Goetz FC, Sutherland DER, *et al*: Progression of diabetic retinopathy after pancreas transplantation for insulin-dependent diabetes mellitus. *N Engl J Med* 1988;318:208.

113. Wang Q, Klein R, Moss SE, *et al*: The influence of combined kidney-pancreas transplantation on progression of diabetic retinopathy. *Ophthalmology* 1994;101:1071.

114. Abouna GM, Al-Adnani MS, Kremer GD, *et al*: Reversal of diabetic nephropathy in human cadaveric kidneys after transplantation into nondiabetic recipients. *Lancet* 1983;2:1274.

115. Abouna GM, Adnani MS, Kumar MSA, *et al*: Fate of transplanted kidneys with diabetic nephropathy. *Lancet* 1986;1:622.

116. Mauer SM: Commentary. *Diabetes Spectrum* 1988;1:110.

117. Tatersall RB: The quest for normoglycaemia: A historical perspective. *Diabetologia* 1994;11:618.

Pancreas Transplantation

David E. R. Sutherland

Rainer W. G. Gruessner

S. Michael Mauer

Angelika C. Gruessner

INTRODUCTION

β-Cell (beta cell) replacement by transplantation of a pancreas either as an immediately vascularized organ or as a free graft of isolated islets is the only treatment of type I diabetes mellitus (T1DM) that can make an afflicted individual independent of exogenous insulin (termed insulin independence). Pancreas transplantation has been able to consistently do so in a large number of patients at many centers throughout the world for more than a decade.[1]

Historically, islet transplantation has been less successful for a variety of reasons,[2] but the gap is narrowing. Recently one center reported achieving insulin independence in several consecutive diabetic recipients by sequential grafting of islets obtained from more than one donor and using a relatively nondiabetogenic steroid-free immunosuppressive regimen.[3] Another center reported achieving insulin independence in a few patients following transplantation of islets obtained from one donor per recipient.[4]

In the latter series at the University of Minnesota,[4] the recipients had a low body mass index (BMI), while the donors had a high BMI. Thus the number of islets transplanted per unit weight in the Minnesota recipients from one donor was similar to that using multiple donors in the other series at the University of Alberta.[3] These series show that pancreatic islet transplantation could eventually supersede vascularized pancreas transplantation as the means for β cell replacement therapy for the majority of diabetic candidates, but the transition will not be complete until islet transplantation mimics the efficiency of pancreas transplantation. One pancreas graft usually suffices to induce insulin independence regardless of the recipient's exogenous regimens. In addition, only a few centers currently possess the infrastructure to do islet isolation on a large scale, while pancreas transplants can be done at most centers with the logistics and infrastructure already developed for solid organ transplantation in general. In the interim, an integrated approach may be possible by selecting low-BMI diabetics for islet transplantation and using high-BMI donors for this population, while high-BMI diabetics receive pancreas grafts from low-BMI donors.

This chapter focuses on pancreas transplantation as an immediately vascularized graft. The rationale and objectives are the same as for islet transplantation. For candidates in whom islet transplantation can replace pancreas transplantation, the main benefit will be in elimination of the surgical complications that are associated with the latter. Currently, both approaches require generalized immunosuppression to prevent rejection. Strategies to induce specific immunologic tolerance are just beginning to be tested in the clinical arena. Nevertheless, advances in pharmacologic immunosuppression and infection prophylaxis have made organ transplantation in general increasingly successful and benign, and thus pancreas (or islet) transplantation will be applied to the extent that organs are available until strategies to prevent or actually treat the pathogenesis of diabetes materialize (for example, preventing autoimmunity before onset in T1DM, or if after onset, coupling such prevention with stimulation of β-cell regeneration[5]).

RATIONALE

The purpose of pancreas (or islet) transplantation is to establish euglycemia and free the diabetic patient of the daily burden of multiple insulin injections or dose or diet adjustments based on multiple fingerstick blood glucose determinations. This burden has to be assumed not only to remain alive (for T1DM) but also to lower the risk for secondary diabetic complications.

The Diabetes Control and Complications Trial (DCCT) conclusively proved that vigorous diabetic control reduces the incidence of secondary complications.[6] The price is the rigorous self-discipline required to lower glycohemoglobin as much toward normal as possible, plus an increased frequency of insulin reactions and hypoglycemic episodes.[7] Even in the DCCT group given intense insulin treatment, mean glycosylated hemoglobin levels were a gram percent above normal. Some individuals developed secondary complications even when glycosylated hemoglobin levels were only moderately elevated. The incidence of secondary complications decreases progressively with decreasing mean glycosylated hemoglobin levels, but the threshold for zero risk is a constantly normal value, something that currently can only be achieved with pancreas transplantation. A closed-loop insulin pump coupled to a glucose sensor should theoretically do the same, but a miniaturized, implantable, practical device is not yet available.

Thus at the moment, perfect diabetic control is only provided by β-cell replacement. The main current drawback of both pancreas and islet transplantation is the need to immunosuppress the recipient, but this can be done with oral drugs without the need for constant dose adjustments. A pancreas transplant requires major surgery, but a successful graft makes the recipient euglycemic and glycosylated hemoglobin levels are normal for as long as the graft functions.[8,9] The need for immunosuppression is only a relative drawback, since it is used for other organ transplants even when alternative treatments are available, such as dialysis for renal failure. Indeed, the modern management of diabetes by exogenous insulin may be as burdensome as dialysis is for renal failure: >4 blood glucose determinations daily and 4 insulin injections or a constantly placed needle adds up to 35–50 needle sticks per week, or approximately 2000 per year (dialysis 3 times per week with 2 needles is only 300 needle sticks per year). If one looks at exogenous insulin needle-intensive treatment as akin to dialysis, immunosuppression for treatment of diabetes by islet or pancreas transplantation is logical.

β-Cell transplants should ideally be performed before complications occur. Because of uncertainty in an individual patient as to whether he or she is complication-prone (even with poor control, not all get complications), as well as the uncertainty over what the individual side effects of immunosuppression will be, only a few institutions do pancreas transplants soon after onset of disease.[10] Antirejection strategies to decrease the side effects of immunosuppression, however, are increasingly available.[11]

During the past decade, pancreas transplants alone were largely employed in patients with very labile diabetes and hypoglycemic unawareness, a syndrome that may emerge many years after onset of diabetes, particularly in patients with neuropathy.[12] In this situation pancreas transplantation is the most effective treatment since it completely obviates insulin reactions. However, for patients who are not labile, but who wish to obviate a lifetime need for insulin injections and glucose monitoring, as well as to absolutely eliminate the risk of secondary diabetic complications by choosing the alternative risk of immunosuppression complications, pancreas transplantation can reasonably be chosen. To fully assess the trade-off and risks of immunosuppression versus the risks of secondary diabetic complications, randomization of candidates, transplantation versus insulin, soon after onset of diabetes would be ideal, but until that is done, a diabetic individual can just as logically choose one approach or the other. Even with emphasis on tight control through intensive glucose monitoring and constant insulin dose adjustments, the diabetes literature continues to show an extremely high rate of secondary complications that are just as morbid,[13] if not more morbid, than those described secondary to chronic immunosuppression in organ allograft recipients.[14,15]

Nevertheless, because of the need for immunosuppression, most pancreas transplants have been done either simultaneous with or subsequent to a kidney transplant in diabetic patients with advanced nephropathy.[16] Nearly everyone agrees that a kidney transplant is preferable to dialysis in the treatment of uremia (particularly in diabetic patients). Thus when a diabetic patient is already obligated to immunosuppression, there is very little reason not to add a β-cell transplant, and only the surgical risks need to be considered. Indeed, simultaneous pancreas-kidney (SPK) transplants have even been done in insulin-treated uremic diabetics meeting criteria for type 2 diabetes mellitus (T2DM).[17]

Unfortunately, in uremic diabetic patients, retinopathy and neuropathy are usually far advanced and the DCCT did not study the effect of maintaining strict control on established lesions. Thus the main value of adding a pancreas to the kidney is the additional improvement of quality of life that accompanies being insulin-independent as well as dialysis-free.[18] This is not to say that there

is no effect of the pancreas transplant on nonrenal secondary complications that are present in the uremic diabetic. Improvement in neuropathy has been documented.[19–21] As expected, recurrence of diabetic nephropathy in a renal transplant is also prevented by successful pancreas transplant.[22,23] Nevertheless, advanced retinopathy and vascular disease are unlikely to be affected,[24] even though a pancreas transplant has been shown to decrease atherosclerotic risk factors and improve endothelial function.[25] It is for this reason that early β-cell replacement should be the goal.

HISTORY

The first clinical pancreas transplant was performed at the University of Minnesota in 1966.[26] During the 1970s a few institutions performed a few cases with low success rates.[27] In 1980, the International Pancreas Transplant Registry (IPTR) was formed,[28] followed by annual reports.[1] By 2000 more than 15,000 pancreas transplants had been reported worldwide (Fig. 55-1), including more than 11,000 in the U.S.[29]

A dramatic improvement in outcome occurred in the 1980s following advances in surgical techniques and the introduction of cyclosporine for immunosuppression. In the United States, the inception of the United Network for Organ Sharing (UNOS) in 1987, facilitating organ procurement and placement, was followed by a steady growth in the number of applicants. By the mid-1990s, more than 1000 pancreas transplants were being done yearly in the U.S.[1]

SPK transplants have predominated in the past, but there is great potential for growth in the solitary β-cell transplant categories since far more cadaver (CAD) organs are available than are being transplanted. There are approximately 5500 CAD donors annually in the U.S., but many cannot be used for an SPK transplant since the majority of renal allograft candidates are nondiabetic. A large number of diabetic renal allograft recipients are available as candidates for pancreas (or islet) transplants after kidney (PAK) transplantation.[30] Likewise, the number of diabetic patients not in need of a kidney transplant in whom immunosuppression would be acceptable to become insulin-independent by a pancreas transplant alone (PTA) or islet transplant greatly exceeds the number of organs available. All should be used.

The historical development of pancreas transplantation has been summarized in detail elsewhere.[31] In brief, the focus during the early years was on refinement of surgical techniques and reduction of surgical complications (many related to the exocrine pancreas), using either a segment (tail) of the pancreas or the entire

FIGURE 55-1. Number of pancreas transplants tabulated by the International Pancreas Transplant Registry (IPTR) from 1966 through 2000.

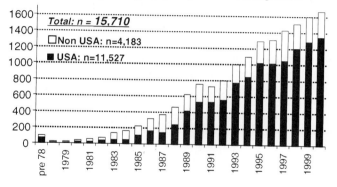

pancreas with attached duodenum. By the mid 1970s three techniques were in use: enteric drainage (ED) (first used by Richard Lillihei in 1967 at the University of Minnesota in Minneapolis), urinary drainage (first into the ureter by Marvin Gliedman at Montefiore Hospital in New York in 1970, and later modified by direct implantation into the bladder by Hans Solligner at the University of Wisconsin in 1982), and duct injection (first used by Jean-Michael Dubernard at Herriot Hospital in Lyon, France in 1974).

During the 1980s bladder drainage (BD) was shown to be safe,[32] and it became the predominant technique in all recipient categories (Fig. 55-2). Some groups, however, continued to use ED,[33] and during the 1990s a shift back to ED occurred for SPK transplants (Fig. 55-3). In SPK recipients, the creatinine level can be used to monitor for kidney rejection, a surrogate marker for pancreas rejection when both organs come from the same donor. For solitary pancreas transplant (PTA or PAK), BD continues to be recommended because of the ability to monitor urine amylase, the most sensitive marker of pancreas rejection alone.[34]

Vascularized management of the pancreas graft has also evolved. Drainage of the graft venous effluent can either be into the systemic or the portal circulation. Portal drainage was used for segmental pancreas grafts in a few patients by four groups in the 1980s.[35–38] Portal drainage using whole pancreatic duodenal grafts began in the 1990s, first coupled with bladder drainage,[39] and then with enteric drainage.[40,41] Rosenlof and colleagues[40] described anastomosis to the recipient splenic vein and Gaber and associates[42] to the recipient superior mesenteric vein (Fig. 55-4). Several groups adapted portal-enteric drainage as their routine or did prospective studies.[43–45] It is more physiological than systemic drainage,[43] and

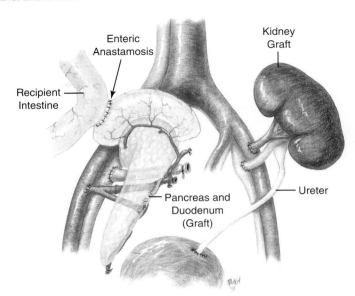

FIGURE 55-3. Enteric-drained (ED) simultaneous pancreas-kidney (SPK) transplant from a cadaver donor with systemic venous drainage.

possibly lowers the incidence of rejection,[46] although not all confirm that claim.[47] About 20% of SPK transplants in the United States have been portal-enteric drained since 1996.[1]

Although segmental grafts were commonly used for pancreas transplants done in the 1970s, during the 1980s techniques for

FIGURE 55-2. Bladder-drained pancreaticoduodenal transplant alone (PTA) from a cadaver donor.

FIGURE 55-4. Enteric-drained SPK transplants with portal venous drainage of the pancreas graft via the superior mesenteric vein.

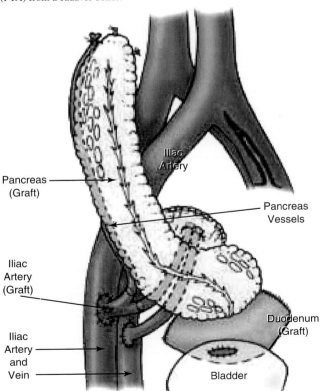

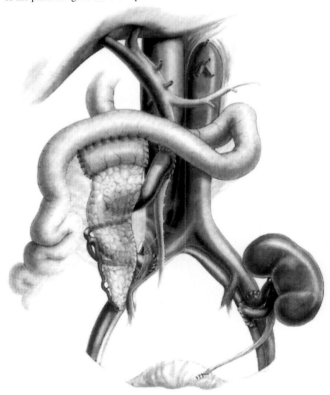

preserving the vascular supply to both the whole pancreas and the liver were developed.[49,50] Thus nearly all groups now use pancreaticoduodenal grafts from CAD donors.[51] Segmental grafts continue to be done, but primarily for pancreata procured from living donors.[52] Pancreas transplants from living donors were first done at the University of Minnesota in 1979,[53] primarily as a solitary procedure at a time when the rejection rate for CAD grafts was high.[54] In the 1990s, living donor pancreas transplants were usually done simultaneously with a kidney (Fig. 55-5), in order to allow a single procedure, eliminate waiting time, and preempt dialysis for SPK recipients.[55–57] Other institutions have also done living donor SPK transplants with good outcome.[58] The pressure to use living donor tissue primarily relates to long waiting times,[59] and once all CAD pancreata are being utilized, the number of applications for solitary pancreas transplants is likely to increase. Recently, the University of Minnesota has begun to do living donor segmental pancreatectomy laparoscopically, as has now become routine for living kidney transplantation.[48]

Another option to shorten waiting time for the uremic diabetic and still perform a single operation is to do a simultaneous living donor kidney with a CAD pancreas transplant, first done in the 1980s,[54] and now applied much more frequently.[60] An interesting sidelight to the Minnesota living donor pancreas experience in the 1980s related to observations in diabetic recipients of segmental grafts from their nondiabetic identical twin donor counterparts. Without immunosuppression, isletitis recurred in the new graft.[61,62] With immunosuppression, β-cell morphology and function were preserved in the identical twin donor graft.[52,63] Thus for pancreas transplants in general to succeed in type 1 diabetic recipients, both rejection and autoimmune isletitis must be prevented. In regard to the latter, the generalized immunosuppressive regimens in use since at least the mid-1980s are adequate, since autoimmune recurrence in pancreas grafts is exceedingly rare,[64] except in the nonimmunosuppressed recipients.[63]

In regard to immunosuppression, in the mid-1990s FK506 (tacrolimus) and mycophenolate mofetil became available, and were quickly applied to pancreas transplantation.[65,66] These drugs have now become mainstays of immunosuppression in pancreas

FIGURE 55-5. Simultaneous segmental pancreas and kidney transplant from a living donor (LD). Either BD or ED can be used, but the BD technique has a lower complication rate and is illustrated. *(Reproduced with permission from Gruessner et al.[56])*

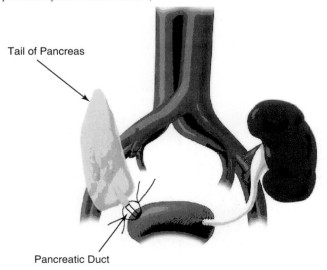

Tail of Pancreas

Pancreatic Duct

transplant recipients and have further improved results,[67,68] particularly in solitary pancreas transplant recipients.[69,70] Other recent additions to the immunosuppression regimens include sirolimus for maintenance and interleukin-2 receptor monoclonal antibody for induction, both yielding favorable results.[71] Steroid withdrawal has also been shown to be associated with low rejection rates in stable pancreas transplant recipients.[72]

Currently, there are more than 100 pancreas transplant programs in the United States[29] Most have come into existence only during the past decade and are relatively small. A few centers have extensive experience.[46,52,73,74] The University of Wisconsin has reported experience with more than 500 SPK transplants,[73] and the University of Minnesota has reported on a total of more than 1000 pancreas transplants.[52] However, the overall recent results of pancreas transplantation are best viewed by compiling a review of the collective data.

In the following section the current results of pancreas transplants from CAD donors as tabulated by the IPTR are given. The results with living donor segmental pancreas transplants at the institution primarily using this approach are summarized in a separate section.

IPTR REPORT OF OUTCOME WITH CADAVER PANCREAS TRANSPLANTATION

Analyses of IPTR data have been published yearly since the mid-1980s, and the results (long-term insulin independence) have continually improved over time.[1] The latest Registry analyses[29] focus on U.S. cases done from 1996–2001, including >4500 SPK, >900 PAK, and >350 PTA cases (Fig. 55-6). The patient survival rates

FIGURE 55-6. Patient (**A**) and pancreas graft (**B**) survival rates from 1996–2001 U.S. cadaver SPK, PAK, and PTA transplants as reported to UNOS and the IPTR. *(Reproduced with permission from Gruessner et al.[29])*

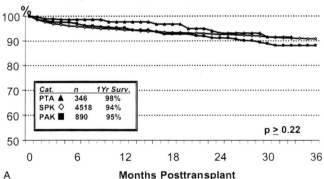

Cat.	n	1Yr Surv.
PTA ▲	346	98%
SPK ◇	4518	94%
PAK ■	890	95%

p ≥ 0.22

A Months Posttransplant

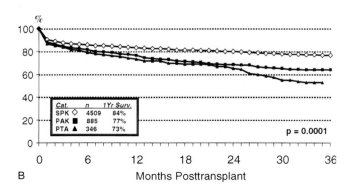

Cat.	n	1Yr Surv.
SPK ◇	4509	84%
PAK ■	885	77%
PTA ▲	346	73%

p = 0.0001

B Months Posttransplant

are not significantly different between the three categories, and are >90% at 3 years posttransplant (Fig. 55-6A). Most deaths are from preexisting cardiovascular disease; the mortality risk of a pancreas transplant *per se* is extremely low (1-year patient survival for PTA recipients is 98%).

Pancreas graft survival rates were slightly higher in the SPK than the PAK and PTA categories, 84% versus 75% and 73%, respectively, at 1 year (Fig. 55-6B). The differences are in part due to the decreased ability to monitor for rejection episodes in enteric-drained solitary pancreas transplant recipients. In the SPK category, 1-year graft survival rates were 85% for BD (n = 1781) versus 83% for ED (n = 2798; p = ns). In the PAK category, the 1-year graft survival rates were 83% for BD (n = 368) versus 74% for ED (n = 328) cases ($p < 0.05$). In the PTA category, the 1-year graft survival rates were 81% for BD (n = 190) versus 73% for ED (n = 133) ($p < 0.05$). Thus with current immunosuppressive protocols (predominantly tacrolimus and mycophenolate mofetil for maintenance), 1-year graft survival rates of over 80% are achieved in all categories with bladder drainage, and in the SPK category with either bladder or enteric drainage.

Kidney graft survival rates in SPK recipients have been higher than for diabetic recipients of kidney transplants alone in all eras.[75] For the 1996–2001 SPK transplants, kidney graft survival rates were >90% at 1 year in both the ED and BD subcategories.

The proportion of older diabetic patients receiving pancreas transplants in the United States increased significantly during the 1990s. In 1988–1989, only 5% of the recipients were >45 years old. In 2000–2001, 75% were >45 years old in all three categories of recipients. Only 2% were <21 years old. The outcomes according to recipient age for 1997–2001 are shown in Figs. 55-7, 55-8, and 55-9. The age of the recipient has had very little impact on outcomes. In the SPK category, patient survival rates were over 90% at 1 year in both age categories (Fig. 55-7A), and 1-year graft survival rates were ≥80% (Fig. 55-7B). In the PAK category, patient survival rates at 1 year were also >90% (Fig. 55-8A), and graft survival rates were again not significantly different (Fig. 55-8B). Interestingly, in the PTA category, the 1-year patient survival rate was 100% in the older age category (Fig. 55-9A), and the graft survival rates were significantly higher in the older PTA recipients, 85% versus 77% at 1 year (Fig. 55-9B). The young, nonuremic PTA recipients tend to have a higher rejection graft loss rate than the PAK and SPK recipients (at 2 years, 12% versus 5% and 3%, respectively). In the older group, the rejection graft loss rate at 2 years is low in all categories: 2%, 5%, and 3%, respectively.

With the increased number of older patients receiving pancreas transplants, it is not surprising that some have been classified as having T2DM. Most of the patients classified as type 2 have been in the SPK category. For 1996–2000 SPK transplants,[1] 1-year insulin-independence rates were 84% in those classified as type 1 (n = 3323) and 83% in those classified as type 2 (n = 157).

The improvement in pancreas graft functional survival rates reflects a decrease in both the technical failure (TF) rate and rejection rates. The TF rate (grafts lost from thrombosis, pancreatitis, or perigraft infection) for 1997–2001 U.S. cases was 8% overall. In the analysis of technically successful cases (death with functioning graft censored), the 1-year rejection loss rate was only 2% for SPK, 6% for PAK, and 8% for PTA cases.

It is apparent that with the generalized immunosuppressive regimes being used currently, there is very little difference in pancreas graft survival rates in SPK and PAK recipients, giving further impetus to the use of living donor kidney in diabetic patients with

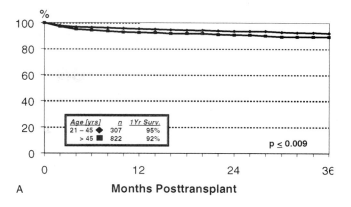

A

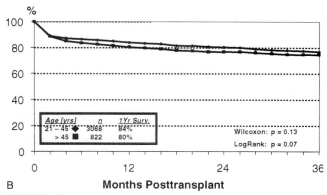

B

FIGURE 55-7. Patient (**A**) and pancreas graft (**B**) functional survival rates for 1997–2001 U.S. cadaver SPK transplants by recipient age.

advanced nephropathy. With a living donor kidney, the need for dialysis can be preempted and a subsequent pancreas transplantation from a CAD donor has nearly the same probability of success as that done simultaneously with a CAD kidney. The only drawback to a PAK is the need for two operations. For those with a suitable living donor, an SPK transplant with a segmental graft is an alternative to sequential transplants, as described in the next section.

LIVING SEGMENTAL DONOR PANCREAS TRANSPLANTS

Of the more than 15,000 pancreas transplants reported to the International Registry, slightly more than 1% have been from living donors (LDs).[29] As for other organ transplants, LDs are used to (1) alleviate the CAD donor shortage, (2) eliminate waiting time, and (3) decrease rejection.

The number of diabetics who would benefit from a pancreas transplant alone (PTA) exceeds the number of CAD donors. The number of nonuremic candidates registered has been well below the potential number of organs available, so waiting times have been relatively short for a solitary pancreas transplant. However, the waiting time for CAD kidney transplants is long. Thus the incentive for an LD pancreas transplant is highest in uremic diabetics, whose waiting time for a CAD simultaneous pancreas kidney (SPK) transplant would otherwise be long and most likely require dialysis. The outcomes of an LD kidney procedure first, followed by a CAD pancreas (PAK) procedure, are good,[30] but this requires two operations. Outcomes are also good in patients who receive a

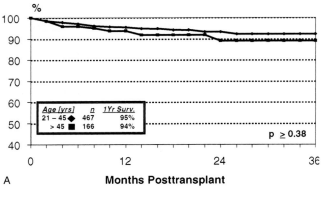

A   **Months Posttransplant**

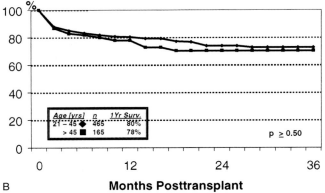

B   **Months Posttransplant**

FIGURE 55-8. Patient (**A**) and pancreas graft (**B**) survival rate for 1997–2001 U.S. cadaver PAK transplants by recipient age.

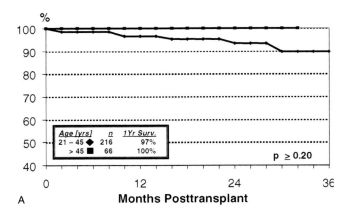

A   **Months Posttransplant**

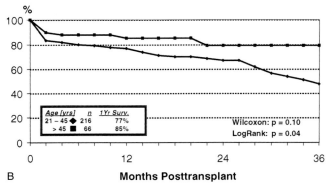

B   **Months Posttransplant**

FIGURE 55-9. Patient (**A**) and pancreas graft (**B**) functional survival rates for 1997–2001 U.S. cadaver PTA transplants by recipient age.

simultaneous CAD pancreas and living donor kidney,[60] but these procedures are logistically difficult for some patients, and waiting time is still involved.

More than 80% of the living donor segmental pancreas transplants in the Registry have been done at the University of Minnesota, and it is the Minnesota experience that is reviewed here. We began to offer LD segmental pancreas transplants in 1979,[53] at a time when the rejection rate of CAD pancreata was high.[54] Initially, we did only solitary pancreas transplants (PAK or PTA) from LDs, with the main aim being an improvement in results. Through the 1980s our solitary pancreas transplant results were superior with living donors.[76]

In the 1990s, the results of solitary pancreas transplants from CAD donors improved dramatically,[52] making a CAD pancreas after an LD kidney an attractive option from an outcome standpoint.[30,55] Nevertheless, some uremic diabetic patients who had an LD wanted to avoid two operations and having to wait for either organ. Thus in 1994 we began to do LD segmental pancreas transplants simultaneously with a kidney transplant for these reasons.[56] An update of our previous reports[59] on the LD SPK experience is summarized below.

The donors have ranged in age from 24–58 years. Pretransplant, LDs had to have normal oral and intravenous glucose tolerance tests, a threefold increase in first-phase insulin release during intravenous stimulation, and a body mass index below 29 kg/m^2. The LD SPK recipients ranged in age from 14–58 years, with diabetes duration of 11–29 years. Twenty-four of the LD SPK recipients were not on dialysis pretransplant. Duct management was with bladder drainage (BD) in 32 and duct injection (DI) in 3.

Actuarial patient, kidney, and pancreas (insulin independence) survival rates at 1 year were 100%, 100%, and 86%, respectively, for the LD SPK transplants (Fig. 55-10).

Of the 35 LD SPK transplants, 4 failed for technical reasons, 3 (BD) from thrombosis, and 1 from primary nonfunction (duct injected). There were two late pancreas graft losses from rejection, and one late kidney loss from hemolytic uremic syndrome. All of the LD SPK recipients are alive. The pancreas graft survival rates are at least as high for LD or for CAD SPK recipients, and the kidney graft survival rates are higher with LDs. Furthermore, two-thirds of the LD recipients avoided pretransplant dialysis, which is usually not possible with CAD transplants.

All 35 of the SPK living donors are alive and insulin-independent. Surgical complications included the need for splenectomy in seven, percutaneous fluid drainage in three, and gastritis in one. Two donors had impaired glucose tolerance; one had a prior history of gestational diabetes, and the other had a BMI above our usual limits. Currently, we exclude individuals from being a segmental pancreas donor who have a history of gestational diabetes. Our current criteria also require segmental pancreas living donors to be less than 60 years old, to have a BMI <29 kg/m^2, to have all glucose values <150 during an oral GTT, and to have an acute insulin response to intravenous glucose and arginine stimulation of >300% above baseline.

Metabolic perturbations can occur in the donors,[77] but all donors meeting the criteria itemized above have remained normoglycemic and insulin-independent.

Currently, the main application of LD pancreas transplant is in uremic diabetic patients who desire to avoid the long wait for a

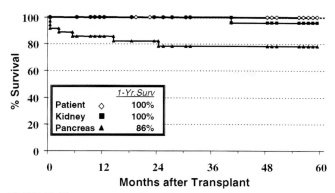

FIGURE 55-10. Patient and graft survival for 35 living related donor simultaneous pancreas and kidney (SPK) transplants at the University of Minnesota (1994–2001).

CAD SPK, and for those who would otherwise have bypassed an LD kidney for a CAD SPK to avoid two operations.

LD pancreas transplantation also has a role as a solitary procedure, particularity in highly sensitized patients with a negative crossmatch against a potential donor. Not all CAD pancreata are currently used for clinical pancreas transplantation, so LDs are not yet needed to alleviate a shortage of organs. This likely will change because the results of CAD solitary pancreas transplantation are now so good.[78] Once a CAD pancreas shortage exists, there will be an incentive to use LDs for solitary as well as SPK transplants.

SURGICAL TECHNIQUE

For solitary organ pancreas transplants, the main choices facing the surgeon are (1) whether to transplant the whole organ or a segment, (2) how to manage the exocrine secretions, and (3) how to establish venous drainage (portal or systemic).

CAD donor grafts are nearly always transplanted as a whole pancreas, since preservation of the blood supply to the entire gland is possible even when the liver is procured.[79] A Y-graft of donor iliac artery can easily be used to join the splenic and superior mesenteric arteries of the graft, allowing for a single arterial anastomosis in the recipient. Thus almost all segmental grafts done today are from living donors. Adequacy of segment transplants has been established by metabolic studies.[9,80] Segmental grafts from CAD donors still have a role when there is a rare anatomic abnormality that does not allow the head of the pancreas to be used, or when there is a compelling reason to split the pancreas into two segments for transplantation to two different recipients, such as when both have a high panel reactive antibody but a negative crossmatch for the same donor.[81] Indeed, as the number of candidates listed for pancreas transplants and waiting times increase, the incentive to split cadaver organs will also increase.

In regard to current management of the exocrine secretions, some groups always use ED,[43,46] some always use BD,[74] and for others the approach is dictated by the recipient category.[52] Both techniques now have a relatively low surgical risk.[82]

BD allows direct measurement of enzyme activity in the pancreatic graft exocrine secretions. A decrease in urine amylase is a sensitive marker of rejection, even though it is not entirely specific.[83] Urine amylase always decreases before hyperglycemia ensues. A rise in serum amylase may precede a decrease in urine

amylase, but serum amylase by itself is less sensitive (it does not always rise, while urine amylase always decreases), and is no more specific for diagnosis of rejection. Thus for solitary pancreas transplants, the rejection loss rate is lower with BD than with other duct management techniques.[29] Rejection episodes are detected early with BD, increasing the probability that the process will be reversed by a temporary increase in immunosuppression. If necessary, a rejection diagnosis can be confirmed by a percutaneous biopsy whether the graft is ED or BD.[84,85]

In the SPK category, isolated rejection of the pancreas is now rare with the immunosuppressants FK506 (tacrolimus) and mycophenolate mofetil (MMF). Rejection episodes affecting both organs are nearly always first manifested by a rise in serum creatinine (easily confirmed by renal graft biopsy). Thus, most transplant centers now use ED for SPK transplants, as has been advocated for years by the Stockholm group.[86] Although the acute surgical complication rate leading to graft loss may be slightly higher with ED (mainly leaks, the graft thrombosis incidence being about the same with all techniques), the chronic complication rate is lower.[87] Between 10% and 20% of recipients of BD grafts are ultimately converted to ED because of chronic complications such as metabolic acidosis from bicarbonate loss secreted directly from the pancreas, urinary tract infections related to the enterovesical anastomosis, dysuria, hematuria, or late leaks.[1]

ED could be the standard duct management technique for all pancreas transplant categories once immunomodulation strategies that completely prevent rejection episodes are devised.[88,89] Currently, a rejection episode–free regimen does not exist, so BD gives an advantage in solitary pancreas transplants. For SPK transplants, ED is justifiably the dominant method of drainage.

Another question is whether to drain the venous effluent of the pancreas graft into the recipient's portal or systemic circulation. Portal drainage is more physiologic than systemic drainage,[90,91] but it is not easily combined with bladder drainage.[39] Thus, most portally drained transplants have been done with ED in SPK recipients, and several groups now make it their standard technique.[44–46,92]

With both systemic and portal drainage, the recipients are euglycemic with a normal glycohemoglobin, but portally drained recipients will have lower systemic insulin levels.[80] However, even with systemic drainage of pancreas grafts, the situation of *de novo* hyperinsulinemia (syndrome X) is not replicated. There is no evidence that there is any detrimental effect of systemic drainage on lipid levels[93] or vascular disease.[24] Most groups have continued to use systemic venous drainage for ED SPK transplants. On the other hand, there is no reason not to mimic nature, and most likely there will be a shift toward portal drainage for ED SPK transplants, particularly if the reports of fewer rejections with portal drainage are confirmed.[43,46]

PREVENTION OF GRAFT REJECTION

Currently, generalized immunosuppression must be given for all organ or cellular transplants.[15] From the mid-1980s through the mid-1990s, cyclosporine in conjunction with either azathioprine or steroids were the mainstays of maintenance immunosuppression.[68] Many protocols included induction immunosuppression with heterologous antibody anti–T-cell agents.[1] Since the mid-1990s, FK 506 (tacrolimus) and mycophenolate mofetil (MMF) have been used widely in pancreas transplants, and both immunosuppressants have been associated with improvement in pancreas graft survival rates.[66,70,78] In addition, steroids have been successfully withdrawn from pancreas transplant recipients without precipitating rejection,[72] or have been avoided altogether.[94]

In the groups at highest risk for rejection, PTA and pretransplant immunosuppression have been associated with a decrease in both rejection episodes and immunologic graft loss.[95] Finally, advances in antimicrobial prophylaxis have also been an important advance in allowing the immunosuppressive drugs to be used so effectively.[96,97]

EFFECTS OF PANCREAS TRANSPLANTATION ON METABOLISM AND SECONDARY COMPLICATIONS OF DIABETES

A successful pancreas transplant nearly always establishes euglycemia and insulin independence in the recipient, with constantly normal glycosylated hemoglobin levels.[8] Minor metabolic perturbations can exist in some pancreas recipients, and are of academic interest,[98] but do not affect day-to-day life. Pancreas graft function has been extremely durable[9] as illustrated by studies in patients followed for more than 10 years (Figs. 55-11 and 55-12). In diabetic patients with impaired hypoglycemic counterregulation, a successful pancreas transplant can permanently restore counterregulatory mechanisms. Pancreas transplantation is the best treatment for diabetic patients afflicted with hypoglycemic unawareness.[99]

As mentioned in the section on surgical techniques, most pancreas transplants are drained via the systemic venous system and thus induce a degree of hyperinsulinemia. Portal drainage of the graft venous effluent avoids this potential problem.[42] On the other hand, a beneficial effect of pancreas transplants on lipid metabolism occurs even with systemic drainage.[93]

In regard to the effect on secondary complications, it is clear that a successful pancreas transplant performed early in the course of diabetes would prevent their occurrence. There is also an effect on established lesions, as summarized in previous reviews.[24,100] The rapidity with which neuropathy improves is quite variable, sometimes occurring early and sometimes evolving over several years[14–21]. Severely neuropathic patients have a very high mortality rate. Remarkably, after a pancreas transplant, the mortality rate is much reduced, independent of the effect on neuropathy.[101,102] The beneficial effect of pancreas transplantation on survival of diabetic

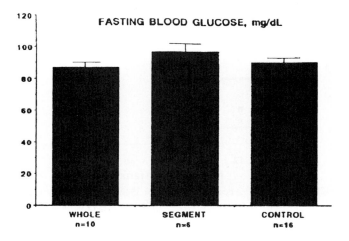

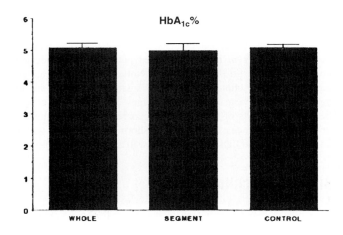

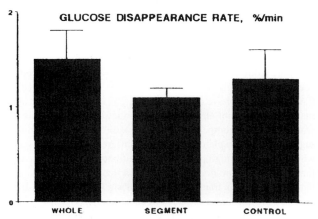

FIGURE 55-11. Fasting blood glucose levels in 16 type 1 diabetic recipients at increasing numbers of years after pancreas transplantation. Lines connect sequential data that were available in 14 of the 16 patients. Inset shows mean ± SE of the data for the group.

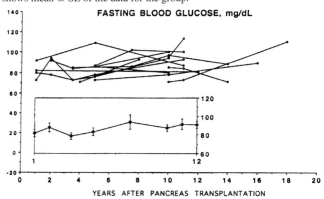

FIGURE 55-12. Levels of fasting blood glucose, HbA$_{1c}$, and intravenous glucose tolerance in type 1 diabetic recipients 10–18 years after whole or segmental pancreas transplantation, compared with age-, sex-, and BMI-matched nondiabetic control subjects. No significant differences were found.

patients, particularly those that are nephropathic, is also well documented.[52,103–108] Pancreas transplantation can prevent the occurrence of diabetic nephropathy in renal allografts.[22,23]

In regard to diabetic nephropathy in native kidneys, remarkably, in long-term PTA recipients, established structural changes of diabetes in the kidney can reverse between 5–10 years after transplant[109] (Figs. 55-13 and 55-14). Thus pancreas transplants alone could be used earlier in the course of diabetic nephropathy to prevent the otherwise inevitable deterioration.

In regard to vascular disease, an improvement in microvascular microangiopathy following pancreas transplantation has been described.[110] Improvement of left ventricular function[111] and a decrease in atherosclerotic risk factors[112] following pancreas-kidney transplantation have also been reported.

Several reviews on the effect of pancreas transplantation on secondary complications have been published, including articles describing a favorable effect on microcirculation.[24,100,113] These reviews also include studies on quality of life. All show that patient satisfaction is higher in SPK and PAK than in kidney transplant alone (KTA) recipients due to many factors, including dietary management, and that there is a positive impact on the recipient's family as well.[18,114] Nearly uniformly, PTA recipients state that management of immunosuppression is easier than management of diabetes.

RECIPIENT SELECTION

Not every diabetic patient can undergo pancreas transplant because of the shortage of suitable CAD donors. It is unlikely that living donors can make up this deficit, because even for kidney transplants, where living donation is widely promoted, the shortage is large. In the United States, there are approximately 30,000 new cases of T1DM each year, and there are only approximately 5000 CAD donors annually. Thus even if every CAD donor was used for a pancreas transplant with the organ split into two parts, the pancreas transplant rate would be only one-third of the new T1DM case rate.

Pancreas transplantation can also establish a euglycemic state in patients with T2DM,[17] making the gap between available donors and potential candidates even greater. Thus a strategy of allocating the available organs to those who would benefit the most (e.g., to alleviate hypoglycemic unawareness) is needed. Pancreas transplantation can be used to prevent secondary complications of diabetes, and those at high risk (if they can be identified) should have priority.

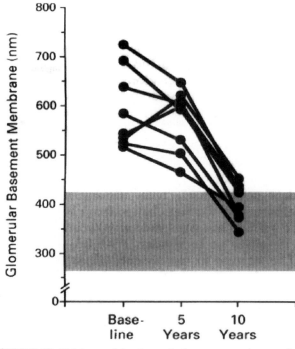

FIGURE 55-13. Thickness of the glomerular basement membrane, at baseline and 5 and 10 years after pancreas transplantation. The shaded area is the normal range. *(Reproduced with permission from Fioretto et al.[109])*

Even though it is late in the course of the disease, the most obvious patients to undergo pancreas transplant are those who also need a kidney transplant and are obligated to immunosuppression. For those who do not have a living donor for the kidney, an SPK transplant from a CAD donor makes sense. For those that have an LD, the ideal approach would be an SPK from this source. If the donor is suitable only for a kidney, it would still be preferable to perform an LD kidney transplant first with either a simultaneous or subsequent CAD pancreas.[60] Long-term graft functional survival rates for LD kidneys have been consistently higher than for CAD donor kidneys, and the insulin-independence rate with PAK transplants are nearly identical to those of SPK transplants.[29,30]

The PAK option is vastly underutilized. An LD kidney followed later by a CAD pancreas avoids long waiting times to get off dialysis or avoids the need for dialysis altogether, and gives the highest probability of remaining dialysis-free long term. Thus for the uremic diabetic the best option would be an LD SPK transplant,

FIGURE 55-14. Photomicrographs of renal biopsy specimens obtained before (**left**) and 10 years after (**right**) pancreas transplantation. Specimens were taken from a 33-year-old woman with type 1 diabetes of 17 years' duration at the time of transplantation. Mesangial matrix expression with nodular lesions seen in a typical glomerulus pretransplant shows resolution of mesangial lesions and more open capillary lumina posttransplant. *(Reproduced with permission from Fioretto et al.[109])*

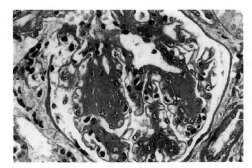

Pretransplant

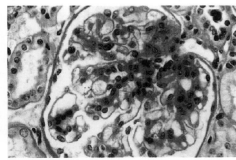

10 years posttransplant

the second best option an LD KTA with a CAD pancreas simultaneously, the third best option an LD KTA followed by a PAK, and the fourth a CAD SPK.

In regard to nonuremic diabetic patients, there are no satisfactory treatments for patients with hypoglycemic unawareness. Thus strict control is really the only alternative strategy, resulting in high glycosylated hemoglobin levels and an increased risk for secondary complications. A successful pancreas transplant allows such patients to avoid hypoglycemia and gives them the freedom of insulin independence.[12,99]

In regard to doing PTA early in the course of diabetes before complication occurs, it is logical to do so. Again, only a small percentage of diabetic patients can take advantage of this approach, so it would be ideal to identify those at high risk for secondary complications. Ideally, randomized studies should be done to compare the long-term complication rate of immunosuppression versus the complication rate of diabetes in comparable populations of patients whose diabetic control is only of average difficulty. However, in patients who have more difficulty with diabetic control and who are not able to maintain nearly normal glycosylated hemoglobin levels, the risk of secondary complications is going to be greater than the risk of immunosuppressive complications. In this situation a PTA is a reasonable choice.[52]

ORGAN ALLOCATION AND FINANCIAL COVERAGE ISSUES FOR PANCREAS AND ISLET TRANSPLANTS

Pancreas or islet transplantation is an expensive treatment for diabetes mellitus, at least for the procedure itself.[115] The organ procurement costs are the same for both. Pancreas transplantation requires surgery and a period of hospitalization, while islet transplantation requires processing of the organ. Once the graft is in place, the cost of maintenance immunosuppression is approximately equivalent to the cost of modern diabetic management on an ongoing basis.[116]

Financial coverage by insurance companies and health maintenance organizations for pancreas transplantation has been variable, but has been provided for all categories by some insurance companies since the 1980s. In general, insurance coverage has been most frequent for SPK transplants and least frequent for PTA transplants, with PAK transplants being intermediate, but the number of insurance companies covering each of the categories has progressively increased. In 1999, Medicare began to cover SPK and PAK transplants, so now virtually every uremic diabetic is financially eligible for a pancreas transplant. PTA coverage is usually decided on a case-by-case basis by the insurance companies that have such a provision.

Pancreas organ allocation from CAD donors is done under the auspices of the United Network for Organ Sharing (UNOS). As for all organs, the pancreas is first offered to patients on a local organ procurement organization (OPO) waiting list; if it is not needed locally, it is next offered regionally, and then nationally. The UNOS policy for local pancreas allocation is based on candidate waiting time. Nationally, allocation is according to match; for multiple candidates with an equivalent match, waiting time is the tiebreaker. Some OPOs have a variance for allocation according to the best match, again with waiting time as the tiebreaker.

In addition, each OPO has to decide whether priority is given first to recipients waiting for a pancreas and kidney transplant, or to those waiting for a solitary pancreas transplant. Since there is an allocation system for kidney transplants that is also based on waiting time and match, some OPOs allocate a pancreas for SPK transplant only if the patient reaches the appropriate level on the kidney transplant waiting list. If the pancreas is not allocated to a diabetic kidney transplant candidate, it is then allocated to the candidate for solitary pancreas transplant.

In regard to allocation for pancreas and islet transplantation, ideally, patients waiting for either should be on a common waiting list. Conceptually, the allocation system should simply be designed for β-cell transplantation, and the technique (islet or immediately vascularized graft) should be tailored to the individual circumstances of the candidate. A pancreas transplant almost always induces insulin independence in the diabetic recipient. Currently, the β-cell mass that engrafts from islet transplantation may not be sufficient to induce islet independence without an additional transplant.[3] On the other hand, single islet transplants have been able to induce insulin independence when done from large donors to small recipients with low insulin requirements.[4]

A utilitarian approach would be to use islets for β-cell replacement therapy in diabetic patients with a low body mass index (BMI) or with low insulin requirements, and to use an immediately vascularized pancreas transplant for those with high insulin requirements. Donors with a high BMI (e.g., 28 kg/m^2) could be used for islet transplantation and the smaller donors for pancreas transplantation. By such an allocation scheme, the largest number of candidates could be made insulin-independent with surgery only as appropriate; high-BMI donors for islets to low-BMI recipients, and low-BMI donors for pancreas transplants to high-BMI candidates or those with high insulin requirements.

Just as there is an insufficient number of CAD organs available to treat all who would benefit from kidney, heart, or liver transplantation, the same is true for pancreas or islet transplantation. The number of new cases of diabetes mellitus exceeds the number of CAD organ donors available. Thus for large-scale treatment of diabetes through β-cell replacement therapy, sources other than CAD (or even living) donors will be needed. Medical priority for those least well served by exogenous insulin replacement may be necessary in the future for fair allocation of the few organs available.

FUTURE OF PANCREAS OR ISLET TRANSPLANTATION

Pancreas transplantation is now performed as a routine treatment for uremic diabetic recipients of kidney transplants, either simultaneously or after the kidney. Such patients are obligated to immunosuppression, and with a successful pancreas transplant can achieve insulin independence as well as a dialysis-free state.

Pancreas transplants alone are less commonly applied because of the need for immunosuppression, but the trade-off to achieve an insulin-independent state is worthwhile for individual patients, particularly those with labile diabetes or hypoglycemic unawareness. A positive effect on secondary complications will occur with early transplantation, and even when done late can have an impact, as has been shown for both neuropathy and nephropathy.[24]

Almost certainly, the side effects of immunosuppression will decrease as new immunomodulation strategies are developed.[88] Unless the need for pancreas transplant diminishes (either through preventive or regenerative strategies), the impetus to alleviate the donor shortage for all organ transplants will continue. Xenotransplantation is the long-range answer, and there are attempts being made to genetically engineer pigs as a source of organs that will not incite the vigorous rejection response that normally occurs.[117]

Not all of the tools necessary to prevent rejection of solid organ xenografts are available. It is likely to be several years before xenotransplantation becomes routine. The generalized immunosuppression necessary to prevent rejection of allografts is relatively mild, preserving host immune defense mechanisms sufficiently to ward off infections. Opportunistic infections are basically xenografts, but are a problem only in allograft recipients who are overimmunosuppressed.[118] For xenograft recipients, the level of immunosuppression needed may predispose to opportunistic infections.

Islet xenografts are touted as having an advantage by using immunomodulation or encapsulation.[119] Although islet encapsulation has succeeded in animal models as isografts or allografts, once it has been done in a xenograft situation, immunosuppression has been necessary. Even as an allograft, immunosuppression has been necessary when done in autoimmune models. Thus, pancreas or islet xenotransplantation is not a likely option in the near future.

Islet allotransplantation remains a goal in an attempt to minimize surgery. With adequate numbers, islet autotransplantation is nearly uniformly successful in preventing diabetes after total pancreatectomy.[120] Islet allotransplantation appears to require a larger number of islets,[3] but can succeed with a single donor under special circumstances.[4]

All available CAD organs should be used for pancreas (or islet) transplantation, and distributed between uremic and nonuremic patients. The number of uremic diabetic patients should diminish as intensive insulin treatment is universally applied and as pancreas (or islet) transplants alone are done to prevent diabetic nephropathy in the first place. Until preventive or regenerative strategies eliminate the need, transplantation will be a major part of the modern diabetologist's armamentarium.

REFERENCES

1. Gruessner AC, Sutherland DER: Pancreas transplant outcomes for United States (US) cases reported to the United Network for Organ Sharing (UNOS) and non-US cases reported to the International Pancreas Transplant Registry (IPTR) as of October, 2000. In: Cecka JM, Terasaki PI, eds. *Clinical Transplantation 2000*. UCLA Immunogenetics Center:2001;45.
2. Hering BJ, Ricordi C: Islet transplantation for patients with type I diabetes. *Graft* 1999;2:12.
3. Shapiro AM, Lakey JR, Ryan EA, et al: Islet transplantation in seven patients with type 1 diabetes mellitus using a glucocorticoid-free immunosuppressive regimen. *N Engl J Med* 2000;343:230.
4. Hering BJ, Kandaswamy R, Harmon JV, et al: Insulin independence after single-donor islet transplantation in type 1 diabetes with hOKT3-1 (ala-ala), sirolimus, and tacrolimus therapy. *Am J Transplant* 2001;1:180.
5. Rafaeloff R, Pittenger GL, Barlow SW, et al: Cloning and sequencing of the pancreatic islet neogenesis associated protein (INGAP) gene and its expression in islet neogenesis in hamsters. *J Clin Invest* 1997; 99:2100.
6. The Diabetes Control and Complications Trial Research Group: The effect of intensive treatment of diabetes on the development and progression of long-term complications in insulin-dependent diabetes mellitus. *N Engl J Med* 1993;329:977.
7. The Diabetes Control and Complications Trial Research Group: Lifetime benefits and costs of intensive therapy as practiced in the Diabetes Control and Complications Trial. *JAMA* 1997;277:372.
8. Morel P, Goetz FC, Moudry-Munns K, et al: Long-term glucose control in patients with pancreatic transplants. *Ann Intern Med* 1991; 115:694.
9. Robertson RP, Sutherland DER, Lanz KJ: Normoglycemia and preserved insulin secretory reserve in diabetic patients 10–18 years after pancreas transplantation. *Diabetes* 1999;48:1737.
10. Sutherland DER, Stratta R, Gruessner A: Pancreas transplant outcome by recipient category: Single pancreas versus combined kidney-pancreas. *Curr Opin Organ Transplant* 1998;3:231.
11. Halloran PF: Development of best immunosuppressive strategies. *Transplant Proc* 2002; in press.
12. Gruessner RWG, Sutherland DER, Najarian JS, et al: Solitary pancreas transplantation for nonuremic patients with labile insulin-dependent diabetes mellitus. *Transplantation* 1997;64:1572.
13. Krolewski AS, Warram JH, Freire MB: Epidemiology of late diabetic complications. A basis for the development and evaluation of preventive programs. *Endocrinol Metab Clin North Am* 1996;25:217.
14. Syndman D: Infection in solid organ transplantation. *Transpl Infect Dis* 1999;1:21.
15. First MR: Current clinical immunosuppressive agents and their actions. *Transplant Proc* 2002; in press.
16. Sutherland DER, Stratta R, Gruessner A: Pancreas transplant outcome by recipient category: Single pancreas versus combined kidney-pancreas. *Curr Opin Organ Transplant* 1998;3:231.
17. Light JA, Sasaki TM, Currier CB, et al: Successful long-term kidney-pancreas transplants regardless of C-peptide status or race. *Transplantation* 2001;71:152.
18. Gross CR, Kangas JR, Lemieux AM, et al: One-year change in quality-of-life profiles in patients receiving pancreas and kidney transplants. *Transplant Proc* 1995;27:3067.
19. Kennedy WR, Navarro X, Goetz FC, et al: Effects of pancreatic transplantation on diabetic neuropathy. *N Engl J Med* 1990;322:1031.
20. Solders G, Tyden G, Persson A, et al: Improvement of nerve conduction in diabetic neuropathy. A follow-up study 4 years after combined pancreatic and renal transplantation. *Diabetes* 1992;41:946.
21. Allen RD, Al Harbi IS, Morris JG, et al: Diabetic neuropathy after pancreas transplantation: Determinants of recovery. *Transplantation* 1997;63:830.
22. Bilous RW, Mauer SM, Sutherland DER, et al: The effects of pancreas transplantation on the glomerular structure of renal allografts in patients with insulin-dependent diabetes. *N Engl J Med* 1989;321:80.
23. Wilczek H, Jaremko G, Tydén G, et al: A pancreatic graft protects a simultaneously transplanted kidney from developing diabetic nephropathy: A 1–6 year follow-up study. *Transplant Proc* 1993;25:1314.
24. Stratta RJ: Impact of pancreas transplantation on complications of diabetes. *Curr Opin Organ Transplant* 1998;3:258.
25. Fiorina P, La Rocca E, Venturini M, et al: Effects of kidney-pancreas transplantation on atherosclerotic risk factors and endothelial function in patients with uremia and type 1 diabetes. *Diabetes* 2001;50:496.
26. Kelly WD, Lillehei RC, Merkel FK: Allotransplantation of the pancreas and duodenum along with the kidney in diabetic nephropathy. *Surgery* 1967;61:827.
27. Sutherland DER: Pancreas and islet transplantation. II. Clinical trials. *Diabetologia* 1981;20:435.
28. Sutherland DE: International human pancreas and islet transplant registry. *Transplant Proc* 1980;12(4 suppl 2):229.
29. Gruessner AC, Sutherland DER: Report of the International Pancreas Transplant Registry. In: Cecka JM, Terasaki PI, eds. *Clinical Transplants 2001*. 2002: in press.
30. Gruessner AC, Sutherland DE, Dunn DL, et al: Pancreas after kidney transplants in posturemic patients with type I diabetes mellitus. *J Am Soc Nephrol* 2001;12:2490.
31. Sutherland DER, Groth CG: History of pancreas transplantation. In: Hakim NS, Stratta RJ, Gray D, eds. *Pancreas and Islet Transplantation*. Oxford University Press 2002: in press.
32. Nghiem DD, Corry RJ: Technique of simultaneous renal pancreatico-duodenal transplantation with urinary drainage of pancreatic secretion. *Am J Surg* 1987;153:405.
33. Groth CG, Collste H, Lundgren G, et al: Successful outcome of segmental human pancreatic transplantation with enteric exocrine diversion after modifications in technique. *Lancet* 1982;2:522.
34. Prieto M, Sutherland DE, Fernandez-Cruz L, et al: Experimental and clinical experience with urine amylase monitoring for early diagnosis of rejection in pancreas transplantation. *Transplantation* 1987;43:73.
35. Calne RY: Paratopic segmental pancreas grafting: A technique with portal venous drainage. *Lancet* 1984;1:595.

36. Tyden G, Lundgren G, Ostman J, et al: Grafted pancreas with portal venous drainage. *Lancet* 1984;1:964.

37. Gil-Vernet JM, Fernandez-Cruz L, Caralps A, et al: Whole organ and pancreaticoureterostomy in clinical pancreas transplantation. *Transplant Proc* 1985;17:2019.

38. Sutherland DE, Goetz FC, Moudry KC, et al: Use of recipient mesenteric vessels for revascularization of segmental pancreas 1987; 19(1 pt 3):2300.

39. Muhlbacher F, Gnant MF, Auinger M, et al: Pancreatic venous drainage to the portal vein: A new method in human pancreas transplantation. *Transplant Proc* 1990;22:636.

40. Rosenlof LK, Earnhardt RC, Pruett TL, et al: Pancreas transplantation. An initial experience with systemic and portal drainage of pancreatic allografts. *Ann Surg* 1992;215:586.

41. Shokouh-Amiri MH, Gaber AO, Gaber LW, et al: Pancreas transplantation with portal venous drainage and enteric exocrine diversion: A new technique. *Transplant Proc* 1992;24:776.

42. Gaber AO, Shokouh-Amiri MH, Hathaway DK, et al: Results of pancreas transplantation with portal venous and enteric drainage. *Ann Surg* 1995;221:613.

43. Stratta RJ, Shokouh-Amiri MH, Egidi MF, et al: A prospective comparison of simultaneous kidney-pancreas transplantation with systemic-enteric versus portal-enteric drainage. *Ann Surg* 2001; 233:740.

44. Cattral MS, Bigam DL, Hemming AW, et al: Portal venous and enteric exocrine drainage versus systemic venous and bladder exocrine drainage of pancreas grafts: Clinical outcome of 40 consecutive transplant recipients. *Ann Surg* 2000;232:688.

45. Bruce DS, Newell KA, Woodle ES, et al: Synchronous pancreas-kidney transplantation with portal venous and enteric exocrine drainage: Outcome in 70 consecutive cases. *Transplant Proc* 1998; 30:270.

46. Philosophe B, Farney AC, Schweitzer EJ, et al: Superiority of portal venous drainage over systemic venous drainage in pancreas transplantation: A retrospective study. *Ann Surg* 2001;234:689.

47. Petruzzo P, DaSilva M, Feitosa LC: Simultaneous pancreas-kidney transplantation: Portal versus systemic venous drainage of the pancreas allografts. *Clin Transplant* 2000;14:287.

48. Gruessner RWG, Kandaswamy R, Denny R: Laparoscopic simultaneous nephrectomy and distal pancreatectomy from a live donor. *J Am Coll Surg* 2001;193:333.

49. Marsh CL, Perkins JD, Sutherland DER, et al: Combined hepatic and pancreaticoduodenal procurement for transplantation. *Surg Gynecol Obstet* 1989;168:254.

50. Delmonico FL, Jenkins RL, Auchincloss H Jr, et al: Procurement of a whole pancreas and liver from the same cadaveric donor. *Surgery* 1989;105:718.

51. Stratta RJ, Taylor RJ, Gill IS: Pancreas transplantation: A managed cure approach to diabetes. *Curr Probl Surg* 1996;33:709.

52. Sutherland DE, Gruessner RWG, Dunn DL, et al: Lessons learned from more than 1000 pancreas transplants at a single institution. *Ann Surg* 2001;233:463.

53. Sutherland DE, Goetz FC, Najarian JS: Living-related donor segmental pancreatectomy for transplantation. *Transplant Proc* 1980;12 (4 Suppl 2):19.

54. Sutherland DE, Gores PF, Farney AC, et al: Evolution of kidney, pancreas, and islet transplantation for patients with diabetes at the University of Minnesota. *Am J Surg* 1993;166:456.

55. Gruessner RW, Sutherland DE: Simultaneous kidney and segmental pancreas transplants from living related donors—the first two successful cases. *Transplantation* 1996;61:1265.

56. Gruessner RW, Kendall DM, Drangstveit MB, et al: Simultaneous pancreas-kidney transplantation from live donors. *Ann Surg* 1997; 226:471.

57. Sutherland DE, Najarian JS, Gruessner R: Living versus cadaver donor pancreas transplants. *Transplant Proc* 1998;30:2264.

58. Benedetti E, Dunn T, Massad MG, et al: Successful living related simultaneous pancreas-kidney transplant between identical twins. *Transplantation* 1999;67:915.

59. Gruessner RWG, Sutherland DE, Drangstveit MB, et al: Pancreas transplants from living donors: Short- and long-term outcome. *Transplant Proc* 2001;33:819.

60. Farney AC, Cho E, Schweitzer EJ, et al: Simultaneous cadaver pancreas living-donor kidney transplantation: a new approach for the type 1 diabetic uremic patient. *Ann Surg* 2000;232:696.

61. Sutherland DE, Sibley R, Xu XZ, et al: Twin-to-twin pancreas transplantation: reversal and reenactment of the pathogenesis of type I diabetes. *Trans Assoc Am Physicians* 1984;97:80.

62. Sibley RK, Sutherland DE, Goetz F, et al: Recurrent diabetes mellitus in the pancreas iso- and allograft. A light and electron microscopic and immunohistochemical analysis of four cases. *Lab Invest* 1985; 53:132.

63. Sutherland DE, Goetz FC, Sibley RK: Recurrence of disease in pancreas transplants. *Diabetes* 1989;38(Suppl 1):85.

64. Tyden G, Reinholt FP, Sundkvist G, et al: Recurrence of autoimmune diabetes mellitus in recipients of cadaveric pancreatic grafts. *N Engl J Med* 1996;335:860.

65. Gruessner RW, Burke GW, Stratta R, et al: A multicenter analysis of the first experience with FK506 for induction and rescue therapy after pancreas transplantation. *Transplantation* 1996;61:261.

66. Stratta RJ: Simultaneous use of tacrolimus and mycophenolate mofetil in combined pancreas-kidney transplant recipients: a multicenter report. The FK/MMF Multi-Center Study Group. *Transplant Proc* 1997;29:654.

67. Gruessner A, Sutherland DER: Pancreas transplants for United States (US) and non-US cases as reported to the International Pancreas Transplant Registry (IPTR) and to the United Network for Organ Sharing (UNOS). In: Cecka JM, Terasaki PI, editors. *Clinical Transplants 1997*. UCLA Tissue Typing Laboratory:1998;45.

68. Stratta RJ: Immunosuppression in pancreas transplantation: progress, problems and perspective. *Transpl Immunol* 1998;6:69.

69. Gruessner AC, Sutherland DE, Gruessner RW: Solitary pancreas transplants: improving results and factors that influence outcome. *Transplant Proc* 1997;29:664.

70. Gruessner RW, Sutherland DE, Drangstveit MB, et al: Mycophenolate mofetil and tacrolimus for induction and maintenance therapy after pancreas transplantation. *Transplant Proc* 1998;30:518.

71. Stratta RJ, Alloway RR, Lo A, et al: A multi-center, open-label, comparative trial of two daclizumab dosing strategies versus no antibody induction in combination with tacrolimus, mycophenolate mofetil, and steroids for the prevention of acute rejection in simultaneous kidney-pancreas transplantation: 6-month interim analysis. *Am J Transplant* 2001;1:159.

72. Gruessner RWG, Sutherland DER, Parr E, et al: A prospective, randomized, open-label study of steroid withdrawal in pancreas transplantation—A preliminary report with 6-month follow-up. *Transplant Proc* 2001;33:1663.

73. Sollinger HW, Odorico JS, Knechtle SJ, et al: Experience with 500 simultaneous pancreas-kidney transplants. *Ann Surg* 1998;228:284.

74. Elkhammas EA, Demirag A, Henry ML: Simultaneous pancreas-kidney transplantation at the Ohio State University Medical Center. Cecka JM, Terasaki PI, eds. *Clinical Transplants 1999*. 2000;211.

75. Sutherland DER, Cecka JM, Gruessner AC: Report from the International Pancreas Transplant Registry (IPTR)—1998. *Transplant Proc* 1999;31:597.

76. Sutherland DE, Gruessner R, Dunn D, et al: Pancreas transplants from living-related donors. *Transplant Proc* 1994;26:443.

77. Seaquist ER, Kahn SE, Clark PM, et al: Hyperproinsulinemia is associated with increased beta cell demand after hemipancreatectomy in humans. *J Clin Invest* 1996;97:455.

78. Gruessner AC, Sutherland DER: Analysis of the United States (US) and non-US pancreas transplants as reported to the International Pancreas Transplant Registry (IPTR) and the United Network for Organ Sharing (UNOS). *Clin Transplant* 1998; :53.

79. Geller D, Dodson S, Corry R: Methods of organ procurement for pancreas transplantation. *Curr Opin Organ Transplant* 1998;3:242.

80. Diem P, Abid M, Redmon JB, et al: Systemic venous drainage of pancreas allografts as independent cause of hyperinsulinemia in type I diabetic recipients. *Diabetes* 1990;39:534.

81. Sutherland DE, Morel P, Gruessner RW: Transplantation of two diabetic patients with one divided cadaver donor pancreas. *Transplant Proc* 1990;22:585.

82. Humar A, Kandaswamy R, Granger DK, et al: Decreased surgical risks of pancreas transplantation in the modern era. *Ann Surg* 2000; 231:269.

83. Benedetti E, Najarian JS, Gruessner AC, et al: Correlation between cystoscopic biopsy results and hypoamylasuria in bladder-drained pancreas transplants. *Surgery* 1995;118:864.

84. Gaber AO, Gaber LW, Shokouh-Amiri MH, et al: Percutaneous biopsy of pancreas transplants. *Transplantation* 1992;54:548.

85. Laftavi MR, Gruessner A, Bland BJ, et al: Diagnosis of pancreas rejection. *Transplantation* 1998;65:528.

86. Tyden G, Tibell A, Sandberg J, et al: Improved results with a simplified technique for pancreaticoduodenal transplantation with enteric exocrine drainage. *Clin Transplant* 1996;10:306.

87. Becker Y, Collins B, Sollinger H: Technical complications of pancreas transplantation. *Curr Opin Organ Transplant* 1998;3:253.

88. Kirk AD: Immunosuppression without immunosuppression? How to be a tolerant individual in a dangerous world. *Trans Infec Dis* 1999; 1:65.

89. Bartlett S: Techniques of pancreatic duct implantation. *Curr Opin Organ Transplant* 1998;3:248.

90. Carpentier A, Patterson BW, Uffelman KD, et al: The effect of systemic versus portal insulin delivery in pancreas transplantation on insulin action and VLDL metabolism. *Diabetes* 2001;50:1402.

91. Bagdade JD, Ritter MC, Kitabchi AE, et al: Differing effects of pancreas-kidney transplantation with systemic versus portal venous drainage on cholesteryl ester transfer in IDDM subjects. *Diabetes Care* 1996;19:1108.

92. Stratta RJ, Gaber AO, Shokouh-Amiri MH, et al: Experience with portal-enteric pancreas transplant at the University of Tennessee-Memphis. In Terasaki, PI, Cecka JM, eds. *Clinical Transplants 1998*. 1999;239.

93. Konigsrainer A, Foger BH, Miesenbock G, et al: Pancreas transplantation with systemic endocrine drainage leads to improvement in lipid metabolism. *Transplant Proc* 1994;26:501.

94. Kaufman DB: A Prospective Study of Rapid Corticosteroid Elimination in Simultaneous Pancreas-Kidney Transplantation. Comparison of two maintenance immunosuppression protocols: Tacrolimus/mycophenolate mofetil versus tacrolimus/sirolimus: *Transplantation* vol. 73, 169-177, no 2. January 27, 2002.

95. Sutherland DER, Gruessner RWG, Humar A, et al: Pretransplant immunosuppression for pancreas transplants alone in nonuremic diabetic recipients. *Transplant Proc* 2001;33:1656.

96. Rubin RH: A new beginning. *Transplant Infect Dis* 1999;1:1.

97. Villacian JS, Paya CV: Prevention of infections in solid organ transplant recipients. *Transplant Infect Dis* 1999;1:50.

98. Robertson RP, Sutherland DER, Kendall DM, et al: Characterization of long-term successful pancreas transplants in type I diabetes. *J Invest Med* 1996;44:549.

99. Paty BW, Lanz K, Kendall DM, et al: Restored hypoglycemic counterregulation is stable in successful pancreas transplant recipients for up to 19 years after transplantation. *Transplantation* 2001;72: 1103.

100. Landgraf R: Impact of pancreas transplantation on diabetic secondary complications and quality of life. *Diabetologia* 1996;39:1415.

101. Navarro X, Kennedy WR, Loewenson RB, et al: Influence of pancreas transplantation on cardiorespiratory reflexes, nerve conduction, and mortality in diabetes mellitus. *Diabetes* 1990;39:802.

102. Navarro X, Kennedy WR, Aeppli D, et al: Neuropathy and mortality in diabetes: influence of pancreas transplantation. *Muscle Nerve* 1996; 19:1009.

103. Tyden G, Bolinder J, Solders G, et al: Improved survival in patients with insulin-dependent diabetes mellitus and end-stage diabetic nephropathy 10 years after combined pancreas and kidney transplantation. *Transplantation* 1999;67:645.

104. Rayhill SC, D'Alessandro AM, Odorico JS, et al: Simultaneous pancreas-kidney transplantation and living related donor renal transplantation in patients with diabetes: Is there a difference in survival? *Ann Surg* 2000;231:417.

105. Becker BN, Brazy PC, Becker YT, et al: Simultaneous pancreas-kidney transplantation reduces excess mortality in type 1 diabetic patients with end-stage renal disease. *Kidney Int* 2000;57:2129.

106. Smets YF, Westendorp RG, van der Pijl JW, et al: Effect of simultaneous pancreas-kidney transplantation on mortality of patients with type-1 diabetes mellitus and end-stage renal failure. *Lancet* 1999;353:1915.

107. Navarro X, Kennedy WR, Aeppli D, et al: Neuropathy and mortality in diabetes: Influence of pancreas transplantation. *Muscle Nerve* 1996; 19:1009.

108. Ojo AO, Meier-Kriesche HU, Hanson JA, et al: The impact of simultaneous pancreas-kidney transplantation on long-term patient survival. *Transplantation* 2001;71:82.

109. Fioretto P, Steffes MW, Sutherland DE, et al: Reversal of lesions of diabetic nephropathy after pancreas transplantation. *N Engl J Med* 1998;339:69.

110. Cheung AT, Chen PC, Leshchinsky TV, et al: Improvement in conjunctival microangiopathy after simultaneous pancreas-kidney transplants. *Transplant Proc* 1997;29:660.

111. Fiorina P, La Rocca E, Astorri E, et al: Reversal of left ventricular diastolic dysfunction after kidney-pancreas transplantation in type 1 diabetic uremic patients. *Diabetes Care* 2000;23:1804.

112. Fiorina P, La Rocca E, Venturini M, et al: Effects of kidney-pancreas transplantation on atherosclerotic risk factors and endothelial function in patients with uremia and type 1 diabetes. *Diabetes* 2001;50:496.

113. Sutherland DE: Pancreas and pancreas-kidney transplantation. *Curr Opin Nephrol Hypertens* 1998;7:317.

114. Bruce DS, Newell KA, Josephson MA, et al: Long-term outcome of kidney-pancreas transplant recipients with good graft function at one year. *Transplantation* 1996;62:451.

115. Gruessner A, Troppmann C, Sutherland DER, et al: Donor and recipient risk factors significantly affect cost of pancreas transplants. *Transplant Proc* 1997;29:656.

116. Stratta RJ: The economics of pancreas transplantation. *Graft* 2000; 3:19.

117. Auchincloss H Jr, Sachs DH: Xenogeneic transplantation. *Annu Rev Immunol* 1998;16:433.

118. Matas AJ, Humar A, Kandaswamy R, et al: Kidney and pancreas transplantation without a crossmatch in select circumstances—it can be done. *Clin Transplant* 2001;15:236.

119. Lanza RP, Chick WL: Transplantation of encapsulated cells and tissues. *Surgery* 1997;121:1.

120. Wahoff DC, Papalois BE, Najarian JS, et al: Autologous islet transplantation to prevent diabetes after pancreatic resection. *Ann Surg* 1995;222:562.

Islet Cell Transplantation

Gina R. Rayat

Ray V. Rajotte

Gregory S. Korbutt

INTRODUCTION

Current methods for treating insulin-dependent (type 1) diabetes mellitus (T1DM) do not prevent transient episodes of hyperglycemia. Recurrent hyperglycemia has been suggested to cause chronic lesions that can culminate in renal failure, blindness, heart disease, neuropathy, or atherosclerosis. The most definitive study in the field, the Diabetes Control and Complications Trial,[1] clearly showed that with intensive insulin therapy, a 2% decrease in HbA_{1c} significantly reduced the risk of microvascular complications. However, this improvement in HbA_{1c} did not result in normalization of the value (median 7%) and was associated with an increased risk of severe hypoglycemia. In addition, the extraordinary effort required in self-monitoring and providing ongoing management for these patients may exceed the capabilities of many individuals and their health care providers. Thus, a predominant focus of human diabetes research has been the development of better methods to achieve optimal glucose control, so that the disabling complications can be reduced or prevented.

Vascularized pancreas transplantation has become accepted as an alternative therapy for individuals receiving simultaneous kidney transplants. Although occasionally used as a solitary pancreas transplant, the significant risks associated with whole organ transplants usually limit its use to cotransplantation with other organs. Furthermore, pancreas transplantation remains associated with significant morbidity in terms of surgical risk, but is also associated with about 86% graft survival.[2] Compared to vascularized pancreatic grafts, transplantation of isolated islets offers a number of advantages. For example, islet transplantation is a much simpler and less invasive procedure, which if performed earlier on can potentially result in excellent glucose control and prevent long-term complications. Islet transplantation also has the potential benefit that the donor tissue can be tested and/or pretreated before implantation, thus allowing the possibility of using grafts with defined metabolic or immunologic characteristics. This chapter reviews the history and current status of islet cell transplantation.

EXPERIMENTAL ISLET TRANSPLANTATION

Pancreatic islets were first described by Paul Langerhans in 1869, when his thesis as a medical student in Virchow's laboratory was published.[3] The possibility of transplanting pancreatic tissue has interested clinicians and scientists since 1889 when Von Mering and Minkowski[4] demonstrated that removal of the canine pancreas resulted in hyperglycemia. However, the concept of separating islet endocrine cells from the exocrine tissue of the pancreas was not examined until 1964, when Hellerstrom used microdissection to isolate islets from the rat pancreas.[5] Since this method was traumatic and islet yield was poor, Moskalewski[6] used the enzyme collagenase to digest guinea pig pancreas in an attempt to improve islet recovery and function. Lacy and Kostianovsky[7] further improved this technique by intraductal distention of the rat pancreas with collagenase to disrupt the exocrine tissue prior to mechanical mincing and enzymatic digestion of the gland. Methods to purify islets from contaminating exocrine tissue began by using centrifugation in sucrose gradients.[8] Later centrifugation on Ficoll gradients proved to be the most effective means to purify islets from contaminating exocrine tissue because it provided a better osmotic environment for the islets.[9] Although numerous methods and gradients for islet purification have been proposed, Ficoll still remains the gradient of choice for both animal and human pancreases.

The first report of transplanting isolated rodent islets was in 1970 by Younoszai and associates.[10] They demonstrated temporary amelioration of chemically induced diabetes in rats. Subsequently, Ballinger and Lacy[11] achieved euglycemia following transplantation of 400–600 islets in the peritoneal cavity or thigh muscle of inbred diabetic Lewis rats. In 1973, Reckard and Barker[12] reported complete normalization of glucose levels in rats for 7 months following intraperitoneal injection of 800–1200 autologous islets. Kemp and colleagues[13] demonstrated that approximately 800 islets could completely normalize plasma insulin and glucose concentrations when embolized to the liver by the portal vein. The physiologic significance of the hepatic portal circulation has been demonstrated by a number of investigators.[14–18] Islets have also been transplanted into the peritoneum,[11–13,19–21] liver,[14,15,21,22] spleen,[23,24] a surgically created peritoneal-omental pouch,[25] the renal subcapsular area,[16–18,26,28,29] the testicles,[30] the ventricles of the brain,[31] and the thymus.[32] With respect to transplantation site, the most consistent results occurred when the graft was placed in a highly vascular bed with portal venous drainage.

The experimental success of islet transplantation in rodents prompted studies in larger animals, including primates, with the overall goal to use this therapy for the treatment of patients with type 1 diabetes. It soon became apparent that the standardized isolation techniques for rodent islets could not be applied to the more compact and fibrous mammalian pancreas, in particular the human pancreas.[33–38] Unlike inbred rodent models, where it is feasible to use multiple donors per recipient, multiple donors could not be used in a population of outbred large animals, such as dogs, since allogeneic islets would be rejected before long-term function of a technically successful graft could be determined. Merkovitch and Campiche,[34] therefore, eliminated the islet purification step and reversed diabetes in 20 of 25 dogs with intrasplenic autografts of dispersed pancreatic fragments isolated from the tail portion of the pancreas. Kretschmer and coworkers[35] improved these results by achieving normoglycemia in 20 of 21 dogs by intrasplenic transplantation of pancreatic fragment autografts prepared from the entire gland. Preparation of the grafts involved mincing the entire pancreas in a mechanical tissue chopper followed by collagenase digestion in a shaking water bath. Using these techniques, or modifications thereof, autografts of dispersed pancreatic fragments prepared by enzymatic digestion and mechanical dispersion were shown by other investigators to reverse the diabetic state in dogs.[39–41]

More efficient means of digesting the large mamalian pancreas were subsequently developed when collagenase was introduced into the duct by direct injection.[42–46] This effective delivery of collagenase to the connective tissue stroma of the islet–acinar interface resulted in a greater separation of the islets from the surrounding exocrine tissue. Using these methods for pancreas digestion, successful intraportal autotransplantation of purified canine islets became a reality. These technical advancements, along with many modifications, also led to their use for the isolation of islets from the human pancreas. Gray and colleagues[47] reported that prewarming the collagenase to 39°C improved digestion of acinar tissue and the use of a mesh filter also improved the islet yield. Ricordi and coworkers[48] modified this method in pigs, by injecting collagenase prewarmed to 24°C, dispersing pancreatic cells with a mechanical macerator, and purifying with mesh filtration and Ficoll density gradient centrifugation. In 1988, Ricordi and colleagues[49] modified this procedure and developed an automated method for isolation of human pancreatic islets. Unfortunately, the lack of consistent and effective lots of enzymes used in the isolation of canine and human islets had prevented the successful recovery of large numbers of viable islets, thus hindering research in this area for many years. A major advance in islet isolation took place recently with the development of Liberase-HI and Liberase-CI (Boehringer-Mannheim). These purified enzyme blends helped eliminate the lot-to-lot variability often associated with crude collagenase and improved the effectiveness of human and canine islet isolation.[50,51] In 1999, based on a technique first described by Horaguchi and Merrell[42] and later modified by Warnock and associates,[45] Lakey and coworkers confirmed that retrograde intraductal delivery of Liberase-HI using a recirculating controlled perfusion system provided superior human islet recovery and survival when compared to syringe loading.[52] By providing controlled perfusion pressures and temperature during loading of the enzyme into the pancreas, the recirculating controlled perfusion system more effectively delivers the collagenase to the islet–acinar interface, resulting in a greater separation of islets from the surrounding exocrine tissue.[45,52]

In an attempt to identify donor factors that can influence islet recovery and function, Lakey and coworkers conducted a retrospective study of 153 human islet isolations over a 3-year period.[53] This multiple regression analysis of postdigestion and postpurification islet recovery identified donor age, body mass index, and local procurement team to be positively correlated with isolation success. Elevated blood glucose levels, frequency and increased dura-

tion of cardiac arrest, and prolonged cold storage of the pancreas prior to islet isolation were identified as factors that were negatively correlated with isolation success.[53] Therefore, rigorous selection criteria of suitable pancreases for processing and potentially individualized isolation protocols based on the several donor variables identified improved consistency in human islet isolation.[22] The ability to consistently isolate a higher quality and quantity of islets from human pancreases has been a key to the development and continuation of experimental and clinical trials in islet transplantation as a realistic treatment option for patients with type 1 diabetes.

CLINICAL ISLET TRANSPLANTATION

According to the International Islet Transplantation Registry,[54] from 1974 to 1989, a total of 90 human islet allografts were conducted. Between 1990 and December 31, 2000, 394 were performed. Recipients of these initial human islet allografts were predominantly type 1 diabetic patients with a kidney graft (either simultaneous or prior to an islet graft), nonuremic type 1 diabetic patients, or pancreatectomized patients receiving a liver graft due to upper abdominal exenteration. Until 1989, virtually all attempts to correct basal hyperglycemia in humans failed.[54] Moreover, of the 267 human islet allografts from 1990 to 1998, only 12.4% resulted in insulin independence for periods of more than 1 week, and only 8.2% have done so for periods greater than 1 year.[54] The poor outcome with the initial attempts at human islet transplantation can be attributed to implantation of an insufficient β-cell mass and the use of nonoptimal immunosuppression. More recently, techniques for isolating large numbers of human islets have improved, permitting renewed attempts at clinical islet transplantation.[55–59] Furthermore, with the increased availability of novel and more specialized immunosuppressive agents, strategies are now available specifically for islet grafts that will provide protection for both allograft rejection and autoimmune destruction as well as avoiding diabetogenic side effects.[60]

In 1999, the Edmonton Group developed a glucocorticoid-free immunosuppressive protocol for use in a clinical islet transplant trial that included patients with brittle type 1 diabetes.[60] This initial trial was conducted in seven patients receiving islet grafts alone as well as exhibiting either severe hypoglycemic unawareness or uncontrolled diabetes despite compliance with an insulin regime. Immunosuppression was initiated immediately before transplantation using sirolimus (Rapamune), low-dose tacrolimus (Prograf), and a monoclonal antibody against the interleukin-2 receptor, daclizumab (Zenapax). No glucocorticoids were given at any time during the trial. As soon as sufficient numbers of islets were available for transplantation, patients were given prophylactic intravenous antibiotics (vancomycin and imipenem) and oral supplementation with vitamin E, vitamin B_6, and vitamin A. Inhaled pentamidine (for PCP prophylaxis) was given once a month after transplantation, and oral ganciclovir was given for 14 weeks to reduce the risk of graft loss and protect against lymphoproliferative disorder. Patients received an average of 800,000 islet equivalents, which were isolated using xenoprotein-free medium and transplanted immediately after isolation via transhepatic injection into the portal vein. Islet donors were matched for blood type and lymphocytotoxic antibodies but not HLA. Insulin therapy was discontinued after each transplantation and not resumed unless serum glucose concentrations rose above 200 mg/dL, in which case another transplant was performed. Blood glucose levels were checked seven times per day. Patients also underwent oral glucose tolerance testing. HbA$_{1c}$ and C-peptide levels were also measured.

All seven patients quickly attained sustained insulin independence after receiving islets from two donor pancreases. One recipient required a third transplant from an additional two donors. The mean HbA$_{1c}$ values were normal in all transplant recipients. The amplitude of blood glucose fluctuations was dramatically decreased, and further episodes of severe hypoglycemia, common before transplantation, did not occur. Detectable C-peptide levels were measurable at 3 and 6 months. Glucose tolerance was not completely normalized; whereas none of the recipients had diabetic oral glucose tolerance tests, five had impaired glucose tolerance, and two had impaired fasting glucose.

In a more recent publication of the results from the Edmonton Group, data were provided on 12 type 1 diabetic patients receiving islet allografts with the same protocol and with a median follow-up of 10.2 months, with the longest at 20 months.[61] Each patient received approximately 850,000 islet equivalents isolated from two to four donor pancreases. In 11 of 12 patients, insulin independence was obtained when a minimum of 9000 islet equivalents/kg were implanted intraportally. The one patient that required daily insulin despite receiving 9000 islet equivalents/kg experienced a thrombosis in a peripheral portal vein, which may have contributed to a partial loss of islet function. All patients, however, discontinued insulin after the final transplant. The pretransplant fasting and meal tolerance–stimulated glucose levels were 12.5 ± 1.9 and 20.0 ± 2.7 mmol/L, respectively, and were shown to significantly decrease, with posttransplant level of 6.3 ± 0. and 7.5 ± 0.6 mmol/L, respectively. All patients were shown to have sustained insulin productions, as indicated by elevated C-peptide levels after a meal tolerance test. Four patients were reported to have normal glucose tolerance, five exhibited impaired glucose tolerance, and three required oral hypoglycemic agents and low-dose insulin (<10 U/day). The most adverse complication observed in these patients was an increase in serum creatinine in two individuals who already had elevated serum creatinine. Other complications included increased blood pressure (four patients) that required antihypertensive therapy and elevated cholesterol where lipid-lowering therapy was required in three of these five patients. Nonetheless, none of the serious surgical complications that are associated with whole-pancreas transplant were evident in any of these 12 patients, and the procedure was simple and well tolerated. Even though these patients have encountered a few complications with these trials, the longer the patients remain off insulin, the more they have significantly improved glucose control, have no episodes of hypoglycemia, and have an enhanced quality of life. Furthermore, this series of clinical transplants is the first to provide a scientific means of assessing the long-term efficacy of functional human islet allografts. In particular, it is now possible to define and, more importantly, optimize graft characteristics with respect to cellular composition and functional viability, which may be critical for long-term graft survival.

SUPPLY OF ISLET TISSUE

A limited supply of human donor pancreas makes it unrealistic for all persons with diabetes to achieve insulin independence through islets from multiple donors. Since it has been estimated that there are approximately 1–1.5 million islets in a human pancreas[62–64]

and the recipients of the Edmonton Protocol have required approximately 800,000 islet equivalents to achieve insulin independence, it is conceivable that a single donor pancreas can be used to treat one recipient. However, in the most optimal isolations, islet recovery is often 40% or lower, thereby necessitating the need for multiple pancreases for each recipient or developing an unlimited supply of insulin-producing tissue.

One significant obstacle for successful, widespread clinical islet transplantation is the limited availability of insulin-producing tissue. Each year in the United States, approximately 5000 organ donors are available, and only a portion of these are suitable for islet transplantation.[65] Yet there are approximately 30,000 new cases of type 1 diabetes each year.[66] Clearly, the demand for insulin-producing tissue is higher than the availability of human islets. In an attempt to overcome the "islet supply" problem, insulin-producing tissue from abundant and readily accessible sources is being considered for clinical transplantation. These sources include (1) porcine and bovine islets,[67–71] (2) fish Brockmann bodies,[72,73] (3) genetically engineered insulin-secreting cell lines,[74,75] and (4) *in vitro* production of human pancreatic islet tissues.[76,77] Most studies have shown there is limited *in vitro* growth of adult islet cells of any species, but several recent reports have found cell proliferation using cultures of islet preparations with extracellular matrix and growth factors. Two recent studies demonstrated that human pancreatic ductal tissue can be expanded in culture and then induced to differentiate into islet tissue *in vitro*.[76,77] Our group has also demonstrated that human pancreatic ductal cells can be successfully differentiated *in vitro* into insulin-positive cells (Fig. 56-1). However, due to the limited availability of the ductal tissue as well as its limited ability to differentiate into pancreatic endocrine cells, further optimization of conditions are needed to generate yields of islet tissue that can make an impact on islet isolation.

Considering that less than 95% of the pancreas is exocrine, it would be extraordinary if this normally discarded majority fraction could be converted to endocrine tissue suitable for transplantation. Indeed, the hypothesis exists that acinar cells have the innate ability to "transdifferentiate" into endocrine islets.[78,79] Remarkably,

FIGURE 56-1. Immunohistochemical localization of insulin-positive cells following tissue culture of human pancreatic ductal tissue. Human pancreatic ductal cells were cultured as monolayers in four-well chamber slides for 16 days. Insulin-positive cells were absent at the beginning of culture and were found scattered throughout the monolayer after 16 days' culture.

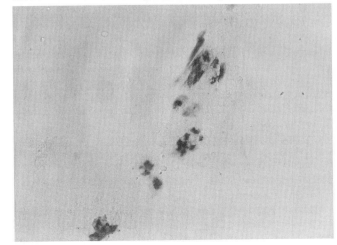

digested human pancreatic acinar cells (amylase-positive, cytoker-atin-19 negative) take on a ductal phenotype (amylase-negative, cytokeratin-19 positive) after only a few days culture.[80] Notably, the possibilities of overgrowth of the acinar population by a ductal subpopulation or selective adherence were excluded in this study. This process is associated with the induction of PDX-1 expression,[81,82] a homeodomain transcription factor believed to be a master regulator of β-cell development. The decisive role of PDX-1 in endocrine differentiation was recently demonstrated in the liver, whereby targeted expression of PDX-1 resulted in insulin gene expression.[83] However, while the exocrine-derived ductal-like cells express PDX-1, little insulin gene expression occurs.[81,82] The loss of insulin expression also occurs in expanded β cells, despite retained PDX-1 expression.[84] Nevertheless, if the differentiation potential of these putative pancreatic stem cells is confirmed, as recently suggested,[76,77,85] this model may have immediate clinical repercussions.

The establishment of pluripotent embryonic stem cells[86,87] and embryonic germ cells[88] introduces a new potential source for cell therapy for the treatment of patients with type 1 diabetes. Glucose-sensitive insulin secreting cells have been produced from mouse embryonic stem cells.[89,90] In one study, which utilizes a gene trap strategy to clone insulin-producing cells, these clones exhibited regulated insulin secretion in vitro and achieved euglycemia following transplantation in diabetic mice.[89] However, 40% (6 of 15) of the recipients of these embryonic stem cells became hyperglycemic at about 12 weeks posttransplant.[89] In a subsequent study, insulin expressing as well as other pancreatic endocrine cells were produced from mouse embryonic stem cells.[90] These endocrine cells were shown to self-assemble into three-dimensional cell clusters similar in morphology to normal pancreatic islets. These cell clusters were responsive to glucose in vitro; however, they were shown to contain 50 times less insulin per β cell than found in normal β cells, thereby suggesting an immature phenotype. When culturing undifferentiated human embryonic stem cells in either adherent or suspension tissue culture, Assady and co-workers[91] observed spontaneous differentiation of numerous insulin-positive cells. These newly differentiated cells were associated with the expression of β-cell–related genes and shown to secrete insulin into the tissue culture medium, but were not shown to be glucose-responsive.[91] Taken together, these studies demonstrate that the engineering of embryonic stem cells to produce an abundant source of islet tissue for transplantation holds a growing promise for finding a solution to the supply of insulin-producing tissue.

Although the production of islet tissue from pancreatic stem cells is exciting and encouraging, there still are ethical concerns associated with embryonic cells as well as the limited potential of adult pancreatic stem cells to generate sufficient quantities of islet tissue for the treatment of patients with diabetes. Thus, porcine islets are still being considered as an unlimited supply of insulin-producing tissue. Pigs are attractive because they have many physiologic similarities to humans and their glucose levels are similar to those of humans. In addition, pigs can be raised in a controlled environment and subjected to genetic manipulation, thus making the use of their organs and tissues as xenografts more acceptable.

The first description of a method for the isolation of adult porcine islets appeared in 1974 when Sutherland and colleagues[36] used a modification of the collagenase technique described for rat isolation to prepare porcine islets for autotransplantation. In 1986, Ricordi and coworkers[48] reported that an average of 80,000 islets could be prepared from adult pigs by an enzymatic and mechanical procedure. Marchetti and colleagues[92] were able to isolate an average of 500,000 islets per adult pig pancreas using a method based on collagenase digestion and filtration of the digested tissue. Warnock and colleagues[93] reported that remarkable purity can be obtained from their isolation technique, but the majority of adult pig islets were lost during the purification stage. These losses, which also occur during subsequent tissue culture, are due predominately to the excessive fragility of the adult porcine islet. In spite of the occasional advance in the isolation of adult pig islets, there still remains serious problems in obtaining intact, viable adult pig islets to provide a source of islet tissue for transplantation.

The use of fetal porcine islets for treating patients with type 1 diabetes was performed by Groth and coworkers[68] in Sweden. Although there was no evidence to indicate engraftment of the fetal cells, all patients in this study tolerated the procedure well and no adverse effects were recorded. Unlike adult pig islets, tissue culture of collagenase-digested fetal porcine pancreas produces viable islet-like cell clusters[94] that have the ability to cure diabetes in nude mice within 2 months posttransplantation.[94] A general finding, however, in rat,[95–98] porcine,[94] and human fetal pancreatic β cells is that they exhibit a poor insulin secretory response to glucose, and the onset of maturation of glucose-induced insulin secretion is more evident in the postnatal period.[95–98] Thus, recent attention has focused on the potential of pancreatic cells obtained from neonatal pigs.[67]

Neonatal porcine islets have the advantage of being more mature than the fetal islets and yet maintain considerable capacity for growth. Korbutt and colleagues[67] developed a simple, standardized procedure for isolating large numbers of neonatal porcine islet cell aggregates with a reproducible and defined cellular composition. After 9 days of culture, the average number of neonatal porcine islet cell aggregates recovered from one pancreas was approximately 50,000. As opposed to adult pig islets, which are known to consist of approximately 80–90% endocrine cells, neonatal porcine islets consist primarily of 35% fully differentiated endocrine cells and 55% epithelial cells or endocrine precursor cells.[67] In vitro viability assessment of the cultured islets showed that in the presence of 20 mmol glucose, the islets were capable of releasing seven-fold more insulin than at 2.8 mmol glucose. When exposed to 20 mmol glucose plus 10 mmol theophylline, the stimulation index increased to 30-fold compared to basal release. Moreover, transplantation of 2000 neonatal porcine islet cell aggregates (consisting of 6×10^5 β cells) under the kidney capsule of alloxan-induced diabetic nude mice corrected hyperglycemia in 100% (20/20) of recipients within 8 weeks posttransplantation.[67] Examination of the neonatal porcine islet grafts revealed that they were largely composed of insulin-positive cells and the cellular insulin content of these grafts was 20- to 30-fold higher than at the time of transplantation. These results indicate that abundant neonatal porcine islets that have the potential for growth can be routinely isolated in the laboratory and may possibly be used for clinical transplantation. Ultimately, the availability of an unlimited supply of insulin-producing tissue would solve the problem of donor supply for the treatment of patients with type 1 diabetes.

PREVENTION OF ISLET GRAFT REJECTION

It has been suggested that the predominant pathway of islet allograft rejection is through direct antigen presentation by donor-type APC.[99–101] Thus, donor tissue has been pretreated to reduce its immunogenicity, placed in immunoisolation devices, or transplanted into immunoprivileged sites. The main rationale for pretreating donor islets is to eliminate the need for continuous immunosuppression. Various methods of pretreating islets prior to allografting have been demonstrated to be successful in rodent models. Isolated islets have been pretreated to eliminate or inactivate major histocompatibility complex (MHC) class II–bearing cells, which are known to exert potent immunostimulatory effects.[102–105] Faustman and colleagues[100,105] demonstrated that islet grafts remained functional in allogeneic recipients preexposed to a cell-specific antibody cytotoxicity reaction, which selectively destroys Ia-expressing or dendritic cells before transplantation. This procedure was marginally successful, however, when used by researchers in other laboratories.[106,107] The use of ultraviolet light to inactivate allostimulatory cells for prolonging rat islet allografts was reported by Lau and coworkers.[108] However, when tested in experiments using rats with a stronger allogeneic response, pretreatment by ultraviolet light required temporary immunosuppression to permit survival of donor tissue.[109] Islets have also been cultured to reduce islet immunogenicity, either at 24°C[110] or at 37°C in the presence of a gaseous phase containing 95% oxygen.[111] Lacy and colleagues[110] demonstrated that culture at 24°C for 7 days prolonged survival of allogeneic rat islets, provided the recipients received a single injection of antilymphocyte serum. Interestingly, Markmann and coworkers[112] showed that the reduced immunogenecity of rat islets cultured at 24°C is correlated to a reduction in endocrine cells' class I MHC antigen expression rather than to the depletion of class II–positive cells. Warnock and associates[113] reported that low-temperature culture of dog islet allografts in combination with low doses of cyclosporine improved survival; however, grafts failed after cessation of cyclosporine treatment. In addition, human islet allografts were also rejected despite the use of immunosuppression and low-temperature culture for 7 days.[114] These studies indicate that although pretreatment can prevent islet allograft rejection in mice and rats, its efficacy in larger animal models is highly dependent on immunosuppressive treatment.

Prevention of experimental islet allograft rejection has also been tested by placing islets in immunoisolation devices constructed of semipermeable membranes separating donor tissue from the recipient's immune system. These devices consist of synthetic membranes that allow diffusion of low-molecular-weight substances (i.e., glucose, insulin) yet exclude cellular contacts between donor and host cells as well as passage of larger-molecular-weight molecules (i.e., immunoglobulins). Islets have been immunoisolated by placing them in biohybrid chamber anastomosed to the vascular system,[115] diffusion chambers,[116,117] and microcapsules.[118,119] Although numerous studies have shown successful reversal of diabetes by transplanting alginate microencapsulated rodent islets in chemically induced diabetic recipients, many of these reports have been difficult to reproduce, and moreover, there has been limited success in the NOD mouse model. More recently, however, Duvivier-Kali, et al. have described a novel microencapsulation technique that provides complete protection of mouse islets against allorejection as well as the recurrence of autoimmune diabetes.[120] This technique utilizes a simple, highly biocompatible barium alginate membrane without a traditional permselective component.

Many sites have also been explored for their potential of providing an immunoprivileged environment for islet grafts. Dispersed pancreatic islet cells were shown to restore normoglycemia following intracerebral allotransplantation in diabetic rats.[31] When implanted into the testes, concordant islet xenografts were shown to exhibit prolonged survival survival.[30] Korbutt and colleagues developed a novel cellular therapeutic approach to engraft and protect islet grafts from immune-mediated destruction. The approach uses Sertoli cells to create an immunologically privileged site that protects rodent islet grafts from allogeneic rejection,[121] as well as autoimmune destruction in NOD mice,[122,123] without requiring chronic immunosuppression. Interestingly, it was shown that Sertoli cell–secreted transforming growth factor-β1, not FasL, was the underlying mechanism that was responsible for protecting the grafts from autoimmune destruction.[123]

Since porcine islets are being considered as a potential source of insulin-producing tissue for clinical transplantation, studies to further understand the rejection process as well as prevention of xenograft rejection have been conducted. In solid organ xenotransplantation, it has been demonstrated that a major barrier to discordant (e.g., pig-to-human) xenotransplantation is the occurrence of hyperacute rejection (HAR). HAR is a process believed to be initiated when naturally occurring xenoreactive antibodies in the recipient's sera binds to antigens present on the surface of endothelial (and other) cells within the xenograft. In turn, antibody binding activates complement, which rapidly destroys the transplanted organ or tissue.[124–129] HAR is characterized pathologically by severe endothelial cell aggregation of platelets to form thrombi, infiltration by neutrophils, edema, and interstitial hemorrhage.[126,130] All of these effects are the result of endothelial cell activation and lysis by the combined action of recipient antibodies and complement.[124,128] The most important target for these antibodies has been identified as the carbohydrate galα(1,3)gal.[131–136] This epitope is present in high concentrations on all porcine endothelial cells,[133,136] and has also been detected on fetal porcine islet cells.[137,138] Rapid destruction of an islet graft has been described in a rabbit-to-primate model,[138] and it has been demonstrated that neonatal porcine islet β cells express galα(1,3)gal and are susceptible to cytolysis mediated by human antibody and complement.[139,140] To develop a strategy to protect porcine islets from this form of destruction, Rayat and coworkers[141] demonstrated that microencapsulating neonatal porcine allows protection of neonatal porcine islets from the cytotoxic effects of human antibody and complement *in vitro*.

In addition to humoral-mediated rejection, T cells are also capable of inducing xenograft rejection and are likely to be the most significant barrier to successful xenotransplantation.[142] It has been suggested that islet xenograft rejection appears to be less dependent on donor APC than allograft rejection.[101] In contrast to allograft rejection where CD8+ T cells play a major role, CD8+ T cells are not required for acute xenograft rejection.[101] Rather, CD4+ T cells appear to be the predominant T-cell subset involved in porcine islet graft rejection.[143–145] Murray and associates[143] demonstrated that neonatal porcine islets do not express sufficiently high levels of costimulatory and/or adhesion molecules to either activate human CD8+ T cells or to be effective targets for activated human cytotoxic lymphocytes. Moreover, this study also suggests that neonatal porcine islets may not be destroyed by a natural killer cell or cytotoxic lymphocyte–mediated lytic mechanisms after transplantation into humans.[143] These studies on the experimental prevention of islet allogeneic and xenogeneic rejection provide novel approaches for permitting long-term graft survival, which stimulate attempts in larger animal models for their ultimate application in patients with type 1 diabetes.

CONCLUSION

In the 1970s, normoglycemia was achieved in rodents with chemically induced diabetes following islet transplantation. Twenty years later, islet transplantation became a clinical reality, resulting in long-term insulin independence in only a few isolated cases. As of January, 2001, 12 patients with type 1 diabetes had received islet transplants using the Edmonton protocol.[60,61] All recipients achieved insulin independence and exhibited significant improvements in their glycemic control and were no longer at risk for severe hypoglycemia. Several lessons have been learned from this experience with the Edmonton protocol. First, prolonged insulin independence is now achievable with a sufficient mass of viable islets and using an appropriate immunosuppressive protocol. Second, functional islet survival appears to be determined by the characteristics of the islet preparation, such that cold-ischemia time of the donor pancreas is an important determinant of islet viability and should be minimized.[61] Finally, these short-term results are extremely encouraging and provide the impetus for continued research in this area.

REFERENCES

1. Diabetes Control and Complications Trial Research Group: The effect of intensive treatment of diabetes on the development and progression of long-term complications in insulin-dependent diabetes mellitus. *N Engl J Med* 1993;329:997.
2. Farney AC, Cho E, Schweitzer EJ, *et al*: Simultaneous cadaver pancreas living-donor kidney transplantation: A new approach for the type 1 diabetic uremic patient. *Ann Surg* 2000;232:696.
3. Langerhans P: Beitrage zur mikroskopischen anatomie der bauchspeicheldruse. Inauguraldissertation, Medizinische Fakultat, Friedrich-Wilhelm-Universitat Berlin, Lange, Berlin, 1869.
4. Minkowski O: Weitere Mittheilungen uber den diabetes mellitus nach extirpation des pankreas. *Berl Klin Wochenschr* 1892;29:90.
5. Hellerstrom C: A method for the microdissection of intact pancreatic islets of mammals. *Acta Endocrinol* 1964;45:122.
6. Moskalewski S: Isolation and culture of the islets of Langerhans of the guinea pig. *Gen Comp Endocrinol* 1965;5:342.
7. Lacy PE, Kostianovsky M: Method for the isolation of intact islets of Langerhans from the rat pancreas. *Diabetes* 1967;16:35.
8. Lindall AW, Steffes MW, Sorensen R: Immunoassayable content of subcellular fractions of rat islets. *Endocrinology* 1969;85:218.
9. Scharp DW, Kemp CB, Knight MJ, *et al*: The use of ficoll in the preparation of viable islets of Langerhans from the rat pancreas. *Transplantation* 1973;16:686.
10. Younoszai R, Sorensen RL, Lindall AW: Homotransplantation of isolated pancreatic islets. *Diabetes* 1970;(suppl 1):406.
11. Ballinger WF, Lacy PE: Transplantation of intact pancreatic islet in rats. *Surgery* 1972;72:175.
12. Reckard C, Barker C: Transplantation of isolated pancreatic islets across strong and weak histocompatibility barriers. *Transplant Proc* 1973;5:761.
13. Kemp CB, Knight MJ, Scharp DW, *et al*: Effect of transplantation site on the results of pancreatic islet isografts in diabetic rats. *Diabetologia* 1973;9:486.
14. Matas AJ, Payne WD, Grotting JC, *et al*: Portal versus systemic transplantation of dispersed neonatal pancreas. *Transplantation* 1977;24:333.
15. Brown J, Mullen Y, Clark W, *et al*: Importance of hepatic portal circulation for insulin action in streptozotocin-diabetic rats transplanted with foetal pancreas. *J Clin Invest* 1979;64:1688.
16. Reece-Smith H, McShane P, Morris PJ: Glucose and insulin changes following a renoportal shunt in streptozotocin diabetic rats with pancreatic islet isografts under the kidney capsule. *Diabetologia* 1982;23:343.
17. Cuthbertson RA, Mandel TE: A comparison of portal versus systemic venous drainage in murine foetal pancreatic islet transplantation. *Aust J Exp Biol Med Sci* 1986;64:175.
18. Lazarow A, Wells LJ, Carpenter AM, Hegre OD: Islet differentiation, organ culture and transplantation. *Diabetes* 1973;22:413.
19. Panijayanaud P, Soroff HS, Monaco AP: Pancreatic islet isografts in mice. *Surg Forum* 1973;24:329.
20. Lorenz D, Peterman J, Beckert R, *et al*: Transplantation of isologous islets of Langerhans in diabetic rats. *Acta Diabetol Lat* 1979;12:30.
21. Rumpf KD, Lohlein D, Pichlmayr R: Multiple transplantations of islets of Langerhans. *Eur Surg Res* 1977;9:40.
22. Henriksson C, Bergmark J, Claes G: Metabolic response to isologous transplantation of small numbers of isolated islets of Langerhans in the rat. *Eur Surg Res* 1977;9:411.
23. Finch DRA, Wise PH, Morris PJ: Successful intrasplenic transplantation of syngeneic and allogeneic isolated pancreatic islets. *Diabetologia* 1977;13:195.
24. Reckard CR, Franklin W, Schulak JA: Intrasplenic vs intraportal pancreatic islet transplantation. Quantitative, qualitative and immunologic aspects. *Trans Am Soc Artif Organs* 1978;24:232.
25. Yasunami Y, Lacy PE, Finke E: A new site for islet transplantation—a peritoneal omental pouch. *Transplantation* 1983;36:181.
26. Reece-Smith H, Du Toit DF, McShane P, Morris PJ: Prolonged survival of pancreatic islet allografts transplanted beneath the renal capsule. *Transplantation* 1981;31:301.
28. Serie J, Hickey GE, Schmitt RV, Hegre OD: Prolongation of cultured isolated neonatal islet xenografts without immunosuppression. *Transplantation* 1983;36:6.
29. Gray DWR, Reece-Smith H, Fairbrother B, *et al*: Isolated pancreatic islet allograftsin rats rendered immunologically unresponsive to renal allografts. The effect of the site of transplantation. *Transplantation* 1984;37:434.
30. Bobzien B, Yasunami Y, Majercik M, *et al*: Intratesticular transplants of islet xenografts (rat to mouse). *Diabetes* 1983;32:213.
31. Tze WJ, Tai J: Successful intracerebral allotransplantation of purified pancreatic endocrine cellsin diabetic rats. *Diabetes* 1983;32:1185.
32. Posselt AM, Barker CF, Tomaszewski JE, *et al*: Induction of donor-specific unresponsiveness by intrathymic islet transplantation. *Science* 1990;249:1293.
33. Scharp DW: Clinical feasibility of islet transplantation. *Transplant Proc* 1984;16:820.
34. Merkovitch V, Campiche M: Intrasplenic autotransplantation of canine pancreatic tissue: Maintenance of normoglycemia after total pancreatectomy. *Eur Surg Res* 1977;9:173.
35. Kretschmer GJ, Sutherland DER, Matas AF, *et al*: The dispersed pancreas: Transplantation without islet purification in totally pancreatectomized dogs. *Diabetologia* 1977;13:495.
36. Sutherland DER, Steffes MW, Bauer GE, *et al*: Isolation of human and porcine islets of Langerhans and islet transplantation in pigs. *J Surg Res* 1974;16:102.
37. Scharp DW, Murphy JJ, Newton WT, *et al*: Transplantation of islets of Langerhans in diabetic rhesus monkeys. *Surgery* 1975;88:100.
38. Scharp DW, Downing R, Merrel RC, Greider M: Isolating the elusive islet. *Diabetes* 1980;29:19.
39. Kolb E, Ruckert R, Largardier F: Intraportal and intrasplenic autotransplantation of pancreatic islets in the dog. *Eur Surg Res* 1977;9:419.
40. Schulak JA, Stuart FP, Reckard CR: Physiologic aspects of intrasplenic autotransplantation of pancreatic fragments in the dog after 24 hours of cold storage. *J Surg Res* 1978;24:125.
41. Mehigan DG, Zuidema GD, Cameron JL: Pancreatic islet transplantation in dogs: Critical factors in technique. *Am J Surg* 1981;141:208.
42. Horaguchi A, Merrel RC: Preparation of viable islet cells from dogs by a new method. *Diabetes* 1981;30:455.
43. Warnock GL, Rajotte RV, Procyshyn AW: Normoglycemia after reflux of islet containing fragments into the splenic vascular bed in dogs. *Diabetes* 1983;32:452.
44. Warnock GL, Rajotte RV: Critical mass of purified islets that induce normoglycemia after implantation into dogs. *Diabetes* 1988;37:467.
45. Warnock GL, Rajotte RV, Ellis D, *et al*: High yield isolatioin of viable large-mammal islet of Langerhans. In: Jaworski MA, Molnar GD, Rajotte RV, Singh B, eds. *The Immunology of Diabetes Mellitus.* Elsevier Science: 1986;207.
46. Warnock GL, Ellis DK, Rajotte RV, *et al*: Studies of the isolation and viability of human islets of Langerhans. *Transplantation* 1988;45:957.

47. Gray DWR, McShane P, Grant A, et al: A method for isolation of islets of Langerhans from the human pancreas. *Diabetes* 1984; 33:1055.

48. Ricordi C, Finke E, Lacy PE: A method for the mass isolation of islets from the adult pig pancreas. *Diabetes* 1986;35:649.

49. Ricordi C, Lacy PE, Finke EH, et al: Automated method for isolation of human pancreatic islets. *Diabetes* 1988;37:413.

50. Lineski E, Bottino R, Lehmann R, et al: Improved human islet isolation using a new enzyme blend, Liberase. *Diabetes* 1997;46:1120.

51. Lakey JRT, Cavanagh TJ, Ziegler MAL, et al: Evaluation of a purified enzyme blend for the recovery and function of canine pancreatic islets. *Cell Transplant* 1998;7:365.

52. Lakey JRT, Warnock GL, Shapiro AMJ, et al: Intraductal collagenase delivery into the human pancreas using syringe loading or controlled perfusion. *Cell Transplant* 1999;8:285.

53. Lakey JRT, Warnock GL, Rajotte RV, et al: Variables in organ donors that affect the recovery of human islets of Langerhans. *Transplantation* 1996;7:1047.

54. Bretzel RG, Brendel MD, Hering BJ, et al: *International Islet Transplant Registry Report.* Justus-Liebis University of Geissen: 2001;8:1.

55. Warnock GL, Rajotte RV: Human pancreatic islet transplantation. *Transplant Rev* 1992;6:1.

56. Hering BJ, Browatzki CC, Schultz A, et al: Clinical islet transplantation—registry report, accomplishments in the past and future research need. *Cell Transplant* 1993;2:269.

57. Hering BJ, Ricordi C: Results, research priorities, and reasons for optimism: Islet transplantation for patients with type 1 diabetes. *Graft* 1999;2:12.

58. Warnock GL, Kneteman NM, Ryan E, et al: Long term follow up after transplantation of insulin-producing pancreatic islets into patients with type 1 diabetes mellitus. *Diabetologia* 1992;35:89.

59. Korbutt GS, Warnock GL, Rajotte RV: Islet transplantation. In: Porte D, Sherwin RS, eds. *Ellenberg & Rifkin's Diabetes Mellitus*, 5th ed. Appleton & Lange: 1997;1281.

60. Shapiro AMJ, Lakey JRT, Ryan EA, et al: Islet transplantation in seven patients with type 1 diabetes mellitus using a glucocorticoid-free immunosuppressive regime. *N Eng J Med* 2000;343:230.

61. Ryan EA, Lakey JRT, Rajotte RV, et al: Clinical outcomes and insulin secretion after islet transplantation with the Edmonton protocol. *Diabetes* 2001;50:710.

62. Hellman B: The frequency distribution of the number and volume of the islets of Langerhans in man. 1) Studies on non-diabetic adults. *Acta Soc Med Upsaliensis* 1959;64:432.

63. Hellman B: The frequency distribution of the number and volume of the islets of Langerhans in man. 2) Studies in diabetes of adult onset. *Acta Pathol Microbiol Scand* 1961;51:95.

64. Hellman B: Actual distribution of the number and volume of the islets of Langerhans in different size classes in non-diabetic humans of varying ages. *Nature* 1959;164:1498.

65. Hauptman PJ, O'Connor KJ: Procurement and allocation of solid organs for transplantation. *N Engl J Med* 1997;336:422.

66. La Porte RE, Matsushima M, Chang Y-F: Prevalence and incidence of insulin-dependent diabetes. In: Harris MI, Cowie CC, Stern MP, et al: eds. *Diabetes in America*, 2nd ed. US Govt. Printing Office: 1995;37 (NIH publ. No 95-1468).

67. Korbutt GS, Warnock GL, Ao Z, et al: Large scale isolation, growth and function of porcine neonatal islet cells. *J Clin Invest* 1996; 97:2119.

68. Groth CG, Korsgren O, Tibell A, et al: Transplantation of porcine fetal pancreas to diabetic patients. *Lancet* 1994;344:1402.

69. Davalli AM, Ogawa Y, Scalia L, et al: Function, mass and replication of porcine and rat islets transplanted into diabetic nude mice. *Diabetes* 1995;44:104.

70. Ricordi C, Socci C, Davalli AM, et al: Isolation of the elusive pig islet. *Surgery* 1989;107:688.

71. Marchetti P, Giannarelli R, Cosimi S, et al: Massive isolation, morphological and functional characterization, and xenotransplantation of bovine pancreatic islets. *Diabetes* 1995;44:375.

72. Wright JR Jr, Polvi S, Maclean H: Experimental transplantation with principal islets of teleost fish (Brockman bodies). Long-term functional of tilapia islet tissue in diabetic nude mice. *Diabetes* 1992; 41:1528.

73. Wright JR Jr, Yang H, Dooley KC: Tilapia—a source of hypoxia-resistant islet cells for encapsulation. *Cell Transplant* 1998;7:299.

74. Ferber S, Beltrandelrio H, Johnson JH, et al: GLUT-2 gene transfer into insulinoma cells confers both low and high affinity glucose-stimulated insulin release. *J Biol Chem* 1994;269:11523.

75. de la Tour DD, Halvorsen T, Demeterco C, et al: β-cell differentiation from a human pancreatic cell line in vitro and in vivo. *Mol Endocrinol* 2001;15:476.

76. Zulewski H, Abraham EJ, Gerlach MJ, et al: Multipotential nestin-positive stem cells isolated from adult pancreatic islets differntiate ex vivo into pancreatic endocrine, exocrine, and hepatic phenotypes. *Diabetes* 2001;50:521.

77. Bonner-Weir S, Taneja M, Weir GC, et al: *In vitro* cultivation of human islets from expanded ductal tissue. *Proc Natl Acad Sci USA* 2000;97:7999.

78. Hughes W: An experimental study of regeneration in the islets of Langerhans with reference to the theory of balance. *Horm Res* 1956; 37:190.

79. Bouwens L: Transdifferentiation versus stem cell hypothesis for the regeneration of islet beta-cells in the pancreas. *Microsc Res Tech* 1998;43:332.

80. Hall PA, Lemoine NR: Rapid acinar to ductal transdifferentiation in cultured human exocrine pancreas. *J Pathol* 1992;166:97.

81. Rooman I, Heremans Y, Heimberg H, et al: Modulation of rat pancreatic acinoductal transdifferentiation and expression of PDX-1 in vitro. *Diabetologia* 2000;43:907.

82. Gmyr V, Kerr-Conte J, Belaich S, et al: Adult human cytokeratin 19-positive cells reexpress insulin promoter factor 1 in vitro: Further evidence for pluripotent pancreatic stem cells in humans. *Diabetes* 2000; 49:1671.

83. Ferber S, Halkin A, Cohen H, et al: Pancreatic and duodenal homeobox gene 1 induces expression of insulin genes in liver and ameliorates streptozotocin-induced hyperglycemia. *Nat Med* 2000;6:568.

84. Beattie GM, Itkin-Ansari P, Cirulli V, et al: Sustained proliferation of PDX-1$^+$ cells derived from human islets. *Diabetes* 1999;48:1013.

85. Kerr-Conte J, Pattou F, Lecomte-Houcke M, et al: Ductal cyst formation in collagen-embedded adult human islet preparations. A means to the reproduction of nesidioblastosis in vitro. *Diabetes* 1996;45:1108.

86. Thomson JA, Itskovotz-Eldor J, Shapiro SS, et al: Embryonic stem cell lines derived from human blastocysts. *Science* 1998;282:1145.

87. Reubinoff BE, Pera MF, Fong Cy, et al: Embryonic stem cell lines from human blastocysts: Somatic differentiation in vitro. *Nat Biotech* 2000;18:399.

88. Shamblott MJ, Axelma J, Wang S, et al: Derivation of pluripotent stem cells from cultured human primordial germ cells. *Proc Natl Acad Sci USA* 1998;95:13726.

89. Soria B, Roche E, Berna G, et al: Insulin-secreting cells derived from embryonic stem cells normalize glycemia in streptozotocin-induced diabetic mice. *Diabetes* 2000;49:157.

90. Lumelsky N, Blondel O, Laeng P, et al: Differentiation of embryonic stem cells to insulin-secreting structures similar to pancreatic islets. *Science* 2001;292:1389.

91. Assady S, Maor G, Amit M, et al: Insulin production by human embryonic stem cells. *Diabetes* 2001;50:1691.

92. Marchetti P, Finke EH, Gerasimidi-Vazeou A, et al: Automated large scale isolation, in vitro function and xenotransplantation of porcine islets of Langerhans. *Transplantation* 1991;52:209.

93. Warnock GL, Katyal D, Okamura J, et al: Studies of the isolation, viability, and preservation of purified islets after surgical pancreatectomy in large pigs. *Xenotransplantation* 1995;2:161.

94. Korsgren O, Jansson L, Eizirik D, et al: Functional and morphological differentiation of fetal porcine islet-like clusters after transplantation into nude mice. *Diabetologia* 1994;34:379.

95. Asplund K, Westman S, Hellerstrom C: Glucose stimulation of insulin secretion from the isolated pancreas of foetal and new born rats. *Diabetologia* 1969;5:260.

96. Asplund G: Dynamics of insulin release from the foetal and neonatal rat pancreas. *Eur J Clin Invest* 1973;3:338.

97. Rhoten WB: Insulin secretory dynamics during development of rat pancreas. *Am J Physiol* 1980;239:E57.

98. Hole RL, Pian-Smith MCM, Sharp GWG: Development of the biphasic response to glucose in fetal and neonatal rat pancreas. *Am J Physiol* 1988;254:E167.

99. Bowen K, Andrew L, Lafferty K: Successful allotransplantation of mouse pancreatic islets to nonimmunosuppressed recipients *Diabetes* 1980;29:98.

100. Faustman DL, Hauptfield V, Lacy PE, et al: Prolongation of murine islet allograft survival by pretreatment of islets with antibody directed to Ia determinants. Proc Natl Acad Sci USA 1981;78:5156.

101. Gill RG: Antigen presentation pathways for immunity to islet transplants. Ann NY Acad Sci 1999;875:255.

102. Klinikert WEF, LaBadie JU, O'Brien JP, et al: Rat dendritic cells function as accessory cells and control the production of a soluble factor required for mitogenic responses of T lymphocytes. Proc Natl Acad Sci USA 1980;77:5414.

103. Lechler RI, Batchelor JR: Restoration of immunogenicity to passenger cell-depleted kidney allografts by the addition of donor strain dendritic cells. J Exp Med 1982;155:31.

104. Knight SC, Mertin J, Stackpoole A, et al: Induction of immune responses in vivo with small numbers of veiled (dendritic) cells. Proc Natl Acad Sci USA 1983;80:6032.

105. Faustman DL, Steinman RL, Gebel HM, et al: Prevention of rejection of murine islet allografts by pretreatment with anti-dendritic cell antibody. Proc Natl Acad Sci USA 1984;81:8864.

106. Gores PF, Sutherland DER, Platt JL, et al: Depletion of donor IA+ cells before transplantation does not prolong islet allograft survival. J Immunol 1986;137:1482.

107. Terasaki R, Lacy PE, Hauptfeld V, et al: The effect of cyclosporin A, low-temperature culture, and anti-Ia antibodies on prevention of rejection of rat islet allografts. Diabetes 1986;35:83.

108. Lau H, Reemtsma K, Hardy MA: Prolongation of rat islet allograft survival by direct ultraviolet irradiation of the graft. Science 1984;223:607.

109. Lau H, Reemtsma K, Hardy MA: The use of direct ultraviolet irradiation and cyclosporin in facilitating indefenite pancreatic allograft acceptance. Transplantation 1984;88:566.

110. Lacy PE, Davie JM, Finke EH: Prolongation of islet allograft survival following in vitro culture (24°C) and a single injection of ALS. Science 1979;204:312.

111. Bowen KM, Prowse SJ, Lafferty KJ: Successful allotransplantation of mouse pancreatic islets to nonimmunosuppressed recipients. Diabetes 1980;29(suppl 1):98.

112. Markmann JF, Tomaszewski J, Posselt AM, et al: The effect of islet cell culture in vitro at 24°C on graft survival and MHC antigen expression. Transplantation 1990;49:272.

113. Warnock GL, Dabbs KD, Cattral MS, et al: Improved survival of in vitro cultured canine islet allografts. Transplantation 1994;57:17.

114. Scharp DW, Lacy PE, Santiago JV, et al: Insulin independence after islet transplantation into type I diabetic patient. Diabetes 1990;39:515.

115. Monaco AP, Maki T, Ozato H, et al: Transplantation of islet allografts and xenografts in totally pancreatectomized diabetic dogs using the hybrid artificial pancreas. Ann Surg 1991;214:889.

116. Altman JJ, McMillan P, Callard P, et al: A bioartificial pancreas prevents chronic complications of diabetes in rats. Am Soc Artif Organs 1986;32:145.

117. Lanza RP, Borland KM, Lodge P, et al: Treatment of severely diabetic pancreatectomized dogs using a diffusion-based hybrid pancreas. Diabetes 1992;41:886.

118. Fritschy WM, Strubbe JH, Wolters GHJ, et al: Glucose tolerance and plasma insulin response to intravenous glucose infusion and test meal in rats with microencapsulated islet allografts. Diabetologia 1991;34:542.

119. Soon-Shiong P, Feldman E, Nelso R, et al: Successful reversal of spontaneous diabetes in dogs by intraperitoneal microencapsulated islets. Transplantation 1992;54:769.

120. Duvivier-Kali VF, Omer A, Parent RJ, et al: Complete protection of islets against allorejection and autoimmunity by a simple barium-alginate membrane. Diabetes 2001;50:1698.

121. Korbutt GS, Elliott JF, Rajotte RV: Cotransplantation of allogeneic islets with testicular cell aggregates allows long-term graft survival without systemic immunosuppression. Diabetes 1997;46:317.

122. Korbutt GS, Suarez-Pinzon WL, Power RF, et al: Testicular Sertoli cells exert both protective and destructive effects on syngeneic islet grafts in non-obese diabetic mice. Diabetologia 2000;43:474.

123. Suarez-Pinzon WL, Korbutt GS, Poer R, et al: Testicular Sertoli cells protect islet β-cells from autoimmune destruction in NOD mice by transforming growth factor-β1-dependent mechanism. Diabetes 2000;49:1810.

124. Schilling A, Land W, Pratschke E, et al: Dominant role of complement in the hyperacute xenograft rejection reaction. Surg Gynecol Obstet 1976;142:29.

125. Auchincloss H Jr: Xenogeneic transplantation: A review. Transplantation 1988;46:1.

126. Platt J, Vercellotti GM, Dalmasso AP, et al: Transplantation of discordant xenografts: A review of progress. Immunol Today 1990;11:450.

127. Platt JL, Bach FH: The barrier to xenotransplantation. Transplantation 1991;52:937.

128. Baldwin WM III, Pruitt SK, Brauer RB, et al: Complement in organ transplantation: Contribution to inflamation, injury, and rejection. Transplantation 1995;59:797.

129. Platt JL, Fischel RJ, Matas AJ, et al: Immunopathology of hyperacute rejection in a swine-to-primate model. Transplantation 1990;52:214.

130. Galili U: Interaction of the natural anti-gal antibody with α-galactosyl epitopes: A major obstacle for xenotransplantation in humans. Immunol Today 1993;14:480.

131. Sandrin MS, Vaughan HA, Dabkowski PL, McKenzie IFC: Anti-pig IgM antibodies in human serum react predominantly with galα(1,3)gal epitopes. Proc Natl Acad Sci USA 1993;90:11291.

132. Oriol R, Ye Y, Koren E, Cooper DKC: Carbohydrate antigens of pig tissues reacting with human natural antibodies as potential targets for hyperacute vascular rejection in pig-to-man organ xenotransplantation. Transplantation 1993;56:1433.

133. Cooper DKC, Good AH, Koren E, et al: Identification of α-galactosyl and other carbohydrate epitope that are bound by human anti-pig antibodies: Relevance to discordant xenografting in man. Transplant Immunol 1993;1:198.

134. Vaughan HA, Loveland BE, Sandrin MS: Galα(1,3)gal is the major xenoepitope expressed on pig endothelial cells recognized by naturally occurring cytotoxic human antibodies. Transplantation 1994;58:879.

135. Sandrin MS: Distribution of the major xenoantigen (galα(1,3)gal) for pig-to-human xenografts. Transplant Immunol 1994;112:293.

136. McKenzie IFC, Koulmanda M, Mandel TE, et al: Pig-to-human xenotransplantation: The expression of Galα(1,3)gal epitopes on pig islet cells. Xenotransplantation 1997;2:1.

137. Rydberg L, Groth CG, Moller E, et al: Is the galα(1,3)gal epitope a major target for xenoantibodies on pig fetal islet cells? Xenotransplantation 1995;2:148.

138. Hamelmann W, Gray DW, Cairns TD, et al: Immediate destruction of xenogeneic islets in a primate model. Transplantation 1994;58:1109.

139. Korbutt GS, Aspeslet LJ, Rajotte RV, et al: Natural human antibody-mediated destruction of porcine neonatal islet cell grafts. Xenotransplantation 1996;3:207.

140. Rayat GR, Rajotte RV, Elliott JF, et al: Expression of galα(1,3)gal on neonatal porcine islet β-cells and susceptibility to human antibody/complement lysis. Diabetes 1998;47:1406.

141. Rayat GR, Rajotte RV, Ao Z, et al: Microencapsulation of neonatal porcine islets: Protection from human antibody/complement-mediated cytolysis in vitro and long-term reversal of diabetes in nude mice. Transplantation 2000;69:1084.

142. Wolfe L, Coulombe M, Gill RG: Donor antigen-presenting cell-independent rejection of islet xenografts. Transplantation 1995;1164.

143. Murray AG, Nelson RC, Rayat GR, et al: Neonatal porcine islet cells induce human CD4+, but not CD8+ lymphocyte proliferation and resist cell-mediated cytolytic injury in vitro. Diabetes 1999;48:1713.

144. Lalain S, Chaillous L, Gouin E, Sai P: Intensity and mecahnisms of in vitro xenorecognition of adult pig pancreatic islet cells by CD4+ and CD8+ lymphocytes from type I diabetic or healthy subjects. Diabetologia 1999;42:330.

145. Friedman T, Smith RN, Colvin RB, Iacomini J: A critical role for human CD4+ T cells in rejection of porcine islet cell xenografts. Diabetes 1999;48:40.

CHAPTER 57

New Treatments for Diabetes Mellitus: Outlook for the Future

Lester B. Salans

INTRODUCTION

The importance of achieving and maintaining normal or near-normal blood glucose levels ("tight" glucose control) in individuals with diabetes mellitus is well established. In the great majority of diabetic patients, however, glycemic levels necessary to completely control the disease and to eliminate chronic complications are not achieved. As a result, the disease progressively worsens over time and complications develop. Research advances have provided new management tools to achieve tight glucose control and treatment of diabetes has improved, but the intensive therapeutic regimens required are neither practical nor feasible for many patients. Even under circumstances in which best current treatment is optimally applied by highly motivated patients, tight control of blood glucose greatly reduces, but does not entirely eliminate, disease progression and complications. While this is a significant advance over past treatments, it is insufficient and limited to too few individuals. Clearly, there is a need for still better treatments and better treatment methods.

This chapter will review some of the major shortcomings of current treatment and treatment approaches for type 1 (T1DM) and type 2 diabetes mellitus (T2DM), and within this context will highlight some of the pharmacologic agents and technologies under investigation and development for the treatment of diabetes in the future. New therapies for prevention and treatment of diabetic complications are also discussed. The focus of the chapter is on blood glucose control, although the importance of controlling other risk factors such as dyslipidemia and hypertension is fully recognized (see Chaps. 47 and 48).

T1DM: TREATMENT SHORTCOMINGS

Insulin is Not Delivered Physiologically

Current methods of insulin replacement do not mimic physiologic glycemic control closely enough. Delivery of insulin by subcutaneous injection and insulin pumps does not adequately imitate the control of blood glucose achieved by normal pancreatic β (beta) cells, which continuously adjust insulin secretion according to the prevailing blood glucose. Subcutaneous administration by injection and pump delivers insulin to the peripheral circulation rather than portally, the physiologic route, thereby bypassing the liver's ability to modulate peripheral insulinemia. As a consequence of bypassing first-pass hepatic extraction, insulin is delivered to the peripheral tissues in pharmacologic doses, causing chronic exposure to excessive levels of insulin, especially in the fasting or basal state. Chronic hyperinsulinemia impairs insulin action and may increase the risk of diabetic complications.

While providing too much insulin during basal or fasting conditions, current practice often does not provide insulin in sufficient amounts or with the appropriate timing and pharmacokinetics to control mealtime and postprandial glucose levels. As a result, mealtime blood glucose excursions are excessive. Administration of insulin after, rather than before, blood glucose is elevated is not only unphysiologic, but it is also inefficient; much less insulin is required to prevent hyperglycemia than to reduce hyperglycemia.[1]

Intensive Treatment Regimens Are Not Readily Applicable

Achievement of levels of blood glucose necessary to prevent or control disease progression and diabetic complications requires strict therapeutic regimens that are neither practical nor feasible for many patients and their families. Intensive therapy requires multiple daily injections of insulin and frequent monitoring of blood glucose. Adherence to stringent dietary practices coupled with the necessity of coordinating food intake and insulin administration is difficult, especially for children and adolescents. No wonder most patients do not use the tools and do not follow the strict regimens of intensive treatment necessary to achieve tight glucose control.

Intensive Therapy Regimens Cause Frequent Episodes of Hypoglycemia

Current therapeutic regimens required to achieve normal or near-normal glycemia cause frequent episodes of hypoglycemia (more than a threefold increased risk of severe hypoglycemia in the DCCT). Hypoglycemia and the accompanying counterregulatory hormone response produced by iatrogenic hypoglycemia are often the major limiting factor in achieving tight glucose control. Frequent hypoglycemia causes hypoglycemic unawareness, a serious clinical problem (see Chap. 31). Avoidance of frequent hypoglycemia restores hypoglycemia awareness.[2]

Health Care Professionals' Experience with Intensive Glycemic Therapy Is Limited

Physicians and other health care professionals may not be adequately trained or experienced in the methods of intensive glycemic therapy. The integrated, multidisciplinary resources required for intensive therapy (e.g., dietitians, nurse educators, etc.) may not be available.

Insufficient Patient Knowledge about Diabetes and Involvement in Self-Management

Many patients do not fully understand their disease, the importance of tight glycemic control, and the principles of diet and exercise, nor are they sufficiently aware of the key role they must play in the treatment of their disease and attainment of good glycemic control.

Limited Awareness and Inadequate Support for Diabetes Care from the Health Care System

Intensive diabetes treatment is costly, beyond the capability of families with limited financial resources, and inadequately reimbursed. The critical need for intensive therapy is not always understood by those who administer health care systems.

CHANGES IN THERAPEUTIC APPROACHES FOR T1DM

New Prevention Approaches

Three targets provide the most obvious points for potential intervention in T1DM: genes, the immune system, and environmental factors.

Genes

The prevention, cure, and effective treatment of T1DM may ultimately come from genetic research that can identify the genes conferring disease susceptibility and delineate the mechanisms by which they produce their effects. This might lead to gene-based therapies. While the major human genes for T1DM could be identified and cloned within the relatively near future, elucidation of how they act to produce susceptibility to T1DM and development of gene-based therapy for this polygenic disease, if ever achievable, is unlikely to be accomplished in the near term.

Immune System

Immune modulation offers another approach for preventing T1DM. Primary prevention clinical trials are, or soon will be, under way to assess whether immune modulation can prevent T1DM in individuals at high risk (see Chap. 15). The NIH-sponsored Diabetes Prevention Trial—Type 1 Diabetes (DPT-1) recently reported that daily parenteral or oral insulin administration to induce immune tolerance to insulin in individuals at high risk did not prevent subsequent development of T1DM.[3] Other means of modulating immune responses and preventing autoimmune β-cell destruction are being pursued, including antigen-, cytokine-, and monoclonal antibody–based interventions. However, applicability of results of trials in high-risk relatives to the general population in which 90% of new cases of T1DM occur is uncertain, and broader population-based trials will be necessary. Nevertheless, prevention of T1DM by immune intervention in high-risk relatives is certainly desirable and may be achievable.

Environment

A third approach to prevention of T1DM would be to block environmental factors that activate or interact with T1DM susceptibility genes. Unfortunately, the offending environmental factors, whether infectious (e.g., viruses), toxins, dietary, or otherwise, are unknown.

New Treatment Options

Noninjectable Routes of Insulin Administration

Oral Insulin

Proteolytic degradation and poor absorption have so far made efforts to produce an orally bioavailable insulin unsuccessful. Efforts to expand oral delivery technologies for controlled release of molecules with predictable activity, e.g., polymer encapsulation and osmotic release technology, and to develop modified insulins that can be orally administered and reliably and reproducibly absorbed through the buccal or intestinal mucosa without loss of biological activity are ongoing, but far from being available for clinical application.[4,5]

Orally Available Insulin Mimetics

An orally bioavailable fungal metabolite that activates the human insulin receptor tyrosine kinase, mimicking the action of insulin and lowering blood glucose in diabetic mice, has recently been discovered.[6]

Inhaled Insulin

Administration of insulin by the pulmonary route is currently in phase III clinical testing (see Chaps. 28 and 29),[7] and may be available for treatment in the near future. Given its short duration of action, for type 1 diabetics inhaled insulin will have to be administered in combination with long- and/or intermediate-acting insulin to meet basal requirements and achieve 24-hour glycemic control. Issues of reproducible absorption, inhalation technology, powder versus liquid formulations, and long-term safety remain to be fully resolved.

Other Routes

While nasal and rectal routes of insulin administration appear unlikely to be successful, transdermal delivery by iontophoresis[8] and via innovative implantation technology is being investigated.

New Injectable Insulin Formulations

Rapid-Onset Short-Acting Insulin

Rapid-onset short-acting lispro insulin has enabled better control of mealtime glucose and improved overall glycemic control in many with T1DM.[9] Insulin aspart is a second rapid-onset short-acting insulin with similar activity to lispro insulin, available for treatment of diabetes.[9] Both of these insulins will be increasingly utilized in clinical practice in the future.

Long-Acting Insulin

Insulin glargine, a new long-acting insulin analog, has become available for clinical use.[9] This acidic insulin analog formulation cannot be mixed in the same syringe with other standard insulins. A second long-acting insulin analog, insulin detemir, is currently in clinical development.[10] Clinical studies indicate that these insulin formulations provide relatively constant levels of basal insulin over 24 hours, and achieve better control of fasting glucose and HbA_{1c}

levels with less nocturnal hypoglycemia than NPH insulin. They could enable significantly better glucose control when combined with injection or inhalation of other forms of insulin before meals.

Hepatoselective Insulin Analogs

A novel hepatoselective insulin analog, $N^{\alpha\beta1}$L-thyroxyl-insulin (B1-T4-Ins), has the potential to provide more physiologic insulin action than current insulin preparations.[11]

Pancreatic Islet Transplantation

The use of islet allografts and novel combinations of immunosuppressive agents in T1DM has recently shown promise,[12] and multicenter trials are underway. A major hurdle is the lack of sufficient numbers of donor islets to meet the needs for successful islet transplantation. Pluripotential stem cells, and genetically engineered somatic cell lines may provide a source of cells and enable successful transplantation without requirement for lifelong immune suppression to prevent rejection and autoimmune destruction of transplanted cells (see Chap. 56). The early promise of xenograft transplanted pig islets appears to be fading because of concerns over possible transmission of infectious porcine microorganisms. Each of these approaches has significant hurdles to overcome before successful clinical application is possible.

The Artificial Pancreas

An implantable "artificial pancreas" that provides continuous, on-line measurement of blood glucose, activating a mechanical device (pump) to deliver insulin directly to the liver, with or without glucagon, would permit more physiologic and readily applicable replacement of insulin (see Chaps. 14 and 29). Such a device is unlikely to become available in the near future. In the meantime, the two components of insulin delivery, the insulin pump and glucose sensor, will be used separately in the management of diabetes.

Implantable Insulin Pumps

Delivery systems that are implantable, able to be regulated with greater precision, and have more safety features are being developed and will be available in the not-too-distant future for treatment of T1DM and T2DM (see Chap. 29). Delivery of insulin directly to the liver, perhaps through an intraperitoneal route, if safe, would be more physiologic than delivery via the currently employed subcutaneous route. Adequate training of health care personnel and of patients and their families is essential for these devices to be used effectively and safely.

Noninvasive Glucose Sensors

The availability of accurate and sensitive, noninvasive glucose sensors for continuous measurement of blood glucose, displaying, downloading, and storing real-time blood glucose levels at a suitable interval and containing reliable hypoglycemia alert alarm systems, will greatly enhance glucose control and reduce the risk of hypoglycemia and hypoglycemia unawareness. Significant improvement in glucose-sensing technology can be anticipated in the not-too-distant future (see Chap. 29).

Control of Mealtime and Postprandial Glucose Levels

Achievement of normal or near-normal glycemia requires control of mealtime and postmeal blood glucose, not only fasting glucose.[13] Treatment of T1DM will focus more on postprandial hyperglycemia than in the past, and will increasingly utilize premeal administration of fast-onset short-acting insulins such as lispro, aspart, and possibly inhaled insulin. An analog of amylin, pramlintide, has been reported to reduce postprandial glucose in both T1DM and T2DM, and is currently being tested in humans.[14] If results show adequate efficacy and safety, this drug may be useful, but the requirement for parenteral administration and the fact that it cannot be mixed with insulin in the same syringe will limit its clinical application.

Treatments to Induce Remission and Ameliorate Autoimmune β-Cell Destruction

Advances in understanding of the immunology of T1DM have laid the foundation for several clinical trials to assess whether immune modulation can prevent T1DM, or slow β-cell destruction and induce remission in newly diagnosed type 1 diabetics (see Chap. 15). As already discussed, the DPT-1 failed to demonstrate that daily parenteral insulin administration altered subsequent development of T1DM in individuals at high risk.[3] Whether this failure means that insulin is not an important antigen in the autoimmune destruction of β cells in T1DM, or is the result of a flawed study design in the clinical trial, is not clear at this time. Other antigen-based approaches utilizing other antigens postulated to play a role in the autoimmune destruction of β cells in T1DM, including IA-2, IA-2b, heat shock proteins (e.g., hsp60, hsp70), and other immune targets (e.g., IL-4 and IL-2 related), are also being evaluated in human type 1 diabetic patients.

Studies in animal models of diabetes such as the nonobese diabetic (NOD) mouse demonstrate that several of these approaches can prevent development of insulitis and diabetes, but the relevance and applicability to the prevention and treatment of human T1DM of these results in mouse type 1 diabetes must await the outcomes of ongoing and future human clinical trials of these agents and approaches. Encouragingly, initial clinical studies of a humanized anti-CD-3 monoclonal antibody have recently reported efficacy in inducing remission or slowing the rate of progression in newly diagnosed type 1 diabetic patients with sufficient remaining β-cell function.[15]

Methods to Stimulate β-Cell Regeneration and Growth and Inhibit β-Cell Apoptosis

Advances in β-cell biology could eventually lead to development of methods to stimulate β-cell regeneration in patients with diabetes (see Chap. 14). Factors such as glucagon-like peptide (GLP-1), exendin-4, insulin-like growth factor (IGF-I), nitric oxide, and certain β-cell transcription factors (e.g., pancreas duodenum homeobox-containing transcription factor-1 [PDX-1]) have been shown to possess stimulatory activity for islet cell growth, but their specificity is unknown.[16,17] In T1DM this approach will have to be coupled with immune suppression to prevent autoimmune destruction of β cells; it may, therefore, be more feasible in patients with T2DM. Advances in this area may enable stimulation of β-cell growth and help to ensure an adequate supply for islet transplantation.

T2DM: TREATMENT SHORTCOMINGS

Limitations in Understanding the Causes and Pathophysiology of T2DM

More effective and safer therapies directed towards specific underlying defects require greater knowledge about the disease gained through intensified biomedical and behavioral research.

Limitations of Existing Oral Hypoglycemic Agents

Current oral agents, at least as currently utilized by most patients, are limited in their ability to achieve normal or near-normal glycemia in most type 2 diabetic patients. Significant side effects such as hypoglycemia, gastrointestinal dysfunction, fluid retention, edema, liver failure, and lactic acidosis compromise proper dosing and limit patient compliance. Both more effective and safer drugs and better use of existing agents are required.

Therapy May Be Initiated Too Late

Treatment of T2DM is usually begun after the disease has progressed significantly, perhaps to the point where intervention can have only limited effect. Numerous studies, most recently the UKPDS,[18] have established that the complications of diabetes often begin before clinical diagnosis of the disease, and before the development of fasting hyperglycemia and elevated HbA_{1c}. Epidemiologic evidence from the UKPDS indicates that increased risk for micro- and macrovascular disease begins at HbA_{1c} levels of 6.5%.

Both underlying defects of T2DM, insulin resistance and defective insulin secretion, exist before fasting hyperglycemia occurs, HbA_{1c} becomes elevated, diagnosis of diabetes is made, and therapy is initiated. Both defects predict subsequent development of overt disease and may be risk factors for complications,[19] and both may be targets for earlier therapeutic intervention. For example, acute-phase insulin secretion is commonly lost at fasting glucose levels between 6.1 and 6.5 mmol/L.[20] Loss of acute phase insulin secretion in response to a meal causes mealtime and postprandial hyperglycemia, reactive hyperinsulinemia, and hypoglycemia, often the earliest clinically detectable abnormalities of T2DM. Isolated mealtime hyperglycemia commonly exists in individuals with normal fasting glucose levels, especially in older adults who make up such a large proportion of the type 2 diabetic population.[21–23] Restoration of early insulin levels has been reported to improve glucose tolerance in type 2 diabetics,[1] yet treatment usually does not begin until the diabetes is diagnosed by fasting hyperglycemia.

Clearly, T2DM needs to be treated earlier, perhaps even before development of fasting hyperglycemia of 7.0 mmol/L as defined by current diagnostic criteria, and the current therapeutic target of HbA_{1c} of 7%. Further downward revision of the new diagnostic criteria established in 1997[24] may be necessary to help address this shortcoming. The results of the recently-concluded NIH-sponsored Diabetes Prevention Program (DPP) strongly support this view.[25] This study demonstrated that in prediabetic patients at high risk for developing T2DM (patients with impaired glucose tolerance), treatment intervention to improve glucose control can significantly reduce progression to overt clinical diabetes.

Therapy Is Too Narrowly Focused

Although, as just described, insulin resistance and defective insulin secretion exist early in the course of the disease, current treatment approaches usually address only one of these two abnormalities. Treatment is likely to be more effective if both defects, insulin resistance and impaired insulin secretion, are addressed, and in the view of this author the earlier the better.

Additionally, current therapy is often focused on managing fasting hyperglycemia and on targeting this endpoint as a measure of adequate glycemic control. Mealtime and postprandial glycemia are often ignored, yet they contribute to overall 24-hour hyperglycemia,[13,23] worsen the underlying defects of insulin secretion and action, and may increase risk of complications. The newly established treatment targets focus on fasting plasma glucose levels and give scant attention to the importance of reducing postprandial hyperglycemia.[24,26] As an additional consideration, several recent epidemiologic studies suggest that mealtime and postprandial blood glucose levels are independent risk factors for cardiovascular disease and mortality.[21,27] It is to be emphasized, however, that controlled clinical studies are needed to confirm this epidemiologic association.

Future treatment of T2DM will be more broadly focused, to address both impaired insulin action and insulin secretion, and to reduce both fasting *and* postprandial hyperglycemia.

Therapy Is Insufficiently Aggressive

Blood glucose levels are often allowed to remain too high for too long because patients are asymptomatic. Combination therapy with oral agents and addition of, or switching to, insulin is too often delayed until the disease is well advanced and glycemic control has deteriorated substantially. Efforts to control body weight, caloric intake, and physical activity are unfortunately often insufficient. Limitations in physician and allied health provider training and experience in the management of diabetes, and inadequate patient self-management, also contribute to the lack of more aggressive therapy.

Limited Awareness and Inadequate Support

T2DM does not receive the priority or attention from governments and the health care system that is required to contain and control what is rapidly becoming a worldwide pandemic (see Chap. 19). The magnitude, medical seriousness, and enormous economic cost of T2DM, as well as the extent to which socioeconomic factors and lifestyle contribute to the disease, remain unrecognized by these agencies. Governments must take the lead in sponsoring programs to enhance public awareness, and introduce public health programs to modify social, cultural, and lifestyle factors that contribute to T2DM.

CHANGES IN THERAPEUTIC APPROACHES FOR T2DM

Prevention

Theoretically, the most obvious means of preventing a large percentage of cases of T2DM is to prevent obesity. Indeed, clinical studies demonstrate that lifestyle intervention, including diet, reduced dietary fat intake, weight loss, and exercise, can significantly improve glucose tolerance in individuals at high risk for T2DM.[25,28] However, societal attitudes, lifestyles, and nutrition tend to increase body weight and reduce physical activity, and preventing obesity or reducing body weight has proven difficult to accomplish and to maintain over time. Unless these lifestyle issues can be addressed more effectively, other interventions, primarily pharmacologic, will be required for the treatment of T2DM.

Prevention of T2DM may ultimately come from identification of the genes responsible for this form of the disease, and discovery of how they function to cause abnormalities of insulin secretion and action. While the major human genes for T2DM might be identified and cloned within a few years, elucidation of how they act, and development of gene-based therapy for this polygenic disease, if ever achievable, is unlikely to be accomplished for many years.

New Treatment Options

A major shift in the approach to the treatment of T2DM is required. Current treatment is often too late, too little, and too narrowly focused. As discussed above, physician and allied health provider education and training must be increased so that diagnosis and therapy are more aggressive.

Earlier Diagnosis and Treatment

Increased efforts to detect and treat asymptomatic patients with fasting hyperglycemia, elevated HbA$_{1c}$, and postprandial hyperglycemia must become standard medical practice for the reasons discussed above. The recent downward revision of the fasting plasma glucose levels diagnostic of diabetes (i.e., ≥ 7 mmol/L [126 mg/dL]),[24] and treatment target levels to HbA$_{1c}$ $\leq 7\%$, will enable earlier diagnosis and treatment, but these levels may not be low enough. The risk of complications appears to begin at significantly lower levels of fasting glucose and HbA$_{1c}$.[18,24,26,27,29,30] Lower diagnostic criteria will enable earlier diagnosis and treatment of abnormalities that contribute to disease progression and complications, with the likelihood of more effective outcomes. However, documentation of such theoretical benefits through controlled clinical trials may be necessary to justify such a change in criteria.

The establishment of the categories of impaired glucose tolerance (IGT) and impaired fasting glucose (IFG) provides another opportunity for a major shift in the management of T2DM by potentially enabling earlier intervention.[24,30] As discussed above, the DPP indicates that treatment during IGT, either with an effective program of diet and exercise or with the oral hypoglycemic drug metformin, can decrease the rate of progression of IGT to frank T2DM.[25] Thus, in all likelihood, future therapy may be directed toward treating individuals with IGT with lifestyle change programs (diet, weight control, and exercise) or with oral hypoglycemic agents capable of overcoming insulin resistance and/or restoring acute insulin secretion and lowering postprandial blood glucose. Drugs with proven safety and very low risk of hypoglycemia will have to be utilized. The thiazolidenediones may offer an opportunity to address the fundamental abnormality of insulin resistance. However, because of their potential for significant side effects (discussed later in this chapter), this class of drugs should not yet be utilized for early intervention in patients with IGT until adequate long-term safety has been clearly demonstrated. Though the DPP suggests that metformin may be sufficiently safe, at this time there is insufficient information from that study about patient tolerability of the drug. The newly emerging fast-acting nonsulfonylurea oral hypoglycemic drugs (discussed later in this chapter), which stimulate first-phase insulin secretion and reduce postprandial glucose, thereby addressing an early type 2 defect, might have a role in treatment of patients with IGT, provided that their long-term safety is established. At this time, lifestyle modification, including better nutrition, weight loss, and maintenance of normal body weight, and an appropriate program of physical activity, appears to be the only intervention with a sufficient level of established safety to be utilized in IGT.

Future therapy may also be directed toward treatment of patients with IFG, again with drugs with proven safety and a very low risk of hypoglycemia. As currently defined, IFG identifies a different group of at-risk patients in the population than does IGT, with perhaps as little as 30–50% overlap with IGT.[29,30] Thus if only VIFG is utilized to determine treatment intervention, large numbers of patients with IGT would go undetected. Since IGT is known to be a significant risk factor for development of cardiovascular disease, detection and treatment of IFG *alone*, without detection and treatment of IGT, would appear to be an undesirable strategy for early detection of risk and early intervention. For this reason, it has been suggested that the fasting glucose level diagnostic of IFG be lowered to ≤ 6 mmol/L (108 mg/dL) in order to identify individuals more similar to those with IGT with regard to risk of cardiovascular disease,[29] and that oral glucose tolerance testing continue, especially in high-risk patients.

Control of Mealtime and Postprandial Blood Glucose

Therapy of T2DM in the future should focus not only on controlling fasting blood glucose and HbA$_{1c}$, but also on control of mealtime and postmeal glucose levels. In some type 2 diabetic patients, reduction of postprandial glucose levels has been shown to contribute to lowering HbA$_{1c}$ at least as much and possibly to a greater degree than reduction of fasting glucose.[31,32] In the future, mealtime and postprandial hyperglycemia may be treated *before fasting hyperglycemia occurs* (i.e., before fasting glucose reaches >7 mmol/L or 125 mg/dL). For example, patients with elevated postprandial glucose levels, but normal fasting glucose, may be treated with oral hypoglycemic agents capable of stimulating early insulin secretion, and lowering postmeal hyperglycemia (discussed later in this chapter). Easier methods to detect patients with postprandial hyperglycemia and to assess efficacy of treatment in a clinical setting are required. Screening of patients at high risk for developing T2DM with oral glucose tolerance tests is cumbersome, but may be desirable. Appropriate targets for postprandial glucose levels will have to be established. Current epidemiologic data on increased cardiovascular risk suggest that a 2-hour postprandial plasma glucose of 11 mmol/L is too high, and that <10 mmol/L or 180 mg/dL may be more appropriate.[27]

Combination Therapy

It is unlikely that a single oral agent will successfully control 24-hour blood glucose levels for very long in most patients with T2DM. Combinations of two or more drugs (see Chaps. 30 and 32) that target *both* underlying defects of T2DM, impaired insulin secretion and action, and *both* fasting and postprandial hyperglycemia, should begin earlier in the course of the disease, perhaps as early as at the time of diagnosis, in order to achieve better overall glycemic control, and perhaps more successfully modify the disease process. At times, three oral hypoglycemic agents or two oral agents and insulin may have to be utilized. Earlier addition or switch to insulin may be required in certain patients in order to more aggressively control blood glucose.

Control of Nonglucose Risk Factors

In addition to control of blood glucose, restoration of normal blood lipids, with statins and other hypolipidemic agents, and blood pressure control are essential in the management of T2DM. Better outcomes in the future demand more aggressive antihyperlipidemic and antihypertensive therapy, if necessary through the use of combinations of multiple drugs (see Chaps. 47 and 48).

New Orally Active Drugs To Stimulate Insulin Action and Overcome Insulin Resistance

Numerous targets for oral agents to enhance insulin action and increase glucose disposal exist, principally insulin-signaling proteins shown to cause insulin resistance in insulin-resistant tissues and laboratory animals (see Chaps. 5 and 22). Although as discussed in those chapters, defects have been demonstrated at several molecular sites in the insulin-signaling pathway, which, if any, account for the insulin-resistant state in human T2DM, and therefore might be viable targets for new drugs to overcome insulin resistance, is unknown. Given the high likelihood that there is a heterogeneity of defects responsible for insulin resistance in T2DM, that the relative contribution of each defect varies among type 2 patients, and that insulin resistance may be the result of additive effects of several interacting genetic and environmental (e.g., nutritional, obesity) factors on several insulin-signaling proteins, a single drug to prevent or correct all forms of insulin resistance in type 2 diabetic populations or even within individual type 2 patients is unlikely. Rather, multiple drugs targeted to different signaling molecules, at times in a "cocktail-like" form, together with lifestyle interventions, may have to be utilized.

Insulin Mimetics, Potentiators, and Sensitizers

Molecules are being developed to act at the insulin receptor or at one or more postreceptor signaling events to either mimic, potentiate, or sensitize cells to insulin action in order to overcome insulin resistance and promote glucose disposal. The orally active fungal derivative mimicking insulin action through phosphorylation of the tyrosine kinase domain of the insulin receptor described earlier is an example.[6] A second orally active nonpeptide agent which induces insulin-dependent activation of the tyrosine kinase domain of the insulin receptor β subunit and reduces blood glucose in diabetic laboratory animals suggests another potentially useful approach for the treatment of insulin resistance in T2DM.[33] Inhibitors of protein tyrosine phosphatase, especially PTP-1B, are currently being evaluated in laboratory animals.[34] They are reported to enhance insulin sensitivity, increase glucose uptake, and improve glucose tolerance. It remains to be seen whether sufficient selectivity and specificity can be achieved with these agents to avoid unacceptable toxicity.

Other molecules involved in the cascade of signaling events that culminate in insulin's metabolic action are being explored as targets for development of drugs to enhance insulin action and increase glucose disposal (e.g., insulin receptor substrate 1 [IRS-1]), second messenger systems such as phosphatidylinositol-3-kinase (PI-3-kinase), glucose transport (stimulation of GLUT-4 translocation to the plasma membrane), and other downstream signaling proteins.[34,35]

Agents Acting Through PPARγ

The thiazolidenedione insulin sensitizers act through the nuclear receptor, peroxisome proliferator activated receptor (PPARγ) (see Chap. 32). They have been welcomed as a step forward in the management of T2DM because they enhance insulin sensitivity and increase glucose disposal, thus addressing insulin resistance, a fundamental abnormality in T2DM. However, because of severe liver toxicity, the first thiazolidenedione, troglitazone, has been withdrawn. Rosiglitazone and pioglitazone, the most recently developed drugs in the class, appear not to cause hepatotoxicity, but more clinical experience is required to be certain of their safety in this regard. On the other hand, both of these drugs can cause significant weight gain, fluid retention, and edema, side effects that may limit their long-term usefulness. Additional thiazolidenedione analogs and nonthiazolidenedione drugs acting through PPARγ with greater efficacy and safety are being sought and developed.[36,37] In this regard, RXR agonists, which act through the PPARγ-RXR heterodimer to increase insulin action and decrease blood glucose, also appear to be associated with significant toxicity, raising doubts about the long-term clinical usefulness of drugs acting on this target.

The recent observations that a PPARγ knockout mouse model with PPARγ deficiency is associated with increased insulin sensitivity,[38] and that a RXR antagonist reduces blood glucose in diabetic laboratory animals,[39] suggests another PPARγ-RXR–based approach to developing insulin sensitizers. Several dual PPAR agonists, targeting both PPARγ for glucose control and PPARα for control of lipids are currently in clinical development.[39] If they are to be successful, it will be necessary to achieve the correct balance of PPARγ and PPARα activity.

β₃-Adrenergic Receptor Agonists

β₃-Adrenergic receptor agonists, which increase energy expenditure through increased thermogenesis in brown and lipolysis in white adipose tissue, and which increase insulin-stimulated glucose disposal and improve glucose tolerance in laboratory animals and humans,[41] have so far been hampered by having modest hypoglycemic efficacy, insufficient selectivity, and significant side effects. These drawbacks must be overcome for this approach to be of use in the management of T2DM.

Inhibition of Fatty Acid Oxidation

It is highly likely that all agents focused on fatty acid oxidation inhibition will have the same unacceptable toxicities as previously developed and tested drugs.[42]

Inhibition of Hepatic Gluconeogenesis and Hepatic Glucose Output

Inhibitors of gluconeogenic enzymes such as PEPCK and F1-6 bisphosphonate have been associated with unacceptable toxicity, especially serious hypoglycemia. New avenues of research in this area include: (1) overexpression of the bifunctional hepatic enzyme 6-phosphofructo-2-kinase/fructose-2-6-bisphosphonate, thereby decreasing gluconeogenesis and increasing glycolysis,[43] and (2) modulation of hepatic nuclear transcription factors that regulate gluconeogenic enzymes,[34] an indirect approach that may lead to therapeutic agents to inhibit gluconeogenesis that are safer than those directly targeting gluconeogenic enzymes in the liver.

Stimulation of Glycogen Synthesis

The demonstration that reduced levels of hepatic glycogen contribute to dysregulated hepatic glucose production in T2DM has led to efforts to seek drugs that increase the capacity of the liver for glycogenesis. Focus has been on molecules that enhance the activity of glycogen synthase, hepatic glucokinase, and protein phosphatase-1 (PP-1). In laboratory animals these approaches have been associated with increased hepatic glucose disposal. Hepatic overexpression of glucokinase reduces blood glucose concentration in diabetic mice, but increases plasma free fatty acids and triglycerides. Increasing expression of other regulated members of the family of glycogen-targeting subunits of hepatic PP-1 to enhance glucose disposal and glycogen storage in diabetic patients, thereby lowering blood glucose levels, are being pursued.[44]

Growth Hormone and IGF-1

Fragments of growth hormone (e.g., hGH 6-13) have been shown to increase insulin action and improve glucose tolerance in laboratory animals, and several analogs are in preclinical development.[45] Adequate oral bioavailability is uncertain. IGF-1 has been demonstrated to substitute for insulin action in rodents and humans, and has been explored for treatment of T2DM.[46] IGF-1 has been associated with side effects, but they can be reduced by combination with IGF-BP3. Inhibition of growth hormone secretion by IGF-1 and somatostatin analogs are also being evaluated. To date they have met with limited success. Inhibition of growth hormone may promote obesity, and thus on balance may be undesirable.

Glucagon Inhibition

Inhibitors of pancreatic glucagon secretion (e.g., glucagon-like peptide [GLP-1], somatostatin, exendin-4[47,48]), and of glucagon action in the liver (e.g., glucagon receptor antagonists[49]), have been shown to reduce blood glucose in laboratory animals. GLP-1 and synthetic exendin-4 have to be made either orally bioavailable or long-acting for large-scale application to treatment of T2DM. Such agents are unlikely to have a major impact on glycemic control unless used in combination with other hypoglycemic agents, but they may have the desirable effect of reducing insulin dosage.

Miscellaneous Approaches To Overcome Insulin Resistance

Among various approaches currently being pursued are TNFα antagonists, resistin antagonists, and adenosine agonists.[34,50]

Obesity-Related Approaches

The most obvious target for increasing insulin action in T2DM and returning blood glucose to normal or near-normal levels is reduction of excess adiposity. Indeed, numerous clinical studies demonstrate that lifestyle intervention can significantly improve glucose tolerance in individuals at high risk for T2DM.[28] Although recent progress in basic research has been great (see Chap. 23), many years will probably be required to develop effective drugs to prevent obesity or achieve and maintain weight loss. It is unlikely that a drug targeted to a single mechanism (e.g., leptin), a neuroendocrine peptide or receptor, or an uncoupling protein, will be successful given the redundancy and complexity of the process regulating eating behavior, energy homeostasis, and the adipose tissue mass. Rather, a combination of agents targeted to different sites in this process is likely to be required.

New Drugs To Stimulate Insulin Secretion

Several approaches to stimulate insulin secretion in a more physiologic manner are currently being pursued, and compounds are being tested in humans, including agents that stimulate first-phase insulin secretion, restore β-cell sensitivity to glucose, and stimulate or mimic gastrointestinal tract incretins such as GLP-1.

Nonsulfonylurea Insulin Secretagogues

A new class of nonsulfonylurea insulin secretagogues are now available for reducing mealtime and postprandial hyperglycemia in type 2 diabetics. This has not been achievable or achievable to only a limited degree by other oral hypoglycemic agents. Two drugs from this class are available: repaglinide, a benzoic acid derivative,[51] and nateglinide, an amino acid derivative.[32] A third agent, KAD 1229, is currently in development with only limited clinical experience at this time.[52]

These drugs stimulate insulin secretion with a rapid onset and short duration of action, thereby reducing excessive mealtime glucose excursions that adversely affect overall glycemic control, and avoiding prolonged elevation of plasma insulin levels and exposure of tissues to hyperinsulinemia, in contrast to even the fast-acting sulfonylureas glipizide, gliclazide, and glimiperide.

The major value of these short-acting nonsulfonylurea insulin secretagogues appears to be their stimulation of early insulin secretion after a meal and control of postprandial glucose, thereby offering the opportunity in certain subsets of type 2 patients to achieve better overall glycemic control and lower HbA$_{1c}$ levels than is achievable with current drugs that focus only on fasting glucose. These drugs appear to be most useful when combined with drugs that enhance insulin action, and control fasting glucose (e.g., metformin or thiazolidenediones). Combination with sulfonylureas appears to have little or no added benefit. As monotherapy, these drugs may be useful for treatment of patients with T2DM who do not respond adequately to diet and exercise, suffer mild degrees of hyperglycemia ($\leq$7mm/L, $\leq$ 126mg/dL), and are either early in the course of their disease, or are elderly, in whom hyperglycemia during (prandial) and after meals (postprandial) is the most pronounced glycemic abnormality, while fasting plasma glucose is either normal or mildly increased. For type 2 patients with more severe degrees of hyperglycemia, monotherapy with these agents is insufficient. To date, drugs of this class appear to be well tolerated and safe, particularly for avoiding hypoglycemia in patients with blood glucose levels below 180 mg/dL (10 mmol/L) and in older adults with T2DM. If proven safe with a low risk of hypoglycemia over the long term, these drugs may have a role in treatment of IGT.

Glucagon-Like Peptide-1 (GLP-1)

GLP-1 agonists and drugs that raise plasma levels of GLP-1 are being developed by several companies as a new approach for improving glycemic control (see Chap. 6).[47,48,53-55] Because of its extremely short half-life and the need for parenteral administration, native GLP-1 itself is unlikely to become a therapeutic agent. Modified GLP-1 molecules with longer half-lives, requiring only once or twice daily injection, are also in clinical development and may soon be available for clinical practice. Since these agents must be administered parenterally on a daily basis, their applicability to the treatment of T2DM may be limited. An orally bioavailable inhibitor of DDP-IV,[55] the enzyme that degrades GLP-1, is currently in clinical development. This agent raises and maintains increased GLP-1 and GIP levels, increases insulin secretion and insulin action, inhibits glucagon secretion, reduces plasma glucose levels, and improves glucose tolerance in animal models of T2DM. Clinical trials have recently been initiated, and if efficacy is demonstrated, and inhibition of DDP-IV and prolonged elevation of GLP-1, GIP, and other peptides is safe, this could be an attractive drug for treatment of T2DM.

Exendin-4 is a 39-amino-acid peptide isolated from the saliva of the Gila monster. It has 53% sequence homology to GLP-1. A synthetic exendin-4 molecule, Ac2993, stimulates insulin secretion, reduces glucagon secretion, enhances insulin action, slows gastric emptying, and reduces plasma glucose in laboratory animals and humans.[48] Like GLP-1, this peptide must be administered parenterally, but unlike GLP-1 it has a prolonged half-life and activity. If ongoing clinical trials demonstrate adequate safety and efficacy in patients with T2DM, and an orally bioavailable formulation or a molecule with an extended half-life not requiring daily injection can be developed for large scale clinical application, exendin-4 could have considerable value in the future treatment of T2DM.

If these drugs become available for clinical use, it is likely that they will be most useful in the treatment of T2DM as combinations of oral and parenteral forms, depending on the stage and severity of the disease, and when combined with other hypoglycemic agents.

Glucokinase

Efforts to restore or enhance β-cell sensitivity to glucose-stimulated insulin secretion by stimulation of β-cell–specific glucokinase activity are currently under investigation.[56] Even if a defect in glucokinase does not exist in the great majority of type 2 diabetics, increased β-cell sensitivity to glucose should be useful. While an agent enhancing glucokinase activity in both the β cell and the liver might appear to be attractive, a β-cell–specific drug may be preferable, given the finding that glucokinase stimulation in the liver of rodents is associated with elevated free fatty acids and triglycerides.[44]

Reduction of Insulin Dosage and Hyperinsulinemia

It has been postulated that hyperinsulinemia contributes to the development of diabetic macrovascular disease. To minimize hyperinsulinemia, drugs that can be co-administered with insulin to reduce insulin dosage, such as the thiazolidenediones, will be increasingly utilized, if such use is not prevented by safety problems. Pramlintide, an analog of amylin, has been reported to reduce insulin dosage in both T1DM and T2DM, and is currently undergoing clinical testing.[14] If safe and effective, this drug may be useful in insulin-treated patients with T1DM and T2DM, but the requirement for parenteral administration and the inability to mix it with insulin in the same syringe will limit its clinical application.

Other New Treatment Options

Methods to stimulate β-cell growth and regeneration, improved glucose sensors, the artificial pancreas, and islet transplantation, discussed earlier under the section on T1DM, are equally applicable to the management of T2DM, and offer opportunities for improved outcomes in the future.

COMPLICATIONS OF DIABETES

Therapies for Prevention and Treatment

Optimal Glycemic Control

Control of blood glucose to normal or near normal levels will continue to be the cornerstone of treatment to prevent and slow the rate of progression of diabetic complications. Methods for achieving this goal have been discussed earlier in this chapter.

Tissue-Specific Therapies

Identification of potential molecular and biochemical mechanisms by which hyperglycemia causes tissue damage gives rise to potential new therapeutic interventions targeted directly at diabetic complications (see Chaps. 1, 40–50, and 55). Many of these approaches are directed towards hyperglycemia-induced alterations in vascular endothelial cells. A few of them are described below.

Inhibitors of AGE, AGE-RAGE Interactions

Inhibitors of advanced glycation end-product (AGE) formation (see Chap. 42) (e.g., aminoguanidine[57]) are being developed, but they have encountered safety and efficacy problems. Inhibition of the AGE-RAGE (receptors for AGEs) interaction by blocking RAGE on endothelial, vascular smooth muscle, neural, mesangial, immune, and inflammatory cells appears more attractive and likely to be successful. Soluble RAGE (sRAGE) is reported to be effective against microvascular disease in laboratory animals, and sRAGE may provide a basis for developing an oral inhibitor of AGE-RAGE interaction or of AGE receptors.[58]

Inhibition of Protein Kinase C (PKC)

PKC is believed to play an important role in the development of the vascular and neurologic complications of diabetes. At least one inhibitor of PKC is currently in phase III clinical studies for treatment of diabetic retinopathy[59] (see Chap. 41). Vitamin E and α-lipoic acid antioxidants have been shown to inhibit PKC.

Inhibitors of Aldose Reductase and Sorbitol Formation

Inhibitors of aldose reductase are in development by several companies for treatment of diabetic neuropathy (see Chaps. 44–46). Most appear to have had limited efficacy and unacceptable toxicity. A new generation of aldose reductase inhibitors is now in development, however at this time it is not known whether these will be more successful than their predecessors.

Inhibition of Angiogenic Growth Factors To Decrease the Formation of New Blood Vessels in Diabetic Retinopathy

A major focus of current drug discovery and development is inhibitors of vascular endothelial growth factor (VEGF) for the treatment of diabetic retinopathy.[60] Other targets receiving attention include growth hormone, TGFβ, IGF-1, bFGF, angiotensin, integrins, and endothelin.[61] Endothelin antagonism may also be applicable to the treatment of macrovascular disease.

Stimulation of Angiogenic Growth and Other Factors

Stimulation of these factors to increase formation of new blood vessels for treatment of coronary and peripheral vascular disease and to treat neuropathy is also under study.[62] Gene therapy approaches to stimulate growth of new blood vessels are currently under investigation. Drugs that stimulate VEGF are also being sought for this indication, but these will have to be highly tissue-specific and selective, since systemic effects could adversely affect retinopathy by stimulating new retinal vessel growth. Agents that stimulate nerve growth factors (e.g., NGF, neurotropins) are also being sought for treatment of diabetic neuropathy.[63]

Antioxidants

Research to develop antioxidants to decrease oxidative stress and free radical formation in cells and tissues of the body is ongoing. A variety of drugs and natural substances such as vitamins C and E, α-lipoic acid, and γ-linolenic acid have been tested with minimal success.[64]

REFERENCES

1. Bruttomesso D, Pianta A, Mari A, et al: Restoration of early rise in plasma insulin levels improves glucose tolerance of Type 2 diabetic patients. *Diabetes* 1999;48:99.
2. Fritsche A, Stefan N, Haring H, et al: Avoidance of hypoglycemia restores hypoglycemia awareness by increasing β-adrenergic sensitivity in Type 1 diabetes. *Ann Intern Med* 2001;134:729.

3. Skyler J: New therapies for the prevention of Type 1 diabetes: Results of the DPT-1. *Diabetes* 2001;50(suppl 2):35.

4. Dandona P, Clement S, Gordon J, *et al*: Effect of an oral modified insulin on blood glucose levels in fasting and fed Type 1 diabetic patients receiving a "basal" regimen of injected insulin. *Diabetes* 2001; 50(Suppl 2):A44.

5. Modi P, Mihic M: Replacement of s.c. injections with Oralin in treatment of diabetes. *Diabetes* 2001;50(suppl 2):A44.

6. Zhang B, Salituro G, Szalkowski D, *et al*: Discovery of a small molecule insulin mimic with antidiabetic activity in mice. *Science* 1999; 284:974.

7. Cefalu WT, Balagtas CC, Landschulz WH, *et al*: Sustained efficacy and pulmonary safety of inhaled insulin during 2-years of outpatient therapy. *Diabetes* 2000;49(suppl 1):A101.

8. Leung FK, Li J, Huang L, *et al*: A new transdermal insulin formulation—results of insulin pharmacokinetics and hypoglycaemic efficacy in comparison to azone and subcutaneous insulin injections in non-diabetic rats. *Diabetes* 2001;50(suppl. 2):A123.

9. Lando H: The new "designer" insulins. *Clin Diabetes* 2000;4:154.

10. Gray RS, Schmitz O, Kristensen A, *et al*: The dose relationship between insulin detemir and NPF: a multicentre, open, two-period cross-over trial in insulin treated Type 2 diabetic patients. *Diabetes* 2001;50(suppl. 2):A115.

11. Shojaee-Moradie F, Powrie JK, Sunderman E, *et al*: Novel hepatoselective insulin analogue: studies with a covalently linked thyroxyl-insulin complex in humans. *Diabetes Care* 2000;23:1124.

12. Shapiro AMJ, Lakey JR, Ryan E, *et al*: Islet transplantation in seven patients with Type 1 diabetes mellitus using a glucocorticoid-free immunosuppressive regimen. *N Engl J Med* 2000;343:289.

13. Avignon A, Radauceanu A, *et al*: Nonfasting plasma glucose is a better marker of diabetic control than fasting plasma glucose in Type 2 diabetics. *Diabetes Care* 1997;20:1822.

14. Whitehouse F, Kruger DF, Fineman M, *et al:* A randomized study and open-label extension evaluating the long-term efficacy of pramlintide as an adjunct to insulin therapy in Type 1 Diabetes. *Diabetes Care* 2002;25:724

15. Herrold KC, Hagopian W, Auger J, *et al*: Treatment with anti-CD3 monoclonal antibody (mAB) HOKT3γ(1(Ala-Ala) improves glycemic control during the first year of Type 1 diabetes mellitus (T1DM). *Diabetes* 2001;50(suppl. 2):A34.

16. Tourel C, Baile D, Meile MJ, *et al*: Glucagon-like peptide and exendin-4 stimulate β-cell neogenesis in streptozotocin-treated newborn rats resulting in persistently improved glucose homeostasis at adult age. *Diabetes* 2001;50:1562.

17. Xu GX, Stoffes DA, Habener JF, *et al*: Extendin-4 stimulates beta cell replication and neogenesis, resulting in increased beta cell, mass and improved glucose tolerance in diabetic rats. *Diabetes* 1999;48:2270.

18. UKPDS Prospective Diabetes Study Group: Intensive blood glucose control with sulfonylureas or insulin compared with conventional treatment and risk of complications in patients with Type 2 diabetes (UKPDS 33). *Lancet* 1998;353:837.

19. Weyer C, Bogardus C, Mott DM: The natural history of insulin secretory dysfunction and insulin resistance in the pathogenesis of Type 2 diabetes mellitus. *J Clin Invest* 1999;104:787.

20. Brunzel JD, Robertson, RP, Lerner RL, *et al*: Relationship between fasting plasma glucose levels and insulin secretion during intravenous glucose tolerance tests. *J Clin Endocrinol Metab* 1976;42:229.

21. Shaw JE, Hodge AM, de Courten M, *et al*: Isolated post-challenge hyperglycemia confirmed as a risk factor for mortality. *Diabetologia* 1999;42:1050.

22. Resnick HE, Harris MI, Brock DB, *et al*: American Diabetes Association diabetes diagnostic criteria, advancing age, and cardiovascular disease risk profiles. Results from the Third National Health and Nutrition Examination Survey. *Diabetes Care* 2000;23:176.

23. Bando Y, Ushiogi Y, Okafuji K, *et al*: The relationship of fasting glucose values and other variables to 2-h postload plasma glucose in Japanese subjects. *Diabetes Care* 2001;24:1156.

24. American Diabetes Association: Report of the Expert Committee on the Diagnosis and Classification of Diabetes Mellitus. *Diabetes Care* 2000;23(suppl 1):4.

25. Diet and exercise dramatically delay Type 2 diabetes: Diabetes medication metformin also effective. Human Health Services Announcement on the results of the Diabetes Prevention Program (DPP). August 8, 2001.

26. American Diabetes Association: Standards of medical care for patients with diabetes mellitus. *Diabetes Care* 2000;23(suppl 1):32.

27. The Decode Study Group: Glucose tolerance and mortality: comparison of WHO and American Diabetes Association diagnostic criteria. *Lancet* 1999;354:617.

28. Tuomilehto J, Lindstrom J, Eriksson JG, *et al*: Prevention of type 2 diabetes by changes in lifestyle among subjects with impaired glucose tolerance. *N Engl J Med* 2001;344:1390.

29. Shaw JE, Zimmet P, Hodge AM: Impaired fasting glucose: how low should it go? *Diabetes Care* 2000;23:34.

30. Alberti KGMM, Zimmet PK: For the World Health Organization. Definition, diagnosis and classification of diabetes mellitus and its complications. *Diabetic Med* 1998;15:539.

31. Bastyr EJ, Stuart CA, Brodows RG, *et al*: Therapy focused on lowering postprandial glucose, not fasting glucose, may be superior for lowering HbA$_{1c}$. *Diabetes Care* 2000;23:1236.

32. Horton ES, Clinkingbeard C, Gatlin M, *et al*: Nateglinide alone and in combination with metformin improves glycemic control by reducing mealtime glucose levels in type 2 diabetes. *Diabetes Care* 2000;23:1160.

33. Manchem VP, Goldfine ID, Kohanski R, *et al*: A novel small molecule that sensitizes the insulin receptor in vitro and in vivo. *Diabetes* 2001; 50:824.

34. Personal communication.

35. Deben DEY, Bishwajt NAG: Mechanism of CLX-0901 action: A novel plant-derived orally active anti-diabetic compound. *Diabetes* 2000;49(suppl 1):A103.

36. Araki K, Yachi M, Hagisawa Y: Antidiabetic characterization of CS-011: A new thiazolenedione with potent insulin-sensitizing action. *Diabetes* 2000;49(suppl 1):A105.

37. Skrumsager BK, Nielsen KK, Pedersen PC: NNC 61-0029 (-)-DRF2725: The multiple dose pharmacokinetics of a novel dual acting PPARα and PPARγ agonist in healthy subjects and Type 2 diabetic patients. *Diabetes* 2001;50(suppl 2):A131.

38. Etgan GJ, Oldham BA, Johnson WT. The dual peroxisome proliferator–activated receptor–α/γ agonist LY465608 ameliorates insulin resistance and diabetic hyperglycemia while improving cardiovascular risk factors in preclinical models. *Diabetes* 2002; 51:1083.

39. Miles PDG, Barak Y, He W, *et al*: Impaired insulin sensitivity in mice heterozygous for PPARγ in mice deficiency. *J Clin Invest* 2000; 105:287.

40. Yamauchi T, Waki H, Komeda K, *et al*: RXR antagonist provides a novel treatment for obesity and Type 2 diabetes. *Diabetes* 2000; 49(suppl 1):A38.

41. Kiso T, Namikawa T, Tokunaga T, *et al*: Anti-obesity and anti-diabetic activities of a new beta-3 adrenergic receptor antagonist, SWR-0342SA, in KK-Ay mice. *Biol Pharm Bull* 1999;22:1073.

42. Foley JE: Rationale and application of fatty acid oxidation inhibitors in treatment of diabetes mellitus. *Diabetes Care* 1992;15:773.

43. Wu C, Okar DA, Newgard CB, *et al*: Overexpression of 6-phosphofructo-2-kinase/fructose-2,6-bisphosphatase in mouse liver lowers blood glucose by suppressing hepatic glucose production. *J Clin Invest* 2001;107:91.

44. Newgard CB, Brady MJ, O'Doherty RM, *et al*: Organizing glucose disposal: Emerging roles of the glycogen targeting subunits of protein phosphatase-1. *Diabetes* 2000;49:1967.

45. Hintz RL: Current and potential therapeutic uses of growth hormone and insulin-like growth factor I. *Endocrinol Metab Clin North Am* 2000;25:759.

46. LeRoith D: Insulin-like growth factors. *N Engl J Med* 1997;336:635.

47. Nauck MA, Holst JJ, Wilms B, *et al*: Glucagon-like peptide-1 (GLP-1) as a new therapeutic approach for Type 2 diabetes. *Exp Clin Endocrinol Diabetes* 1997;105:187.

48. Buse J, Fineman M, Gottlieb A, *et al:* Effects of five-day dosing of synthetic exendin-4 (Ac2993) in people with Type 2 diabetes. *Diabetes* 2000;29(suppl):A100.

49. Bjerre Knudsen L, Brand CI, Sidelman UG, *et al*: NNC 25-2504, a potent glucagon receptor antagonist. *Diabetes* 2001;50(supp 2): A309.

50. Way JM, Gorgun CZ, Tong Q, *et al*: Adipose tissue resistin expression is severely suppressed in obesity and stimulated by peroxisome proliferator-activated receptor gamma agonists. *J Biol Chem* 2001; 276:25651.

51. Goldberg RB, Einhorn D, Lucas C: A randomised placebo-controlled trial of repaglinide in the treatment of Type 2 diabetes. *Diabetes Care* 1998;21:1897.

52. Ohnota H, Koizumi T, Kobayashi M, *et al*: Normalisation of impaired glucose tolerance by the short-acting hypoglycaemic agent calcium (2s)-2-benzyl-3-(cis-hexahydro-2-isoindolinylcarbonyl) propionate dihydrate (KAD-1229) in non-insulin dependent diabetes mellitus rats. *Can J Physiol Pharmacol* 1995;73:1.

53. Juhl CB, Hollingdal M, Porksen N, *et al*: Evidence of a substantial reduction in fasting and postprandial glycemia in Type 2 diabetes after bedtime administration of a long-acting GLP-1 derivative, NN2211. *Diabetes* 2001;50(suppl 2):A118.

54. Myers SR, Baker J, Broderick C, *et al*: LY315902: An analog of GLP-1 with enhanced activity and time action in vivo. *Diabetes* 1998; 48(suppl 1):A193.

55. Ahren B, Simonsson E, Efendic S, *et al*: Inhibition of DPPIV by NVP DPP728 improves metabolic control over a 4-week period in Type 2 diabetes. *Diabetes* 2001;50(suppl 2):A104.

56. Cuesta-Munoz AI, Boettger CW, Davis E, *et al*: Novel pharmacological glucokinase activators partly or fully reverse the catalytic defects inactivating glucokinase missense mutants that cause MODY-2. *Diabetes* 2001;50(suppl 2):A109.

57. Yu PH, Zuo DM: Aminoguanidine inhibits semicarbizide-sensitive amine oxidase activity: Implications for advanced glycation and diabetic complications. *Diabetologia* 1997;40:1243.

58. Herrold KC, Ziang HP, Liu E, *et al*: Prevention of recurrent autoimmune diabetes by blockade of receptor for advanced glycation end product (RAGE). *Diabetes* 2001;50(suppl 2):A33.

59. Idris I, Gray S, Donnelly R, *et al*: Protein kinase C activation isoenzyme-specific effects on metabolic and cardiovascular function. *Diabetologia* 2001;44:659.

60. Aiello L, Pierce EA, Foley ED, *et al*: Inhibition of vascular endothelial growth factor (VEGF) suppresses retinal neovascularization in vivo. *Proc Natl Acad Sci USA* 1995;92:10457.

61. Hopfner RL, Gropalakrishnan V: Endothelin: Emerging role in diabetic vascular complications. *Diabetologia* 1999;42:1383.

62. Schratzberger P, Walter DH, Rittig K, *et al*: Reversal of experimental diabetic neuropathy by VEGF gene transfer. *J Clin Invest* 2001;107:1083.

63. Riaz S, Malcangio M, Miller M: A vitamin D(3) derivative (CB1093) induces nerve growth factor and prevents neurotrophic deficits in streptozotocin-diabetic rats. *Diabetologia* 1999;42:1308.

64. Packer L, Roy S, Dyck P: Alpha lipoic acid is bioavailable in nerve: Implications for treatment of diabetic polyneuropathy. *Diabetes* 1999; 48(suppl 1):A150.

CHAPTER 58

Hypoglycemia

Pierre J. Lefèbvre

André J. Scheen

Strictly speaking, the definition of hypoglycemia is biochemical; i.e., hypoglycemia is present when the blood glucose level is lower than the lowest limit of normal physiologic fluctuations. Using a specific assay on whole blood, this limit is approximately 50 mg/dL or 2.8 mmol/L (45 mg/dL or 2.5 mmol/L for some authors). Such a limit is based on the fact that numerous studies have indicated that a blood glucose level of about 55 mg/dL (3 mmol/L) induces impairment of cognitive function in most subjects tested, suggesting that it may represent the threshold for brain damage (see below). During the first 48 hours of life, in the full-term neonate, this limit is 30 mg/dL or 1.7 mmol/L, whereas values below 20 mg/dL (1.1 mmol/L) are defined as hypoglycemia for small-for-date newborns. Thus, use of the term *hypoglycemia* to characterize a clinical symptomatologic entity is not entirely appropriate. Nevertheless, in clinical practice, one observes a constellation of symptoms and signs that point to the diagnosis.

CLINICAL SYMPTOMS SUGGESTING HYPOGLYCEMIA

In the adult, the symptoms of hypoglycemia[1,2] are due to:

1. Adrenergic reaction, the symptoms of which predominate when the fall in blood glucose is rapid; they include pallor, sweating, tachycardia and palpitations, sensation of hunger, restlessness, and anxiety.
2. Cellular malnutrition at the neurological level, producing what Marks and Rose[3] have called *neuroglycopenia*, or "the signs and symptoms which develop when the supply of metabolizable carbohydrates to the neuron is inadequate for normal function." The symptoms are variable from one subject to another; they are generally more severe and occur at higher blood glucose levels in the elderly than in the young. These symptoms, which are more prominent when hypoglycemia develops slowly, include fatigue, irritability, headache, loss of concentration, somnolence, psychiatric or visual disorders (e.g., diplopia), transient sensory or motor defects, confusion, convulsions, and coma. If hypoglycemia remains untreated, death may supervene. Angina pectoris (and very rarely actual myocardial infarction) may also result from cellular malnutrition. In a given patient, the symptoms associated with hypoglycemia tend to be repetitive and stereotyped. Weinger and associates[4] have reported that many patients make clinically serious errors

in glucose estimation and use symptoms that do not differentiate hyperglycemia from hypoglycemia.

It should be noted that recurrent episodes of severe hypoglycemia may result in cumulative and permanent cognitive impairment,[5,6] although this has recently been challenged.[7] Furthermore, repetitive episodes of hypoglycemia, particularly at night, have been recognized to induce *hypoglycemia unawareness*, a situation in which the patient with diabetes does not experience appropriate autonomic warning symptoms before development of neuroglycopenia.[8] Several recent studies have shown that glycemic thresholds for hypoglycemic cognitive dysfunction, like those for autonomic and symptomatic responses to hypoglycemia, shift to lower plasma glucose levels after recent antecedent hypoglycemia in patients with type 1 diabetes (T1DM).[9–11] Interestingly, antecedent hypoglycemia also induces blunting of the hormonal and metabolic responses to physical exercise.[12]

In the newborn, the symptoms of hypoglycemia may be more difficult to recognize. They include a high-pitched cry, skin pallor or cyanosis, respiratory distress, apnea, sluggishness, irritability, hypotonia, or intermittent twitching and occasionally grand mal seizures.[3] In the older child, the following symptoms may arouse suspicion: frequent yawning, episodic staring, bizarre behavior, twitching, pallor, remoteness, paresthesias, visual disturbances, and loss of concentration. These symptoms are often mistaken for petit mal attacks.

ETIOLOGY OF HYPOGLYCEMIA

There are two principal forms of hypoglycemia: exogenous hypoglycemia attributable to injection or ingestion of a hypoglycemic compound, and endogenous hypoglycemia, which will be considered later (Table 58-1).

Exogenous Hypoglycemia

Insulin

Insulin is by far the most frequent cause of hypoglycemia, and it can occur in both diabetic and nondiabetic patients. The EURO-DIAB IDDM Complications Study indicated that the proportion of patients with one or more severe hypoglycemic attacks in 1 year averaged 32%, with a minimum of 12% in one center and as many as 48% in another.[13] Predictors of severe hypoglycemia in patients

TABLE 58-1. Etiology of Hypoglycemia

Exogenous Hypoglycemia	*Endogenous Hypoglycemia*	*Functional Hypoglycemias*
Insulin	Organic hypoglycemias	Alimentary hypoglycemia
Oral antidiabetic agents	Insulinomas and related disorders	Spontaneous reactive hypoglycemia
Alcohol	Insulinoma	Alcohol-promoted reactive hypoglycemia
Other exogenous agents	Nesidioblastosis and β-cell hyperplasia	Posthyperalimentation hypoglycemia
Salicylates	Extrapancreatic neoplasms	Endocrine deficiency states
Hypoglycins	Inborn errors of metabolism	Hypoglycemia due to glucocorticoid deficiency
Pentamidine	Hereditary fructose intolerance	Hypoglycemia in GH deficiency
Perhexilin	Fructose-1,6-diphosphatase deficiency	Hypoglycemia and catecholamine deficiency
Quinine	Galactosemia	Hypoglycemia and glucagon deficiency
β-Receptor blocking drugs	Phosphoenolpyruvate carboxykinase deficiency	Severe liver deficiency
Other drugs	Inborn errors in glycogen metabolism	Profound malnutrition
		Prolonged muscular exercise
		Autoimmune insulin syndrome
		Antibodies against the insulin receptor
		Functional or transient hypoglycemia in infancy
		Transient neonatal hypoglycemia
		Infants of diabetic mothers
		Erythroblastosis fetalis
		Leucine-induced hypoglycemia
		Ketotic hypoglycemia
		Maple syrup urine disease
		Adrenal hyporesponsiveness

with T1DM have been described by Gold and colleagues[14] and Mülhauser and coworkers.[15]

In diabetic patients, hypoglycemia may result from administration of an overdose or from the concomitant administration of drugs that when given alone favor hypoglycemia. The overdose may be absolute or relative: mistake in the evaluation of the dose, injection repeated by mistake (by the patient or by the nursing staff), poor comprehension of medical instructions, lack of sufficient food intake (gastrointestinal problems, ritual or presurgery fast, etc.), unusual physical exercise, or abrupt decrease in the insulin requirements (immediate postpartum, certain cases of insulin resistance). Hypoglycemia unawareness has been claimed to be more frequent with human than with porcine insulin, but this has not been confirmed in subsequent studies.

To prevent excessive insulin-induced decrements in plasma glucose levels, the glucoregulatory hierarchy is as follows: (1) The primary counterregulatory role is played by *glucagon*, which stimulates hepatic glucose production; (2) *epinephrine*, which is not normally critical, but plays an essential role when glucagon is deficient, acts by reducing glucose utilization and stimulating hepatic glucose production; (3) *growth hormone* and *cortisol* contribute late in glucose recovery from prolonged hypoglycemia by increasing rates of glucose production and decreasing rates of glucose utilization; and (4) *hepatic glucose autoregulation*, independent of hormonal and neural regulation, which is demonstrable only during very severe hypoglycemia.[16] The major role of the hypothalamus in mediating the counterregulatory response to hypoglycemia has been evidenced by the demonstration that such counterregulation was completely lost in a patient with hypothalamic sarcoid infiltration.[17] Recent studies have shown that the counterregulatory response of type 1 diabetic women is decreased compared to that of type 1 diabetic men.[18] Furthermore, the epinephrine response to hypoglycemia is markedly reduced during sleep.[19] Finally, the counterregulatory response to the short-acting insulin analogue lispro has been found to be identical to that to human or porcine insulin.[20] It is now well demonstrated that glucagon secretory responses to plasma glucose decrements become deficient early in the course of T1DM in the vast majority of patients, often within the few years following diagnosis. However, because epinephrine compensates for deficient glucagon secretion, counterregulation is adequate in many of these patients. Nevertheless, the epinephrine secretory response to plasma glucose decrements becomes deficient typically later in the course of the disease and this defect has generally been attributed to autonomic neuropathy. Those patients with combined glucagon and epinephrine deficiencies are at substantially increased risk of severe hypoglycemia, at least during intensive therapy.

Particularly severe hypoglycemia has been reported in some patients treated with continuous subcutaneous insulin infusion (CSII). During CSII, the incidence of severe hypoglycemic episodes ranges between 0.1 and 1.2 per patient per year. As shown by White and associates,[21] patients having defective counterregulatory responses to insulin-induced hypoglycemia have a 20- to 25-fold greater chance of developing severe hypoglycemia than those who counterregulate correctly. In the Diabetes Control and Complications Trial (DCCT), the incidence of severe hypoglycemia was approximately three times higher in the intensive therapy group than in the conventional-therapy group.[22] In fact, in the intensive therapy group, there were 62 hypoglycemic episodes per 100 patient-years in which assistance was required in the provision of treatment, as compared to 19 such episodes per 100 patient-years in the conventional therapy group. This included 16 and 5 episodes of coma or seizure per 100 patient-years in the respective groups.

A recent meta-analysis of the effect of insulin lispro on severe hypoglycemia in patients with T1DM has shown a slight but significant reduction in the incidence of severe hypoglycemia as compared with regular insulin therapy; out of 2327 patients receiving lispro, 72 (3.1%) had a total of 102 severe episodes, compared to a group of 2339 receiving regular human insulin in which 102 (4.4%) had a total of 131 episodes ($p = 0.024$).[23]

The hypoglycemic effect of insulin can be exacerbated by the simultaneous ingestion of ethanol (see later) or of numerous drugs. These include sulfonylureas, biguanides, nonselective β-receptor blocking agents like propranolol, monoamine oxidase inhibitors,

ACE inhibitors, salicylates, and tetracyclines. When β-receptor blockade is needed in diabetics for cardiocirculatory reasons, selective β₁-receptor blocking agents like atenolol, metoprolol, bisoprolol, or acebutolol should be used. Potentiation of the hypoglycemic effect of insulin in diabetic patients can be observed in coexisting adrenocortical or pituitary insufficiency. Pituitary ablation, irradiation, and cryoablation have been used in the past for the treatment of advanced diabetic retinopathy. These procedures always result in increased insulin sensitivity and a potential danger of hypoglycemia.

In nondiabetic as well as in diabetic patients, insulin has been used for homicidal or suicidal purposes (reviewed in Marks and Teale[24]). Severe unexplained hypoglycemia in a nondiabetic individual should always raise the possibility of exogenous insulin administration, either suicidal or criminal. Such cases are more frequently encountered in the medical milieu or in the family or neighborhood of diabetics. Inadvertent insulin administration to a hospitalized nondiabetic patient has also been reported. In psychiatric patients, intentionally induced insulin shock therapy sometimes leads to prolonged hypoglycemia and irreversible brain damage. Factitious hypoglycemia due to clandestine self-administration of insulin must always be considered in the differential diagnosis of hypoglycemia. Again, this situation is more frequently encountered in the relatives of diabetic patients, in the medical or paramedical professions, and sometimes in diabetic patients themselves.

Oral Antidiabetic Agents

These drugs not infrequently cause hypoglycemia in diabetic patients, particularly if used inappropriately. Hypoglycemia is observed more frequently in patients taking long-acting sulfonylureas such as chlorpropamide and glibenclamide[25] or in those taking the highly potent sulfonylureas such as glibenclamide, glyburide, or glipizide. Overdose or insufficient food intake often explains the occurrence of hypoglycemia. Patients with renal or hepatic insufficiency, which may interfere with excretion or metabolism (or both) of these drugs, are especially susceptible to hypoglycemia.

As with insulin, oral antidiabetic agents can be involved in the pathogenesis of hypoglycemia in nondiabetic patients through inadvertent administration, accidental ingestion (mainly in children), a suicide attempt, and clandestine ingestion (a variety of factitious hypoglycemia). Over recent years, potentiation of the hypoglycemic properties of sulfonylureas by alcohol or by various drugs has been recognized as a major source of hypoglycemia. Table 58-2 summarizes the various mechanisms involved, and Table 58-3 gives the pharmacologic classes of the drugs to consider.[26] In contrast to sulfonylureas, biguanides, when taken alone, essentially never cause hypoglycemia, except in the case of simultaneous prolonged fasting or severe caloric and carbohydrate restriction. Hypo-

TABLE 58-2. Mechanisms by which Various Drugs Increase the Hypoglycemic Effect of Sulfonylureas

1. Increase in half-life due to inhibition of metabolism or excretion rate: ethanol, phenylbutazone, coumarin anticoagulants, chloramphenicol, doxycycline, antibacterial sulfonamides, phenyramidol, allopurinol
2. Competition for albumin binding sites: phenylbutazone, salicylates, antibacterial sulfonamides
3. Inhibition of gluconeogenesis, increase in glucose oxidation, or stimulation of insulin secretion: ethanol, β-adrenergic drugs, monoamine oxidase inhibitors, tranylcypromine, tromethamine.

TABLE 58-3. List of Main Drugs Capable of Inducing Hypoglycemic Episodes in Diabetic Patients Treated with Sulfonylureas

Antibacterial sulfonamides: sulfaphenazole, sulfamethoxime, sulfadimidine, sulfathiazole, sulfadiazone, sulfisoxazole, etc.
Analgesics and anti-inflammatory drugs: salicylates, phenylbutazone, oxyphenbutazone
Drugs affecting plasma lipoprotein concentration: clofibrate, fenofibrate
Antibiotics: chloramphenicol, novobiocin, tetracyclines, doxycycline
Miscellaneous: allopurinol, probenecid, phenyramidol, monoamine oxidase inhibitors, tromethamine, isoniazid, sulfinpyrazone, angiotensin-converting enzyme (ACE) inhibitors

glycemia is not caused by α-glucosidase inhibitors or glitazones used in monotherapy.

Alcohol

The ability of ethanol to induce hypoglycemia has long been recognized. In this section we will deal only with alcohol-induced fasting hypoglycemia; the so-called alcohol-promoted reactive hypoglycemia will be discussed later, in the section on functional hypoglycemias. Alcohol-induced fasting hypoglycemia characteristically develops in chronically malnourished or more acutely food-deprived individuals within 6–36 hours of ingesting a moderate to large amount of alcohol. Alcohol-induced fasting hypoglycemia results essentially from decreased hepatic glucose output due to impairment of liver gluconeogenesis, but other mechanisms such as ethanol-induced abnormalities in hypothalamic-pituitary-adrenal or hypothalamic-pituitary growth hormone secretions may be involved. Accidental ingestion of alcohol in children can also lead to severe hypoglycemia. As seen previously, alcohol also markedly potentiates the hypoglycemic effects of insulin and oral antidiabetic agents. According to Marks,[27] alcohol-induced fasting hypoglycemia often develops slowly and insidiously in the comatose person who has overindulged, and probably accounts for at least some of the deaths that occur in vagrants and others who are put unsupervised into police cells to sober up overnight and are found dead in the morning.

Other Exogenous Agents

Numerous other exogenous agents or drugs may cause hypoglycemia (see review in Marks and Teale[28]).

Salicylates

Salicylic acid, salicylate, and their derivatives have been recognized as potential hypoglycemic agents for more than 100 years, and the beneficial effect of sodium salicylate in diabetes mellitus was reported in the nineteenth-century pharmacopeia. The mechanism of their hypoglycemic properties is not fully elucidated, but involves increased utilization of glucose by peripheral tissues and reduction of gluconeogenesis. In salicylate poisoning, particularly in children below the age of 2 years, hypoglycemia may be observed together with the more common alteration of the acid–base equilibrium: initial respiratory alkalosis due to stimulation of the respiratory center and subsequent metabolic acidosis caused by the drug itself. Children with fever and dehydration are particularly prone to intoxication from relatively small doses of salicylate. Salicylates potentiate the hypoglycemic effects of sulfonylureas. Aspirin can also induce hypoglycemia in adults, mainly under exceptional circumstances such as when large doses are given to patients with renal failure.

Hypoglycins

Hypoglycins are compounds found in the unripe tropical fruit *Blighia sapida*. They are responsible for the Jamaican vomiting sickness, a syndrome characterized by vomiting, shock, and hypoglycemic coma; death is common. Hypoglycemia results from inhibition of liver gluconeogenesis and increased peripheral glucose utilization; these alterations apparently result from inhibition of long-chain fatty acid oxidation caused by the toxic agent.

Quinine

Severe hypoglycemia and hyperinsulinemia can occur in patients with *Plasmodium falciparum* malaria treated with intravenous quinine. The hypoglycemia is due to massive stimulation of insulin by quinine. The risk of hypoglycemia is particularly high in patients with cerebral malaria. These patients require frequent blood glucose monitoring, and massive intravenous glucose infusion.

β-Receptor Blocking Agents

As already mentioned, nonselective β-receptor blocking agents potentiate the hypoglycemic action of both insulin and sulfonylurea-type drugs. Furthermore, β-blockers may favor hypoglycemia by their inhibitory effect on adipose tissue lipolysis, which provides alternative fuels when the glucose concentration is low. Consequently, hypoglycemia due to β-blockers has been observed in young children, usually after a 6- to 10-hour fast. Maternal therapy with β-blockers may affect the fetus and exaggerate neonatal hypoglycemia.

Pentamidine

Used in the treatment of *Pneumocystis carinii* infection, an opportunistic infection frequently seen in patients with the acquired immunodeficiency syndrome (AIDS), pentamidine has been reported to induce massive cytolysis of the β cells of the islets of Langerhans, a process leading to temporary hyperinsulinemia and hypoglycemia followed by insulinopenic diabetes.

Other Drugs

Ouabain, mebendazole, isoproterenol, tris(hydroxymethyl) aminomethane (THAM), mesoxalate, disopyramide, tranylcypromine, and possibly monoamine oxidase inhibitors may cause hypoglycemia by stimulating insulin release. Potassium para-aminobenzoate, haloperidol, propoxyphene, anabolic steroids, perhexilin, and guanethidine have been incriminated as possible causes of hypoglycemia through unknown mechanisms. Clofibrate and angiotensin-converting enzyme inhibitors have been reported to potentiate the hypoglycemic properties of oral antidiabetic agents.

Endogenous Hypoglycemia

Endogenous hypoglycemia may be organic (insulinoma, extrapancreatic neoplasms, or due to inborn errors of metabolism) or functional.

Organic Hypoglycemias

Insulinomas and Related Disorders

Insulinoma   Insulinomas are uncommon neoplasms that derive from the β cells of the islets of Langerhans.[29,30] The majority of these tumors, 68–85% according to published series, are single, benign adenomas; multiple adenomas or scattered microadenomas

are observed in 10–19% of the cases; and islet cell carcinomas are less frequent (2–11% of cases). Islet cell adenoma can be part of the pluriglandular syndrome. It has sometimes been reported to coexist with the pancreatic gastrinoma of the Zollinger-Ellison syndrome.

Nesidioblastosis and β-Cell Hyperplasia   Nesidioblastosis, now called persistent hyperinsulinemic hypoglycemia of infancy (PHHI), is a rare disease leading to persistent hypoglycemia of infancy. It is histologically characterized by the budding off from duct epithelium of endocrine cells and by the presence in the pancreas of microadenomas. The onset of symptoms of β-cell hyperplasia may occur during the first days of life, but most commonly appears within the first 6 months. A few cases with symptoms beginning later than 1 year of age have been reported. The group of Saudubray in Paris[31] has recently reported the features of 52 neonates with hyperinsulinism. Thirty neonates had diffuse β-cell hyperfunction, and 22 had focal adenomatous islet cell hyperplasia. Among the latter, the lesions were in the head of the pancreas in nine, the isthmus in three, the body in eight, and the tail in two. Partial pancreatectomy has been successful in curing the 19 out of the 22 neonates in whom this procedure has been attempted. Recent studies (reviewed in Thomas[32]) have shown that congenital hyperinsulinism with focal or diffuse nesidioblastosis can be associated with several mutations affecting the β cell, such as the genes encoding for the sulfonylurea receptor, glucokinase, or glutamate dehydrogenase.

Extrapancreatic Neoplasms

In a review on tumor hypoglycemia, Kahn[33] stated that it was likely that non–islet cell tumors would be second only to islet cell tumors as a cause of chronic fasting hypoglycemia in the adult. Most of these neoplasms are large and present as masses in the mediastinum or the retroperitoneal space. According to Kahn,[33] 45% of the tumors have a mesenchymal origin (Doege-Potter syndrome), 23% are hepatomas (Nadler-Wolfer-Elliott syndrome), 10% are adrenocortical carcinomas (Anderson's syndrome), 8% are gastrointestinal tumors, 6% are lymphomas and leukemias, and 8% miscellaneous. Tumor hypoglycemia may occur in any age group, but is most common in adults between 40 and 70 years of age. The pathogenesis of the hypoglycemia in these tumors has been investigated by numerous groups in the past 20 years. Among the many theories that have been advanced to explain hypoglycemia, the production of an insulin-like substance has been considered likely by many investigators.[34–36] A large form of insulin-like growth factor II, known as big IGF-II, has now been recognized to be responsible for the hypoglycemia by direct insulin-like action on nonhepatic tissues and the suppression of growth hormone secretion. Severe hypoglycemia caused by elevated IGF-II levels has also been reported in patients with acinar cell carcinoma of the pancreas,[37] solitary fibrous tumor of the pleura,[38] metastasis from a meningeal hemangiopericytoma,[39] and disseminated breast cancer.[40]

Inborn Errors of Metabolism

One may argue against our choice to classify the inborn errors of metabolism as a cause of organic hypoglycemia. We certainly agree that some of these syndromes may also be considered as functional, e.g., when the symptoms occur only after ingestion of a single sugar, like fructose in the hereditary fructose intolerance syndrome. We think, however, that in many respects, these syndromes, characterized by a well-defined enzymatic defect, are really organic at the molecular level (see review in Lteif and Schwenk[41]).

Hereditary Fructose Intolerance (HFI)

Hereditary fructose intolerance, initially described as idiosyncratic to fructose, is a rare, autosomal recessively inherited, inborn error of metabolism characterized by an almost total lack of liver fructose-1-phosphate aldolase. Ingestion of fructose leads to intracellular accumulation of large amounts of fructose-1-phosphate. This in turn induces a decreased intracellular level of inorganic phosphorus, a derangement of the phosphate potential, and secondary enzyme inhibition by fructose-1-phosphate. These secondary enzymatic blocks are (1) an inhibition of further phosphorylation of fructose by fructokinase, leading to fructosemia and fructosuria; (2) an inhibition of liver phosphorylase; and (3) an inhibition of the remaining fructose-1,6-diphosphate liver aldolase activity. Inhibition of phosphorylase impairs glycogenolysis, a phenomenon that is favored by the low inorganic phosphorus concentrations. Inhibition of fructose-1,6-diphosphate liver aldolase, the enzyme that should perform the condensation of trioses to fructose-1,6-diphosphate, results in impairment of liver gluconeogenesis. Simultaneous inhibition of liver glycogenolysis and gluconeogenesis explains why fructose administration in HFI induces profound hypoglycemia, accompanied by convulsions and coma. Clinical manifestations at onset of symptoms can be rather unspecific, but usually the first signs of the disease start with exposure to saccharose. Besides hypoglycemia, the symptoms involve vomiting, poor weight gain, anorexia, various degrees of liver dysfunction, and perturbations of renal tubular function.

Fructose-1,6-Disphosphatase Deficiency

In this rare autosomal recessive disease, the lack of functioning fructose-1,6-phosphatase has little consequence as long as the liver glycogen stores are sufficient. When liver glycogen is depleted (e.g., after 12- to 24-hour fasting), hypoglycemia occurs, often accompanied by severe lactic acidosis. Hypoglycemia results from impairment in liver gluconeogenesis, and lactic acidosis is due to the transformation of various gluconeogenic precursors (glycerol, amino acids) or of fructose into lactic acid.

Galactosemia

Although hypoglycemia is the rule in hereditary fructose intolerance, it is less frequent in galactosemia. In this autosomal recessively transmitted disease, the missing enzyme is galactose-1-phosphate uridyl transferase, the enzyme permitting the transformation of galactose-1-phosphate into UDP-galactose. The major symptoms of galactosemia (jaundice, hepatomegaly, cirrhosis, kidney function alterations, cataracts, and mental retardation) seem to result from the accumulation of galactose-1-phosphate. Hypoglycemia, occurring after galactose exposure, would be the result of inhibition of liver glucose output due to inhibition of phosphoglucomutase by galactose-1-phosphate.

Phosphoenolpyruvate Carboxykinase Deficiency

Phosphoenolpyruvate carboxykinase (PEPCK) is a key enzyme in gluconeogenesis. This defect has been reported in a few cases of infants with severe fasting hypoglycemia.

Inborn Errors of Glycogen Metabolism

Among the 11 varieties of glycogen storage diseases now recognized, only some lead to hypoglycemia. Type I glycogen storage disease, or von Gierke's disease, is due to a lack of liver glucose-6-phosphatase. Without this enzyme, the liver cannot produce glucose either from glycogenolysis or by gluconeogenesis (glucose-6-phosphate is an obligatory pathway in both processes). Unless carbohydrates are frequently given, severe hypoglycemia occurs, accompanied by excessive production of lactic acid. The clinical picture consists of small stature, puppet face, increased subcutaneous fat tissue, and massive hepatomegaly. Type II glycogen storage disease, or Pompe's disease, results from a deficiency in the lysosomal enzyme α-1,4-glucosidase, as demonstrated in 1963 by Hers. Lysosomal accumulation of glycogen causes cardiomegaly and heart failure, macroglossia, and hypotonia of voluntary muscles. This disease does not lead to hypoglycemia. Type III glycogen storage disease, or Forbe's disease, is characterized by accumulation of structurally abnormal glycogen in all tissues. It is due to various degrees of enzymatic defect at the level of the debranching enzyme (or enzymes). The debranching enzymes control the hydrolysis of glucose moieties at the branch points of glycogen where they are joined in a 1:6 linkage. When these enzymes are deficient, hydrolysis of the glycogen molecule at the level of the 1:4 linkages is possible. Partial hydrolysis of glycogen and intact mechanisms of gluconeogenesis explain why hypoglycemia is usually mild and occurs only under conditions of prolonged food deprivation. Type IV glycogen storage disease, due to a defect in the branching enzyme that leads to accumulation of an abnormal glycogen (starchlike amylopectin), causes liver cirrhosis and premature death; there is no hypoglycemia. Type V glycogen storage disease, or MacArdle's disease, is due to an absence of muscle phosphorylase that leads to the occurrence of muscular cramping upon exertion; here again, there is no hypoglycemia. Type VI glycogen storage disease, or Hers' disease, is an autosomal recessive disorder due to low overall liver phosphorylase activity that leads to hepatomegaly; it has been reported to be associated with mild to moderate hypoglycemia that occurs with fasting in young infants. Type VII glycogen storage disease results from deficient muscle phosphofructokinase activity. The symptoms are similar to those of McArdle's disease; no hypoglycemia is recorded. Type VIII glycogen storage disease is a rare disorder in which incomplete activation of the adenylate cyclase system leads to low phosphorylase activity and accumulation of glycogen in the liver and the central nervous system. Type IX glycogen storage disease exists in two forms. In type IXa, an autosomal recessive disease, a partial defect in phosphorylase kinase leads to accumulation of glycogen in the liver and secondary hepatomegaly. In type IXb, the recessive trait is sex-linked, affecting only males; the phosphorylase kinase defect is relatively severe and leads to accumulation of liver glycogen; and fasting hypoglycemia is observed. Type X glycogen storage disease is an extremely rare condition in which excessive liver and muscle glycogen storage is due to deficient activity of the cyclic AMP–dependent protein kinase, with the result that all phosphorylase would be in the β (or inactive) form, and therefore glycogen would not be degraded.

Functional Hypoglycemias

Alimentary Hypoglycemia

Consumption of carbohydrates by individuals who have had a gastrectomy may lead to severe hypoglycemia within 1–2 hours after the meal. This disorder is occasionally seen in patients who have not had a gastrectomy, but who for various other reasons have rapid gastric emptying. Rapid gastric emptying is frequently encountered in hyperthyroidism. It had been thought that the rapid dumping of carbohydrate into the upper small intestine and the consequent early hyperglycemia cause reactive hyperinsulinemia and alimentary hypoglycemia. It is now generally accepted that, in addition, several gut factors are released after glucose ingestion, and act in concert with glucose, or even prior to glucose, to stimulate insulin secretion. Among these factors, secretin, glucagon-like peptide 1 (GLP-1), and cholecystokinin may be involved, as is gastric inhibitory polypeptide (GIP).[42] A recent study has suggested that *Helicobacter pylori*–induced gastritis may contribute to the occurrence of postprandial symptomatic hypoglycemia, since *H. pylori* eradication is associated with a reduction in number and severity of postprandial hypoglycemic attacks.[43]

Spontaneous Reactive Hypoglycemia

This entity is poorly defined. The term is usually applied to a syndrome with the following features: (1) symptoms that resemble those seen in insulin-induced hypoglycemia (diaphoresis, tachycardia, tremulousness, and headache, among others), but these are often accompanied by other symptoms less typical of hypoglycemia, such as fatigue, drowsiness, feelings of incipient syncope, depersonalization, irritability, and lack of motivation; (2) symptoms that may be episodic, and are sometimes aggravated by carbohydrate-rich meals; and (3) plasma glucose concentrations that drop to 45 mg/dL (2.5 mmol/L) or less at one or more of the half-hourly samples taken in a 5- to 6-hour glucose tolerance test. Abnormal insulin secretory patterns have been reported in certain patients, presenting as reactive hypoglycemia associated with impaired glucose tolerance (delayed and sometimes excessive insulin response), obesity (excessive insulin response), or renal glycosuria (excessive insulin response in about half the cases). Excessive insulin response has also been observed in about 50% of patients with isolated reactive hypoglycemia.

This entity has become widespread, particularly in the United States, over the past 30 years, but is more rarely diagnosed elsewhere in the world. The American Diabetes Association and the Endocrine Society have issued a joint statement to the effect that this entity is probably overdiagnosed. Indeed, the very existence of this condition is now called into question following several studies that have demonstrated that 25–30% of apparently healthy individuals without any hypoglycemic symptoms may exhibit low plasma glucose values when given a glucose load. Furthermore, the similarity of the symptoms to those of hyperventilation, and indeed with other functional syndromes, emphasizes the need to reevaluate the very existence of so-called functional or reactive hypoglycemia. The question of cause and effect has not been settled. It would be reasonable at present to restrict the diagnosis of reactive hypoglycemia to individuals in whom hypoglycemic blood glucose levels are demonstrated in samples taken after the sort of meals that are said to induce their symptoms. As shown by Palardy and associates,[44] these samples should preferably be taken at the time of symptoms and not only after a glucose load, which, as noted above, often produces low blood glucose values in normal people. Abnormalities in counterregulatory hormones have not been conclusively demonstrated to be associated with idiopathic reactive hypoglycemia. Increased insulin sensitivity has been documented in a euglycemic hyperinsulinemic glucose clamp in 10 out of 16 patients investigated by Tamburrano and colleagues.[45] Furthermore, and as discussed by Lefèbvre,[46] some patients have adrenergic responses after a meal or during OGTT *without* hypoglycemia. Such "adrenergic hormone postprandial syndrome"

probably results from an altered glycemic threshold (a higher glucose level) for generating an adrenergic response, which results in confusion.[47]

A critical analysis of the reactive hypoglycemia syndrome can be found in the proceedings of an international symposium held in Rome in September 1986.[48,49]

Alcohol-Promoted Reactive Hypoglycemia

O'Keefe and Marks[50] have demonstrated that alcohol given in moderate doses (50 g) increases the insulin response elicited by the ingestion of insulinotropic carbohydrates, like saccharose, but not of noninsulinotropic ones, like fructose. They emphasized that drinks that contain both alcohol and glucose or saccharose (beer, gin and tonic, rum and cola, whisky and ginger ale, among others) are more likely to provoke hypoglycemia on an empty stomach than those containing only alcohol and saccharin or alcohol and fructose. Flanagan and colleagues[51] have confirmed that in otherwise healthy individuals, a combination of gin and regular tonic can induce reactive hypoglycemia. Furthermore, they have shown that acute ingestion of alcohol impairs the epinephrine response and markedly suppresses the release of growth hormone in response to a fall in blood glucose levels.

Posthyperalimentation Hypoglycemia

Hypoglycemia has been reported following discontinuation of total parenteral alimentation. It is considered to be secondary to residual effects of insulin from chronically stimulated islets of Langerhans.

Endocrine Deficiency States

Hypoglycemia Due to Glucocorticoid Deficiency   Glucocorticoid deficiency may induce fasting hypoglycemia due to defective gluconeogenesis.[52] This condition may be encountered in acute or chronic adrenal insufficiency (Addison's disease), in congenital adrenal hyperplasia, as a consequence of removal or destruction of the adrenals, in panhypopituitarism, in isolated ACTH deficiency, and other conditions. Spontaneous hypoglycemia in patients with glucocorticoid deficiency mainly occurs if other precipitating factors such as alcohol ingestion, pregnancy, or prolonged fasting are present. It is important to recall here the danger of insulin or sulfonylurea administration to any patient with adrenal insufficiency.

Hypoglycemia in Growth Hormone Deficiency   Growth hormone deficiency leads to hypoglycemia during a prolonged fast. This situation is accompanied by a marked sensitivity to both exogenous and endogenous insulin. Growth hormone deficiency may be isolated or part of panhypopituitarism (removal or destruction of the hypophysis). As reviewed by Gerich and Campbell,[53] the prevalence of fasting hypoglycemia is approximately 20% in children with hypopituitarism. Hypoglycemia occurs with equal frequency in children with isolated growth hormone deficiency and those with multiple pituitary defects. As noted previously, hypophysectomy results in increased insulin sensitivity, and therefore reduced insulin requirements.

Hypoglycemia and Catecholamine Deficiency   For many years epinephrine deficiency has been considered as a possible cause of hypoglycemia in children. The so-called Zetterström syndrome is observed predominantly in male infants of low birthweight who do not increase their urinary catecholamine excretion in response to insulin-induced hypoglycemia.

Hypoglycemia and Glucagon Deficiency Attempts to isolate a glucagon deficiency syndrome have been disappointing. Glucagon deficiency has been suspected, but not definitively proven, in some cases of neonatal hypoglycemia. In 1977, Vidnes and Øyasaeter[54] reported a patient with severe neonatal hypoglycemia with impairment of gluconeogenesis, in whom circulating glucagon levels were low (but not zero), and in whom treatment with glucagon resulted in a marked clinical improvement. Bleicher and colleagues[55] reported a case in whom arginine infusion induced hyperinsulinemia and hypoglycemia with unmeasurable plasma glucagon, an observation that supports the concept that the role of stimulation of glucagon by amino acids is to prevent hypoglycemia from the associated insulin release. The suggestion that glucagon deficiency may play a role in the pathogenesis of certain cases of reactive hypoglycemia seems to be ruled out.

Severe Liver Disease

Fasting hypoglycemia may result from severe liver damage caused by hepatitis (hepatitis fulminans), various poisons (carbon tetrachloride, chloroform, benzene derivatives, *Amanita phalloides* toxin, hypoglycins, and others), primary carcinoma of the liver, or thrombosis of the subhepatic veins (Budd-Chiari syndrome). Hypoglycemia results from insufficient liver glucose output.

Profound Malnutrition

Extreme malnutrition leads to hypoglycemia. It is also found with relative frequency in kwashiorkor. In infants, hypoglycemia may result from acute or chronic diarrhea.

Prolonged Exercise

In prolonged exercise, the glucose turnover is markedly increased because of simultaneously increased production and utilization. If exercise is too prolonged, too severe, and if nutrient intake and carbohydrate stores are insufficient, hypoglycemia can occur.

Autoimmune Insulin Syndrome

Since the description of the first case of autoimmune insulin syndrome in 1970, more than 200 patients with this syndrome have been reported, mainly in Japan.[56] The main clinical feature of the syndrome is the presence of hypoglycemic attacks associated with the presence of spontaneous antibodies against insulin (see review in Redmon and Nuttall[57]). The mechanism whereby spontaneous antibodies against insulin are generated remains obscure. At least one-third of the patients with the syndrome have been treated with some drug containing a sulfhydryl group, like methimazole or penicillamine. These patients usually have huge amounts of extractable insulin in their plasma. The affinity constant of the antibodies of patients with the autoimmune insulin syndrome, as tested in Scatchard plots, is usually much smaller than that of insulin-treated diabetes. Hypoglycemia is considered to be the consequence of inappropriate release of insulin from the insulin-antibody complexes.

Antibodies Against the Insulin Receptor

Autoantibodies against the insulin receptor are usually observed in patients with type B extreme insulin resistance associated with acanthosis nigricans. As reviewed recently,[57] in some of

these patients the hyperglycemia remitted and the patients developed fasting hypoglycemia. Furthermore, some patients have been reported in whom fasting hypoglycemia was the initial presenting sign, suggesting the presence of autoantibodies against the insulin receptor. The hypoglycemia is attributed to an insulinomimetic action of the antibody. The reasons that some patients develop insulin resistance and hyperglycemia and others develop hypoglycemia are not yet clear. Remissions can be obtained by plasmapheresis, immunosuppression with alkylating agents, or glucocorticoid therapy.

Functional or Transient Hypoglycemia in Infancy

An encyclopedic review of hypoglycemia at birth and in infancy has been presented by Lteif and Schwenk.[41] Many of the causes of infant hypoglycemia have already been mentioned. Other causes of neonatal or infant hypoglycemia will be briefly considered next.

Transient Neonatal Hypoglycemia Transient neonatal hypoglycemia is common[58]; it can be observed in about 10% of live births, will be symptomatic in 30% of these cases, and occurs only during the first 3 days of life. It may be due to insufficient supply (delayed feeding), insufficient hepatic glycogen stores (prematurity, intrauterine malnutrition, dysmaturity, and perinatal stress), anaerobic energy production (secondary to hypoxia), or increased heat production (secondary to hypothermia).

Infants of Diabetic Mothers Infants of diabetic mothers frequently develop severe hypoglycemia during their first hours of life. It results from hyperinsulinemia caused by the β-cell hyperplasia, itself induced by fetal hyperglycemia of maternal origin. Relative hypoglucagonemia may be a contributing factor.

Erythroblastosis Fetalis Hypoglycemia is frequently associated with erythroblastosis fetalis, a consequence of rhesus immunization. As in the infants of diabetic mothers, hypoglycemia results from hyperinsulinemia caused by hyperplasia of the islets of Langerhans.

Leucine-Induced Hypoglycemia Certain infants develop hypoglycemia when given leucine or leucine-containing food. It should be emphasized that cow's milk is richer in leucine than mother's milk. Excessive insulin response to leucine is characteristic of the syndrome, and relative basal hyperinsulinism is also found when fasting hypoglycemia is present. Hypertrophy and hyperplasia of the islets of Langerhans are frequently found. In most cases, the onset of symptoms takes place prior to 6 months of age. Severe hypoglycemic attacks may occur postprandially or after short periods of fasting. Severe mental retardation occurs if diagnosis is delayed.

Ketotic or Ketogenic Hypoglycemia This form of childhood hypoglycemia is classically considered to be one of the most common forms of hypoglycemia of childhood. It is characterized by sporadic attacks of hypoglycemia and ketosis that occur preferentially after food deprivation between the ages of 1 and 8 years, usually with spontaneous recovery before 10 years of age. Hypoglycemia is consistently evoked within 24 hours by a hypocaloric ketogenic diet, but normal children exposed to the same diet may show glucose levels equally as low as those of patients with ketotic hypoglycemia. As reviewed recently,[41] more data accumulate indicating that ketotic hypoglycemia is not a specific entity, but may represent a metabolic derangement in the presence of various biochemical abnormalities; one of the main derangements leading to hypoglycemia and ketosis seems to be any disturbance of the gluconeogenic mechanisms, due either to an enzymatic block or due to a diminished availability of substrate. In addition to the idiopathic form, ketotic or ketogenic hypoglycemia has been reported in fructose-1,6-diphosphatase deficiency, hypoalaninemia, growth hormone deficiency, adrenal medullary hyporesponsiveness, adrenal cortical insufficiency, branched-chain aminoacidemia, glucose-6-phosphatase deficiency, and amylo-1,6-glucosidase deficiency.

Maple Syrup Urine Disease Hypoglycemia is frequently encountered in patients with maple syrup urine disease. Its mechanism is still obscure. It usually clears with appropriate dietary treatment.

Adrenal Hyporesponsiveness Hypoglycemia with adrenal hyporesponsiveness is a distinct clinical entity found most frequently in children born small for dates after a complicated pregnancy. The hypoglycemic attacks, occurring between 0.5 and 5 years of age, are sporadic and occur without pallor or perspiration. The insufficient rise in urinary epinephrine during hypoglycemia often associated with insufficient cortisol rise has been interpreted as evidence for a dysfunction of the hypothalamic hypoglycemia center.

INVESTIGATION OF A PATIENT WITH POSSIBLE HYPOGLYCEMIA

Hypoglycemia should be suspected in all patients exhibiting the following signs and symptoms:

1. Presenting with the symptoms already noted
2. With seizures or episodic psychiatric syndromes
3. With coma of unknown origin
4. Presenting with stereotyped symptom patterns relative to similar or identical circumstances, such as in the fasting state, after muscular exercise, or a few hours after a meal
5. Any patient at risk of developing hypoglycemia (diabetic patients treated with insulin or sulfonylureas, alcoholics, and others).

However, before a detailed investigation is carried out, hypoglycemia must always be confirmed by an accurate measurement of the blood glucose concentration.

History

A complete history is essential in patients with possible hypoglycemic disorders. Relief of symptoms after ingesting food or sugar suggests the general diagnosis, whereas the relation of the symptoms to other events suggests the etiology. If the symptoms occur after a meal, the hypoglycemia is probably alimentary or reactive, whereas signs occurring in the fasting state or after exercise suggest organic hypoglycemia.

In diabetics receiving insulin, particular attention should be paid to the true dose of insulin injected, the site of injection (it has been claimed that insulin is more rapidly absorbed from an exercising limb than a resting site), the nature and quantity of food ingested, the importance of physical activity prior to the hypoglycemic episode, and the ingestion of alcohol or of various drugs. In diabetic patients on oral medications, the nature of the drug used should be documented, and the number of tablets ingested should be assessed. One of the major aims of the anamnesis should be to detect any drug that may have been simultaneously ingested and may have potentiated the hypoglycemic properties of the oral antidiabetic agents. Here also, alcohol should not be forgotten.

In a patient suspected of an insulinoma, the history frequently reveals that hypoglycemic symptoms are precipitated by fasting or exercise and relieved by food or sugar ingestion. This situation is also encountered in patients with extrapancreatic tumor hypoglycemia. In these patients, however, the discovery of the tumor often precedes the symptoms of hypoglycemia, but the reverse has been reported. Symptoms occurring early after food ingestion suggest alimentary hypoglycemia, while symptoms occurring 90 minutes to 5 hours after the meal suggest reactive hypoglycemia. The nature of the drink mixtures and cocktails consumed will permit diagnosis of alcohol-promoted reactive hypoglycemia. The interrogation of parents of infants presenting with hypoglycemia may lead to the diagnosis. For instance, symptoms occurring after ingestion of milk suggest leucine-induced hypoglycemia or galactose intolerance, whereas the abrupt occurrence of vomiting and hypoglycemia when a child who is breastfed is given his first drink of orange juice or is changed over to a diet containing fructose strongly suggests fructose intolerance. By definition, the history is often misleading in factitious hypoglycemia.

In a patient suspected of an autoimmune insulin syndrome, previous intake of drugs containing sulfhydryl groups (methimazole, penicillamine, and related compounds) should be carefully probed.

Physical Examination

As seen previously, when hypoglycemia is present, the symptoms result from both neuroglycopenia and the counterregulatory adrenergic reaction. In case of doubt, the prompt cessation of symptoms upon ingestion or injection of glucose is an easy means to confirm the diagnosis. It is important to recall here the fundamental rule that a blood sample must always be drawn to authenticate the hypoglycemia before glucose is administered. Between crises, the physical examination may be completely normal.

One should pay special attention to the following signs:

- A weight gain may occur in certain patients if hypoglycemic episodes are frequent; this has been reported in both organic (e.g., insulinoma) and functional (e.g., alimentary or reactive) hypoglycemia.
- A weight loss can be seen in nonpancreatic tumor hypoglycemia as well as in hypoglycemia associated with pituitary or adrenal insufficiency.
- Injection sites should be sought in factitious, suicidal, or criminal hypoglycemia.
- Acanthosis nigricans may be present in patients presenting with hypoglycemia due to antibodies against the insulin receptor with insulinomimetic properties.

- Hepatomegaly is usually present in the Nadler-Wolfer-Elliott syndrome and in various hypoglycemias of childhood (e.g., galactosemia and types I, VI, IX, and X glycogenosis).
- Abdominal and thoracic masses should be sought in tumor-associated hypoglycemia.
- Psychoneurotic symptoms are frequently associated with reactive hypoglycemia.

Laboratory and Technical Investigations in Endogenous Hypoglycemia

In this section, we briefly survey the main laboratory and technical investigations available at present to diagnose the most frequently encountered causes of endogenous hypoglycemia.

How to Explore a Patient Suspected of Presenting with an Insulinoma

An insulinoma should be suspected in any patient presenting with the triad described by Whipple: symptoms precipitated by fasting or exercise, hypoglycemia associated with symptoms, and relief of symptoms by glucose. However, as emphasized in all reviews on the subject, the demonstration of endogenous plasma insulin levels inappropriate to the prevailing blood glucose levels is the cornerstone of the diagnosis. Simultaneous determination of blood glucose and plasma insulin after an overnight fast or during a 24- to 48-hour fast is one of the best procedures to demonstrate relative hyperinsulinism. Various insulin suppression or stimulation tests are also helpful. Finally, when one is convinced of the diagnosis of insulinoma, every effort should be made to attempt to localize the tumor before sending the patient to surgery.

Basal Plasma Levels of Glucose and Insulin

Relative basal hyperinsulinism can often be demonstrated by the repeated (5–12 times), simultaneous determination of blood glucose and plasma insulin after an overnight fast. In normal individuals, fasting plasma glucose concentration is usually 70–110 mg/dL (3.9–6.1 mmol/L), with plasma insulin concentrations usually ranging between 5 and 15 μU/mL. In obese individuals, basal plasma insulin is usually increased due to insulin resistance, and values up to 40–50 μU/mL have been reported.

Circulating Levels of Glucose, Insulin, and C Peptide During a Prolonged Fast

A 24- to 48-hour fast in normal individuals is accompanied by a modest decline in blood glucose and a significant decline in plasma insulin and C peptide. The decrease in plasma insulin is usually 30–40%, relative to the values measured after an overnight fast. In patients with insulinoma, blood glucose declines markedly during fasting, while insulin and C-peptide plasma levels remain stable or decline only very moderately; relative hyperinsulinism therefore appears. If fasting has to be interrupted due to the occurrence of clinical hypoglycemia, a sample for blood glucose and plasma insulin determinations should always be taken before interrupting the fast or injecting glucose. According to Service and colleagues, a C-peptide plasma level above 0.2 nmol/L at the end of a prolonged fast is highly suggestive of the presence of an insulinoma.[59] In most patients with an insulinoma, symptomatic hypoglycemia will occur within a few hours of food deprivation.[60] In some, however, continuation of the fast for up to 72 hours may be necessary.[61] Continuous nocturnal blood glucose monitoring has been used to gather evidence of episodes of nocturnal hypoglycemia in insulinoma patients.

Insulin Suppression Tests

Suppression of endogenous insulin secretion by hypoglycemia induced by exogenous insulin administration is an elegant means to differentiate between insulin secretion under physiologic control and uncontrolled insulin release by tumoral tissue. In normal subjects, insulin-induced hypoglycemia induces a more than 50% reduction of plasma C-peptide circulating levels, indicating inhibition of endogenous insulin secretion by hypoglycemia (and maybe partly by insulin itself). Such inhibition is not observed in 90% of the insulinoma cases. The diazoxide infusion (600 mg over 1 hour in 500 mL saline) or oral (600 mg) administration tests can be confirmatory in showing a suppression of insulin and a correction of fasting hypoglycemia. These tests may be useful in foreseeing the effectiveness of chronic diazoxide therapy when surgical removal of the tumor cannot be realized. The response of basal and glucose- or glucagon-stimulated insulin release to an intravenous infusion of somatostatin is heterogeneous in the small series of patients studied with benign or malignant insulinoma. This test seems of little value in the diagnosis of insulinoma.

Other Determinations

In normal subjects, plasma proinsulin represents only 10–15% of the total immunoreactive insulin. In 85% of patients with insulinoma, the proinsulin component has been found to be elevated and exceeded 25% of total fasting insulin immunoreactivity. Values up to 80% have been reported in malignant insulinomas. Plasma levels of glucagon and pancreatic polypeptide may be elevated in insulinoma. Low levels of HbA$_{1c}$ have been reported in 25% of the patients with insulinoma.

Localization of the Tumor

Diagnosis of an insulinoma on radiologic evidence is often difficult due to the usually small size of the tumor (see review in Grant[62]). Selective arteriography via the celiac axis and the superior mesenteric artery localizes the tumor(s) in approximately 50% of the cases, but occasionally false localizations have been suggested by the arteriography. Tomodensitometry and ultrasonography help in the diagnosis of relatively large tumors whose diameter exceeds 2–3 cm. Magnetic resonance imaging using a high gradient power 0.5-T magnet has recently been shown most useful in the preoperative localization of insulinomas.[63] Percutaneous transhepatic catheterization of the splenic and portal veins can be used for selective retrograde venous angiography and for selective blood sampling and subsequent insulin plasma measurements: Higher plasma insulin levels are found in the vein or veins draining the tumor. One should always remember that in about 10% of cases there is more than one insulin-secreting tumor. External scanning of the liver following intravenous administration of technetium sulfur colloid or radiolabeled octreotide[64] can detect hepatic metastasis of malignant insulinomas. Günther and associates[65] have reported their experience in the pre- and perioperative localization of small (<2-cm diameter) islet cell tumors. Of 31 small tumors, 27 were correctly localized using a combined diagnostic approach: ultrasound was successful in 12 of 20 tumors, tomodensitometry in 9 of 21, angiography in 20 of 31, intra-arterial digital subtraction angiography in 1 of 2, and pancreatic venous sampling in 13 of 16. The smallest tumor found by ultrasound was 7 mm in diameter. Intraoperative ultrasound demonstrated all nine insulinomas examined. Rösch and associates[66] have shown that endoscopic ultrasonography is a highly sensitive and specific procedure for the localization of pancreatic endocrine tumors. Using this procedure, they were able to localize 32 of 39 tumors (sensitivity 82%), and no tumor was incorrectly localized. Among 22 patients who underwent both angiography and endoscopic ultrasonography, ultrasonography was significantly more sensitive than angiography for tumor localization (sensitivity 82% versus 27%). Among 19 control patients without pancreatic exocrine tumors, endoscopic ultrasonography was negative in 18 (specificity 95%). Proye and colleagues[67] have recently reported the potential of combining endoscopic ultrasonography and somatostatin receptor scintigraphy. Glucose-controlled insulin and glucose infusions (by an artificial pancreas) during surgical manipulation of the gland may help in localizing the tumor[68] as will the intra-arterial infusion of calcium.[69,70] Like others,[71] we have observed that intraoperative ultrasensitive pancreas echotomography is also a most valuable procedure for localizing the tumor(s).[72] In view of the performance of the combination of surgical operation and intraoperative ultrasonography, several groups now consider that preoperative localization of insulinomas is not necessary.[73,74]

How to Investigate a Patient Suspected of Presenting with Non–Islet Cell Tumor Hypoglycemia

Basal and Fasting Levels of Glucose and Insulin

As in patients with insulinoma, patients with non–islet cell large tumor hypoglycemic syndrome usually have low fasting blood glucose, and in a starvation test, blood glucose continuously falls. In contrast to patients with insulinoma, insulin plasma levels are low and decrease to almost zero during fasting.

Dynamic Tests

Insulin suppression and stimulation tests are of little help. Insulin is usually markedly suppressed by the prevailing hypoglycemia. In provocative tests (with tolbutamide, glucagon, or leucine), the insulin response is usually low. In the OGTT, abnormal glucose tolerance with low insulin response is frequently found. The glycemic response to glucagon is usually normal, indicating the persistence of significant amounts of glycogen stores.

Other Determinations

As stated previously, hypoglycemia results from increased circulating levels of insulin-like growth factors, recently identified to be a large form of insulin-like growth factor II (big IGF-II).

Localization of the Tumor

Most of these tumors are large or very large and easy to localize on the basis of careful clinical examination, routine x-ray investigation (chest or abdominal roentgenogram), magnetic resonance imaging (MRI), or ultrasonography.

How to Investigate a Patient Suspected of Alimentary or Reactive Hypoglycemia

As stated earlier, there is little doubt that it would be ideal to restrict the diagnosis of alimentary or reactive hypoglycemia to individuals in whom hypoglycemic blood glucose levels (below 45 mg/dL or 2.5 mmol/L) can be demonstrated in blood samples taken in everyday life,[44–46] preferably with the use of a memory glucometer,[46] or after the sort of meals that are said to induce the

symptoms. For practical reasons, however, this is rarely the case, and the oral glucose tolerance test (OGTT) is still widely (if not wildly) used as a routine tool for the diagnosis of the various sorts of postprandial hypoglycemia.

The Oral Glucose Tolerance Test

In the standard OGTT, using 100 g glucose, or as more recently recommended by various authorities, 75 g glucose, one or more blood glucose values below 45 mg/dL are found in these patients. The glucose nadir may occur early, at 90 or 120 minutes, and when this occurs it is usually preceded by an excessive early rise in alimentary hyperglycemia. In reactive hypoglycemia, the glucose nadir is usually found 3, 4, or even 5 hours after the ingestion of glucose. As already mentioned, excessive insulin response due to the rapid dumping of glucose into the upper small intestine is likely to be the cause of alimentary hypoglycemia. In reactive hypoglycemia, delayed and sometimes excessive insulin response is observed when the glucose tolerance is reduced; excessive insulin response is found associated with obesity or with half the cases of renal glycosuria. Excessive insulin response has also been observed in about 50% of patients with isolated reactive hypoglycemia. In 50% of patients with renal glycosuria and in 50% of patients with the syndrome, the insulin response is normal in time and magnitude.[75] In the late phase of the OGTT, an unequivocal rise in cortisol, glucagon, and growth hormone occurs following the glucose nadir.

Investigation of Gastric Emptying

Rapid gastric emptying, the causative factor in alimentary hypoglycemia, can be demonstrated by x-ray or isotopic studies of the upper gastrointestinal tract.

How To Deal with a Patient Suspected of Factitious Hypoglycemia

Surreptitious self-administration of insulin or sulfonylureas is not easy to detect[24] and can lead to a false diagnosis of islet cell disease.

C Peptide Measurements

The association of low blood glucose, high plasma insulin, and low C-peptide levels strongly suggests exogenous administration of insulin,[76] in contrast with endogenous insulin overproduction, in which low blood glucose and high plasma insulin levels are accompanied by normal or high C-peptide levels.

Detection of Factitious Hypoglycemia Due to Sulfonylurea Ingestion

Clandestine ingestion of sulfonylurea compounds may mimic an insulinoma both clinically and biologically. Screening plasma and urine for sulfonylurea compounds may establish the diagnosis.

How To Recognize Hormone Deficiency as a Cause of Hypoglycemia

Routine endocrinologic investigations will easily confirm a suspected diagnosis of glucocorticoid or growth hormone (GH) deficiency, panhypopituitarism, and catecholamine deficiency. Apparently extremely rare, the syndrome of glucagon deficiency could be diagnosed on the basis of a lack of glucagon rise during the insulin tolerance test, as well as in response to an alanine or arginine intravenous infusion. The insulin tolerance test is the most commonly used procedure for revealing a state of increased insulin sensitivity, as well as for measuring the responses of the various counterregulatory hormones. The test is performed after an overnight fast, and the amount of soluble insulin given corresponds to 0.1 U/kg body weight in adults and 4 U/m² in children. Plasma samples are taken at 20, 30, 45, 60, 90, and 120 minutes after injection for measurements of ACTH, cortisol, and 18-OH desoxy-corticosterone, adrenaline and noradrenaline, and growth hormone and glucagon. Urinary catecholamine excretion during the 3 hours following insulin administration gives an overall picture of the sympathicoadrenomedullary responsiveness, mainly in young children. In adults suspected of presenting with GH or glucocorticoid deficiency, a first test can be performed using 0.05 U/kg body weight of insulin to avoid severe hypoglycemia.

How To Investigate Neonatal and Childhood Hypoglycemia

Neonatal hypoglycemia is often transient and will disappear spontaneously within the first 3–4 days of life. Priority should be given to careful monitoring of both infants who are known to be at risk (in a manner similar to that used for infants of diabetic mothers or those suffering from erythroblastosis) and infants who manifest clinical signs that could be due to hypoglycemia. Continuous monitoring, and if necessary intravenous glucose infusion, should be performed prior to any diagnostic investigation. If hypoglycemia persists after 3–4 days, organic hyperinsulinism or hereditary defects of carbohydrate or amino acid metabolism should be suspected.[41]

In neonatal hyperinsulinism, as in the insulinoma syndrome of the adult, the clue to diagnosis is the demonstration of excessive circulating insulin levels (in the peripheral or the portal blood) in the face of baseline blood glucose. In 22 neonates with focal hyperinsulinism, fasting plasma glucose averaged 1 ± 0.2 mmol/L and plasma insulin 20 ± 11 µU/mL; 30 neonates with diffuse hyperinsulinism exhibited similar biochemical features: plasma glucose 1 ± 0.2 mmol/L and plasma insulin 22 ± 19 µU/mL.[31] In these infants, the insulin response to intravenous glucose is usually relatively small, suggesting that the β cells are already secreting maximally in the basal state; the glucose rise after glucagon injection is usually present, indicating the ability of glucagon to mobilize the glycogen stores.

In glycogen storage diseases, the most useful test is the glucagon test, in which 0.03 mg/kg of glucagon is injected intravenously. A normal blood glucose response is observed in types II, IV, V, VII, VIII, IXa, and X; in type I (von Gierke's disease), the injection of glucagon does not induce any rise in blood glucose, but does induce a rise in lactate; in type III, the response to glucagon is normal after food, but poor in the fasting state; in type VI, in which liver phosphorylase activity is absent, there is no glycemic response to glucagon; and in type IXb the response is poor. In all these cases, the diagnosis can be established with certainty by detailed enzymatic measurements on tissue (liver, muscle) biopsy specimens. The same applies for rare disorders such as hereditary fructose intolerance, fructose-1,6-diphosphatase deficiency, galactosemia, and phosphoenolpyruvate carboxykinase deficiency.

In hereditary fructose intolerance, the intravenous infusion of fructose (0.25 g/kg) invariably induces marked hypoglycemia, contrasting with the modest rise in blood glucose usually seen in normal children; in these patients, the blood glucose response to glucagon is normal, providing the test is not performed immediately after giving fructose. In fructose-1,6-diphosphatase deficiency, fasting induces hypoglycemia with simultaneous hyperlactacidemia and often ketosis, hyperuricemia, and hyperalaninemia. In galactosemia, a significant fall in blood glucose after oral galactose (1.25–1.75 g/kg body weight) is observed in about two-thirds of the galactosemic patients, but in view of the toxicity of this sugar in these patients, this test is not recommended. Impaired oxidation of $[1\text{-}^{14}C]$ galactose by the red cells of these patients can be demonstrated *in vitro*. For establishing the diagnosis of leucine-induced hypoglycemia, a drop of the blood glucose level below 50% of the fasting level during the first 45 minutes of an oral leucine test (0.15 g/kg body weight) is required; an excessive insulin response is usually observed. The response to tolbutamide is abnormal in more than 80% of these patients. The leucine and tolbutamide tests should not be performed if the initial blood glucose is already low. For the diagnosis of ketogenic hypoglycemia, a hypocaloric high-fat diet (ketogenic provocative test) is commonly used. Urine should be tested every 2 hours for ketones, and blood glucose (and if possible plasma alanine) determined every 3–4 hours. For the diagnosis of growth hormone or epinephrine deficiency in children, the lack of increase in plasma growth hormone or in urinary epinephrine during an insulin tolerance test (0.1 U/kg intravenously) is the best criterion. The test should not be performed if the fasting blood glucose is not above 50 mg/dL (about 2.8 mmol/L).

TREATMENT OF HYPOGLYCEMIA

Prevention of Hypoglycemia

In many circumstances, the prevention of hypoglycemia is possible. In insulin-treated patients with diabetes, appropriate education is of paramount importance; they should know how to adjust their insulin regimen according to their daily needs, their food intake, and their physical activity (see Chap. 29). In adolescents, the use of continuous subcutaneous insulin infusion has been advocated to lower the risk of severe hypoglycemia, improve metabolic control, and enhance coping.[77,78] Knowledge by the physician of the pharmacologic interactions of many drugs with both insulin and oral antidiabetic agents will permit the necessary adjustments of the doses of hypoglycemic agents when interfering compounds are simultaneously prescribed. Alcohol-induced fasting hypoglycemia can be prevented by advising the patient to consume an adequate amount of carbohydrate within 6–36 hours of ingesting moderate or large amounts of alcohol. In susceptible subjects suffering from alcohol-provoked reactive hypoglycemia, the incidence and severity of symptoms are reduced by decreasing the amount of sucrose (or glucose) ingested and by replacing it with either saccharin or fructose. Finally, the administration of acetylsalicylic acid in children below the age of 2 years should be avoided, and the daily dose, if used, should not exceed 10–20 mg/kg body weight every 6 hours. One must be particularly cautious in dehydrated children. Prevention of neonatal hypoglycemia implies the prenatal identification of infants at risk, such as infants of diabetic mothers or those suffering from erythroblastosis, as well as those who are small for dates, preterm, or the smaller of twins. Prophylaxis consists of reducing nonessential caloric expenditure, effecting heat conservation by nursing the infant in the appropriate thermal environment, and ensuring adequate caloric intake through a regimen of early feeding. Adequate and specific dietary changes prevent hypoglycemic attacks in patients with fructose intolerance (removal of sucrose, fruit, and fruit juices), galactosemia (galactose-free diet), and leucine-induced hypoglycemia. In children prone to ketotic hypoglycemia, attacks can be avoided by insisting on a nighttime carbohydrate-rich snack and consumption of frequent small-to-moderate amounts of carbohydrate-rich foods, particularly during periods of mild illness. Finally, frequent feeding (every 2–3 hours) prevents severe hypoglycemia in type I glycogen storage disease; portacaval transposition performed in a few cases gave promising results. Hypoglycemia following total parenteral nutrition is prevented by starting an IV infusion of 10% glucose at the time of discontinuation and gradually decreasing the IV glucose load over 12 hours.

Management of Acute Hypoglycemia

When the patient remains conscious, ingestion of some form of sugar by mouth (soft drinks containing saccharose, sugar cubes, glucose tablets, or solution equivalent to 5–20 g of carbohydrate) is usually followed by rapid relief of symptoms. In the unconscious patient, intravenous injection of glucose should be given, approximately 0.5 g/kg body weight in children. In diabetics with severe hypoglycemia, glucose doses in the range of 25–50 mL of 30–50% solution should be given. Intravenous glucose should be maintained as long as necessary (possibly days in hypoglycemia due to long-acting sulfonylureas) until persistent euglycemia or slight hyperglycemia is present. Intravenous, subcutaneous, or intramuscular glucagon (0.5–1.0 mg) can be used to treat severe hypoglycemic reactions of insulin-treated diabetic patients. The patient will often become conscious in 5–20 minutes; if not, a second dose may be given. Glucagon is not effective for much longer than 1–1.5 hours, and the patient should eat a snack or a meal of at least 20 g of carbohydrates as soon as he or she becomes conscious to prevent hypoglycemia from occurring again. Glucagon is less suitable for treating hypoglycemic attacks in sulfonylurea-treated patients because hypoglycemia in this circumstance is much more prolonged. The symptoms of hypoglycemia yield almost immediately to intravenous glucose unless hypoglycemia has been sufficiently prolonged to induce organic changes in the brain. If the patient remains unconscious after prolonged hypoglycemic coma despite blood glucose levels in the range of 200 mg/dL, the blood glucose should be maintained at that level by a glucose drip to which 100 mg hydrocortisone should be added every 4 hours for the first 12 hours to minimize cerebral edema. Sufficient insulin should be given to prevent ketosis. Finally, rapid recovery of consciousness has been described in cases refractory to glucose and hydrocortisone following slow intravenous infusion of 200 mL of a 20% solution of mannitol. The possible side effects of this treatment should be kept in mind.

Etiologic Management and Particular Cases

Insulinoma

Single benign adenomas are most common and their removal by pancreatic surgery is the first and obvious choice of treatment.[62,79] Preoperative localization of the tumor is recommended. The risk of the operation is related to the location of the tumor, being minimal with enucleation of the adenoma or distal pancreatic resection, and increasing if subtotal pancreatectomy or particularly if pancreatoduodenectomy is performed. Laparoscopic excision has been reported. Medical management of a benign tumor is reserved for patients who do not accept surgery or in whom major contraindications for the operation exist. In those cases, the management will often include diet with frequent meals, diazoxide,

which directly inhibits the release of insulin by β cells and also has extrapancreatic hyperglycemic effects, and a thiazide diuretic. Diazoxide daily doses range from 150–600 mg. High doses induce sodium retention and edema, which are counteracted by thiazides. In some cases of insulinoma, the anticonvulsant diphenylhydantoin (300–600 mg/d) has been used successfully for controlling refractory hypoglycemia.

Neonatal Hyperinsulinism Due to Nesidioblastosis

The initial treatment consists of glucose (up to 15–25 mg/kg/min), hydrocortisone (10 mg/kg/d), and diazoxide (20 mg/kg/d), as well as intermittent glucagon injections (0.1 mg/kg IM). If the situation is unstable with this therapy, removal of 75%, and sometimes in a second operation, of 95–100%, of the pancreas may be necessary to prevent severe hypoglycemia and secondary mental retardation. De Lonlay-Debeney and associates[31] have recently reported that among 52 neonates with hyperinsulinism, 22 had focal adenomatous islet cell hyperplasia that was successfully treated with partial pancreatectomy. These neonates had been identified through pancreatic catheterization and intraoperative histologic studies. Striking beneficial effects of long-acting protamine somatostatin treatment have also been reported.[80]

Autoimmune Insulin Syndrome

The drugs accelerating the production of insulin antibodies include methimazole, thiopronin, glutathione, and penicillamine. Definitive withholding of those drugs is mandatory because immediate recurrence of the syndrome has been reported after readministration of the incriminated drug.

Anti–Insulin Receptor Antibodies

Prognosis is poor in patients presenting with fasting hypoglycemia due to antibodies against the insulin receptor having insulinomimetic properties. In some patients, high doses of prednisolone (120 mg/d) have improved the situation. Other therapeutic approaches include plasmapheresis or immunosuppression with alkylating agents.

Malignant Tumors

Streptozocin, in association with fluorouracil or doxorubicin,[81] is the most effective antitumor agent for treating metastatic malignant insulinoma, possibly after surgical reduction of the tumor mass and/or removal of liver metastases.[82] Streptozocin causes selective destruction of the pancreatic β cell. It is often capable of controlling hypoglycemia, and in about half of cases causes a measurable decrease in tumor size. Renal tubular toxicity resulting in proteinuria is the most significant side effect. The treatment schedule is most often 1–2 g/m^2 administered every week. Medical treatment often involves diazoxide and a thiazide diuretic, the doses required often being higher than in benign tumors. Other compounds capable of alleviating hypoglycemia include glucocorticoids, which increase gluconeogenesis and insulin resistance, and high doses of propranolol or chlorpromazine, which in a small number of patients reduce plasma insulin levels. Besides streptozocin, other tumoricidal drugs have been used in a small number of cases: chlorozotocin,[81] L-asparaginase, 5-fluorouracil, tubercidin, doxorubicin, and mithramycin. A few studies have indicated that some patients with malignant insulinoma can be improved by the use of the somatostatin analogue octreotide at 3–4 daily doses of 50–100 μg[83,84] or by radiotherapy.[85]

Alimentary and Reactive Hypoglycemia

Diet is the first treatment of alimentary and reactive hypoglycemia.[86] Simple sugars should be omitted and replaced by complex carbohydrates. Alcohol consumption should also be limited. If symptoms persist, small but frequent meals (usually 6) of a high-protein, low-carbohydrate diet should be tried. When dietary management is insufficient, dietary fiber or anticholinergic drugs (such as atropine or propantheline) or both can be used to retard gastric emptying and the carbohydrate absorption rate. This is often necessary in patients who have had gastric surgery. The dose of propantheline is 7.5 mg 30 minutes before meals. Biguanides (such as metformin) may help some patients. In our experience the treatment of choice is acarbose, an α-glucosidase inhibitor that delays carbohydrate digestion and intestinal glucose absorption. With a dose of 50–100 mg at the beginning of the meal, acarbose significantly reduces postprandial hypoglycemia.[87] Similar results have been reported with miglitol, another α-glucosidase inhibitor.[88]

Leucine-Sensitive Hypoglycemia

The treatment of leucine-sensitive hypoglycemia consists of frequent feeding and a low-leucine diet. In some cases, it is necessary to prescribe diazoxide, at doses ranging between 5 and 10 mg/kg/d. Hirsutism may complicate long-term treatment with diazoxide.

REFERENCES

1. Amiel SA: Hypoglycaemia in diabetes mellitus—protecting the brain. *Diabetologia* 1997;40:S62.
2. Amiel SA: Cognitive function testing in studies of acute hypoglycaemia: Rights and wrongs? *Diabetologia* 1998;41:713.
3. Marks V, Rose FC: *Hypoglycemia*, 2nd ed. Blackwell Scientific:1981.
4. Weinger K, Jacobson AM, Draelos MT, *et al*: Blood glucose estimation and symptoms during hyperglycemia and hypoglycemia in patients with insulin-dependent diabetes mellitus. *Am J Med* 1995;98:22.
5. Wredling R, Levander S, Adamson U, *et al*: Permanent neuropsychological impairment after recurrent episodes of severe hypoglycaemia in man. *Diabetologia* 1990;33:152.
6. Langan SJ, Deary IJ, Hepburn DA, *et al*: Cumulative cognitive impairment following recurrent severe hypoglycaemia in adult patients with insulin-treated diabetes mellitus. *Diabetologia* 1991;34:337.
7. Kramer L, Fasching P, Madl B, *et al*: Previous episodes of hypoglycemic coma are not associated with permanent cognitive brain dysfunction in IDDM patients on intensive insulin treatment. *Diabetes* 1998;47:1909.
8. Veneman T, Mitrakou A, Mokan M, *et al*: Induction of hypoglycemia unawareness by asymptomatic nocturnal hypoglycemia. *Diabetes* 1993;42:1233.
9. Fanelli CG, Pampanelli S, Porcellati F, *et al*: Shift of glycaemic thresholds for cognitive function in hypoglycaemia unawareness in humans. *Diabetologia* 1998;41:720.
10. Fanelli CG, Paramore DS, Hershey T, *et al*: Impact of nocturnal hypoglycemia on hypoglycemic cognitive dysfunction in Type 1 diabetes. *Diabetes* 1998;47:1920.
11. Ovalle F, Fanelli CG, Paramore DS, *et al*: Brief twice-weekly episodes of hypoglycemia reduce detection of clinical hypoglycemia in Type 1 diabetes mellitus. *Diabetes* 1998;47:1472.
12. Davis SN, Galassetti PG, Wasserman DH, *et al*: Effects of antecedent hypoglycemia on subsequent counterregulatory responses to exercise. *Diabetes* 2000;49:73.
13. The EURODIAB IDDM Complications Study Group: Microvascular and acute complications in IDDM patients: The EURODIAB IDDM complications study. *Diabetologia* 1994;37:278.
14. Gold AE, Frier BM, MacLeod KM, *et al*: A structural equation model for predictors of severe hypoglycaemia in patients with insulin-dependent diabetes mellitus. *Diabet Med* 1997;14:309.
15. Mülhauser I, Overmann H, Bender R, *et al*: Risk factors of severe hypoglycaemia in adult patients with Type I diabetes—a prospective population based study. *Diabetologia* 1998;41:1274.
16. Cryer PE, White NH, Santiago JV: The relevance of glucose counterregulatory systems to patients with insulin-dependent diabetes mellitus. Review. *Endocrinol Rev* 1986;7:131.
17. Fery F, Plat L, van de Borne P, *et al*: Impaired counterregulation of glucose in a patient with hypothalamic sarcoidosis. *N Engl J Med* 1999;339:852.
18. Davis SN, Fowler S, Costa F: Hypoglycemic counterregulatory responses differ between men and women with Type 1 diabetes. *Diabetes* 2000;49:65.
19. Jones TW, Porter P, Sherwin RS, *et al*: Decreased epinephrine responses to hypoglycemia during sleep. *N Engl J Med* 1998;338:1657.
20. Jacobs MAJM, Salobir B, Popp-Snijders C, *et al*: Counterregulatory hormone responses and symptoms during hypoglycaemia induced by porcine, human regular insulin, and Lys (B28), Pro(B29) human insulin analogue (Insulin Lispro) in healthy male volunteers. *Diabet Med* 1997;14:248.
21. White NH, Skor DA, Cryer PE, *et al*: Identification of type 1 diabetic patients at increased risk for hypoglycemia during intensive therapy. *N Engl J Med* 1983;308:485.
22. The Diabetes Control and Complications Trial Research Group: The effect of intensive treatment of diabetes on the development and progression of long-term complications in insulin-dependent diabetes mellitus. *N Engl J Med* 1993;329:977.
23. Brunelle RL, Llewelyn J, Anderson JH Jr, *et al*: Meta-analysis of the effect of insulin Lispro on severe hypoglycemia in patients with Type 1 diabetes. *Diabetes Care* 1998;21:1726.
24. Marks V, Teale JD: Hypoglycemia: Factitious and felonious. *Endocrinol Metab Clin North Am* 1999;28:579.
25. Stahl M, Berger W: Higher incidence of severe hypoglycaemia leading to hospital admission in Type 2 diabetic patients treated with long-acting versus short-acting sulphonylureas. *Diabet Med* 1999;16:586.
26. Scheen AJ, Lefèbvre PJ: Antihyperglycemic agents. Drug interactions of clinical importance. *Drug Saf* 1995;12:32.
27. Marks V: Alcohol hypoglycaemia: Forensic aspects. In: Andreani D, Marks V, Lefèbvre PJ, eds. *Hypoglycaemia*. Raven Press:1987;211.
28. Marks V, Teale JD: Drug-induced hypoglycaemia. *Endocrinol Metab Clin North Am* 1999;28:555.
29. Marks V, Teale JD: Tumours producing hypoglycaemia. *Diabetes Metab Rev* 1991;7:79.
30. Service FJ, McMahon MM, O'Brien PC, *et al*: Functioning insulinoma—incidence, recurrence and long-term survival of patients: A 60-year study. *Mayo Clin Proc* 1991;66:711.
31. De Lonlay-Debeney P, Poggi-Travert F, Fournet JC, *et al*: Clinical features of 52 neonates with hyperinsulinism. *N Engl J Med* 1999;340:1169.
32. Thomas PM: Genetic mutations as a cause of hyperinsulinemic hypoglycemia in children. *Endocrinol Metab Clin North Am* 1999;28:647.
33. Kahn R: The riddle of tumor hypoglycemia. *Clin Endocrinol Metab* 1980;9:335.
34. Shapiro ET, Bell GI, Polonsky KS, *et al*. Tumor hypoglycemia: Relationship to high molecular weight insulin-like growth factor-II. *J Clin Invest* 1990;85:1672.
35. Hizuka N, Fukuda I, Takano K, *et al*: Serum insulin-like growth factor II in 44 patients with non-islet cell tumor hypoglycemia. *Endocr J* 1998;45:S61.
36. Hodzic D, Delacroix L, Willemsen PH, *et al*: Characterization of the IGF system and analysis of the possible molecular mechanisms leading to IGF-II overexpression in a mesothelioma. *Horm Metab Res* 1997;29:549.
37. Mizuta Y, Isomoto H, Futuki Y, *et al*: Acinar cell carcinoma of the pancreas associated with hypoglycemia: Involvement of "big" insulin-like growth factor-II. *J Gastroenterol* 1998;33:761.
38. Fukusawa Y, Takada A, Tateno M, *et al*: Solitary fibrous tumor of the pleura causing recurrent hypoglycemia by secretion of insulin-like growth factor II. *Pathol Int* 1998;48:47.
39. Grunenberger F, Bachellier P, Chenard MP, *et al*: Hepatic and pulmonary metastases from a meningeal hemangiopericytoma and severe hypoglycemia due to abnormal secretion of insulin-like growth factor. *Cancer* 1999;85:2245.

40. Bessell EM, Selby C, Ellis IO: Severe hypoglycaemia caused by raised insulin-like growth factor II in disseminated breast cancer. *J Clin Pathol* 1999;52:780.

41. Lteif AN, Schwenk WF: Hypoglycemia in infants and children. *Endocrinol Metab Clin North Am* 1999;28:619.

42. Toft-Nielsen M, Madsbad S, Holst JJ: Exaggerated secretion of glucagon-like peptide-1 (GLP-1) could cause reactive hypoglycemia. *Diabetologia* 1998;41:1180.

43. Acbay O, Celik AF, Kadioglu P, *et al*: *Helicobacter pylori*-induced gastritis may contribute to occurrence of postprandial symptomatic hypoglycemia. *Dig Dis Sci* 1999;44:1837.

44. Palardy J, Havrankova J, Lepage R, *et al*: Blood glucose measurements during symptomatic episodes in patients with suspected postprandial hypoglycemia. *N Engl J Med* 1989;321:1421.

45. Tamburrano G, Leonetti F, Sbraccia P, *et al*: Increased insulin sensitivity in patients with idiopathic reactive hypoglycemia. *J Clin Endocrinol Metab* 1989;69:885.

46. Lefèbvre PJ: Hypoglycemia or non-hypoglycemia. In: Rifkin H, Colwell JA, Taylor SI, eds. *Diabetes 1991*. Excerpta Medica:1991;757.

47. Berlin I, Grimaldi A, Landault C, *et al*: Suspected postprandial hypoglycemia is associated with β-adrenergic hypersensitivity and emotional distress. *J Clin Endocrinol Metab* 1994;79:1428.

48. Andreani D, Marks V, Lefèbvre PJ, eds.: *Hypoglycemia*. Raven Press: 1987.

49. Lefèbvre PJ, Andreani D, Marks V: Statement on "post-prandial" or "reactive" hypoglycaemia. *Diabetologia* 1988;31:68; *Diabet Med* 1988:5:200; *Diabetes Care* 1988;11:439.

50. O'Keefe SJD, Marks V: Lunchtime gin and tonic a cause of reactive hypoglycemia. *Lancet* 1977;i:1286.

51. Flanagan D, Wood P, Sherwin R, *et al*: Gin and tonic and reactive hypoglycemia: What is important—the gin, the tonic, or both? *J Clin Endocrinol Metab* 1998;83:796.

52. McMahon M, Gerich J, Rizza R: Effects of glucocorticoid on carbohydrate metabolism. *Diabetes Metab Rev* 1988;4:17.

53. Gerich JE, Campbell PJ: Overview of counterregulation and its abnormalities in diabetes mellitus and other conditions. *Diabetes Metab Rev* 1988;4:93.

54. Vidnes J, Øyasaeter S: Glucagon deficiency causing severe neonatal hypoglycemia in a patient with normal insulin secretion. *Pediatr Res* 1977;11:943.

55. Bleicher SJ, Levy LJ, Zarowitz J, et al: Glucagon-deficient hypoglycemia: A new syndrome. *Clin Res* 1970;18:355.

56. Hirata Y: Autoimmune insulin syndrome "up to date." In: Andreani D, Marks V, Lefèbvre P, eds. *Hypoglycemia*. Raven Press:1987;105.

57. Redmon JB, Nuttall FQ: Autoimmune hypoglycemia. *Endocrinol Metab Clin North Am* 1999;28:603.

58. Stanley CA, Baker L: The causes of neonatal hypoglycemia. *N Engl J Med* 1999;340:1200.

59. Service FJ, O'Brien PC, McMahon MM, *et al*: C-peptide during the prolonged fast in insulinoma. *J Clin Endocrinol Metab* 1993;76:655.

60. Hirschberg B, Livi A, Bartlett DL, *et al*: Forty-eight-hour fast: The diagnostic test for insulinoma. *J Clin Endocrinol Metab* 2000;85:3222.

61. Service FJ, Natt N: The prolonged fast. *J Clin Endocrinol Metab* 2000;85:3973.

62. Grant CS: Surgical aspects of hyperinsulinemic hypoglycemia. *Endocrinol Metab Clin North Am* 1999;28:533.

63. Catalano C, Pavone P, Laghi A, *et al*: Localization of pancreatic insulinomas with MR imaging at 0.5 T. *Acta Radiologica* 1999;39:644.

64. Lamberts SWJ, Krenning EP, Reubi JC: The role of somatostatin and its analogs in the diagnosis and treatment of tumors. *Endocrinol Rev* 1991;12:450.

65. Günther RW, Klose KJ, Ruckert K, *et al*: Localization of small islet-cell tumors. Preoperative and intraoperative ultrasound, computed tomography, arteriography digital subtraction angiography, and pancreatic venous sampling. *Gastrointest Radiol* 1985;10:145.

66. Rösch T, Lightdale CJ, Botet JF, *et al*: Localization of pancreatic endocrine tumors by endoscopic ultrasonography. *N Engl J Med* 1992; 326:1721.

67. Proye C, Malvaux P, Pattou F, *et al*: Noninvasive imaging of insulinomas and gastrinomas with endoscopic ultrasonography and somatostatin receptor scintigraphy. *Surgery* 1998;124:1134.

68. Gin H, Catargi B, Rigalleau V, *et al*: Experience with the Biostator for diagnosis and assisted surgery of 21 insulinomas. *Eur J Endocrinol* 1998;139:371.

69. Doppman JL, Miller DL, Chang R, *et al*: Intraarterial calcium stimulation test for detection of insulinomas. *World J Surg* 1993;17:439.

70. Iwanaka T, Matsumoto M, Yoshikawa Y, *et al*: Accurate localization of an insulinoma by preoperative selective intra-arterial calcium injection and intraoperative glucose monitoring. *Pediatr Surg Int* 2000; 16:118.

71. Huai JC, Zhang W, Niu HO, *et al*: Localization and surgical treatment of pancreatic insulinomas guided by intraoperative ultrasound. *Am J Surg* 1998;175:18.

72. Jacquet N, Scheen AJ, Lefèbvre PJ: Localization of insulinoma by intraoperative ultrasonography[letter]. *J Roy Soc Med* 1989;82:317.

73. Hashimoto LA, Walsh RM: Preoperative localization of insulinomas is not necessary. *J Am Coll Surg* 1999;189:368.

74. Boukhman MP, Karam JM, Shaver J, *et al*: Localization of insulinomas. *Arch Surg* 1999;134:818.

75. Luyckx AS, Lefèbvre PJ: Plasma insulin in reactive hypoglycemia. *Diabetes* 1971;20:435.

76. Lebovitz MR, Blumenthal SA: The molar ratio of insulin to C-peptide. An aid to the diagnosis of hypoglycemia due to surreptitious (or inadvertent) insulin administration. *Arch Intern Med* 1993;153:650.

77. Boland EA, Grey M, Oesterle A, *et al*: Continuous subcutaneous insulin infusion. A new way to lower risk of severe hypoglycemia, improve metabolic control, and enhance coping in adolescents with type 1 diabetes. *Diabetes Care* 1999;22:1779.

78. Kaufman FR, Klein M, Halvorson M, *et al*: Nocturnal hypoglycemia in children and adolescents with Type 1 diabetes: Attempt at prediction and prevention. *Endocrinologist* 1999;9:342.

79. Bliss RD, Carter PB, Lennard TWJ: Insulinoma: A review of current management. *Surg Oncol* 1997;6:49.

80. Tauber MT, Harris AG, Rocchioli P: Clinical use of the long-acting somatostatin analogue octreotide in pediatrics. *Eur J Pediatr* 1994; 153:304.

81. Moertel CG, Lefkopoulo M, Lipsitz S, *et al*: Streptozotocin-doxorubicin, streptozotocin-fluorouracil, or chlorozotocin in the treatment of advanced islet-cell carcinoma. *N Engl J Med* 1992;326:519.

82. Que FG, Nagorney DM, Batts KP, *et al*: Hepatic resection for metastatic neuroendocrine carcinomas. *Am J Surg* 1995;169:36.

83. Boden G: Insulinoma and glucagonoma. *Semin Oncol* 1987;14:253.

84. Diem P, Peyer T, Köchli HP, *et al*: Malignant insulin-producing islet-cell tumor: Treatment of severe hypoglycemia with octreotide acetate. *Diabetes Nutr Metab* 1991;4:221.

85. Torrisi JR, Treat J, Zeman R, *et al*: Radiotherapy in the management of pancreatic islet cell tumors. *Cancer* 1987;60:1226.

86. Lefèbvre PJ: Hypoglycemia: Post-prandial or reactive. In: Bardin CW, ed. *Current Therapy in Endocrinology and Metabolism*, Vol. 3. Dekker:1988;339.

87. Gérard J, Luyckx AS, Lefèbvre PJ: Acarbose in reactive hypoglycemia: A double blind study. *Int J Clin Pharmacol* 1984;22:25.

88. Renard E, Parer-Richard C, Richard JL, *et al*: Effect of Miglitol (Bay m1099), a new alpha-glucosidase inhibitor, on glucose, insulin, C-peptide and GIP responses to an oral sucrose load in patients with postprandial hypoglycaemic symptoms. *Diabetes Metab* 1991;17:355.

CHAPTER 59

Economic Aspects: Insurance, Employment And Licensing

Christopher D. Saudek

Shereen Arent

Diabetes mellitus imposes significant social and financial as well as medical burdens. In 1997, diabetes cost the United States an estimated $98 billion.[1] Interestingly, only $7.7 billion of this was for acute glycemic care. The vast majority of the cost of diabetes is related to specifically related chronic complications ($11.8 billion), excess prevalence of general medical conditions ($24.6 billion) and attributable indirect costs (totaling $54.1 billion, including $37.1 billion for disability and $17 billion for premature death).

At an individual level, even the person who is well adjusted and free of significant diabetic complications is affected financially by the disease. He or she may be blocked from purchasing adequate health, disability, and life insurance at an affordable price, because diabetes imposes a potentially high cost of medical care and risk of premature death. There may be hardship caused by unfair exclusion from employment opportunities. Employers may even terminate a person or seriously restrict opportunities for advancement because of perceived disabilities attributed to diabetes.

This chapter will address the economic dilemmas encountered by people with diabetes, insurers, and employers. The underlying theme is that the interests of all three can be reconciled within the law, and that the health care practitioner should know enough to help in this reconciliation process.

THE HEALTH CARE SYSTEM IN TRANSITION

Universal, all-inclusive health care reform has hardly been mentioned since the early 1990s.[2] But there is no doubt that the financing as well as the organization of health care is undergoing fundamental change in the United States. The shift toward managed care may be receding, with early signs of re-emphasis on patients' rights and broadening coverage. But even without knowing how it will all turn out, it is clear that many pitfalls as well as opportunities exist for people with diabetes. It therefore behooves health care professionals to understand and deal effectively with the forces at work.

Driving Forces of Health Care Reform

Two major forces drive every discussion of health care reform: the spiraling cost of health care in the United States and its inconsistent quality. While some moderation in expenditure growth was enforced in the first few years of managed care, costs again appear to

be spinning out of control,[3] most recently at a rate of about 6.5% per year, with further acceleration predicted.[4] Some 28% of the Medicare budget goes to health care for people with diabetes. Furthermore, Americans continue to spend a far higher fraction of the gross domestic product on health than any other industrialized nation. Moreover, indices of quality are not encouraging. There have been few international comparisons of the quality of care,[5, 6] but it is clear that we have a long way to go as a nation before all people with diabetes receive quality care. It is understandable, therefore, that patients, employers, providers of care, and third-party payers all have an interest in the economic consequences of diabetes.

Organization of Health Care

One reason our costs are so high and our quality so variable may be that in fact there is no health care "system" in the United States; rather, there is an almost unbelievably complex patchwork of different systems. Physician providers may practice alone or in a group. The traditional model of a physician earning a living by billings is far less prevalent than it was decades ago. In fact, while practitioner earnings based on billing may still be the majority approach, a great many health care professionals are now salaried, whether working in full-time academic positions, as military or public health service employees, working for large companies, or in health maintenance organizations (HMOs), or any combination of these. The certified diabetes educator has become a widely accepted profession, existing in a wide variety of practice settings.

Delivery sites also vary tremendously. They may be single offices, hospitals, or clinics operated by profit or nonprofit corporations; they may be university clinics, or federal, state, or local government facilities. It would be nice to think that people with diabetes are rationally triaged along a sequence of practice settings, with the most stable patients receiving basic, primary care, and the most difficult-to-manage receiving the attention of specialists. But such rational use of manpower is not the rule.

Payment mechanisms, too, are diverse and often without sound rationale. Examples abound of nonsensical decisions about "medical necessity" or "clinically indicated care." Therefore, an understanding of the various reimbursement systems in place and under development is necessary if we are to operate effectively in this consummately pluralistic environment, and bring some rationality or reform to it.

Methods of Coverage

Fee for Service Payment

This time-honored system is the equivalent of piece work, and the incentives are roughly the same: the provider is paid by the number of visits, tests, and particularly, procedures. Knowingly or not, providers often orient their practice toward a high volume of remunerative procedures. Insurance premiums escalate as the payouts to providers increase, making these "indemnity" insurance plans less price competitive. The only way to control the outlays is to discourage volume and hold down reimbursement, particularly of hospital days and procedures. Insurers who reimburse providers on a fee-for-service basis, then, initiate utilization review, preauthorization, and other means of reducing the volume of payments.

Prepaid Capitated Payment

Under capitated payment plans, an organization (for-profit or not-for-profit) is paid up front premiums and contracted to provide, not just pay for, the total care for enrolled individuals. Having already collected the fee, the delivery system loses, rather than gains, from every service it provides. The incentives, then, are the exact opposite of those operating in a fee-for-service mode: capitated systems profit by enrolling healthy people. The "staff model" HMO, first popularized in the 1970s, is the prototype capitated payment system. Professionals are hired by the corporation to provide care, and the corporation profits to the extent that cost per patient remains under the capitated rate.

Hybrid Systems

Virtually every imaginable permutation exists of pure fee-for-service, indemnity insurance, and the staff model HMO. HMOs open their panel, for example, to negotiate with outside physicians, offering a high volume of patients in return for a reduced per-service fee. Indemnity plans develop lists of "preferred providers" who, again, agree to accept a reduced per-service fee in exchange for volume. Physicians may be added to or cut from these lists based on the cost of their practice style. A system popular in the mid-1990s was the "point of service" approach, which allows enrolled patients to go outside a closed list of approved doctors, but the patient pays more out-of-pocket or a co-pay to do so.

It may be oversimplified to think that professionals respond only to the basic (and base) economic incentives described above—that fee-for-service physicians provide unneeded services just to increase income, and prepaid systems withhold needed services to increase their profit. But it also seems naive to imagine that physicians and managed care systems are immune to financial incentives. There is little doubt, for example, that capitated systems try to enroll healthy, low-risk people (known as "lives" in the industry), and there is little doubt that fee-for-service providers deliver more services to people with insurance coverage.

Competition in Health Care Delivery

A prevalent notion, popular among legislators and deeply rooted in the American psyche, holds that competition among providers will contain cost. There are basic flaws in this notion as applied to health care, however. For example, if "consumer" is taken to mean "patient," then shopping for the best deal is among the least likely behaviors when someone is sick.

The consumer need not be the individual patient, however, and indeed negotiations now occur much more effectively between providers and professionals who represent large consumers of health care, such as corporations, unions, or government. As providers, not only physicians, but hospitals, HMOs, and indemnity insurance plans are all in fierce competition with each other. Competition is now a fundamental part of the health care landscape.

Even sophisticated negotiators in the diverse arena of health care finance are often ignorant of the needs of individual people with chronic diseases like diabetes. How may coverage negotiators, faced with decisions on open heart surgery sites, PET scanning facilities, or neonatal intensive care units, think a great deal about glucose monitoring strips or the importance of routine foot care? Professionals who are aware of these issues must speak out, demanding coverage of needed services for their patients.

Navigating the System for People with Diabetes

Availability of Health Insurance

Given the competitive incentives noted above, people with diabetes can find themselves excluded from insurance coverage, provided with minimal care, or forced to pay out-of-pocket for a substantial part of their health care costs. To prepaid and capitated providers, people with diabetes are a predictably high expense; there is no incentive for HMOs to enroll them or to retain them once enrolled. Insurers who pay fee-for-service and are concerned about the cost of premiums, can also do better simply by excluding from coverage preexisting conditions like diabetes.

Health insurance for people with diabetes will be more available, and the costs of caring for diabetes will be more equitably distributed, if these disincentives are rectified. Assuring that capitated plans take their share of sick people would help, as would prohibition of noncoverage for preexisting conditions. But the best way out of the quagmire may be to change the incentives themselves, through a process called risk adjustment.

Risk Adjustment

The arcane process of risk adjustment gauges how sick a particular group is and pays the provider a capitated rate according to the risk of the population covered. A managed care organization enrolling predominantly Medicare patients over 65 would receive more, per enrollee, than would one enrolling a young, working population. Without risk adjustment, as described, there is no incentive to care for the sick since it is cheaper to care for the well. In theory, resources are distributed according to the amount of care required and provided. Risk adjustment may therefore be the ultimate mechanism that will allow a pluralistic delivery system to survive in the United States. It is very much in the interest of people with diabetes to assure adequate compensation for quality care to people with known chronic disease.

Quality of Care Issues

Particularly with the benefits of glycemic control now well-proven, significant quality issues are raised. What supplies are reimbursed? What counseling services are provided? When should an endocrinologist be involved? A podiatrist? Self-management training? The case can and must be made that good self-care yields long-term financial savings, but this case may not be enough, when providers look at annual balance sheets. Even "outcomes research" can be misleading if it does not factor in the long-term consequences of poor care.

Standards of care should be disseminated and enforced, with all payers made aware that quality care is the right of all people with diabetes. Evidence should be gathered and summarized for the various aspects of quality care. "Medical necessity" should cover all elements of care proven to have benefit, not just those needed to allow the person to survive another day or year.

OBTAINING HEALTH INSURANCE

Harris and associates have compared the health insurance status of adults with diabetes versus those without.[7] They concluded that 8% of adults with diabetes were without any health insurance. This is the same figure estimated much earlier by Krall.[8] Harris and associates went on to find that the percentage of the sample covered by insurance was nearly equal for those with diabetes and for those without. Because having diabetes increases the likelihood of high medical expenses, however, it is particularly risky not to have adequate coverage. There is also evidence that the uninsured population with diabetes is increasing. In California, the number of uninsured people with diabetes increased 50% between 1979 and 1986. Many of these uninsured people were neither poor nor unemployed. Thus, finding adequate, affordable health insurance remains a major problem for people with diabetes.

Health insurance is obtained either through the private sector or by qualifying for a government-funded plan. While qualification criteria for government programs are relatively specific, there is, as summarized above, an enormous array of private health insurance options available.

Options for Health Insurance Coverage

For people with diabetes it is most important to have some form of health care coverage, and a prospective employer's insurance options may legitimately become the driving force when a person with diabetes chooses a job. While in large employer and "entitlement" programs, a series of choices are often available ("cafeteria" style), small employers may offer little or no health care coverage, and temporary or part-time work may be the worst option. In general, people with diabetes are well advised to look for work with a large company or the government.

Public Entitlement Programs

The federal government is the single largest provider of health insurance, and federal entitlement programs are often the most reliable source of health insurance coverage. Indeed, over 57% of Americans with diabetes are covered by federal programs.[7] In addition to Medicare and Medicaid, the Department of Veterans Affairs and the Indian Health Service also provide care for large numbers of people with diabetes.

Generally, eligibility for public sector coverage is established as an "entitlement"—a right to coverage under law—if the person meets certain defined characteristics. Legislatures and federal or state agencies define exactly who is entitled to coverage under a given program, and the extent of that coverage. Medicare eligibility, for instance, is established mainly on the basis of age, disability, or end-stage renal disease. Receipt of veterans' medical benefits depend upon the person having served on active military duty. Medicaid is meant mainly for low-income people.

There may be, as with Medicare, a significant monthly fee to the enrollee, and often copayment is required. There may also be enormous coverage gaps, exemplified by the longstanding failure of Medicare to cover pharmaceuticals or long-term care, both of which are clearly major health care needs of the elderly. These gaps in coverage spawned the market for supplemental, or "Medigap" insurance. "Medigap" policies are sold with the specific purpose of covering items government plans leave uncovered. However, there are two pitfalls: the policies may be redundant, re-covering what is already covered, and the price may be excessive (a judgment made by comparison shopping or by an independent insurance expert).

Principles of Private "Indemnity" Health Insurance

The principles which govern privately obtained coverage are quite different from those of public programs. In theory, private health insurance provides a risk-sharing approach: the cost of illness in a few is spread among many subscribers. As long as they comply with state laws, private insurers are free to offer whatever coverage they choose, to whomever they choose, at whatever price they choose. This freedom may allow the private insurer to refuse coverage, offer it only at a high price, limit benefits, or select their covered population by more subtle means such as targeted marketing campaigns.

Group Coverage

Over 80% of private health insurance is sold on a group basis, because actuarial calculations are more accurate if based upon relatively large populations. As few as ten subscribers may qualify as a group. Usually, group policies are obtained through employment, although associations such as unions and fraternal or professional organizations often offer group insurance. Until the day when portability becomes the rule (i.e., when a person's policy is not tied to the employer, but can be transported from job to job), it is crucial for people with diabetes to seek employment where group health insurance is offered, or to be sure they have access to a group policy elsewhere. The best option for keeping coverage after leaving a given employer is called COBRA.

COBRA is an acronym for Consolidated Omnibus Budget Reconciliation Act, and it has provided important protections since its passage in 1986. COBRA permits a person and their dependents to continue in a previous employer's group health plan after that person retires, quits, is fired, or has work hours reduced. Continuation coverage also extends to surviving, divorced, or separated spouses, and dependent children. COBRA continuation coverage generally lasts 18–36 months. A person may be eligible if the employer has 20 or more employees, but the person must pay the full premium him- or herself.

Group insurance is priced either by "experience rating" or "community rating."

Experience rating refers to the adjustment of rates based upon the health claims experience of a given group. This practice can work to the disadvantage of people with diabetes, especially if a small employer is singled out for rate increases because of a single sick employee. There may be pressure on the person with diabetes to leave employment or be removed from the company policy. For this reason, "community rating" is far more desirable. It adjusts rates based on the wider community, spreading risk broadly rather than penalizing subscribers for legitimate health care claims.

Individual Coverage

Policies rated and issued on an individual basis to people with diabetes are contrary to insurance theory, since they amount to collecting high premiums and paying out predictably high expenses, rather than sharing the risk of illness broadly. Individuals, who have limited economic clout or a chronic disease such as diabetes, are thus at a great disadvantage in the individual coverage insurance market. This is the primary reason why a person with diabetes is best served when he or she is part of a large group. The person with diabetes is unattractive to the insurer and to the subscriber, and it may be impossible for that person to obtain coverage at a reasonable cost.

Pooled Risk Plans

Some states provide pooled risk plans to cover otherwise uninsurable risks. People can usually only apply if they have been rejected for standard individual policies. Although the programs vary from state to state, the cost of coverage is commonly 150% of the standard individual rate, sometimes with a deductible as high as $2000. This price is far preferable to going without adequate insurance or paying exorbitant individual rates. Physicians and their patients can contact their state insurance commissioner to find out what is offered in their state. For more information, go to the website of the National Association of Insurance Commissioners at http://www.naic.org/1regulator/.

HIPA

A more recent protective law is the 1996 Health Insurance Portability and Accountability Act or HIPA, which is intended to make it easier for people with preexisting conditions to get or keep health insurance, or to change from one health plan to another. This law sets national standards for all health plans. It also requires the consumer to meet very specific conditions for continuing to acquire insurance. Since states can pass different reforms for the health plans they regulate (fully insured group health plans and individual health plans), protections may vary from state to state. While the statute has provided assurances that people—even those with diabetes and other chronic conditions—must be able to purchase insurance, it unfortunately did not offer any price protections. Thus premiums offered may be quite high. However, for the person with diabetes, high premiums are often preferable to no insurance.

For more information on HIPA and other insurance issues, go to Georgetown University: http://www. healthinsuranceinfo. net/.

Community Health Centers: Help for the Uninsured

Harris pointed out in 1994 that almost 600,000 people with diabetes did not have any insurance coverage at all[7]. While 93% of all adults with diabetes had some form of insurance, there was marked variability based on ethnicity with, for example, 34% of Mexican-Americans uncovered.[9]

The nation's community health center (CHC) system currently provides health care to some 12 million people. Of these, about 25% or 4 million have no insurance at all. The two most frequently diagnosed conditions among those using the CHCs are hypertension and diabetes. The number of people served by community health centers is expected to increase dramatically, and federal funding for CHCs is also increasing significantly. The majority of community health centers receive partial funding from the Health Resources and Services Agency (HRSA). HRSA and the Centers for Disease Control (CDC) have collaborated on a program to improve diabetes care among those CHCs that do receive HRSA funding, and this has resulted in dramatic improvements in the frequency and results of the HbA$_{1c}$ test. As part of the social safety net, CHCs are required by law to see anyone seeking medical assistance and cannot turn away the uninsured.

Specific Issues in Health Insurance Coverage

In addition to physician and hospitalization fees, a number of expenses are part of necessary diabetes care. Indeed, the per capita medical costs for the person with diabetes is $10,071 versus just $2669 for the person without diabetes.[1] Among the individual costs may be durable equipment such as blood glucose meters and insulin pumps, orthotic shoes, or even prostheses. Diabetes care of course also often requires insulin, syringes, testing strips, or oral hypoglycemic agents. Yet, incredibly, these basic elements of self-management may not be reimbursed, while more expensive and less easily justified expenses such as hospitalization for diabetic control are well reimbursed.

Comprehensive patient education and access to the supplies and equipment needed to manage the disease are all integral to good diabetes care. In 1997, Congress passed a bill mandating that Medicare pay for blood glucose monitors and strips as well as diabetes self-management training. Passage of the legislation resulted from years of advocacy on the part of the American Diabetes Association (ADA) and other associations interested in improved care for diabetes. In 1998, the Health Care Financing Administration (HCFA) established rules to implement the glucose meter and strip coverage portion of the legislation. In February of 2001 Medicare established final rules for diabetes education programs, and reimbursement is now available for all the quality diabetes education programs recognized by the ADA.

Medicare coverage policy does not assure coverage by other insurance mechanisms, although the federal program is traditionally seen as the leader in coverage policy. And while the Medicare changes for diabetes coverage were going into effect, states were also improving coverage for people with diabetes. At this writing, thanks in large part to the American Diabetes Association and its partners, 44 states and the District of Columbia have enacted laws requiring state-regulated insurance plans to include coverage for diabetes supplies, equipment, and education as part of the basic coverage offered to all purchasers (Table 59-1). As many as one-third of people with diabetes get their insurance coverage from state-regulated plans. More information about coverage in a particular state is available through employers human resources departments, or through the ADA at 1-800-DIABETES.

Conclusion: Advising a Patient on Health Insurance

The following points should be emphasized in discussing health insurance with patients with diabetes:

1. Adequate insurance coverage for people with diabetes is essential. The adequacy of coverage should often be a significant factor in job selection.
2. Government entitlement programs, group health insurance policies, or pooled risk plans are usually far more cost effective than purchasing an individual insurance policy.
3. Insurance policies should be evaluated for specific covered benefits the individual with diabetes may require: specialist care, meters, glucose test strips, insulin, etc.
4. Reimbursement for diabetes self-management training is becoming more readily available, and is an important addition to the financing of diabetes care.

TABLE 59-1. Impact of Diabetes Legislative Initiatives

State	Year Enacted	Residents with Diabetes*
Wisconsin	1987	319,006
New York	1993	1,222,283
Minnesota	1994	273,409
Florida	1995	1,104,972
New Jersey	1996	534,990
West Virginia	1996	150,997
Maine	1996	78,096
Oklahoma	1996	251,944
Rhode Island	1996	67,088
New Mexico	1997	100,865
Arkansas	1997	182,161
Indiana	1997	433,535
Maryland	1997	367,508
Vermont	1997	34,942
Washington	1997	312,796
Texas	1997	1,211,149
Tennessee	1997	381,067
Connecticut	1997	212,826
Louisiana	1997	315,814
Missouri	1997	368,592
North Carolina	1997	539,837
Nevada	1997	94,585
New Hampshire	1997	65,722
Georgia	1998	490,715
Kentucky	1998	284,011
Colorado	1998	199,617
Arizona	1998	213,092
Kansas	1998	142,270
Illinois	1998	786,815
Mississippi	1998	209,319
Pennsylvania	1998	874,355
Virginia	1999	420,642
South Dakota	1999	42,335
Iowa	1999	191,673
Nebraska	1999	105,065
South Carolina	1999	259,191
California	1999	2,096,337
Utah	2000	91,146
Massachusetts	2000	383,946
Alaska	2000	28,510
Hawaii	2000	75,103
District of Columbia	2000	40,582
Delaware	2000	52,189
Michigan	2001	702,485
Wyoming	2001	24,326
Total:		16,337,908[1]

*United States Centers for Disease Control and Prevention (diagnosed and undiagnosed).

Approximately 33% of Americans are covered by private health insurance plans regulated by state laws. The remainder either have plans not regulated by state law (e.g., Medicare, ERISA-exempt, Federal Employees Health Benefit Plan) or have no coverage at all.

LIFE INSURANCE

Diabetes, despite its variability in clinical outcome, does increase the risk of premature death. For this reason, life insurance may be difficult to obtain and relatively expensive. However, life insurance policies are available, even for the individual with type 1 diabetes. Two points are worth noting. First, the patient and the physician must be honest in recording significant, known diagnoses on any application. Hiding a diagnosis of diabetes may invalidate a policy if payment becomes necessary, and may also leave the physician open to charges of providing (by omission) false information. Second, if the actual diagnosis is not in fact diabetes mellitus, but impaired glucose tolerance with borderline or high risk of developing diabetes, then the word "diabetes" should *not* appear, lest the person be saddled with the economic penalties of a disease he or she does not have.

EMPLOYMENT

Potential employers, employees, and society at large have fundamentally different employment priorities. Employers want to hire the person who will accomplish a job with optimal reliability, and minimal absenteeism, disability, or cost to the company. Employers may act with little understanding of, and less concern for, diabetes. The job applicant wants the job. Society wants to minimize accidents while practicing fair and nondiscriminatory employment practices.

Job discrimination law balances the needs of the employer with those of the employee and society. For example, the employer can legitimately take into account whether a person's disabilities or limitations will interfere with specific job performance. Poor vision due to diabetes may disqualify a person from a secretarial job just as surely as would poor typing skills. Peripheral vascular disease with claudication may disqualify a person from a job that requires extensive walking. But it is not permissible for an employer to assume that just because someone has diabetes, he or she has poor vision or claudication. Moreover, simply having these complications of diabetes does not disqualify a person for a job if, with reasonable accommodations, that person can perform the essential functions of the job.

Physicians are often asked to evaluate a person for employment, acting as the intermediary between the patient, the employer, and society. Whether paid by the individual patient or the employer, it is necessary to understand what constitutes employment discrimination, which areas are most problematic for people with diabetes, and what the physician should look for in performing a medical evaluation. The first issue, then, is whether the person is medically qualified for the job (i.e., whether the diabetes or its complications would keep him or her from doing the work safely and well).

Assessment of the ability to do the job is not always as straightforward as it seems, since there is a requirement that employers make a "reasonable accommodation." Checking blood glucose, access to a snack, or taking insulin would generally be considered reasonable accommodations, easily accomplished at almost any workplace. Other less obvious but applicable accommodations could include a large-print computer screen for a secretary with retinopathy, or permitting a cashier with neuropathy to sit while on the job. Whatever accommodation is required, it must be provided unless the employer can show that doing so would cause undue hardship.

Safety is often another contentious issue. An employer may require that the individual not pose a "direct threat" to his or herself or to others in the workplace. The risk of hypoglycemia is frequently cited, often with the most severe hypoglycemic reactions described. But under this standard, an employer is not permitted to deny employment opportunity because of a slightly increased risk, a speculative risk, or a judgment based on stereotypes about people with diabetes.

To summarize, in evaluating a person for a given job, that person must first be deemed medically able to perform the job safely, with reasonable accommodations by the employer. In such a case, federal law specifically prohibits discrimination.

Laws Prohibiting Discrimination on the Basis of Disability

The Americans with Disabilities Act of 1990 is the most comprehensive federal law prohibiting discrimination on the basis of disability. The goal of the Americans with Disabilities Act is to eliminate discrimination against persons with disabilities in employment, education, and recreation, and to require equal access to a broad range of facilities and services.

The act prohibits employment discrimination by state and local governments and by private employers that employ over 15 employees. The earlier Rehabilitation Act of 1973 had similar prohibitions against employment discrimination, but applied only to the federal government and employers that either receive federal funding or that contract with the federal government.

Both laws prohibit discrimination in hiring, firing, promotion, training, compensation, or any other term or condition of employment, and both laws generally use the same standards to determine what constitutes unlawful discrimination. The Americans with Disabilities Act, the federal law, prohibits discrimination against a "qualified individual with a disability."

However, it is far from clear exactly what is and what is not a "disability." Unless a person with diabetes meets the legal definition of having a disability, there is little under federal law to stop a employer from refusing to hire a person, or taking other adverse employment action against that person simply because he or she has diabetes.

Legally, the term "disability" is defined as follows:

1. A physical or mental impairment that substantially limits one or more of the major life activities of such an individual;
2. A record of having such an impairment; or
3. Being regarded as having such an impairment.

"Major life activities" could include eating, sleeping, working, learning, seeing, walking, and many others. To be "substantially" limited under the law means to be unable to perform the major life activity or to be significantly restricted in its performance *when compared to the average person*.

Recent Supreme Court decisions have made it more difficult for people with diabetes to establish that they are protected under antidiscrimination laws. In 1999, the Court ruled that a person must be viewed in his or her "mitigated" state, which means taking into account the positive and negative effects of any medications or aids the person uses. Thus, for a person with insulin-treated diabetes, the court must evaluate whether or not the person is disabled *when taking medications*; the need for insulin itself does not amount to a disability.

Dietary requirements may qualify a person with diabetes as being covered by the Americans with Disabilities Act. The intricacies of balancing food and insulin, for instance, may be considered a significant restriction when compared with people who do not have diabetes.

Three more important points: First, it is not acceptable for an employer to make a class decision (for example, that taking insulin does not qualify as a disability). Disability decisions must be the result of an *individual* inquiry, based on up-to-date medical information. Second, the physician's report should not be the sole basis of a disability decision. Other important factors include the individual's employment history as well as medical history. Finally, it is not legal for an employer to base the disability decision on whether insurance rates will increase or on the fact that the employer does not want to provide reasonable accommodations.

In addition to the federal laws, each state has its own antidiscrimination laws. Some, like those in New York and California, provide broader coverage than the federal law, so that people with diabetes are unquestionably covered against employment discrimination on the basis of having diabetes.

Another federal law that is often useful to people with diabetes is the Family and Medical Leave Act (FMLA). This law permits most government workers and employees of private companies with over 50 employees to take up to a total of 12 weeks of unpaid medical leave each year to deal with their own, or an immediate family member's, serious health condition, without losing their job.

The Employment Policy of the American Diabetes Association

The American Diabetes Association has worked hard and effectively to reduce discrimination against people with diabetes. A position was adopted in 1990 (based on a policy formulated in 1984), and is consistent with the Americans with Disabilities Act. It provides that: "People with diabetes should be individually considered for employment based on the requirements of the specific job. Factors to be weighed include the individual's medical condition, treatment regime (medical nutrition therapy alone, oral agents, and/or insulin) and medical history . . . . Any person with diabetes, whether insulin-dependent or non-insulin-dependent, should be eligible for any employment for which he/she is otherwise qualified."

Thus, the American Diabetes Association's policy, consistent with federal law, opposes any blanket exclusion of an individual with diabetes from a particular job or line of work. The diagnosis of diabetes should not, *per se*, make a person ineligible for any job. This does not, of course, imply that every person with diabetes is qualified for every job, or that physical limitations imposed by diabetes cannot be a factor in determining someone's ability to perform a job. It simply states that each case must be considered on its own merits, on a case-by-case basis.

Employment Discrimination in Practice

Despite federal and state laws that should provide protection for people with diabetes, discrimination is still pervasive, and may begin with unlawful preemployment inquiries. "Do you have diabetes?" for example, is not a permissible interview question. By law, the employer is permitted to ask only those questions necessary to determine the applicant's eligibility to be considered for employment in a particular position.

An employer's ability to make disability-related inquiries or require medical examinations is analyzed in three stages: preoffer, postoffer, and during employment. Prior to an offer of employment, an employer cannot require a medical examination or make any disability-related inquiries. Once an applicant has been given a job offer conditional upon passing a physical examination, an employer may make disability-related inquiries and conduct medical examinations, as long as all incoming employees are treated equally. After the person becomes employed, an employer may make disability-related inquiries and require medical examinations only if there is a job-related reason for doing so.

The Health Professional's Medical Evaluation of a Person for Employment

The health care professional is best thought of as working on behalf of the patient, the employer, and society, reconciling the needs and rights of each. The medical evaluation yields only a recommendation, without the force of law or the authority of a licensing agency. We know of no cases in which physicians have been held legally liable for the results of a recommendation to hire a person with diabetes, so the examining physician need not be excessively concerned about his or her own liability. Nor should the positive qualities be forgotten, since people with diabetes may as a group have many favorable employment characteristics that are well worth emphasizing. Disciplined behavior, reliability, a healthy diet, and a generally health-conscious lifestyle may translate into above-average work habits.

The possibility of complications occurring at some later time should not be used to keep someone out of a job. Complications progress at such variable rates that it is medically unsound to assume, for example, that background retinopathy will progress to visual impairment, or that mild neuropathy will become severe. Long-term complications are relevant only when, at the time in question, they interfere with performance of the job or safety on the job.

Clinical or laboratory evaluation of a patient's blood glucose control as assessed by a given blood glucose or hemoglobin HbA_{1c} level is not usually relevant to a job evaluation. An exception might be that extremely poor control can cause generalized fatigue or the need for frequent urination. But mild to moderate hyperglycemia is rarely a significant risk to job performance. The immediate risk posed by an insulin reaction is usually the primary issue.

Considering hypoglycemia specifically, adrenergic symptoms, or even profuse diaphoresis and tachycardia are also generally of little concern if these conditions are reliably self-treated before a threat is perceived. But when there is a relatively recent history of altered mentation requiring the assistance of another competent person, the risk of a threat increases.

Evaluation of the Job

Is a particular job suitable for a given person with diabetes? As noted, a job should be considered suitable unless the person cannot perform the job adequately or will create a direct threat to others.

In the particular job, would even brief periods of confusion or loss of reflexes have serious consequences? In jobs involving driving or operating heavy machinery, the person's likelihood of having a serious hypoglycemic episode must be carefully assessed. Given that the past is the most accurate predictor of the future, a history of confusion during hypoglycemic reactions may be the most important historical point. Various specific regulations (see section on driving, below) have been devised to try to codify the assessment of risk, and most require a minimum period of freedom from severe hypoglycemia.

Existing complications of diabetes must be considered. For example, microelectronics assembly work may require perfect vision, and night watch work may require good night vision. A high level of physical activity may be unsuitable for a person with unstable coronary artery disease. Long-distance driving may not be advisable for a person with hypoglycemic unawareness.

Will a given job adversely affect the person's health? For instance, irregular shift work may be detrimental if a person has unstable diabetes and does not practice good self-care. In these cases, a physician may advise the patient about what is in their medical best interest, although if the person chooses to apply for a given job, they cannot be discriminated against solely on the basis of paternalistic concern for their own health.

Problem Areas in Employment

Historically, the rationale for discriminating against people with diabetes has usually been based on the chance that a severe hypoglycemic incident could create an immediate danger to other people. There has been across-the-board discrimination in jobs that require driving, flying, law enforcement, and all positions in the military. These blanket prohibitions, however, were created when there were fewer and less effective management tools, and severe hypoglycemia was a greater risk. Individuals must be carefully evaluated by licensing bodies, employers, and physicians asked to make an objective risk assessment.

Trucking

Regulations of the United States Department of Transportation (DOT) presently disqualify anyone with diabetes requiring insulin treatment from driving a commercial motor vehicle in interstate or foreign commerce. Thus, if a person needs insulin, he or she must either leave driving as a profession (or give up the chance to make it a profession), avoid taking insulin despite clinical need, or cover up the need for insulin. Despite this federal blanket ban, however, most states have waiver programs that, under various conditions, allow some people with insulin-treated diabetes to drive some commercial vehicles within the state.

In 1998, the DOT was ordered by Congress to consider allowing certain individuals with insulin-treated diabetes to operate commercial motor vehicles interstate. As of this writing, the details of any new policy are not clear, but it is possible that by following a strict set of guidelines designed to minimize the chance of a serious hypoglycemic episode, people treated with insulin may be able to obtain a commercial license to drive interstate.

Opening the door to interstate commercial driving is being accomplished by the concerted efforts of the American Diabetes Association and others. As with so many other "test cases," it can have reverberations well beyond the drivers themselves, since many government agencies and private companies look to DOT for guidance in this area.

Law Enforcement

Evaluation of the job and the person is especially important when considering law enforcement work. Physical demands and irregular meal schedules make these jobs difficult. Confusion caused by severe hypoglycemia could have serious consequences. But none of these factors are absolute contraindications for employment in law enforcement, and many people with diabetes have performed in an exemplary fashion as law enforcement officers.

Law enforcement agencies may be under local, county, state, or federal jurisdiction. While all are subject to federal antidiscrimination laws, both written regulations and actual practices vary widely from place to place. Some law enforcement agencies disqualify all those taking insulin, some have no written policy but *de facto* exclusion of people with diabetes if the physician who clears recruits has a personal bias, and still others have a protocol to individually assess whether a given candidate with diabetes is qualified for the job.

Key federal law enforcement agencies used to automatically disqualify anyone with insulin-treated diabetes. As a result of a lawsuit against the Department of Treasury, it was forced to abandon its hiring policy of automatic disqualification and now considers hiring individuals with insulin-dependent diabetes on a case-by-case basis. Similarly, the Federal Bureau of Investigation U.S. Marshal's Service, the Bureau of Prisons, the Drug Enforcement Administration, and the Immigration and Naturalization Service have all been banned from discriminating on the basis of diabetes as such. Unfair individual cases of discrimination may still exist, but the changes in federal law enforcement policy are an important step in removing the unwarranted discrimination often faced by people with diabetes.

Military

The U.S. armed forces are a major employer, and diabetes still makes a person ineligible for employment in the military, regardless of insulin use or not, duration, or status of complications. In addition, a new diagnosis of diabetes may well cause termination of current employment in the U.S. military. By contrast, in Israel, even insulin use does not disqualify a person from active combat duty. Appeals can be made to medical boards in the various branches of the military, and in at least one test case pursued with the army, such an appeal was successful. In general, though, a pre-existing diagnosis of diabetes will keep a person out of the military, and new onset of diabetes during military service may be cause for discharge.

In evaluating military employees and applicants, physicians should bear in mind that the diagnosis of impaired glucose tolerance is not a diagnosis of diabetes[11], and should not disqualify a person from holding any job. Physicians should also be especially mindful of the fact that early termination can seriously affect a person's retirement benefits.

LICENSING ISSUES

License to Drive

Driver's licenses are issued by states, and except with regard to commercial drivers licenses, medical standards for licensure are established on a state-by-state basis. Laws and regulations may therefore vary widely. In every case, though, the physician's role is that of advisor to the state agency, not a guarantor that any given patient drives safely. The medical evaluation form in California, for example, states "The Department of Motor Vehicles is solely responsible for any decision regarding the patient's driving qualification and license." It is the health care professional's job, then, not to guarantee that a person is a safe driver, but to consider facts that may affect whether or not to recommend that a person should drive a motor vehicle.

The data are few and inconclusive regarding whether, overall, people with diabetes have more motor vehicle accidents than others. One study suggested that women with diabetes may have an increased accident rate,[10] but controversy still exists. Clarke and colleagues[12,13] suggested that people with diabetes often choose to

drive when their blood glucose is too low.[19] Certainly in aggregate, the number of accidents caused by medical conditions are small compared to those caused by alcohol abuse or negligent driving.

State policies vary widely in their treatment of issuing driver's licenses to diabetics.[20] An absurd example is that until relatively recently, the criteria for determining whether a government employee who had diabetes could drive on the job in some Maryland counties was whether he or she took more than 25 units of insulin per day! Routinely, driver's license applicants are asked directly if they have diabetes. If so, a statement from a physician is required. If a person with diabetes is involved in an accident, a report is prepared that usually indicates that the driver has diabetes, and in some states, his or her license is suspended immediately pending a hearing, whether or not hypoglycemia caused the accident.

In considering whether to support a person's application for a driver's license, the same issues discussed above would apply: Does the applicant have severe long-term complications such as impaired vision, impaired night vision, severe peripheral neuropathy, or impairments from cerebrovascular accidents? Do they have a history of hypoglycemic unawareness coupled with prior incidents of severe hypoglycemia? Do they have good self-care practices, and a thorough understanding of, ability to anticipate, and the means to self-treat hypoglycemia?

In summary, no state automatically disqualifies people with diabetes from obtaining a noncommercial driver's license. States do rely heavily on the treating physician for a recommendation, but the physician is not the final arbiter, and a good medical evaluation is not a guarantee of safe driving. States generally have the authority to impose conditions or restrictions on the license issued, such as requiring the driver to submit a medical report on a regular basis.

Other Licenses

Beyond driver's licenses, there are a number of other licenses that are important to people, and these may be restricted by the diagnosis of diabetes. Intrastate commercial driving such as driving a school bus may be restricted by state laws. People with insulin-treated diabetes in the past were categorically denied a license to fly both commercial or noncommercial airplanes. However, in 1996, the Federal Aviation Administration (FAA) changed its policy to allow people with insulin-treated diabetes who want to fly private non-commercial airplanes to be able to do so. The FAA set up a protocol for the effective screening, monitoring, and managing of pilots with insulin-treated diabetes.

REFERENCES

1. American Diabetes Association: Economic consequences of diabetes mellitus in the U.S. in 1997. *Diabetes Care* 1998;21:296.
2. Schroeder SA: Health Policy 2001: Prospects for Expanding Health Insurance Coverage. *N Engl J Med* 2001;344:847.
3. Blumenthal D: Controlling health care expenditures. *N Engl J Med* 2001;344:766.
4. Smith S, AUTHOR?, AUTHOR?, *et al*: The next ten years of health spending: what does the future hold? The Health Expenditures Projection Team. *Health Aff (Millwood)* 1998;17:128.
5. Songer TJ, AUTHOR?, AUTHOR?, *et al*: International comparisons of IDDM mortality. Clues to prevention and the role of diabetes care. *Diabetes Care* 1992;15(Suppl 1):15

6. Tajima, N., AUTHOR?, AUTHOR?, *et al:* A comparison of the epidemiology of youth-onset insulin-dependent diabetes mellitus between Japan and the United States (Allegheny County, Pennsylvania). *Diabetes Care* 1985;8(Suppl 1):17.

7. Harris MI, Cowie CC, Eastman R: Health-insurance coverage for adults with diabetes in the U.S. population. *Diabetes Care* 1994; 17:585.

8. Krall LP, Entmacher PS, Drury TF: Life cycle in diabetes: socioeconomic aspects. *Joslin's Diabetes Mellitus,* 12 ed. [AQ 8]PUBLISHER?:1985.

9. Harris MI: Racial and ethnic differences in health insurance coverage for adults with diabetes. *Diabetes Care* 1999;22:1679.

10. American Diabetes Association. Position Statement: Hypoglycemia and Employment/Licensure. *Diabetes Care* 2002.25:S132.

11. American Diabetes Association. Report of the expert committee on the diagnosis and classification of diabetes mellitus. *Diabetes Care,* 1998. 21 [Suppl.2]:B1-167, 1998.

12. Clarke WL, *et al:* Hypoglycemia and the decision to drive a motor vehicle by persons with diabetes. *JAMA* 1999;282:750.

13. Gower IF, et al: Epidemiology of insulin-using commercial motor vehicle drivers. Major variability of state licensing requirements in the U.S. *Diabetes Care* 1992;15:1464.

CHAPTER 60

Health Education for Diabetes Self-Management

Elizabeth A. Walker

Judith Wylie-Rosett

Harry Shamoon

It has long been recognized that persons with diabetes have much to learn about self-care, as well as lifestyle changes to adopt and maintain, in the ongoing management of this chronic disease.[1–3] Traditional models of the educational process, however, do not adequately address *how* to teach persons with chronic disease, so that when making informed choices they can learn and sustain changes in behavior related to health over their lifespan.[4] Learning for lifestyle change is a complex process that requires assessment, coordinated planning, and individualized implementation, with both process and outcome evaluations.[5] This chapter addresses *health education* for self-management of diabetes as a more broad topic than either patient education or diabetes education.

We will provide an overview of teaching–learning principles for health education, including several behavioral models applicable to diabetes self-management. The phases of the education process for both individual patients and groups will be examined in the context of practice settings, followed by a description of the new revised content areas related to diabetes self-management education. Information about practical aspects of creating a diabetes education team, educational program structure, and resources for educational materials will assist health care professionals to provide access to health education for diabetes self-management for their patients.

APPLYING PRINCIPLES OF TEACHING AND LEARNING

Education: Teaching and Learning

These three concepts take on special meaning when applied to patients with diabetes, their families, and support systems. *Teaching* involves an interaction between two or more persons or systems; *learning* denotes a change in attitude, knowledge, or capability, persisting over time (i.e., a change in behavior). The word *education* generally describes the total process, encompassing the various modes of teaching and the many styles of learning.[5–7] A basic and tremendously important educational principle is that *teaching does not necessarily lead to learning.* Additionally, knowledge is a necessary component, but knowledge is not sufficient for learning and behavior change. For example, a simple demonstration of the procedure to test blood glucose does not guarantee that patients will understand how to do it or why they should test their blood glucose, or that they will consistently perform this behavior. Education is a process requiring assessment, planning, implementation, and evaluation for successful outcomes, especially when daily diabetes self-management and adoption of lifestyle changes are among the goals.

Cognitive, Affective, and Psychomotor Learning

Bloom[8] and others described three major domains of learning: cognitive, affective, and psychomotor. Briefly stated, the cognitive is the domain of information or knowledge; the affective domain can be described as the domain of attitude and belief; and the psychomotor domain encompasses skill acquisition and performance. Acknowledging and discriminating among these three domains can remind health care professionals of the complexity of the teaching–learning process for a chronic disease like diabetes. In the following example the utility of considering domains of learning is highlighted.

A capable 23-year-old man, newly diagnosed with type 1 diabetes, must learn to administer insulin to maintain independence. Thus information about the need for insulin and the timing of injections, as well as the procedures for the drawing up and injection of insulin, are part of the cognitive domain. However, the person's attitudinal response (e.g., his fear, negativity, intention to follow medical advice) to the recommendation for self-injecting insulin is part of the affective domain. The psychomotor domain involves this person's physical ability, coordination, and skill in completing the process of insulin administration.

If the educational assessment and planning for this young man were based on any one of these three domains and not the others, the desired outcome would likely not be achieved or maintained over time. The interaction between patient and health professional in the health education process emerges as various elements of diabetes self-management skills are assessed.

Optimizing the Learner's Experience

Table 60–1 provides examples of characteristics of adult learners[6,7,9,10] that may be helpful to clinicians and educators in planning health education. Using these principles in practice, for example, when there are several topics to be discussed, encourages patients

TABLE 60-1. Selected Characteristics of Adult Learners Applied to Diabetes Education

- Adults must have a "felt need to know" the information presented: Begin with a brief rationale for the content.
- Problem-oriented learning is more acceptable to adults: Frame the diabetes education as problems to be solved or challenges to be overcome in collaboration with their health professionals.
- Self-directed learning enhances the person's sense of autonomy: Allow choices when feasible—in the mode of learning, time spent on specific topics, and the order of the information to be addressed.
- Incorporating the person's life experiences will enhance adult motivation to learn: Allow time in educational interaction for patients to share their past experience or current knowledge of this diabetes care topic.
- Learning can be threatening to the learner: Assess for fear as a barrier to learning diabetes self-management skills.
- Active participation of the learner is essential for a change in behavior to take place: Speaking, reading, writing, demonstrating, or problem-solving activities should be incorporated into the educational plan.

to verbalize what they see as a learning priority. Recent literature on teaching and learning strongly emphasizes individualization of the process as imperative for learning and sustained behavior changes. In many cases the process cannot be rushed, and health professionals have the challenge of planning their time to incorporate these principles.

BEHAVIORAL MODELS RELEVANT TO SELF-MANAGEMENT EDUCATION

Because of the chronicity and complexity of therapeutic regimens for diabetes, models to help explain human behavior in coping with diabetes can be useful to clinicians in teaching both individuals and groups. Models are also used to plan programs or systems for delivery of diabetes care. The following selected behavioral models have been considered useful by health care professionals for designing learning experiences and enhancing adherence to diabetes regimens.

Self-Efficacy

Self-efficacy is a construct of Social Learning Theory, which posits that self-efficacy is predictive of outcome and that persons are more likely to perform behaviors if they feel confident that they are *able to perform* the particular behavior.[11] For example, exercise self-efficacy has been found to be predictive of weight loss.[12] In practice, instructing a middle-aged man with type 2 diabetes about increasing his exercise by walking 1 mile each day may be effective only if he is *confident* that he can walk that far and can actually adopt this change from his current lifestyle.

A practical application of the self-efficacy construct is for health professionals to ask patients, "Do you think you can do this?" "How confident are you that you can . . . ?" The query should be made specific for each health behavior under consideration. A broad, "Can you take care of your diabetes?" may not be helpful for diagnosing a behavioral challenge. If a patient replies, "Not at all," "I probably can't do it," or "No way!," then the planning and nego-

tiation process must continue until the stated goal is feasible and mutually acceptable, and the action phase can begin.[13,14]

Stages of Change

A more recently developed model for the process of changing behavior is the Stages of Change (or Transtheoretical) Model.[15,16] This model has been widely studied in persons with addictive behaviors such as smoking,[17] and it has been found to be predictive of change for some self-care behaviors such as exercise, weight control, and mammography screening. The model describes five cyclical stages in readiness for behavior change. These stages include: precontemplation, contemplation, preparation, action, and maintenance.

After assessing for the particular stage, health professionals can develop and plan interventions relevant to the patient's current stage of change.[15] For example, if a person who smokes cigarettes has not even considered quitting smoking, it is probably premature to encourage them to enroll in an action-oriented smoking-cessation program. Rather than immediate action, providing information relevant to smoking cessation may be more beneficial at this stage. Specific application of these five stages of change to diabetes education and care[18] is described in this chapter under the assessment phase of the health education process.

Autonomy and Patient Empowerment

A model incorporating the construct of autonomy would highlight issues related to an individual's desire to be competent and self-determining related to his or her environment, including a chronic disease like diabetes. There is some evidence that patients with diabetes who have providers who support their autonomy may have improved outcomes.[19] The model of patient empowerment[20] in health education assumes the perspective that persons with a chronic disease like diabetes should learn about self-management options, so that they can make informed choices about their care and their lives. Assisting patients to assume responsibility for diabetes self-management is a priority. Success in the patient empowerment model is linked to the collaboration between patients and health care professionals in formulating the individual's plan of care. However, the responsibility for diabetes self-management behaviors remains with the person with diabetes, depending on their developmental stage or current health status.

The Health Belief Model

The Health Belief Model has been useful in diabetes care and education to elucidate the variables that may have an impact on a patient's adherence to a therapeutic regimen. The perceived threat of diabetes (its severity and the patient's susceptibility to this disease) interacts with cues from the environment and a balance of the barriers versus the benefits of performing health behaviors.[21] For example, if an elderly woman with type 2 diabetes is following few of the recommended exercise or dietary behaviors, it could be that she considers her condition as "only a touch of sugar" and so does not consider herself vulnerable to complications of diabetes. The Health Belief Model can prompt health care professionals to explore possible reasons for nonadherence to recommended regimens so that interventions can be altered. In summary, behavioral models have been beneficial in guiding diabetes education for interventions to promote and sustain changes in behavior.

THE HEALTH EDUCATION PROCESS FOR DIABETES

The educational process (Fig. 60-1) is cyclical, not necessarily sequential, and it involves at least four phases: assessment, planning (goal setting), implementation, and evaluation.[5] The complexity of self-management activities for diabetes, especially when optimal metabolic control is a priority, necessitates the use of an education plan as a road map, a heuristic for both educator and for learner.

Assessment

Assessment is the data-gathering phase of the educational process, during which individualization of the content and the process for teaching is addressed. What to teach? How to teach it? Is the patient ready to learn? Is the patient able to make lifestyle changes? What are the desired outcomes of this education experience? Assessment takes time and reflective listening by the provider, especially when the learner is a new patient for the health care professional. Establishing good communication patterns with a patient is paramount for optimal diabetes care and for the subsequent educational process.[22,23] Listening skills and being able to ask questions to elicit information are necessary skills for providers.

Areas to be explored for a comprehensive assessment include current level of understanding of diabetes self-management, family/social support, literacy level, health beliefs and cultural differences, past experience with the health care delivery system, coping skills and self-efficacy, and current health behaviors, among others. Though some health care settings have found paper-and-pencil as-

sessment surveys to be efficient ways of collecting information, others are developing computer software for assessment. Health professionals can also use targeted interview questions to assess a patient's knowledge, motivation, and readiness to learn about specific topics. See Table 60-2 for examples. The data derived from these and other questions regarding diabetes self-management knowledge and skills must be used in moving the process forward to the planning phase.

Planning

This phase uses the assessment data to develop a collaborative plan with the patient for the educational process. For example, information about the patient's stage of readiness to change behavior can help to define the plan. Table 60-3 portrays the Stages of Change model[18] applied to diabetes as a guide to plan interventions appropriate for the assessed stage. Using this behavioral model, for example, once a patient is assessed as being in the *preparation* stage for changing a particular behavior, specific behavioral guidelines should be given for this planned change in behavior. Other assessment data will be used to decide on one-to-one teaching sessions or group classes; involvement of family; or appropriate printed, video, or computer-assisted educational materials or age-related games. Educational sessions may not always be the first priority; some patients may need counseling for coping with a new diagnosis of diabetes or other life stressors prior to any teaching–learning occurring.

The *goal-setting* process can be part of the planning phase, as it specifies, first, a particular behavior in measurable terms; second, a

FIGURE 60-1. The process of health education is cyclical and moves through four main activities: assess, plan, implement, and evaluate.

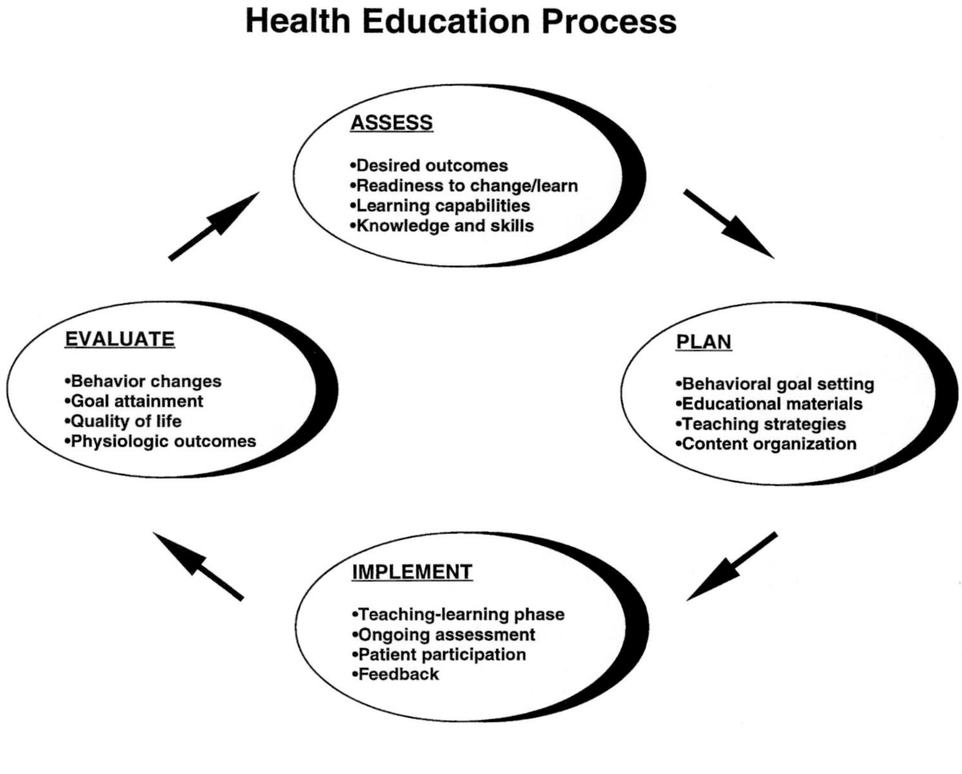

Health Education Process

TABLE 60-2. Targeted Interview Questions

Weight Loss
- Why do you believe weight loss is important? Why or why not?
- Are you ready to try to lose some weight?
- What would you have to do to begin dieting for a small amount of weight loss?

Increasing Routine Exercise
- In what ways do you think exercise might benefit your diabetes control?
- Are you prepared to make time for an exercise program?
- What changes in your lifestyle will exercise require?

Blood Glucose (BG) Monitoring
- How do you think BG monitoring can be helpful for your diabetes control?
- Can you imagine yourself checking your BG at home at least two times each day?
- Are you able to start testing at least once a day this week?

time frame for attaining the goal; and finally, an appropriate reward for achieving the goal. When there is mutual agreement on a specific goal, then possible obstacles to achieving the goal are explored with the patient, with discussion of strategies to overcome the obstacles. Goal setting can be useful for specific diabetes management behaviors, for example, waiting 20–30 minutes after injecting regular insulin to begin eating a meal in order to match insulin action with food intake. Goal setting assures that both patient and professional have defined a mutually acceptable, reasonable goal, and since it is measurable, they will also know when it has been achieved. A goal-setting "contract" should be written down, with copies for both patient and provider.

The following is an example of a typical behavioral, goal-setting statement focused on decreasing the risk of hypoglycemia[24] when intensifying therapy in type 1 or type 2 diabetes to improve metabolic control.

Until my visit next month, I will increase my blood sugar testing to four times each day (before each meal and before bed) and will record the results to discuss with my doctor, nurse, or dietitian.

The patient had identified an obstacle to reaching this goal, that is, falling asleep while watching TV before testing at night. To overcome this obstacle, the patient and provider discussed placing the monitoring equipment at the bedside after testing her blood glucose before dinner, as a reminder of the need to do another test before getting into bed. It is important to define specific behavior changes, so that the challenges of the complex diabetes regimen can be viewed as realistic mutual goals and incremental change can be recognized and rewarded.

Although behavioral learning objectives for diabetes education are well established,[25] a variety of techniques and strategies should be considered in the planning phase. For example, in the Diabetes Control and Complications Trial (DCCT),[26] the goals for metabolic control were standardized, but the blood glucose management and nutrition management approaches were individualized within the protocols. The planned nutrition approaches included carbohydrate counting, the Total Available Glucose (TAG) system, and exchange lists for meal planning to optimize metabolic control.[27] The planning phase builds on the assessment phase for individualizing interventions to meet the needs of diverse populations with materials appropriate and sensitive to their cultures.[28]

TABLE 60-3. General Guidelines for Applying Stages of Change to Diabetes Care

Stage of Readiness	Key Factors Associated with Movement to Next Stage	Treatment Do's at This Stage	Treatment Don'ts at This Stage
Precontemplation	Increased information and awareness, emotional acceptance	Provide personalized information. Allow patient to express emotions about his or her disease.	Do not assume patient has knowledge or expect that providing information will automatically lead to behavior change. Do not ignore patient's emotional adjustment to the disease, which could override ability to process relevant information.
Contemplation	Increased confidence in one's ability to adopt recommended behaviors	Encourage support networks. Give positive feedback about a patient's abilities. Help to clarify ambivalence about adopting behavior, and emphasize expected benefits.	Do not ignore the potential import of family members and others on patient's ability to comply. Do not be alarmed by or critical of a patient's ambivalence.
Preparation	Resolution of ambivalence, firm commitment and specific action plan	Encourage patient to set specific, achievable goals (e.g., walk briskly for 15 min at least 3 times a week). Reinforce small changes that patient may have already achieved.	Do not recommend general behavioral changes (e.g., "Get more exercise"). Do not refer to small changes as "not good enough."
Action	Behavioral skill training and social support	Refer to education program for self-management skills. Provide self-help materials.	Do not refer patients to "information-only" classes.
Maintenance	Problem-solving skills and social and environmental support	Encourage patient to anticipate and plan for potential difficulties (e.g., maintaining dietary changes on vacation). Collect information about local resources (e.g., support groups, shopping guides). Encourage patient to "recycle" if he or she has a lapse or relapse.	Do not assume that initial action means permanent change. Do not be discouraged or judgmental about a lapse or relapse.

Source: Reprinted with permission from Curry SJ: Commentary on In Search of How People Change. *Diabetes Spectrum* 1993;6:34.

Implementation

The action phase of the educational process is when the individualized teaching plan is implemented. Some well-known challenges or barriers to implementation of the educational plan include:

- Lack of clarity about *who* will do the teaching.
- Lack of communication/documentation related to progress.
- Lack of time or priority assigned to the teaching–learning process by either educator or patient.

Strategies to enhance the patient's learning process incorporate many principles of adult education previously described.[7–10] Active participation for the patient, incorporation of their life experiences, and allowing mastery of one topic before moving on to the next are examples of educational strategies in the implementation phase.[4]

Evaluation

Health education for diabetes self-management must focus on both *process and outcome evaluations*.[29] A *process* (or *formative*) *evaluation* is an ongoing assessment to provide valuable information for refining or altering the educational intervention. Patient attitudes, behaviors, knowledge, and skills should be evaluated to make adjustments in either the content or the teaching strategy. When barriers to achieving the educational goals are identified early, the educational program can be modified to overcome the barriers. The results of process evaluations should be shared; receiving timely feedback on individual progress is important to adult learners. Process evaluations for group education programs should be shared with all members of the diabetes education team, so that program improvements can be implemented by all educators.

An *outcome* (or *summative*) *evaluation* assesses goals attained or appropriate endpoints. These may include physiologic parameters, such as weight or metabolic control, as well as self-management skills, self-efficacy, coping skills, and knowledge.[30,31] If goal setting has been used in the process, the endpoint has already been agreed upon by patient and health professional. When goals have not been met, the educational process cycles back to the assessment phase.

Ongoing evaluation of diabetes self-management skills and knowledge is very important. Patients may remember the utility information, for example, how to correctly draw up insulin, but they may forget the particulars of other, less frequently used information, for example, urine testing for ketones when ill. Reinforcement of information or redemonstration of self-care skills may be (and probably are) needed. Finally, the evaluation process in health education should recognize and provide positive reinforcement for even the seemingly small, incremental changes in behavior to promote long-term success.[18]

Documentation and Communication

The educational process should be continuous rather than episodic; it is simply a matter of the intensity of the process. This continuity of the process is supported when the education is documented and shared with all health care professionals interacting with the patient. When used consistently, computer records, chart forms, or checklists designed to easily document diabetes self-management education for individual patients can orient health professionals to the patient's progress in knowledge and skill for self-management.[6,25]

Current level of motivation for self-management and specific health behaviors must also be documented to fully describe the education process.

CREATING A TEAM: EDUCATIONAL RESOURCES AND PROGRAM DEVELOPMENT

Content of Diabetes Self-Management Education

The goals and content of health education for diabetes self-management must be adapted to individual patient needs. Goals for diabetes education[25] can be described in two broad levels: initial or survival level education, and in-depth or continuing education and counseling. These broad levels are then delineated for type 1 diabetes, type 2 diabetes, and both gestational diabetes and pregnancy with preexisting diabetes. The *initial* educational goals are designed to address the most basic skills and knowledge needed to cope with newly diagnosed diabetes without a medical crisis. The *continuing* education goals are gradually introduced after the basic survival goals are achieved.

According to the recently revised national standards for diabetes self-management education programs, there are 10 content areas for consideration in educational program planning and for individualized education.[25] These include:

- Describing the *diabetes disease process* and treatment options
- Incorporating appropriate *nutritional management*
- Incorporating *physical activity* into lifestyle
- Utilizing *medications* (if applicable) for therapeutic effectiveness
- *Monitoring* blood glucose and urine ketones (when appropriate), and using the results to improve control
- Preventing, detecting, and treating *acute complications*
- Prevention (through *risk reduction* behavior), detecting, and treating chronic complications
- *Goal setting* to promote health, and *problem solving* for daily living
- Integrating *psychosocial adjustment* into daily life
- Promoting *preconception care*, management during *pregnancy*, and *gestational diabetes management* (if applicable)[25]

Beyond the more traditional diabetes education programs, several new behaviorally oriented programs have been developed and continue to be studied, with promising results. Among these are Blood Glucose Awareness Training,[32,33] coping skills training for diabetes,[34] and a patient empowerment program for those who have had basic self-management education.[20]

Structure for Education Programs

Patient education can be provided through on-site services in health care facilities and medical offices or through external referral to health professional educators for specific services. The structure of the educational experience can vary widely within each model. Both models can be used to achieve educational goals for patients in a coordinated manner.[2]

Communication between the health care providers, the educators, and the patient must be maintained so a team approach to the education and care is not lost. The strength of a team approach, whatever the model, is that multiple perspectives are drawn on to provide the education. But the challenge to the team is in delivering a consistent message to patients. Consistency is more likely to occur if providers and educators are familiar with the educational materials in use in their settings. If differences in opinion occur between the health care professionals (e.g., site selection for insulin injections or amount of carbohydrate to treat mild hypoglycemia), then they should resolve differences rather than confuse patients. Good verbal and written communication are the key to creating a health care team, whether or not the physical location is the same.

Data from the 1990 National Institutes of Health physician survey indicate that endocrinologists referred the vast majority of patients with diabetes to a nurse or dietitian. Over 80% reported that a formal diabetes education program was necessary for diabetes self-management. Only 41% felt that they could provide adequate dietary counseling for their patients with diabetes.[35] Glasgow and colleagues[36] suggested that active recruitment of patients into intensive education programs may not be a successful strategy for providing diabetes education, and they proposed incorporating diabetes self-management education into the medical office setting. Consideration of health education as a process may emphasize the need for careful planning to achieve a quality educational program in the office setting. Perceived sources of information about diabetes were reported by individuals over 18 years of age, as seen in Table 60-4. The largest proportion perceived their physicians as a source of information about diabetes.[37]

Attempting to link education program targets (goals) and the interventions to meet those targets is an important example of the assessment and planning phases in a continuum. Peyrot[38] portrays some of these potential linkages in Table 60-5, based on various studies in health education. This provides a basis for planning interventions; however, definitive associations of interventions with targets has rarely been accomplished in the complexity of educational research.

Assessment of Needs and Resources

The health care delivery setting and health care financing can play major roles in decisions regarding whether diabetes education will be on-site or by external referral. Health professionals who may be

TABLE 60-4. Sources of Information about Diabetes Reported by Diabetic Individuals ≥ 18 Years of Age

Source	Patients (%)
Any source	97.1
Physician in physician's office	86.3
Nurse in physician's office	17.8
Dietitian or nutritionist	28.0
Physician or nurse in a hospital	25.2
Relative or friend	14.0
Another person with diabetes	10.1
Diabetes education class	12.2
Diabetes organization	12.2
Newspaper	11.6
Library	5.3
Diabetes support group	4.4
Health department	2.9
Other	15.1

Sources were options listed for the question, "Where have you obtained information about diabetes?"
Source: Reprinted from Coonrod et al.[37]

TABLE 60-5. Linkage of Education Targets and Interventions

Target	Intervention
Knowledge, beliefs	*Didactic education*: Increasing awareness of risks and benefits; helping patients know how to make appropriate self-care decisions.
Skill	*Demonstration/feedback*: Showing how to execute skills; observing performance, correcting errors.
Intentions	*Goal setting*: Establishing specific and appropriate goals that are ambitious but realistic; behavioral contracting to increase commitment.
Barriers	*Problem solving*: Helping patients find ways to overcome barriers to implementing intentions.
Self-efficacy, burnout	*Support/counseling*: Helping patients maintain positive emotional well-being.

Source: Reprinted with permission from Peyrot.[38]

involved in patient education include nurses, dietitians, physicians, social workers, psychologists, pharmacists, or exercise physiologists, among others. Hospitals and other larger institutions are more likely to have a wider range of disciplines and educational resources available. However, as the size of the institution increases, the task of coordinating the patient education effort may become more complex.

Third-party reimbursement for patient education varies by state and type of insurance, adding to both health professional and patient confusion.[2,39] In some regions, diabetes education or "self-management skills training" that is linked to medical care may not be billable as a separate service. In other instances, when education is provided in a nonhospital setting, the coverage may be limited or nonexistent. Coverage inconsistencies have led to efforts at the state and national level to mandate coverage for diabetes education and supplies, and by 2000 the majority of states had passed such legislation with varying results. These laws should assist patients seeking coverage for specific diabetes supplies and education by a provider of a quality diabetes self-management education program or service.

On-Site Education

Selecting the on-site (clinic, medical practice) education option involves a number of organizational decisions, including how educational services will be financed, the role and scope of practice of the educator, and the logistics of program planning. The diabetes education staff may be employed by the health care facility or provide educational programs and consultations on a fee-for-service basis. Smaller medical practices may find the consultative option more fiscally viable. Group practices, especially those specializing in diabetes, are more likely to find employing a full- or part-time diabetes educator feasible.

When diabetes education is provided on site, the medical group must consider many factors, such as mutually agreeable financial arrangements for the fee-for-service arrangement. Having a written contract often clarifies fee schedules that may be ambiguous. When diabetes education is offered on an on-site basis, there may still be a need for external consultation for patients with special needs. For example, many practices may be unable to include an exercise physiologist as part of the diabetes education and care team, but some patients with diabetes will need an external referral for such education. Patients with complications (e.g., visual impairment) are also likely to need specialized educational services or social services.[6] Communication and documentation of the educational process may be somewhat easier in the on-site model, as documentation can be placed in the patient's record immediately and various members of the diabetes care team (e.g., physician, nurse, dietitian) can collaborate with greater ease.

Referral for Education

Referring patients for diabetes education that is outside the medical practice setting is well suited to the needs of many medical practices providing care to patients with diabetes. The medical practice would not have to be organized to provide additional services requiring physical space and expansion of staff on site. The external referral model provides a wide range of options that vary from hospital-based programs to diabetes educators in private practice with a variety of backgrounds and expertise (e.g., nursing, nutrition, counseling). Hospitals may have freestanding units devoted to outpatient education, whereas other programs are located within the hospital complex. Much thought must be given, however, to assessing the quality of the educational services, as well as to the methods for receiving feedback about patient progress to enhance continuity of care. Educational services provided by referral must be thought of as a necessary extension of the diabetes team, and sharing records of these services will enhance continuity of care for patients.

Individual versus Group Education

Programs may be offered as group classes, individual consultation, or a combination of both. In one-on-one consultation, the identified needs of an individual patient can be addressed more easily than in a group setting. The patient's knowledge, skills, and beliefs can be assessed, and families and significant others can be included when beneficial. The content and time allotted to individual topics can be adjusted to needs. The evaluation can be by return demonstration of skills or discussion of topics.

Group learning, on the other hand, provides support and a shared learning experience.[40] Support groups usually focus more on emotional issues, whereas topical classes are more likely to address skills and knowledge. However, group education programs can be designed to address both areas. The patient mix in group programs needs to be considered, though there is in reality often not a choice. Patients newly diagnosed with diabetes may be overwhelmed if they are in a group with other patients who have advanced complications. When the treatment priorities differ greatly in a group, patients may feel isolated and confused rather than sharing a common bond. An adolescent who is facing difficulty adjusting to diabetes may feel little in common with older adults who may focus on coping with chronic complications. Overweight patients may focus on hypoglycemia rather than weight management, even when they are on dietary therapy alone. However, group classes are a vehicle for the peer support sought by many patients.[41]

ASSESSING QUALITY DIABETES EDUCATION PROGRAMS

New national standards for diabetes self-management education programs have been developed.[25] These standards have been used to establish criteria to evaluate the quality of formal diabetes education

programs for recognition by the American Diabetes Association (ADA). This recognition process involves a comprehensive written application, which is then peer-reviewed, to document that a program and institution comply with the standards. The following areas are included: needs assessment, planning, program management, communication/coordination, patient access, content/curriculum, educator qualifications, follow-up, and evaluation and documentation, among others. As of 2000, there were over 1000 diabetes education programs recognized by the ADA as meeting the national standards. Recognition is currently granted for a 3-year period. Requirements for renewal include an update of the application and documentation of staff participation in continuing education related to the diabetes education content areas or of a diabetes educator who maintains credentials as a certified diabetes educator (CDE). Other agencies besides the American Diabetes Association may soon also be authorized providers of recognition for diabetes self-management education.

Many practice settings, especially solo or small group practices, may find that referral to a quality diabetes education program is not feasible owing to location and other factors. However, there are other options available to assure that patients have access to diabetes self-management education. In such settings, patient education can be included with diabetes office visits. Careful planning for appropriate length of patient visits and educational resources, both print materials and audiovisuals, is necessary. Also, referral to outside qualified diabetes educators may be possible. An educational needs assessment can facilitate decision making regarding inclusion of education within a practice setting or planning for outside referral. The criteria used in the assessment should be based on needs of the patient, qualifications of the educator, the educational goals and techniques used, and systems for follow-up and communication about patient progress.

Qualifications and Scope of Practice for Diabetes Educators

The complex education and counseling needs of a patient with diabetes may be met by the skills of a variety of health care disciplines. Generally, diabetes educators are nurses and dietitians, but health education is also provided by physicians, pharmacists, social workers, psychologists, and podiatrists, among others. The credentials of any diabetes educator must be assessed on knowledge and experience in diabetes education, as well as discipline-specific qualifications. The certification program of the National Certification Board for Diabetes Educators assures that candidates are qualified to be certified diabetes educators (CDEs) by virtue of passing a certification examination, completion of at least 2000 hours of clinical experience in diabetes education, and having credentials in one of the clinical disciplines described previously or a master's degree in a health-related field. Recertification is required for CDEs every 5 years by retesting with the certification examination. In 2000, CDEs in the United States numbered over 10,000 health care professionals.

Factors that determine a diabetes educator's scope of practice include licensure and discipline-specific practice, individual knowledge and skills, liability concerns, and practice setting.[42] Registered nurses (RNs) include those prepared by 2- and 3-year nursing programs and by university-based 4-year degree programs. There are also master's-prepared advanced practice nurses (clinical nurse specialists and nurse practitioners). A registered dietitian (RD) has a bachelor's or master's degree with course requirements in biochemistry, physiology, foods, nutrition, and psychology. Registration for dietitians is regulated by the Commission of Dietetic Registration of the American Dietetic Association and is on a voluntary basis. A growing number of states have licensure for dietitians, generally based on the criteria used for dietetic registration. Medical nutrition therapy for diabetes should be sought from RDs specializing in diabetes nutritional management.

Although the number of independent diabetes education practices have increased, educators' concerns about inclusion in third-party reimbursement, scope of practice, and liability tend to limit the number. Dietitians may be more likely to have independent practices, but many are not certified diabetes educators.

CDEs will vary in type and level of expertise. For example, some CDEs will be very familiar with insulin infusion pump therapy and adjustment of therapy to achieve metabolic control, whereas others may have more experience in teaching the visually impaired or in coordinating a hospital-wide inpatient program. Expertise in weight control techniques and behavioral interventions can also vary widely. An interview with a diabetes educator is beneficial to ascertain specific areas of expertise and philosophy of practice.

Education Program Materials

A program assessment must include assessing the needs of the target patient population for diabetes educational materials. The National Diabetes Information Clearinghouse maintains a directory of diabetes educational materials that are available from a variety of sources. A directory of patient education materials is also published by the National Diabetes Education Program (NDEP), the American Diabetes Association, and the University of Michigan Diabetes Research and Training Center, as well as by The Joslin Diabetes Center in Boston or The International Diabetes Center in Minneapolis.

The assessment of need for educational materials should address the following questions:

1. *What are the educational needs of the target patient population?* Programs designed for the elderly,[43,44] for children, [45,46] for adolescents, [47], or for disadvantaged populations have different content, as well as presentation, tone, and format.
2. *Is the information contained in the material accurate, up-to-date, and motivating in tone?* Consider the actions a patient may take based on the message. Minor misinterpretations may not pose difficulty, but other errors could have greater impact and result in increased risks for patients.
3. *Is the presentation appealing and acceptable to the target population?* Patients may find the layout and format unappealing. Some material may be unsuitable because it fails to consider how culture influences lifestyle. Other material may appear to be judgmental or condescending. Sources for appropriate materials are available.[48]
4. *Is the information presented in a clear, concise manner?* Many materials provide too much information and may be overwhelming, whereas other materials may include more than one interpretation.
5. *Is the material practical and feasible to use?* Materials must be incorporated into the flow of the educational or medical program. For example, having educational videotapes available may not be feasible if no one is available to load or rewind the tapes.

6. *Is there a disparity in the targets for patient education materials, such that some populations in need are not addressed?*

HEALTH EDUCATION FOR DIABETES SELF-MANAGEMENT: PRESENT AND FUTURE

The challenges of living well with complex diabetes regimens have directed patient teaching toward the more comprehensive health education process for diabetes self-management that is prevalent today. Recognizing that provider teaching does not necessarily equal patient learning or a change in behavior has been an important step.

After the success of the DCCT,[26,49] the importance of the team approach to diabetes care, education, and counseling has been widely discussed. However, the practicalities of delivering a team approach had to be worked through and resolved. Still, behavioral strategies place the patient in the center of the team: assisting patients to develop problem-solving skills; encouraging increased communication during office visits,[50,4] through recordkeeping, and by telephone; and providing a forum for mutual goal setting between patient and provider. Although the diabetes care team need not be in one physical location, the delivery of integrated diabetes care through good communication among the medical, nursing, nutrition, behavioral, and other educational services is the important feature.[1,2] The cyclical process (assess, plan, implement, evaluate) of diabetes self-management education may seem unrealistic for a busy practicing physician; however, the emerging educational technologies, innovative educational materials, and models for creating a team provide opportunities for diabetes patients and their health care professionals to work together toward optimal glycemic control and improved quality of life.

Acknowledgment.   We are ever grateful for the early guidance of Dr. Harold Rifkin in the development of the diabetes education team at the Diabetes Research and Training Center of the Albert Einstein College of Medicine.

REFERENCES

1. Clement C: Diabetes self-management education. *Diabetes Care* 1995;18:1204.
2. Report of the Task Force on Diabetes Self-Management Education. *Diabetes Spectrum* 1999;12:44.
3. American Diabetes Association: *ADA Complete Guide to Diabetes*, 2nd ed. American Diabetes Association:1999.
4. Walker EA: Characteristics of the adult learner. *Diabetes Educator* 1999;25:16.
5. Redman BK: *The Process of Patient Education*, 7th ed. Mosby:1993.
6. Funnell MM, ed.: *A Core Curriculum for Diabetes Education*, 3rd ed. American Association of Diabetes Educators:1999.
7. Brookfield SD: *Understanding and Facilitating Adult Learning*. Jossey-Bass:1986.
8. Bloom BS, ed.: *Taxonomy of Educational Objectives*. McKay:1956.
9. Knowles M: *The Adult Learner*, 4th ed. Gulf Publishing Co:1990.
10. Wlodkowski RJ: *Enhancing Adult Motivation to Learn*. Jossey-Bass: 1985.
11. Bandura A: *Self-Efficacy: The Exercise of Control*. WH Freeman & Co:1997.
12. Bernier M, Avard J: Self-efficacy, outcomes, and attrition in a weight reduction program. *Cognitive Ther Res* 1986;10:319
13. Hurley AC, Shea CA: Self-efficacy: Strategy for enhancing diabetes self-care. *Diabetes Educator* 1992;18:146.

14. Strecher VJ, DeVellis BM, Becker MH, *et al*: The role of self-efficacy in achieving health behavior change. *Health Ed Q* 1986;13:73.

15. Ruggiero L, Prochaska JO, eds.: Readiness for change: Application of the Transtheoretical Model to diabetes. *Diabetes Spectrum* 1993;6:21.

16. Ruggiero L: Helping people with diabetes change behavior: From theory to practice. *Diabetes Spectrum* 2000;13:125.

17. Prochaska JO, DiClemente CC, Norcross JC: In search of how people change: Application to addictive behaviors. *Am Psychol* 1992; 47:1102.

18. Curry SJ: Commentary: Application of the Transtheoretical Model to diabetes. *Diabetes Spectrum* 1993;6:34.

19. Williams GC, Freedman ZR, Deci EL: Supporting autonomy to motivate patients with diabetes for glucose control. *Diabetes Care* 1998; 21:1644.

20. Funnell MM, Anderson RM: *The Art of Empowerment: Stories and Strategies for Diabetes Educators.* American Diabetes Association: 2000.

21. Strecher VJ, Rosenstock IM: The Health Belief Model. In: Glanz K, Lewis FM, Rimer BK, eds. *Health Behavior and Health Education*, 2nd ed. Jossey-Bass;1997:41.

22. Anderson LA: Health care communication and selected psychosocial correlates of adherence in diabetes management. *Diabetes Care* 1990; 13(suppl 1):66.

23. Kaplan SH, Greenfield S, Ware JE Jr: Assessing the effects of physician-patient interactions on the outcomes of chronic disease. *Med Care* 1989;27:S110.

24. Cryer PE, Fisher JN, Shamoon H: Hypoglycemia: Technical review. *Diabetes Care* 1994;17:734.

25. Mensing C, Boucher J, Cypress M, *et al*: National Standards for Diabetes Self-Management Education. *Diabetes Care* 2000;23:682.

26. The Diabetes Control and Complications Trial (DCCT) Research Group: The effect of intensive treatment of diabetes on the development and progression of long-term complications in insulin-dependent diabetes mellitus. *N Engl J Med* 1993;329:977.

27. Delahanty L, Halford B: The role of diet behaviors in achieving improved glycemic control in intensively treated patients in the DCCT. *Diabetes Care* 1993;16:1453.

28. Brown SA, Hanis CL: A community-based culturally sensitive education and support-group intervention for Mexican Americans with NIDDM: A pilot study of efficacy. *Diabetes Educator* 1995;21:203.

29. Haire-Joshu D: The process of evaluation in diabetes. In: Haire-Joshu D, ed. *Management of Diabetes Mellitus: Perspectives of Care Across the Life Span.* Mosby:1992:593.

30. Glasgow RE, Osteen VL: Evaluating diabetes education: Are we measuring the most important outcomes? *Diabetes Care* 1992; 15:1423.

31. Brown SA: Meta-analysis of diabetes patient education research: Variations in intervention effects across studies. *Res Nurs Health* 1992;15:409.

32. Cox DJ, Gonder-Frederick LA, Julian D, *et al*: Intensive versus standard blood glucose awareness training (BGAT) with insulin-dependent diabetes: Mechanisms and ancillary effects. *Psychosom Med* 1991;53:453.

33. Cox DJ, Gonder-Frederick L, Julian DM, *et al*: Long-term follow-up evaluation of blood glucose awareness training. *Diabetes Care* 1994; 17:1.

34. Rubin RR, Peyrot M, Saudek C: The effect of a diabetes education program incorporating coping skills training on emotional well-being and diabetes self-efficacy. *Diabetes Educator* 1993;19:210.

35. Prospect Associates Final Report: Survey of physician practice behaviors related to the treatment of people with diabetes mellitus (endocrinologists). Doc # NO1DK82233. National Institutes of Diabetes, Digestive, and Kidney Diseases (NIDDK), National Institutes of Health:1991.

36. Glasgow RE, Toobert DJ, Hampson SE: Participation in outpatient diabetes education programs: How many patients take part and how representative are they? *Diabetes Educator* 1991;17:376.

37. Coonrod BA, Betschart J, Harris MI: Frequency and determinants of diabetes patient education among adults in the United States population. *Diabetes Care* 1994;17:852.

38. Peyrot M: Behavior change in diabetes education. *Diabetes Educator* 1999;25:62.

39. Hill EH, Fischer CG: *ADA Guide to Diabetes Coding.* American Diabetes Association:1999.

40. Campbell EM, Redman S, Moffitt PS, *et al*: The relative effectiveness of educational and behavioral instruction programs for patients with NIDDM: A randomized trial. *Diabetes Educator* 1996;22:379.

41. Arseneau DL, Mason AC, Bennett-Wood O, *et al*: A comparison of learning activity packages and classroom instruction for diet management of patients with NIDDM. *Diabetes Educator* 1994;20:509.

42. American Association of Diabetes Educators: The 1999 Scope of Practice and Standards of Practice for Diabetes Educators. *Diabetes Educator* 2000;26:519.

43. Glasgow RE, Toobert DJ, Hampson SE, *et al*: Improving self-care among older patients with type II diabetes: The "sixty something . . ." study. *Patient Educ Counseling* 1992;19:61.

44. Funnell MM, Arnold MS, Fogler J, *et al*: Participation in a diabetes education and care program: Experience from the diabetes care for older adults project. *Diabetes Educator* 1998;24:163.

45. McNabb W, Quinn MT, Murphy D, *et al*: Increasing children's responsibility for diabetes self-care: The *In Control* Study. *Diabetes Educator* 1994;20:121.

46. Wolanski R, Sigman T, Polychonakos C: Assessment of blood glucose monitoring skills in a camp for diabetic children: Effects of individualized feedback counseling. *Patient Educ Counseling* 1996;29:5.

47. Boardway RH, Delamater AM, Tomakowsky J, *et al*: Stress management training for adolescents with diabetes. *J Pediatr Psychol* 1993; 18:29.

48. http://www.diabetes.org; www.aadenet.org; www.NDEP.nih.gov

49. Walker EA: ". . . Not just more insulin." *Diabetes Spectrum* 1993; 6:220.

50. Kaplan SH, Greenfield SW, Ware JE: Assessing the effects of physician-patient interactions on the outcomes of chronic disease. *Med Care* 1989;27:5110.

INDEX

NOTE: A *t* following a page number indicates tabular material and an *f* following a page number indicates a figure. Drugs are listed under their generic names. When a drug trade name is listed, the reader is referred to the generic name.

A-box elements, in insulin gene transcription regulation, 30–31, 30*f*
A cells. *See* Alpha cells (A cells/α cells)
A chain, insulin, 23, 24*f*, 482–483, 482*f*
AA messenger system. *See* Arachidonic acid messenger system
Aarhus studies, 912*t*, 914
AAV. *See* Adeno-associated virus
ABC proteins. *See* ATP-binding cassette (ABC) proteins
Abdominal pain
    acarbose/miglitol therapy and, 546
    in hyperglycemic hyperosmolar syndrome, 596*t*
ABPM. *See* Ambulatory blood pressure monitoring
Acanthosis nigricans
    hypoglycemia and, 966
    with insulin resistance, 267, 347, 355, 392–393, 897–898, 898*f*
Acarbose, 543
    for alimentary and reactive hypoglycemia, 971
    clinical use and efficacy of, 544, 544*f*
    in combination therapy, 544
        with insulin, 558
        with sulfonylurea or metformin, 555–556, 557*t*
    diabetic nephropathy and, 545, 739
    dosage recommendations and, 545
    drug interactions and, 546
    in dumping syndrome, 545
    lipid levels affected by, 545, 806–807
    mechanism of action of, 543
    pharmacokinetics of, 543–544
    in prevention of type 2 diabetes, 545
    in reactive hypoglycemia, 545
    side effects of, 545–546
    in type 1 diabetes, 544
    weight loss and, 545
Accelerated starvation, in pregnancy, 621
ACE gene, polymorphism in, diabetic retinopathy and, 705
ACE inhibitors. *See* Angiotensin-converting enzyme inhibitors
Acesulfame K, in nutritional management, 440, 440*t*
Acetoacetate, enzymatic pathway for production of, 18–20, 18*f*
Acetoacetyl CoA thiolase, in fatty acid metabolism, 18
Acetohexamide, 531, 532*t*
    clinical use/efficacy of, 533
    pharmacokinetics of, 533*t*
Acetone, in diabetic ketoacidosis, 578–579
Acetyl CoA, in ketogenesis, 18, 18*f*, 19, 20, 21*f*
Acetyl LDL receptor, 167
Acetylcholine, in insulin release, 49*t*, 50
ACh. *See* Acetylcholine
Acid-base disorders, in diabetic ketoacidosis, 575, 576, 576*t*
    therapy and, 581–582
Acidosis, metabolic
    in diabetic ketoacidosis, 576, 582
    in hyperglycemic hyperosmolar syndrome, 587, 590
Acinar cells, conversion of to endocrine tissue for transplantation, 943–944
Acomys cahirinus (spiny mice), diabesity in, 246–247
Acquired perforating dermatosis, 903–904, 903*f*

Acquired (metabolic/hemodynamic) theory, of diabetic nephropathy, 702–704, 725–726, 725*t*, 726*f*, 727–728, 727*f*
Acromegaly, glucose intolerance/diabetes associated with, 267, 426
ACTH, hypoglycemia recovery and, 132
Activities of daily living (ADL), assessment of in older patient with diabetes, 418
Activity. *See* Exercise/physical activity
Actos. *See* Pioglitazone
Acute coronary syndromes, 833
Acute illnesses
    nutritional management and, 446–447
    in older diabetic, 422
Acute insulin response (AIR)
    to glucose, 53*t*, 54–55, 55*f*
        in type 2 diabetes, 333, 334*f*, 336*f*
    to nonglucose stimuli, 53*t*, 55–56
        in type 2 diabetes, 334, 336*f*
Acyl CoA
    carnitine, in alloxan- and STZ-treated animals, 234
    long-chain
        in insulin release, 48
            molecular studies of, 201, 206–207
        in insulin resistance, 407
Acylation stimulating protein (ASP), in insulin resistance, 407
ADA. *See* American Diabetes Association
Adaptive immunity, 219, 220*f*
Adeno-associated virus (AAV), as gene transfer vector, 198–199
Adenovirus, recombinant, as gene transfer vector, 198, 199*f*
Adhesion molecules, in atherosclerotic fatty streak formation, 166
Adipocytes, hormones secreting, insulin resistance in obesity and, 407, 408*f*
Adipose tissue
    distribution of
        insulin resistance and, 379–380, 391
        in type 2 diabetes, 402
    in fat metabolism
        in fasted state, 3, 5*f*, 6*f*
        in fed state, 4, 5*f*
    in glucose metabolism, 3, 3*f*
    insulin action in, exercise/physical activity affecting, 474
    in ketogenesis, liver and, 16–17
    thiazolidinediones affecting, 549–550, 550*f*
"Adipose-tissue homunculus," 154
Adiposity. *See also* Body weight
    food intake regulation and, 154–159
        circulating (adiposity) signals and, 154–156, 155*f*, 156*f*, 158–159, 159*f*
    in offspring of diabetic mothers, 623, 641, 642, 646
Adiposity signals, 154–156, 155*f*, 156*f*
    insulin as, 155–156, 155*f*
    interaction with signals controlling meal size and, 158–159, 159*f*
    leptin as, 156, 156*f*
Adipsin (factor D), in insulin resistance, 407
ADL. *See* Activities of daily living
Adolescents. *See also* Children
    type 1 diabetes in
        developmental and family issues and, 566*t*, 568–569
        intensive therapy and, 918
        nutritional management and, 445
    type 2 diabetes in, 287, 287*f*
        nutritional management and, 445–446
        obesity and, 409–410
Adrenal hyporesponsiveness, hypoglycemia and, 966, 968–969

ISBN 0-8385-2178-9

90000

9 780838 521786

PORTE/DIABETES, 6E